# Fetal and Neonatal Neurology and Neurosurgery

Third Edition

Commissioning Editor: Deborah Russell
Project Development Manager: Paul Fam
Project Manager: Scott Millar
Designer: Jayne Jones
Illustrations Manager: Mick Ruddy
Illustrator: Sandie Hill

# Fetal and Neonatal Neurology and Neurosurgery

## Third Edition

*Edited by*

**Malcolm I Levene** MD FRCP FRCPH FMedSc

Professor of Pediatrics, Division of Pediatrics & Child Health, Leeds General Infirmary, UK

**Frank A Chervenak** MD

Given Foundation Professor, Department of Obstetrics and Gynecology, The New York Presbyterian Hospital, New York, USA

**Martin J Whittle** MD FRCOG FRCP(Glas)

Head of Division of Reproductive Child Health, Birmingham Women's Hospital, Birmingham, UK

*Associate Editors*

**Michael J Bennett** MD CHB FRCO(SA) FRCOG DDU

Professor and Head of School, University of New South Wales, School of Obstetrics & Gynecology, Royal Hospital for Women, Randwick, Australia

**Jonathan Punt** FRCS

Queen's Medical Centre, Academic Division of Child Health, Nottingham, UK

*Foreword by*
Jerry Lucey
Professor
Fletcher Allen Healthcare, Burlington, Vermont, USA

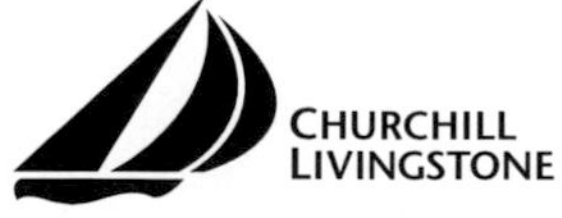


London • Edinburgh • New York • Philadelphia • St Louis • Sydney • Toronto 2001

CHURCHILL LIVINGSTONE
An imprint of Elsevier Science Limited



First edition 1988
Second edition 1995
Third edition 2001
Reprinted 2002

ISBN 0 443 06379 6

**British Library Cataloguing in Publication Data**
A catalogue record for this book is available from the British Library

**Library of Congress Cataloging in Publication Data**
A catalog record for this book is available from the Library of Congress

Note
Medical knowledge is constantly changing. Standard safety precautions must be followed, but as new research and clinical experience broaden our knowledge, changes in treatment and drug therapy may become necessary or appropriate. Readers are advised to check the most current product information provided by the manufacturer of each drug to be administered to verify the recommended dose, the method and duration of administration, and contraindications. It is the responsibility of the practitioner, relying on experience and knowledge of the patient, to determine dosages and the best treatment for each individual patient. Neither the Publisher nor the authors assume any liability for any injury and/or damage to persons or property arising from this publication.

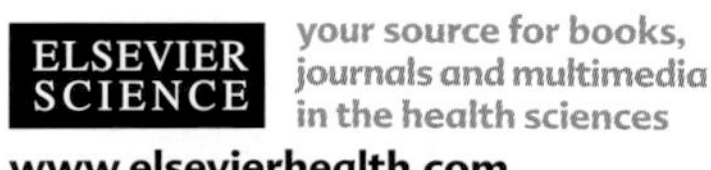

**www.elsevierhealth.com**

Typeset by Phoenix Photosetting, Chatham, Kent
Printed in China by RDC Group Limited

The Publisher's policy is to use **paper manufactured from sustainable forests**

# Contents

*Foreword* xi
*Preface to Third Edition* xiii
*Acknowledgements* xiv
*Preface to First Edition* xv
*Contributors* xvii

SECTION I

**Structural Development of the CNS**

1. Genetic and Epigenetic Control of the Early Brain Development 3
*Hugo Lagercrantz, T Ringstedt*

2. Early Embryonic Development of the Brain 11
*G Moscoso*

3. Anatomical Development of the CNS 21
*MA England*

4. Three-dimensional Ultrasonography of the Embryonic Brain 39
*Harm-Gerd K Blaas, Sturla H Eik-Nes*

5. Ultrasound Assessment of Normal Fetal Brain Development 45
*Harm-Gerd K Blaas, Sturla H Eik-Nes*

6. Imaging the Neonatal Brain 57
*R Arthur, Luca A Ramenghi*

SECTION II

**Functional Assessment of CNS Development**

7. Functional Assessment of the Fetal CNS 89
*Ilse Nijhuis, Jan G Nijhuis*

8. Clinical Assessment of the Infant Nervous System 99
*Claudine Amiel-Tison*

9. Doppler Assessment of the Fetal and Neonatal Brain 121
*M Kilby, Karen Brackley, David Evans*

10. CBF and Metabolism of the Developing Brain 139
*G Greison*

11. Neonatal Electroencephalography 155
*Fabrizio Ferrari, Enrico Biagioni, Giovanni Cioni*

12. Evoked Potentials in the Neonatal Brain 181
*P Eken, Linda S de Vries*

SECTION III

**Anomalies**

13. Congenital Structural Defects of the Brain 199
*Stephen Ashwal*

14. Genetics of Neurodevelopmental Anomalies 237
*Mohnish Suri, Ian D Young*

15. Functional Teratogenic Effects of Chemicals on the Developing Brain 251
*DF Swaab, K Boer*

16. Antenatal Screening for Neurologic Disorders 267
*HS Cuckle, Jennifer Murray*

17. Antenatal Assessment of CNS Anomalies, including NTDs: Abdominal Ultrasound 275
*Karim Kalache, Lyn Chitty*

18. Transvaginal Fetal Neuroscan 297
*Ilan Timor-Tritsch, Ana Monteagudo*

19. Epidemiology and Prevention of NTDs 317
*NC Nevin*

SECTION IV

**Hemorrhagic and Ischemic Lesions**

20. Fetal Cerebral Pathology of Hypoxic–Ischemic Origins 323
*Waney V Squier*

21. Neonatal Intracranial Hemorrhage 339
*Malcom I Levene, Linda S de Vries*

22. Cerebral Ischemic Lesions 373
*Linda S de Vries, Malcom I Levene*

SECTION V

Perinatal Asphyxia

23. Pathophysiology of Asphyxia 407
*Laura Bennet, Jenny A Westgate, Peter D Gluckan, Alistair J Gunn*

24. Antenatal Prediction of Asphyxia 427
*KA Sorem, Maurice A Druzin*

25. Intrapartum Monitoring for Asphyxia 443
*David Miller, Richard H Paul*

26. Prediction of Asphyxia with Fetal Blood Gas Analysis 459
*Sergio De La Fuente, Peter W Soothill*

27. The Asphyxiated Newborn Infant 471
*Malcolm I Levene*

28. Neuroprotection of the Fetal and Neonatal Brain 505
*Hendrick Hagberg, C Mallard, K Blomgren*

29. Medico-legal Issues: The UK Perspective 521
*Roger V Clements*

30. Medico-legal Issues: The US Perspective 527
*Barry S Schifrin, Kristi A Schifrin*

SECTION VI

Infection of the CNS

31. Toxoplasmosis 543
*Yyves Ville, J Nizard*

32. Viral Infections 553
*Catherine Peckham, Marie-Louise Newell*

33. Bacterial and Fungal Infections 573
*Patrick McMaster, David Isaacs*

SECTION VII

Metabolic Disorders

34. Prenatal Diagnosis of Inborn Errors of Metabolism 595
*JW Wraith*

35. Inborn Errors of Metabolism, Postnatal Diagnosis and Management 605
*JW Wraith*

36. Degenerative Disorders of the Infant CNS 623
*SH Green, RGF Gray*

SECTION VIII

Seizure Disorders

37. Seizure Disorders of the Neonate and Infant 647
*A Arzimanoglou, Jean Aicardi*

SECTION IX

The Special Senses

38. Disorders of Vision 659
*Alistair R Fielder*

39. Disorders of Hearing 683
*VE Newton*

SECTION X

Disorders of the Nerve and Muscle

40. Disorders of the Spinal Cord, Cranial and Peripheral Nerves 695
*Malcolm I Levene*

41. Neuromuscular Disorders 709
*Eugenio Mercuri, J Heckmatt, Victor Dubowitz*

SECTION XI

Hydrocephalus and Neurosurgery

42. Fetal Neurosurgical Interventions 729
*Michael Chan, Russell Jennings, Bettina Westerburg*

43. Neonatal Hydrocephaus – Clinical Assessment and Non-Surgical Management 739
*Andrew Whitelaw*

44. Neurosurgical Management of Hydrocephalus 753
*Jonathan Punt*

45. Neurosurgical Management of NTD 763
*Jonathan Punt*

46. Congenital Defects, Vascular Malformations and Other Lesions 775
*Jonathan Punt*

## SECTION XII

### Epidemiology of Neurologic Disability

47. Epidemiology of Cerebral Palsy 791
*Eve Blair, Fiona Stanley*

48. Epidemiology of Mental Retardation 799
*Maureen Durkin, Nicole Schupf, Zena Stein, Mervin Susser*

## SECTION XIII

### Ethical Dilemas

49. Issues for the Obstetrician 821
*Frank Chervenak, Laurence McCullough*

50. Issues for the Neonatologist 829
*Terence Stephenson*

Index 833

# Foreword

This is the Third edition of this monumental tome, which first appeared in 1988. It is a worthy successor to the first two editions. Fifty internationally know experts in the field have created a very valuable, comprehensive, source book. It contains a wealth of current information; well organized and carefully evaluated by critical research workers who are leaders in their fields. It's very useful to have all of this information in one place. It's also inspiring to see the increasing use of 'evidence-based medicine' concepts in this field.

Newborn survival rates are higher than ever before in history, but unfortunately 'intact survival' often eludes us. Recent obstetrical and surgical advances covered in this book are very promising. The whole field is poised to begin the testing of several promising new neuro-protective strategies and therapies for brain care.

Who knows, the next volume (2010?) might even contain attempts not just to prevent brain damage, but actually improve brain functions!?

Jerold F. Lucey, MD, FAAP
Professor of Pediatrics and University Scholar,
University of Vermont
Harry Wallace Professor of Neonatology,
University of Vermont
Editor, *Pediatrics*

# Preface to the Third Edition

Understanding the processes involved in the developing brain remains one of the great challenges to clinicians and neuroscientists alike. In recent years great strides have been made in understanding the control of early brain development, assessment of the fetal central nervous system and diagnosis and management of neonatal brain disorders. In the third edition of this book we have attempted to include an up-to-date overview of the neurobiology of the developing brain and in particular that which is relevant to the field of perinatal medicine. A major new area is in our understanding (albeit still fairly basic) of the genetic and epigenetic influence on early brain development and this is the subject of a new introductory chapter in the book. Major advances in both fetal and neonatal anatomical and functional analysis have been made and these are reflected in new and revised chapters. Other novel and exciting areas introduced for the first time in this edition are in the area of fetal and neonatal brain protection (a field that is sure to grow rapidly in future years) and the speciality of fetal neurosurgery which also offers great promise for reducing disability in the future.

This edition has been further strengthened by the collaboration of two new Senior Editors who bring to bear their expertise in fetal medicine and ethical issues raised by developments in this field. We feel that we have further consolidated the original aims of this book firstly to produce a truly international overview of the subject (there are now contributors from eleven countries) and to present a seamless scientific and clinical overview of the developing brain from the first evidence of neural tissue at 18 days after conception until the end of the neonatal period.

We dedicate this book to the children of the future in the hope that more will develop free of disability or at least with their potential for optimal outcome enhanced.

MIL, FC, MW
Leeds 2001

*We are grateful to the support of our colleagues in producing this book. In particular Miss Mandy Jones for co-ordinating the vast network of contributors from Leeds and Mr Paul Fam for his support and encouragement throughout the project.*

# Preface to the First Edition

Neurological disability is the most feared complication of pregnancy, labour and the early months of life. The earliest recognizable neural tissue develops approximately 18 days after fertilization and development of the central nervous system proceeds to maturity some six years later. The developing brain is an extremely vulnerable organ and is subject to a wide range of insults that may alter structure or function. Problems affecting the immature brain may come under the care of the obstetrician, neonatologist, general pediatrician or pediatric neurologist and neurosurgeon. Investigations may encompass a wide range of other specialists including radiologists, physicists, pharmacologists, microbiologists, physiologists, pathologists, biochemists and ophthalmologists. These major cross-specialty links make it difficult to consider the developing central nervous system (CNS) for what it is: a complex but continuous process rather than a series of loosely related parts.

The basic aim of this book is to consider the developmental neurology and pathology of the developing CNS from conception to the end of the first year of life. We have approached the subject as specialists representing obstetrics, pediatrics and neurosurgery but with a particular interest in the immature brain. We have attempted to break down the constraints of our respective specialty training to produce a book that crosses these divisions and brings together all the aspects of brain development and pathology during the critical stages of early development. We have been supported in this aim by our 55 contributors who represent a wide range of disciplines and the experience of 10 different countries within Europe, Australia and North America.

The book is presented in three parts: morphological development, methods of investigation and management. Part 1 is a comprehensive review of embryology and developmental anatomy of the CNS and provides the basic foundation necessary to understand much of the pathology that may occur. Part 2 incorporates methods of investigating the immature brain, both fetal and neonatal. The rapid advance in our understanding of cerebral pathology is directly related to the recent introduction of these methods. We have drawn upon the experience to discuss their role and limitations. Some of these methods are already used in routine clinical practice and others are state-of-the-art and unlikely to ever come into routine use but give important information on both structure and function. Part 3 involves the management of disorders of the developing brain and this is further subdivided into sections related to particular areas of clinical interest.

We hope that this book will provide all those involved in the management of the fetus and infant with the information necessary to understanding better the delicate mechanisms that exist within the central nervous system. Perhaps better understanding of these fragile tissues will, in the future, enable more effective treatment or prevention of neurological handicap.

M I L, M J B, J P
Leicester, 1988

# List of Contributors

**Jean Aicardi** MD, FRCP
Honorary Professor of Child Neurology
Institute of Child Health, London
Consultant
Hôpital Robert-Debré
Paris
France

**Claudine Amiel-Tison** MD
Emeritus Professor of Paediatrics
Hôpital Cochin
Department of Paediatrics
Maternité Baudelocque
Paris
France

**Rosemary Arthur** BSc, MBCHB, FRCP, FRCR
Consultant Paediatric Radiologist
Leeds General Infirmary
Leeds
UK

**Alexis Arzimanoglu** MD
Head of the Epilepsy Programme
Child Neurology and Metabolic Diseases Dept.
Hôpital Robert-Debré
Paris
France

**Stephen Ashwal** MD
Chief, Division of Pediatric Neurology
Department of Pediatrics
Loma Linda University School of Medicine
Loma Linda, CA
USA

**Laura Bennet** PhD
Senior Lecturer
University of Auckland
Department of Paediatrics
Auckland
New Zealand

**Michael J Bennett** MD, CHB, FRCO(SA), FRCOG, DDU
Professor and Head of School
University of New South Wales
School of Obstetrics & Gynaecology
Royal Hospital for Women
Randwick
Australia

**Enrico Biagioni** MD
Senior Researcher
Stella Maris Scientific Institute
Division of Child Neurology & Psychiatry
Pisa
Italy

**Harm-Gerd K Blaas** MD, PhD
Consultant
Department of Obstetrics and Gynaecology
National Center for Fetal Medicine
St Olavs Hospital
Trondheim
Norway

**Eve Blair** BSc (Hons), PhD
Senior Research Officer
TVW Telethon Institute for Child Health Research
West Perth WA
Australia

**Klas Blomgren** MD, PhD
Perinatal Center
Department of Physiology
University of Göteborg
Göteborg
Sweden

**Karen Brackley** MRCOG, DM
Consultant in Fetal Medicine
Wessex Maternal and Fetal Medicine Unit
The Princess Anne Hospital
Southampton
UK

**Michael Chan**
Children's Hospital
300 Longwood Avenue
Boston MA
USA

**Frank A Chervenak** MD
Given Foundation Professor and Chairman
The New York Presbyterian Hospital – Weill Medical College
Department of Obstetrics and Gynecology
New York NY
USA

**Lyn Chitty** PhD, MRCOG
Consultant in Genetics and Fetal Medicine
Fetal Medicine Unit
Obstetric Hospital
University College Hosptial
London
UK

**Giovanni Cioni** MD
Professor of Child Neurology and Psychiatry
Stella Maris Scientific Institute
Division of Child Neurology & Psychiatry
Pisa
Italy

**Roger V Clements** BM, BCH, FRCS, FRCOG
Consultant Obstetrician and Gynaecologist
Harley Street
London
UK

**Howard S Cuckle** BA, MSc, DPhil
Professor of Reproductive Epidemiology
Reproductive Epidemiology
University of Leeds
Leeds

**Maurice L Druzin**
Stanford University
Department of Obstetrics & Gynecology
Stanford CA
USA

**Victor Dubowitz** MD, PhD, FRCP, DCH
Hammersmith Hospital
Dept Paediatrics/Neonatal Medical
Royal Postgraduate Medical School
London
UK

**Maureen S Durkin** PhD, DrPH
Associate Professor of Clinical Public Health
Colombia University
Sergievsky Center
New York NY
USA

**Sturla H Eik-Nes** MD, PhD
Professor
Department of Obstetrics and Gynaecology
National Center for Fetal Medicine
St Olavs Hospital
Trondheim
Norway

**Paula Eken** MD, PhD
Research Physician
Department of Neonatology
Wilhelmina Kinderziekenhuis
Utrecht
The Netherlands

**Marjorie A England** BA, PhD
University of Leicester
Department of Pre-Clinical Sciences
Leicester
UK

**David J Evans** BM, BCh, MA, MRCP, FRCPCH
Consultant Neonatologist
Neonatal Intensive Care Unit
Southmead Hospital
Bristol
UK

**Fabrizio Ferrari** MD
Professor of Neonatology
Department of Obstetrics, Gynaecology and Paediatrics
Division of Neonatology
University Hospital
Modena
Italy

**Alistair R Fielder** FRCP, FRCS, FRCOphth
Kennerley Bankes Professor of Ophthalmology
Department of Ophthalmology
The Western Eye Hospital
Imperial College School of Medicine
London
UK

**Sergio De La Fuente**
Department of Obstetrics and Gynaecology
St Michael's Hospital
Bristol

**Peter D Gluckman** MBChB, DSc, FRACP
Dean, Faculty of Medicine & Health Science
University of Auckland
Auckland
New Zealand

**R George F Gray** BSc, MSc, PhD
Principal Biochemist
Department of Clinical Chemistry
Birmingham Children's Hospital
Birmingham
UK

**Stuart H Green** MA, MB, BChiv, FRCP, FRCPCH
Senior Lecturer
Institute of Child Health
Birmingham Children's Hospital
Birmingham
UK

**Gorm Greison** MD, Dr Med Sci
Professor of Paediatrics
Department of Neonatology
Rigshospitalet
Copenhagen
Denmark

**Alistair J Gunn** MBChB, PhD, FRACP
Senior Lecturer
Department of Paediatrics
Faculty of Medicine & Health Science
University of Auckland
Auckland
New Zealand

**John Heckmatt** MBChB, FRCP, MD, FRCPCH
Consultant Paediatrician
Child Development
Peace Childrens Centre
Peace Prospect
Watford
UK

**David Isaacs** FRACP
Associate Professor of Paediatric Infectious Diseases and Immunology
The Childrens Hospital at Westmead
Parramatta
Australia

**Russell Jennings**
The Fetal Treatment Center, Children's Hospital, Boston
Boston
USA

**Karim Kalache**
University College Hospital, Obstetrics Hospital
London
UK

**Mark Kilby** MRCOG, DM
Honorary Consultant in Fetal Medicine
Division of Reproductive and Child Health
University of Birmingham
Birmingham
UK

**Henrik Hagberg** MD, PhD
Professor of Obstetrics & Perinatal Medicine
Perinatal Center
Sahlgrenska University Hospital
Göteborg
Sweden

**Hugo Largercrantz** MD, PhD
Professor of Paediatrics
Karolinska Institute
Neonatal Program
Astrid Lindgren Children's Hospital
Stockholm
Sweden

**Malcolm I Levene** MD, FRCP
Division of Pediatrics & Child Health
Leeds General Infirmary
Leeds
UK

**Carina Mallard** PhD
Assistant Professor
Perinatal Center
Department of Physiology
University of Göteborg
Göteborg
Sweden

**Laurence B McCullough** PhD
Professor of Medicine & Medical Ethics
Center for Medical Ethics and Health Policy
Baylor College of Medicine
Houston TX
USA

**Paddy McMaster** MRCP
Fellow in Paediatric Infectious Diseases
The Children's Hospital at Westmead
Parramatta
Australia

**Eugenio Mercuri** MD, PhD
Lecturer in Paediatric Neurology
Department of Paediatrics
Hammersmith Hospital
London
UK

**David Miller** MD
Associate Professor of Clinical Obstetrics and Gynecology
University of Southern California School of Medicine
LAC & USC Women's & Childrens' Hospital
Los Angeles CA
USA

**Ana Monteagudo** MD
Associate Professor of Obstetrics & Gynecology
New York University
School of Medicine
New York NY
USA

**Gonzalo Moscoso-Alvarino** MB, BS, MD, PhD
Senior Lecturer
Department of Physiology
St George's Hospital
UK

**Jennifer Y Murray** BSc, MSc
Research Fellow
Reproductive Epidemiology
University of Leeds
Leeds
UK

**Norman C Nevin** BSc, MB, BCh, BAO, MD, FRPHM, FRCPath, FRCPed, FRCP
Professor of Medical Genetics
Department of Medical Genetics
Belfast City Hospital
Belfast
UK

**Marie-Louise Newell** MSc, MB, PhD
Reader in Epidemiology
Institute of Child Health
London
UK

**Valerie E Newton** MD, MSc, FRCP FRCPCH
Professor of Audiological Medicine
The University of Manchester
Centre for Human Communication and Deafness
Manchester
UK

**Ilse J M Nijhuis** MD, PhD
Register in Paediatrics
Beatrix Children's Hospital
University Hospital Groningen
Groningen
Netherlands

**Jan G Nijhuis** MD, PhD
Professor and Head of Obstetrics
Department of Obstetrics and Gynaecology
University Hospital Maastricht
Maastricht
The Netherlands

**J Nizard**
Specialist Registrar
Université Paris
Poissy
France

**Richard H Paul**
Pasadena CA
USA

**Catherine Peckham** MD, FRCP, FFPHM
Professor of Paediatric Epidemiology
Institute of Child Health
London
UK

**Jonathan Punt** FRCS
Queen's Medical Centre
Academic Division of Child Health
Nottingham
UK

**Luca A Ramenghi** MD
Consultant Neonatologist
Neonatal Department
Clinica Mangiagalli
Instituti Clinici di Perfezionamento
Milan
Italy

**Thomas Ringstedt** PhD
Research Fellow
Karolinska Institute
Neonatal Program
Astrid Lindgren Children's Hospital
Stockholm
Sweden

**Barry S Schifrin** MD
Director, Department of Maternal-Fetal Medicine
Director of OBGYN Residency Program
Glendale Adventist Hospital
Glendale CA
USA

**Kristi A Schifrin**
Associate
Miracle, Pruzan, Pruzan & Baker
Seattle WA
USA

**Nicole Schupf** PhD, DrPH
Research Scientist
Laboratory of Epidemiology
NYS Institute of Basic Research in Developmental Disabilities
Staten Island NY
USA

**Peter W Soothill** MBBS, BSc, MD, MRCOG
Professor of Maternal & Fetal Medicine
St Michael's Hospital
Bristol University
Bristol
UK

**Waney V Squier** BSc, MBChB, MRCP, FRCPath
Consultant Neuropathologist and Clinical Lecturer
Department of Neuropathology
Radcliffe Infirmary
Oxford
UK

**Fiona J Stanley** MB, BS, MSc, MD, FRACP, FRACOG, FASSA
Director
The Telethon Institute for Child Health Research
West Perth WA
Australia

**Zena A Stein** MA, MB, BCh
Professor of Public Health and Psychiatry Emerita
Colombia University
Sergievsky Center
New York NY
USA

**Terence Stephenson** BSc (Hons), BM, BCh, DM, FRCP, FRCPCH
Professor of Child Health
School of Human Development
University Hospital
Queen's Medical Centre
Nottingham
UK

**Mohnish Suri** MD, MRCP
Consultant Clinical Geneticist
Clinical Genetic Service
City Hospital
Nottingham
UK

**Mervin W Susser** MB, BCh, FRCP(E)
Colombia University
Sergievsky Center
New York NY
USA

**Dick F Swaab** MD, PhD
Director, Professor of Neurobiology
Netherlands Institute for Brain Research
Amsterdam
The Netherlands

**Ilan E Timor-Tritsch** MD
Professor of Obstetrics & Gynecology
New York University
School of Medicine
New York NY
USA

**Yves G Ville**
Professor of Obstetrics and Gynecology
Université Paris
Poissy
France

**Linda S de Vries** MD, PhD
Professor of Neonatal Neurology
Dept of Neonatology
Wilhelmina Kinderziekenhuis
Utrecht
The Netherlands

**Bettina Westerburg**
University of California
San Francisco CA
USA

**Jennifer A Westgate** MBChB, DipObs, FRANZCOG
Associate Professor of Obstetrics and Gynaecology
The University of Auckland
National Womans Hospital
Auckland
New Zealand

**Andrew Whitelaw** MD, FRCPCH
Professor of Neonatal Medicine
Division of Child Health
University of Bristol
Medical School
Southmead Hospital
Bristol
UK

**Martin J Whittle** MD, FRCOG, FRCP(Glas)
Head of Division of Reproductive Child Health
Birmingham Women's Hospital
Department of Fetal Medicine
Birmingham
UK

**James W Wraith** MB, CLB, MRCP(UK), FRCP
Director
Willink Biochemical Genetics Unit
Royal Manchester Children's Hospital
Manchester
UK

**Ian D Young** MSc, MD, FRCP
Professor/Consultant Clinical Genetecist
Departent of Clinical Genetics
Leicester Royal Infirmary
Leicester
UK

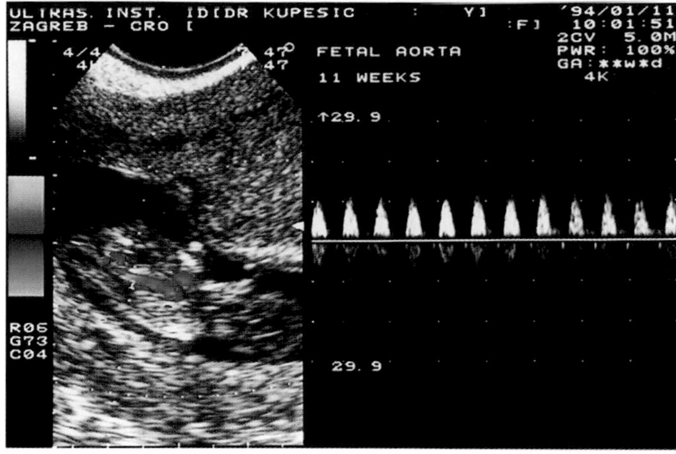


**Plate 4.1** Fetal aorta displayed in color at 11 weeks' gestation. The pulsed Doppler signals show absence of diastolic flow, typical of the fetal aorta at this gestational age.

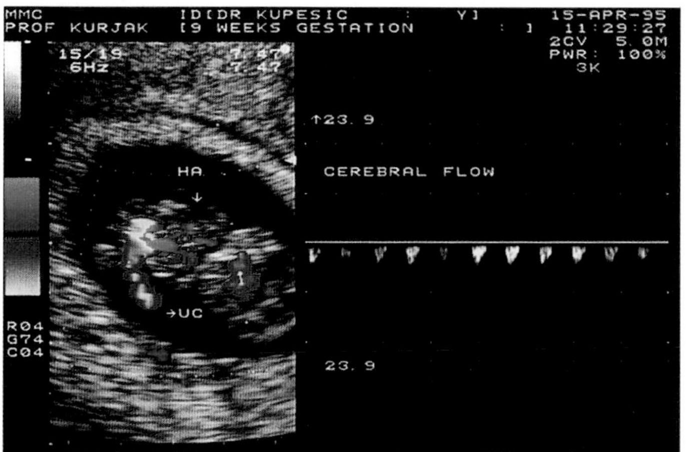


**Plate 4.2** Cerebral flow, characterized by absent diastolic flow at 8 weeks' gestation.

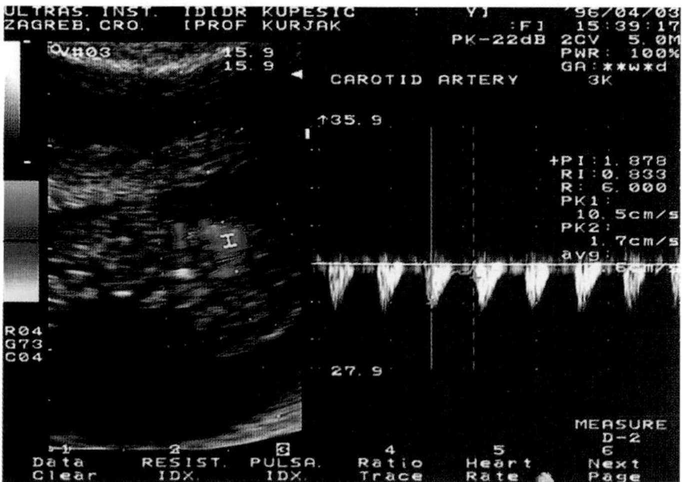


**Plate 4.3** The internal carotid artery at 9/10 weeks' gestation (left). The pulsed Doppler waveform analysis demonstrates inconsistent end-diastolic flow (right).

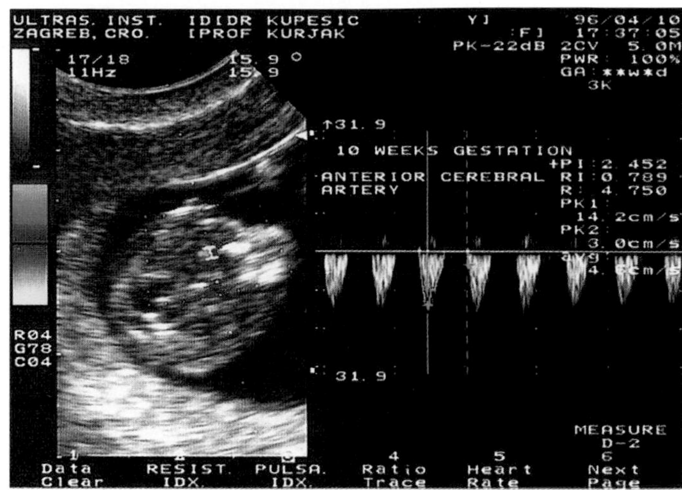


**Plate 4.4** Absent diastolic flow in the anterior cerebral artery at 10 weeks' gestation.

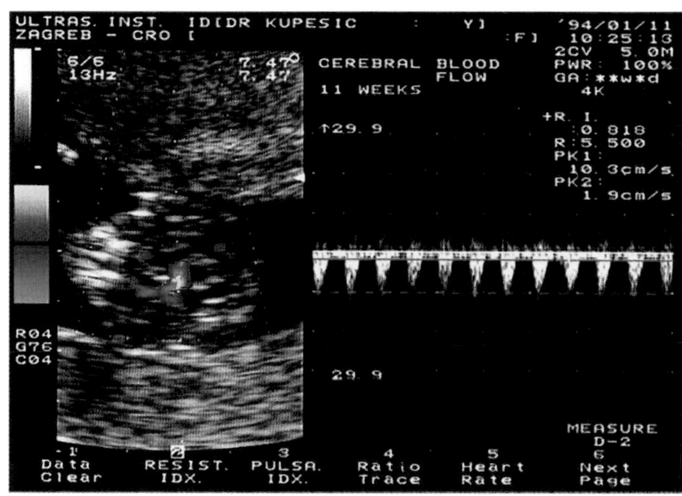


**Plate 4.5** The cerebral artery at 11 weeks' gestation (left). The pulsed Doppler waveform analysis indicates permanent diastolic flow and significantly lower impedance to flow (right) than in other fetal vessels.

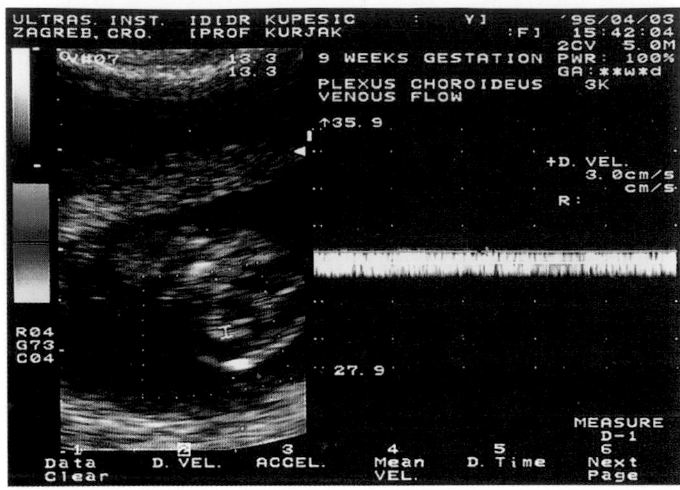


Plate 4.6 Transvaginal scan demonstrating the choroid plexus at 10 weeks' gestation (left). Continuous venous blood flow signals were easily obtainable (right).

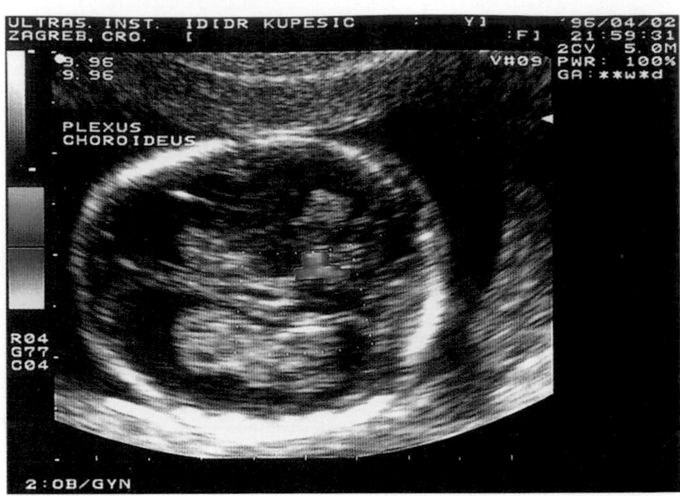


Plate 4.8 Choroid plexuses filling more than one third of the lateral ventricles at 13 weeks' gestation.

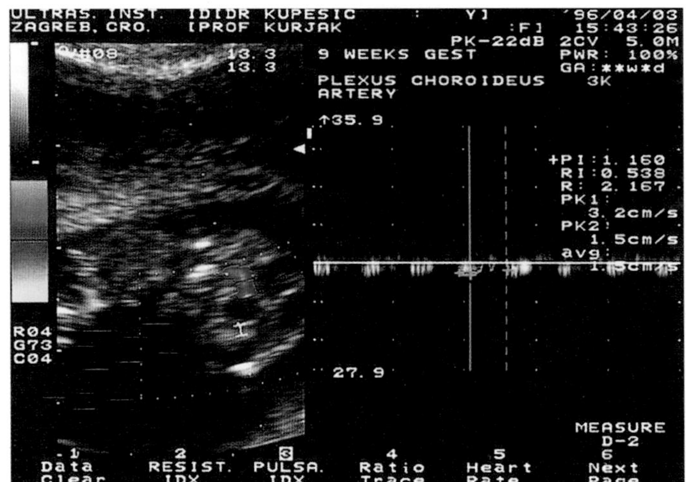


Plate 4.7 The same patient as in Fig. 6. The pulsed Doppler waveform analysis of the choroid plexus arteries demonstrates absence of end-diastolic blood flow (right).

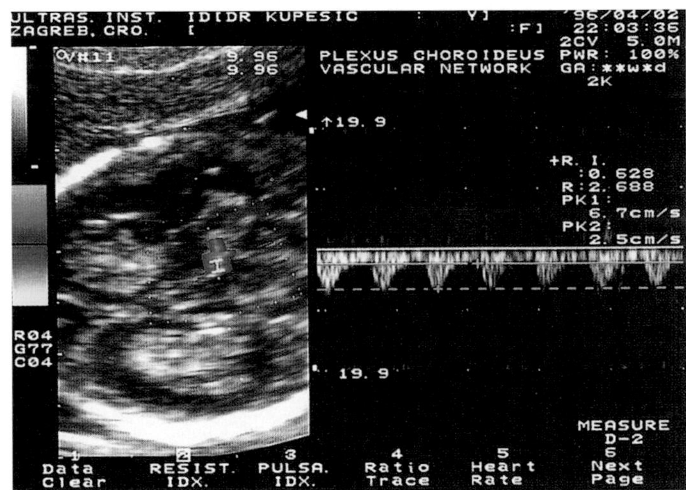


Plate 4.9 The same patient as in Figure 8. Color signals were obtained at the inner edge of the plexus (left). Low vascular impedance (RI = 0.63) is typical for these arteries.

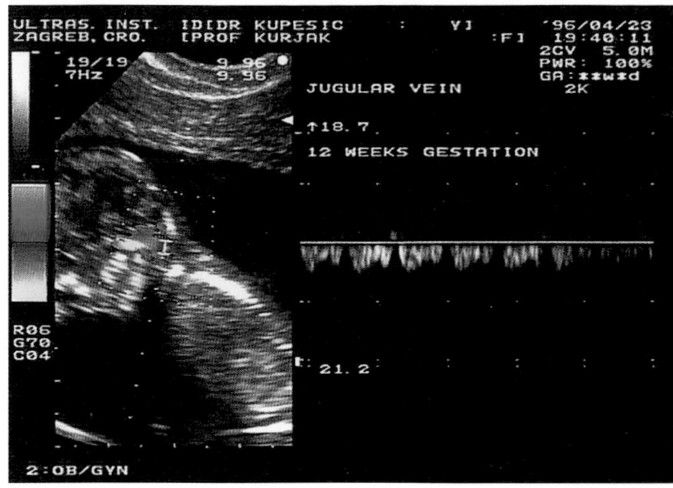


Plate 4.10 Color image of the internal jugular vein (left). The pulsed Doppler waveform analysis demonstrates irregular blood flow (right).

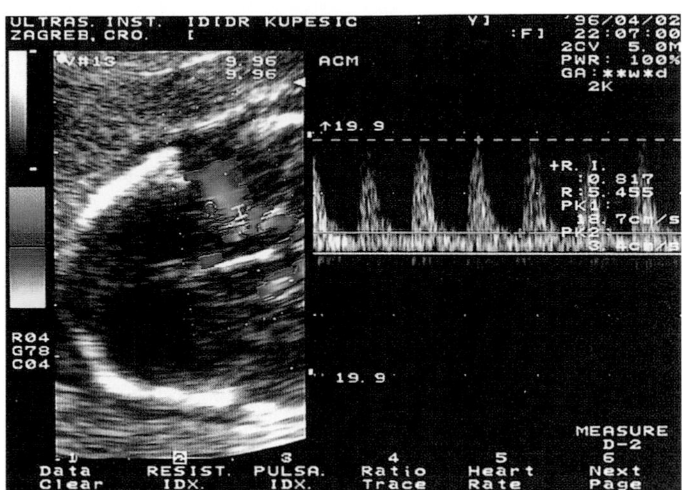


Plate 4.12 The same patient as in Figure 11. Continuous diastolic flow and high vascular resistance (RI = 0.82) are obtained from the anterior cerebral artery. Vascular impedance of the cerebral arteries obtained from 11th gestational week demonstrate a gradual decrease towards the 16th week.

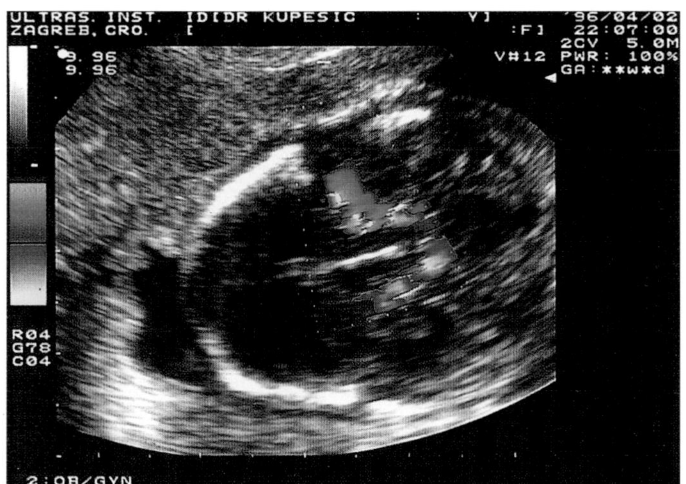


Plate 4.11 Entire cerebral circulation at 14 weeks' gestation as depicted by color Doppler ultrasound.

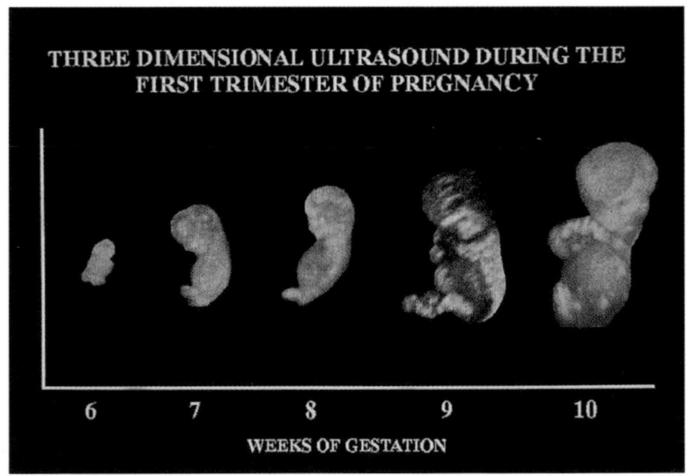


Plate 4.13 Embryonic and fetal development as seen by 3D ultrasound during the first trimester of pregnancy.

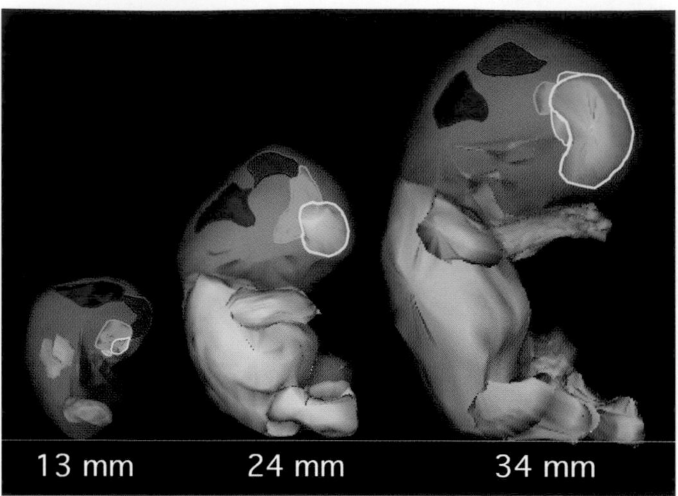


**Plate 4.4** 3D reconstructions of two embryos, 13 mm ≈ 7 weeks, 24 mm ≈ 9 weeks, and one fetus, 34 mm ≈ 10 weeks. The cavities of the brain are coloured: blue = rhombencephalon, red = mesencephalon, green = diencephalon, yellow = lateral ventricles.

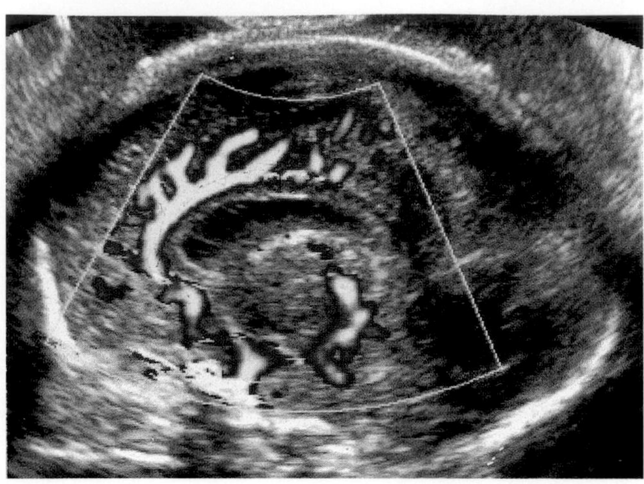

**Plate 18.4** The corpus callosum at 23 postmenstrual weeks. (A) Median section demonstrating the C-shaped corpus callosum. Under it the anterior cavum septi pellucidi (long arrow) and cavum vergae (short arrow) are seen. T, thalamus. (B) Power Doppler study of the pericallosal artery above the corpus callosum.

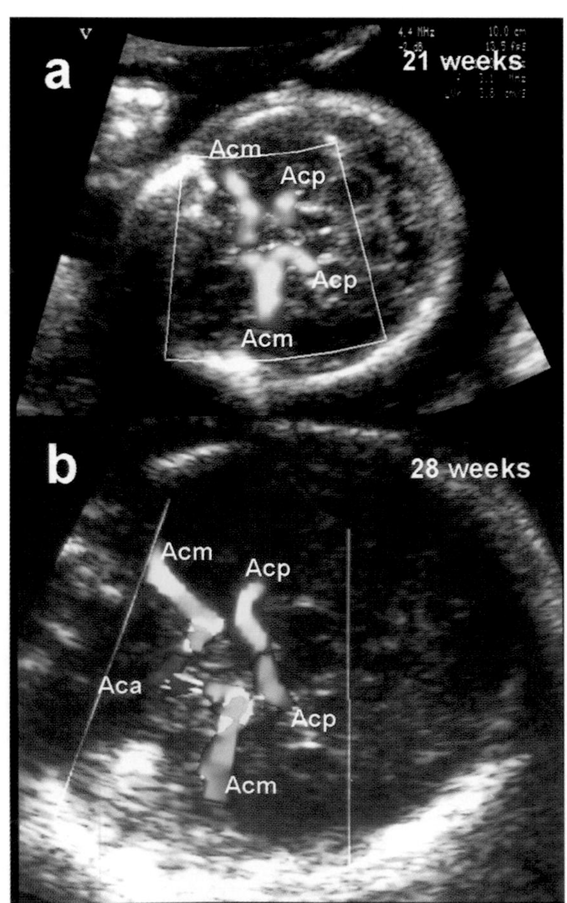


**Plate 5.13** (a) Power Doppler image of the circulus Willisii at 21 weeks. (b) Color Doppler image of the circulus Willisii at 28 weeks; Aca = arteria cerebri anterior; Acm = arteria cerebri media; Acp = arteria cerebri posterior

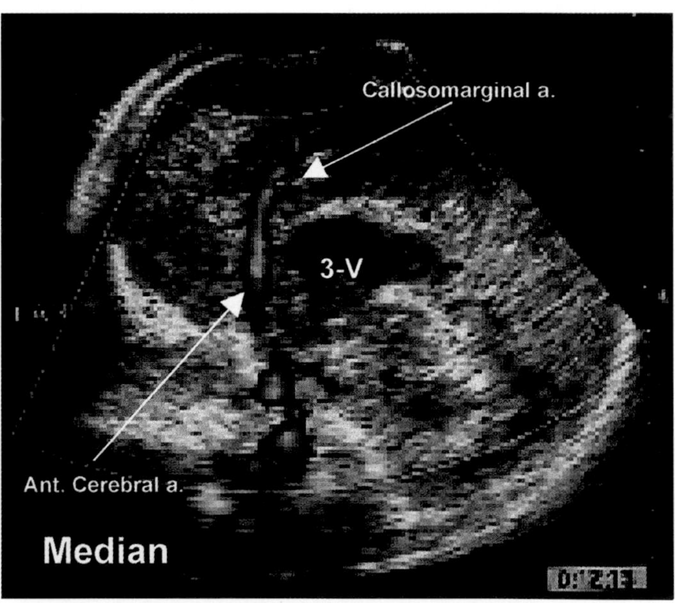


**Plate 18.13** Total agenesis of the corpus callosum at 23 postmenstrual weeks. (A) MC-2, Mid-coronal-2 section with the 3rd ventricle (3-V) communicating with the lateral ventricles (LV) without the presence of the corpus callosum or the cavum septi pellucidi. The two median sections (B, C) and practically the same showing the upward displaced 3rd ventricle above the thalamus (T), however part (C) is a power Doppler image of the anterior cerebral and the callosomarginal arteries without the presence of the pericallosal artery.

# Section I
# Structural development of the CNS

Chapter 1

# Epigenetic and functional organization of the neuronal circuits in the CNS during development

H. Lagercrantz & T. Ringstedt

## INTRODUCTION

The development of the CNS proceeds through a series of milestones, from induction of the neuroectoderm to formation of the neural tube, cephalic folding, proliferation of neurons, migration, synaptogenesis, and wiring (Table 1.1). The first steps are probably strictly genetically controlled, but it is difficult to understand how about 30 000 genes involved in the formation of the human brain can control the organization of about 100 billion neurons and their trillions of synapses. Changeux (2001) has pointed out that there is a striking parsimony of genetic information to code for human brain complexity compared with, for example, nematodes (Table 1.2). One possible solution is multiple combinations of gene activity in time and space (Changeux 1983); another is that the genes are just involved in the scaffolding of the brain and only impose certain genetic constraints (Edelman 1996). Environmental mechanisms should then be responsible for the more detailed wiring. Alternatively, there may be a redundancy of neuronal circuits in the immature brain – a jungle, which is successively organized due to functional requirements by the so-called group selection mechanism or neuronal Darwinism (Edelman 1996).

**Table 1.1 Milestones of CNS development**

| | |
|---|---|
| 3–4 weeks | Formation of the neural tube |
| 5–10 weeks | Prosencephalic phase, formation of the hemispheres |
| 8–18 weeks | Neuronal proliferation |
| 12–24 weeks | Migration |
| 25– weeks | Wiring of the brain |
| | Arborization of the neurons |
| | Synaptogenesis |
| | Apoptosis |
| 40– weeks | Myelination |

**Table 1.2 The simplicity of the genome and the complexity of the brain**

| | | |
|---|---|---|
| Nematode | 19 099 genes | 302 neurons |
| Drosophila | 12 000 genes | 250 000 neurons |
| Mouse | 100 000 genes | 40 million neurons |
| Man | 100 000 genes | 100 billion neurons |

*Source*: From Changeux (2001).

## PATTERNING OF THE FETAL HUMAN BRAIN

The development of the human brain cannot be understood without considering that it derives by evolutionary tinkering from prior ancestral brains (see Changeux 2001). A number of genes involved in the early formation of the brain have been retained during evolution, from 600 million years ago, when the insects and the vertebrates started to develop along separate evolutionary branches. These genes are called homeotic genes and are involved in controlling the Cartesian coordinates of the embryo, the segmentation of the body and identity of its segments. They may be used and reused in different ways during both phylogenesis and ontogenesis (Fig. 1.1).

The brain originates from the neuroectoderm which may comprise about half of the whole ectoderm (see Jacobson 1991; Wolpert 1998). The neuroectoderm is developed by a default pathway, i.e. the formation of non-neuronal ectoderm on each side is achieved by blocking signals at either side (see Frisén *et al.* 1998). The neural groove is made by bending the neural plate and by the action of the notochord. (For further description on the formation and closure of neural tube see Chapter 2.)

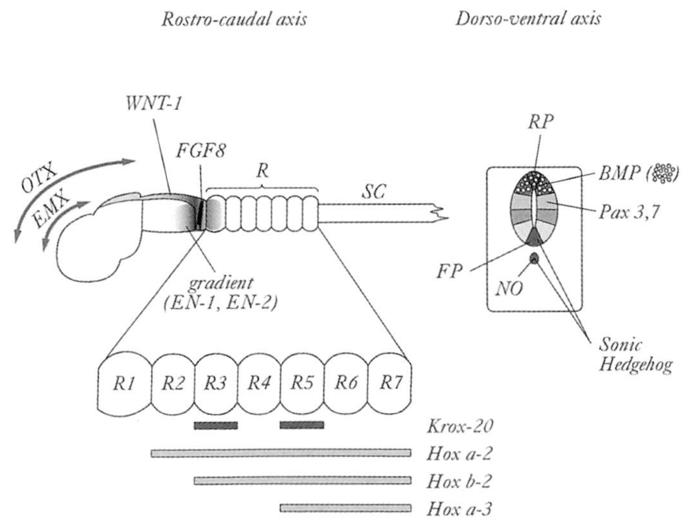


**Figure 1.1** Some genes involved in the patterning of the rostro-caudal and dorso-ventral axis of the mammalian CNS. RP: roof plate, FP: floor plate, NO: notochord, R: rhombomeres, SC: spinal chord (with permission from V. Lendahl)

To form the rostro-caudal axis in the embryo the HOX genes (clustered homeobox-containing genes) are important. They are homologous to the homeotic gene complex (HOM-C) in the fruit fly (Fig. 1.1). The Hox gene clusters (A–D) differentiate the segments. According to the so-called Hox code, cells expressing many Hox proteins develop posterior structures, while those with lower levels form the anterior part of the axis. Knocking out these genes results in replacement of more posterior segments (Krumlauf 1994). Excess doses of retinoic acid, which affects the expression of more posterior Hox genes, disrupt the order of the rhombomeres. Engrailed (En) genes are required for the formation of the tectum (dorsal midbrain) and the cerebellum. EMX and OTX are expressed in the forebrain and midbrain region. Mutation of the EMX gene leads to severe malformation of the cortex – schizencephaly.

Krox-20 is necessary for the development of the cranial nerves in the hindbrain. The Sonic Hedgehog genes serve several functions dependent on timing and spacing. The hedgehog genes encode for proteins that determine, for example, which neurons should develop into motor neurons controlling muscle movements in the spinal cord. If this gene is knocked out all neurons will become sensory neurons by a default pathway. Furthermore, the phenotype will develop a cyclopic eye. Mutation of this gene in the human results in holoprosencephaly (see Chapter 13).

Another important family of genes are the so called Pax genes, the name is derived from paired box, first identified in the fruit fly. They encode for transcription factors and also seem to be important for the formation of the dorso-ventral axis. Mutations of the PAX3 gene in the human results in Wardenburg's syndrome and PAX6 in Peter's anomaly (aniridia). How do these early immature nerve cells know how to differentiate? The concentration of the inducing substance seems to be important. For example, high concentrations of the Sonic Hedgehog proteins induce the formation of most of the ventral cells of the neural plate while lower levels induce specifically motor neurons. Thus if undifferentiated cells are exposed to a high concentration of the substance they will become other cells than if they are exposed to low levels (Wolpert 1997).

## PROLIFERATION OF NEURONS

After formation of the neural tube and prosencephali, proliferation of new neurons takes place. New neurons originate from the pseudostratified ventricular epithelium (PVE). Cells in the pseudostratified epithelium become neurons first by elongation during the G phase and enter the S phase maximally elongated with the nucleus in the other half of the epithelium. The cells proliferate asynchronously, i.e. after mitotic cell division, one will migrate and not proliferate further, while the other returns to the PVE and undergoes a new cell cycle. The pace of neuron production is dependent on the exit rate of cells from the PVE (Caviness *et al.* 1995). Young, newly formed neurons migrate and form the neocortex.

To determine the rate of proliferation the proliferative cells in the epithelium are labeled with the thymidine analog BrdU which will be incorporated into DNA. By using this cumulative labeling, all parameters like the duration of the cell cycle or neurogenetic interval can be calculated. In the mouse there are 11 cell cycles over a 6 day period. About 200 000 new neurons are formed every minute between the 8th and 18th gestational weeks. The fact that most nerve cells are formed after the 8th and before the 18th gestational week was first established by Dobbing & Sands (1970) who analyzed DNA in aborted fetuses. We also learned this in a tragic way: fetuses that were exposed to the first atom bombs in Hiroshima and Nagasaki during this period of pregnancy became microcephalic, a condition which did not affect fetuses who were younger or older at the time of these events (Miller & Blot 1972).

Based on a series of very careful studies in primates, Rakic postulated that there is no neurogenesis after birth in the human (Rakic 1985, 1995). Other animals, like male canary birds, generate new nerve cells in the singing center during the mating season. The number of syllables in their song seems to be directly related to the number of neurons (Nottebohm & Arnold 1976). Recent studies indicate that some new neurons can be formed even in the human adult. Terminally ill patients with cancer were given radioactively labeled thymidine, and after their death a few hundred nuclei of hippocampal neurons were found to be labeled, i.e. newly formed neurons (Eriksson *et al.* 1998). Whether these neurons are of functional significance remains to be elucidated.

## MIGRATION

During formation of the neocortex, the first postmitotic neurons, born in the ventricular zone, will migrate radially to form the primitive plexiform zone or the preplate. Cells born later migrate into the preplate and split it into an outer marginal zone or future layer I, and an inner subplate. These neurons migrate along a fan-like scaffold of glial threads. Newly born cells will migrate past those cells that arrived earlier. The neocortex therefore has an 'inside-out' pattern with the latest born cells in layer II, and the first born (excepting those in the subplate and the marginal zone) in layer VI. Migration occurs mainly between embryonic day 12 and the first postnatal days in the rat and mouse, and between the 12th and 24th weeks of gestation in the human fetus.

The neurons find their way by climbing the radial glial cells. These glial guides correspond to a protomap present in the germinative zone and the cortical areas (Rakic 1985). Integrin receptors play a critical role. The fascicles of glial fibers form corridors filled with glycogen providing energy to the migrating neurons. About 20% of the new neurons migrate horizontally without the support of radial glia. Some of the early born neurons in the marginal zone, the Cajal–Retzius cells, secrete reelin. This substance is essential for correct cortical lamination. It might act by inhibiting the migrating neurons, instructing them to leave the radial glia and assume their final position. Thus reelin would act as a stop signal for the successive waves of cortical neurons.

Neuronal migration can be affected by glutamate. *N*-methyl-D-aspartate antagonists were found to retard the migration or result in the formation of heterotopias and arrest of migrating neurons (see Gressens 1998). Neurotropic factors like NT-4 or brain derived neurotrophic factor can also affect neuronal migration. Severe disturbance of migration can be seen in the Zellweger cerebro-hepato-renal syndrome which is a peroxisomal disease (p. 634). A disorder of migration is also involved in schizencephaly (p. 213) (Evrard *et al.* 1997).

## AXONAL GUIDANCE

The crucial question is how the neurons find their way to their targets. Navigating the interstates from New York to San Francisco is relatively easy compared with what the neurons of the developing nervous system must do in order to reach their goals, or so it was expressed in *Science* (Travi 1994).

In 1892 the Spanish anatomist Ramon y Cajal discovered that axons have special growth cones on their tips. These growth cones behave like immune cells sniffing out chemical scents released by different tissues. This has now been confirmed. The target seems to release a diffusible substance that promotes its own innervation – attractant molecules. Given that the distance between the target and the origin of the axon can be quite long, mechanisms other than simple attraction are involved as well. By analogy with a traveler crossing continental USA, the axons divide its path into several steps, maneuvring between choice points along more or less established routes. The signals that guide a growing axon along its way can, based on their function, be subdivided into four categories: chemo-attractive, chemo-repellent, contact-attractive and contact-repellent. While the chemo-attractive and chemo-repellent signals are diffusible molecules that act over longer distances, the contact-attractive and contact-repellent molecules are bound to cell membranes or to the extracellullar matrix. Repulsive signals seem to be particularly important in axonal pathfinding, because they can be used to outline a permissive path for the growing axons. The complicated task of navigating long distances through the CNS is eased by following routes established by pioneer axons that found their targets early during development, when the brain was smaller and its structure considerably less complex. Axons that grow along these routes are bundled together in fascicles. At the various choice points they have to de-fasciculate in order to change route. Therefore molecules that modulate fasciculation are important in axonal guidance.

Certain structures in the brain are of particular importance to navigating axons. An example of this is the floor plate, an area with mainly non-neuronal cells in the ventral part of the developing spinal cord. The floor plate seems to express several guidance cues. Among these is netrin, which attracts commissural neurons in the upper part of the spinal cord. Netrin is evolutionarily conserved and is also found in the fruit-fly (Drosophila). The midline of the fly's nervous system is, similarly to the spinal cord floor plate, an important landmark for axons. Axons are attracted towards the midline by netrin. The midline also expresses the diffusible ligand Slit, which repulses axonal growth cones carrying the Slit receptor (Robo), thereby preventing these from entering the midline. For axons destined to cross over the midline the situation becomes very complicated, as once they have entered the midline they cannot leave it (on the other side) unless repulsed by Slit. This paradox is solved by the expression of another gene, Comm, in the midline. Comm down-regulates Robo expression on the neurons growing towards the midline, thus enabling them to enter despite the presence of Slit. After they have entered the midline, the axons lose their sensitivity to Comm; Robo is upregulated and they are forced to leave the midline by the repellant activity of Slit. The combined activity of Netrin, Slit and their receptors with Comm thus guides the axons across the midline, and ensures that they do not re-cross it (Kidd *et al.* 1999). Like Netrin, Slit and Robo are also found in mammals (including humans); their functions are just starting to be revealed, but it is already clear that they are involved in axonal guidance in several systems in the brain and spinal cord.

Several other ligand- and receptor families are known in addition to those mentioned above. Among these are the Semaphorins with over 30 members, some of which are secreted, while others are membrane bound. Semaphorins can signal both attraction and repulsion, and in at least some cases, the same ligand can serve both functions. The semaphorin ligands also seem to have different biological specificities. Classes of membrane-bound molecules that mediate contact-inhibition and attraction include the immunoglobulin cell adhesion molecules (Ig Cams), the Cadherins and the Eph receptors (Cook *et al.* 1998). The Ephs constitute the largest subgroup within the receptor tyrosine kinases. Their ligands, the ephrins, are also quite numerous, and the receptor–ligand interaction is quite promiscuous. Like their receptors, the ephrins are membrane-bound, and it is possible that they can have a receptor function as well.

A growth cone is likely to carry receptors for several classes of axon guidance molecules. The inputs from these are integrated into a 'decision' (Stoeckli & Landmesser 1998). One way that this could be achieved is by intracellular signaling mechanisms affecting the growth cone's $Ca^{2+}$ level. It has recently been demonstrated that restricted elevation of $[Ca^{2+}]$ on one side of the growth cone induces either turning towards that side (attraction), or away from it (repulsion), depending on the extracellular $Ca^{2+}$ level (Zheng 2000). Many axonal guidance molecules have also been shown to induce both attraction and repulsion, even if this is dependent in at least some cases on the type of receptor involved (Bashaw & Goodman 1999).

Some ligands involved in axonal guidance, for example

Slit, also affect cell migration. It has become increasingly clear that axonal guidance and cell migration have many mechanisms in common. The migrating cell sends out a 'leading process' that trails ahead of the cell soma, and probably orientates towards the target like an axonal growth cone.

## NEUROTROPHIC AGENTS

The nerve growth factor (NGF) was discovered by Rita Levi-Montalcini and Viktor Hamburger in 1951. They found that sensory and also sympathetic ganglia grow better in the vicinity of sarcoma tumors and they postulated that this was due to a secreted agent. To characterize this factor they used snake venom to inactivate the postulated protein. To their surprise this resulted in a better stimulation of nerve growth, because the salivary glands contain high amounts of NGF. Salivary glands were then used to isolate NGF. (See the fascinating autobiography by Rita Levi-Montalcini 1988.)

A number of other nerve growth factors or neurotrophic agents have since been discovered (see Davies 1994). The neurotrophin family comprises nerve growth factor (NGF), brain derived neurotrophic factor (BDNF), neurotropin-3 (NT-3) and neurotropin 4 (NT-4). They are diffusible peptide factors active in the form of homodimers. They act through two classes of receptors: the p75 neurotropin receptor (p75 NTR) and the tropomyosin kinase receptors (trkA, trkB, and trkC).

The role of the neurotrophins is better understood in the peripheral than in the central nervous system. In the peripheral nervous system they mainly act as target derived neurotrophic agents, ensuring the survival of axons that innervate the target correctly. However, they seem to be important also in the CNS, although studies on mice with neurotrophin ligand and receptor genes deleted showed, contrary to expectations, that most of the cell populations in the CNS were retained, indicating that their function there is a different one (Snider 1994). As an example, embryonic overexpression of BDNF in the brain of transgenic mice resulted in a striking and unexpected phenotype with clustering of the Cajal–Retzius cells and a reduced expression of reelin. The normal inside-out lamination of the neocortex was disturbed. On the basis of these findings it is assumed that BDNF acts as an intrinsic determinant of cortical maturation (Ringstedt *et al.* 1998).

## NEUROTRANSMITTERS

Although the development of the scaffold of the CNS is mainly determined by genes, the detailed wiring of the neuronal circuits is more self-generated, being dependent on the action of neurotransmitters and neuromodulators. They can promote, amplify, block, inhibit, or attenuate the microelectric signals that are passed on to them and through them, and thereby give rise to the signaling patterns between myriads of neuronal networks providing the physical networks of cerebral neurons. Catecholamines appear in the embryos of vertebrate and invertebrate animals even before neurons are differentiated. Possibly they then function as morphogenes or trophic factors. Some of the cells in the neuronal crest contain from the beginning noradrenaline, but become cholinergic due to enivronmental influences.

A neuroactive agent can be expressed in high amounts during certain stages of development, but then remains only in a few synapses. Either this agent only has a transitory role at a critical phase during development or it may remain mostly as an evolutionary residue, with minor functions in, for example, the mammals (see Lagercrantz & Herlenius 2001).

It is interesting to note that if the synthesis of some of these neurotransmitters/modulators is blocked pharmacologically or knocked-out by transgenic techniques the apparent effect may be minimal. This illustrates the plasticity of the brain during early development. Other neuroactive agents seem to be able to take over.

Noradrenaline and acetylcholine are regarded as classical neurotransmitters and dominate in the peripheral nervous system. They appear at an early stage during both phylogenesis and ontogenesis. Many of the neuropeptides were first identified in the gastrointestinal tract and probably appear also early during development. They act slowly since they have to be synthesized and packaged in the cell soma and carried to the terminals before they can be released. The more developed sophisticated mammalian brain requires more fast-switching neurotransmitters acting directly on ion-channels like the excitatory and inhibitory amino acids, which seem to dominate in the mature CNS, whilst the monoamines and neuropeptides may act more as neuromodulators.

In the immature brain, synaptic transmission is weak, extremely plastic and mediated to a large extent by *N*-methyl-D-aspartate (NMDA) receptors. The AMPA receptors are more or less silent at resting membrane potentials (Fox *et al.* 1999). During maturation many NMDA receptors are substituted by AMPA receptors. Dark rearing or blocking the activity with tetrodotoxin results in preservation of the NMDA receptors. Dark rearing also preserves the immature form of the NMDA receptors containing NR2B, and the expression of NR2A is delayed. This subunit switch is essential for rapid synaptic transmission. Thus NMDA receptors are important for the experience-dependent synaptic traffic.

Another amino acid, $\gamma$-aminobutyric acid (GABA), is known as an inhibitory neuorotransmitter in the mature brain, but is actually excitatory in the developing brain. This is due to the fact that the $Cl^-$ concentration is high in the nerve cells. When GABA opens the $Cl^-$ channels a depolarization occurs (i.e. excitation). During maturation the $Cl^-$ concentration decreases intracellularly resulting in an opposite effect of GABA i.e. $Cl^-$ ions are pumped out and the cells become hyperpolarized (Miles 1999). In this way GABA switches from being an excitatory neurotransmitter in the fetus to becoming an inhibitory one after birth.

## SYNAPTOGENESIS

Five 'waves' of synaptogenesis have been identified in the primate by Bourgeois (1997) who studied the primary visual cortex of the macaque monkey (Fig. 1.2). Based on studies of the human occipital cortex (Zecevic 1998) a tentative timetable can be drawn up for the human:

- *Phase 1* begins around 6–8 weeks of gestation at the same time as the onset of neuron proliferation. This early synaptogenesis is limited to lower structures like the subplate.
- *Phase 2* begins after 12–17 weeks and is also relatively sparse. It occurs in the cortical plate. These early synapses form contacts on the dendritic shafts of the neurons.
- *Phase 3* is much more rapid and is assumed to start around midgestation (20–24 weeks) and persists up to 8 months after birth. The rate of this synaptogenesis has been estimated to 40 000 new synapses per second in each striate cortex of the macaque. It occurs at the same time as the arborization of axons and dendrites.
- *Phase 4* lasts until puberty and occurs also at a very high rate.
- *Phase 5* Synaptogenesis continues up to the age of 70 years, but there are also considerable losses during this phase.

The first two phases are not at all affected by lack of sensory stimulation, while the third phase may be partially dependent on sensory input. This has been demonstrated by visual stimulation or ablation in the macaque. Synaptogenesis during the third phase is partially intrinsic and partially dependent on sensory stimulation. Thus it coincides with the critical periods. Many of the sensory, motor and cognitive skills function very early after birth when the synaptoarchitecture is still being laid down.

Synaptogenesis during the fourth phase is even more dependent on experience. During this phase there is a reorganization and fine tuning of neuronal circuits. When this phase has ended during puberty there seems to be a 'freezing' of the personality and the end of several basic learning capacities such as learning to talk a new language without accent. There is some evidence that learning induces formation of new synapses. However, learning during life would then result in continuous brain growth. Recently, it has actually been demonstrated that associative learning does not increase the number of synapses in the hippocampus (Geinisman *et al.* 1999).

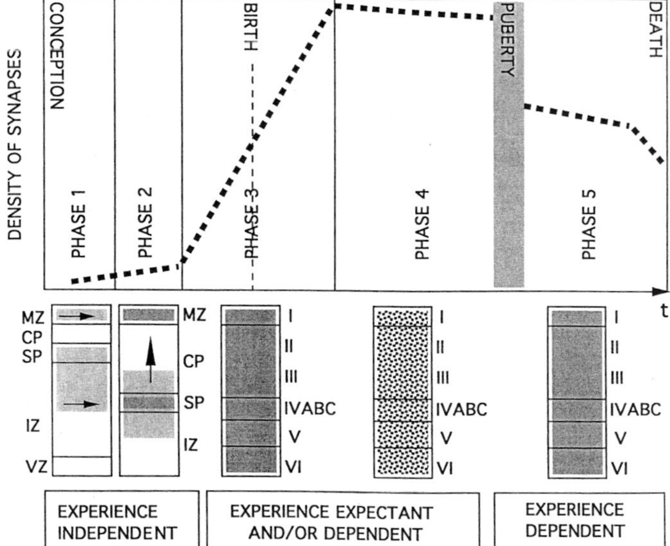


Figure 1.2 Changes in the relative densities of synapses, expressed on a log scale fron the abscissa. The figure is based on studies of the visual cortex of the macaque monkey, but can be extrapolated to the human. During phase 1 synapses appear first in the Marginal Zone (MZ), SubPlate (SP) and Intermediate Zone (IZ). During phase 2 they also appear in the Cortical Plate (CP). (From Bourgeois 1997.)

## WIRING THE BRAIN

The wiring of the precise neural circuits seems to be dependent on neuronal activity which could be stimulated either by sensory input or by endogenously driven activity. Redundant numbers of neuronal pathways and circuits are formed in the fetal brain. About half of the neurons disappear before birth by apoptotic processes. This was found already in the 1930s by Hamburger, who observed that the number of neurons innervating the chicken wing decreased during maturation (see Purves & Lichtman 1985).

The importance of sensory stimulation was discovered by Hubel & Wiesel who found in the 1960s that closing one eye in the kitten or baby monkey resulted in blindness in that eye and disruption of the ocular dominance columns in the visual cortex (see Hubel 1995). This occurred between the fourth week and fourth month in the kitten, while the sensitive period began earlier in the monkey.

This process has been discovered to occur also before birth (Penn & Shatz 1998) by studying the lateral geniculate bodies in ferret fetuses. The optic nerves from the two eyes grow into the geniculate body and spread out through all layers. During maturation these structures become organized and layers are formed. This process is dependent on spontaneous firing in the retina. If it is blocked with tetrodotoxin, the segregation into layers is disturbed.

The spontaneous activity begins at some focus of the retina and spreads out in waves. This could be visualized by a fluorescence imaging technique in whole-mounted retinae from newborn ferrets. It seems to be generated by cholinergic amacrine cells, as it could be reversibly blocked by a nicotinic acetylcholine receptor antagonist (Feller *et al.* 1996). Each wave lasts several seconds followed by a minute long interval. Neighboring cells seem to fire in synchrony, and this local retinal synchrony forms the basis for the layering of the geniculate bodies and the ocular dominance

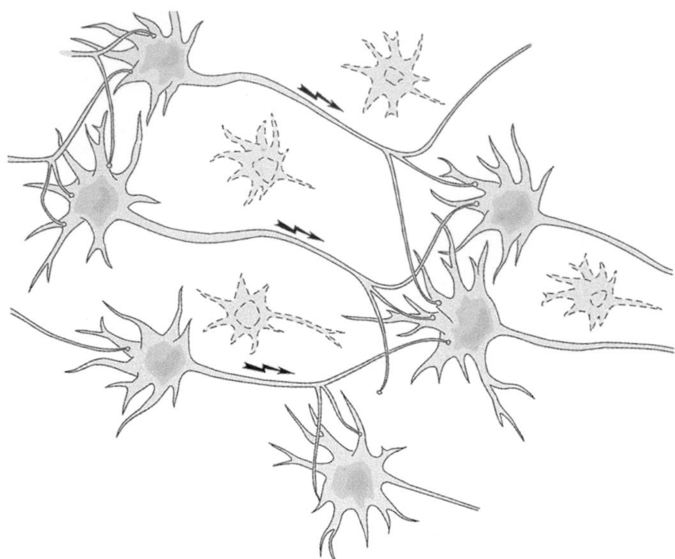

Figure 1.3 Neurons which fire together wire together, neurons which don't won't (see Penn & Shatz).

columns in the cortex. Shatz coined the expression: 'Cells that fire together wire together while those which don't won't' (Fig 1.3). However, recent studies by Crowley & Katz (1999) have shown that ocular dominance columns can be formed without electrophysiological stimulation and are thus genetically determined, but they admit that visual stimulation is important for the refinement of the ocular dominance columns and thus the vision.

## ORGANIZATION OF THE BRAIN (Fig. 1.4)

Changeux in *Neuronal Man* (1985) wrote that 'Recognizing the power of the genes in no way forces us to submit to their supreme authority'. To claim that complex behaviors are mainly genetically determined has been strongly refuted by Rose (1995) who is one of the strongest critics of 'neurogenetic determinism'. The discovery of a number of genes determining diseases and human behavior may result in some social defeatism, according to Rose (1995). The genome is relatively simple while the brain, particularly the human brain, is very complex. Genetic determinism assumes that genes directly control development, morphology and behavior. Development, in this view, would be purely a process of programmed maturation, contaminated perhaps occasionally by a certain amount of noise (Edelman & Tononi 1996). Development is viewed instead as epigenetic, that is many different components must come together at the right time and at the right place. The idea that the genes provide the 'blueprint' should probably be rejected. Genes certainly matter but development is more a form of 'jazz with improvization' than a fixed musical score (Bateson & Martin 1999).

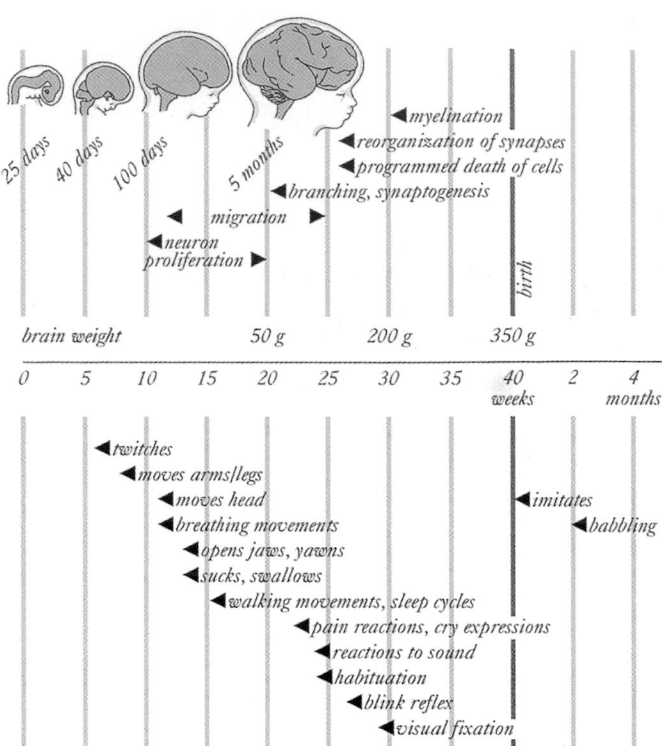


Figure 1.4 Overview of the morphological and functional development of the CNS.

Environmental instructionism cannot explain the formation of the neuronal circuits. The view that the newborn brain may be regarded as a tabula rasa has been abandoned and it is now well established that the human baby is born with the ability to recognize the human face and voice, etc. The idea whether there is an innate grammar is controversial, but there is probably a general agreement that some kind of language ability is innate (Pinker 1994).

Edelman has proposed the idea of neuronal Darwinism or the theory of neuronal group selection to explain how the brain is constructed with regard to the limited number of genes encoding the formation of the human brain. The theory of neuronal group selection (TNGS) consists of three tenets. The first is that dynamic primary processes lead to the formation of the neuroanatomy. This anatomy possesses enormous variation due to the 'stochastic fluctuation of cell movement, cell process extension and cell death during development.' The entire process is a selective one based on topobiological competition. The second tenet states that a variety of functioning circuits are carved out i.e. strengthening of the synapses. In the third tenet physiology and psychology are combined. A number of maps are formed in the brain by sensory impressions. New impressions reinforce the neuronal wiring of certain maps. Neurotransmitters like acetylcholine and dopamine have been proposed to be involved in this selection mechanism.

According to Edelman particularly the developing brain is jungle. It is not a question of creating novel connections, rather eliminating pre-existing ones (Changeux 1996). Neuronal Darwinism or the theory of neuronal group selection has been challenged by Purves *et al.* (1996). He claims that there is no selective elimination of an initial excess of dendrites and synapses. Although there is essentially a very small increase of the number of neurons after birth, the existing neurons grow and develop synapses throughout life. Growing neurons gain synapses rather than lose them. Spontaneous activity stimulates formation of synapses and elaborates the synaptoarchitectonic organization. Losses of neurons, axons, and synapses are just epiphenomena (Purves *et al.* 1996).

According to Changeux, Purves favors a kind of Lamarckian constructivism: 'the function would create the organ'. One example in favor of Purves is how well the tongue and the thumb are represented in the human brain corresponding to the importance of these organs for the human being. On the other hand associative learning does not seem to increase the number of synapses and stimulate brain growth, which speaks against the idea of constructivism (see above).

## ACKNOWLEDGMENT

A similar article entitled: 'A brief review on the organization of the neuronal circuits in the CNS during development' will be published in Acta Paediatrica by permission of the publishers.

## REFERENCES


Bashaw G J & Goodman C S (1997) Chimeric axon guidance receptors: the cytoplasmic domains of Slit and Netrin receptors specify attraction versus repulsion. *Cell* 97:917–926.

Bateson P & Martin P (1999) *Let them think cake.* London: Jonathan Cape.

Berger-Sweeney J (1997) Behavioral consequences of abnormal cortical development: insights into developmental disabilities. *Behav Brain Res* 86:121–142.

Bourgeois J P (1997) Synaptogenesis, heterochrony and epigenesis in the mammalian neocortex. *Acta Paediat Suppl* 422:27 33.

Caviness V S, Takahashi T & Nowakoski R S (1995) Numbers, time and neocortical neurogenesis: a general developmental and evolutionary model. *Trends Neurosci* 18:379–383.

Changeux J-P (1983) *Neuronal man* (new edn, 1997). Princeton, NJ: Princeton University Press.

Changeux J-P (2001) Reflexions on the origins of the human brain. In: Lagercrantz H, Evrard P, Hanson M, Rodeck C (eds) *The newborn brain – scientific basis and clinical applications.* Cambridge: Cambridge University Press.

Cook G, Tannahill D & Keynes R (1998) Axon guidance to and from choice points. *Curr Opin Neurobiol* 8:64–72.

Crair M C (1999) Neuronal activity during development: permissive or instructive? *Curr Opin Neurobiol* 9:88–93.

Crowley J C & Katz L C (1999) Development of ocular dominance columns in the absence of retinal input. *Nat Neurosci* 2:1125–1130.

Davies A M (1994) Neurotrophic factors. Switching neurotrophin dependence. *Curr Opin Cell Biol* 4:273–276.

Dobbing J & Sands J (1970) Timing of neuroblast multiplication in developing human brain. *Nature* 226:639–640.

Dubowitz L & Dubowitz V (1981) The neurological assessment of the preterm and full-term newborn infant. *Clin Dev Med* No. 79. London: SIMP/Heinemann.

Edelman G M (1996) Neural Darwinism: selection and reentrant signalling in higher brain function. *Neuron* 10:1–20.

Edelman G M & Tononi G (1996) Selection and development: the brain as a complex system. In: Magnusson D *et al.* (ed) *Behavioral, neurobiological and psychosocial perspectives.* Cambridge: Cambridge University Press; pp. 107–138.

Eriksson P S, Perfilieva E, Björk-Eriksson T *et al.* (1998) Neurogenesis in the adult human hippocampus. *Nat Med* 4:1313–1317.

Evrard P, Marret S & Gressens P (1997) Environmental and genetic determinants of neural migration and postmigratory survival. *Acta Paediat Suppl* 422:20–26.

Feller M B, Wellis D P, Stellwagen D *et al.* (1996) Requirement for cholinergic synaptic transmission in the propagation of spontaneous retinal waves. *Science* 272:1182–1187.

Fox K, Henley J & Isaac J (1999) Experience-dependent development of NMDA receptor transmission. *Nat Neurosci* 2:297–299.

Frisén J, Johansson C B, Lothian C & Lendahl U (1998) Central nervous system stem cells in the embryo and adult. *Cell Mol Life Sci* 54:935–945.

Geinisman Y, Disterhof J F, Gunderson H J G *et al.* (2000) Remodelling of hippocampal synapses hippocampus-dependent associative learning. *J Comp Neurol* 417:49–59.

Gressens P (1998) Mechanisms of cerebral dysgenesis. *Curr Opin Pediat* 10:556–560.

Hubel DH (1995) *Eye, brain, and vision.* New York, NY: Scientific American Library.

Jacobson M (1991) *Developmental neurobiology.* New York, NY: Plenum Press; 776pp.

Johnston M V & Silverstein F S (1998) Development of neurotransmitters. In: Polin R A, Fox W W (eds) *Fetal and neonatal physiology.* Philadelphia, PA: W B Saunders Company; pp. 2110–2117.

Kidd T, Bland K S & Goodman C S (1999) Slit is the midline repellent for the Robo receptor in Drosophila. *Cell* 96:785–794.

Krumlauf R (1994) Hox genes in vertebrate development. *Cell* 78:191–201.

Lagercrantz H & Herlenius E (2000) Neurotransmitters and neuromodulators. In: Lagercrantz H, Evrard P, Hanson M, Rodeck (eds) *The newborn brain – scientific basis and clinical applications.* Cambridge: Cambridge University Press (in press).

Le Douarin N M (1981) Plasticity in the development of the peripheral nervous system. *CIBA Symposium* 83:19–46.

Levi-Montalcini R (1988) *My life and work.* New York, NY: Basic books.

Miles R (1999) A homeostatic switch. *Nature* 397:215–216.

Miller R W, Blot W J (1972) Small head size after in-utero exposure to atomic radiation. *Lancet* 14:784–787.

Nottebohm F, Arnold A P (1976) Sexual dimorphism in vocal control areas of the songbird brain. *Science* 194:211–213.

Parnavelas J G, Stern C D & Stirling R V (1988) *The making of the nervous system,* London: Oxford University Press.

Penn A A & Shatz C J (1999) Brain waves and brain wiring: the role of endogenous and sensory-driven neural activity in development. *Pediatr Res* 45:447–456.

Pinker S (1994) *The Language Instinct.* London: Penguin.

Purves D & Lichtman JW (1985) *Principles of neural development.* Sunderland, Mass: Sinauer Associates.

Purves D, White L E & Riddle D R (1996) Is neuronal development Darwinian? *Trends Neurosci* 19:460–464.

Rakic P (1985) Limits of neurogenesis in primates. *Science* 227:1054–1055.

Rakic P (1995) A small step for the cell, a giant leap for mankind: a hypothesis of neocortical expansion during evolution. *Trends Neurosci* 18:383–388.

Ringstedt T, Linnarsson S, Wagner J *et al.* (1998) BDNF regulates reelin expression and cajal-Retzius cell development in the cerebral cortex. *Neuron* 21:305–315.

Rose S (1995) The rise of neurogenetic determinism. *Nature* 373:380–382.

Snider W D (1994) Functions of the neurotrophins during nervous system development: what the knockouts are teaching us. *Cell* 77:627–638.

Smith C U M (1986) *Elements of molecular neurobiology,* 2nd edn. Chichester: John Wiley & Sons.

Stoeckli E T & Landmesser L T (1998) Axon guidance at choice points. *Curr Opin Neurobiol* 8:73–79.

Travi J (1994) Wiring the nervous system. *Science* 266:568–570.

Wolpert L (1997) *Principles of development.* Oxford: Oxford University Press.

Zecevic N (1998) Synaptogenesis in layer I of the human cerebral cortex in the first half of gestation. *Cerebral Cortex* 8:245–252.

Zheng J Q (2000) Turning of nerve growth cones induced by localized increases in intracellular calcium ions. *Nature* 403:89–93.

# Chapter 2 Early embryonic development of the brain

G. Moscoso

## INTRODUCTION

The human brain is a unique organ that subordinates every organ system in the body. It generates the mind, a complex framework that tells us that 'we are' or that 'we exist', and also that we are different from the surroundings. To the capacity of learning, the brain adds the emotional component that comes into play at some point during development. Thus the individual can feel pleasure, pain, aggression, or fear. The combination of intellectual and emotional reactions will determine behavior commonly exteriorized as 'actions'. Today, humans can modify the environment in such a way that no other living creature has ever been capable of since the creation of the universe.

At present neuropathology, adult psychopathology and child psychiatry are actively revisiting developmental neurobiology in an effort to identify the origins of neurologic and psychological disorders. There are two main reasons for this effort. The first is the concept that factors affecting brain development, which could start operating early during pregnancy, may play a central role in the pathogenesis of neurologic and psychiatric illness. Based on good experimental evidence, an organic basis for schizophrenia and major depressive illness has been put forward by more than one team of researchers (Weinberger *et al.* 1982, 1987; Weinberger 1987; Suddath *et al.* 1990). The second reason is the development of new tools for research at molecular, cell and organ-system levels using genetically modified animal models, thereby providing the investigator with clearer variables to study the emergence of form and function of the CNS in health and disease, from the earliest stages of development until well after birth.

Brain development proceeds according to intrinsic and extrinsic influences. Intrinsic influences are given by the genetic code that modulates the development of form and symmetry and primes neural circuits for function. The extrinsic influences start *in utero* and will continue until the death of the individual. At organ level, brain development starts with the formation of the neural tube or neurulation, followed by neuronal migration and neuritic differentiation with synapse formation and controlled neural 'pruning' (Bourgeois *et al.* 1989). The last two stages have become areas of great interest in recent years. More importantly, it is now well accepted that environmental influences condition brain development.

This chapter describes the development of the CNS at organ level from the start of embryonic life to the end of the first trimester of pregnancy. In addition, some data on gene expression during brain development observed in some animal models will be presented, suggesting that similar patterns of gene expression may operate in humans.

## ORGANOGENESIS

In the human as in higher vertebrates, the development of the CNS starts with the formation of the neural plate at about the 18/19th day postfertilization (Carnegie's stage 8). The neural plate develops cranial to the primitive streak along the midsagittal line (Fig. 2.1). It is shortly followed by the emergence of two neural folds which fuse at the level of the first pair of somites during days 20th and 21st (Carnegie's stages 9–10) (O'Rahilly & Muller 1999). As a result of this fusion, the embryonic disk adopts a tubular shape, when the crown–rump length is about 3.3 mm (Fig. 2.2). Closing of the neural tube proceeds in a zip-up action from day 20th to day 25th when the anterior neuropore closes (Fig. 2.3); 2 days later the caudal neuropore closes at the level of somite 31 or where the 2nd sacral segment will differentiate. In this fashion the neural tube becomes isolated from the amniotic environment.

Observations in mutant mice lacking laminin $\alpha 5$ chain showed multiple developmental defects including failed closure of the anterior neuropore (exencephaly) (Miner *et al.* 1998). Therefore, absence of laminin, a non-collagen glycoprotein and normal constituent of the basal lamina, appears to play an important role during closure of the neural tube. From the initial stages of neural tube closing, a population of neural crest cells emerges at the level of the fusing neural crests, and migrate, following chemical cues, along the lateral sides of the embryo's body to specific target organs. Their role during morphogenesis and organogenesis, however, is ample and complex and beyond the scope of this chapter.

In the early twenties, whilst studying early Drosophila embryos, Bridges & Morgan (1923) identified a cluster of homeotic selector genes, the HOM complex, which participate in modulating the development and orientation of specific body segments and limbs (Dolle *et al.* 1989; Oliver *et al.* 1989). Today, it is known that mammals and other vertebrates have homeoboxes containing tightly linked clusters or HOM complexes, for example, Hox-1, Hox-2, Hox-3 and Hox-5 genes that are expressed in early mouse embryos. Similarly, HOX genes that modulate the development of the

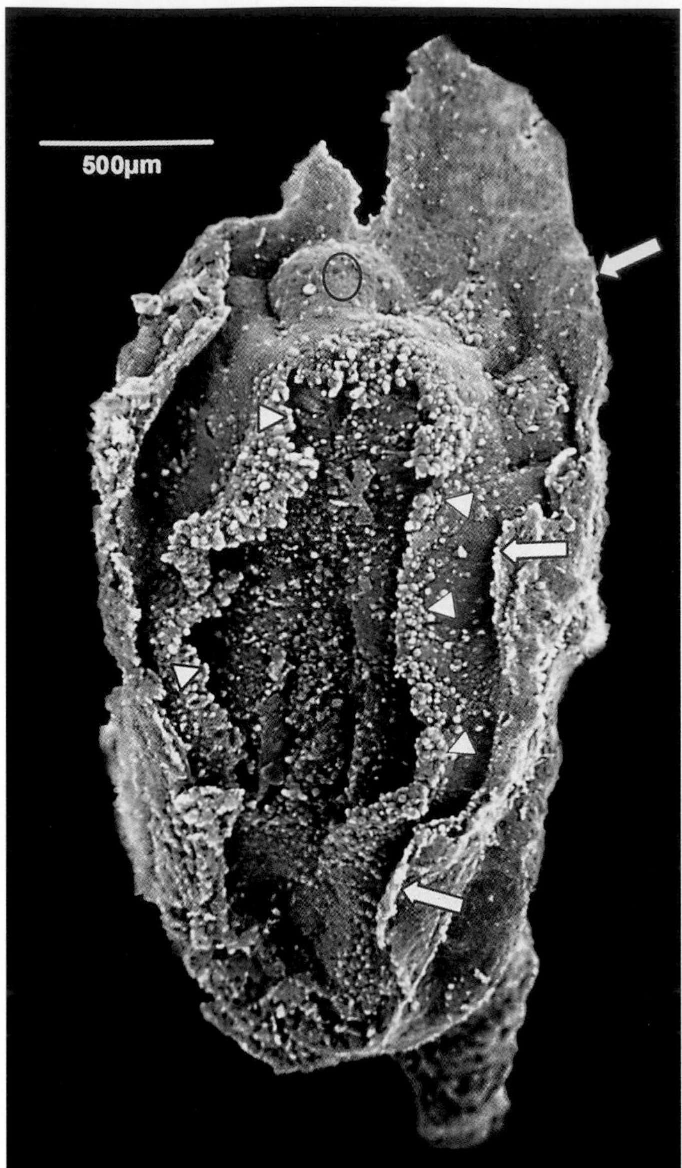


Figure 2.1 Human embryo at 19 days postfertilization (stage 8). There are prominent marginal lobulations at the cephalic end (circled). Some ectoderm has been removed (arrow heads) to reveal a midline triangular ridge and two flaking grooves. These formations are beneath the primitive streak. The amnion (arrows) has been partially removed to expose the embryonic disk. SEM ×180.

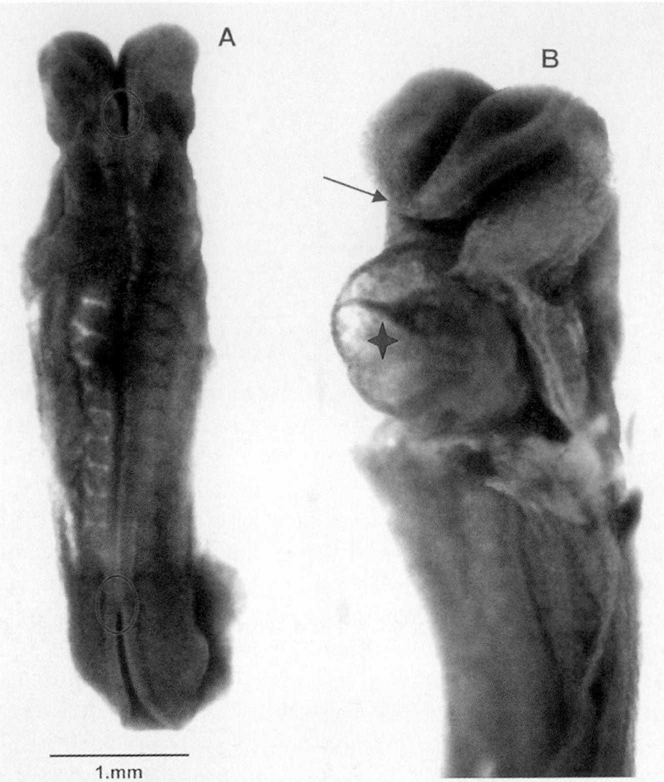


Figure 2.2 Human embryo at 23 days postfertilization (stage 11). (A) Posterior view. Note the tubular shape of the embryo's body. The anterior and caudal neuropores are open (circles). (B) Left lateral view. The cephalic end of the neural tube (arrow) and the cardiac loop (star) are very close to each other at this stage. This will facilitate neural crest cell migration to selected areas of the developing heart.

CNS also are expressed in early embryonic stages (Holland & Hogan 1988). This is discussed in detail in Chapter 1.

When examined at the appropriate time of development, the hind brain of the chicken presents eight bulges known as rhombomeres, limited by constrictions (Lumsden & Keynes 1989). In-situ hybridization has shown selective expression first of Krox-20 gene in rhombomere 3 followed by expression in rhombomere 5. Downregulation occurred in the same order, and these observations indicate that segmentation of the hindbrain occurs in an antero-posterior direction (Wilkinson *et al.* 1989). Furthermore, histological examination at these levels showed a neuronal organization in these segments, directly related to cranial sensory ganglia and cranial nerve roots connecting branchial and pharyngeal arches. Thus, patterning of the body axis and of the CNS seems to be dependent on a specific set of HOM genes if normal development is to be achieved.

The Sonic Hedgehog gene (p. 4) is also expressed during early embryogenesis and the peptides it generates will assist in the formation of the notochord and neural tube (neurulation). Later on, it will induce the differentiation of spinal motor neurons (Roelink *et al.* 1994), midbrain dopaminergic neurons (Hynes *et al.* 1994; Wang *et al.* 1995) and dorsal forebrain dopaminergic neurons (Ericson *et al.* 1995) (Fig. 2.4). Interestingly, the Sonic Hedgehog gene has a protective effect on neurones when challenged with specific neurotoxins, i.e. MMP$^+$ (Miao *et al.* 1997), and contributes to determining the body axis (Tanabe & Jessel 1996).

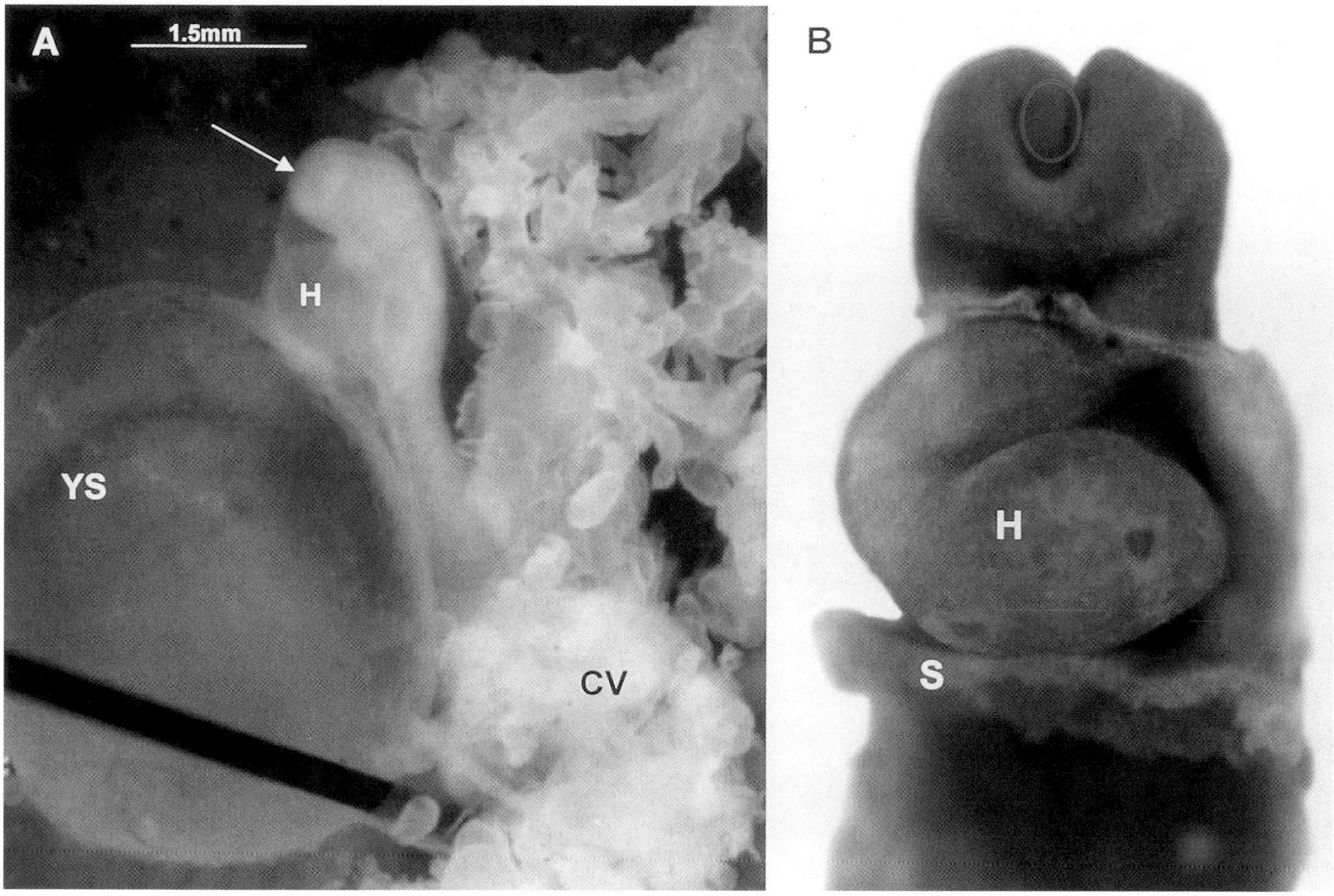

Figure 2.3 Human embryo at 25 days postfertilization (stage 11). (A) Left lateral view. Note the tubular shape of the embryo's body and the attached secondary yolk sac (YS). The cardiac loop is larger than the head. (B) Frontal view of the embryo in (A). The rostral neuropore (circle) is about to close. The cardiac loop shows a transverse (H) and an ascending segments (outflow portion). S = septum transversum.

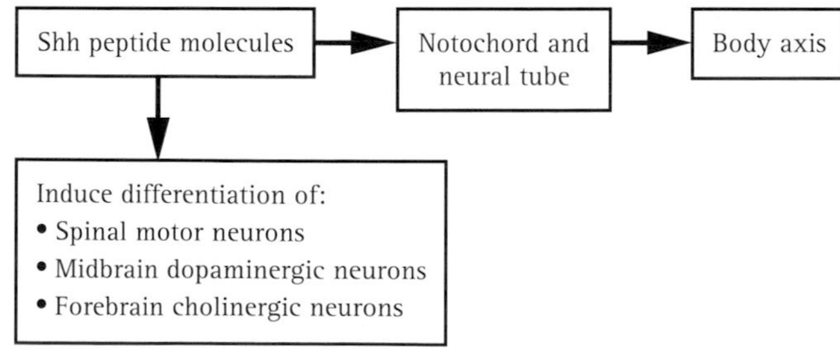


Figure 2.4 Neural development and the Sonic Hedgehog gene.

The almost straight 'tubular' embryo at 22 days, gradually folds into a 'C'-shape embryo already apparent at 29±1 days postfertilization (stage 12) (Fig. 2.5) and remains so through to the end of the embryonic period (8th week gestation) when the body axis 'unfolds' slightly whilst the head stays bent forwards over the chest.

Following closure of the neuropores, the brain enters into a stage of rapid differential growth, and the gentle cervical flexure, already evident at stage 12, becomes more prominent at 35 days postfertilization (stage 15) when, on external examination, a midbrain flexure and the pontine flexure can be observed (Fig. 2.6A). However, a mid-saggital histological section shows four bending points (Fig. 2.6B). The morphogenetic mechanisms, at gene, cell, and tissue levels, determining and modulating the appearance and roles of these four 'bearing' points have yet to be elucidated.

The appearance of flexures in the body of the embryo is associated with segmentation of the CNS. These become more apparent following closure of the neural tube. At 29 days postfertilization (stage 13), three brain vesicles or neuromeres can be clearly identified on close examination: the prosencephalon, the mesencephalon, and the rhombencephalon (Fig. 2.5). At 32 days postfertilization (stage 13), each segment will develop subsegments expected to emerge at given stages of development (Table 2.1).

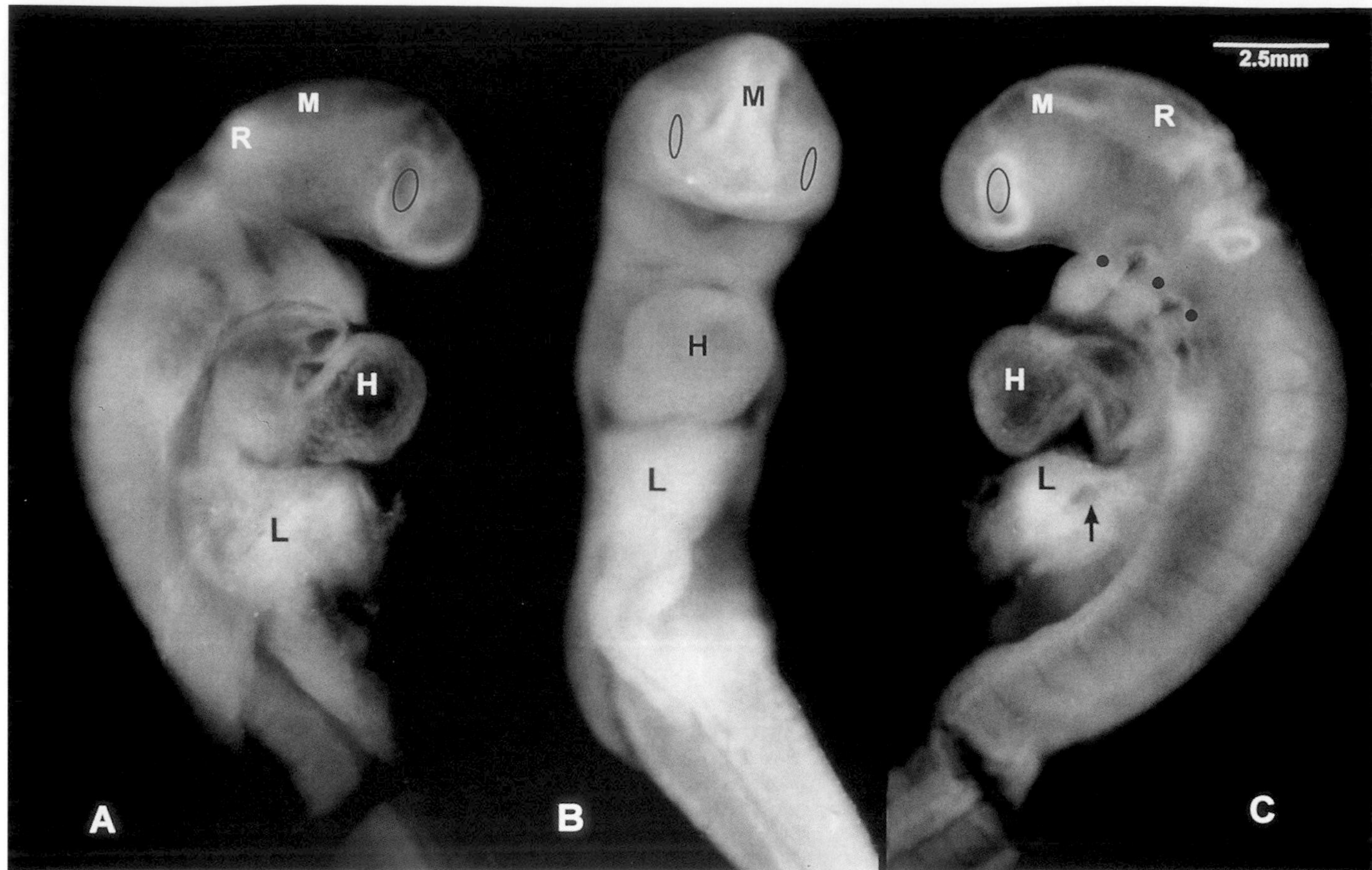


**Figure 2.5** Human embryo at 29 days postfertilization (stage 13). On a frontal view (B), the telencephalic vesicles are clearly seen (open circles). These are also seen lateraly in (A) and (C). The head is now larger than the cardiac loop. M = mesencephalon, R = rhombencephalon. The dots point to three pharyngeal arches. The black arrow in (C) points to the stomach containing some fluid seen by translucency. H = heart; L = rhombic lips.

**Table 2.1 Neuromeres in the human embryo**

| Primary neuromeres | | | Secondary neuromeres | |
|---|---|---|---|---|
| Prosencephalon | | | Telencephalon | |
| | | | Diencephalon 1 | S10 |
| | | | Diencephalon 2 | |
| | | | Parencephalon rostralis | S14 |
| | | | Parencephalon caudalis | |
| | | | Synecephalon--------- | S13 |
| Mesencephalon | | | Mesencephalon 1 | S12 |
| | | S9 | Mesencephalon 2 | |
| | | | Isthmic neuromere------- | S13 |
| Rhombomeres | Rh. A | | Rhombomeres: Rh. 1 | |
| | | | Rh. 2 | |
| | | | Rh. 3 | |
| | Rh. B | | Rh. 4 | S11 |
| | Rh. C | | Rh. 5 | |
| | | | Rh. 7 | |
| | Rh. D | | Rh. 8 | |

S = Developmental stage.
*Source*: From R. O'Rahilly & F. Müller 1999 with permission.

The prosencephalon or forebrain is the most anterior neuromere which presents two small telencephalic vesicles at 29±1 days postfertilization (stage 13) (Fig. 2.5). By the end of the 38th day (stage 16), the telencephalic vesicles have gone past the level of the eye when observed on a lateral view (Fig. 2.7). Towards the end of the embryonic period (8 weeks gestation), the telencephalic vesicles can be recognized as developing brain hemispheres. Their outer surface appears smooth and will remain so for the first 12 weeks of gestation (Fig. 2.8). However, at 12 weeks, their medial sagittal aspect, facing the falx cerebri, show emerging gyri, suggesting a faster growth on their medial aspect (Fig. 2.9).

At the histological level, the differential growth of the brain segments is accompanied by significant changes in the histological architecture of each segment and in the topology of the gray and white matter. Here it should be remembered that the anterior neuropore closes at the level where the rhombencephalon will develop. At this point, as the neural tube closes, neuroblasts start to differentiate from neuroepithelial cells generating first the ventricular layer. From it, neurons will originate and migrate towards the pia creating the second or mantle layer later to become the gray

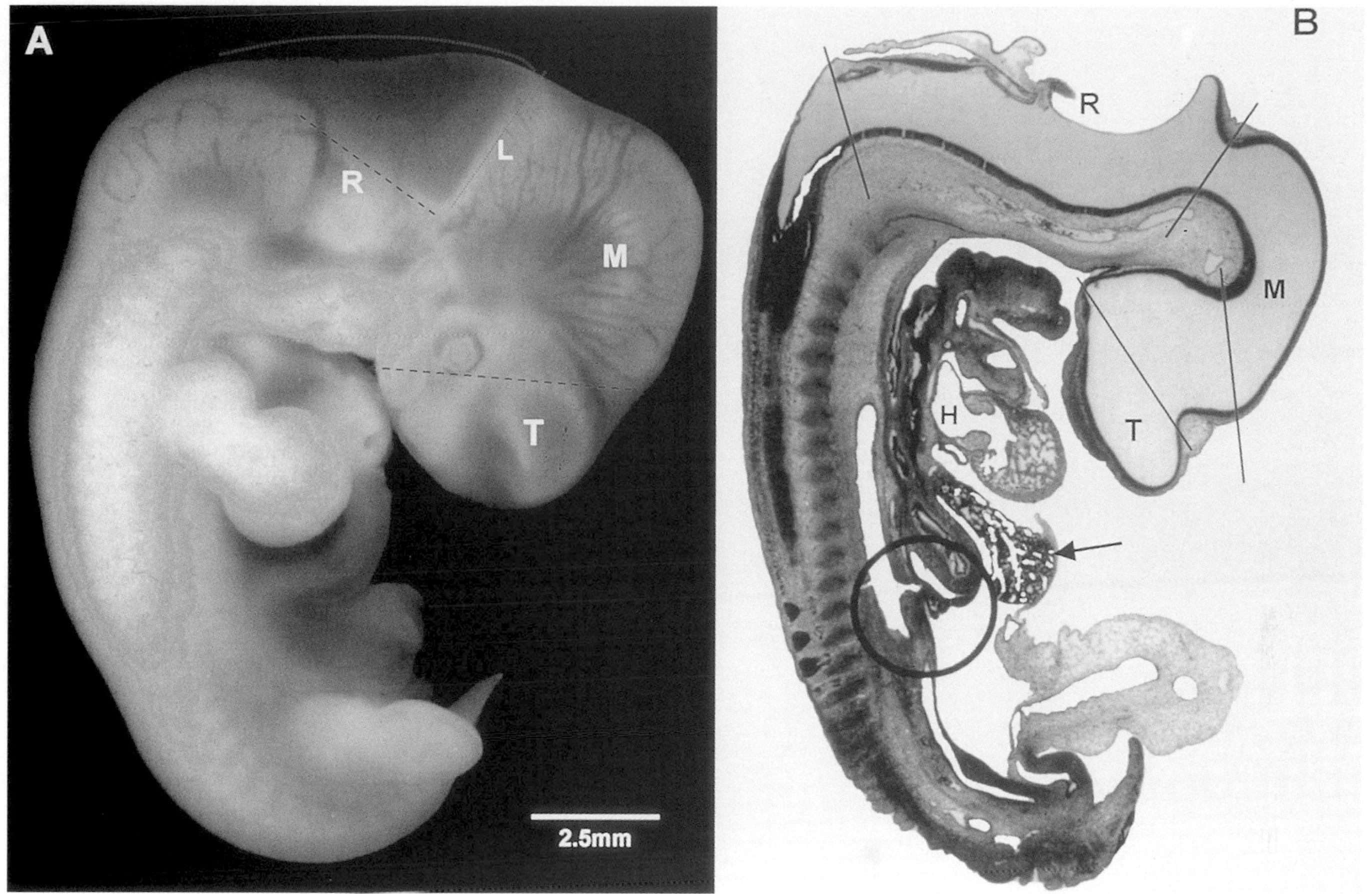


Figure 2.6 (A) Human embryo at 35 days postfertilization (stage 15). Note the pronounced flexion of the head over the chest. The telencephalic vesicles are approaching the level of the pigmented eye (lower dashed line). The mesencephalon (M) is a predominant brain segment. The pontine flexure appears as a straight angle made up by the rhombic lips (L) and the floor of the IVth ventricle. The space (curved red dotted line) thus created contains water-clear fluid. Brain blood vessels appear to emerge at the level of the temporal region to spread radially. R = rhombencephalon. (B) Paramedial sagittal section of the human embryo in (A). There are four bending points (lines). Note the attenuated epidermal and neural tissue (R) making together a thin membrane covering the pontine flexure. The heart (H) shows unfused atrioventricular cushions. Liver (arrow). M = mesencephalon; T = telencephalic vesicle.

matter. A third, outermost acellular layer of the brain will be formed by interconnecting neural fibers which later become the white matter. In the prospective brain hemispheres, the marginal layer or primordial plexiform lamina appears at 33 days (stage 15) according to O'Rahilly *et al.* (1984). Although Marin-Padilla (1983) finds it at 42 postovulatory days (stage 18), this is followed nevertheless by the appearance of the cortical plate at about 50 days postfertilization (stage 21). Neuronal migration is assisted by radial glia which extend from the ventricular walls to the pia mater. The glial processes are present at 12 weeks of gestation (Choi 1986) and can be demonstrated immunohistochemically using glial fibrillary acid protein (GFAP). In the ensuing months, the telencephalic vesicles will grow at spectacular speed to form the brain hemispheres. According to Mikhailets (quoted by Blinkov and Glezer 1968), half-way through pregnancy the brain has over 400% of the volume of the embryo's body but by the end of gestation the volume is only about 42%.

Studies of gene expression in the hippocampus of some animal models show that morphogenesis and neuronal differentiation depends in part on the LIM Homeobox gene Lhx5 (Zhao et al 1999) encoding a transcription factor present in a region containing the earliest differentiated Cajal–Retzius (C-R) cells (Soriano *et al.* 1994). These C-R cells guide neural migration during the development of the hippocampus (D'Arcangelo *et al.* 1995; Nakajima *et al.* 1997). In mutant mice, absence of Lhx5 is associated with a malformed hippocampus, agenesis of the choroid plexus in both the lateral and 3rd ventricles and absent callosal axons crossing the midline. Furthermore, several Homeobox genes, including Lhx2, Emx2 and Otx1, are needed during morphogenesis of the telencephalic choroid plexus (Pellegrine *et al.* 1996; Porter *et al.* 1997; Yoshida *et al.* 1997). Absence of Lhx5 in mutant mouse embryos is associated with poor expression of Wnt5, Bmp4 and Bmp7, resulting in abnormal patterning of the midtelencephalic wall from which the

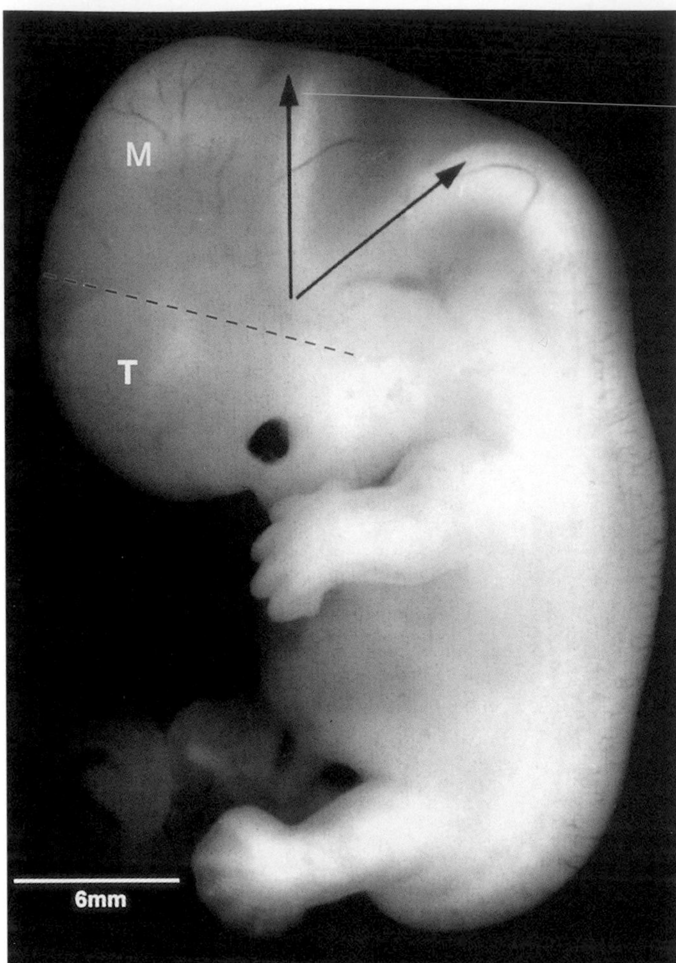


Figure 2.7 Human embryo at 46 days postfertilization (stage 18). The left telencephalic vesicle (T) is beyond the eye level. The mesencephalon (M) still predominates in size over the other brain segments. The pontine flexure (between the arrows) has an angle less than 90 degrees.

hippocampus will differentiate (Zhao *et al.* 1995). Moreover, there is rapidly accumulating evidence indicating that hippocampal cells maintain the capability for generating neurons from progenitor cells in the adult human brain (Roy *et al.* 2000). Therefore, the hippocampus appears to hold a potential for neuron regeneration believed to be impossible once brain development is completed. The therapeutic potential, perhaps including memory improvement among others, is of much relevance (Gould *et al.* 1999).

The mesencephalon or second neuromere, once prominent shortly after closure of the neural tube (Fig. 2.5) undergoes less changes than the other two primary neuromeres: the forebrain and the rhombencephalon. Its main contribution is in the formation of the cerebral aqueduct. It is also associated with the brain peduncles, the origin of the tegmentum and the substantia nigra which appear to be derived from the basal plate of the mesencephalon.

A family of transcription factors containing the fork head (fkh) domain, a region-specific homeotic gene, has been identified in Drosophila. Deficient fkh-5, the homolog gene in mice, is responsible for dysgenesis in the caudal midbrain and hypothalamic mamillary body (Wehr *et al.* 1997).

From the early stages in embryogenesis the rhombo-encephalon shows increasing complexity. At 20 days postfertilization (stage 9) it reaches its peak of prominence making up to 51–67% of the neural plate (Muller & O'Rahilly, 1983; O'Rahilly *et al.* 1984). At 34 days postfertilization, the pontine flexure is a prominent feature made up by the rhombic lips at its cephalic end and by the developing floor of the 4th ventricle at its caudal end. The 'roof' of the pontine flexure is made up of attenuated neural and ectodermic layers (Fig. 2.5B). The pontine 'chamber' thus created at 34 days, is a large space within the central neural system at this stage. It contains clear watery fluid which, presumably, is a type of cerebrospinal fluid (CSF). The pontine 'angle' decreases with continuing growth and becomes significantly reduced to a few degrees by the end of the embryonic period.

The rhombic lips contribute significantly to the formation of the cerebellum whose rate of growth accelerates towards the end of the embryonic period. At this point, the rhombic lips resemble the roof-top of an oriental temple (Fig. 2.10). As the embryo approaches the end of the first trimester, the cerebellar hemispheres showing a smooth outer surface are clearly defined, and the vermis is developing as a medial raphe (Fig. 2.11). Cerebellar foliation will not form until the 14th week. Precursors of Purkinje cells form a thin lamina separated from the granular layer by a clear zone named lamina dissecans (Rakic & Sidman 1970). The granular layer forms from germinal cells of the rhombic lip. Cerebellar morphogenesis is slow and will be completed after the 2nd year of life.

The floor of the 4th ventricle in the brain stem appears as an unfolded lily (Fig. 2.10). Tanaka *et al.* (1987) have identified a set of supra-ependymal cells and supra-ependymal fibers. Some of the latter appear to penetrate the ependymal layer but their role is unknown.

At 11 weeks gestation, the choroid plexus crosses freely the 4th ventricular space between the cerebellum and the floor of the IVth ventricle (Fig. 2.11). During this time, the foramina of Lushka and Maggendi communicate the IVth ventricle with the subarachnoidal space.

Cell communication and its pattern together with timing with reference to brain organogenesis, is now gradually being unraveled. Tyrosine kinases, peptide growth factors for receptor tyrosine kinase, are known to play important roles during neuron migration, axon guidance, and neuron cell differentiation (Schlessinger & Ukkrich 1992; Fantl *et al.* 1993). Furthermore, neural cell activity has been documented shortly before the end of the first trimester. At this time brain cells are proliferating at a rate approaching 250 000/min (Rakic 1995; Shatz 1996).

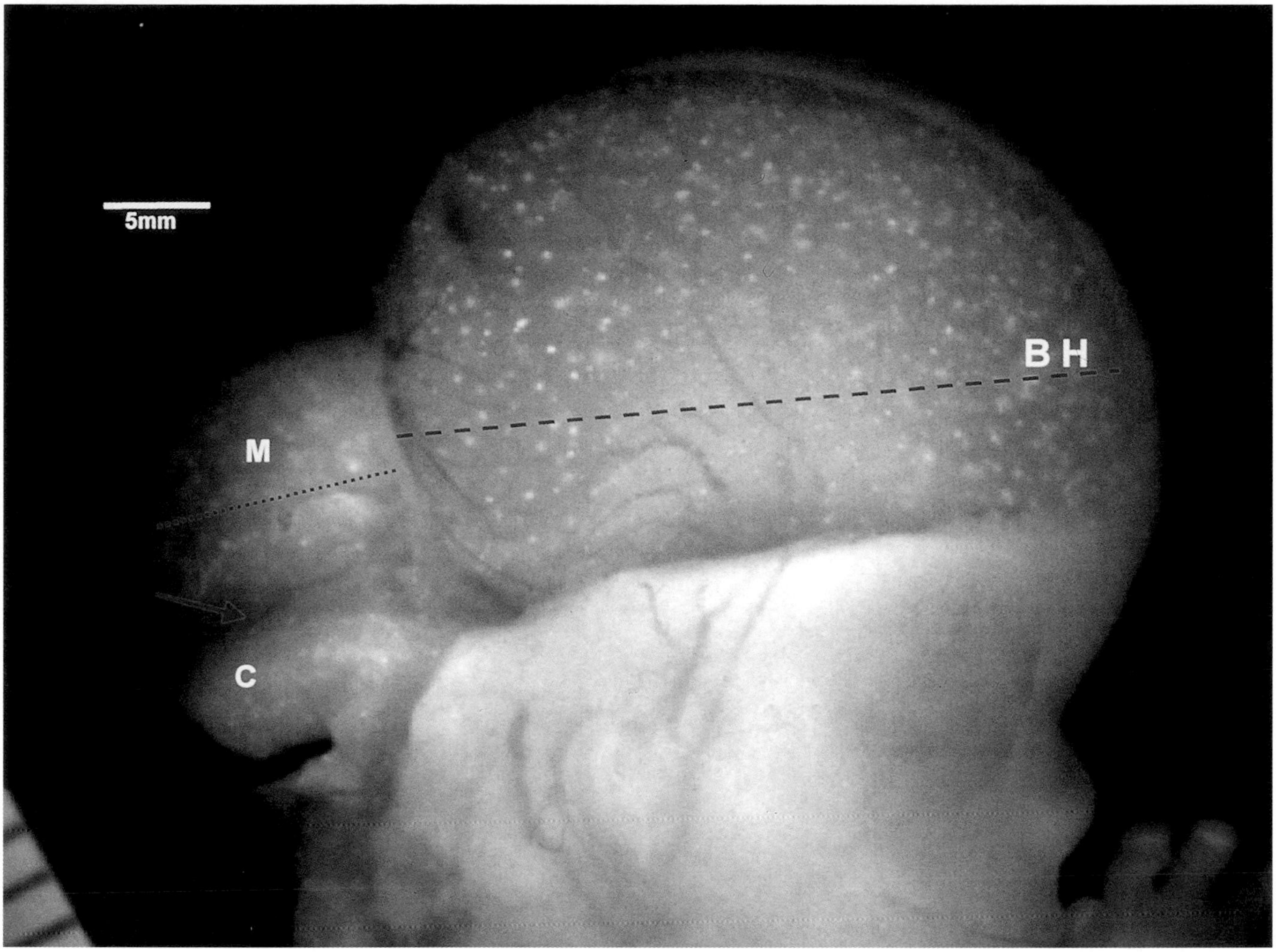

Figure 2.8 Human fetus at 10 weeks gestation. The outer surface of the right brain hemisphere appears smooth. The caudal end of the mesencephalon (M) is in contact with the tentorium (arrow). The right cerebellar hemisphere has a smooth surface (C).

## FUTURE PROSPECT

Whilst much of the rapidly accumulating new knowledge, at gene and molecular levels, on brain development, appears to be oriented to the understanding of brain pathology after birth, the application of diagnostic ultrasound at ever earlier stages of gestation is making possible the accurate imaging of the developing human brain (Blass 1999). This together with other tests based on the isolation of fetal cells from maternal blood, may assist, in the not-too-distant future, in diagnosing and perhaps treating neurologic disorders.

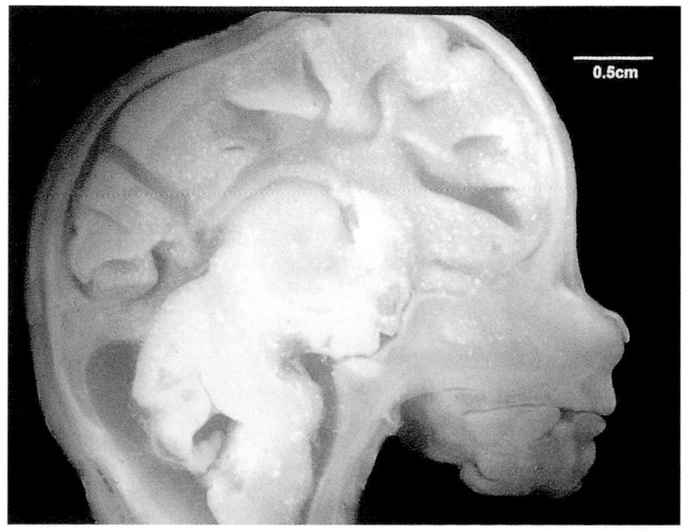


Figure 2.9 Fetal brain at 12 weeks gestation. Sagittal view of the developing left hemisphere of the brain facing the flax cerebri. Note the emerging gyri suggestive of a faster growth on this side when compared with its smooth parietal brain surface.

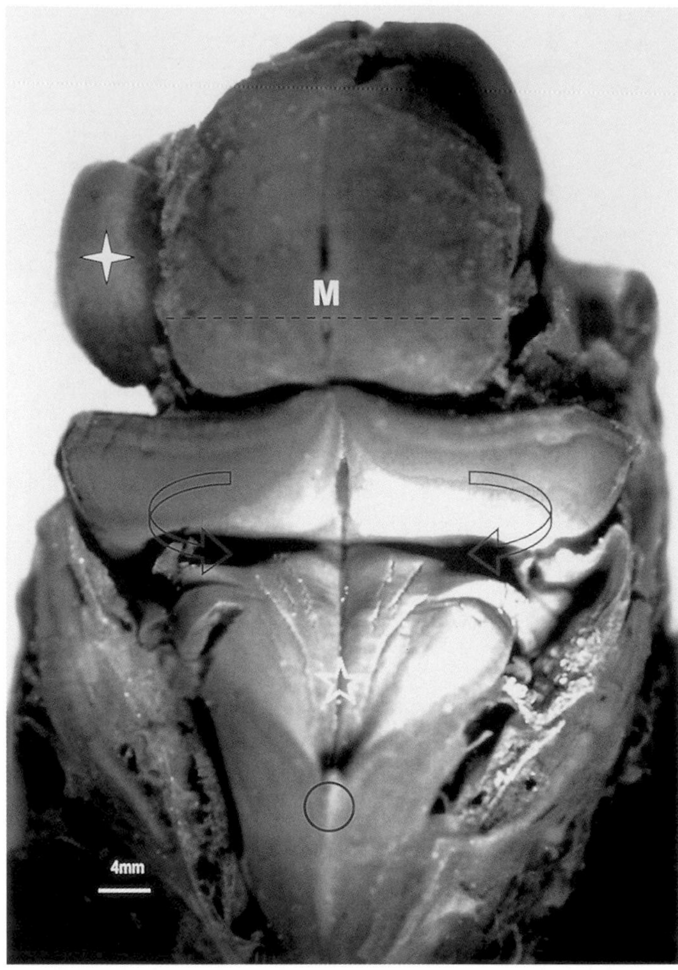


Figure 2.10 A posterior view of the CNS of a human fetus at 8 weeks gestation. Note the prominent mesencephalon and the characteristic 'winged' shape of the rhombic lips. The curved arrows indicate their convergence during growth. The cerebellar vermix has not yet differentiated. The brain stem (circle) has a lily-like shape. The brain hemispheres (star) have not covered the mesencephalon.

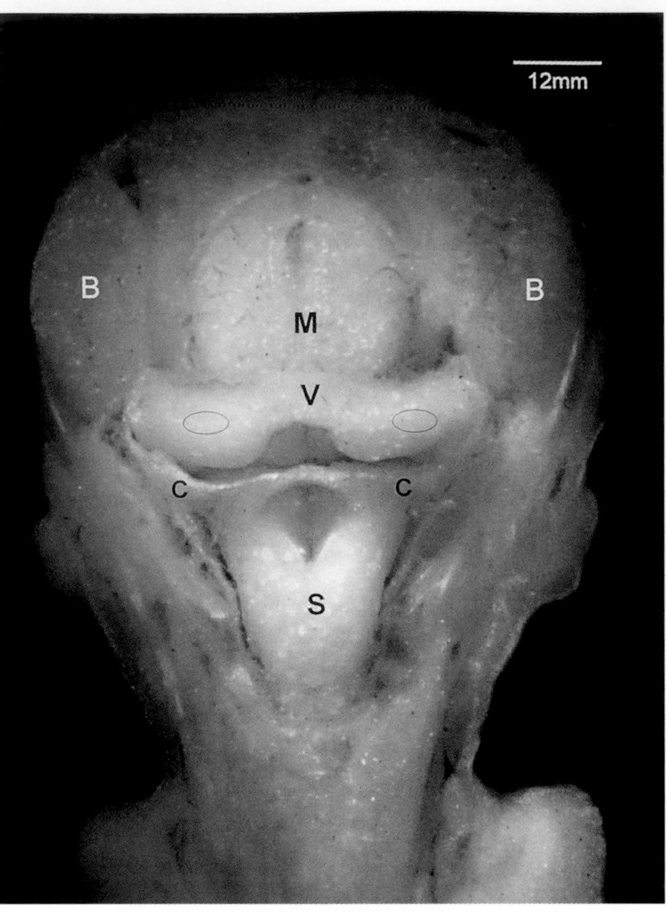


Figure 2.11 A view of the posterior fossa of a human fetus at 11 weeks gestation. The rhombic lips (circles) have fused (V) in the midline. Thus the cerebellum can be recognized. The choroid plexus (C) crosses freely the 4th ventricle. B = brain hemispheres; M = mesencephalon; S = brain stem.

## REFERENCES


Blass H-G K (1999) The embryonic examination: ultrasound studies on the development of the human embryo. Thesis, Norwegian University of Science and Technology. Tapir trykkeri, ISBN 82-519-1515-5.

Blinkov S M, Glezer II (eds) (1968) *The human brain in figures and tables.* New York: Plenum Press, pp. 126–334.

Bourgeois J P, Jastreboff P J & Rakic P (1989) Synaptogenesis in visual cortex of normal and preterm monkeys: evidence for intrinsinc regulation of synaptic overproduction. *Proc Natl Acad Sci USA* 86:4297–4301.

Bridges C B & Morgan T H (1923) The third-chromosome group of mutant characters of *Drosophila melanogaster. Carnegie Inst Washington* 251pp., roy 8.

Choi B H (1986) Glial fibrillary acid protein in radial glia of early human fetal cerebrum: a light and electron microscopy immunoperoxidase study. *J Neuropathol Exp Neurol* 45:408–418.

D'Arcangelo G, Miao G G, Chen S C *et al.* (1995) A protein related to extracellular matrix proteins deleted in the mouse mutant reeler. *Nature* 374:719–723.

Dolle P, Izpisua-Belmonte J C & Falkestein H (1989) Coordinate expression of the murine Hox-5 complex homeobox-containing genes during limb pattern formation. *Nature* 342:767–772.

Ericson J, Muhr J, Placzek M *et al.* (1995) Sonic hedgehog induces differentiation of ventral forebrain neurons: a common signal for ventral patterning within the neural tube. *Cell* 81:747–756.

Fantl W J, Johnson D E, Williams L T (1993) Signalling by receptor tyrosine kinases. *Annu Rev Biochem* 62:453–481.

Gould E, Beylin A, Tanapat P *et al.* (1999) Learning enhances adult neurogenesis in the adult hippocampal formation. *Nature Neurosci* 2:260–265.

Holland P W & Hogan B L (1988) Expression of homeobox genes during mouse development: a review. *Genes Dev* 2773–2782.

Hynes M A, Porter J A, Chiang C *et al.* (1995) Induction of midbrain dopaminergic neurons by sonic hedgehog. *Neuron* 15:35–44.

Lumsden A & Keynes R (1989) Segmental patterns of neuronal development in the chick hindbrain *Nature* 337:424–428.

Marin-Padilla M (1983) Structural organization of the human cerebral cortex prior to the appearance of the cortical plate. *Anat Embryol* 168:21–40.

Miao N, Wang M, Ott J A *et al.* (1997) Sonic hedgehog promotes the survival of specific CNS neuron populations and protects these cells from toxic insult *in vitro. J Neurosci* 17:5891–5899.

Miner J H, Cunningham J & Sanes J R (1998) Roles for laminin in embryogenesis: exencephaly, syndactily and placentopathy in mice lacking the laminin α5 chain. *J Cell Biol* 143:1713–1723.

Muller F & O'Rahilly R (1983) The first appearance of the major divisions of the human brain at stage 9. *Anat Embryol* 168:419–432.

Nakajima K, Mikoshiba K, Miyata T *et al.* (1997) Disruption of hippocampal development in vivo by CR-50mAb against reelin. *Proc Natl Acad Sci USA* 94:8196–8201.

Oliver G, Sidell N, Fiske W *et al.* (1989) Complementary homeoprotein gradients in developing limb buds. *Genes Dev* 3:641–650.

O'Rahilly R & Muller F (eds) (1999) *The embryonic human brain: an atlas of developmental stages*, 2nd edn. New York, Chichester, Singapore, Toronto: Wiley-Liss.

O'Rahilly R, Muller F, Hutchins G M & Moore G W (1984) Computer ranking of the sequence of appearance of 100 features of the brain and related structures in staged human embryos during the first 5 weeks of development. *Am J Anat* 171:243–257.

Pellegrine M, Mansouri A, Simeoni A *et al.* (1996) Dentate gyrus formation requires Emx2. *Development* 122:3898–3993.

Porter F D, Drago J, Xu Y *et al.* (1997) Lhx2, a LIM homeobox gene, is required for eye, forebrain and definitive erythrocyte development. *Development* 124:2935–2944.

Rakic P & Sidman R L (1970) Histogenesis of cortical layers in human cerebellum, particularly the lamina dissecans. *J Comp Neurol* 139:473–500.

Rakic P (1995) The development of the frontal lobe. A view from the rear of the brain. *Adv Neurol* 66:1–6.

Roelink H, Porter J A, Chiang C *et al.* (1994) Floor plate and motor neuron induction by Vhh-1, a vertebrate homolog of hedgehog expressed by the notochord. *Cell* 76:761–775.

Roy N S, Wang S, Jian L (2000) In-vitro neurogenesis by progenitor cells isolated from the adult human hippocampus. *Nat Med* 6:271–277.

Schlessinger J & Ukkrich A (1992) Growth factor signalling by receptor tyrosine kinases. *Neuron* 9:383–391.

Shatz C J (1996) Emergence of order in visual system development. *J Physiol* 90:141–150.

Soriano E, Del Rio J A, Martinez H & Super O O (1994) Organization of the embryonic and early postnatal murine hippocampus. I. Immunocytochemical characterization of neuronal populations in the subplate and marginal zone. *J Comp Neurol* 342:571–595.

Suddath R L, Christison G W, Torrey F E *et al.* (1990) Anatomical abnormalities in the brain of monozygotic twins discordant for schizophrenia. *New Engl J Med* 322:789–794.

Tanabe, Y & Jessell T M (1996) Diversity and pattern in the developing spinal cord. *Science* 274:1115–1123.

Tanaka O, Otani H & Fujimoto K (1987) Fourth ventricular floor in human embryos: scanning electron microscopy observations. *Am J Anat* 178:193–203.

Wang M Z, Jin P, Bumcrot D A *et al.* (1995) Induction of dopaminergic neuron phenotype in the midbrain by sonic hedgehog protein. *Nature Med* 1:1184–1188.

Wehr R, Mansouri A, de Maeyer T & Gruss P (1997) Fkh5-deficient mice shows dysgenesis in the caudal midbrain and hypothalamic mammillary body. *Development* 124:4447–4456.

Weinberger D R, DeLisi L E, Perman G P *et al.* (1982) Computed tomography in schizophreniform disorder and other acute psychiatric disorders. *Arch Gen Psychiatry* 39:778–783.

Weinberger D R (1987) Implications of normal brain development for the pathogenesis of schizophrenia. *Arch Gen Psychiatry* 44:660–669.

Weinberger D R, Berman K G & Illowsky B P (1988) Physiological dysfunction of dorsolateral prefrontal cortex in schizophrenia. III. A new cohort and evidence for a monoaminergic mechanism. *Arch Gen Psychiatry* 45:609–615.

Wilkinson D G, Bhatt S & Chavrier P (1989) Segment specific expression of a zinc-finger gene in the developing nervous system of the mouse. *Nature* 337:461–464.

Yoshida M, Suda Y, Matsuo I *et al.* (1997) Emx1 and Emx2 functions in development of the dorsal telencephalon. *Development* 124:101–111.

Zhao Y, Sheng H Z, Amini R *et al.* (1999) Control of hippocampal morphogenesis and neuronal differentiation by the LIM Homeobox gene Lhx5. *Science* 284:1155–1158.

# Chapter 3

# Anatomical development of the CNS

M. A. England

## INTRODUCTION

At birth, the brain and spinal cord are already highly developed and exhibit considerable functional ability, although anatomical development continues for a further 2 years after birth (Dobbing & Sands 1973). The newborn brain weighs 300–400 g at full-term and lies in a head whose circumference averages 35 cm (males). Male brains weigh slightly more than those of females but, in either case, constitute 10% of the body weight at birth (Crelin 1973). Early embryonic development of the CNS is described in Chapter 2 and the genetic interaction with brain development in Chapter 1. This chapter describes in some detail development of the CNS after the early embryonic period until birth. For further reading, the excellent book by Lemire *et al.* (1975) is recommended.

Unfortunately, the aging and subsequent staging of embryos and fetuses is a source of confusion amongst embryologists. The age of the developing child has been referred to in postconceptual and postmenstrual (gestational) weeks or lunar months. Crown–rump (CR) length is also commonly described. A more accurate method of assessing maturity is based on a series of developing external and internal features combined with CR measurements. Streeter (1942, 1948) presented a series of horizons, 1–23, which described embryos until day 47 after fertilization. When true age is based on a fertilization date, full-term is at week 38 (266 completed days of gestation). O'Rahilly (1973) has made slight alterations to Streeter's horizons. These comprise modifications between stages 14 and 23, and these have been incorporated in the Carnegie staging system and extend to 56 days. Tables 3.1 and 3.2 indicate the relationship between stages, CR length and age of the embryo and fetus. Throughout this chapter, wherever possible, the postconceptual age of the embryo (up to 56 days) is given, and thereafter the postmenstrual (gestational) age. In some cases it is not possible to know from the authors' original descriptions whether they were referring to postconceptual or gestational age, and some confusion between these two is inevitable.

**Table 3.1 Embryological development of the CNS. Relationship between postconceptual age of the embryo and the Carnegie stage. The CR length and somite stages are also included**

| | Postconceptual age (days) | Carnegie stage | CR length (mm) | Somite stage |
|---|---|---|---|---|
| Neurulation | 18–19 | 8 | 1.0–3.0 | |
| | 20–21 | 9 | 1.5–3.0 | 1–3 |
| | 22–23 | 10 | 2.0–3.5[a] | 4–12 |
| | 24–25 | 11 | 2.5–4.5[a] | 13–20 |
| | 26–27 | 12 | 3–5 | 21–29 |
| Secondary canalization | 28–30 | 13 | 4–6 | 30–35 |
| | 31–32 | 14 | 5–7[1] | |
| | 33–36 | 15 | 7–9 | |
| | 37–40 | 16 | 8–11 | |
| | 41–43 | 17 | 11–14 | |
| | 44–46 | 18 | 13–17 | |
| | 47–48 | 19 | 16–18 | |
| | 49–51 | 20 | 18–22 | |
| Retrogressive differentiation (to 80 days) | 52–53 | 21 | 22–24 | |
| | 54–55 | 22 | 23–28 | |
| | 56 | 23 | 27–31 | |

[a]Refers to greatest length rather than CR length.

**Table 3.2 Fetal growth. The approximate CR length of gestational (postmenstrual) age in weeks is shown**

| Gestational age (weeks) | CR length (mm) |
|---|---|
| 9 | 50 |
| 10 | 61 |
| 12 | 87 |
| 14 | 120 |
| 16 | 140 |
| 18 | 160 |
| 20 | 190 |
| 22 | 210 |
| 24 | 230 |
| 26 | 250 |
| 28 | 270 |
| 30 | 280 |
| 32 | 300 |
| 36 | 340 |
| 38 | 360 |

## GENERAL DEVELOPMENT

Brain development can be classified into a number of stages which are discussed in detail in Chapter 2.

1. Early development, days 18–27 (neurulation)
2. Secondary caudal neural tube formation (or secondary canalization), days 30–50
3. Retrogressive differentiation, days 50–80

### DEVELOPMENT OF THE SPINAL CORD

The spinal cord extends into the tail of the embryo until stages 18–20 (44–51 days) and the beginning of retrogressive differentiation. Once the filum terminale and conus medullaris have formed, the conus assumes a higher and higher position within the vertebral canal (Fig. 3.1). This phenomenon is believed to be due to the fact that the vertebrae are growing more rapidly than the spinal cord. As a result, the spinal cord 'ascends' in the canal and may reach its adult level of $L_1$–$L_2$ as early as week 31. There is a great deal of variation, however, and more usually the $L_1$–$L_2$ level is reached within 2 weeks postnatally.

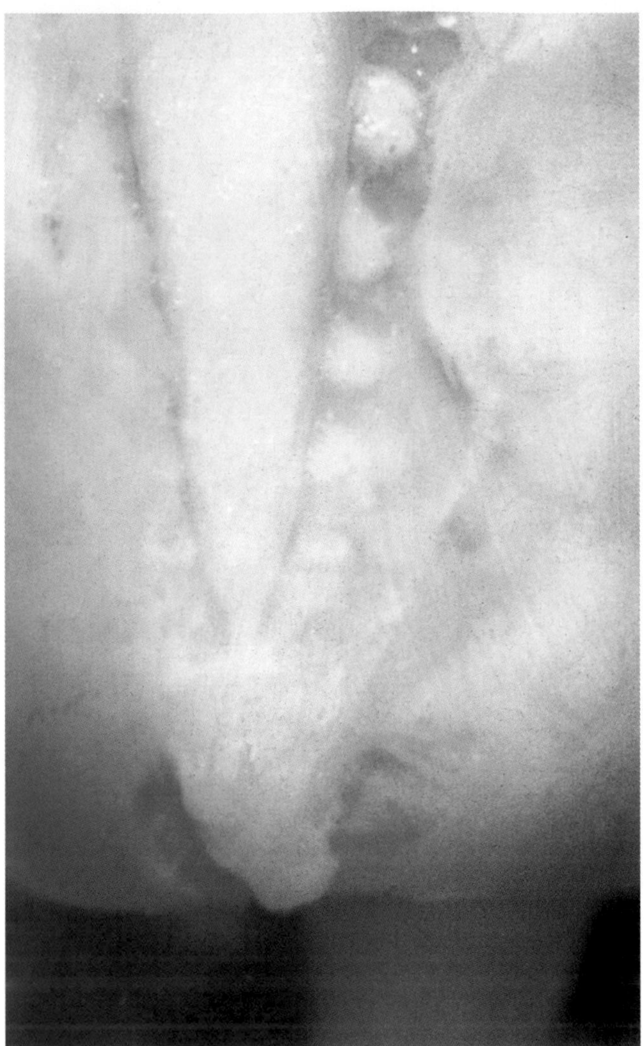

Figure 3.1 The caudal spinal cord in a 60 mm CR fetus.

#### Histology of the early embryo

The development of the spinal cord has been studied extensively because it is the simplest model. As the neural folds first fuse to form a tube, the walls are composed of a single layer of columnar epithelium. These cells proliferate rapidly so that the neural tube walls soon become thickened and composed of a pseudostratified columnar epithelium. The central canal initially is relatively large, but later, when the white and gray matter increase, it will become smaller. The epithelial layer is called the ventricular zone (germinal or ependymal layer or matrix) (Boulder Committee 1970). All of these cells synthesize DNA at this stage of development. At 17–21 days, each cell is approximately wedge shaped and attached at both ends to the outer and luminal surfaces of the neural tube (Sauer 1936; Sidman & Rakic 1973). During week 4, the cells successively retract to the luminal margin of the neural tube and divide. The daughter cell nuclei then migrate back into the layer, and reconnect to the outer margin of the neural tube. The process is repeated so that these cells eventually give rise to all the neural and macroglial cells in the CNS.

Once the neural tube has closed, this ventricular layer will give rise to the immature neurons (neuroblasts or primitive neurons) (Fujita 1973). These cells, unlike the neuroepithelial cells, are not connected to the luminal surface. While the neuroepithelial cells are producing immature neurons, they are also producing glioblasts (spongioblasts or primitive neuroglia). As the earliest immature neurons migrate from the neuroepithelial layer they are accompanied by glia.

Radial glia are also present from the earliest stages and form the glia limitans. They may also guide neurons. During the early stages, neuron production predominates. Even when the neurons cease dividing, glia production continues throughout life (Sturrock 1982a). The most rapid increase in glial number occurs just before and during early myelination. This increase in glial cells is brought about by division of the glial cells already present in white matter (Sturrock 1982b). Finally, the neuroepithelial cells produce ependymal cells. Ultimately, these cells will line the ventricular system of the brain, choroid plexuses, and central canal of the spinal cord.

Soon (stages 15–17, 33–43 days) a second layer, the marginal zone (subpial or molecular layer) appears outside the ventricular zone. This relatively acellular layer is composed of the outer parts of the neuroepithelial cells and will eventually form the white matter (Boulder Committee 1970). By 26–38 mm CR the marginal zone surrounds the entire cord (Lemire *et al.* 1975).

As the neuroepithelial cells proliferate, the lateral walls of the spinal cord thicken, but the roof and floor plates remain thin. At stages 15–17 (33–43 days) a shallow groove (sulcus limitans) appears between the dorsal and ventral parts of the spinal cord. The dorsal part of the spinal cord becomes the alar plate (lamina) and the ventral part the basal plate (lamina). The alar and basal plates extend throughout the spinal cord as long columns (Fig. 3.2). The alar plates form the dorsal gray columns comprised of groups of afferent nuclei. The basal plates form the ventral and lateral gray columns. Axons from unipolar neurons in the spinal ganglia enter the spinal cord and form the dorsal roots of the spinal nerves, whilst axons from ventral horn cells grow out of the spinal cord and form the ventral roots of the spinal cord. The relative thickness of the three layers of the spinal cord changes: by 38–55 mm CR, the ependymal layer is thinner, and by 55–75 mm CR, the marginal zone is increasing in thickness at a greater rate than the mantle zone. The posterior median septum is now evident as a thin glial layer (Lemire *et al.* 1975). By 75–105 mm CR, there is a greater volume of white matter than gray matter, and by 180–265 mm CR the thoracic cord is composed of over 60% white matter (Lemire *et al.* 1975).

Beginning in week 12, ascending, descending and propriospinal fibers invade the marginal zone (FitzGerald 1985).

The third layer of the neural tube, the intermediate layer (middle or mantle layer), is present by 10 mm CR (38–40 days), and is located between the ventricular and marginal zones. This layer forms from neuroblasts which have arisen in the ventricular zone and then move outwards. This thick, cellular middle layer begins at stage 18 (44–46 days) and is destined to form the gray matter. The cells migrating to form this layer do not do so uniformly; there is a difference in pattern and intensity of migration from various parts of the neural tube (Kallen 1977). As a result, migration occurs in waves (Berquist & Kallen 1954). The ventral cells acquire their positions in the basal plate prior to the dorsal cells

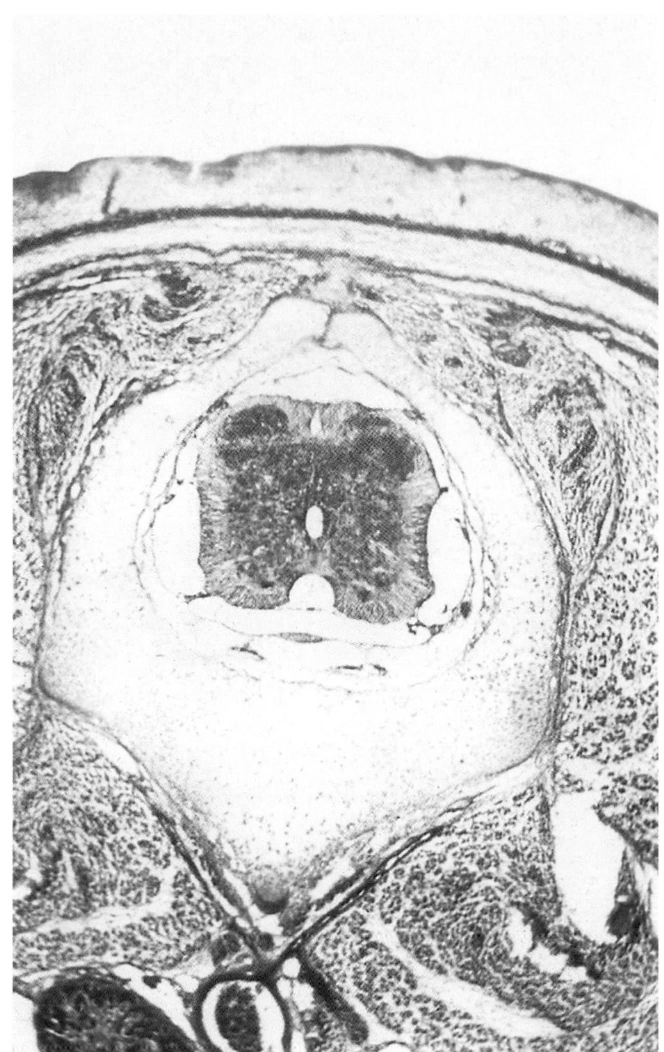

**Figure 3.2** The 120 mm CR lumbar spinal cord. The alar and basal plates are evident.

forming the alar plates (His 1888; Kallen 1977). Initially the neuroblasts are apolar and lack processes. Later they develop processes at the opposite poles and are referred to as bipolar. Finally, the processes directed towards the lumen regress and the neuroblasts become unipolar. The remaining process becomes the axon and grows towards the periphery of the neural tube to contribute to the marginal layer. Subsequently, a group of outgrowths (primordial dendrites) form at the pole opposite the axon, so becoming a multipolar cell. The multipolar neuron cytoplasm is initially homogeneous, although later large amounts of RNA and neurofibrils are present. The axon grows actively and either contacts other cells in the neural tube wall, usually via the marginal zone, or becomes motor by passing out of the neural tube to an effector organ. The dendrites become more complex by establishing contacts with adjacent nerve cells or their processes. Initially the axons and dendrites arise independently, but there is an interaction and correlation between dendritic tree formation and synaptic contacts. By stage 18 (44–46 days) the processes of the intermediate zone grow outwards into the narrow marginal zone.

Okado & Kojima (1984) have reported that by 7 mm CR (32 days) the primary afferents, interneurons and motor neurons are identifiable, but not, as yet, connected. By 10–12 mm CR (38–42 days) the motor cell columns in the cervical region are large and the first synapses are present in the motor nucleus between the motor neurons, dendrites, and the interneurons.

The first association neurons appear in the alar plate at 10 mm CR (Okado & Kojima 1984). By 22 mm CR (51–52 days) connections develop between sensory fibers and interneurons. When the fibrous components of the spinal reflex arc are complete at 22 mm CR, there is a rapid increase in the density of synapses in the motor nucleus at the level of the cervical spinal cord. Wozniak *et al.* (1980) reported that synaptogenesis proceeds craniocaudally.

### Histology of the late embryo and fetus

Okado & Kojima (1984) have identified three periods of synaptogenesis which coincide with descriptions of behavioral responses by other authors. These include: spinal reflex activities at 8 weeks (Fitzgerald & Windle 1942), when the fibrous connections of the spinal reflex arc are complete; the onset of local activities (Humphrey 1964a,b) with a rapid increase in axodendritic synapses (9.5 weeks); and multiple responses at 13–15 weeks with a rapid increase in axosomatic synapses (Humphrey & Hooker 1959). Ultrasound studies (de Vries *et al.* 1982) have shown that the first observable movements are at 7.5 weeks.

The spinal cord, like the brain, develops in identifiable spurts of growth and differentiation. Two periods have been identified in the first half of fetal development at 9.5–10.5 weeks and at 17.5–21 weeks (Okado & Yokota 1980).

## NEUROGLIA

### Macroglia

The supporting cells of the CNS form from the neuroepithelial cells of the ventricular zone. During the production of immature neurons, the supporting cells (glioblasts or spongioblasts) are also produced and migrate into the intermediate and marginal zones. Here they will differentiate to form astroblasts and then astrocytes (for a review, see Sturrock 1986); or oligodendroblasts and then oligodendrocytes. There is some controversy as to whether astrocytes and oligodendrocytes are two distinct cell types. Choi *et al.* (1983) proposed that oligodendrocytes in the human fetal spinal cord form (with an intermediate astroglial form) from radial glial cells.

### Microglia

There has been some controversy concerning the origins of the microglia. It was previously reported that they form from mesenchyme cells outside the CNS and then invade after the blood vessels form in the late fetal period (Barr 1979). However, microglia, which are small neuroglial cells, have been demonstrated in the human CNS from 5 to 8 weeks postconception by light microscopy (Kershman 1939), electron microscopy (Sturrock 1984), and by histochemical methods (Fujimoto & Mizoguti 1985). Blood vessels are present in the CNS from very early developmental stages. Embryonic human optic nerve has well-formed blood vessels, complete with tight junctions present at 8 weeks.

## REGIONAL DEVELOPMENT

## FOREBRAIN (TELENCEPHALON)

The timing of the major events in human neocortical ontogenesis during the embryonic period is schematically illustrated in Fig. 3.3. The early stages of telencephalon development are discussed in Chapter 2 (p. 14).

### Histology of the cerebral cortex

The adult cerebral neocortex has six layers when examined histologically (Fig. 3.4). They are numbered I–VI when looked at from superficial to deep. These layers are thought to arise from within and grow out towards the external surface. Autoradiographic studies have shown that the neurons first formed comprise the deepest layers of the neocortex, while the most superficial layers are made from the last formed cells. The cortical layers are formed in an 'inside-out' manner in higher mammals (McConnell 1988). Three successive waves of cell migration are thought to form the neocortex: the earliest layers to form are layer V (ganglionic) and layer VI (multiform) in the first wave, followed by layer IIIa (pyramidal) and layer IV (inner granular) in the second wave, and layer I (plexiform) and layer II (outer granular) in the final wave (Warwick & Williams 1973).

Marin-Padilla (1984, 1988b), however, in a series of studies has presented a noteworthy exception to this rule. While studying the formation of layer I, he found that the undifferentiated telencephalic vesicle is first penetrated by primitive corticipital fibers which extend throughout the layer. These fibers are believed to be monoaminergic and are possibly of mesencephalic origin. They course horizontally and establish a superficial or external white matter which is termed the marginal zone (Boulder Committee 1970) or primordial plexiform layer (Marin-Padilla 1978, O'Rahilly *et al.* 1987, 1988). Neurones from the original marginal zone may only be a transient population as they are rarely found in the adult cortex.

Larroche (1981) in a report on a 20 mm CR embryo observed that the cerebral hemisphere at this time is approximately 1 mm in thickness and is composed of two layers. The inner (ventricular) or matrix layer is a pseudostratified epithelium with numerous mitoses near the luminal (ependymal) surface. The outer, marginal or plexiform layer has an appreciable cell density whose nuclei are lighter than those of the matrix (ventricular zone). Neurones, stimulated

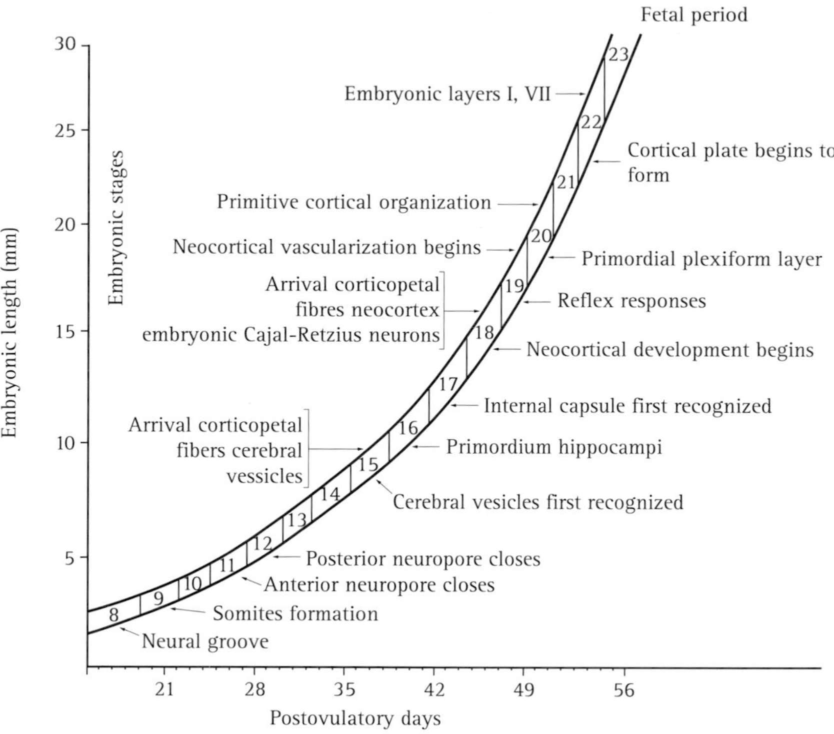


**Figure 3.3** Summary of the major events in human cortical ontogenesis. (Reproduced with permission of Dr Marin-Padilla.)

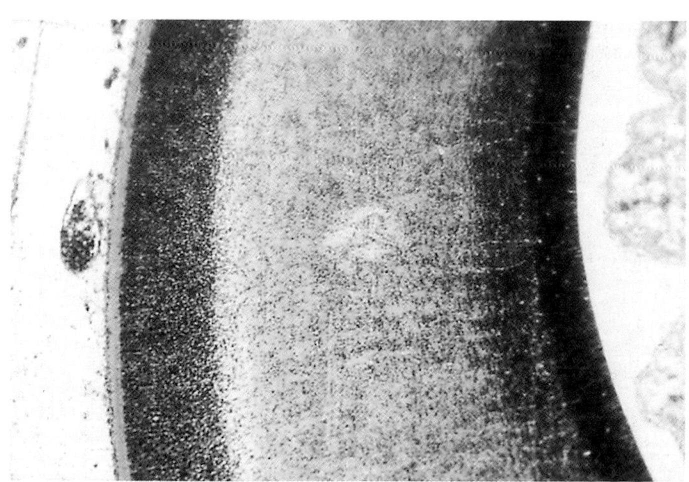

**Figure 3.4** The layers of the developing cerebral cortex of a 35 mm CR embryo. The choroid plexus appears at the right.

by the presence of corticipital fibers, appear and develop in this external white matter or marginal zone. Larroche (1981) describes them as large, well-differentiated neurons, which she interpreted as Cajal–Retzius cells. This primitive layer is called the primordial plexiform layer (Marin-Padilla 1971, 1990; Larroche & Houcine 1982; O'Rahilly *et al.* 1987, 1988) and is well established by stage 20 (50 days) (Marin-Padilla 1983) and is of short duration. O'Rahilly *et al.* (1984) report this layer as early as stage 15 (33–36 days) near the corpus striatum. The primordial plexiform layer is functionally active, as shown by the fact that it is the first to contain synapses, so confirming its precocious development. At this stage the layer is 40 μm thick. The Cajal–Retzius cells form a special class whose maturation and development are in advance of the rest of the brain (Larroche 1981; Marin-Padilla & Marin-Padilla 1982). Duckett & Pearse (1968) reported that these cells are the first site of cholinesterase activity.

The cortical plate (pyramidal cell plate) is next to develop at stage 22 (25 mm CR, 54 days) as migrating neuroblasts guided by radial glial fibers (Rakic 1981) penetrate the primordial plexiform layer and accumulate *within it* (Marin-Padilla 1984, 1988b, 1990). The cortical plate divides the primordial plexiform layer into a superficial layer I (external white matter) and a deep subplate layer VII (Marin-Padilla 1978). This finding has been corroborated by Larroche *et al.* (1981). The neurons remaining in layer I will form the embryonic, horizontally oriented Cajal–Retzius neurons.

Most of the subplate neurons are transient and are eliminated by programmed cell death (apoptosis). It is unclear whether this is also true of the upper marginal zone (presumptive layer I) (McConnell 1988). Evidence implies that subplate neurons may act as a temporary target for afferents and may help to stabilize axons or assist in the selection of the correct cortical target (McConnell 1991). Axons from

**Table 3.3 Development of the cerebral cortex during the fetal period: the thickness and differentiation of various laminations (layers I and VII as well as the cortical plate)**

| Age (WG) | Length (mm) | Layer I (μm) | Cortical plate (μm) | Development cortical plate | Layer VII (μm) |
|---|---|---|---|---|---|
| 7 | 22 CR | PPL, 30 | No CP | – | PPL |
| 11 | 40 CR | 25–35 | 100–120 | Undifferentiated CP | 30–50 |
| 15–16 | 80–100 CH | 50–60 | 300–500 | Layers VI, V, undifferentiated CP | 250–300 |
| 18–20 | 140–160 CH | 90–100 | 700–800 | Layers VI, V, IV, undifferentiated CP | Undetermined[a] |
| 24–26 | 200–250 CH | 125–135 | 900–1000 | Layers VI, V, IV, IIIC, undifferentiated CP | Undetermined[a] |
| 28–30 | 280–320 CH | 150–170 | 1300–1500 | Layers VI, V, IV, IIIC, IIIB, undifferentiated CP | Undetermined[a] |
| 38–40 | 420–460 CH | 250–300 | 1800–2100 | Layers VI, V, IV, IIIC, IIIB, IIIA, IIB, undifferentiated CP | Undetermined[a] |

*Source*: Reproduced, with permission, from Marin-Padilla (1988b).

*Key*: WG, weeks of gestation; PPL, primordial plexiform layer; CP, cortical plate; CH, crown-heel; CR, crown-rump.

[a]As layer VII becomes progressively intermingled and incorporated into the expanding cortical white matter, its dimensions and limits are no longer recognizable.

various areas, including ipsilateral and contralateral cortex and thalamus, wait in the subplate for several weeks before invading their targets in the cortical plate (Rakic 1983; Ghose *et al.* 1989; McConnell 1991).

Just as the cortical plate divides the primordial plexiform layer into two layers, so it also divides the primitive corticopetal fibers into two plexuses. One plexus is superficial to the cortical plate and the other lies below it. The first synapses that appear occur in relation to these two plexuses (Molliver *et al.* 1973; Larroche 1981) and are believed to be functional at this stage.

The differentiation of the various cortical layers during the fetal period of human development is reproduced in Table 3.3.

### Diencephalon

The posterior part of the forebrain is called the diencephalon. Its lumen is continuous with the lumen of the anterior part of the forebrain, and together their lumena form the third ventricle.

Three swellings form on each side of the diencephalon: the future thalamus, epithalamus, and the hypothalamus in the floor. Caudal to the thalamus, the lateral and medial geniculate bodies form. The epithalamus gives rise to the pineal body, the posterior commissure, and the nucleus habenulae. The mammillary bodies, the tuber cinereum, and part of the hypophysis (pituitary) arise in the hypothalamus.

The pineal body and subcommissural organ form at the junction of the diencephalon and mesencephalon.

The optic vesicles and second cranial nerve also form from the diencephalon.

The amygdaloid area arises in stages 14–15 (31–36 days) and joins with the telencephalic part of the basal nuclei at stages 15–16 (33–40 days) (O'Rahilly *et al.* 1987). This area greatly differentiates in stages 16–17 (37–43 days).

*Thalamus.* The thalamus is located in the superior portion of the diencephalon. It contains the main afferent relay nuclei projecting on to the cerebral cortex. The auditory and visual pathways relay in the medial and lateral geniculate bodies, respectively. The thalamic region can be identified as early as stage 10 (22–23 days) (Muller & O'Rahilly 1985).

The thalamus is further subdivided into a dorsal and a ventral part. The dorsal part forms the main portion of the thalamus. Although the epithalamus, ventral thalamus, and hypothalamus differentiate first, and all four structures are present by stage 15 (33–36 days) (Lemire *et al.* 1975), the growth of the dorsal thalamus overshadows that of the other three after stage 20 (49–51 days). The dorsal thalamus develops from two bulges, one on either side of the third ventricle, which grow rapidly (stages 20–21, 49–53 days). In approximately 80% of brains, the two bulges fuse in the midline, forming a bridge of gray matter across the third ventricle called the massa intermedia. This is always present by 14–15 weeks of gestation and almost fills the third ventricle (Lemire *et al.* 1975). Although by 50–60 mm CR, parts of the major subdivisions of the thalamus have appeared, the cephalic region of the dorsal thalamus remains undifferentiated (Lemire *et al.* 1975).

The pulvinar appears at 70–90 mm CR, and by 110–130 mm CR it overhangs the geniculate bodies. As the dorsal thalamus grows caudally the geniculate bodies are carried both caudally and ventrally, and eventually by 250 mm CR (26 weeks' gestational age) the lateral geniculate body has rotated into its final position. With further growth of the dorsal thalamus, the ventral thalamus is displaced laterally and away from the third ventricle (Kuhlenbeck 1948), which itself is reduced to a narrow canal (45–125 mm CR) and eventually a slit.

Also, as the thalamus grows, the lateral part of its superior surface fuses with the thin wall of the cerebral vesicle overlying it. This part of the thalamus (diencephalon) is brought into close proximity to the corpus striatum (telencephalon) and eventually the two regions become continuous and provide a route for projection fibers to and from the cortex via the internal capsule.

The ventral thalamic nucleus gives rise to several nuclei. By mid-term the major nuclear subdivisions are identifiable (Lemire *et al.* 1975).

The sulci separating the parts of the diencephalon appear in stage 18 (44–46 days), although two later fuse to form the hypothalamic sulcus of the adult brain (Lemire *et al.* 1975).

The development of the thalamocortical connections has been described by Rakic (1981) as occurring in three phases. Initially, thalamic fibers grow into the intermediate zone of the cerebral wall and collect below the cortical plate. This is followed by the fibers entering the appropriate cortical region in a diffuse manner. In the final phase the fibers are distributed into specific terminal fields (Rakic 1981), e.g. the somatic sensory pathways (touch, pain, temperature, conscious proprioception) relay in the ventral posterior nuclei of the thalamus and project to somatic sensory areas of the cortex, particularly the postcentral gyrus.

*Epithalamus.* The epithalamus forms in the caudal part of the roof and the dorsal lateral walls adjoining this region. Initially this swelling appears to be large, but with later development it becomes smaller in relative terms. Whilst the epithalamus can be identified early in development (stage 15, 33–36 days), it is shifted caudally by the tremendous growth of the dorsal thalamus.

*Pineal gland (epiphysis cerebri).* The pineal gland develops from the midline in the caudal part of the roof of the diencephalon. High concentrations of serotonin and melatonin are present in this gland. The pineal gland first becomes distinguishable at stage 14 (31–32 days) (O'Rahilly 1968; O'Rahilly *et al.* 1982, 1984) and appears at stage 15 (33–36 days) (Bartelmez & Dekaban 1962) as a thickening in the ependyma between the rostral habenular commissure and the caudal posterior commissure. By stages 16–17 (days 37–43), follicles appear in the epiphysis cerebri (O'Rahilly *et al.* 1987), and the thickening in the ependyma is followed by the appearance of a slight recess. After approximately 10–15 weeks, the gland begins to increase in size (Dooling *et al.* 1983a), and at the end of the first trimester consists of irregular tubules separated by loose mesenchymal cells (Dooling *et al.* 1983a). By 16–23 weeks, numerous large and small nests of epithelial cells are present and, at the end of the second trimester (24–27 weeks), there are numerous solid cords of cells. Melanin pigment cells are present at this time, particularly at the periphery, although they are also dispersed throughout the gland. At the beginning of the third trimester (28–31 weeks) the gland has an alveolar appearance, but as the parenchymal cells enlarge, the pigment cells are not as conspicuous (Dooling *et al.* 1983a). From 32–39 weeks there is an increase in small hyperchromic cells. At term, the pineal contains large vesicular cells mixed with small hyperchromic cells (Dooling *et al.* 1983a) but few pigment granules are present.

*Posterior and habenular commissures.* The posterior commissure is present at stage 15 (33–36 days) (O'Rahilly *et al.* 1984) (stage 23, 56 days according to Dekaban 1954), and is formed when fibers invade the caudal part of the pineal recess from both sides (Warwick & Williams 1973). The nucleus habenulae forms in the lateral wall of the diencephalon. Originally it lies close to the geniculate bodies, but as the thalamus grows it becomes separated. The habenular commissure first appears at stages 18–19 (44–48 days) (O'Rahilly *et al.* 1988) in the cranial pineal recess.

*Hypothalamus.* The hypothalamus is a suprasegmental area responsible for integrating autonomic and endocrine gland control. It lies in the inferior portion of the diencephalon ventral to the hypothalamic sulci, where it is formed by proliferating immature neurons of the intermediate layer. Later, nuclei concerned with homeostasis and endocrine functions develop, and a pair of nuclei (mammillary bodies) develop on the ventral surface in stages 16–17 (37–43 days). The mammillary bodies originally arise as a single thickening which in the third month is divided by a furrow into two structures (Warwick & Williams 1973). The tuber cinereum develops anterior to the mammillary bodies.

*Globus pallidus.* The globus pallidus also forms from the diencephalon (Sidman & Rakic 1973, O'Rahilly & Gardner 1977), although others have thought that it is a derivative of the telencephalon. It arises as a longitudinally oriented bulge in the hypothalamus (Kuhlenbeck & Haymaker 1949). This region will give rise to the globus pallidus and subthalamic nucleus (Hewitt 1958, 1961). As the cerebral hemispheres enlarge, the globus pallidus shifts laterally (Sidman & Rakic 1973; O'Rahilly & Gardner 1977), and eventually comes to lie medial to the putamen.

*Pituitary gland (hypophysis cerebri).* The hypophysis is attached to the floor of the hypothalamus by the pituitary stalk. The pituitary gland has a dual origin: an anterior pituitary or glandular portion and a posterior pituitary or nervous portion. The anterior pituitary (also called the adenohypophysis) arises as a shallow diverticulum (Rathke's pouch) from the oral ectoderm and will contribute to the pars anterior (distalis), pars tuberalis, and pars intermedia. The posterior pituitary (also called the neural lobe, pars neuralis, or neurohypophysis) arises as an evagination (infundibulum) from the floor of the hypothalamus and is therefore a derivative of the neuroectoderm. This neural portion of the pituitary will form the pars nervosa, the infundibular stem, and the median eminence.

The first indications of the adenohypophysis are evident at stage 10 (22–23 days) (Muller & O'Rahilly 1985), while Rathke's pouch appears during stage 12 (26–27 days) rostral to the notochord, and during the next two stages (28–32 days) this pouch deepens and contacts the floor of the diencephalon (Lemire *et al.* 1975). However, the first evagination of the diencephalic floor (the infundibulum) does not occur until stages 16 (37–40 days), and this region then assumes the appearance of a 'wrinkled sac' (Lemire *et al.* 1975). By stage 21 (52–53 days) it is a deep sac whose lumen remains connected to the third ventricle. Tilney (1936), in a study of the hypophysis from the 11 mm CR embryo to the adult, presents a clear and comprehensive study of the development and appearance of this gland. O'Rahilly (1983) has claimed that instead of this interpretation, the hypophysis forms from a single locus.

*Adenohypophysis (anterior pituitary) and the stalk of Rathke's pouch.* At stage 17 (41–43 days) the stalk which connects Rathke's pouch with the stomodeal roof (primitive mouth cavity) begins to constrict in places, so that the lumen is no longer continuous. Between stages 19 and 21 (47 and 53 days) the lumen of the stalk connecting Rathke's pouch with the foregut becomes largely obliterated, and the stalk which is initially thick and solid becomes thinner, and then threadlike. Finally, the center portion of the stalk disappears, leaving only a remnant at each end (Wislocki 1937). According to O'Rahilly *et al.* (1988), the separation of the adenohypophysis from the oral cavity occurs much earlier at stage 18 (44–46 days). In the following stage the cranial portion disappears as the sphenoid cartilage appears, but the caudal portion persists in the posterior nasopharynx as the pharyngeal hypophysis (Melchionna & Moore 1938; Boyd 1956; Lemire *et al.* 1975).

The anterior pituitary is divided into three regions: the pars tuberalis, the pars intermedia, and the pars anterior (distalis). The first indications of the pars tuberalis are seen late in stage 16 (37–40 days). Two lateral lobes (or tuberal processes) arise from Rathke's pouch near the mouth epithelium, and in the following stage (stage 17, 41–43 days) surround the infundibulum laterally. The bilateral lobes then begin to curve medially. By the end of stage 23 (56 days), the two pars tuberalis meet in the midline (behind the optic chiasma) and continue caudally to invest the median tuber cinereum by 45 mm CR (Lemire *et al.* 1975), fuse with it at 55 mm CR, and completely invest the infundibulum between 120 and 170 mm CR.

By stage 18 (44–46 days) the second region, the pars intermedia, becomes identifiable as the anterior lobe cells adjacent to the infundibulum. In stage 19 (47–48 days) the pars intermedia grows laterally around the posterior lobe of the pituitary. The third region, the pars anterior, enlarges in the midline dorsally at the stage when the stalk of Rathke's pouch becomes threadlike (stage 21, 52–53 days). As a result the lumen of Rathke's pouch becomes reduced in size and is eventually reduced to a cleft (Rathke's cleft). This is not usually identifiable in the adult, but cysts may form in its remnants.

At the same time (stages 19–21, 47–53 days), the floor of the third ventricle is becoming wider. By 55 mm CR, 'vascular grooves' in this region have formed blood vessels which have penetrated the pars distalis and pars tuberalis (Lemire *et al.* 1975). All three regions of the adenohypophysis have now become glandular.

*Neurohypophysis (posterior pituitary).* The neurohypophysis develops early functional activity as evidenced by the detection of its hormones after 10 weeks (Dicker & Tyler 1953; Skowsky & Fisher 1973). Both the neurovascular contacts and the neurosecretory granules appear around 10 weeks. By 8.5 weeks (45 mm CR) the axon profiles contain accumulations of granular vesicles (Okado & Yokota 1980). Later in development these granular vesicles store hormones, but it is not clear whether this is so at the earlier stages.

At 15.5–19 weeks there is a further increase in the number of vesicles; this is associated with an increase in the neurosecretory materials in the hypothalamic supraoptic and/or paraventricular nuclei which send axons into the neural lobe (Okado & Yokota 1980).

Between 170 and 200 mm CR (19–21 weeks) the posterior pituitary differentiates further and the proximal cells resemble neuroglial cells while the distal cells are oval or fusiform in shape. Nerve fibers from the hypothalamus grow into the pars nervosa. Generally, the entire pituitary gland is well formed by 110 days (Dicker & Tyler 1953).

*Infundibular stem.* During the fetal period (120 mm CR) the stem elongates and forms a backward angle of 20° with the ventricular floor. By 170 mm CR the stalk assumes an angle of 45°, and by birth is nearly perpendicular (Lemire *et al.* 1975).

*Subcommissural organ.* The subcommissural organ appears at the junction of the diencephalon and mesencephalon. This organ was originally described by Dandy & Nichols (1910) as two bands of columnar epithelium united in the shape of a groove. Although this organ is present in the fetus (Wislocki & Roth 1958), it is vestigial at birth and disappears in the early adult (Rakic 1965). Dooling *et al.* (1983a) describe the organ as a prominent secretory structure at 12–24 weeks, gradually becoming less distinct by 25–40 weeks. This change is brought about by atrophy and by the loss of specialized epithelial cells. However, it has been suggested that this rudiment is still an active cell population (Kelly 1982).

## MIDBRAIN (MESENCEPHALON)

The midbrain originally has relatively thin walls and its lumen is a continuation of the third ventricle. As a result of the walls thickening, the lumen of the midbrain is eventually reduced to the narrow cerebral aqueduct (of Sylvius). This aqueduct connects the third and fourth ventricles. The dorsal midbrain roof (tectum) enlarges as two pairs of protuberances form, the rostral or superior colliculi and the inferior colliculi (Lund 1978). The superior colliculi are concerned with visual reflexes and the inferior colliculi with auditory transmission. Several nuclear groups also develop from the basal plates in the midbrain floor (tegmentum): the midbrain reticular formation, the red nucleus, the substantia nigra, and the oculomotor (III) and trochlear (IV) motor nuclei. The floor is additionally thickened by the base consisting of the cerebral peduncles, two large tracts conveying fibers from the cerebral cortex to subcortical areas.

In the early embryo (stage 10, 22–23 days) the rostral limit of the mesencephalon is a narrowing caudal to the optic primordium called the promesencephalic sulcus. The caudal limit is termed the isthmus rhombencephali (Warwick & Williams 1973). Later in development, the rostral limit is the mesmetencephalic sulcus (the future isthmus).

### Neuromeres

As the rostral neuropore closes, two midbrain neuromeres appear in the midbrain floor, a large rostral one and a smaller caudal one. These landmarks are linked with the cephalic flexure which appears in this region (stage 12, 26–27 days), and caudal to the second neuromere is the mesmetencephalic sulcus.

### Colliculi

The colliculi (tectum or corpora quadrigemina) form from cells that migrate from the alar plates. The primordium of the colliculi is the collicular plate, which appears at stage 11 (24–25 days). The two neuromeres described above have been equated with Streeter's pretectal and collicular areas (Bartelmez & Dekaban 1962). When the sulcus limitans appears (stages 13–14, 28–32 days), the corpora are separated from the tegmentum. Also during stage 14 (31–32 days) the isthmus grows rapidly. The tectum then thickens (7–9 mm CR), and the collicular plate is approximately equal in thickness throughout its area. In stage 16 (37–40 days) the borders of the colliculi are further established rostrally and caudally as the posterior commissure and the dorsal decussation of the trochlear nerve (IV) assume their positions in the midbrain. During stage 17 (41–43 days) the primordia of the paired bilateral superior colliculi and the paired bilateral inferior colliculi become visible as the collicular plate thickens. They become distinct by stage 18 (44–46 days).

### Red nucleus

By stage 15 (33–36 days) the basal laminae are distinctly larger than the alar laminae of the same region. As the basal plate grows, the relative size of the midbrain lumen becomes smaller. At stage 16 (37–40 days) the two somatic efferent columns are present in the basal plate. The midventral region between the two columns contains collections of neuroblasts which will form the midventral proliferation. This structure is well formed by stage 18 (44–46 days), and by stage 20 (49–51 days) some of its lateral cells will separate and form the red nucleus, together with cells from the lateral angle of the basal lamina. Fibers arrive from the cerebellum and contribute to the formation of the tegmentum. Fibers from the cerebellum running in the brachium conjunctivum (superior cerebellar peduncle) also arrive and invade the midventral proliferation. By the middle of week 9 (40 mm CR), they clearly demarcate the capsule of the red nucleus (Morrell 1985). The brachium conjunctivum is finely myelinated by 180 mm CR, and by the eighth month it is heavily myelinated.

From stages 20–21 (49–53 days) up until stage 23 (56 days), several structures become evident in the red nucleus. By stage 20–21 the fasciculus retroflexus is seen passing through the medial aspect of the red nucleus, followed in stages 21–22 (52–55 days) by the appearance of the mamillotegmental tract. In stage 23, clusters of cells (pars magnocellularis) appear in the red nucleus at approximately the same time as the functionally linked dentate nucleus appears in the cerebellum. By the end of month 3, the red nucleus is clearly defined (Warwick & Williams 1973) and will reach its full size at 5 years of age.

### Substantia nigra

The substantia nigra forms as cells from the ventrolateral aspect of the midventral proliferation spread and form a crescent-shaped mass (Cooper 1946, 1950; Lemire *et al.* 1975) (stages 20–21, 49–53 days). This broad layer of gray matter is located adjacent to the cerebral peduncle. The basis pontis also forms from the midventral proliferation, and by stage 23 (56 days) its cells have established a continuity with the nigral cells. Later, at 60 mm CR, two zones are established in the substantia nigra: the corpus and the cauda. By 90 mm CR (12 weeks) the substantia nigra is pyramidal in shape, and by 190 mm CR (20 weeks) a third zone appears called the caput. It is possible to find some brown pigmentation at this stage, but it is not visible in gross specimens until 5 years of age. The 'adult' appearance is assumed at puberty (Lemire *et al.* 1975).

By the eighth month (300 mm CR), myelinated fibers extend from the substantia nigra to the contralateral substantia nigra. They also extend to the subthalamic nucleus, into the medial lemniscus, descending corticospinal fibers and temporopontine pathway.

### Cerebral peduncles

The cerebral peduncles develop as small thickenings from the ventral laminae. In the fourth month they increase rapidly in size and become more prominent as their fiber tracts appear in the marginal zone (Warwick & Williams 1973). These tracts are passing through the midbrain to the brainstem and spinal cord and they include the corticopontine, corticobulbar, and corticospinal tracts.

## HINDBRAIN (METENCEPHALON)

The metencephalon is composed of a dorsal tissue mass, the cerebellum, forming the roof and a ventral tissue mass, the pons, forming the floor. The fourth ventricle lies between these two masses.

### Cerebellum

The cerebellum (little brain) is an outgrowth of the hindbrain (metencephalon) and is located rostral to the developing trigeminal nerve (sensory). It appears at the same time as the pontine flexure. The flocculonodular lobes are the first to form and differentiate. They also are the first to have a mature cell population and to myelinate.

Initially the rhombencephalic region in the early embryo (stage 12, 26–27 days) has a very thin roof oriented longitudinally. With the appearance of the pontine flexure (stage 13–14, 28–32 days) the rhombencephalon is re-oriented from a longitudinal axis to a horizontal one. In this process, the very thin roof creases (plica chorioidea). Cranial to this landmark the cerebellum will develop, while the choroid plexus will form at its site.

The rhombencephalon is now diamond shaped, and at its most lateral part (the alar plates) there is a burst of mitotic activity during week 4. This neuroblast activity causes the dorsal portion of the alar plates to enlarge and form the rhombic lips. The rhombic lips are a proliferative zone which contributes cells ventrally to the brainstem (pontine nuclei and inferior olive) and dorsally to the cerebellum (Muller & O'Rahilly 1990). Initially the lips are small swellings which bulge into the fourth ventricle (40–90 mm CR) (Fig. 3.5). The cerebellum, which now has a large number of neuroblasts, bulges externally. This area continues to grow at the expense of the intraventricular portion. By stage 17 (41–43 days) the rhombic lips have differentiated rostrally from the level of the vestibular nuclei to the rostral end of the rhombic roof. Because the mitotic rate is high in the rhombic lips, and neuroblasts migrate into the lips, the pontine flexure continues to deepen. As a result, the rhombic lips fuse to the ventral portion of the alar plates. Initially, these areas are parallel to the longitudinal axis of the neural tube. Then as the pontine flexure forms, the rhombic lips come to run in an oblique line rostrally towards the midline. Eventually, they fuse in the midline to form a dumb-bell-shaped cerebellum. The lateral regions grow rapidly and form the lateral lobes.

The first fissure (posterolateral) appears early in month 4 (50 mm CR), separating the nodule from the vermis, the floccules, and the hemispheres. This fissure separates the most primitive phylogenetic portion, the flocculonodular lobe (archicerebellum), from the remainder (trigeminal-spinal portion). The second fissure to appear is the primary fissure at 75 mm CR, separating the culmen from the declive. Later, secondary fissures appear in the vermis and flocculonodular lobes which eventually extend into the hemispheres and give rise to the adult folia.

The dumb-bell shape of the cerebellum is acquired when the middle portions ultimately proliferate more than the rostral or caudal portions (Fig. 3.6). Then the hemispheres grow and almost obscure the vermis. The vermian lobules are present at 150 mm CR and their folia are beginning to form. Finally, the cerebellum overgrows the fourth ventricle, the pons, and medulla. In the neonate, the cerebellum weighs 18–20 g and comprises 5–6% of the weight of the entire brain (Crelin 1973). Although by birth the cerebellum has the same shape as the adult, cellular differentiation, migration, and myelination continue.

*Histology of the cerebellum.* In the embryo, the cerebellar wall consists of three identifiable layers: the ventricular,

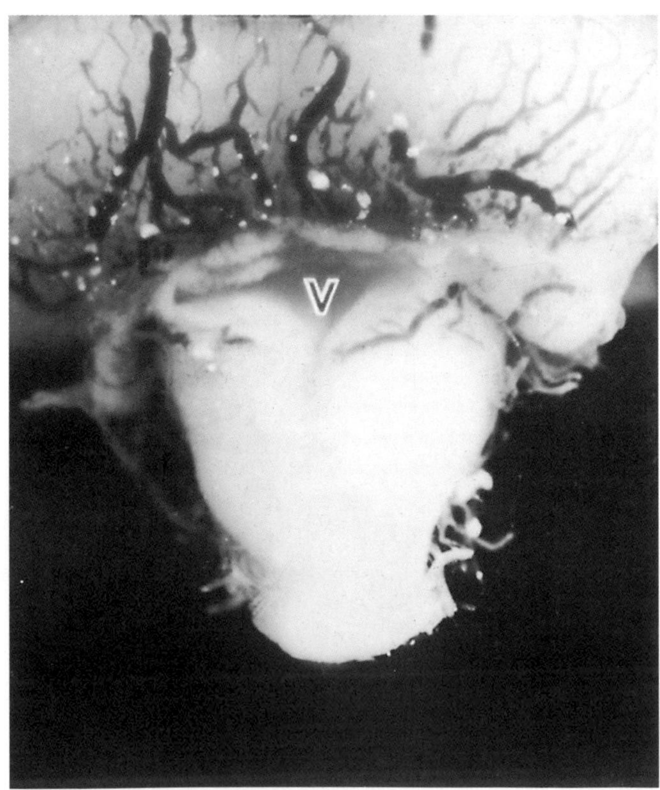


**Figure 3.5** The developing cerebellum. V, fourth ventricle.

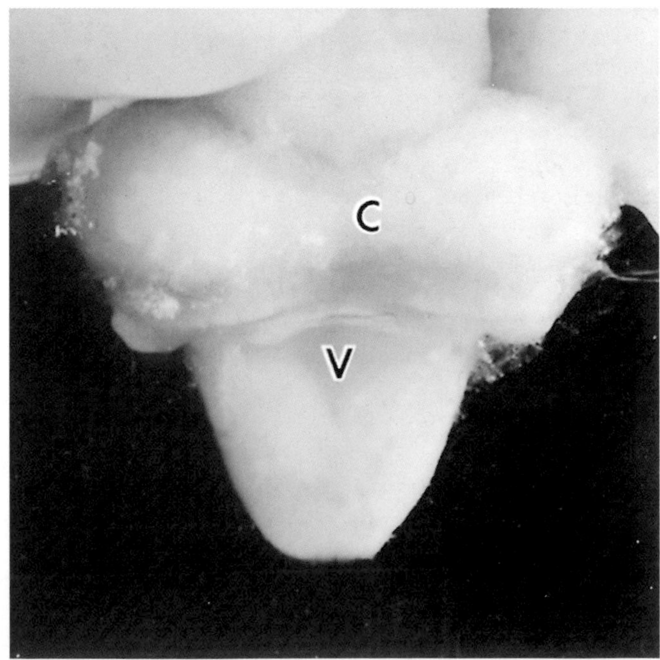


**Figure 3.6** The cerebellum of the week 15 fetus. C, cerebellum; V, fourth ventricle.

intermediate, and marginal zones. The first indications of the future cerebellar cortex are the development of Purkinje cells generated in the roof of the fourth ventricle (intermediate cells of the alar plates) (Muller & O'Rahilly 1990). These cells then migrate externally at 9–10 weeks, until they come to lie in the most superficial part of the marginal zone. At the same time, a subventricular zone forms (particularly prominent in the rhombic lip), and by 10–11 weeks granule cells derived from this layer migrate over the external surface of the cerebellum and form a transient layer, the external granular layer. Once the cells to which this layer gives rise are postmitotic they migrate inwards, trailing a perpendicular axon, and develop dendrites upon reaching their position below (internal to) the Purkinje cell layer. A transient layer, the lamina dissecans, separates the internal granular layer from the Purkinje cells. Ultimately, this is filled by migrating granule cells and disappears (Rakic & Sidman 1970). At the same time as the postmitotic granule cells migrate inwards (16–25 weeks), the Purkinje cells enlarge and develop dendritic trees. Shortly following the appearance of the internal granular layer, basket cells also start to form.

The transient external granular layer normally regresses markedly between 2 and 4 months after birth (Friede 1973). It becomes progressively thinner as the number of cells in the layer decreases. By 18 months after birth the adult appearance is reached (Larroche 1966). Medulloblastoma, a brainstem tumor of childhood, is thought to originate in malignant external granule cells (Kadin *et al.* 1970).

Other intermediate layer cells which did not migrate give rise to the dentate nucleus at stage 18 (44–46 days) (O'Rahilly *et al.* 1988) and fastigial nuclei, both of which are apparent at an early stage, as well as the globose and emboliform nuclei.

### Pons

The pons forms from the basal lamina in the ventral metencephalon. Three groups of motor cells arise from the basal lamina. From medial to lateral these are: (1) somatic efferents giving rise to the nucleus of nerve VI; (2) the special visceral efferent (branchiomotor) nucleus of nerve VII (caudally); and (3) nerve V (cranially), and general visceral efferent (superior salivary nucleus) of nerve VII.

The nuclei pontis of the basilar part of the pons are formed by a contribution from the alar plate of the myelencephalon, as well as from cells of the metencephalon. Later, their axons grow transversely in the marginal zone to the cerebellum of the opposite side. These comprise the transverse fibers of the pons and the brachium pontis (middle cerebellar peduncle) (Hamilton & Mossman 1972).

## HINDBRAIN (MYELENCEPHALON)

The myelencephalon forms the medulla (medulla oblongata) and is continuous cranially with the pons and caudally with the spinal cord. It is arbitrarily divided into two areas: the rostrally 'open' part of the medulla and the caudally 'closed' part continuous with the spinal cord (Moore 1982).

The 'open' part of the medulla is wide and flat due to the pontine flexure, causing the walls to splay outwards. As a result the roof is thinned and the medullary walls containing the alar plates flatten out and come to lie lateral to the basal plates. The cavity of the fourth ventricle is therefore diamond shaped. As a result of the alar plates lying lateral to the basal plates, the motor nuclei, which are derivatives of the basal plates, form medially. The sensory nuclei from the alar plates generally form laterally. The motor nuclei form three columns. From medial to lateral these are the general somatic efferent, the special visceral (branchial) efferent, and the general visceral efferent. The sensory nuclei form four columns. From medial to lateral these are the general visceral afferent, the special visceral afferent, the general somatic afferent, and the special somatic afferent. The olivary nuclei form when some cells from the alar plates migrate ventrally.

The caudal 'closed' portion of the myelencephalon resembles the spinal cord structurally, but unlike the spinal cord, islands of gray matter form in the marginal zone. These are principally the gracile nuclei, located medially, and the cuneate nuclei, located laterally. The pyramids containing the corticospinal fibers descending from the cerebral cortex are in the ventral area.

## ASSOCIATION FIBERS, COMMISSURES, AND THE PYRAMIDAL TRACT

Association fibers connect adjacent areas of the brain, while commissures connect equivalent areas on the opposite side of the brain. The pyramidal tract is the only tract to span the entire length of the CNS without synaptic relay.

*Association fibers.* The development and growth of the association fibers in the cerebral cortex is poorly understood.

*Commissures.* The forebrain roof is thickened by bundles of fibers crossing between the two hemispheres. The most important commissures cross the rostral end of the forebrain in the lamina terminalis. They extend from the roof plate of the diencephalon to the optic chiasma. Bartelmez & Dekaban (1962) divided the embryonic lamina terminalis (stage 22, 54–55 days) into four regions: (1) a ventral primordium for the optic chiasma (chiasmatic plate); (2) a short, membranous portion dorsal to the chiasmatic plate which will become the adult lamina terminalis; (3) a commissural plate for the anterior and hippocampal commissures and corpus callosum; and (4) a membrane to the velum transversum that is dorsal to the commissural plate.

The first commissures to form from the commissural plate are the anterior and hippocampal commissures (Rakic & Yakolev 1968). The commissural plate enlarges caudally, and axons from the cerebral cortex of each hemisphere begin to grow through the plate to form the commissures. The anterior commissure (week 10, 40 mm CR) has a large temporal component, and connects the olfactory bulbs and areas related to it, while the hippocampal (or fornix) commissure (weeks 10–11, 45–55 mm CR) connects the hippocampal formations (Brown 1983). These are phylogenetically older regions of the brain. After these commissures form, the corpus callosum begins to form and connects neocortical regions. Initially, the corpus callosum, the largest commissure to form from the commissural plate, lies in the lamina terminalis above the hippocampal commissure. As the cortex enlarges, more and more fibers are added and the corpus callosum gradually extends beyond the lamina terminalis, and at birth extends over the diencephalic roof (pineal). As it spreads caudally it overrides the hippocampal commissure. The crossing over of the callosal fibers begins in the first trimester (50–60 mm CR, weeks 10–11), becomes distinct by 60–80 mm CR (weeks 12–13) and continues throughout most of the fetal period (Rakic & Yakovlev 1968; O'Rahilly & Gardner 1977).

While the cerebral commissures are forming, other commissures are also developing: the optic chiasma (stages 15–17, days 33–43), the habenular (or superior) commissure (O'Rahilly *et al.* 1987, 1988; Muller & O'Rahilly 1990) and the posterior commissure (stage 15, 33–36 days) (O'Rahilly 1968; O'Rahilly *et al.* 1984, 1987). The habenular commissure first appears in stages 18–19 (days 44–48) (O'Rahilly *et al.* 1988) and develops immediately rostral to the stalk of the pineal, while the posterior develops behind the stalk at the junction of the dimesencephalic boundary. At 54 mm CR (9 weeks) the anterior and posterior commissures and the corpus callosum are present.

As the corpus callosum connects the two hemispheres, the fornix is cut off from the rest of the hemisphere, as well as the tela choroidea, a horizontal sheet of pial mesenchyme adhering to a thin, ependyma-only area of the brain wall. This results in the choroid plexus of the lateral ventricle lying peripherally at the edge of the tela choroidea and the choroid plexus of the third ventricle lying on the ventral surface of the tela. The choroid plexus of the third ventricle lies in the roof of the third ventricle. The septum pellucidum may form from part of the medial hemispherical wall ventral to the corpus callosum.

*Pyramidal tract.* The pyramidal tract grows through an organized brainstem and spinal cord (Humphrey 1960). Pyramidal fibers have been identified in the cerebral peduncles at 32 mm CR and the pyramidal decussation is complete by 17 weeks (Humphrey 1960). Well-myelinated fibers are scattered above the pyramidal decussation by 23 weeks (220 mm CR), and some are also apparent below the decussation in the anterior and lateral corticospinal tracts. Well-differentiated glial cells are also identifiable among the tracts (Wozniak & O'Rahilly 1982). From 29 weeks on, an adult arrangement is apparent in the distal part of the tract. Yakovlev & Rakic (1966) have published a detailed account of the distribution and pattern of these fibers in the fetal and neonatal spinal cord. All of the tract's fibers are myelinated by 18 months of life. It should be remembered, however, that the presence of incoming fibers from the brainstem to the spinal cord does not necessarily indicate that they are functional (Okado & Kojima 1984).

## SYNAPTIC DEVELOPMENT

Excitatory amino acids (EAAs), which are estimated to be the primary neurotransmitter in approximately 50% of mammalian synapses, have a wide range of activities and functions in the development of the CNS. Under normal circumstances they participate both in neuronal signal transduction and exert trophic influences on neuronal development. They directly affect neuronal differentiation, growth and survival, as well as neuronal circuitry. During development, receptors for EAAs undergo marked ontogenic changes in their biochemical and electrophysiologic properties (McDonald & Johnston 1990). Markers for their pathways also undergo marked changes; in particular they are overproduced during times when synaptic plasticity is greatest. EAAs are also responsible for neuronal demise under other circumstances (see p. 418).

By the end of the embryonic period, the brainstem is more highly developed than more rostral structures (O'Rahilly & Gardner 1977). Monoamine synthesizing neurons are present at this time in the brainstem, and will have assumed a near-adult distribution in the spinal cord, cerebellum, and forebrain by midterm (Olson *et al.* 1973). Generally, the cell bodies of noradrenaline synthesizing neurons are located in the medulla oblongata (ventral and ventrolateral portions, dorsal and dorsomedial portions) and in the locus coeruleus and nucleus subcoeruleus. Dopamine neurons are present in the substantia nigra (pars compacta), in the tegmentum of the caudal mesencephalon and rostral pons, and in the hypothalamus (arcuate nucleus).

Cell bodies of indoleamine synthesizing neurons (5-hydroxytryptamine) are present cephalocaudally in the lateral reticular formation of the caudal portion of the mesencephalon, the rostral part of the pons, and the raphe of the pons and medulla oblongata.

## CRANIAL NERVES

The 12 pairs of cranial nerves appear between weeks 5 and 6. O'Rahilly *et al.* (1984) in an extensive study of 100 features of the brain and related structures reported that the cranial nerves of the rhombencephalon, with one exception (abducent), develop more rapidly than those associated with the midbrain and forebrain. They reported that in stages 12 and 13 (26–30 days) the order of development of efferent, afferent, or both types of fibers is as follows: nerves XII, V, VII, VIII, IX/X and XI. Then the following nerves appear: in stage 13 (28–30 days), nerve III; in stage 14 (31–32 days), nerve IV; and in stage 15 (33–36 days), nerve VI. Late in stage 15, the first olfactory (nerve I) fibers develop and in stages 19–20 (47–51 days) the optic (nerve II) fibers are found.

## NUCLEI

The motor nuclei appear much earlier (stage 12, 26–27 days) than the sensory nuclei (stage 17, 41–43 days). This pattern of motor before sensory is true in the rhombencephalon, mesencephalon, and diencephalon (O'Rahilly *et al.* 1984). A detailed analysis of the cranial nerves and nuclei is reported by O'Rahilly *et al.* (1984) and is recommended for a more detailed account.

## SULCI AND GYRI FORMATION

Initially the cerebral hemispheres are smooth (Fig. 3.7), but, as they grow, complex patterns of sulci and gyri develop. These patterns permit an increase in cerebral cortical volume without a concomitant increase in cranial volume. Hofman (1985) in a recent study of mammalian brains suggests that in addition to considerations of volume, there are also limitations on the degree of cortical folding based on the thickness of the cortex. By birth the total surface area of the cerebral cortex buried in the sulci and fissures is approximately twice that of the visible surface area of the cerebral cortex (Larroche 1966).

The sulci and fissures develop in a repeatable and recognizable pattern that can serve as an indicator of both developmental age and of normal development. The fetal brain increases dramatically in weight at 24–25 weeks (Dooling *et al.* 1983b), and many gyri become well defined between 26 and 28 weeks. Fujimura & Seryu (1977), however, state that brain growth (weight) is a smooth progression until week 33, in contrast to the findings of Dooling *et al.* (1983b). Secondary and tertiary gyration occurs late in gestation (weeks 40–44). The frontal and temporal areas become increasingly complex, and a few weeks later similar changes occur in the orbital and occipital gyri.

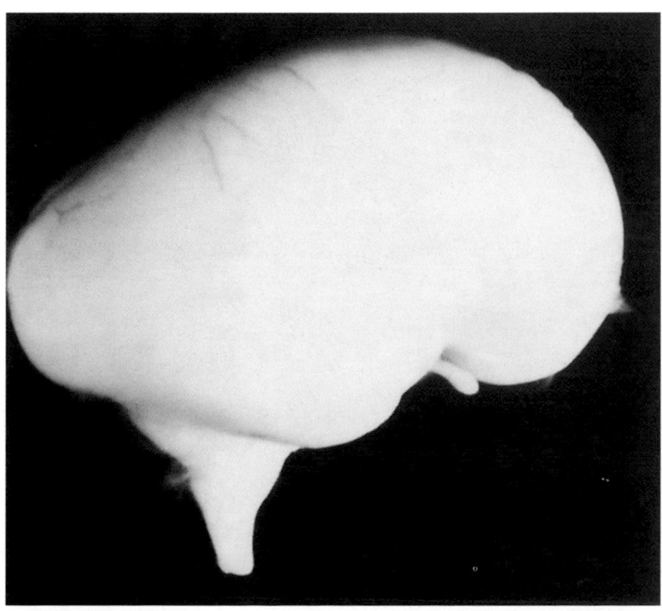

**Figure 3.7** External appearance of the cerebral hemisphere in a fetus at 130 mm CR length. Note the smooth cerebral surface.

The sulci begin to appear during month 4, with the lateral and central fissures among the earliest to form along with the pre- and postcentral sulci and the posterior portion of the superior temporal sulcus (Rorke & Riggs 1969). The first primary fissure to appear is the longitudinal fissure at 8 weeks, and is very distinct by week 10. The transverse fissure and the hippocampal sulcus are evident at 9–10 weeks (Hines 1922; Humphrey 1967).

By week 14 the lateral sulcus (Sylvian fissure) appears as a shallow depression on the lateral surface of the hemispheres. This depression deepens as the surrounding frontal, parietal and temporal areas grow rapidly, and by week 19 the tissue of the depression forms the insula (Fig. 3.8). There is also an associated thickening of the pia-arachnoid and an increasingly rich blood supply. As the insula remains exposed throughout most of gestation (Dooling *et al.* 1983b) many other sulci and fissures are better indicators of gestational age.

The callosal sulcus appears around week 14, together with the corpus callosum. The olfactory sulcus appears as a shallow depression at week 16 and gradually becomes distinct at week 25. The parieto-occipital fissure appears at week 16. As it forms, a distinctive layer of cells appears in the molecular layer of the isocortex at the future site of the fissure. As the fissure develops, this layer of cells is carried down into the walls of the fissure and eventually disappears.

By week 16 the calcarine fissure is also present and appears on the right before the left. By week 27 this fissure indents the occipital horn of the lateral ventricle.

At 20 weeks the central sulcus (Rolandic sulcus) is a distinct groove and by 22–23 weeks a distinct sulcus. The right central sulcus appears before the left. It is of interest that many areas appear on the right side of the brain before they appear on the left. Secondary gyri also appear earlier on the right side than on the left side.

At birth the sulci and gyri are similar in arrangement to that of the adult. The central sulcus, however, is slightly more rostral and the lateral sulcus more oblique than in the adult (Fig. 3.9).

## CHOROID PLEXUSES

Four choroid plexuses develop in the brain: one in the medial wall of each lateral ventricle, one in the roof of the third ventricle, and one in the roof of the fourth ventricle (Streeter 1912, 1951). These plexuses secrete cerebrospinal fluid (CSF).

The primordium of the choroid plexus of the fourth ventricle forms first at stage 17 (41–43 days) (O'Rahilly *et al.* 1987) and is easily distinguishable at stage 18 (44–46 days). As the pontine flexure occurs, the thin rhombic roof of the fourth ventricle changes its greatest dimension from a longi-

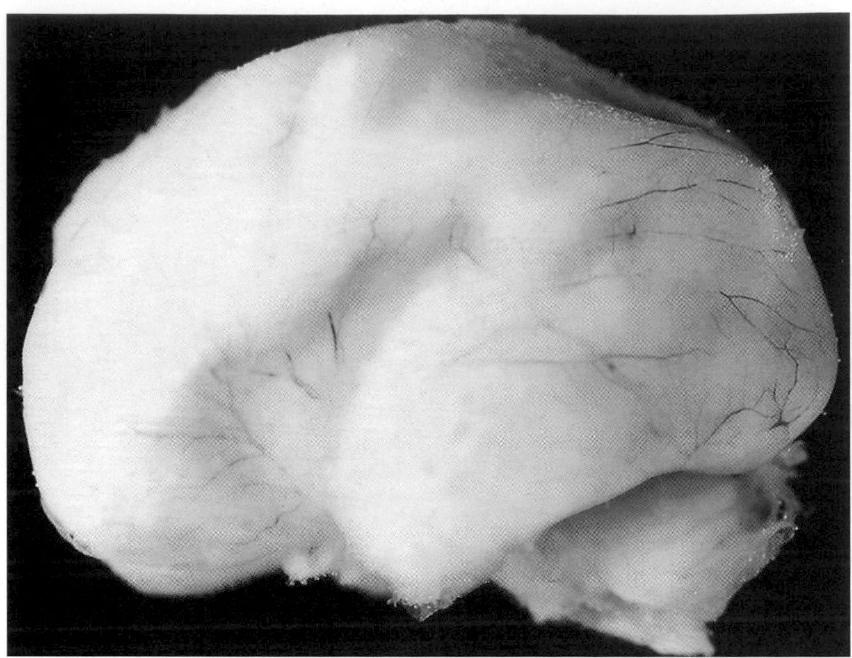

**Figure 3.8** The early insula. Note the central sulcus.

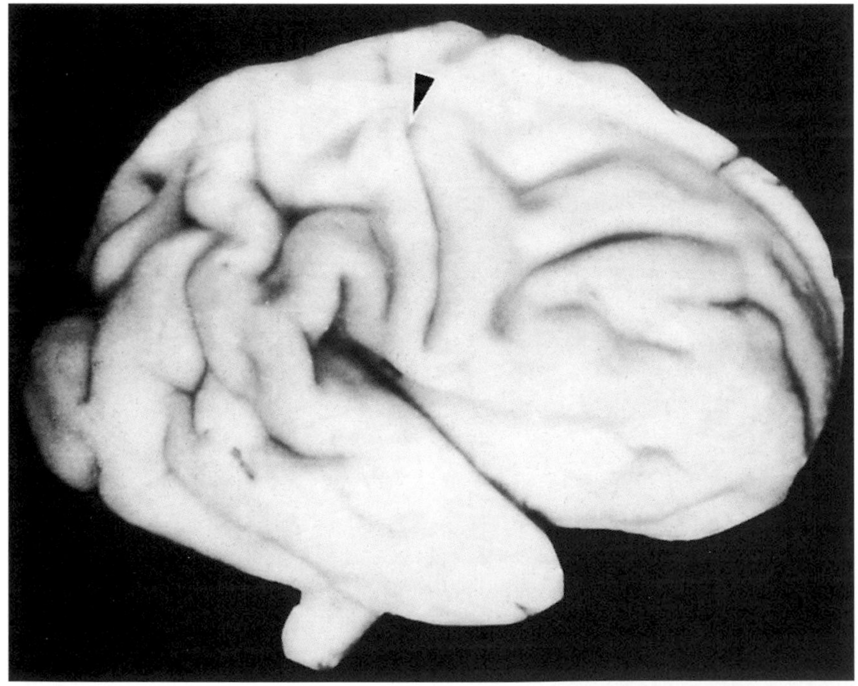

**Figure 3.9** Week 28. Note the clearly defined central sulcus (arrow) and the patterns of sulci and gyri. (Reproduced by permission of Wolfe Medical Publications, London.)

tudinal to a horizontal one. The transverse crease or plica choroidea that forms is where the choroid plexus will develop in the roof of the fourth ventricle. Initially, the choroid plexus has a horizontal orientation, and this position ultimately corresponds to the location of the foramina of Luschka.

The final position of the choroid plexus is determined by the subsequent changes that occur in the rhombic roof (see

'Cerebellum', p. 29). As the thin ependyma roof of the fourth ventricle loses its mitotic activity it forms a single epithelial layer. This layer has an external covering of very vascular pia mater, which together with the epithelial layers is known as the tela choroidea. As the pia mater proliferates rapidly, the tela choroidea invaginates into the fourth ventricle (Brocklehurst 1969) to form the choroid plexus. In the 37 mm CR embryo the epithelium is columnar but by 59 mm CR it has become cuboidal (Hoyes & Barber 1976). The cellular elements of the choroid plexus become granulated and appear as a secretory epithelium. The histologic structure of the fetal and adult choroid plexus is, therefore, different (Larroche 1966).

The first perforation to appear in the roof of the fourth ventricle is the midline foramen of Magendie. This foramen occurs as the result of an active process of differentiation which occurs before the choroid plexus begins to function; perforation is not a result of the build-up of CSF pressure. Shortly after CSF appears outside the fourth ventricle, the thin arachnid trabeculae differentiate. Laterally, two additional foramina (of Luschka) appear in the roof of the fourth ventricle, adjacent to cranial nerves VII and VIII. Although these foramina have been described as patent as early as 195 mm CR (week 21), their exact time of opening is not known. At birth, all three foramina are patent, although Alexander (1931) found that 20% of the population had no foramina of Luschka.

The first signs of the choroid plexuses of the lateral ventricles appear in stage 17 (days 41–43) (O'Rahilly *et al.* 1987), and form in a similar manner (stage 19, 47–48 days), whilst those of the third ventricle develop last (stage 21, 52–53 days) (Lemire *et al.* 1975).

## MYELINATION

The rate of myelination varies with the anatomical structure and developmental age. According to Yakovlev & Lecours (1967), myelination of a region or fiber system is an important indicator of regional maturation. Cycles of myelination progress at different rates and may not be complete for some structures until several years after birth (Fig. 3.10). For example, the medial lemniscus begins myelination during the sixth month of fetal life and continues until early into the second year of postnatal life. Those which function first tend to be myelinated first (Hamilton & Mossman 1972; Gilles *et al.* 1983). Those with long phases of myelination are particularly at risk (Gilles *et al.* 1983). One of the most rapid myelination cycles is that of the statoacoustic system, which begins in the fifth fetal month and is completed by the middle of the ninth fetal month. In general, myelin accumulates slowly in the third trimester followed by a sudden and marked increase in deposition, particularly in the thalamus, pallidum, field of Forel and the subthalamic region (Gilles *et al.* 1983).

Myelin is formed in the CNS by oligodendrocytes. Immediately before the beginning of myelin deposition, there is a marked proliferation of oligodendrocytes and an increased vascularization of the area (Lemire *et al.* 1975). Myelin is laid down first on the fiber close to the nerve cell body and then deposition proceeds along its axon (Keene & Hewer 1931; Gilles *et al.* 1983). The oligodendrocyte wraps its lipoprotein plasma membranes repeatedly around the axon to produce the myelin sheath. An oligodendrocyte myelinates more than one axon (Bunge *et al.* 1961). Generally, myelination proceeds in the direction of the major flow of information (Gilles *et al.* 1983). The only major exception inside the CNS is the myelination of transpontine fibers and the middle cerebellar peduncle before the cortico-pontine fibers myelinate in the mesencephalic cerebral peduncle (Gilles *et al.* 1983).

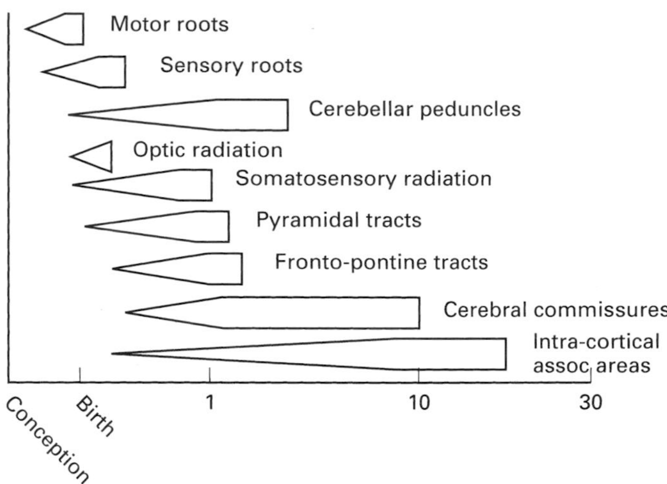


Figure 3.10 Cycles of myelination in the developing brain indicating when myelination commences and is complete for different structures. (Modified from Yakovlev & Lecours 1967.)

### SPINAL CORD

As the cell tracts and columns differentiate, their interrelationships change constantly. The formation of myelin in the spinal cord begins during the middle of the fetal period (11–14 weeks, 75–105 mm CR) (Hamilton & Mossman 1972) and continues until 1 year after birth. Yakovlev & Lecours (1967) described several tracts in their study, but generally concluded that in the peripheral nervous system the motor roots of the spinal nerves are myelinated in a short cycle between the fourth and ninth fetal months, while the sensory root fibers have a longer cycle from the end of the fifth fetal month to several months after birth. Myelination begins in the cervical cord and proceeds caudally. Okado & Kojima (1984) showed that myelination begins at 12 weeks, but the growth patterns of the myelinated tracts and myelin deposition are labile and variable (Gilles *et al.* 1983). Okado & Kojima's (1984) study also demonstrated that myelination and synaptogenesis occur simultaneously in some periods of development. Previously, it had been thought that synaptogenesis preceded myelination (Bodian 1970).

Gilles *et al.* (1983) reported that, with the exception of the cranial and spinal roots which were not examined, the earliest myelin in the CNS is deposited before week 20 in the rhombencephalic portion of the medial longitudinal fasciculus. They also observed that there are selected systems in the lower brainstem and rostral spinal cord which myelinate by mid-gestation and are heavily myelinated by birth. They include the fasciculus cuneatus, the caudal medial lemniscus, the trapezoid body and the lateral lemniscus, the inferior cerebellar peduncle, and the spinal trigeminal tract.

## BRAIN

Myelination reaches the cerebral hemispheres by birth and is finally complete by 2–3 years after birth. Yakovlev & Lecours (1967) reported that there are no myelinated fibers in the CNS before the end of the fifth fetal month. Interestingly, there is no myelination of the forebrain until the seventh fetal month, which continues in some parts through the years of maturity. The greatest quantity of myelin is deposited in the telencephalon during the third trimester and postnatally (Gilles *et al.* 1983). The first to acquire myelin sheaths are neurons in the olfactory, optic and acoustic cortical areas and the motor cortex (pyramidal cells) (Crelin 1973). The last to be myelinated are the projection, commissural and association neurons of the cerebral hemispheres (Crelin 1973). The projection fibers begin myelination before the association fibers, whose myelination continues through adulthood.

Wozniak & O'Rahilly (1982) observe that myelination is in progress in the pyramidal tract at the level of the pyramidal decussation in a week 23 fetus (220 mm CR). Gilles *et al.* (1983) report the optic tract is myelinated in week 29, the chiasma at 32 weeks, and the radiation in weeks 38–39. Myelination occurs in the posterior limb of the internal capsule at week 32, the corona radiata at week 34, the cingulum and the cerebral peduncle medial to the corticospinal tract at week 38, and the fornix at week 39. Later at week 46, the corpus callosum and anterior commissure become myelinated, with the mammilothalamic tract at either week 48 (Gilles *et al.* 1983) or week 36 (Yakovlev & Lecours 1967).

The cranial nerves of the midbrain, pons and medulla have been reported to begin myelination during the sixth fetal month (Crelin 1973). Yakovlev & Lecours (1967), however, reported that myelination of the cranial nerves begins earliest with cranial nerve VIII in the latter part of the fifth fetal month. At about the same time, the roots of nerves III, IV, and V, and the motor division of the trigeminal nerve undergo myelination. Late in the fifth fetal month the intermedullary roots of the facial nerve and glossopharyngeal and hypoglossal root fibers have a short myelination cycle while the sensory roots have a longer cycle.

The cerebellar connections are myelinated and the afferent thalamic pathways are myelinated as far as the thalamus in the seventh month.

By 32 weeks of gestation (300 mm CR), myelinated fibers are found extending from the substantia nigra to the subthalamic nucleus, to the contralateral substantia nigra to the medial lemniscus, descending cerebrospinal fibers and the temporopontine pathway (Lemire *et al.* 1975).

However, it is clear when comparing the findings of different authors that there is a great deal of biologic and methodologic variation (Langworthy 1933; Larroche 1966; Yakovlev & Lecours 1967; Gilles *et al.* 1983). In a more recent study, Brody *et al.* (1987) reported on the sequence of CNS myelination at 62 sites in 162 infants from birth through to the second postnatal year. Generally, the anatomical features studied at birth (36 weeks of postconceptual age to 2 years of postnatal age) are very close to those reported by Yakovlev & Lecours (1967). One notable exception was the corpus callosum, which was reported to myelinate slowly by Yakovlev & Lecours and not be complete until 4 years of age. By contrast, Brody *et al.* (1987) reported that myelination was complete in this structure by 2 years.

## ACKNOWLEDGMENTS

The author is deeply grateful to Professor M. Marin-Padilla (Dartmouth College, USA) who generously read and commented upon this text. He also suggested the use of and contributed Fig. 3.3 and Table 3.3. Dr A. R. Lieberman (University College London, UK) also generously read the chapter and made extensive comments. Dr R. R. Sturrock and Dr I. H. M Smart (University of Dundee, UK) and Dr J. Wakely (Leicester University, UK) also made useful and constructive comments which are much appreciated.

The author would also like to express her gratitude to Dr G. Batcup (Leeds General Infirmary, UK), to Dr E. C. Blenkinsopp (Watford General Hospital, UK) and to Mr P. A. Runicles (The Middlesex Hospital Medical School, London, UK) for allowing photography of materials.

Professor K. Carr (Department of Anatomy) generously allowed me to photograph Fig. 3.2 from The Belfast Collection, the Queen's University of Belfast, Northern Ireland.

The photographers whose assistance was invaluable are Mr K. Garfield (Central Photographic Unit) and Mr G. L. C. McTurk, both of Leicester University, UK. Figure 3.9 was photographed from the Royal Free Hospital School of Medicine, London, UK.

## REFERENCES


Alexander L (1931) Die Anatomie der Seitentaschen der vierten Hirnkammer. *Zeitschrift für die Gesamte Anatomie* 95:531–707.

Barr M L (1979) *The human nervous system, an anatomic viewpoint*, 3rd edn. Hagerstown, MD: Harper & Row.

Bartelmez G W, Dekaban A S (1962) The early development of the human brain. *Contrib Embryol* 37:13–32.

Berquist H & Kallen B (1954) Notes on the early histogenesis and morphogenesis of the central nervous system in vertebrates. *J Comp Neurol* 100:627–660.

Bodian D (1970) A model of synaptic and behavioural ontogeny. In: Schmitt F O (ed) *The neurosciences second study program*. New York, NY: Rockefeller University Press; pp. 129–140.

Boulder Committee (1970) Embryonic vertebrate central nervous system: revised terminology. *Anat Rec* 166: 257–262.

Boyd J D (1956) Observations on the human pharyngeal hypophysis. *J Endocrinol* 14:66–77.

Brocklehurst G (1969) The development of the human cerebrospinal fluid pathways with particular reference to the roof of the fourth ventricle. *J Anat* 105:467–475.

Brody B A, Kinney H C, Kloman A S & Gilles F H (1987) Sequence of central nervous system myelination in human infancy. I. An autopsy study of myelination. *J Neuropathol Exp Neurol* 46:283–301.

Brown J W (1983) Early prenatal development of the human precommissural septum. *J Comp Neurol* 215:331–350.

Bunge M B, Bunge R P & Ris H (1961) Ultrastructural study of remyelination in an experimental lesion in adult cat spinal cord. *J Biophys Biochem Cytol* 10:67–94.

Choi B H, Kim R C & Lapham L W (1983) Do radial glia give rise to both astroglial and oligodendroglial cells? *Dev Brain Res* 8:119–130.

Cooper E R A (1946) The development of the human red nucleus and corpus striatum. *Brain* 69:34–44.

Cooper E R A (1950) The development of the thalamus. *Acta Anat* 9:201–226.

Crelin E A (1973) *Functional anatomy of the newborn*. London: Yale University Press.

Dandy A & Nichols G E (1910) On the occurrence of a mesocoelic recess in the human brain, and its relation to the subcommissural organ of lower vertebrates; with special reference to the distribution of Reissner's fibre in the vertebrate series and its possible function. *Proc R Soc Lond* 82:515–529.

De Vries J I P, Visser G H A & Prechtl H F R (1982) The emergence of fetal behaviour I: qualitative aspects. *Early Hum Dev* 7:301–322.

Dicker S E & Tyler C (1953) Vasopressor and oxytocic activities of the pituitary glands of rats, guinea pigs and cats and of human foetuses. *J Physiol* 121:206–214.

Dobbing J & Sands J (1973) The quantitative growth and development of the human brain. *Arch Dis Child* 48:757–767.

Dooling E C, Chi J G & Gilles F H (1983a) Dorsal mesodiencephalic junction: pineal, subcommissural organ, and mesocoelic recess. In: Gilles F H, Leviton A & Dooling E C (eds) *The developing human brain: growth and epidemiologic neuropathology*. London: Wright; pp. 105–112.

Dooling E C, Chi J G & Gilles F H (1983b) Telencephalic development: changing gyral patterns. In: Gilles F H, Leviton A & Dooling E C (eds) *The developing human brain: growth and epidemiologic neuropathology*. London: Wright; pp. 94–104.

Duckett S & Pearse A G E (1968) The cells of Cajal–Retzius in the developing human brain. *J Anat* 102: 183–187.

FitzGerald J E & Windle W F (1942) Some observations on early human fetal movements. *J Comp Neurol* 76:159–167.

Fitzgerald M J T (1985) *Neuroanatomy basic and applied*. London: Baillière Tindall.

Friede R L (1973) Dating the development of human cerebellum. *Acta Neuropathol (Berlin)* 23:48–58.

Fujimoto E & Mizoguti H (1985) The first appearance of microglia in human embryonic pallium. Abstracts of the XIIth International Anatomical Congress, A218.

Fujimura M & Seryu J I (1977) Velocity of head growth during the perinatal period. *Arch Dis Child* 52:105–112.

Fujita S (1973) Genesis of glioblasts in the human spinal cord as revealed by Feulgen cytophotometry. *J Comp Neurol* 151:25–34.

Gilles F H, Shankle W & Dooling E C (1983) Myelinated tracts: growth patterns. In: Gilles F H, Leviton A & Dooling E C (eds) *The developing human brain: growth and epidemiologic neuropathology*. London: Wright; pp. 117–183.

Hamilton W & Mossman H W (1972) *Hamilton, Boyd and Mossman's human embryology: prenatal development of form and function*, 4th edn. Cambridge: Heffer.

Hines M (1922) Studies in the growth and differentiation of the telencephalon in man. The fissura hippocampi. *J Neurol* 34:73–171.

His W (1888) Zur Geschichte des Gehims sowie der centralen und periferischen Nervenbahnen beim menschlichen Embryo. *Abh math-phys Kl Kgl Sachs Ges Wiss* 14:339–392.

Hofman M A (1985) Size and shape of the cerebral cortex in mammals I. The cortical surface. *Brain Behav Evol* 27:28–40.

Hoyes A D & Barber P (1976) Ultrastructure of the epithelium of the human fetal choroid plexus. *J Anat* 122: 743.

Humphrey T (1960) The development of the pyramidal tracts in human fetuses, correlated with cortical differentiation. In: Tower D B & Schade J P (eds) *Structure and function of the cerebral cortex*. Amsterdam: Elsevier; pp. 93–103.

Humphrey T (1964a) Some correlations between the appearance of human fetal reflexes and the development of the nervous system. In: Purpura D P, Schade J P (eds) *Growth and maturation of the brain*. Amsterdam: Elsevier; pp. 93–133.

Humphrey T (1964b) Some correlations between the appearance of human fetal reflexes and the development of the nervous system. *Prog Brain Res* 4:93–135.

Humphrey T (1967) The development of the human hippocampal fissure. *J Anat* 101:655–676.

Humphrey T (1968) The development of the human amygdala during early embryonic life. *J Comp Neurol* 132:135–166.

Humphrey T & Hooker D (1959) Double simultaneous stimulation of human fetuses and the anatomical patterns underlying the reflexes elicited. *J Comp Neurol* 112:75–102.

Kadin M E, Rubinstein L J & Nelson J S (1970) Neonatal cerebellar medulloblastoma originating from the fetal external granular layer. *J Neuropathol Exp Neurol* 29:583–600.

Kallen B (1977) Errors in the differentiation of the central nervous system. In: Vinken P J, Bruyn G W (eds) *Handbook of clinical neurology*. New York, NY: North Holland; vol 30; pp. 41–83.

Keene M F L & Hewer E E (1931) Some observations on myelination in the human central nervous system. *J Anat* 66:1–13.

Kelly (1982) Circumventricular organs In: Haymaker & Adams (eds) *Histology and histopathology of the nervous system*. Charles C Thomas, Springfield, IL, vol II, pp. 1735–1800.

Kershman J (1939) Genesis of microglia in the human brain. *Arch Neurol Psychiatry* 41:24–50.

Kuhlenbeck H (1948) The derivatives of the thalamus ventralis in the human brain and their relation to the so-called subthalamus. *Military Surgery* 102:433–447.

Langworthy O R (1933) Development of behavioural patterns and myelinations of the nervous system in the human fetus and infant. *Contrib Embryol* 24:1–57.

Larroche J C (1966) Development of the nervous system in early life. Part II: The development of the central nervous system during intrauterine life. In: Falkner F (ed) *Human development*. Philadelphia, PA: Saunders; pp. 257–276.

Larroche J C (1981) The marginal layer in the neocortex of a 7-week-old human embryo. *Anat Embryol* 162:301–312.

Larroche J C & Houcine O (1982) Le neo-cortex chez l'embryon et le foetus humain: apport du microscope electronique et du Golgi. *Reprod Nutr Dev* 22:163–170.

Lemire R J, Loeser J D, Leich R W & Alvord E C (1975) *Normal and abnormal development of the human nervous system*. London: Harper & Row.

Lund R D (1978) *Development and plasticity of the brain. An introduction*. New York, NY: Oxford University Press.

McConnell S K (1988) Development and decision-making in the mammalian cerebral cortex. *Brain Res Rev* 13:1–23.

McConnell S K (1991) The generation of neuronal diversity in the central nervous system. *Annu Rev Neurosci* 14:269–300.

McDonald J W & Johnston M V (1990) Physiological and pathophysiological roles of excitatory amino acids during central nervous system development. *Brain Res Rev* 15:41–70.

Marin-Padilla M (1971) Early prenatal ontogenesis of the cerebral cortex (neocortex) of the cat (*Felis domesticus*): a Golgi study. I. The primordial neocortical organization. *Zeitschrift für Anatomie und Entwicklungsgeschichte* 134:117–145.

Marin-Padilla M (1978) Dual origin of the mammalian neocortex and evolution of the cortical plate. *Anat Embryol* 152:109–126.

Marin-Padilla M (1983) Structural organization of the human cerebral cortex prior to the appearance of the cortical plate. *Anat Embryol* 168:21–40.

Marin-Padilla M (1984) Neurons of layer I. A developmental analysis. In: Peters A & Jones E G (eds) *Cerebral cortex: cellular components of the cerebral cortex*. London: Plenum Press, vol I; ch 14; pp. 447–478.

Marin-Padilla M (1988) Early ontogenesis of the human cerebral cortex. In: Jones E G & Peters A (eds) *Cerebral cortex: cellular components of the cerebral cortex*. New York: Plenum Press; Vol VII.

Marin-Padilla M (1990) Three dimensional structural organization of Layer I of the human cerebral cortex: a Golgi study. *J Comp Neurol* 299:89–105.

Marin-Padilla M & Marin-Padilla M T (1982) Origin, prenatal development and structural organization of layer 1 of the human cerebral (motor) cortex: a Golgi study. *Anat Embryol* 164:161–206.

Melchionna R H & Moore R A (1938) The pharyngeal pituitary gland. *Am J Pathol* 14:763–771.

Molliver M E, Kostovic I & Van Der Loos H (1973) The development of synapses in cerebral cortex of the human fetus. *Brain Res* 50:403–407.

Moore K L (1982) *The developing human: clinically oriented embryology*, 3rd edn. London: W B Saunders.

Morrell N W (1985) The development of the human midbrain tegmentum with particular reference to the red nucleus. *J Anat* 140:544.

Muller F & O'Rahilly R (1985) The first appearance of the neural tube and optic primordium in the human embryo at stage 10. *Anat Embryol* 172:157–169.

Muller F & O'Rahilly (1990) The human brain at stages 18–20, including the choroid plexuses and the amygdaloid and septal nuclei. *Anat Embryol* 182:285–306.

Okado N & Kojima T (1984) Ontogeny of the central nervous system: neurogenesis, fiber connection, synaptogenesis and myelination in the spinal cord in continuity of neural functions from prenatal to postnatal life. *Clin Dev Med* 94.

Okado N, Yokota N (1980) An electron microscopic study on the structural development of the neural lobe in the human fetus. *Am J Anat* 159:261–273.

Olson L, Boreus L O & Seiger A (1973) Histochemical demonstration and mapping of 5-hydroxytryptamine and catecholamine-containing neuron systems in the human brain. *Zeitschrift für Anatomie und Entwicklungsgeschichte* 139:259–282.

O'Rahilly R (1968) The development of the epiphysis cerebri and the subcommissural complex in staged human embryos. *Anat Rec* 160:488–489.

O'Rahilly R (1973) *Developmental stages in human embryos including a survey of the Carnegie Collection. Part A: embryos of the first three weeks (stages 1–9)*. Washington, DC: Carnegie Institution of Washington.

O'Rahilly R (1983) The timing and sequence of events in the development of the human endocrine system during the embryonic period proper. *Anat Embryol* 166:439–451.

O'Rahilly R & Gardner E (1977) The developmental anatomy of the human central nervous system. In: Vinken R J, Bruyn G W (eds) Handbook of clinical neurology: congenital malformations of the brain and skull. Myrianthopoulos N C (ed), Amsterdam, i, pp. 15–40.

O'Rahilly R & Muller F (1984) Embryonic length and cerebral landmarks in staged human embryos. *Anat Rec* 209:265–271.

O'Rahilly R, Muller F & Bossy J (1982) Atlas des stades du developpement du systeme nerveus chez l'embryon humain intact. *Archives d'Anatomie, d'Histologie et d'Embryologie Normales et Experimentales* 65:57–76.

O'Rahilly R, Muller F, Hutchins G M & Moore G W (1984) Computer ranking of the sequence of appearance of 100 features of the brain and related structures in staged human embryos during the first 5 weeks of development. *Am J Anat* 171:243–257.

O'Rahilly R, Muller F, Hutchins G M & Moore G W (1987) Computer ranking of the sequence of appearance of 73 features of the brain and related structures in staged human embryos during the sixth week of development. *Am J Anat* 180:69–86.

O'Rahilly R, Muller F, Hutchins G M & Moore G W (1988) Computer ranking of the sequence of appearance of 40 features of the brain and related structure in staged human embryos during the seventh week of development. *Am J Anat* 182:295–317.

Rakic P (1965) Mesocoelic recess in the human brain. *Neurology (Minneapolis)* 15:708–715.

Rakic P (1981) Developmental events leading to laminar and areal organization of the neocortex. In: Schmitt F O, Worden F G (eds) *Organization of the cerebral cortex*. London: MIT Press.

Rakic P & Sidman R L (1970) Histogenesis of cortical layers in human cerebellum, particularly the lamina dissecans. *J Comp Neurol* 139:473–500.

Rakic P & Yakovlev P I (1968) Development of the corpus callosum and cavum septi in man. *J Comp Neurol* 132:45–72.

Rorke L B & Riggs H E (1969) *Myelination of the brain in the newborn*. Philadelphia, PA: Lippincott.

Sauer F C (1936) The interkinetic migration of embryonic epithelial nuclei. *J Morphol* 60:1–11.

Sidman R L & Rakic P (1973) Neuronal migration with special reference to the developing human brain: a review. *Brain Res* 62:1–35.

Skowsky R & Fisher D A (1973) Immunoreactive arginine vasopressin (AVT) in the fetal pituitary of man and sheep. *Clin Res* 21:205.

Streeter G L (1912) The development of the nervous system. In: Keibel F & Mall F P (eds) *Manual of human embryology*. Philadelphia, PA: J B Lippincott, Vol II; pp. 1–156.

Streeter G L (1942) *Carnegie Institution of Washington Publications* 30:211–245.

Streeter G L 1948 *Carnegie Institution of Washington Publications* 32:133–203.

Streeter G L (1951) Developmental horizons in human embryos, age groups XI-XXIII. Embryology Reprint, vol II, Carnegie Institute of Washington, Washington, DC. Contributions of Embryology 34:165–196.

Sturrock R R (1982a) Changes in cell number in the central canal ependyma and in the dorsal grey matter of the rabbit thoracic spinal cord during fetal development. *J Anat* 135:635–647.

Sturrock R R (1982b) Cell division in the normal central nervous system. *Adv Cell Neurobiol* 3.

Sturrock R R (1984) Microglia in the human embryonic optic nerve. *J Anat* 139:81–91.

Sturrock R R 1986 Postnatal ontogenesis of astrocytes. Astrocytes, London: Academic Press vol. 1.

Tilney F (1936) The development and constituents of the human hypophysis. *Bull Neurol Inst NY* 5:387–436.

Warwick R & Williams P L (1973) *Gray's anatomy*, 35th edn. London: Longman.

Wislocki G B (1937) The meningeal relations of the hypophysis cerebri. II. An embryological study of the meninges and blood vessels of the human hypophysis. *Am J Anat* 61:95–129.

Wislocki G B & Roth W D (1958) Selective staining of the human subcommissural organ. *Anat Rec* 130:125–133.

Wozniak W & O'Rahilly R (1982) An electron microscopic study of myelination of pyramidal fibers at the level of the pyramidal decussation in the human fetus. *Journal für Hirnforschung* 23:331–342.

Wozniak W & O'Rahilly R & Olszewski B (1980) The fine structure of the spinal cord in human embryos and early fetuses. *Journal für Hirnforschung* 21:101–124.

Yakovlev P I & Lecours A (1967) The myelogenetic cycles of regional maturation of the brain. In: Minkowski A (ed) *Regional development of the brain in early life*. Oxford: Blackwell.

Yakovlev P I & Rakic P (1966) Patterns of decussation of bulbar pyramids and distribution of pyramidal tracts on two sides of the spinal cord. *Trans Am Neurol Assoc* 91:366–367.

# Chapter 4 Three-dimensional ultrasonography of the embryonic brain

H-G. K. Blaas and S. H. Eik-Nes

## INTRODUCTION

One of the pioneers of classic human embryology was Wilhelm His Senior (His 1880–85), who systematically described embryonic development by means of macroscopic and microscopic analyses. His soon realized the need for magnified three-dimensional (3D) imaging to understand the complexity of embryonic development. Therefore, he made solid wax 3D reconstructions from freehand drawings of histologic slices (His 1887) after the method 'Die Plattenmodellirmethode', which had been described earlier by Born (Born 1883). In 1921, Jenkins carried out a study on the developing human brain on the basis of such solid 3D reconstructions (Jenkins 1921). He estimated the volumes of embryonic and fetal brain compartments of a few specimens from the Carnegie collection. Three-dimensional imaging by graphic reconstructions with the help of special devices (Forster 1967) has often been used in modern human embryology (O'Rahilly & Müller 1994). Recently, very clear 3D images of the embryonic central nervous system obtained from embryos of the Carnegie collection have been presented by using magnetic resonance imaging (Smith 1999).

While the above quoted studies and methods are based on examinations of aborted specimens, modern ultrasound technology has made it possible to examine living embryos and fetuses. The transvaginal approach should be preferred because of the small size of the embryo. Only by this approach can the transducer be placed near the structure of interest; high frequencies can be used to improve the resolution and thus the quality of the ultrasound images.

Two-dimensional (2D) ultrasonography, however, has its limitations. The position of the embryo or fetus in the uterus is not always suitable to obtain measurements or describe the anatomy. In particular, the reduced mobility of the transducer at transvaginal examination limits the access of 2D scan planes. Thus, the information obtained from the images depends on the angle of insonation through the embryo, and the diagnostic insight and imagination of the sonographer.

Since 3D ultrasonography is an imaging mode that can remedy some of these problems, the interest in 3D imaging has been setting the tone for technologic efforts to develop 3D ultrasonographic systems that can be used in clinical situations over the past 20 years (Brinkley *et al.* 1982). The basis for 3D ultrasonography is the original 2D ultrasound image. Acquiring 3D data involves making a set of consecutive 2D ultrasound slices by moving the transducer and continuously storing the images. To obtain 3D images of good resolution and sufficient quality, which is essential when imaging tiny embryonic CNS structures, the width between the tomograms should be narrow (Baba & Okai 1997), and the original 2D ultrasound tomograms (slices) must be thin (Blaas *et al.* 2000a). In the 3D volume, new ultrasound tomograms can be obtained in any desirable direction – so-called anyplane slices or multiplanar images (Figs 4.1–4.3). Thus, brain structures can be depicted in the optimal direction. One must be aware that the resolution of the ultrasound 'anyplane' image in the 3D volume can never be as good as that of the original scan planes. In other

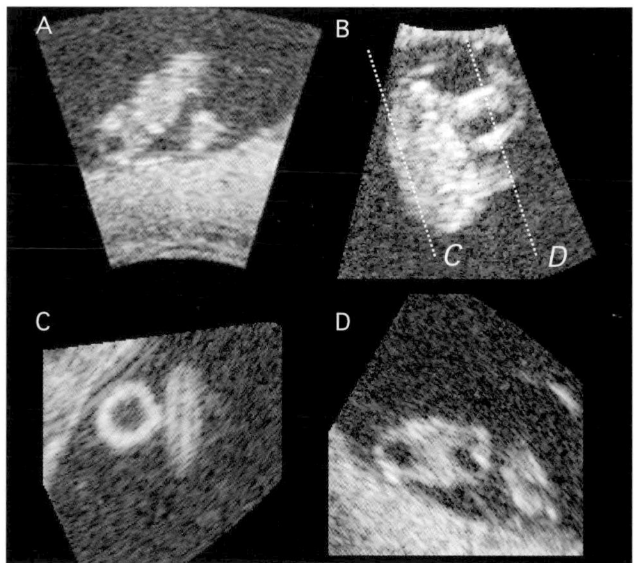


**Figure 4.1** A) Original transvaginal scan of an embryo at seven weeks, crown-rump length (CRL) 13 mm. (B-D) Anyplane slices (new ultrasound tomograms) through the 3D data set: (B) Sagittal section through the embryo, showing the rhombencephalic cavity in the top of the head, which leads to the right into the curved mesencephalic cavity and further into the future third ventricle. Dotted lines = sections of C and D. (C) The future spine is depicted as parallel lines; the 'ring' to the left is the yolk sac with a diameter of approximately 4 mm. (D) Oblique section through the rhombencephalic cavity, the future third ventricle and the evaginations of the future lateral ventricles.

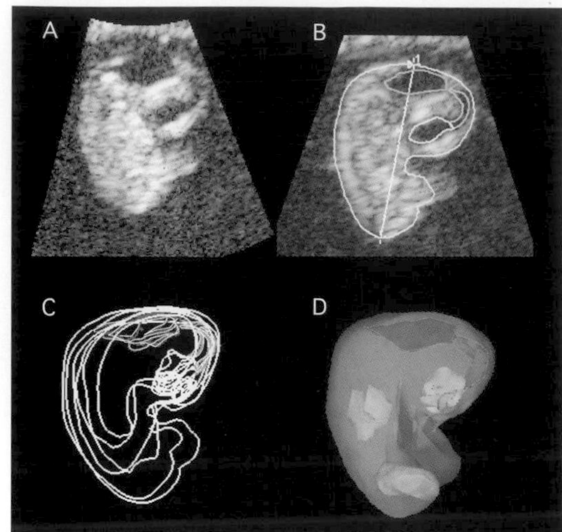


Figure 4.2 Illustration of the segmentation process in the same data set as Figure 4.1. (A) Anyplane slice sagittal through the embryo at seven weeks, crown-rump length (CRL) 13 mm. (B) 2D measurement of the greatest length; straight line 1. The outer contours of the embryo and the inner contours of its brain cavities are drawn. (C) Solely the contours of the embryonic body and the brain cavities are shown. (D) 3D volume rendering of the embryo and its brain cavities, see also Figure 4.4.

words, if we want to have a good resolution in the 3D volume, we have to ensure that the original recordings are of very high quality. If the original ultrasound tomograms are blurred, the 3D reconstructions will be even more blurred.

In the technique of creating new ultrasound tomograms in the 3D data set, several other modes of 3D imaging have been developed, such as volume rendering (e.g. transparency mode), geometry visualization with volume calculations (Figs 4.2 & 4.4), and surface rendering (Figs 4.5 & 4.6). Two-dimensional measurements (Fig. 4.2B) and volume calculations are of interest in the evaluation of the embryonic brain. For volume reconstruction of the brain from the 3D data set, the object of interest needs to be delineated or segmented from its surroundings. Segmentation is usually done manually by drawing contours around the object in a number of 2D slices (Fig. 4.2B,C). The reconstructed geometric objects can then be visualized as a 3D image by rendering its surface using different colors and different opacity values (Fig. 4.4). Such volume reconstructions and calculations of embryonic and young fetal brain cavities have been published (Blaas *et al.* 1998; Berg *et al.* 2000).

In this chapter we present our experience with 3D sonoembryology of the normal embryonic brain. The overview is based on *in vivo* 3D ultrasound studies using the

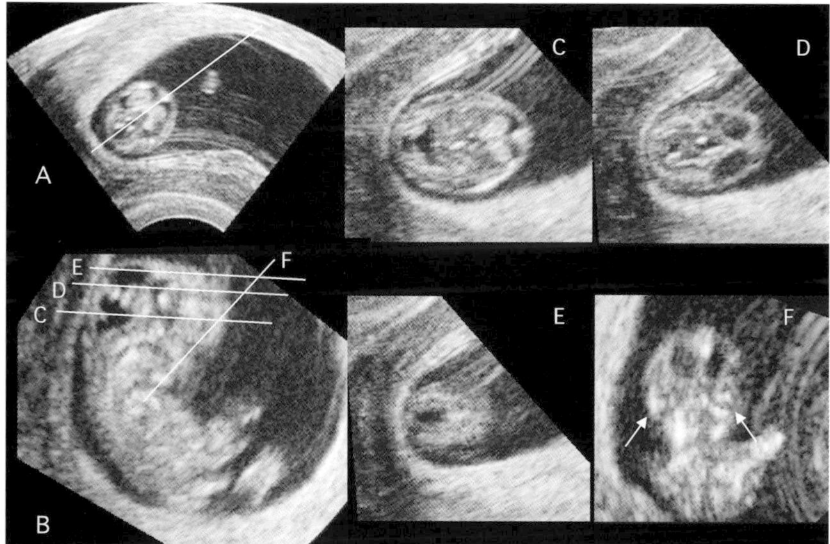


Figure 4.3 Original ultrasound image (A) and anyplane slices (new ultrasound tomograms, B-F) through the head of a specimen of 32 mm CRL, gestational age approximately 9 weeks 6 days. (B) Sagittal section through the head and body. On the left side, the future fourth ventricle can be seen, with the echogenic choroid plexus at the roof. The narrow isthmus rhombencephali leads into the relatively large mesencephalic cavity. To the right, the isthmus prosencephali leads into the third ventricle. The echogenic area in the third ventricle corresponds to the dorsal thalamus. (C–E) represent new horizontal sections: (C) Section through the choroid plexuses of the fourth ventricle posteriorly (left) and the echogenic choroid plexuses of the lateral ventricles (right). (D) Section through the mesencephalic cavity (future Sylvian aqueduct) and the third ventricle. (E) Section through the mesencephalic cavity. (F) Coronal section through the face; there is a 'physiological' hypertelorisme of the eyes (arrows).

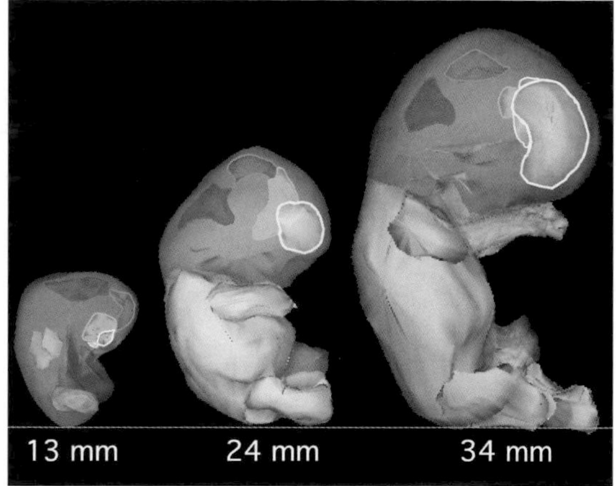


Figure 4.4 3D reconstructions of two embryos, 13 mm ≈ 7 weeks, 24 mm ≈ 9 weeks, and one fetus, 34 mm ≈ 10 weeks. The cavities of the brain are coloured: blue = rhombencephalon, red = mesencephalon, green = diencephalon, yellow = lateral ventricles. (Please see the plate section pp. 5 for colour figure.)

anyplane mode and the geometry visualization mode (Blaas *et al.* 1995, 1998; Blaas 1999b); the overview confirms the descriptions of human brain development from classic embryology. We also describe examples and provide images of early brain anomalies visualized with the help of 3D ultrasonography.

In order to use a uniform terminology, all statements of time in this chapter are based on the last menstrual period, expressed in completed weeks and completed days, assuming a regular cycle with ovulation at 2 weeks 0 days. This means that both the length of the pregnancy and the age of the embryo are expressed in the same way in order to simplify the comparison of embryonic development with first trimester ultrasound (obstetric) descriptions.

## ANATOMIC DEVELOPMENT FROM 7 TO 10 WEEKS

### 7 WEEKS, 0–6 DAYS; CROWN–RUMP LENGTH (CRL) 9–14 MM

Using a 7.5-MHz transvaginal transducer, the brain cavities become visible at 7 weeks, when they appear as large holes in the embryonic head (Figs 4.1, 4.2 & Fig. 4.4). They can easily be delineated in the 3D segmentation process. The lateral ventricles are small evaginations located laterally and rostrally from the cavity of the diencephalon, shaped like small round balls. The broad cavity of the diencephalon continues directly into that of the mesencephalon. The isthmus rhombencephali represents the connection to the rhombencephalic cavity and future fourth ventricle. The cavity of the rhombencephalon is located superiorly in the head as a rather broad and shallow cavity, representing the largest brain ventricle. The future spine appears as two parallel bright lines (Fig. 4.1C).

### 8 WEEKS, 0–6 DAYS; CRL 15–22 MM

The lateral ventricles gradually change shape from small round vesicles via thick round slices originating anterocaudally from the third ventricle into a crescent shape in larger embryos. The future foramina of Monro become distinct at 8.5 weeks. The connections between the third ventricle, the mesencephalic cavity and the lateral ventricles are wide. The cavity of the mesencephalon is relatively large in all embryos. With the increasing size of embryos, the mesencephalic cavity changes its position. It will later be posterior in the head. The rhombencephalic cavity deepens gradually with the growth of the embryo, at the same time decreasing in length. Its position in the head changes with the increasing size of the specimen, moving posteriorly. The rhombencephalic cavity (future fourth ventricle) has a pyramid-like shape, where the central deepening of the pontine flexure represents the peak of the pyramid.

### 9 WEEKS, 0–6 DAYS; CRL 23–31 MM

The size of the lateral ventricles increases quickly Fig. 4.4). While the third ventricle is still relatively wide at the beginning of this week, its anteromedial part narrows during this

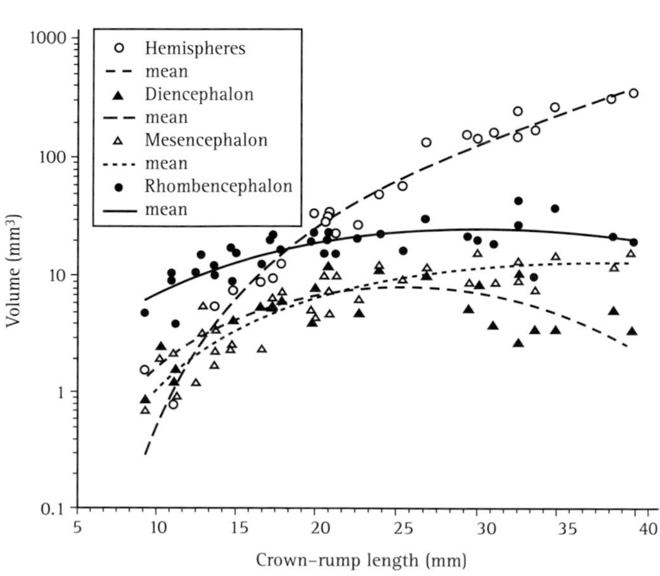


Figure 4.5 Measurements and mean volume of lateral ventricles, cavities of diencephalon, mesencephalon and rhombencephalon. (Reproduced with permission from Blaas *et al.* (1998), with permission from Elsevier Science).

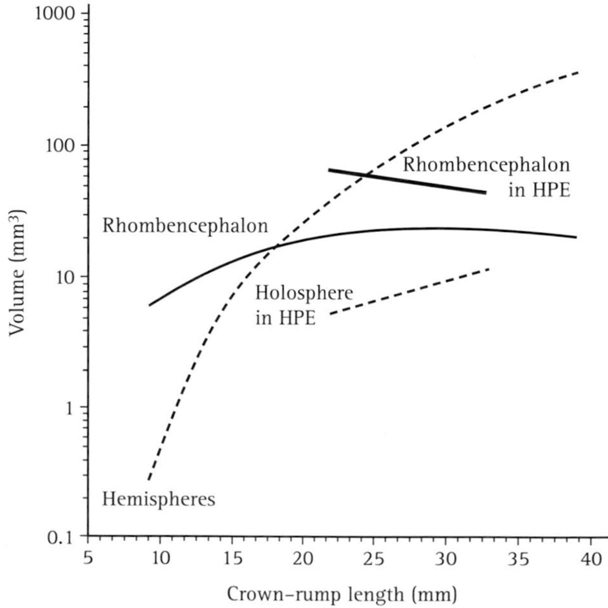


Figure 4.6 Mean volumes of cavities of rhombencephalon and hemispheres, and corresponding cavities, in a case of alobar holoprosencephalon (HPE) with CRL of 22 and 33 mm; compare also with Figure 4.5.

week as a result of the growth of the thalami (Fig. 4.3B,D). In fetuses with a CRL of 25 mm or more there is a clear gap between the rhombencephalic and the mesencephalic cavity owing to the growing cerebellum. The isthmus rhombencephali is narrow; often it is not visible in its entire length. The width of the diencephalic cavity decreases at the end of the embryonic period and becomes narrow, especially at its upper anterior part. The eyes can be identified; there is physiologic hypertelorism (Fig. 4.3F). The spine is still characterized by two echogenic parallel lines.

## EARLY POSTEMBRYONIC PERIOD

### 10 WEEKS, 0–6 DAYS; CRL 32–42 MM

The cavity of the diencephalon has become too narrow to be outlined correctly on the 2D anyplane slices. Both rostrally and caudally, the cavity of the mesencephalon is connected to the neighboring cavities by narrow isthmuses. The cavities of the mesencephalon and rhombencephalon are located posteriorly, while the cavities of the hemispheres occupy the anterior and superior part of the head (Fig. 4.4). The thick crescent lateral ventricles fill the anterior part of the head and conceal the diencephalic cavity, which becomes smaller. The gap between the mesencephalic and the rhombencephalic cavity filled with the growing cerebellum becomes clear.

#### Measurements

Table 4.1 and Fig. 4.5 show volume calculations of the brain cavities of 34 7–10-week-old embryos/fetuses (Blaas *et al.* 1998; Blaas & Eik-Nes 2002). These volume estimations of embryonic brains represent new insight into embryonic development with information that could not be obtained from aborted specimens. When we look at the 3D images and volume estimations of the specimens in Fig. 4.4 & Fig. 4.5, we clearly perceive the dynamic process that alters the appearance of the brain within a few weeks. The brain compartments change rapidly in their form, size and relation to one another; for example, the telencephalon develops from two tiny balls into large crescent-shaped cavities, dominating the brain at the end of the first trimester. The cavity of the rhombencephalon alters, too. Initially, at 7 weeks, it lies as a large, shallow and broad cavity in the top of the head. Later, it becomes deeper and shorter, as is also reflected by the change of the angle of the pontine flexure, and it is 'pushed' posteriorly; see also Figs 2.6 and 2.7 in Chapter 2 (Moscoso 2001). The ultrasound volume estimations of the brain (Table 4.1) correspond well with Jenkins' solid 3D reconstructions of two embryos (Jenkins 1921). Jenkins calculated the volume of the brain to be 41 mm3 in an embryo with a CRL of 16 mm, and 126 mm3 in an embryo with a CRL of 25 mm.

Interestingly, Fig. 4.4 & Fig. 4.5 give way to considerations regarding evolution, as the 3D ultrasound measurements of the brain cavities reflect the evolutive process of brain compartments (see also Ch. 5): The 'old' rhombencephalon is large during the early phase of development, while the 'young' hemispheres are very small. Within a few weeks, this size correlation becomes dramatically reversed.

## EMBRYONIC ANOMALIES

Our 3D ultrasound study has demonstrated the potential for embryologic research by showing the normal development of brain compartments, and it may be used as a basis for the evaluation of abnormal brain development. There are case reports concerning embryonic CNS anomalies obtained by 2D ultrasound diagnoses – of specimens younger than 10 weeks based on the last menstruation. These studies conclude that if the cerebral ventricles are abnormally enlarged, or if the brain ventricles cannot be identified, anomalous development must be suspected (Blaas & Eik-Nes 1996, 1999; Blaas 1999a; Becker *et al.* 2000).

Three-dimensional ultrasound reports about CNS anomalies of embryos are still exceptions. However, the clinical significance of our 3D brain study (Blaas *et al.* 1998) could be shown in one case of alobar holoprosencephalon (Blaas *et al.* 2000b). A 2D ultrasound examination revealed this anomaly as early as 9 weeks 2 days, the CRL being 22 mm. Three-dimensional recordings were performed at 9 and

**Table 4.1 Mean (± 2SD) volumes of embryonic body and cavities of the brain (n = 34)**

| CRL* (mm) | Body ($mm^3$) | Total brain ($mm^3$) | Hemispheres ($mm^3$) | Diencephalon ($mm^3$) | Mesencephalon ($mm^3$) | Rhombencephalon ($mm^3$) |
|---|---|---|---|---|---|---|
| 10 | 96 (209; 26) | 5.2 (18.2; 0.1) | 0.5 (2.7; 0.0) | 1.7 (4.8; 0.2) | 1.1 (3.3; 0.1) | 7.3 (15.9; 2.0) |
| 15 | 402 (611; 237) | 25.6 (49.4; 9.5) | 6.7 (15.1; 2.2) | 4.4 (9.0; 1.5) | 3.6 (7.1; 1.3) | 13.4 (24.4; 5.7) |
| 20 | 918 (1222; 657) | 61.3 (96.1, 34.3) | 25.9 (44.6; 13.4) | 6.7 (12.1; 2.8) | 6.6 (11.2; 3.2) | 18.8 (31.6; 9.4) |
| 25 | 1644 (2044; 1288) | 112.4 (158.1; 74.4) | 65.7 (98.7; 41.0) | 7.5 (13.3; 3.4) | 9.4 (14.7; 5.3) | 22.6 (36.4; 12.0) |
| 30 | 2581 (3076; 2129) | 178.8 (235.3; 129.9) | 133.4 (184.8; 92.6) | 6.7 (12.1; 2.9) | 11.5 (17.3; 6.9) | 23.9 (38.1; 13.0) |
| 35 | 3727 (4318; 3180) | 260.5 (328.0; 200.7) | 236.6 (310.4; 175.5) | 4.5 (9.1; 1.5) | 12.5 (18.6; 7.7) | 22.7 (36.5; 12.1) |

In the 3D segmentation process, the brain cavities were outlined at the inner surfaces of the ventricular walls. The choroid plexus was included in the measurements.
*Approximate gestational age based on last menstrual period: crown–rump length (CRL) 10 mm, 7 weeks 2 days; CRL 15 mm, 8 weeks 0 days; CRL 20 mm, 8 weeks 5 days; CRL 25 mm, 9 weeks 2 days; CRL 30 mm, 9 weeks 6 days; CRL 35 mm, 10 weeks 2 days.
*Source*: From Blaas & Eik-Nes (2002), with permission from Cambridge Press.

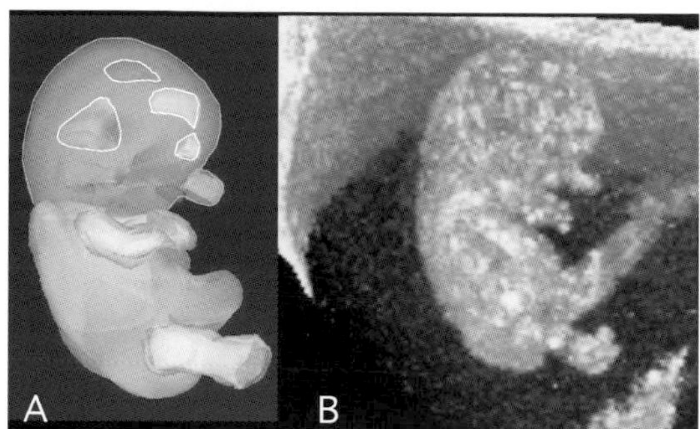


Figure 4.7 (A) Geometric 3D reconstruction of an embryo with holoprosencephaly, CRL 22 mm. The proboscis, and the single holosphere behind the forehead are outlined. (B) Surface rendering of the same embryo. The proboscis and the umbilical cord can be seen. (Reproduced with permission from Blaas, Eik-Nes *et al.* 2000b).

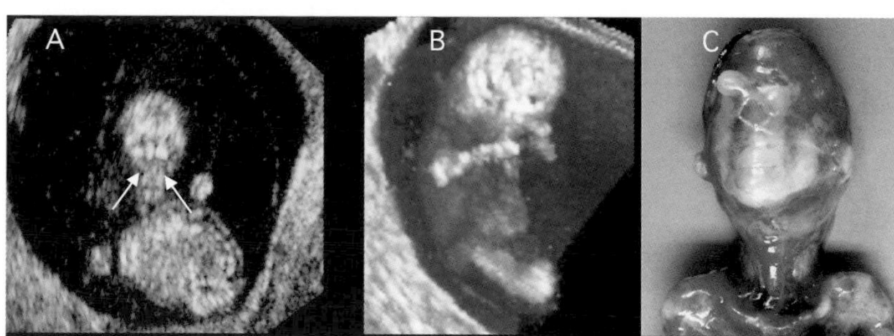


Figure 4.8 The same specimen as in Figure 4.7, at the age of 10 weeks, CRL 33 mm. (A) Coronal section (anyplane slice) through the face, showing two eye-anlagen (arrows); compare with normal embryo in Figure 4.3. (B) Surface rendered image showing the proboscis. (C) The same specimen after termination of the pregnancy. There were two eye-anlagen behind the cyclopia (not identifyable on this photo). (A and C reproduced with permission from Blaas, Eik-Nes *et al.* 2000b: with permission from Blackwell Publishing)

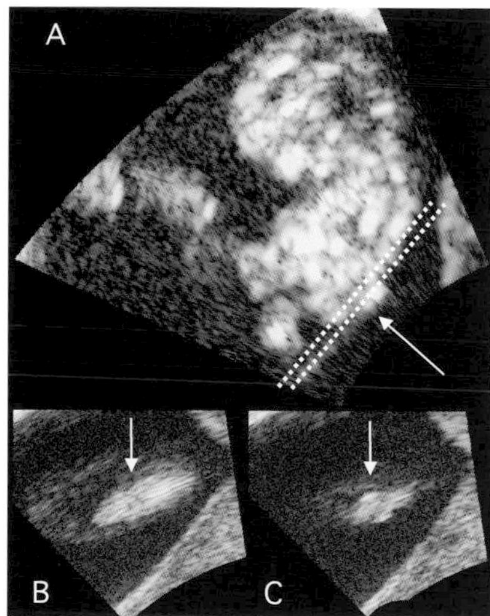


Figure 4.9 (A) Sagittal section in a 3D ultrasound data set from an embryo of 22 mm CRL. There is an irregularity at the lumbal part of the back (arrow). The dotted lines indicate new 2D tomograms (B and C). B and C are new ultrasound tomograms, which show the round irregular myelomeningocele of the spine (arrows). (Reproduced with permission from Blaas, Eik-Nes *et al.* 2000c: with permission from Blackwell Publishing)

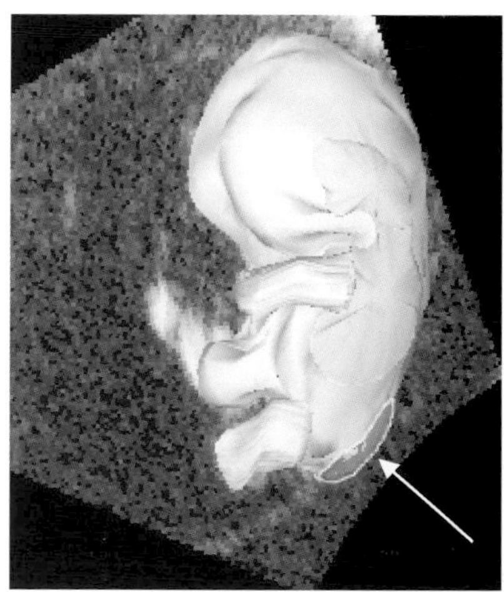

Figure 4.10 Geometrical 3D reconstruction of the same embryo, CRL 22 mm. The arrow points at the myelomenigocele. (Reproduced with permission from Blaas, Eik-Nes *et al.* 2000c: with permission from Blackwell Publishing)

10 weeks, and the volumes of the brain cavities, especially of the endbrain and the hindbrain (Figs 4.6 and 4.7A), revealed the abnormal proportions of these compartments compared with normal brain development (Blaas *et al.* 2000b). Although volumetry was not necessary for confirmation of this specific anomaly, it showed the potential of this visualization mode. We also performed anyplane slicing through the abnormal face in the 3D data set. By doing so, we were able to show two eye anlagen lying close together in an ultrasound tomogram that we had not seen in the original transvaginal scan (Fig. 4.8A). The surface rendering of the specimen additionally illustrated the presence of a proboscis (Figs 4.7B & 4.8B).

Another embryonic anomaly described by 3D ultrasonography was an embryo with a bifid spine (Blaas *et al.* 2000c). We used high-frequency 2D ultrasonography to detect this malformation by recognizing irregular contours of the spine. We then imaged the anomaly by 3D ultrasonography using the anyplane slicing mode and volume reconstruction (Figs 4.9 & 4.10), and enhanced the information about the diagnosis.

## Summary

High-quality 2D ultrasound tomograms achieved by using high-frequency transvaginal transducers are the basis for good 3D reconstructions of the human embryonic brain. So far, 3D ultrasonography has shown its potential in the research of embryonic brain development and in imaging early CNS anomalies. Three-dimensional ultrasound technology, and probably magnetic resonance technology, is improving, and promises important new insights into very early development. We are at the threshold being able to study the developing central nervous system longitudinally in very small detail – features with a size of only 1 mm – and to describe its normal and abnormal development.

## REFERENCES

Baba K & Okai T. (1997) *Basis and principles of three-dimensional ultrasound.* In: Baba K & Jurkovic D (eds). Three-dimensional ultrasound in obstetrics and gynaecology. London: Parthenon; pp. 1-19.

Becker R, Mende B, Stiemer B, Entezami M. (2000) Sonographic markers of exencephaly at 9 + 3 weeks of gestation. *Ultrasound Obstet Gynecol* 16:582–584.

Berg S, Torp H, Blaas H-GK. (2000) Accuracy of *in-vitro* volume estimation of small structures using three-dimensional ultrasound. *Ultrasound Med Biol* 26:425–432.

Blaas H-G K. (1999a) The examination of the embryo and early fetus: how and by whom? (editorial) *Ultrasound Obstet Gynecol* 14(3):153–158.

Blaas H-G K. (1999b) *The embryonic examination. Ultrasound studies on the development of the human embryo* (thesis). Department of Obstetrics and Gynecology, National Center for Fetal Medicine, Trondheim, Norwegian University of Science and Technology.

Blaas H-G & Eik-Nes S H. (1996) Ultrasound assessment of early brain development. In: *Ultrasound and early pregnancy.* Jurkovic D & Jauniaux E (eds) New York: Parthenon; pp. 3–18.

Blaas H-G & Eik-Nes S H. (1999) Das Zentralnervensystem. Die normale Entwicklung und die Entwicklung von Anomalien – Ultraschalldiagnostik in der Frühschwangerschaft. *Gynäkologe* 32:181–191.

Blaas H-G & Eik-Nes S H. (2002) The description of the early development of the human central nervous system using two- and three-dimensional ultrasound. In: *The new born brain - neuroscience and clinical applications.* Hanson M & Lagercrantz H (eds) Cambridge: Cambridge University Press; 278–288.

Blaas H-G, Eik-Nes S H, Kiserud T. (1995) Three-dimensional imaging of the brain cavities in human embryos. *Ultrasound Obstet Gynecol* 5:228–232.

Blaas H-G, Eik-Nes S H, Berg S, Torp H. (1998). *In-vivo* three-dimensional ultrasound reconstructions of embryos and early fetuses. Lancet 352(9135):1182–1186.

Blaas H-G K, Eik-Nes S H, Berg S. (2000a) Three-dimensional fetal ultrasound. *Baillieres Clin Obstet Gynecol* 14:611–627.

Blaas H-G K, Eik-Nes S H, Vainio T, Isaksen CV. (2000b) Alobar holoprosencephaly at 9 weeks' gestational age visualized by two- and three-dimensional ultrasound. *Ultrasound Obstet Gynecol* 15:62–65.

Blaas H-G K, Eik-Nes S H, Isaksen CV. (2000c) The detection of spina bifida before 10 gestational weeks using 2D- and 3D ultrasound. *Ultrasound Obstet Gynecol* 16:25–29.

Born G. (1883) Die Plattenmodellirmethode. *Arch Mikr Anat* 22:584–599.

Brinkley JF, McCallum WD, Muramatsu SK, Liu DY. (1982) Fetal weight estimation from ultrasonic three-dimensional head and trunk reconstructions: evaluation *in vitro. Am J Obstet Gynecol* 144(6):715–721.

Forster F. (1967) Perspektomat P-40, ein selbstzeichnender Apparat für Parallelperspektive. *Mitt Naturforsch Ges Schaffhausen* 28:251–274.

His W. (1880–85) *Anatomie menschlicher Embryonen*, vols 1–3. Leipzig: Vogel.

His W. (1887) Über Methoden plastischer Rekonstruktion und über deren Bedeutung für Anatomie und Entwicklungsgeschichte. *Anat Anz* 2:382–394.

Jenkins G B. (1921) Relative weight and volume of the component parts of the brain of the human embryo at different stages of development. *Contrib Embryol Carneg Inst* 13:41–60.

Moscoso G. (2002) Early embryonic development of the brain. In: Levene M I, Chervenak F A & Whittle M (eds) *Fetal and neonatal neurology and neurosurgery.* London: Churchill Livingstone; pp. 11–19.

O'Rahilly R & Müller F. (1994) *The embryonic human brain. An atlas of developmental stages.* New York: Wiley-Liss.

Smith B R. (1999) Visualizing human embryos. *Sci Am* 280:58–63.

# Chapter 5 Ultrasound assessment of normal fetal brain development

H-G. Blaas and S. H. Eik-Nes

## INTRODUCTION

The technical development of ultrasound equipment has made possible major advances in the imaging of the developing fetal brain. In the 1960s, with the help of the A-scan, the fetal head, the skull, and the falx could be identified. Today, the use of high frequency transvaginal transducers has improved the image quality to such an extent that a detailed anatomical description of the living embryo has become possible. The large hypoechogenic cavities of the embryonic brain have, naturally, attracted the attention of ultrasound examiners (Timor-Tritsch *et al.* 1988; Warren *et al.* 1989; Bree & Marn 1990; Cullen *et al.* 1990; Timor-Tritsch *et al.* 1990; Achiron & Achiron 1991; Timor-Tritsch *et al.* 1991; Takeuchi 1992). Two-dimensional measurements of the embryonic brain have been made to describe the normal development and dimensions of the cavities of the hemispheres, the diencephalon, the mesencephalon (Blaas *et al.* 1994, 1995a), and the rhombencephalon (Blaas *et al.* 1995a; van Zalen-Sprock *et al.* 1996). Three-dimensional ultrasound allows the off-line analysis of a recorded ultrasound volume in any plane making it possible to measure the diameters and volumes of interest more precisely as well as to make more precise diagnoses (Blaas *et al.* 1995b, 1998).

In this chapter we review the development of the brain as described by embryologists and anatomists, and compare this with sonoanatomic descriptions. The anatomic descriptions are limited to details that are of interest for the understanding of ultrasound examinations. The most dramatic changes of size and shape take place in early pregnancy; therefore, the embryonic period is described week by week.

The ultrasound descriptions of the brain development until 12 weeks are based on longitudinal two-dimensional (2-D) and three-dimensional (3-D) studies (Blaas *et al.* 1994, 1995a, 1998; Blaas 1999a). All statements of gestational age are based on the last menstrual period (LMP), expressed in completed weeks and completed days, assuming a regular cycle with ovulation at 2 weeks 0 days. Though the term 'trimester' is imprecise (Blaas 1999b), it is used in this review as a rough subdivision of the pregnancy.

## CHOICE OF TRANSDUCER AND APPROACH

During 38 weeks, from the unicellular stage at 2 weeks LMP-based gestational age to the newborn at 40 weeks, the conceptus goes through extensive changes of size and appearance, and various ultrasound techniques and approaches are needed to image the brain in this period.

The very small size and the constantly changing anatomical appearance of the brain in the embryonic and early fetal period are well suited to the transvaginal approach with high frequency transducers such as 7.5 MHz. Phased and annular array transducers may be used. Because of the symmetric focusing, annular array technology produces very thin ultrasound tomograms. Such mechanical transducers make it possible to image the tiny embryonic brain structures, so that features of clinical interest can be identified. Three-dimensional (3-D) ultrasound may be used to obtain new ultrasound images in planes not available in the original scan plane, to present form and shape of an object of interest, and to calculate volume. The basis and prerequisite for all 3-D imaging are clear 2-D tomograms.

The embryonic/early fetal brain with its large ventricles can easily be imaged by the transvaginal approach, and is well suited to 3-D imaging (Blaas 1999a). The increasing size of the early fetus at the end the first and the beginning of the second trimesters makes the transvaginal approach for the CNS examination more difficult in breech presentations. Then, lower frequencies, usually 5 MHz, for the transabdominal route have to be chosen. However, this will often lead to poor resolution of the images because of more acoustic noise and attenuation when the ultrasound beam has to pass the abdominal wall of the mother.

During mid-pregnancy, the transabdominal route with a 5 MHz transducer usually gives acceptable images of the growing fetal brain. In vertex presentations, the transvaginal approach makes it possible to obtain very detailed information of the neuroanatomy (Timor-Tritsch & Monteagudo 1996).

At the end of the pregnancy, the increasing ossification of the skull impairs the examination of the brain, especially when the head is positioned low down in the maternal pelvis. Low frequencies such as 3.5–5 MHz have to be used for the transabdominal approach. As always in vertex presentations, the transvaginal route improves the imaging (Timor-Tritsch & Monteagudo 1996), though it may be very difficult to obtain the classic standard scan planes for the neuroanatomic examination as it is done in the newborn (Cremin *et al.* 1983). Because of the relatively large size of the head, lower frequencies are appropriate. The access through the fetal fontanelle as an optic window can be difficult in the asynclitic position of the head.

## FIRST TRIMESTER, <14 WEEKS

### 2 WEEKS, 0 DAYS TO APPROXIMATELY 6 WEEKS, 6 DAYS

#### Embryology

The first five postovulatory weeks of embryonic development are described by Carnegie stages 1 to 15 (see p. 21). The embryo develops from the unicellular stage 1 through stages characterized by the bilaminar and trilaminar disc into a cylindric body by a folding process. This folding process takes place during week 5 (LMP-based) and is completed at stage 12. The knowledge about normal neural development is important for the understanding of the early ultrasound images of the embryonic brain: the occurrence of the primitive streak in the epiblast of the two-cellular layer embryonic disc at stage 6 (O'Rahilly & Müller 1987) initiates the developmental phase 'gastrulation'. Cells from the organizer tissue (Spemann & Mangold 1924) in the primitive node migrate anteriorly along the midline and establish the notochord and the prechordal plate. Molecular signals from these midline structures induce the overlying ectoderm to differentiate into a plate of neuroepithelium (Rubenstein *et al.* 1998). The primordium of the CNS, the neural tube, develops from this ectodermal neural plate after a transitional stage of neuroectodermal folding. The closure of the caudal neuropore, creating the ventricular system, takes place at Carnegie stage 12, i.e. ≈5 weeks 6 days (Streeter 1948; O'Rahilly *et al.* 1984; O'Rahilly & Müller 1990). At Carnegie stages 14 (≈6 weeks, 4 days) and 15 (≈6 weeks 5 days) the forebrain divides into the telencephalon, with the cerebral hemispheres as small evaginations, and into the diencephalon (Yokoh 1975; O'Rahilly & Müller 1994). Then, the ventricular system is divided into five brain regions on its cranial pole: the telencephalon (future hemispheres) and the diencephalon (future between-brain) derive from the prosencephalon (forebrain); the mesencephalon (midbrain) remains undivided, and the metencephalon (future cerebellum and pons) and the myclencephalon (medulla oblongata) derive from the rhombencephalon (hindbrain). Successively, the brain compartments enlarge, changing their proportions and positions to each other, and developing their specific shapes.

#### Ultrasound

The pregnancy becomes detectable after 4.5 weeks as a ring structure lying in the decidua. Not before the end of week 6 do the first brain structures become identifiable. The hypoechogenic oblong cavity of the rhombencephalon is found at the top of the embryonic head/body (Fig. 5.1 a–c).

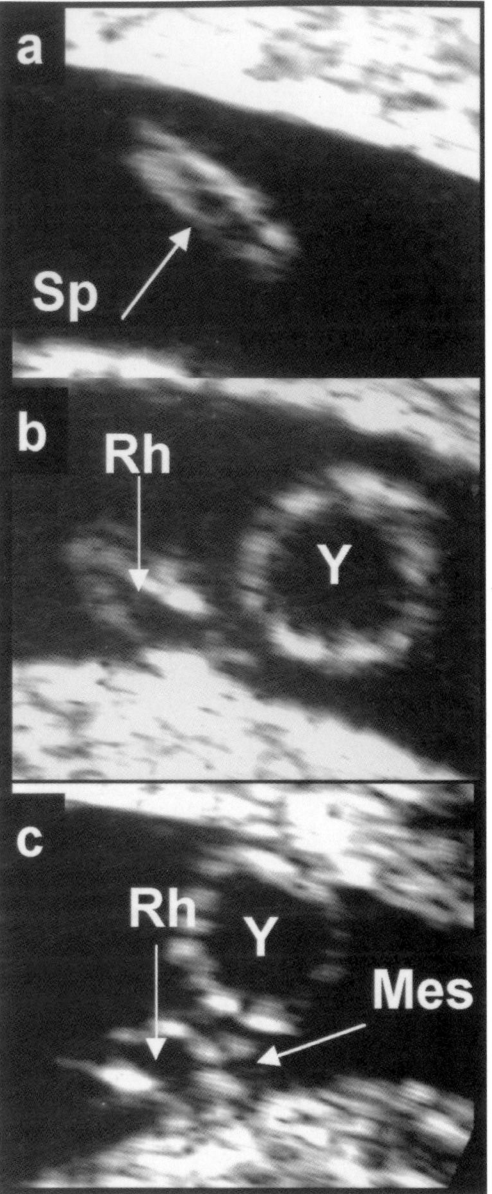


Figure 5.1 Ultrasound sections through a 7-week 0-day-old embryo, CRL 8 mm. (a) Coronal section through the spine (Sp). (b) Horizontal section through the head, the arrow points at the rhomboid cavity of the rhombencephalon (Rh); Y = yolk sac. (c) The section is tilted slightly anteriorly, in order to see the isthmus rhombencephali leading into the mesencephalic cavity (Mes); Y = yolk sac.

### 7 WEEKS, 0–6 DAYS; CRL 9–14 mm

#### Embryology

No longitudinal fissure is found between the laterally bulging cerebral hemispheres at this Carnegie stage. At the end of the week, at Carnegie stage 17 (≈7 weeks 5 days), the interventricular foramen is delimited by the corpus striatum and the ventral thalamus. The cerebellar primordium grows and the isthmus rhombencephali is evident.

#### Ultrasound

The hypoechogenic brain cavities can be identified, including the separated cerebral hemispheres (Fig. 5.2 a–c). The lateral ventricles are shaped like small round vesicles. The cavity of the diencephalon (future third ventricle) runs

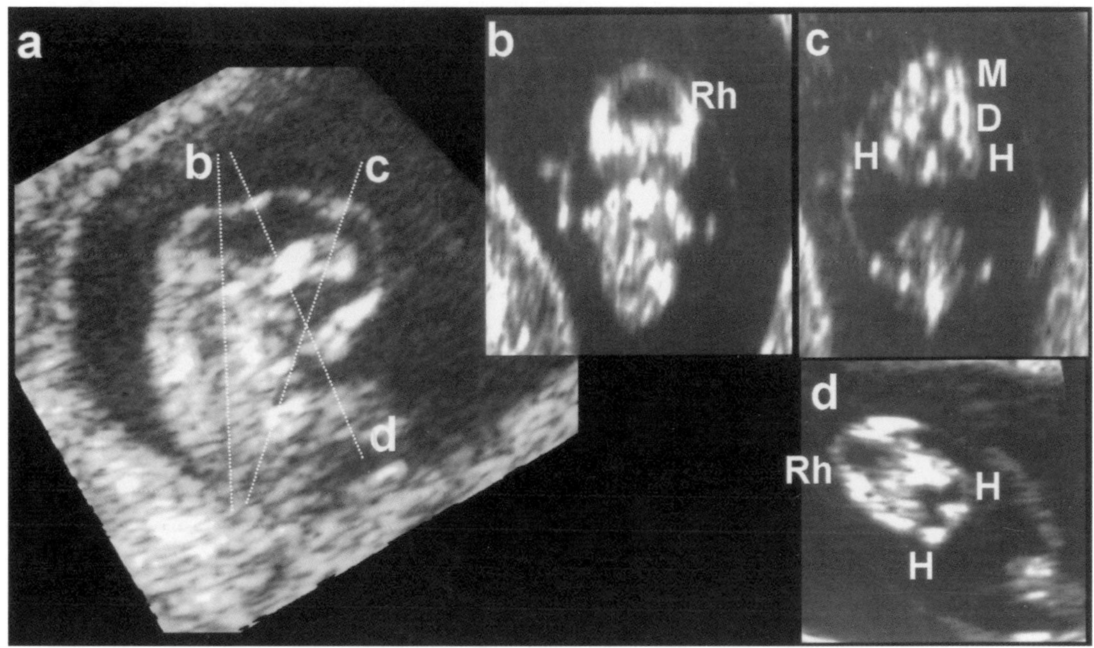


Figure 5.2 Images of an embryo at the end of week 7, CRL 13 mm. (a) Sagittal section, showing the continuum of the brain cavities from the shallow fourth ventricle in the top of the head, via the bent mesencephalic cavity (to the right) into the third ventricle (down to the left); the lines indicate the sections in parts (b–c). (b) Posterior coronal section, showing the typical 'hole in the head', which is the fourth ventricle. (c) Anterior coronal section through the mesencephalon (M), diencephalon (D) and hemispheres (H). (d) This section shows the rhombencephalic cavity (Rh) and the forebrain divided into two hemispheres (H).

posteriorly. The medial telencephalon forms a continuous cavity between the lateral ventricles. The future foramina of Monro are wide during week 7. In the sagittal plane, the height of the cavity of the diencephalon (future third ventricle) is slightly greater than that of the mesencephalon (future Sylvian aqueduct). Thus, the wide border between the cavities of the diencephalon and the mesencephalon is indicated. The curved tube-like mesencephalic cavity lies anteriorly, its rostral part pointing caudally. It straightens considerably during the subsequent weeks. By week 8 it is regularly identified. The rather broad and shallow rhombencephalic cavity is always visible. It has a well-defined rhombic shape in the cranial pole of the embryo. The future spine appears as two parallel lines (Fig. 5.1a).

## 8 WEEKS, 0–6 DAYS; CRL 15–22 mm

### Embryology

Half of the diencephalon is covered by the hemispheres. The mesencephalon is on the top of the brain (O'Rahilly & Müllet 1987). The choroid plexuses of the lateral ventricles and of the fourth ventricle develop at stage 18 (O'Rahilly & Müller 1994).

### Ultrasound

The brain cavities are easily seen as large 'holes' in the embryonic head (Figs 5.2 and 5.3). The hemispheres enlarge, developing via thick round slices originating anterocaudally from the third ventricle into a crescent shape. The choroid plexus in the lateral ventricles becomes visible as tiny echogenic areas. The future foramina of Monro become

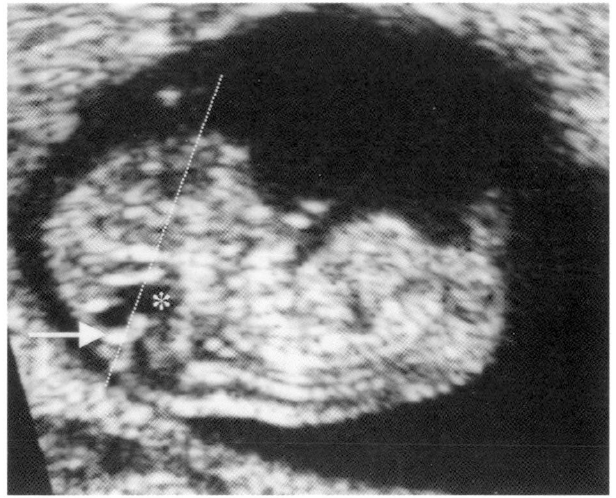

Figure 5.3 Sagittal section through an embryos, CRL 23 mm; the arrow points at the choroid plexus in the roof of the fourth ventricle (*); the pontine flexure is deep (cf. Fig. 5.2 a).

more accentuated. The third ventricle is still wide, as is the mesencephalic cavity. At this time, the mesencephalon lies on top of the head. The rhombencephalic cavity (future fourth ventricle) has a pyramid-like shape with the central deepening of the pontine flexure as the peak of the pyramid. The first signs of the bilateral choroid plexuses are lateral echogenic areas originating near the branches of the medulla oblongata caudal to the lateral recesses. Within a short time, the choroid plexuses traverse the roof of the fourth ventricle, meeting at the midline and dividing the roof into two portions; about two-thirds are located rostrally and one-third caudally. In the sagittal section, the choroid plexuses are identified as an echogenic fold of the roof.

## 9 WEEKS, 0–6 DAYS; CRL 23–31 mm

### Embryology

The chondrocranium and the skeletogenous layer of the head become recognizable. At the end of the embryonic period, the falx cerebri starts to develop from the skeletogenous layer. The cerebral hemispheres nearly conceal the diencephalon. Fusion of the medial walls of the hemispheres does not occur during the embryonic period. The foramina of Monro reduce to dorso-ventral slits. The insula appears. The thalami are thickening. The cavity of the mesencephalon is still wide. The rhombic lips have developed into cerebellar hemispheres. The choroid plexuses of the fourth ventricle divide the roof into the pars membranacea superior and inferior.

### Ultrasound

The lateral ventricles are always visible. Their size increases rapidly. They are best seen in the parasagittal plane, where the C-shape becomes apparent. The cortex is smooth and hypoechogenic. The bright choroid plexuses of the lateral ventricles are regularly detectable at 9 weeks 4 days (Figs 5.4 and 5.5c). They show rapid growth, similar to the hemispheres, and soon fill most of the ventricular cavities.

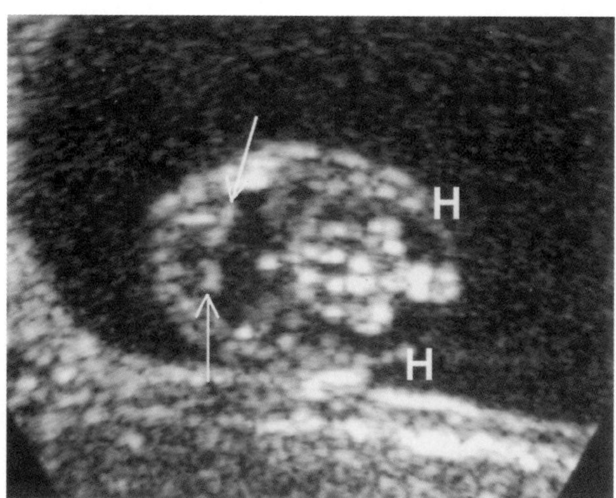


Figure 5.4 Section (stippled line in Fig. 5.3) through the head of a 9-week-old embryo, CRL 23 mm; the arrows point at the choroid plexuses of the fourth ventricle (cf. Fig. 5.2 d); the echogenic choroid plexuses of the hemispheres (H) can be seen.

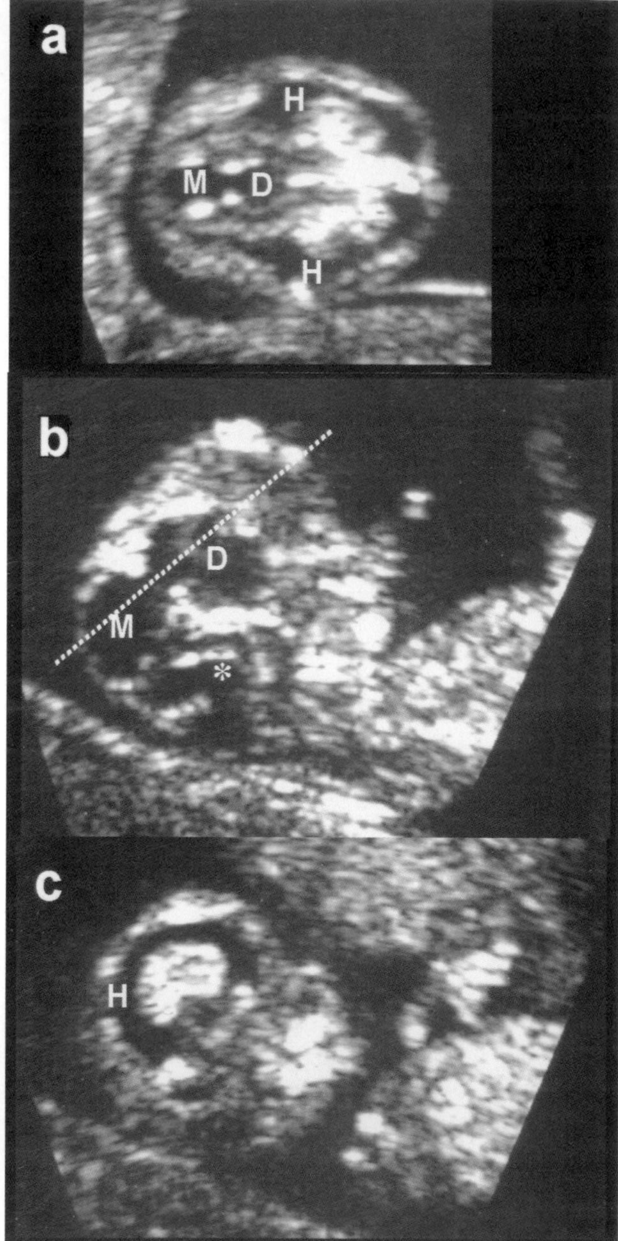


Figure 5.5 Ultrasound images of an embryo at the end of the embryonic period, CRL 31 mm. (a) Horizontal section through the mesencephalon, diencephalon, and hemispheres (cf. part b, stippled line). (b) Sagittal section through the head, the stippled line indicates the section of part a; anterior to the fourth ventricle (*) lies the pons; D = diencephalon, M = mesencephalon. (c) Parasagittal section through a hemisphere (H); the cortex is thin, the echogenic choroid plexus lies in the hypoechogenic ventricle.

In the 2-D image, the width of the diencephalic cavity narrows gradually while the width of the mesencephalon remains wide (Fig. 5a). The wall of the diencephalon, initially very thin, thickens considerably starting from week 8 to 9. The volume of the third ventricle decreases during week 9 and the cavity becomes narrow, especially at its upper anterior part due to the growing thalami. A distinct border ('isthmus prosencephali') has developed between the cavity of the mesencephalon and the third ventricle.

The cavity of the mesencephalon remains relatively large (Fig. 5a, b), especially the posterior part. The height and the width are about equal in size. The isthmus rhombencephali is always distinct.

During weeks 8 and 9, the rhombic fossa becomes deeper due to the progressive flexure of the pons (Figs 5.2a, 5.3, and 5.5b). The lateral corners of the rhombencephalic cavity, called the lateral recesses (Fig. 5.4), are easily identified at 7 and 8 weeks. During this period, the distance between these recesses increases (rhombencephalon width). Later, during weeks 9 and 10, the lateral recesses often become covered by the enlarging cerebellar hemispheres. Thus only the central part of the hypoechogenic fourth ventricle, which is divided by the choroid plexuses, is visible. The choroid plexuses of the fourth ventricle are bright landmarks dividing the ventricle into a rostral and a caudal compartment (Fig. 5.6a). There is a clear gap between the rhombencephalic and the mesencephalic cavity due to the growing cerebellum, which is easily detectable. The primordia of cerebellar hemispheres are clearly separated in the midline during the embryonic period. The isthmus rhombencephali is narrow; in most cases it is not visible in its complete length. The spine is still characterized by two echogenic parallel lines.

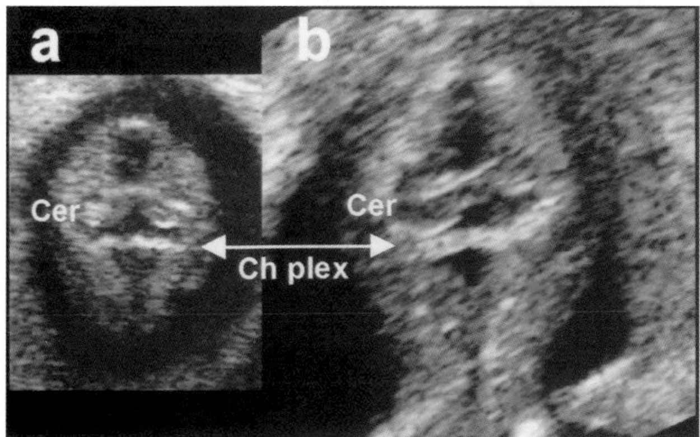


Figure 5.6 (a) Coronal section through the posterior head of a 9-week-old embryo, CRL 25 mm; the choroid plexuses (Ch plex) divide the roof of the fourth ventricle into an area membranacea superior and inferior. (b) Coronal section through the posterior head of an 11-week-old fetus, CRL 45 mm; the choroid plexuses lie close to the caudal border of the cerebellar hemispheres; the double-headed arrow points at the echogenic choroid plexuses; Cer = cerebellum.

## EARLY POSTEMBRYONIC PERIOD, 10 AND 11 WEEKS, CRL 32–54 mm

### Anatomic development

A staging system for the fetal period is not available. Among the most noticeable external changes of the brain are the apparent union of the cerebellar hemispheres with the development of the upper vermis and the increasing concealment of the diencephalon and mesencephalon by the cerebral hemispheres. The cerebellum enlarges, drawing the roof of the fourth ventricle beneath its caudal border. The mesencephalic cavity is still wide.

Various 2-D measurements for the embryonic/fetal brain and brain cavities have been proposed (Day 1959; Westergaard 1971; O'Rahilly & Müller 1990), but no systematic standardized measurements of the embryonic brain have been adopted. The development of the form of the brain compartments was demonstrated by 3-D reconstructions from histological slices as shown by Hochstetter (Hochstetter 1919; Kostovic 1990) using the technique described by Born (1883), or by 3-D casts from the lateral ventricles of aborted specimens (Woolam 1952; Westergaard 1971; Day 1959). Jenkins calculated the volumes of embryonic and fetal brain compartments obtained from 3-D reconstructions of a few specimens from the Carnegie collection (Jenkins 1921).

### Ultrasound

The thick crescent lateral ventricles fill the anterior part of the head and conceal the diencephalic cavity. The thickness of the cortex is about 1 mm at the end of the first trimester. The diencephalon lies between the hemispheres, and the mesencephalon gradually moves towards the center of the head. The width of the third ventricle definitely becomes narrow towards the end of the first trimester. There is a gap between the mesencephalic and the rhombencephalic cavity which is filled with the growing cerebellum. The cerebellar hemispheres seem to meet in the midline during weeks 11 to 12. After 10 weeks 3 days, the choroid plexuses of the fourth ventricle can always be seen. The distance between the choroid plexuses and the cerebellum becomes shorter during weeks 9 to 11 (Figure 6b). At the end of the first trimester the choroid plexuses are found close to the caudal border of the cerebellum. Successively, the ossification of the spine appears.

The reference points for measuring the head of the second trimester fetus (biparietal diameter, BPD, occipito-frontal diameter, OFD, and head circumference, HC) such as the cavum septi pellucidi and thalami are not formed in the first trimester. The shape of the embryonic head and the position of the intracranial structures change significantly during the early development, as described in the embryologic literature (Streeter 1942, 1945, 1948, 1949; O'Rahilly & Müller 1987, 1994). At 7 weeks, at Carnegie stages 16 and 17, the horizontal plane through the embryonic head includes the rhombencephalon and the posterior part of the mesencephalon. This plane lies above the diencephalon and the hemispheres. The largest width is found at the height of the rhombic lips, the future cerebellum. The greatest length extends from the cervical flexure to the anterior wall of the bent mesencephalon. Owing to the development of the brain, characterized by uneven growth of the brain compartments and by the 'deflection' of the brain, the greatest width alters its position during the embryonic and early fetal period. At the beginning of week 9, Carnegie stages 21 and 22, the plane for the measurement of the head size includes the hemispheres anteriorly, the diencephalon in the middle of the head, and the cerebellum posteriorly. At the end of the embryonic period, at Carnegie stage 23, the measurement plane comprises the hemispheres, the diencephalon and the upper part of the cerebellum. In the early fetal period, the future cranium becomes successively distinguishable. Thus, the terms BPD and OFD are basically not suitable for the embryonic period, and it would be more correct to use terms like 'width of the head' and 'antero-posterior diameter'. There is a sliding transition from the embryonic 'head width' to the fetal 'biparietal diameter', therefore the historically oldest term BPD should be kept.

The 2-D and 3-D ultrasound measurements of the embryonic brain compartments reflect, so to speak, the phylogenetic development of the brain: the 'old' rhombencephalon is large during the early phase, while the 'young' hemispheres are very small. During a few weeks, this correlation becomes reversed. Ultrasound also reveals another embryonic feature: the cavities of the diencephalon (third ventricle) and mesencephalon (Sylvian aqueduct) are relatively very large. The mean diameter of the mesencephalic cavity even has a similar diameter in the early postembryonic period, as it is found in children and adults (Flyger & Hjelmquist 1957)

## LATE FIRST TRIMESTER, 12 AND 13 WEEKS, BPD ≈ 20–29 mm

### Anatomic development

The lateral ventricle has an anterior and an inferior horn. From approximately 11 weeks on (CRL >40 mm), the posterior horn becomes visible (Westergaard 1971). The hippocampal formation and its subdivisions are identifiable in fetuses of CRL 70 mm (Lemire 1975). The massa intermedia is a tissue bridge of gray matter which develops between the dorsal thalami and crosses the third ventricle in most individuals (Lemire 1975). The development of the corpus callosum begins at about 12–13 weeks, thus creating one of the main landmarks for the ultrasound evaluation of the head, namely the cavum septi pellucidi. Whether the cavum septi pellucidi initially is an open pocket that is bridged by the corpus callosum, or is formed by necrosis within the massa commissuralis, is not certain (O'Rahilly & Müller 1994). The aqueduct is still relatively large, and the corpus callosum is still limited to the rostral region (O'Rahilly & Müller 1994).

### Ultrasound

The smooth hemispheres dominate the brain. The thickness of the cortex is between 1 and 2 mm. The lateral ventricles are large and filled by the echogenic choroid plexuses. The insula appears as a slight depression on the lateral surface. The third ventricle has become a narrow slit (Fig. 5.7). In early hydrocephaly, the massa intermedia may be detected in a dilated third ventricle (Blaas & Eik-Ness 1999b). The cavity of the mesencephalon is still wide. The choroid plexuses of the fourth ventricle are 'pulled' to the lower border of the cerebellar hemispheres, the fourth ventricle is found covered by the cerebellum.

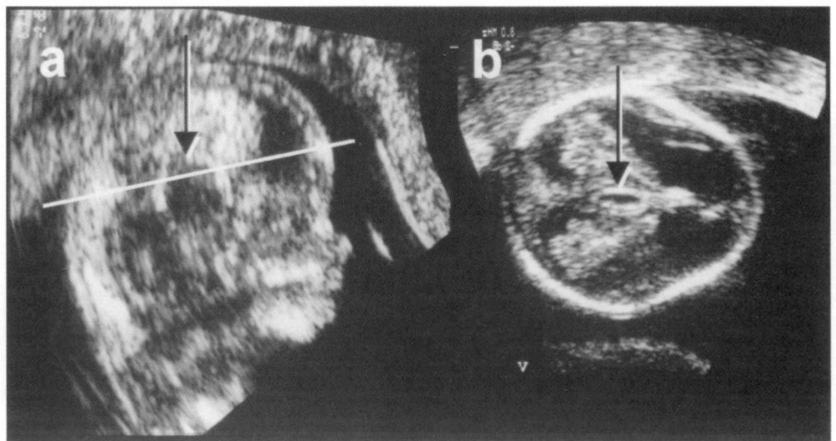


**Figure 5.7** (a) Sagittal section through the head of a 13 week-old fetus; the third ventricle lies relatively high in the middle of the head (arrow).
(b) Horizontal section as indicated in part a; the arrow points at the third ventricle, which should not be taken for the cavum septi pellucidi.

## SECOND TRIMESTER

### APPROXIMATELY 14 TO 27 WEEKS, BPD ≈ 30–74 mm

#### Anatomic development

The cavum septi pellucidi becomes a landmark in the horizontal imaging of the brain. Its width increases slowly from 3.4 mm at 19–20 weeks to 6.4 mm at 27–28 weeks (Jou *et al.* 1998). The posterior horns of the lateral ventricles gradually become more elongated as shown in casts from fetal ventricles (Westgaard 1971; Kier 1977). The hippocampus in the human temporal lobe projects into the temporal horn (Kier 1977). Sulci begin to appear on the surface of the cerebral hemisphere at about the middle of prenatal life (Dorovini-Zis & Dolman 1977; O'Rahilly & Müller 1994). Chi and coworkers have described the chronological development of the gyri and sulci (Chi *et al.* 1976): together with the development of the corpus callosum, the corresponding callosal sulcus appears at the 14th week. The corpus callosum forms the roof of a cavity, which is the cavum septi pellucidi et Vergae. This cavity usually closes postnatally when the infant is 2 months old (Shaw & Alvord 1969). During 16 to 19 weeks the cingulate gyrus appears on the medial surface of the hemispheres. At the same time, the parieto-occipital fissure appears and delineates the primitive occipital lobe from the parietal lobe, while the calcarine fissure gradually indents the occipital horn of the lateral ventricle. By 27 weeks, the adjacent cuneus and lingual gyrus have become distinct. Between 20 and 23 weeks, the central sulcus and the superior temporal sulcus appear. Before the end of the second trimester, additional sulci become visible, such as the pre- and postcentral sulcus, the middle temporal sulcus, the interparietal sulcus, superior frontal sulcus, and lateral occipital sulcus. The cavity of the mesencephalon becomes gradually reduced, particularly because of the growth of the tectum (Kier 1977). The cerebellar development is not completed at the beginning of the second trimester: the midline fusion of the cerebellar primordia gives rise to the vermis, which progressively grows caudally and dorsally with the cerebellar hemispheres, but at a relatively slower rate (Lemire 1975; Müller & O'Rahilly 1990). Primary and secondary folia of the vermis and the cerebellar hemispheres appear during the first half of the second trimester (Lemire 1975).

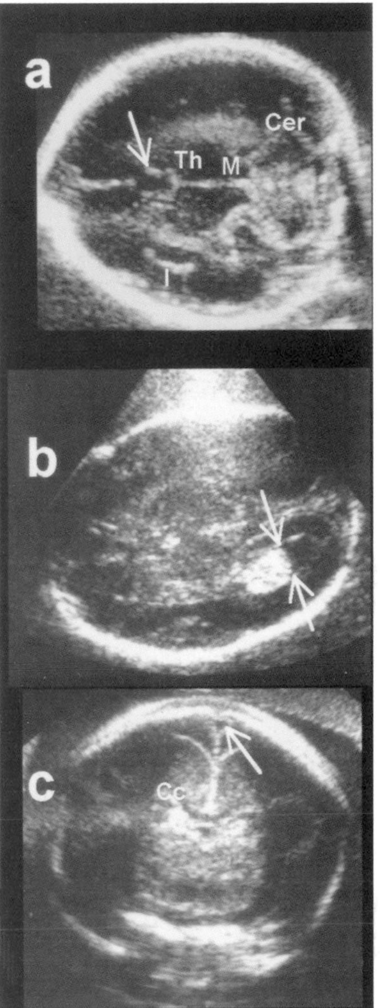


Figure 5.8 Ultrasound sections through the head of fetuses between 22 and 25 weeks. (a) Horizontal section through the cavum septi pellucidi (arrow), thalami (Th), mesencephalon (M) and cerebellum (Cer), I = insula and lateral sulcus.
(b) Horizontal section through the lateral ventricle with emphasis on the atrium; the arrows indicate where to measure the lateral ventricular atrium width. (c) Coronal section, showing the superior sagittal venous sinus (arrow) and the corpus callosum (Cc).

#### Ultrasound

By scanning in different planes, it is possible to evaluate the shape of the brain and its ventricles (Figs 5.8 and 5.9). Since ultrasound has been introduced, many biometric parameters and ratios have been proposed to evaluate the fetal brain and its ventricular system. Examples of such parameters are cerebro-frontal horn distance (Goldstein *et al.* 1988), cerebro-atrial distance (Pilu *et al.* 1989), posterior horn width, cerebro-posterior horn distance (Goldstein *et al.* 1990), occipital horn height, thalamus-to-tip-of-occipital-horn distance, midline-to-edge of lateral ventricle (Monteagudo *et al.* 1993), and many others. A variety of these parameters have been presented and discussed in a comprehensive outline by Monteagudo and coworkers (Monteagudo *et al.* 1996). For the clinical practice simple measurements are preferable. The atrial width of the lateral ventricle (Fig. 5.8b) has shown to have a constant value throughout the second and third trimesters as shown by Cardoza and coworkers (7.6 ± 0.6 mm) and Pilu and co-workers (6.9 ± 1.3 mm) (Cardoza *et al.* 1988; Pilu *et al.* 1989). Therefore, atrial diameters above 10 mm should raise the suspicion of ventriculomegaly (Cardoza *et al.* 1988). The surface of the cortices can be evaluated by tangential (oblique) sections (Fig. 5.9c),

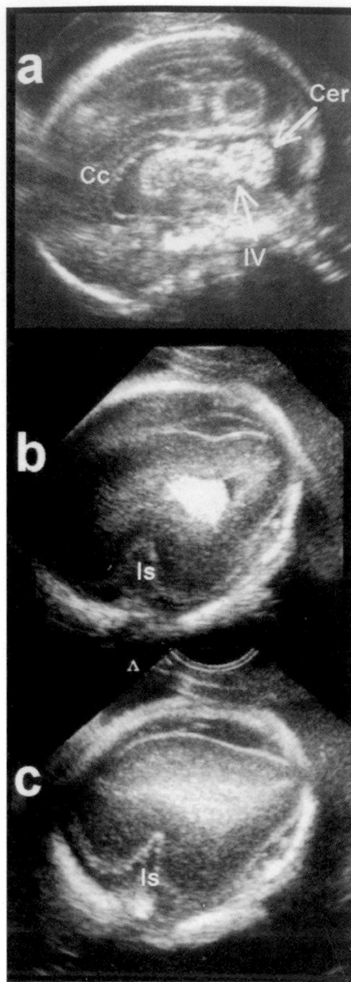


Figure 5.9 Ultrasound sections through the head of fetuses between 22 and 25 weeks. (a) Sagittal section through the corpus callosum (Cc), cavum septi pellucidi, diencephalon, mesencephalon, cerebellum (Cer) and fourth ventricle (IV). (b) Oblique section through the posterior of the lateral ventricle with its echogenic choroid plexus; ls = lateral sulcus. (c) Further oblique section through the smooth cortex and the lateral sulcus.

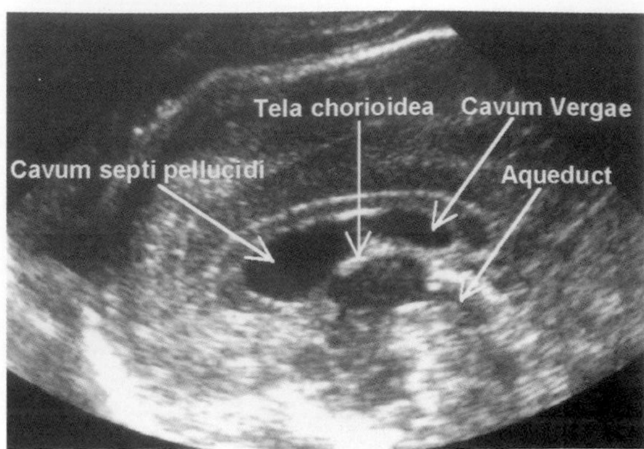


Figure 5.10 Sagittal image zoomed-in on the central brain, showing the rather large corpus callosum, the cavum septi pellucidi and cavum Vergae at 28 weeks (cf. Fig. 5.9a). The roof of the third ventricle consists of the echogenic tela chorioidea. The Sylvian aqueduct can easily be identified.

which is not easy, or by sections perpendicular to the surface of the brain. In a study involving 262 normal fetuses, the gestational age at which fissures and sulci were first detected was 14 weeks for the callosal sulcus, 18 weeks for the lateral sulcus, the parieto-occipital and calcarine fissures, and 26 weeks for the cingulate sulcus (Monteagudo & Timor-Tritsch 1997). The third ventricle is relatively well imaged in the early second trimester, but it narrows as gestation progresses, and develops into a virtual space between the thalami (Fig. 5.8a) (Timor-Tritsch & Monteagudo 1996). The corpus callosum, the cavum septi pellucidi and the cavum Vergae are easily depicted in the sagittal section (Figs 5.9a, 5.10, and 5.11a). The cerebral aqueduct of Sylvius develops into a narrow tube during the early second trimester and

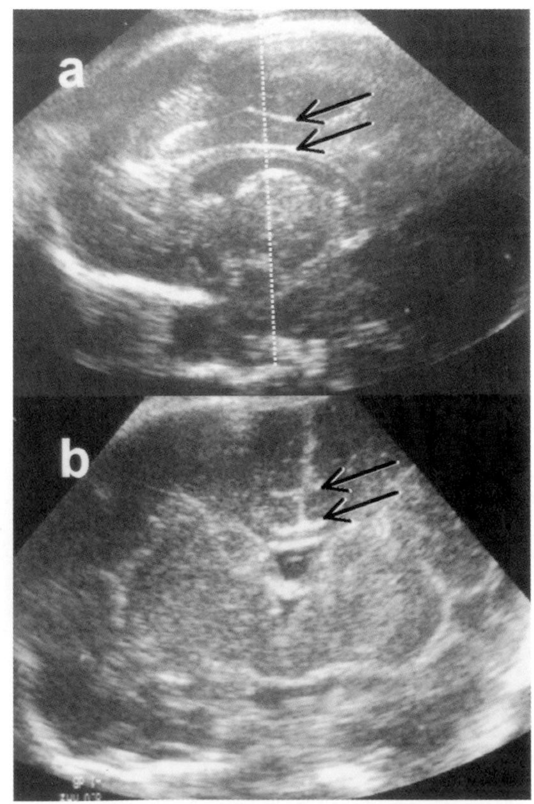


Figure 5.11 (a) Sagittal section through the brain at 30 weeks: the echogenic lines above the cavum septi pellucidi and corpus callosum are the pericallosal and cingulate sulci; between them lies the cingulate gyrus; the stippled line indicates the section of part b. (b) The arrows point at the pericallosal and cingulate sulci in the coronal section.

looks like an echogenic line in the longitudinal axis of the midbrain (Fig. 5.10). The lower cerebellar vermis may still be small until 16–18 weeks (Bromley *et al.* 1994; Babcook *et al.* 1996). There are no normative data on the size of the fetal fourth ventricle at 12–24 weeks of gestation. Bronshtein and colleagues noted that the lateral diameter of the fourth ventricle comprises less than half of the lateral cerebellar width, while the postero-anterior diameter of the fourth ventricle is less than two-thirds of the cerebellar postero-anterior diameter (Bronshtein *et al.* 1998). Measurements of the transverse diameter of the cerebellum have shown that the value of this parameter expressed in millimeters corresponded approximately to the gestational age expressed in weeks during the second trimester (Goldstein *et al.* 1987; Hata *et al.* 1989). Thus, the mean transverse diameter was found to be 14 mm at 15 weeks, increasing to 30–31 mm at 27 weeks (Goldstein *et al.* 1987; Hill *et al.* 1990). The depth of the cisterna magna is measured as the midline diameter from the inner table of the occiput to the posterior aspect of the cerebellum in the standard horizontal plane of the cerebellum. The mean depth of the cisterna magna in normal second and third trimester fetuses is 5 ± 3 mm, with a maximum of 10 mm (Mahony *et al.* 1984).

## THIRD TRIMESTER

### APPROXIMATELY 28 WEEKS TO TERM, BPD ≥ 75 mm

#### Anatomic development

At 28 weeks, the appearance of the superior temporal sulcus is a constant feature (Dorovini-Zis & Dolman 1977). A great growth spurt occurs between the 28th and 30th weeks: numerous sulci and gyri develop, and the brain assumes a much more ‘finished’ appearance. After 30 weeks, the assessment of gestational age by looking at the external brain becomes more difficult (Dorovini-Zis & Dolman 1977). By the 40th week, tertiary sulci have made their appearance (Dorovini-Zis & Dolman 1977). The insula remains smooth until 28–29 weeks, after which the frontal, temporal, and parietal opercula begin to override it (Chi *et al.* 1976).

#### Ultrasound

The diameter of the cavum septi pellucidi decreases from 6.1 mm at 29–30 weeks to 5.5 mm at 41–42 weeks (Jou *et al.* 1998). The transverse diameter of the cerebellum increases from 31–33 mm at 28 weeks to 52 mm at 40 weeks (Goldstein *et al.* 1987; Hill *et al.* 1990). In principle, it is possible to depict all hemispherical sulci by ultrasound. Still, the complexity of the cerebral surface makes the correlation of a sonographically described sulcus with the correct definition on the anatomical map difficult (Fig. 5.12). Therefore, usually only the main sulci may be identified, especially those on the median surfaces of the hemispheres, which are rather easily identifiable by sagittal and coronal sections (Fig. 5.11) (Timor-Tritsch & Monteagudo 1996). The increased ossification of the skull at the end of the pregnancy impedes the accessibility for the ultrasound imaging of the brain, such that the transfontanelle approach becomes essential.

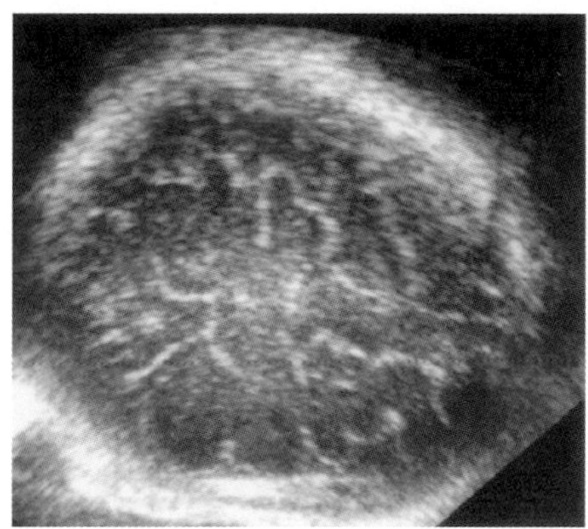

**Figure 5.12** Oblique section of the cortex at 36 weeks showing numerous sulci (echogenic lines) and gyri.

## VASCULATURE OF THE BRAIN

The blood supply of the brain originates from an anterior circulation through the internal carotid arteries, and a posterior circulation through the vertebral arteries via the common single basilar artery. These arterial circulations communicate with each other through the circulus arteriosus of Willis (Fig. 5.13a,b). The main components of the circulus arteriosus are present at Carnegie stage 16, and the circle is complete at Carnegie stage 19 (O'Rahilly & Müller 1994). The middle cerebral artery (MCA) is the largest branch of the circle and runs laterally in the Sylvian fissure as a direct continuation of the internal carotid artery. The two MCAs supply most of the cerebral cortex on the convexity of the hemispheres, and the deep parts of the cerebrum, such as the basal ganglia and the internal capsule. The brain stem and cerebellum are supported from the vertebral arteries and their branches. The venous circulation drains the blood into dural sinuses (Fig. 5.8c), which meet in the confluence of the sinuses at the occipital pole. From here, the blood passes into the jugular veins. Pulsed Doppler and color Doppler (Fig. 5.13b) have been used to image and evaluate the cerebral arterial blood flow. One of the first studies on cerebral blood flow was measurements of the carotid arteries (Marsál *et al.* 1984). Especially the fetal middle cerebral artery has been the object of Doppler measurements and studies as a representative blood vessel of the cerebral circulation (Maesel 1996). Power Doppler angiography (Fig. 5.13a) has demonstrated that many vessels of both arterial and venous circulation can be imaged by this ultrasound application (Pooh & Aomo 1996). These authors showed clear power Doppler images of the main anterior and posterior arterial circulation as early as at the end of the first trimester (Pooh & Aomo 1996).

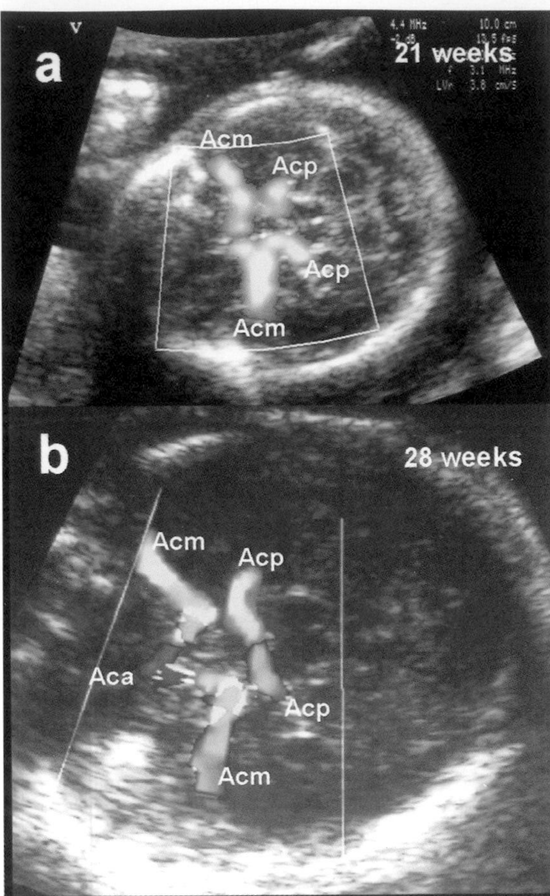


Figure 5.13 (a) Power Doppler image of the circulus Willisii at 21 weeks. (b) Color Doppler image of the circulus Willisii at 28 weeks; Aca = arteria cerebri anterior; Acm = arteria cerebri media; Acp = arteria cerebri posterior

## CONCLUSION

In the growing embryo, the brain is the first organ system to develop in such a way that it can be imaged with ultrasound technology at a level where the diagnosis of malformations can be made. Due to its nature, holoprosencephaly is probably the first condition that can be recognized with ultrasound in the developing embryo. At present, we are at the borderline of being able to diagnose holoprosencephaly when the embryo is 7–8 weeks. At 9 weeks, significant diagnoses such as holoprosencephaly (Blaas *et al.* 2000a), spina bifida (Blaas *et al.* 2000b), acrania (Blaas & Eik-Nes 1996), encephalocele (Blaas & Eik-Nes 1999b), and Meckel Gruber (Blaas & Eik-Nes 1999a) have been made. These malformations may be imaged in greater detail during the subsequent few weeks of pregnancy. From 12 weeks and onwards, additional conditions such as Arnold Chiari malformation (Blaas *et al.* 2000b) and Dandy Walker malformation (Achiron *et al.* 1993) may be diagnosed. Later in pregnancy most of the structural maldevelopments of the CNS may be recognized and have been described. Thus, women at risk for having a fetus with brain anomalies may have early examination at the specific time when the diagnosis can be made.

To utilize the potential of ultrasound diagnosis in the embryonic/fetal period, it is important to have a basic knowledge of the normal development. It is also essential to establish the time when the various diagnoses can be made with adequate certainty, in order to offer women at risk an examination at the appropriate time.

We have come so far that the expected development of the ultrasound technology will probably not make it possible to make diagnosis of brain anomalies significantly earlier than at present, but will increase reliability. We may expect the rapidly developing 3-D technology, with the option of any-plane slicing, to help us establish diagnoses in the future. Such multiplane presentations of a diagnosis will contribute to increasing the diagnostic accuracy.

## REFERENCES


Achiron R & Achiron A (1991) Transvaginal ultrasonic assessment of the early fetal brain. *Ultrasound Obstet Gynecol* 1:336–344.

Achiron R, Achiron A & Yagel S (1993) First trimester transvaginal sonographic diagnosis of Dandy-Walker malformation. *J Clin Ultrasound* 21 (Jan):62–64.

Babcook C J, Chong B W, Salamat M S *et al.* (1996) Sonographic anatomy of the developing cerebellum: normal embryology can resemble pathology. *Am J Roentgenol* 166:427–433.

Blaas H-G K (1999a) The embryonic examination. Ultrasound studies on the development of the human embryo [Thesis]. Trondheim: Norwegian University of Science and Technology.

Blaas H-G K [Editorial] (1999b) The examination of the embryo and early fetus: how and by whom? *Ultrasound Obstet Gynecol* 14(3):153–158.

Blaas H-G, Eik-Nes S H, Kiserud T, Hellevik L R (1994) Early development of the forebrain and midbrain: a longitudinal ultrasound study from 7 to 12 weeks of gestation. *Ultrasound Obstet Gynecol* 4:183–192.

Blaas H-G, Eik-Nes S H, Kiserud T, Hellevik L R (1995a) Early development of the hindbrain: a longitudinal ultrasound study from 7 to 12 weeks of gestation. *Ultrasound Obstet Gynecol* 5:151–160.

Blaas H-G, Eik-Nes S H, Kiserud T *et al.* (1995b) Three-dimensional imaging of the brain cavities in human embryos. *Ultrasound Obstet Gynecol* 5:228–232.

Blaas H-G & Eik-Nes S H (1996) Ultrasound assessment of early brain development. In: Jurkovic D, Jauniaux E, eds. *Ultrasound and early pregnancy.* New York, London: Parthenon Publishing Group; pp. 3–18.

Blaas H-G, Eik-Nes S H, Berg S & Torp H (1998) *In vivo* three-dimensional ultrasound reconstructions of embryos and early fetuses. *Lancet* 352(9135):1182–1186.

Blaas H-G & Eik-Nes S H (1999a) First-trimester diagnosis of fetal malformations. In: Rodeck, Whittle, eds. *Fetal medicine: basic science and clinical practice.* London: Harcourt Brace; pp. 581–597.

Blaas H-G & Eik-Nes S H (1999b) Das Zentralnervensystem. Die normale Entwicklung und die Entwicklung von Anomalien – Ultraschalldiagnostik in der Frühschwangerschaft. *Gynäkologe* 32:181–191.

Blaas H-G K, Eik-Nes S H, Vainio T & Isaksen C V (2000a) Alobar holoprosencephaly at 9 weeks gestational age visualized by two- and three-dimensional ultrasound. *Ultrasound Obstet Gynecol* 2000;15:62–65.

Blaas H-G K, Eik-Nes S H & Isaksen C V (2000b) The detection of spina bifida before 10 gestational weeks using 2D- and 3D ultrasound. *Ultrasound Obstet Gynecol* 16:25–29.

Born G (1883) Die Plattenmodellirmethode. *Arch Mikr Anat* 22:584–599.

Bree R L & Marn C S (1990) Transvaginal sonography in the first trimester: embryology, anatomy, and hCG correlation. *Semin Ultrasound CT MRI* 11:12–21.

Bromley B, Nadel A S, Pauker S, Estroff J A & Benacerraf B R (1994) Closure of the cerebellar vermis: evaluation with second trimester US. *Radiology* 193:761–763.

Bronshtein M, Zimmer E Z & Blazer S (1998) Isolated large fourth ventricle in early pregnancy – a possible benign transient phenomenon. *Prenat Diagn* 18:997–1000.

Cardoza J D, Goldstein R B & Filly R A (1988) Exclusion of fetal ventriculomegaly with a single measurement: the width of the lateral ventricular atrium. *Radiology* 169:711–714.

Chi J G, Dooling E C & Gilles F H (1976) Gyral development of the human brain. *Ann Neurol* 1:86–93.

Cremin B J, Chilton S J & Peacock W J (1983) Anatomical landmarks in anterior fontanelle ultrasonography. *Br J Radiol* 56:517–526.

Cullen M T, Green J, Whetham J *et al.* (1990) Transvaginal ultrasonographic detection of congenital anomalies in the first trimester. *Am J Obstet Gynecol* 163(2):466–476.

Day R W (1959) Casts of foetal lateral ventricles. *Brain* 82:109–115.

Dorovini-Zis K & Dolman C L (1977) Gestational development of brain. *Arch Pathol Lab Med* 101:192–195.

Flyger G & Hjelmquist U (1957) Normal variations in the caliber of the human cerebral aqueduct. *Anat Record Philad* 127:151–162.

Goldstein I, Reece A, Pilu G *et al.* (1987) Cerebellar measurements with ultrasonography in the evaluation of fetal growth and development. *Am J Obstet Gynecol* 156:1065–1069.

Goldstein I, Reece E A, Pilu, G, Hobbins J C & Bovicelli L (1988) Sonographic evaluation of the normal developmental anatomy of fetal cerebral ventricles. I. The frontal horn. *Obstet Gynecol* 72:588–592.

Goldstein I, Reece E A, Pilu G & Hobbins J C (1990) Sonographic evaluation of the normal development anatomy of fetal cerebral ventricles. IV. The posterior horn. *Am J Perinat* 7(1):79–83.

Hata K, Hata T, Senoh D *et al.* (1989) Ultrasonographic measurement of the fetal transverse cerebellum *in utero*. *Gynecol Obstet Invest* 28:111–112.

Hill L M, Guzick D, Fries J *et al.* (1990) The transverse cerebellar diameter in estimating gestational age in the large for gestational age fetus. *Obstet Gynecol* 75:983–992.

Hochstetter F (1919) *Beiträge zur Entwicklungsgeschichte des menschlichen Gehirns.* Wien: Franz Deuticke.

Jenkins G B (1921) Relative weight and volume of the component parts of the brain of the human embryo at different stages of development. *Contr Embryol Carneg Instn* 13:41–60.

Jou H-J, Shyu M-K, Wu S-C *et al.* (1998) Ultrasound measurement of the fetal cavum septi pellucidi. *Ultrasound Obstet Gynecol* 12:419–421.

Kier E L, ed. (1977) *The cerebral ventricles: a phylogenetic and ontogenetic study.* Anatomy and pathology. St Louis, MO: Mosby.

Kostovic I (1990) Zentralnervensystem. In: Hinrichsen KV, ed. *Humanembryologie.* Berlin: Springer-Verlag; pp. 381–448.

Lemire R J (1975) *Deep cerebral nuclei.* In: Lemire R J, ed. Normal and abnormal development of the human nervous system. Hagerstown, MD: Harper & Row; pp. 169–195.

Müller F & O'Rahilly R (1990) The human brain at stages 21–23, with particular reference to the cerebral cortical plate and the development of the cerebellum. *Anat Embryol* 182:375–400.

Maesel A (1996) *Human fetal cerebral circulation. Perinatal Doppler velocimetry and fetal pulse oximetry studies.* (Thesis) Malmö University Hospital Lund: Malmö; pp. 1–86.

Mahony B S, Callen P W, Filly R A & Hoddick W K (1984) The fetal cisterna magna. *Radiology* 153:773–736.

Marsál K, Lingman G & Giles W (1984) Evaluation of the carotid, aortic and umbilical blood velocity waveforms in the human fetus. In: 11th Annual Conf Soc Study of Fetal Physiology; 1984; Oxford; Abstr No. C33.

Monteagudo A, Timor-Tritsch I E & Moomjy M (1993) Nomograms of the fetal lateral ventricles using transvaginal sonography. *J Ultrasound Med* 5:265–269.

Monteagudo A, Haratz-Rubinstein N & Timor-Tritsch I E (1996) Biometry of the fetal brain. In: Timor-Tritsch I E, Monteagudo A, Cohen H L, editors. *Ultrasonography of the prenatal and neonatal brain.* Stamford, CT: Appleton & Lange.

Monteagudo A & Timor-Tritsch I E (1997) Development of fetal gyri, sulci and fissures: a transvaginal sonographic study. *Ultrasound Obstet Gynecol* 9:222–228.

O'Rahilly R & Müller F (1987) *Developmental stages in human embryos.* Washington, DC: Carneg Instn Publ.

O'Rahilly R & Müller F (1990) Ventricular system and choroid plexuses of the human brain during the embryonic period proper. *Am J Anat* 189:285–302.

O'Rahilly R & Müller F (1994) *The embryonic human brain. An atlas of developmental stages.* New York: Wiley-Liss.

O'Rahilly R, Müller F, Hutchins G M & Moore G W (1984) Computer ranking of the sequences of appearance of 100 features of the brain and related structures in staged human embryos during the first 5 weeks of development. *Am J Anat* 171:243–257.

Pilu G, Reece E A, Goldstein I *et al.* (1989) Sonographic evaluation of the normal developmental anatomy of the fetal cerebral ventricles. II. The atria. *Obstet Gynecol* 73:250–256.

Pooh R K & Aomo T (1996) Transvaginal power Doppler angiography of the fetal brain. *Ultrasound Obstet Gynecol* 8:417–421.

Rubenstein J L R, Shimamura K, Martinez S & Pelles L (1998) Regionalization of the prosencephalic neural plate. *Annu Rev Neurosci* 21:445–477.

Shaw C-M & Alvord E C (1969) Cava septi pellucidi et Vergæ: their normal and pathological states. *Brain* 92:213–224.

Spemann H, Mangold H (1924) Über Induktion von Embryonenanlagen durch Implantation artfremder Organisatoren. *Arch mikr Anat Entw mech* 100:599–638.

Streeter G L (1942) Developmental horizons in human embryos. *Contr Embryol Carneg Inst* 197(30):211–245.

Streeter G L (1945) Developmental horizons in human embryos. *Contr Embryol Carneg Inst* 199(31):27–63.

Streeter G L (1948) Developmental horizons in human embryos. *Contr Embryol Carneg Inst* 211(32):133–203.

Streeter G L (1949) Developmental horizons in human embryos (fourth issue). A review of the histogenesis of cartilage and bone. *Contr Embryol Carneg Inst* 220(33):150–173.

Takeuchi H (1992) Transvaginal ultrasound in the first trimester of pregnancy. *Early Hum Dev* 29:381–384.

Timor-Tritsch I E, Farine D & Rosen M G (1988) A close look at the embryonic development with the high frequency transvaginal transducer. *Am J Obstet Gynecol* 159:678–681.

Timor-Tritsch I E, Peisner D B & Raju S (1990) Sonoembryology: an organ-oriented approach using a high-frequency vaginal probe. *J Clin Ultrasound* 18:286–298.

Timor-Tritsch I E, Monteagudo A & Warren W B (1991) Transvaginal ultrasonographic definition of the central nervous system in the first and early second trimesters. *Am J Obstet Gynecol* 164:497–503.

Timor-Tritsch I E & Monteagudo A (1996) Normal neurosonography of the prenatal brain. In: Timor-Tritsch I E, Monteagudo A, Cohen H L, editors. Ultrasonography of the prenatal and neonatal brain. Stamford, Connecticut: Appleton & Lange pp. 11–88.

van Zalen-Sprock R M, van Vugt J M G, van Geijn H P (1996) First-trimester sonographic detection of neurodevelopmental abnormalities in some single-gene disorders. *Prenat Diagn* 16:199–202.

Warren W B, Timor-Tritsch I E, Peisner D B *et al.* (1989) Dating the pregnancy by sequential appearance of embryonic structures. *Am J Obstet Gynecol* 161:747–753.

Westergaard E (1971) The lateral cerebral ventricles of human foetuses with a crown–rump length of 26–178 mm. *Acta Anat* 79:409–421.

Woollam D (1952) Casts of the ventricles of the brain. *Brain* 75:259–267.

Yokoh Y (1975) Early development of the cerebral vesicles in man. *Acta Anat* 91:455–461.

# Chapter 6 Imaging of the neonatal brain

R. Arthur and L. Ramenghi

## INTRODUCTION

Technological advances in diagnostic imaging over the last 25 years have made a major contribution to the understanding of disorders of the neonatal brain. Improvements in imaging have resulted in more accurate diagnoses and helped to clarify the nature and pathogenesis of perinatal brain injury, and to predict the long term outlook with regard to the development of neurologic deficit. Imaging also plays an important role in screening for congenital malformations and other significant intracranial abnormality in infants with clinical suspicion of an underlying neurologic disorder.

## IMAGING MODALITIES

### CARE OF THE INFANT

Consideration of the well being of the neonate should be paramount in any discussions concerning the choice of imaging modality. In many situations a compromise will be needed, taking into consideration the clinical status of the infant, suspected pathology and imaging modalities available. Although ultrasound examinations can be performed at the bedside, even minimal disturbance of the very sick neonate may provoke apneic episodes and bradycardia during ultrasound examinations (Boyer 1994). The baby may be receiving respiratory support, i.e. mechanical ventilation or supplemental inspired oxygen requiring close monitoring of heart rate, blood pressure, oxygen saturation, and fluid balance. In a few situations the potential benefit from magnetic resonance imaging (MRI) or computerized axial tomography (CT) will outweigh the additional risks of transferring the infant receiving intensive care to the radiology department. Great care must be taken not to dislodge in-dwelling catheters, endotracheal tubes and chest drains when moving a baby who will need to be well swaddled in order to maintain body temperature.

Most CT and MRI examinations can be performed in the newborn infant without sedation, particularly if the baby is well enough to have a feed beforehand. The longer examination times for MRI increase the requirement for sedation, particularly after the first few weeks of life, and it is essential that MRI units have the facilities for monitoring pulse and blood oxygen saturation during the examination. Local protocols giving advice on the administration and supervision of sedation are essential.

### ULTRASOUND

The potential value of real time ultrasound of the neonatal head was realized early, following its introduction in the late 1970s. For the first time intracranial anatomy could be clearly visualized and intraventricular hemorrhage, cerebral infarction and ventricular dilatation diagnosed without moving the infant to the imaging department for a CT scan. Further technological improvements now allow us not only to image gross structural anatomy, but also the development of spectral, color and power Doppler imaging permit detailed assessment of the vascular anatomy of the brain (see Chapter 9).

Cranial ultrasound is usually performed through the anterior fontanelle which acts as an acoustic window. Directly following birth the fontanelle may be very small, on account of molding of the sutures and this may limit the visualization of the intracranial anatomy. The anterior fontanelle remains open for much of the first year of life and begins to close at about 9 months, although as the infant grows the scalp tissues thicken and detailed imaging of the infant brain gradually becomes more difficult. The posterior fontanelle can also be used as an acoustic window, particularly to examine the posterior periventricular white matter and the occipital horns of the lateral ventricles. Taylor has recently described the advantages of scanning through the mastoid fontanelle for evaluation of the cerebellum and brain stem and has suggested that these views should be routinely incorporated into the standard imaging protocol (Taylor 1998). Scanning through the thin squamous temporal bone may be useful in certain clinical situations, particularly for Doppler assessment of the middle cerebral artery and branches of the circle of Willis. The transtemporal and the mastoid approaches also provide an axial view of the brain comparable with CT images and permit better visualization of the peripheral regions of the parietal lobes which are often not well visualized through the anterior fontanelle.

An ultrasound scanner for use on the neonatal unit should be easily maneuverable, have a good range of transducers to image both the extremely premature and term infant, and have facilities for image documentation, including video recording and hardcopy images. Both gray scale and color Doppler imaging should be available; in the future, power Doppler imaging may become an important asset. The choice of transducer frequency is a compromise between resolution and penetration; high frequency transducers give better resolution but may have relatively poor penetration. In general

7–10 MHz sector transducers are appropriate for scanning the brain of the very preterm infant, whereas a 5 MHz transducer will be more appropriate for the term infant. Even lower frequency, e.g. a 3.5 MHz transducer may be necessary to adequately visualize the posterior fossa in an older infant. High frequency, e.g. 10 MHz, linear or curved linear transducers are particularly valuable to examine the extra-axial space and the peripheral cerebral cortex immediately below the fontanelle, which can be useful for evaluation of the superior sagittal sinus in conjunction with color Doppler imaging. In addition most modern scanners have sophisticated post-processing software to optimize the image and it is important that the unit is appropriately set-up for the range of clinical applications to be examined.

A full description of the examination technique and normal anatomy is outside the scope of this chapter but is well described elsewhere (Siegel 1995; Taylor 1998; Teele & Share 1991). Generally, scans are performed in both the coronal and sagittal plane angling as far forward, backward and as laterally as possible to interrogate the intracranial contents. It may be necessary to change transducers or scan through other acoustic windows to clarify the nature of any pathology detected. The images and reports for all ultrasound examinations should be recorded in the clinical records as these may be valuable at a later date to help time any intracranial injury, and possibly provide crucial evidence with regard to the timing of brain injury in any subsequent litigation.

Recognition of the limitations of neurosonography should indicate where additional imaging using other modalities is necessary to answer specific clinical problems. Although imaging in the near field has improved in recent years with the advent of high frequency linear transducers, small convexity subdural collections may not be well demonstrated. In addition ultrasound is generally considered to be relatively insensitive in the detection of abnormalities in the peripheral regions of the brain and posterior fossa, and further imaging with MRI or CT will be required to exclude a significant abnormality in these regions (Fig. 6.1). It is difficult to evaluate the echogenicity of the white matter objectively other than by comparison with that of the choroid plexus. It is important to recognize the normal peritrigonal blush in the white matter and not confuse this with increased echodensity due to hypoxic ischemic injury. This area of mildly increased echogenicity may be related to the white matter fibers that course radially from the cortex to the subependymal layer of the lateral ventricle, or possibly may be a reflection of the high water content of the white matter in this region (Di Pietro *et al.* 1986) (Fig. 6.2).

Image acquisition and interpretation in ultrasound is operator dependent and subject to inter-observer error. It is crucial when performing any ultrasound examination to be meticulous with the gain settings to ensure that areas of altered echogenicity are not simply due to artifact. Scanning off-center through the anterior fontanelle may give rise erroneously to the impression of unilateral increased

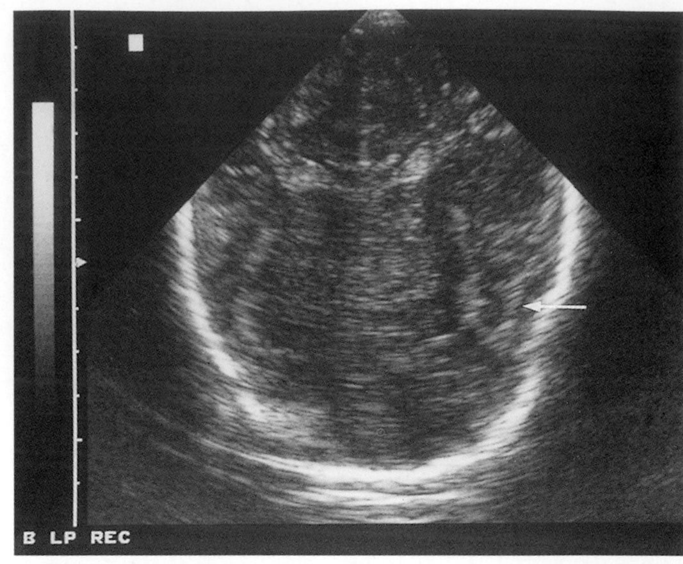


(a)

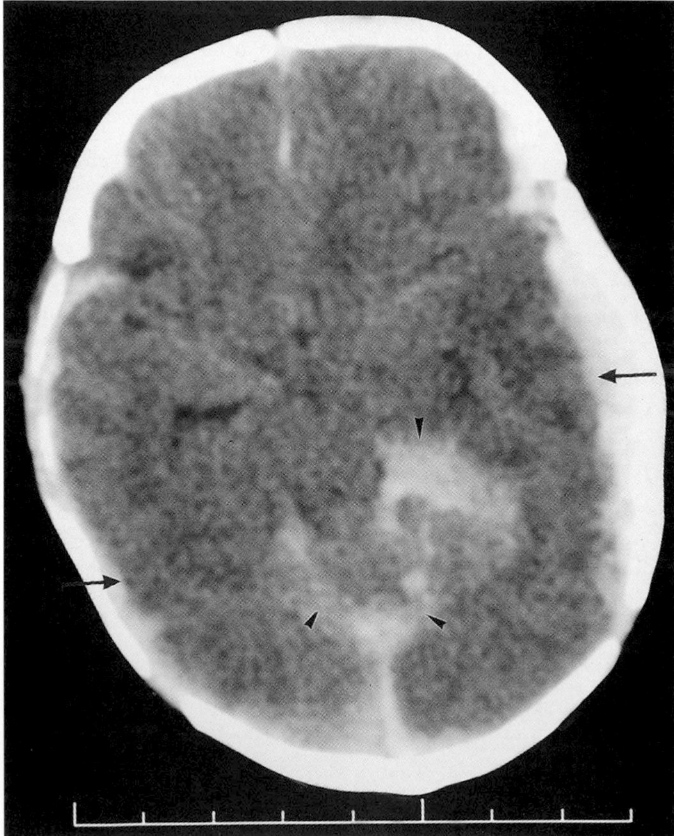

(b)

**Figure 6.1** Acute extra-axial (subdural and subarachnoid) hemorrhages. (a) Coronal ultrasound scan from the posterior fontanelle showing subtle widening of the extra-axial space along the left parieto-occipital bone (white arrow) compared to the right. (b) Unenhanced CT scan at 1 day of age demonstrating bilateral extra-axial hemorrhages (arrows) and further hemorrhage in the region of the tentorium (arrowheads). Shift of the midline to the right is also noted.

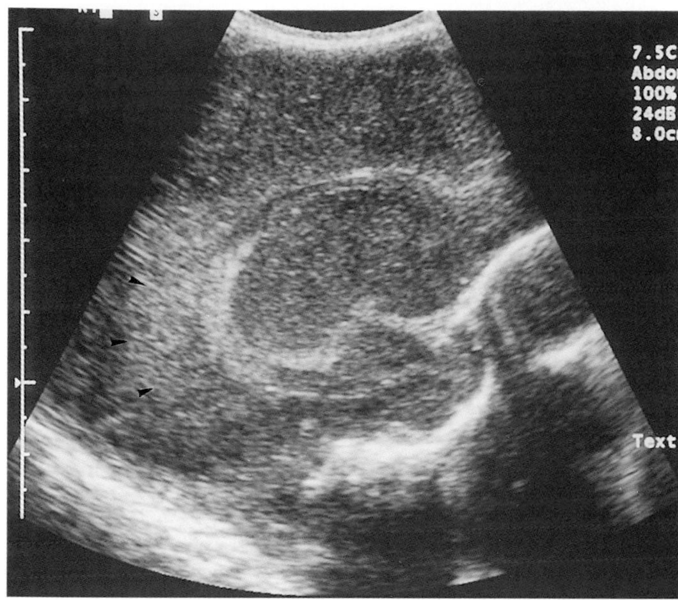


Figure 6.2 Sagittal ultrasound examination demonstrating the normal peritrigonal blush (arrowheads).

echodensity in the parenchyma. Similarly, misdiagnosis of transient echodensity/flare may be made if the gain settings are too high or the slope of the time gain compensation (TGC) is inappropriate. Conversely, abnormality may be overlooked when the gain is too low. It is important to ensure that the focus is set at an appropriate level which may need to be altered during the scanning sequence, to examine both the periventricular regions and the structures of the posterior fossa. Subtle findings, such as mild echodensity, may not be easily reproduced on hard copy images and this may be a particular problem when the images are reported by radiologists and clinicians who have not performed the examination.

## DOPPLER APPLICATIONS (see also Chapter 9)

The anterior fontanelle provides the best window for evaluation of the anterior cerebral, pericallosal and basilar arteries, whereas the transtemporal approach is more suited to insonation of the middle and posterior cerebral circulation. The availability of color Doppler imaging in addition to spectral Doppler imaging helps with vessel identification and choice of optimal angle for insonation. The major veins and venous sinuses can be assessed by Doppler imaging through the mastoid fontanelle (Taylor 1998). Color Doppler imaging is particularly valuable in identifying arteriovenous malformations, e.g. vein of Galen aneurysm and dural fistulae, although further imaging will be necessary for full evaluation. A number of clinical applications have been developed for spectral and color flow Doppler imaging (McMenamin & Volpe 1983; Archer *et al.* 1986; Blankenberg *et al.* 1997) and these are discussed in detail in Chapter 9.

Power Doppler imaging is a more recent development whereby a significant proportion of the electronic noise associated with color and spectral Doppler imaging is eliminated and the dynamic range and sensitivity of the system are increased three to five times. Power Doppler imaging is sensitive to body motion which may be a problem when scanning neonates. Power Doppler is superior to standard color and spectral Doppler imaging and is able to detect low velocity flow. Taylor has shown the feasibility of developing regional perfusion cerebral flow maps in animal studies, and future developments may see ultrasound techniques capable of assessing cerebral perfusion at the cotside (Taylor 1998).

A further development in ultrasound technology has seen the emergence of 3-D imaging. This has been shown to be useful particularly in evaluating fetal craniofacial anomalies, but a definite role in neonatal imaging has not yet been established.

## COMPUTERIZED TOMOGRAPHY

The indications for CT have decreased over the last 10 years following the more widespread use of MRI, but CT still has a role in the evaluation of neurologic disorders in the neonate. The total examination time is shorter for CT than for MRI and it is generally easier to monitor the infant during a CT examination. Reduction in scan times, often down to 1–2 seconds for CT has reduced the need for sedation or general anesthesia in this age group. Most infants can be examined during sleep following a feed or wrapped in a blanket to reduce motion artifact. Injection of contrast agents is rarely indicated for the evaluation of common pathologies in the neonatal age range but may be necessary for the evaluation of suspected cerebral abscess, ventriculitis, vascular malformation and neoplasia. It is wise to insert the cannula prior to the scan being performed and light sedation may be useful to reduce patient movement precipitated by the injection.

Detailed attention to technique is essential to optimize any CT examination (Barkovich 1995; Flodmark 1995). In general, axial sections at a thickness of 5 mm are necessary in the neonate, although thinner sections may be appropriate, particularly where subtle pathology in the posterior fossa is suspected. A field of view appropriate to the size of the infant's head should be chosen to maximize resolution, but care should be taken to ensure that the infant's head is positioned in the centre of the gantry and that the entire intracranial contents are included in the scan (Flodmark 1995).

Interpretation of a CT scan in the neonate requires familiarity with the normal appearances on account of the higher water content of the neonatal brain. The white matter of the normal neonatal brain will be of lower attenuation compared with an older child and should not be erroneously misinterpreted as showing evidence of white matter edema. The window width should be set between 60–80 HU and the images viewed at a level of 25–35 HU (Barkovich 1995; Flodmark 1995).

The risk from exposure to ionizing radiation during a CT scan should be considered. The skull vault contains a third of the bone marrow in the neonate and thus the absorbed dose from a cranial CT may be disproportionately higher than for a body or chest CT (Chan *et al.* 1999). The estimated lifetime risk for the induction of fatal cancer is estimated to be 1:5000 for a child of up to 10 years of age compared to a risk of 1:1 000 000 for a chest X-ray. Several studies have shown that patients undergoing CT examinations receive a wide range in radiation dose which depends upon both the model of CT scanner used and the radiographic and examination technique employed (Shrimpton & Wall 1995). Thus the examination protocol should be tailored to suit the diagnostic requirements of the examination. In the majority of neonates the radiographic exposure can be reduced considerably below the standard adult setting of 200–250 Mas to 125–150 Mas, thereby reducing the dose by 40% (Chan *et al.* 1999). In addition the dose to the orbit can be significantly reduced by altering the scanning plane to 20 degrees above the orbito-meatal line (Casselden 1988).

## MAGNETIC RESONANCE IMAGING

The potential clinical value of magnetic resonance imaging (MRI) in the neonate was soon realized in the early 1980s. The greater soft tissue contrast inherent in MRI compared with CT permitted much better differentiation between gray and white matter and for the first time allowed us to assess the impact of pathological processes on the developing brain. Although the difficulties of performing an MRI scan are greater than for CT scanning, it is superior for most clinical indications at this age and has now become the definitive modality for imaging the neonatal brain. A full description of the basic principles of MRI scanning, choice of sequences and recognition of artifacts is available (Barkovich 1995; Boyer 1994; Huppi & Barnes 1997).

High field-strength units are preferable for neonatal scanning on account of the faster scan times, ability to obtain thinner sections using a smaller field of view, better signal-to-noise ratio and improved soft tissue contrast with better differentiation of gray from white matter. The precise choice of sequences will depend on the model and field strength of the scanner, the age of the baby and suspected pathology. Scanning protocols will generally be based on conventional T1- and T2-weighted spin echo, fast spin echo, inversion recovery or 3-D gradient echo sequences. Slice thickness between 3–5 mm is usually appropriate in the neonatal period. Although routine imaging of the brain in the adult and older child may require a single axial T2-weighted sequence, the complex changes and signal alterations associated with the developing brain require that both T1- and T2-weighted axial images are performed in most cases. A T1-weighted sagittal sequence is also useful as malformations of the brain may be associated with midline abnormalities which are well demonstrated in this plane. An additional coronal sequence may also be helpful to evaluate congenital malformations of the brain and other abnormalities in the cerebellum and around the tentorium.

Some abnormalities may be difficult to detect on standard T2-weighted images as the high water content of the premature brain may mask edema or cystic lesions at this age; T1- and T2-weighted sequences should be heavily weighted to account for this (Boyer 1994). Other sequences may be worth considering in specific clinical situations. Fluid attenuated inversion recovery (FLAIR) sequences null the signal from cerebrospinal fluid and give heavily weighted T2 images. This is of potential value in the neonate to help differentiate the high signal seen on standard T2-weighted images due to cystic periventricular leukomalacia (PVL) from the more chronic changes of PVL, i.e. gliosis (Okuda *et al.* 1998). T2* gradient echo sequences are particularly sensitive towards the detection of subtle areas of old hemorrhage as may be found in association with arterio-venous malformations, and may also be helpful in confirming the presence of previous hemorrhage which may not be evident on standard imaging.

Although it has been suggested that higher quality images are obtained when scanning the neonatal head using a knee coil, our experience supports that of Boyer who found the image quality superior using a standard quadrature head coil (Boyer 1994). Currently there are no commercially available head coils specifically designed for neonatal use.

There are few clinical indications for the administration of intravenous MRI contrast agents in the neonate. Gadopentetate dimeglumine is safe in the neonate and can be useful for the evaluation of inflammatory and neoplastic diseases, suspected phakomatoses and MR angiography, particularly venography.

The further development of gradient echo techniques and echo planar imaging has led to the development of fast and ultrafast sequences for imaging the brain which have resulted in the emergence of new MR applications of diffusion-weighted imaging and perfusion imaging.

### Normal anatomy and development

Development of the human brain is incomplete at birth in both the preterm and term newborn infant and continues for many months following birth. Although the normal development of the gyral pattern has been well documented on both ultrasound and MRI there is no doubt that MRI is superior in the comprehensive assessment of brain maturation, because the progressive stages of myelination, regression of the germinal matrix and extent of glial cell migration can all be visualized and followed on MRI (Fig. 6.3). The process of myelination has been studied most extensively. Early changes due to myelination tend to be better seen on T1-weighted images as evidenced by an increase in signal intensity due to the primary process of myelination. This increase in signal intensity on the T1-weighted images generally precedes the decrease in intensity of the T2-weighted images and probably reflects changes in water loss (Barkovich 1998). The T2-weighted images are superior to T1-weighted images to assess early maturation in the basal ganglia, cerebellum, and brainstem (Barkovich 1998, 2000a;

Martin *et al.* 1991; Van der Knapp *et al.* 1991). In a group of neurologically normal preterm and term neonates myelin appeared on MRI in the lateral part of the posterior limb of the internal capsule and in the central part of the corona radiata between 34 and 46 weeks of postconceptional age. The rapid process of cortical folding between 24 and 40 weeks can be readily followed on MRI. Before 24 weeks of gestation the brain is essentially agyric with the exception of the Sylvian fissure, which is initially very wide and appears vertically orientated. From 24 to 28 weeks the cortex shows the developing central Rolandic, pericallosal and intraparietal sulci; by 32–33 weeks an increased number of gyri and shallow sulci appear; from 34 weeks further thickening of the cerebral cortex is accompanied by the development of a nearly normal adult sulcal pattern by term (Barkovich 2000a).

In the very premature infant the distribution of the germinal matrix and migrating bands of glial cells can be followed

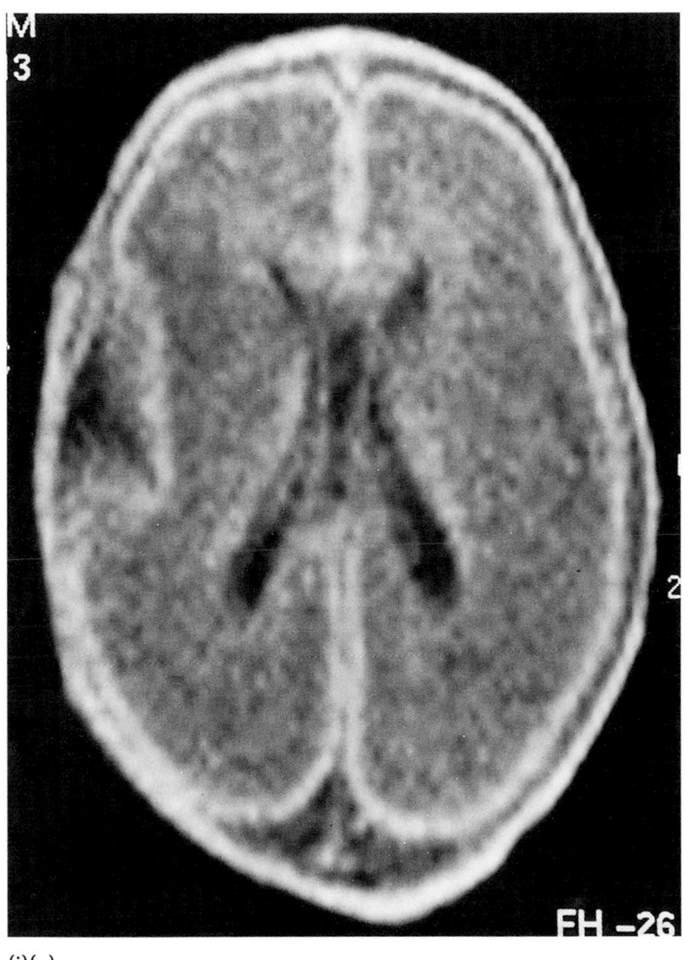


(i)(a)

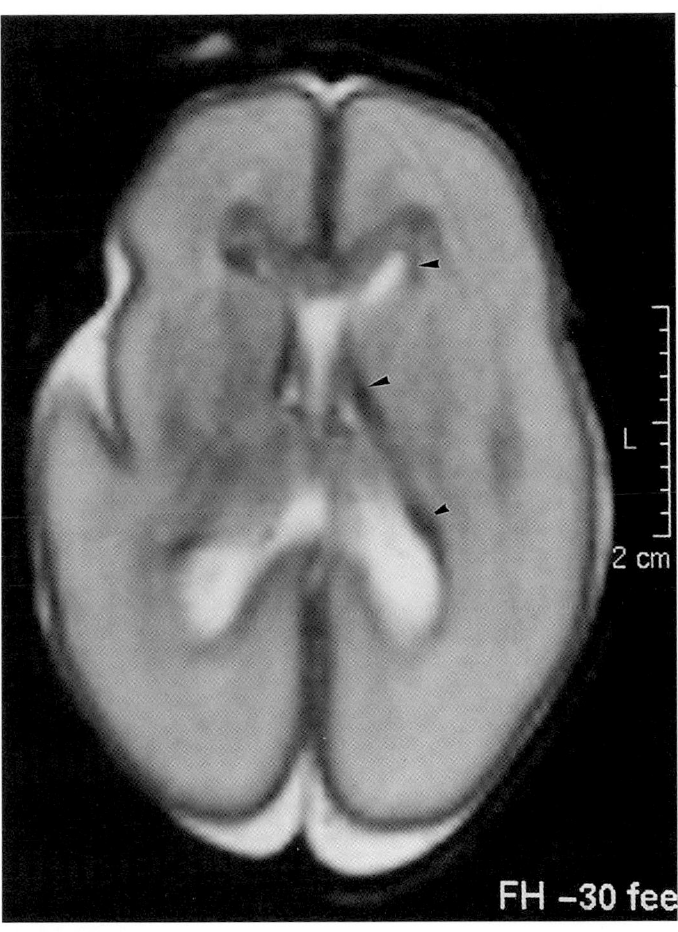


(i)(b)

**Figure 6.3** Progression of maturation as seen at the level of the basal ganglia and lateral ventricles at the level of the Foramen of Monroe. Series showing changes at increasing postmenstrual ages. (i) At *24 weeks gestation.* (a) T1- and (b) T2-weighted images showing the smooth cortex and wide open insula. No myelination of the basal ganglia is visible. The germinal matrix is evident on the T2-weighted image as a low intensity strip adjacent to the lateral ventricle around the frontal horns, caudo-thalamic notch, and posterior horn (arrowheads). (ii) *At 32 weeks gestation.* (a) T1- and (b) T2-weighted images showing the developing sulcation. Myelination is now seen as increased signal on T1-weighted image and decreased signal on T2-weighted image in the globus pallidus and ventrolateral thalamus (arrows). Germinal matrix is less evident, being mainly visible around the frontal horn and at the caudo-thalamic notch. Discrete bands of low signal noted in the frontal white matter on T2-weighted images are thought to represent bands of migrating glial cells (arrowheads). A small GMH-IVH is present on the left. (iii) At 37 weeks gestation. (a) T1- and (b) T2-weighted images showing further development of sulcation and some infolding of the insula. Myelination is visible in the posterior limb of the internal capsule (arrow). Germinal matrix is faintly visible around the frontal horns. The bands of migrating glial cells are becoming less prominent. (iv) At 44 weeks gestation. (a) T1- and (b) T2-weighted images showing mature sulcal pattern, with gray/white matter of isointensity on T1-weighted images. Myelination is visible in the anterior (arrow) and posterior limbs (arrowhead) of the internal capsule and optic radiation (long arrow). Germinal matrix and bands of migrating glial cells are no longer visible.

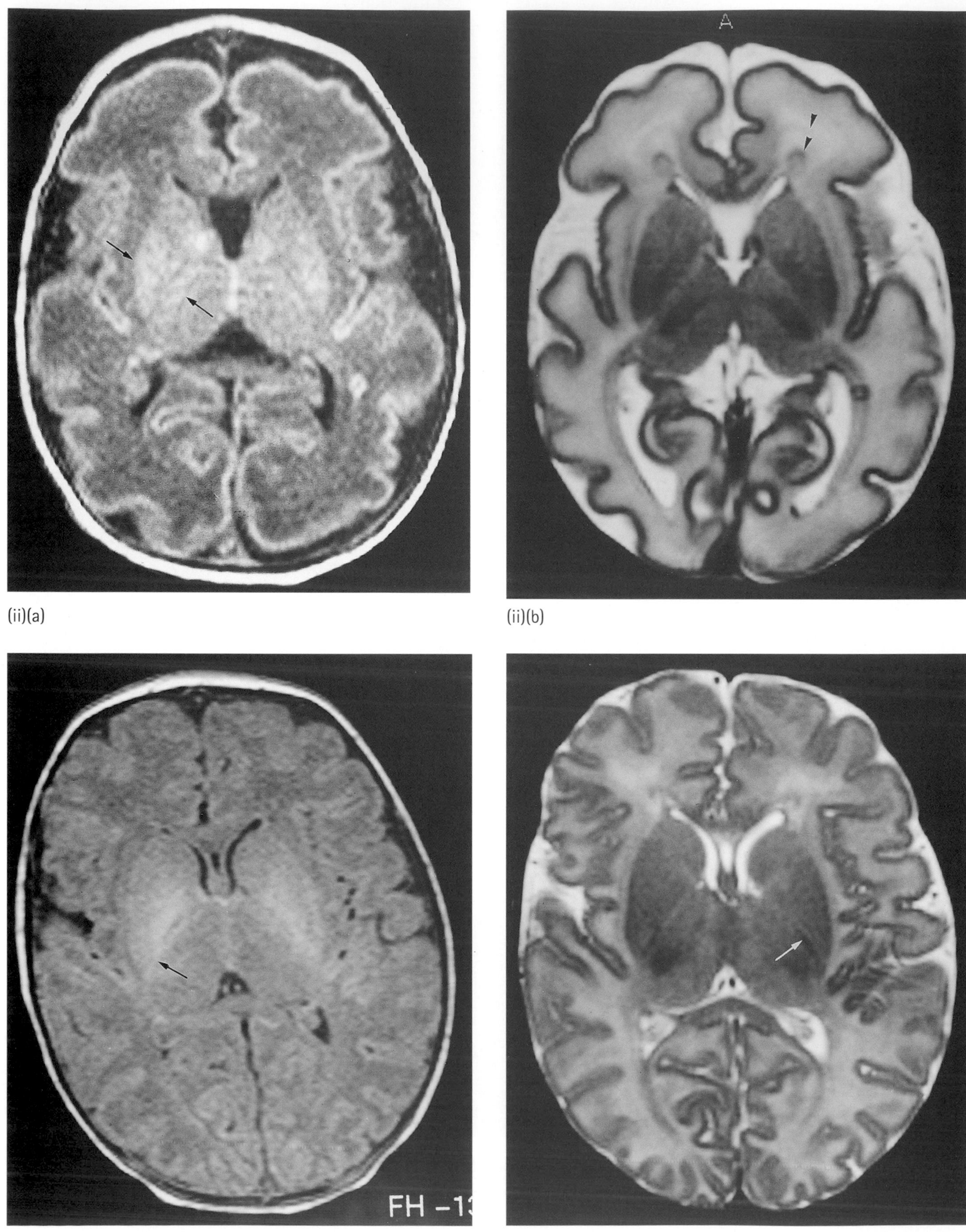


(ii)(a)

(ii)(b)

(iii)(a)

(iii)(b)

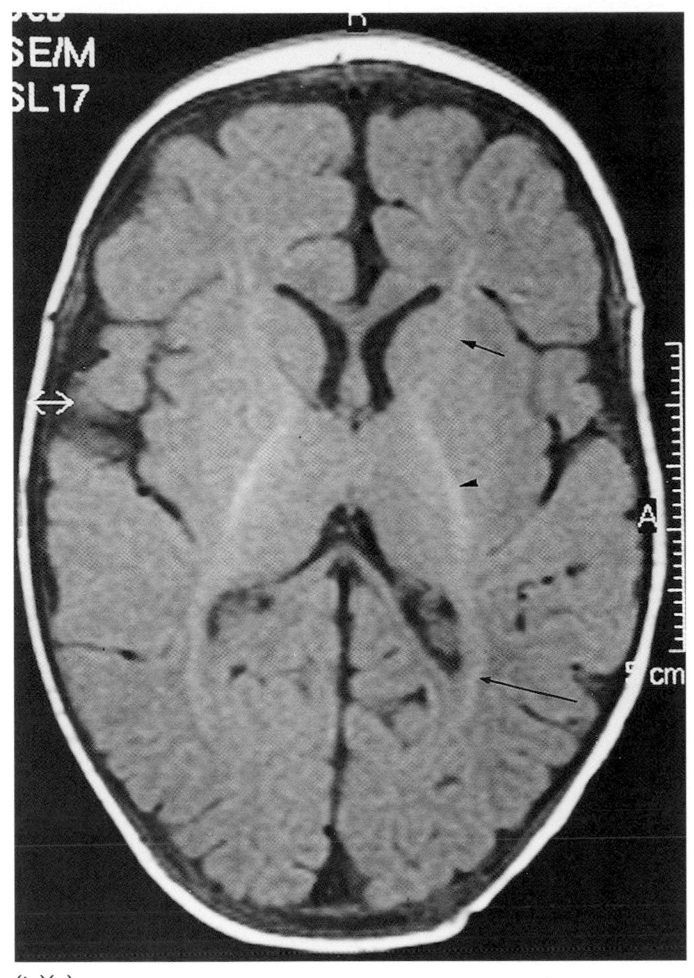


(iv)(a)

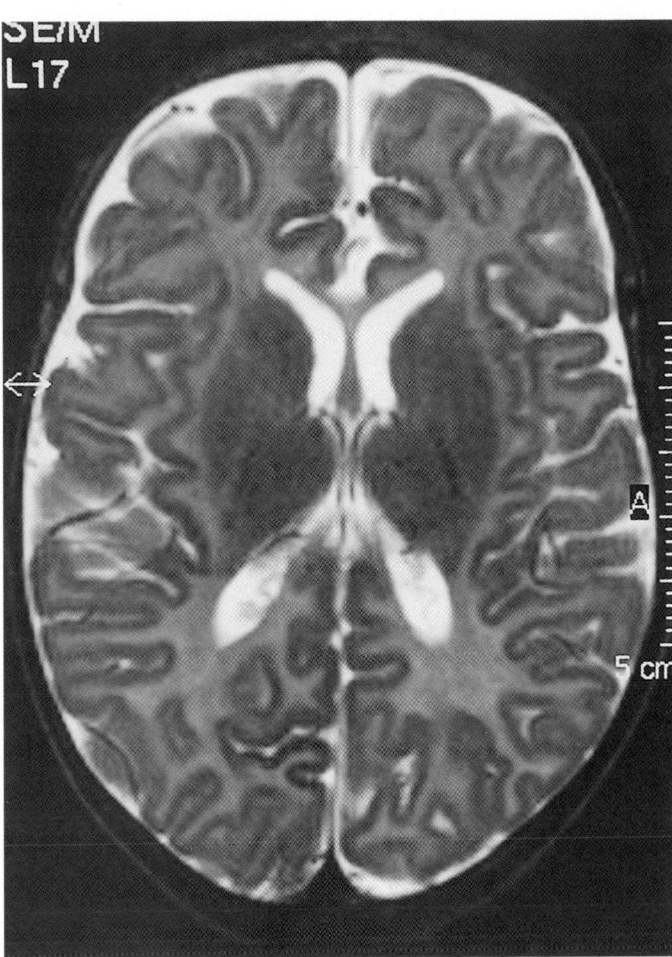


(iv)(b)

on high quality MRI images (Battin *et al.* 1998; Childs *et al.* 1998) (Fig. 6.3). The germinal matrix appears as a strip of low signal intensity on T2-weighted images lateral to the ventricles. Its anatomical representation is inversely related to gestational age and it can be visualized throughout the subependymal areas around 24–25 weeks postconceptual age. The germinal matrix gradually regresses with the last remnants being seen around the frontal areas of the lateral ventricles, often as late as nearly 40 weeks of postconceptual age (Evans *et al.* 1997). Discrete bands of altered signal intensity (high signal on T1-weighted images, low signal on T2-weighted images) have been described in the frontal white matter and are thought to represent bands of migrating glial cells (Childs *et al.* 1998). These bands become more diffuse and eventually disappear towards term and may also be used as a marker of increasing maturation.

## DIFFUSION WEIGHTED IMAGING

Diffusion weighted imaging (DWI) of the brain measures the diffusion of water molecules in the brain tissue. This allows ADC (apparent diffusion coefficient) maps of the brain to be generated to demonstrate areas of differing water diffusivity. On DWI, regions of low diffusivity appear hyperintense and thus areas of acute ischemia which demonstrate decreased water diffusion, possibly as a result of the development of cytotoxic edema, will appear as areas of increased intensity compared with the surrounding brain parenchyma. These changes may be apparent on DWI prior to any abnormality being detected on conventional sequences (Cowan *et al.* 1994; Huppi & Barnes 1997; Beaulieu *et al.* 1999; Inder *et al.* 1999). Following the acute insult the ADC values begin to rise due to increased diffusion of water possibly related to cell lysis (Fig. 6.4). ADC maps may change with age due to the decreasing water content of the developing brain and to increasing myelination and these changes must be taken into account when interpreting DWI (Tanner *et al.* 2000). Although further evaluation is required, DWI promises to be a valuable tool in the early assessment of hypoxic ischemic brain injury, particularly for focal lesions, in the neonate.

## MAGNETIC RESONANCE ANGIOGRAPHY AND VENOGRAPHY

MR angiography (MRA) and MR venography (MRV) are now established non-invasive techniques for the evaluation of

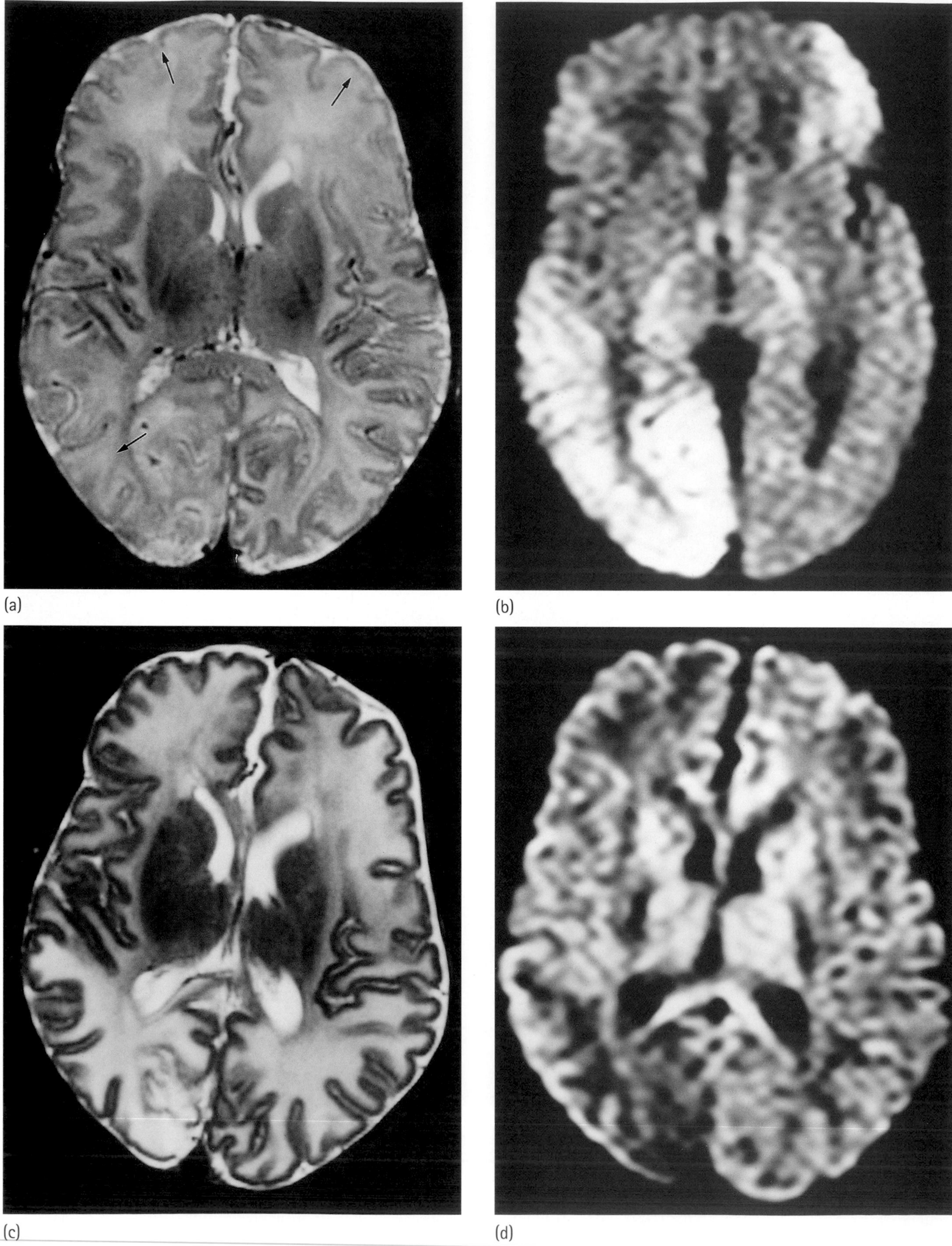
(a)
(b)
(c)
(d)

both intracranial and extracranial vascular disorders in adults. Experience with children is more limited and there are only occasional reports of its use in the neonate (Boyer 1994; Lee *et al.* 1995; Huppi & Barnes 1997). 3-D time of flight techniques are generally used to examine the arterial anatomy and 2-D time of flight for the venous anatomy, although other techniques using phase contrast methods have been used. Arterial and venous 'maps' are subsequently reconstructed from the raw data using maximal intensity projections at a workstation. Image quality is generally considered to be good, but the resolution is inferior to that of conventional angiography. MRA is generally good at detecting major stenoses or displacement of vessels, but currently cannot replace angiography for the evaluation of small vessel disease. Lee *et al.* (1995) have shown that these techniques are particularly useful in demonstrating the arterial and venous anatomy related to congenital malformations, in particular with regard to the patency and course of the superior sagittal sinus in relation to an occipital encephalocele. MRV was considered superior to conventional angiography in the assessment of thrombosis and compression of the dural venous sinuses.

Other MRI techniques have also been developed including perfusion imaging, functional imaging and MR spectroscopy (Logan 1999; Shevell *et al.* 1999). MR spectroscopy is proving to be a valuable tool in the diagnosis of metabolic disorders (see Chapter 10) of the brain and is likely to become increasingly important in the future, although the technology and expertise is not yet widely available for routine clinical use (Huppi & Barnes 1997; Shevell *et al.* 1999; Zinnermann & Wang 1997). Perfusion imaging and functional MRI imaging are still mainly research tools in the neonate. Both applications are technically demanding at this age, and very much at the development stage. As yet there are no established clinical applications for these techniques.

## RADIONUCLIDE IMAGING (see also Chapter 10)

Modern radionuclide imaging techniques are becoming increasingly important in the investigation of neurologic disorders in both adults and children, although currently their role in imaging the neonatal brain is confined to research applications. Cerebral single photon emission computerized tomography (SPECT) imaging assesses brain perfusion following the intravenous injection of $^{99m}$Tc-labeled hexamethyl-propylene amine oxime and is particularly valuable in the evaluation of suspected cerebrovascular disease (Bloom *et al.* 1996; Peter 1996). Positron emission tomography (PET) scanning is a relatively non-invasive method for studying brain activity which involves the intravenous injection of a tracer labeled with an unstable positron emitting isotope which can be subsequently mapped by the sensors in the PET scanner. In the neonatal age group, PET scanning is largely used as a research tool. In older children clinical applications for PET scanning include the identification of focal cortical abnormalities and epileptogenic foci in the investigation of intractable epilepsy, particularly when the MRI is normal (Kuzniecky 1996; Shulkin 1997; Mohan *et al.* 1999).

## RADIOGRAPHIC PATHOLOGY

### INTRACRANIAL HEMORRHAGE

Although the majority of intracranial hemorrhages seen in the neonate affect the low birth weight, premature infant, intracranial hemorrhage may also occur in the term infant, particularly in response to birth trauma. Hemorrhage into the germinal matrix and ventricular system is a particular feature of the neonate with a gestational age of less than 32 weeks. Term infants are more likely to suffer extra-axial hemorrhage in the subdural and subarachnoid compartments, but bleeding into the choroid plexus and subsequently the ventricles may occur. Other sites for neonatal intracranial hemorrhage include the cerebellum, basal ganglia, and cerebral hemispheres (see Chapter 21).

#### Ultrasound

Acute intracranial hemorrhage is very echogenic on ultrasound and will generally appear much more echogenic than the choroid plexus in the first week following the bleed (Fig. 6.5). Acute hemorrhage into the ventricular system may be difficult to see if the scan is performed immediately before the blood consolidates to form a clot. Between 1 and 2 weeks the degree of echogenicity begins to reduce with the center of the hematoma becoming more sonolucent than the rim, after which time the clot gradually becomes smaller and retracts from the margins of the brain or ventricular wall; the clot will usually have completely resorbed by 2–3 months (Siegel 1995).

#### CT scanning

Acute hemorrhage is clearly visualized immediately on CT whether the bleeding has occurred into the cerebral sub-

**Figure 6.4** Diffusion weighted imaging (DWI). Term baby with (a) T2-weighted image on day 4 demonstrating diffuse hyperintensity of the white matter, with subtle loss of differentiation between the cortex and subcortical white matter in both frontal and right parieto-occipital regions (arrows). (b) DWI performed the same day demonstrating corresponding areas of markedly increased signal intensity due to low diffusivity. (c) At 14 days later, T2-weighted image shows diffuse increased signal intensity of the white matter, most marked in the right parieto-occipital region. (d) DWI demonstrates regions of decreased signal intensity, due to increased diffusivity, in both frontal as well as the right posterior-parietal area.

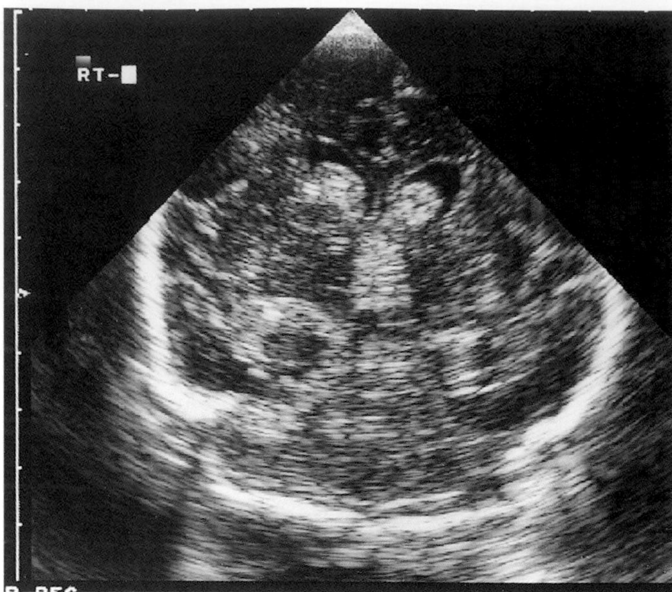


Figure 6.5 Coronal ultrasound image showing increased echogenicity due to bilateral intraventricular hemorrhages, with further hemorrhage evident in the third ventricle.

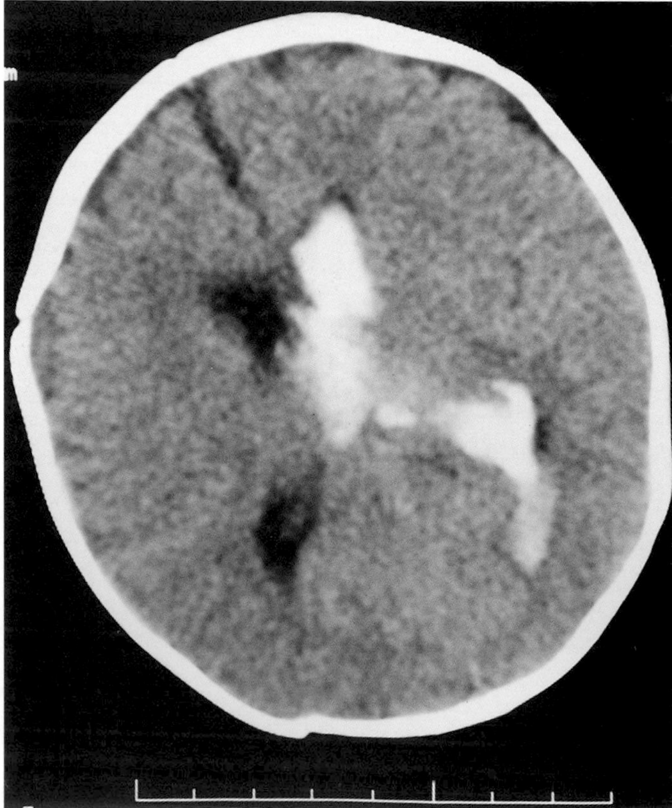

Figure 6.6 A 3-month-old infant with hemorrhagic disease of the newborn. Unenhanced axial CT scan demonstrating acute left-sided intraventricular hemorrhage.

stance or into the cerebrospinal fluid on account of the increased density of fresh haemorrhage (Fig. 6.6). Hemorrhage generally becomes isointense between 1 and 2 weeks on CT, and may make the presence of an old hemorrhage difficult to detect in the absence of any associated parenchymal damage. Thus ultrasound scanning is more sensitive than CT for the detection of subacute hemorrhage after the first week, as the hemorrhage should still be visible on ultrasound scanning after it has become isointense on CT.

## Magnetic resonance imaging

The appearances of intracranial hemorrhage are quite complex and have been extensively discussed in the literature, particularly in the mature brain (Barkovich 1995; Zuerrer *et al.* 1991; Huppi & Barnes 1997). A number of factors affect the appearance of hemorrhage on MRI scanning including the site of bleeding, i.e. whether the bleeding is intracerebral or into cerebrospinal fluid (CSF), the magnetic field strength and the level of T1- and T2-weighting of the scans and the age of the patient (Zuerrer *et al.* 1991; Huppi & Barnes 1997). The changes of the MRI appearances of hemorrhage as imaged on lower field strength MRI scanners (<1.5 T) are summarized in Table 6.1. In the hyperacute stage, intracerebral hemorrhage appears indistinguishable from water or edema at most field strengths. At higher field strength acute hemorrhage may appear iso- to hypointense on T1-weighted images and iso- to hypointense on T2-weighted images due to the enhanced susceptibility of deoxyhemoglobin, which is proportional to the strength of the magnet. Over the next few days, as intracellular oxyhemoglobin is deoxygenated to deoxyhemoglobin, the hemorrhage becomes very hypointense on T2-weighted images caused by selective shortening of T2. After approximately 7 days intracellular deoxyhemoglobin metabolizes to paramagnetic methemoglobin, which causes T1 shortening, i.e. high signal intensity on T1-weighted images. Lysis of erythrocytes then begins and hemorrhage becomes hyperintense on both T1- and T2-weighted images. In the chronic stages methemoglobin is metabolized to ferritin and hemosiderin, which appear as iso- or hypointense on T1-weighted images and hypointense on T2-weighted images.

The pattern of signal intensity change differs for hemorrhage into CSF, e.g. ventricular fluid compared to intracerebral bleeding. The deoxygenation of oxyhemoglobin is slower on account of the higher $PO_2$ in the CSF compared with the white matter, and the pattern of signal changes appears more slowly (Zuerrer *et al.* 1991).

Thus with lower field strengths MRI is less sensitive than CT scanning in the detection of hyperacute and acute hemorrhage, as hemorrhage is indistinguishable from water or edema (Boyer 1994). However, MRI is very sensitive in the detection of subacute and chronic hemorrhage, and is a valuable tool in helping to determine the age of a hemorrhage. Hemosiderin staining occurs after about one month and may remain visible for many months (Boyer 1994).

**Table 6.1 Outline of MRI signal changes following intracranial hemorrhage**

| | Time from hemorrhage | T1 | T2 |
|---|---|---|---|
| Hyperacute | <24 hours | Iso or hypointense | Iso-hyperintense[a] |
| Acute | 24–72 hours | Iso or hypointense | Hypointense |
| Subacute | 4 days - 2 weeks | Hyperintense | Hypointense |
| Early chronic | 2–8 weeks | Hyperintense | Hyperintense |
| Late chronic | >8 weeks (hemosiderin) | Iso or hypointense | Hypointense |

[a]T2 shortening may occur after a few hours with higher field strength magnets and acute hemorrhage may appear hypointense even in the early acute phase on T2-weighted images (Fig. 6.7).
*Source*: Adapted from Huppi & Barnes (1997).

## GERMINAL MATRIX HEMORRHAGE–INTRAVENTRICULAR HEMORRHAGE (GMH–IVH)

This is the most frequent and important cause of intracranial hemorrhage in the neonate (pp 339–356). Ultrasound is now accepted as the primary modality for the diagnosis of GMH-IVH and full descriptions of the ultrasonic findings are well reported (Hay *et al.* 1989; Teele & Share 1991; Siegel 1995). GMH can be recognized as a globular area of intense increased echogenicity beneath the floor of the lateral ventricle, just anterior to the caudothalamic notch. The abnormality should be demonstrated in two planes and should be distinguished from other normal echogenic structures such as the normal choroid plexus. Larger hemorrhages may rupture into the lateral ventricle and when acute appear as an echogenic clot within the ventricle which may distend the ventricular lumen. Approximately 10–20% of neonates with large GMH-IVHs subsequently develop an associated parenchymal echodensity due to the development of venous infarction (Shankaran *et al.* 1982; Levene & de Vries 1984; Volpe 1997). Venous infarction should be distinguished from periventricular echodensity which is caused by hypoxic ischemic injury. The echodensity associated with periventricular leukomalacia is generally bilateral and may or may not be associated with IVH, whereas the echodensity of venous infarction is usually unilateral and associated with a large IVH that distends the lateral ventricle (Takashima *et al.* 1986; Trounce *et al.* 1986; Gould *et al.* 1987; Siegel 1995). However, GMH-IVH and periventricular leukomalacia can coexist and in some cases it may be difficult to differentiate between the two conditions by ultrasound scanning. (McMenamin *et al.* 1984; Grant & Schellinger 1985; Goetz *et al.* 1995).

The appearance of GMH-IVH and venous infarction change with time. GMHs resolve leaving a small subependymal cyst or a linear echodense line. The margins of a clot within the lateral ventricles remain echogenic whilst the more central region gradually becomes increasingly echopoor and smaller until the hemorrhage finally resolves by approximately 12 weeks of age. Resolution of an area of venous infarction is generally accompanied by the formation of a porencephalic communication with the lateral ventricle as the area of hemorrhage retracts and is absorbed. Mild ventricular dilatation commonly occurs following IVH but will become static or resolve in approximately 65% of these infants (Roland & Hill 1997). Careful monitoring will be necessary in these infants to determine whether ventricular decompression occurs.

Several grading systems have been proposed to classify GMH-IVH, the majority of which are based on the extent of bleeding into the germinal matrix and lateral ventricle, the development of venous infarction and the presence of ventricular dilatation (Papile *et al.* 1978, de Vries *et al.* 1985, 1998). However, the grades do not correlate closely with long-term outcome, which may be influenced to a greater extent by coexisting periventricular leukomalacia (Flodmark 1995). The classification proposed by de Vries is given in Table 6.2.

The accuracy of ultrasound imaging in the diagnosis of GMH-IVH is reported to be approximately 90% which is comparable to diagnosis by CT (Dewbury and Bates 1981; Babcock *et al.* 1982; Pape *et al.* 1983; Trounce *et al.* 1986b). Thus ultrasound imaging has now become the imaging modality of choice for the detection of GMH-IVH, as it can be performed on a daily basis if necessary, with no risk of exposure to ionizing radiation or the need to move the infant to the imaging department. Nevertheless, CT is very accurate for the diagnosis of hemorrhage and may detect

**Table 6.2 Grading system for the classification of GMH-IVH**

| | |
|---|---|
| Grade I | Small germinal matrix hemorrhage (GMH) |
| Grade IIa | GMH plus intraventricular hemorrhage (IVH) filling the ventricle <50% |
| Grade IIb | Large IVH distending lateral ventricle in the acute phase >50% |
| Grade III | IVH associated with unilateral parenchymal involvement |

*Source*: de Vries *et al.* (1998).

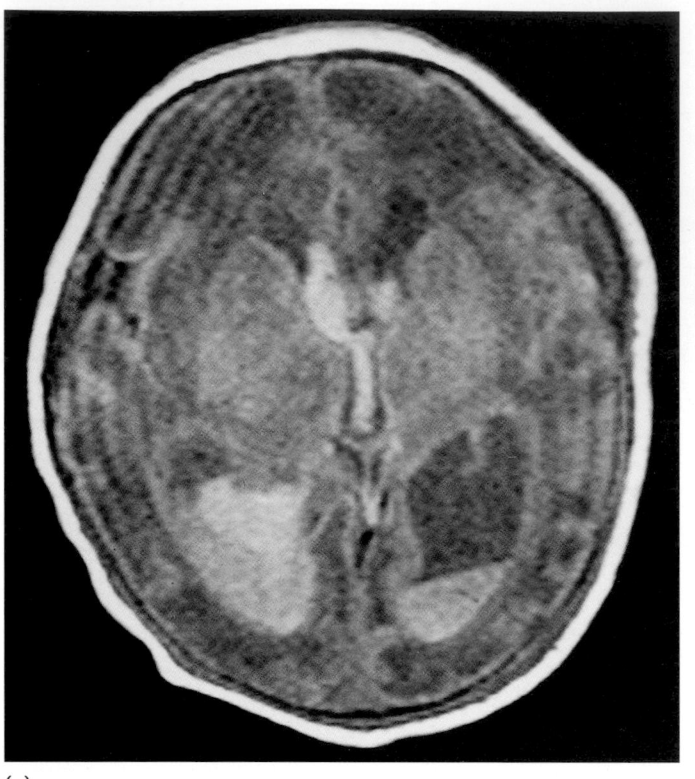

(a)

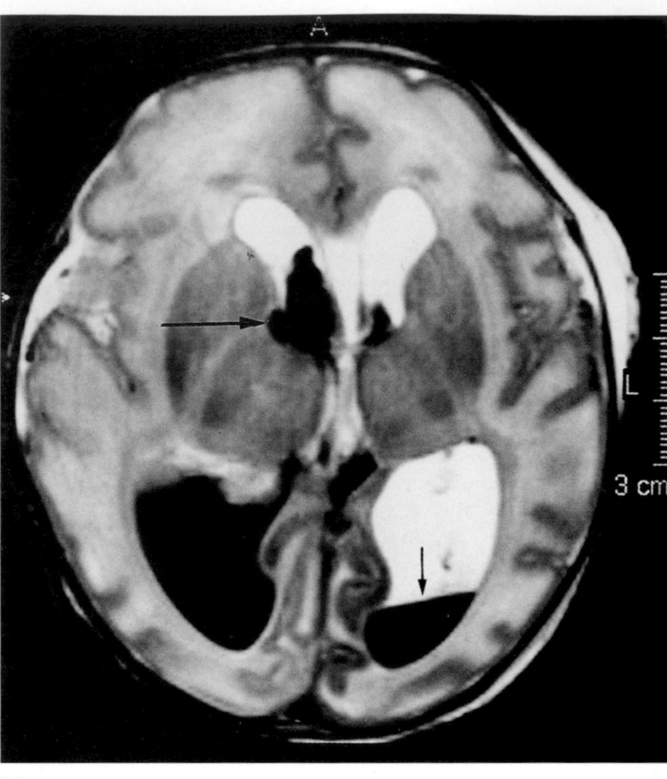


(b)

**Figure 6.7** (a) T1- and (b) T2-weighted images acquired with at 1.5T magnet demonstrating large bilateral intraventricular hemorrhages extending into the third ventricle, with fluid–fluid level within the lateral ventricles (arrow). Subependymal extension of the hemorrhage is noted on the right (long arrow). The hemorrhage is slightly hyperintense on T1-weighted and hypointense on T2-weighted images despite being less than 72 hours old. This reflects the earlier changes seen with higher field strength magnets. (Some movement artifact is noted on the images.)

small areas of parenchymal hemorrhage in the acute phase, in the periphery of the brain, which are not easily visualized on an ultrasound examination (Flodmark *et al.* 1980a,b). MRI scanning is not appropriate for scanning the sick unstable neonate because of both the practical difficulties and the lack of sensitivity in the detection of hemorrhage in the acute phase (see above). MRI, however, may have a role to assess the full extent of any parenchymal injury once the infant's general condition has stabilized. Keeney demonstrated that MRI performed between 29 and 44 weeks postconceptual age, was superior to ultrasound and CT in both the assessment of the extent of any parenchymal injury and for differentiating parenchymal injury associated with GMH-IVH (Keeney *et al.* 1991).

## INTRAPARENCHYMAL HEMORRHAGE (p. 362)

Intracerebral, cerebellar, or thalamic hemorrhages may occur as a primary event although hemorrhage into an area of infarction particularly associated with GMH-IVH is more common. Primary hemorrhage (Fig. 6.8) may occur as a result of a birth trauma, clotting disorder, or possibly an underlying arterio-venous malformation. In general, ultrasound scanning should be chosen as the first imaging modality, but if the ultrasound scan is normal and there is a strong clinical suspicion of acute hemorrhage, a CT scan should be considered. Hemorrhage occurring peripherally in the brain or in the cerebellum may not be easy to visualize by ultrasound, particularly if the anterior fontanelle is relatively small (Hay *et al.* 1989, Boyer 1994). In the subacute stage, MRI scanning is generally more sensitive than CT scanning (see above) and should be substituted for CT, if available, where hemorrhage is thought to be more than a week old.

## SUBDURAL AND SUBARACHNOID HEMORRHAGE (see also p. 356 and p. 359)

Extra-axial hemorrhage is best evaluated in the acute phase by CT scanning (Fig. 6.1), although ultrasound scanning can be useful to assess the size of any subdural collection on follow-up. MRI scanning is particularly valuable at detecting older hemorrhage in the extra-axial space. The multiplanar capability of MRI scanning also increases its sensitivity, since scanning in the sagittal and coronal planes may be helpful in demonstrating hemorrhage around the tentorium. If MRI is not available, CT scanning may need to be performed in a direct coronal or clival-perpendicular plane to

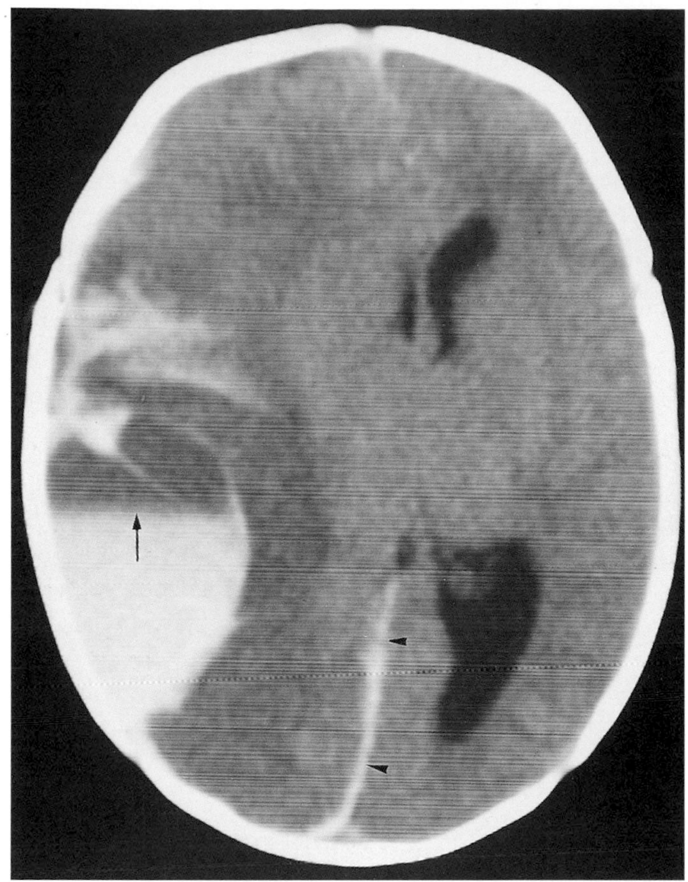

Figure 6.8 Unenhanced CT scan demonstrating a large acute intracerebral hemorrhage in a 1-month-old infant. A fluid–fluid level is noted centrally within the hematoma (arrow). There is a marked peripheral region of decreased attenuation due to edema contributing to the mass effect, with midline shift to the left and effacement of the right lateral ventricle. Extra-axial hemorrhage is also noted in the interhemispheric fissure (arrowheads).

demonstrate tentorial and cerebellar hemorrhage well (Boyer 1994). An acute subdural hemorrhage may be detected as an echogenic fluid collection in the extra-axial space on an ultrasound scan. The fluid collections result in easier visualization of the cortical surface of the brain and separation of the interhemispheric fissure. The gyri may become flattened and the ventricles compressed. An increased echogenicity of the extra-axial fluid should be considered suspicious for hemorrhage. Subarachnoid hemorrhage is poorly demonstrated by ultrasound although large acute presentations may be visualized as echogenic fluid collections over the convexities.

## HYPOXIC ISCHEMIC BRAIN INJURY

### Preterm infant

The response of the neonatal brain to hypoxic ischemic injury is variable and depends upon both the gestational age of the infant at the time of the insult and the severity of the hypoxic ischemic episode. In the preterm infant the deep white matter of the periventricular regions are most at risk. Increased periventricular echodensity in the frontal or peritrigonal white matter may be the first indication on cranial sonography of an ischemic injury to the brain in a preterm infant. This usually occurs within 24–48 hours of the insult, and may represent areas of both hemorrhagic and non-hemorrhagic infarction occurring in the vascular watershed regions of the premature infant's brain. These echodensities may be transient and disappear over the course of the next few days or weeks, persist unchanged, or undergo cystic degeneration to give rise to the classical-ultrasonic appearances of cystic periventricular leukomalacia (PVL) (Trounce *et al.* 1986a; de Vries *et al.* 1988a,b; Ringleberg & van der Bor 1993) (Fig 6.9). In some cases the early echodensity may resolve and the ultrasound scan become normal prior to the later development of cystic PVL (Dubowitz *et al.* 1985). The spectrum of PVL abnormalities detected by ultrasound scan is graded by de Vries *et al.* (1992) and is shown in Table 6.3.

**Table 6.3 Grading system for PVL lesions detected on ultrasound imaging**

| | |
|---|---|
| Grade I | Periventricular echodense area, present for >7 days or more |
| Grade II | Periventricular echodense areas evolving into localized frontoparietal cysts |
| Grade III | Periventricular echodense areas evolving into multiple cysts in the parieto-occipital white matter |
| Grade IV | Echodense areas in the deep white matter, with evolution into multiple subcortical cysts |

*Source*: de Vries *et al.* (1992).

Cystic changes usually occur 2–4 weeks after the initial insult but may take much longer to appear (Goetz *et al.* 1995). Cysts may be of varying sizes which may change over time, with some coalescing to become larger and others disappearing. In time, the cysts become less apparent and may not be seen on ultrasound scans, particularly 3 months after the initial insult. As the cysts disappear, evidence of white matter injury may become apparent on subsequent ultrasound scans, as indicated by ventricular dilatation, the development of an irregular wavy outline to the ventricular margins, and widening of the interhemispheric fissure and cortical sulci (Bozynski *et al.* 1985; Dubowitz *et al.* 1985; Volpe 1997).

It is now well accepted that the presence of periventricular echodensity without subsequent cystic degeneration may be a marker for hypoxic ischemic injury (Appleton *et al.* 1990; Trounce *et al.* 1986b; de Vries *et al.* 1988a; Ringleberg & van de Bor 1993; de Vries & Levene 1995). The echodensity may only be present for a few days and probably represents edema and congestion, without necessarily indicating permanent injury. Echodensities which persist beyond 7 days but do not become cystic are thought to represent the milder end of the spectrum of PVL (PVL grade 1) and are generally referred to as transient parenchymal echodensities or flares. Pathological echodensity can usually be differentiated from the normal physiological peritrigonal blush as the margins of an echodensity are usually more discrete and the echodensity more intense and inhomogeneous than the diffuse area of relatively mild echodensity that characterizes the normal peritrigonal blush (Figs 6.2 and 6.9a). In coronal section pathological echodensity is generally triangular in shape, with the apex pointing towards the angle of the lateral ventricle (Grant *et al.* 1983; Di Pietro *et al.* 1986).

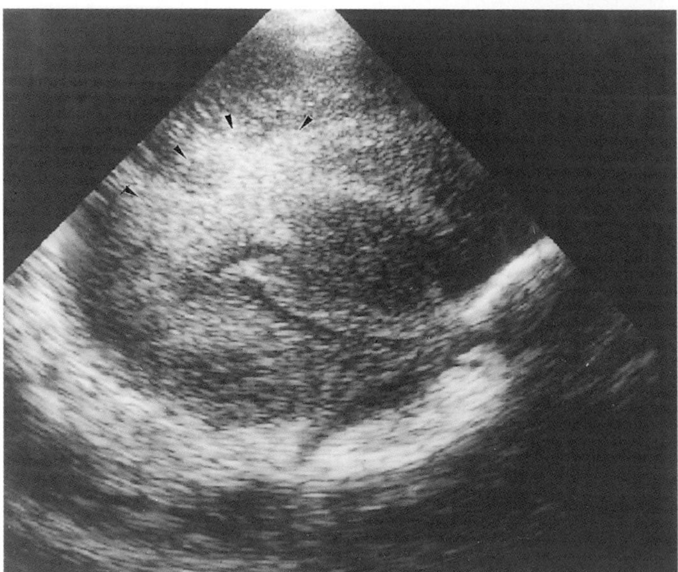

(a)

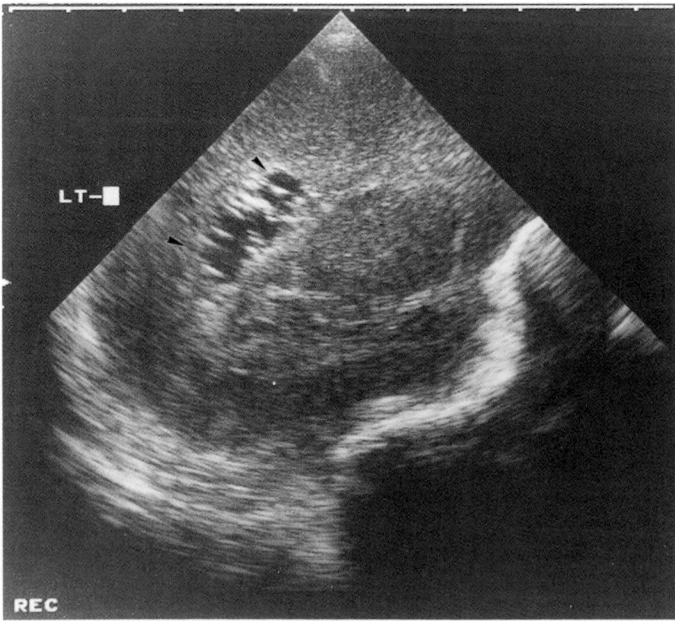


(b)

**Figure 6.9** Hypoxic ischemic injury in a premature infant. Sagittal ultrasound scans showing (a) pathological increased echodensity in the posterior parietal region (arrowheads), and (b) cavitational PVL (arrowheads).

Although some authors have reported a high sensitivity and specificity for the detection of PVL, this has been questioned by others. Hope *et al.* demonstrated a sensitivity of 28% and specificity of 86% compared with Trounce who reported an accuracy of 90%, sensitivity 91%, and specificity 93% (Trounce *et al.* 1986a; Hope *et al.* 1988). The presence of cystic change and hemorrhage within the area of infarction is said to increase the detection of PVL on ultrasound examination (Nwaesei *et al.* 1984; Baarsma *et al.* 1987; de Vries *et al.* 1988b; Paneth *et al.* 1990). False negative ultrasound examinations can be associated with failure to detect small areas of PVL and areas of gliosis in the periventricular white matter (Di Pietro *et al.* 1986; Baarsma *et al.* 1987; Skranes *et al.* 1993; Goetz *et al.* 1995).

CT is of little value in further investigation of hypoxic ischemic injury in the premature infant. Ischemic lesions will appear as low density areas in the deep white matter but do not show well due to the normal low attenuation of the white matter in this age group (Flodmark *et al.* 1980a; Boyer 1994; Barkovich 1997). The role of CT scanning in these babies is reserved for the exceptional case where there is poor correlation between the ultrasound findings and clinical examination, and MRI scanning is not available.

The high soft tissue contrast inherent in MRI scanning is an excellent modality for detecting all stages of PVL (de Vries *et al.* 1993, Boyer 1994, Barkovich 1997). However, its use is generally reserved for the evaluation of the extent of injury during the recovery phase on account of the practical difficulties of scanning the very sick neonate during its first few days of life. Signal abnormality due to brain injury may be shown within 2–3 days of the insult as areas either punctate or more extensive areas of T1 shortening (high signal intensity on T1-weighted images and low signal on T2-weighted sequences) (Barkovich 1997) (Fig. 6.10).

Punctuate (or petechial) lesions are predominately seen in preterm neonates; most commonly they are linearly organized and border the lateral ventricles. Their origin is most probably hemorrhagic, and they may represent a mild form of PVL. Caution is needed when interpreting isolated punctate lesions seen on MRI as their clinical significance with regard to long-term outlook is uncertain (Cornette *et al.* 2000). Early reports suggest that diffusion-weighted imaging may have the potential to demonstrate abnormality in the diffusion of water in the cerebral white matter before abnormality can be detected by conventional MRI (Inder *et al.* 1999). Thus MRI has the potential to confirm the presence of brain injury prior to the detection of cystic PVL on ultrasound examination, although its potential clinical value in the management of the critically ill neonate has not yet been fully evaluated.

Later changes include the development of cystic PVL, as

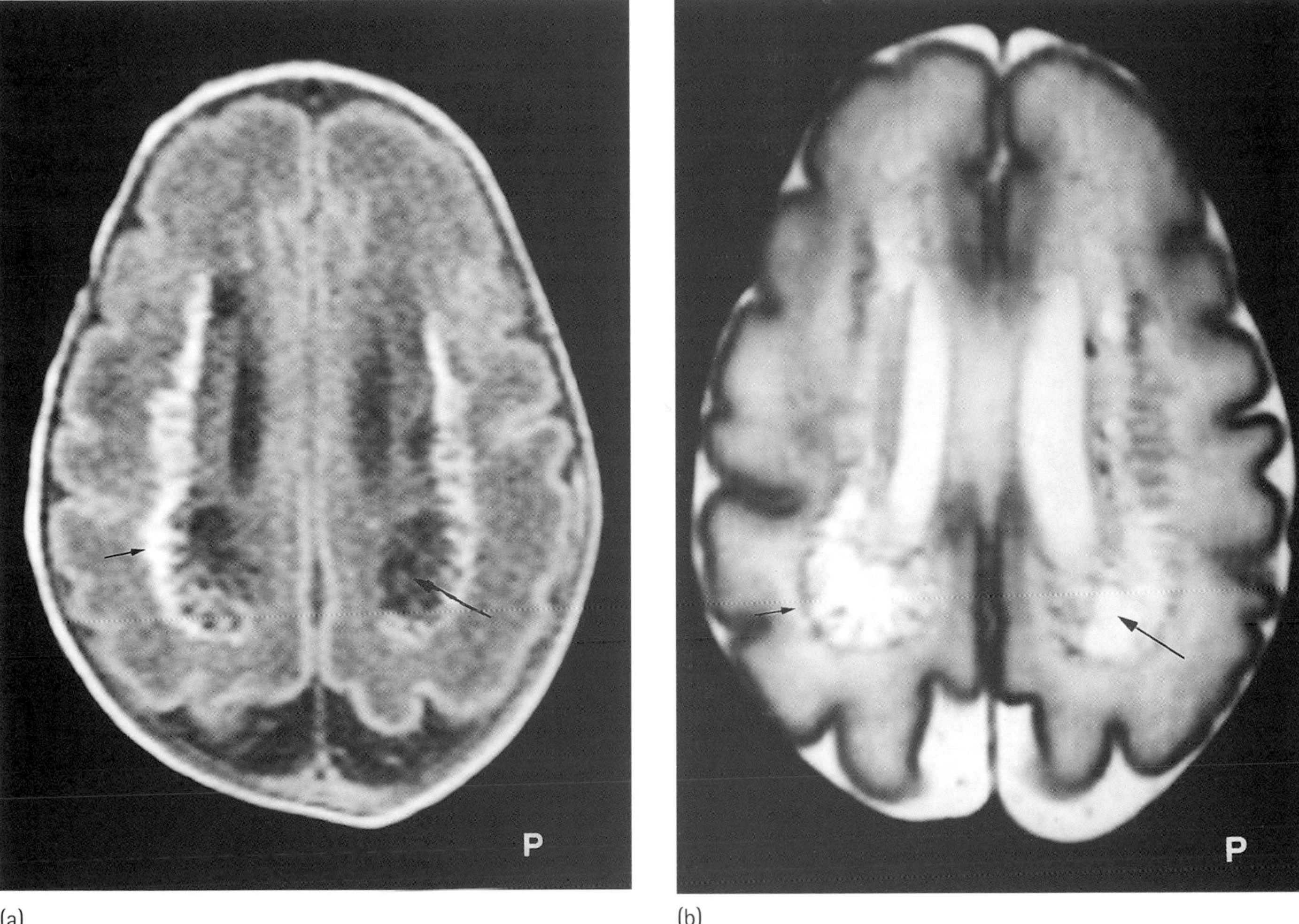


(a) (b)

**Figure 6.10** PVL in a preterm infant. (a) Axial T1- and (b) T2-weighted images. Bilateral signal abnormality secondary to hypoxic ischemic injury is noted in the deep white matter with increased signal on T1-weighted and decreased signal on T2-weighted images in a linear distribution (short arrows). More centrally, the changes of cystic PVL are well established with multiple small cysts developing showing signal characteristics similar to that of CSF (long arrows). There is mild ventricular dilatation.

demonstrated by the development of multiple cysts in the periventricular white matter (Fig. 6.10). The longer term sequelae of PVL are well demonstrated on MRI scans. The most frequent abnormality, seen in older children with PVL, is high signal intensity on T2-weighted images in a periventricular distribution, thought to represent gliosis. Other features include thinning of the white matter and corpus callosum, enlargement of the lateral ventricles and the development of irregular ventricular outlines.

Many studies have reported the sensitivity and specificity of periventricular infarction and cavitational periventricular leukomalacia detected by both ultrasound and more recently by MRI to predict long-term outcome in preterm babies. However, the data from different studies are often difficult to compare on account of varying terminology and recruitment. The prediction of outcome based on imaging findings is fully discussed in Chapter 22.

### Term infant

Brain injury in term babies with clinical evidence of hypoxic ischemic encephalopathy (HIE) arising from perinatal asphyxia tends to affect the basal ganglia, particularly the ventro-lateral thalami and posterior putamen. Less frequently injury may occur to the hippocampi, the cerebral cortex and subcortical white matter, particularly the perirolandic region (Banker & Laroche 1962; Leech & Ellsworth 1977; Takashima & Tanaka 1978; Babcock & Ball 1983; Pasternak *et al.* 1991, 1998; Barkovich 1992, 2000b; Connolly *et al.* 1994; Cowan *et al.* 1994; Rutherford *et al.* 1994; Grant & Barkovich 1998/1999; Roland *et al.* 1998). Injury to the brainstem nuclei is most commonly associated with severe hypoxic ischemic encephalopathy although these lesions have also been described in association with less severe injury to the basal ganglia (Leech & Ellsworth 1977; Barkovich 2000b).

It is unclear why certain regions of the brain are preferentially damaged. A combination of different factors have been suggested including the severity and duration of the hypotensive asphyxial event, the presence of relatively avascularized areas (watershed zones) in the white matter, the level of metabolic activity in certain areas compared to others (higher during active myelination), and the distribution of *N*-methyl-D-aspartate (NMDA) receptors. Whilst changes due to HIE are well documented on both ultrasound and CT, MRI is now considered the imaging of choice for the evaluation of extent and distribution of injury (Barkovich 2000b).

### Ultrasound

In the very acute phase the brain may appear normal on ultrasound imaging even following a significant episode of HIE. Cerebral edema and raised intracranial pressure may be suspected by demonstrating a subtle generalized increase in echogenicity of the white matter, in association with slit-like ventricles. Areas of infarction, particularly when associated with hemorrhage in the cerebral cortex, deeper white matter and basal ganglia may be detected as areas of abnormal increase in echogenicity (Fig. 6.11). In the chronic phase, ultrasound scanning may demonstrate the development of periventricular or multicystic encephalomalacia.

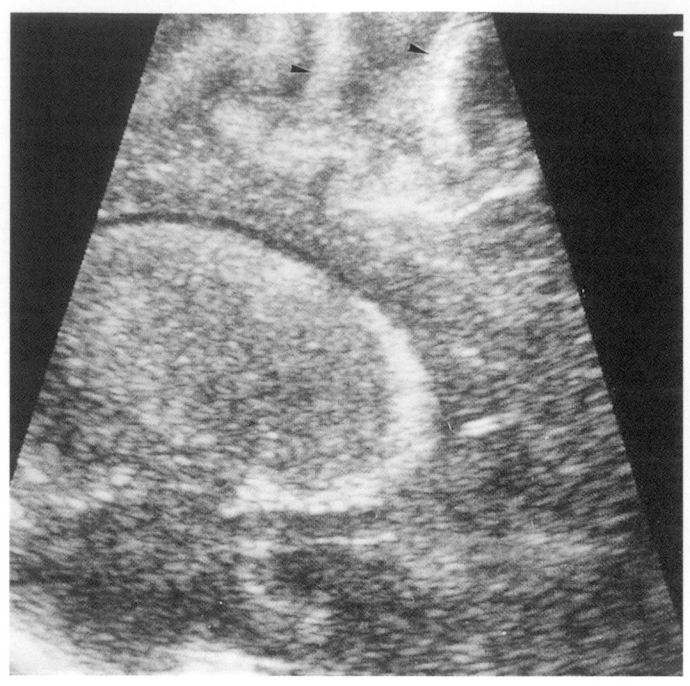

**Figure 6.11** Parasagittal ultrasound scan showing increased echogenicity within the gyri in keeping with cortical infarction (arrowheads).

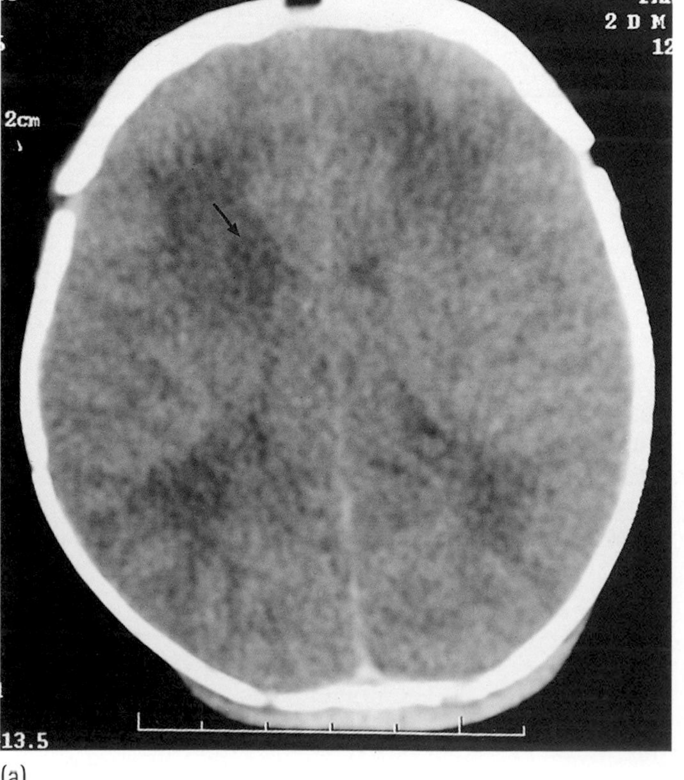


(a)

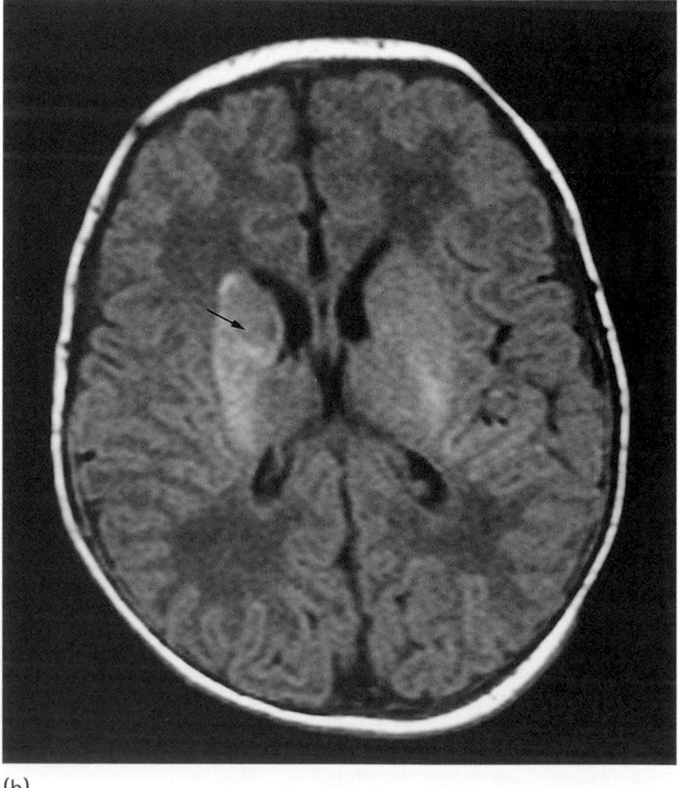

(b)

**Figure 6.12** Hypoxic ischemic encephalopathy. (a) Axial unenhanced CT scan at 2 days demonstrating reduced white matter attenuation in both cerebral hemispheres extending into region of the putamen on the right (arrow). (b) T1-weighted axial MRI more clearly demonstrating increased signal in both basal ganglia, particularly in the putamina and generalized decreased signal in the deep white matter secondary to cerebral edema.

### Computed tomography

Hemorrhagic infarction and extra-axial hemorrhage is well demonstrated on CT but non-hemorrhagic lesions, particularly in the cerebral cortex and deep white matter, are less well seen especially in the acute phase, as edema may be difficult to differentiate from the physiologically normal low attenuation seen in the frontal and occipital regions in the newborn infant (Cowan *et al.* 1994) (Fig. 6.12). CT is also relatively insensitive for the detection of injury involving the brain stem nuclei which are known to be associated with an adverse outcome.

### Magnetic resonance imaging

MRI is thought to be the most appropriate technique to image brain injury following perinatal asphyxia in the term newborn infant (Barkovich 2000b). Although a number of pathological features of HIE may be demonstrated on MRI, abnormal signal in the basal ganglia is the most characteristic lesion (Fig. 6.13). These lesions have a variable appearance relating to the time following the insult as summarized in Table 6.4.

In the acute phase MRI shows areas of diffuse increase in signal on T1-weighted images which become more discrete, patchy or globular areas of altered signal in the subacute phase. Initially T2-weighted images demonstrate a subtle alteration in signal intensity which may be isointense with white matter, before evolving into a more heterogeneous appearance with patchy areas of both high and low signals developing in the basal nuclei. Selective injury to the basal ganglia is not specific and may be associated with injury

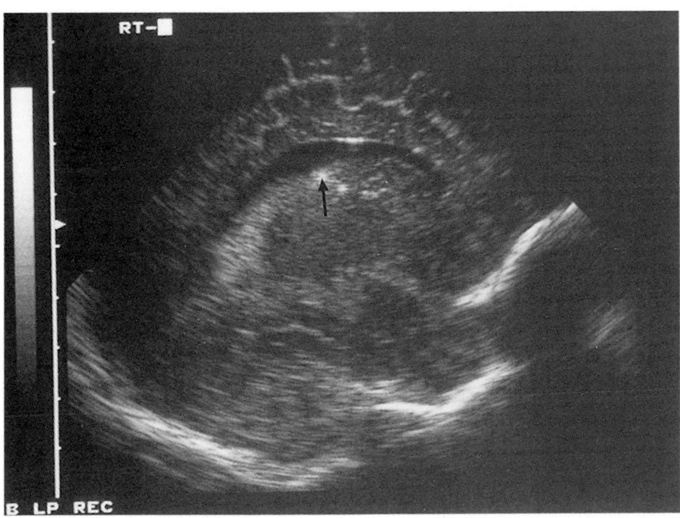


(a)

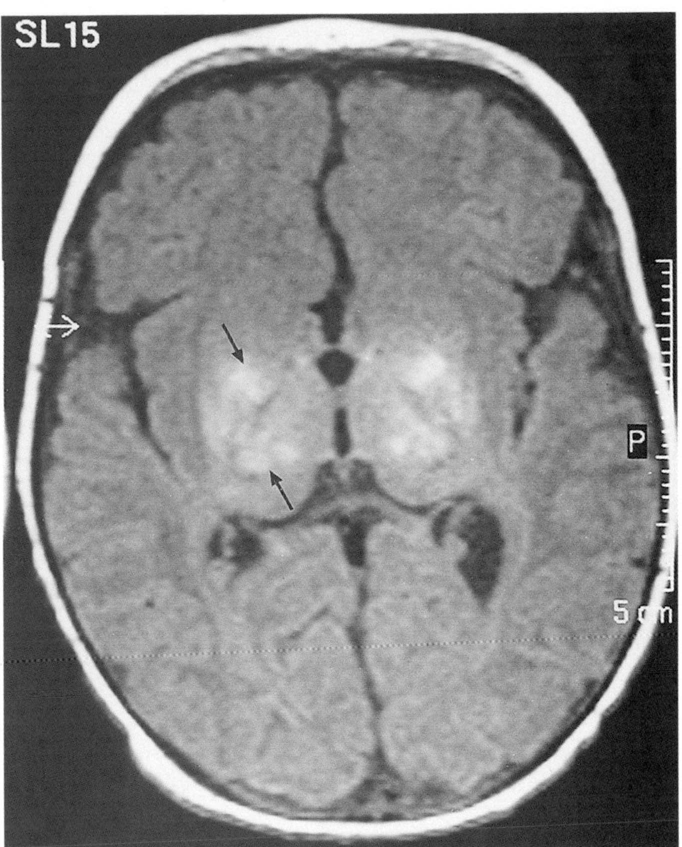


(b)

(c)

**Figure 6.13** Hypoxic ischemic encephalopathy. (a) Sagittal ultrasound examination at 26 days of age, demonstrating punctate echogenic lesions in the head of the caudate nucleus (arrow). (b) T1-weighted axial MRI (on the same day) showing patchy high signal and (c) T2-weighted axial MRI showing patchy low signal in the basal ganglia (arrows).

**Table 6.4 Summary of changes seen on MRI in the basal ganglia in infants with hypoxic ischemic encephalopathy**

| Timing | MRI T1 | MRI T2 | Diffusion weighted MRI | CT | Ultrasound |
|---|---|---|---|---|---|
| 0–24 h | Normal | Normal | Not known, likely to be abnormal | Normal | Diffuse hyperechogenicity or normal |
| 2–3 days | Subtle, diffuse high signal | Subtle, isointense with white matter | Abnormal, areas of increased signal | Low attenuation or normal | Diffuse hyperechogenicity |
| 7–10 days | More globular, patchy high signal | Patchy high and low signal | Abnormal or normal | Increased attenuation or normal | Better definition of echodensities |

related to a variety of metabolic insults in addition to hypoxic ischemic injury. When abnormalities are exclusively located in the basal ganglia, the involvement of the other gray nuclei in addition to the posterior putamen and thalamus should raise the suspicion of an underlying genetic or metabolic cause (Hoon *et al.* 1997).

Other abnormalities that may be detected following significant asphyxia include focal infarction, cortical highlighting (Fig. 6.14), and evidence of subdural and subarachnoid hemorrhage. Single or multiple punctate lesions of high signal on T1-weighted images and low signal on T2-weighted images may be demonstrated in the deep white matter in addition to more generalized alteration in signal intensity due to cerebral edema.

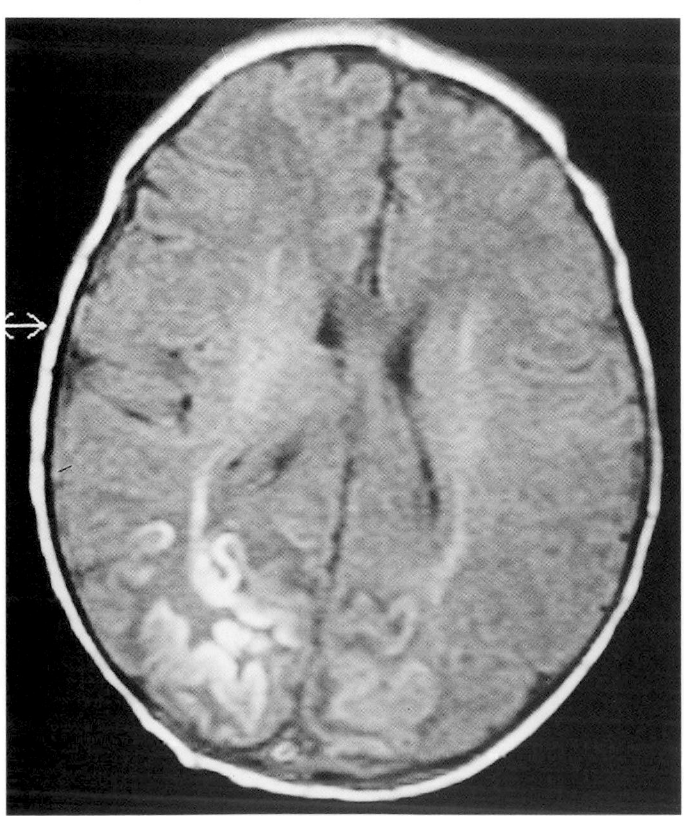

Figure 6.14 T1-weighted axial image showing cortical highlighting with high signal following the line of the gyri.

In the subacute-to-chronic phase, MRI may demonstrate cystic lesions in the white matter which may involve both the subcortical and deeper periventricular white matter (Fig. 6.15). These lesions typically affect the premature infant although they were originally described by Banker and Larroche in a group of mainly term babies suffering hypoxic insults following birth asphyxia (Banker & Larroche 1962). Multiple cystic lesions are usually bilateral in distribution and represent multicystic encephalomalacia. Although frequently associated with diffuse injury following a hypoxic ischemic insult it may also be seen following severe infection, hemorrhage, and trauma.

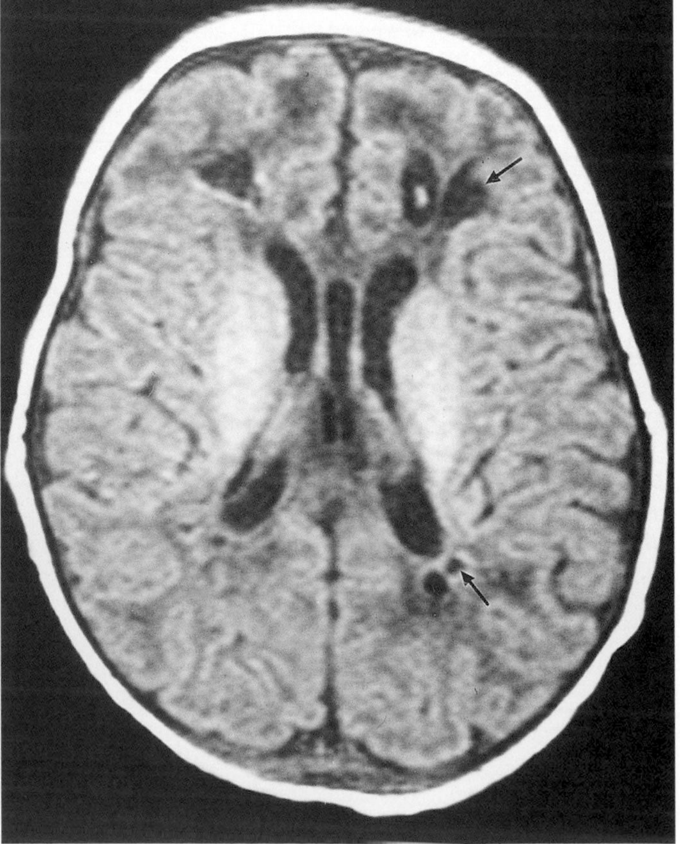

Figure 6.15 T1-weighted axial image demonstrating cystic leukomalacia in the deep white matter 'watershed' regions in a term infant with HIE (arrows).

In the acute phase, ultrasound will show increased diffuse echogenicity usually persisting for up to 5–7 days of life followed by cystic degeneration which may develop between 7 and 30 days (Frigieri *et al.* 1996). It is difficult to date the timing of the insult with accuracy, since the precise timing of cystic degeneration varies and is influenced by the severity of the injury (Barkovich 2000b). Ultrasound is the most sensitive technique to demonstrate the development of cystic degeneration as the glial septae, which develop following a diffuse reactive astrocytosis, are particularly well seen by this modality.

Initially the white matter will appear as a diffuse area of low attenuation on CT which may be difficult to distinguish from the normal appearances in the newborn infant. Once cystic degeneration has developed the cysts will be readily visualized on subsequent CT examinations due to the low attenuation of the fluid filled cavities. However, it may be difficult to differentiate cystic degeneration of encephalomalacia from the development of a porencephalic cyst on CT.

MRI is superior to both ultrasound imaging and CT in the complete assessment of encephalomalacia (Barkovich 2000b). In the acute phase, MRI shows areas of diffuse signal alteration probably due to the presence of white matter edema (low signal on T1-weighted images and high signal on T2-weighted images). In time the white matter degenerates to form the typical appearances of cystic encephalomalacia as clearly demarcated fluid-filled cavities which show prolongation of T2 (high signal on T2-weighted images and low signal on T1-weighted images). The prediction of outcome based on brain imaging is discussed on p. 492.

## FOCAL ISCHEMIC LESIONS (see p. 393)

Infarction of the major or minor branches of the cerebral arteries can be revealed by ultrasound, CT, and MRI. There is insufficient evidence in the literature to confirm which is the most appropriate imaging modality. MRI and diffusion-weighted imaging seem to be the most promising especially in the earliest stages of the disease. Areas of asymmetrical echogenicity will be detected on ultrasound in the first 12–36 hours following the onset of seizures. The areas of abnormality often only show a subtle increase in echogenicity at first and may be overlooked on account of their more peripheral position (Fig. 6.16). The lesions may appear as low attenuation areas of infarction on CT scanning although hemorrhagic areas may be noted within the region of the infarction. On conventional MRI, areas involved by the infarction will show low signal on T2-weighted images and sometimes an increase on T1-weighted images secondary to hemorrhagic reperfusion. However, the MRI scan may be

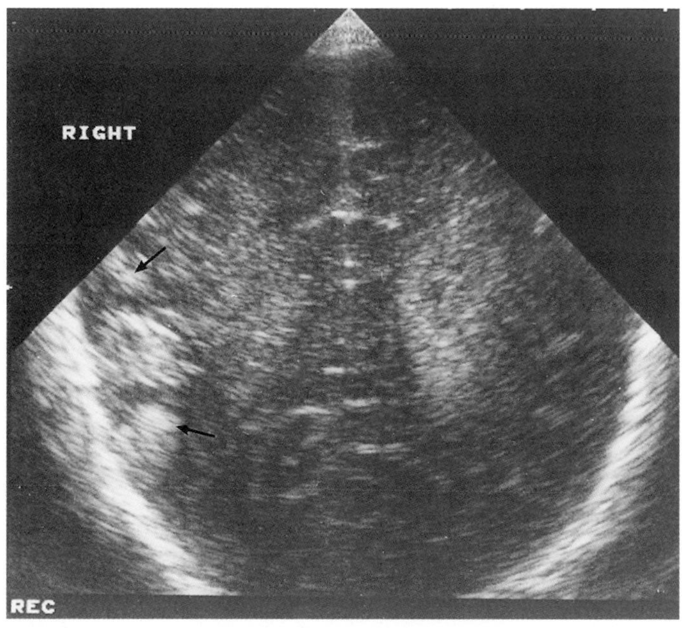


(a)

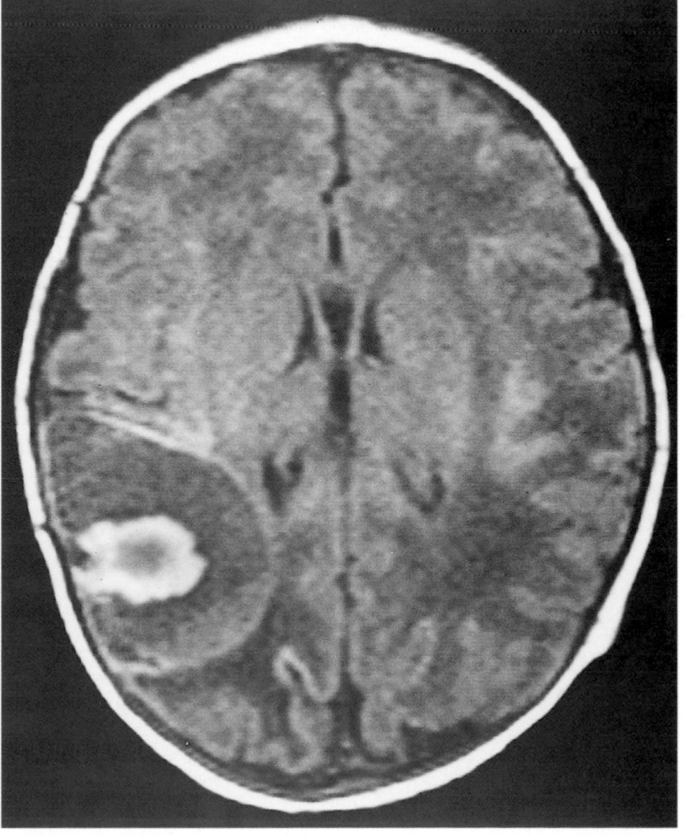

(b)

Figure 6.16 Focal hemorrhagic infarction. (a) Coronal ultrasound image at 3 days of age showing increased echodensity peripherally in the right parietal-occipital region (arrows). (b) T1-weighted axial MRI scan performed at 3 weeks of age showing evidence of a resolving hemorrhagic infarction with clot retraction and cystic degeneration in the middle cerebral artery territory.

normal in the first few hours following the infarction. Diffusion-weighted imaging is particularly valuable as it may demonstrate the area of signal alteration secondary to infarction when conventional MRI imaging is still normal (Cowan *et al.* 1994; Baird *et al.* 1997; D'Arceuil *et al.* 1998; Tuor *et al.* 1998). In our experience, ultrasound is often adequate to suggest the diagnosis of a middle cerebral artery infarction. The cavitational phase of the infarcted area is equally recognizable with all techniques and it occurs at a variable time after the initial insult. The majority of these focal lesions tend to affect term babies, although they can affect premature infants. Lesions in the subcortical regions are often difficult to demonstrate by ultrasound scanning, and are most appropriately imaged by MRI.

## CEREBRAL VEIN THROMBOSIS (see p. 365)

This is a rare condition, but increasingly diagnosed in neonates since the introduction of MRI. The infant often presents with seizures but the diagnosis may be overlooked when the only clinical sign is mild drowsiness On conventional MRI the abnormality appears as an increased signal on T1-weighted images and decreased signal on T2-weighted images along the vessels involved due to the thrombotic lesion (Fig. 6.17). Cerebral vein thrombosis usually affects the major venous sinuses of the brain but can involve the deep venous system up to the inner small veins draining the blood from the germinal matrix and periventricular white matter. It has been associated with parenchymal lesions and can be associated with thrombophilic disorders such as protein C, S, and factor V Leiden (p. 365). The diagnosis with CT scanning is possible but difficult and requires administration of intravenous contrast medium. Although color flow Doppler can be useful in identifying thrombosis in the sagittal sinus it is difficult to visualize the other major venous sinuses and any associated infarction using this modality (Rivkin *et al.* 1992; Grossman *et al.* 1993; Bakac & Wardlaw 1997; De Veber *et al.* 1998; Nowak-Gottl *et al.* 1997; Becker *et al.* 1998; Debus *et al.* 1998; Pohl *et al.* 1998).

## MACROCRANIA AND VENTRICULAR DILATATION (see also Chapter 43)

It is important to differentiate ventricular dilatation due to hydrocephalus from ventricular dilatation secondary to cerebral atrophy where the lateral ventricular margins may show some irregularity and the extra-axial space and interhemispheric fissure may be widened (Hay *et al.* 1989). Findings that favor the diagnosis of hydrocephalus include dilatation of the temporal horns to the same extent as the bodies of the lateral ventricles, enlargement of the anterior

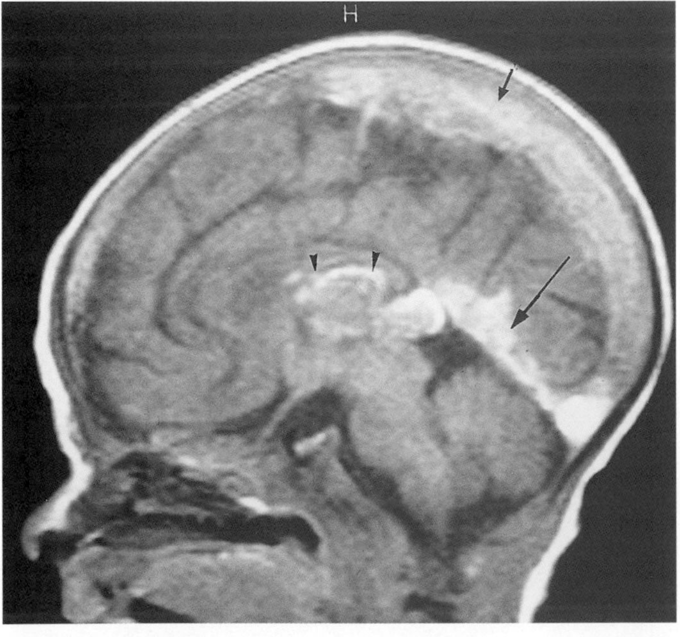


(a)

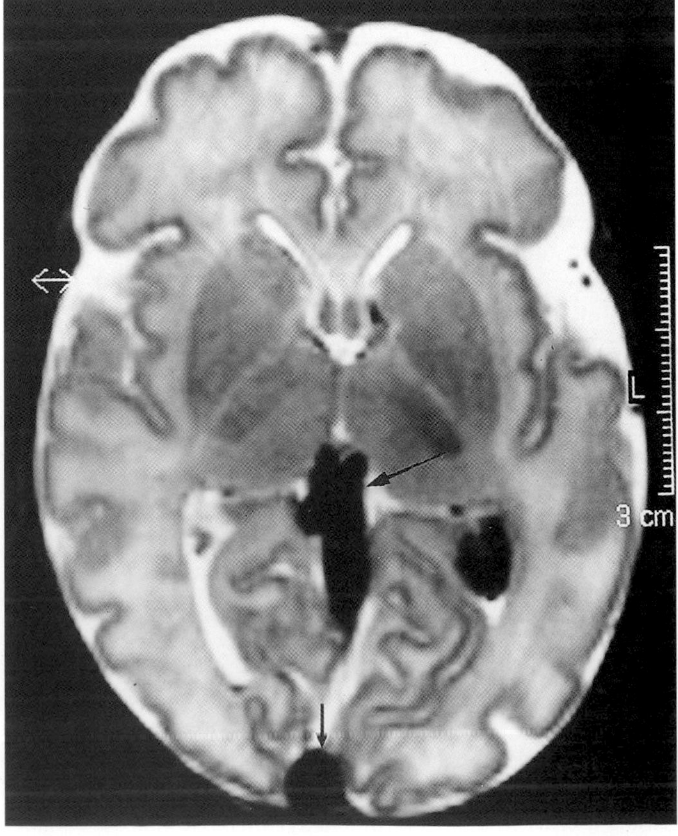


(b)

Figure 6.17 Cerebral vein thrombosis. (a) T1-weighted sagittal MRI image demonstrating high intensity signal within the sagittal sinus (short arrow), straight sinus (long arrow) and deep veins of the basal ganglia (arrowheads). (b) T2-weighted axial image showing a signal void in the sagittal sinus (arrows) and straight sinus (long arrows). Small left GMH-IVH is present.

and posterior recesses of the 3rd ventricle, effacement of the cortical sulci and the presence of interstitial edema in the periventricular white matter (Barkovich & Edwards 1992). The distinction between hydrocephalus or cerebral atrophy by imaging alone may be difficult and knowledge of the infant's clinical status including rate of rise of head circumference must also be taken into account. In some very low birth weight infants with evidence of previous IVH the etiology of ventriculomegaly may be complex and related to both the previous hemorrhage and hypoxic ischemic white matter injury (Leviton & Gilles 1996; Roland & Hill 1997).

Transient ventricular dilatation commonly develops after intraventricular hemorrhage, in up to 35% of cases, often commencing within 2–3 days of the initial hemorrhage, but in the majority the degree of dilatation resolves or becomes static within 4 weeks (Rumack & Johnson 1984; Siegel 1995; Roland & Hill 1997). The degree of ventricular dilatation is related to the severity of the hemorrhage, with dilatation invariably associated with large IVH (Papile *et al.* 1978). It is necessary to closely monitor those infants in whom the dilatation has become static since up to 5% of these infants may subsequently develop progressive dilatation requiring treatment over the course of the first year (Roland & Hill 1997).

Other causes of hydrocephalus include congenital malformations, e.g. aqueduct stenosis, infection, and more rarely neoplasia (posterior fossa hamartoma or choroid plexus papilloma) and arterio-venous malformations, e.g. vein of Galen aneurysm (p. 781). The role of imaging is to confirm the presence of ventriculomegaly and monitor ventricular size, to identify the etiology, and to assess the cerebral white matter for evidence of hypoxic ischemic injury. Detailed anatomical assessment of the ventricular system by MRI is becoming increasingly important in preoperative planning and postoperative assessment of neuroendoscopic third ventriculostomy (Laitt *et al.* 1999).

Ultrasound is the most appropriate imaging modality for the initial assessment of ventricular size in an infant with an enlarged head circumference. Ventricular size can be measured and monitored equally by ultrasound, CT and MRI but ultrasound is clearly more accessible and cost-effective. Doppler ultrasound has been reported to be of some value in the monitoring of infants with progressive hydrocephalus, although there is some debate with regard to the reproducibility of the results and thus the clinical usefulness (Siegel 1995; Taylor *et al.* 1998). The addition of gentle compression of the fontanelle whilst performing a Doppler examination may be of value in identifying those infants with limited intracranial compliance to small increases in the ventricular cerebrospinal fluid (CSF) volume (Taylor *et al.* 1998).

Further imaging should be undertaken to establish the cause of the ventriculomegaly in those cases where the etiology is unclear after the initial ultrasound assessment. In most cases MRI would be most appropriate, since this modality is superior to CT in the assessment of the posterior fossa and the exclusion of a posterior fossa tumor compressing the aqueduct or 4th ventricle (Paakko *et al.* 1994). MRI is also superior to both CT and ultrasound imaging in the demonstration of old intraventricular and extra-axial hemorrhage which may no longer be evident on ultrasound scanning or CT.

CSF flow studies have become increasingly important in the assessment of hydrocephalus prior to surgical intervention (Enzmann & Pelc 1991; Barkovich & Edwards 1992; Quencer 1992). Early studies were based on the characteristic signal void from CSF in regions where CSF flow is fast or turbulent on standard spin echo sequences. More sophisticated sequences are now available based on gradient echo imaging, cine MR imaging and phase contrast velocity MR imaging which can quantitate flow of CSF through the foramen of Monroe and other foraminae and indicate the probable site of obstruction or to assess the patency following third ventriculostomy (Fig. 6.18). Following placement of a ventriculo-peritoneal shunt or access device for the intermittent drainage of CSF, ultrasound imaging should be the first modality of choice in the assessment of a ventricular catheter position and possible malfunction. Further imaging by MRI or CT can then be arranged if appropriate.

Ultrasound imaging of a term infant with increased head circumference may demonstrate minimal enlargement of ventricular size in association with an increase in extra-axial fluid. This condition – given a variety of names including benign extra-axial fluid collections of infancy, external hydrocephalus, or benign macrocephaly of infancy – is generally self-limiting and associated with normal development (Babcock *et al.* 1988; de Vries *et al.* 1990; Barkovich & Edwards 1992). Most infants can be monitored by regular clinical examination and ultrasound assessment, although further imaging including MRI and CSF flow studies may be appropriate in a minority of infants with abnormal clinical signs (de Vries *et al.* 1990). If there is any suspicion of trauma the possibility of a subdural collection should also be considered and a CT or MRI obtained without delay.

## CONGENITAL MALFORMATIONS

A wide range of developmental and congenital abnormalities of the brain may occur (Chapter 13). Whilst an ultrasound examination of the brain can identify many of the major congenital abnormalities such as agenesis of the corpus callosum (Fig. 6.19), holoprosencephaly, hydrocephalus, and hydranencephaly (Siegel 1995), MRI is necessary for full evaluation and has a considerably higher exclusion value than either ultrasound examination or CT scanning (Barkovich 1995). Congenital brain disorders are often complex and may be associated with a number of other abnormalities that will be better demonstrated by MRI, e.g. disordered neuronal migration (Fig. 6.20), gray matter heterotopias, intracerebral lipomas and posterior fossa abnormalities. MRI spectroscopy is likely to become of increasing importance in the differentiation of congenital metabolic

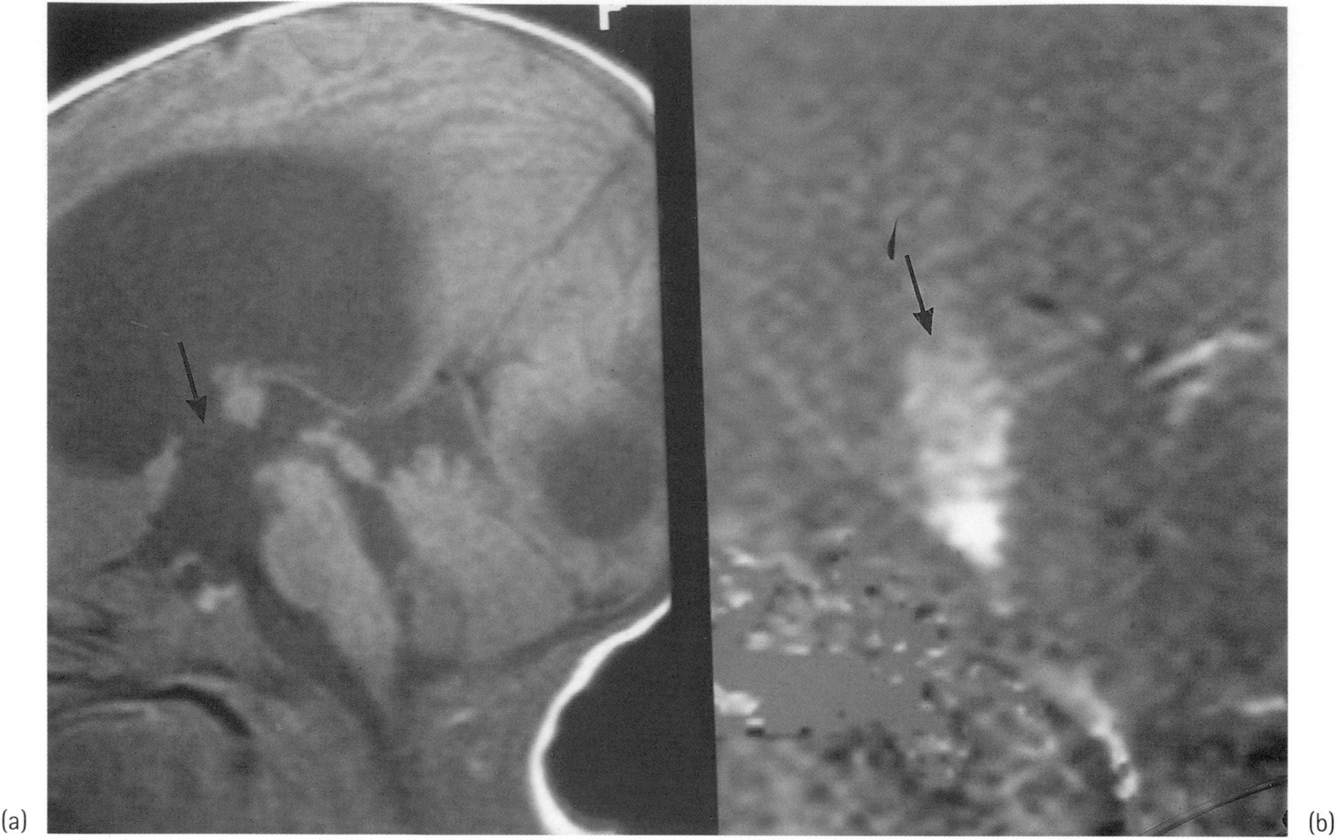

Figure 6.18 CSF flow studies. (a) Sagittal T1-weighted image for orientation and (b) sagittal CSF flow studies show high signal confirming CSF flow during systole at the site of the 3rd ventriculostomy (arrow).

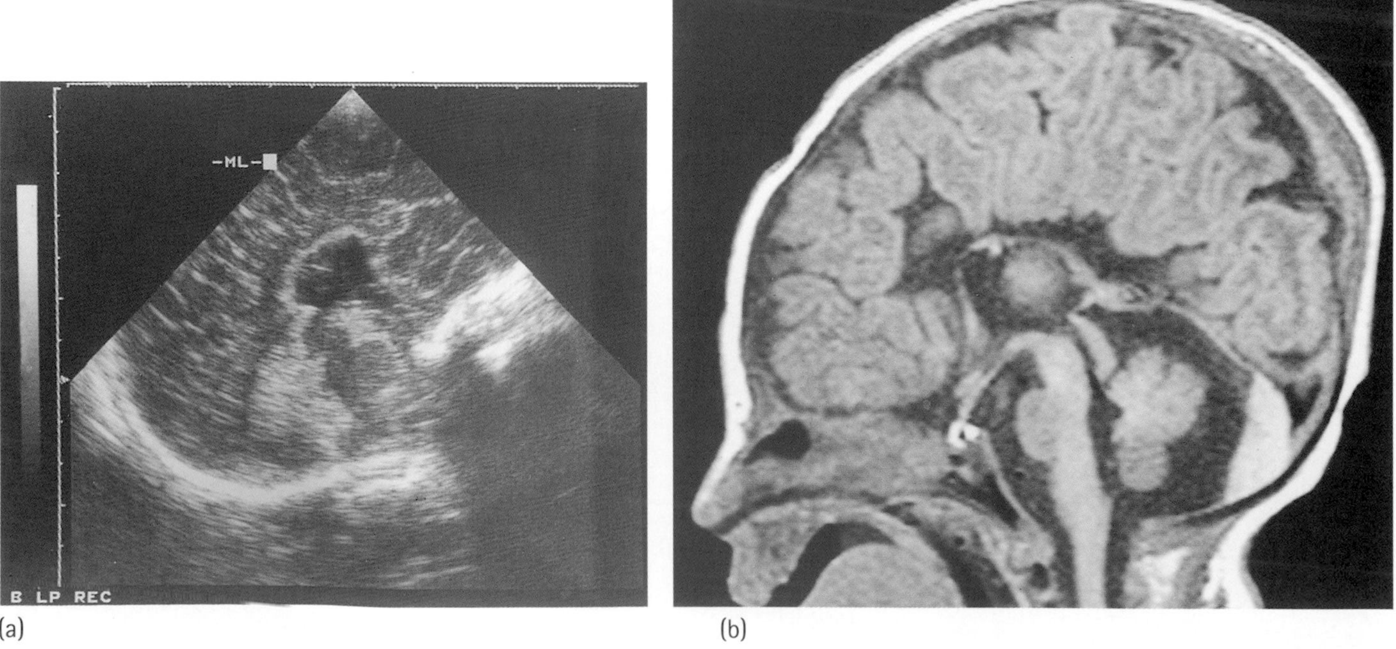


Figure 6.19 Agenesis of the corpus callosum. (a) Sagittal ultrasound scan showing absence of the corpus callosum. (b) T1-weighted sagittal MRI scan confirming malformation and demonstrating a coincidental and asymptomatic extra-axial hemorrhage in the posterior fossa.

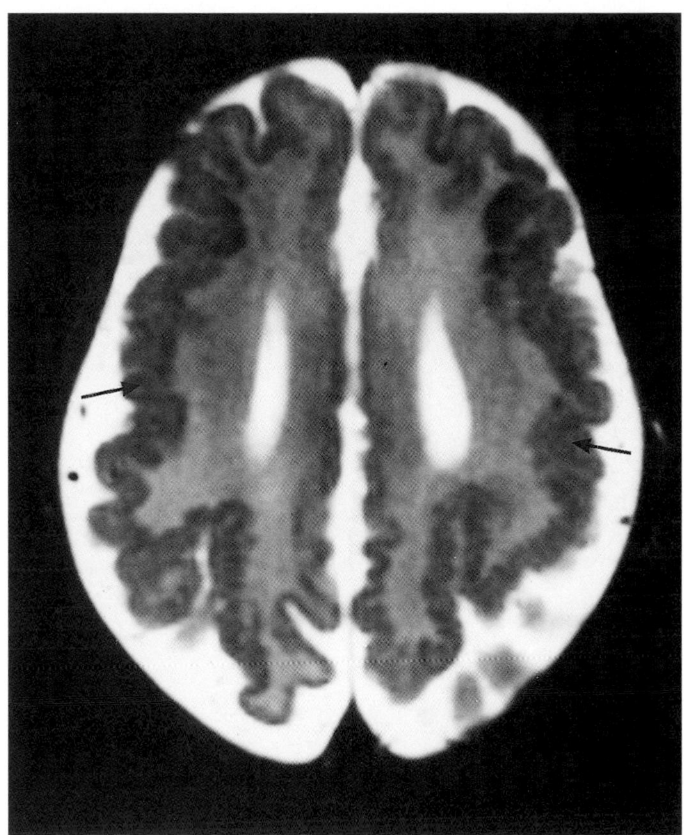

Figure 6.20 Polymicrogyria of unknown aetiology despite exhaustive investigations in a term infant presenting at one day of age with seizures. T2-weighted axial MRI scan showing diffuse cortical dysplasia (long arrows).

encephalopathies (Huppi & Barnes 1997), e.g. $^{31}$P-MRI spectroscopy has been shown to be useful in the diagnosis of inheritable disorders of oxidative phosphorylation, and $^{1}$H-MR spectroscopy useful to detect high levels of cerebral lactate associated with pyruvate dehydrogenase deficiency and other mitochondrial disorders.

## VASCULAR MALFORMATIONS

A number of congenital vascular anomalies in the brain may present in the neonatal period, either following prenatal diagnosis on routine ultrasound scanning or as the result of clinical abnormality, including hydrocephalus and the development of congestive cardiac failure. The vein of Galen aneurysm is the best known and includes a wide spectrum of vascular anomalies which have the common feature of a dilated vein of Galen (Horowitz *et al.* 1994). Ultrasound imaging with color Doppler analysis is an invaluable tool for screening for intracranial arterio-venous malformations and for monitoring the effect of therapy (Ciricillo *et al.* 1990; Siegel 1995). Whilst contrast enhanced CT scanning can be used for further evaluation, MRI is superior. Multiplanar scanning and the facility for MR angiography allows the radiologist to assess not only the site and size of the malformation, the presence of any hypoxic ischemic injury and the degree of hydrocephalus, but also helps to identify vascular access routes suitable for subsequent angiography (Fig. 6.21). Angiography remains essential for full evaluation of

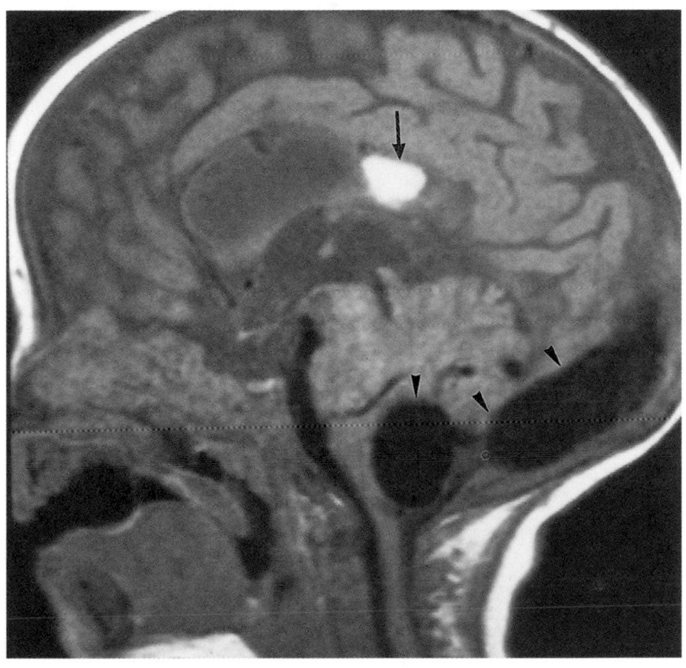

(a)

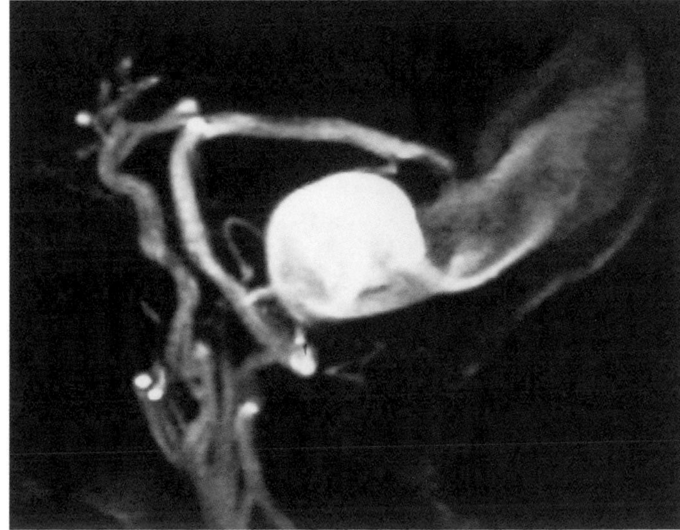

(b)

Figure 6.21 Cerebral arterio-venous malformation. (a) MRI; sagittal T1-weighted scan showing hyperintense lesion (arrow) at the level of the internal cerebral vein and large veins in the posterior fossa (arrows) displacing the cerebellum, due to an extensive arterio-venous malformation. (b) Magnified angiography of the posterior fossa showing basilar artery and its branches directly feeding into the large draining veins of the arterio-venous malformation.

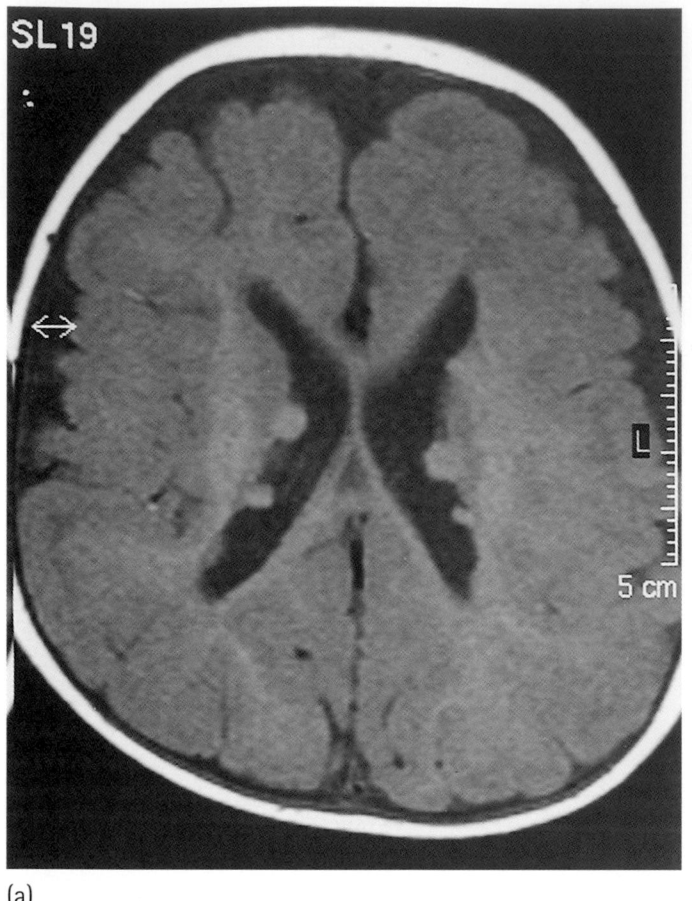

(a)

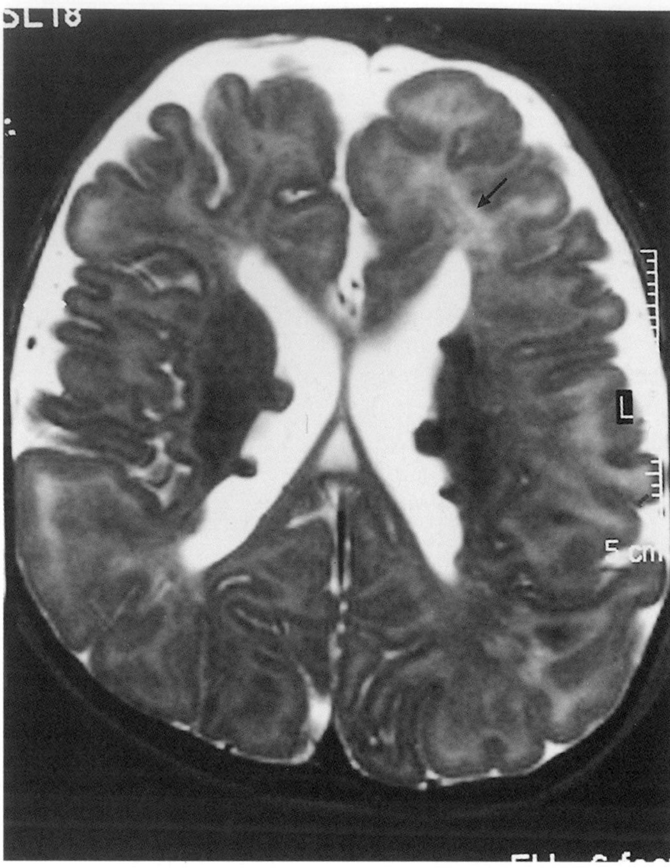

(c)

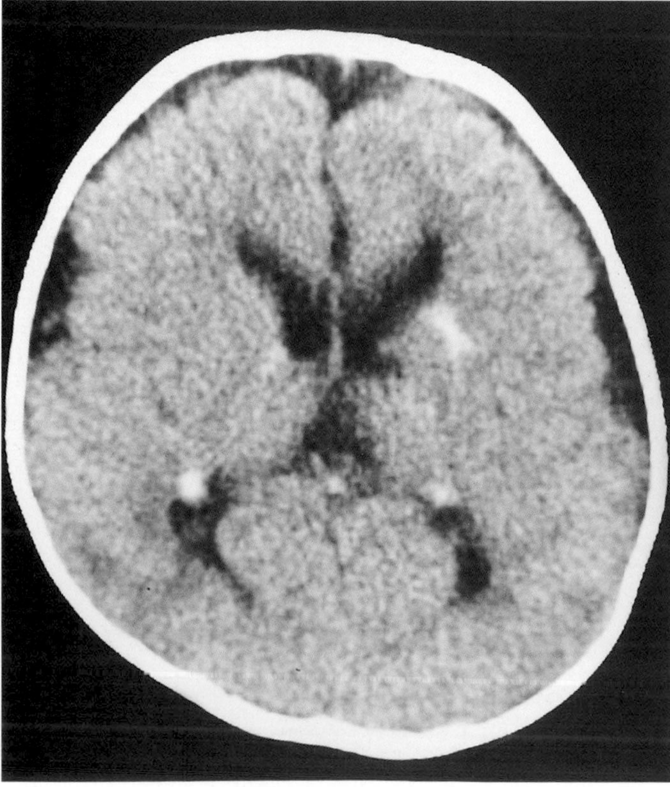
(b)

**Figure 6.22** Tuberous sclerosis. (a) Unenhanced axial CT scan, (b) MRI axial T1-weighted and (c) T2-weighted images demonstrate multiple subependymal nodules. Abnormal signal in the frontal white matter is also seen on T2-weighted images (arrow).

the arterial and venous components of the malformations prior to treatment, which is generally by endovascular embolization (Lasjaunias *et al.* 1991; Barkovich 1995; Brunelle 1997).

## PHAKOMATOSES

The phakomatoses represent a group of congenital disorders that mainly affect tissues of ectodermal origin and are characterized by the development of tumor-like malformations in the brain. Von Hippel–Lindau disease and tuberous sclerosis may present in the neonatal period with seizures that may be difficult to control, although tuberous sclerosis more commonly presents in the young infant with cardiac rhabdomyomas and brain tumors (Miller *et al.* 1998). Other phakomatoses, e.g. neurofibromatosis types I and II and Sturge–Weber disease do not usually present at this age. Criteria for diagnosis of tuberous sclerosis have recently been revised on the basis of new information derived from molecular genetic studies (Roach *et al.* 1998). No single clinical sign or radiological abnormality is now considered specific for confirmation of diagnosis. In the neonatal period, imaging may detect subependymal nodules and cortical tubers both of which are considered as major diagnostic criteria. Other diagnostic features include the presence of giant cell tumors in the subependymal region, abnormal regions in the white matter due to islands of gray matter heterotopia, and cerebral white matter radial migration lines (Braffman *et al.* 1992; Roach *et al.* 1998). Although subependymal tubers may be demonstrated by ultrasound examination as echogenic nodules in the walls of the lateral ventricles, small foci of calcification and parenchymal tubers are more difficult to identify. In the past, CT was considered the imaging modality of choice as it was more sensitive than MRI in the detection of calcified subependymal nodules (Flodmark 1995). However, these nodules are frequently not calcified in the first few months of life and may be more apparent on MR scanning. The nodules often are seen as protrusions into the ventricular lumen, and although most commonly are seen close to the Foramen of Monroe may be seen anywhere along the ventricular margins of the lateral, 3rd, and 4th ventricles (Fig. 6.22).

Hamartomas are also found in the cerebral cortex and cause enlargement of the gyri. These lesions commonly calcify with increasing age but may show no calcification in the neonate and may be difficult to detect on CT. On MRI they are seen as enlarged gyri which show increased intensity on T1-weighted images and decreased signal on T2-weighted images, although the characteristic signal changes with age as the white matter myelinates (Barkovich 1995; Miller *et al.* 1998).

## CEREBRAL INFECTION

The clinical and radiological manifestations of intracranial infection are quite different in those infants who acquire the infection prenatally from those in whom the infection occurs in the neonatal period, and the extent of subsequent injury is related to the age of the fetus at the time of infection.

Ultrasound imaging is useful in the initial assessment of an infant with possible prenatally acquired infection (Fig. 6.23). Intracerebral calcifications are seen as dense echogenic foci, which may or may not demonstrate acoustic shadowing in the periventricular white matter, basal ganglia, or in the gyri due to cortical involvement. The extent, nature and distribution of intracranial calcification varies according to the infecting organism (Flodmark 1995). Abnormal linear densities may be demonstrated in the basal ganglia in the line of normal vascular channels and are thought to represent a thalamo-striate vasculopathy (Teele *et al.* 1988). This finding is not specific for prenatal infection and has also been demonstrated following hypoxic ischemic injury and in association with a number of chromosomal abnormalities. In addition to ventricular dilatation, ultrasound imaging may also show evidence of a ventriculitis by demonstrating evidence of echogenic debris and septae within the lateral ventricles (Carey *et al.* 1987). Whilst ultrasound imaging is an important screening tool, MRI offers the potential for a comprehensive assessment of the extent of injury. Although small foci of calcification may not be as evident as on CT or ultrasound scanning, MRI has the advantage of better demonstration of the extent of white matter injury and its effect on myelination, gyration, and neuronal migration.

Herpes simplex infection acquired during delivery may result in a very severe necrotizing encephalitis in the first few weeks of life with devastating consequences. Ultrasound imaging may demonstrate massive foci of calcification. Both

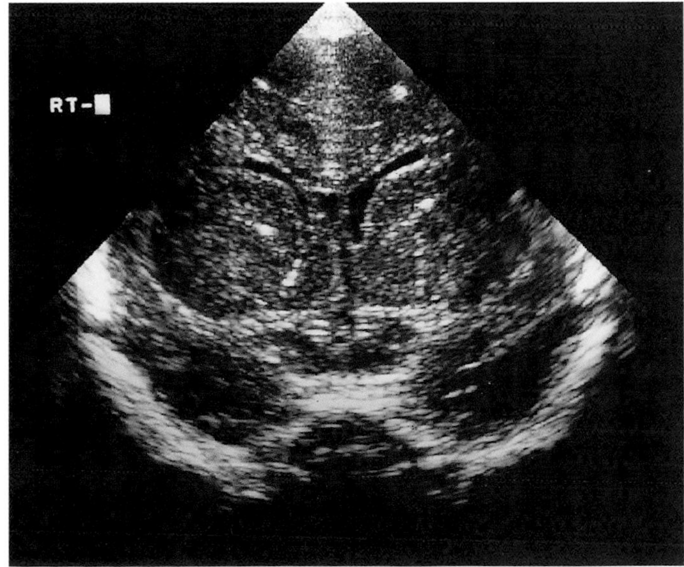


**Figure 6.23** Prenatal *Toxoplasma gondii* infection. Coronal ultrasound image demonstrating punctate lesion in the basal ganglia, periventricular regions and white matter due to foci of calcification.

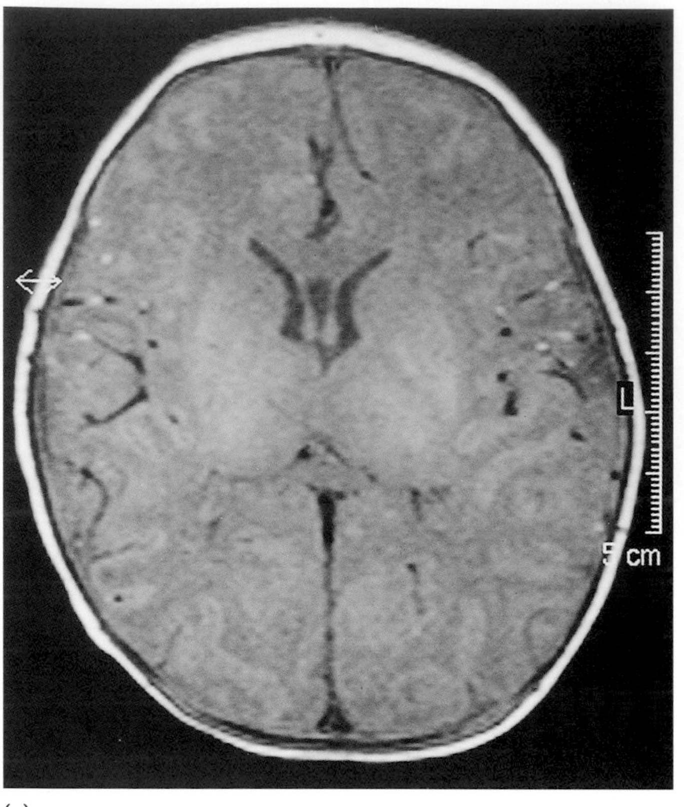

(a)

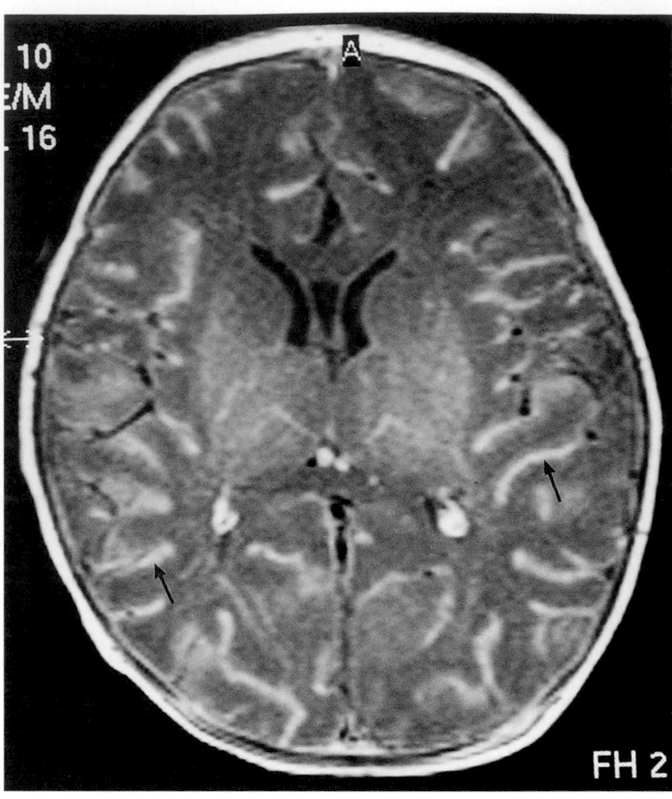

(b)

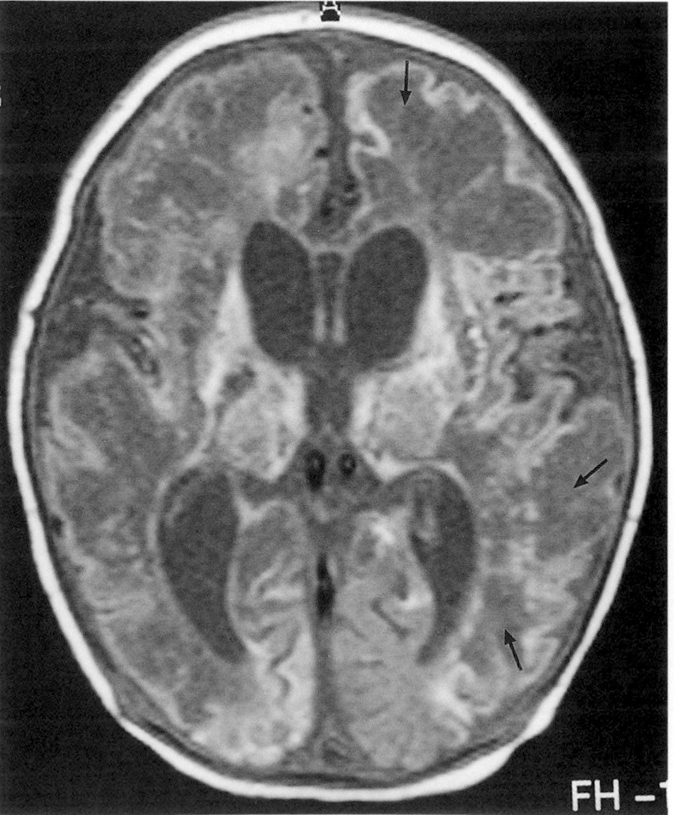

(c)

**Figure 6.24** Herpes encephalitis presenting with seizures at 21 days of age. (a) MRI axial T1-weighted image at 22 days of age demonstrating effacement of the sulcal outline, possibly indicating cerebral edema. (b) Contrast enhanced T1-weighted image demonstrating abnormal meningeal enhancement (arrows). (c) T1-weighted image at 5 weeks of age demonstrating multicystic encephalomalacia (arrows).

CT and MRI demonstrate widespread white matter edema in the acute phase. There is prominent meningeal enhancement following the injection of intravenous contrast agents, which together with the white matter abnormalities are suggestive of herpes simplex infection (Fig. 6.24).

Cerebral infection may be acquired postnatally, most commonly from infection by Gram negative organisms, which may give rise to meningitis, ventriculitis, cerebritis, and abscess formation. Ultrasound imaging is useful to monitor for the development of ventricular dilatation and subdural effusions. Ultrasound may also demonstrate the development of ventriculitis by the demonstration of echogenic CSF and the development of ventricular septae. Whilst the development of subdural collections and abscess formation may be suspected on an ultrasound examination, contrast enhanced CT or MRI are usually necessary where a cerebral abscess is suspected (Barkovich 1995).

## CHOICE OF TECHNIQUE

Ultrasound has become established as the first line imaging modality in all sick infants with suspected intracranial pathology. The accuracy in diagnosis of germinal matrix and intraventricular hemorrhage is well established, and at present there is no convincing evidence to suggest that there is any clinical benefit from performing an early MRI examination in these infants.

On the other hand, there are a number of limitations to an ultrasound examination where additional information from cross-sectional imaging may be helpful. This applies particularly in the term infant with hypoxic ischemic encephalopathy and in the evaluation of the posterior fossa. MRI has now largely replaced CT scanning in these infants, although a CT examination will detect the most important pathological abnormalities that are likely to have an immediate impact on clinical management. CT is of little value in the early assessment of the brain of a premature infant with suspected hypoxic ischemic injury, apart from the detection of acute hemorrhage, and cross-sectional imaging should probably be deferred until an MRI scan can be obtained. MR angiography and CSF flow studies are likely to become increasingly important in the evaluation of more complex neurologic problems. The clinical role of MR spectroscopy, PET and SPECT scanning in routine clinical practice is still to be established in the neonatal population.

The role of neuroradiological imaging in clinical management is specific to the neonate. In older children and adults, imaging is frequently directed towards informing the decision-making process with regard to treatment options, e.g. approach to tumor excision or treatment of hydrocephalus. In the neonate, most neurologic imaging is directed towards the identification of brain injury, hemorrhage, and congenital malformations for which there are currently few treatment options. Nevertheless, the identification of these lesions is crucial in developing a better understanding of their pathogenesis and helping the clinical team inform the parents of their long term consequences. This is particularly true in the very preterm and unwell babies mechanically ventilated in whom prolongation of the intensive care may not be appropriate.

## REFERENCES


Appleton R E, Lee R E J & Hey E N (1990) Neurodevelopmental outcome of transient neonatal intracerebral echodensities. *Arch Dis Child* 65:27–29.

Archer L N J, Levene M I & Evans D H (1986) Cerebral artery Doppler ultrasonography for prediction of outcome after perinatal asphyxia. *Lancet* 2(8516):1116–1117.

Baarsma R, Laurini R N, Baerts W & Okken A (1987) Reliability of sonography in non-hemorrhagic periventricular leukomalacia. *Pediatr Radiol* 17:189–191.

Babcock D S, Bove K E & Han B K (1982) Intracranial hemorrhage in premature infants: sonographic pathologic correlation. *Am J Neuroradiol* 3:309–317.

Babcock D S & Ball W S (1983) Postasphyxial encephalopathy in full term infants: ultrasound diagnosis. *Radiology* 148:417–423.

Babcock D S, Han B K & Dine M S (1988) Sonographic findings in infants with macrocrania. *Am J Radiol* 150:1359–1365.

Baird A E, Benfield A, Schlaug S *et al.* (1997) Enlargement of human cerebral ischemic lesion volumes measured by diffusion weighted magnetic resonance imaging. *Ann Neurol* 41:581–589.

Bakac G & Wardlaw J M (1997) Problems in the diagnosis of intracranial venous infarction. *Neuroradiology* 39:566–570.

Banker B Q & Larroche J C (1962) Periventricular leukomalacia of infancy. *Arch Neurol* 7:386–410.

Barkovich A J, Edwards M S B (1992) Applications of neuroimaging in hydrocephalus. *Pediatr Neurosurg* 18:65–83.

Barkovich A J (1992) MR and CT evaluation of profound neonatal and infantile asphyxia. *Am J Neuroradiol* 13:959–972.

Barkovich A J (1995) *Pediatric neuroimaging*. New York, NY: Raven Press.

Barkovich A J (1997) The encephalopathic neonate: choosing the proper imaging technique. *Am J Neuroradiol* 18:1816–1820.

Barkovich A J (1998) MR of the normal neonatal brain, assessment of deep structures. *Am J Neuroradiol* 19:971–976.

✪ Barkovich A J (2000a) Normal development of the neonatal and infant brain, skull, and spine. In: *Pediatric neuroimaging*, 3rd edn. Philadelphia, PA: Lippincott Williams & Wilkins, pp. 13–69.

✪ Barkovich A J (2000b) Brain and spine injuries in infancy and childhood In: *Pediatric neuroimaging*, 3rd edn. Philadelphia, PA: Lippincott Williams & Wilkins; pp. 157–250.

Battin M R, Maalouf E F, Counsell S J *et al.* (1998) Magnetic resonance imaging of the brain in very preterm infants: visualization of the germinal matrix, early myelination and cortical folding. *Pediatrics* 101:957–962.

Beaulieu C, D'Arceuil H, Hedahus M *et al.* (1999) Diffusion-weighted magnetic resonance imaging: theory and potential applications to child neurology. *Semin Pediatr Neurol* 6:87–100.

Becker S, Heller C, Gropp F *et al.* (1998) Thrombophilic disorders in children with cerebral infarction. *Lancet* 352:1756–1757.

Blankenberg F G, Loh N N, Norbash A M *et al.* (1997) Impaired cerebrovascular autoregulation after hypoxic-ischemic injury in extremely low birth weight neonates: detection with power and pulsed wave Doppler US. *Radiology* 205:563–568.

Bloom M, Jacobs S, Pile-Spellman J *et al.* (1996) Cerebral SPECT Imaging: effect on clinical management. *J Nuclear Med* 37:1070–1073.

Boyer R S (1994) Neuroimaging of premature infants. *Neuroimag Clin N Am* 4:241–259.

Bozynski M E, Nelson M N, Matalon T A S (1985) Cavitatory periventricular leukomalacia: incidence and short term outcome in infants weighing <1200 g at birth. *Dev Med Child Neurol* 27:572–577.

✪ Braffman B H, Bilaniuk L T, Naidich T P (1992) MR imaging of tuberous sclerosis: pathogenesis of this phakomatosis. Use of gadopentetate dimeglumine and literature review. *Radiology* 183:227–238.

Brunelle F (1997) Arterio-venous malformation of the vein of Galen in children. *Pediatr Radiol* 27:501–513.

Carey B, Arthur R J & Houlsby W T (1987) Ventriculitis in congenital rubella: ultrasound demonstration. *Pediatr Radiol* 17:415–416.

Casselden P A (1988) Ocular lens dose in cerebral vascular imaging. *Br J Radiol* 61:202–204.

Chan C, Wong Y, Chau L *et al.* (1999) Radiation dose reduction in pediatric CT. *Pediatr Radiol* 29:770–775.

Childs A M, Ramenghi L A, Evans D J *et al.* (1998) MR features of developing periventricular white matter in preterm infants: evidence of glial cell migration. *Am J Neuroradiol* 19:971–976.

Ciricillo S F, Schmidt K G, Silverman N H *et al.* (1990) Serial ultrasonographic evaluation of neonatal vein of Galen malformations to assess the efficacy of interventional neuroradiological procedures. *Neurosurgery* 27:544–548.

Connolly B, Kelehan P, O'Brien N *et al.* (1994) The echogenic thalamus in hypoxic-ischaemic encephalopathy. *Pediatr Radiol* 24:268–271.

Cornette L, Toh V, Ramenghi L *et al.* (2000) Characteristics of punctate lesions in neonatal brain magnetic resonance imaging. *Child Nerv Syst* 16:49 [Abstr].

Cowan F M, Pennock J M, Hanrahan J D, Manji K P, Edwards A D (1994) Early detection of cerebral infarction and hypoxic ischaemic encephalopathy in neonates using diffusion weighted magnetic resonance imaging. *Neuropediatrics* 25:172–175.

D'Arceuil H E, de Crespigny A J, Rother J *et al.* (1998) Diffusion and perfusion magnetic resonance imaging of the evolution of hypoxic ischemic encephalopathy in the neonatal rabbit. *J Magn Reson Imag* 8:820–828.

Debus O, Koch H G, Kurlemann *et al.* (1998) Factor V Leiden and genetic defects of thrombophilia in childhood porencephaly. *Arch Dis Child* 78:F121–F124.

De Veber G, Monagle P, Chan A *et al.* (1998) Prothrombotic disorders in infants and children with cerebral thromboembolism. *Arch Neurol* 55:1539–1543.

De Vries L S, Dubowitz L M S, Dubovitz V *et al.* (1985) Predictive value of cranial ultrasound in the newborn baby: a reappraisal. *Lancet* 2(8447):137–140.

De Vries L S, Regev R, Pennock J M *et al.* (1988a) Ultrasound evolution and later outcome of infants with periventricular densities. *Early Hum Dev* 16:225–233.

De Vries L S, Wigglesworth J S, Regev R & Dubowitz L M S (1988b) Evolution of periventricular leukomalacia during the neonatal period and infancy: correlation of imaging and postmortem findings. *Early Hum Dev* 17:205–219.

De Vries L S, Smet M, Ceulemans B *et al.* (1990) The role of high resolution ultrasound and MRI in the investigation of infants with macrocephaly. *Neuropediatrics* 21:72–75.

De Vries L S, Eken P & Dubowitz L M S (1992) The spectrum of leukomalacia using cranial ultrasound. *Behav Brain Res* 49:1–6.

De Vries L S, Eken P, Groenendaal F *et al.* (1993) Correlation between the degree of periventricular leukomalacia diagnosed using cranial ultrasound and MRI later in infancy in children with cerebral palsy. *Neuropediatrics* 24:263–268.

De Vries L S & Levene M I (1995) Cerebral ischaemic lesions. In: *Fetal and neonatal neurology and neurosurgery*, 2nd edn. Levene M I L & Lilford R J, eds. Edinburgh: Churchill Livingstone; pp. 367–386.

De Vries L S, Rademaker K J, Groenedaal F *et al.* (1998) Correlation between neonatal cranial ultrasound, MRI in infancy and neurodevelopmental outcome in infants with a large intraventricular haemorrhage with or without unilateral parenchymal involvement. *Neuropediatrics* 29:180–188.

Dewbury K C & Bates R I (1981) The value of transfontanellar ultrasound in infants. *Br J Radiol* 54:1044–1052.

Di Pietro M A, Brody B A & Teele R L (1986) Peritrigonal echogenic 'blush' on cranial sonography: pathologic correlates. *Am J Roentgenol* 146:1067–1072.

Dubowitz L M S, Bydder G M & Mushin J (1985) Development sequence of periventricular leukomalacia. *Arch Dis Child* 60:349–355.

Enzmann D & Pelc N (1991) Normal flow patterns of intracranial and spinal cerebrospinal fluid defined with phase-contrast cine MR imaging. *Radiology* 178:467–474.

Evans D J, Childs A M, Ramenghi L A *et al.* (1997) Magnetic resonance imaging of the brain of premature infants. *Lancet* 2(9076):350.

Flodmark O, Becker L E, Harwood Nash D C *et al.* (1980a) Correlation between computed tomography and autopsy in premature and full-term neonates that have suffered perinatal asphyxia. *Radiology* 137:93–103.

Flodmark O, Fitz C R & Harwood-Nash D C (1980b) CT diagnosis and short term prognosis of intracranial hemorrhage and hypoxic/ischemic brain damage in neonate. *J Comput Assist Tomog* 4:775–787.

Flodmark O (1995) Imaging of the neonatal brain. In: Fetal and neonatal neurology and neurosurgery, 2nd edn. Levene M I L & Lilford R J, eds. Edinburgh: Churchill Livingstone; pp. 105–128.

Frigieri G, Guidi B, Costa Zacarelli S *et al.* (1996) Multicystic encephalomalacia in term infants. *Child Nerv Syst* 12:759–764.

Goetz M C, Gretebeck R J, Sang Oh S *et al.* (1995) Incidence, timing, and follow-up of periventricular leukomalacia. *Am J Perinatol* 12:325–327.

Gould S J, Howard S, Hope P L & Reynolds E O (1987) Periventricular intraparenchymal cerebral haemorrhage in preterm infants: the role of venous infarction. *J Pathol* 151:197–202.

Grant E G, Schellinger D, Richardson J D *et al.* (1983) Echogenic periventricular halo: normal sonographic finding or neonatal cerebral hemorrhage. *Am J Roentgenol* 140:793–796.

Grant E G & Schellinger D (1985) Sonography of neonatal periventricular leukomalacia: recent experience with a 7.5 MHz scanner. *Am J Neuroradiol* 6:781–785.

✪ Grant P E & Barkovich A J (1998/1999) MRI in cerebral palsy. *Clin MRI/Dev MR* 8:105–114.

Grossman R, Novak G, Patel M *et al.* (1993) MRI in neonatal dural sinus thrombosis. *Pediatr Neurol* 9:235–338.

Hay T C, Rumack C M & Horgan J G (1989) Cranial sonography: intracranial hemorrhage, periventricular leukomalacia and asphyxia. *Clin Diagn Ultrasound* 24:25–42.

Hoon A H, Reinbardt E M, Kelley R I *et al.* (1997) Brain magnetic resonance imaging in suspected extrapyramidal cerebral palsy: observations in distinguishing genetic-metabolic from acquired causes. *J Pediatr* 131:240–245.

Hope P J, Gould S J, Howard S *et al.* (1988) Ultrasound diagnosis of pathologically verified lesions in the brains of very preterm infants. *Dev Med Child Neurol* 30:457–471.

Horowitz M B, Jungreis C A, Quisling R G & Pollack I (1994) Vein of Galen aneurysms: a review and current perspective. *Am J Neuroradiol* 15:1486–1496.

✪ Huppi P S & Barnes P D (1997) Magnetic resonance techniques in the evaluation of the newborn brain. *Clin Perinatol* 24:693–723.

Inder T, Huppi P S, Zientara G P (1999) Early detection of periventricular leukomalacia by diffusion-weighted magnetic resonance imaging techniques. *J Pediatr* 134:631–634.

Keeney S E, Adcock E W & McArdle C B (1991) Prospective observations of 100 high-risk neonates by high field (1.5 Tesla) magnetic resonance imaging of the central nervous system: 1. Intraventricular and extracerebral lesions. *Pediatrics* 87:421–430.

Kuzniecky R I (1996) Neuroimaging in pediatric epilepsy. *Epilepsia 37* Suppl 1:S10–S21.

Laitt R D, Mallucci C L, McConachie N S *et al.* (1999) Constructive interference in steady-state 3-D Fourier-transform MRI in the management of hydrocephalus and third ventriculostomy. *Neuroradiology* 41:117–123.

Lasjaunias P, Garcia-Monaco R, Rodesch G *et al.* (1991) Vein of Galen malformation: endovascular treatment of 43 cases. *Child Nerv Syst* 7:360–367.

✪ Lee B C P, Park T S & Kaufmann B A (1995) MR angiography in pediatric neurologic disorders. *Pediatric Radiology* 25:409–419.

Leech R W & Ellsworth C A (1977) Anoxic-ischemic encephalopathy in the human neonatal period. The significance of brain stem involvement. *Arch Neurol* 34:109–113.

Levene M I & de Vries L S (1984) Extension of neonatal intraventricular haemorrhage. *Arch Dis Child* 59:631–636.

Leviton A & Gilles F (1996) Ventriculomegaly, delayed myelination, white matter hypoplasia, and 'periventricular' leukomalacia: how are they related? *Pediatr Neurol* 15:127–136.

Logan W J (1999) Functional magnetic resonance imaging in children. *Semin Pediatr Neurol* 6:78–86.

Martin E, Krassnitzer S, Kaelin P & Boesch C (1991) MR imaging of the brainstem: normal postnatal development. *Neuroradiology* 33:391–395.

McMenamin J B & Volpe J J (1983) Doppler ultrasonography in the determination of neonatal brain death. *Ann Neurol* 14(3):302–307.

McMenamin J B, Shackleford G D & Volpe J J (1984) Outcome of neonatal intraventricular haemorrhage with periventricular echodense lesions. *Ann Neurol* 15:285–290.

Miller S P, Tasch T, Sylvain M *et al.* (1998) Tuberous sclerosis complex and neonatal seizures. *J Child Neurol* 13:619–623.

Mohan K K, Chugani D C & Chugani H T (1999) Positron emission tomography in pediatric neurology. *Semin Pediatr Neurol* 6:111–119.

Nowak-Gottl U, von Kries R & Gobel U (1997) Neonatal symptomatic thromboembolism in Germany: two year survey. *Arch Dis Child* 76:F163–F167.

Nwaesei C G, Pape K E, Martin D J *et al.* (1984) Periventricular infarction diagnosed by ultrasound: a postmortem correlation. *J Pediatr* 105:106–110.

Okuda T, Korogi Y, Ikushima I (1998) Use of fluid-attenuation recovery (FLAIR) sequences in perinatal hypoxic-ischaemic encephalopathy. *Br J Radiol* 71(843):282–290.

Paakko E, Lopponen T L, Saukkonen A-L *et al.* (1994) Information value of magnetic resonance imaging in shunted hydrocephalus. *Arch Dis Child* 70:530–535.

Paneth N, Rudelli R, Monte W *et al.* (1990) White matter necrosis in very low birth weight infants: neuropathologic and ultrasonographic findings in infants surviving six days or longer. *J Pediatr* 116:975–984.

Pape K E, Bennett-Britton S, Szymonowicz W (1983) Diagnostic accuracy of neonatal brain imaging: a postmortem correlation of computed tomography and ultrasound scans. *J Pediatr* 102:275–280.

Papile L A, Burstein J, Burstein R & Koffler H (1978) Incidence and evolution of subependymal and intraventricular hemorrhage: a study of infants with birth weights less than 1500 gm? *J Pediatr* 92:529–534.

Pasternak J F, Predley T A & Mikhael M A (1991) Neonatal asphyxia: vulnerability of basal ganglia, thalamus and brainstem. *Pediatr Neurol* 7:147–149.

Pasternak J F & Gorey M T (1998) The syndrome of acute near total intrauterine asphyxia in the term neonate. *Pediatr Neurol* 18:391–398.

Peter B M (1996) Brain SPECT gets favourable review from neuroradiology panel. *J Nuclear Med* 37:14N.

Pohl M. Zimmerhackl L B, Heinen F *et al.* (1998) Bilateral renal vein thrombosis and venous sinus thrombosis in a neonate with factor V mutation (FV Leiden). *J Pediatr* 132:159–161.

Quencer R M (1992) Intracranial CSF flow in pediatric hydrocephalus: evaluation with cine-MR imaging. *Am J Neuroradiol* 13:601–608.

Ringelberg J & van de Bor M (1993) Outcome of transient echodensities in preterm infants. *Neuropediatrics* 24:269–273.

Rivkin M J, Anderson M L & Kaye E M (1992) Neonatal idiopathic cerebral venous thrombosis: an unrecognised cause of transient seizures or lethargy. *Annals Neurol* 32:51–56.

Roach E S, Gomez M R & Northrup H (1998) Tuberous sclerosis complex consensus conference: Revised clinical diagnostic criteria. *J Child Neurol* 13:624–628.

✪ Roland E H & Hill A (1997) Intraventricular haemorrhage and posthaemorrhagic hydrocephalus. Current and potential interventions. *Clinics in Perinatology* 24:589–605.

Roland E H, Poskitt K, Rodriguez E *et al.* (1998) Perinatal hypoxic-ischemic thalamic injury: clinical features and neuroimaging. *Ann Neurol* 44:161–166.

Rumack C & Johnson M (1984) *Perinatal and infant brain imaging.* Chicago: Year Book Medical Publishers.

✪ Rutherford M A, Pennock J M & Dubowitz L M S (1994) Cranial ultrasound and magnetic resonance imaging in hypoxic-ischaemic encephalopathy: a comparison with outcome. *Dev Med Child Neurol* 36:813–825.

Shankaran S, Slovis T L, Bedard M P & Poland R L (1982) Sonographic classification of intracranial hemorrhage: a prognostic indicator of mortality, morbidity and short-term neurologic outcome. *J Pediatr* 100:469–475.

Shevell M I, Ashwal S & Novonty E (1999) Proton magnetic resonance spectroscopy: clinical applications in children with nervous system diseases. *Semin Pediatr Neurol* 6:68–77.

✪ Siegel M J (1995) Pediatric sonography Brain. 29–101 2nd edn. ed. Siegel C M J. New York: Raven Press Ltd.

Shrimpton P C & Wall B F (1995) The increasing importance of X-ray computed tomography as a source of medical exposure. *Rad Protect Dosim* 57:413–415.

Shulkin B L (1997) PET applications in pediatrics. *Q J Nuc Med* 41:281–291.

Skranes J S, Vik T, Nilsen G *et al.* (1993) Cerebral magnetic resonance imaging (MRI) and mental and motor function of very low birth weight infants at one year of corrected age. *Neuropediatrics* 24:256–262.

Takashima S & Tanaka K (1978) Subcortical leukomalacia, relationship to development of the central sulcus, and its vascular supply. *Arch Neurol* 35:470–476.

Takashima S, Mito T & Ando Y (1986) Pathogenesis of periventricular white matter hemorrhages in preterm infants. *Brain Dev* 8:25–30.

Tanner S F, Ramenghi L A, Ridgeway J P *et al.* (2000) Quantitative comparison of the intra brain diffusion in adults versus pre-term and term neonates and infants. *Am J Radiol* 174(6):16643–16649.

✪ Taylor G A (1998) Recent advances in neonatal cranial ultrasound and Doppler techniques. *Clin Perinatol* 24:677–689.

Taylor G A, Soul J S & Dunning P S (1998) Sonographic ventriculography: a new potential use for sonographic contrast agents in neonatal hydrocephalus. *Am J Neuroradiol* 19:1931–1934.

Teele R, Hernanz-Schulman M & Sotrel A (1988) Echogenic vasculature in the basal ganglia of neonates: a sonographic sign of vasculopathy. *Radiology* 169:423–427.

Teele R & Share J (1991) *Ultrasonography of infants and children.* Philadelphia, PA: WB Saunders & Co.

Trounce J Q, Rutter N & Levene MI (1986a) Periventricular leukomalacia and intraventricular haemorrhage in the preterm neonate. *Arch Dis Child* 61:1196–1202.

Trounce J Q, Fagan D & Levene M I (1986b) Intraventricular haemorrhage and periventricular leukomalacia: ultrasound and autopsy correlation. *Arch Dis Child* 61:1203–1207.

Tuor U I, Kozlowski P, Del Bigio M R *et al.* (1998) Diffusion and T2-weighted increases in magnetic resonance images of immature brain during hypoxia-ischemia: transient reversal posthypoxia. *Exp Neurol* 150:321–328.

Van der Knapp M S, Valk J, de Neeling N & Nauta J J P (1991) Pattern recognition in MRI of white matter disorders in children and young adults. *Neuroradiology* 33:478–493.

Volpe J J (1997) Brain injury in the premature infant. Neuropathology, clinical aspects, pathogenesis, and prevention. *Clin Perinatol* 24:567–587.

Zinnermann R A & Wang Z J (1997) The value of proton MR spectroscopy in pediatric metabolic brain disease. *Am J Neuroradiol* 18:1872–1879.

Zuerrer M, Martin E & Boltshauser E (1991) MR imaging of intracranial haemorrhage in neonates and infants at 2.35 Tesla. *Neuroradiology* 33:223–229.

Section II

# Functional assessment of CNS development

Chapter 7

# Functional assessment of the fetal CNS

I. J. M. Nijhuis and J. G. Nijhuis

## INTRODUCTION

Both in obstetrics and pediatrics there is growing interest in the assessment of the integrity and activity of the fetal CNS. As it is not yet possible to test the fetal nervous system directly, a lot of attention has been focussed on fetal behavior as a measure for the neurologic maturation. Fetal behavior can be studied by investigating fetal heart rate (patterns), and ultrasonic observations of fetal gross body movements and eye movements, or combinations of the above variables. Recent studies have shown that the use of valid reference ranges appropriate for the gestation duration (Nijhuis *et al.* 1998) and an objective analysis with strict application of techniques (Nijhuis *et al.* 1999; ten Hof *et al.* 1999) are prerequisites for studying fetal behavior. Without them, comparisons with former or future measurements or among groups of patients and studies cannot be made.

In this chapter we will review the most important data on fetal behavioral states and on isolated fetal behavioral variables such as fetal body, eye, breathing, and mouth movements, and fetal heart rate patterns (FHRP). This will be followed by paragraphs on fetal neurology and the consequences of the concept of fetal behavior in clinical practice. Finally, a description of fetal behavior in twins will be given.

**Table 7.1** First appearance of several fetal movement patterns in postmenstrual weeks in both singleton and twin gestations.

| Fetal movement pattern | Singletons | Twins‡ |
|---|---|---|
| Fetal heart activity* | 5.5–6.5 | |
| Just-discernible movement | 7.5–8.5 | |
| Startle | 8.0–9.5 | 8.0–10.5 |
| General movement | 8.5–9.5 | |
| Hiccup | 8.5–10.5 | 8.0–11.0 |
| Breathing movement | 10.5–11.5 | 9.0–14.5 |
| Hand/face contact | 10.0–12.5 | 8.5–11.0 |
| Jaw opening | 10.5–12.5 | 8.0–12.0 |
| Stretch | 10.5–15.5 | 11.5–15.5 |
| Yawn | 11.5–15.5 | 11.5–15.5 |
| Sucking and swallowing | 12.5–14.5 | 10.0–13.5 |
| Eye movements** | | |
| Slow | 16.0 | |
| Rapid | 23.0 | |
| *Movement patterns only in twins‡* | | |
| Touch without reaction | | 9.5–13.0 |
| First reaction | | 10.0–13.5 |
| Slow body contact | | 9.0–16.0 |
| Fast body contact | | 11.0–15.0 |
| Complex contact: 'embrace' | | 12.0–16.0 |
| Complex mouth contact: 'kiss' | | 13.0–18.5 |

*Source*: Adapted from De Vries *et al.* (1982), *van Heeswijk *et al.* (1990), **Birnholz (1981) and ‡Arabin *et al.* (1998).

## FETAL BODY MOVEMENTS

Fetal body movements yield important information on the condition of the fetus. Ever since the introduction of ultrasound, researchers have focussed on both the quantitative and qualitative aspects of fetal movements. Most types of movement patterns emerge between 7 and 15 weeks gestation. From then onwards, 15 distinct patterns can be distinguished (Table 7.1). These movements, once observed, remain present during the course of pregnancy and their appearance hardly changes (de Vries *et al.* 1982).

Comparison of the quantitative parameters of movements between different studies is hampered by the various fetal movement definitions used and by methodological differences. One aspect which makes it difficult to compare results is the use of different procedures to smooth the data by inclusion of a certain time interval between single movements that compose a burst of movement. This effect is enhanced early in gestation due to the larger number of movements separated by short intervals while episodes of fetal quiescence develop gradually, especially after 30 weeks gestation. These different smoothing procedures explain a large part of the discrepancy in results between different studies (ten Hof *et al.* 1999). The percentage incidence and the number of movements decrease curvilinearly from 24 weeks of gestation. This overall decline in movement incidence appears to be a developmental phenomenon, rather than just the result of the emergence of rest–activity cycles with progressively increasing episodes of fetal quiescence. During episodes of quiescence the fetus moves less than during active periods. But towards term, movements gradually disappear almost completely during these quiet episodes.

Up till now, the quality of movements might be a better indicator of the integrity of the fetal nervous system. Normal quality of general movements is defined, for both the pre- and postnatal periods, as spontaneous, gross movements involving the whole body, lasting from a few seconds to a few minutes, with a variable sequence of arm, trunk, head and leg movements, a waxing and waning in intensity, force and speed, and a gradual onset and end (Prechtl & Einspieler 1997).

### ABNORMAL FETAL BODY MOVEMENTS

A delay of the appearance of fetal movement patterns by 1 to 2 weeks has been found in generally well-controlled studies in women with type-1 diabetes mellitus. Abnormal movement patterns have been found in fetuses with several abnormalities, e.g. chromosomal anomalies, anencephaly, and growth-retardation. The abnormal movement patterns are indicative of altered brain and/or muscular development and are most commonly due to changes in the quality of the movements (e.g. abrupt, forceful movements or slow, monotonous movements). In some fetuses this coincides with a change in the quantity of the movements, mostly a decrease (Visser *et al.* 1992). Absent fetal movements have been found in fetuses with the fetal akinesia deformation sequence. Unfortunately, it is still not feasible to use quality of movements in a single case as an instrument for clinical decision-making.

### INTRAFETAL CONSISTENCY IN FETAL BODY MOVEMENTS

The intrafetal consistency for body movements is low and is probably a feature of the normal development of movements. This high inter- and intrafetal variation makes the sole measurement of fetal movements an inappropriate tool to assess the fetal condition. Nevertheless, a percentage incidence of movements below the lower range of normality (2.5–4.0% after 30 weeks) would warrant further investigations.

## FETAL EYE MOVEMENTS

Fetal eye movements (EM) can be observed from 16–18 weeks gestation onwards (Bots *et al.* 1981; Birnholz 1981). Overall frequency of EM increases up to 30–33 weeks, after which frequency remains constant up to term. From about 30 weeks onwards, consolidation into long-term clusters of EM occur. Episodes with and without (mainly rapid) EM become closely linked with the other two state variables (fetal body movements and fetal heart rate) at about 36 weeks gestation and then represent behavioral states (Nijhuis *et al.* 1982).

### ABNORMAL FETAL EYE MOVEMENTS

The frequency of EM is significantly lower in hydrocephalic fetuses than in normal fetuses, while growth-retarded fetuses show less rapid EM. In fetuses with dysmorphic brain structure, EM of a different nature or no EM can be found (Birnholz 1981). Fetuses in breech and cephalic presentations show no difference in the EM incidence, although differences in EM directions are found.

## FETAL HEART RATE

Antenatal fetal heart rate (FHR) monitoring is widely used to assess the fetal condition. Normal basal FHR is around 70–80 beats per minute (bpm) at 7–8 weeks gestation, has a peak of around 180 bpm at 10 weeks gestation and decreases thereafter (van Heeswijk *et al.* 1990). Before 20 weeks gestation the normal FHR pattern sometimes resembles the 'terminal' patterns as found during late gestation before fetal uterine death. In general, good bandwidth or (beat-to-beat) variability and accelerations are indicative of a good fetal condition and a silent pattern (small bandwidth, no accelerations) is indicative of fetal distress, certainly in the presence of severe variable or late decelerations. During gestation, both FHR variability and the number of accelerations increase. FHR decelerations regularly occur before 28 weeks gestation, but rapidly decrease thereafter. They should not occur in the third trimester of pregnancy.

An objective analysis of FHR and FHR variability can be obtained by using a computer [e.g. Sonicaid System (Dawes *et al.* 1994)]. The numerical FHR analysis is preferred over visual analysis, which is associated with considerable inter- and intraobserver variation.

Nomograms for basal FHR and its long-term (LTV) and short-term (STV) variation show that, with increasing gestational age, basal FHR decreases linearly and FHR variability increases curvilinearly (Fig. 7.1A–C) (Nijhuis *et al.* 1998). The lower limit (P2.5) of the normal range of FHR variability increases till 30 weeks of gestation and stabilizes thereafter, despite an overall increase in FHR variability and a widening of the normal range (Nijhuis *et al.* 1998).

Besides gestation, many other conditions influence FHR and its variability, such as fetal and maternal diseases, medication, fetal diurnal rhythm, cardiac abnormalities and fetal hypoxia (for an overview see van Geijn 1996). Also fetal behavioral states and fetal movements like regular mouth movements and sucking can influence FHR and its variation considerably, as explained below (van Woerden & van Geijn 1992). Moreover, differences in FHR variation can be explained by about 50% by differences in heart rate, with FHR and FHR variation having a negative relationship.

FHR variation has a diurnal rhythm with lowest values in the early morning and highest values around midnight (Visser *et al.* 1982). So, the time of recording also influences the heart rate parameters. During the day, FHR decreases by 0.45 bpm every hour and LTV and STV increase by about 0.8–0.1 ms/h, respectively (Nijhuis *et al.* 1998). The diurnal variation might, to a great extent, be explained by differences in the occurrence of the distinct FHR patterns and fetal behavioral states during the day. Reference ranges based on 1-h recordings and those based on shorter recordings show considerable differences, with the reference ranges being lower when based on recordings of a shorter duration. The validity of normal ranges based on recordings of varying or shorter durations should therefore be reviewed (Dawes *et al.* 1994; Nijhuis *et al.* 1998). Furthermore, recent investigations

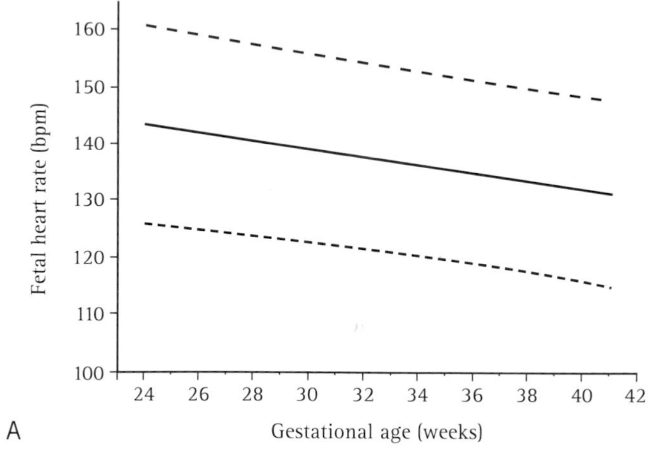


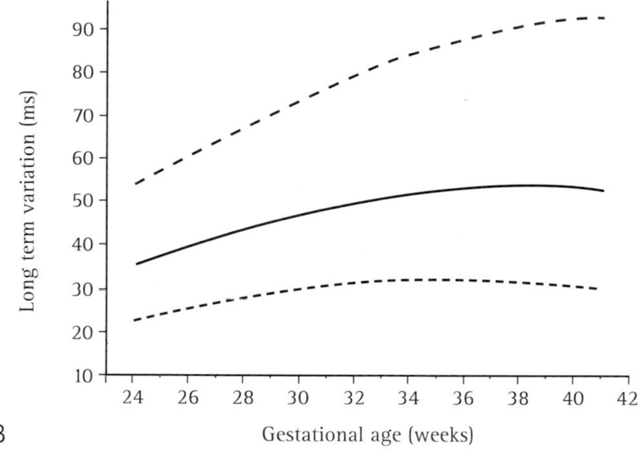


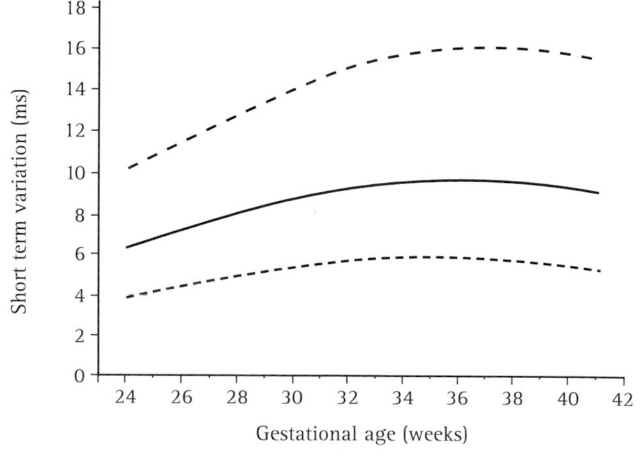


**Figure 7.1** Normal ranges of (A) fetal heart rate (FHR), (B) long term FHR variation and (C) short term FHR variation with gestational age. Given are the P50 (solid line), the P2.5 and P97.5 (dashed lines). (From Nijhuis 1998.)

have shown that, near term, normal baseline FHR varies between 110 and 150 bpm (Nijhuis *et al.* 1998), and not between 120 and 160 bpm, as is reported by others.

## INTRAFETAL CONSISTENCY IN FHR

Intrafetal differences in FHR are less than interfetal differences. The FHR of the individual fetus is on average 19–55% of the total variability between fetuses (Fig. 7.2) (Nijhuis *et al.* 1998). This intrafetal consistency is also present in growth-retarded fetuses with a low FHR variation.

For monitoring of trends and/or the detection of small changes, each fetus should therefore be its own control using recordings of standardized duration and appropriate reference ranges (Nijhuis *et al.* 1998). A recording duration of 1 h is preferred to avoid too much intrafetal variation induced by the developing sleep states. In addition, standardization for the time of the day may prevent variation induced by fetal diurnal rhythms (Visser *et al.* 1982; Nijhuis *et al.* 1998).

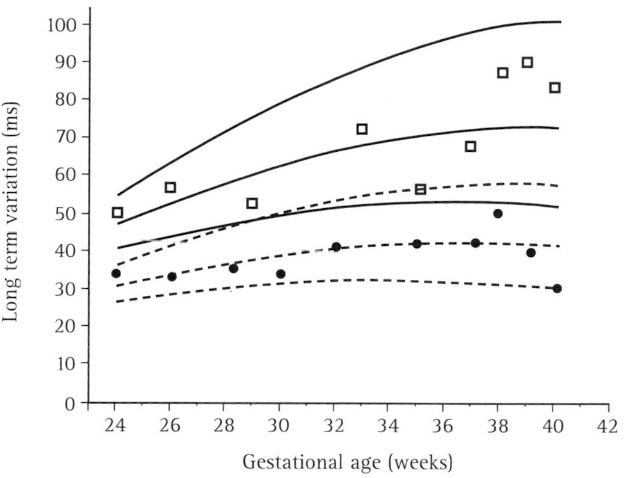


**Figure 7.2** Intrafetal consistency in long term FHR variation as shown for two fetuses by their regression lines and 90% confidence intervals, together with the original data points. In one fetus LTV was consistently high (solid lines; □), while the other fetus showed a consistently low variation (dashed lines; •). (Reproduced from Nijhuis *et al.* (1998), with permission from Parthenon Publishing Ltd.)

## FETAL HEART RATE IN GROWTH-RETARDED FETUSES

In intrauterine growth-retarded fetuses, LTV is about 25% less than in age-matched appropriately grown fetuses, and gradually decreases with progressive compromise of the fetal condition. This reduced FHR variation is not caused by a change in the rest–activity cycles, but it coincides with an increase in basal heart rate. However, correction for basal heart rate in growth-retarded fetuses does not result in a significant change in the number of recordings that are identified as having a FHR variation below the normal range, and will therefore not result in significant changes in the population identified as being at the highest risk. This correction is therefore not necessary.

## FETAL HEART RATE PATTERNS

In the course of pregnancy there is a progressive patterning of FHR into low and high variation during fetal rest and activity periods, respectively. When pregnancy progresses the amount of time spent in low variation gradually increases (Nijhuis *et al.* 1982). As a consequence, the existence of these rest–activity cycles has to be taken into account when interpreting the FHR tracing.

Using predefined criteria, FHR patterns (FHRP) can be classified as A, B, C, or D, corresponding to different fetal rest–activity states, the fetal behavioral states 1F through 4F (Fig. 7.3) (Nijhuis *et al.* 1982). These behavioral states develop during pregnancy and are generally well developed at about 36 weeks postmenstrual age. FHRP A–D are defined as follows: FHRP A has a stable heart rate, with a narrow oscillation bandwidth. Isolated accelerations occur that are strictly related to body movements; FHRP B has a wider oscillation bandwidth with frequent accelerations during movements; FHRP C is stable with a wider oscillation bandwidth than pattern A and there are no accelerations; FHRP D is unstable, with large and long-lasting accelerations, which are frequently fused into a sustained tachycardia – 'the jogging fetus'. This pattern D might easily be misinterpreted as a 'tachycardia with decelerations' if the observer is not alert to the presence of the motor activity and its effect on the FHR (Tas & Nijhuis 1992).

During gestation, normal basal FHR decreases in both FHRP A and B. FHR variation increases during FHRP B and decreases slightly during FHRP A near term. FHRP A is therefore 'flatter' near term than at earlier gestation, with FHR variability being below the normal range of overall FHR variation in 50% of cases. This may falsely suggest the presence of hypoxemia or acidemia, but in fact reflects a mature fetus with fully developed behavioral states in which state 1F (and FHRP A) is seldom interrupted by fetal movements and FHR accelerations (Table 7.2A). For an adequate assessment of the fetal condition it is therefore important to include B patterns in the analysis.

## FETAL BEHAVIORAL STATES

Fetal behavioral states are identified by the coincidence of specific combinations of FHRP A through D with presence or absence of body and eye movements (Fig. 7.3) (Nijhuis *et al.* 1982). Simultaneous occurrence of specific combinations of the three parameters is classified as 'periods of coincidence 1F–4F'. If none of the specified combinations can be applied this is defined as 'no-coincidence'. Fetal behavioral states are fully developed when the parameters of the three state variables show close linkage or association for prolonged periods and change in concert (i.e. within 3 min) during transitions between behavioral states. Fetal behavioral state profiles can be drawn up for each recording, indicating the on and off time of each variable and the (no-)coincidence of the three variables (Fig. 7.4) (Nijhuis *et al.* 1982). Fetal states develop during pregnancy and are almost always present from

| State criteria | State 1F | State 2F | State 3F | State 4F |
|---|---|---|---|---|
| Body movements | Incidental | Periodic | Absent | Continuous |
| Eye movements | Absent | Present | Present | Present |
| Heart rate pattern | A | B | C | D |

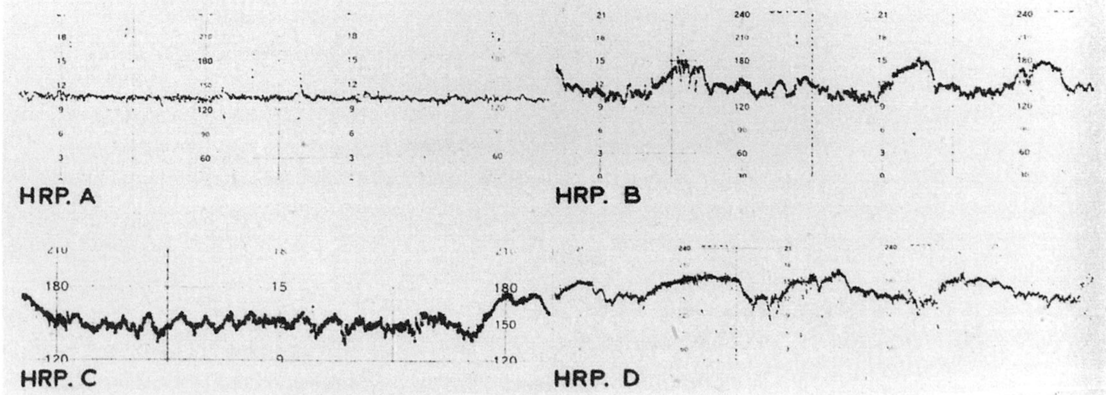


Figure 7.3 Criteria for fetal behavioral states, with examples of the four distinct fetal heart rate patterns (HRP A-D) at a paper speed of 3 cm/min. (Reproduced from van Vliet *et al.* (1985), with permission from Elsevier Science Ltd.)

**Table 7.2 Differential diagnosis and proposed management in case of a silent fetal heart rate pattern (A) or a sinusoidal fetal heart rate pattern (B).**

| Differential diagnosis | Management |
|---|---|
| **A. The silent fetal heart rate pattern** | |
| State 1F/FHRP A | Extension of the recording time |
| Effect of medication | Exclusion of use of medication |
| Tachycardia | Inspection of the baseline |
| Anomalies | Ultrasonographic examination |
| | Behavioral study |
| Hypoxia | Contraction stress test (CST) |
| Brain death | Cordocentesis |
| Very premature fetus | Verification of gestational age |
| **B. The sinusoidal fetal heart rate pattern** | |
| Fetal mouth movements: | |
| Sucking ('major' or 'marked') | Behavioral study |
| Regular mouthing ('minor') | Behavioral study |
| Effect of medication | Exclusion of use of medication |
| Congenital anomalies | Ultrasonographic examination |
| Fetal asphyxia | Biophysical profile testing |
| Fetal anemia | Cordocentesis |

around 36 weeks gestation onwards (Nijhuis *et al.* 1982). The development of states is generally similar in fetuses of nulli- and multiparous women, although states appear at a somewhat later gestational age in the fetuses of nulliparae (Van Vliet *et al.* 1985a). The frequency of the occurrence of state 3F and 4F has been found to be relatively low, e.g. with the incidence of 3F being so low that Pillai & James (1990) questioned its very existence. The duration of state 1F and absence of fetal movements can be as long as 45 min in the near-term fetus. This emphasizes again that the fetal age should be taken into account: what is abnormal in a fetus at 20 weeks may be normal in the same fetus at 38 weeks!

Variables like fetal breathing movements, fetal micturition, and (regular) mouthing movements are called state concomitants, because they are state dependent and occur more frequently and/or more regularly during one specific state (Nijhuis *et al.* 1982). In the fetus, breathing episodes during fetal state 1F tend to have a much more regular rhythm than during 2F, while the breathing activity is generally higher during 2F than during 1F. This is in contrast to the continuously breathing neonate, where regular breathing is a state criterion for state 1 and irregular breathing for state 2.

Also fetal blood flow in various fetal vessels is influenced by the different behavioral states and the (Doppler) measurements in these vessels should therefore be 'standardized for states'. Doppler flow measurements in the umbilical artery are fetal behavioral state-independent (van Eyck & Wladimiroff 1992).

The specific sequence of change of state variables during transitions is also used to define the neurologic maturation of the fetus (Groome *et al.* 1996; Nijhuis *et al.* 1998). In normal term fetuses, FHRP is the first variable to change during 1F to 2F transitions and the last variable during 2F to 1F transitions.

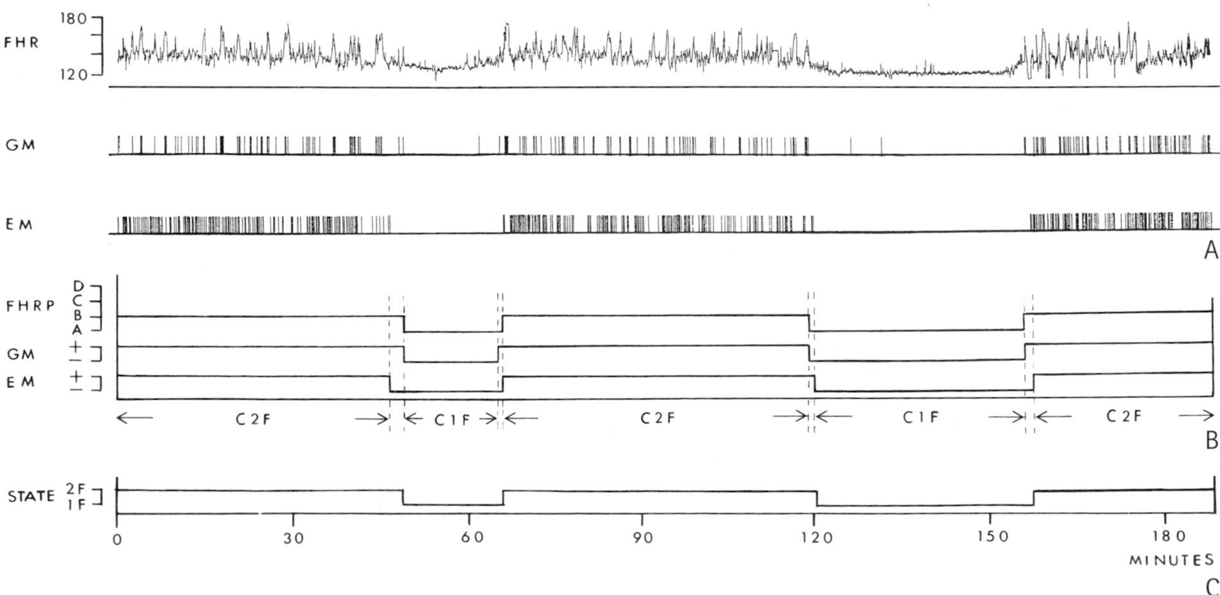


**Figure 7.4** Fetal behavioral state profile of a 3-h recording of a healthy fetus at 38 weeks gestation. It shows from the top (A) the fetal heart rate (FHR) tracing, and the presence or absence of body (GM) and eye (EM) movements, (B) the on/off time of the three variables and the periods of (no-)coincidence, and (C) the presence of behavioral states 1F and 2F. (Reproduced from Mulder *et al.* (1993) with permission from S. Karger AG, Basel.)

Periods of no-coincidence bounded on both sides by the same behavioral state or by different behavioral states have been called insertions and transitions, respectively (Nijhuis *et al.* 1982; Groome *et al.* 1996).

In normal post-term fetuses (> 41 weeks gestation), the development of the fetal CNS continues, resulting in an increasing percentage of 'fetal wakefulness', i.e. an increasing percentage of states 3F and 4F. The sequence of change of state variables during transitions in these post-term fetuses differs among the various studies during both 1F to 2F transitions and 2F to 1F transitions. These equivocal results may be due to the generally small numbers of transitions analyzed among the studies and to methodologic differences (Nijhuis *et al.* 1999). Linkage of pairs of state variables and coincidence of the three parameters, higher than expected by chance, can already be found from around 28–30 weeks gestation before true states can be identified Nijhuis *et al.* 1982, 1989).

## ABNORMAL FETAL BEHAVIOR

Delayed behavioral state development has been found both in growth-retarded fetuses [e.g. Van Vliet *et al.* (1985b)] and in fetuses of insulin-dependent diabetic women (Mulder 1993). Abnormal state development has been found in a fetus with multiple congenital anomalies with normal FHR and in a case of prolonged rupture of membranes from 26–35 weeks gestation. The abnormal behavioral patterns of three fetuses did correlate with lesion sites in the CNS as found after birth.

Growth-retarded fetuses show longer transitional periods than healthy fetuses and a random order in which state variables change during transitions (e.g. Nijhuis *et al.* 1999). Many drugs administered to the mother have effects on fetal behavior (for reviews see Groome & Watson 1992; Kisilevsky & Low 1998). But also other influences are of importance. Abnormal fetal state cycling has been found in fetuses of cocaine addicted mothers, a fetus exposed to maternal alcohol abuse, and, temporarily, in fetuses whose mothers drank two glasses of white wine. Furthermore, the fetus has been described to respond to touch, temperature, (maternal) sound, vibration, chemical stimuli and perhaps light from 24 weeks of gestation onwards or even earlier (Hepper & Shahidullah 1992).

Corticosteroids, given to the mother to enhance fetal lung maturation, are found to have several effects. Betamethasone significantly decreases both long and short term FHR variation, while short term FHR variation seems to increase after administration of dexamethasone (Mulder *et al.* 1997). Furthermore, the decrease in FHR variation after betamethasone administration did not coincide with an increase in FHR, so that the relation of FHR with FHR variation changed; this was not the case with dexamethasone. Betamethasone also reduces body movement, and it is known to disturb the coordination between eye and body movements (Mulder *et al.* 1997).

Also the influence of maternal emotions or stress on the fetus has gained interest in fetal behavioral research. Evidence has been supplied that maternal emotions do affect brain development and fetal behavior *in utero* and that they might form a risk factor for the development of psychological problems in childhood. The mechanisms by which maternal emotions cause behavioral changes are still speculative and largely unexplained but might also be mediated by hormonal changes in cortisol or catecholamine levels.

## FETAL BREATHING MOVEMENTS AND HICCUPS

Both fetal breathing movements and fetal hiccups can be observed from 8–10 weeks gestation onwards (Table 7.1) (de Vries *et al.* 1982). Breathing movements, defined as a paradoxical inward movement of the chest wall with outward movement of the abdominal wall, are considered a normal feature of fetal life and are necessary for the development of the fetal lungs. However, breathing movements are episodic in nature, subjected to diurnal and ultradian rhythms and influenced by a number of internal and external factors. They are therefore highly variable within and between individual fetuses, even under normal physiological conditions (e.g. Kisilevsky & Low 1998). For example, the postprandial increase in breathing movements, which can be found from 20 to 22 weeks onward, causes much variance. This high inter- and intra-individual variability makes the use of fetal breathing, as an indicator of fetal health or compromise, of little clinical value. Due to their episodic character, breathing movements can also not be used as a state variable in the fetus. Fetal hiccups are short and powerful contractions of the diaphragm which can easily be differentiated from breathing movements. In the first trimester, periods with hiccups can be observed very regularly, while in the third trimester only 2–4 episodes with hiccups per 24 hours will be noticed.

## FETAL MOUTH MOVEMENTS

The fetal mouth is easy to visualize using ultrasound; sucking and swallowing can be observed from 12 weeks gestation onward (Table 7.1). Recurrent clusters of 'regular mouthing movements' can be observed during the quiet state 1F, while during state 3F 'sucking movements' can be observed (for an overview, see Van Woerden & van Geijn 1992). Both regular mouthing and sucking may result in 'sinusoidal-like' fetal heart rate patterns which may be confused with underlying pathology like severe fetal anemia (Table 7.2B). The fetus also swallows the amniotic fluid, and a normal amount of amniotic fluid is the resultant between fetal swallowing and fetal micturition.

## FETAL MICTURITION

The fetal bladder (and kidneys) can be visualized from 10 to 11 weeks gestation onward. Based on ultrasound measurements of the filling of the bladder, fetal urine production seems to increase linearly from a few till 25–50 ml/h in the term fetus. In the post-term fetus, a reduction of the micturition may be observed. In term fetuses, voiding often occurs quickly after a transition from behavioral state 1F to 2F.

In certain diseases (mainly where kidneys are involved), significant decreases and increases in urine production are found. However, in clinical practice, presence or absence of bladder filling is of great importance, while measurements of bladder volume or of filling rate are not frequently used.

## FETAL SEX

Recently, several studies appeared, in both singleton and twin pregnancies, describing a difference in one of the fetal behavioral variables between the two sexes, or no difference at all. So, although the data are not conclusive, there might be differences between male and female fetal behavior.

## CLINICAL IMPLICATIONS OF FETAL BEHAVIOR

Insight into fetal behavior has influenced the interpretation of CTGs. The 'silent' and the 'sinusoidal' heart rate pattern are the two most important examples. Obviously, a 'silent' FHR pattern may indicate fetal distress, but it may also reflect a physiologic behavioral state 1F. It is therefore crucial to consider a differential diagnosis if such a pattern is recorded (Table 7.2A) (Tas & Nijhuis 1992). The most extreme example of a silent heart rate pattern is that of the 'intrauterine brain death fetus'. Intrauterine brain death is thought to be the result of a severe hypoxic accident with subsequent fetal recovery. The fetus does not move and has a heart rate which is persistently silent, with a somewhat elevated baseline. The absence of decelerations excludes asphyxia and a cordocentesis would reveal a normal pH-value. At birth – usually via a Cesarean section because of 'fetal distress' – a floppy infant is born and artificial ventilation will be needed for this neonate. An electroencephalogram will be isoelectric and then a diagnosis of 'brain-death' will finally be made.

As already mentioned, a 'sinusoidal-like' heart rate pattern can be found in the sucking and the mouthing fetus. However, this heart rate pattern can also be recorded in combination with severe fetal anemia. So, also for this heart rate a differential diagnosis is of importance (Table 7.2B).

For clinical practice, the studies of Mulder *et al.* (1997) are of great consequence. They showed a clear effect of betamethasone on fetal behavior. This drug, which is used for the stimulation of fetal lung maturation, decreases heart rate variability and the number of movements. Dexamethasone, which is used for the same purpose, seems to increase especially short term FHR variability (Mulder *et al.* 1997). Moreover, Visser *et al.* have nicely considered the change of consecutive variables in a deteriorating fetal condition, and they proposed that changes in fetal behavior and quality of fetal movements is among the first signs, while a terminal heart rate pattern is of course the final step (Visser *et al.* 1995).

## FETAL NEUROLOGY

Fetal behavior reflects the activity of the fetal CNS. More direct insight in the fetal CNS and the development of an intrauterine neurologic investigation is a main goal when studying fetal behavior.

A global assessment of the fetal condition might be made by using the biophysical profile, where 0–2 points are given to each of the five aspects FHR-accelerations, amount of amniotic fluid, fetal body- and breathing movements, and fetal tone. However, the correlation of the biophysical profile with acidemia is much better than with hypoxemia, most likely because the latest three aspects only deteriorate late with worsening fetal condition.

So far, direct assessment of the nervous system has been difficult. Fetuses with congenital anomalies may show bizarre behavior or dissociation of heart rate and movements (Tas & Nijhuis 1992). Other fetuses may show disrupted behavioral states or state transitions, or a delayed development of states [e.g. (Mulder 1993; Nijhuis *et al.* 1999)]. Nevertheless, it is still difficult to draw conclusions from a single behavioral recording in a single fetus. Tas *et al.* (1993) were able to evoke an intercostal-to-phrenic-inhibitory reflex (IPIR): a reflex that is elicited by manual compression of the fetal ribcage, resulting in an apnea. This seemed an interesting approach, but they were not able to find a different result in a group of growth-retarded fetuses. Fetal habituation, i.e. the cessation of response to a repeated stimulus, is another test. For example, Hepper & Shahidullah (1992) demonstrated that fetuses with Down's syndrome take longer to habituate than normal fetuses.

It still remains difficult to perform a prenatal neurologic examination. In future, it seems possible that no single, isolated aspect of behavior alone will evolve to conduct a fetal neurologic investigation, but rather a combination of behaviors/tests.

## TWINS

Multiple pregnancies allow us to analyze specific twin behavior, with possible passive and active interactions between the two fetuses. When studying twins, note that the two fetuses must always be reliably distinguished.

From early gestation onward several distinct movement patterns have been demonstrated (Table 7.1). Complex movements, lasting more than 5 s, are described to emerge somewhat later in pregnancy (Arabin *et al.* 1998). Investigations into whether contacts between the twins are preferably initiated by one of the multiplets have, up to now, not revealed a 'dominant' twin. Furthermore, studies could not show differences in the frequency and sensitivity in reaction towards touch between the two twin fetuses and thus no 'dominant' position was found. Monochorionic twins are described to have earlier and more numerous contacts, and greater coincidence of behavior. Yet, it seems impossible to define zygoticity by studying fetal heart rate and fetal behavior in twin pregnancies.

The inter-twin contacts have been supposed to cause increased simultaneous activities. So far, conflicting results have been described. In one study, for example, FHR-accelerations were more often associated within the members of a twin pair (57%) than statistically expected, while in another study FHR-accelerations were simultaneous in just 36%. However, in this last study, synchronous behavioral patterns were exhibited 95% of the time. A third study, assessing fetal movements by ultrasound, demonstrated simultaneous fetal movements in only 26% of the time.

When analyzing the studies assessing twin behavior, several (methodologic) problems appear. At first, not all studies distinguish between mono- and dizygotic and between mono- and dichorionic twins. Second, the definition of synchronic is not consistent. In some studies, simultaneous movements are defined by the beginning of one movement within 15 seconds of the beginning of another, while other studies use synchronic movements for movements occurring exactly at the same time. Furthermore, in most of the studies fetuses are monitored for only 20 or 30 minutes, which makes synchronic (not) moving by chance during one specific state more likely. This is even more the case in term fetuses where active states might last for as long as 80 minutes (Van Vliet *et al.* 1985). Finally, at advanced gestation most investigators use the fetal actocardiograph to simultaneously monitor FHR and fetal movements in twins. Without it, investigation of these two parameters simultaneously in two fetuses is quite difficult, needing two separate cardiotacographs and two ultrasound transducers. Despite that, the use of the actocardiograph might give less reliable results, especially when one wants to differentiate between active and passive movements. In addition, it might be possible that the actocardiograph, mentioned to record movements of the first twin, also measures (some) movements of the second twin.

Inter-twin differences are especially of importance when studying (early) growth differences and twins discordant for fetal anomalies (Arabin *et al.* 1998).

### Key Points

- Insight into fetal behavior is crucial for the understanding of normal fetal well-being and in the evaluation of the possibly compromised fetus. It has introduced a completely different way of looking at the developing human being. However, it is very time-consuming to study fetal behavior as a routine screening method.
- Although the patterns of development of fetal behavior exist for most healthy fetuses, there is a wide normal range that makes the identification of the compromised fetus very complex (Nijhuis *et al.* 1999). It is therefore difficult to differentiate between normal and impaired neurologic maturation.
- The large normal ranges are mainly caused by considerable inter-individual differences, but the influence of factors complicating pregnancy (maternal and fetal) and drug-induced effects also play a role in this.
- Much more investigation is needed to unravel the possible effects of specific drugs on human fetal behavior.
- When assessing the fetus it is essential to use appropriate reference ranges, to analyze objectively with strict application of techniques and, even more importantly, to be aware of the influence of fetal behavior and fetal behavioral patterns.

## REFERENCES


Arabin B, Mohnhaupt A & Van Eyck J (1998) Intrauterine behavior of multiplets. In: Kurjak A, ed. *Textbook of perinatal medicine*, Part 2. London: Parthenon Publishing; pp. 1506–1531.

Birnholz J C (1981) The development of human fetal eye movements patterns. *Science* 213:679–681.

Bots R S G M, Nijhuis J G, Martin C B, Jr. & Prechtl H F R (1981) Human fetal eye movements: detection *in utero* by ultrasonography. *Early Hum Dev* 5:87–94.

Dawes G S, Meir Y J & Mandruzzato G P (1994) Computerized evaluation of fetal heart-rate patterns. *J Perinat Med* 22:491–499.

De Vries J I P, Visser G H A & Prechtl H F R (1982) The emergence of fetal behavior. I. Qualitative aspects. *Early Hum Dev* 7:301–322.

Groome L J & Watson J E (1992) Assessment of *in utero* neurobehavioral development. 1. Fetal behavioral states. *J Matern-Fetal Invest* 2:183–194.

Groome L J, Benanti J M, Bentz L S & Singh K P (1996) Morphology of active sleep-quiet sleep transitions in normal human term fetuses. *J Perinat Med* 24:171–176.

Hepper P G & Shahidullah S (1992) Habituation in normal and Down's syndrome fetuses. *Q J Exp Psychol B* 44:305–317.

Kisilevsky B S & Low J A (1998) Human fetal behavior: 100 years of study. *Dev Review* 18:1–29.

Mulder E J H (1993) Diabetes in pregnancy as a model for testing behavioural teratogenicity in man. *Dev Brain Dysfunct* 6:210–228.

Mulder E J H, Derks J B & Visser G H A (1997) Antenatal corticosteroid therapy and fetal behavior: a randomised study of the effects of betamethasone and dexamethasone. *Br J Obstet Gynecol* 104:1239–1247.

Nijhuis I J M. Nomograms for F H R, L T V and S T V for all recording times. In: ten Hof J, Nijhuis I J M, editors. Ph.D. Thesis: Development of fetal heart rate and behavior. Utrecht University, The Netherlands; pp. 178–186.

Nijhuis J G, Prechtl H F R, Martin C B, Jr., Bots R S G M (1982) Are there behavioural states in the human fetus? *Early Hum Dev* 6:177–195.

Nijhuis I J M, ten Hof J, Mulder E J H *et al.* (1998) Numerical fetal heart rate analysis: nomograms, minimal duration of recording and intrafetal consistency. *Prenat Neonat Med* 3(3):314–322.

Nijhuis I J M, ten Hof J, Nijhuis J G *et al.* (1999) Temporal organization of fetal behavior from 24 weeks gestation onwards in normal and complicated pregnancies. *Dev Psychobiol* 34(4):257–268.

Pillai M & James D (1990) Behavioural states in normal mature human fetuses. *Arch Dis Child* 65:39–43.

Prechtl H F R & Einspieler C (1997) Is neurologic assessment of the fetus possible? *Eur J Obstet Gynecol Reprod Biol* 75:81–84.

Tas B A P J & Nijhuis J G (1992) Consequences for fetal monitoring. In: Nijhuis J G, ed. *Fetal behavior. Development and perinatal aspects*, 1st edn. Oxford: Oxford University Press; pp. 258–67.

Tas B A, Nijhuis J G, Nelen W & Willems E (1993) The intercostal-to-phrenic-inhibitory reflex (IPIR) in normal and intrauterine growth-retarded (IUGR) human fetuses from 26 to 40 weeks of gestation. *Early Hum Dev* 32:177–182.

Ten Hof J, Nijhuis I J M, Mulder E J H *et al.* (1999) Quantitative analysis of fetal generalised movements: methodological considerations. *Early Hum Dev* 56:57–73.

van Geijn H P (1996) Developments in CTG analysis. *Bailliere's Clin Obstet Gynaecol* 10(2):185–209.

Van Eyck J & Wladimiroff J W (1992) Doppler flow measurements. In: Nijhuis J G, ed. *Fetal behavior.*

*Developmental and perinatal aspects*, 1st edn. Oxford: Oxford University Press; pp. 227–240.

van Heeswijk M, Nijhuis J G, Hollanders H M (1990) Fetal heart rate in early pregnancy. *Early Hum Dev* 22:151–156.

Van Vliet M A T, Martin C B, Jr., Nijhuis J G & Prechtl H F R (1985a) Behavioural states in the fetuses of nulliparous women. *Early Hum Dev* 12:121–135.

Van Vliet M A T, Martin C B, Jr., Nijhuis J G & Prechtl H F R (1985b) Behavioural states in growth-retarded human fetuses. *Early Hum Dev* 12:183–197.

Van Woerden E E & van Geijn H P (1992) Heart-rate patterns and fetal movements. In: Nijhuis J G, ed. *Fetal behavior. Development and perinatal aspects.* 1st edn. Oxford: Oxford University Press; pp. 41–56.

Visser G H A, Mulder E J H & Prechtl H F R (1992) Studies on developmental neurology in the human fetus. *Dev Pharmacol Ther* 18:175–183.

Visser G H A, Goodman J D S, Levine D H & Dawes G S (1982) Diurnal and other cyclic variations in human fetal heart rate near term. *Am J Obstet Gynecol* 142:535–544.

Visser G H A, Ribbert L S M & Bekedam D J (1994) Sequential changes in Doppler waveform, fetal heart rate and movements patterns in IUGR fetuses. In: van Geijn H P & Copray F J A, eds. *A critical appraisal of fetal surveillance*. Amsterdam: Elsevier Science; pp. 193–200.

# Chapter 8 Clinical assessment of the infant nervous system

C. Amiel-Tison

## HISTORICAL BACKGROUND

Cerebral function in infants received minimal scientific attention in the early 1900s. Obstetricians were concerned with the problems of labor and delivery while pediatricians focussed on the role of diet in infancy. Advances in perinatology were measured by infant survival rates. By the 1950s and early 1960s, clinicians were focussing their attention on function of the CNS in the neonatal period. These pioneers included André-Thomas and Saint-Anne Dargassies in Paris (André-Thomas *et al.* 1952, 1960), Peiper in Leipzig (Peiper 1963), Prechtl and Beintema in Groningen (Prechtl & Beintema 1964). Each developed a type of assessment based on their own scientific expertise: adult neurology for André-Thomas, pediatrics for Peiper, ethology for Prechtl.

These developments in clinical assessment occurred at the same time that care for the sick neonate became more sophisticated. Neonatologists, however, were unable to fully incorporate these clinical methods of assessment into their routine practice because of certain practice limitations. There was already too much physical handling of sick neonates, physicians were busy with new priorities and had less time for clinical assessment, and most pediatricians lacked the self-confidence to practise methods that they considered exceedingly complex.

Later, in the 1970s, technical apparatus for artificial ventilation and monitoring of vital functions made any clinical approach even more difficult and limited the clinician to observation in the acute stage. On the other hand, remarkable advances occurred, including bedside brain imaging and the development of neurophysiological studies such as electroencephalography (Chapter 11) and brainstem auditory evoked responses (Chapter 12). At this time, there was a temptation among physicians to give up clinical assessment and rely only on imaging and other investigations in order to obtain information on neurologic impairment. This tendency is still apparent in recent literature in which radiologists and neurophysiologists compete in the early prediction of adverse late outcome.

Despite this greater reliance on diagnostic technology, two significant trends emerged in the 1970s that strengthened the usefulness of clinical assessment. First, clinicians became more aware of the importance of behavioral organization of the neonate and how to take into account interaction between neonates and their caretakers. Brazelton (1973) and his followers included these data in their assessment instruments. The influence of behavioral studies has enriched the field of neonatal neurology, with some overlap in the item content of the assessment instruments. Second, clinicians began to recognize a high incidence of transient neurologic signs in the neonatal period during the first 2 months which did not affect late outcome. They subsequently became more interested in early definition of optimal CNS function.

In the 1980s, clinical evaluation in the neonatal intensive care units improved due to (i) a better understanding of anatomical and physiological correlates of neurologic early development, as reviewed by Sarnat (1984); (ii) perinatal epidemiologists became more effective partners in neonatal intensive care units, leading to increased precision in research design (Amiel-Tison & Gosselin 2001).

It is clear from this historical overview that the evolution of newborn neurology as a field has been influenced and strengthened by other scientific disciplines and technological advances and approaches (from psychiatry to the most sophisticated brain imaging and electrophysiology). A systematic approach to reaching a clinical judgment about neurologic status and outcome will be outlined, based on a methodology derived from André-Thomas's school of neurology. This approach encompasses regular assessment of neurologic maturation in the neonate along with a basic assessment of neurologic optimality at 40 weeks of gestation and repeated assessments if abnormalities are detected.

Given that neurological examination of the newborn infant is difficult to learn and pitfalls are many, it is important that the neonatologist should build up his or her self-confidence in this field by very careful study of the procedures involved and by repeated practice. It is only when self-confidence in carrying out the examination has been achieved that the full value of a neonatal clinical examination will become evident. As a step towards this end, the first section of the present chapter aims to provide a precise description of each observation and manipulation. Later, several steps involved in reaching a clinical judgment are considered: (1) the estimated maturity and the presence or absence of concordance between obstetrically determined and neurologically determined ages; (2) the optimality or non-optimality of CNS function at term; (3) the clustering of abnormal findings indicative of one or other of the known etiologies of perinatal damage.

# PHYSIOLOGICAL BASIS FOR BRAIN MATURATION AND FUNCTION

## ANATOMICAL AND PHYSIOLOGICAL CORRELATES

In order to recognize normal or abnormal neurologic function, the clinician needs a basic understanding of the motor pathways, the timing and direction of their myelination, and their role in determining motor patterns (Sarnat 1984). There are two major motor pathways: (1) the earlier (subcorticospinal) pathways (Fig. 8.1) derive from the reticular formation, vestibular nuclei and tectum; (2) the later (corticospinal) pathways originate in the motor and premotor cortex. The major component of the corticospinal pathways is the pyramidal tract which crosses to the opposite side of the brain in the medulla. Basal ganglia are also functionally linked to this corticospinal system. The subcorticospinal pathways (brainstem) will be referred to as the 'lower system', and the corticospinal pathways (cerebral hemispheres) as the 'upper system'.

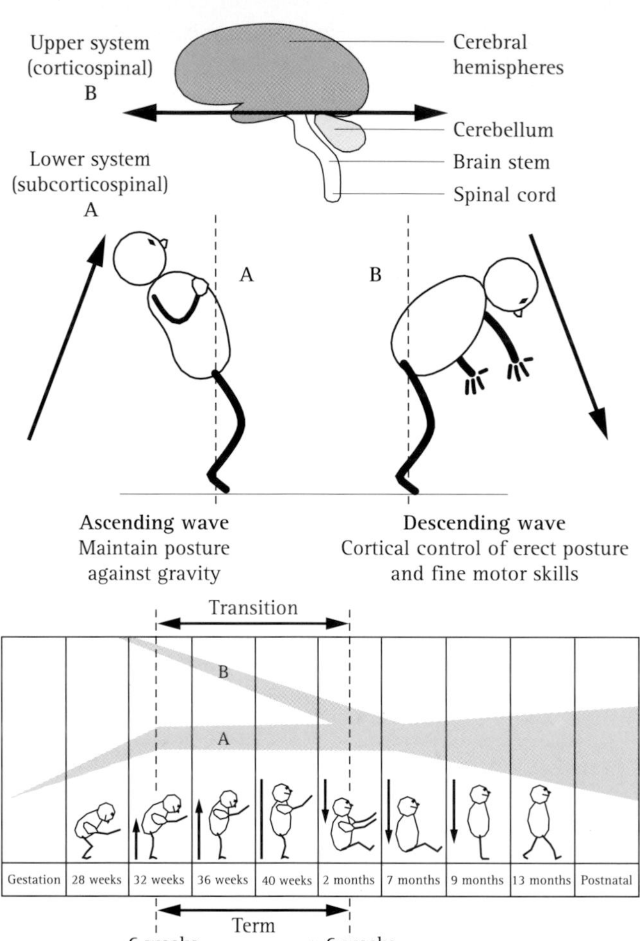


**Figure 8.1** Maturation in motor control from fetal life through infancy. The *subcortical pathways* (lower system or extrapyramidal) derive from the brain stem with myelination taking place between 24 and 32 weeks of gestation and proceeding upward, starting in the spinal cord. Their essential role is to maintain posture against gravity. The *corticospinal pathways* (upper system or pyramidal) originate in cerebral hemispheres. Their myelination starts around 32 weeks of gestation, proceeds downward from the pons to the spinal cord, reaching completion at about 2 years of age. They are responsible for control of erect posture and for movements of the extremities including fine motor skills. From term onward, corticospinal control takes over, allowing development of mature head control, sitting, and walking.

## TIMING AND DIRECTION OF MYELINATION

Myelin is easily visible and therefore used as an approximate indicator of maturation of these neuromotor pathways. In the lower system, myelination takes place and is completed during fetal life (between 24 and 34 weeks) and proceeds in an *upward* direction, from the spinal cord (Fig. 8.1). In the upper system, myelination starts later, at 32 weeks of gestation, and proceeds much more slowly *downward* to the spinal cord, reaching completion only at about 2 years of postnatal age.

## FUNCTIONS OF THE TWO SYSTEMS

The lower (subcortical) system, which originates in the phylogenetically oldest cerebral structures, is mainly homolateral and has important connections with the cerebellum. Its essential role is to maintain posture against gravity (Fig. 8.1). The upper (corticospinal) system is, phylogenetically speaking, a more recently developed structure. It is responsible for control of erect posture and for movements of the extremities, including fine motor skills. In this hierarchical organization, optimal neurologic maturation requires intact and mutually dependent motor systems.

# CLINICAL ASSESSMENT OF CNS FUNCTION

In describing each observation and maneuver, the convention adopted is that 'normal' refers to the response expected at full term (40 weeks). The examination as described evolves from observation to manipulation, more and more activity being demanded from the infant as the examination progresses. In individual cases this order may need to be changed, depending on the infant's state of arousal. When a poor response to some procedure is obtained, it should be repeated and the best response taken as the right one.

## STATES OF ALERTNESS: CRYING PATTERN

The most favorable time for a neurologic examination is when the infant is quiet but alert, having wakened spontaneously from a 2 h sleep after a feed. However, it is often difficult to choose such a favorable moment, and the clinician is faced with waking a sleeping baby or quieting a disturbed one in the hope of obtaining a few minutes of quiet alertness. It is important that the alertness level should be specified, because this information is required both for interpretation of the neurologic examination and also helps in the assessment of the infant's clinical status. For these purposes it is customary to use the following scale derived by Prechtl & Beintema (1964).

*State 1*: eyes closed, regular respiration, no movements.
*State 2*: eyes closed, irregular respiration, no gross movements.
*State 3*: eyes open, no gross movements.
*State 4*: eyes open, gross movements, no crying.
*State 5*: eyes open or closed, crying.

It is only when a few minutes of state 3 can be obtained that the neurologic examination can be completed and the infant shown to be normal. If states 4 and 5 predominate with no period of quiet alertness, it may be because the infant is abnormally hyperexcitable. This conclusion is supported by the presence of tremulous movements, a high-pitched cry, and a record of inadequate sleep.

In contrast, if state 2 predominates and no contact can be established with the infant despite several attempts, the infant can be considered to be abnormally lethargic. Finally, persistence of state 1 can be designated as coma and the level further specified by noting the presence or absence of response to stimuli. The pattern of sleep and wakefulness should be noted. In term infants it starts with periods of sleep lasting about 50 minutes and of wakefulness lasting about 10 minutes. These periods gradually lengthen during the neonatal period to 2 hours of sleep and 20–30 minutes of wakefulness.

*The infant's crying pattern* may provide diagnostic clues. Short bursts of high-pitched cry are characteristic of meningitis or birth asphyxia. An incessant high-pitched cry is heard in the infant of the addicted mother. A cry that the infant cannot sustain, and that may be associated with tachypnea and cyanosis or pallor, may draw attention to an underlying cardiac or pulmonary disorder. The acoustic features of the cry have been shown to vary with neuromaturational development.

## VISUAL AND AUDITORY COMMUNICATION; CONSOLABILITY

Vision and hearing are dealt with elsewhere in this book (Chapters 38 and 39). Here we are concerned with communication involving these modalities.

### Fix and track

It is easy to test 'fix and track' in a healthy full-term infant. When the baby is held at a distance of about 30 cm, an intense look appears to be fixed on the observer. This eye-to-eye contact is usually present soon after birth. When the infant is in an incubator, the best way to obtain a visual response is to use the 'bull's eye' method described by Daum *et al.* (1980). This uses a round piece of cardboard printed with glossy black and white concentric circles (Fig. 8.2) which is held some 20–30 cm from the infant's face. When the infant has fixed his or her gaze in this target, it is moved to one side and then to the other. When the response is normal, the eyes and then the head follow movements of the card. The test is easy to perform and it is reproducible by different observers. Indeed, with this technique, visual fixation and following (track) can be detected from 34 week's

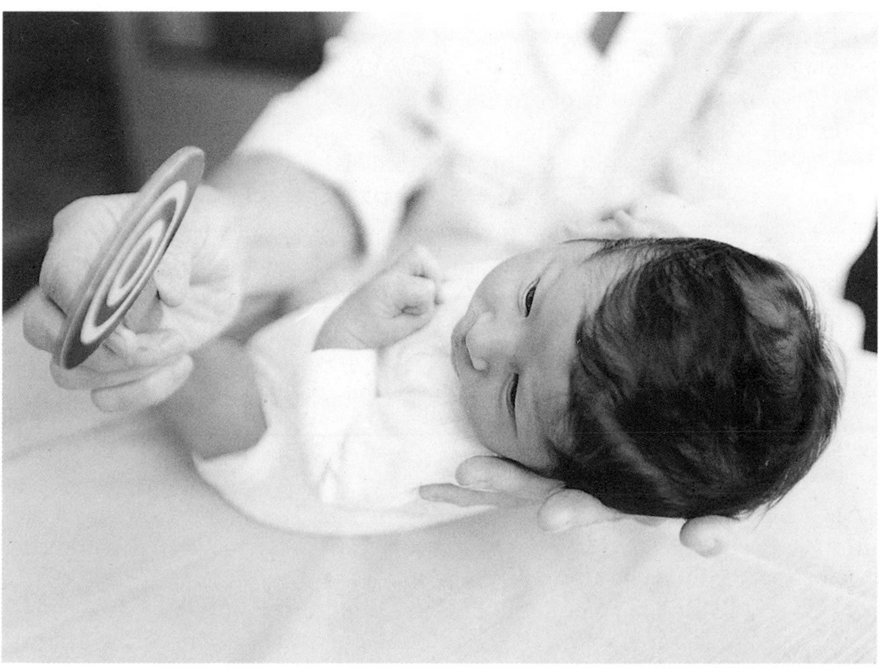

Figure 8.2 Testing for fixing and tracking with the 'bull's eye'. Note the testing position, head able to rotate on the examiner's hand.

gestation. It constitutes one of the best neurologic tests at this early gestational age, as it implies a state of quiet alertness.

### Response to sound

Response to sound has been shown to be present from early in fetal life by observing a change in fetal heart rate in response to sound. After birth, a response to sound in the form of a facial grimace or turning of the head can be evoked by a voice, a bell or, with greater precision, an acoustic stimulator producing 'white' noise. It can be impossible to use the simple clinical form of testing responses to sound in the noisy conditions of a neonatal intensive care unit.

### Consolability

Consolability, which is defined by the response of the crying infant to voice or soothing maneuvers, has been widely used as a test of communication (Brazelton 1973; Brazelton & Nugent 1995). With the infant supine and crying, soothing tactile stimuli are applied to the arms and chest. If this is not enough to quiet the infant, he or she is gently rocked to and fro, either in the supine or, preferably, the prone position. Consolability can be classified in three grades: (1) easily obtainable, (2) obtainable with difficulty within 1 min, or (3) unobtainable.

## HEAD AND FACE: CRANIAL NERVES

### Head circumference

Measurement of the maximum occipito-frontal circumference of the head provides a simple, reproducible measurement of head size that correlates very well with sophisticated radiological measurement of head volume. When the caput succedaneum has subsided after 3 days, a more valid measurement can be obtained than at birth. When comparing a given finding with normal by the use of growth charts, it is important to take the birth weight percentile into account, particularly when assessing the significance of a small or large value. There is also a familial tendency towards small or large heads which may explain a slightly abnormal value, particularly at the upper end of the range. The use of appropriate growth charts, such as the UK growth charts, is essential (Child Growth Foundation 1995).

### Cranial shape and sutures

Evaluation of the head includes observation of the shape; cranial deformities can be due to intrauterine or intrapartum compression (Graham 1988). The flattened head typical of breech pregnancies is caused by pressure from the uterine fundus, whereas conventional molding, leading to extreme dolichocephaly in some cases, is the commonest of the skull deformities due to vaginal delivery in cephalic presentation. Limitation of the normal growth stretch at a suture during fetal life may result in craniostenosis: the constrained suture tends to develop a bony ridge; the expanding brain will then distort the calvarium into aberrant shape (e.g. scaphocephaly, oxycephaly). The most common cause of craniostenosis is considered to be constraint of the fetal head *in utero*. A deficit in brain growth may also result in a severe primary microcephaly with every suture being stenotic (p. 211). The size of the anterior fontanelle is very variable. A full, pulsating or bulging, tense fontanelle is an important sign of increased intracranial pressure. Lumbar puncture can be performed despite this. Areas of unossified membrane (craniotabes), usually affecting the parietal bone, are not uncommon.

Detailed examination of the sutures provides further information. Normally, they are overlapping immediately after a vaginal delivery then separated a few hours later, due possibly to slight cerebral edema.

### Cephalhematoma and caput succedaneum

The presence of one or more cephalhematomas, which cause a fluctuant swelling due to subperiosteal bleeding limited at the suture lines, is certainly to be noted, but these lesions are quite common and are not an indication of significant trauma. A large caput succedaneum is of more significance. It consists of subcutaneous edema created by pressure at the circumference of the presenting part and it is a sign of prolonged, mechanically difficult labor. Detection of its presence early in labor can be a warning sign to the obstetrician, and its localization after birth can provide a retrospective clue to the nature of a mechanical difficulty in labor. Unlike cephalhematoma, the presence of a large caput is linked statistically to abnormal neurologic signs in the newborn infant (Amiel-Tison & Stewart 1994).

### Examination of the mouth and tongue

Examination of the mouth and tongue should be included in the neurologic examination. A narrow, high-arched palate is a sign of abnormal motor function of the fetal tongue during a period of several weeks at least (it is the movements of tongue and oropharynx in swallowing that determine the growth and form of the fetal palate). Fasciculation of the tongue may be seen in spinal muscular atrophy (such as Werdnig–Hoffmann's disease), which occasionally presents in the neonatal period. It also occurs in cases of 12th nerve damage and in some cases of hypoxic–ischemic brain injury. However, fasciculation, which is relatively rare, must be distinguished from tremulous tongue movements during crying. These latter movements are common and not abnormal. To be meaningful, fascicular movements have to be observed at rest and at the periphery of the tongue (Volpe 1995). If sucking is absent, it is important to test the gag reflex, which is done by stimulating the soft palate gently with a small spatula.

### Cranial nerve examination

The infant of 28 weeks' gestation blinks when a bright light is shone into the eyes (cranial nerves II and VII). The term infant retains this reflex and, in addition, when alert may fixate on a face or large object and track it (cranial nerves II, III, IV, and VI, see above). The pupillary reaction to light appears between 28 and 32 weeks of gestation (cranial nerves II and III). Funduscopic examination may reveal atrophy or hypoplasia of the optic disc or defects of the retina, indicating congenital malformations involving the optic nerve or retina. Retinitis may identify an intrauterine infection. Retinal hemorrhages are not uncommon in the neonate and do not necessarily indicate clinically significant intracranial hemorrhage. Disconjugate gaze is common in normal newborn infants when they are not fixating. The corneal reflex and withdrawal to pinprick on the face (cranial nerve V) are present in the term infant. The symmetry and amplitude of facial movements (cranial nerve VII) are observed during spontaneous and evoked facial movements, including crying (see below). Hearing (cranial nerve VIII) is assessed by eliciting a blink to a loud sound such as a hand clap. The sucking reflex is used to evaluate the function of cranial nerves V, VII, and XII. The swallowing reflex is used to evaluate cranial nerves IX and X (see below). The strength of the suck and coordination of sucking and swallowing change with increasing gestational age (Hack *et al.* 1985). Abnormalities of sucking and swallowing are manifested by the inability to feed adequately or even to handle saliva. Severe gastroesophageal reflux leading to aspiration may accompany disorders of swallowing. The tongue (cranial nerve XII) is observed for atrophy or fasciculations (see above) and sternocleidomastoid muscle (cranial nerve XI) for atrophy or contracture.

## POSTURE AND SPONTANEOUS MOTOR ACTIVITY

### Posture

The spontaneous posture of a full-term infant delivered with a cephalic presentation is one of full flexion of all four limbs and of moderate axial flexion in lateral decubitus. However, this posture is usually modified in very low birth weight (VLBW) and sick infants by the various constraints of intensive care. At any age, arching of the trunk is abnormal, and if the neck extensor muscles are hypertonic the infant cannot lie flat. Lying with the neck extended and the head turned to one side is described as 'retrocollis'. When the arching involves the whole body axis, the posture is described as 'opisthotonos'.

### Spontaneous movements

A growing interest has risen regarding the analysis of qualitative aspects of spontaneous movements as an assessment for normality or abnormality of CNS function in the newborn. Characteristically, the spontaneous movements of the infant are smooth, symmetrical, and varied. They stop briefly when the infant's attention is caught by a noise or other external stimulus. In contrast to the normal pattern of varied movement referred to above, slow stereotyped movements are abnormal. A global judgement based on clinical observation of the movement pattern is helpful (Ferarri *et al.* 1990; Prechtl 1990; Touwen 1990; Cioni *et al.* 1997). Persistent tremors (high frequency, low amplitude) and burst of clonic movements (low frequency, high amplitude) with the infant at rest are also abnormal when observed after the first 2–3 days of life. Chewing movements and repetitive in-and-out movements of the tongue are also abnormal.

### Facial motility

Facial movements are of special interest as the facial nerve may be compressed during cephalic delivery or during late fetal life. The resulting facial palsy is usually unilateral and of the peripheral type, involving both the upper and lower parts of the face. Hence the palpebral fissure is wider and the nasolabial fold flattened on the affected side. There is often some asymmetry of the mouth, sometimes associated with dribbling, but sucking is usually normal. These signs are most obvious on crying, when the eye may not close completely on the affected side. It is important, however, to distinguish facial palsy from congenital hypoplasia of one of the minor muscles of facial expression – the depressor angulae oris (see p. 697). Absence of this muscle produces virtually no abnormality at rest, but there is an asymmetry on crying, the affected side of the mouth not being pulled down as on the normal side. However, in these cases the upper part of the face is not involved as it is in 7th nerve paralysis. The diagnosis of facial paralysis is more difficult in bilateral than in unilateral involvement (as in the Moebius sequence) which presents with an immobile, expressionless, but symmetrical facial appearance.

### Movements of the fingers

Movements of the fingers, which should be observed throughout the examination, become independent, more elegant, and more controlled as term is approached. The ability to abduct the thumbs is particularly important as persistent adduction indicates a lesion involving the corticospinal tract.

## PASSIVE TONE IN LIMBS AND AXIS

### Definition

The extensibility of muscles, which reflects their passive tone, is examined by evaluating the amplitude of slow passive movement carried out by the observer when the infant is at rest (André-Thomas *et al.* 1960; Amiel-Tison & Grenier 1986). Passive movement is performed slowly and gently while the observer notes the degree of resistance. The angle through which the articulation can be moved provides an objective measurement of extensibility and hence of passive tone. Alternatively, extensibility can be evaluated by reference to certain anatomical landmarks as in the 'scarf' sign, or by an estimation of gross curvature in the case of the whole trunk. In carrying out all these examinations, the examiner must carefully control the force applied to find the limit of passive movement without causing discomfort. It is also important to keep the infant's head in the midline during these maneuvers in order to avoid eliciting the asymmetric tonic neck reflex.

Passive tone in the limbs evolves from global hypotonia at 28 weeks' gestation to strong flexor tone in all four limbs at 40 weeks' gestation. This development takes place in an upward direction, starting in the lower limbs and proceeding subsequently to the upper limbs. This changing pattern of passive tone in late gestation means that abnormal hypotonia or hypertonia has to be defined with strict reference to the normal finding at a given GA. Abnormalities may be of various kinds – global hypotonia, global hypertonia, or abnormal distribution of tone. The last of these may be of various kinds; for example, an excess of extensor as compared to flexor tone in the axis, or relative hypotonicity of the upper limbs only, or lateral asymmetry of tone.

Six specific maneuvers allow relatively precise estimation of passive tone by measurement of the degree to which it limits movement or restores a spontaneously adopted posture. These maneuvers include measurement of the popliteal and foot dorsiflexion angles, the scarf sign, forearm recoil, the ventral flexion, and dorsal extension of the body axis. These are specified below.

### Popliteal angle

The examiner flexes the infant's thighs laterally beside the abdomen and then extends the knee to its limit. The angle formed between the leg and the thigh, which is the popliteal angle, is then measured (Fig. 8.3).

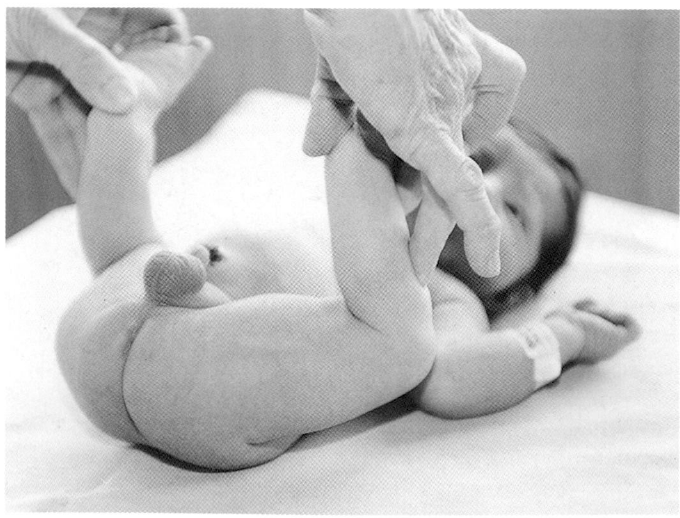

Figure 8.3 Popliteal angle. Very tight in the full-term infant (90° or less). Note the testing position, pelvis flat on the table.

### Foot dorsiflexion angle

With the knee extended, the examiner dorsiflexes the ankle by applying pressure with a thumb on the sole of the foot. The angle measured is between the dorsum of the foot and the anterior aspect of the leg. In fact this angle depends on the progressive restriction of space *in utero* up to term and therefore has to be interpreted as a physical criterion of GA.

### Scarf sign

With one hand the examiner supports the infant in a semi-reclining supine position, keeping the head straight. One of the infant's hands is then pulled across the chest towards the opposite shoulder and the position of the elbow noted (Fig. 8.4). Three positions corresponding to states of decreasing muscle tone are described: (1) the elbow does not reach the midline; (2) it passes the midline; (3) the arm encircles the neck.

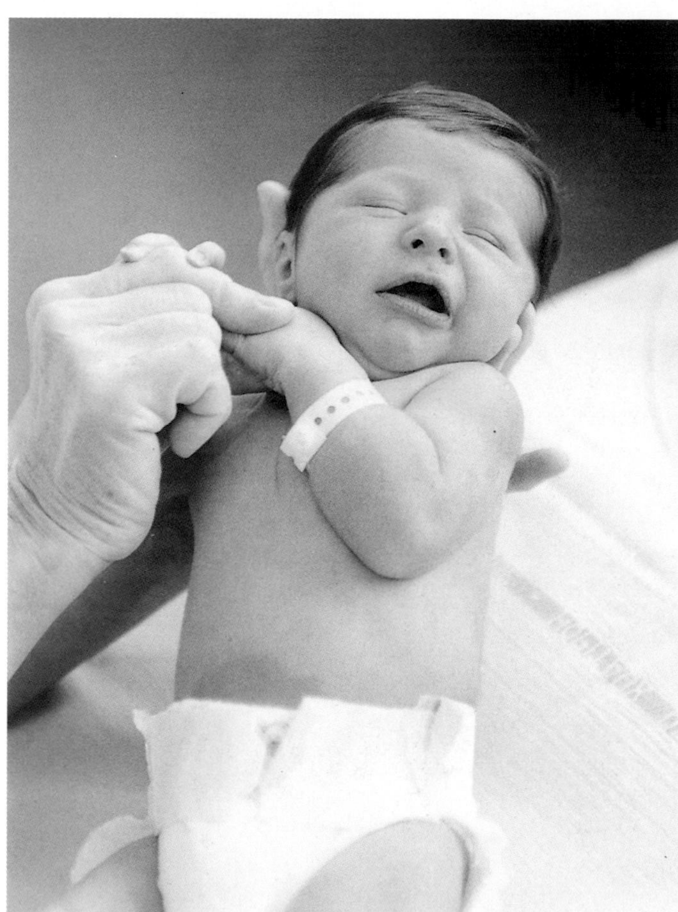

Figure 8.4 Scarf sign. The elbow does not reach the midline in the full-term infant (position 1). Note the testing position, head maintained in the axis.

### Forearm recoil

This can be elicited only when the infant is in a spontaneously flexed position. It is tested by extending the arm passively at the elbow by pulling on the hand. The hand is then immediately released and the speed of recoil of the forearm to its former position is observed. If the forearm recoils normally, the test can be repeated after holding the forearm in extension for 20–30 seconds (usually not inhibited in the full-term).

### Ventral flexion in the axis

With the child supine, the lower limbs are grasped and both legs and pelvis are pushed towards the head in order to achieve the maximum curvature of the spine. Some passive flexion of the trunk is normally present (Fig. 8.5a).

### Dorsal extension in the axis

With the infant lying on his or her side, the flat of the palm of one hand is placed on the lumbar region and both legs pulled backwards with the other hand. Extension is normally minimal or absent (Fig. 8.5a). There is a lot of individual variation in the extent of flexion and extension at all ages, but in the normal individual, flexion always exceeds extension (Fig. 8.5a). An abnormal balance is observed when there is no ventral flexion and moderate or excessive extension (Fig. 8.5b). A global hypotonia is defined by unlimited flexion and extension (Fig. 8.5c).

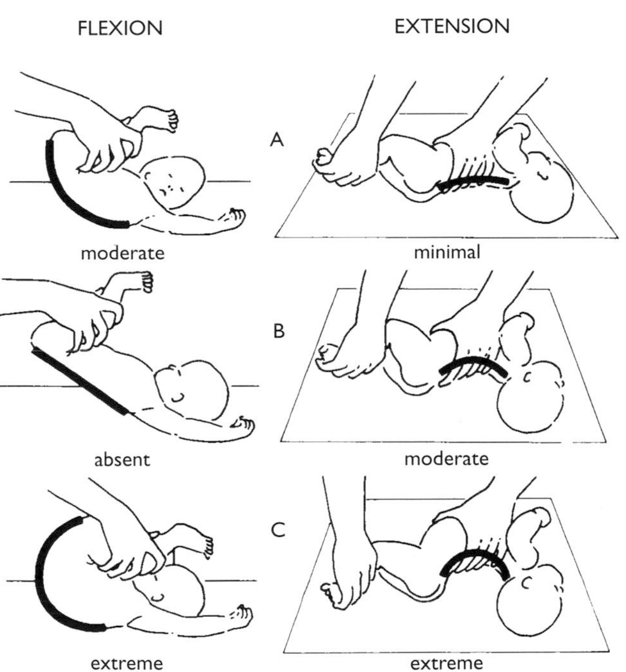


Figure 8.5 Passive tone in the body axis. (a) Ventral flexion normally exceeds dorsal extension. (b) Dorsal extension exceeding ventral flexion and (c) global hypotonia are both abnormal findings.

## ACTIVE TONE

### Definition

This term refers to the tone observable when the infant makes an active movement in reaction to certain situations defined later in this section. It can be assessed by means of three reactions: the righting reaction, the 'raise to sit' maneuver, and the reverse ('back to lying'). These three reactions are the only way to make a rough assessment of muscle strength at this early age.

### Righting reaction

To elicit this reaction the examiner places the infant in the standing position, with the feet on a horizontal surface while supporting the trunk with one hand. A normal mature response consists of contraction of the extensor muscles of the legs and trunk so that the infant supports his or her own weight (Fig. 8.6).

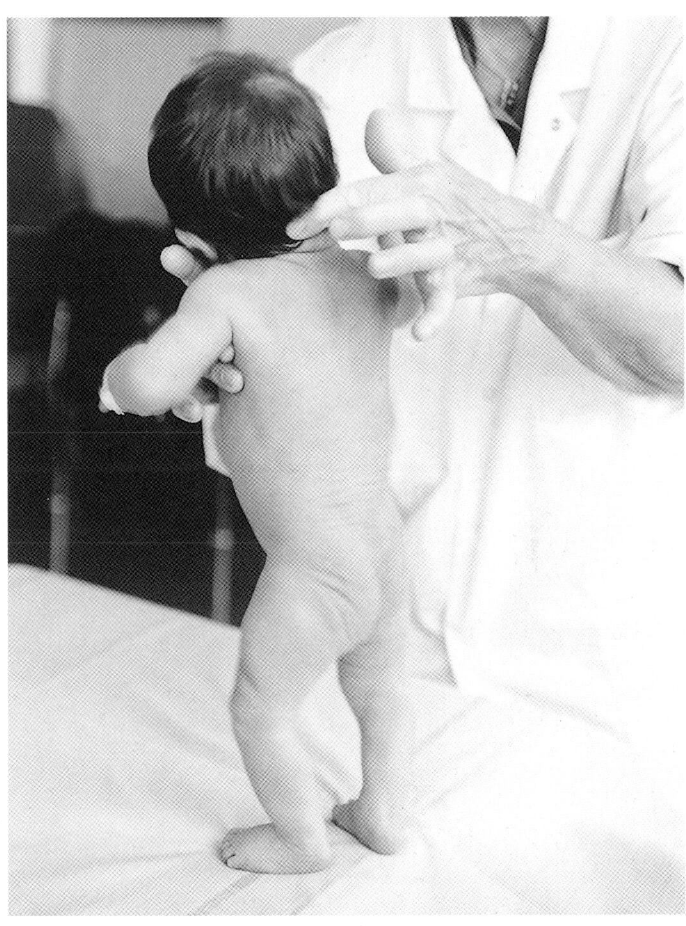

Figure 8.6 Righting reaction. When placed in the standing position, a strong contraction of the antigravity muscles is observed; the infant is able to support himself/herself for a few seconds.

### Neck flexor tone tested by the 'raise to sit' maneuver

The examiner holds the infant's shoulders and pulls him or her from the lying to the sitting position, the relationship between the head and the trunk being noted. The forwards movement elicits active contraction of the neck flexor muscles in an attempt to raise the head to a vertical position (Fig. 8.7).

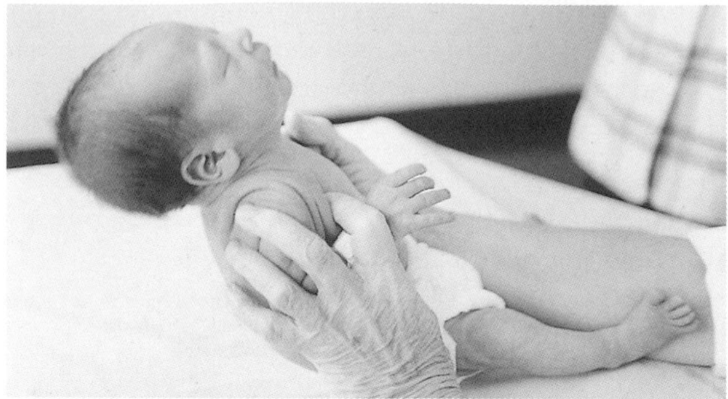
A

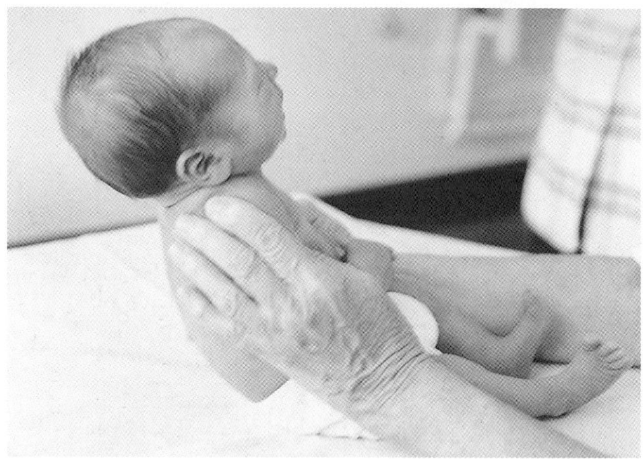
B

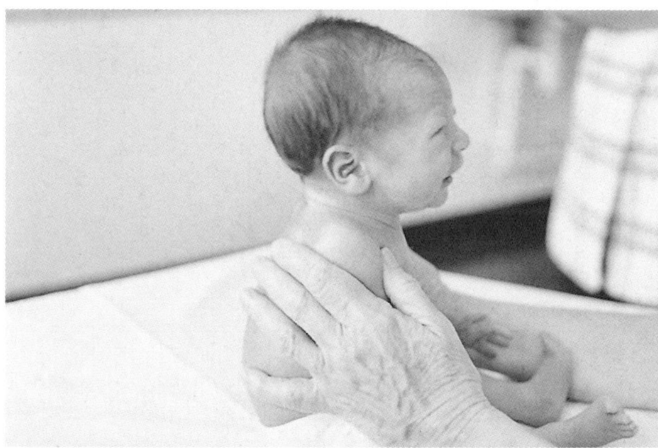
C

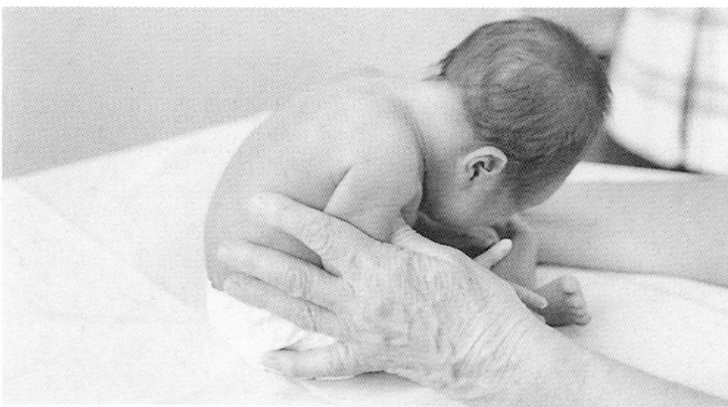
D

**Figure 8.7** Active tone in flexor and extensor muscles of the neck. The 'raise-to-sit' response is shown in reading the pictures A to D (note the head in the axis before the trunk is vertical). The 'back-to-lying' response is shown in reading the pictures D to A. Both responses are identical in the term infant.

### Neck extensor tone tested by the reverse maneuver 'back to lying'

With the infant held in the sitting position and the head hanging forwards on the chest, the examiner moves the trunk gently backwards (Fig. 8.7) while observing the reaction of the head extensor muscles. A normal reaction consists of a contraction of the neck extensor muscles in an attempt to raise the head to a vertical position. In the term infant, gentle movements of the trunk around the vertical position evoke active and symmetrical movements, which show a perfect balance between the two sets of muscles and only minimal lag. With maturation, the progressive equalization of flexor and extensor muscle activity is measurable by comparison of the responses obtained by these two maneuvers, 'raise to sit' and 'back to lying' (see Table 8.1).

In testing the neck muscles, three distinct abnormalities can be detected: (1) abnormal tone may be detectable by the weakness or absence of both flexor and extensor responses (Fig. 8.8a); (2) there may be weakness or absence of flexor muscle activity, insufficient to lift the head forwards (Fig. 8.8b); (3) there may be excessive action of the extensor muscles, which pull the head back too soon and too far when the trunk is moved backwards from the sitting position (Fig. 8.8c). The position of the chin poking forwards at the end of the 'raise to sit' maneuver is easy to identify.

## PRIMARY REFLEXES

### Definition

Primary (or primitive) reflexes are automated responses that appear during the second half of pregnancy and are present at birth; controlled by the lower motor system (brainstem), they are later suppressed by higher cortical function before 6 months of age. These reflexes are a source of fascination for most observers of the newborn infant. The walking reflex is the best known to parents and it is also the reflex which has been most written about, particularly by André-Thomas and Saint-Anne Dargassies (1952) and by Peiper (1963). The fascination is easily explained by the clear demonstration of CNS preprogramming which determines neonatal behaviour. They are a useful screening tool: when they cannot be elicited in the newborn infant, this indicates CNS depression; when persisting beyond the normal limits this indicates damage of the upper motor control. Only a few are used in routine evaluation and therefore described here.

### Moro's reflex

Holding both hands of the infant in abduction, the examiner lifts the infant's shoulders a few centimeters off the bed and then releases the hands briskly. The normal response is a rapid abduction and extension of the arms, followed by complete opening of the hands.

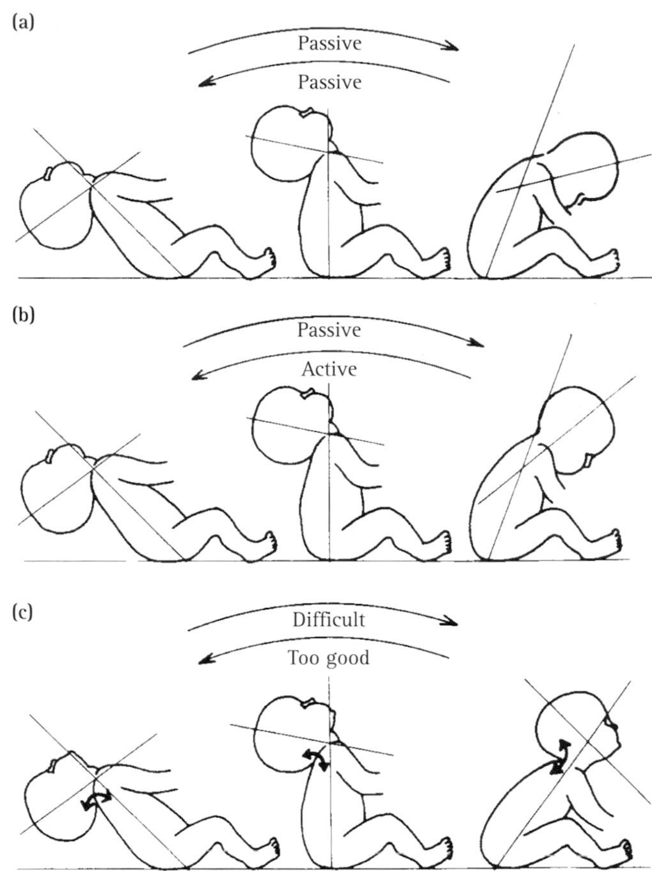


Figure 8.8 Three patterns of abnormal responses in neck muscles. (a) Weakness or absence of both flexor and extensor responses. (b) Weakness or absence of response of the flexor muscles. (c) Excessive action of the extensor muscles. Note the position of the chin poking forwards at the end of the 'raise-to-sit' maneuver.

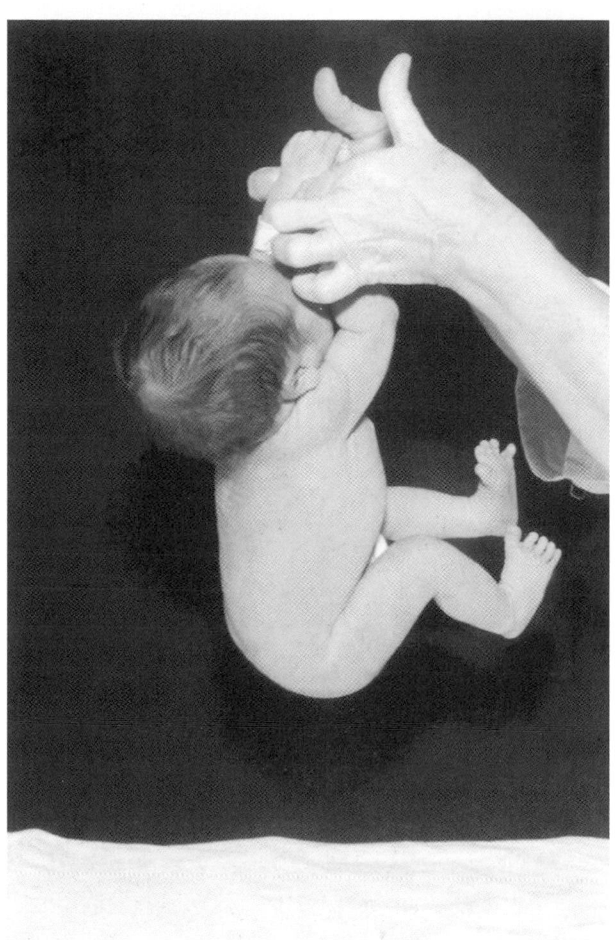

Figure 8.9 Finger grasp and response to traction. The full-term newborn infant lifts his or her whole body weight for a few seconds, the head moving forwards at the same time.

## Finger grasp and response to traction

The examiner inserts his or her index fingers into the hands of the infant to obtain flexion of the infant's fingers amounting to a palmar grasp which is sufficiently strong to take the infant's weight when the examiner lifts the index fingers. This 'response to traction' provides a very good estimate of the strength of active tone (Fig. 8.9).

## Automatic walking

The examiner holds the infant upright with his or her feet on a table in a standing position to obtain a supporting reaction by the infant. When the infant is tilted forwards slightly, he or she should make a step.

## Crossed extension

With one leg held in extension, the plantar surface of the foot is stroked gently, which produces a sequence of three movements of the opposite leg (Fig. 8.10): (1) a rapid move-

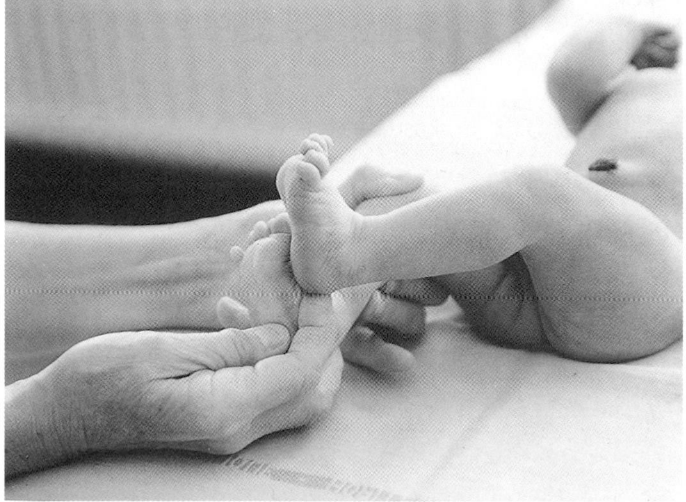

Figure 8.10 Crossed extension reflex. The three components are shown here: extension, fanning of the toes, and adduction. In the full-term infant the free foot immediately crosses to the stimulated foot.

ment of withdrawal followed by extension of the leg; (2) fanning of the toes; (3) adduction of the leg towards the stimulated side. The first two parts of this response are present at all the gestational ages in question, whereas the third component shows a distinct maturational change, first appearing at 36 weeks and becoming fully developed at 40 weeks.

### Suck–swallow reflex

The examiner places a clean finger in the infant's mouth and notes the strength and rhythm of sucking and its synchrony with swallowing. One can roughly estimate the number of movements in a burst (eight or more in the full-term infant) and the negative pressure perceived.

### Asymmetric tonic neck reflex (ATNR)

The ATNR is often observed spontaneously or elicited by turning the infant's head to one side (Fig. 8.11). The limbs on the facial side should extend and the limbs on the occipital side should flex. ATNR is normally present (but not necessarily) in the neonate and will disappear later. To avoid the consequences of the ATNR when testing passive tone in limbs, the child's head has to be maintained in the midline, particularly for comparing extensibility in the upper limbs.

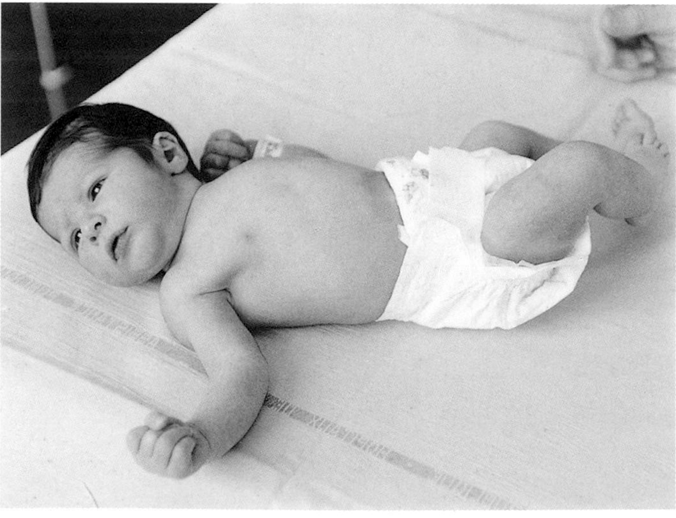

**Figure 8.11** Asymmetric tonic neck reflex. Limbs extended on the facial side and flexed on the occipital side are often observed at rest in the neonatal period (fencing position).

## DEEP TENDON REFLEXES

The deep tendon reflexes are not very helpful in the neonatal period except to confirm the presence of asymmetry. The biceps and patellar tendon jerks are easily elicited. Ankle clonus is frequently detectable and has no pathological significance. In the case of damage to the lower motor neurone, dorsal root or peripheral nerve, the tendon reflexes may be absent or depressed. In disorders of the neuromuscular junction they may be present or diminished during the early months.

## PLANTAR RESPONSES

This polysynaptic nociceptive response, elicited by stroking the lateral part of the sole of the foot from heel to toe, is mediated by the lower spinal roots ($L_5$–$S_2$). The immature response is usually said to be extensor but, in fact, the neonatal response depends on the strength of the stimulus applied, a flexor response often being obtainable by gentle stroking with a thumbnail. By the age of 1 year it becomes definitely flexor, even in response to a noxious stimulus.

## NURSING REPORTS ON ACUTE EVENTS

Education of the nursing staff in observation of the newborn infant in the neonatal intensive care unit is of paramount importance, otherwise many acute events relating to the CNS can be missed. Seizures, which are discussed in Chapter 37, may be difficult to recognize in the full-term infant and even more difficult in the VLBW infant. Rhythmic movements restricted to the hands or to the face may be the only expression of a fit. The associated signs, apnea and color change, may be masked when the infant is on a ventilator. An exact description of the event, including whether it was spontaneous or provoked, is of great value in diagnosis. The report of an apneic spell, in fact, may relate to the end of a seizure, not recognized as such. In contrast, intense synchronous movement of all four limbs may be wrongly interpreted as a seizure and, in these circumstances, a normal EEG may be particularly useful in excluding this interpretation.

Similarly, observation of the states of sleep and wakefulness should be recorded and deviations from the normal pattern for gestation should be recorded. Behavior during feeding is also relevant, as fatigue, choking, and changes of color may be signs of neurologic abnormality. Repetitive yawning is observed in cases of intracranial hypertension, although occasional yawning is normally a sign of health.

## RECORDS OF NEUROLOGIC OBSERVATIONS; CHECK LISTS

To record a detailed description of the results of the analytical part of the neurological assessment would be unduly time-consuming, especially as the signs may change rapidly. A check list is therefore indispensable for any infant not labeled as perfectly normal.

## OTHER CLINICAL ASSESSMENTS

In the recent literature, clinical descriptions are repeatedly refined and revised, such as the Dubowitz Assessment (Dubowitz *et al.* 1999); reliability and validity of the standardized assessments are studied and compared (Majnemer & Mazer, 1998). Most of the tests have enormous overlap and each clinician will have more experience with one than another. However if use is made of any of these, it is important to remember that, historically, they were all devised for some specific purpose and that, when used out of context, serious pitfalls may appear. Scoring systems are dangerous because they suggest a level of accuracy which does not really exist and because they are often performed mechanically. Their use, therefore, should be restricted to carefully defined research purposes. Three types of assessments are considered below, as examples.

### Neonatal Behavioral Assessment Scale (NBAS)

A repertoire of neonatal behavioral capacities has been progressively built up in the past 40 years. To this has been added, relatively recently, an awareness of the significance of this repertoire in social interaction with the care-giver. The most comprehensive method for making an assessment, including all these elements, is the NBAS proposed by Brazelton (1973). The basic score includes 28 behavioral items and 18 elicited responses. The procedure takes 30–40 minutes and requires special training. The NBAS is intended as a means of scoring interactive behavior and is not a formal neurologic evaluation. Many 'allied health professionals' are using the concept of the scale in their work with parents (Brazelton & Nugent 1995). This approach has helped both parents and care-givers to develop more warmth and sensitivity in communicating with the newborn infant. Brazelton's Boston school has contributed widely to the creation of the multidisciplinary field of environmental neonatology in which concern is focussed on the well-being of the infant within the highly technical world of the modern hospital. Als *et al.* (1982) and Als & Gilkerson (1997) have adapted the NBAS for use in the neonatal intensive care unit where, in particular, it helps to persuade the carer to respect signs of fatigue or distress in the infant. These include autonomic stress as shown by changes in color and heart rate, self-regulatory changes in 'state', which are believed to be an adaptation by the infant designed to shut out the obnoxious hospital unit environment, and changes described as 'behavioral' such as yawning, sneezing, hiccoughing, and alterations in tone.

### Neurologic and Adaptive Capacity Score (NACS)

We have described this score for use in full-term newborn infants in the delivery room, again for research projects by obstetricians and anesthesiologists (Amiel-Tison *et al.* 1982). It is based on 20 criteria, each given a score of 0, 1, or 2, which are selected from five general areas (adaptive capacity, passive tone, active tone, primary reflexes, and observation of general alertness including crying and spontaneous motor activity). Repeated assessments allow consideration of the recovery pattern. For example, when CNS depression is linked to a drug effect, the score can be expected to improve in parallel with the falling plasma level of the drug, whereas when the depression is due to birth asphyxia the score may well worsen in the following days due to secondary brain edema.

### Complementary neuromotor examination

An alternative approach to the use of scores has been provided by Grenier (1986), whose neurologic assessment is based on a very intense state of communication, named a 'liberated state', which aims to create a window through the archaic motor activity of the newborn. As Grenier shows, there is no limit to the fascination of communicating with the newborn infant.

# ASSESSMENT OF MATURATION

## VARIOUS TYPES OF ASSESSMENT

At a time when duration of pregnancy is known with accuracy for most infants born in developed countries, clinical assessment of neurologic maturation (Amiel-Tison 1968; Dubowitz *et al.* 1970; Dubowitz & Dubowitz 1977; Ballard *et al.* 1991) may appear obsolete; moreover, an assessment based on physical criteria (Farr *et al.* 1966a, b) is more feasible than one based on neurologic criteria due to intensive care apparatus. However, in many respects, failure to repeatedly assess neurologic maturation can be detrimental. The measurement of maturational stages at 2-week intervals contributes first to early identification of neurologic abnormalities in premature newborns and second to the identification of the possible phenomenon of accelerated maturation in some at-risk pregnancies.

### Neurological maturation measured at 2-week intervals

Table 8.1 describes the progression of 10 items divided into 2-week stages: 4 passive tone items (popliteal angle, scarf sign, forearm recoil, dorsiflexion of the foot), 3 active tone items (righting reaction, neck flexor tone, neck extensor tone), and 3 primary reflexes (finger grasp and response to traction, crossed extension, sucking–swallowing). The passive tone items and righting reactions assess the upward wave of maturation of the subcortical system described earlier. The development of active tone in the neck flexor muscles allows the assessment of the upper system control beginning at the neck level. Presence of primary reflexes is linked with the function of the lower system; some of them, however, including crossed extension reflex and sucking, clearly change between 35 and 40 weeks of gestation as upper system control develops.

**Table 8.1 Neurologic criteria described at 2-week intervals from 32 to 40 weeks of gestation, without scoring. Periods of rapid modification are highlighted, indicating the most discriminative period for each observation. Asterisk indicates that the items are not appropriate for maturational assessment performed after several weeks of postnatal life: sucking is modified as a result of practice; the foot dorsiflexion angle remains as it was at the time of premature birth.**

| Weeks gestation | Below 32 | 32–33 | 34–35 | 36–37 | 38–39 | 40–41 |
|---|---|---|---|---|---|---|
| POPLITEAL ANGLE | 130° or more | 120°-110° 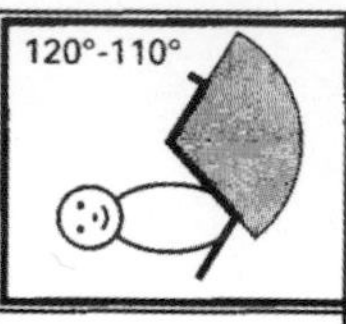 | 110°-100° 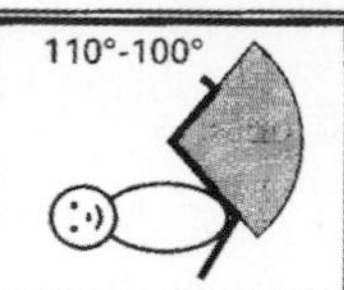 | 100°-90° 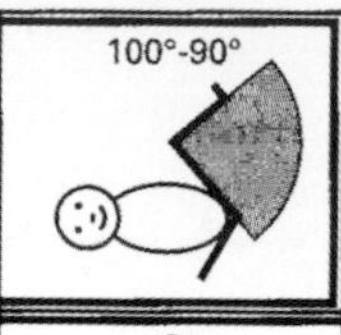 | 90° 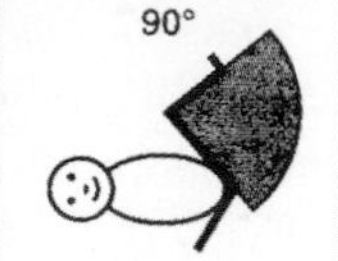 | 90° or less 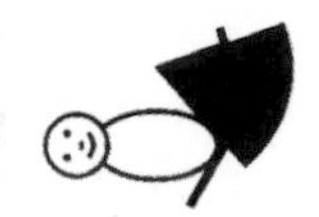 |
| SCARF-SIGN | no resistance | very weak resistance | 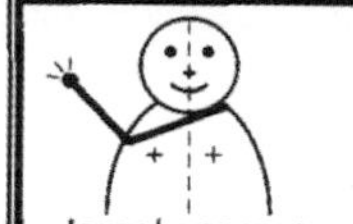 largely passes midline | 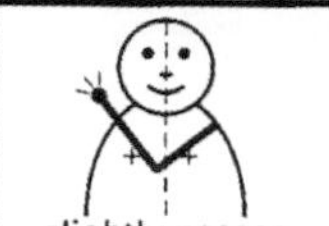 slightly passes midline | 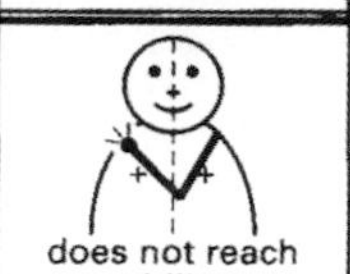 does not reach midline | 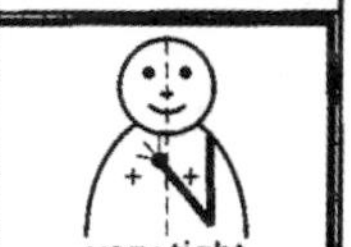 very tight |
| RETURN TO FLEXION OF FOREARMS | posture in extension most of the time | | weak or absent | present, less than 4 times | 4 times or more brisk but inhibited | 4 times or more very strong & not inhibited |
| FINGER GRASP | present | | present | present | present | present |
| RESPONSE TO TRACTION | absent | | very weak or absent | able to lift part of the body weight | able to lift all body weight for 1 sec. | maintains 2 to 3 sec with head passing forwards |
| RIGHTING REACTION lower limbs and trunk | no support | 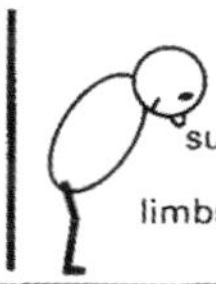 brief support lower limbs only | begins to maintain trunk | 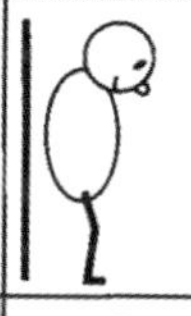 trunk more firm | begins to raise head | 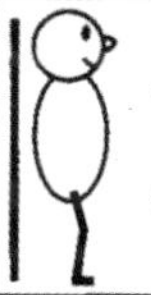 complete righting for a few secs. |
| RAISE-to-SIT (neck flexor muscles) | no movement of the head forwards | | 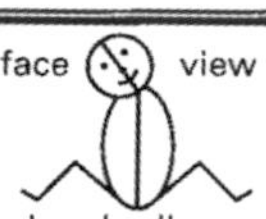 face view head rolls on the shoulder | 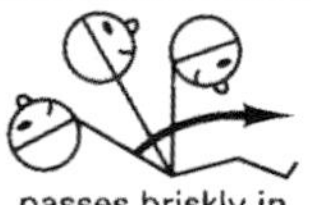 passes briskly in the axis | 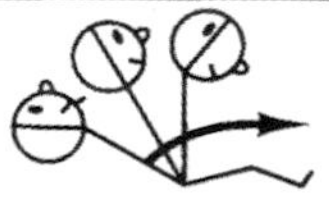 more poweful | 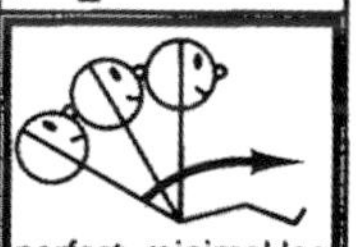 perfect, minimal lag |
| | | | BETTER BACKWARDS | PROGRESSIVE EQUALISATION | | SYMMETRICAL |
| BACK-to-LYING (neck extensor muscles) | no movement of the head backwards | head begins to lift but cannot pass backwards | 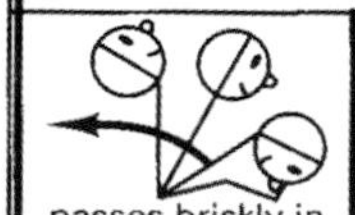 passes briskly in the axis | 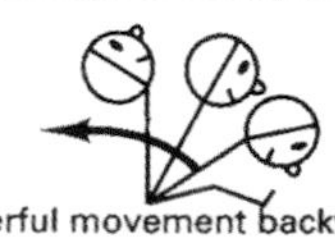 powerful movement backwards | | 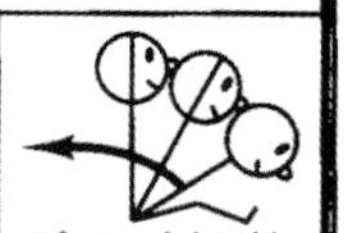 perfect, minimal lag |
| CROSSED EXTENSION | good extension but no adduction | | | tendency to adduction | reaches the stimulated foot | crosses immediately |
| *SUCKING | n° mvts in a burst<br>rate of mvts<br>negative pressure<br>interburst time | 3 or less<br>1/sec.<br>weak or none<br>15–20 sec. | 4 to 7<br>1, 5/sec.<br>intermediate<br>5 to 10 sec. | 8 or more<br>2/sec.<br>high<br>5 to 10 sec. | idem | idem |
| *FOOT-DORSIFLEXION ANGLE | ≥ 50° 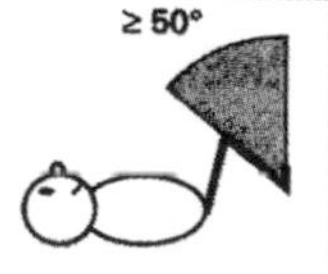 | 40°–30° 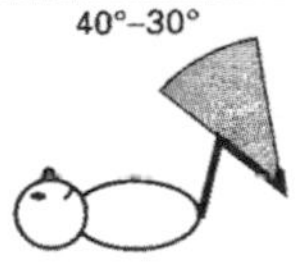 | | 20°–1 0° 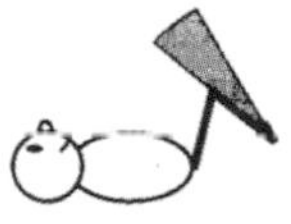 | | nul 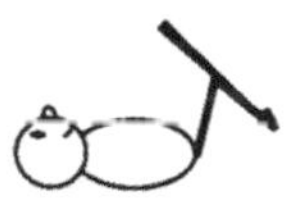 |

A definite conclusion on neurologic maturation can be reached from this assessment only if 7 out of the 10 responses correspond to the same 2-week gestation period (i.e. they are arranged in a line on the chart of 2-week gestation groups). This defines the 'neurologic age'. When more than three responses are out of line, which happens in some 10% of cases, it is wisest to reach no firm conclusion on neurologic maturation. Scattered results of this kind may also suggest the probability that some neurologic abnormality is present (see below).

### Physical maturation (non-CNS)

In very sick infants, when a neurologic examination cannot be carried out, it is possible to rely on non-neurological physical features for estimation of GA. These features are represented in Table 8.2.

**Table 8.2 (a). Scoring system on external physical characteristics.**

| | Score | | | | |
|---|---|---|---|---|---|
| External sign | 0 | 1 | 2 | 3 | 4 |
| Oedema | Obvious oedema of hands and feet; pitting over tibia | No obvious oedema of hands and feet; pitting over tibia | No oedema | | |
| Skin texture | Very thin, gelatinous | Thin and smooth | Smooth; medium thickness; rash or superficial peeling | Slight thickening; superficial cracking and peeling, especially of hands and feet | Thick and parchment-like; superficial or deep cracking |
| Skin colour | Dark red | Uniformly pink | Pale pink; variable over body | Pale; only pink over ears, lips, palms, or soles | |
| Skin opacity (trunk) | Numerous veins and venules clearly seen, especially over abdomen | Veins and tributaries seen | A few large vessels clearly seen over abdomen | A few large vessels seen indistinctly over abdomen | No blood vessels seen |
| Lanugo (over back) | No lanugo | Abundant; long and thick over whole back | Hair thinning, especially over lower back | Small amount of lanugo and bald areas | At least half of back devoid of lanugo |
| Plantar creases | No skin creases | Faint red marks over anterior half of sole | Definite red marks over > anterior half; indentations over < anterior third | Indentations over > anterior third | Definite deep indentations over > anterior third |
| Nipple formation | Nipple barely visible; no areola | Nipple well defined; areola smooth and flat, diameter < 0.75 cm | Areola stippled, edge not raised, diameter < 0.75 cm | Areola stippled, edge raised, diameter > 0.75 cm | |
| Breast size | No breast tissue palpable | Breast tissue on one or both sides, < 0.5 cm diameter | Breast tissue on both sides, one or both 0.5–1.0 cm | Breast tissue on both sides, one or both > 1 cm | |
| Ear form | Pinna flat and shapeless, little or no incurving of edge | Incurving of part of edge of pinna | Partial incurving of whole of upper pinna | Well-defined incurving of whole of upper pinna | |
| Ear firmness | Pinna soft, easily folded, no recoil | Pinna soft, easily folded, slow recoil | Cartilage to edge of pinna but soft in places, ready recoil | Pinna firm, cartilage to edge, instant recoil | |
| Genitals: male | Neither testis in scrotum | At least one testis high in scrotum | At least one testis right down | | |
| Genitals: female (with hips half abducted) | Labia majora widely separated, labia minora protruding | Labia majora almost cover labia minora | Labia majora completely cover labia minora | | |

Adapted by Dubowitz *et al.* (1970) from Farr *et al.* (1966).

**Table 8.2 (b). Conversion of total maturity score to predicted gastational age.**

| Score | Gestational age (weeks) | Score | Gestational age (weeks) | Score | Gestational age (weeks) |
|---|---|---|---|---|---|
| 5 | 28.1 | 15 | 35.9 | 25 | 40.3 |
| 6 | 29.0 | 16 | 36.5 | 26 | 40.6 |
| 7 | 29.9 | 17 | 37.1 | 27 | 40.8 |
| 8 | 30.8 | 18 | 37.6 | 28 | 41.0 |
| 9 | 31.6 | 19 | 38.1 | 29 | 41.1 |
| 10 | 32.4 | 20 | 38.5 | 30 | 41.2 |
| 11 | 33.2 | 21 | 39.0 | 31 | 41.3 |
| 12 | 33.9 | 22 | 39.4 | 32 | 41.4 |
| 13 | 34.6 | 23 | 39.7 | 33 | 41.4 |
| 14 | 35.3 | 24 | 40.0 | 34 | 41.4 |

### Scores combining neurological and physical criteria

The most popular scores combining neurological and physical findings are the Dubowitz (Dubowitz *et al.* 1970; Dubowitz and Dubowitz 1977) and the Ballard (Ballard *et al.* 1991). The selected criteria in these scores mostly emphasize passive tone, which is chosen because it shows less interobserver variability and is easier to test in the intensive care situation than active tone. But this bias in favor of passive tone has had the effect of introducing an element of unreliability into these assessments, because passive tone can be affected, or 'contaminated', by non-neurologic intrauterine constraints on movement such as occur in oligohydramnios, multiple pregnancy and uterine malformation. Moreover, information derived from these types of score, while useful as a check on or replacement for obstetric data, provides no information about the CNS maturational state or the CNS function.

## INTERPRETATION OF FINDINGS: CONCORDANCE OR DISCORDANCE WITH GESTATIONAL DATA

The concordance or discordance of clinical and gestational ages (calculated from the last menstrual period and/or early fetal ultrasound measurements) is examined. In most neonates, these ages are concordant; that is, the clinical stage is what is expected from GA. Sometimes, however, they are discordant, thereby implying that the maturational clock is not independent of adverse gestational circumstances (see below).

### Identification of acceleration of maturation

Advanced neurological maturation by 4 weeks or more was reported in a small series of publications (Gould *et al.* 1977; Amiel-Tison 1980) in the late 1970s and early 1980s. The concept of advanced maturation in cases of multiple pregnancies and of pregnancy-induced hypertension was not well accepted until electrophysiological data (brain auditory evoked potentials) were presented in 1985 to support these clinical observations (Pettigrew *et al.* 1985; Amiel-Tison & Pettigrew 1991). Adaptive phenomena in these at-risk pregnancies have only been recognized quite recently. Since there are no longer taboos against accepting that the maturational clock can be flexible and that environmental circumstances can affect the speed of maturation (Denver, 1999), further corroboration will very likely blossom in cases including placental insufficiency and multiple pregnancies.

### Superimposed fetal distress

Doppler velocimetry has taught us much about the two successive stages recognized in the fetus in case of pregnancy-induced hypertension (Amiel-Tison 1999). The process of redistribution of the fetal blood flow (described as the brain-sparing effect) helps to explain the protective mechanisms when the fetus is first deprived of nutrients and oxygen (see Chapter 9). We also know, however, that the compensatory mechanisms can be overwhelmed and that a secondary deterioration may ensue, accompanied by a high risk of hypoxic–ischemic lesions in the brain. For these reasons, our view of adaptive phenomena such as accelerated fetal maturation is clouded when the outcome of those fetuses born during the adaptive period and of those born during the secondary deterioration period are studied together. Moreover, intrauterine growth restriction may be, but is not necessarily, present during the compensatory phase; in other words, growth restriction is associated with, but is not the cause of accelerated maturation. Unpublished data show that growth restriction does not influence the extent of acceleration of maturation in multiple pregnancies. Similar results have been obtained for pregnancy-induced hypertension by using BAERs to measure maturation of conduction velocity (Amiel-Tison & Pettigrew 1991).

The widespread use of scores to assess neurologic maturation unfavorably affects the identification of these adaptive phenomena. A common pitfall is illustrated by the situation encountered in many intrauterine growth-restricted neonates; due to inadequate nutrition, transient neurologic signs may be present within the first days of life (hypotonia, hypoactivity, and poor alertness). The use of a one-time score in the first 48 hours has the effect, first, of underestimating clinical maturation and, second, of improperly interpreting transient neurologic signs. Using clustered responses at 2-week intervals initially shows scattered criteria without a maturational profile; some days later, when the 10 criteria are aligned, the profile allows us to define a neurologic age (using corrected age to include postnatal days elapsed) and then shows accelerated maturation compared to GA.

## NEUROLOGIC OPTIMALITY AT 40 WEEKS OF GESTATION

## CHOICE OF OBSERVATIONS FOR BASIC ASSESSMENT

Despite the gap between sophisticated developmental research and routine clinical assessment, pediatricians must

**Table 8.3 Clinical criteria defining optimality of CNS function around term**

| Observations or tests | Optimal responses | Significance |
|---|---|---|
| (1) Head circumference ... cm | Same range as birth weight | Adequate hemispheric growth |
| (2) Cranial sutures | Edge-to-edge, squamous included | |
| (3) Visual pursuit | Easily obtainable | No CNS depression |
| (4) Social interaction | Eager | |
| (5) Sucking reflex | Efficient, rhythmic | |
| (6) 'Raise-to-sit' & reverse | Active flexor muscles (balance with extensor m.) | Upper motor control integrity |
| (7) Passive tone in the axis | More flexion than extension | |
| (8) Passive tone in limbs | Within normal limits for GA and symmetrical | |
| (9) Fingers and thumbs | Independent movements and abduction of thumbs | |
| (10) Autonomic control during assessment | No disturbance | Brain stem integrity |

be confident in their clinical abilities to identify optimal CNS function at 40 weeks of gestation. By the choice of variables we have tried to fulfil the need for basic neurologic assessment at 40 weeks for all infants (Amiel-Tison 1996). It is not a score and it avoids the normal–abnormal dichotomy.

A simple 10 item neonatal neurologic assessment is presented in Table 8.3. This assessment measures optimal neurologic function and can be performed during the first 48 hours of life for term infants or at 40 corrected weeks for premature neonates in newborn nurseries, neonatal intensive and intermediate care units, or in follow-up clinics.

The selection of each of the 10 variables included in the assessment was intended to cover the main areas of CNS function at term: hemispheric growth, alertness and communication, motor control, and brainstem activity. Alertness is judged by visual pursuit and social interaction (eye-to-eye contact and facial expression). Primary reflexes are reduced to one, the sucking reflex. Passive tone is judged by the flexor tone in limbs with symmetrical quadriflexion due to the lower system. Passive tone in the axis is tested by comparison of passive flexion and extension (the upper system inhibits the excess of extension caused by the lower system). Active tone is judged by the balance between flexor and extensor muscle responses elicited by the 'raise to sit' maneuver and reverse, and by independent movements of fingers and thumb (including abduction of thumbs). Most of these observations demonstrate the presence of upper control functioning, the prerequisite for predicting a normal outcome. Finally, during the assessment, signs of autonomic disturbance are constantly checked through observation of items such as changes in color, cardiac or respiratory patterns and hiccups.

The rationale for this screening assessment is based on the fact that perinatal brain damage is most predominantly located in the hemispheric structures. Although these lesions are likely to be expressed in the long-term by deficits in upper motor neurone control, they may first be expressed as disharmony between the two motor systems or by a complete supremacy of the subcortical system. The assessment was simplified by limiting the number of items to ten, which improves efficiency while maintaining accuracy. The literature is replete with assessments containing redundant items. Several observations in these assessments in fact explore the same function and can therefore be reduced to one without losing any information. For example, as primary reflexes reflect brain stem activity, they will either all be perfect, all be depressed, or all be absent. Therefore, testing sucking is enough to define optimality. Another example is to be found in spontaneous motor activity: because movements of fingers and thumbs are the best markers for the upper motor function, quantitative and qualitative descriptions of the whole motor activity are unnecessary in a screening assessment. Furthermore, deficit in spontaneous motor activity is most frequently (but not always) associated with other clinical signs. Finally, sophisticated observations of states are not formally present in the assessment. However, the state of quiet alertness is a prerequisite for visual pursuit, which cannot be obtained if a child is persistently lethargic or hyperexcited.

## FEASIBILITY AND BENEFITS

Optimal responses for each of the 10 selected variables allows the examiner to define overall cerebral function for an individual infant without using a score. As no complicated scoring is required, the assessment is both time-efficient and cost-effective.

This assessment has five major advantages:

1. It is quick to perform (less than 5 minutes), which, although certainly not a goal in itself, implies that it

can be performed in the course of the pediatric assessment of every neonate.
2. It is easy to teach to pediatricians, if the rationale for the choices of items is well understood and the technique is adequate, particularly for the 'raise to sit' maneuver.
3. When responses are adequate, the probability of a favorable outcome is high, although the predictive value of an optimal assessment has not yet been demonstrated on a large cohort. In our experience when responses are optimal for each of the 10 variables, the risk for later contradiction has been very low when dealing with full-term neonates with appropriate growth.
4. This assessment provides useful information to the parents about how their neonate responds. In the absence of any noxious stimuli, the spectacular demonstration of visual pursuit, for instance, makes the assessment pleasant to watch. Moreover, when a neonate is properly held and manipulated during the assessment, and passive shaking of the head is avoided, his or her ability to communicate is enhanced. This aptitude for interaction has been present since birth but may be discovered on this occasion by inexperienced parents. Observing such an interaction in person may positively influence mother and infant bonding and mutual pleasure. Moreover, when parents have been worried by risk factor during pregnancy or birth, observing their child's responses helps to relieve their anxiety. This assessment also provides early feedback to the obstetric team.
5. The assessment can be helpful in cases of litigation. Birth asphyxia is often poorly defined, and the neurologic signs present early in life are necessary to establish causative links between birth circumstances and sequelae. *A contrario*, an optimal neurologic assessment at birth eliminates asphyxia as the etiology of later problems (MacLennan 1999). If the assessment has not been completed or has not been written up in detail, this lack of information can be very damaging to the obstetrician in case of later litigation.

### PREDICTIVE VALUE AT 40 WEEKS CORRECTED

Clinical data gathered at 40 corrected weeks in a cohort of VLBW infants born at a corrected age below 33 weeks (Stewart *et al.* 1988) have shown that, when ultrasound imaging and the clinical assessment on discharge are normal, the probability estimates for any disorder and for a major disorder at 1 year of age are 2% and 0%, respectively. This is not the case for ultrasound imaging alone. In other words, when ultrasound imaging is normal and neurologic assessment optimal, prediction for an optimal outcome becomes more powerful and the need for rigorous clinical follow-up becomes less important. It is therefore advisable to subdivide the group of children with normal imaging into two groups, according to optimal and non-optimal clinical findings.

## CLINICAL CLUES TO THE MOST COMMON DISORDERS

### NON-SPECIFICITY AND LABILITY OF EARLY NEUROLOGIC SIGNS

In the early stages of extrauterine adaptation, it is difficult to separate the transient effects of cardiorespiratory and metabolic problems from the specific expression of brain damage. Repeated assessment provides the only good way of resolving the difficulty posed by the lability of clinical signs. When the acute phase of adaptation is complete, the clinical assessment really becomes contributory. For instance, if a lack of alertness, poor reactivity, and hypotonia are found repeatedly, they are likely to be due to CNS damage, whereas the same signs, if transient or variable, may be due to disturbances in the infant's general condition from almost any cause.

### CLUES TO FETAL BRAIN DAMAGE

Much litigation could be avoided by a careful neurologic assessment within the first days of life as it may provide specific clues to dating brain damage as prenatal: the presence of a high-arched palate, non-reducible adduction of thumbs in a tightly clenched fist, and suture ridges indicate an insult that took place some weeks (or more) earlier (Fig. 8.12). These signs are not specific; their diagnostic value is linked with their presence at birth. If not identified soon after birth, they will be of no value later in dating the insult, because an intrapartum insult will provoke identical signs after a few weeks. An early (within the first days of life) computerized tomography (CT) scan or magnetic resonance imaging (MRI) would confirm the clinical dating in showing that a cerebral atrophy is already organized in these cases of prenatal damage.

Subnormal head size, suspected prenatally or discovered at birth is also significant. Head growth is so rapid in the last 3 months of gestation that a subnormal head size (compared to weight and height on normative curves) may indicate fetal brain damage. This finding is rarely an isolated one and a careful clinical assessment will often reveal subtle neurologic abnormalities. Investigations of toxic (i.e. fetal alcohol syndrome) and viral exposures should be undertaken in the presence of subnormal head size at birth.

### CLINICAL PROFILE AS A DIAGNOSTIC CLUE

When neurologic signs and symptoms are found at the first assessment, clinical assessments repeated daily or every other day can distinguish two different types of profiles: evolving or stable. *An evolving profile* is typical of very recent insult, most often intrapartum (Fig. 8.13). The signs of CNS depression increase until day 3. There are associated signs of hemodynamic lability (cyanosis or pallor around the upper lips and nose, etc.) that indicate autonomic nervous system disturbances. In these cases, by day 5, CNS function

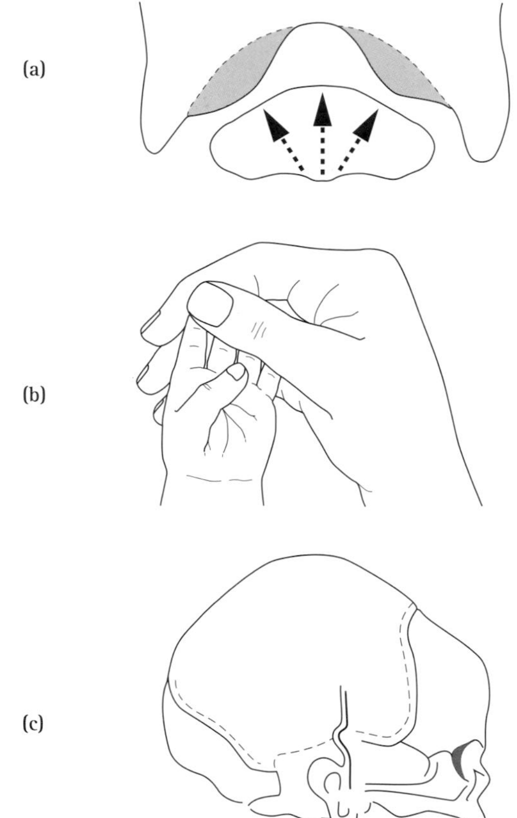


Figure 8.12 Early signs of fetal brain damage. (a) Persistence of prominent lateral ridges results in a high-arched palate, due to insufficient molding forces of the tongue (dotted lines indicate normal palate shaped by normal tongue movements. (b) Non-reducible adduction of the thumb in a clenched fist due to absence of spontaneous motor activity. (c) Cranial ridges on every suture, or restricted to the squamous suture, due to severe or moderate impairment of hemispheric growth. (From Amiel-Tison 1999, with permission.)

improves markedly, alertness, motor activity and sucking progressively getting better.

*A stable profile* is typical of a prenatal insult that occurred several weeks earlier and implies that the pattern just described has ended before birth; the signs at birth are what remain after stabilization *in utero* (Fig. 8.13).

## CLINICAL PATTERNS OF CNS INJURY

At the end of the first week, severity of neurologic deficit should be estimated by clusters of signs and symptoms. The following clusters may be recognized.

### Seizures and hyperexcitability

Seizures may be isolated (one or two episodes) or repeated for more than 30 minutes. Hyperexcitability includes a restless sleep pattern, abnormal movements, a lowered threshold for the primary reflexes, excessive hypertonia, persistent 'fisting', and excessive crying.

### CNS depression of various degrees

The deficit in alertness may range from lethargy to coma. The infant may be sleepy and difficult to awake, have reduced spontaneous movements, infrequent crying, or poor or absent primary reflexes. Hypotonia is often seen in CNS depression. It may be global or confined to the upper part of the body.

### Severe global hypotonia

This is defined as the absence of both passive and active tone in the axis and limbs, a condition sometimes referred to as 'rag doll'. It is a common, non-specific finding in the early stages of any type of perinatal brain damage such as hypoxic–ischemic encephalopathy (HIE), intracranial haemorrhage, or kernicterus. Global hypotonia is also seen after sedative drugs given to the mother or infant and in systemic infections. It is also seen in cases of damage to the spinal

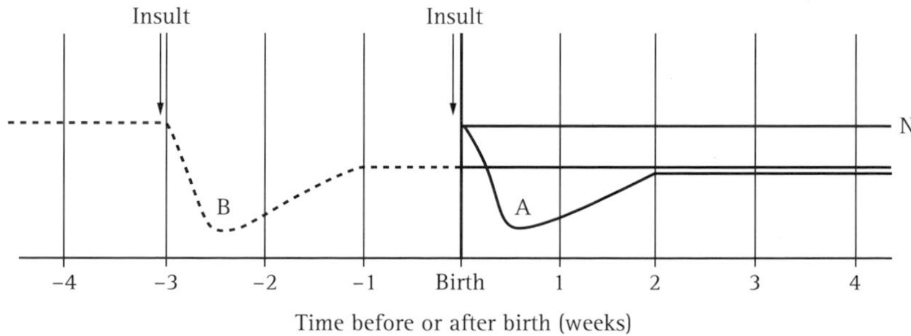


Figure 8.13 Profiles of CNS depression in the first postnatal weeks. N = normal CNS function (based on alertness, tone, primary reflexes and spontaneous motor activity). A = evolving profile following an intrapartum insult. B = stable profile indicating a prenatal insult going back 2–3 weeks before birth, after acute changes and stabilization *in utero*. (From Amiel-Tison 1999, with permission.)

cord, in cases of spinal muscular atrophy such as Werdnig-Hoffmann's disease, and in primary muscular disorders. In these cases there may be a history of diminished fetal movements and of polyhydramnios, and there is no obvious lethargy, such as usually occurs when the hypotonia is of central origin. Other features suggesting one of these diseases include the absence of tendon reflexes, and the typical distribution of muscle weakness in proximal muscle groups. A definitive diagnosis can be confirmed by electrophysiological and other laboratory based investigations.

### Asymmetric tone

When an asymmetry of muscular tone can be unequivocally demonstrated, the difficulty remains, curiously enough, to decide which is the abnormal side, the hypotonic or hypertonic. In recent years, repeated comparison with the results of new imaging methods has shown the following:

1. When the primary reflexes are depressed on the hypotonic side, this is the abnormal side; the abnormality is due to a recent lesion, not yet visible, in the opposite hemisphere.
2. 'Fisting' and an adducted thumb on the hypertonic side indicate that this is the abnormal side. In such cases the lesion may be several weeks old or more and sufficiently organized to be visible on a CT scan.

Indeed, the association of flaccidity with a recent lesion, and of spasticity with an older one, appears to follow the well known sequence observed in adult hemiparesis. Early asymmetry is also sometimes seen in cases of periventricular leukomalacia (PVL), reflecting inequality in the two sides of this essentially bilateral lesion.

### INTEGRATION OF NON-CLINICAL INVESTIGATIONS IN THE ASSESSMENT

Special investigations are performed according to indications provided by the clinical history and findings on examination. These frequently include lumbar puncture, ultrasound imaging via the fontanelle, non-invasive measurement of intracranial pressure, and skull radiography. An early CT or MR imaging may have indications in the search for cerebral malformations, HIE or subdural hematoma. These imaging methods are, however, usually more useful after a lapse of several weeks in evaluating brain damage due to HIE or PVL. Electrophysiological studies may be performed, depending on the facilities and expertise of the neonatal intensive care unit. In any case, repeated EEG recordings are virtually indispensable when seizures are present or suspected (p. 167). Brain auditory evoked responses are also very useful, particularly in order to evaluate the extension of HIE to the brainstem (p. 187). Appropriate non-neurologic investigations are required in cases of suspected chromosomal abnormality, inborn errors of metabolism, muscle disorders, and viral infections of the CNS.

### TENTATIVE DIAGNOSIS

Table 8.4 summarizes the essential characteristics of the most typical forms of perinatal brain damage. It is greatly oversimplified. The diversity of risk factors and presentations at this age often leave the clinician with a large margin for personal interpretation. In the full-term infant, in which the susceptibility to tissue damage is less and morphological investigation not so contributory as in the preterm infant, accumulated clinical experience allows the following general empirical conclusions to be reached:

1. Clinical estimation of severity at the end of the first week is useful in the full-term newborn infant. For this purpose it is helpful to define the following three grades of severity:
   *Mild*: Abnormalities of tone and hyperexcitability, no CNS depression, no seizures.
   *Moderate*: Abnormalities of tone with signs of CNS depression and up to two isolated seizures.
   *Severe*: Repeated seizures and overt CNS depression.
2. The full-term neonate possesses the means to produce symptoms related to perinatal neurologic damage and it is therefore unreasonable to attribute damage discovered later in life to obstetric factors if no neurologic signs appeared during the first week of life.
3. In about a third of cases, the cause of the symptoms remains unknown despite evaluation of all obstetric and pediatric factors.
4. In recent years there has been a change in the pattern of perinatal brain damage. On one hand, in well staffed, well equipped maternity units, cases of damage due to obstetric factors have become uncommon. On the other hand, various possible causes of antenatal brain damage are nowadays better identified, with the increasing skills of many disciplines. This is a hot topic, due to the increasing incidence of litigation (MacLennan 1999) and is discussed in detail in Chapters 29 and 30. A more precise terminology concerning fetal status before birth and during labor will be hopefully the first step to achieving an international consensus, to replace the loose concept of 'fetal distress' and 'birth asphyxia'.

## RECOVERY PERIOD

### PARENTS' QUESTIONS ON OUTCOME

In the acute stages of a neonatal neurologic disorder, the parents are usually too preoccupied with the immediate outcome to ask many questions about long-term disability. These often begin to arise in the convalescent stage when they are still difficult to answer. On the medical side there is usually a great deal of uncertainty as to outcome except at the two extremes of the spectrum: the perfectly normal and the seriously damaged. For the cases in between, the statistical approach to the probability of any given outcome is not tolerable to the vast majority of parents. There are evidently

**Table 8.4 Diagnostic clues in four common types of perinatal neurological disorder and a few congenital diseases**

| Various types | Hypoxic-ischemic encephalopathy | Periventricular leukomalacia | | Intraventricular hemorrhage | Infarction of arterial territory | CNS malformations genetic diseases | Congenital myopathy myotonic dystrophy |
|---|---|---|---|---|---|---|---|
| *Gestational history* | IUGR or post term (often negative) | S.G.A.<br>Mat. hyper-tension<br>Multiple pr. | A.G.A.<br>very preterm birth | very preterm birth < 33 weeks | usually negative | often IUGR<br>fetal U.S. abnormalities? | weak fetal mvts<br>polyhydramnios |
| *Obstetric history* | Birth process markedly abnormal (often negative) | Rarely contributive | Rarely contributive | Breech delivery is a risk factor | Not contributive | ○ | ○ |
| *Neonatal risk factors or associated conditions* | Meconium aspiration<br>Secondary anuria | Not specific | RDS<br>Apneic spells<br>Cardiac arrest<br>Low B.P. | RDS; hemodynamic instability | Usually absent | ○ | ○ |
| *Timing of damage* | Prenatal or intrapartum (often uncertain) | Prenatal | Postnatal | Postnatal | Prenatal | | |
| *Alertness and seizures* | | | | | | | |
| Coma | In severe grade | ○ | | ± | ○ | • Low state of alertness is common (except in Werdnig-Hoffman)<br>• If seizures, check for inborn errors of metabolism | Dissociation between good eye contact and low activity |
| Lethargy | In moderate grade | + | | ± | + | | |
| Seizures (meningitis excluded) | In severe grade | ○ | | ± | + | | |
| Hyperexcitability (hypoglycemia excluded) | In mild grade | ○ | | ± | ○ | | |
| *Abnormalities of tone* | | | | | | | |
| Global hypotonia (drug effect excluded) | In severe grade | ○ | | + | ○ | Rag-doll<br>plus tongue fasciculation and areflexia<br>→ Werdnig-Hoffman type I<br>plus height more than 54 cm at birth | |
| Hypotonia upper part of the body | In moderate and mild grades | + | | ○ | ○ | → gigantism de Sotos<br>plus facial diplegia and arthrogryposis<br>→ myotonic dystrophy (Steinert)<br>plus nystagmus | |
| Hypertonia in axial muscle extensor | Indicates intracranial hypertension at the acute stage | ○ | | Present in Gr III, with distension | ○ | → [CNS] malformation<br>plus no suck and swallow<br>→ Prader-Willi | |
| Asymmetry Left-right | ○ | frequent | | ○ | initially – contralateral hypotonia<br>later – contralateral spasticity | plus facial weakness and acute respiratory failure<br>→ transient myasthenia gravis neostigmine test required | |
| *Cranial findings* | | | | | | | |
| Size and shape | Already abnormal at birth if due to cerebral atrophy of prenatal origin | ○ | | ○ | ○ | Often abnormal size and/or shape (compare centiles of HC, weight and length) | ○ |
| Skull and sutures | Caput succedaneum, facial ecchymosis, separation of sutures associated to birth trauma | ○ | | Initial separation of sutures or later hydrocephalus | ○ | ridges<br>lacunae | ○ |
| *Other findings or comments* | high-arched palate and/or cortical thumb at birth indicates prenatal origin | Gliosis or cavitations visible at 1 month postnatal are associated with a poor outcome | | Prognosis depending on associated leukomalacia | Septicemia and multiple pregnancy are risk factors | Dysmorphic features, familial history may provide orientation | Presence of deep tendon reflexes does not exclude muscular diseases |

quite large cultural differences in the types of question asked and in the answers usually provided. In some countries the pediatrician aims to provide comprehensive information on the evidence of damage and potential risks, whereas in others he or she tends to remain vague but encouraging. In considering these various approaches it is appropriate to ask what purpose is served by providing an early prognosis. When this is definitely bad, the parents will often complain if they are told too early because they were unprepared to receive this information. If they are told too late, they may develop a retrospective feeling of mistrust linked to the fear that early intervention might also have been delayed. In either case the messenger of ill-tidings must expect to be blamed, which is less than satisfactory for the child and his or her parents who continue to have need of medical support. However, parental dissatisfaction with the way they are given bad news does not seem inevitable.

In our Maternity Hospital, we systematically follow a plan designed to help the parents and infant to convalesce from the period of acute stress. In doing so, we hope to provide a breathing space of potentially life-long importance for the infant, during which interaction and bonding can proceed. During this convalescent period, we do not provoke questions and emphasize the importance of respecting the need for a quiet recovery period. When asked about intellectual outcome, we tend to remain vague, emphasizing the extent of our ignorance and also the extent of individual variations. Unconsidered comments about head size or other individual items are as far as possible avoided. We emphasize that assessments during the convalescent period are carried out to measure progress and not, at this stage, to reach a definitive prognosis. As often as possible, the assessments are made in the presence of the mother and emphasis is placed on demonstrating newly acquired abilities. When information has to be transmitted to the parents, even if not very optimistic, it seems best to do so at the bedside with both parents present, if possible.

For all children suspected of neurologic damage, however mild, we provide early physiotherapy to prevent deformities and to stimulate interactions. This helps the parents to accept that something useful has been done even when the outcome is very poor. We also aim to follow the infant's progress in our pediatric clinic where neurologic assessments are carried out as part of general pediatric care. Parents usually begin to ask serious questions about development at 8–10 months when they see that other children of the same age have developed abilities, such as being able to sit independently, which their own child has not developed. This is the time to carry out any investigations, such as MR imaging, which might be helpful in clarifying the picture.

## THE FIRST 3 MONTHS IN THE FOLLOW-UP CLINIC

It is generally agreed that it is necessary to wait until the corrected postnatal age of 3 months before a prediction of neurologic development is possible. The abnormalities observed within the first 2–3 months are of the same nature as those observed in the early neonatal period, as expected during the transitional stage of maturation described above. Except for a few cases in which abnormalities disappear in the first week, the course observed in the first 2 months is fairly static. However, in the majority of cases with only moderate neurologic dysfunction, the signs disappear abruptly during the third month. The most striking transformation is in the acquisition of head control, the infant becoming able to sustain his or her head vertically for 30 seconds or longer. At the same time, postural tone begins to relax in the upper limbs, the grasp and Moro reflexes disappear, and the infant begins to develop the capacity for cheerful interaction. Some mothers tell how all these changes take place quite rapidly within a few days. It cannot be too strongly emphasized that for preterm infants it is very important to use corrected age (i.e. age after 40 weeks' gestation) in relation to these postnatal aquisitions.

The most important early sign, however, is simply head growth. During the first 3 months of life the head circumference normally increases at about 3 cm per month – not far short of a centimeter per week – and the commonest severe abnormality in CNS findings at this age is insufficient head growth. When recorded on charts showing the normal statistical limits of head circumference, it is found, in very severe cases of cerebral atrophy following HIE, that over a period of 2–3 months the head circumference gradually reaches a value 2 standard deviations below the mean, where it tends to stabilize. At the same time all the cranial sutures develop a prominent ridge, mimicking the findings in craniosynostosis. In moderate cases, head growth is sometimes, but not always, affected and a ridge may become evident at the site of the squamous sutures but not elsewhere. Indeed, this ridge may remain as a marker of moderate perinatal brain damage (Amiel-Tison & Stewart 1994). A commonly observed but worrying pattern at 3 months is the combination of evidence of poor head growth, neurologic signs (particularly imbalance between axial extensor and flexor tone and persisting primary reflexes), together with delayed developmental acquisitions such as the social smile, cooing and head control. When all these signs are present, a full recovery rarely takes place, and if these signs are severe the deficit will involve all aspects of neurologic development: motor, intellectual, sensory and behavioral. When they are mild, development may appear normal or only slightly abnormal in the first few years, but learning disabilities may become evident by 7–9 years.

## CONCLUDING COMMENTS

The prediction of neonatal neurologic outcome at the time of discharge from the neonatal intensive care unit is all too often based exclusively on ultrasound findings without taking into account clinical assessment. A simplistic dichotomy is implemented that equates abnormal imaging findings with bad outcome, requiring follow-up. In contrast, normal imaging is equated with good outcome and no follow-up is required.

Although the first statement is rarely contradicted later on, the second often is. From experience and from literature, we daily encounter that ultrasound consistently detects only severely destructive cellular damage; i.e. periventricular cerebral atrophy, mainly in the group of premature newborn infants with a birth weight below 1500 g. Moderate hypoxic–ischemic damage is frequently missed when clinical assessment is neglected. Who pays the price for this neglect? It is not the extremely low birth weight group, also called the 'new survivors', because they are carefully followed in a systematic way. Those who suffer are the heaviest group of premature newborns (1500–2500 g), those who might be called 'macropremies' or 'old-fashioned survivors' and who are supposed to do well but sometimes fail; and also full-term neonates with no risk circumstances identified before birth.

Several types of clinical neurologic assessment in neonatal units can identify abnormalities at an early stage and allow clinicians to make more accurate indications for early intervention. It will also reduce the expense of following the large cohort of neonates who were considered at risk during pregnancy or first days of life but who demonstrated optimal CNS function soon after.

### Key Points

- A basic understanding of chronology and direction of maturation in brainstem versus cerebral hemispheres provides helpful clinical markers when assessing the infant nervous system.
- Palpation of each cranial suture is an integral part of neurological assessment, overlapping or distention often being more contributive than HC values alone.
- Repeated assessments within the first week of life in a fullterm neonate may provide the best diagnostic clues: an evolving profile in the case of recent damage, a stable profile in the case of prenatal insult.
- In a former premature infant optimal neurological function at 40 weeks corrected is a better predictor of a favorable outcome than normal imaging data.
- Preventive postural managements are essential in the NICU: if neglected, muscle shortening and osteocartilaginous deformities will soon occur and can be misleading in the interpretation of neurological findings.

## REFERENCES


Als H, Lester B, Tronick E & Brazelton T B (1982) Toward a research instrument for preterm infants behavior (APIB). In: Fitzgerald H, Lester B & Yogman M, eds. *Theory and research in behavioral pediatrics.* New-York: Plenum Press. vol 1, pp. 35–131.

Als H & Gilkerson L (1997) The role of relationship-based developmentally supportive newborn intensive care in strengthening outcome of preterm infants. *Seminars Perinatol* 21:178–89.

Amiel-Tison C (1968) Neurological evaluation of the maturity of newborn infants. *Arch Dis Child* 43:89–93.

Amiel-Tison C (1980) Possible acceleration of neurological maturity following high risk pregnancy. *Am J Obstet Gynecol* 138:303–306.

Amiel-Tison C (1996) Does neurological assessment still have a place in the NICU? *Acta Paediatrica* Suppl 416:31–38.

Amiel-Tison C (1999) Correlations between hypoxic–ischemic events during fetal life and outcome. In: Arbeille P, Maulik D & Laurini R (eds.) *Fetal hypoxia.* Carnforth, UK: Parthenon; pp. 123–140.

Amiel-Tison C, Barrier G, Shnider S M, *et al.* (1982) A new neurologic and adaptive capacity scoring system for evaluating obstetric medications in full-term newborns. *Anesthesiology* 56: 340–350.

✪ Amiel-Tison C & Grenier A (1986) *Neurological assessment during the first year of life.* New-York: Oxford University Press.

Amiel-Tison C & Stewart A (1994) *The newborn infant: one brain for life.* Paris: INSERM-Doin.

Amiel-Tison C & Pettigrew A G (1991) Adaptive changes in the developing brain during intrauterine stress. *Brain Dev* 13:67–76.

Amiel-Tison C, Gosselin J (2001) *Neurologic development from birth to six years.* Baltimore: Johns Hopkins University Press. In press.

André-Thomas & Saint-Anne-Dargassies S (1952) *Etudes neurologiques sur le nouveau-né et le jeune nourrisson.* Paris: Masson.

André-Thomas, Chesni Y & Saint-Anne Dargassies S (1960) *The neurological examination of the infant.* Clinics in Developmental Medicine No. 1. London: SIMP.

Ballard J L, Khoury J C, Wedig K *et al.* (1991) New Ballard score expanded to include extremely premature infants. *J Pediatr* 19:417–423.

Brazelton T B (1973) *Neonatal behavioural assessment scale.* Clinics in Developmental Medicine No. 50. Philadelphia: SIMP with Heinemann.

Brazelton T B & Nugent J K (1995) *Neonatal Behavioral Assessment Scale.* 3rd edn. Clinics in Developmental Medicine No. 137. MacKeith Press. London.

Child Growth Foundation (1995) *Growth Charts: United Kingdom Cross-Sectional Reference Data.* 1995/I, London: Child Growth Foundation.

Cioni G, Ferrari F, Einspieler C, Paolichelli P B, Barbani M T, Prechtl H F R (1997) *Journal of Pediatrics* 130:704–711.

Daum C, Kurtzberg D, Ruff H & Vaughan H (1980) Preterm development of visual and auditory orienting in very low birth weight infants. *Pediatric Res* 14: Abstr. 41.

Denver R J (1999) Evolution of the corticotropin-releasing hormore signaling system and its role in stress-induced phenotypic plasticity. *An New-York Academy of Sciences* 897:46–53.

Dubowitz L M & Dubowitz V (1977) *Gestational age of the newborn.* London: Addison-Wesley.

Dubowitz L M, Dubowitz V, Goldberg C (1970) Clinical assessment of gestational age in the newborn infant. *J Pediatrics* 77:1–10.

Dubowitz L, Dubowitz V & Mercuri E (1999) *The neurological assessment of the preterm and full-term newborn infant.* 2nd edn. Mac Keith Press. London.

Farr V, Mitchell R G, Neligan G A & Parkin J M (1966a) The definition of some external characteristics used in the assessment of gestational age in the newborn infant. *Dev Med Child Neurol* 8:507–511.

Farr V, Kerridge D F & Mitchell R G (1966b) The value of some external characteristics in the assessment of gestational age at birth. *Dev Med Child Neurol* 8: 657–660.

Ferrari F, Cioni G & Prechtl H F R (1990) Qualitative changes of general movements in preterm infants with brain lesions. *Early Human Development* 23:193–231.

Gould J B, Gluck L & Kulovich M V (1977) The relationship between accelerated pulmonary maturity and accelerated neurological maturity in certain chronically stressed pregnancies. *Am J Obstet Gynecol* 127:181–186.

Graham J M (1988) *Smith's recognizable patterns of human deformation,* 2nd edn. Philadelphia: W B Saunders.

Grenier A (1986) Complementary neuromotor examination: early affirmation of normalcy. In: Amiel-Tison C & Grenier A, eds. *Neurological assessment during the first year of life.* New-York: Oxford University Press. pp. 96–145.

Hack M, Estabrook M M & Robertson S S (1985) Development of sucking rhythm in preterm infant. *Early Human Development* 11:133–140.

MacLennan A, for the International Cerebral Palsy Task Force (1999) A template for defining a causal relation between acute intrapartum events and cerebral palsy: international consensus statement. *B M J* 319:1054–1059.

Majnemer A & Mazer B (1998) Neurologic evaluation of the newborn infant: definition and psychometric properties. *Dev Med Child Neurol* 40:708–715.

Peiper A (1963) *Cerebral function in infancy and childhood* (translation of the 3rd revised German edition by Nagler B & Nagler H). New-York: Consultants Bureau.

Pettigrew A G, Edwards D A & Henderson-Smart D J (1985) The influence of intrauterine growth retardation on brainstem development of preterm infants. *Dev Med Child Neurol* 27:467–472.

Prechtl H F R (1990) Qualitative changes of spontaneous movements in fetus and preterm infant as a marker of neurological dysfunction. *Early Human Development* 23:151–158.

Prechtl H F R & Beintema D J (1964) *The neurological examination of the fullterm newborn infant.* Clinics in Developmental Medicine No. 12. London: SIMP with Heinemann.

✪ Sarnat H B (1984) Anatomic and physiologic correlates of neurologic development in prematurity. In: Sarnat H B, ed. *Topics in neonatal neurology.* New-York: Grune & Stratton pp. 1–24.

Stewart A, Hope P L, Hamilton P, *et al.* (1988) Prediction in very preterm infant of satisfactory neurodevelopmental progress at 12 months. *Dev Med Child Neurol* 30:53–63.

Touwen B C L (1990) Variability and stereotypy of spontaneous motility as a predictor of neurological development of preterm infants. *Developmental Medicine and Child Neurology* 32:501–508.

Volpe J J (1995) *Neurology of the newborn.* 3rd edn. Philadelphia: W B Saunders.

# Chapter 9 Doppler assessment of the fetal and neonatal brain

K. Brackley, M. Kilby and D. Evans

## INTRODUCTION

Doppler ultrasound has been used to investigate the human circulation since 1957 (Satomura 1957), but it was in 1977 that Fitzgerald & Drumm developed a Doppler system to obtain velocity waveforms from the umbilical artery and suggested its use in the evaluation of the fetal condition in cases with pre-eclampsia and intrauterine growth restriction. Since that time Doppler ultrasound has become increasingly utilized as a non-invasive tool to evaluate the hemodynamics of the uteroplacental and fetoplacental circulations. Continuing technical developments in Doppler ultrasound equipment, particularly highly sensitive color flow imaging techniques, have made it possible to study the fetal circulation in even greater detail. Neonatal Doppler studies date from 1979 (Bada *et al.* 1979). Doppler ultrasound has mainly been used as a research tool, but a number of clinical applications have been recognized.

Doppler ultrasound is a non-invasive method of measuring blood flow velocity, which detects hemodynamic changes instantly. Repeated measurements can conveniently be made at the bedside or cotside. However, it is important to understand the limitations of the method before considering its uses in obstetric and neonatal practice.

## DOPPLER MEASUREMENTS

When an ultrasound signal is directed towards a moving object (e.g. red blood cells within a vessel) the frequency of the reflected signal is altered. The size of this change or Doppler shift is directly proportional to the velocity of the moving object (Doppler 1842):

$$D = \frac{2Fv \, \mathrm{Cos}\Theta}{C}$$

where $D$ is the Doppler shift, $F$ is the transmitted frequency, $v$ is the blood flow velocity (m/s), $\Theta$ is the angle of insonation and $C$ is the velocity of sound in tissue, which is a constant (1540 m/s). The Doppler-shifted frequencies received by the same ultrasound probe are within the audible range and can be displayed in real-time as a spectral display of repeated flow velocity waveforms. The maximum frequencies of the waveform envelope or outline are proportional to the maximum velocities of erythrocytes within the vessel, usually in the center of the blood vessel. The accuracy of the technique is partly operator dependent, including uniform insonation of vessels and the correct setting of hi-pass filters. Doppler waveforms can be assessed either quantitatively or qualitatively.

## QUANTITATIVE MEASUREMENT

Accurate quantitative assessment of the blood flow depends upon several variables.

### Angle of insonation

The measurement of the blood flow velocity depends upon the angle between the Doppler beam and the longitudinal axis of the vessel studied. The angle of insonation should be kept as small as possible. The greater the angle, the less accurate the velocity measurement becomes, and an angle of greater than 60° should not be used. In neonatal cerebral studies the angle should be kept as close to zero as possible. Duplex or color Doppler equipment can be used to measure the angle of insonation to correct blood flow velocity measurements (Eik-Nes *et al.* 1980; Griffin *et al.* 1983).

### Vessel cross-sectional area

The volume flow depends upon the radius of the vessel studied. Errors in vessel diameter measurement will be doubled in the calculation of absolute blood flow, which is a particular problem when measuring smaller blood vessels such as fetal cerebral arteries. The blood vessel is also assumed to be circular with a constant diameter but this is known to vary with arterial pressure during each cardiac cycle (Eik-Nes *et al.* 1984):

$$\text{volume flow} = v\,\Pi r^2,$$

where $v$ is the time average mean velocity and $r$ is the radius of the vessel studied.

There is evidence that the neonatal cerebral arteries do change in diameter (Mchedlishvili 1985; Sonesson & Herin 1988). However, if the angle of insonation is fixed, Doppler ultrasound may give a reliable measure of changes in cerebral hemodynamics but this may not be directly comparable between infants.

## QUALITATIVE MEASUREMENT

Methods of extracting hemodynamic information from Doppler signals that avoid the problems associated with measurement of absolute velocity and flow have been developed. These methods include the calculation of simple ratios or indices using certain points on the maximum frequency outline of the waveforms. They have the advantage that they are angle independent, as the angle of insonation appears in both the numerator and the denominator of the ratio and its effect is cancelled out.

The three main indices used in clinical studies are (Fig. 9.1):

*A*/*B* (S/D ratio) (Stuart *et al.* 1980)

$$= \frac{\text{peak systolic velocity}}{\text{end-diastolic velocity}}$$

PI (pulsatility index) (Gosling *et al.* 1971)

$$= \frac{\text{peak systolic velocity} - \text{end-diastolic velocity}}{\text{mean velocity}}$$

RI (resistance index) (Pourcelot 1975)

$$= \frac{\text{peak systolic velocity} - \text{end-diastolic velocity}}{\text{peak systolic velocity}}$$

These Doppler indices are generally used as a measure of downstream resistance in the circulation, values increasing with a reduction in end-diastolic flow or higher downstream resistance. When there is absent end-diastolic velocity (AEDV), PI provides the most useful information since the *A*/*B* ratio will be infinity and the RI unity ($A/B = A/0 =$ infinity, RI $= (A-0)/A = 1$). It should also be noted that completely different alterations in the waveform shape can result in the same change in ratio. Central circulatory changes can contribute to alterations in waveform shape, particularly as all the indices are dependent on heart rate or length of the cardiac cycle (Mires *et al.* 1987; Maulik *et al.* 1992). It is important to recognize that with acute hemodynamic changes, the measurement of PI can yield misleading results. In a recent report Gunnarson *et al.* (1998) used cerebral Doppler blood flow velocimetry to study central hemodynamics in the ovine fetus during conditions of hypoxemia and acidemia. An increase in blood velocities occurred within a cerebral vessel during hypoxemia and hypoxic-acidotic periods, whereas PI remained unchanged due to the effects of a reduced heart rate. This highlights the potential problems with the interpretation of PI.

*In vitro* studies and *in vivo* cerebral studies in neonates and animals have shown a good correlation between Doppler velocity measurements and cerebral blood flow measured by other techniques (Hansen *et al.* 1983; Greisen *et al.* 1984, Smith 1984; Raju *et al.* 1987). The RI is the index favored by neonatologists and has been shown to be of clinical value in asphyxiated infants (see below). Although it may be assumed to be a measure of cerebral vascular resistance, this has been disputed and its correlation with resistance in animal models is not good.

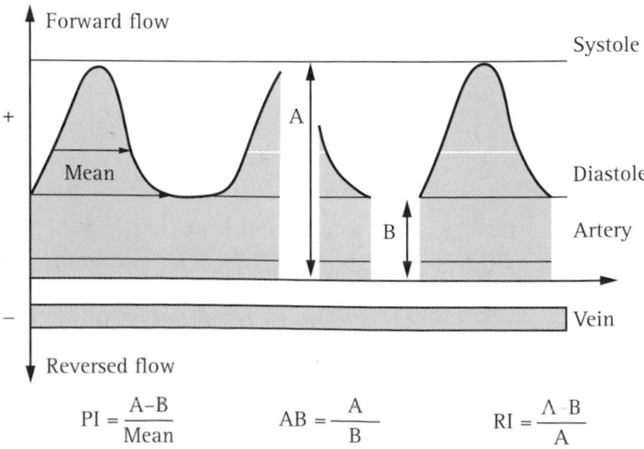


**Figure 9.1** Calculation of Doppler velocity waveform indices.

## DOPPLER EQUIPMENT

Continuous-wave Doppler probes transmit ultrasonic waves and receive the Doppler-shifted frequencies continually. Doppler signals are therefore obtained blindly from all moving structures in the line of the Doppler beam. Visualization of the vessels cannot be achieved using this equipment, which excludes its use in the fetal cerebral circulation. In neonatal cerebral studies the two main acoustic windows are transfontanellar for the anterior cerebral arteries and transtemporal for the middle cerebral arteries (Figs 9.2 and 9.3). Continuous-wave Doppler will sample all vessels in the path of the ultrasound beam, which may confuse the origin of the signal. Also, the angle of insonation may be impossible to estimate. These problems reduce the reproducibility of the technique and pulsed-wave Doppler is preferred.

Duplex Doppler ultrasound is a combination of pulsed-wave Doppler and real-time ultrasound in which the same transducer is used both to transmit repetitive ultrasound pulses and receive the echoes. The depth of the signals can

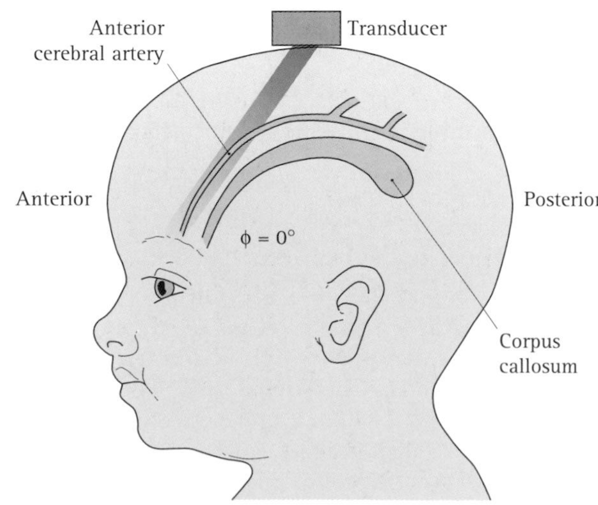


**Figure 9.2** The transfontanellar approach to the anterior cerebral artery in a neonate. (Reproduced with permission from Anthony & Levene 1993.)

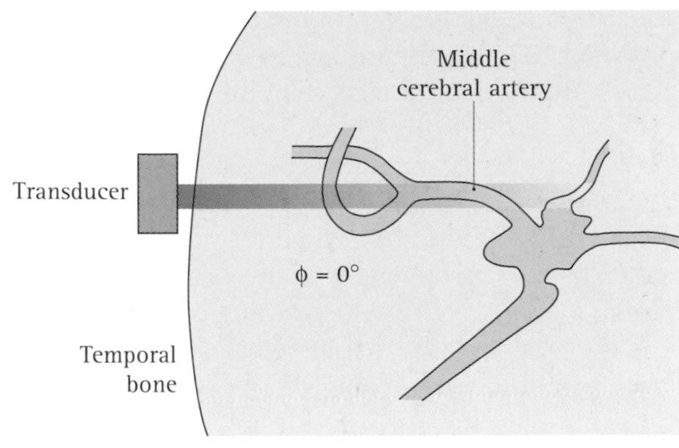


**Figure 9.3** The transtemporal approach to the middle cerebral artery in a neonate. (Reproduced with permission from Anthony & Levene 1993.)

be adjusted to allow visualization and targeting of the vessel studied, enabling Doppler assessment in a number of fetal and neonatal vessels including the descending aorta, renal artery, common carotid artery, internal carotid artery, and anterior, middle, and posterior cerebral arteries.

Duplex systems can be rather large and cumbersome for neonatal studies and pulsed-wave probes without real time may offer a good alternative. The facility for altering the depth of the signal acquisition 'gate' allows a defined tissue sample to be taken. As the vessels are very small it is possible to sample across the whole artery, providing more complete velocity profiles. Ideally, a fixed probe should be used to maintain a constant angle of insonation during a study, in which case a change in the frequency shift will reflect a change in velocity (assuming vessel diameter remains the same). This is not possible in the fetus. Absolute velocity values can only be measured if the angle of insonation is known (see above). Velocity signals are subject to very marked physiological variations and therefore the recordings should be gathered over as many cardiac cycles as possible.

Using color flow imaging, blood flow information is color-coded, in terms of direction, velocity and turbulence, and superimposed on the gray-scale real-time image. This equipment offers major advantages, especially in the study of small vessels such as in the fetal cerebral circulation. It allows rapid visualization and accurate identification of the desired vessel, which minimizes examination time with reduced exposure to ultrasound energy. It also allows a more accurate estimation of the angle of insonation.

More recently, a new technique of detecting blood flow has been introduced called power Doppler imaging or angiography. Power Doppler displays the intensity or energy of the returning Doppler signal. Although power Doppler provides no information on flow direction, velocity, or flow character, it has improved sensitivity compared to color Doppler imaging in demonstrating slower flow, perfusion in smaller vessels, and continuous imaging of tortuous vessels as it is angle independent. Its potential value in the investigation of fetal cerebral blood flow including intracranial hemorrhage (Guerriero *et al.* 1997), microcephaly (Pilu *et al.* 1998), vascular malformations (Paladini *et al.* 1996), and tumors has been suggested, although the increased sensitivity to tissue motion can be problematic in the fetus (Pooh & Aono 1996).

## SAFETY OF ULTRASOUND USED IN DOPPLER INVESTIGATIONS

The three main potential mechanisms for damage using ultrasound are heating and cavitation effects and possible sister chromatid exchange:

1. The heating effect arises from the absorption of the ultrasound energy by the tissues through which it passes (Nyborg 1985). Different tissues have varying acoustic absorption coefficients, bone having the highest. All of the studies have been carried out *in vitro* and they do not take into account the cooling effect that occurs in perfused tissues. Nevertheless, the high intensity of pulsed-wave Doppler used in certain circumstances, such as by vaginal probes in early pregnancy, have the potential to cause significant heating in tissues, a fact underlining the need for care (Ter Haar *et al.* 1989).
2. Cavitation is the formation of small, gas-filled cavities caused by the negative pressures in the acoustic field. Both stable and unstable cavitation are theoretically possible although evidence of their effects is not available *in vivo*. However, cavitation is potentially harmful, and *in vitro* models may cause tissue disruption (O'Brien *et al.* 1979). No studies suggest that the phenomenon occurs at diagnostic intensities *in vivo*.
3. Sister chromatid exchange remains a theoretical risk; no adverse clinical results have yet been reported.

Follow-up studies of infants scanned *in utero* have not shown any detrimental neurodevelopmental outcome (Salvesen *et al.* 1992; Carstensen & Gales 1983), although one report suggests an increased incidence of non-right-handedness in those infants exposed to ultrasound *in utero* (Salvesen *et al.* 1993).

## PRACTICAL GUIDANCE FOR SAFE USE OF DOPPLER ULTRASOUND

1. The acoustic power and pulse amplitude should be kept to a minimum commensurate with the production of waveforms which can be accurately measured. The output intensity, $I_{SPTA}$, should be kept below 100 mW/cm$^2$, as advised by the American Institute of Ultrasound in Medicine (1984).
2. The lowest pulse repetition frequency (PRF) which still allows measurement of the highest velocities should be used.

3. If the output of the machine used is not known, the local medical physics service should be asked to obtain such information.
4. The maximum temperature that may be reached by the transducer should be ascertained.
5. Particular caution should be taken if the patient has an elevated body temperature.
6. When using duplex Doppler equipment the Doppler beam should be turned-off until the vessel required is identified.
7. The Doppler beam should not be directed towards a particular point for longer than 1 min.
8. Exposure of tissue–bone interfaces should be minimized as much as possible.
9. The total duration of exposure to the ultrasound beam should be minimized.

## TECHNIQUE OF MEASURING FETAL CEREBRAL BLOOD FLOW

All the cerebral blood flow velocity (CBFV) waveforms should be obtained using a 3.5 MHz transducer, during fetal apnea and in the absence of fetal movements (see below). The pressure exerted on the maternal abdomen by the ultrasound transducer should be kept to a minimum. The fetal head is readily compressed and a significant positive correlation between pressure and PI in the middle carotid artery (MCA) and internal carotid artery (ICA) has been noted (Vyas *et al.* 1990a), potentially giving rise to spurious results. The vessels studied should be the closest to the Doppler transducer, the angle of insonation always being less than 60°, and the Doppler sample gate length always being 4 mm or less, both to minimize the interference from other small cerebral vessels and to ensure the production of waveforms that can be accurately measured. It is important to identify correctly each cerebral vessel using color flow imaging, as significant fetal regional cerebral blood flow differences are present *in utero* (Mari 1994). Downstream resistance is highest in the MCA and lowest in an intracerebellar artery. In the majority of published fetal cerebral circulation studies, data have been obtained from the most easily accessible MCA.

Using transabdominal ultrasound, the fetal basal cerebral arteries are visualized in an axial view of the fetal head at the level of the brain stem. An angled horizontal section of the brain including the thalami and cavum septum pellucidum is obtained initially (plane where biparietal diameter is usually measured). If the transducer is moved caudally in a parallel plane, the anterior, middle, and posterior fossae are seen and the circle of Willis can be clearly identified using color flow imaging. This consists of an anastomosis (anterior and posterior communicating arteries) between the paired internal carotid arteries and the basilar artery.

The ICA divides into the anterior and middle cerebral arteries (Fig. 9.4A). The use of duplex Doppler equipment allows detection of the ICA pulsations, but color flow Doppler facilitates visualization and confirmation of the vessel identity as it branches immediately after its exit from the bony canal (Fig. 9.4B).

The MCA is the largest branch of the ICA supplying approximately 80% of the blood flow to the cerebral hemisphere. It passes anterolaterally from the circle of Willis in the Sylvian fissure, to supply the corpus striatum, basal ganglia, cortex of the insula, and the inferior frontal gyrus. The greater wings of the sphenoid bone, between the anterior and middle fossae are good reference points for locating the MCA. As the fetal head is often in a lateral position, an acute angle of insonation (which may reach zero) can be achieved to produce a clear waveform, an advantage for velocity measurements. Locci *et al.* (1992) demonstrated that PI values obtained from the proximal MCA are significantly lower

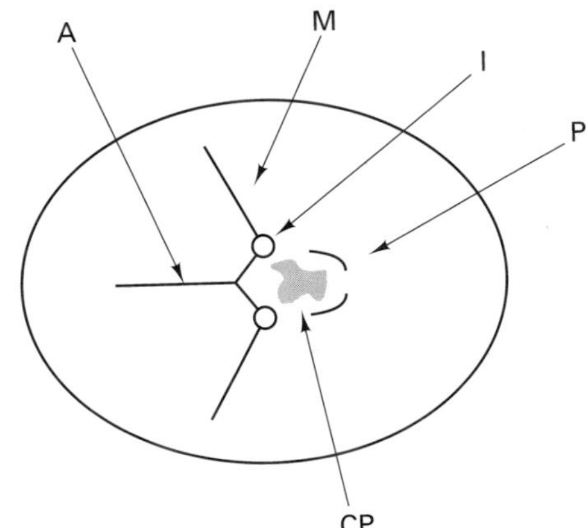


A

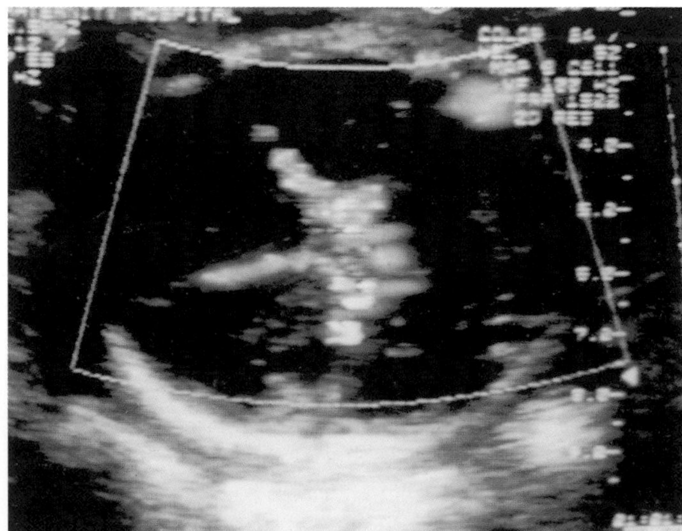

B

**Figure 9.4** (A) Diagramatic representation of the cerebral arteries through a cross-section of the fetal head showing the cerebral peduncles (CP), internal carotid (I), and the anterior (A), middle (M) and posterior (P) cerebral arteries. (B) Fetal cerebral circulation shown by color flow Doppler.

than from the distal segment. The MCA is recognized to consist of four segments: M1, M2, M3, and M4 (Aaslid 1986). The M1 segment maintains a more constant diameter and is the preferable site for Doppler studies.

The anterior cerebral artery (ACA) leaves the ICA at the anterior perforating substance and passes forwards, above the optic nerve towards the orbital surface of the frontal lobe. With color flow imaging the vessel can be easily identified as it leaves the anterior boundary of the circle of Willis and tracks towards the frontal lobe (Fig. 9.4B). Accurate measurements of the ACA can sometimes be difficult as the angle of insonation would be greater than 60° when the fetal head is in the lateral position.

The posterior cerebral artery (PCA) is the terminal branch of the basilar artery and curls back around the cerebral peduncles before passing backwards above the tentorium towards the occipital lobe. The superior cerebellar arteries (SCA) originate from the basilar artery, just before it terminates into the PCAs. The SCA can be localized running parallel and caudal to the PCA (Uerpairojkit *et al.* 1996).

Transvaginal Doppler assessment has been shown to have some advantages over transabdominal scanning in that a coronal section of the fetal brain is produced, allowing better distinction between the ICA and MCA and producing signals of equal quality from both cerebral hemispheres (Lewinsky *et al.* 1991). In addition, it may be superior at early gestations (Kurjak *et al.* 1992), in obese patients, and when the fetal head is deeply engaged in the pelvis (Lewinsky *et al.* 1991).

## PHYSIOLOGICAL VARIABLES AFFECTING FETAL CEREBRAL BLOOD FLOW

A number of physiological variables will influence Doppler measurements in the fetal cerebral arteries.

### GESTATIONAL AGE

Transvaginal color Doppler imaging has made it possible to visualize the fetal intracranial circulation earlier in gestation than with transabdominal ultrasound (Kurjak *et al.* 1992). Fetal intracranial blood flow has been detected as early as 8 weeks' gestation. End-diastolic frequencies in the Doppler waveform become more common with advancing gestational age, being constantly present after 13 weeks' gestation. Therefore, a significant decrease occurs in the PI during the early weeks of pregnancy (Kurjak *et al.* 1992).

Earlier cross-sectional studies noted a weak parabolic correlation of PI with gestational age from intracerebral arteries in normal pregnancy. There was a slight rise in PI between 15 and 20 weeks' and a fall towards term (van den Wijngaard *et al.* 1989; Arduini & Rizzo 1990; Vyas *et al.* 1990b; Mari & Deter 1992). This is in contrast to changes in the umbilical artery (UA), which indicate a steady fall in the vascular resistance with increasing gestation (Trudinger *et al.* 1985). However, in a longitudinal study Veille *et al.* (1993) found that **although the diameter of the** MCA, the time velocity integral and the peak flow velocity all increased progressively with gestational age, the standard Doppler indices did not demonstrate a significant decrease. Only PI showed a weak correlation with gestational age. Blood flow within the MCA ranged between 23 ml/min at 19 weeks' gestation to 133 ml/min at term, paralleling the increase in fetal weight and total cardiac output. Therefore, the proportion of the cardiac output received by each MCA remained constant throughout gestation, between approximately 3 and 7%.

Other studies have noted a downward trend, but not always reaching levels of statistical significance, in Doppler resistance indices within the ICA (Wladimiroff *et al.* 1986, 1987) and the MCA (Meerman *et al.* 1990; Rizzo & Arduini 1991; Harrington *et al.* 1995; Kurmanavicius *et al.* 1997) in the third trimester. However, an increase in cerebral blood flow velocity with advancing gestational age is a consistent finding (Meerman *et al.* 1990; Vyas *et al.* 1990b; Mari *et al.* 1995). In a cross-sectional study Joern *et al.* (1996) calculated maximum systolic, mean and maximum end-diastolic velocities in the MCA after correcting for the angle of insonation. The maximum end-diastolic velocity increased to a relatively greater extent than the maximum systolic velocity throughout the third trimester and this was interpreted as a constant decrease in cerebral vascular resistance up to 42 weeks' gestation. This illustrates the problems associated with Doppler waveform analysis in the interpretation of changing downstream resistance or impedance in terms of absolute blood velocity or actual blood flow and vice versa. However, it is apparent that under normal circumstances the MCA is a low-resistance, high-capacitance bed, even early in gestation (Wladimiroff *et al.* 1992).

### FETAL BREATHING MOVEMENTS

Wladimiroff (1989) recorded a wide range of PI values in the ICA in the presence of fetal breathing movements, demonstrating measurements taken during that time are unreliable. Therefore, all studies of cerebral and other fetal vessels should be made during fetal apnea.

### FETAL HEART RATE

Measurements of the Doppler velocity waveforms have been shown to be inversely correlated with fetal heart rate due to the alteration in end-diastolic frequencies with length of cardiac cycle. Calculation of the indices can be standardized for a particular heart rate of 140 bpm (Mires *et al.* 1987). A decrease in the PI was found with increased fetal heart rates in the ICA, descending aorta and UA in appropriately grown and growth-restricted fetuses (van Eyck *et al.* 1985, 1986). When the heart rate is within the normal range (110–150 bpm), its influence on the waveform indices is of little clinical importance. However, fetal heart rate decelerations (Mari *et al.* 1991) or a fetal tachycardia secondary to ritodrine (Rasanen 1990) will have a significant effect.

## FETAL BEHAVIORAL STATES (see p. 92)

Nijhuis *et al.* (1982) provided clear evidence for the existence of fetal behavioral states in the human fetus, during the last few weeks of pregnancy. Four states were defined based on fetal heart rate patterns, eye movements, and body movements. Van Eyck *et al.* (1987) studied the ICA and the UA in relation to fetal behavioral states in normal pregnancy at 37–38 weeks' gestation. The PI in the ICA was found to be significantly lower during the 2F state (active sleep) compared with the IF state (quiet sleep) whereas the PI in the UA did not significantly change. The reduction in PI was not related to differences in fetal heart rate and was interpreted as representing an increase in cerebral blood flow. In pregnancies complicated by intrauterine growth restriction (van Eyck *et al.* 1988), this behavior dependency during the 1F and 2F states disappeared in the ICA, the PI being constantly lower.

Interestingly, when Kofinas *et al.* (1996) investigated the effect of vibroacoustic stimulation on fetal MCA waveforms in 160 normal pregnant women at various gestations, they noted a reduction in PI values in fetuses over 28 weeks. The influence of fetal heart rate changes was thought to be negligible and an explanation for the response is not clear.

## TECHNIQUE OF MEASURING NEONATAL CBFV

As described above, the ACA and MCA are the most commonly studied vessels. A pulsed-wave transducer which may be securely fixed over the anterior fontanelle or temporal area to give a constant angle of insonation is preferred. Collection of data continuously for up to a minute will allow assessment of beat-to-beat and cycling variability (see below).

Other vessels which have been studied are the PCA, basilar artery and the circle of Willis. Color flow mapping has also made it possible to study the internal cerebral veins, the vein of Galen and the sagittal sinus.

## PHYSIOLOGICAL VARIABLES AFFECTING NEONATAL CBFV

### GESTATIONAL AGE AND POSTNATAL AGE

Several studies of the MCA and ACA have shown that cerebral blood velocity increases with increasing gestational age and with each postnatal day, but for each day after birth a wide range of velocity values has been reported. The major change occurs within the first 12 h of life and is associated with a fall in the RI (Archer *et al.* 1985; Deeg & Rupprecht 1988; Horgan *et al.* 1989, Fenton *et al.* 1990). These physiological changes must be taken into account in recordings between babies or in repeated measurements made in the same baby (see Table 9.1).

**Table 9.1 Mean velocities for postnatal age in the ACA and MCA in term and preterm infants (Fenton *et al.* 1990: with permission from Elsevier Science)**

| | Velocity (cm/s) | | | |
|---|---|---|---|---|
| | ACA | | MCA | |
| Age (hours) | Term | Preterm | Term | Preterm |
| 12 | 6.3 | | 5.5 | |
| 24 | 8.4 | 3.3 | 10.0 | 4.7 |
| 48 | 8.8 | 4.6 | 11.5 | 6.5 |
| 72 | 9.7 | 6.3 | 11.8 | 8.1 |
| 120 | 11.5 | | 15.0 | |
| 196 | 11.0 | | 13.9 | |

*Source:* Reproduced, with permission, from Anthony & Levene (1993).

### CYCLING VARIATION AND BEAT-TO-BEAT VARIABILITY

Marked beat-to-beat variability of the velocity signal has been recognized for many years (Perlman *et al.* 1983a). When recordings were made over periods of one or more minutes, it became apparent that the cycling variations occur at several frequencies (Anthony *et al.* 1991). Both preterm and healthy full-term infants show similar patterns of variation (Anthony *et al.* 1991). One of the major components of this variability appears to be respiration (Bignall *et al.* 1988). The influence of respiration is greatest in preterm infants who are artificially ventilated, presumably representing entrainment to that of the ventilator frequency (Coughtrey *et al.* 1993). The influence of respiration is accentuated in hypovolemic states (Rennie 1989).

Ferrari *et al.* (1994) observed slow frequency CBFV variations of significantly greater amplitude during quiet sleep compared with active sleep, in full-term infants. The frequency was similar to that described in preterm babies and adults, at a similar frequency to Lundberg B waves in intracranial pressure. These may represent vasomotor waves in the small autoregulatory arteries of the brain. Greater variability in CBFV has also been described during rapid eye movement sleep than non-rapid eye movement sleep in both full-term and preterm infants (Cowan 1985; Rehan *et al.* 1996). Rehan *et al.* (1996) also describe greater CBFV variability with periodic and apneic breathing than with regular breathing.

Therefore, it is important to be aware of such influences upon CBFV so that observed changes are not necessarily ascribed to pathological states.

### OXYGEN, CARBON DIOXIDE AND ARTERIAL PRESSURE

Transient hyperoxia has been shown to induce a small but consistent reduction in CBFV (Niijima *et al.* 1988), approximately 3% per 1 kPa rise in $PO_2$ (Menke *et al.* 1993). The effect of carbon dioxide upon CBFV, however, is much greater than that of oxygen. There is an approximate rise of 30% per 1 kPa rise in $PCO_2$ (Menke *et al.* 1993). Hypercapnia in full-term healthy neonates provokes a rise in diastolic velocity, due to cerebral vasodilatation (Archer *et al.* 1986a). On the first day of life, sick preterm infants show a blunted

CBFV response to increasing carbon dioxide tension, which becomes exaggerated after 24 h of age (Levene *et al.* 1988). The CBFV response to carbon dioxide changes on the first day of life appears largely dependent on the concomitant change in arterial pressure (Fenton *et al.* 1992).

The effects of carbon dioxide changes and changes in arterial blood pressure upon CBFV are difficult to untangle as there is usually interdependence. Using regression analysis on observations of arterial pressure, $PCO_2$, and $PO_2$ in 16 ventilated preterm infants, Menke *et al.* (1993) suggest there is an 8% rise in CBFV per 1 kPa rise in arterial pressure. The change is greater in infants below 30 weeks gestation, implying that these infants have immature autoregulatory control of cerebral blood flow (Jorch & Jorch 1987).

### PLASMA VISCOSITY

In both adults and neonates, it is known that a low hematocrit is associated with an increased velocity, and the hematocrit should therefore be noted in each study (Rosenkrantz & Oh 1982; Brass *et al.* 1988). Hemodilution in nine neonates resulted in a significant decrease in hematocrit, an increase in cardiac output and 20% increases in blood flow velocities of the internal carotid artery and the celiac artery (Mandelbaum *et al.* 1994).

## CEREBRAL BLOOD FLOW IN COMPLICATED PREGNANCIES

### FETAL INTRAUTERINE GROWTH RESTRICTION

In intrauterine growth restriction (IUGR) secondary to placental insufficiency there is an increase in downstream resistance in the fetoplacental circulation, with reduced, absent or even reversed end-diastolic flow in the UA Doppler waveforms (Trudinger *et al.* 1985; Morrow *et al.* 1989; Battaglia *et al.* 1993). Conversely, in the cerebral circulation, early studies noted an increase in end-diastolic flow suggesting a reduction in downstream resistance (Wladimiroff *et al.* 1986, 1987; van den Wijngaard *et al.* 1989). These findings are consistent with the phenomenon of 'brain-sparing' or redistribution of blood flow in response to fetal hypoxia demonstrated in animal models. Flow is preferentially increased in favor of the vital organs such as the brain, heart, and adrenal glands to maintain adequate oxygen supply, with a decrease in the blood flow to the gut, kidneys, and carcass (Cohn *et al.* 1974, Peeters *et al.* 1979). During acute fetal lamb asphyxia, induced by obstruction of the maternal aortic blood flow, Malcus *et al.* (1991) observed significant changes in vessel diameter using ultrasound. A decrease in the aortic diameter and aortic blood flow occurred with fetal acidemia whereas in the common carotid artery, vessel diameter and blood flow significantly increased, i.e. there was apparent vasodilatation. In the chronic hypoxic state of the growth-restricted fetus, a preservation of head growth at the expense of the abdominal circumference or liver size is well recognized. In a recent longitudinal study of fetuses that developed IUGR, Harrington *et al.* (1999) demonstrated that a reduction in abdominal circumference mirrored the rise in UA PI and preceded waveform changes in the MCA and thoracic aorta. Interestingly, when growth restriction was associated with either a structural or chromosomal abnormality, Wladimiroff *et al.* (1988) noted that PI in the ICA was always within the normal range (suggesting the absence of circulatory redistribution) whereas the PI was raised in 33% of cases in the UA.

In growth-restricted fetuses the MCA PI demonstrates a significant inverse correlation with the degree of fetal hypoxemia, measured by cordocentesis (Vyas *et al.* 1990b; Akalin-Sel *et al.* 1994). Simultaneous intrapartum pulse oximetry has also shown significantly higher blood flow velocity in the MCA in the presence of reduced oxygen saturation (Sutterlin *et al.* 1999). However, with severe degrees of hypoxemia (>4 SD below the mean for gestation), Vyas *et al.* (1990b) noted a tendency for PI to rise (Fig. 9.5). This has been attributed to increased intracranial pressure due to cerebral edema. There appears to be a limit to the adaptive mechanism present in that the severely compromised fetus may lose its ability to vasodilate the cerebral circulation.

Arduini *et al.* (1992a) performed Doppler velocimetry on 36 growth-restricted fetuses at weekly intervals after the diagnosis of a 'brain-sparing' effect, until the onset of antepartum late fetal heart rate decelerations were observed. In the cerebral circulation a nadir of vasodilatation was reached 2 weeks before the onset of decelerations, whereas a further dramatic increase in PI occurred within the UA and descending aorta close to the development of the abnormal heart rate tracing. These results are consistent with data

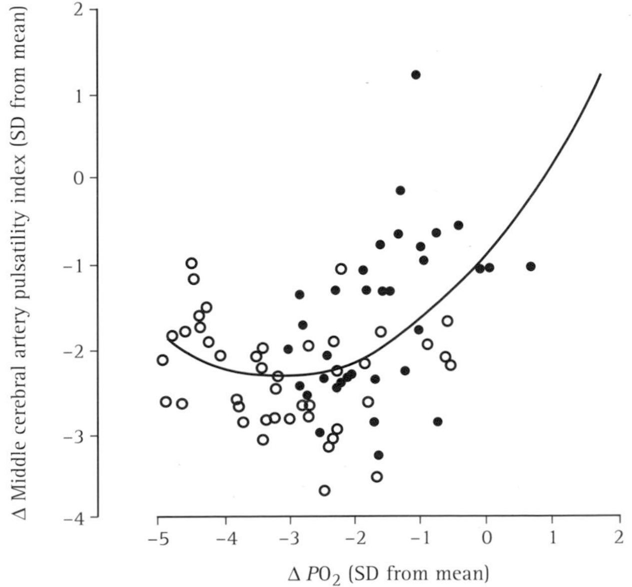


**Figure 9.5** Fetal hypoxia and the PI in the MCA. Open circles represent acidemic fetuses and closed circles represent non-acidemic fetuses. (Reproduced with permission from Vyas *et al.* 1990b: with permission from Elsevier Science.)

from fetal lamb experiments, showing that changes in the cerebral circulation take place at an early stage of fetal hypoxemia when only slight alterations in peripheral blood flow are detected (Peeters *et al.* 1979). However, in more severe hypoxemia, there are marked increases in peripheral vascular resistance and minimal increases, or even decreases, in cerebral blood flow. Individual values of PI may be difficult to interpret due to this variable effect. Indeed, as discussed above, studies on the cerebral circulation have shown that velocity is better correlated with brain blood flow than is PI (Rosenberg *et al.* 1985; Martin *et al.* 1990; Gunnarsson *et al.* 1998).

The possibility that a reduction in MCA PI can predict adverse perinatal outcome, such as preterm delivery, growth restriction, Cesarean section for fetal distress and neonatal complications, has been investigated. Several studies have used a ratio of Doppler indices, comparing the MCA or ICA to the umbilical artery or descending thoracic aorta, as a better indicator of centralization of the fetal circulation and subsequent perinatal problems (Arduini & Rizzo 1992b; Gramellini *et al.* 1992; Scherjon *et al.* 1992; Hecher *et al.* 1995a; Chan *et al.* 1996; Luzi *et al.* 1996; Ozcan *et al.* 1998; Harrington *et al.* 1999; Ott 1999; Ozeren *et al.* 1999). In an ovine model of acute fetal hypoxia secondary to reduced umbilical or maternal aortic flow, Arbeille *et al.* (1995) found the cerebroplacental ratio (cerebral RI : umbilical RI) to be the hemodynamic parameter that most closely followed the changes in $PO_2$. Bahado-Singh *et al.* (1999) evaluated the screening efficiency of the cerebroplacental ratio for the prediction of IUGR and associated perinatal complications in 203 at-risk fetuses. A highly significant increase in perinatal morbidity and mortality was observed in cases with an abnormal ratio (Fig. 9.6). The cerebroplacental ratio appeared superior to umbilical artery Doppler in predicting perinatal complications. There was a progressive increase in screening efficiency as the interval between Doppler study and delivery fell. An unexplained finding of the study was that the ratio did not appear to correlate significantly with outcome in fetuses over 34 weeks' gestation. An immaturity of the mechanisms that autoregulate cerebral blood flow in preterm fetuses was postulated to explain the difference in results.

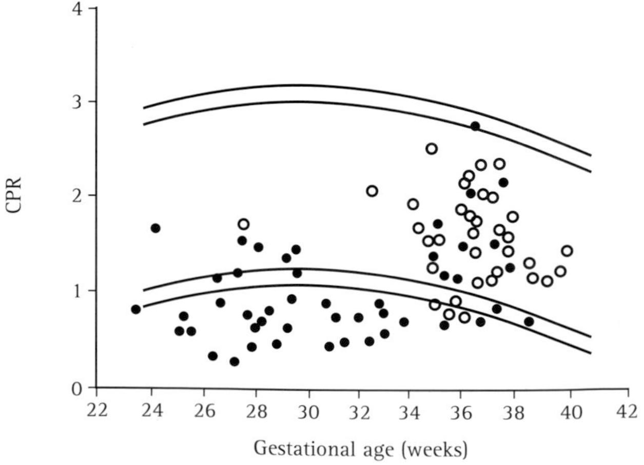


**Figure 9.6** Fifth, 10th, 90th and 95th percentile values for cerebroplacental ratio (CPR) morbidity and perinatal complications (Doppler imaging-to-delivery interval <2 weeks). Open circles, <10th percentile, no morbidity; filled circles, <10th percentile, with morbidity. (Reproduced with permission from Bahado-Singh *et al.* 1999.)

The hemodynamic effect appears to be a protective mechanism to prevent fetal brain hypoxia, as follow-up studies to date have not shown an increase in neurologic problems in the neonate or up to 3 years of age (Scherjon *et al.* 1993; Chan *et al.* 1996; Scherjon *et al.* 1998). Interestingly, Scherjon *et al.* (1996) recorded shorter visual-evoked potential latencies at 6 months of age in infants with abnormal ratios. They postulated that this accelerated neurophysiologic maturation could be the result of a beneficial adaptation to severe fetal growth restriction. In a cohort of 77 growth-restricted fetuses, Yoshimura *et al.* (1998) found no relationship between abnormal MCA : UA PI ratios and follow-up growth at 6 and 12 months of age, despite initially lower birth weight, increased admission, and length of stay in the neonatal unit. The available evidence suggests that an abnormal cerebroplacental ratio is not an indication to intervene too early and deliver a preterm fetus, but that increased surveillance is required. However, the value of cerebral Doppler velocimetry in improving clinical outcome has not yet been assessed by a randomized controlled trial. Neither has the issue of cost-effectiveness in clinical practice been addressed.

With increasingly adverse conditions there is a preferential shift in cardiac output in favor of the left ventricle (Al Ghazali *et al.* 1989) with increasing right ventricular afterload (Rizzo & Arduini 1991). This has prompted investigators to assess the venous side of the fetal circulation as well as the arterial vessels. As pressure in the right atrium increases, 'a' wave decelerations are seen in the ductus venosus and there is an increase in reversed flow within the inferior vena cava (Hecher *et al.* 1995b). Such abnormalities in venous flow are associated with metabolic acidemia whereas arterial redistribution affecting only the MCA does not appear to be associated with acidemia in IUGR (Rizzo *et al.* 1995). Longitudinal observations in preterm growth-restricted fetuses have demonstrated that abnormal venous waveforms precede abnormally reduced short-term variation of fetal heart rate (Hecher & Hackeloer 1997). Short-term heart rate variation, assessed by computer analysis, is itself considered a better predictor of acidemia compared to decelerations (Guzman *et al.* 1996).

Using arterial and venous Doppler velocimetry in a prospective study of 19 severely growth-restricted fetuses, Ozcan *et al.* (1998) found that absent or reversed flow in the ductus venosus was the only significant parameter associated with perinatal death and 5 min Apgar scores. Randomized controlled trials are needed to determine whether additional venous Doppler assessment will enable obstetricians to assess more accurately the optimal time for delivery before the development of abnormal cardiotocography (Hecher *et al.* 1995a; Black & Campbell 1997; Hecher & Hackeloer 1997). This is particularly important in the management of the very preterm or growth-restricted fetus, aiming to minimize perinatal morbidity and any subsequent complications. It must always be appreciated that there is a variation in fetal responses to adverse intrauterine conditions (Hecher & Hackeloer 1997). Long-term follow-up studies are indicated to assess minor differences in neurologic development. It is also possible that the combined use of arterial and venous Doppler assessment may allow more women to be monitored as outpatients. However, because of the requirement for expensive color flow Doppler equipment and technical expertise, they are likely to be of limited value as a screening tool in normal pregnancy.

## TWIN PREGNANCY

Twin–twin transfusion syndrome (TTTS) is a specific complication of monochorionic diamniotic twin pregnancies associated with extremely high perinatal morbidity and mortality. A hemodynamic mismatch is thought to occur between the twins because of placental vascular communications between their circulations (Bajoria *et al.* 1995). Cardiac and venous Doppler studies of the fetal circulation in TTTS are consistent with hypovolemia and increased placental resistance in the smaller donor twin and hypervolemic congestive heart failure in the larger recipient twin (Hecher *et al.* 1995c). Significantly decreased PI was found in the MCA of the larger recipient twin but not in thc smaller donor twin (Hecher *et al.* 1995c). Mean blood flow velocity in the MCA of both twins was normal for gestational age whereas it was decreased in the thoracic aorta.

In contrast, small-for-gestational-age fetuses of monochorionic diamniotic twin pregnancies unaffected by TTTS are more likely to demonstrate the 'brain-sparing effect' (with decreased resistance in the MCA) compared to diamniotic dichorionic twins of similar low birth weights (Gaziano *et al.* 1998). Joern *et al.* (1997) compared a non-stress cardiotocograph, ultrasound biometry and Doppler ultrasound from the fetal descending aorta, UA and MCA in the prediction of placental insufficiency in 130 multiple pregnancies. Doppler results from all three vessels rather than a single vessel was the best predictor of IUGR (sensitivity 75.9%) and of an adverse fetal outcome in terms of Apgar score, UA pH < 7.20 and neonatal unit admission.

## ABNORMAL AMNIOTIC FLUID VOLUME

Doppler velocity waveforms of the ICA were studied in pregnancies complicated with prolonged severe oligohydramnios due to bilateral renal agenesis (van den Wijngaard *et al.* 1988). The end-diastolic velocity was reduced, absent or even reversed with a raised PI (>2 SD), suggesting very high peripheral vascular resistance, which Van den Wijngaard and colleagues postulated was due to head compression. The same mechanism was applicable in the newborn when Newton & Gooding (1975) demonstrated that molding of the skull compressed the superior sagittal sinus, resulting in decreased cerebral blood flow.

In post-term fetuses with oligohydramnios, Weiner *et al.* found the MCA PI was lower compared to post-term fetuses with normal amniotic fluid volume or compared to term fetuses, but this was associated with a reduced left cardiac output and normal PI in the UA and abdominal aorta (Weiner *et al.* 1996).

Mari *et al.* (1992) noted a significant decrease in fetal MCA PI after decompression amniocentesis for symptomatic polyhydramnios in twin pregnancies, suggesting a possible improvement in cerebral perfusion.

## FETAL ANEMIA

Vyas *et al.* (1990c) studied 24 red cell isoimmunized pregnancies and found mean blood flow velocity in the fetal MCA to be increased with anemia. Although PI was decreased in anemic fetuses, there was no significant association with the difference in hemoglobin concentration. These hemodynamic changes were not significantly associated with the difference in blood $PO_2$. Therefore, the hyperdynamic circulation was considered to be a consequence of the reduced blood viscosity. Mari *et al.* (1997) noted a decrease in MCA peak systolic velocity with an increase in fetal hematocrit after intrauterine transfusion.

The value of blood flow velocity measurements in the MCA for the non-invasive diagnosis of fetal anemia due to maternal red cell alloimmunization has been recently addressed in a prospective multicenter study involving 111 at-risk fetuses (Mari 2000). All of the fetuses with moderate or severe anemia had peak systolic velocity values above 1.5 times the median (Fig. 9.7). The multiple of the median of peak systolic velocity was a strong predictor of anemia regardless of the presence or absence of hydrops. Measurements of the peak systolic velocity were found to predict the presence of moderate or severe anemia with a sensitivity of 100% and a false positive rate of 12%. Potentially, this could decrease the number of fetuses subjected to invasive amniocentesis or cordocentesis for this condition.

## FETAL BLOOD SAMPLING

A significant decrease in PI occurs within the MCA as well as the UA and descending aorta following cordocentesis but not amniocentesis, even when performed transplacentally (Capponi *et al.* 1996; Chitrit *et al.* 1997). This may reflect the release of vasoactive substances (Rizzo *et al.* 1996a).

## LABOR

Conflicting results have been published using MCA Doppler in normal labor with some investigators reporting

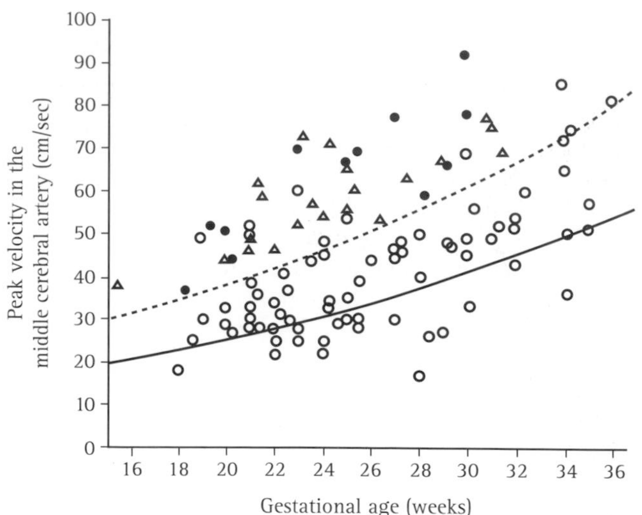


Figure 9.7 Peak velocity of systolic blood flow in the middle cerebral artery in 111 fetuses at risk for anemia due to maternal red-cell alloimmunization. Open circles indicate fetuses with either no anemia or mild anemia (> = 0.65 multiples of the median hemoglobin concentration). Triangles indicate fetuses with moderate or severe anemia (<0.65 multiples of the median hemoglobin concentration). The solid circles indicate the fetuses with hydrops. The solid curve indicates the median peak systolic velocity in the middle cerebral artery, and the dotted curve indicates the 1.5 multiples of the median. (Reproduced, with permission, from Mari 2000 – for the collaborative group for Doppler assessment of the blood velocity in anemic fetuses © Massachusetts Medical Society. All Rights Reserved.)

no significant change in PI (Maesek *et al.* 1990, 1994; Kurjak *et al.* 1996) and others noting decreased values (Yagel *et al.* 1992; Chen *et al.* 1999). Decreased impedance to cerebral blood flow may be a protective mechanism to prevent fetal hypoxia during labor, although no significant difference was detected between downstream resistance in the MCA during uncomplicated labor and in labor with variable decelerations (Yagel *et al.* 1992). Contrary to their findings during spontaneous labor, Chen *et al.* (1999) found no significant change in MCA Doppler indices when labor was induced with prostaglandin $E_1$. It may therefore be significant that these induced labors were more frequently associated with abnormal UA pH values.

In pregnancies complicated by preterm labor, significantly lower MCA PI values were also noted in fetuses delivered within 24–48 h compared to fetuses delivered later or at term (Ghezzi *et al.* 1995; Rizzo *et al.* 1996b). Recent randomized trials involving tocolysis with sulindac or terbutaline (Kramer *et al.* 1999) and indomethacin or magnesium sulfate (Parilla *et al.* 1997) have reported no significant effects of the drug therapy on downstream resistance in the MCA.

## CLINICAL ASSOCIATION OF CEREBRAL BLOOD FLOW IN THE NEONATE

There have been many studies describing the association of certain disease states and drugs with changes in CBFV measurements. Few studies have addressed the clinical consequences and relevance of the associations described.

## CBFV AND DRUGS

### SURFACTANT ADMINISTRATION

The literature describing the effects of surfactant administration on neonatal CBFV gives conflicting results, with increased, unchanged, and decreased states being described. These differences may arise from the different types of surfactant studied (natural versus synthetic), the different methods of delivery (bolus versus slower administration), and the timescale of CBFV measurements.

Jorch *et al.* (1989a) found no change in CBFV when measured every 10 minutes following bovine surfactant administration to preterm infants in a controlled study. Van de Bor *et al.* (1991) studied 25 preterm infants given synthetic Exosurf for respiratory distress syndrome and found that mean CBFV increased by 33% at 5 minutes, returning to baseline by 30 minutes. Cowan *et al.* (1991) used continuous CBFV measurement of 10 preterm infants and found a 36% reduction in CBFV and a 16% reduction in mean arterial pressure, within 2 minutes of administering natural Curosurf. There was also loss of the end-diastolic velocity, thought to be due to ductal shunting following the fall in the pulmonary vascular resistance. Van Bel *et al.* (1992) noted a fall in CBFV during the instillation of prophylactic natural Curosurf but the velocities rose to above baseline values 10 minutes after administration.

Endotracheal suction and disconnection from the ventilator are common procedures during the administration of surfactant. Transient airway obstruction will lead to a rapid rise in carbon dioxide, a potent cerebral vasodilator, thereby increasing cerebral blood flow. Surfactant acts to improve lung compliance and ventilation, leading to a subsequent fall in carbon dioxide and cerebral blood flow. Could the effects of surfactant on CBFV be due to fluctuations in carbon dioxide? Bell *et al.* (1994) used the Xenon clearance technique to measure cerebral blood flow and concluded that the observed reduction following natural Curosurf was due to the fall in carbon dioxide levels. Saliba *et al.* (1994) studied different rates of instillation of synthetic Exosurf (5 versus 15 minutes) and, although increases in CBFV and $PCO_2$ were observed following more rapid instillation, the increase in CBFV could not wholly be explained by the fluctuation in $PCO_2$. In this study, there was no evidence that CBFV changes were mediated by alterations in cardiac output, blood pressure, and ductal patency. Rey *et al.* (1994) demonstrated that the fall in CBFV following natural Curosurf was more marked at higher doses (200 mg/kg versus 100 mg/kg). This dose-related effect has also been seen using near-infrared spectroscopy (NIRS) (Dorrepaal *et al.* 1993).

The literature therefore suggests that synthetic surfactant is associated with increases in CBFV (van de Bor *et al.* 1991; Saliba *et al.* 1994), whereas natural surfactants appear to reduce CBFV (Cowan *et al.* 1991; Rey *et al.* 1994; van Bel *et al.* 1992). This was tested by Murdoch & Kempley (1998) in a randomized controlled trial of 20 ventilated preterm infants undergoing surfactant treatment (synthetic Exosurf versus natural Curosurf). There was a slow and sustained rise in CBFV with synthetic surfactant. In contrast, with natural surfactant, there was an abrupt fall in CBFV. This was maximal at 1 minute and had largely resolved by 15 minutes. The rapid recovery in CBFV may explain why other groups using NIRS have not observed such changes (Edwards *et al.* 1992), as the technique requires that stability in oxygenation is achieved before measurements are carried out.

Most investigators who claim surfactant has an effect on cerebral blood flow independent of changes in $PCO_2$ and arterial blood pressure have endeavored to measure these parameters. However, fluctuations in $PCO_2$ and arterial pressure may be rapid and go undetected (Halley *et al.* 1995).

The observed changes in CBFV following surfactant instillation have led to fears that surfactant therapy may be associated with an increased risk of intraventricular hemorrhage (IVH). The evidence suggests that these fears are unfounded. A meta-analysis of the randomized controlled trials evaluating the efficacy of surfactant therapy in the treatment of respiratory distress syndrome shows a reduction in the risk of all IVH (relative risk 0.88; 95% CI 0.77 to 0.99) (Soll 1999).

## ANALGESIA, SEDATION, AND PARALYSIS

A bolus of 0.1 mg/kg midazolam produces a minor reduction in CBFV, associated with a transient fall in blood pressure (Harte *et al.* 1997; van Straaten *et al.* 1992). Diazepam also appears only to produce minor changes in CBFV (Jorch *et al.* 1989b). Neuromuscular blockade and, to a lesser extent, morphine sedation decrease fluctuations in CBFV in preterm infants (Perlman *et al.* 1985; Colditz *et al.* 1989). Perlman *et al.* (1985) suggest that using paralysis to reduce CBFV fluctuations results in a decreased risk of intraventricular hemorrhage in ventilated preterm infants.

## SEIZURES AND ANTICONVULSANTS

Seizures in adults and children produce a substantial increase in cerebral blood flow. Perlman & Volpe (1983b) studied clinical seizures in 12 preterm infants and found that CBFV, blood pressure, and intracranial pressure all rose during seizure activity. The increase in CBFV appears independent of motor activity, as it has also been observed in EEG seizures during paralysis (Bode 1992). Boylan *et al.* (1999) found an increase in CBFV during both electroclinical and electrographic (clinically silent) seizures; regression analysis suggested that the increase in CBFV was not wholly explained by changes in blood pressure or $PCO_2$ during the seizure. A regional increase in cerebral perfusion has been demonstrated by SPECT, but it was not possible to correlate the area of hyperperfusion with the epileptiform focus (Borch *et al.* 1998).

Phenobarbitone does not produce any significant change in CBFV when given as a 20 mg/kg loading dose (Saliba *et al.* 1991a) and appears not to reduce CBFV fluctuations (Kuban *et al.* 1988).

## INDOMETHACIN

When used as treatment for patent ductus arteriosus (PDA) at doses of 0.1 and 0.2 mg/kg, indomethacin is associated with a 20–50% reduction in mean CBFV. The effect appears maximal around 30–40 minutes after giving indomethacin and persists for 120 minutes (Laudignon *et al.* 1988; van Bel *et al.* 1989b; Saliba *et al.* 1991b; Austin *et al.* 1992; van Bel *et al.* 1993). A slow infusion over 30 minutes produces a more gradual fall but the overall magnitude is similar to bolus administration (Austin *et al.* 1992). Other methods, such as NIRS and Xe clearance, show a similar magnitude and timescale of reduced cerebral blood flow (Pryds *et al.* 1988, Edwards *et al.* 1990).

A PDA can have profound effects upon CBFV. It is associated with a raised RI and a decrease in CBFV (Lipman *et al.* 1982, Martin *et al.* 1982). In some cases retrograde cerebral blood flow velocities can occur (Perlman *et al.* 1981). Nevertheless, the action of indomethacin appears to be a direct effect of the drug. There is no evidence of ductal closure in studies that have used echocardiographic assessment (Austin *et al.* 1992) and surgical ligation tends to increase CBFV by increasing end-diastolic flow (Saliba *et al.* 1991c). Indomethacin given prophylactically for intraventricular hemorrhage prevention, i.e. in the absence of a patent ductus, causes a reduction in CBFV end-diastolic flow (Yanowitz *et al.* 1998). Indomethacin leads to a reduction in vascular reactivity to changes in $CO_2$ (Levene *et al.* 1988, Saliba *et al.* 1991b) and its effect appears not to be mediated by alterations in prostaglandin concentration (van Bel *et al.* 1993).

## METHYLXANTHINES

In adults, cerebral blood flow is known to decrease after a single bolus injection of aminophylline. Rosenkrantz & Oh (1984) demonstrated a 21% reduction in anterior cerebral artery CBFV, 60 minutes following aminophylline administration to nine infants. A substantial reduction in $PCO_2$ was also seen, suggesting that CBFV changes may be mediated via $CO_2$ changes. Two studies also demonstrated a fall in CBFV following aminophylline but the magnitude of the fall was too great to be explained solely by $CO_2$ changes (Chang & Gray 1994, Goven *et al.* 1995). These findings have been confirmed by NIRS (McDonnell *et al.* 1992; Bucher *et al.* 1994) and Xe clearance (Pryds & Schneider 1991).

Aminophylline at steady state, therapeutic concentrations does not appear to alter CBFV (Ghai *et al.* 1989).

Caffeine therapy has not been shown to reduce CBFV, despite causing a reduction in $CO_2$ (Saliba *et al.* 1989a, b; van Bel *et al.* 1989c), although it has not been compared directly with aminophylline.

### DEXAMETHASONE

Cabanas *et al.* (1997) measured CBFV around the first, third, and fifth doses of dexamethasone given to ten ventilated infants with chronic lung disease. There was a short-term increase in CBFV over one to two hours, accompanied by a rise in mean arterial pressure. Progressive doses of dexamethasone produced larger increases in CBFV. Using NIRS, the same group confirmed the increase in CBFV and found that the effect was independent of changes in mean arterial pressure and $CO_2$ (Pellicer *et al.* 1998).

## CBFV AND PREDICTION

### HYDROCEPHALUS

Many investigators have documented the association between higher CBFV resistivity index (RI) values and hydrocephalus in neonates and children (Hill & Volpe 1982; Alvisi *et al.* 1985). Following CSF drainage in neonates with hydrocephalus, the RI falls and the mean CBFV rises (Hill & Volpe 1982; van Bel *et al.* 1988; Seibert *et al.* 1989; Goh *et al.* 1991a, b, 1992; Kempley & Gamsu 1993).

These findings have prompted several groups to identify a value of RI, above which would be an indication of the requirement for CSF drainage. Pople *et al.* (1991) studied children with shunted hydrocephalus. An abnormally raised RI predicted a blocked shunt with a sensitivity of 56% and a specificity of 97%. The RI correlated with intracranial pressure in patients with confirmed shunt blockage. These results were not confirmed in infants. Anderson & Mawk (1988) studied infants with hydrocephalus and found that RI was raised in 31% of those who subsequently required a shunt and in 36% of those who did not. Seibert *et al.* (1989) found wide variation in RI values in infants with hydrocephalus that limited predictive ability.

When compared with intracranial pressure (ICP) measurement, there is an association between a raised RI and raised ICP (Goh *et al.* 1991a, b, 1992). The change in RI occurs early in the evolution of hydrocephalus (Quinn *et al.* 1992) and thus, the correlation between RI and ICP is too weak for RI to be predictive (Goh *et al.* 1991a; Quinn *et al.* 1992; Kempley & Gamsu 1993).

In infants with hydrocephalus, compression of the anterior fontanelle (using the ultrasound transducer) during Doppler ultrasound examination for a brief period (3–5 seconds) was found to result in a transient increase in RI only in those infants who subsequently required surgical intervention. An increase in RI during compression of >40% from baseline was predictive of subsequent shunt placement (Taylor & Madsen 1996). Westra *et al.* (1998) applied this technique to infants and children referred for possible tapping or shunt placement. Using an RI > 0.90 during transducer pressure, they predicted raised ICP with a specificity of 100% and sensitivity of 76%.

### PRETERM BRAIN INJURY

Calvert *et al.* (1988) undertook serial CBFV measurement in 29 preterm infants. Three infants, who had evidence of intraventricular hemorrhage on cranial ultrasound, had similar CBFV compared with the infants with no evidence of hemorrhage. Two infants died with evidence of periventricular leukomalacia at autopsy, both of whom had had a prolonged period of low CBFV.

Shortland *et al.* (1990) studied 120 preterm infants and found no association between CBFV and intracranial lesions. Van Bel *et al.* (1989a) found that preterm infants who were later found to have major impairment at two years of age had a consistently higher RI in the first week of life, although the predictive ability of RI was not formally tested. Rennie *et al.* (1995) performed CBFV measurements in 74 very low birth weight infants and found no association with subsequent outcome when formally assessed at 18 months of age.

Thus, the absolute values of RI or CBFV do not appear useful in the prediction of preterm brain injury or neurodevelopmental outcome. Baenziger *et al.* (1999) found no correlation with outcome when cerebral blood flow was measured during the neonatal period using Xe clearance. The lack of predictive ability when considering the absolute values of CBFV has prompted investigators to examine the relationship between fluctuations in CBFV and outcome. Perlman *et al.* (1983a) studied 50 preterm infants and concluded that a fluctuating pattern of CBFV was associated with a risk of developing intraventricular hemorrhage (likelihood ratio 8; 95% CI 2 to 31). No such association was seen by Coughtrey *et al.* (1997) or Kuban *et al.* (1988). The reactivity of CBFV to a $CO_2$ challenge was also found not to be associated with ultrasound evidence of neurologic injury (Fenton *et al.* 1992).

Therefore, CBFV measurement is not a proven and reliable method of predicting brain injury or long-term outcome in preterm infants.

### HYPOXIC–ISCHAEMIC INJURY IN TERM INFANTS

The original Doppler study in neonates after intrapartum hypoxic–ischaemic injury demonstrated a low RI, due to an increase in end-diastolic velocity, which was thought to represent impairment in cerebrovascular autoregulation (Bada *et al.* 1979). Archer *et al.* (1986b) performed repeated Doppler measurements on infants after intrapartum hypoxia–ischemia and related the findings to the neurodevelopmental outcome at follow-up. Of the 18 infants with an abnormal RI (<0.55), 12 died or were severely handicapped. All the abnormal results were apparent between 24 and 62 hours of age. All the infants with normal RI values were normal at follow-up. A RI < 0.55 gives a likelihood ratio of 5.1 (95% CI 2.5 to 10.6) for the prediction of death or neurodevelopmental handicap. The association of reduced RI and poor outcome after hypoxia–ischemia has been confirmed by other workers (Deeg *et al.* 1990; Stark & Seibert 1994).

The abnormalities in Doppler waveform take 24 hours to emerge and are usually normal in the first 6 hours, despite significant injury (Eken *et al.* 1995). Levene *et al.* (1989) have shown that an increase in CBFV (absolute value as opposed to RI) in the second 24 hours and a lack of reactivity to $PCO_2$ predicted a poor outcome. An increase in global cerebral blood flow has also been demonstrated with Xe clearance (Pryds *et al.* 1990) and NIRS techniques (Meek *et al.* 1999).

Therefore, measurement of CBFV and estimation of RI can be of some prognostic value, provided it is performed 24 hours after the hypoxic–ischemic insult.

## CONCLUSION

It is possible that Doppler assessment of the fetal cerebral circulation could identify the extent of fetal compromise and aid in judging the time of delivery of such pregnancies. However, the problem of implementing such a policy is substantial. Not only is the equipment expensive, but the measurements are sometimes difficult, even in skilled hands. Nevertheless, tertiary referral centers may eventually establish that abnormal venous Doppler in the presence of redistributed cerebral blood flow is a clear indication for delivery. Further long-term follow-up studies must be performed to ensure that by this time cerebral damage has not already occurred.

The limitations in using Doppler indices to assess cerebral hemodynamics, particularly acute changes in blood flow, should be recognized. However, the potential of peak systolic velocity measurements in the MCA to predict fetal anemia will hopefully improve our management of alloimmunized pregnancies.

In the neonate, Doppler measurements have been shown to have a clinical role in the prediction of outcome following hypoxic–ischemic injury in term infants. There is no convincing proof that CBFV measurements are likely to be of clinical use in the prediction of outcome in preterm infants. Although initially promising, the use of CBFV assessment to detect infants with raised intracranial pressure likely to require surgical CSF drainage procedures has been difficult to apply in the clinical arena. There are many studies reporting CBFV changes with different physiological states and pharmacological interventions. As yet, these remain research interests with little clinical application. Techniques for continuous measurement of the CBFV and analysis of variability may be a useful non-invasive research tool for studying neonatal cerebral hemodynamics.

### Key Points

- The interpretation of changes in Doppler indices and cerebral blood flow velocity in terms of actual cerebral blood flow has certain limitations.
- The observation of trends rather than individual Doppler measurements from the MCA may be of more clinical value.
- An increase in end diastolic flow occurs in the MCA Doppler waveform during fetal and neonatal hypoxia.
- An abnormal cerebroplacental ratio is associated with a significant increase in perinatal morbidity and mortality but the value of cerebral Doppler velocimetry in improving clinical outcome has not yet been assessed by a randomized controlled trial.
- The non-invasive measurement of peak systolic velocity in the MCA has been shown to predict moderate or severe fetal anemia in maternal red cell alloimmunization. The potential to decrease the number of invasive procedures performed for this condition requires further study.
- Following intrapartum hypoxia–ischemia, an abnormal Resistance Index (RI < 0.55) in the term neonate is predictive of adverse outcome (death or neurodevelopmental handicap), when the examination is performed 24–60 hours of age (Likelihood ratio 5.1; 95% CI 2.5 to 10.6).
- Doppler CBFV measurement is not a proven and reliable method for the prediction of neurodevelopmental outcome following preterm brain injury.

## REFERENCES


Aaslid R (1986) *Transcranial Doppler Sonography.* New York: Springer Verlag; pp. 42–59.

Akalin-Sel T, Nicolaides K H, Peacock J & Campbell S (1994) Doppler dynamics and their complex interrelation with fetal oxygen pressure, carbon dioxide pressure, and pH in growth-retarded fetuses. *Obstet Gynecol* 84:439–444.

Al-Ghazali W, Chita S K, Chapman M G & Allan L D (1989) Evidence of redistribution of cardiac output in symmetrical growth retardation. *Br J Obstet Gynaecol* 96:697–704.

Alvisi C, Cerisoli M, Giulioni M *et al.* (1985) Evaluation of cerebral blood flow changes by transfontanelle Doppler ultrasound in infantile hydrocephalus. *Child Nerv Sys* 1:244–247.

American Institute of Ultrasound in Medicine Bioeffects Committee (1984) Safety considerations for diagnostic ultrasound. *J Ultrasound Med* p. 316.

Anderson J C & Mawk J R (1988) Intracranial arterial duplex Doppler waveform analysis in infants. *Child Nerv Syst* 4:144–148.

Anthony M Y, Evans D H & Levene M I (1991) Cycling variations in cerebral blood flow velocity. *Arch Dis Child* 66:12–16.

Anthony M Y & Levene M I (1993) Doppler of the neonatal brain. In: Cosgrove D, Meire H, Dewbury K, eds. *Clinical Ultrasound: Abdominal and general ultrasound.* Edinburgh: Churchill Livingstone; pp. 945–956.

Arbeille P, Maulik D, Fignon A *et al.* (1995) Assessment of the fetal $pO_2$ changes by cerebral and umbilical Doppler on lamb fetuses during acute hypoxia. *Ultrasound Med Biol* 21(7):861–870.

Archer L N J, Evans D H & Levene M I (1985) Doppler ultrasound examination of the anterior cerebral arteries of normal newborn infants: the effect of postnatal age. *Early Hum Dev* 10:255–260.

Archer L N J, Evans D H, Patton J Y & Levene M I (1986a) Controlled hypercapnia and neonatal cerebral artery Doppler ultrasound wave forms. *Pediatr Res* 20:218–221.

✪ Archer L N J, Levene M I & Evans D H (1986b) Cerebral artery Doppler ultrasonography for prediction of outcome after perinatal asphyxia. *Lancet* ii:1116–1118.

Arduini D & Rizzo G (1990) Normal values of pulsatility index from fetal vessels: a cross-sectional study on 1556 healthy fetuses. *J Perinatal Med* 18:165–171.

✪ Arduini D, Rizzo G & Romanini C (1992a) Changes of pulsatility index from fetal vessels preceding the onset of late decelerations in growth-retarded fetuses. *Obstet Gynecol* 79:605–610.

Arduini D & Rizzo G (1992b) Prediction of fetal outcome in small for gestational age fetuses: comparison of Doppler measurements obtained from different fetal vessels. *J Perinat Med* 20:29–38.

Austin N C, Pairaudeau P W, Hames T K & Hall M A (1992) Regional cerebral blood flow velocity changes after indomethacin infusion in preterm infants. *Arch Dis Child* 67:851–854.

Bada H S, Hajjar W, Chua C & Sumner D S (1979) Non-invasive diagnosis of neonatal asphyxia and intraventricular hemorrhage by Doppler ultrasound. *J Pediatr* 95:775–779.

Baenziger O, Mueller A M, Morales C G *et al.* (1999) Cerebral blood flow and neurological outcome in the preterm infant. *Eur J Pediatr* 158:138–143.

✪ Bahado-Singh R O, Kovanci E, Jeffres A *et al.* (1999) The Doppler cerebroplacental ratio and perinatal outcome in intrauterine growth restriction. *Am J Obstet Gynecol* 180:750–756.

Bajoria R, Wigglesworth J & Fisk N (1995) Angioarchitecture of monochorionic placentas in relation to the twin-twin transfusion syndrome. *Am J Obstet Gynecol* 172:856–863.

Battaglia C, Artini P G, Galli P A *et al.* (1993) Absent or reversed end-diastolic flow in umbilical artery and severe intrauterine growth retardation. An ominous association. *Acta Obstet Gynecol Scand* 72:167–171.

Bell A H, Skov L, Lundstrom K E, Saugstad O D & Greisen G (1994) Cerebral blood flow and plasma hypoxanthine in relation to surfactant treatment. *Acta Paediatr* 83:910–914.

Bignall S, Bailey P C, Rivers R P A & Lissauer T J (1988) Quantification of cardiovascular instability in premature infants using spectral analysis of wave-forms. *Pediatr Res* 23:398–401.

✪ Black R S, Campbell S (1997) Cardiotocography versus Doppler. *Ultrasound Obstet Gynecol* 9:148–151.

Bode H (1992) Intracranial blood flow velocities during seizures and generalized epileptic discharges. *Eur J Pediatr* 151:706–709.

Borch K, Pryds O, Holm S *et al.* (1998) Regional cerebral blood flow during seizures in neonates. *J Pediatr* 132:431–435.

Boylan G B, Panerai R B, Rennie J M (1999) Cerebral blood flow velocity during neonatal seizures. *Arch Dis Child Fetal Neonat Edn* 80:F105–F110.

Brass L M, Pavlakis S G, De Vivo D (1988) Transcranial Doppler measurements of the middle cerebral artery. Effect of the hematocrit. *Stroke* 19:1466–1469.

Bucher H U, Wolf M, Keel M, von Siebenthal K & Duc G (1994) Effect of aminophylline on cerebral hemodynamics and oxidative metabolism in premature infants. *Eur J Pediatr* 153:123–128.

Cabanas F, Pellicer A, Garcia-Alix A *et al.* (1997) Effect of dexamethasone therapy on cerebral and ocular blood flow velocity in premature infants studied by color Doppler flow imaging. *Eur J Pediatr* 156:41–46.

Calvert S A, Ohlsson A, Hosking M C *et al.* (1988) Serial measurements of cerebral blood flow velocity in preterm infants during the first 72 hours of life. *Acta Paediatr Scand* 77:625–631.

Capponi A, Rizzo G, Rinaldo D *et al.* (1996) The effects of fetal blood sampling and placental puncture on umbilical artery and fetal arterial vessels blood flow velocity waveforms. *Am J Perinatol* 13(3):185–190.

Carstensen E L & Gales A H (1983) University of Rochester New York electrical engineering technical report, No GM 09933 21R. University of Rochester, New York

✪ Chan F Y, Pun T C, Lam P *et al.* (1996) Fetal cerebral Doppler studies as a predictor of perinatal outcome and subsequent neurologic handicap. *Obstet Gynecol* 87:981–988.

Chang J & Gray P H (1994) Aminophylline therapy and cerebral blood flow velocity in preterm infants. *J Paediatr Child Health* 30:123–125.

Chen W H, Lai H C, Tang Y H & Liu H S (1999) Fetal Doppler hemodynamic changes in spontaneous versus prostaglandin E1-induced active labor. *Acta Obstet Gynecol Scand* 78(7):599–604.

Chitrit Y, Caubel P, Boulanger M C *et al.* (1997) Changes in umbilical artery, middle cerebral artery and aorta blood flow Doppler waveform pulsatility indices after funisocentesis. *J Ultrasound Med* 16(5):359–364.

Cohn H E, Sacks E J, Heymann M A & Rudolph A M (1974) Cardiovascular responses to hypoxemia and acidemia in fetal lambs. *Am J Obstet Gynecol* 120(6):817–824.

Colditz P B, Williams G L, Berry A B & Symonds P J (1989) Variability of Doppler flow velocity and cerebral perfusion pressure is reduced in the neonate by sedation and neuromuscular blockade. *Aust Paediatr J* 25:171–173.

Coughtrey H, Rennie J M & Evans D H (1997) Variability in cerebral blood flow velocity: observations over one minute in preterm babies. *Early Hum Dev* 47:63–70.

✪ Coughtrey H, Rennie J M, Evans D H & Cole T J (1993) Factors associated with respiration induced variability in cerebral blood flow velocity. *Arch Dis Child* 68:312–316.

Cowan F (1985) Cerebral blood flow velocities and their variability in different sleep states in the newborn infant. *Pediatr Res* 19:Abstr. 1084.

Cowan F, Whitelaw A, Wertheim D & Silverman M (1991) Cerebral blood flow velocity changes after rapid administration of surfactant. *Arch Dis Child* 66:1105–1109.

Deeg K H & Rupprecht T H (1988) Doppler sonographic measurement of normal values for flow velocities in the internal carotid arteries of healthy infants. *Monatsschrift Kinderheilkunde* 136: 193–199 [in German; English Abstr.].

Deeg K H & Scharf J (1990) Color Doppler imaging of arteriovenous malformation of the vein of Galen in a newborn. *Neuroradiology* 32:60–63.

Deeg K H, Rupprecht T H & Zeilinger G (1990) Doppler sonographic classification of brain edema in infants. *Pediatr Radiol* 20:509.

Doppler C J (1842) Uber das farbige Licht der Doppelsterneund einiger und ever gestern des himmels. *Abhandlung Konglich Bohmisch Gessellschaft-Wissenchaft* 2:465–482.

Dorrepaal C A, Benders M J, Steendijk P, van de Bor M, van Bel F 1993 Cerebral hemodynamics and oxygenation in preterm infants after low- vs. high-dose surfactant replacement therapy. *Biol Neonate* 64:193–200.

Edwards A D, McCormick D C, Roth S C *et al.* (1992) Cerebral hemodynamic effects of treatment with modified natural surfactant investigated by near infrared spectroscopy. *Pediatr Res* 32:532–536.

Edwards A D, Wyatt J S, Richardson C *et al.* (1990) Effects of indomethacin on cerebral hemodynamics in very preterm infants. *Lancet* 335:1491–1495.

Eik-Nes S, Brubakk A O & Ulstein M (1980) Measurement of human fetal blood flow. *BMJ* i:283–284.

Eik-Nes S, Marsal K, Kristofferson K (1984) Methodology and basic problems related to blood flow studies in the human fetus. *Ultrasound Med Biol* 10:329–338.

✪ Eken P, Toet M C, Groenendaal F & de Vries L S (1995) Predictive value of early neuroimaging, pulsed Doppler and neurophysiology in full term infants with hypoxic-ischaemic encephalopathy. *Arch Dis Child Fetal Neonat Edn* 73:F75–F80.

Fenton A C, Shortland D B, Papathoma E (1990) Normal range for blood flow velocity in cerebral arteries of newly born infants. *Early Hum Dev* 22(2):73–79.

Fenton A C, Woods K L, Evans D H & Levene M I (1992) Cerebrovascular carbon dioxide reactivity and failure of autoregulation in preterm infants. *Arch Dis Child* 67:835–839.

Ferrarri F, Kelsall A W, Rennie J M & Evans D H (1994) The relationship between cerebral blood flow velocity fluctuations and sleep state in normal newborns. *Pediatr Res* 35:50–54.

Fitzgerald D E & Drum J E (1977) Non-invasive measurement of human fetal circulation using ultrasound: a new method. *BMJ* ii:1450–1451.

Gaziano E, Gaziano C & Brandt D (1998) Doppler velocimetry determined redistribution of fetal blood flow: correlation with growth restriction in diamniotic monochorionic and dizygotic twins. *Am J Obstet Gynecol* 178:1359–1367.

Ghai V, Raju T N, Kim S Y & McCulloch K M (1989) Regional cerebral blood flow velocity after aminophylline therapy in premature newborn infants. *J Pediatr* 114:870–873.

Ghezzi F, Ghidini A, Romero R *et al.* (1995) Doppler velocimetry of the middle cerebral artery in patients with preterm labor and intact membranes. *J Ultrasound Med* 14:361–366.

Goh D, Minns R A & Pye S D (1991a) Transcranial Doppler (TCD) ultrasound as a non-invasive means of monitoring cerebrohemodynamic changes in hydrocephalus. *Eur J Pediatr Surg* 1(Suppl. 1):14–17.

Goh D, Minns R A, Pye S D & Steers A J (1991b) Cerebral blood flow velocity changes after ventricular taps and ventriculoperitoneal shunting. *Child Nerv Syst* 7:452–457.

Goh D, Minns R A, Hendry G M *et al.* (1992) Cerebrovascular resistive index assessed by duplex Doppler sonography and its relationship to intracranial pressure in infantile hydrocephalus. *Pediatr Radiol* 22:246–250.

Gosling R G, Dunbar G, King D H *et al.* (1971) The quantitative analysis of occlusive peripheral arterial disease by a non-intrusive technique. *Angiology* 22:52–55.

Govan J J, Ohlsson A, Ryan M L *et al.* (1995) Aminophylline and Doppler time-averaged mean velocity in the middle cerebral artery in preterm neonates. *J Paediatr Child Health* 31:461–464.

Gramellini D, Folli M C, Raboni S *et al.* (1992) Cerebral-umbilical Doppler ratio as a predictor of adverse perinatal outcome. *Obstet Gynecol* 79:416–420.

✪ Greisen G, Johansen K, Ellison P A *et al.* (1984) Cerebral blood flow in the newborn infant: comparison of Doppler ultrasound and 133-xenon clearance. *J Pediatr* 104:411–413.

Griffin D, Bilardo K, Diaz J & Teague M (1983) The measurement of human fetal blood flow with linear array pulsed Doppler duplex. *Eur J Obstetrics Gynaecol Reprod Biol* 15:426–430.

Guerriero S, Ajossa S, Mais V *et al.* (1997) Color Doppler energy imaging in the diagnosis of fetal intracranial hemorrhage in the second trimester. *Ultrasound Obstet Gynecol* 10:205–208.

Gunnarsson G O, Gudmundsson S, Hokegard K *et al.* (1998) Cerebral Doppler blood flow velocimetry and central hemodynamics in the ovine fetus during hypoxemia-acidemia. *J Perinat Med* 26(2):107–114.

Guzman E, Vintzileos A & Martins M (1996) Prediction of umbilical artery and vein pH in intrauterine growth restricted fetuses based on fetal and maternal Doppler velocimetry and computer fetal heart rate. *Am J Obstet Gynecol* 172(1 pt 2):269.

Haar G T, Duck F, Starritt H & Daniels S (1989) Biophysical characterisation of diagnostic ultrasound equipment preliminary results. *Phys Med Biol* 34:1533–1542.

Halley G C, Stenson B J, Laing I A & McIntosh N (1995) Acute blood pressure response to surfactant administration. *Arch Dis Child* 73:F197.

Hansen M B, Stonestreet B S & Rosenkrantz T S (1983) Validity of Doppler measurements of anterior cerebral artery blood flow velocity. Correlation with brain blood flow in piglets. *Pediatr Res* 72:526–531.

Harrington K, Carpenter R G, Nguyen M & Campbell S (1995) Changes observed in Doppler studies of the fetal circulation in pregnancies complicated by pre-eclampsia or the delivery of a small-for-gestational-age baby. I. Cross-sectional analysis. *Ultrasound Obstet Gynecol* 6:19–28.

Harrington K, Thompson M O, Carpenter R G *et al.* (1999) Doppler fetal circulation in pregnancies complicated by pre-eclampsia or delivery of a small for gestational age baby. 2. Longitudinal analysis. *Br J Obstet Gynaecol* 106:453–466.

Harte G J, Gray P H, Lee T C *et al.* (1997) Hemodynamic responses and population pharmacokinetics of midazolam following administration to ventilated, preterm neonates. *J Paediatr Child Health* 33:335–338.

✪ Hecher K, Campbell S, Doyle P *et al.* (1995a) Assessment of fetal compromise by Doppler ultrasound investigation of the fetal circulation. Arterial, intracardiac and venous blood flow velocity studies. *Circulation* 91:129–138.

Hecher K, Snijders R, Campbell S & Nicolaides K (1995b) Fetal venous, intracardiac and arterial blood flow measurements in intrauterine growth retardation: relationship with fetal blood gases. *Am J Obstet Gynecol* 173(1):10–15.

Hecher K, Ville Y, Snijders R & Nicolaides K (1995c) Doppler studies of the fetal circulation in twin-twin transfusion syndrome. *Ultrasound Obstet Gynecol* 5:318–324.

✪ Hecher K & Hackeloer B-J (1997) Cardiotocogram compared to Doppler investigation of the fetal circulation in the premature growth-retarded fetus: longitudinal observations. *Ultrasound Obstet Gynecol* 9:152–161.

Hill A & Volpe J J (1982) Decrease in pulsatile flow in the anterior cerebral arteries in infantile hydrocephalus. *Pediatrics* 69:4–7.

Horgan J G, Rumack C M, Hay T (1989) Absolute intracranial blood-flow velocities evaluated by duplex Doppler sonography in asymptomatic preterm and term neonates. *Am J Roentgenol* 152:1059–1064.

Joern H, Funk A, Goetz M *et al.* (1996) Development of quantitative Doppler indices for uteroplacental and fetal blood flow during the third trimester. *Ultrasound Med Biol* 22(7):823–835.

Joern H, Schroeder W, Sassen R & Rath W (1997) Predictive value of a single CTG, ultrasound and Doppler examination to diagnose acute and chronic placental insufficiency in multiple pregnancies. *J Perinat Med* 25(4):325–332.

Jorch G & Jorch N (1987) Failure of autoregulation of cerebral blood flow in neonates studied by pulsed Doppler ultrasound of the internal carotid artery. *Eur J Pediatr* 146:468–472.

Jorch G, Rabe H, Garbe M *et al.* (1989a) Acute and protracted effects of intratracheal surfactant application on internal carotid blood flow velocity, blood pressure and carbon dioxide tension in very low birth weight infants. *Eur J Pediatr* 148:770–773.

Jorch G, Rabe H, Rickers E *et al.* (1989b) Cerebral blood flow velocity assessed by Doppler technique after intravenous application of diazepam in very low birth weight infants. *Dev Pharmacol Ther* 14:102–107.

Kempley S T & Gamsu H R (1993) Changes in cerebral artery blood flow velocity after intermittent cerebrospinal fluid drainage. *Arch Dis Child* 69:74–76.

Kofinas A D, Cabbad M & Kofinas G D (1996) The effect of vibratory acoustic stimulation on fetal middle cerebral artery impedance and instantaneous fetal heart rate: a prospective cross-sectional study from 20 to 42 weeks' gestational age. *J Maternal–Fetal Invest* 6:19–22.

Kramer W B, Saade G R, Belfort M *et al.* (1999) A randomized double-blind study comparing the fetal effects of sulindac to terbutaline during the management of preterm labor. *Am J Obstet Gynecol* 180:396–401.

Kuban K C K, Skouteli H, Cherer A *et al.* (1988) Hemorrhage, phenobarbital, and fluctuating cerebral blood flow velocity in the neonate. *Pediatrics* 82:548–553.

Kurjak A, Predanic M, Kupesic-Urek S *et al.* (1992) Transvaginal color Doppler study of middle cerebral artery blood flow in early normal and abnormal pregnancy. *Ultrasound Obstet Gynecol* 2:424–428.

Kurjak A, Dudenhausen J W, Kos M *et al.* (1996) Doppler information pertaining to the intrapartum period. *J Perinat Med* 24(3):271–276.

Kurmanavicius J, Florio I, Wisser J *et al.* (1997) Reference resistance indices of the umbilical, fetal middle cerebral and uterine arteries at 24–42 weeks' gestation. *Ultrasound Obstet Gynecol* 10:112–120.

Laudignon N, Chemtob S, Bard H & Aranda J V (1988) Effect of indomethacin on cerebral blood flow velocity of premature newborns. *Biol Neonate* 54:254–262.

Levene M I, Shortland D, Gibson N & Evans D H (1988) Carbon dioxide reactivity of the cerebral circulation in extremely premature infants: effects of postnatal age and indomethacin. *Pediatr Res* 24:175–179.

✪ Levene M I, Fenton A C, Evans D H *et al.* (1989) Severe birth asphyxia and abnormal cerebral blood-flow velocity. *Dev Med Child Neurol* 131:427–434.

Lewinsky R M, Farine D & Ritchie J W (1991) Transvaginal Doppler assessment of the fetal cerebral circulation. *Obstet Gynecol* 78(4):637–640.

Lipman B, Senver G & Brazy J E (1982) Abnormal cerebral hemodynamics in preterm infants with patent ductus arteriosus. *Pediatrics* 69:778–781.

Locci M, Nazzaro G, De Placido G *et al.* (1992) Fetal cerebral hemodynamic adaptation: a progressive mechanism? pulsed and color Doppler evaluation. *J Perinat Med* 20: 337–343.

Luzi G, Coata G, Caserta G *et al.* (1996) Doppler velocimetry of different sections of the fetal middle cerebral artery in relation to perinatal outcome. *J Perinat Med* 24(4):327–334.

McDonnell M, Ives N K & Hope P L (1992) Intravenous aminophylline and cerebral blood flow in preterm infants. *Arch Dis Child* 67:416–418.

Maesel A, Lingman G & Marsal K (1990) Cerebral blood flow during labor in the human fetus. *Acta Obstet Gynecol Scand* 69:493–495.

Malcus P, Kjellmer I, Lingman G *et al.* (1991) Diameters of the common carotid artery and aorta change in different directions during acute asphyxia in the fetal lamb. *J Perinat Med* 19:259–267.

Mandelbaum V H, Guajardo C D, Nelle M & Linderkamp O (1994) Effects of polycythaemia and haemodilution on circulation in neonates. *Arch Dis Child Fetal Neonat Edn* 71:F53–F54.

Mari G, Moise K J, Deter R L (1991) Fetal heart rate influence on the pulsatility index in the middle cerebral artery. *J Clin Ultrasound* 19:149–153.

Mari G & Deter R L (1992) Middle cerebral artery flow velocity waveforms in normal and small-for-gestational-age fetuses. *Am J Obstet Gynecol* 166:1262–1270.

Mari G, Wasserstrum N & Kirshon B (1992) Reduction in middle cerebral artery pulsatility index after decompression of polyhydramnios in twin gestation. *Am J Perinatol* 9: 381–384.

Mari G (1994) Regional cerebral flow velocity waveforms in the human fetus. *J Ultrasound Med* 13:343–346.

Mari G, Adrignolo A, Abuhamad A Z *et al.* (1995) Diagnosis of fetal anemia with Doppler ultrasound in the pregnancy complicated by maternal blood group immunization. *Ultrasound Obstet Gynecol* 5:400–405.

Mari G, Rahman F, Olofsson P *et al.* (1997) Increase of fetal hematocrit decreases the middle cerebral artery peak systolic velocity in pregnancies complicated by rhesus alloimmunization. *J Maternal–Fetal Med* 6(4):206–208.

✪ Mari G (2000) Noninvasive diagnosis by Doppler ultrasonography of fetal anemia due to maternal red-cell alloimmunization. *New Engl J Med* 342:9–14.

Martin CG, Snider S, Katz S M *et al.* (1982) Abnormal cerebral blood flow patterns in preterm infants with large patent ductus arteriosus. *J Pediatr* 101:587–593.

Martin C, Hansen T, Goddard-Finegold J *et al.* (1990) Prediction of brain blood flow using pulsed Doppler sonography in newborn lambs. *J Clin Ultrasound* 18: 487–495.

✪ Maulik D, Arbeille P & Kadado T (1992) Hemodynamic foundation of umbilical artery Doppler waveform analysis. *Biology of the Neonate* 62:280–289.

Mchedlishvili G (1985) Principles of cerebral blood flow control: a deductive approach. In: Bevan J A, ed. *Arterial behaviour and blood circulation in the brain.* New York: Consultants Bureau; pp. 17–41.

Meek J H, Elwell C E, McCormic D C *et al.* (1999) Abnormal cerebral hemodynamics in perinatally asphyxiated neonates related to outcome. *Arch Dis Child Fetal Neonat Edn* 81:F110–F115.

Meerman R J, van Bel F & van Zwieten P H T *et al.* (1990) Fetal and neonatal cerebral blood velocity in the normal fetus and neonate: a longitudinal Doppler ultrasound study. *Early Hum Dev* 24:209–217.

✪ Menke J, Michel E, Rabe H *et al.* (1993) Simultaneous influence of blood pressure, $PCO_2$, and $PO_2$ on cerebral blood flow velocity in preterm infants of less than 33 weeks' gestation. *Pediatr Res* 34:173–177.

Mires G, Dempster J, Patel N B & Crawford J W (1987) The effect of fetal heart rate on umbilical artery flow velocity waveforms. *Br J Obstet Gynaecol* 94:665–669.

Mitchell D G, Merton D A, Desai H *et al.* (1988) Neonatal brain: color Doppler imaging. Part II. Altered flow patterns from extracorporeal membrane oxygenation. *Radiology* 176:307–310.

Mitchell D G, Merton D A, Mirsky P J & Needleham L (1989) Circle of Willis in newborns: color Doppler imaging of 53 healthy full term infants. *Pediatr Radiol* 172:201–205.

Morrow R J, Adamson S L, Bull S B & Knox Ritchie J W (1989) Effect of placental embolization on the umbilical arterial velocity waveform in fetal sheep. *Am J Obstet Gynecol* 161:1055–1060.

Murdoch E & Kempley S T (1998) Randomized trial examining cerebral hemodynamics following artificial or animal surfactant. *Acta Paediatr* 87:411–415.

Newton T H & Gooding C A (1975) Compression of superior sagittal sinus by neonatal calvarial molding. *Radiology* 115:635–639.

Niijima S, Shortland D B, Levene M I & Evans D H (1988) Transient hyperoxia and cerebral blood flow velocity in infants born prematurely and at full term. *Arch Dis Child* 63:1126–1130.

Nijhuis J G, Prechtl H F R, Martin C B J & Bots R S G M (1982) Are there behavioural states in the human fetus? *Early Hum Dev* 6:177.

Nyborg W L (1985) Optimization of exposure conditions for medical ultrasound. *Ultrasound Med Biol* 11(2):245–260.

O'Brien W D J, Brady K K & Dunn F (1979) Morphological changes to mouse testicular tissue from *in vivo* ultrasonic radiation. *Ultrasound Med Biol* 5:35–43.

Ott W J (1999) Comparison of the non-stress test with the evaluation of centralization of blood flow for the prediction of neonatal compromise. *Ultrasound Obstet Gynecol* 14:38–41.

Ozcan T, Sbracia M, d'Ancona J *et al.* (1998) Arterial and venous Doppler velocimetry in the severely growth-restricted fetus and associations with adverse perinatal outcome. *Ultrasound Obstet Gynecol* 12:39–44.

Ozeren M, Dinc H, Ekmen U *et al.* (1999) Umbilical and middle cerebral artery Doppler indices in patients with pre-eclampsia. *Eur J Obstet Gynaecol Reprod Biol* 82(1):11–16.

Paladini D, Palmieri S, D'Angelo A & Martinelli P (1996) Prenatal ultrasound diagnosis of cerebral arteriovenous fistula. *Obstet Gynaecol* 88:678–681.

Parilla B V, Tamura R K, Cohen L S & Clark E (1997) Lack of effect of antenatal indomethacin on fetal cerebral blood flow. *Am J Obstet Gynecol* 176:1166–1171.

Peeters L L H, Sheldon R E, Jones M D *et al.* (1979) Blood flow of fetal organs as a function of arterial oxygen content. *Am J Obstet Gynecol* 135:637–646.

Pellicer A, Gaya F, Stiris T A *et al.* (1998) Cerebral hemodynamics in preterm infants after exposure to dexamethasone. *Arch Dis Child Fetal & Neonat Edn* 79:F123–F128.

Perlman J M, Hill A & Volpe J J (1981) The effects of patent ductus arteriosus on flow velocity in the anterior cerebral arteries; ductal steal in the preterm newborn infant. *J Pediatr* 99:767–771.

Perlman J M, McMenamin J B & Volpe J J (1983a) Fluctuating cerebral blood flow velocity in respiratory distress syndrome. *New Engl J Med* 309:204–209.

Perlman J M & Volpe J J (1983b) Seizures in the preterm infant: effects on cerebral blood flow velocity, intracranial pressure, and arterial blood pressure. *J Pediatr* 102:288–293.

Perlman J M, Goodman S, Kreusser K L & Volpe J J (1985) Reduction in intraventricular hemorrhage by elimination of fluctuating cerebral blood flow velocity in preterm infants with respiratory distress syndrome. *New Engl J Med* 312:1353–1357.

Pilu G, Falco P, Milano V (1998) Prenatal diagnosis of microcephaly assisted by vaginal sonography and power Doppler. *Ultrasound Obstet Gynaecol* 11:357–360.

Pooh R K & Aono T (1996) Transvaginal power Doppler angiography of the fetal brain. *Ultrasound Obstet Gynecol* 8:417–421.

Pople I K, Quinn M W, Bayston R & Haywood R D (1991) The Doppler pulsatility index as a screening test for blocked ventriculo-peritoneal shunts. *Eur J Paediatr Surg* I (suppl 1):27–29.

Pourcelot L (1975) Application clinique de l'examen Doppler transcutane. In: Peronneau P, ed. *Velocimetri ultrasonore.* Paris: Inserm; pp. 213–240.

Pryds O, Greisen G & Johansen K H (1988) Indomethacin and cerebral blood flow in preterm infants treated for patent ductus arteriosus. *Eur J Pediatr* 147:315–316.

Pryds O, Greisen G, Lou H & Friis-Hansen B (1990) Vasoparalysis associated with brain damage in asphyxiated term infants. *J Pediatr* 117:119–125.

Pryds O & Schneider S (1991) Aminophylline reduces cerebral blood flow in stable, preterm infants without affecting the visual evoked potential. *Eur J Pediatr* 150:366–369.

Quinn M W, Ando Y & Levene M I (1992) Cerebral arterial and venous flow velocity measurements in post haemorrhagic ventricular dilatation and hydrocephalus. *Dev Med Child Neurol* 34:863–869.

Raju T N K, Ryva J C & Schmidt D J (1987) Common carotid artery flow velocity measurements in the newborn period with pulsed Doppler technique. *Biol Neonate* 52:241–249.

Raju T N K, Kim S Y & Chapman L (1989) Circle of Willis blood flow patterns in healthy newborn infants. *J Pediatr* 114:455–458.

Rasanen J (1990) The effect of ritodrine infusion on myocardial function and fetal hemodynamics. *Acta Obstet Gynecol Scand* 69:487–492.

Rehan V K, Fajardo C A, Haider A Z (1996) Influence of sleep state and respiratory pattern on cyclical fluctuations of cerebral blood flow velocity in healthy preterm infants. *Biol Neonate* 69:357–367.

Rennie J M (1989) Cerebral blood flow velocity variability after cardiovascular support in premature babies. *Arch Dis Child* 64:897–901.

✪ Rennie J M, Coughtrey H, Morley R & Evans D H (1995) Comparison of cerebral blood flow velocity estimation with cranial ultrasound imaging for early prediction of outcome in preterm infants. *J Clin Ultrasound* 23:27–31.

Rey M, Segerer H, Kiessling C & Obladen M (1994) Surfactant bolus instillation: effects of different doses on blood pressure and cerebral blood flow velocities. *Biol Neonate* 66:16–21.

Rizzo G & Arduini D (1991) Fetal cardiac function in intrauterine growth retardation. *Am J Obstet Gynecol* 165:876–882.

✪ Rizzo G, Capponi A, Arduini D & Romanini C (1995) The value of fetal arterial, cardiac and venous flows in predicting pH and blood gases measured in umbilical blood at cordocentesis in growth retarded fetuses. *Br J Obstet Gynaecol* 102(12):963–969.

Rizzo G, Capponi A, Rinaldo D *et al.* (1996a) Release of vasoactive agents during cordocentesis: differences between normally grown and growth-restricted fetuses. *Am J Obstet Gynecol* 175:563–570.

Rizzo G, Capponi A, Arduini D *et al.* (1996b) Uterine and fetal blood flows in pregnancies complicated by preterm labor. *Gynecologic Obstet Invest* 42(3):163–166.

Rosenberg A A, Narayanan V & Jones M D (1985) Comparison of anterior cerebral artery blood flow velocity and cerebral blood flow during hypoxia. *Pediatr Res* 19:67–70.

Rosenkrantz T S & Oh W (1982) Cerebral blood flow velocity in infants with polycythaemia and hyperviscosity: effects of partial exchange transfusion with plasmanate. *J Pediatr* 101:94–98.

Rosenkrantz T S & Oh W (1984) Aminophylline reduces cerebral blood flow velocity in low birthweight infants. *Am J Dis Child* 138:489–491.

Saliba E, Autret E, Gold F *et al.* (1989a) Effect of caffeine on cerebral blood flow velocity in preterm infants. *Biol Neonate* 65:198–203.

Saliba E, Autret E, Gold F *et al.* (1989b) Caffeine and cerebral blood flow velocity in preterm infants. *Dev Pharmacol Ther* 13:134–138.

Saliba E, Autret E, Khadiry L *et al.* (1991a) Effects of phenobarbital on cerebral hemodynamics in preterm neonates. *Dev Pharmacol Ther* 17:133–137.

Saliba E, Chantepie A, Autret E *et al.* (1991b) Effects of indomethacin on cerebral hemodynamics at rest and during endotracheal suctioning in preterm neonates. *Acta Paediatr Scand* 80:611–615.

Saliba E, Chantepie A, Marchand M *et al.* (1991c) Intra-operative measurements of cerebral hemodynamics during ductus arteriosus ligation in preterm infants. *Eur J Pediatr* 150:362–365.

Saliba E, Nashashibi M, Vaillant M-C *et al.* (1994) Instillation rate effects of Exosurf on cerebral and cardiovascular hemodynamics in preterm neonates. *Arch Dis Child* 71:F174–F178.

Salvesen K A, Bakketeig L S, Eik-Nes S H *et al.* (1992) Routine ultrasonography *in utero* and school performance at 8–9 years. *Lancet* 339:85–89.

Salvesen K A, Vatten L J, Eik-Nes S H *et al.* (1993) Routine ultrasonography *in utero* and subsequent handedness and neurological development. *BMJ* 307:159–164.

Satomura S (1957) Ultrasonic Doppler method for the inspection of cardiac functions. *J Acoustic Soc Am* 29:1181–1185.

Scherjon S A, Kok J H, Oosting H *et al.* (1992) Fetal and neonatal cerebral circulation: a pulsed Doppler study. *J Perinat Med* 20:79–82.

Scherjon S A, Smolders-Dettas H, Kok J H & Zondervan H A (1993) The 'Brain sparing' effect: antenatal cerebral Doppler findings in relation to neurologic outcome in very preterm infants. *Am J Obstet Gynecol* 169(1):169–175.

Scherjon S A, Oosting H, de Visser B W *et al.* (1996) Fetal brain sparing is associated with accelerated shortening of visual evoked potential latencies during early infancy. *Am J Obstet Gynecol* 175(6):1569–1575.

✪ Scherjon S A, Oosting H, Smolders-DeHaas H *et al.* (1998) Neurodevelopmental outcome at three years of age after fetal 'brain sparing'. *Early Hum Dev* 52(1):67–79.

Seibert J J, McCowan T C, Chadduck W M *et al.* (1989) Duplex pulsed Doppler ultrasound versus intracranial pressure in the neonate: clinical and experimental studies. *Radiology* 171:155–159.

Shortland D B, Levene M, Archer N *et al.* (1990) Cerebral blood flow velocity recordings and the prediction of intracranial hemorrhage and ischaemia. *J Perinatal Med* 18:411–417.

Smith H J (1984) Quantitative Doppler flowmentry II. Reliability of duplex scanning system under *in vitro* conditions. *Acta Radiologia (Diag)* 25:535–543.

Soll R F (1999) Synthetic surfactant for respiratory distress syndrome in preterm infants (Cochrane Review). *The Cochrane Library*, Issue 4. Oxford: Update Software.

Sonesson S-E & Herin P (1988) Intracranial arterial blood flow velocity and brain blood flow during hypocarbia and hypercapnia in newborn lambs: a validation of range-gated Doppler ultrasound flow velocimetry. *Pediatr Res* 24:423–426.

Stark J E & Seibert J J (1994) Cerebral artery Doppler ultrasonography for prediction of outcome after perinatal asphyxia. *J Ultrasound Med* 13:595–600.

Stuart B, Drumm J, Fitzgerald D E & Duignan N M (1980) Fetal blood velocity waveforms in normal pregnancy. *Br J Obstet Gynaecol* 87:780–785.

Sutterlin M W, Seelbach-Gobel B, Oehler M K *et al.* (1999) Doppler ultrasonographic evidence of intrapartum brain-sparing effect in fetuses with low oxygen saturation according to pulse oximetry. *Am J Obstet Gynecol* 181:216–220.

Taylor G A & Madsen J R (1996) Neonatal hydrocephalus: hemodynamic response to fontanelle compression – correlation with intracranial pressure and need for shunt placement. *Radiology* 201:685–689.

Ter Haal G, Duck F, Starritt H & Daniels S (1989) Biophysical characterisation of diagnostic ultrasound equipment – preliminary results. *Phys Med Biol* 34(11):1533–1542.

Trudinger B J, Giles W B & Cook C M (1985) Flow velocity waveforms the maternal uteroplacental and fetal umbilical placental circulations. *Am J Obstet Gynecol* 152:155–163.

Uerpairojkit B, Chan L, Reece A E *et al.* (1996) Cerebellar Doppler velocimetry in the appropriate- and small-for-gestational age fetus. *Obstet Gynecol* 87:989–993.

Van Bel F, Van de Bor M, Baan J *et al.* (1988) Blood flow velocity pattern of the anterior cerebral arteries. Before and after drainage of posthemorrhagic hydrocephalus in the newborn. *J Ultrasound Med* 7:553–559.

✪ Van Bel F, den Ouden L, Van de Bor M *et al.* (1989a) Cerebral blood flow velocity during the first week of life of preterm infants and neurodevelopment at two years. *Dev Med Child Neurol* 31:320–328.

Van Bel F, Van de Bor M, Stijnen T *et al.* (1989b) Cerebral blood flow velocity changes in preterm infants after a single dose of indomethacin: duration of its effect. *Pediatrics* 84:802–807.

Van Bel F, Van de Bor M, Stijnen T *et al.* (1989c) Does caffeine affect cerebral blood flow in the preterm infant? *Acta Paediatr Scand* 78:205–209.

Van Bel F, de Winter P J, Wijnands H B *et al.* (1992) Cerebral and aortic blood flow velocity patterns in preterm infants receiving prophylactic surfactant treatment. *Acta Paediatr* 81:504–510.

Van Bel F, van Zoeren D, Houdkamp E & Berger H M (1993) Is there a relationship between indomethacin-induced reduction in neonatal cerebral blood flow velocity and prostaglandin production? *Dev Pharmacol Ther* 20:45–53.

Van de Bor M, Ma E J & Walther F J (1991) Cerebral blood flow velocity after surfactant instillation in preterm infants. *J Pediatr* 118:285–287.

Van den Wijngaard J A G W, Wladimiroff J W, Reuss A & Stewart P A (1988) Oligohydramnios and fetal cerebral blood flow. *Br J Obstet Gynaecol* 95:1309–1311.

Van den Wijngaard J A G W, Wladimiroff J W & Hop W C J (1989) Cerebral Doppler ultrasound of the human fetus. *Br J Obstet Gynaecol* 96:845–849.

Van Eyck J, Wladimiroff J W, Noordam M J *et al.* (1985) The blood flow velocity waveform in the fetal descending aorta; its relationship to fetal behavioural states in normal pregnancy at 37–38 weeks. *Early Hum Dev* 12:137–143.

Van Eyck J, Wladimiroff J W, Noordam M J *et al.* (1986) The blood flow velocity waveforms in the fetal descending aorta; its relationship to behavioural states in the growth-retarded fetus at 37–38 weeks of gestation. *Early Hum Dev* 14:99–107.

Van Eyck J, Wladimiroff J W, van den Wijngaard J A G W *et al.* (1987) The blood flow velocity waveform in the fetal internal carotid and umbilical artery; its relation to fetal behavioural states in normal pregnancy at 37–38 weeks of gestation. *Br J Obstet Gynaecol* 94:736–741.

Van Eyck J, Wladimiroff J W, Noordam M J *et al.* (1988) The blood flow velocity waveform in the fetal internal carotid and umbilical artery; its relation to fetal behavioural states in the growth retarded fetus at 37–38 weeks gestation. *Br J Obstet Gynaecol* 95:473–477.

Van Straaten H L, Rademaker C M & de Vries L S (1992) Comparison of the effect of midazolam or vecuronium on blood pressure and cerebral blood flow velocity in the premature newborn. *Dev Pharmacol Ther* 19:191–195.

Veille J-C, Hanson R & Tatum K (1993) Longitudinal quantitation of middle cerebral artery blood flow in normal human fetuses. *Am J Obstet Gynaecol* 169:1393–1398.

Vyas S, Campbell S, Bower S & Nicolaides K H (1990a) Maternal abdominal pressure alters fetal cerebral blood flow. *Br J Obstet Gynaecol* 97:740–747.

✪ Vyas S, Nicolaides K H, Bower S & Campbell S (1990b) Middle cerebral artery flow velocity waveforms in fetal hypoxaemia. *Br J Obstet Gynaecol* 97:797–803.

Vyas S, Nicolaides K H & Campbell S (1990c) Doppler examination of the middle cerebral artery in anemic fetuses. *Am J Obstet Gynecol* 162:1066–1068.

Weiner Z, Farmakides G, Schulman H *et al.* (1996) Central and peripheral hemodynamic changes in post-term fetuses: correlation with oligohydramnios and abnormal fetal heart rate pattern. *Br J Obstet Gynaecol* 103:541–546.

Westra S J, Lazareff J, Curran J G *et al.* (1988) Transcranial Doppler ultrasonography to evaluate need for cerebrospinal fluid drainage in hydrocephalic children. *J Ultrasound Med* 17:561–569.

Wladimiroff J W, Tonge H M & Stewart P A (1986) Doppler ultrasound assessment of cerebral blood flow in the human fetus. *Br J Obstet Gynaecol* 93:471–475.

Wladimiroff J W, van den Wijngaard J A G W, Degani S *et al.* (1987) Cerebral and umbilical artery blood flow velocity waveforms in normal and growth retarded pregnancies. *Obstet Gynecol* 69:705–709.

Wladimiroff J W, Noordam M J, van den Wijngaard J A G W & Hop W C L (1988) Fetal internal carotid and umbilical artery blood flow velocity waveforms as a measure of fetal well-being in intrauterine growth retardation. *Pediatr Res* 24:609–613.

Wladimiroff J W (1989) Fetal cerebral blood flow. *Clin Obstet Gynaecol* 32:710–718.

Wladimiroff J W, Huisman T W A & Stewart P A (1992) Intracerebral, aortic and umbilical artery flow velocity waveforms in the late-first-trimester fetus. *Am J Obstet Gynecol* 166:46–49.

Yagel S, Anteby E, Lavy Y *et al.* (1992) Fetal middle cerebral artery blood flow during normal active labour and in labour with variable decelerations. *Br J Obstet Gynaecol* 99:483–485.

Yanowitz T D, Yao A C, Werner J C *et al.* (1998) Effects of prophylactic low-dose indomethacin on hemodynamics in very low birth weight infants. *J Pediatr* 132:28–34.

Yoshimura S, Masuzaki H, Miura K *et al.* (1998) Fetal blood flow redistribution in term intrauterine growth retardation (IUGR) and postnatal growth. *Int J Obstet Gynaecol* 60(1):3–8.

# Chapter 10 Cerebral blood flow and energy metabolism in the developing brain

G. Greisen

## INTRODUCTION

Cerebral perfusion may be quantitated as blood flow in milliliters per 100 grams brain weight per minute (ml/100 g/min). This quantity is commonly termed cerebral blood flow (CBF) and relates to the brain as a whole or to a specified region, depending on the method of measurement.

CBF was first estimated in a few newborn infants by Garfunkel *et al.* in 1954. However, only during the last 20 years did the interest in neonatal CBF increase, when it was hypothesized that some important types of perinatal brain damage may be caused by perturbation of CBF. Observing proportionality between arterial blood pressure and CBF in eight distressed infants shortly after birth (Fig. 10.1), Lou *et al.* (1977) proposed that the normal pressure–flow autoregulation may be abolished after asphyxia. This may allow moderate arterial hypotension to cause ischemia as well as moderate hypertension to be transmitted to the capillary bed and cause rupture and cerebral hemorrhage.

The principal role of cerebral perfusion is to provide substrates for the cerebral energy metabolism, with the final purpose of maintaining normal cellular concentrations of the high-energy phosphate metabolites adenosine triphosphate (ATP) and phosphocreatine (PCr) (Fig. 10.2). Cerebral metabolic rate (CMR) may be quantitated as the consumption of oxygen and glucose as CMR-$O_2$ or CMR-Glu, respectively, in μmol/100 g/min. In hypoglycemia, alternatives to glucose, primarily lactate, may help supporting CMR, and in hypoxemia or ischemia anaerobic glycolysis will speed up CMR-Glu. Hence, it should be noted that although oxygen and glucose consumption are closely linked and reflect energy metabolism in the normal state, this might not be so in pathologic states.

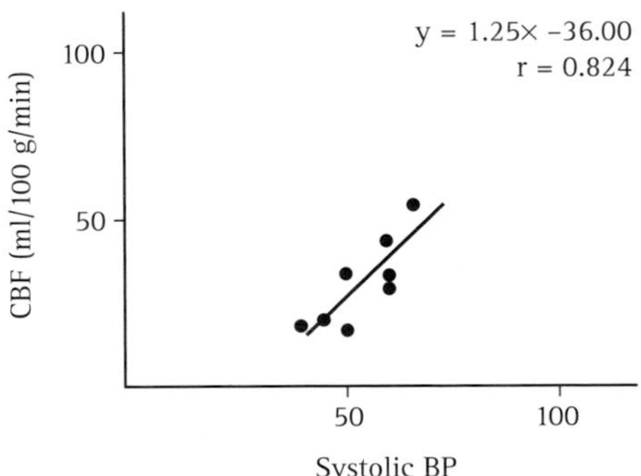


Figure 10.1 Relationship between CBF and systolic blood pressure in eight stressed newborn infants, a few hours after birth. CBF was estimated by the intra-arterial $^{133}$Xe clearance method, using an early slope index, reflecting mainly flow to gray matter. (Reproduced with permission from Lou *et al.* 1977 © Munksgaard International Publishers Ltd, Copenhagen, Denmark.)

The main problem for experimental animal studies is the differences among species in cerebrovascular anatomy and physiology, in cerebral development, and to a much lesser degree in cellular energy metabolism. The main problem in clinical research is the methodologic limitations imposed by the need to limit patient risk. Risks may be associated with the measurement itself, with transportation to the laboratory, or with manipulation of physiological variables. Therefore, this chapter describes the clinical research methods briefly, to allow critical interpretation of the available data. Furthermore, an outline of the regulation of CBF is given along with a review of the available data concerning human perinatal CBF and cerebral energy metabolism.

## CLINICAL RESEARCH METHODS

CBF as well as CMR are complex variables. CBF may change within seconds in hypoxia or with abrupt changes in blood pressure. CBF and CMR vary from one part of the brain to the other and among brain structures. During functional activation, or during stress, the distribution may change markedly. The methods available for use in human newborns provide only crude measures of those complexities.

### THE KETY–SCHMIDT METHOD

This method is based on Fick's principle for metabolically inert tracers, stating that the change of the mean tracer concentration in a tissue equals the perfusion rate multiplied by the arterio-venous concentration difference. All CBF methods using tracers build on variations of this principle, therefore it will be presented in some detail here. Nitrous oxide, a freely diffusible inert gas, is administered by inhalation. The tracer concentration in arterial and jugular venous blood is followed by taking six to eight precisely timed blood samples over 10 minutes after the start of inhalation of 15% nitrous oxide. The tissue concentration is estimated at equilibrium as the venous concentration multiplied by the tissue–blood partition coefficient.

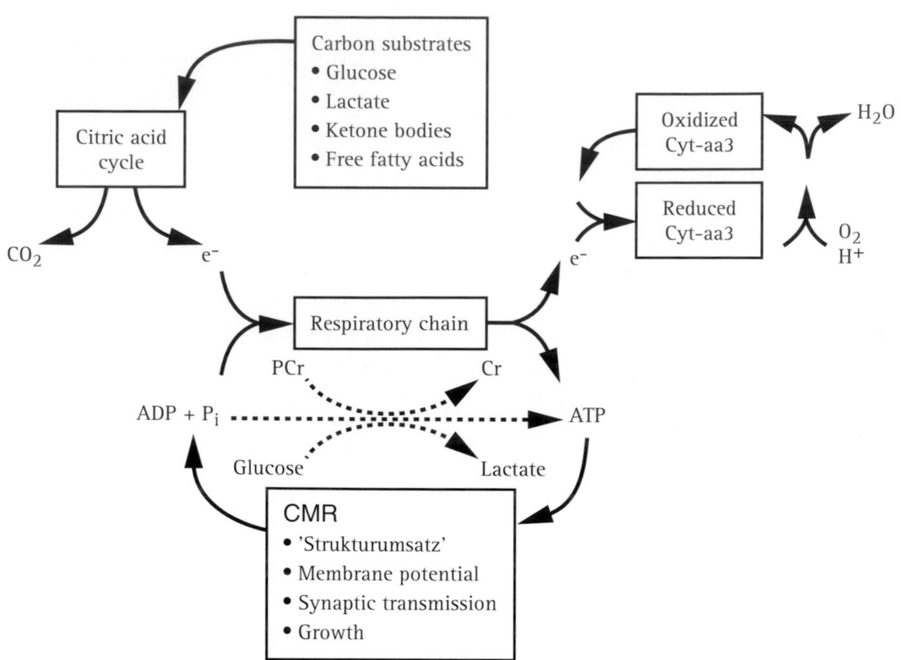


**Figure 10.2** A simple, qualitative scheme of cerebral energy metabolism. Carbon passes through the citric acid cycle, yielding electrons. The passage of electrons through the respiratory chain results in phosphorylation of ADP to ATP, driving the energy consuming processes of the brain cells. The electrons are transferred to protons and oxygen by the terminal member of the respiratory chain, cytochrome-$aa_3$ to yield water. If this oxidative phosphorylation fails, use of the phosphocreatine pool as well as anaerobic glycolysis to lactate may help to maintain ATP concentrations for some time.

The assumption of equilibration may not hold if parts of the brain are perfused at low rates and therefore remain unsaturated, which often occurs in infants (Sharples *et al.* 1991). In this situation the wash-in must be followed for 15 minutes. Completely unperfused regions of the brain will never be represented. If counter-current exchange of nitrous oxide from artery to vein takes place, the difference between venous concentration and tissue concentration will be even greater. The result is overestimation of CBF.

The value of CBF obtained by the Kety–Schmidt method is a mean over the wash-in period and relates to the part of the brain drained by the jugular vein at the sampling site; even at the jugular bulb there may be a small admixture of extracerebral blood. The Kety–Schmidt method was used in newborn infants by Garfunkel *et al.* in 1954, and recently by Frewen *et al.* (1991) and Sharples *et al.* (1991). It was made possible by the development of a micromethod for analysis of nitrous oxide (total volume of blood samples is 2–3 ml) but the application is strictly limited by the need for arterial and jugular venous blood sampling. Catheterization of the jugular bulb in infants of less than 2.5 kg is likely to be more difficult, and to carry greater risks than catheterization in larger infants and children.

The advantage is that once the jugular vein is catheterized it is possible to measure global CMR-$O_2$ and CMR-Glu by multiplying the CBF by the cross-brain extraction of oxygen or glucose.

## $^{133}$Xe CLEARANCE

Measurement of CBF by $^{133}$Xe clearance is based on a modification of the Kety–Schmidt method. If instantaneous equilibration between brain and venous blood is assumed, the venous concentrations can be derived from tissue concentrations as measured by external detection of the $\gamma$-radiation emitted by the $^{133}$Xe in the brain. In this way the need for jugular vein catheterization can be circumvented. In the small neonatal brain $^{133}$Xe clearance provides a measure of global CBF, as the detector samples from a brain volume of about 200 ml and gives an average over 5–10 minutes (Greisen & Pryds 1988).

## SINGLE PHOTON EMISSION TOMOGRAPHY

Tomographic images of radiotracer localization may be obtained by methods similar to computed X-ray tomography. $\gamma$-emitting decays (photons) across the brain are detected by a number of collimated detectors from a large number of angles around the circumference. The image is constructed by backprojection and usually subjected to various smoothing procedures (filters). There is no theoretical limit to the spatial resolution, but the narrow collimation required for high resolution reduces the sensitivity, and at the same time more counts are needed to fill the larger number of pixels (image elements). Furthermore, Compton scatter tends to mask 'cold' areas, whereas small high flow structures will be underrated owing to partial volume effects. Spatial resolution is 6–12 mm FWHM (full width at half-maximum). Slowly rotating gamma cameras may image the distribution of radioactively labeled substances, which are fixed in the brain tissue during the first passage, such as $^{131}$I-iodoamphetamine (Rubinstein *et al.* 1989) or $^{99m}$Tc-HMPAO (Hexamethyl-propylene amine oxime) (Denays *et al.* 1992). The advantage of these compounds is that they may be injected intravenously in an acute clinical situation, e.g. a seizure, whereas the imaging may take place several hours later. The disadvantage is that only the distribution, no absolute levels, of flow is obtained. Equipment rotating in 5–10 seconds may follow the local uptake and clearance of $^{133}$Xe (Chiron *et al.* 1992).

## STABLE XENON-ENHANCED COMPUTED TOMOGRAPHY

This method is also a variant of the Kety–Schmidt method. Detection of tracer in the brain is based on the high density of xenon to X-rays. By repeated X-ray CT scans during inhalation of 35% stable (non-radioactive) xenon, brain saturation can be followed. In principle the spatial resolution is as good as for conventional CT scanning, unfortunately, the low brain–blood partition coefficient of xenon in newborn brain results in a low signal-to-noise ratio. Very low levels of CBF, however, have been documented in young, brain-dead infants (Ashwal *et al.* 1989).

## POSITRON EMISSION TOMOGRAPHY

Positron emission tomography (PET) is similar to single photon emission CT (SPECT) in image reconstruction, but differs in that it utilizes the fact that positron annihilation results in two photons emitted always at an angle of 180°. Therefore localization is done by accepting only counts occurring simultaneously at two oppositely positioned detectors and collimation is not needed. Hence the sensitivity is better than SPECT at high resolution. The resolution now approaches the theoretical minimum (3 to 5 mm) which is the average positron movement before annihilation. Existing studies, however, have been done with much less spatial resolution, typically 10–14 mm, which for instance is insufficient for imaging of the preterm infant's cortex.

Biologically relevant positron emitting isotopes exist, e.g. $^{11}$C, $^{13}$N, and $^{15}$O and many biochemical substances can be labeled. PET is ideally suited for receptor studies, as imaging and quantification can be done with picomoles of tracer. The positron emitting isotopes are very short-lived (2 min to 2 h) and hence PET requires a nearby cyclotron facility.

CBF, CMR-$O_2$, cerebral blood volume, cerebral oxygen extraction fraction, and CMR-Glu may all be measured by PET (Volpe *et al.* 1983, Powers & Raichle 1985, Chugani *et al.* 1987, Altman *et al.* 1993).

## NEAR INFRARED SPECTROPHOTOMETRY

Near infrared spectrophotometry (NIRS) is of great potential value, as it may be used at the bedside and is potentially without risks, quantitative, continuous, automated, and low cost.

For *in vivo* NIRS, light of 3 to 6 wavelengths between 760 and 910 nm produced by laser diodes is delivered to the scalp of the infant by optical fibers. Transmitted light is picked up from another area of the scalp, at a 4 to 8 cm distance, by another optical fiber. Optical pathlength, however, is not simply the distance between the fibers; actually photons are scattered several times per millimeter of tissue. The propagation of light may be likened to a diffusion process; the tissue volume interrogated by NIRS is roughly the shape of a banana; the effective pathlength in human neonatal brain has been measured at 4 to 5 times the distance between the optodes, on average (Wyatt *et al.* 1990a). The variant part of the optical density is assumed to be due to varying tissue concentrations of three absorbers. These are deoxyhemoglobin, oxyhemoglobin (their sum being proportional to variations in cerebral blood volume), and change in cytochrome aa3, the terminal member of the mitochondrial respiratory chain, from a reduced to an oxidized state [$CytO_2$] (Wyatt *et al.* 1986).

Small, induced changes in arterial oxygen saturation, $SaO_2$, may be used to quantify cerebral blood volume, CBV in ml/100 g brain weight (Wyatt *et al.* 1990b) and CBF in ml/100 g/min (Edwards *et al.* 1988). CBF can also be determined by rapid injection of indocyanine green, an intravascular tracer, although a light guide must be inserted through an umbilical artery to trace the arterial concentration (Patel *et al.* 1998). The values for global CBF obtained in newborn infants compare well to those obtained by the $^{133}$Xe clearance (Skov *et al.* 1991), although it was not possible to use the NIRS CBF technique in all the infants tested. The values obtained for CBV have not yet been compared to a reference method in babies, although the typical values (2–4 ml/100 g) are reasonable.

When infants are tilted head-down, or the jugular veins are compressed, a rapid increase in optical density over the brain is seen in most, but not all, infants. If it is assumed that the increased optical density is due exclusively to pooling of cerebrovenous blood in the brain, then the proportional increase in [$HbO_2$] to [$HbO_2$] + [Hb] estimates the cerebrovenous oxygen saturation, $SvO_2$ (Skov *et al.* 1993, Yoxall *et al.* 1995). The $SvO_2$ is a very basic physiological variable, being firmly regulated in health and a good indicator of (global) cerebral oxygen sufficiency in disease. At present the only alternative way of measuring $SvO_2$ is by direct blood sampling from the sagittal sinus or the internal jugular vein.

A number of advanced NIRS techniques have been developed to obtain absolute quantification of mean cerebral hemoglobin saturation, that is a mean of the oxygen saturation of arterial, capillary, and venous blood, i.e. tissue oximeters. Because of the nature of absorption of light in heterogeneous media, blood in larger vessels is underrepresented in such a mean value. There are two major problems in this development. First, tissue is not homogenous so the algorithms used are unlikely to provide exact values, and second, there is no standard method to compare with. In animal experiments comparison has been done to a weighted average of arterial and venous saturation in a ratio 1:2 (Brun *et al.* 1997), but it is unlikely that this ratio remains constant during physiological stress.

Quantification of changes in cytochrome-aa3 oxidation is much more difficult than quantification of changes in the hemoglobins, as the cytochrome signal is one order of magnitude smaller.

## MAGNETIC RESONANCE SPECTROSCOPY

The nucleus of certain elements, e.g. $^{31}P$ and $^{1}H$, are stable but magnetically asymmetric and hence behave like magnetic dipoles. Subjected to a strong magnetic field (0.5 to 2 Tesla) they will tend to align with the field, longitudinal magnetization, or rather to rotate around the axis of the field. The rotation (precession, like a spinning top) occurs at a frequency proportional to the field strength, and specific to the nucleus (about 26 MHz for $^{31}P$ at 1.5 T), with small differences (typically ± 1 kHz) according to its chemical environment, 'chemical shift'. Exposed to a pulse of electromagnetic energy of the proper frequencies, at 90° angle, the rotation may be synchronized, resulting in a transverse magnetization. When the pulse is discontinued the synchrony continue, and hence emit electromagnetic energy, and decay in a complex pattern due to the interference of the several slightly different resonance frequencies. Fourier analysis can transform the decay pattern into a frequency spectrum with a number of peaks, each of which represents the nucleus in a particular chemical constellation.

The height of each peak is proportional to the molar

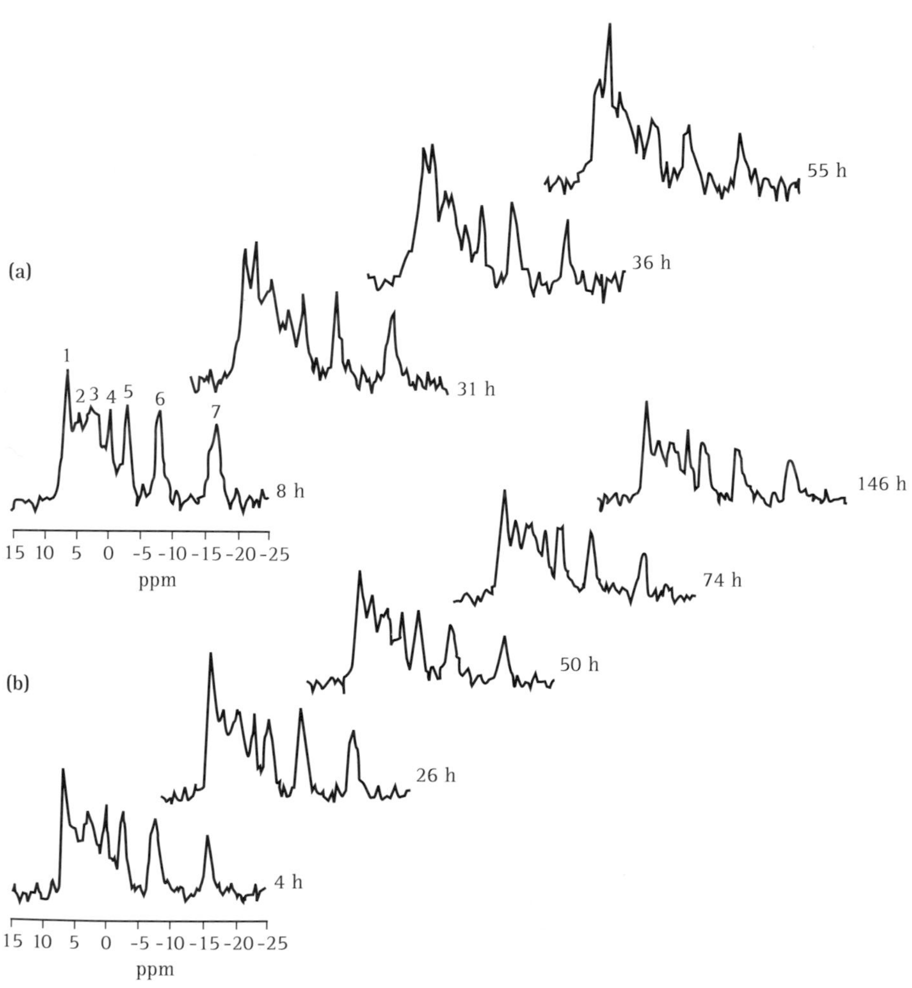


**Figure 10.3** Repetitive $^{31}P$-MRS spectra obtained from two severely asphyxiated neonates from 4 to 146 hours after the asphyxic insult. The peaks in the spectra reflect the concentration of phosphorus atoms in various chemical environments. The 'chemical shifts' indicate the resonance frequency in parts per million of the base frequency (80.5 MHz) relative to the phosphocreatine peak. The numbers in the first spectrum in part (a) indicate: 1, phosphomonoesters; 2, inorganic phosphate, $P_i$; 3, phosphodiesters; 4, phosphocreatine, PCr, and 5, 6, and 7, $\gamma$- $\alpha$-, and $\beta$-ATP. The most direct information lies in the PCr/$P_i$ peak area ratio, as well as the chemical shift of $P_i$ relative to PCr, from which intracellular pH may be calculated. In part (a) the PCr ratio is initially normal, but subsequently deteriorates. In part (b) the deterioration at 50 hours recovers at 146 hours.

concentration, but due to imperfections, e.g. inhomogeneity of the magnetic field, a certain broadening of the peaks is seen, hence the area beneath may be more informative. In order to obtain an acceptable signal-to-noise ratio, only elements of concentrations in the millimolar range are measurable and it is necessary to use high field strengths, e.g. 1.5 Tesla or above and to sum many spectra, e.g. 128 or more. If the times in between pulses are insufficient (<10 s) for complete decay (relaxation) the peak height will be underestimated.

The first use of MRS in human brain was reported by Cady *et al.* (1983). $^{31}$P spectra were obtained from a rather large hemispheric tissue volume using a 5 or 7 cm surface coil for excitation as well as resonance detection. This allowed spectra of good signal-to-noise ratio to be obtained in less than 20 minutes. The peaks which have been used subsequently are β, α, and γ adenosine triphosphate, phosphocreatine (PCr), phosphodiesters, inorganic orthophosphate ($P_i$), and surprisingly prominent phosphomonoesters. The interest in the present context focuses on the PCr/$P_i$ ratio, which is a sensitive indicator of the cellular energy charge (Fig. 10.3), as well as on intracellular pH, which may be calculated from the frequency difference (chemical shift) between $P_i$ and PCr.

It is a problem that such spectra are derived from a poorly defined and large tissue volume, even including some scalp and skull. Doing MRS on imaging equipment (superimposing small magnetic gradients in the X, Y, and Z-plane on the main field, and hence delineating an excitable volume) may allow localization, but the relative low abundancy of phosphorus, and the low signal intensity from phosphorus precludes use of sample volumes smaller than several cubic centimeters and makes metabolic imaging impractical in patients.

Proton MRS, using $^1$H, was made very useful by the invention of 'pre-saturation' pulse sequences, suppressing the large peak from water and retaining the spatial localization. Well defined peaks became apparent: *N*-acetyl aspartate (NAA), a marker of neurons, choline (Ch) and its derivatives, and creatine + phosphocreatine associated with all types of cells (Peden *et al.* 1990). Hence a low focal NAA/Ch ratio may prove a convenient marker of neuronal loss. Furthermore, lactate may be demonstrated by using long echo times, a strong tool in the investigation of marginal brain hypoxia/ischemia. Because of the better signal intensity from $^1$H, smaller sample volumes may be examined, and metabolic imaging with sub-centimeter resolution is practical.

Metabolite concentrations can be expressed in mmol/l by dividing their peak areas with that of the unsupervised water signal and using an estimate of the concentration of water in the brain (Toft *et al.* 1994).

Deoxyhemoglobin is paramagnetic, and hence a change in the amount of deoxyhemoglobin in tissue, e.g. as induced by a change in blood volume or in oxygen extraction can be assessed (creating the BOLD contrast – blood oxygenation label dependence). This is termed functional magnetic resonance imaging (fMRI).

Finally, global CBF may be estimated by imaging the four arteries on the neck and multiplying their cross-sectional area with blood flow velocity, estimated by the loss of magnetization caused by fresh blood water flowing into the plane of imaging.

## DOPPLER ULTRASOUND

The use of Doppler ultrasound for estimation of cerebral blood flow in ml/100 g/min has not yet been reported. The major problem is related to estimation of vessel diameter (see Chapter 9). Power Doppler can image the density of moving blood, without weighing for flow velocity; thus it provides an image of CBV rather than of CBF. The mean transit time (= CBV/CBF) of ultrasound contrast can be measured easily and methods based on this are likely to be tried in newborn babies.

## OTHER TECHNIQUES USED IN NEWBORN INFANTS

Venous occlusion plethysmography is a standard method for measurement of limb blood flow and has been used to estimate jugular blood flow (Cross *et al.* 1979). In spite of its virtues of technical simplicity and low risk in healthy infants, the method has fallen into disuse, mostly because of concern that low skull compliance yields falsely low values of cranial blood flow.

The transcephalic impedance, as measured by applying a small alternating electrical current, is slightly pulsatile. The pulsatility is correlated to CBF (Colditz *et al.* 1988), although the precise basis of the impedance pulsatility is unclear. This method has theoretical risks only but gives qualitative information only and is sensitive to movement. It appears well suited for long-term monitoring, but has been little used.

*A note on radiation and risk of cancer* Radiation to patients from X-rays or various isotopes may be compared by calculation of the 'whole body dose', the effective dose equivalent. This is the dose of X-rays, which if absorbed evenly in all parts of the body will result in an identical risk of cancer or genetic damage in germ cells. In this approximation, the affinity of some tracers for certain organs is considered, and organs of high vulnerability are weighed accordingly. Recently, the International Committee of Radiation Protection reviewed the evidence, mainly from Hiroshima and Nagasaki, and increased the estimate to 5% lifetime risk of fatal cancer per Sievert (1 Sv = 100 Rad = 1 J/kg) in adults. In the last trimester and in young children the risk is estimated three times greater. This means that the added lifetime risk in an infant receiving 1 mSv as a result of an investigation is 0.00015, or 1 per 7000 compared to the average lifetime risk in western populations of 0.25 or 1 in 4. The yearly radiation from all sources averages 3 mSv. Estimated doses from the various methods described above are listed in Table 10.1.

**Table 10.1 Typical patient radiation doses (effective dose equivalent) resulting from various techniques in use for the study of cerebral blood flow or metabolism in neonates.**

| Technique | Isotope | Activity used (MBq/kg) | Effective dose equivalent (mSv) |
|---|---|---|---|
| Xenon clearance, global CBF | $^{133}$Xe | 40 | 0.2 |
| SPECT, Xenon | $^{133}$Xe | 60–200 | 0.3–1 |
| SPECT, HMPAO | $^{99m}$Tc | 4–50 | 1.5–20 |
| SPECT, iodo-amphetamine | $^{131}$I | 2–10 | 1.5–8 |
| Xenon-enhanced tomography | X-rays | 20 mSv in field | 1 |
| PET, CBF | $^{15}$O | 30 | 1 |
| PET, CMR-$O_2$ | $^{15}$O | 110 | 5 |
| PET, CMR-Glu | $^{18}$F | 5 | 3 |

[a] For comparison the mean annual dose equivalent for the population in general is 3 mSv.

## PHYSIOLOGICAL REGULATION OF CBF

### COUPLING OF CBF TO CEREBRAL ENERGY METABOLISM

Through a wide range of functional states, from deep hypothermia to electrical seizures, CBF increases in proportion to the increase in cerebral metabolic rate (CMR). The precise mechanism of this coupling is not known (Lou *et al.* 1987), nor is it known when in fetal life it develops. Proportionality between local CBF and local glucose metabolism is present in newborn puppies, which are rather immature at birth.

CBF, as estimated by venous occlusion plethysmography, is increased during active sleep as compared with quiet sleep (Milligan 1979; Rahilly 1980a; Mukhtar *et al.* 1982). Using $^{133}$Xe clearance after intravenous injection in preterm infants of 32 to 35 weeks postconceptional age, Greisen *et al.* (1985) found CBF increased in the awake state when compared with quiet or active sleep. This is evidence of flow–metabolism coupling, the action of which is also suggested by the increase in CBF seen during seizures, and the strong relation between CBF and blood hemoglobin concentration (Younkin *et al.* 1987; Pryds *et al.* 1990a).

Recently, the cerebrovascular response to functional activation by visual stimulation has been studied by MRI (Born *et al.* 1998; Martin *et al.* 1999) and NIRS (Meek *et al.* 1998) and found non-existent or inconsistent in infants before term or within the first weeks of life. One possible explanation for this is that visual cortical projections are not well developed at term.

### PERFUSION PRESSURE–FLOW AUTOREGULATION

Cerebral blood flow is hemodynamically determined by the perfusion pressure (the arterial blood pressure minus the intracranial pressure) and by the cerebrovascular resistance. The cerebrovascular resistance is partly determined by the degree of contraction of the precapillary arterioles, partly by the pre-arteriolar arteries (Farachi & Heistad 1990).

Pressure–flow autoregulation has been widely investigated since the original observation of direct proportionality of CBF to systolic blood pressure in a group of neonates during stabilization after birth (Lou *et al.* 1977). An adequate autoregulatory plateau, shifted to the left to match the lower perinatal blood pressure, has been demonstrated in several animal species before and after birth (Hernandez *et al.* 1980; Tweed *et al.* 1983; Papile *et al.* 1985; Pasternak & Groothuis 1985). Autoregulation was abolished by hypoxemia (arterial oxygen saturation about 50%) for 20 min (Tweed *et al.* 1986), to return after 4 to 7 hours.

Unfortunately this issue is much less well investigated in the human neonate, the main reason being lack of controlled manipulation of blood pressure. All studies of global CBF in stable neonates without evidence of major brain injury suggest that autoregulation is intact (Greisen 1986; Greisen & Trojaborg 1987; Younkin *et al.* 1987; Pryds *et al.* 1989; Pryds *et al.* 1990a, b; Tyszczuk *et al.* 1998). From the mean arterial blood pressure that was reported in these studies it is suggested that the lower limit of autoregulation is below 30 mmHg.

Based on SPECT estimates of CBF distribution during arterial hypotension in 24 preterm infants with persistently normal brain ultrasound it has been suggested that CBF to the periventricular white matter may be selectively reduced at blood pressures below 30 mmHg (Børch & Greisen 1997). Although this data supports the concept of periventricular white matter being a 'watershed area' it must be realized that the statistical relation was based on differences among infants, which may have many causes.

Three studies have provided evidence of loss of autoregulation either following severe birth asphyxia (Pryds *et al.* 1990b) or preceding major germinal layer hemorrhage (Milligan 1980; Pryds *et al.* 1989).

### CARBON DIOXIDE–CBF REACTIVITY

Carbon dioxide is a strong cerebral vasodilator. In normocapnic adults, small changes in arterial carbon dioxide

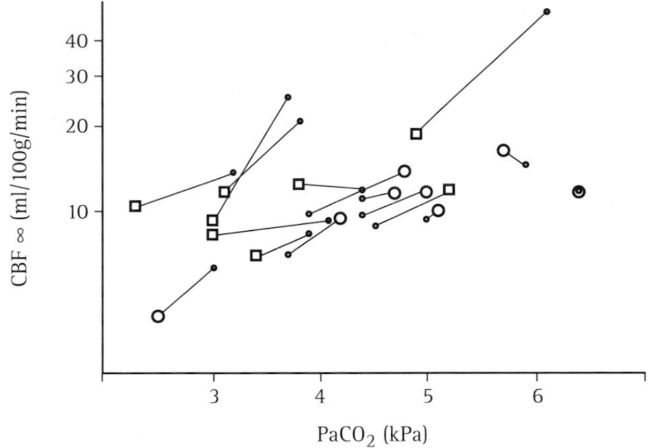


**Figure 10.4** The relationship between changes in CBF, estimated by intravenous [133]Xe clearance, and changes in $PaCO_2$ in 16 mechanically ventilated, preterm infants. In eight infants the change occurred spontaneously (○), whereas in the other eight infants the $PaCO_2$ changed after a change in the ventilator settings (□). The intra-individual reactivity to acute changes, represented by the lines, is clearly greater than the inter-individual differences, which reflect, among other factors, more long-lasting changes in $PaCO_2$. (Reproduced with permission from Greisen & Trojaborg 1987.)

tension ($PaCO_2$) result in a change in CBF by 30%/kPa (4%/mmHg). Adaptation, with return of CBF to normal values, occurs within 24 hours after a chronic change of $PaCO_2$. Similar reactivity has been demonstrated in the normal human neonate by venous occlusion plethysmography (Leahy *et al.* 1980; Rahilly 1980b) and in stable preterm ventilated infants without major germinal layer hemorrhage by [133]Xe after intravenous injection (Greisen & Trojaborg 1987, Fig. 10.4). Reactivity was less than 30%/kPa during the first 24 hours (Pryds *et al.* 1989).

## NEUROGENIC REGULATION OF CBF

From animal studies it appears that the sympathetic system may play a more marked role in the perinatal period compared to later life (Hernandez *et al.* 1982; Hayashi *et al.* 1984; Wagerle *et al.* 1986; Kurth *et al.* 1988; Goplerud *et al.* 1991). This is perhaps so because of a relative immaturity of the nitric oxide-induced vasodilatation (Wagerle *et al.* 1995). The mechanism is in part a constriction of larger cerebral arteries. The observation of a 30–40% decrease in CBF after a feed in full-term newborn infants using venous occlusion plethysmography (Dear 1980; Rahilly 1980a) may suggest a neurogenic mechanism, although hardly mediated by increased sympthetic tone.

## CBF, CEREBRAL OXYGEN DELIVERY AND CMR IN NORMAL NEONATES

The three infants studied by Garfunkel *et al.* (1954) were all abnormal (one with myelomeningocele, one with microcephaly, and one with hydrocephalus) – CBF ranged from 15 to 23 ml/100 g/min, as estimated by the Kety-Schmidt method. The CMR-$O_2$ ranged from 50 to 94 μmol/100 g/min (1.1–2.1 ml $O_2$). These values were surprisingly low compared with normal adult values of 150 μmol/100 g/min.

Few entirely normal human neonates have been investigated by reliable techniques. Values of CMR-$O_2$ in normal human neonates are not available, although $SvO_2$ was entirely normal (64± 5%) as estimated by NIRS and jugular occlusion in 11 healthy, term infants, 3 days after birth (Buchvald *et al.* 1999). The average value of global CBF measured by [133]Xe clearance in 11 preterm, healthy infants during the first week of life was 20 ml/100 g/min (Greisen 1986). The contrast between flow to white and gray matter is high compared to experimental perinatal animals (Børch & Greisen 1998).

The value of global CBF increases with postnatal age (Younkin *et al.* 1982), and probably also with increasing gestational age. The dramatic increase from the perinatal period to 3 years of postnatal age, and later decrease to adult values (Fig. 10.5) matches maturational changes in CMR-Glu, as estimated from PET studies of patients (Chugani *et al.* 1987), who later turned out to be free of neurologic disease (Fig. 10.6). This pattern of development also matches the number of synapses per cubic millimeter of visual cortex (Huttenlocher *et al.* 1982).

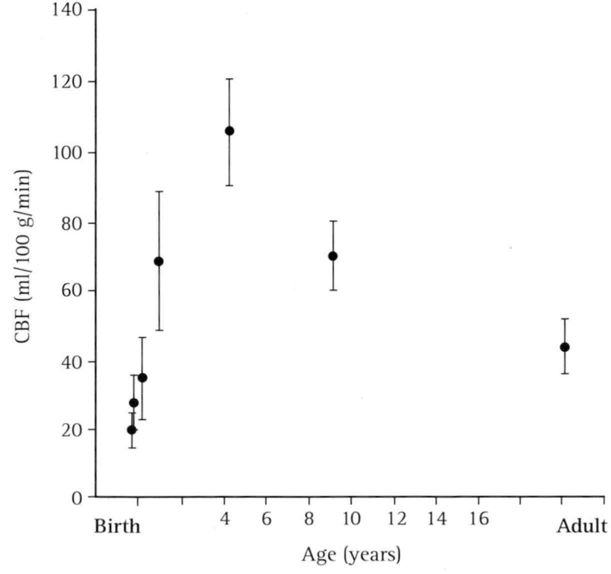


**Figure 10.5** Values of CBF obtained in healthy, apparently normal humans from 10 weeks before term to adulthood. (From Kennedy & Sokoloff 1957; Settergren *et al.* 1976; Meyers *et al.* 1978; Cross *et al.* 1979; Younkin *et al.* 1982; Lou *et al.* 1984; Greisen 1986.)

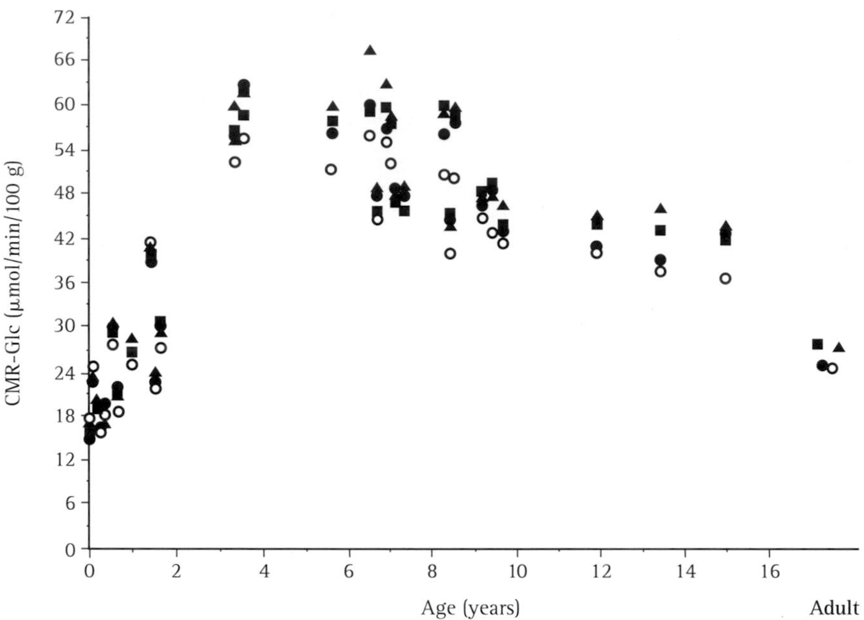


Figure 10.6 Cortical glucose uptake in patients investigated for neurologic abnormality, but subsequently considered normal. There are no values for preterm neonates but the general developmental pattern is quite similar to that of CBF. (Reproduced with permission from Chugani *et al.* 1987. Wiley-Liss inc., Jossey-Bass inc. a subsidiary of John Wiley & Sons, inc.)

## PATHOPHYSIOLOGY

### ACUTE HYPOXIA–ISCHEMIA

The basic physiological quantity in hypoxic–ischemic brain injury is cerebral oxygen delivery, which is the product of CBF and arterial oxygen content. When oxygen delivery becomes insufficient to meet the cellular demands for oxygen, a sequence of events will be triggered, starting with anaerobic glycolysis and lactacidosis, proceeding to membrane pump failure, efflux of potassium, influx of sodium and calcium. This leads to microstructural damage and cell death, possibly several days later through a process of apoptosis (see below and Chapter 23).

During arterial hypoxemia, the normal cerebrovascular reaction leads to rising CBF and the oxygen extraction fraction increases (Fig. 10.7). CBF may maximally increase two to threefold. Oxygen extraction can increase until the critical level of venous oxygen saturation ($SvO_2$), which corresponds to the minimal oxygen tension providing a sufficient diffusion gradient from the venous end of the capillary to the mitochondrion. In the newborn puppy $SvO_2$ may decrease from 75 to 40% without significant elevation in lactate production (Reuter & Disney 1986). The exact minimum value will depend on the oxygen dissociation curve, and hence among other factors be increased by alkalosis and a high fraction of fetal hemoglobin.

Decrease of CBF below a threshold, when oxygen supply is no longer sufficient, is termed ischemia. In the cerebral cortex of adult baboon and adult man, the threshold of blood flow sufficient to maintain tissue integrity depends on time of exposure; for a duration of a few hours, the limit is in the range of 10 ml/100 g/min (Jones *et al.* 1981). In acute, localized brain ischemia the concept of a border-zone or

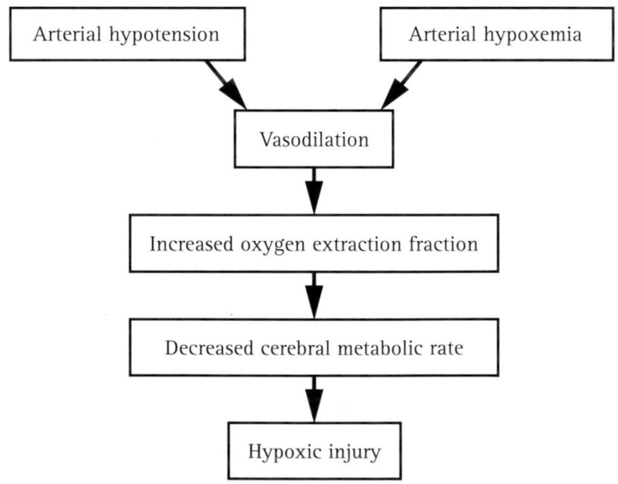


Figure 10.7 Buffering mechanisms protect the brain against hypoxic–ischemic injury. Vasodilation leads to decreased cerebrovascular resistance. Oxygen extraction fraction increases until the oxygen tension at the venous ends of the capillaries is minimized. When oxygen is no longer sufficient the metabolic rate begins to fall. Only when the metabolic rate falls markedly, is injury likely to occur.

'penumbra' has been proposed, i.e. a state in which the blood flow is sufficient to maintain the '*strukturumsatz*' membrane potentials but fails to sustain electrical activity (Astrup 1982). The brain tissue in such a zone is electrically silent. In progressing ischemia, electrical failure is a prewarning of permanent tissue injury. This concept has been used in EEG-monitoring during carotid surgery. In adult human brain cortex, electrical function ceases at about 20 ml/100 g/min. In subcortical gray matter and the brainstem of the adult baboon the values are 10–15 ml/100 g/min (Branston *et al.* 1984).

The threshold values for neonates are not known but in view of the low resting levels of CBF and the comparatively much longer survival in total ischemia or anoxia, the thresholds are likely to be considerably below 10 ml/100 g/min. Thus, in ventilated preterm infants visual evoked responses were unaffected at global flow levels below 10 ml/100 g/min corresponding to a cerebral oxygen delivery of 50 μmol/100 g/min (Greisen & Trojaborg 1987; Pryds & Greisen 1990).

Periventricular white matter is thought of as particularly vulnerable to hypoxic–ischaemic injury in preterm infants, although it has been difficult to find direct evidence that periventricular leukomalacia is a hypoxic–ischemic lesion.

## THE POST-ASPHYXIATED STATE

The loss of cellular energy charge during an asphyxial event can be studied by $^{31}$P-MRS in animals (Hope *et al.* 1987). For logistic reasons it has not been demonstrated in human neonates; it is presumably corrected during resuscitation.

The early recovery phase lasts 4–12 hours and is not well studied in human infants. From animal studies of acute asphyxia–ischaemia it is expected that CBF, CMR-$O_2$ and CMR-Glu is low, as witnessed by reduced EEG activity. Clearly, in clinical practice an asphyxial event may be intermittent or subacute during the last hours before delivery or during gradual cardio-respiratory decompensation due to severe postnatal illness. As a result, the early phase may be short or missing in some infants.

After the most severe, global injury follows a delayed phase, which lasts for several days. The PCr/$P_i$ which has normalized in the early phase declines again (Fig. 10.3, Hope *et al.* 1984) and intracellular pH rises above normal, whereas the NAA/Cho ratio by $^1$H-MRS is typically normal (Fig. 10.8). This carries a poor prognosis (Fig. 10.9, Azzopardi *et al.* 1989), and gives more precise prediction of handicap compared to a clinical score (Martin *et al.* 1996). High levels of CBF in the delayed phase has been well documented (Friis-Hansen 1985; Pryds *et al.* 1990b; Frewen *et al.* 1991; Leth *et al.* 1996), and is associated with low oxygen extraction (Frewen *et al.* 1991; Skov *et al.* 1993). A similar 'luxury perfusion' (Lassen 1966) has been described following head trauma, particularly in young individuals (Obrist *et al.* 1984; Cohan *et al.* 1989). Loss of cerebrovascular tone is suggested by the loss of reactivity to $CO_2$ as well as to changes in blood pressure (Fig. 10.10). In parallel, abnormally high CBV has been demonstrated by NIRS associated with a reduced reactivity of CBV to changes in $PaCO_2$ (Meek *et al.* 1999a). The low oxygen extraction contrasts with the increased cerebral lactate concentration as shown by $^1$H-MRS (Groenendaal *et al.* 1994; Hanrahan *et al.* 1996; Leth *et al.* 1996) and increased CMR-Glu by PET (Blennow *et al.* 1995). Each of these findings has been shown to predict later handicap and together they indicate mitochondrial failure.

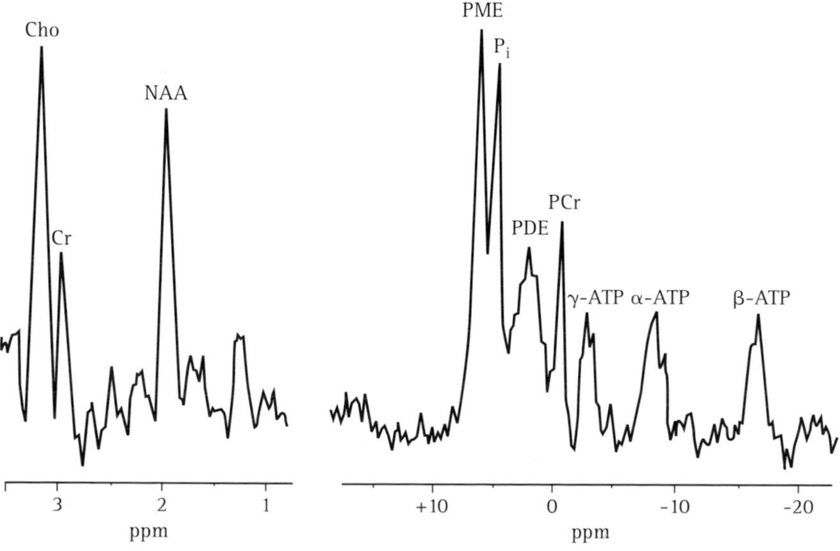


**Figure 10.8** $^1$H (left) and $^{31}$P (right) spectrum from a term, asphyxiated infant 48 hours after birth. The NAA/Cho ratio is 0.8, probably within normal range. The PCr/$P_i$ ratio was 0.5, severely abnormal. The infant subsequently developed subcortical cysts. (Reproduced with permission from Peden *et al.* 1990.)

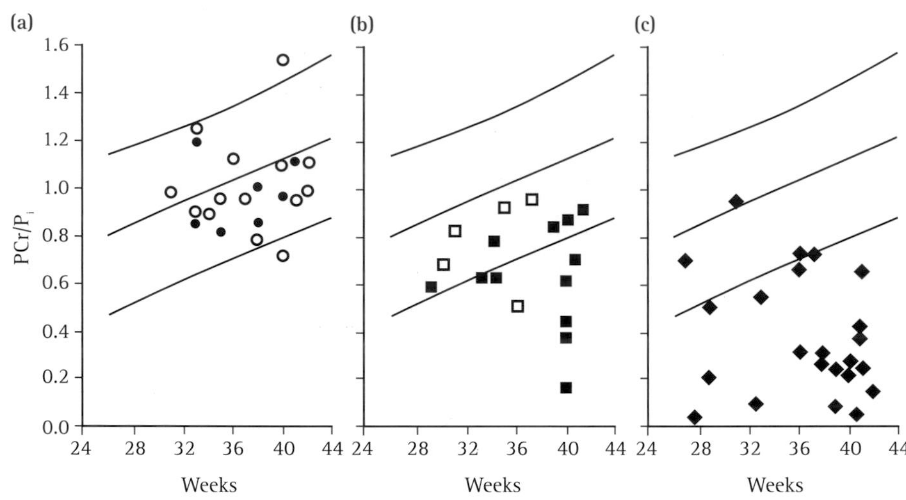


**Figure 10.9** Relationship between minimum values of $PCr/P_i$ ratio in 61 infants with hypoxic–ischemic brain injury and 1 year outcome. The regression line, 5 and 95 centiles for $PCr/P_i$ as a function of gestational age in normal babies are indicated in each of the three panels. (a) ○, normal progress; ●, minor impairment; (b) □, major neuromotor impairment; ■, multiple major impairments; (c) ◆, death. Whereas the $PCr/P_i$ ratio is specific, since only one normal child had a low ratio, the ratio has a rather low sensitivity for neurodevelopmental impairment. (Reproduced with permission from Azzopardi *et al.* 1989.)

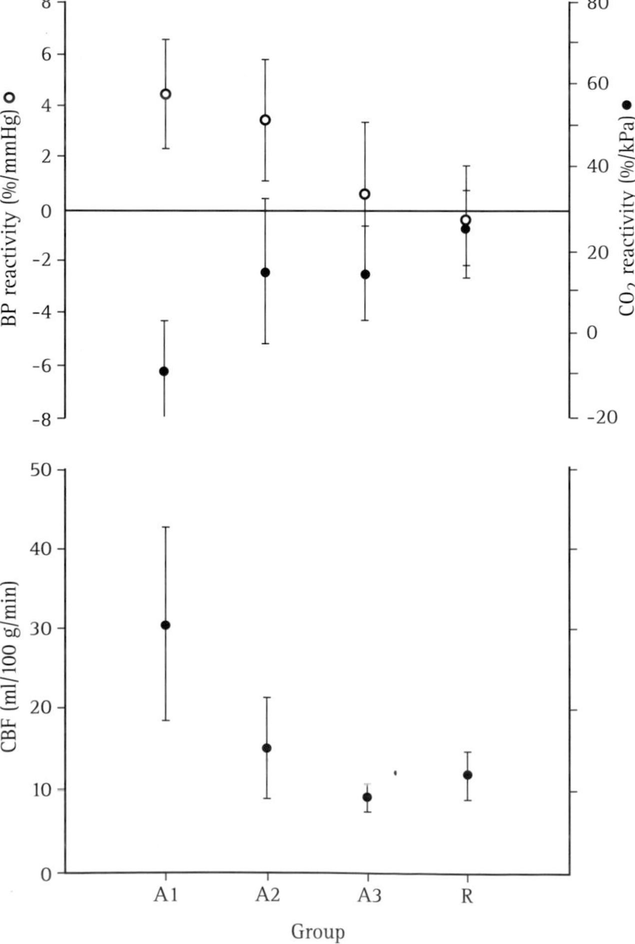


In infants who develop neurologic signs of focal brain damage only, slightly low levels of global CBF with abnormal pressure–flow reactivity and near-normal CBF-$CO_2$ reactivity has been demonstrated (Pryds *et al.* 1990b, Fig. 10.10).

In the slightly longer term, Volpe *et al.* (1985) reported local decrease in CBF, as estimated by PET, in the parasagittal regions 3 to 20 days after the insult corresponding to a decreased CMR-Glu in asphyxiated term neonates with poor later outcome (Suhonen-Polvi *et al.* 1993; Thorngren-Jerneck *et al.* 1999). The $PCr/P_i$ ratio normalizes, whereas the *N*-aspartate/acetate concentration fails to develop normally (Fig. 10.11) as evidenced by $^1$H-MRS (Peden *et al.* 1990). Considering all these techniques relate to a given volume, the results do not indicate brain 'atrophy' but rather transformation of brain tissue into a 'scar' tissue of lower energy metabolism and possibly

**Figure 10.10** Global CBF (●, lower panel) and its reactivity to changes in $PaCO_2$ (●, upper panel) and mean arterial blood pressure (○, upper panel) in 3 groups of severely asphyxiated infants (A1, A2, A3) and a reference group of term infants similarly mechanically ventilated for cardiorespiratory or surgical illness (R). The asphyxiated infants were grouped according to the extent of resulting brain damage: severe and global (A1), focal (A2), and none (A3). The horizontal axis for the vascular reactivities indicates the normal value of 0%/mmHg for arterial blood pressure and 30%/kPa for $PaCO_2$. (Redrawn from Pryds *et al.* 1990b.)

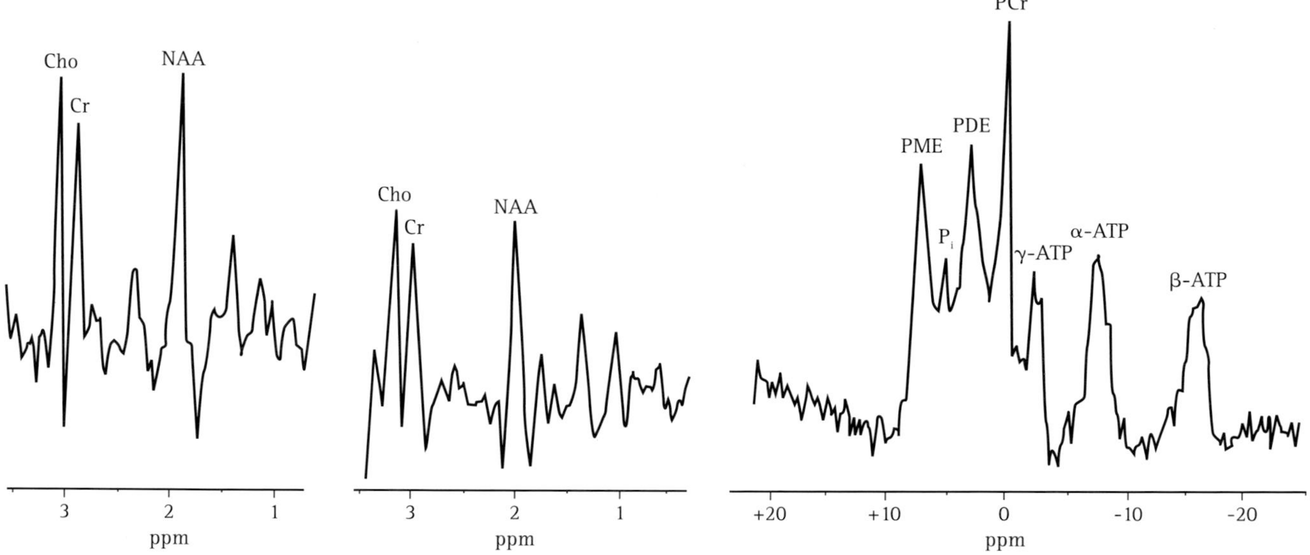


**Figure 10.11** $^1$H spectrum (left) at 5 months of age, and $^1$H spectrum (middle) and $^{31}$P spectrum (right) at 14 months of age from an infant with thalamic echodensities and subcortical cysts on cerebral ultrasound in the perinatal period. At 5 months the NAA/Cho ratio was 1.1 only, in the normal range of infants at birth. At 14 months, presenting cerebral palsy and global delay, the NAA/Cho ratio had still not developed (the normal adult range is 3.5–4.5), whereas in the $^{31}$P spectrum the PCr/$P_i$ was quite normal, 2.5. (Reproduced with permission from Peden *et al.* 1990.)

containing fewer neurons. Interestingly, the lactate/creatine ratio appears to remain elevated for months (Hanrahan *et al.* 1998) as well as the intracellular pH (Robertson *et al.* 1999).

## HYPOGLYCEMIA

Severe hypoglycemia lasting hours may cause brain damage by substrate insufficiency. The significance of moderate or brief hypoglycemia is less clear. Perinatal animals (Belik *et al.* 1989) and human neonates (Kraus *et al.* 1974) may to a large extent depend on alternative carbon sources during hypoglycemia (Fig. 10.2), but probably not fully. Furthermore, although in some situations substitutes for glucose are abundant, e.g. lactate after asphyxia or ketone bodies in fasting, in other situations they may be scarce, e.g. following a sudden discontinuation of intravenous glucose infusion.

Cerebral glucose uptake has not been studied during hypoglycemia, which is associated with increased CBF in preterm infants a few hours after birth (Fig. 10.12, Pryds *et al.* 1988b). The increase is apparent at a blood glucose slightly below 2 mM. At the lowest levels of glucose, CBF increases to maximal values. The mechanism of this increase, as well as its effect on glucose uptake is unclear. Monitoring of preterm infants with NIRS during bolus glucose administration for hypoglycemia suggests that cerebral blood volume decreases (normalises?) in the course of the first few minutes (Skov & Pryds 1992), suggesting capillary recruitment. This would increase the permeability-surface product and hence increase glucose flux across the blood–brain barrier. The concept of capillary recruitment, however, has been seriously questioned (Kuschinsky & Paulson 1992).

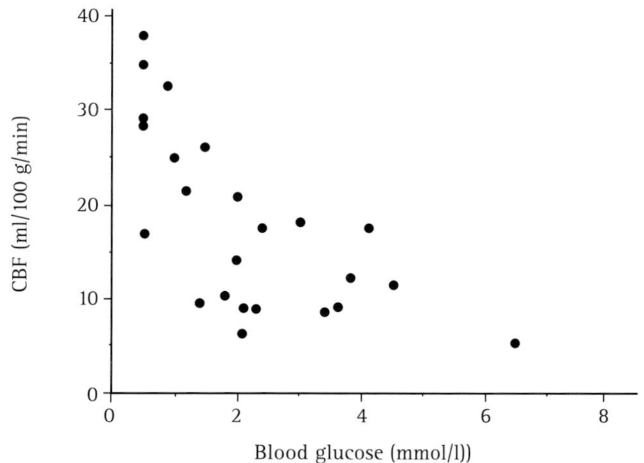


**Figure 10.12** CBF as a function of blood glucose concentrations a few hours after birth in 24 preterm neonates. (Reproduced with permission from Pryds *et al.* 1988b.)

## HYPERVENTILATION

Hyperventilation causes hypocapnic cerebral vasoconstriction and has been found associated with brain injury in preterm infants (Calvert *et al.* 1987; Greisen *et al.* 1987; Graziani *et al.* 1992 and see p. 380) but not in term infants (Ferrara *et al.* 1984) or adults. It is questionable whether hypocapnia alone can cause ischemia, or if it may work in combination with other factors, such as hypoxemia, hypoglycemia, sympathetic activation or seizures.

## SEIZURES

The clinical relevance of the flow–metabolism coupling is most clearly appreciated by considering focal electrical seizures. PET (Perlmann *et al.* 1985) and SPECT (Børch *et al.* 1998) has demonstrated increase in local CBF. The increases were less than the increase during seizures in adult experimental animals but the difference may be due to volume averaging. If the flow–metabolism coupling is insufficient, the highly increased local metabolic demands may not be met and neuronal injury may ensue. Ictal MRS showed a drop in PCr/$P_i$ ratio in four infants with seizures (Younkin *et al.* 1986). Evidence of damaging effects of seizures *per se* is of crucial importance for the indication of aggressive anticonvulsive therapy.

## RESPIRATORY DISTRESS, OXYGEN EXPOSURE AND ARTIFICIAL VENTILATION

Respiratory distress syndrome is characterized by several circulatory features of which decreased visceral blood flow is one. It is possible that brain blood flow is affected similarly. Thus, among 42 preterm infants (Fig. 10.13) artificial ventilation was associated with low levels of CBF which could not be explained by the $PaCO_2$, arterial blood pressure, or gestational age in the group of mechanically ventilated infants (Greisen 1986). This reduction of CBF may possibly increase the exposure to ischemia. Overexposure to oxygen in preterm infants in the delivery room was associated with a reduction of CBF by 23% two hours later (Lundstrøm *et al.* 1995).

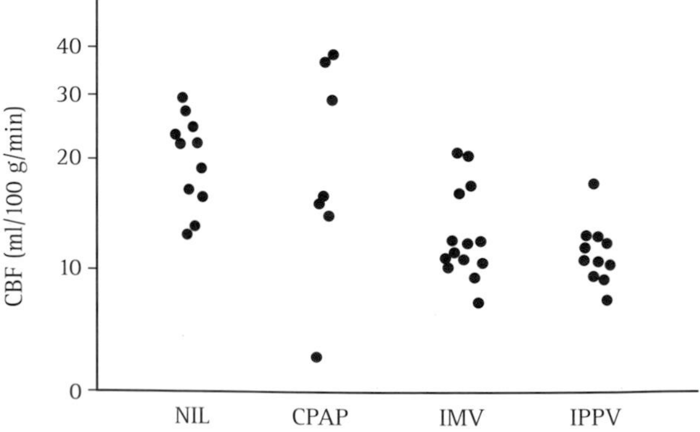


**Figure 10.13** CBF in 42 preterm infants less than 5 days of age, estimated by the intravenous $^{133}$Xe method. Of these infants 11 required no respiratory assistance (NIL), 6 had continuous positive airway pressure (CPAP), 14 were mechanically ventilated at a rate <20/min (IMV), whereas 11 required a faster rate (IPPV). (Reproduced with permission from Greisen 1986.)

## INTRACRANIAL HEMORRHAGE (see also Chapter 21)

Decreased levels of CBF (Pryds *et al.* 1989, Meek *et al.* 1999b) and impaired pressure–flow autoregulation as well as CBF-$CO_2$ reactivity was demonstrated in preterm infants, who went on to develop severe germinal layer hemorrhage (Pryds *et al.* 1989). It is unknown whether the CBF abnormality did contribute to the causation of the hemorrhage, or whether it was just another manifestation of a primary injury. It should be noted that the germinal layer, the typical origin of hemorrhage in preterm infants, is characterized by an atypical vascularization, and that this small region will contribute little to measurements of global CBF. Thus, further progress on the pathogenesis of germinal layer hemorrhage may have to await methods for measurement of blood flow to the germinal layer itself.

Once a severe hemorrhage is established, it is possible that the presence of extravascular blood induces vasospasm, leading to ischemia in the periphery (Volpe *et al.* 1983). Alternatively, a widespread hypoperfusion may indicate a more extensive ischemic injury than evidenced by the extent of the hemorrhage or simply reflect diaschisis, i.e. far-away reduction in neuronal activity due to loss of connectivity (Børch & Greisen 1994). It is not known if the widespread perturbations of CBF that are seen in some cases of severe hemorrhage can help identifying infants at particular risk of extensive handicap.

## EFFECT OF DRUGS

Indomethacin reduces CBF in experimental animals, in adults, and in preterm neonates treated for persistence of the arterial duct (Pryds *et al.* 1988a). The loss of normal CBF-$CO_2$ reactivity has also been demonstrated in preterm infants (Fig. 10.14; Edwards *et al.* 1990). The crucial question of whether indomethacin may actually reduce CBF to ischemic levels and cause brain injury has not yet been addressed. Interestingly ibuprofen (ibobrufen) does not have significant cerebrovascular effects (Mosca *et al.* 1997; Patel *et al.* 2000).

Aminophylline reduces CBF and $PaCO_2$ in experimental animals, in adults, and in preterm infants (Pryds & Schneider 1991). It is not yet clear whether the reduction of CBF is a direct effect of aminophylline or rather just a result of the fall in $PaCO_2$.

Dopamine increases blood pressure and thereby may affect CBF. It does not appear to have a specific (dilatory) effect on brain vessels (Seri *et al.* 1998; Zhang *et al.* 1999; Lundstrøm *et al.* 2000).

# MEASUREMENT OF CBF AND CMR IN CLINICAL PRACTICE

At present there is little place for evaluating CBF or cerebral energy metabolism in the perinatal period. Low CBF or cere-

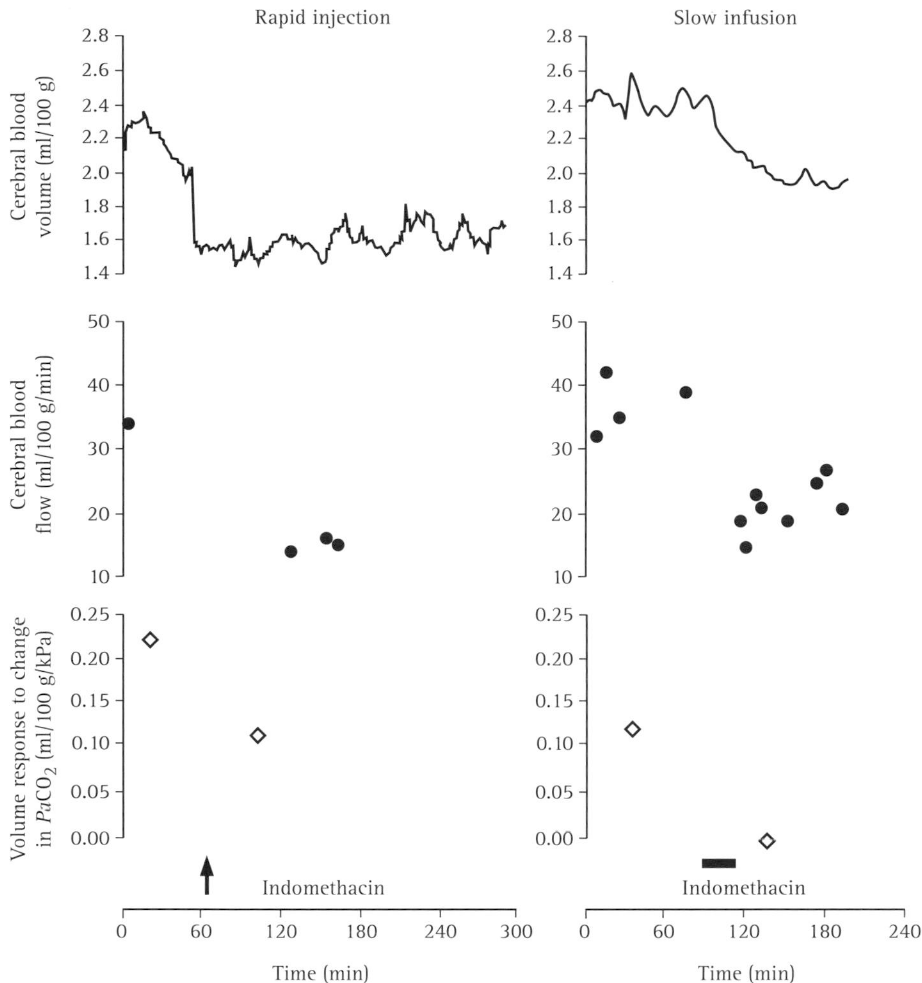


Figure 10.14 The effect of indomethacin on cerebral haemodynamics as monitored and quantified by near-infrared spectrophotometry in two preterm infants treated for persistence of the arterial duct. (Reproduced with permission from Edwards *et al.* 1990 © the Lancet Ltd.)

bral oxygen delivery as estimated by $^{133}$Xe clearance carried a risk of later death, cerebral atrophy or neurodevelopmental deficit (Lou & Skov 1979; Ment *et al.* 1983; Pryds 1994; Krageloh-Mann *et al.* 1999). We do not know, however, with any precision the lower limit of acceptable CBF and furthermore it is uncertain whether management to increase CBF can improve the outcome.

It is likely that abnormal CBF reactivity may be a forerunner of cerebral hemorrhage but it has not been demonstrated that hemorrhage may be prevented by identifying such abnormality.

The demonstration of luxury perfusion, vasoparalysis and increased cerebral lactate by $^{1}$H-MRS and abnormality in the PCr/$P_i$ ratio by $^{31}$P-MRS, provides supportive evidence of severe asphyxial vascular and neuronal injury, and may contribute to the decision to discontinue intensive care. Unfortunately, detection of these abnormalities is likely to be too late to be helpful in the selection of patients for anti-apoptotic therapy. They may be useful for the evaluation of its effectiveness.

## Key Points

The avoidance of brain damage is a principal task for those caring for ill, newborn infants. Cerebral oxygen delivery is an important variable, which due to lack of clinically applicable monitoring methods currently has to be managed 'blind' by the clinician. The following considerations are appropriate:

- Marginal hypoxia–ischaemia takes time (30 minutes to some hours) to cause brain injury.
- In a minority of ill babies pressure–flow autoregulation may be deficient and this may make them more sensitive to moderate arterial hypotension.
- It is customary to try to limit blood pressure rise in very preterm babies, e.g. by correcting hypovolemia gradually, but the effect must be monitored and treatment accelerated if needed.
- Rapid lowering of $PCO_2$ is a most potent way to reduce CBF; adaptation to a new level of $PCO_2$ takes several hours.
- There is no situation where CBF should be reduced.

- The advantage of a higher blood hemoglobin for increasing oxygen carrying capacity is nearly balanced out by greater viscosity. Optimal Hb may be 8–10 mmol/l.
- Combinations of factors adverse to cerebral energy sufficiency, e.g. low CBF, low blood glucose, combined with seizures may add up.
- Future research will aim to help in refining the above advice. The most directly useful monitoring equipment would be a tissue oximeter.

## REFERENCES


Altman D I, Perlman J M, Volpe J J *et al.* (1993) Cerebral oxygen metabolism in newborns. *Pediatrics* 92:99–104.

Ashwal S, Schneider S & Thompson J (1989) Xenon computed tomography measuring blood flow in the determination of brain death in children. *Ann Neurol* 25:539–546.

Astrup J (1982) Energy-requiring cell functions in the ischaemic brain. *J Neurosurg* 56:482–497.

Azzopardi D, Wyatt J S, Cady E B *et al.* (1989) Prognosis of newborn infants with hypoxic-ischaemic brain injury assessed by phosphorus magnetic resonance spectroscopy. *Pediatr Res* 25:445–451.

Belik J, Wagerle L C, Stanley C A *et al.* (1989) Cerebral metabolic response and mitochondrial activity following insulin-induced hypoglycemia in newborn lambs. *Biol Neonate* 55:281–289.

Blennow M, Ingvar M, Lagercrantz H *et al.* (1995) Early [18F]FDG positron emission tomography in infants with hypoxic-ischaemic encephalopathy shows hypermetabolism during the postasphyctic period. *Acta Paediatr Scand* 84:1289–1295.

Børch K & Greisen G (1994) Widespread regional cerebral blood flow disturbances in preterm infants with intracerebral haemorrhages. *Pediatr Res* 36:24 [Abstr].

Børch K & Greisen G (1997) Regional cerebral blood flow during hypotension and hypoxaemia in preterm infants *Pediatr Res* 42:389 [Abstr.].

Børch K & Greisen G (1998) Blood flow distribution in the normal human preterm brain. *Pediatr Res* 43:28–33.

Børch K, Pryds O, Holm S *et al.* (1998) Regional cerebral blood flow during seizures in neonates. *J Pediatr* 132:431–435.

Born P, Leth H, Miranda M J, *et al.* (1998) Visual activation in infants and young children studied by functional magnetic resonance imaging. *Pediatr Res* 44:578–583.

Branston N M, Ladds A, Symon L & Wang A D (1984) Comparison of the effects of ischaemia on early components of somatosensory evoked potentials in brainstem, thalamus, and cerebral cortex. *J Cerebr Blood Flow Metab* 4:68–81.

Brun N C, Moen A, Borch K *et al.* (1997) Near-infrared monitoring of cerebral tissue oxygen saturation and blood volume in newborn piglets. *Am J Physiol* 273:H682–H686.

Buchvald F F, Keshe K & Greisen G (1999) Measurement of cerebral oxyhaemoglobin saturation and jugular blood flow in term healthy newborn infants by near-infrared spectroscopy and jugular venous occlusion. *Biol Neonate* 75:97–103.

Cady E B, Costello A M de L, Dawson M J *et al.* (1983) Non-invasive investigation of cerebral metabolism in newborn infants by phosphorus nuclear magnetic resonance spectroscopy. *Lancet* i:1059–1062.

Calvert S A, Hoskins E M, Fong K W & Forsyth S C (1987) Etiological factors associated with the development of periventricular leucomalacia. *Acta Paediatr Scand* 76:254–259.

Chiron C, Raynaud C, Maziere B *et al.* (1992) Changes in regional cerebral blood flow during brain maturation in children and adolescents. *J Nuc Med* 33:696–703.

Chugani H T, Phelps M E & Mazziotta J C (1987) Positron emission tomography study of human brain functional development. *Ann Neurol* 22:487–497.

Cchan S L, Mun S K, Petite J P *et al.* (1989) Cerebral blood flow in humans following resuscitation from cardiac arrest. *Stroke* 20:761–765.

Colditz P, Greisen G & Pryds O (1988) Comparison of electrical impedance and $^{133}$Xe clearance for the assessment of cerebral blood flow in the newborn infant. *Pediatr Res* 24:461–464.

Cross K W, Dear P R F, Hathorn M K S *et al.* (1979) An estimation of intracranial blood flow in the newborn infant. *J Physiol* 289:329–345.

Dear P R F (1980) Effect of feeding on jugular venous blood flow in the normal infant. *Arch Dis Child* 55:365–370.

Denays R, Ham H, Tondear M *et al.* (1992) Detection of bilateral and symmetrical anomalies in technecium-99 HMPAO brain SPECT studies. *J Nuc Med* 33: 485–490.

Edwards A D, Wyatt J S, Richardson C *et al.* (1988) Cotside measurements of cerebral blood flow in ill newborn infants by near infrared spectrocopy. *Lancet* ii:770–771.

Edwards A D, Wyatt J S, Richardson C *et al.* (1990) Effects of indomethacin on cerebral haemodynamics in very preterm infants. *Lancet* i:1491–1495.

Farachi F M & Heistad D D (1990) Regulation of large cerebral arteries and cerebral microvascular pressure. *Circulat Res* 66:8–17.

Ferrara B, Johnson D E, Chang P-N & Thompson T R (1984) Efficacy and neurologic outcome of profound hypocapneic alkalosis for the treatment of persistent pulmonary hypertension in infancy. *J Pediatr* 105:457–461.

Frewen T C, Kissoon N, Kronick J *et al.* (1991) Cerebral blood flow, cross-brain oxygen extraction, and fontanelle pressure after hypoxic-ischemic injury in newborn infants. *J Pediatr* 118:265–271.

Friis-Hansen B (1985) Perinatal brain injury and cerebral blood flow in newborn infants. *Acta Paediatr Scand* 74:323–331.

Garfunkel J M, Baird H W & Siegler J (1954) The relationship of oxygen consumption to cerebral functional activity. *J Pediatr* 44:64–72.

Goplerud J M, Wagerle L C & Delivoria-Papadopoulos M (1991) Sympathetic nerve modulation of regional cerebral blood flow during asphyxia in newborn piglets. *Am J Physiol* 260:H1575–H1580.

Graziani L J, Spitzer A R, Mitchell D G *et al.* (1992) Mechanical ventilation in preterm infants: neurosonographic and developmental studies. *Pediatrics* 90:515–522.

Greisen G, Hellstrom-Westas L, Lou H *et al.* (1985) Sleep-waking shifts and cerebral blood flow in stable preterm infants. *Pediatr Res* 19:1156–1159.

Greisen G (1986) Cerebral blood flow in preterm infants during the first week of life. *Acta Paediatr Scand* 75:43–51.

Greisen G & Trojaborg W (1987) Cerebral blood flow, $PaCO_2$ changes, and visual evoked potentials in mechanically ventilated, preterm infants. *Acta Paediatr Scand* 76:394–400.

Greisen G, Munck H & Lou H (1987) Severe hypocarbia in preterm infants and neurodevelopmental deficit. *Acta Paediatrica Scandinavica* 76:401–404.

Greisen G & Pryds O (1988) Intravenous $^{133}$Xe clearance in preterm neonates with respiratory distress. Internal validation of CBF-infinity as a measure of global cerebral blood flow. *Scand J Clin Lab Invest* 48:673–678.

Groenendaal F, Veenhoven R H, van der Grond J *et al.* (1994) Cerebral lactate and *N*-acetyl-aspartate/choline ratios in asphyxiated full-term neonates demonstrated *in vivo* using proton magnetic resonance spectroscopy. *Pediatr Res* 35: 148–151.

Hanrahan J D, Sargentoni J, Azzopardi D *et al.* (1996) Cerebral metabolism within 18 hours of birth asphyxia: a proton magnetic resonance spectroscopy study. *Pediatr Res* 39:584–590.

Hanrahan J D, Cox I J, Edwards A D *et al.* (1998) Persistent increases in cerebral lactate concentration after birth asphyxia. *Pediatr Res* 44:304–311.

Hayashi S, Park M K & Kuelh T J (1984) Higher sensitivity of cerebral arteries isolated from premature and newborn baboons to adrenergic and cholinergic stimulation. *Life Sci* 35: 253–260.

Hernandez M J, Brennan R W & Bowman G S (1980) Autoregulation of cerebral blood flow in the newborn dog. *Brain Res* 184:199–201.

Hernandez M J, Hawkins R A & Brennan R W (1982) Sympathetic control of regional cerebral blood flow in the asphyxiated newborn dog. In: Heistad D D, Marcus M L, eds. *Cerebral blood flow, effects of nerves and neurotransmitters.* New York: Elsevier; pp. 359–366.

Hope P L, Costello A M deL, Cady E B *et al.* (1984) Cerebral energy metabolism studied with phosphorus NMR spectroscopy in normal and birth-asphyxiated infants. *Lancet* ii:366–370.

Hope P L, Cady E B, Chu A *et al.* (1987) Brain metabolism and intracellular pH during ischaemia and hypoxia: an *in vivo* $^{31}$P and $^{1}$H nuclear magnetic resonance study in the lamb. *J Neurochem* 49:75–82.

Huttenlocher P R, de Courten C, Garey L J & van der Loos H (1982) Synaptogenesis in the human visual cortex – evidence for synapse elimination during normal delopment. *Neurosci Lett* 33:247–254.

Jones T H, Morawetz R B, Crowell R M *et al.* (1981) Thresholds of focal cerebral ischaemia in awake monkeys. *J Neurosurg* 54:773–782.

Kennedy C & Sokoloff L (1957) An adaptation of the nitrous oxide method to the study of the cerebral circulation in children: normal values for cerebral blood flow and cerebral metabolic rate in childhood. *J Clin Invest* 36:1130–1137.

Krageloh-Mann I, Toft P, Lunding J *et al.* (1999) Brain lesions in preterms: origin, consequences and compensation. *Acta Paediatr* 88:897–908.

Kraus H, Schlenker S & Schwedesky D (1974) Developmental changes of cerebral ketone body utilisation in human infants. *Zeit Physiol Chemie* 355: 164–170.

Kurth C D, Wagerle L C & Delivoria-Papadopoulos M (1988) Sympathetic regulation of cerebral blood flow during seizures in newborn lambs. *Am J Physiol* 255:H563–H568.

Kuschinsky W & Paulson O B (1992) Capillary circulation in the brain. *Cerebrovasc Brain Metab Rev* 4:261–286.

Lassen N (1966) The luxury-perfusion syndrome and its possible relation to acute metabolic acidosis localised within the brain. *Lancet* ii:1113–1115.

Leahy F A N, Cates D, MacCallum M & Rigatto H (1980) Effect of $CO_2$ and 100% $CO_2$ on cerebral blood flow in preterm infants. *J Appl Physiol* 48:468–472.

Leth H, Toft P B, Peitersen B *et al.* (1996) Use of brain lactate levels to predict outcome after perinatal asphyxia. *Acta Paediatr* 85:859–864.

Lou H C, Lassen N A & Friis-Hansen B (1977) Low cerebral blood flow in hypotensive perinatal distress. *Acta Neurol Scand* 56:343–352.

Lou H C & Skov H (1979) Low cerebral blood flow: a risk factor in the neonate. *J Pediatr* 95:606–609.

Lou H C, Henriksen L & Bruhn P (1984) Focal cerebral hypoperfusion in children with dysphasia and/or attention deficit disorder. *Arch Neurol* 41:825–829.

Lou H C, Edvinsson L & MacKensie E T (1987) The concept of coupling blood flow to brain function: revision required? *Ann Neurol* 22:289–294.

Lundstrøm K, Pryds O & Greisen G (1995) Oxygen at birth and prolonged cerebral vasoconstriction in preterm infants. *Arch Dis Child* 73:F81–F86.

Lundstrøm K, Pryds O & Greisen G (2000) The haemodynamic effect of dopamine and volume expansion in sick preterm infants. *Early Hum Dev* 57:157–163.

Martin E, Buchli R, Ritter S *et al.* (1996) Diagnostic and prognostic value of cerebral $^{31}$P magnetic resonance spectroscopy in neonates with perinatal asphyxia. *Pediatr Res* 40: 749–758.

Martin E, Joeri P, Loenneker T *et al.* (1999) Visual processing in infants and children studied using functional MRI. *Pediatr Res* 46:135–140.

Meek J H, Firbank M, Elwell C E *et al.* 1998 Regional hemodynamic responses to visual stimulation in awake infants. *Pediatr Res* 43:840–843.

Meek J H, Elwell C E, McCormick D C *et al.* (1999a) Abnormal cerebral haemodynamics in perinatally asphyxiated neonates related to outcome. *Ach Dis Child* 81:F110–F115.

Meek J H, Tyszczuk L, Elwell C E, Wyatt J S (1999b) Low cerebral blood flow is a risk factor for severe intraventricular haemorrhage. *Arch Dis Child* 81:F15–F18.

Ment R L, Scott D T, Lange R C *et al.* (1983) Postpartum perfusion of the preterm brain: relationship to neurodevelopmental outcome. *Child Brain* 10: 266–272.

Meyer J S, Ishihara N, Deshmukh V D *et al.* (1978) Improved method for measurement of regional cerebral blood flow by $^{133}$-xenon inhalation. I. Description of method and normal values obtained in healthy volunteers. *Stroke* 9:195–205.

Milligan D W A (1979) Cerebral blood flow and sleep state in the normal newborn infant. *Early Hum Dev* 3: 321–328.

Milligan D W A (1980) Failure of autoregulation and intraventricular haemorrhage in preterm infants. *Lancet* i: 896–899.

Mosca F, Bray M, Lattanzio M *et al.* (1997) Comparative evaluation of the effects of indomethacin and ibuprofen on cerebral perfusion and oxygenation in preterm infants with patent ductus arteriosus. *J Pediatr* 131:549–554.

Mukhtar A I, Cowan F M & Stothers J K (1982) Cranial blood flow and blood pressure changes during sleep in the human neonate. *Early Hum Development* 6:59–64.

Obrist W D, Langfitt T W, Jaggi J L *et al.* (1984) Cerebral blood flow and metabolism in comatose patients with acute head injury. *J Neurosurg* 61:241–253.

Papile L A, Rudolp A M & Heyman M A (1985) Autoregulation of cerebral blood flow in the preterm fetal lamb. *Pediatr Res* 19:159–161.

Pasternak J F & Groothuis D R (1985) Autoregulation of cerebral blood flow in the newborn beagle puppy. *Biol Neonate* 48: 100–109.

Patel J, Marks K, Roberts I *et al.* (1998) Measurement of cerebral blood flow in newborn infants using near infrared spectroscopy with indocyanine green. *Pediatr Res* 43:34–39.

Patel J, Roberts I, Azzopardi D *et al.* (2000) Randomised double-blind controlled trial comparing the effects of ibobrufen with indomethacin on cerebral hemodynamics in preterm infants with patent ductus arteriosus. *Pediatr Res* 47:36–42.

Peden C J, Cowan F M, Bryant D J *et al.* (1990) Proton MR spectroscopy of the brain in infants. *J Comput Assist Tomog* 14:886–894.

Perlman J M, Herscovitch P, Kreusser K *et al.* (1985) Positron emission tomography in the newborn: effect of seizure on regional cerebral blood flow in an asphyxiated infant. *Neurology* 35:244–247.

Powers W J & Raichle M E (1985) Positron emission tomography and its application to the study of cerebrovascular disease in man. *Stroke* 16:361–376.

Pryds O (1994) Low neonatal cerebral oxygen delivery is associated with brain injury in preterm infants. *Acta Paediatrica* 83:1233–1236.

Pryds O, Greisen G & Johansen K (1988a) Indomethacin and cerebral blood flow in preterm infants treated for patent ductus arteriosus. *Eur J Pediatr* 147:315–316.

Pyrds O, Greisen G & Friis-Hansen B (1988b) Compensatory increase of CBF in preterm infants during hypoglycaemia. *Acta Paediatr Scand* 77:632–637.

Pryds O, Greisen G, Lou H & Friis-Hansen B (1989) Heterogeneity of cerebral vasoreactivity in preterm infants supported by mechanical ventilation. *J Pediatr* 115:638–645.

Pryds O, Andersen G E & Friis-Hansen B (1990a) Cerebral blood flow reactivity in spontaneously breathing, preterm infants shortly after birth. *Acta Pediatr Scand* 79:391–396.

Pryds O, Greisen G, Lou H & Friis-Hansen B (1990b) Vasoparalysis is associated with brain damage in asphyxiated term infants. *J Pediatr* 117:119–125.

Pryds O & Greisen G (1990) Preservation of single flash visual evoked potentials at very low cerebral oxygen delivery in sick, newborn, preterm infants. *Pediatr Neurol* 6:151–158.

Pryds O & Schneider S (1991) Aminophylline induces cerebral vasoconstriction in stable, preterm infants without affecting the visual evoked potential. *Eur J Pediatr* 150: 366–369.

Rahilly P M (1980a) Effects of sleep state and feeding on cranial blood flow of the human neonate. *Arch Dis Child* 55:265–270.

Rahilly P M (1980b) Effects of 2% carbon dioxide, 0.5% carbon dioxide and 100% oxygen on cranial blood flow of the human neonate. *Pediatrics* 66:685–689.

Reuter J H & Disney T A (1986) Regional cerebral blood flow and cerebral metabolic rate of oxygen during hyperventilation in the newborn dog. *Pediatr Res* 20:1102–1106.

Robertson N J, Cox I J, Cowan F M *et al.* (1999) Cerebral intracellular lactic alkalosis persisting months after neonatal encephalopathy measured by magnetic resonance spectroscopy. *Pediatr Res* 46:287–296.

Rubinstein M, Denays R, Ham H R *et al.* (1989) Functional imaging of brain maturation in humans using iodine $^{123}$Iodoamphetamine and SPECT. *J Nuc Med* 30:1982–1985.

Seri I, Abbasi S, Wood D C & Gerdes J S (1998) Regional hemodynamic effects of dopamine in the sick preterm neonate. *J Pediatr* 133:728–734.

Settergren G, Lindblad B S & Persson B (1976) Cerebral blood flow and exchange of oxygen, glucose, ketone bodies, lactate, pyruvate and amino acids in infants. *Acta Pediatr Scand* 65:343–353.

Sharples P M, Stuart A G, Aynsley-Green A *et al.* (1991) A practical method of serial bedside measurement of cerebral blood flow and metabolism during neurointensive care. *Arch Dis Child* 66:1326–1332.

Skov L, Pryds O & Greisen G (1991) Estimating cerebral blood flow in newborn infants: comparison of near infrared spectroscopy and $^{133}$Xe clerance. *Pediatr Res* 30:570–573.

Skov L & Pryds O (1992) Capillary recruitment for preservation of cerebral glucose influx in hypoglycemic, preterm newborns: evidence for a glucose sensor? *Pediatrics* 90:193–195.

Skov L, Pryds O, Greisen G & Lou H (1993) Cerebral mixed venous oxygen saturation and cerebral blood flow. *Pediatr Res* 32: 52–55.

Suhonen-Polvi H, Kero P, Korvenrante H *et al.* (1993) Repeated fluoroeoxyglucose positron emission tomography of the brain in infants with suspected hypoxic-ischaemic brain injury. *Eur J Nuc Med* 29:759–765.

Thorngren-Jerneck K, Ohisson T, Sandell A *et al.* (1999) Cerebral glucose metabolism measured by positron emission tomography in term newborn infants with hypoxic-ischaemic encephalopathy *Pediatr Res* 45:905 [Abstr.].

Toft P, Christiansen P, Pryds O, Lou H C & Henriksen O (1994) T1, T2 and concentrations of brain metabolites in neonates and adolescents estimated with H-1 MR spectroscopy. *J Magn Res Imag* 4:1–5.

Tweed W A, Cote J, Pash M & Lou H (1983) Arterial oxygenation determines autoregulation of cerebral blood flow in the fetal lamb. *Pediatr Res* 17:246–249.

Tweed W A, Cote J, Lou H *et al.* (1986) Impairment of cerebral blood flow autoregulation in the newborn lamb by hypoxia. *Pediatr Res* 20:516–519.

Tyszczuk L, Meek J, Elwell C & Wyatt J S (1998) Cerebral blood flow is independent of mean arterial blood pressure in preterm infants undergoing intensive care. *Pediatrics* 102:337–341.

Volpe J J, Herscovitch P, Periman J M & Raichle M E (1983) Positron emission tomography in the newborn. Extensive impairment of regional cerebral blood flow with intraventricular hemorrhage and hemorrhagic cerebral involvement. *Pediatrics* 72:589–601.

Volpe J J, Herscovitch P, Periman J M *et al.* (1985) Positron emission tomography in the asphyxiated term newborn: parasagittal impairment of cerebral blood flow. *Ann Neurol* 17:287–296.

Wagerle L C, Kumar S P & Delivoria-Papadopoulos M (1986) Effect of sympathetic nerve stimulation on cerebral blood flow in newborn piglets. *Pediatr Res* 20:131–135.

Wagerle L C, Moliken W & Russo P (1995) Nitric oxide and $\alpha$-adrenargic mechanisms modify contractile responses to norepinephrine in ovine fetal and newborn cerebral arteries. *Pediatr Res* 38:237–242.

Wyatt J S, Delpy D T, Cope M *et al.* (1986) Quantifications of cerebral oxygenation and haemodynamics in sick newborn infants by near infrared spectrophotometry. *Lancet* ii:1063–1066.

Wyatt J S, Cope M, Delpy D T *et al.* (1990a) Measurement of optical pathlength for cerebral near-infrared spectrocopy in newborn infants. *Dev Neurosci* 12:140–144.

Wyatt J S, Cope M, Delpy D T *et al.* (1990b) Quantitation of cerebral blood volume in human infants by near-infrared spectroscopy. *J Appl Physiol* 68:1086–1091.

Younkin D P, Delivoria-Papadopoulos M, Maris J *et al.* (1986) Cerebral metabolic effects of neonatal seizures measured with *in vivo* $^{31}$P NMR spectroscopy. *Ann Neurol* 21:513–519.

Younkin D P, Reivich M, Jaggi J *et al.* (1982) Noninvasive method of estimating newborn regional cerebral blood flow. *J Cereb Blood Flow Metab* 2:415–420.

Younkin D P, Reivich M, Jaggi J L *et al.* (1987) The effect of haematocrit and systolic blood pressure on cerebral blood flow in newborn infants. *J Cereb Blood Flow Metab* 7:295–299.

Yoxall C W, Weindling A M, Dawani N H & Peart I (1995) Measurement of cerebral venous oxyhemoglobin saturation in children by near-infrared spectroscopy and partial jugular venous occlusion. *Pediatr Res* 38:319–323.

Yoxall C W & Weindling A M (1998) Measurement of cerebral oxygen consumption in the human neonate using near infrared spectroscopy: cerebral oxygen consumption increases with advancing gestational age. *Pediatr Res* 44:283–290.

Zhang J, Penny D J, Kim N S *et al.* (1999) Mechanisms of blood pressure increase induced by dopamine in hypotensive preterm neonates. *Arch Dis Child* 81: F99–F104.

Chapter 11

# Neonatal electroencephalography

F. Ferrari, E. Biagioni and G. Cioni

## INTRODUCTION

Over the last few decades neonatal electroencephalography has developed into a valuable non-invasive technique for the evaluation of neurologically compromised neonates. In newborn infants, the electroencephalogram (EEG) provides a particularly useful assessment of brain functioning in many cases of brain damage. The procedure requires good equipment, skilled technicians, and highly trained and experienced interpreters of neonatal EEG. Only specific training combined with an accurate knowledge of the maturational evolution of the neonatal EEG enables the operator to distinguish between normal and abnormal neonatal traces. Criteria have been established for normal patterns in preterm and full-term infants (Parmelee *et al.* 1968; Monod & Tharp 1977). Maturation of spontaneous EEG activity has been usually studied in combination with studies of sleep states.

The two most widely used recording techniques are traditional EEG-polygraphic recordings and EEG monitoring. In addition to EEG, a few units benefit from more sophisticated equipment such as video-EEG, which is particularly useful in distinguishing epileptic from non-epileptic paroxysmal events (Mizrahi & Kellaway 1987). A simplified EEG monitoring technique, so-called cerebral function monitoring (CFM), has been adopted in many neonatal units. The need for continuous EEG monitoring and for quick and easy interpretation of the EEG are the reasons for the success of CFM: it provides a simplified, compressed single-lead, heavily filtered EEG trace suitable for continuous recordings. Its advantages and shortcomings will be discussed below.

In this chapter we review the method of recording the neonatal EEG, normal and abnormal aspects, and of the behavioral states, EEG and brain lesions in the preterm and full-term infant, paroxysmal non-epileptic phenomena, neonatal status epilepticus and EEG monitoring.

## NORMAL APPEARANCES

### EEG IN PRETERM VS. FULL-TERM NEWBORN INFANTS

When confronted with a neonatal EEG it must be remembered that the clinical indications in full-term infants, as well as EEG diagnostic and prognostic values, are different from those of preterm infants.

Most authors agree with the high prognostic significance of EEG-polygraphic recordings performed in a standardized environment in the full-term infant with perinatal complications, whereas no consensus exists regarding the definition of EEG abnormalities of the preterm infant. Moreover, it is hard to establish the borderline between normal and abnormal EEG in the preterm period or, indeed, the differences between active and quiet sleep, for variations occur not only between infants but also within each individual. An explanation for the different diagnostic and prognostic impact of EEG in preterm as distinct from full-term infants is based on the different types, etiopathogenesis, and development of the cerebral damage in the two populations.

In full-term infants the brain insult is usually perinatal, sudden and acute: the state of vasoparalysis and cerebral hyperemia as well as the cascade of the metabolic disorder that follows the primitive hypoxic–ischemic insult develop typically during the first hours of life, reach a plateau, and then attenuate in the following hours and days. The EEG is therefore particularly helpful during the first hours of life to document changes in brain function: EEG abnormalities such as depression of voltage and discontinuity of the background activity (burst–suppression pattern) start to occur a few minutes after the hypoxic–ischemic insult. Recent studies based on early and prolonged EEG monitoring have confirmed the extraordinary power of the EEG in assessing the severity of the brain lesion and its usefulness in determining early monitoring and therapeutic interventions in full-term infants affected by hypoxic–ischemic encephalopathy (HIE).

Adverse events that contribute to the brain lesions peculiar to preterm infants, including periventricular leukomalacia (PVL), germinal matrix-intraventricular hemorrhage (GMH-IVH) and periventricular hemorrhagic infarction (PVHI), may occur pre-, peri- or postnatally. No patterns have so far been recognized in the timing of these events; the onset of acute brain compromise is both variable and unpredictable most the times. Moreover, acute or insidious cerebral insults may occur on a background of an already damaged or compromised brain earlier in development. Cystic PVL takes a number of weeks to develop fully (p. 374), and it is therefore important to differentiate between acute and chronic-stage EEG abnormalities (Ferrari 1981; Watanabe *et al.* 1999). No general rules as to the best timing for a neonatal EEG can therefore be laid down, although it is true that EEG is more sensitive if performed as soon as possible after the brain insult has occurred. Clinical data and ultrasound scan results may be of help in choosing the optimum time for an EEG in individual preterm infants, but only serial EEGs beginning immediately after birth can afford reliable information regarding the timing, mode, and development of brain lesions in preterm infants. Accurate EEG-polygraphic interpretation is still restricted to just a few centers. While it is true that EEG is a sensitive tool for measuring electrical activity in the cerebral cortex, it does not perform so well for other brain structures. Cortical and subcortical areas are most often involved in the hypoxic–ischemic insult of full-term infants, whereas they are hardly affected by PVL and GMH-IVH of preterm infants.

## NEONATAL EEG AS A DIAGNOSTIC AND PROGNOSTIC TOOL

Many studies have emphasized the prognostic implications of EEG findings. Whereas traditionally EEG was essentially regarded as a diagnostic tool for epileptic disorders, in the neonatal period it does have a definite prognostic value, although there are important limitations.

Normal and severely abnormal EEGs have important prognostic value. Normal traces almost invariably predict a normal outcome, while persistent severely abnormal traces predict a poor outcome. The prognostic value of mild-to-moderate EEG abnormalities, on the other hand, is less certain. This is not surprising if we remember that developmental changes in the brain may lead to recovery from dysfunction; in fact, most of the at-risk infants affected by definite brain lesions and clear neurologic symptoms in the neonatal period tend to normalize during the first months of life and look normal at 1 year of age and later.

The sensitivity of neonatal EEG is therefore high and the number of false negatives is low. Conversely, specificity is low and the number of false positives is high. The specificity of neonatal EEG – as with other types of functional neurologic assessment performed in the neonatal period (e.g. neurologic examination, Chapter 8; somatosensory and visual, evoked potentials, Chapter 12) – is increased by means of serial assessments.

Therefore, EEG appears to be diagnostic rather than a prognostic tool: it reflects the severity of the brain disorder in the neonatal period and may (or may not) predict the final outcome. But in several pathological conditions, especially those of preterm infants with mild-to-moderate EEG abnormalities, it has little or no power to predict the individual outcome.

## BEHAVIORAL STATES AND THE NEONATAL EEG

Polygraphic recording explores behavioral states and sleep-cycle organization and EEG maturation from 26 to 44 weeks of postmenstrual age (PMA) proceeds in parallel with the development of sleep and wakefulness: EEG maturation is largely a function of PMA, with minimal alterations as a function of extrauterine existence. Therefore, EEG maturation of the preterm infant is not accelerated or retarded by the extrauterine environment (Ferrari *et al.* 1992). In turn, the link between behavioral states and EEG patterns increases with increasing PMA (Nolte & Haas 1978).

Thus, interpretation of the EEG, once the PMA of the patient is determined, starts from recognition of the infant's actual state and of the behavioral states observed during the EEG recording. Sleep–wake differentiation is difficult before 32 weeks PMA: indeterminate sleep predominates in early prematurity; brief periods of active sleep and quiet sleep can be recognized as early as 30–32 weeks PMA, and wakefulness is definite from 34 to 36 weeks. Active sleep is prominent in the preterm age (60% of total sleep time at 34 weeks PMA), whereas with maturation quiet sleep increases so that at 8 months post-term age its duration in the sleep cycle is double that of active sleep.

The next step is to recognize maturational features of the actual EEG (see later), which may or may not be consistent with the PMA, and then to check whether the EEG patterns are consistent with the behavioral states, i.e. quiet sleep, active sleep, and wakefulness. EEG patterns consistent with the PMA and the behavioral states and good sleep-state organization are signs of brain integrity. Alternatively, EEG patterns that are inconsistent with the PMA and the behavioral states, poor or absent sleep-state organization, and abnormal states are signs of brain dysfunction.

Sleep-state organization is therefore another window on the development and integrity of the CNS. Completing the cycle of physiological variables of the sleep states involves coordinating the multiple physiological systems that, at different CNS levels, subserve neonatal sleep patterns. The coordination of EEG activity and of other physiological parameters reflects the capacity of specific neuronal systems to work as a net, integrating interdependent biological functions. Moreover, some EEG abnormalities may be apparent only in quiet sleep. Since quiet sleep is the state that requires the closest integration between the cortex and other parts of the brain, it is usually the most sensitive state for the detection of minor EEG abnormalities (Lombroso 1985; Ferrari *et al.* 1992). Periods of quiet sleep should therefore be included in the EEG evaluation of the newborn.

EEG maturation patterns, corresponding to younger and older gestational age, may coexist in individual infants. Younger EEG codes are more frequent in preterm infants affected by brain lesions than in healthy preterm infants and full-term infants at the same PMA. These young EEG codes are more often present in quiet sleep than in active sleep (Fig. 11.1) and may be found in one part but not all subsequent quiet–active sleep epochs of the same recording. Therefore, the so-called 'bioelectrical' age of the EEG may be different, depending on the specific quiet–active sleep epochs being considered (Ferrari *et al.* 1992). Accordingly, most authors recommend polygraphic EEG recordings, including various episodes of quiet sleep and active sleep. Anders *et al.* (1971) suggest 3–4 hours' recording in polygraphic studies of the normal newborn, to ensure a representative sample of the entire sleep–wake cycle. Stockard-Pope *et al.* (1992) state that recordings should be

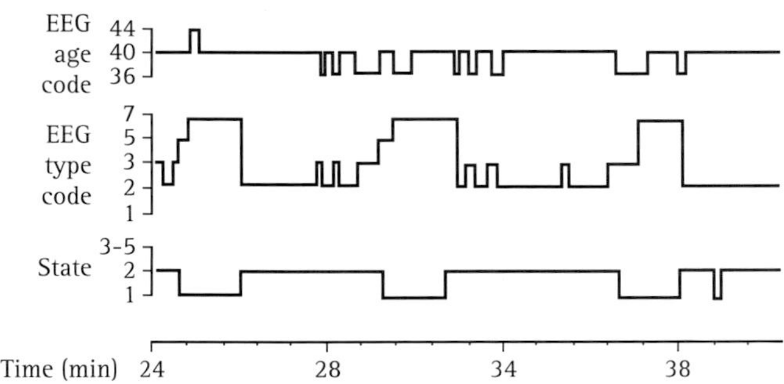


Figure 11.1 EEG and state profile in a normal fullterm infant, PMA at the time of recording 39.4 weeks. Younger (36 weeks) EEG maturation patterns (EEG age code) defined according to Nolte & Haas (1978), are present in the second and third quiet sleep (state 1) epoch but not in the first. (Reprinted from Ferrari *et al.* 1992, with permission from Elsevier Science.)

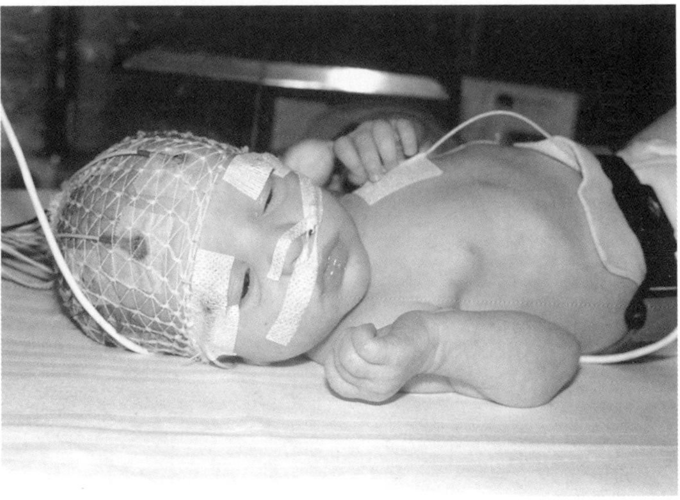

Figure 11.2 Electrode locations for EEG eye movements and ECG; thermistor placed in front of the infant's nostril for nasal respiration; band around the abdomen for detection of the diaphragmatic excursions.

of sufficient duration to yield information about the infant's sleep–wake cycle: the average duration of the total cycle in the fullterm newborn is approximately 50–60 minutes.

## RECORDING THE NEONATAL EEG: TECHNICAL ASPECTS

Nowadays, it is much easier to perform EEGs in neonatal intensive care units than it was some years ago. In particular, the advent of computer-aided portable electroencephalographs, equipped with battery-operated head-boxes including amplifiers and A/D converters, have significantly improved the general quality and reliability of recordings. Although it is possible to apply a larger number of leads, not more than 8–10 active electrodes are often used. They generally include Fp1–2, C3–4, O1–2, and T3–4 of the International 10–20 System. In order to be able to detect vertex localized physiological and pathological features, midline leads (Fz, Cz) have also been recommended.

Since silver chloride cup electrodes, applied by means of ring-shaped double-adhesive plasters, permit reliable recordings without restricting the neonate's freedom of movement and without using toxic substances, more invasive techniques (needle electrodes, use of collodion, etc.) do not seem justified. Electrodes can also be applied by means of adhesive/conductive paste, which is as reliable and more convenient but is not suitable for lengthy recording. Cup electrodes are kept in contact with the skin of the head by means of a soft net, identical to that used in surgery to keep dressings in place (Fig. 11.2), that covers the neonate's skull. For prolonged EEG monitoring fresh conductive cream needs to be applied beneath the cup electrodes once or twice a day.

In addition to conventional scalp EEG recording, other physiological parameters are needed for recording sleep states. The measurement of eye movements (EOG) requires a piezoelectric accelerometer placed on one eyelid or disc electrodes placed at the outer canthi of the eyes, 0.5 cm above the left and 0.5 cm below the right. Respiration may be recorded by means of a thermocouple/thermistor taped under the nostril that detects nasal airflow or through a strain gauge transducer inserted in a band around the chest for detection of chest/diaphragmatic excursions. Submental muscle activity (EMG) is recorded by means of a pair of skin electrodes placed under the chin; heart activity is recorded using electrocardiography (ECG).

For most routine EEG recordings, chin EMG and ECG are not essential: an alert technician can note gross and subtle distal body movements. Not more than 10–15 extra minutes, in expert hands, are needed for the placement of the EOG and respiration devices. As for the polygraphic recording in preterm infants, it is necessary at least to record EEGs during quiet sleep and active sleep. Recordings of about 40 minutes, including discontinuous and more continuous patterns, are advisable in infants under 32–34 weeks of PMA, when quiet sleep and active sleep are still not fully differentiated.

In full-term infants, *reactivity* must be studied systematically at the end of the recording by auditory (hand-clapping) or tactile stimulation. Electrical responses consist of flattening of the EEG activity (rare before 36 weeks of PMA), bouffées of EEG activity (usually a negative sharp wave often followed by a slow wave at the vertex) or diffuse bursts of theta or delta rhythms. These EEG reactions are a characteristic of quiet sleep but are rare in active sleep and wakefulness, in which reactivity consists essentially in behavioral responses such as startles, grimaces, stretches, or general movements (Monod & Tharp 1977).

## MATURATIONAL CHANGES OF NEONATAL EEGs

Rapid and dramatic transformation of EEG patterns takes place in the period between 28 and 44 weeks PMA (Table 11.1).

## LESS THAN 31 WEEKS OF PMA

The EEG of the very premature infant is characterized by constantly discontinuous patterns (Fig. 11.3): 'bursts', consisting of high-voltage delta (0.5–3 Hz) activity, alternating with long-lasting, low-activity intervals (Nolte &

**Table 11.1 Maturational changes of EEG and behavioral states during ontogenesis**

| PMA (weeks) | Basic EEG pattern | Behavioural states | Specific maturational features and EEG patterns |
|---|---|---|---|
| <31 | Discontinuous | Indeterminate state | High voltage delta waves (0.5–3 Hz, 200–400 or > 400 μV) with some faster frequencies (delta brush) superimposed (8–22 Hz) more frequent in occipital and rolandic areas, alternating with long-lasting low activity (<5–10 μV) intervals<br>Temporal theta (sawtooth): high voltage (up to 350 μV) 4–7 Hz rhythmic activities in temporal regions; occipital sawtooth predominate before 27 weeks PMA |
| 31–32 | Continuous activity periods with bursting tendency<br>Discontinuous in rest periods | Rest activity periods<br>Brief periods of poorly differentiated AS and QS | Continuous mixed-frequency activities<br>Discontinuous activity with occipital delta waves (no more than 250 μV wide) and a mixture of delta, theta and alpha rhythms in centro-temporal areas<br>Frequent and high amplitude (up 200–250 μV) delta brush<br>Less frequent and smaller amplitude temporal theta |
| 33–34 | Continuous in AS (no more bursting tendency)<br>Discontinuous in QS | More definite AS and QS periods: AS periods predominate | Delta brush increases in number and synchrony and it is various in amplitude (up to 300 μV)<br>No more temporal theta<br>Immature high voltage (up to 250 μV) polyphasic sharp waves in frontal regions (FST) |
| 35–37 | Continuous in AS and W<br>Discontinuous in QS | Well established QS and AS periods, definite W | Continuous mixed activity (M): medium-high voltage theta-delta activities with superimposed delta brush<br>Continuous low voltage theta activities with superimposed very low amplitude 8–22 Hz rhythms (LVI)<br>FST are better defined in morphology and increase in frequency; they are often associated with anterior slow dysrhythmia (ASD) that appears at the beginning of this period<br>Increased number of delta brush during burst periods |
| 38–42 | Discontinuous during the TA phase of QS | QS sleep periods increase: AS sleep periods reduce<br>Fully developed sleep cycles | Five basic EEG patterns are present:<br>(1) *Activité moyenne*: continuous 0.5 to 10–12 Hz activity at 25–50 μV in W and in AS following QS<br>(2) LVI: low voltage irregular in AS<br>(3) Mixed: *activité moyenne* with superimposed delta-theta activity in AS<br>(4) HVS: continuous medium voltage delta waves activity in QS<br>(5) *Tracé alternant* (TA): discontinuous 1–3 Hz, 50–100 μV activity mixed with lower-amplitude beta and theta activity in 3–5 s bursts occurring at 3–10 s intervals in QS<br>Prominent FST and ASD |
| 43–44 | Discontinuous during the TA phase of QS | QS sleep prevails to AS | M, TA, FST and ASD begin to disappear<br>EEG pattern in QS predominantly consists of HVS |

*Key:* PMA; postmenstrual age; AS; active sleep; QS; quiet sleep; W, wakefulness; HVS; high voltage slow; TA, *tracé alternant*; LVI; low-voltage irregular; M: mixed EEG; FST; frontal sharp transient; ASD; anterior slow dysrhythmia. Activity periods are characterized by repeated general movements and other movement patterns, whereas rest periods by marked decrease in spontaneous motility.

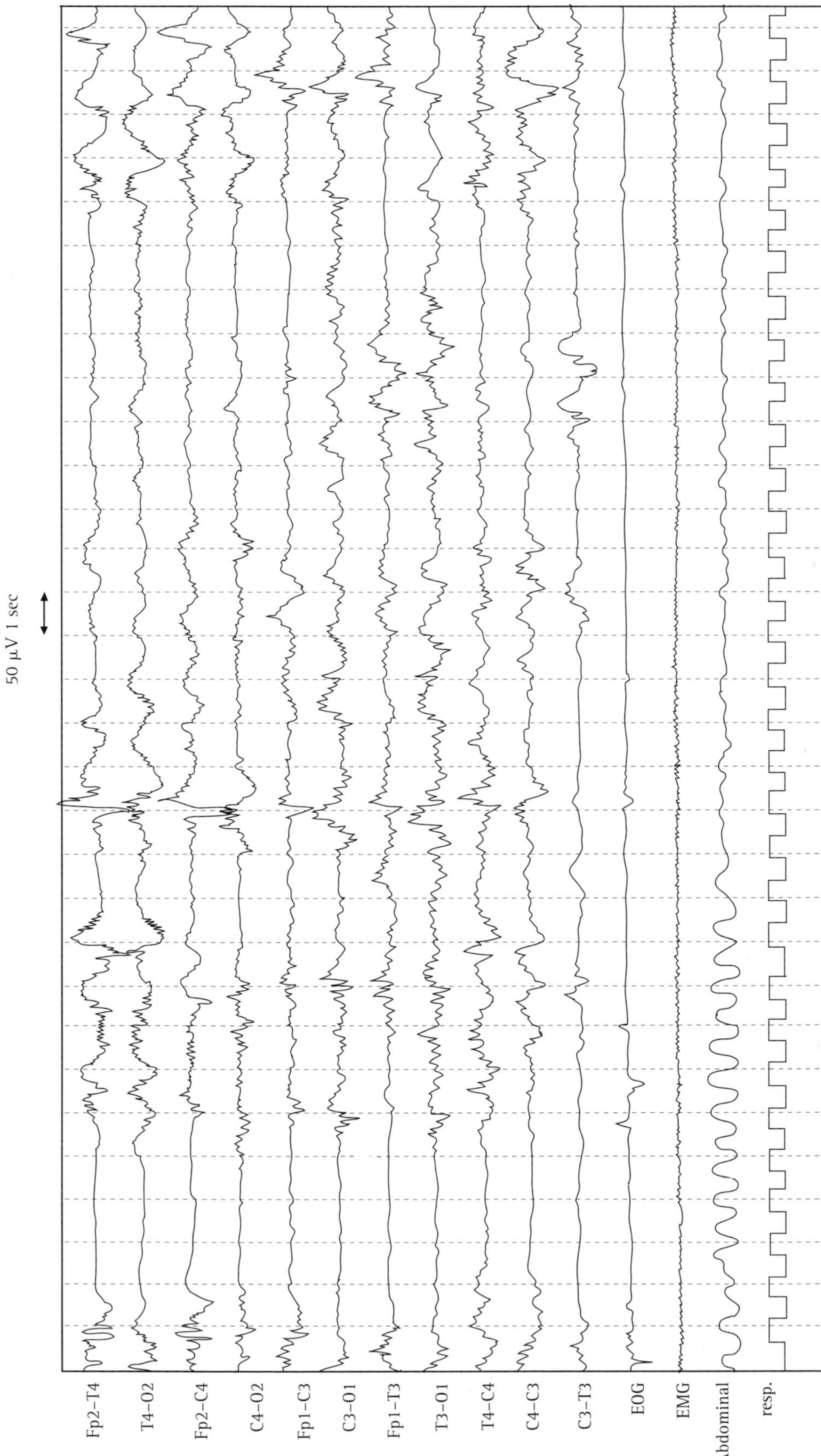


**Figure 11.3** At 28 weeks PMA: discontinuous EEG with asynchronous bursts of high voltage delta waves and 8–22 Hz frequencies (brush) superimposed, synchronous and asynchronous rhythmic temporal theta activities (sawtooth). The bursts alternate with low voltage periods.

Haas 1978; Anderson *et al.* 1985). The bursts last for 1–12 seconds and the intervals last for 1 second to more than 1 minute. The delta waves within the bursts can exceed 400 μV, whereas the intervals are very flat (less than 5 or 10 μV). Although no real continuous pattern is seen, bursts may be longer with short intervals and higher activity (up to 30 μV). This variability of discontinuous patterns is a prelude to that differentiation between continuous and discontinuous EEG activity that will take place later.

Within bursts, faster frequencies are often superimposed on the delta waves. Rapid 8–22 Hz rhythms are sporadically seen at very low PMA. The combination of these activities with the underlying slow waves is called 'delta brush'. Between 27 and 30 weeks of PMA the prevalent faster rhythm superimposed on delta waves is the 'temporal sawtooth', also called 'preterm theta' or 'temporal theta'. It consists of a 4–7 Hz rhythmic activity following a regular pattern, usually located in the temporal regions. Temporal theta is high in amplitude (up to 350 μV), symmetrical and often asynchronous on the two hemispheres and present in half (or more) of the bursts. At this age, bilateral temporal theta is a strong marker for normal EEG. Before 27 weeks of PMA, this pattern is rather unusual in the temporal regions but common in the occipital ones, hence the term 'occipital sawtooth' (Biagioni *et al.* 1994).

## 31–32 WEEKS OF PMA

Continuous EEG activity now appears, mainly in activity periods. It consists of delta waves with superimposed faster rhythms as well as of bursts of discontinuous patterns; the slow and fast activities are lower in amplitude than the bursts, the delta waves being no more than 250 μV wide. Continuous EEG activity is sometimes interrupted by short (1–3 s) periods of flat activity, known as 'bursting tendency'. During the rest periods the EEG remains constantly discontinuous. At 30 weeks or later, intervals are generally shorter than 20 s and bursts are constantly longer than 1.5 s. Temporal sawtooth is less frequent and of a smaller amplitude, whereas delta brushes are more frequent and reach high amplitudes (up to 200–250 μV). Delta brushes of higher amplitude actually show a brush-like or, better a comb-like appearance while high frequency (13–22 Hz) activities may present sharp peaks (Biagioni *et al.* 1994).

## 33–34 WEEKS OF PMA

The bursting tendency is no longer present, continuous EEG activity being observed during the activity periods (Fig. 11.4A, B). This continuous EEG pattern is characterized by medium–high voltage delta waves with superimposed medium–low amplitude 8–22 Hz rhythms. During the rest periods, discontinuous EEG consists of bursts lasting at least 2 s, intervals are usually shorter than 18 s. Rapid 8–22 Hz activity can be very high within bursts (up to 300 μV), whereas temporal sawtooth is no longer observed.

## 35–37 WEEKS OF PMA

At this age, the behavioral states are well structured. Phases of wakefulness, active sleep and quiet sleep are now recognized. Two kinds of continuous pattern are present; one is called mixed (M), the other low voltage irregular (LVI). The former, observed in those active sleep periods that precede quiet sleep, consists of medium–high voltage theta–delta activities with superimposed low amplitude 8–22 Hz rhythms. The latter, seen during wakefulness and active sleep periods following quiet sleep, consists of predominant low voltage theta activities with superimposed very low amplitude 8–22 Hz rhythms. Periods of wakefulness (eyes open and LVI EEG pattern) alternate with sleep states. In quiet sleep the EEG is still discontinuous; bursts consist of high amplitude delta waves (up to 300 μV) with superimposed 8–22 Hz activities (up to 180 μV).

Some polyphasic high amplitude (up to 250 μV) sharp waves appear on the frontal regions. These transients are generally symmetrical and synchronous on the two hemispheres and tend to spread to the posterior regions. This latter characteristic allows them to be distinguished from ocular artifacts even when an EOG is not included in the recording: they are called 'frontal sharp transients' (FST) or '*encoches frontales*'. Immature forms of FST are present at lower PMA (Stockard-Pope *et al.* 1992).

## 38–42 WEEKS OF PMA

At term age, EEG activity in the different phases of the sleep/wakefulness cycle is fully differentiated. In wakefulness, the EEG is characterized by low voltage (less than 60 μV) mixed theta–delta activity (*activité moyenne*); 8–22 Hz rhythms (brushes) are no longer detected. In the active sleep periods that precede quiet sleep, a mixed, medium voltage (up to 100 μV) delta–theta activity is observed; delta brushes are still observed within this pattern until 39 weeks of PMA, after which they disappear. Active sleep following quiet sleep (Fig. 11.5A) shows low voltage (less than 70 μV) predominantly theta activity, often in runs of low voltage, irregular 4–5 Hz activity; no superimposed rhythm is present. During quiet sleep a discontinuous pattern (*tracé alternant* or TA) (Fig. 11.5B) alternates with a high voltage continuous delta pattern (high voltage slow or HVS). The former is characterized by bursts of delta waves (up to 250 μV), still with superimposed low voltage (less than 60 μV) 8–22 Hz activities; intervals are shorter than 10 s and relatively high in amplitude (up to 45 μV). The latter shows delta waves of smaller amplitude than those observed in TA bursts (less than 220 μV). They are not accompanied by faster rhythms. *Encoches frontales* are relatively frequent.

## 43–44 WEEKS OF PMA

At the end of the neonatal period, the wakefulness EEG is characterized by theta-band activities. The mixed EEG pattern tends to disappear unlike the LVI EEG pattern, which remains unchanged, and for the first time newborn infants drift into quiet sleep. The TA of quiet sleep disappears and within the HVS pattern 11–16 Hz low-voltage rhythms (prespindles) are now observed. *Encoches frontales* disappear after 42 weeks.

## THE ABNORMAL EEG

Abnormal EEG features may be classified as background abnormality, ictal abnormalities, abnormal transients, abnormalities in the organization of states and in EEG maturational indices. Ictal EEG abnormalities will not be dealt with as they are described in Chapter 37 on neonatal seizures.

### BACKGROUND EEG ABNORMALITY

The background EEG is the best indicator both of the severity of brain damage and of prognosis in newborn infants with perinatal asphyxia. Depending on the amplitude, continuity and morphology of the EEG patterns, the background of the EEG activity of the newborn infant may be classified under three main headings: extremely abnormal, moderately abnormal, normal or slightly abnormal activity. While most authors accept this grading, the type and definition of individual EEG abnormalities vary slightly from author to author. We propose the classification originally adopted by Pezzani *et al.* (1986) for full-term infants as it is simple and clear and, with modifications, also seems suitable for preterm infants (Table 11.2). It implies the knowledge of normal, previously described developmental changes. Long experience in assessing neonatal EEG and normative data on individual EEG maturational patterns at the various PMAs are mandatory when dealing with moderately or mildly abnormal EEGs.

#### Isoelectric EEG and extreme low voltage (≤5 µV for all states)

No background activity or no EEG activity over 2 µV is recorded; the term 'inactive' EEG is also used when the activity is continuously below 5–10 µV with maximum amplification and long inter-electrode distances (Monod *et al.* 1972; Lombroso 1985). Most of the isoelectric EEGs are non-reactive. Isoelectric or absent electrical activity is known to be invariably associated with a poor prognosis; infants with isoelectric EEG either die in the newborn period or develop severe neurologic sequelae.

Depression of background activity is usually accompanied by the disappearance of normal maturational features and their spatial location. These EEG abnormalities are usually due to generalized insults, such as severe hypoxic–ischemic insult. Diffuse encephalomalacia and neuronal necrosis may be found at autopsy. Persistence of electrocerebral silence for 72 hours or more, in the absence of barbiturates, hypothermia, or severe cerebral malformation, is indicative of cerebral death. Electrocerebral silence indicates cerebral cortical death, not necessarily brainstem death (Volpe 1995).

**Table 11.2 Classification of EEG abnormalities**

**A. Extremely abnormal EEG activity**

1. Electrical discharges
2. Inactive EEG: background activity of less than 5 µV
3. Excessively slow background without the maturational features characteristic of PMA
4. Permanent discontinuous activity: bursts of activity are less than ten seconds in duration and consist of spikes, slow waves, theta or beta rhythms
   'Risk factors' in the EEG:
   - the longest interburst interval is longer than 40 s
   - the shortest interburst interval is greater than 2 s
   - the longest burst length is shorter than 6 s
   - absent normal physiological patterns
   - background amplitude between bursts less than 5 µV

   Factors with a good prognosis:
   - presence of some normal physiological activity
5. Transitory discontinuous activity: periods of continuous activity interrupted by periods of discontinuous activity
6. Frequent type A positive rolandic sharp waves
7. Severe dysmaturity
8. Severe asymmetry (>50%) persisting through all states

**B. Moderate abnormalities**

Continuous activity with physiological patterns of maturation but with an excess of slow waves, theta fast rhythms, spikes, low voltage activity (less than 10–25 µV during QS, below 5–15 µV during W and AS), absent or poor spatial organization; interburst periods of TA and of discontinuous EEG in preterm infants are too flat and too long for PMA (interburst periods typically exceeding 45 s for PMA <30 weeks or 30 s for PMA ≥ 30 weeks); mild and/or transient dysmaturity; excessive asynchrony for PMA age; asymmetry <50%

**C. Normal or slightly abnormal activity**

Isolated temporal spikes, mild interhemispheric asynchrony, poor or excessive ASD, mild focal abnormalities (i.e. excessive sharp waves in temporal or central regions), poor concordance between physiological and behavioural variables of the two sleep states

*Key*: TA, *tracé alternant*; ASD; anterior slow dysrhythmia; PMA; postmenstrual age; QS, quiet sleep; AS; active sleep; W; wakefulness.

#### Burst–suppression (paroxysmal) and permanent/transitory discontinuous EEG

The burst-suppression pattern, also called paroxysmic or paroxysmal, presents long periods (usually >10 s) of inactivity interrupted by bursts of abnormal activity. The bursts are <10 s in duration and consist of spikes, slow waves, theta or beta rhythms (Fig. 11.6). This pattern is most frequently seen in hypoxic–ischemic encephalopathy. Absent or poor reactivity, no regular periodicity, no spatial organization, no lability and absent or poor sleep state organization characterize these recordings. If this EEG abnormality is invariant during prolonged and/or subsequent recordings, the outcome is poor (Monod *et al.* 1972;

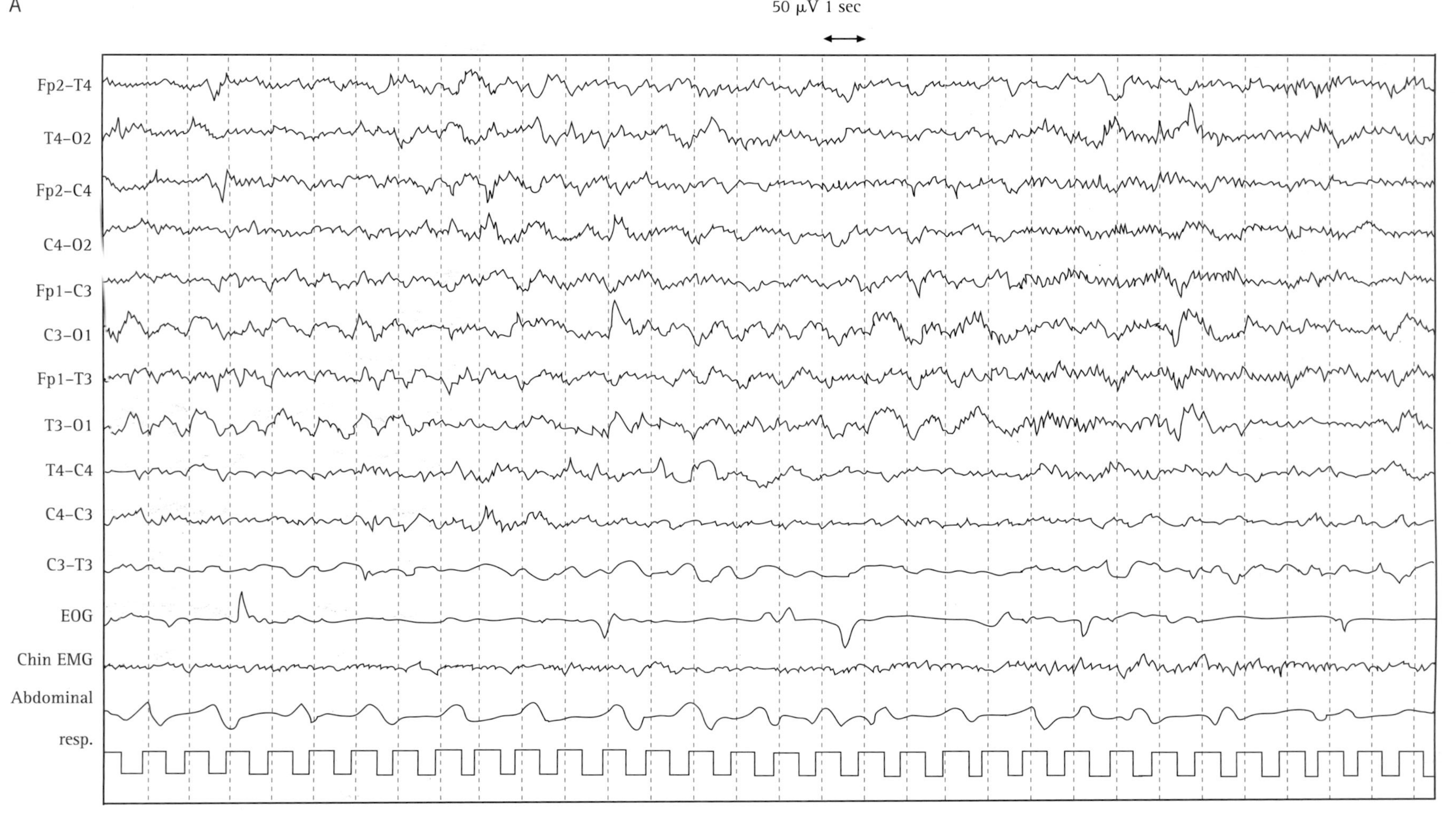
A
50 μV 1 sec
Fp2–T4
T4–02
Fp2–C4
C4–02
Fp1–C3
C3–01
Fp1–T3
T3–01
T4–C4
C4–C3
C3–T3
EOG
Chin EMG
Abdominal
resp.

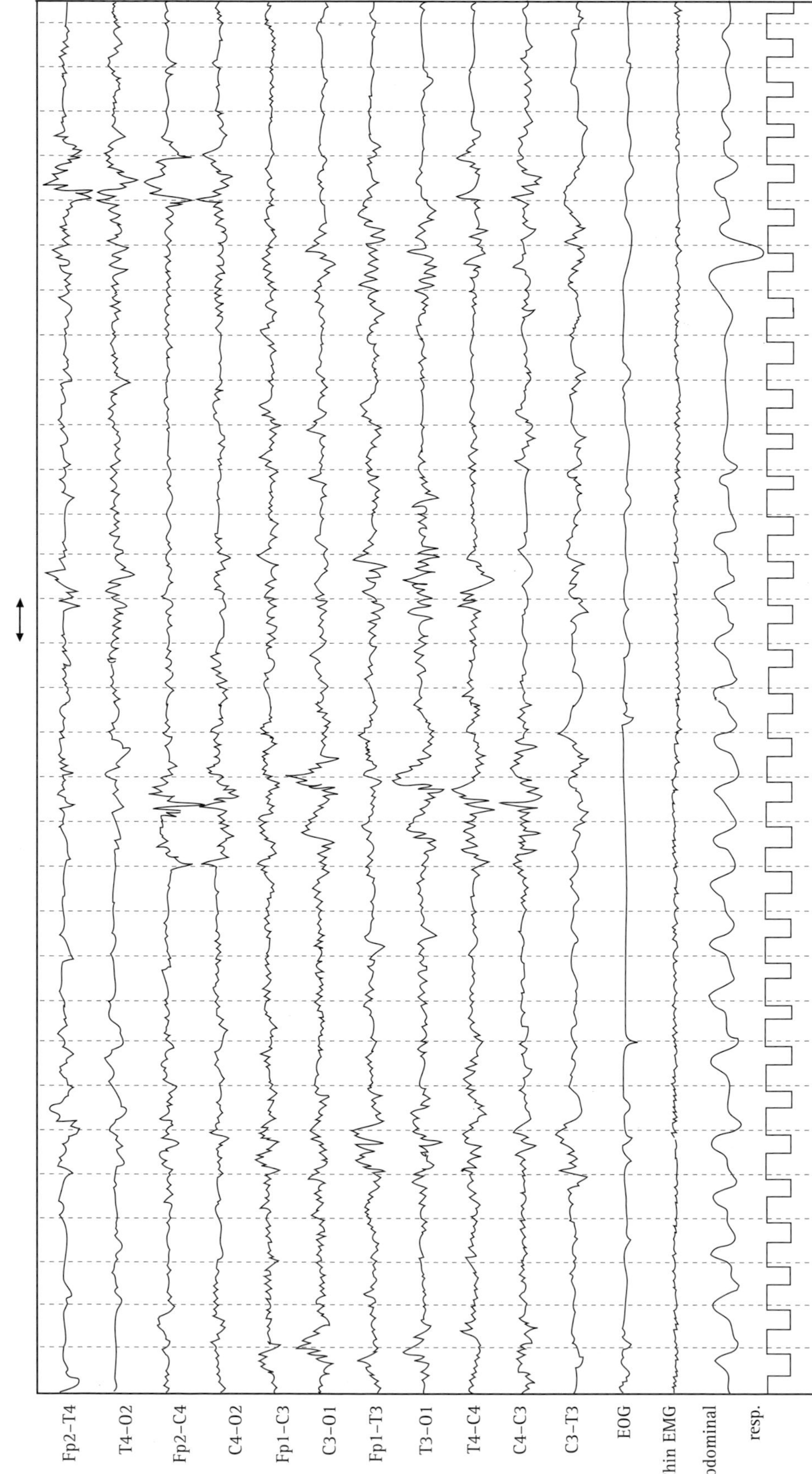


**Figure 11.4** Sleep state in an infant at 34 weeks PMA. (A) Active sleep: continuous EEG with plenty of delta brush, no more temporal theta activities. (B) Quiet sleep: discontinuous EEG with delta brush bursts, a few theta activities are still present in the temporal areas.

A

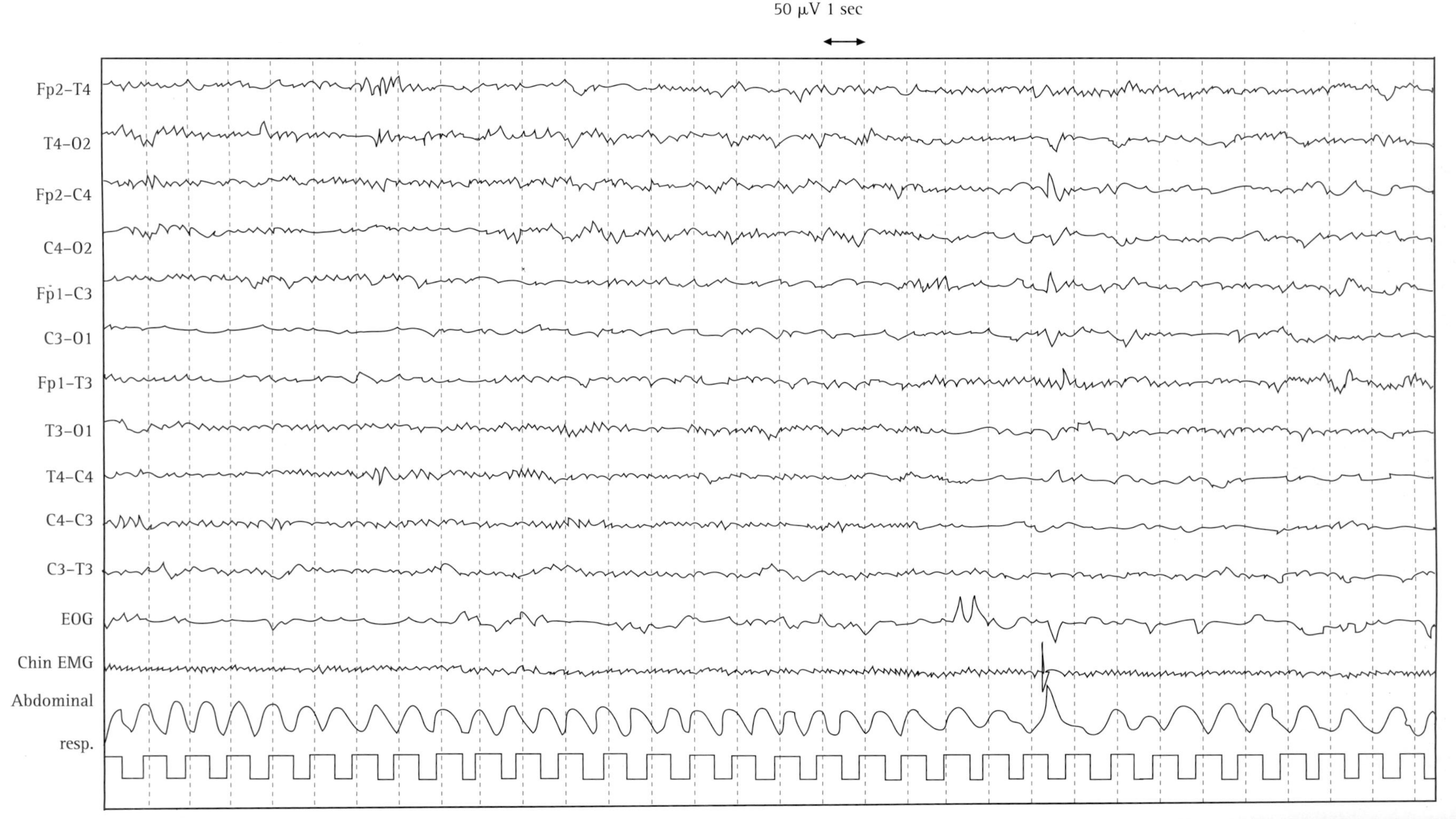
50 μV 1 sec
Fp2–T4
T4–O2
Fp2–C4
C4–O2
Fp1–C3
C3–O1
Fp1–T3
T3–O1
T4–C4
C4–C3
C3–T3
EOG
Chin EMG
Abdominal
resp.

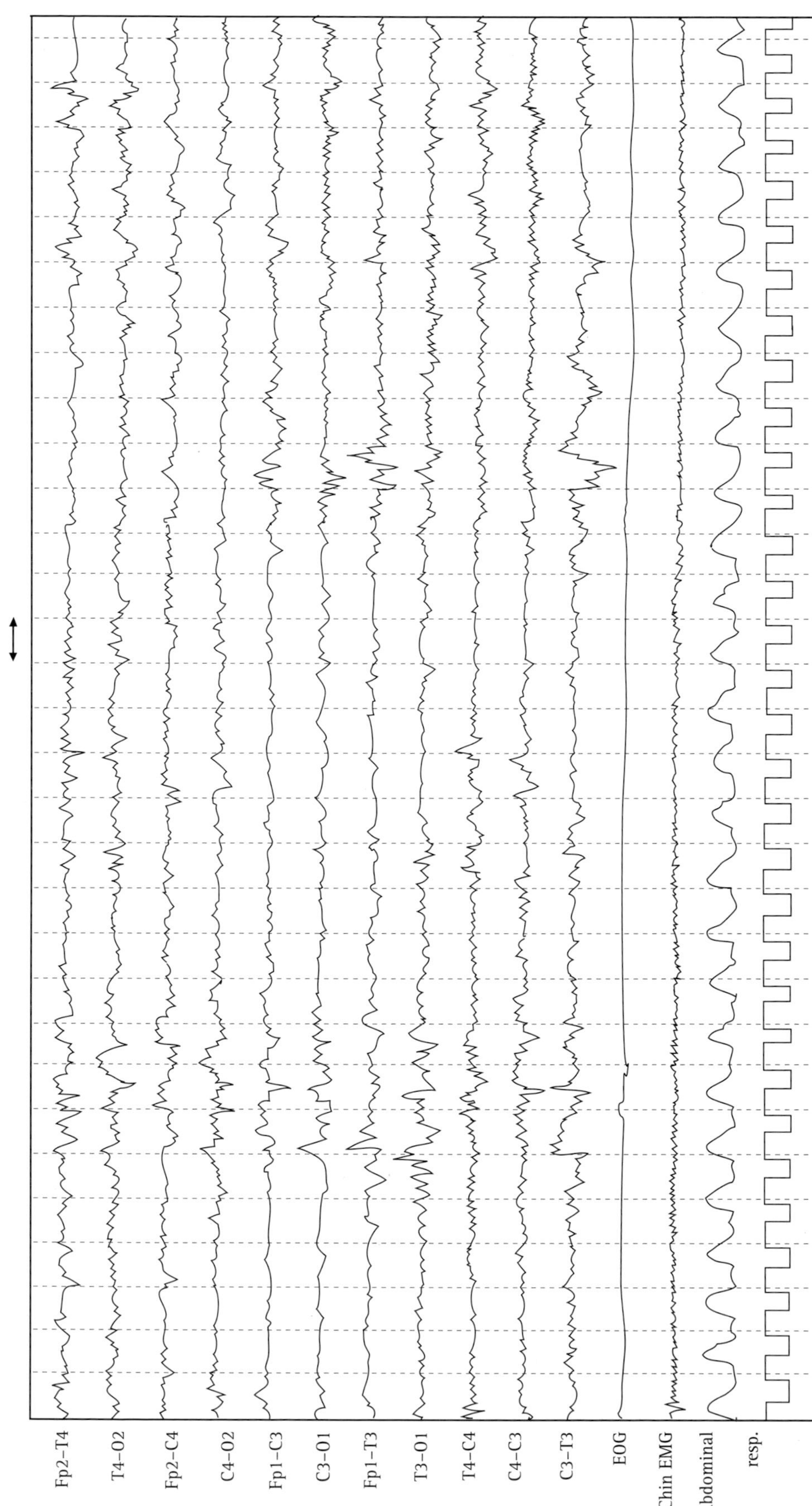


**Figure 11.5** Sleep state in an infant at 39 weeks PMA. (A) Active sleep: continuous EEG, low-voltage irregular activity EEG pattern. (B) Quiet sleep: *tracé alternant* with synchronous and asynchronous bursts of slow waves and theta activities. Intervals between bursts are shorter than 10 seconds.

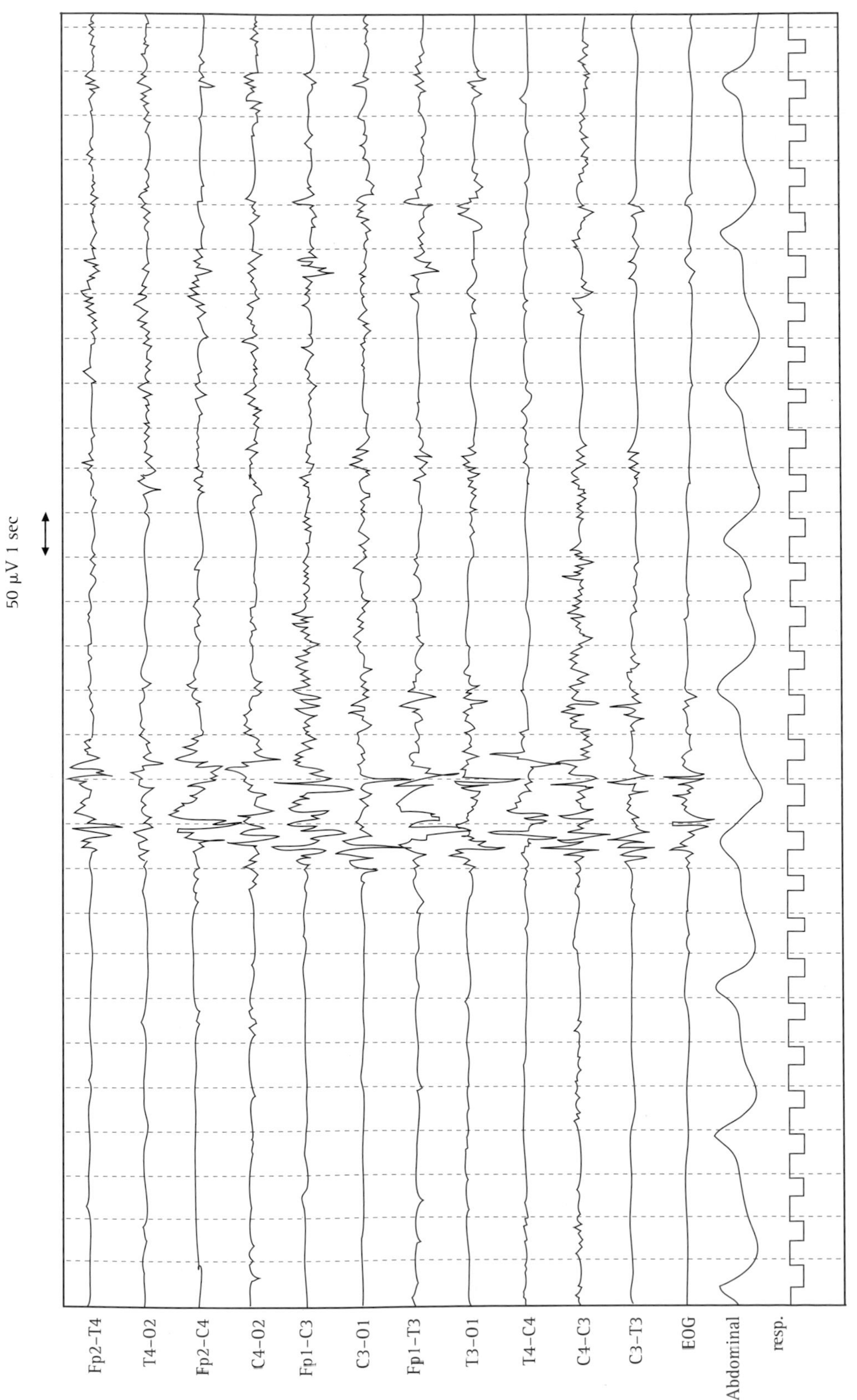


**Figure 11.6** Severe perinatal asphyxia (HIE grade 3) in a term infant. EEG-polygraphic recording on the first day of life showing burst-suppression pattern. Short bursts of spikes, sharp waves and slow waves alternate with long periods of flat or low voltage activity.

Pezzani *et al.* 1986; Holmes & Lombroso 1993; Biagioni *et al.* 1999). If some reactivity is present, the outcome may occasionally be favorable. Pezzani *et al.* (1986) use the term 'permanent discontinuous' activity which refers to those 'permanently discontinuous records having less than thirty seconds of continuous activity of >10 μV'. The outcome is generally poor with death and major sequelae predominating, but cases with only minor sequelae or normal development are also observed. Risk factors that imply a poor prognosis are:

- long interburst intervals (the longest being more than 40 s)
- brief length of the burst (the shortest being less than 6 s)
- small amplitude of the interburst activity (amplitude <5 μV).

By contrast, the presence of some physiological activity, such as age-characteristic EEG patterns may predict a good prognosis. Transitory discontinuous activity consists of periods of continuous activity interrupted by periods of discontinuous activity; usually distinct criteria of maturation are present. Outcome is either normal or severely abnormal.

Permanent discontinuous recordings are normal features in tiny preterm infants of less than 30 weeks PMA. Discontinuous background activity is classified as a major abnormality only when the bursts lack all maturational features normal for PMA, and are invariant and nonreactive (Tharp *et al.* 1981).

Depressants of the CNS, such as anesthetic, diazepam, and other anticonvulsant drugs (Scavone *et al.* 1985; Pezzani *et al.* 1986) and severe acidosis (Murdoch-Eaton *et al.* 1994) may induce a transitory discontinuous EEG trace. A constantly discontinuous EEG pattern, always accompanied by several EEG discharges, can also be observed in some specific, severe, early epileptic encephalopathies. Similar findings can also be observed in the CNS and in metabolic, genetic or degenerative disorders of the CNS.

### Interhemispheric asymmetry

Mild interhemispheric asymmetry is normal in the newborn infant. Amplitude in one hemisphere should be at least 20–30% higher than in the other. In young preterm infants, asymmetry of less than 50% is considered non-significant (Anderson *et al.* 1985). Scalp edema and cephalohematoma should be discounted as possible causes of hemispheric or focal attenuation. If the asymmetry is marked, persistent and present in all behavioral states it may be due to a unilateral lesion such as hemorrhage, infarct (Fig. 11.7), or unilateral subdural hematoma. These lesions may also induce an attenuation of the ipsilateral EEG. Conversely, congenital malformations such as cortical dysplasia (Wertheim *et al.* 1994) and hemimegalencephaly may produce high and slow ipsilateral activity. In asymmetric recordings normal EEG features such as delta brush may be lacking (Lombroso 1985).

### Interhemispheric asynchrony

Synchrony between hemispheres is assessed by monitoring the TA bursts in five consecutive minutes of well-established quiet sleep, and Lombroso (1979) described a progressive increase in interhemispheric synchrony with increasing PMA. By term age, virtually all bursts during TA are synchronous. Excessive, marked and persistent asynchrony (Figs 11.7 and 11.8), with synchrony of less than 25%, is related to a poor outcome (Tharp *et al.* 1981). Mild-to-moderate neuropathologic abnormalities, including lesions of the corpus callosum and of the white matter, have been found in patients with excessive asynchrony (Aso *et al.* 1993). A minor degree of asynchrony is often found in EEG dysmaturity (Ferrari *et al.* 1992). Surprisingly, an almost complete interhemispheric synchrony may be seen in very young (PMA <30 weeks) preterm infants (Holmes & Lombroso 1993).

## ABNORMAL EEG TRANSIENTS

Normal transients, such as temporal theta, delta brush and frontal sharp transients, have been described under the EEG maturational changes and need to be distinguished from abnormal EEG transients, such as positive rolandic (Figs 11.7 and 11.9) and temporal sharp waves (Fig. 11.8), prolonged sequences of delta, theta, alpha and beta activity, and abnormal spikes and sharp waves.

### Positive rolandic sharp waves (PRSWs)

Despite the fact that these EEG transients have been widely investigated, their diagnostic and prognostic value remains uncertain. Positive rolandic sharp waves are broad-based sharp transients of up to 500 ms duration observed over the rolandic areas (C3–C4). Two types of PRSW have been distinguished (Dreyfus-Brisac & Monod 1972). Type A occurs singly or at intervals of 1 s or more (Figs 11.7, 11.8), while type B consists of bursts (3–7 s) of rolandic transients. PRSWs have been associated with a number of brain lesions such as germinal matrix–intraventricular hemorrhages, intraparenchymal or subarachnoid bleeding, periventricular leukomalacia, hydrocephalus, and asphyxia. They have also been demonstrated in healthy, apparently neurologically intact preterm infants younger than 32 weeks PMA. We agree with Holmes & Lombroso (1993) who state that 'in spite of their paroxysmal features that might suggest an epileptic form signature, PRSWs do not correlate with ictal phenomena ... the consensus at present is that they are more directly associated with pathologies that induce deep white-matter lesions'. Recent studies on these characteristics identify PRSWs as an early and very specific marker of PVL in preterm infants (Marret *et al.* 1992; Baud *et al.* 1998).

### Positive temporal sharp waves (PTSWs)

PTSWs are EEG transients with a similar morphology to PRSWs but with a different, midtemporal, location (Fig. 11.9).

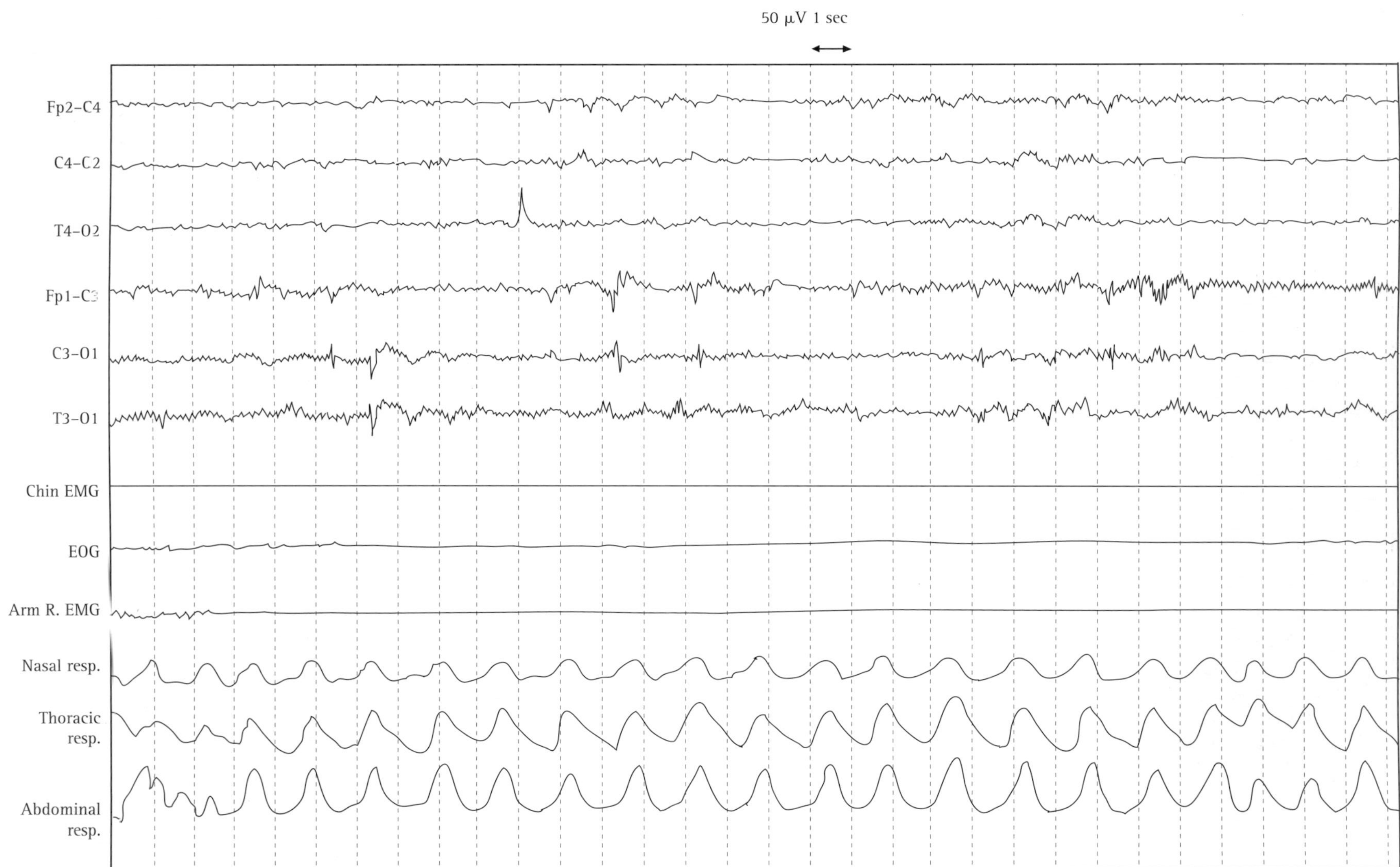


**Figure 11.7** Infant at 32 weeks gestational age: 1.4 kg body weight, respiratory distress syndrome, intermittent positive pressure ventilation for 3 days. By ultrasound: GMH-IVH grade 3, left white matter increased echogenicity (infarction). Outcome at 3 years of age: right hemiplegia. EEG-polygraphic recording at 7 days of life: low voltage EEG, numerous small amplitude left PRSWs, marked inter-hemispheric asymmetry (lower voltage on the right side) and asynchrony; poverty of maturational features.

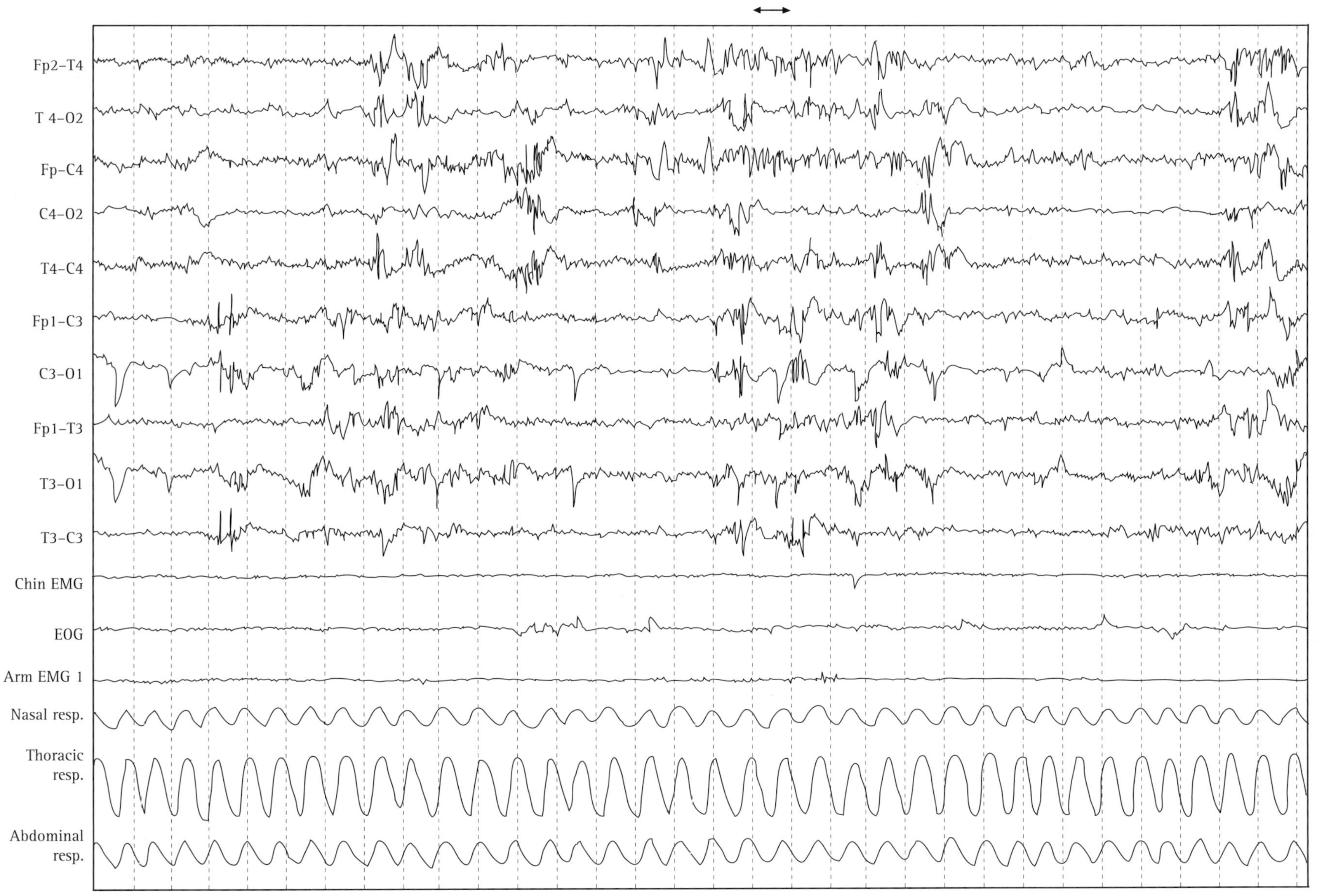


**Figure 11.8** Infant at 29 weeks gestational age: 1.3 kg body weight, severe respiratory distress syndrome, intermittent positive pressure ventilation for 4 days. Apathy in the 2nd and 3rd weeks of life. Bilateral temporo-parietal-occipital cystic PVL on imaging. Outcome: spastic diplegia. EEG at 33 weeks PMA: PRSWs and PTSWs in quiet sleep, excess of high voltage brush, interhemispheric asynchrony. The EEG-polygraphic trace refers to quiet sleep: a few eye movements are present on the EOG (poor interrelationship between physiological parameters of quiet sleep).

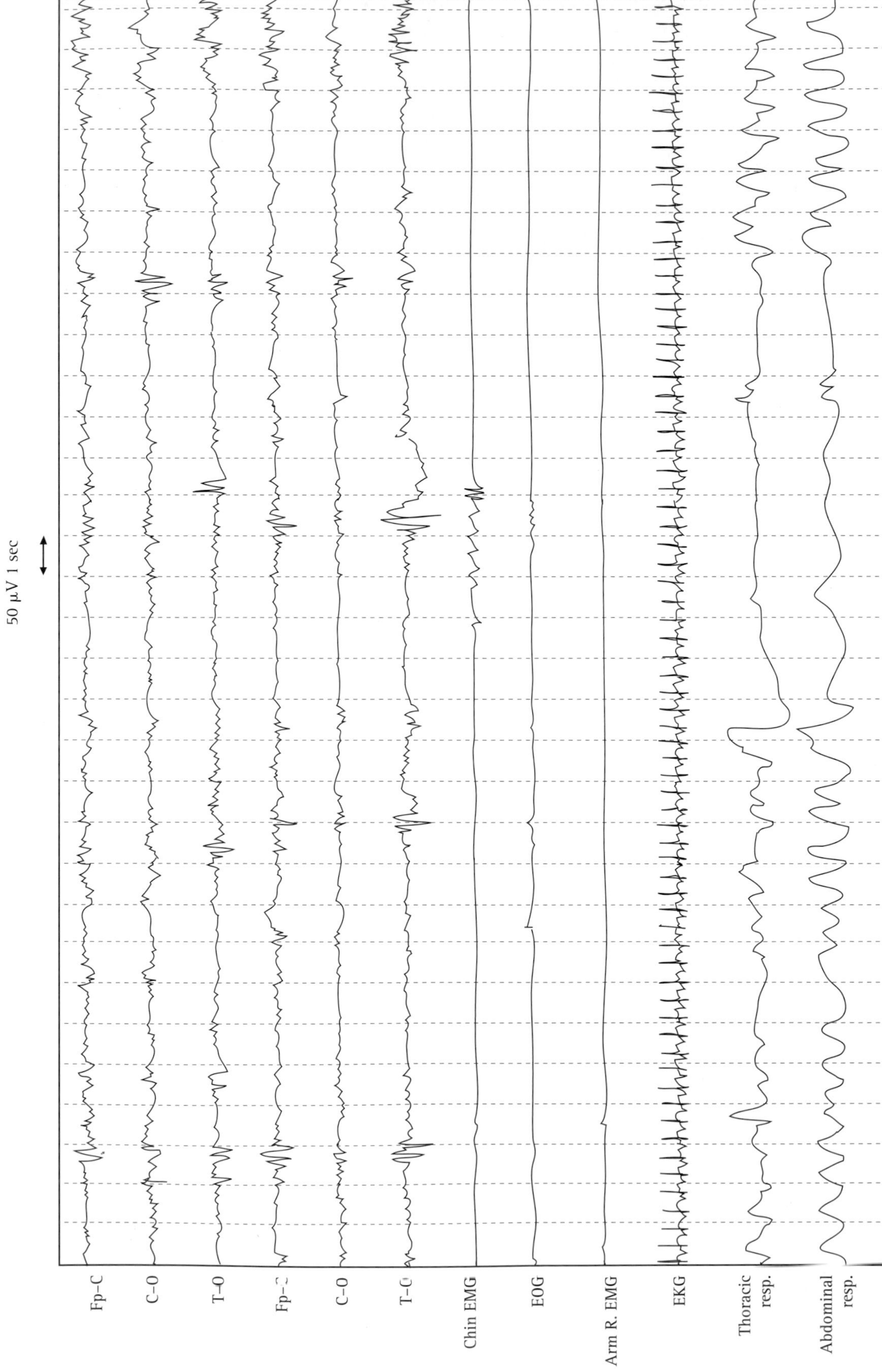


**Figure 11.9** Infant at 28 weeks gestational age: 1.2 kg body weight, intubation at birth, respiratory distress syndrome, continuous positive pressure ventilation (1st–4th days), recurrent apneas (5th–6th days), severe hypoxic episode on the 7th day, seizures (8th day). Bilateral diffuse cystic PVL on scanning. Outcome: spastic quadriplegia and mental retardation. EEG at 35 weeks PMA: abnormal maturational features (severe dysmaturity) with monotonous anachronistic frontal and temporal theta bursts. No other EEG pattern, no maturational features.

They have been associated with perinatal asphyxia and hypoxic–ischemic lesion in full-term infants. Both PRSWs and PTSWs are usually accompanied by other background abnormalities (Figs 11.7 and 11.9), but this association leaves unanswered the diagnostic and prognostic significance of these EEG transients.

### Abnormal paroxysmal rhythmic activity

Delta, theta and alpha rhythmic activity in brief runs are observed predominantly in normal full-term infants but also in abnormal infants (Stockard-Pope *et al.* 1992), and their significance is therefore uncertain. To be accepted as normal they must be brief in duration, sporadic, without persistent focality, with a temporal or occipital rather than a rolandic location, and be superimposed on a normal background EEG. A theta/alpha burst seen in the midline frontal area, often with a spiky shape, is considered one of the normal EEG components in the alternating trace of quiet sleep. Prolonged sequences of rhythmic activity in the beta, alpha, theta, or delta bands, either associated with or without clinical seizures, are truly abnormal; most often they are electrical discharges themselves. Some authors claim that even brief intermittent rhythmic discharges (BIRDS), as well as prolonged periodic discharges, must be considered as ictal phenomena. Rhythmic fast, beta-band activity in prolonged sequences must be distinguished from delta brushes, and this distinction is easy when the location and morphology of delta brushes is abnormal.

### Spikes and sharp waves

Sharp transients occurring in a random and sporadic fashion in a long EEG recording are considered a normal feature of neonatal EEG (Monod *et al.* 1972). What constitutes the borderline between normal and abnormal spikes and sharp waves remains a matter of debate. With increasing PMA, normal transients are most often seen within the bursts of TA; they are rarely located in the rolandic regions. Abnormal characteristics are:

- persistent focality
- repetitiveness (excessive frequency)
- spiky shape (150 ms or less)
- occurrence in either wakefulness or sleep.

Multifocal sharp transients on a depressed background have less favorable diagnostic and prognostic significance than when on a normal or moderately abnormal EEG.

## ABNORMALITIES IN ORGANIZATION OF BEHAVIORAL STATES AND IN EEG MATURATIONAL INDICES

### Behavioral states

Several authors have pointed out that newborn infants at neurologic risk have difficulty in organizing behavioral states, more specifically in developing and maintaining proper sleep-cycle organization and sleep states. Quite a wide range of states and sleep disorder has been detected in high-risk infants. A definite lack of sleep has been observed in infants affected by brain malformations, while the absence of cyclic organization or the absence of recognizable states have been seen in comatose infants, affected by severe hypoxic–ischemic encephalopathy (HIE) and convulsions. Poor interrelationships between behavioral and EEG characteristics of sleep states have been observed in various pathologies (Monod *et al.* 1972; Pezzani *et al.* 1986) (Fig. 11.8). One state may prevail over the others: for example, excess of wakefulness and/or of indeterminate sleep is quite common among at-risk infants (Prechtl *et al.* 1973). One single physiological variable may be lacking or poorly represented for example, few or no eye movements may be seen in the active sleep of infants affected by HIE. The EEG patterns may be inappropriate for the state such as discontinuous EEG in active sleep. In general these abnormalities of the states are non-specific as no definite relationship has been found between state abnormality and type of pathology. Disturbance of sleep cycles, however, correlates with the background EEG. Cycles are slightly disturbed in infants with minimally depressed EEG and are increasingly disrupted in infants whose background EEG is moderately to markedly depressed. Serial recordings have disclosed that the cycles are more affected but normalize more quickly than the background EEG (Watanabe *et al.* 1980).

In general, it has to be said that sleep state organization is very fragile, as it can be disrupted by a number of neurologic and non-neurologic conditions. As quiet sleep is the state with the highest degree of homeostasis, it is usually the first to show alterations under pathological conditions. As for the effect of drugs on sleep states, anti-epileptic drugs induce a higher number of quiet sleep episodes of longer duration.

### Dysmature EEG

A neonatal EEG is generally considered as dysmature when it shows abnormal maturational features. This finding is also known as age-inadequate patterns, EEG regression to early maturational levels, or EEG immaturity. The term 'dysmature EEG' is probably preferable, as immature EEG indicates an EEG with maturational features overlapping those of a younger age. Dysmature EEG usually displays immature features along with abnormal ones (Fig. 11.9); therefore the term immature is not fully appropriate. Hence, EEG dysmaturity is defined as the occurrence of maturational features that do not reflect those expected for the PMA (Lombroso 1985; Biagioni *et al.* 1996). EEG normal patterns are well known at term age and criteria of normality have also been defined for preterm infants at different PMAs. Therefore, once the maturational features of neonatal EEGs have been evaluated, it is possible to define as dysmature any trace not fulfilling the established criteria for the PMA at the time of recording. EEG dysmaturity is not frequently observable in full-term patients, and in them it probably constitutes a minor anomaly. On the other hand, it is a frequent finding in preterm infants and can be interpreted in them as a sign

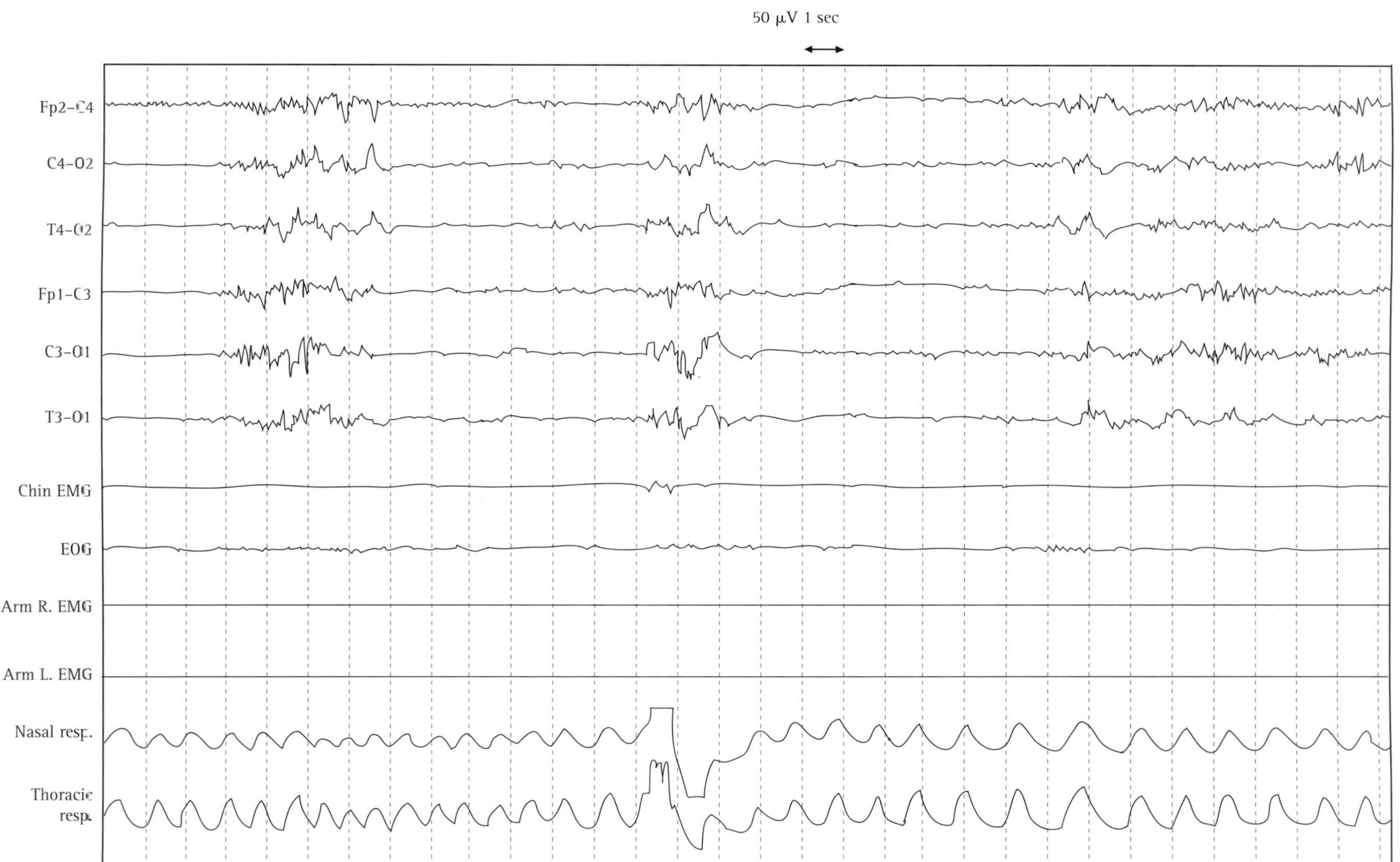


**Figure 11.1C** Infant at 40 weeks gestational age, 3.2 kg, fetal bradycardia, poor condition at birth, intubated, cardiac massage, hyperexcitability (1st–2nd day), apathy (3rd–8th day). Moderate diffuse increased white matter echogenicity. Outcome at 2 years of life was normal. EEG-polygraphic recording on the first day of life: moderate abnormalities with long and overly flat interburst periods (mild dysmaturity).

of brain compromise (Ferrari 1981; Biagioni *et al.* 1996; Hayakawa *et al.* 1997). Some authors report that, in the acute phase, modifications of the general organization of EEG activity, such as absence of continuous pattern and increased discontinuity, are more frequently observable (Watanabe *et al.* 1999), and these findings are distinguished from the general concept of dysmaturity. Other reports include EEG parameters as maximum interval duration, minimum burst length, synchrony of the TA, theta activity in the burst phase of TA as maturational features (Ferrari *et al.* 1992; Biagioni *et al.* 1996) (Fig. 11.10), together with the occurrence and the incidence of specific waveforms, such as temporal sawtooth or delta brush. In the post-acute and recovery phases, modifications of the latter features can constitute the only abnormal background EEG finding.

The diagnostic and prognostic value of dysmature EEG also depends on the severity of dysmaturity, evaluated according to precise criteria (Biagioni *et al.* 1996) and on its transient or persistent character. A severe dysmaturity (Fig. 11.9) has a negative diagnostic and prognostic value (Ferrari *et al.* 1992), especially when persistent in subsequent recordings whereas transient and/or mild dysmaturity (Fig. 11.10) in full-term as well in preterm infants indicates a favorable outcome.

## CLINICAL APPLICATIONS OF NEONATAL EEG

### EEG IN PRETERM INFANTS WITH WHITE MATTER LESIONS

Although improved neonatal care over the last few decades seems to have been effective in reducing the incidence of white matter insults in preterm infants, these lesions, which are usually detected by means of ultrasound or magnetic resonance scans, still account for the vast majority of subsequent neurologic disabilities. As reported above, there is no general agreement on the effective value of the EEG in the diagnosis of brain lesions in preterm infants, and it is probably true that the EEG abnormalities we encounter in these patients are not the direct expression of the insult we observe at neuroimaging scans but, rather, the signs of more generalized cerebral involvement. Indeed, it has already been pointed out that the electrical activity we record on the EEG originates in the cortex, while the lesions observed in these infants mainly involve the white matter. Nevertheless, as in other clinical conditions occurring at later ages, the activity of the cortex can be modified by an alteration of the underlying structures, mainly through changes in the electrical afferences.

According to many authors, the role of the EEG in the diagnosis of white matter lesions of preterm infants mainly relies on the recognition of some abnormal transients, such as positive rolandic sharp waves (Marret *et al.* 1992; Baud *et al.* 1998) (Figs 11.7 and 11.8). In recent years, EEG background abnormalities, such as dysmaturity (Fig. 11.9), have also been taken into account (Biagioni *et al.* 1996; Hayakawa *et al.* 1997; Watanabe *et al.* 1999). As reported above, a distinction is made between abnormalities of the acute phase, mainly consisting of changes in continuity and amplitude, and those of the chronic stage, consisting of modifications of the specific age-related patterns (such as temporal sawtooth and delta brush). These background abnormalities are probably not characteristic of leukomalacia, but should rather be interpreted as a common response of the preterm infant's electrical activity to different insults.

Despite its controversial diagnostic value, EEG plays an important role in the prognosis of white matter lesions of preterm infants, especially for persistent periventricular echodensities and cystic PVL. This point is particularly important in the first few days after birth, when the ultrasound outcome of periventricular echodensities (i.e. their resolution or evolution into cysts) is still uncertain. Clinical studies comparing ultrasound, EEG and neurologic outcome in preterm infants with white matter lesions (Connell *et al.* 1987; Biagioni *et al.* 1996) have shown that early EEG findings may indicate which infants are most at risk of developmental disorders, despite rapid disappearance of the echodensities. Moreover, a normal EEG may suggest a favorable outcome, even in infants with more severe white matter lesions (Fig. 11.11).

Cranial ultrasound findings

| EEG Dysmaturity | | Score 0 | Score 1 | Score 2 |
|---|---|---|---|---|
| | Score 0 | ○ ○ ○ ○ ○ ○ ○ ○ ○ ○ ○ | ○ ○ ○ ○ ○ ○ ○ ○ ○ ○ ○ ○ | ○ ○ ◑ |
| | Score 1 | ○ ○ ○ ○ ○ ○ ○ ○ ○ ○ ○ ○ ◑ | ○ ○ ○ ○ ○ ○ ○ ○ ○ ◑ ◑ ● | ◑ ◑ ◑ |
| | Score 2 | ○ ○ ◑ ◑ ◑ | ○ | ◑ ● ● |

**Figure 11.11** Correlation between severity of ultrasound abnormalities (graded from 0 = normal, 1 = persistent periventricular flare, 2 = severe white matter lesions) and background EEG maturational codes (0 = normal, 1 = mild dysmaturity, 2 = severe dysmaturity). ○, indicates cases with normal outcome; ◑, indicates cases with mildly abnormal outcome; ●, indicates cases with severely abnormal outcome. (Reprinted from Biagioni *et al.* 1996, with permission from Georg Theime Verlag).

## EEG IN PRETERM INFANTS WITH INTRAVENTRICULAR AND PERIVENTRICULAR HEMORRHAGES

Germinal matrix hemorrhages and intraventricular hemorrhages without ventricular dilatation do not imply, by definition, any involvement of the cerebral tissue (Volpe 1995), and no relationship between these findings and any specific EEG abnormalities is therefore to be expected. Obviously, when the hemorrhage is accompanied by an enlargement of the ventricle or by an intraparenchymal infarction due to vein obstruction, the EEG can show signs of cerebral suffering. Positive sharp waves have also been interpreted as indexes of intracranial hemorrhages in preterm infants since the 1970s (Cukier *et al.* 1972), although other authors have more recently denied their value in this field (Aso *et al.* 1993). Background abnormalities, such as significant interhemispheric asymmetries (Fig. 11.7), or dysmaturity (Fig. 11.9) can also occur in these patients, possibly with a higher prognostic value.

## EEG AND HYPOXIC–ISCHEMIC ENCEPHALOPATHY IN FULL-TERM INFANTS

In full-term infants, perinatal asphyxia is still a major concern and the incidence of hypoxic–ischemic encephalopathy (HIE) has remained unchanged over recent decades. The so-called 'therapeutic window' is limited and an early and accurate identification of birth asphyxia is therefore important (Toet *et al.* 1999; see also Chapter 28).

The EEG is a sensitive and precocious index of brain hypoxia; the severity of background EEG abnormalities provides valuable information concerning the severity of the brain insult in HIE. The infants who experience intrauterine asphyxia may not show clear neurologic signs during the first hours of life (Volpe 1995) and conversely, infants with early neurologic signs, such as increase or decrease in tone and reactivity may be without documented brain injury. Yet the use of potentially therapeutic drugs and strict neurologic monitoring are justified only in the presence of clear neurologic dysfunction. EEG in the first hours of life may resolve the question as to whether these infants have significant brain dysfunction and therefore need to be treated. This is one major application of neonatal EEG.

When confronted with an infant with HIE who has been treated with anti-epileptic drugs, it should be borne in mind that these drugs affect EEG and sleep states. Scavone *et al.* (1985) recommend prolonged EEG-polygraphic recordings and interpretation of the EEG combined with the knowledge of the dosages, the time of administration and the plasma levels of the drug. Diazepam induces a flattening of the EEG that lasts 30 to 60 minutes, while phenobarbital loading doses induce transient increased discontinuity of background EEG. This effect seems to correlate with the severity of brain damage: the more severe the damage, the longer and more severe the effect (Toet *et al.* 1999). A definitely abnormal EEG in the first few hours after birth in infants with HIE suggests the need for brain protection, even if the neurologic examination is not severely abnormal and the infant is still free of seizures. On the other hand, a normal EEG suggests the need for strict surveillance but not for protective drugs, whether or not neurologic signs are present.

The more precocious the EEG, the clearer the diagnostic and prognostic indications (Pezzani *et al.* 1986). Scavone *et al.* (1985), studying the EEG in 20 full-term infants who had asphyxia at birth and were in a comatose state for 4 to 15 days, found that the prognosis did not correlate with the onset or duration of the coma, or with the presence of intermittent or continuous electrical discharges. It only correlated with the initial EEG tracing on the first day. On the other hand, an improvement in the EEG on the second or the third day did not necessarily correlate with a favorable outcome. During the following days, only an inactive EEG maintained a clearly negative prognostic value, once the possibility of an overdose of anticonvulsant therapy had been discounted.

Moreover, a close correlation has been found between sleep states and EEG patterns in newborn infants with perinatal hypoxia; the sleep states become progressively disrupted as the severity of the background EEG increases (Watanabe *et al.* 1980). Phenobarbital affects sleep states by inducing longer periods of quiet sleep at the expense of active sleep periods.

## PAROXYSMAL NON-EPILEPTIC PHENOMENA

A number of paroxysmal events may be confused with clinical seizures in the newborn infant. Mizrahi & Kellaway (1987) have shown using video-EEG techniques that some focal or multifocal clonic jerks and myoclonic jerks are epileptic in nature.

Startles look like sudden generalized jerks in quiet sleep and are isolated in time often occurring at regular intervals. Sometimes startles are so vigorous as to awaken the newborn infant and/or make him or her to cry. Myoclonic jerks also occur in sleep and they are actually innocent physiological sleep-state dependent phenomena. Benign myoclonic jerks appear mainly during quiet sleep, occasionally in a dramatic fashion. They may be isolated but can also occur as rhythmical bilateral jerks, mimicking myoclonic or clonic epileptic jerks. With benign myoclonic jerks there is no clinical history of perinatal asphyxia, the infant is free of other neurologic symptoms, the jerks stop when the infant is awakened and they may be suppressed by restraint of the limbs. The EEG-polygraphic recording shows no electrical discharge in coincidence with myoclonic jerks.

Tremors and cloni of 'jitteriness' are also easily distinguished from epileptic jerks. They occur in brief bouts, are non-rhythmical in sequence and, unlike epileptic jerks, may be stopped by flexion of the limbs (Volpe 1995). Physiological tonic posturing of the limbs or abnormal posture with hyperextension of the neck and trunk, such as in opisthotonos, may respectively mimic focal and generalized tonic seizures. Whereas the former is clinically identical to a focal tonic seizure (and only an EEG recording can testify as to the epileptic or non-epileptic nature of the event), the latter, being predominantly continuous and non-paroxysmal, is easier to identify.

Subtle or atypical seizures may consist of one or more of the following phenomena:

- chewing, sucking and swallowing automatisms
- pedalling and swimming movements
- rhythmic eye opening, blinking, eye jerks and/or random eye movements
- fixed gaze with open eyes, tonic deviation of the eyes
- outbursts of crying, apneas, dyspnea–tachypnea, diaphragmatic contractions,
- cardiac acceleration and deceleration.

Most often these phenomena occur in combinations, which may either remain fixed or undergo variation in subsequent paroxysmal episodes.

EEG is mandatory for diagnosis of the convulsive nature of these phenomena, especially when they are seen in infants with a neurologic syndrome and/or interictal background EEG abnormalities. Hyperexplexia, or stiff-baby syndrome, is a familiar disorder that is characterized by a marked increase in flexor muscle tone and attacks of hypertonia provoked by slight sensory stimuli. Excessive startle responses, quite common in these infants, and hypertonic attacks may mimic seizures. Ictal and interictal EEG recordings show no electrical discharge.

### NEONATAL STATUS EPILEPTICUS AND ELECTROCLINICAL CORRELATIONS

Seizures represent the most distinctive sign of neurologic disorder in the neonatal period. It has been suggested that several neonatal seizures have undesirable physiological, metabolic, excitotoxic and genetic effects on the developing brain. It is likely that the more frequent the occurrence of seizures is, and the longer the seizure state lasts, the worse these undesirable effects become. Clinical observation is of little or no value in recognizing most neonatal seizures, whereas EEG has proved increasingly important for their diagnosis, quantification and treatment. The pioneers of EEG in Paris (Dreyfus-Brisac & Monod 1972; Monod *et al.* 1972) have repeatedly stressed the importance of recognizing neonatal status epilepticus (NSE). The main reasons for this are that NSE predicts a worse outcome than isolated seizures, and that the seizures themselves may play a role in further brain injury.

There is no consensus regarding the definition of NSE. According to Dreyfus-Brisac & Monod (1972), NSE consists of 'clinical and/or infraclinical seizures recurrent for at least one hour in infants with interictal neurological symptoms'. An aggressive therapy would therefore seem reasonable, and in fact most, but not all, authors have proposed it. Just how aggressive anticonvulsant therapy should be in the neonatal period is controversial. If seizures themselves may cause brain injury it is also true that the drugs used to treat seizures may have a detrimental effect on development.

Clinical diagnosis of NSE is particularly difficult because a large number of neonatal seizures are clinically irrelevant or even consist of subclinical EEG discharges; electroclinical correlation is often poor in neonatal seizures. Biagioni *et al.* (1998) observed that the more frequent the EEG discharges (i.e the more severe the status epilepticus) the poorer the electroclinical correlations in neonatal seizures are (Fig. 11.12A,B). Increasing efforts are now being directed at the diagnosis and early monitoring of neonatal convulsions (Toet *et al.* 1999), and EEG monitoring, preferably supplemented by simultaneous videorecording, is clearly crucial not only to the diagnosis and prognosis of NSE but also to the choice of therapy.

The use of continuous recording EEG and CFM (see below) may be of great help to the clinician in detecting the changes in background EEG activity, the electrical discharges and the effect of drugs.

## TECHNIQUES FOR PROLONGED EEG MONITORING

### CASSETTE EEG

Since the 1980s, the technique of EEG recording on standard audiocassettes, running at a very reduced speed, has been successfully used. The recorder is similar to that of Holter electrocardiograms and includes recording up to ten channels. It is later examined by introducing the cassette into a reader which shows the polygraphic recording on a monitor.

The main advantages of this apparatus are:

- very long recordings (up to 24 hours with a single cassette), with a very portable electroencephalograph (it can be worn by the patient like a bag)
- an uncompressed complete EEG or polygraphic trace
- its reduced dimensions are convenient in the restricted space of a neonatal intensive care unit (it can be placed directly in the incubator), although its portability is less important, as examined patients are generally not displaced.

The main shortcomings are:

- recording quality is often poor, usually because of the intrusive noise of the oscillations of the tape
- a long time is necessary to examine the cassette with the reader
- correctness of recording cannot be followed on-line, so that the occurrence of an artifact or the malfunction of one or more electrodes are not detectable by the EEG technician.

In more recent years, with the capacity increase of portable microcomputer hard disks, now capable of containing 24–48 hours of high-quality recording (and of being followed on-line), the use of cassette-EEG finds fewer applications. Nevertheless, the technique gave rise to relevant

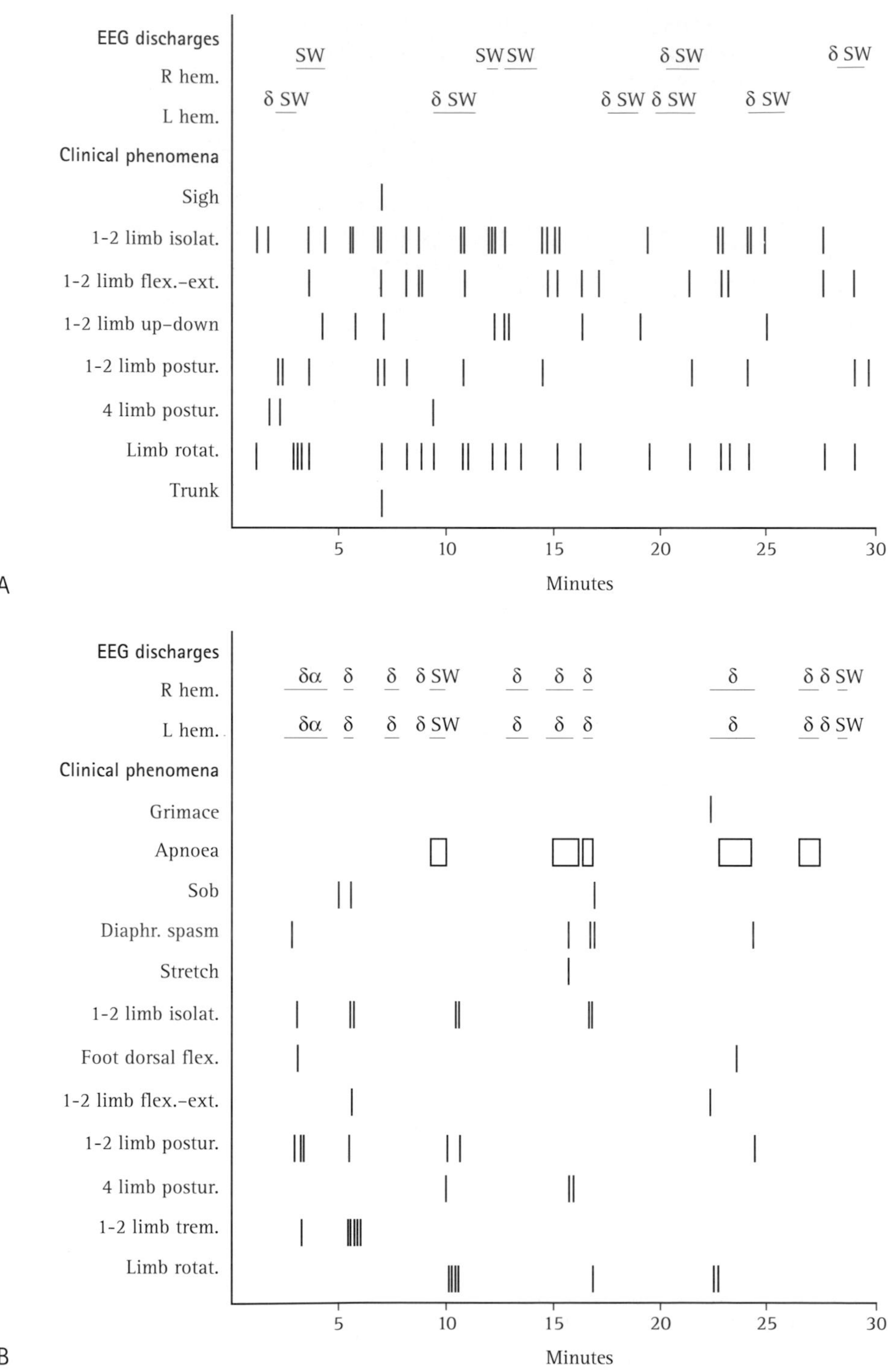


**Figure 11.12** Detailed graphic representation of EEG discharges and clinical phenomena for 30 minutes of the video-EEG recording of two newborn infants with HIE and status epilepticus, respectively. **Infant A**: limbs and trunk movements occur completely unrelated to EEG discharges. **Infant B**: electrical discharges are accompanied in some cases of apnea. R hem: right hemisphere; L hem: left hemisphere; SW: trains of sharp waves; δ, rhythmic sharp delta activities; 1–2 limb isolat: isolated movements of one or two limbs; 1–2 limb flex-ext: monotonous flexion–extension of one to two limbs; 1–2 and 4 limb posture: tonic posturing of one to two, four limbs; limb rotat: rotational movements of the limbs; trunk, trunk movements; alpha discharges; diaphr spasm: sudden contraction of the diaphragmatic muscle; foot dorsal flex: foot dorsal flexion; 1–2 limb trem: tremors of one to two limbs. (Reprinted, from Biagioni *et al.* 1998, with permission).

contributions in the literature and afforded insights into the EEGs of preterm and full-term neonates (Connell *et al.* 1987; Murdoch-Eaton *et al.* 1994; Wertheim *et al.* 1994).

## CEREBRAL FUNCTION MONITORING

Another method of neurophysiological assessment, suitable for very long recordings, has been introduced in neonatal intensive care units, namely, cerebral function monitoring (CFM), also known as amplitude-integrated EEG. It consists of an amplitude-integrated electroencephalogram, characterized by a single-lead trace (generally P3–P4 of the International 10–20 System). Normal cup electrodes are attached to the scalp by means of adhesive paste as in traditional EEGs or, more commonly, are replaced by needle electrodes. The latter procedure is obviously more invasive but allows a more reliable recording, especially when very prolonged. Signal processing consists of amplification, frequency filtration, and amplitude compression and rectification (Thornberg & Thiringer 1990). Frequencies below 2 Hz and above 20 Hz are eliminated and, within this same range, higher frequencies are enhanced. The final result of this process is a very compressed trace (the commonly used paper speed is 1 mm/min but it can be increased to at least 5 mm/min). The lower edge of the tracing reflects a possibly stable measurement of non-rhythmic activities, the so-called 'minimum level of cerebral activity', whereas the upper edge reflects both rhythmic and non-rhythmic activities (i.e. the so-called 'maximum level of cerebral activity'). The width of the trace indicates the variability of the signal. Amplitudes are reported in a semi-logarithmic scale and are included between 0 and 100 μV.

### Normal patterns in full-term and preterm infants

The normal neonatal CFM tracing usually shows periods characterized by different amplitudes. This finding is also observable in preterm infants but it is more evident at term age (Thornberg & Thiringer 1990) when it is easy to distinguish between phases of broad bandwidth, corresponding to periods of quiet sleep, and phases of narrow bandwidth, corresponding to active sleep or wakefulness. Similar variations are observable from the 31st or the 32nd week of PMA and again probably reflect modifications of the sleep–wake condition (Fig. 11.13). By comparing CFM traces of full-term and preterm infants, it can be observed that at low PMAs the bandwidth is generally broader and the minimum level of cerebral activity is located at a lower level (1.9±0.5 μV in the low PMA preterm infant). Approaching term age, the CFM trace becomes narrower, especially due to a raising of the lower edge, and well-defined, state-related amplitude variations are detectable (Thornberg & Thiringer 1990). Obviously, it is not possible to recognize in the CFM tracing the maturational patterns that characterize the EEG of preterm infants, such as temporal sawtooth or delta brushes. This technique of recording rather reflects the development of the general organization of brain electrical activities, such as the differentiation of state-related patterns, the increase in minimum level of cerebral activity (which probably relates to increased amplitudes within inter-burst intervals of discontinuous EEG patterns), and the progressive reduction of maximum voltages.

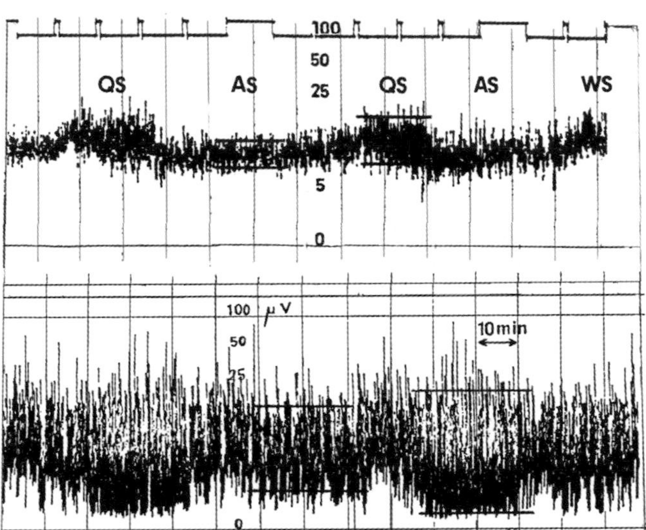


Figure 11.13 Example of CFM traces recorded in a term (upper trace) and a preterm (lower trace) infant. Horizontal lines superimposed on the traces indicate the measurement of maximum and minimum cerebral activity. QS, quiet sleep; AS, active sleep; WS, wake state. (Reprinted from Thornberg & Thiringer 1990, with permission).

### Abnormal patterns and clinical applications

CFM is now widely used in neonatal intensive care units, probably because the technique is easy to use (nurses can easily learn to apply electrodes and start the recording without complex training) and it permits a compressed online overview of cerebral activity. Its interpretation is also easy, even without specific knowledge of clinical neurophysiology, and therefore it is suitable for pediatricians and neonatologists. Despite the simplification of this recording technique, research results indicate a high diagnostic and prognostic value of CFM in neonates, in particular, in full-term patients with hypoxic–ischemic encephalopathy (Eken *et al.* 1995; Hellstrom-Vestas *et al.*, 1995; Naqeeb *et al.* 1999; Toet *et al.* 1999).

Specific abnormalities of full-term CFM have been described by various authors; the classification used by Toet *et al.* (1999) is described here:

- Isoelectric (flat) tracing: very low voltage, mainly inactive, with activity below 5 μV.
- Continuous extremely low voltage: continuous pattern of very low voltage (around or below 5 μV).
- Discontinuous burst–suppression pattern: periods of very low voltage are intermixed with bursts of higher amplitude.

- Discontinuous normal voltage: discontinuous trace where the voltage is predominantly above 5 μV.

Isoelectric tracings and continuous low voltage patterns consistently relate to a very poor outcome, whereas burst–suppression is also compatible with a normal evolution (Hellstrom-Vestas *et al.* 1995), especially when non-persistent in subsequent recordings (Toet *et al.* 1999).

Other authors (al Naqeeb *et al.* 1999) applied a quantitative classification, based on the voltage of the upper and lower edges of the trace. Moderately abnormal amplitudes (upper margin >10 μV and lower margin ≤5 μV) relate to a negative outcome in most cases, whereas suppressed amplitudes (upper edge <10 μV and lower edge <5 μV) never result in a normal evolution (Fig. 11.14).

Fewer reports are available on CFM background abnormalities in preterm infants. Indeed, while the most frequent anomalies of the fullterm infant's background electrical activity (i.e. what is observable on the EEG as a constant low voltage or a burst–suppression) are recognizable by means of the CFM, the specific alterations of maturational features that characterize the EEG of pathological preterm infants do not seem able to modify the CFM; nor can specific abnormal transients, such as positive sharp waves, be distinguished on such a compressed trace. Nevertheless, there is some evidence that the occurrence of a continuous CFM activity and the appearance of differentiated state-related patterns indicate a positive prognosis in low PMA preterm infants, whereas low voltage traces relate to an unfavorable evolution (Hellstrom-Vestas *et al.* 1991).

As far as the recognition of neonatal epileptic phenomena is concerned, some descriptions of specific CFM patterns are available in the literature. Al Naqeeb *et al.* (1999) reported that seizures are characterized by a sudden increase in

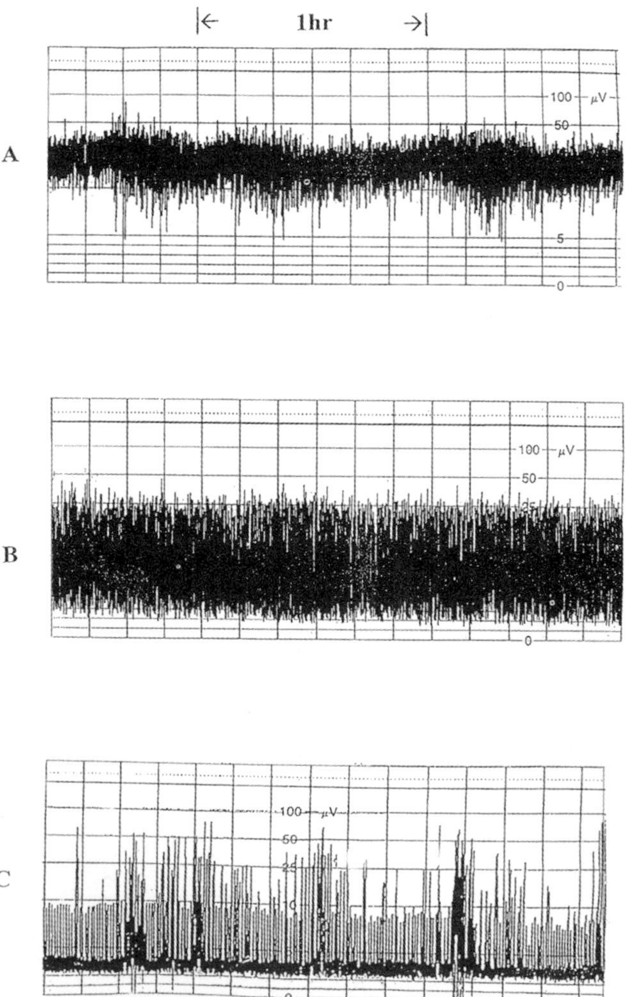


Figure 11.14 Examples of CFM background abnormalities. (A) normal amplitude; (B) moderately abnormal; (C) suppressed amplitude. (Reprinted from al Naqeeb *et al.* 1999, with permission.)

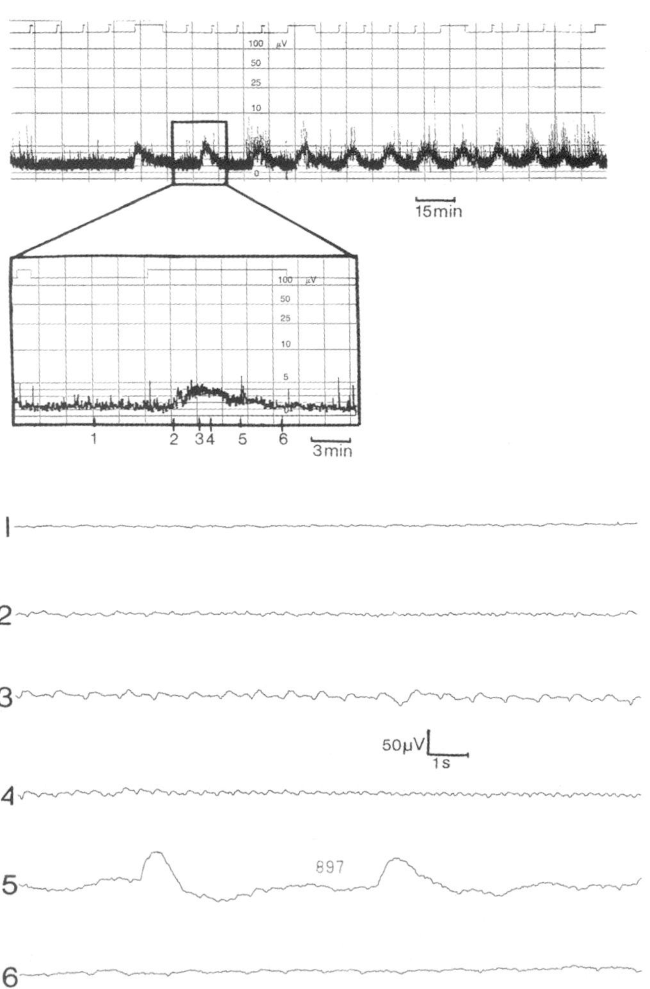


Figure 11.15 Example of saw-pattern in the CFM, consisting of repetitive low-voltage activity on an inactive background, with corresponding EEG trace in a full-term infant with HIE. (Reprinted from Hellstrom-Westas 1992, with permission.)

voltage, accompanied by a narrowing of the bandwidth and followed by a period of suppression. Hellstrom-Vestas (1992), in one of the very few available studies on the comparison between EEG and CFM, described repetitive periods of increased voltage activity on CFM, consisting of the so-called saw-tooth pattern (Fig. 11.15). This feature, which corresponded to low-voltage discharges on the EEG, is, of course, completely unrelated to the temporal theta activities of preterm EEG. Another possible CFM correlate of prolonged EEG discharges is constituted by long-lasting plateaux of high-voltage in both the lower and the upper edges (Fig. 11.16). Nevertheless, in the same paper the author reports that only 15/48 discharges observed on the EEG were also detectable by CFM, mainly due to their short duration but also because 'the integrated voltage of seizure activity did not differ markedly from the cerebral activity before and after the seizure'. Considerable caution is therefore recommended, also considering the fact that epileptic discharges that do not affect parietal regions are presumably unable to modify the one-lead bipolar (P3–P4) CFM tracing.

On balance, given that it is an easy-to-use, easy-to-interpret device, CFM is certainly useful, particularly in those neonatal units where an EEG apparatus is not available, and it finds its main field of application in the neurologic assessment of full-term infants with hypoxic-ischemic encephalopathy. For other purposes, such as the assessment of preterm infants or the recognition of neonatal seizures, CFM can provide useful information but does not seem able to completely replace standard EEG. In these cases, as also recommended by Hellstrom-Vestas (1992), a combination of continuous CFM and intermittent EEG is probably optimal for a correct electrophysiological assessment of the neonate.

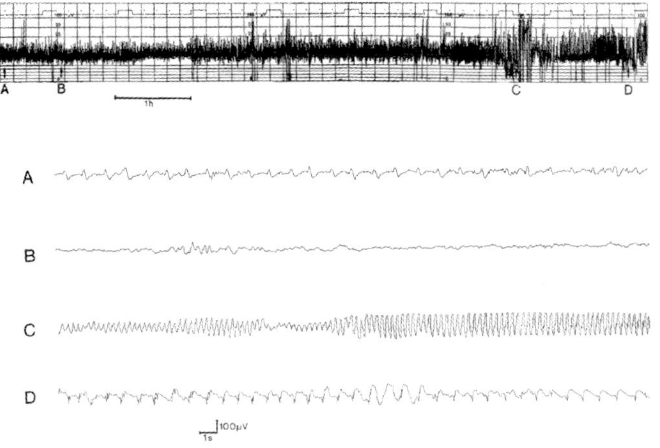


Figure 11.16 CFM recording in a fullterm infant with OTC deficiency. (A) In the first parts of the trace 20 min of subclinical seizure activity is observable, undetected by CFM; (B,C) high-voltage EEG discharges with corresponding apneic spells. (D) New seizures appeared preceded by movement artifacts. (Reprinted from Hellstrom-Westas 1992, with permission.)

## ACKNOWLEDGMENTS

The authors gratefully acknowledge Luca Ori and Rossella Pieri, who perform EEG polygraphic recordings in Modena and Pisa, respectively, and the staff of the neonatal intensive care units of the University of Modena and Pisa, where the infants are observed. We also thank Professor G. B. Cavazzuti, Director of the Institute of Paediatrics and Neonatal Medicine of Modena University, for his continuous support in the field of EEG research, and Maria Guerra and M. Federica Roversi for reviewing manuscript, tables and figures. Fabrizio Ferrari is supported by Italian MURST (grant 40% 1998), Enrico Biagioni and Giovanni Cioni by the Italian Ministry of Health (grant RC 1/99).

### Key Points

- Neonatal electroencephalography (EEG) has developed into a valuable, non-invasive technique for the evaluation of neurologically compromised neonates.
- The two most widely used recording techniques are traditional EEG-polygraphic recordings and EEG monitoring. In addition, a few units benefit from more sophisticated equipment such as video-EEG, which is particularly useful in distinguishing epileptic from non-epileptic paroxysmal events.
- The normal EEG development in the neonatal age is characterized by rapid transformation of represented patterns between 28 and 44 weeks of postmenstrual age.
- Background EEG abnormalities and disturbance of sleep cycles are the best indicators both of the severity of the brain damage and of prognosis in newborn infants, whereas the diagnostic and prognostic role of abnormal EEG transients appears more controversial.
- The occurrence of EEG maturational features that do not reflect those expected for the PMA (dysmaturity) represents an unfavorable prognostic sign in preterm infants' early postnatal period.
- Cerebral function monitoring (CFM), consisting of a single-lead, amplitude-integrated electroencephalogram has been recently introduced in neonatal intensive care unit: it is suitable for very long recordings and it is easy to use and easy to interpret.
- The CFM finds its main field of application in the neurological assessment of fullterm infants with hypoxic–ischemic encephalopathy; for other purposes, such as the assessment of preterm infants or the recognition of neonatal seizures it does not seem able to fully replace standard EEG.
- New computer-aided portable electroencephalograph allows long lasting standard EEG-polygraphic recording and high quality EEG signal fast review without interruption of the recording and video-EEG.

## REFERENCES


Al Naqeeb N, Edwards A D, Cowan F M, Azzopardi D (1999) Assessment of neonatal encephalopathy by amplitude-integrated electroencephalography. *Pediatrics* 103: 1263–1271.

Anders T, Emde R, Parmelee A, eds (1971) A manual of standardized terminology, technique and criteria for scoring of the states of sleep and wakefulness in newborn infants. UCLA Brain Information Service/BRI Publications Office, NINDS Neurological Infant Network

Anderson C M, Torres F, Faoro A (1985) The EEG of the early premature. *Electroencephalog Clin Neurophysiol* 60: 95–105.

Aso K, Abdab-Barmada M & Scher M S (1993) EEG and the neuropathology in premature neonates with intraventricular hemorrhage. *J Clin Neurophysiol* 10: 304–306.

Baud O, d'Allest A M, Lacaze-Masmonteil T *et al.* (1998) The early diagnosis of periventricular leukomalacia in premature infants with positive rolandic sharp waves on serial electroencephalography. *J Pediatr* 132: 813–817.

Biagioni E, Bartalena L, Boldrini A *et al.* (1994) Background EEG activity in preterm infants: correlation of outcome with selected maturational features. *Electroencephalog Clin Neurophysiol* 91: 154–162.

Biagioni E, Bartalena L, Biver P *et al.* (1996) Electroencephalographic dysmaturity in preterm infants: a prognostic tool in the early postnatal period. *Neuropediatrics* 27: 311–316.

Biagioni E, Ferrari F, Boldrini A *et al.* (1998) Electroclinical correlation in neonatal seizures. *Eur J Paediatr Neurol* 2: 117–125.

Biagioni E, Bartalena L, Boldrini A *et al.* (1999) Constantly discontinuous EEG patterns in full-term neonates with hypoxic-ischemic encephalopathy. *Clin Neurophysiol* 110: 1510–1515.

Connell J, Oozeer R, Regev R *et al.* (1987) Continuous four-channel EEG monitoring in the evaluation of echodense ultrasound lesions and cystic leucomalacia. *Arch Dis Child* 62: 1019–1024.

Cukier F, André M, Monod N & Dreyfus-Brisac C (1972) Apport de l'E.E.G. au diagnostic des hémorragies intraventricularies du prématuré. *Revue E.E.G.* 3:318–322.

Dreyfus-Brisac C, Monod N (1972) The electroencephalogram of fullterm newborns and premature infants. In: Remon A, ed. *Handbook of electrencephalography and clinical neurophysiology.* Amsterdam: Elsevier; vol. 6B; pp. 6–23.

Eken P, Toet M C, Groenendaal F & de Vries L S (1995) Predictive value of early neuroimaging, pulsed Doppler and neurophysiology in full-term infants with hypoxic-ischaemic encephalopathy. *Arch Dis Child Fetal Neonat Edn* 73: F75–F80.

Ferrari F (1981) Diagnostic contribution of the electroencephalogram in the premature infant: personal casuistry. *Med Surg Ped* 3: 495–506.

Ferrari F, Torricelli A, Giustardi A *et al.* (1992) Bioelectrical brain maturation in fullterm infants and in healthy and pathological preterm infants at term post-menstrual age. *Early Hum Dev* 28: 37–63.

Hayakawa F, Okumura A, Kato T *et al.* (1997) Disorganized patterns: chronic-stage EEG abnormality of the late neonatal period following severely depressed EEG activities in early preterm infants. *Neuropediatrics* 28: 272–275.

Hellstrom-Vestas L, Rosen I & Svenningsen N W (1991) Cerebral function monitoring during the first week of life in extremely small low birthweight (ESLBW) infants. *Neuropediatrics* 22: 27–32.

Hellstrom-Vestas L (1992) Comparison between tape-recorded and amplitude-integrated EEG monitoring in sick newborn infants. *Acta Paediatr Scand* 81: 812–819.

Hellstrom-Vestas L, Rosen I, Svenningsen N W (1995) Predictive value of early continuous amplitude integrated EEG recordings on outcome after severe birth asphyxia in full-term infants. *Arch Dis Child Fetal Neonat Edn* 72: F34–F38.

Holmes G L & Lombroso C T (1993) Prognostic value of background patterns in the neonatal EEG. *J Clin Neurophysiol* 10: 323–352.

Lombroso C T (1979) Quantified electrographic scales on 10 pre-term healthy newborns followed-up to 40–43 weeks of conceptional age by serial polygraphic recordings. *Electroencephalogr Clin Neurophysiol* 46: 460–474.

Lombroso C T (1985) Neonatal polygraphy in full-term and premature infants: a review of normal and abnormal findings. *J Clin Neurophysiol* 2: 105–155.

Marret S, Parain D, Jeannot E *et al.* (1992) Positive rolandic sharp waves in the EEG of the premature newborn: a five years prospective study. *Arch Dis Child* 67: 948–951.

Mizrahi E M & Kellaway P (1987) Characterization and classification of neonatal seizures. *Neurology* 37: 1837–1844.

Monod N, Pajot N & Guidasci S (1972) The neonatal EEG: statistical studies and prognostic value in full-term and pre-term babies. *Electroencephalogr Clin Neurophysiol* 32: 529–544.

Monod N & Tharp B (1977) Activité électro-encéphalographique normale du nouveau-né et du prématuré au cours des étas de veille et de sommeil. *Rev EEG Neurophysiol* 7: 302–315.

Murdoch-Eaton D G, Wertheim D, Oozeer R *et al.* (1994) Reversible changes in cerebral activity associated with acidosis in preterm neonates. *Acta Paediatr Scand* 83: 486–492.

Nolte R & Haas G (1978) A polygraphic study of bioelectrical brain maturation in preterm infants. *Dev Med Child Neurol* 20: 167–182.

Parmelee A H, Schulte F J, Akiyana Y *et al.* (1968) Maturation of EEG activity during sleep in premature infants. *Electroencephalogr Clin Neurophysiol* 24: 319–329.

Pezzani C, Radvanyi-Bouvet M F, Relier J P & Monod N (1986) Neonatal electroencephalography during the first twenty-four hours of life in full-term newborn infants. *Neuropediatrics* 17: 11–18.

Prechtl H F R, Theorell K & Bair A W (1973) Behavioural state cycles in abnormal infants. *Dev Med Child Neurology* 15: 606–615.

Scavone C, Radvanyi-Bouvet M F, Morel-Khan F & Dreyfus-Brisac C (1985) Coma après souffrance foetale aigue chez le nouveau-ne a terme: evolution electro-clinique. *Rev EEG Neurophysiol* 15: 279–288.

Stockard-Pope J, Werner S S & Bickford R G (1992) *Atlas of neonatal electroencephalography*, 2nd edn. New York: Raven Press

Tharp B R, Cukier F & Monod N (1981) The prognostic value of the elecroencephalogram in premature infants. *Electroencephalogr Clin Neurophysiol* 51: 219–236.

Toet M C, Hellstrom-Vestas L, Groenendaal F *et al.* (1999) Amplitude integrated EEG 3 and 6 hours after birth in full-term neonates with hypoxic-ischaemic encephalopathy. *Arch Dis Child Fetal Neonat Edn* 81: F19–F23.

Thornberg E & Thiringer K (1990) Normal pattern of the cerebral function monitor trace. *Acta Paediatr Scand* 79: 20–25.

Volpe J J (1995) *Neurology of the newborn*, 3rd edn. Philadelphia, PA: W.B. Saunders Company.

Watanabe K, Miyazaki S, Hara K & Hakamada S (1980) Behavioral state cycles, background EEGs and prognosis of newborn with perinatal hypoxia. *Electroencephalogr Clin Neurophysiol* 49: 618–625.

Watanabe K, Hayakawa F & Okumura A (1999) Neonatal EEG: a powerful tool in the assessment of brain damage in preterm infants. *Brain Dev* 21: 361–372.

Wertheim D, Mercuri E, Faundez J C *et al.* (1994) Prognostic value of continuous electroencephalographic recording in full term infants with hypoxic-ischaemic encephalopathy. *Arch Dis Child Fetal Neonat Edn* 71: F97–F102.

# Chapter 12 Evoked potentials in the neonatal period

P. Eken and L. S. de Vries

## INTRODUCTION

An increasing number of very preterm infants surviving the neonatal period is causing a rise in the prevalence of long-term disabilities (Hagberg *et al.* 1989), in spite of concurrent scientific and technological advances in perinatal care. The incidence of infants suffering from hypoxic–ischemic encephalopathy (HIE) is relatively stable, but the sequelae may be far-reaching. Therefore, it is essential to identify those infants who have sustained damage to the immature nervous system at an early stage to reduce the severity of neurologic injury as well as to instigate remedial action. For this purpose, attempts have been made to improve early prediction of neurodevelopmental outcome in at-risk infants.

An objective source of evidence for whether an infant's CNS function is normal is the study of evoked potentials (EPs), which are averaged electrical responses to a repetitive sensory stimulus that can be either auditory, visual, or sensory. EPs are providing information on both peripheral and central aspects of the sensory pathways within the CNS. The responses are recorded from the electroencephalogram (EEG), where they can be identified by their consistent temporal relationship to the stimulus event. The EEG is of higher amplitude than the EP, but it is random to the applied stimulus, whereas the EP is of small amplitude but constant relative to the stimulus. Averaging a number of responses will cause the EP to emerge from the EEG. Age-appropriate norms have to be established, as latencies of the different components of the response decrease rapidly with age in the neonatal period. Changes in latency or amplitude of the EP waveform may indicate involvement of the sensory pathway. EPs have been shown to be of great value when trying to predict neurodevelopmental outcome during the neonatal period, along with clinical, EEG, and neuroimaging data.

This chapter reviews the methodology, the maturational changes, and the clinical applications for neonatal EPs.

## METHODOLOGY AND MATURATION

Over the last decades, there has been an increasing interest in recording EPs, both in preterm infants as well as in asphyxiated full-term babies. The brainstem auditory evoked potentials (BAEPs) and the visual evoked potentials (VEPs) are technically more easy to perform than the somatosensory evoked potentials (SEPs). Initially, a high failure rate was reported in normal neonates, most likely due to the fact that the recording technique had not been adjusted from the adult settings. Only when the filter settings, stimulation rate, and number of stimuli are adapted to the immature nervous system, will the success rate be sufficient.

Applying Ag/AgCl disc electrodes to the scalp should be performed without causing irritation of the vulnerable skin and without disturbing the infant. Either hypo-allergenic tape or adhesive paste with gauze may be used after gentle abrasion of the skin and instillation of electrolyte gel. Restless infants should better be tested in the prone position. During registration of EPs it is standard procedure to repeat the test to ensure reproducibility. When in doubt about the reliability it is important to perform an extra trial, sampling the raw EEG without administering the stimulus. When the noise level is as high as the supposed response, the result should be discarded. Following the stimulus, a series of positive and negative deflections can be measured. In some laboratories the components of the SEPs and VEPs are named according to the order of appearance, e.g. N1 for the first negative peak, or P1 for the first positive one; others use a denomination according to the mean latency of a specific age group, e.g. N19, the first scalp-derived component in adult SEPs, or P200, a positive deflection in the VEP of term neonates. In BAEPs, all laboratories use the same nomenclature (roman numerals) to indicate the different positive peaks.

### BRAINSTEM AUDITORY EVOKED POTENTIALS (BAEPs)

BAEPs are responses generated within the auditory brainstem pathway following an acoustic stimulus. They are the far-field reflection of sequentially activated neurons at successively higher levels of the auditory pathway. They are used to assess both the peripheral sensitivity as well as the neurologic integrity of the auditory brainstem. The response consists of a sequence of seven positive waves of which the first two (waves I and II) represent the action potentials of the distal and rostral portions of the VIIIth nerve; wave III is derived from the cochlear nucleus; wave IV arises from the superior olivary complex, and wave V from the lateral lemniscus. Waves VI and VII are thought to arise from the inferior colliculus (Jewett & Williston 1971). The I–V peak latency is considered to be a measure of central auditory conduction time. The waves arise in the first ten milliseconds after the acoustic stimulus. Middle latency responses, between 20 and 100 ms, have no clinical relevance in the neonatal unit.

To record the response, the active electrode is best positioned on the mastoid bone or earlobe ipsilateral to the stimulus; the reference electrode is placed on the vertex, and the forehead or the contralateral ear is grounded (Stuart *et al.* 1996). Impedance must be below 5 K. Most laboratories use rarefaction broadband click stimuli with a peak power of 2–4 kHz, because they produce clearer wave morphologic features than do condensation clicks (Pope-Stockard & Sharbrough 1992). The rectangular pulses have a duration of 100 μs and usually are presented at a repetition rate of 10 per second. Increasing the repetition rate increases the latencies and decreases the amplitude of the response (Lasky 1984; Klein *et al.* 1992). The pulse is calibrated in decibels above the hearing threshold of normally hearing subjects (dBnHL). The signals are presented monaurally through a special cushioned earphone (TDH-39 pediatric earphones) which may be held over the ear. Ideally, when stimulating at 80 dBnHL or higher, constant white noise should be used to mask the contralateral ear to prevent cross-hearing by bone conduction.

BAEPs are best recorded in a quiet area of the nursery. BAEP latencies are not affected by behavioral state, but they can be obtained more reliably during a period of quiescence (McCall & Ferraro 1991). Also, the responses are not influenced by general anesthetics or drugs. Since the BAEPs are very small compared with the electrical background noise, it is necessary to average at least 1000 individual sweeps to improve the signal-to-noise amplitude ratio. Automatic artifact rejection may be used to reduce the inclusion of high-amplitude muscular activity in the averaged response (Jiang 1995). Analysis-time for the signal averager is usually between 15 and 20 ms, the EEG-amplifier filter bandpass is preferably 30–3000 Hz (Spivak 1993; Stuart & Yang 1994; Sininger 1995). This relatively high-pass recording filter of 30 Hz reveals a larger amplitude and enhances the overall signal-to-noise ratio, as BAEPs from neonates comprise greater low frequency spectral components than do adult BAEPs.

With high-intensity stimuli presented at a low rate it is possible to recognize the presence of waves I, III, and V in infants from as early as 25 weeks of gestation onwards (Fawer & Dubowitz 1982; Despland 1985; Lary *et al.* 1985; Cox *et al.* 1993). The peak latencies decrease progressively with increasing gestational age, and subsequently waves II and IV will appear (Vles *et al.* 1985). The maximal change is between 29 and 36 weeks of gestational age. The latency of wave V decreases more rapidly with age than that of wave I, resulting in a wave I–V peak interval also decreasing with age. Whether preterm birth affects the maturation of the auditory system is still equivocal. Several authors reported that extrauterine preterm exposure to acoustical stimuli does not affect maturation (Schulte *et al.* 1977; Starr *et al.* 1977; Fawer & Dubowitz 1982; Despland 1985; Jiang 1995). However, other groups reported prolonged wave and interpeak latencies (Pasman *et al.* 1992), as well as shorter wave and interpeak latencies (Delorme *et al.* 1986; Collet *et al.* 1989). Eggermont & Salamy (1988) found longer latencies for waves I, III, and V, but normal interpeak latencies. They attributed this mild conductive hearing loss to the higher incidence of otitis media in preterm infants.

At term age, the morphology of the BAEP is similar to that of adults, but with longer latencies (Picton *et al.* 1992). At the age of 2 years, near adult values are reached. Slight gender differences are reported, with shorter latencies and higher amplitudes in females, as well as a significant right-ear advantage in males and females attributed to cerebral laterality in auditory function (Eldredge & Salamy 1996). A high interindividual variability has been reported in several cross-sectional studies, but intraindividual maturation is consistent (Vles *et al.* 1985, Mercuri *et al.* 1994). To rate the maturational changes at their true value, age-specific normative data should be obtained for each laboratory. Auditory thresholds improve significantly with age (Lary *et al.* 1985). Establishing amplitude norms in neonates is difficult, since the overall amplitudes are low, and amplitude is influenced by the low frequency cut-off. Only the wave V:I amplitude ratio is being used for clinical purposes in neonates.

Two neonatal screening techniques have been developed in the 1980s. One is an automated auditory brainstem response (AABR) machine, developed for automated screening on hearing impairment from birth to approximately 6 months old. A machine-based decision is made on the presence or absence of waveforms. A high sensitivity and specificity have been reported (Jacobson *et al.* 1990; Hermann *et al.* 1995; van Straaten 1999). This technique may even be used in Well Baby Clinics or at home (Oudesluys-Murphy & Harlaar 1997). Evoked otoacoustic emissions (EOAE) can be elicited in response to clicks presented to the ear via a small probe also containing a microphone which picks up the acoustic energy generated by the cochlea and transmitted back through the middle to the outer ear (Bamford *et al.* 1998). EOAEs are also feasible in the neonatal unit, and a high sensitivity is reported. However, different failure rates, especially in infants with lower gestational ages and low specificity, have been reported (Kennedy *et al.* 1991; Salamy *et al.* 1996; Watkin 1996).

## VISUAL EVOKED POTENTIALS (VEPs)

The VEP is a gross electrical signal generated by the occipital area of the cortex, in response to a visual stimulus. The stimulus may either be a diffuse flashing light or a patterned visual stimulus. Analysis of VEPs has been used widely for 40 years (Ellingson 1960) in the evaluation of maturational processes in both preterm and term infants, because of the ease with which they can be applied in longitudinal studies. VEPs show systematic changes in electrographical characteristics with advancing gestational age, which are thought to reflect the progress in myelination in the developing human brain (Tsuneishi & Casaer 1997). In adults, the N70 and P100 peaks are the most important features, while in neonates and infants the P200 and N300 peaks are the major components. Monocular stimulation, using a combination of electroretinography and VEP measurement, will allow, by comparison of the response elicited at the two separate visual cortices, differentiation between pre- and postchiasmatic lesions.

Flash-VEPs (FVEPs) are not suitable for neurophysiological measurement of visual acuity. For this purpose the pattern-VEPs (PVEPs) are better, because they are a sensitive and quantitative measure of visual function, especially in the distinction between cortical and subcortical visual function. However, in the neonatal unit PVEPs have not been widely used, as they can only be elicited in infants who are able to fixate on a stimulus during a period of alertness.

## Flash-VEPs

In the neonatal unit, light-emitting diode (LED) goggles or small LED screens which can be placed inside the incubator are most feasible to use as a stimulus source. A stroboscopic flashlight has to be placed outside the incubator, thus producing variable stimulus intensities, and has also been shown to produce more complex waveforms (Mushin *et al.* 1984). FVEPs are recorded from a single midline channel, the positive electrode being placed on Oz, referenced to Fz, and using the forearm as a ground. The analysis time should be 1000 ms, as the components emerge between 200 and 500 ms. The stimulus with a duration of 10 ms has to be delivered sufficiently infrequently to allow the visual system to return to its resting state between the successive stimuli, usually 0.5 Hz.

The recommended filter bandpass is 1–100 Hz, and the impedance needs to be below 5 K. At least two series of 40–60 trials have to be collected to ensure reproducibility, although reproducible VEPs can easily be obtained with a few trials using a long interstimulus interval (Pryds 1992). Several authors emphasized the need for looking at the behavioral state of the infant during the VEP recording, since the P200 was noted to decrease in amplitude and increase in latency in both active and quiet sleep states (Watanabe *et al.* 1973; Whyte *et al.* 1987; Apkarian *et al.* 1991).

FVEPs can be elicited as early as 23, 24, and 25 weeks of gestational age (Hrbek *et al.* 1973; Purpura 1975; Chin *et al.* 1985; Taylor *et al.* 1987). At this early stage, the response consists mainly of a large negative wave occurring at approximately 300 ms (N300). The N300 shortens in latency as the infant matures by a rate of 4.6–5.5 ms a week (Tsuneishi *et al.* 1995; Pike *et al.* 1999). Tsuneishi & Casaer (1997) have, however, demonstrated a stepwise decrease of the latency with 'acceleration weeks', during which the latency decreases at a rate of more than 6 ms a week. These acceleration weeks occur most prominently at 37 weeks postmenstrual age, and this was attributed to an initiation of myelination in the optic radiation. Likewise, Minami *et al.* (1996) reported a faster decrease in latency of the N300 from 35 to 38 weeks, compared with 32 to 35 weeks. After 27 weeks a late positive component is present (P400), but this wave has a variable latency and morphology.

A smaller positive peak, preceding the N300, will emerge at around 34 weeks of gestational age (P200) and become the most consistent feature of the VEP (Ellingson 1970; Umezaki & Morell 1970; Taylor *et al.* 1987). The latency of the P200 also decreases rapidly until term age. At term, the response consists of a negative–positive–negative complex, which will transform into the more complex adult waveform over the next few months.

The N300 peak is supposed to arise from the basilar dendrites of the pyramidal cells in the visual cortex, while the P200 is suggested to arise from the apical dendrites, which develop in the last trimester (Taylor *et al.* 1987). Subcortical components may also be present, since a negative wave has also been reported in infants with severe occipital lesions (Dubowitz *et al.* 1986).

Comparison of FVEPs recorded in preterm infants with those from term infants at equivalent postconceptional ages suggests faster maturation of particularly the P200 peak in the extrauterine versus the intrauterine environment (Taylor *et al.* 1987; Leaf *et al.* 1995). Tsuneishi *et al.* (1995), however, reported that extrauterine life may accelerate the maturation of the N300 waveform, but does not affect the absolute peak latencies. Inter- and even intra-subject variability of the FVEP latencies is high, inducing a wide normal range, but Apkarian *et al.* (1991) stressed that careful control of state during the recording reduces inter and intra-subject variability.

The rapid maturational changes in both preterm and term born infants, the differences in recording technique among various laboratories, and the differences found in intrauterine versus extrauterine development, require the establishment of normative values ideally taking both postmenstrual and gestational age at birth into consideration.

## Pattern VEPs

Several stimulation techniques may be used like flashed checkerboards, steady-state stimulation, and pattern-sweep, but most studies in infants use pattern-reversal checkerboard stimulation where black and white squares exchange places with a constant luminance (McCulloch & Taylor 1994). The first reports on PVEPs in preterm infants were published by Harding's group (Grose *et al.* 1989; Harding *et al.* 1989) and Birch *et al.* (1990). They obtained PVEPs in healthy preterm infants at 33 and 36 weeks of gestation, respectively. Kos-Pietro *et al.* (1997) were able to elicit a response as early as 32 weeks of gestation, but stressed that, even in low-risk infants, they managed to obtain a PVEP to large check sizes in only 11% of their infants at 34 weeks of gestation.

PVEPs in preterm infants show a similar morphology to that of the full-term infant. The waveform morphology becomes more reproducible with larger check sizes and increasing gestational age. As in FVEPs, a gradual decrease in latency of the PVEP components is observed during development in preterm (Grose *et al.* 1989) and in term infants (Marg *et al.* 1975; Kurtzberg & Vaughan 1985; McCulloch & Skarf 1991).

Promising results considering the establishment of cortical visual maturation have been obtained by Mercuri *et al.* (1998), who used a combination of orientation reversal VEP, which is a pure cortical property and can be obtained from 6 weeks postnatally using slow reversal rates, and phase reversal VEP, which requires a lesser degree of cortical maturation and is already present at birth (Wattam-Bell 1983).

## SOMATOSENSORY EVOKED POTENTIALS (SEPs)

Somatosensory evoked potentials (SEPs) are technically the most difficult to perform and more time consuming, compared to the auditory brain stem evoked responses and visual evoked potentials and they require sophisticated electronic equipment. Following the sensory stimulus, usually to the median nerve or the posterior tibial nerve, a series of positive and negative potentials can be detected and measured. The main neuraxis of the tract from periphery to cortex contains the peripheral nerve, brachial plexus, dorsal root, posterior column, cuneate nucleus and, following decussation, medial lemniscus, thalamus, and parietal cortex. After median nerve stimulation, the first negative wave which can be recorded from an electrode placed over Erb's point (brachial plexus) is the N9. Negative waves N11 and N13 can be measured over the lower cervical vertebrae. At the scalp, contralateral to the site of stimulation and overlying the primary somatosensory cortex, wave N19 is recorded, which is considered to be cortically generated. In the newborn this component is usually referred to as the N1.

There has been a lot of discussion about the origin of the N1. According to Chiappa (1985) the component is partially derived from the thalamus. Using principal component analysis, Karniski (1992) was, however, able to show in preterm infants, that the N1 represents a tangential dipole located in the postcentral gyrus. In adults the N19 is followed by a positive component, the P22. This component is usually not yet present in the preterm infant, but can be present at term age. Following stimulation of the posterior tibial nerve, N19 and P22 can be recorded over the lumbar spine. The P35 is recorded over the somatosensory cortex.

SEPs are usually elicited following an electrical stimulus applied over the median or the posterior tibial nerve (see Fig 12.1). Stimulation of the median nerve is better tolerated than stimulation of the posterior tibial nerve. The newborn infant can be tested without the use of sedation following a feed. The cortical SEP after median nerve stimulation has been found to be dependent upon the state of alertness (Desmedt & Manil 1970; Laget 1982). Desmedt & Manil (1970) found no differences in N19 (1) peak latencies between infants who were quietly awake or in REM sleep, but they observed a difference between the N19 (1) peak latencies of infants in REM and in slow wave sleep. Bongers-

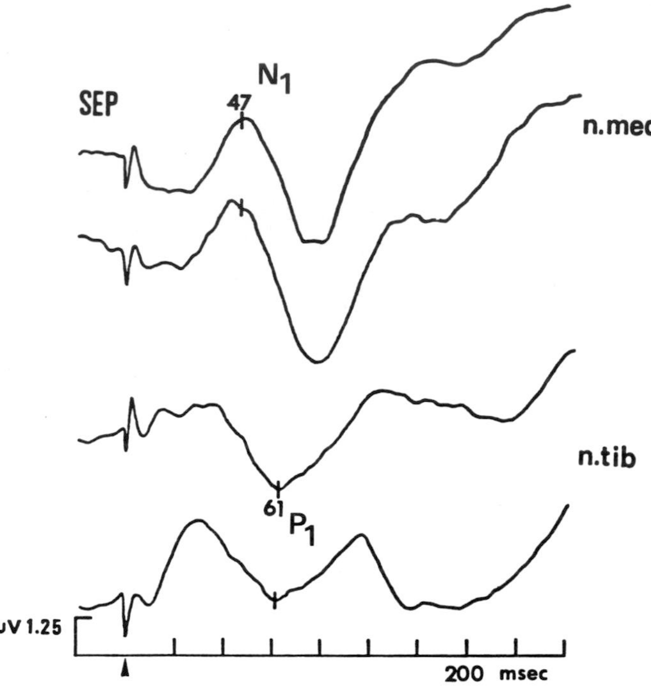


Figure 12.1 A normal response following stimulation of the median nerve (n. med) and posterior tibial nerve (n. tib) in a normal preterm infant with gestational age of 31 weeks. $N_1$, first negative wave; $P_1$, first positive wave; arrowhead, moment of stimulus. (Reproduced from Pierrat *et al.*, 1997.)

Schokking *et al.* (1989) found that the curves of SEPs changed when the infants went from non-quiet into quiet sleep with a bilobed curve in quiet sleep. George & Taylor (1991) showed longer latencies and lower amplitudes of the cortical median nerve SEP with deep sleep. It is known that the cortical response to tibial nerve stimulation is altered with stage II sleep in older children (Gilmore *et al.* 1987). In preterm infants, sleep does not appear to adversely affect the SEPs. Gilmore *et al.* (1987) found the lower limb SEPs easier to obtain in a third of preterm infants when they were sleeping, although occasionally the cortical response disappeared with sleep. Klimach & Cooke (1988a), White & Cooke (1989) and Pike *et al.* (1997) recorded all of their preterm SEPs whilst the baby was asleep.

The negative electrode is placed over the somatosensory area for the upper extremities on C3′, which is 2 cm posterior to C3 in the 10–20 system, or over pCz-L/R, just lateral to pCz for the posterior tibial nerve SEP. The reference electrode is placed in the midfrontal position on Fz and the neutral electrode on the lower arm.

### Median nerve SEPs

Some of the earlier studies of SEPs in neonates were unable to identify components in a percentage of normal infants (30% in Willis *et al.* 1984; 15% in Laureau *et al.* 1988). This is mainly due to the fact that adult filter settings and stimulation rates were used. There is no agreement in the literature about stimulation rate and bandpass; however, studies using slow stimulation rates, long sweep times and lower filters appeared to be most successful in obtaining SEPs in infants (Desmedt *et al.* 1976; Laget *et al.* 1976; Araki *et al.* 1999).

Bongers-Schokking *et al.* (1989) investigated combinations of these factors and recommended a low bandpass (1–100 Hz) and few stimuli (25–50) for recording cortical SEPs. George & Taylor (1991) found two different bandpasses (5–1500 Hz, 30–3000 Hz) to be useful. Gibson *et al.* (1992a) also recorded SEPs with a higher bandpass (10–3000 Hz). Scalais *et al.* (1998) compared different filter settings and showed a longer latency of the N1 when a low bandpass (1–100 Hz) was used compared to a higher bandpass (30–3000 Hz). The impedance should be less than 2 K. Electrical stimuli of 0.1 ms in duration may be delivered at a rate of 0.5 Hz, using a hand-held device placed over the ventral wrist overlying the median nerve. The stimulation intensity needs to be higher than that used in children and adults in order to produce a motor response. It is now however widely accepted that, given modification in testing procedures, SEPs can be reliably recorded in all normal neonates.

It is possible to record SEPs in preterm neonates from 25 weeks gestational age onward (Klimach & Cooke 1988a; Karniski 1992; Taylor *et al.* 1996a), using a low bandpass (1–100 Hz) and an analysis time between 100 and 500 ms. Taylor *et al.* (1996a) were able to study very preterm infants (gestational age 27–32 weeks), with the first test being performed at an average of 5 days of age. Identifiable cortical SEPs were found in all cases studied by Taylor *et al.* (1996a) but not in a small percentage of preterm infants (10–12%) studied by others (Klimach & Cooke 1988a; Karniski 1992).

In preterm neonates the latency of the cortical peaks decreases as the infants mature. At 27 weeks of gestational age the N1 has a latency of over 75 ms which decreased to the value observed in term neonates at 40 weeks postmenstrual age. No differences have been found between term and preterm infants tested at the same conceptional age (Klimach & Cooke 1988a; Karniski 1992; Taylor *et al.* 1996a). Gibson *et al.* (1992a) also reported increased waveform complexity with increasing gestational age. Karniski (1992), however, found that the late components and their scalp topography changed little over the preterm period except for the amplitude.

### Posterior tibial nerve SEPs

Recording posterior tibial nerve SEPs was noted to be more difficult in neonates. Most of the studies reported difficulties in obtaining responses, with success rates varying between 55 and 73% (Gilmore *et al.* 1987; Laureau & Marlot 1990). In preterm neonates, White & Cooke (1989) using a lower bandpass, as already described for median nerve SEPs, recorded SEPs following posterior tibial nerve stimulation in 93% of preterm neonates born between 26 and 41 weeks of gestational age. Good responses were also obtained by Pike *et al.* (1997).

## CLINICAL APPLICATIONS OF BAEPS

### ASSESSMENT OF AUDIOLOGICAL DISORDERS (see also Chapter 39)

When the diagnosis of congenital or perinatally acquired hearing loss is made before the age of 3 months, and treatment using amplification and communication therapy is started before the age of 6 months, there are better chances for language and speech development (Davis *et al.* 1986; Markides 1986; Ramkalawan & Davis 1992; Yoshinaga-Itano *et al.* 1998). As infants who have graduated from neonatal intensive care units have a higher prevalence of moderate-to-severe hearing impairment than healthy newborns, it is important to carry out screening during the neonatal period in those with risk factors associated with sensorineural and/or conductive hearing loss (Joint Committee on Infant Hearing 1994, Position Statement 1995).

BAEPs using broad-band clicks, either performed by a skilled technician using conventional equipment, or performed by a research nurse using automated equipment, is regarded as the most objective and reliable method of evaluating peripheral auditory function in neonates. A prolonged latency of wave I, associated with a normal I–V interpeak latency is suggestive of an audiological abnormality, while a normal wave I latency, associated with a prolonged I–V interpeak latency indicates a delay in central conduction time (Guinard *et al.* 1988). In a recent large multicenter trial in Germany using automated ABR, familial hearing loss, bacterial infections, and craniofacial abnormalities were found to be significant risk factors in a cohort of 777 neonates with risk factors for hearing disorders (Meyer *et al.* 1999) (Table 12.1).

When BAEP threshold abnormalities are found (i.e. absent responses at 30–40 dBnHL at term age), the test should be repeated 3 months later, preferably using frequency-specific

**Table 12.1 Risk factors for hearing impairment and for which BAEP screening is recommended**

- Family history of hearing loss
- *In utero* infections
- Craniofacial anomalies
- Birth weight <1500 g
- Severe hyperbilirubinemia
- Ototoxic medications
- Bacterial meningitis
- Perinatal asphyxia
- Mechanical ventilation >5 days
- Stigmata suggestive of a syndrome associated with hearing loss

*Source*: Joint Committee on Infant Hearing 1994, Position Statement (1995).

and bone conduction BAEPs. Frequency-specific techniques may be used to evaluate hearing thresholds at different frequencies, whereas bone conduction BAEPs are useful to assess the extent of a conductive loss (Picton *et al.* 1994).

## ASSESSMENT OF OTHER DISORDERS

### Prediction of outcome in high-risk neonates

Given that BAEPs assess the integrity of the ascending neuraxis projecting through the brainstem, abnormalities may reflect more diffuse injury to the CNS structures along the auditory pathway (Jewett & Williston 1971). This assumption has instigated several attempts to correlate neonatal BAEP with neurologic outcome. The results of these studies are not always in agreement, possibly because of significant variations in the methodology used and the different samples tested. In high-risk infants it is recommended to perform BAEPs as close to discharge as possible. Both peripheral and central abnormalities may be transient and will have resolved at term age in a number of cases, thus increasing the positive predictive power for the development of neurologic sequelae (Stockard *et al.* 1983).

Hecox & Cone (1981) studied BAEPs in 126 infants who suffered an acute anoxic insult, including 13 full-term neonates with HIE, and found that a decreased amplitude of wave V, and subsequently decreased V:I amplitude ratio, was always related to severe neurologic impairment. Prolonged wave I–V interpeak latencies were also noted and they stressed that normal amplitude ratios did not ensure normal neurologic outcome. Features associated with neurodevelopmental impairment in both preterm and term infants include absent later peaks (waves II to V), significantly depressed wave V amplitudes, and persistence of prolonged interwave latencies (Fig. 12.2). These are signs of increased central conduction time (for a review of 32 studies, see Murray *et al.* 1985). A high specificity is reported by Majnemer, but approximately half of their high-risk infants with an abnormal neurodevelopment at 1 year had normal neonatal BAEPs (Majnemer *et al.* 1988). A more recent study of 56 very low birth weight infants showed that bilateral abnormalities in predischarge BAEPs were predictive of subsequent performance on measures of intelligence quotient, language, and reading at the age of eight years, whereas there was no correlation with unilateral BAEP abnormalities (Cox *et al.* 1992).

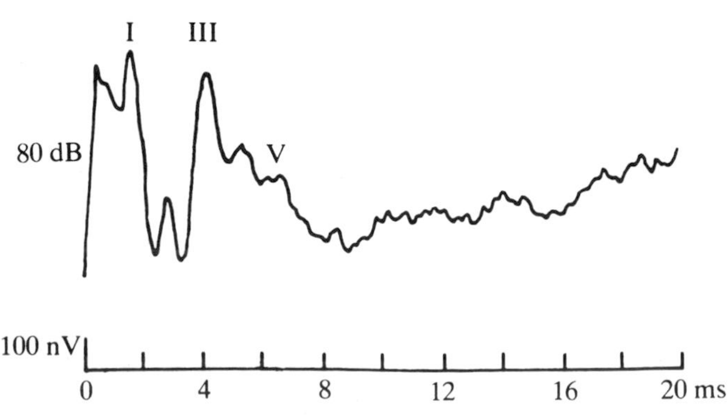


Figure 12.2 BAEP on day 3 of a full term infant who developed HIE stage III. A decreased wave V:I ratio is found.

The high incidence of severe neurologic sequelae in asphyxiated infants who had a normal neonatal BAEPs may be explained by the anatomical site of the lesions observed in infants sustaining HIE. Usually, neuroimaging techniques like cranial ultrasound and magnetic resonance imaging show that the periventricular and subcortical areas are involved more than the brainstem and auditory nuclei (Mercuri *et al.* 1994). Since VEPs and SEPs have proven to be more reliable predictors of neurological outcome, BAEPs have largely fallen into disuse for this purpose.

### BAEPs in hemorrhages and hydrocephalus

There is discussion in the literature as to whether BAEP latencies change in infants with periventricular and/or intraventricular hemorrhages (PVH/IVH). Beverley did not find significantly different latencies and amplitudes in preterm infants with severe PVH/IVH (Beverley *et al.* 1990). Karmel found abnormal waveforms and prolonged latencies, but this study did not discriminate between hemorrhagic and/or ischemic lesions (Karmel *et al.* 1988). Earlier, Fawer *et al.* (1983) had found three of four preterm infants who were shunted for post-hemorrhagic hydrocephalus to have shortened interpeak latencies. Other groups studying infants with hydrocephalus reported a decrease of the wave V:I amplitude ratio associated with elevated thresholds (Edwards *et al.* 1985; Lary *et al.* 1989).

### BAEPs in myelomeningocele

In infants with myelomeningocele, often associated with Arnold Chiari malformation, the BAEPs may have predictive power as to the severity and emergency of clinical brainstem symptoms, as the brainstem is distorted and elongated due to the downward dislocation of the pons, medulla oblongata, and the fourth ventricle. Many reports consider data in infants beyond the neonatal period: infants with normal BAEPs do not develop symptomatic Arnold Chiari malformation, whereas abnormal BAEPs have been reported to be associated with neurologic symptoms. These findings were confirmed in neonates (Mori *et al.* 1988; Worley *et al.* 1994; Taylor *et al.* 1996b).

### Effect of intrauterine growth restriction on BAEPs

Considering the effects of intrauterine growth restriction (IUGR) on BAEPs, infants who were small for gestational age showed shorter wave V latencies and interpeak latencies relative to those appropriate for gestational age infants (Pettigrew *et al.* 1985; Eldredge & Salamy 1996). These studies lend support to the view that infants with IUGR show accelerated neurologic maturation, but Soares posed the idea that the changes may be due to immaturity of the basal cochlea (Soares *et al.* 1992).

Sarda *et al.* (1992) compared the BAEPs of IUGR infants born to hypertensive and non-hypertensive mothers. IUGR infants of the hypertensive mothers showed significantly shortened interpeak latencies. These authors suggest that the reduced interpeak latencies may have been caused by a change in the development of neurotransmitters and catecholaminergic systems due to a major chronic stress.

#### BAEPs in hyperbilirubinemia

The major reason for performing BAEPs in infants with hyperbilirubinemia is the possibility to study the correlation of BAEP abnormalities with changes in bilirubin levels and thus assess the effect of exchange transfusions, keeping in mind that careful management of hyperbilirubinemia may reduce the incidence of sensorineural deafness. De Vries *et al.* (1987b) found sensorineural deafness to be strongly associated with the duration of hyperbilirubinemia. Most abnormalities disappear when the serum bilirubin decreases (Hung 1989), but Soares did not find significant abnormalities in neonates sustaining either mild or severe hyperbilirubinemia (Soares *et al.* 1989). This supports the hypothesis that additional risk factors like acidosis may be operating.

#### BAEPs in extracorporeal membrane oxygenation (ECMO)

A new hazard in neonatology is the sequelae of ECMO, a rescue therapy in severe respiratory failure in term neonates. Since hypoxia and ischemia are related to their underlying illness and the invasive ECMO-procedure, they are at risk of neurologic impairment and sensorineural deafness. Desai *et al.* (1997) found a sensitivity of only 42% and a specificity of 76% for elevated thresholds in neonatal BAEP to predict subsequent hearing loss in a sample of 80 neonates. However, abnormal neonatal BAEPs increased the probability of developing a receptive language delay, even when the BAEP subsequently normalized. Their high abnormality rate may be due to the threshold criteria as to what is considered to be a normal BAEP. Other studies reported abnormal BAEPs in 16–75% of infants treated with ECMO, which was associated with either sensorineural hearing loss and/or developmental delay (Hofkosh *et al.* 1991; Schumacher *et al.* 1991; Kawashiro 1994, Lasky *et al.* 1998). In the latter report it was striking that 7/9 ECMO survivors with hearing loss passed their newborn BAEP screen, although high false-negative rates were found in the other reports as well. The risk of progressive hearing loss warrants a repeated test at the age of 3–4 months (Desai *et al.* 1997).

#### BAEPs in cytomegalovirus (CMV) infection

CMV infection is a well-known cause of severe neurologic handicap. Sensorineural hearing loss, especially when the infection occurs in early pregnancy, is well recognized, but hearing deficits and minor neurologic handicap may occur in late infections (Steinlin *et al.* 1996). Recent reports show that among children with documented asymptomatic congenital CMV, associated with hearing loss, further deterioration occurred in 50% or more of the cases; a delayed onset of sensorineural hearing loss was observed in 18%. Infants with symptomatic congenital CMV infection show an even higher and also cumulating incidence of sensorineural hearing loss (Fowler *et al.* 1997, 1999). This progressive nature of the hearing loss emphasizes the need for continued monitoring of the hearing status in these infants.

## CLINICAL APPLICATIONS OF VISUAL EVOKED POTENTIALS

### ASSESSMENT OF OPHTHALMOLOGIC DISORDERS (see also Chapter 38)

The development of visual function is usually not the major concern for infants in the neonatal intensive care unit, although early application of rehabilitation programs may reduce the consequences of a visual handicap. However, when the infant has stabilized, there are several possibilities to obtain information about the visual system. Absence of fixation and following, absent blink reflex, or nystagmus may indicate disturbance of vision and these require further investigation. Although FVEPs are not suitable for measurement of visual acuity, they may be used to test the light sensitivity of the visual system, even when ophthalmologic disorders such as congenital cataract or optic nerve hypoplasia are present. PVEPs are a sensitive and quantitative indicator of lesions in the visual pathway and have the advantage that they show less intra- and inter-subject variability of latency and waveform than do FVEPs. The use of a psychophysical method like the acuity card procedure (McDonald *et al.* 1985), which can easily be performed in stable, alert neonates, in combination with a VEP-modality may be very useful, for example in infants with delayed visual maturation (Lambert *et al.* 1989; Russell-Eggitt *et al.* 1998).

#### FVEPs as predictor for cerebral visual impairment

FVEPs are good predictors of cerebral visual impairment (CVI) following perinatal asphyxia as shown by McCulloch & Skarf (1991), Wong (1991) and McCulloch & Taylor (1992), who reported a strong association between neonatal FVEPs and visual outcome at 2.5–4.5 years. Others found a high predictive value of abnormal or absent FVEPs for the development of CVI in infants who showed extensive cystic leukomalacia on cranial ultrasound (de Vries *et al.* 1987a), especially when this was associated with abnormal findings using the acuity card procedure (Eken *et al.* 1996).

### ASSESSMENT OF OTHER DISORDERS

#### Prediction of outcome in high-risk neonates

From the late 1970s onward, several authors assessed the predictive value of FVEPs for neurodevelopmental outcome in neonates. The first reports, however, did not make a distinction between term and preterm infants, but assessed heterogeneous groups of high-risk infants including those who had sustained asphyxia, respiratory distress, neurologic disorders, etc. Permanent VEP-abnormalities at repeated investigations were considered to be a serious prognostic sign in 57 term and preterm newborns with different degrees of perinatal asphyxia studied by Hrbek *et al.* (1977). However, no correlation could be drawn between FVEPs and long-term prognosis, given that the serial examinations were conducted over a 3-week period. Hakamada *et al.* (1981) studied BAEPs and FVEPs in 41 infants with a gestational age of 36–41 weeks who had various perinatal disorders, including 21 infants with perinatal asphyxia, during the first year of life. Absent responses or abnormal waveforms were associated with severe neurologic damage. In infants with cerebral palsy or mental retardation, initially abnormal VEPs recovered within 2–3 months of age.

Placzek *et al.* (1985) found delayed maturation of FVEPs in the neurologically abnormal infants of a cohort of 70 preterm infants, 26 of whom had germinal layer or periventricular hemorrhage on cranial ultrasound, but they had a short follow-up period. Häkkinen *et al.* (1987) assessed the predictive value of FVEPs in 109 high-risk term and preterm infants with a variety of risk factors for adverse neurologic outcome at the age of 1 year. They reported absent FVEPs or an abnormal waveform to predict a poor outcome, but they were not able to predict moderate abnormality.

### Preterm infants

FVEPs were not found to be a good prognostic indicator of neurodevelopmental outcome in 62 preterm infants longitudinally studied up to the age of 18 months by Beverley *et al.* (1990). Pryds & Greisen (1990) observed rapid and consistent attenuation of single FVEPs in 32 preterm infants during hypoxic episodes, with an instantaneous recovery of the response after normalization of the $PaO_2$. Low cerebral blood flow, severe hypocapnia or severe arterial hypotension were not found to affect the VEP, provided there was a normal oxygen tension.

Ekert *et al.* (1997a) were not able to predict abnormal developmental outcome in 123 preterm infants on the basis of abnormal FVEPs. In a recent study of 81 preterm infants, a sensitivity and specificity of 60% and 92% respectively were found for abnormal FVEPs in the subsequent development of cerebral palsy (Shepherd *et al.* 1999). A delayed negative wave N300 before term and an absent positive wave P200 at term age were associated with adverse outcome.

### Term infants

In groups of term infants, very high correlation of FVEP and outcome was found. This was especially reported by Taylor's group, who found a high correlation of FVEPs with neurodevelopmental outcome in several groups of full-term asphyxiated infants studied from birth to 24 months of age (Whyte *et al.* 1986; McCulloch & Skarf 1991; Muttitt *et al.* 1991; Taylor *et al.* 1992). Repeated FVEPs were recorded during the first week of life. Absent FVEPs carried a poor prognosis, while persistently abnormal FVEPs also predicted an abnormal outcome. Normal FVEPs before the end of the first week had an accuracy rate of 87% for a normal outcome for the whole group and up to 93% for infants who sustained HIE Sarnat stage II. When comparing SEPs with VEPs, the VEPs appeared to be more resistant to an insult than SEPs, as normal VEPs were not always associated with a normal outcome. The association of SEPs and VEPs increases the prognostic reliability. Still, Taylor *et al.* (1992) recommend VEPs to be conducted first, as they are the most easy to record, and to perform SEPs only when in doubt about the prognosis. Similar findings have been reported by Scalais *et al.* (1998) who analyzed the degree of EP (either BAEP, VEP, or SEP) abnormality by using a scoring system. Eken *et al.* (1995) studied 34 full term asphyxiated infants within the first six hours of life, to be able to select infants at risk of developing a major handicap who might benefit from treatment with neuro-protective agents. FVEPs were found to have a lower predictive value (PPV 77%) than did cerebral function monitoring (PPV 84.2%) and SEPs (PPV 81.8%) at this early stage.

We compared the predictive value of SEPs and VEPs for adverse neurologic outcome in all stages of HIE (Table 12.2), and separately for HIE stage II (Table 12.3), as prediction of outcome in this subgroup is more difficult than in either stages I or III. The predictive value in HIE stage II is lower than in the group as a whole. SEPs predict adverse outcome better than VEPs.

**Table 12.2 Predictive value (%) of SEP and VEP on days 1 and 3 in all stages of HIE**

| Stage | SEP | | VEP | |
|---|---|---|---|---|
| I-II-III | Day 1 (126) | Day 3 (82) | Day 1 (126) | Day 3 (82) |
| Sensitivity | 90 | 87 | 90 | 78 |
| Specificity | 78 | 91 | 64 | 77 |
| PPV | 80 | 83 | 70 | 70 |
| NPV | 89 | 91 | 87 | 84 |

PPV, positive predictive value; NPV, negative predictive value.

**Table 12.3 Predictive value (%) of SEP and VEP on days 1 and 3 in stage II HIE**

| | SEP | | VEP | |
|---|---|---|---|---|
| Stage II | Day 1 (43) | Day 3 (47) | Day 1 (43) | Day 3 (47) |
| Sensitivity | 80 | 77 | 70 | 69 |
| Specificity | 70 | 85 | 61 | 73 |
| PPV | 44 | 67 | 35 | 50 |
| NPV | 92 | 91 | 87 | 86 |

PPV, positive predictive value; NPV, negative predictive value.

### FVEPs in hydrocephalus

Ehle & Sklar (1979) found delayed latencies, fatigability, and asymmetries in 15 infants with documented hydrocephalus. The abnormalities improved in the post-shunt period, whereas VEPs worsened in cases of clinical progression of the hydrocephalus. Significant changes in the maturation curve of the P200 latency were noted by Guthkelch *et al.* (1982, 1984), particularly when the hydrocephalus was associated with an enlarged head or with infection. However, Placzek *et al.* (1985) found no relation between the presence of ventricular dilatation and the delay in maturation of the FVEPs. In infants who were successfully shunted, FVEP abnormalities improved rapidly, although the abnormalities did not correlate with head circumference or clinical status (George & Taylor 1987; Taylor 1992; see also Fig. 12.3). FVEP was not found to be a valuable prognostic tool for neurologic outcome in infants with myelomeningocele (Taylor *et al.* 1996b).

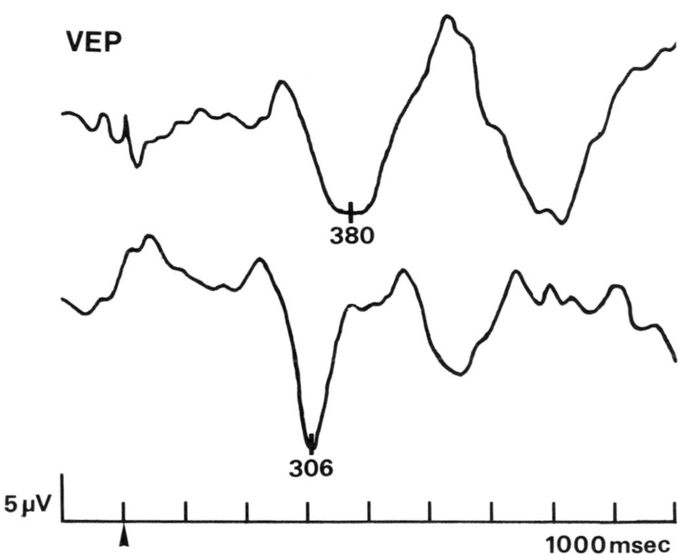


Figure 12.3 FVEPs in a preterm infant born at 28 weeks gestational age, who showed a large grade III hemorrhage with subsequent development of a large porencephalic cyst and posthemorrhagic ventricular dilatation on cranial ultrasound. At 30 weeks gestational age, a Rickham reservoir was inserted, and cerebrospinal fluid was removed twice daily. FVEPs were recorded before the insertion of the reservoir, showing a broad and delayed N300 (upper trace), and 2 weeks later, showing normalization of the N300 (lower trace). Arrowhead, moment of stimulus.

### Effect of IUGR on FVEPs

FVEPs have been used widely to assess the influence of IUGR on the development of the nervous system, but the results are not always in agreement. In 1972, Watanabe *et al.* compared the FVEPs of appropriate for gestational age (AGA) infants and small for gestational age (SGA) infants and noted no differences in latencies and waveforms. In contrast, Hrbek *et al.* (1982) reported a tendency towards longer latencies in SGA infants. They also noted late slow waves, which they attributed to neurologic immaturity. Pryds *et al.* (1989) studied single flash VEPs in 8 SGA infants and found no differences between VEP parameters compared with AGA infants. On the other hand, Petersen *et al.* (1990) found shorter latencies in SGA infants, which they attributed to the smaller head circumference rather than to stress-induced maturation. Stanley *et al.* (1991) reported normal short latency components and delayed long latency negative components and suggested that IUGR may affect the development of secondary activity in the striate cortex.

### FVEPs in hyperbilirubinemia

Usually, BAEPs are recorded in infants with hyperbilirubinemia. However, Chen & Kang (1995) studied the effect of hyperbilirubinaemia on serial visual evoked potentials up to 8 weeks after birth and found prolonged latencies and lower amplitudes in the infants with moderate or severe hyperbilirubinemia.

### FVEPs in infant respiratory distress syndrome

The FVEPs of 13 infants who sustained severe respiratory disorders were studied by Graziani *et al.* (1972). During periods of severe hypoxemia decreased amplitudes and even complete loss of VEPs were found and these changes could be reversed following resuscitation in 4 of 6 infants. However, 11 of the 13 infants subsequently died. Gambi *et al.* (1980) compared the FVEPs of 13 neonates who suffered from respiratory distress with those of 35 healthy term and preterm newborns and found delayed peaks and inverse polarity in the infants who sustained moderate and severe respiratory distress. In the infants with slight anoxic damage, the VEPs normalized quickly; however, in some cases with severe respiratory distress, the changes were still present at 9 months of age. Pryds *et al.* (1989) studied 11 infants who were mechanically ventilated and 75 infants who were assisted by continuous positive airway pressure and found normal VEP parameters in both groups. Of the 86 infants, 18 had a radiological diagnosis of respiratory distress syndrome, of whom only 3 needed mechanical ventilation. These data suggest that the infants suffered from mild respiratory distress.

### FVEPs and dietary long-chain polyunsaturated fatty acids

Over the last few years attention has been drawn to the influence of dietary long-chain polyunsaturated fatty acids (LCP) on the rapid maturation of the nervous system and photoreceptors. Preterm infants may be LCP deficient, and both FVEPs and PVEPs have been used to assess the effect of LCP suppletion. Faldella *et al.* (1996) found morphological differences and significantly longer latencies in infants who were fed on traditional preterm formula, as compared to infants who were fed on breast milk or a preterm formula supplemented with LCP. Makrides *et al.* (1995) found higher

PVEP acuities in breast-fed and LCP supplemented formula-fed infants at 16 and 30 weeks of age, than in traditional formula-fed infants. However, it still has to be determined whether these changes are transient (Neuringer *et al.* 1994).

### FVEPs in substance use

The effect of prenatal substance use on FVEPs was investigated by Scher *et al.* (1998). Maternal alcohol use during the first trimester was associated with prolonged positive wave P200 latencies at 1 month of age, while tobacco use in any trimester was associated with prolonged P200 latencies at birth and at 18 months.

## CLINICAL APPLICATIONS OF SOMATOSENSORY EVOKED POTENTIALS

As there is a close proximity between the somatosensory and motor tracts, it was expected that abnormal SEPs in the neonatal period would be most predictive for an abnormal neurodevelopment.

### PRETERM INFANTS

#### Intracranial lesions

SEPs have been used in preterm babies to identify children at risk of adverse neurologic sequelae. Klimach & Cooke (1988b) found a close relation between SEPs recorded around term and the outcome at 6–16 months. In this study the SEP findings at discharge were more predictive of outcome than those at the first test. All children with bilateral abnormalities in negative wave N1 latency had a developmental delay. Majnemer *et al.* (1987, 1990) presented data of 34 low birth weight infants and those with an absent or persistently delayed N1 latency were found to have a major handicap. At reassessment aged 5 years of age they showed a high sensitivity (100%) and specificity (80%) for early SEP in relation to the long-term outcome (Majnemer and Rosenblatt 1995). Willis *et al.* (1989) studied 39 very low birth weight preterm infants with periventricular hemorrhage at 2, 4, and 6 months of age corrected for prematurity. A delayed N1 latency was predictive of an abnormal outcome but a single normal SEP predicted normal motor development in only 19 of 36 infants. Scalais *et al.* (1992) studied VEPs and SEPs in preterm neonates suffering from perinatal asphyxia and demonstrated a good correlation between VEPs and SEPs and subsequent neurologic outcome.

In a larger series, de Vries *et al.* (1992), found SEPs recorded around term in preterm babies to be less reliable than cranial ultrasonography. A normal N1 latency was no guarantee of a normal outcome as 14 of the 25 infants who developed cerebral palsy had a normal N1 latency at, or even before, 40 weeks postmenstrual age. Pierrat *et al.* (1993) studied 33 infants with extensive cystic leukomalacia: 27 had cysts in the periventricular white matter and 6 developed extensive cysts in the deep white matter. All but two of the 27 surviving infants had a reproducible N1 at discharge; in only 11 was it delayed, and normal in 14 infants. No N1 peak could be recorded in any of the infants with cysts in the deep white matter. All surviving infants developed cerebral palsy, irrespective of the N1 latency.

Ekert *et al.* (1997b) hypothesized that SEPs performed at a very early stage would be more predictive than SEPs performed at discharge, and therefore studied 88 preterm infants twice during their first 3 weeks of life. They were able to show a significant correlation between the early SEP appearance and subsequent development of cerebral palsy, but found a high number of false positives. In this study SEPs were less accurate than cranial ultrasound in the prediction of cerebral palsy. However, a normal early SEP, even in the presence of periventricular echogenicity on ultrasound, predicted a normal outcome in all but 1 of the 9 cases.

As preterm infants tend to develop spastic diplegia rather than quadriplegia, it was subsequently hypothesized that posterior tibial nerve SEPs would be more predictive than median nerve SEPs. White & Cooke (1994) were the first to test this hypothesis in preterm infants. They were indeed able to show a highly significant relation between bilaterally abnormal posterior tibial nerve SEPs and the presence of cerebral palsy at 3 years of age in a group of 50 neonates at risk of future neurodevelopmental impairment. Normal posterior tibial nerve SEPs were associated with a normal outcome in 24 of 25 infants. In this group of neonates posterior tibial nerve SEPs were more predictive of outcome than late cranial ultrasonography. Pierrat *et al.* (1997) subsequently compared the predictive value of SEPs following stimulation of both the median as well as the posterior tibial nerve with that of cranial ultrasound in 39 preterm infants. A normal posterior tibial nerve response almost guaranteed a normal outcome, but the test was very time consuming and the number of false positives was very high (sensitivity 95.6%, specificity 50%). The presence of a parenchymal lesion on ultrasound predicted cerebral palsy with a sensitivity of 95.6% and a specificity of 68.5%. The combination of an abnormal posterior tibial response and the presence of parenchymal brain lesions had the best predictive value, with a sensitivity of 91.3% and a specificity of 81.2%.

#### Hydrocephalus

George & Taylor (1987) recorded VEPs and median nerve SEPs in hydrocephalic neonates of less than 10 weeks of age and found that 83% had abnormal VEPs while less than half had abnormal SEPs. No correlation was found in this study between EP abnormalities and head circumference or clinical status, but the abnormalities improved dramatically within days of shunting in those infants in whom the shunting procedure was successful. De Vries *et al.* (1990) were able to show a decrease in N1 latency within 1 week following shunt insertion in 7 cases.

#### Hypothyroidism

Smit *et al.* (1998) measured median nerve SEPs in 200 preterm infants (gestational age <30 weeks) who were randomized to receive thyroxine or a placebo during the first 6 weeks of life. SEPs were recorded at 2 weeks of age, at term and at 6 months corrected age. No effect of thyroxine administration was noted on the N1 latency.

### Small for gestational age

Only a few studies have so far looked at the influence of IUGR on SEPs. Kjellmer *et al.* (1992) recorded SEPs and VEPs in a group of SGA infants. A high frequency of abnormal recordings were obtained in SGA babies and they had significantly longer latency periods for the primary SEPs than appropriately grown controls. Pierrat *et al.* (1996), performing median nerve SEPs in a large cohort of SGA preterm neonates, found a persistently delayed N1 latency in 25 out of 56 infants. None of these infants had ultrasound abnormalities and none developed cerebral palsy at follow-up. There was a trend for a higher developmental quotient in the infants with a normal SEP, but this did not reach statistical significance.

## FULL-TERM INFANTS

### Birth asphyxia

Hrbek *et al.* (1977) was the first to investigate the value of median nerve SEPs as a means of assessing cortical damage and predicting outcome in the asphyxiated newborn. In this study, however, neonates and infants were included. Asphyxia was defined according to Apgar score only and the duration of follow-up was variable. Lütschg *et al.* (1983), Majnemer *et al.* (1987) and Willis *et al.* (1987) reported SEPs to be reliable predictors of neurologic outcome in term and preterm infants but recorded SEPs after the early neonatal period. Gibson *et al.* (1992b) recorded SEPs during the first week of life in a population of term asphyxiated neonates. They found that the sensitivity of SEPs for adverse outcome was 100% with a specificity of 76%. De Vries *et al.* (1991, 1993) demonstrated that the predictive value of median nerve SEPs was better after the first few days of life. On day 3, SEPs had a sensitivity and a specificity of 89.6% and 86% respectively, and at discharge the value of both sensitivity and speci-



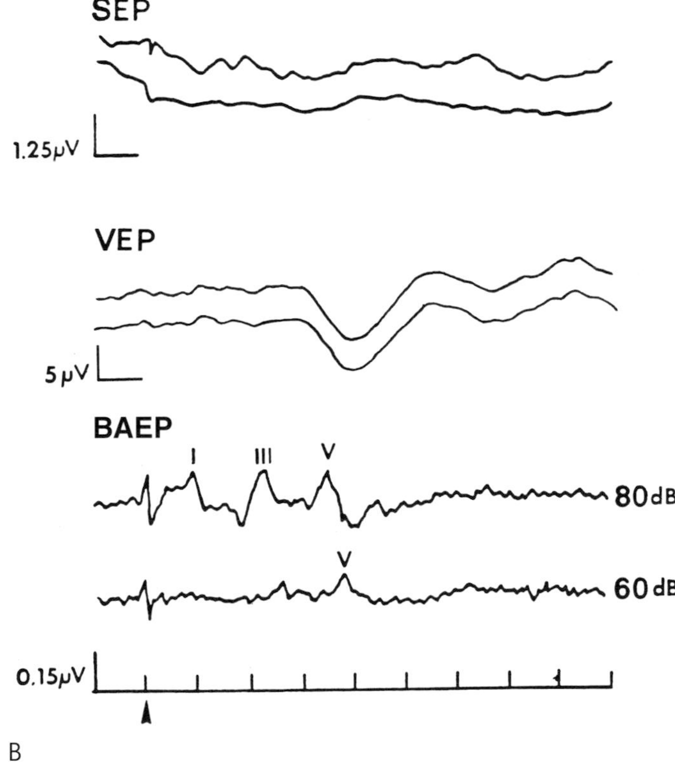


Figure 12.4 Effects of HIE on evoked potentials. (A) Normal SEP, FVEP, and BAEP on day 3 in a full-term infant with HIE stage I. Subsequent neurodevelopmental outcome was normal. (B) Absent SEP, delayed latencies and abnormal waveform in the FVEP, and increased threshold in the BAEP on day 3 in a full-term infant with HIE stage III. The infant subsequently died. Arrowheads, moments of stimuli.

ficity was 91%. Others studied the prognostic value of multimodality evoked potentials in asphyxiated babies. Taylor *et al.* (1992) recorded SEPs and VEPs several times in the first week and found SEPs to be more variable than VEPs but stated that normal SEPs in the first week were virtually always associated with a normal neurologic outcome (Fig. 12.4A).

Consistently abnormal SEPs were associated with a poor neurologic outcome in 85% of the cases (Fig. 12.4B). Scalais *et al.* (1998) recorded SEPs and VEPs in a group of 40 term infants with perinatal asphyxia. SEPs and VEPs demonstrated a good correlation with neurodevelopmental outcome, but SEPs proved to be superior to VEPs with an accuracy of 96% for SEPs and 86% for VEPs. A combination of the two techniques gave a higher predictive power; abnormal SEPs and VEPs were also more accurate in prediction of neurologic outcome compared with the Sarnat score. Of the 24 infants with a Sarnat stage II hypoxic–ischemic encephalopathy (HIE), 5 had a normal outcome and all had a normal SEP, while none of the 18 with a mild (3), moderate (4), or severe (11) handicap had a normal SEP within the first 72 hours of life. We also calculated the predictive value of SEPs and VEPs in HIE stage II on day 1 and day 3, but found lower predictive values than Scalais *et al.* (Table 12.4).

Most of these studies were performed beyond the first 24–48 hours (Hrbek *et al.* 1977; Gibson *et al.* 1992b; de Vries *et al.* 1991, 1993; Taylor *et al.* 1992). With the introduction of medical intervention trials, selection of infants who might benefit from early intervention should be carried out as soon as possible after delivery. Eken *et al.* (1995) therefore decided to study 34 full-term infants with HIE within 6 hours after delivery. Besides SEPs they also performed cranial ultrasonography, the resistance index of the middle cerebral artery, obtained with Doppler ultrasonography, VEPs, and amplitude integrated EEG (aEEG, see p. 175) recordings. The SEP and the aEEG had the best predictive value, with the SEP being slightly more predictive compared with the VEP. As might be expected, the role of cranial ultrasound and Doppler studies was very limited at this early stage. As the aEEG is a quicker and easier tool to use, this technique is now mainly used to select infants.

### Hypothyroidism

Bongers-Schokking *et al.* (1991) studied SEPs in neonates with primary congenital hypothyroidism during the first week of therapy. A maturational delay was found for all SEP parameters in neonates with congenital hypothyroidism. However, a delay of the N1 latency was not related to the initial T4 level nor to the T4 level at the time of examination. The comparison of the results of the SEPs with bone age suggested that SEPs are superior to bone age as parameter for the evaluation of neurologic maturation in infants with congenital hypothyroidism.

### Hyperbilirubinemia

Neonatal hyperbilirubinemia can lead to serious neurologic sequelae and auditory impairment (Johnston *et al.* 1967). However, the toxicity of bilirubin on the neonatal CNS depends on many factors, and outcome cannot be accurately predicted. One study (Bongers-Schokking *et al.* 1990) investigated SEPs in normal term neonates with neonatal jaundice, on the day the highest bilirubin values were reached, 2–3 days later, and at 5 weeks. In this study the central conduction time correlated positively with the bilirubin level, and both the peripheral and the central components of the SEPs were affected by neonatal jaundice. Full recovery was not yet obtained at 5 weeks. They suggested the use of SEPs to monitor daily the effect of bilirubin on the CNS.

### Hypoglycemia

There is controversy over both the definition of hypoglycemia in neonates and children and its significance when there are no symptoms. Koh *et al.* (1988) measured EPs, either SEPs or BAEPs, in relation to blood glucose concentration in 17 neonates and infants. With hypoglycemia they

**Table 12.4 Predictive values of different tests < 6hrs of age (n = 34) (Eken et al 1995)**

| | US | RI | SEP | VEP | CFM |
|---|---|---|---|---|---|
| Sensitivity | 42 | 24 | 95 | 89 | 94 |
| Specificity | 60 | 100 | 73 | 67 | 79 |
| PPV | 57 | 100 | 82 | 77 | 84 |
| NPV | 45 | 54 | 92 | 83 | 92 |

US: ultrasound; RI: resistance index; CFM: cerebral function monitor; PPV: positive predictive value; NPV: negative predictive value.

**Table 12.5 Summary of the clinical value of EPs in management of neonates**

| | |
|---|---|
| BAEPs | Reliable in screening for hearing loss in high-risk neonates<br>Record as near to term as possible<br>Repeated at 3 months post-term.<br>Predictive value for subsequent neurological outcome both in term and preterm infants is limited. |
| VEPs | Most convenient of the EPs to perform.<br>Poor predictor of outcome in preterm infants (FVEPs identify infants with extensive cystic PVL likely to develop cortical visual impairment)<br>High predictive value for adverse outcome in asphyxiated fullterm infants (abnormal or absent VEPs) |
| SEPs | Highest predictive value for adverse outcome in asphyxiated full-term infants.<br>May predict cerebral palsy in infants with preterms with PVL (only when recorded in the second week of life).<br>Posterior tibial nerve SEPs are difficult to record, but may be better predictor of outcome in PVL than median nerve SEP. |

were able to show that the latency to the peak of N1 became prolonged and that the waveform was less well defined. They concluded that the blood glucose concentration should be maintained above 2.6 mmol/l to ensure normal EP function in children, irrespective of the presence or absence of abnormal clinical signs.

## CONCLUSIONS

A summary of the clinical value of EPs is shown in Table 12.5.

### Key Points

- BAEP assessment at term is of clinical value in the diagnosis of hearing impairment
- BAEP in the neonatal period has limited positive predictive value for neurologic impairment
- Flash VEP is good predictor of cerebral visual impairment following perinatal brain injury in term infants
- Consistently abnormal SEP is the best predictor of poor neurologic outcome in term asphyxiated infants

## REFERENCES


Apkarian P, Mirmiran M & Tijssen R (1991) Effects of behavioural state on visual processing in neonates. *Neuropediatrics* 22: 85–91.

Araki A, Takada A, Yasuhara A & Kobayashi Y (1999) The effects of stimulus rates on the amplitude of median nerve somatosensory evoked potentials: the developmental change. *Brain Dev* 21: 118–121.

Bamford J, Davis A & Stevens J (1998) Screening for congenital hearing impairment: time for a change. *Arch Dis Child* 79: F73–F76.

Beverley D W, Smith I S, Beesley P *et al.* (1990) Relationship of cranial ultrasonography, visual and auditory evoked responses with neurodevelopmental outcome. *Dev Med Child Neurol* 32: 210–222.

Birch E E, Birch D G, Petrig B & Uauy R (1990) Retinal and cortical function of very low birthweight infants at 36 and 57 weeks postconception. *Clin Vis Sci* 5: 363–373

Bongers-Schokking C J, Colon E J, Hoogland R A *et al.* (1989) The somatosensory evoked potentials of normal infants: influence of filter bandpass, arousal state and number of stimuli. *Brain Dev* 11: 33–39.

Bongers-Schokking C J, Colon E J, Hoogland R A *et al.* (1990) Somatosensory evoked potentials in neonatal jaundice. *Acta Paediatr Scand* 79: 148–155.

Bongers-Schokking C J, Colon E J, Hoogland R A *et al.* (1991) Somatosensory evoked potentials in neonates with primary congenital hypothyrodism during the first week of therapy. *Pediatr Res* 30: 34–39.

Chen Y J & Kang W M (1995) Effects of bilirubin on visual evoked potentials in term infants. *Eur J Pediatr* 154: 662–666.

Chiappa K H (1985) Evoked potentials in clinical medicine: short latency somatosensory evoked potentials. In: Baker A B, Joynt R J eds *Clinical neurology*. Philadelphia, PA: JB Lippincott; pp. 26–55.

Chin K C, Taylor M J, Menzies R & Whyte H (1985) Development of visual evoked potentials in neonates. *Arch Dis Child* 60: 1166–1168.

Collet L, Soares I, Morgon A & Salle B (1989) Is there a difference between extrauterine and intrauterine maturation on BAEP? *Brain Dev* 11: 293–296.

Cox C, Hack M, Aram D & Borawski E (1992) Neonatal auditory brainstem response failure of very low birth weight infants: 8-year outcome. *Pediatr Res* 31: 68–72.

Cox L C, Martin R J, Carlo W A & Hack M (1993) Early ABRs in infants undergoing assisted ventilation. *J Am Acad Audiol* 4: 13–17.

Davis J M, Elfenbein J, Schum R & Bentler R A (1986) Effects of mild and moderate hearing impairments on language educational and psychosocial behavior of children. *J Speech Hear Disord* 51: 53–62.

Delorme C, Collet L, Morgon A & Salle B (1986) Study of auditory evoked potentials in preterm newborns with same conceptional ages at birth. In: Gallai V (ed.) *Maturation of the CNS and evoked potentials.* Amsterdam: Elsevier; pp. 352–355.

Desai S, Kollros P R, Graziani L J *et al.* (1997) Sensitivity and specificity of the neonatal brain-stem auditory evoked potential for hearing and language deficits in survivors of extracorporeal membrane oxygenation. *J Pediatr* 131: 233–239.

Desmedt J E & Manil J (1970) Somatosensory evoked potentials of the normal human neonate in REM sleep, in slow wave sleep and waking. *Electroencephalogr Clin Neurophysiol* 29: 113–126.

Desmedt J E, Brunko E & Debecker J (1976) Maturation of the somatosensory evoked potentials in normal infants and children with special reference to the early N1 component. *Electroencephalogr Clin Neurophysiol* 40: 43–58.

Despland P A (1985) Maturation changes in the auditory system as reflected in human brainstem evoked responses. *Dev Neurosci* 7: 73–80.

De Vries L S, Connell J A, Dubowitz L M S *et al.* (1987a) Neurological, electrophysiological and MRI abnormalities in infants with extensive cystic leukomalacia. *Neuropediatrics* 18: 61–66.

De Vries L S, Lary S, Whitelaw A G & Dubowitz L M (1987b) Relationship of serum bilirubin levels and hearing impairment in newborn infants. *Early Hum Dev* 15: 269–277.

De Vries L S, Pierrat V, Minami T & Casaer P (1990) Short latency cortical somatosensory evoked potentials in infants with hydrocephalus. *Neuropediatrics* 21: 136–139.

De Vries L S, Pierrat V, Eken P *et al.* (1991) Predictive value of early somatosensory evoked potentials in full term infants with birth asphyxia. *Brain Dev* 13: 320–325.

De Vries L S, Eken P, Pierrat V *et al.* (1992) Prediction of neurodevelopmental outcome in the preterm infant: short latency cortical somatosensory evoked potentials compared with cranial ultrasound. *Arch Dis Child* 67: 1177–1181.

De Vries L S (1993) Somatosensory evoked potentials in term neonates with postasphyxial encephalopathy. *Clin Perinatol* 20: 463–482.

Dubowitz L M S, Mushin J, de Vries L S & Arden G B (1986) Visual function in the newborn infant, is it cortically mediated? *Lancet* ii: 1139–1141.

Edwards C G, Durieux-Smith A & Picton T W (1985) Auditory brainstem response audiometry in neonatal hydrocephalus. *J Otolaryngol* 14: 40–46.

Eggermont J J & Salamy A (1988) Maturational time course for the ABR in preterm and fullterm infants. *Hearing Res* 33: 35–48.

Ehle A & Sklar F (1979) Visual evoked potentials in infants with hydrocephalus. *Neurology* 29: 1541–1544.

Eken P, Toet M C, Groenendaal F & de Vries L S (1995) Predictive value of early neuroimaging, pulsed Doppler and neurophysiology in full term infants with hypoxic-ischaemic encephalopathy. *Arch Dis Child* 73: F75–F80.

Eken P, de Vries L S, van Nieuwenhuizen O *et al.* (1996) Early predictors of cerebral visual impairment in infants with cystic leukomalacia. *Neuropediatrics* 27: 16–25.

Ekert P G, Keenan N K, Whyte H E *et al.* (1997a) Visual evoked potentials for prediction of neurodevelopmental outcome in preterm infants. *Biol Neonate* 71: 148–155.

Ekert P G, Taylor M J, Keenan N K *et al.* (1997b) Early somatosensory evoked potentials in preterm infants: their prognostic utility. *Biol Neonate* 71: 83–91.

Eldredge L & Salamy A (1996) Functional auditory development in preterm and fullterm infants. *Early Hum Dev* 45: 215–228.

Ellingson R J (1960) Cortical electrical responses to visual stimulation in the human infant. *Electroencephalogr Clin Neurophysiol* 12: 663–677.

Ellingson R J (1970) Variability of visual evoked responses in the human newborn. *Electroencephalogr Clin Neurophysiol* 29: 10–19.

Faldella G, Govoni M, Alessandroni R *et al.* (1996) Visual evoked potentials and dietary long chain polyunsaturated fatty acids in preterm infants. *Arch Dis Child* 75: F108–F112.

Fawer C L & Dubowitz L M S (1982) Auditory brainstem response in neurologically normal preterm and full term infants. *Neuropediatrics* 13: 200–206.

Fawer C L, Dubowitz L M S, Levene M I & Dubowitz V (1983) Auditory brainstem responses in neurologically abnormal infants. *Neuropediatrics* 14: 88–92.

Fowler K B, McCollister F P, Dahle A J *et al.* (1997) Progressive and fluctuating sensorineural hearing loss in children with asymptomatic congenital cytomegalovirus infection. *J Pediatr* 130: 624–630.

Fowler K B, Dahle A J, Boppana S B & Pass R F (1999) Newborn hearing screening: will children with hearing loss caused by congenital cytomegalovirus infection be missed? *J Pediatr* 135: 60–64.

Gambi D, Rossini P M, Albertini G *et al.* (1980) Follow-up of visual evoked potential in full-term and preterm control newborns and in subjects who suffered from perinatal respiratory distress. *Electroencephalogr Clinical Neurophysiol* 48: 509–516.

George S R, Taylor M J (1987) VEPs and SEPs in hydrocephalic infants before and after shunting. *Clin Neurol Neurosurg* (Suppl) 1: Abstr. 96.

George S R & Taylor M J (1991) Somatosensory evoked potentials in neonates and infants: developmental and normative data. *Electroencephalogr Clin Neurophysiol* 80: 94–102.

Gibson N A, Brezinova V & Levene M I (1992a) Somatosensory evoked potentials in the term newborn. *Electroencephalogr Clin Neurophysiol* 84: 26–31.

Gibson N A, Graham M, Levene M I (1992b) Somatosensory evoked potentials and outcome in perinatal asphyxia. *Arch Dis Child* 67: 393–399.

Gilmore R L, Brock J, Hermansen M C & Baumann R (1987) Development of lumbar and spinal cord and cortical evoked potentials after tibial nerve stimulation in the preterm newborns: effects of gestational age and other factors. *Electroencephalogr Clin Neurophysiol* 68: 28–39.

Graziani L J, Weitzman E D & Pineda G (1972) Visual evoked responses during neonatal respiratory disorders in low birth weight infants. *Pediatr Res* 6: 203–210.

Grose J, Harding G F A, Wilton A Y & Bissenden J G (1989) The maturation of the pattern reversal VEP and flash ERG in pre-term infants. *Clin Vis Sci* 4: 239–246.

Guinard C, Fawer C L, Despland P A & Calame A (1988) Auditory brainstem responses and ultrasound changes in a high-risk infants population. *Helvet Pediatr Acta* 43: 377–388.

Guthkelch A N, Sclabassi R J & Vries J K (1982) Changes in the visual evoked potentials of hydrocephalic children. *Neurosurgery* 11: 599–602.

Guthkelch A N, Sclabassi R J, Hirsch R P & Vries J K (1984) Visual evoked potentials in hydrocephalus: relationship to head size, shunting, and mental development. *Neurosurgery* 14: 283–286.

Hagberg B, Hagberg G & Zetterstrom R (1989) Decreasing perinatal mortality – increase in cerebral palsy morbidity? *Acta Paediatr Scand* 78: 664–670.

Hakamada S, Watanabe K, Hara K & Miyazaki S (1981) The evolution of visual and auditory evoked potentials in infants with perinatal disorder. *Brain Dev* 3: 339–344.

Häkkinen V K, Ignatius J, Koskinen M (1987) Visual evoked potentials in high-risk infants. *Neuropediatrics* 18: 70–74.

Harding G F A, Grose J, Wilton A & Bissenden J G (1989) The pattern reversal VEP in short-gestation infants. *Electroencephalogr Clin Neurophysiol* 74: 76–80.

Hecox K E, Cone B (1981) Prognostic importance of brainstem auditory evoked responses after asphyxia. *Neurology* 31: 1429–1434.

Hermann B S, Thornton A R & Joseph J M (1995) Automated infant hearing screening using the ABR: development and validation. *Am J Audiol* 4: 6–14.

Hofkosh D, Thompson A, Nozza R *et al.* (1991) Ten years of extracorporeal membrane oxygenation: neurodevelopmental outcome. *Pediatrics* 87: 549–555.

Hrbek A, Karlberg P & Olsson T (1973) Development of visual and somatosensory evoked responses in pre-term newborn infants. *Electroencephalogr Clin Neurophysiol* 34: 225–232.

Hrbek A, Karlberg P, Kjellmer I *et al.* (1977) Clinical application of evoked electroencephalographic responses in newborn infants. I. Perinatal asphyxia. *Dev Med Child Neurol* 19: 34–44.

Hrbek A, Iversen N & Olsson T (1982) *Clinical applications of evoked potentials in neurology.* New York, NY: Raven Press.

Hung K L (1989) Auditory brainstem responses in patients with neonatal hyperbilirubinaemia and bilirubin encephalopathy. *Brain Dev* 11: 297–301.

Jacobson J T, Jacobson C A & Spahr R C (1990) Automated and conventional ABR screening techniques in high-risk infants. *J Am Acad Audiol* 1: 187–195.

Jewett D L & Williston J S (1971) Auditory-evoked far fields averaged from the scalp of humans. *Brain* 94: 681–696.

Jiang Z D (1995) Maturation of the auditory brainstem in low risk preterm infants: a comparison with age-matched full term infants up to 6 years. *Early Hum Dev* 42: 49–65.

Johnston W H, Angara V, Baumal R *et al.* (1967) Erythroblastosis fetalis and hyperbilirubinemia: a five year follow-up with neurological psychological and audiologic evaluation. *Pediatrics* 39: 88–92.

Joint Committee On Infant Hearing 1994, Position Statement (1995) *Pediatrics* 95: 152–156.

Karmel B Z, Gardner J M, Zappulla R A *et al.* (1988) Brain-stem auditory evoked responses as indicators of early brain insult. *Electroencephalogr Clin Neurophysiol* 71: 429–442.

Karniski W (1992) The late somatosensory evoked potential in premature and term infants. I. Principal component topography. *Electroencephalogr Clin Neurophysiol* 84: 32–43.

Kawashiro N, Tsuchihashi N, Koga K, Ito Y, Kawano H (1994) Idiopathic deafness or hearing loss of unknown etiology following discharge from the NICU. *Acta Otolaryngol* Suppl 514: 81–84.

Kennedy C R, Kimm L, Cafarelli Dees D *et al.* (1991) Otoacoustic emissions and auditory brainstem responses in the newborn. *Arch Dis Child* 66: 1124–1129.

Kjellmer I, Thordstein M, Sultan B & Wennergen M (1992) Cerebral function in the growth-retarded fetus and neonate. *Biol Neonate* 62: 265–270.

Klein A J, Alvarez E D & Cowburn C A (1992) The effects of stimulus rate on detectability of the auditory brain stem response in infants. *Ear Hear* 13: 401–405.

Klimach V J & Cooke R W I (1988a) Maturation of the neonatal somatosensory evoked response in preterm infants. *Dev Med Child Neurol* 30: 208–214.

Klimach V J & Cooke R W I (1988b) Short latency somatosensory cortical evoked responses of preterm infants with ultrasound abnormalities. *Dev Med Child Neurol* 30: 215–221.

Koh T H H G, Aynsley-Green A, Tarbit M & Eyre J A (1988) Neural dysfunction during hypoglycemia. *Arch Dis Child* 63: 1353–1358.

Kos-Pietro S, Towle V L, Cakmur R & Spire J-P (1997) Maturation of human visual evoked potentials: 27 weeks conceptional age to 2 years. *Neuropediatrics* 28: 318–323.

Kurtzberg D & Vaughan H G (1985) Electrophysiological assessment of auditory and visual function in the newborn. *Clin Perinatol* 12: 277–299.

Laget P, Raimbault J, D' Allest A M *et al.* (1976) La maturation des potentiels évoqués somesthésiques (PES) chez l'homme. *Electroencephalogr and Clin Neurophysiol* 40: 499–415.

Laget P (1982) Clinical applications of cerebral evoked potentials in pediatric medicine: maturation of the somesthetic evoked potentials in normal children. In: Chiarenza G A & Papakostopoulos D (eds) *Proceedings of international conference on clinical application of cerebral evoked potentials in pediatric neurology.* Amsterdam: Excerpta Medica; pp. 185–206.

Lambert S R, Kriss A & Taylor D (1989) Delayed visual maturation. A longitudinal clinical and electrophysiological assessment. *Ophthalmology* 96: 524–529.

Lary S, Briassoulis G, de Vries L S *et al.* (1985) Hearing threshold in preterm and term infants by auditory brainstem responses. *J Pediatr* 107: 593–599.

Lary S, de Vries L S, Kaiser A *et al.* (1989) Auditory brain stem responses in infants with posthaemorrhagic ventricular dilatation. *Arch Dis Child* 64: 17–23.

Lasky R E (1984) A developmental study on the effect of stimulus rate on the auditory evoked brain-stem response. *Electroencephalogr Clin Neurophysiol* 59: 411–419.

Lasky R E, Wiorek L, Becker T R (1998) Hearing loss in survivors of neonatal extracorporeal membrane oxygenation (ECMO) therapy and high-frequency oscillatory (HFO) therapy. *J Am Acad Audiol* 9: 47–58.

Laureau E, Majnemer A, Rosenblatt B & Riley P (1988) A longitudinal study of short latency evoked responses in healthy newborns and infants. *Electroencephalogr Clin Neurophysiol* 71: 100–108.

Laureau E & Marlot D (1990) Somatosensory evoked potentials after median and tibial nerve stimulation in healthy newborns. *Electroencephalogr Clin Neurophysiol* 76: 453–458.

Leaf A A, Green C R, Esack A *et al.* (1995) Maturation of electroretinograms and visual evoked potentials in preterm infants. *Dev Med Child Neurol* 37: 814–826.

Lütschg J, Hänggeli C & Huber P (1983) The evolution of cerebral hemispheric lesions due to pre- or perinatal asphyxia (clinical and neuroradiological correlation). *Helvet Paediatr Acta* 38: 245–254.

McCall S & Ferraro J A (1991) Pediatric ABR screening: pass-fail rates in awake versus asleep neonates. *J Am Acad Audiol* 2: 18–23.

McCulloch D L, Taylor M J & Whyte H E (1991) Visual evoked potentials and visual prognosis following perinatal asphyxia. *Arch Ophthalmol* 109: 229–233.

McCulloch D L & Skarf B (1991) Development of the human visual system: monocular and binocular pattern VEP latency. *Invest Opthalmol Vis Sci* 32: 2372–2381.

McCulloch D L & Taylor M J (1992) Cortical blindness in children: utility of flash VEPs. *Pediatr Neurol* 8: 156 [Brief commun].

McCulloch D L & Taylor M (1994) Early maturation of the visual evoked potential (VEP): comparison of flash and pattern. *Invest Ophthalmol Vis Sci* Abstr. 35: 2028.

McDonald M A, Dobson V, Sebris S L, Baitch L, Varner D, Teller D Y (1985) The acuity card procedure: a rapid test of infant acuity. *Invest Ophthalmol Vis Sci* 26: 1158–1162.

Majnemer A, Rosenblatt B, Riley P *et al.* (1987) Somatosensory evoked response abnormalities in high-risk newborns. *Pediatr Neurol* 3: 350–355.

Majnemer A, Rosenblatt B & Riley P (1988) Prognostic significance of the auditory brainstem evoked response in high-risk neonates. *Dev Med Child Neurol* 30: 43–52.

Majnemer A, Rosenblatt B & Riley P S (1990) Prognostic significance of multimodality evoked response testing in high-risk newborns. *Pediatr Neurol* 6: 367–374.

Majnemer A & Rosenblatt B (1995) Prediction of outcome at school entry in neonatal intensive care unit survivors, with use of clinical and electrophysiologic techniques. *J Pediatr* 127: 823–830.

Makrides M, Neumann M, Simmer K *et al.* (1995) Are long-chain polyunsaturated fatty acids essential nutrients in infancy? *Lancet* 345: 1463–1468.

Marg E, Freeman D N, Peltzman P & Goldstein P J (1975) Visual acuity development in human infants: evoked potential measurements. *Invest Ophthalmol Vis Sci* 15: 150–153.

Markides A (1986) Age at fitting of hearing aids and speech intelligibility. *Br J Audiol* 20: 165–167.

Mercuri E, von Siebenthal K, Daniels H *et al.* (1994) Multimodality evoked responses in the neurological assessment of the newborn. *Eur J Pediatr* 153: 622–631.

Mercuri E, Braddick O, Atkinson J *et al.* (1998) Orientation-reversal and phase-reversal visual evoked potentials in full term infants with brain lesions: a longitudinal study. *Neuropediatrics* 29: 169–174.

Meyer C, Witte J, Hildmann A *et al.* (1999) Neonatal screening for hearing disorders in infants at risk: incidence, risk factors, and follow-up. *Pediatrics* 104: 900–904.

Minami T, Kukita J, Nakayama H & Ueda K (1996) Maturational changes of VEPs in normal premature neonates: a longitudinal study. *Brain Dev* 18: 46–49.

Mori K, Uchida Y, Nishimura T & Eghwrudjakpor P (1988) Brainstem auditory evoked potentials in Chiari-II malformation. *Child Nerv Syst* 4: 154–157.

Murray A D, Javel E & Watson C S (1985) Prognostic validity of auditory brainstem evoked response screening in newborn infants. *Am J Otolaryngol* 6: 120–131.

Mushin J, Hogg C R, Dubowitz L M S *et al.* (1984) Visual evoked responses to light emitting diode (LED) photostimulation in newborn infants. *Electroencephalogr Clin Neurophysiol* 58: 317–320.

Muttitt S C, Taylor M J, Kobayashi J S & Whyte H E (1991) Serial visual evoked potentials and outcome in full-term birth asphyxia. *Pediatr Neurol* 7: 86–90.

Neuringer M, Reisbick S & Janowsky J (1994) The role of n-3 fatty acids in visual and cognitive development: current evidence and methods of assessment. *J Pediatr* 125: S39–S47.

Oudesluys-Murphy A M & Harlaar J (1997) Neonatal hearing screening with an automated auditory brainstem response screener in the infant's home. *Acta Paediatr* 86: 651–655.

Pasman J W, Rotteveel J J, de Graaf R *et al.* (1992) The effect of preterm birth on brainstem, middle latency and cortical auditory evoked potentials (BMC AERs). *Early Hum Dev* 31: 113–129.

Petersen S, Pryds O, Trojaborg W (1990) Visual evoked potentials in term light-for-gestational age infants and infants of diabetic mothers. *Early Human Development* 23: 85–91.

Pettigrew A G, Edwards D A & Henderson-Smart D J (1985) The influence of intrauterine growth retardation on brainstem development of preterm infants. *Dev Med Child Neurol* 27: 467–472.

Picton T W, Taylor M J & Durieux-Smith A (1992) Brainstem auditory evoked potentials in pediatrics. In: Aminoff M (ed.) *Electrodiagnosis in clinical neurology*, 3rd edn. New York, NY: Churchill Livingstone; pp. 537–567.

Picton T W, Durieux-Smith A & Moran L M (1994) Recording auditory brainstem responses from infants. *Int J Pediatr Otorhinolaryngol* 28: 93–110.

Pierrat V, Eken P, Duquennoy C *et al.* (1993) Prognostic value of early somatosensory evoked potentials in neonates with cystic leukomalacia. *Dev Med Child Neurol* 35: 683–690.

Pierrat V, Eken P, Truffert P *et al.* (1996) Somatosensory evoked potentials in children with intrauterine growth retardation. *Early Hum Dev* 44: 17–25.

Pierrat V, Eken P & de Vries L S (1997) The predictive value of cranial ultrasound and of somatosensory evoked potentials after nerve stimulation for adverse neurological outcome in preterm infants. *Dev Med Child Neurol* 39: 398–403.

Pike A A, Marlow N & Dawson C (1997) Posterior tibial somatosensory evoked potentials in very preterm infants. *Early Hum Dev* 47: 71–84.

Pike A A, Marlow N & Reber C (1999) Maturation of the flash visual evoked potential in preterm infants. *Early Hum Dev* 54: 215–222.

Placzek M, Mushin J & Dubowitz L M S (1985) Maturation of the visual evoked response and its correlation with visual acuity in preterm infants. *Dev Med Child Neurol* 27: 448–454.

Pope-Stockard J E & Sharbrough F W (1992) Brainstem auditory evoked potentials in neurology: methodology, interpretation, and clinical application. In: Aminoff M (ed.) *Electrodiagnosis in clinical neurology*, 3rd edn. New York, NY: Churchill Livingstone.

Pryds O, Trojaborg W, Carlsen J & Jensen J (1989) Determinants of visual evoked potentials in preterm infants. *Early Hum Dev* 19: 117–125.

Pryds O & Greisen G (1990) Preservation of single-flash visual evoked potentials at very low cerebral oxygen delivery in preterm infants. *Pediatr Neurol* 6: 151–158.

Pryds O (1992) Stimulus rate-induced VEP attenuation in preterm infants. *Electroencephalogr Clin Neurophysiol* 84: 188–191.

Purpura D P (1975) Morphogenesis of visual cortex in the preterm infant. In: Brazier M A B (ed.) *Growth and development of the brain.* New York, NY: Raven Press.

Ramkalawan T W & Davis A C (1992) The effects of hearing loss and age of intervention on some language metrics in young hearing-impaired children. *Br J Audiol* 26: 97–107.

Russell-Eggitt I, Harris C M & Kriss A (1998) Delayed visual maturation: an update. *Dev Med Child Neurol* 40: 130–136.

Salamy A, Eldredge L & Sweetow R (1996) Transient evoked otoacoustic emissions: feasibility in the nursery. *Ear Hear* 17: 42–48.

Sarda P, Dupuy R P, Boulot P & Rieu D (1992) Brainstem conduction time abnormalities in small for gestational age infants. *J Perinat Med* 20: 57–63.

Scalais E, François-Adant A, Langhendries J P *et al.* (1992) Multimodality evoked potentials assessment in hypoxic-ischemic preterm infants. *Ann Neurol* Abstr. 32: 480.

Scalais E, Francois-Adant A, Nuttin C *et al.* (1998) Multimodality evoked potentials as a prognostic tool in term asphyxiated newborns. *Electroencephalogr Clin Neurophysiol* 108: 199–207.

Scher M S, Richardson G A, Robles N *et al.* (1998) Effects of prenatal substance exposure: altered maturation of visual evoked potentials. *Pediatr Neurol* 18: 236–243.

Schulte F J, Stennert E, Wulbrand H *et al.* (1977) The ontogeny of sensory perception in preterm infants. *Eur J Pediatr* 126: 211–224.

Schumacher R E, Palmer T, Roloff D *et al.* (1991) Follow-up of infants treated with extracorporeal membrane oxygenation for newborn respiratory failure. *Pediatrics* 87: 451–457.

Shepherd A J, Saunders K J, McCulloch D L & Dutton G N (1999) Prognostic value of flash visual evoked potentials in preterm infants. *Dev Med Child Neurol* 41: 9–15.

Sininger Y S (1995) Filtering and spectral characteristics of averaged auditory brain-stem response and background noise in infants. *J Acoust Soc Am* 98: 2048–2055.

Smit B J, Kok J H, de Vries L S *et al.* (1998) Somatosensory evoked potentials in very preterm infants in relation to L-thyroxine supplementation. *Pediatrics* 101: 865–869.

Soares I, Collet L, Delorme C *et al.* (1989) Are click-evoked BAEPs useful in case of neonate hyperbilirubinaemia? *Int J Pediatr Otorhinolaryngol* 17: 231–237.

Soares I, Collet L, Desreux V *et al.* (1992) Differential maturation of brainstem auditory evoked potentials in preterm infants according to birthweight. *Int J Neurosci* 64: 259–266.

Spivak L G (1993) Spectral composition of infant auditory brainstem responses: implications for filtering. *Audiology* 32: 185–194.

Stanley O H, Fleming P J, Morgan M H (1991) Development of visual evoked potentials following intrauterine growth retardation. *Early Hum Dev* 27: 79–91.

Starr A, Amlie R N, Martin W H & Sanders S (1977) Development of auditory function in newborn infants revealed by auditory brainstem potentials. *Pediatrics* 60: 831–839.

Steinlin M I, Nadal D, Eich G F *et al.* (1996) Late intrauterine cytomegalovirus infection: clinical and neuroimaging findings. *Pediatr Neurol* 15: 249–253.

Stockard J E, Stockard J J, Kleinberg F & Westmoreland B F (1983) Prognostic value of brainstem auditory evoked potentials in neonates. *Arch Neurol* 40: 360–365.

Stuart A & Yang E Y (1994) Effect of high-pass filtering on the neonatal auditory brainstem response to air- and bone-conducted clicks. *J Speech Hear Res* 37: 475–479.

Stuart A, Yang E Y & Botea M (1996) Neonatal auditory brainstem responses recorded from four electrode montages. *J Commun Disord* 29: 125–139.

Taylor M J, Menzies R, MacMillan L J & Whyte H E (1987) VEPs in normal full-term and premature neonates: longitudinal versus cross-sectional data. *Electroencephalogr Clin Neurophysiol* 68: 20–27.

Taylor M J (1992) *The neurophysiological examination of the newborn infant.* London: MacKeith Press.

Taylor M J, Murphy W J & Whyte H E (1992) Prognostic reliability of somatosensory and visual evoked potentials of asphyxiated term infants. *Dev Med Child Neurol* 34: 507–515.

Taylor M J, Boor R & Ekert P G (1996a) Preterm maturation of the somatosensory evoked potential. *Electroencephalogr Clin Neurophysiol* 100: 448–452.

Taylor M J, Boor R, Keenan N K *et al.* (1996b) Brainstem auditory and visual evoked potentials in infants with myelomeningocele. *Brain Dev* 18: 99–104.

Tsuneishi S, Casaer P, Fock J M & Hirano S (1995) Establishment of normal values for flash visual evoked potentials (VEPs) in preterm infants: a longitudinal study with special reference to two components of the N1 wave. *Electroencephalogr Clin Neurophysiol* 96: 291–299.

Tsuneishi S & Casaer P (1997) Stepwise decrease in VEP latencies and the process of myelination in the human visual pathway. *Brain Dev* 19: 547–551.

Umezaki H & Morrell F (1970) Developmental study of photic evoked responses in premature infants. *Electroencephalogr Clin Neurophysiol* 28: 55–63.

van Straaten H L (1999) Automated auditory brainstem response in neonatal hearing screening. *Acta Paediatr* Supplement 88(432): 76–79.

Vles J S H, Casaer P, Kingma H *et al.* (1985) A longitudinal study of brainstem auditory evoked potentials of preterm infants. *Dev Med Child Neurol* 29: 577–585.

Watanabe K, Iwase K & Hara K (1972) Maturation of visual evoked responses in low-birthweight infants. *Dev Med Child Neurol* 14: 425–435.

Watanabe K, Iwase K & Hara K (1973) Visual evoked responses during sleep and wakefulness in pre-term infants. *Electroencephalogr Clin Neurophysiol* 34: 571–577.

Watkin P M (1996) Neonatal otoacoustic emission screening and the identification of deafness. *Arch Dis Child* 74: F16–F25.

Wattam-Bell J (1983) Analysis of infant visual evoked potentials (VEPs) by a phase sensitive statistic. *Perception* 14: A33.

White C P & Cooke R W I (1989) Maturation of the cortical evoked response to posterior nerve stimulation in the preterm neonate. *Dev Med Child Neurol* 31: 657–664.

White C P & Cooke R W I (1994) Somatosensory evoked potentials following posterior tibial nerve stimulation predict later outcome. *Dev Med Child Neurol* 36: 34–41.

Whyte H E, Taylor M J, Menzies R *et al.* (1986) Prognostic utility of visual evoked potentials in term asphyxiated neonates. *Pediatr Neurol* 2: 220–223.

Whyte H E, Pearce J M & Taylor M J (1987) Changes in the VEP in preterm neonates with arousal states, as assessed by EEG monitoring. *Electroencephalogr Clin Neurophysiol* 68: 223–225.

Willis J, Seales D & Frazier E (1984) Short latency somatosensory evoked potentials in infants. *Electroencephalogr Clin Neurophysiol* 59: 366–373.

Willis J, Duncan C & Bell R (1987) Short-latency somatosensory evoked potentials in perinatal asphyxia. *Pediatr Neurol* 3: 203–207.

Willis J, Duncan M C, Bell R *et al.* (1989) Somatosensory evoked potentials predict neuromotor outcome after periventricular haemorrhage. *Dev Med Child Neurol* 31: 435–439.

Wong V C N (1991) Cortical blindness in children: a study of etiology and prognosis. *Pediatr Neurol* 7: 178–185.

Worley G, Erwin C W, Schuster J M *et al.* (1994) BAEPs in infants with myelomeningocele and later development of Chiari II malformation-related brainstem dysfunction. *Dev Med Child Neurol* 36: 707–715.

Yoshinaga-Itano C, Sedey A L, Coulter D K, Mehl A L (1998) Language of early- and later-identified children with hearing loss. *Pediatrics* 102: 1161–1171.

# Section III
# Developmental anomalies

Chapter 13

# Congenital structural defects of the brain

S. Ashwal

## INTRODUCTION

Remarkable progress in developmental and molecular neurobiology has occurred in the past decade (Reid & Walsh 1996; Anderson 1997; Lendahl 1997; Levitt *et al.* 1997). The extraordinary and ever-increasing information about the sequence of molecular and structural events controlling this development, and likewise the effects of gene dysregulation in the pathogenesis of many well-recognized malformations, is emerging at an ever-accelerating pace (see Chapter 1). Neural embryogenesis is described in detail in Chapters 2 and 3. Of particular value has been the contribution of neuroimaging, especially magnetic resonance imaging, to define new syndromes and provide more refined correlations between clinical symptoms and brain dysgenesis (see Chapter 6). This chapter highlights selected aspects of these topics, and several recent monographs on developmental neuropathology (Sarnat 1992; Norman et al 1995), neonatal neurology (Volpe 2000), developmental neurobiology (Mize & Erzurumlu 1996), and pediatric neuroimaging (Barkovich 1995; Ball 1997) provide additional information.

## PATHOGENESIS

Malformations of the brain and spinal cord form during nervous system development. In theory, malformations result from 'an intrinsically abnormal developmental process' within the CNS (Spranger *et al.* 1982); however, malformations may also arise from extrinsic factors, such as teratogens and infections (see Table 13.1). Approximately 3% of newborns have serious multiple or localized malformations, including those of the CNS. These malformations account for 70% of fetal deaths and 40% of deaths within the first year of life (Freeman 1985; Evrard *et al.* 1989a).

Selective defects of morphogenesis may result in readily recognizable malformations. Some may be classified by the initial morphologic phase of development responsible for the defect (see Table 13.2) (DeMyer 1971). These abnormalities of morphogenesis include a primary mesodermal abnormality, failure of neural tube closure (neurulation), abnormal segmentation and sulci formation (sulcation), faulty proliferation, and migration of neurons and precursor cells, and agenesis-hypoplasia (Cohen & Lemire, 1982). This classification does not designate cause, as many malformations cannot be ascribed to known abnormal patterns of development; malformation processes may also span more than one developmental stage.

**Table 13.1 Etiology of human nervous malformations**

| |
|---|
| TERATOGENS |
| **Physical agents *in utero*** |
| Trauma |
| Fetal position or crowding |
| Hyperthermia |
| Radiation |
| **Infectious agents *in utero*** |
| Rubella virus |
| Herpesvirus types 1 and 2 |
| Cytomegalovirus |
| Mumps virus |
| Varicella virus |
| *Treponema pallidum* |
| *Toxoplasma gondii* |
| **Maternal metabolic derangement** |
| Phenylketonuria |
| Diabetes mellitus |
| Toxemia of pregnancy |
| Malnutrition |
| Hypoxia |
| Iodine deficiency |
| **Maternal toxin and drug exposure** |
| Carbon monoxide |
| Ethyl alcohol |
| Cocaine; other substance abuse |
| Antimetabolites |
| Antiepileptic drugs (phenytoin, trimethadione, valproic acid) |
| Isotretinoin (Accutane) |
| Vitamin excess or deficiency |
| Methyl mercury (Minamata disease) |
| GENETIC CONDITIONS |
| **Chromosomal abnormality** |
| **Single-gene inheritance** |
| Autosomal-recessive |
| X-linked recessive |
| Autosomal-dominant |
| **Multifactorial inheritance** |

**Table 13.2 Congenital defects related to embryonic stages**

| |
|---|
| **Neural tube formation** |
| Chiari syndrome |
| Cranioschisis (anterior neuropore) |
| Anencephaly |
| Encephalocele |
| Exencephaly |
| Meningocele |
| Rachischisis (posterior neuropore) |
| Meningocele |
| Myelomeningocele |
| Spina bifida |
| **Segmentation and cleavage** |
| Basilar impression |
| Holoprosencephaly |
| Klippel-Feil syndrome |
| Sprengel deformity |
| **Sulcation, proliferation, neuronal migration, organization** |
| Callosal agenesis |
| Cerebellar anomalies |
| Heterotopias |
| Lissencephaly |
| Macrogyria |
| Microgyria |
| Neuronal migration defects |
| Schizencephaly |
| **Myelination** |
| White matter hypoplasia |
| **Mesodermal development** |
| Craniosynostosis |
| Fibrous dysplasia |

The etiology of CNS malformations is unknown in more than 60% of patients. Hereditary factors that cause nervous system malformations include autosomal- and X-linked conditions (7.5%) and chromosome abnormalities (6%) (Carter 1976; Buckton *et al.* 1980). Single mutant genes may cause localized malformations (Holmes 1974). Multifactorial inheritance originates from several gene abnormalities and environmental factors, and may explain up to 20% of malformations (Carter 1976; Holmes *et al.* 1976).

Teratogens, such as trauma, hypoxia, hyperthermia (Layde *et al.* 1980), chemical toxins (Marsh *et al.* 1980), and drugs (Schardein, 1985); infections; radiation (Schull, 1997); maternal diabetes mellitus; phenylketonuria; and intrauterine conditions, such as constricted fetal position, account for 3.5% of nervous system malformations. Malformations associated with teratogens depend on the mechanism of action and specific time and duration of exposure during gestation. For example, isotretinoin (Accutane), a vitamin A analog used to treat acne, or high oral vitamin A intake (more than 10 000 IU per day) is a well-recognized human teratogen that acts during the first trimester (Lammer *et al.* 1985; Rothman *et al.* 1995). Defective neural crest migration and embryogenesis produce ear anomalies, posterior fossa cysts, microcephaly, heterotopias, Dandy–Walker syndrome, hydrocephalus, cranial nerve dysfunction, and congenital heart disease.

Fetal infections may lead to morphologic alterations, dysfunction without histologic change, and latent infection with subsequent abnormality (Catalans & Sever 1971; Evrard *et al.* 1989b). *Toxoplasma gondii*, rubella, herpes simplex, and cytomegalovirus infections can all cause malformations (Friede, 1989), as can fetal exposure to maternal human immunodeficiency virus infection (Belman *et al.* 1988). Functional teratogenicity is discussed in Chapter 15.

## NEURAL TUBE DEFECTS

### SPINAL DYSRAPHISM AND ASSOCIATED MALFORMATIONS

Spinal dysraphism may involve multiple germ layers with variable clinical manifestations. The condition includes lesions varying from a flat dermal aberration to a gross malformation of a region of the spinal canal and cord (Norman *et al.* 1995; French 1983). Approximately 4000 pregnancies are affected by spina bifida and anencephaly in the United States each year. The subtlest defect, spina bifida occulta, arises when the vertebral arches fail to fuse. When this abnormality is associated with an underlying malformation of the spinal cord, the condition is known as *occult spinal dysraphism*; accompanying abnormalities of the overlying skin and soft tissue usually occur (e.g. dermal sinus or dimple, skin tag, tuft of hair, port-wine stain) (Anderson 1975). When the meninges alone protrude through the defect, the malformation is termed a *meningocele*. Myelomeningocele, in which a portion of the spinal cord or nerve roots are displaced through the spina bifida defect into a sac, is the most complex and usually symptomatic condition. Other classifications of neural tube defects (NTDs) categorize the lesions as being either open or closed (McComb 1997; Norman *et al.* 1995).

#### Pathogenesis

Several hypotheses have been suggested to explain the evolution of myelodysplasia (Marin-Padilla 1991; George & McLone 1995; Norman *et al.* 1995). The most plausible theory is that the neural tube fails to close during embryogenesis (Laurence 1964; Osaka *et al.* 1978). Since the neural tube in humans has multiple sites of closure, the ultimate morphologic appearance is likely to depend on the specific site where failure of fusion occurs. Each of these sites is likely to be controlled at distinct gene loci (Van Allen *et al.* 1993). Multiple mechanisms have been described in animal models at the gene level that affect timing, location, and the process of neural formation that could account for the formation of such defects (Copp *et al.* 1990; Sarnat 1992; Van Allen 1996). Lack of closure of the posterior neuropore, the terminal location of normal neural tube fusion, may explain the reason lumbosacral malformations frequently accompany the disorder. Primary failure of neural tube closure does not account for other dysplastic characteristics of myelodysplasia unless an associated defect of neural induction in the mesoderm is involved.

Spinal dysraphism may be caused by a teratogenic agent acting before neural tube closure, which occurs during the fourth week of gestation. Teratogens capable of inducing myelodysplasia in experimental animals or human beings include radiation, maternal hyperthermia (Shiota 1982), gestational diabetes mellitus, vitamin A deficiency, or excess D-mannose or excess glucose in embryo culture, and valproic acid, carbamazepine, and folic acid deficiency (Kallen 1994; Holmes 1994; Sever 1995).

The role of folic acid is now recognized as important in the pathogenesis of spina bifida, although the specific mechanism remains unknown. This is discussed in detail in Chapter 19.

A variety of genetic models of neural tube defects (NTDs) have also been reported (George & McLone 1995). F52 is a myristoylated, alanine-rich substrate for protein kinase C, and F52-deficient mice manifest severe NTDs (Wu *et al.* 1996). Likewise, NTDs in mice have been reported in chimeric models deficient in expression of the fibroblast growth factor receptor-1 gene (Deng *et al.* 1997), in the splotch (Sp) mouse mutant with mutations in the Pax-3 gene (Epstein *et al.* 1993), in mice with allelic mutations of the breast and ovarian cancer susceptibility gene (BRCA1) (Gowen *et al.* 1996), and in mice lacking the platelet-derived growth factor receptor alpha (PDGFR-$\alpha$) gene that is associated with somite mesodermal development (Payne *et al.* 1997). In children with NTDs, isolated cases of mutations in the PAX1 and PAX3 gene have been reported (Hol *et al.* 1995, 1996).

## SPINA BIFIDA OCCULTA

Spina bifida occulta occurs in at least 5% of the population but is most often asymptomatic. Accompanying associated features may include dermal hyperpigmentation, a patch of hair, a lump, or a dermal sinus. This defect is located most often in the lower lumbar area involving the lamina of $L_5$ and $S_1$. When associated neurologic involvement is present, the condition is occult spinal dysraphism.

## OCCULT SPINAL DYSRAPHISM (see also Chapter 45)

The spectrum of occult spinal dysraphism includes distortion of the spinal cord or roots by fibrous bands and adhesions, intraspinal lipomas, dermoid or epidermoid cysts, fibrolipomas, subcutaneous lipomas (lipomyelomeningoceles), tethered cord, and diastematomyelia (Anderson 1975; Byrd *et al.* 1991). A tethered cord is the most common condition (McLone & La Marca 1997).

Symptoms of occult spinal dysraphism may be absent, minimal, or severe, depending on the degree of neural involvement. The patient may exhibit static or slowly progressive weakness or sensory loss in the legs or feet, gait difficulty, and foot deformity. Bowel and bladder dysfunction, such as incontinence, repeated bladder infection, and enuresis, may also occur. Symptoms are caused by abnormally formed neural tissue or pressure on the spinal cord or nerve roots. Common findings include diminished Achilles tendon reflexes, contracted heel cords, high arches, equinovarus deformity of the feet, decreased rectal sphincter tone, unequal leg or foot length, scattered sensory loss, Babinski signs, and trophic ulcers. Because many of these patients have associated posterior fossa or cervical cord malformations; neurologic involvement of the upper extremities may occur (Jansen *et al.* 1991). Ophthalmologic complications, usually observed when hydrocephalus is present, are also common and require careful evaluation and follow-up (Biglan 1990). Ultrasonography and MRI have greatly facilitated the diagnosis and management of these occult lesions (Fig. 13.1) (Gundry and Heithoff, 1994). A tethered spinal cord or lipoma can be detected without invasive myelography. Ultrasonography can demonstrate a poorly pulsatile, low-lying, or thickened conus medullaris in infants (Korsvik & Keller 1992). Surgical management is described on p. 764.

Recurrent meningitis from external contamination of CSF may result from occult congenital malformations along the spinal canal and neuraxis. These external connections include midline dermal sinus; temporal bone fistula to the middle ear, eustachian tube, or nasopharynx; neurenteric fistula; and basal encephalocele or meningocele involving the cribriform plate, sphenoid bone, or clivus (Hemphill *et al.* 1982). An MRI scan should be obtained, followed by appropriate surgical treatment.

## MENINGOCELE

Meningocele, a protrusion of meninges without accompanying nervous tissue, is not associated with neurologic deficit. The mass is usually evident as a fluid-filled protrusion covered by skin or membrane in the midline. Membranous lesions are found rostrally, and skin-covered lesions are more evenly distributed along the neuraxis. Very small subcutaneous lesions may remain undetected for prolonged periods.

When careful examination of patients with suspected meningocele reveals significant neurologic abnormality (e.g., equinovarus deformity, gait disturbance, abnormal bladder function) (Laurence 1964), the diagnosis of myelomeningocele is appropriate. These patients have entrapped nerve roots within the defect that can be identified during surgery.

A meningocele in the cranial or high cervical area may coexist with aqueductal stenosis, hydromyelia, or an Arnold–Chiari malformation. Membrane-covered meningoceles are more likely to be accompanied by severe abnor-

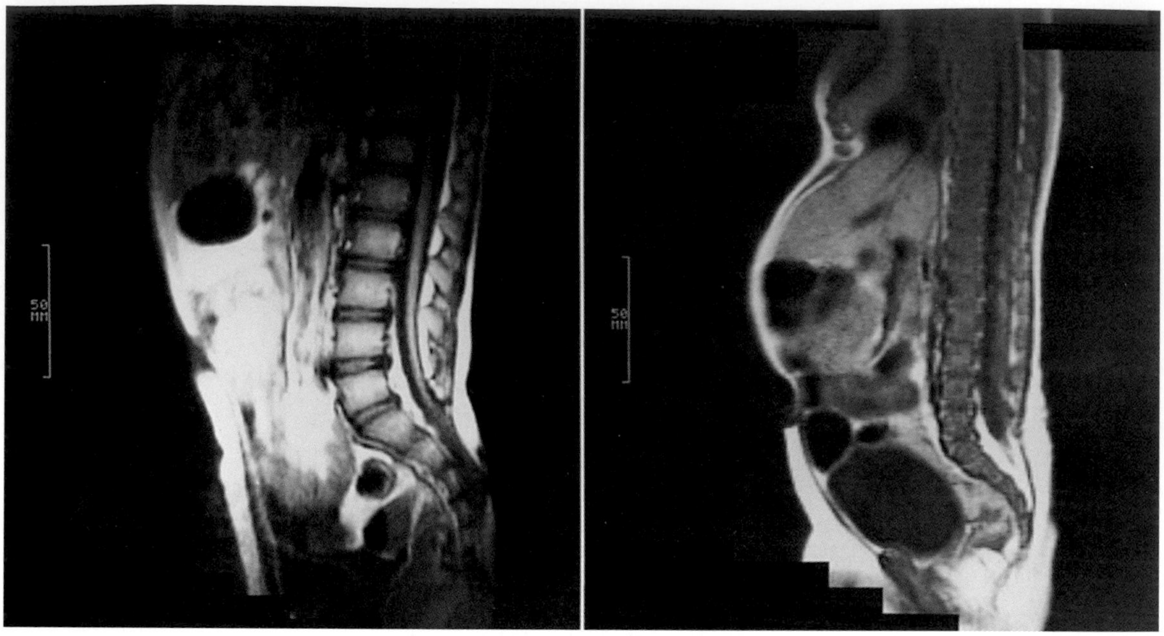

A B

Figure 13.1 (A) Tethered spinal cord. MRI scan demonstrates a low-lying spinal cord that ends at $S_1$–$S_2$. (A normal spinal cord terminates at $L_1$–$L_2$.) (B) Intraspinal lipoma: this MRI scan demonstrates a tethered spinal cord associated with a lipoma. (A, Courtesy Westchester County Medical Center, Valhalla, NY; B, Courtesy Division of Neurosurgery, New York Medical College, New York.)

malities; lesions covered with normal skin are often free of associated abnormalities (Fig. 13.2). Elective surgical treatment is recommended except for very small lesions (Steinbok & Cochrane 1991).

## MYELOMENINGOCELE

Myelomeningocele, the most complex of congenital spinal deformities, involves all underlying layers (i.e. spinal cord, nerve roots, meninges, vertebral bodies, skin). The spinal cord may be exposed because of complete failure of neural closure (myeloschisis). The birth-prevalence rate for spina bifida, which has steadily declined because of improved methods of prenatal diagnosis, has been estimated at 4.6 cases per 10 000 births (Lary & Edmonds, 1996). Antenatal diagnosis is discussed in Chapters 16, 17, and 18.

### Clinical characteristics

The mortality rate of myelomeningocele is approximately 50% in the absence of therapy; surgical intervention is required because death results from hydrocephalus, meningitis, and renal failure. The last complication is induced by chronic urinary tract infections, abnormal urodynamic function, and genitourinary tract abnormalities, such as progressive hydronephrosis (Liptak *et al.* 1988).

Myelomeningoceles may be situated at any longitudinal level of the neuraxis. The location and extent of the defect determines the nature and degree of neurologic impairment; rating scales have been developed in an attempt to standardize the evaluation of affected children (Oi & Matsumoto 1992). Lumbosacral involvement is most common. Thoracic defects are the most complex and are frequently associated with serious complications. Cervical cord involvement is different from myelomeningocele of the lower spine and is characterized by two types of abnormalities: the myelocystocele herniating posteriorly into a meningocele and a meningocele with or without an underlying split cord malformation (Steinbok 1995). The protuberant and fluctuant lesion is readily observable and palpable. Varying degrees of paresis of the legs, usually profound, and sphincter dysfunction are the major clinical manifestations. Congenital dislocation of the hips or deformities of the feet may also occur. Severe sensory loss and accompanying trophic ulcers may complicate the condition. Occasionally, only sphincter disturbances are present. Radiographs reveal the primary defect of the vertebral arch.

Hydrocephalus, a frequently associated defect, is the result of the Arnold–Chiari malformation; there may be associated aqueductal stenosis. Hydrocephalus, present in about 70% of patients with myelomeningocele, occurs most frequently when the lesion is situated in the thoracolumbar area, which is the case in 90% of patients (Lorber 1971). Although hydrocephalus was believed to be present at birth in only 25% of patients, modern imaging techniques almost always reveal the lesion to be present at birth. Lesions located more rostrally than others produce less lower motor unit paralysis and sphincter involvement. Caudal lesions in the neuraxis are typically associated with bladder and sphincter involve-

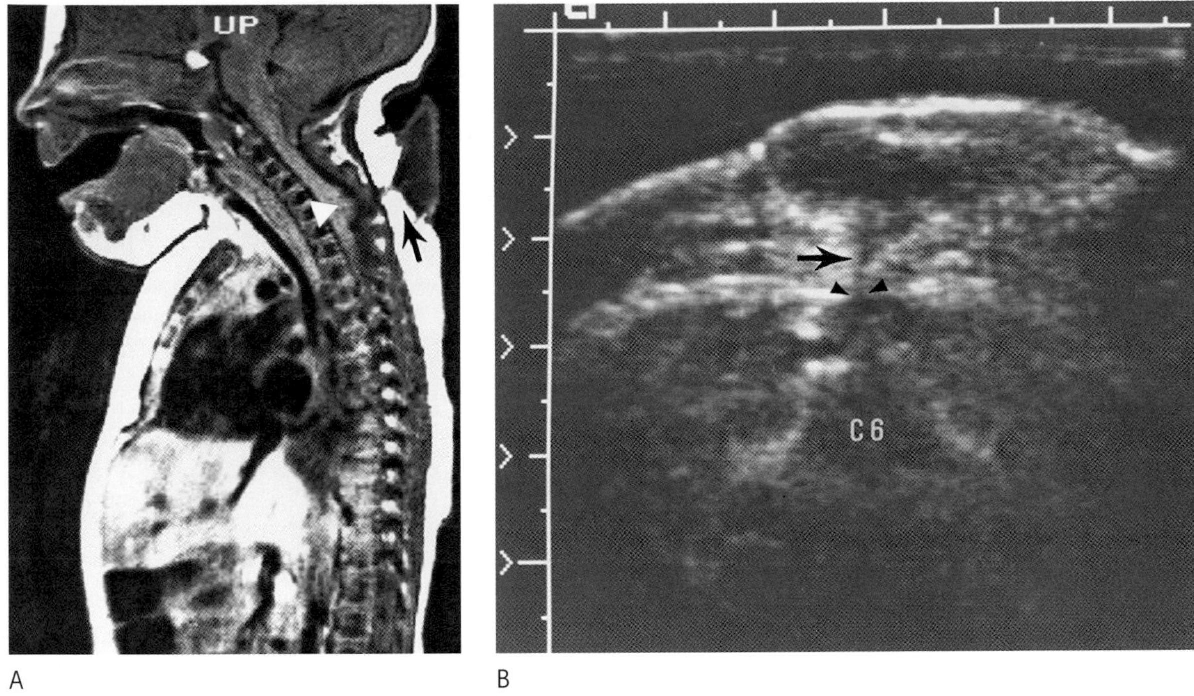


Figure 13.2 Cervical meningocele in a 3-day-old female infant. (A) $C_6$ meningocele (arrow) extending through small dorsal rachischisis, which is demonstrated on this T1-weighted sagittal MRI scan. Spinal cord is deformed (arrowhead) within focally widened thecal sac but does not extend into the dorsal cyst. (B) Small meningocele tract (arrow) and overlying meningocele are revealed well with transaxial sonogram. Note how the cord is tented toward dorsal opening (arrowheads). (Courtesy Joseph R. Thompson, Department of Radiation Sciences, Loma Linda University School of Medicine, Loma Linda, CA.)

ment. The profound paralysis that accompanies caudal involvement often prevents the patient from walking.

Myelomeningocele may be transmitted as an autosomal-recessive or dominant trait, although recurrence risk statistics suggest a polygenic or environmental etiology. This is discussed in detail in Chapter 14.

## Management

Management of a child with a myelomeningocele requires the efforts of many specialists (Colgan 1981; Liptak *et al.* 1988; Park 1992; McDonald 1995; Chambers *et al.* 1996). Treatment includes prevention of infection, surgical reduction and covering of the myelomeningocele, control of hydrocephalus, management of urinary dysfunction, and treatment of the paralysis and abnormalities of the hips and feet.

**Neurosurgical management**, antenatal and postnatal, is discussed in Chapters 42 and 45.

**Seizures** have been reported in up to 17% of patients with meningomyelocele and almost always occur in those with shunted hydrocephalus (Talwar *et al.* 1995). EEG abnormalities are non-specific. Additional CNS abnormalities seen in these patients are believed to explain the cause of seizures and include encephalomalacia, previous stroke, malformations, and intracranial calcifications. Seizures may be difficult to control, and frequently, exacerbation of seizures is associated with shunt malfunction or ventriculitis.

**Bladder dysfunction and urinary incontinence** pose major management problems and may be present at birth (Stone 1995; Boemers *et al.* 1996). Interruption of sacral nerve roots and fiber connections between the brainstem and sacral cord causes the dysfunction. Loss of sphincter tone, overflow incontinence, sacral and rectal loss of sensation, and loss of detrusor activity on cystometry are seen. In other patients with higher lesions, dyssynergia of reflex pathways results in irregular contractions of the bladder in conjunction with outlet obstruction. Normal bladder control occurs in 10% of children with myelomeningocele. Prevention of bladder infection requires intermittent catheterization to maintain low residual urine volumes and prophylactic antibacterial drugs (Buyse *et al.* 1995). Vesicoureteral reflux often develops during the second and third year of life and must be evaluated. Reimplantation of the ureters into the bladder or external drainage of the ureters either directly or through an ileal conduit may be helpful. Transurethral resection of the external sphincter has been recommended when ureteral dilatation occurs. The use of prosthetic devices emulating sphincters holds promise, as does selective sacral rhizotomy (Schneidau *et al.* 1995).

**Constipation and fecal incontinence** are common problems in children with spinal dysraphism and usually can be managed medically (Loening Baucke 1996). Dietary manipulation, oral and rectal laxatives, and manual evacuation are common treatments. Retrograde colonic enemas may also be successful (Scholler Gyure *et al.* 1996).

**Orthopedic defects** associated with paralysis, muscle imbalance, and spasticity may be severe and necessitate early intervention (Karol 1995; Locke & Sarwark 1996). Hip subluxation is usually treated with prosthetic splints or plaster casting (Alman *et al.* 1996). Sensory deficits of the casted skin areas frequently enhance the likelihood of skin ulcers. Severe foot deformities are seen in up to 80% of children and are treated with splinting or casting (de Carvalho *et al.* 1996). Physical therapy may help to preserve and extend the range of motion of the joints (McDonald 1995).

In infants and children, progressive leg or foot deformity, weakness, pain, or deterioration of gait or bladder function suggest restricted growth or tethering of the spinal cord. However, cord tethering may be found in many older children with spina bifida who are neurologically stable (McEnery *et al.* 1992). Stridor, retrocollis, weakness of the vocal cords, periodic breathing, episodes of desaturation, and apnea suggest a brainstem malformation (Ward *et al.* 1986). Evidence of brainstem dysfunction may be recorded by doing respiratory pneumograms with a carbon dioxide challenge (Petersen *et al.* 1995) or by using brainstem auditory-evoked response testing (Docherty *et al.* 1987; Sarnat 1992). These signs and symptoms indicate the possibility of an Arnold–Chiari malformation or a tethered spinal cord. The differential diagnosis of delayed deterioration in a child with repaired meningomyelocele includes a malfunctioning or infected shunt, seizures, scoliosis, hydrocephalus, hydromyelia, or an undetected second lesion of occult spinal dysraphism, such as a dermoid, epidermoid, or arachnoid cyst. Surgical repair of a tethered spinal cord and shunting or fenestration of large hydromyelic cysts can prevent decline of function (Charney *et al.* 1987; Sakamoto *et al.* 1991; Iskander *et al.* 1994).

### Outcome

Virtually all infants and children born with NTDs are provided with surgical and medical treatment. Previous studies reported that the 5-year survival rate for children with sacral lesions was 97%; for lumbar lesions, 93%; and for thoracic lesions, 75% (Welch & Winston 1987). These data suggest that selective criteria for surgical treatment offer the optimal outcome for the less severely affected child and less suffering and distress for the more handicapped patients with myelomeningocele. This is also discussed in detail in Chapter 45, p. 768.

### Counseling

Counseling is essential to ensure that parents understand the nature and severity of the deformities and the necessary surgical and long-term rehabilitative efforts (Liptak *et al.* 1988). Parents should also be aware of the patient's potential for intellectual and physical development. Also, awareness of the higher incidence of latex allergy in children with spina bifida is important to communicate to the family and others involved in their care (Konz *et al.* 1995).

## DIASTEMATOMYELIA

In diastematomyelia a midline septum divides the spinal cord longitudinally into two usually unequal portions extending up to 10 thoracolumbar segments (Bradford *et al.* 1991; Pang 1992). The septum may span the entire width of the spinal canal and is anchored to the ventral dura mater on the posterior aspect of the vertebral bodies. It may be attached posteriorly to the vertebral arch or dura mater. The septum is derived from mesoderm and it is composed of fibrous tissue, cartilage, or bone. The etiology of diastematomyelia is currently unknown.

### Clinical characteristics

Patients with diastematomyelia present with a congenital scoliosis or cutaneous lesion such as hairy patch, dimple, hemangioma, subcutaneous mass, or teratoma (Kothari & Bauer, 1997). They may also develop a progressive myelopathy with deformities of the feet, scoliosis, kyphosis, or discrepancy in leg length. Resection of the spur frequently does not result in clinical improvement. Resection of the spur should be performed in patients who have progressive neurologic manifestations; those without worsening symptoms should be observed until progression occurs and then resection performed (Miller *et al.* 1993). Diastematomyelia can be detected prenatally by ultrasonography (Anderson *et al.* 1994; Sepulveda *et al.* 1997). MRI is the preferred neuroimaging study for the evaluation of patients suspected of having this condition. Although most lesions occur in the lumbosacral region, presentations involving the cervical cord are reported. Diastematomyelia is also much more common in females (McLone & La Marca 1997). Urodynamic and electrophysiological studies are abnormal in about 80% of patients (Kothari & Bauer 1997).

## DIPLOMYELIA

Diplomyelia is a side-by-side or antero-posterior duplication or splitting of the spinal cord (Dias & Pang 1995; Norman *et al.* 1995). Two central canals are usually present, each surrounded by gray and white matter arranged in the normal pattern. The two cords are often completely reunited caudally but may remain separated to the tip of the conus medullaris. A bony septum may partly intervene. The two cords are often unequal, may be side-by-side (the most common position), or one may be dorsal to the other. These malformations are compatible with normal function; deterioration suggests the presence of diastematomyelia or tethering. The etiology of this condition also remains unknown.

More recently the term *split cord malformations* (SCMs) has been applied to diastematomyelia (SCM I) and diplomyelia (SCM II) (Dias & Pang 1995). SCMs can be divided into two types, based on the composition of the dural coverings and intervening mesenchymal tissue. Type I malformations are composed of two dural sacs and a bony or fibrocartilaginous spur; type II malformations are composed of a single dural sac and intradural fibrous bands. In either case the intervening mesenchymal elements contribute to progressive neurologic, urologic, and orthopedic deterioration from spinal cord tethering. The natural history of these lesions supports an early and aggressive operative approach to untether the spinal cord before clinical deterioration begins.

## SACRAL AGENESIS (see also p. 771)

Sacral agenesis, or caudal regression syndrome, is the complete or partial absence of the sacrum, hemisacrum, coccyx, and lower vertebrae, and often includes genitourinary and anorectal anomalies (Davidoff *et al.* 1991; Towfighi & Housman 1991). Although most cases are sporadic, maternal diabetes mellitus (Miller *et al.* 1981) and an autosomal-dominant form associated with chromosome 7q36 deletion are recognized (Schrander-Stumpel *et al.* 1988; Chatkupt *et al.* 1994; Lynch *et al.* 1995). The hallmark of this autosomal-dominant condition is the presence of partial sacral agenesis with an intact first sacral vertebra, a presacral mass, and an anorectal malformation.

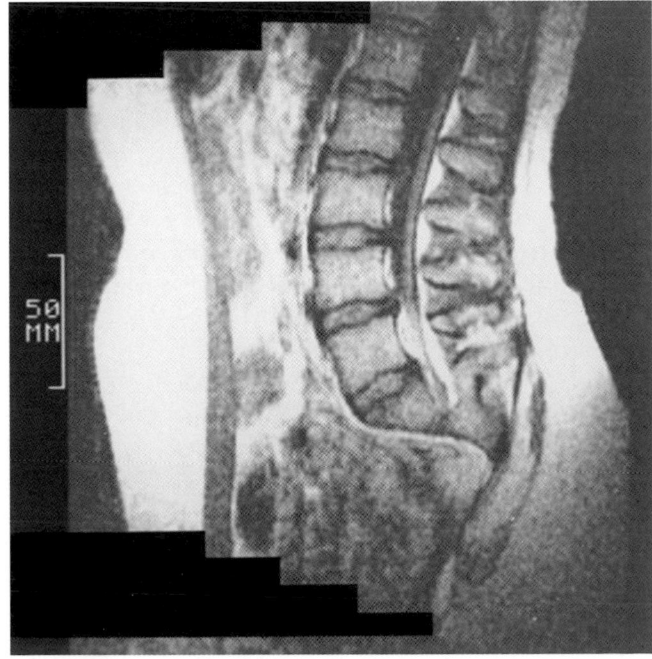


**Figure 13.3** Sacral agenesis. This MRI scan demonstrates a tethered spinal cord that ends at $L_5$ and is associated with sacral agenesis. (Courtesy Westchester County Medical Center, Valhalla, NY.)

The neurologic findings are similar to those of myelomeningocele, ranging from a minimal deficit to equinovarus deformity of the feet to more extensive sensory and motor deficits of the lower extremities. The level of bone anomaly corresponds well with the level of weakness but not to sensory loss; sensation is usually preserved. The caudal spinal cord is often truncated, dysraphic, and tethered (Estin & Cohen, 1995). Most patients have neurogenic urinary tract and bowel impairment, visceral abnormalities, flattened buttocks, and prominent iliac crests (Sarnat, 1992). Constipation and perianal sepsis are common complaints. Ascending infection resulting in bacterial meningitis has also been reported.

Some patients experience progressive neurologic deficits, demonstrating that sacral agenesis is not always a static disability (O'Neill *et al.* 1995). Slow deterioration of neurologic function may masquerade as an orthopedic or urologic problem unless the potential for progressive lesions is appreciated. Dural sac stenosis, tethered spinal cord, diastematomyelia, and cauda equina lipomas and dermoids have also been associated with sacral agenesis (Brooks *et al.* 1981). Although plain radiographs demonstrate the degree of sacral agenesis, CT or MRI is necessary to delineate the underlying spinal cord anomalies (Fig. 13.3) (Gundry & Heithoff 1994). Surgical management is discussed on p. 771.

## ARNOLD–CHIARI MALFORMATION

Four variations of the Arnold–Chiari malformation exist (Table 13.3) (Norman *et al.* 1995; Cai & Oakes 1997). In type 2, the most frequently encountered, the cerebellum and medulla oblongata are shifted caudally; resultant packing into the cervical spinal canal results in deformation. Because of kinking, the thinned and elongated medulla may actually be positioned side-by-side with the upper segments of the dwarfed and deformed cervical spinal cord. Curiously, the abnormal positioning causes the upper cervical roots to course upward before leaving the vertebral foramina (Fig. 13.4). The pons is thin and narrow. By definition, type 2 Arnold–Chiari malformation is associated with myelomeningocele. Hydrocephalus occurs in most patients secondary to aqueductal stenosis or obstruction to CSF flow around the medulla.

Hydromyelia and syringomyelia of the cervical spinal cord occur in 20–50% of patients (Friede 1989; Breningstall *et al.* 1992). Vascular lesions, including hemorrhage and infarction, are often present in the tegmentum of the medulla in children, with resultant altered respiratory control (Papasozomenos & Roessman 1981). Other CNS defects, such as small increased numbers of gyri, heterotopias, Klippel–Feil syndrome, craniolacunae, and bony anomalies at the base of the skull, often accompany the Arnold–Chiari malformation.

Type 1 Arnold–Chiari malformation is similar to type 2, but the malformation is milder. The cerebellum is displaced into the cervical spinal canal. Although it is characteristi-

**Table 13.3 Classification of Arnold–Chiari malformations**

| Type | Anatomic abnormalities | Neurologic findings |
|---|---|---|
| 1 | Downward displacement of the cerebellum and cerebellar tonsils, elongated brainstem fourth ventricle | Mild and delayed onset of headache and brainstem symptoms usually beginning in adolescence. Symptoms secondary to hydrocephalus or syringomyelia |
| 2 | Downward displacement of the cerebellar vermis and cerebellar tonsils; thinned and elongated medulla may actually be positioned side-by-side with the upper segments of the atrophic cervical spinal cord | Associated with myelomeningocele in more than 95% of patients; symptoms resulting from progressive hydrocephalus and secondary brainstem dysfunction; feeding and respiratory complications are common including apnea |
| 3 | Encephalocervical meningocele with spina bifida over the cervical area and protrusion of the cerebellum through the posterior encephalocele | Features similar to Arnold-Chiari, type 2, without the same degree of association with myelomeningocele |
| 4 | Hypoplasia of the cerebellum | Variable findings from asymptomatic to classical cerebellar dysfunction |

*Source*: From Norman *et al.* (1995); Sarnat (1992), Friede (1989).

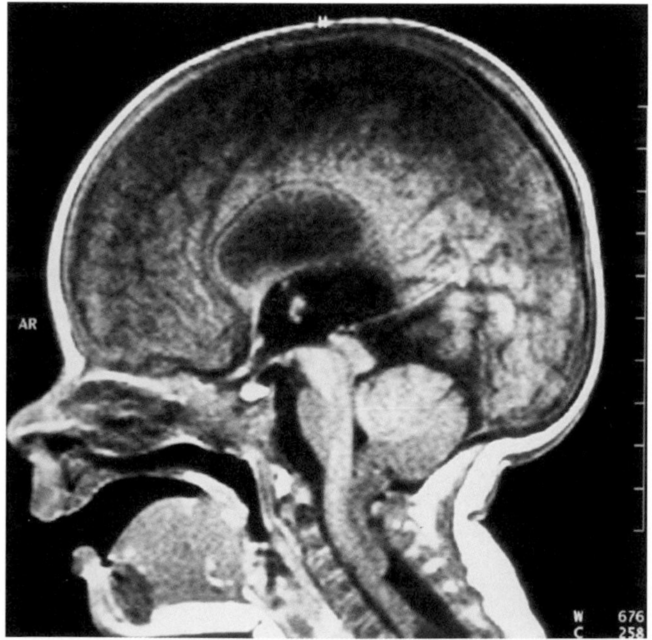


**Figure 13.4** A 2-month-old male with spinal dysraphism. The mid sagittal T1-weighted MRI of the brain demonstrates a small posterior fossa, extension of the cerebellar tissue through the foramen magnum into the upper cervical spinal thecal sac, small and vertically oriented fourth ventricle, and an enlarged third ventricle. The axial images, not seen, depicted enlargement of the lateral ventricles. These are classic findings of Arnold–Chiari type 2 malformation. Incidental note is made of the uppermost aspect of a cervical spinal cord syrinx, also a finding of Arnold–Chiari type 2 malformation. (Courtesy of Shahrokh Toranji, Department of Radiation Sciences, Loma Linda University School of Medicine, Loma Linda, CA.)

cally long and thin, the medulla does not have a side-by-side relationship with the cervical cord. No associated myelomeningocele exists. Type 3 is essentially an encephalocervical meningocele and consists of spina bifida over the cervical area with protrusion of the cerebellum through the opening. Type 4 consists of a single abnormality, hypoplasia of the cerebellum, and may be a variation of the Dandy–Walker syndrome (Caviness 1976).

## Pathophysiology

The precise mechanism causing Arnold–Chiari malformation is unknown (Gilbert *et al.* 1986; Sarnat 1992; Norman *et al.* 1995; Cai & Oakes 1997). At least five explanations have been proposed: (1) tethering at the brainstem–cervical cord junction; (2) altered CSF dynamics causing excessive localized brainstem pressure and distortion; (3) a primary brainstem and cerebellar malformation; (4) birth trauma; and (5) hypoplasia of the posterior cranial fossa bony structures (Nishikawa *et al.* 1997).

## Clinical characteristics

Type 1 Arnold–Chiari malformation may not be associated with clinical manifestations for many decades (Archer *et al.* 1977). The initial symptoms are recurrent occipital and frontal headaches, neck pain, unsteady gait, progressive ataxia, and difficulty in swallowing (McClone & LaMarca 1997). The headaches are typically worsened by coughing, exertion, positional changes, or Valsalva maneuvers. Various functions of cranial nerves IX to XII are compromised. The gag reflex may be unelicitable and the soft palate paretic. Cerebellar impairment, evidenced by ataxia and nystagmus, may be apparent. Downbeat nystagmus and periodic alternating nystagmus are characteristic of craniocervical anomalies, such as the Arnold–Chiari malformation. Extensor toe signs and deep tendon reflexes are present, and the latter are pathologically increased. The posterior columns are usually involved with compromised vibration and position sense. Increased intracranial pressure may also develop. Occasionally children with Arnold–Chiari type I malformations may present with severe spinal cord injury or death after minor injury (McClone & LaMarca, 1997).

### Management

Careful monitoring of infants with known Arnold–Chiari malformations is advocated (Venes *et al.* 1986; Charney *et al.* 1987; Cai & Oakes 1997). Evaluation with MRI is now the procedure of choice (Gundry & Heithoff, 1994). In patients with Arnold–Chiari type 1 malformations, MRI studies have demonstrated that syringomyelia was present in 70%; the remaining patients had evidence of frank herniation of the cerebellar tonsils below the foramen magnum (Amer & el-Shmam, 1997). The neurosurgical management is discussed in Chapter 44.

## ENCEPHALOCELE

A cephalocele is a herniation of intracranial contents through a skull defect. Cephaloceles are classified by their contents and location (Martinez-Lage *et al.* 1996). Cranial meningoceles contain only leptomeninges and CSF, whereas encephaloceles also contain brain (Norman *et al.* 1995). A ventriculocele is an encephalocele in which the herniated brain contents also contain portions of the ventricle. The incidence of cephaloceles is approximately 0.8 to 3.0 per 10 000 live births with encephaloceles being the most common form.

Encephaloceles are usually located in the occipital areas (75%) or frontal areas (25%). The latter condition occurs most frequently among Asians. Basal and trans-sphenoidal encephaloceles are rare; they may appear between the ethmoid and sphenoid bones and extend into the upper pharynx (Harley 1991). Encephaloceles that extend from the area of the orbit, nose, or forehead are termed *sincipital encephaloceles*; those in the occipital region are termed *notencephaloceles*. Exencephaly consists of a large out-pouching of brain tissue with surrounding thick walls. This defect may involve the spinal cord, forming an encephalo-myelocele. Cranial encephalocele may contain a combination of meninges, ventricles, and brain parenchyma (Wininger & Donnenfeld 1994).

The pathogenesis of encephalocele formation is incompletely understood but is likely related to defects in the development of the skull base (Chapman *et al.* 1989; Marin-Padilla 1991).

### Clinical characteristics

A fluctuant, round, balloon-like mass that protrudes from the cranium, usually posteriorly, is the most typical manifestation of encephaloceles. The mass may pulsate and be covered by an erythematous, translucent, or opaque membrane, or by normal skin. The covering may not be uniform throughout its surface. The amount of compromised and deformed neural tissue determines the extent of cerebral dysfunction (Mealey *et al.* 1970). Brain tissue not extending into the encephalocele may be deformed and functionally impaired.

Severe intellectual and motor delays typically occur in association with microcephaly; motor delay is accompanied by weakness and spasticity. Intellectual impairment is more prevalent in patients with posterior rather than anterior encephaloceles (Hockley *et al.* 1990). However, some patients may have completely normal development. Occipital lobe destruction is associated with various degrees of visual impairment. When the deformity includes a ventricle, hydrocephalus is almost inevitable. Because of increased pressure, the encephalocele may become stretched until the covering is infarcted, with resultant infection and rupture.

Other malformations may accompany encephaloceles, including Dandy–Walker syndrome, Klippel–Feil syndrome, Arnold–Chiari malformation, porencephaly, agenesis of the corpus callosum, myelodysplasia, optic nerve dysplasia, and cleft palate (Cohen & Lemire 1982; Bindal *et al.* 1991; Norman *et al.* 1995). Although ultrasonography may be helpful, the clinical diagnosis is confirmed by CT or MRI (Fig. 13.5).

Neuroendocrine disturbances occur, particularly with basal encephaloceles that involve the sella turcica or sphenoid sinus (Ellyn *et al.* 1980). These conditions may be undetectable by gross inspection. Intranasal mass or endocrine dysfunction the cardinal features.

Encephaloceles are seen with a variety of chromosomal disorders (e.g., trisomy 13, 18; 13q or 16q deletion) and syndromes (Table 13.4). They can be inherited in an autosomal-recessive mode (Cohen & Lemire 1982). Occipital encephalocele, microcephaly, cleft palate or lip, polydactyly, holoprosencephaly, and polycystic kidneys constitute Meckel–Gruber syndrome (McKusick 1994). Retinal degeneration with detachment and occipital encephalocele (Knobloch syndrome) is another autosomal-recessive condition (Knobloch & Layer 1971).

Nasal glioma, a congenital tumor, appears as a fronto-nasal mass that mimics an encephalocele (Lemire *et al.* 1975; Younus & Coode 1986). The tumor is derived from herniated brain tissue that has lost its connection to the brain; this relationship can be demonstrated by neuroimaging techniques.

**Management and prognosis** of encephaloceles are discussed in Chapter 45.

## ANENCEPHALY

Anencephaly is a congenital malformation in which both cerebral hemispheres are absent. The cranial vault defect is an extensive cranioschisis (Medical Task Force on

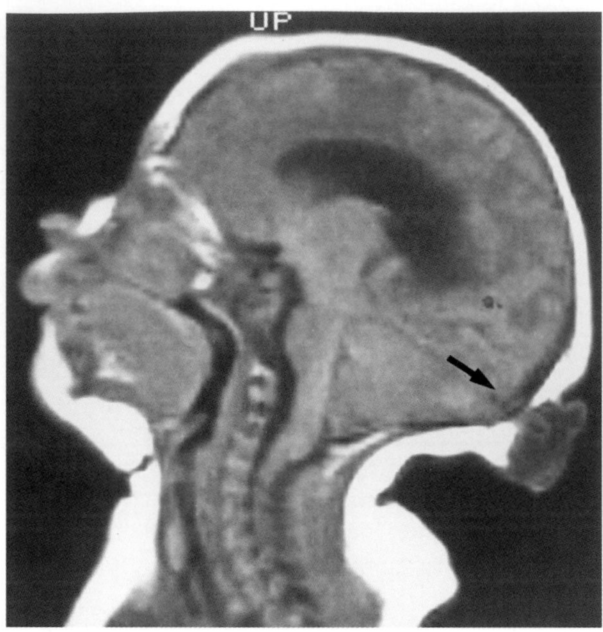


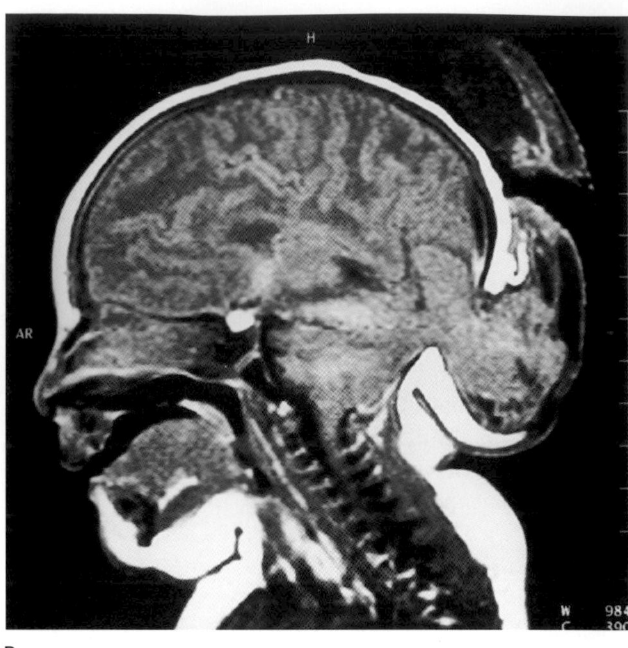

A B

Figure 13.5 Meningoencephalocele in a 4-day-old female infant. (A) Small nubbin of brain tissue (arrow) extending into small occipital meningoencephalocele; these defects are better demonstrated with this T1-weighted sagittal MRI than with axial CT. (B) Large meningoencephalocele in a newborn infant seen on a sagittal T1-weighted image of the brain that also demonstrates a large occipital midline bony defect. (Courtesy of Shahrokh Toranji MD, Department of Radiation Sciences, Loma Linda University School of Medicine, Loma Linda, CA.)

**Table 13.4 Selected syndromes associated with encephaloceles**

| Syndrome | Clinical features |
|---|---|
| Walker–Warburg syndrome | Hydrocephalus, severe neurologic impairment, vermian agenesis, type 2 lissencephaly, autosomal recessive |
| Meckel–Gruber syndrome | Polycystic kidney, sloping forehead, polydactyly, hepatobiliary fibrosis, cleft lip and palate, autosomal recessive |
| Dandy–Walker syndrome | Hydrocephalus, partial or complete absence of the cerebellar vermis, posterior fossa cyst contiguous with the fourth ventricle, cranial nerve palsies, nystagmus, truncal ataxia, sporadic occurrence |
| Joubert syndrome | Cerebellar vermian aplasia, episodic hyperpnea, abnormal eye movements, rhythmic protrusion of the tongue, ataxia, retardation, coloboma, retinal dystrophy, renal cysts, autosomal recessive |
| Goldenhar–Gorlin syndrome | Orofacial abnormalities, preauricular tags, epibulbar dermoids, sporadic occurrence |
| Knobloch syndrome | Vitreoretinal degeneration with retinal detachment, high myopia, and occipital encephalocele, normal intelligence, chromosome 21q22.3 |
| Robert's syndrome | Anterior encephalocele, autosomal recessive |
| Median cleft face syndrome | Anterior encephalocele, autosomal dominant |

*Source*: From OMIM (2000).

Anencephaly 1990). Most anencephalic infants are stillborn. Those infants born alive die shortly after birth (Botkin 1988).

Epidemiologic studies demonstrate a striking variation in prevalence rates. The highest incidence is in Great Britain and Ireland, and the lowest incidence is in Asia, Africa, and South America. Other countries have intermediate rates of incidence. Anencephaly occurs six times more frequently in whites than in blacks. Females are more often affected than males.

Antenatal diagnosis is possible using assays of α-fetoprotein or acetylcholinesterase, which is increased in maternal serum and amniotic fluid (Seller *et al.* 1974; Brock *et al.* 1975; Chan *et al.* 1995; Brennand *et al.* 1998). Antenatal diagnosis is also feasible through the use of fetal ultrasonography (Goldstein & Filly 1988; Johnson *et al.* 1997). In the past two decades, prenatal screening with ultrasound, which is near 100% accurate, and maternal α-fetoprotein determinations have resulted in earlier detection of anencephaly (Sabbagha *et al.* 1985). Earlier detection has resulted in a dramatic decrease in the average gestational age at birth from 35.6 weeks in the 1970s to 19.6 weeks in 1988–90 with virtually no term live-born anencephalic infants born after 1990 in those pregnancies in which a prenatal diagnosis of anencephaly had been made (Limb & Holmes, 1994).

### Pathogenesis

Anencephaly follows failure of closure of the anterior neural tube (Lemire 1987). The critical period during which the neural tube closes is from approximately day 21 to day 26 of gestation; the embryonic defect probably occurs before closure of the anterior neuropore on day 26. Supportive data of multiple sites of anterior neural tube closure in infants with anencephaly have recently been reported (Golden & Chernoff 1995). Two mechanisms leading to anterior NTDs were proposed. Anencephaly could result from failure of neural tube closure to occur at a discrete site, or if there was failure of two closure sites to meet.

The cause of anencephaly remains unknown. Various agents have been incriminated, including perinatal infections, folic acid antagonists, drinking water minerals, maternal hyperthermia, chromosomal abnormalities, and an unidentified agent in blighted potato tubers (Renwick 1972; Kurent & Sever 1973; Miller *et al.* 1978; Lemire 1987). These allegations of causal relationship remain unproven. As noted in the earlier section on spina bifida, evidence suggests a potential genetic etiology. Mutations of the BRCA1 gene in mice embryos are associated with a 40% incidence of spina bifida and anencephaly (Gowen *et al.* 1996). Also, mice homozygous for a deficiency in the paired class Hox gene, Cart 1, may have a form of anencephaly (meroanencephaly) at birth (Zhao *et al.* 1996). Prenatal treatment of these mice with folic acid suppressed NTD formation. Likewise, disruption of the MacMARCKS gene prevents cranial neural tube closure and results in anencephaly (Chen *et al.* 1996). The MacMARCKS gene is a member of the MARCKS family of protein kinase C substrates that integrate calcium and kinase dependent signals to regulate actin structure at the cell membrane.

### Pathology

The cranial vault is defective over the vertex, exposing a soft, angiomatous mass of neural tissue covered by a thin membrane continuous with the skin (Lemire *et al.* 1978). The cranial abnormality may extend inferiorly to the cervical region with formation of a complete spina bifida. The extremely thin and flattened spinal cord (craniorachischisis) is readily observed. The optic globes are usually protuberant because of inadequate bony orbits.

### Clinical characteristics

Anencephaly is a lethal condition (Lemire *et al.* 1978; Melnick & Myrianthopoulous 1987). No specific treatment is available. Neuroendocrine defects are frequent, with failure of endocrine end-organ development secondary to a hypoplastic pituitary gland. Adrenal insufficiency may be associated with adrenocortical hypoplasia. The posterior pituitary is also hypoplastic and may cause clinical diabetes insipidus.

Recent studies have demonstrated that anencephalic infants can exhibit a wide variety of behaviors and that these can be detected prenatally (Ashwal *et al.* 1990; Luyendijk & Treffers 1992; Kurauchi *et al.* 1995). Term infants with anencephaly who live for several days may respond to auditory, vestibular, and painful stimuli that are mediated by brainstem, diencephalic, and spinal pathways without cerebral involvement (Ashwal *et al.* 1990; Medical Task Force on Anencephaly, 1990). Described behaviors include jitteriness, hyperirritability, stiffening, spontaneous or stimulus-induced myoclonus of the extremities, opisthotonic posturing, and smiling (Ashwal *et al.* 1990; Luyendijk & Treffers 1992).

By definition, anencephalic infants are permanently unconscious (Medical Task Force on Anencephaly 1990). Although some concerns have been raised that consciousness may be preserved in the brainstems of such infants, because this is a developmental rather than an acquired brain lesion (Shewmon *et al.* 1989), medical evidence to support this contention has not been published (Lemire *et al.* 1978; Ashwal *et al.* 1990). Several studies have demonstrated that brainstem structures are rudimentary, hypoplastic, and virtually devoid of neurons, fiber tracts, neural networks, or any evidence of primitive functional organization that could support conscious behaviors (Vare & Bansal 1971; Nakamura *et al.* 1972; Walters *et al.* 1997).

The diagnosis of brain death in anencephalic infants is problematic because of the severe CNS malformations that are present, particularly in the brainstem (Ashwal *et al.* 1990). However, brain death can be diagnosed and depends on determining the absence of brainstem function including apnea. Difficulties in performing the examination have been previously described (Ashwal *et al.* 1990). Serial examinations demonstrating the loss of any previously detectable cranial nerve reflexes and the performance of repeated apnea challenge studies documenting the absence of respiratory effort with a $PCO_2$ above 60 torr over 24–48 hours are confirmatory. In anencephalic infants, in contrast to neonates with other etiologies of suspected brain death, there is no need for confirmatory laboratory studies (e.g. electroencephalography or determination of CBF), as these cannot be performed for technical reasons.

In the United States, regulations do not permit organ donation from anencephalic infants because brain death criteria are not fulfilled (Peabody *et al.* 1989). This policy is controversial, as demonstrated by the recent action of the American Medical Association's Council on Ethical and Judicial Affairs' withdrawal of its initial opinion calling for the direct procurement of organs from anencephalic infants (Walters *et al.* 1997).

**Iniencephaly** is a rare, lethal, axial dysraphic malformation diagnosed on the basis of three cardinal features: deficiency of the occipital bone, cervicothoracic spinal retroflexion, and rachischisis (Scherrer *et al.* 1992). Iniencephaly differs from anencephaly in that the cranial cavity is present and skin covers the head and retroflexed region (Lemire *et al.* 1972; Norman *et al.* 1995). Severe retroflexion of the neck present on fetal ultrasound may suggest the diagnosis (Meizner *et al.* 1992). The majority of the patients also have visceral and other severe CNS malformations. Another related condition is **meroanencephaly** (Isada *et al.* 1993), a rare form of anencephaly characterized by malformed cranial bones and a median cranial defect through which protrudes the area cerebrovasculosa.

## CLEAVAGE AND DIFFERENTIATION DEFECTS

### HOLOPROSENCEPHALY

Holoprosencephaly (HPE) results from failure of separation of the embryonic forebrain, or prosencephalon, into symmetric cerebral hemispheres. The defect arises before day 23 of gestation. Only a single lobe is present (holosphere). There is no distinct sagittal division of the brain by an interhemispheric fissure in either the anlage of the telencephalon or of the diencephalon (Norman *et al.* 1995; Leech & Shuman 1986). The prosencephalic ventricle remains undivided and persists as a single ventricle.

The cleavage defects vary in severity. Manifestations range from a minor change, such as a single central incisor or a choroid fissure coloboma, to HPE, a devastating structural aberration. The deformities in HPE are categorized into three major types as follows in order of decreasing severity: alobar, semilobar, and lobar (DeMyer 1971). The failure of prosencephalon division and subsequent formation of paired hemispheres determines the extent of the abnormality and the level of classification. Leptomeningeal glioneuronal heterotopias are commonly found in patients with HPE (Mizuguchi *et al.* 1994).

HPE has a prevalence of 1:250 during embryogenesis and 1:16 000 newborn infants (Roessler *et al.* 1996). The molecular basis underlying HPE is unknown. Teratogens, nonrandom chromosomal anomalies, and familial forms with autosomal-dominant and autosomal-recessive inheritance have been described (Balci *et al.* 1993; Roessler *et al.* 1996). HPE occurs more commonly in infants born to diabetic mothers (Kalter 1993). The genetics of HPE is discussed on p. 242, Chapter 14.

#### Clinical characteristics

The majority of patients with HPE have severe delayed development, spastic quadriplegia, failure to thrive, and seizures. Microphthalmia, ocular hypotelorism and colobomas, midface hypoplasia, single central upper incisor, and cleft lip and palate are frequently present. Neuroendocrine dysfunction results from defects of the anterior and posterior pituitary and secondary hypoplasia of endocrine end organs (Takahashi *et al.* 1995; de Zegher *et al.* 1992). Cranial ultrasonography, CT, and MRI demonstrate the malformation (Fitz, 1994). Some patients with HPE have partial development of the posterior corpus callosum (Rubenstein *et al.* 1996). The EEG is usually suppressed over the holoprosencephalic region, whereas in other patients asynchronous sharp waves and spikes are seen over the frontal regions with a decreasing gradient occipitally (Shah *et al.* 1992). Children with lobar HPE usually have significant developmental delays; some children with normal or near normal development and long-term survival have been reported (Elias *et al.* 1992; Pensler *et al.* 1993).

**Alobar holoprosencephaly** arises from the rudimentary development of the prosencephalon, which includes lack of delineation of an interhemispheric fissure. The undivided telencephalon persists as a solitary lobe without olfactory bulbs or tracts (DeMyer 1975).

Various combinations of median facial defects are associated with the holoprosencephalic brain. The precordial mesoderm is the anlage of the median facial bones. Facial anomalies accompany HPE because the induction process that eventually shapes the neural ectoderm and precordial mesoderm is flawed. When the precordial mesoderm is defective, the midline bones may be deformed. Division of the prosencephalon may be discontinued at various points during the process of formation. Conditions subsumed under alobar HPE, such as cyclopia, ethmocephaly, cebocephaly, and premaxillary agenesis, are associated with identifiable facial abnormalities.

**Cyclopia**, a condition incompatible with life, is characterized by a single median eye and a small, grotesquely shaped nose (proboscis) that arises from the supraorbital area (Liu *et al.* 1997a). No optic chiasm exists. A single optic nerve traverses a solitary optic foramen to reach the brain; it may then separate into right and left branches.

**Ethmocephaly** is associated with exaggerated orbital hypotelorism; however, there are two orbits. The proboscis protrudes from the region between the eyes.

In **cebocephaly**, the facial features include orbital hypotelorism and a proboscis with a single midline, nasal opening. No cleft lip is present. Although the karyotype is virtually always normal, the condition has accompanied trisomies 13 and 15.

**In premaxillary agenesis**, facial features consist of hypotelorism, a flat nose, and a midline cleft upper lip. The hard palate is normally developed. There is no nasal septum. A median angle-like protrusion of the frontal bones may occur. The calvarium may be microcephalic. Failure to thrive, delayed development, poor temperature control, and seizures are common symptoms of premaxillary agenesis. Poor visual acuity, synophrys, colobomas, and spastic quadriparesis are also evident. Most infants do not survive the first year of life.

In **semilobar holoprosencephaly**, prosencephalic cleavage is discernible, mostly posteriorly, with a hypoplastic intermaxillary segment. However, the separated cerebral lobes are grossly underdeveloped. The uncleaved cerebral neocortex is continuous from one side to the other, and the olfactory bulbs and tracts are undeveloped.

Facial abnormalities include a flattened nose, bilateral cleft lip and palate, a midline protrusion (the remnant of the premaxillary anlage), and orbital hypotelorism. Both trigonocephaly and microcephaly have been reported. Profound intellectual retardation usually occurs. Occasionally, patients live beyond infancy.

**Lobar holoprosencephaly** is associated with frontal lobes that are well developed and of normal weight. Normal cleavage implements formation of a normal interhemispheric fissure; however, when the frontal neocortex continues across the midline, the interhemispheric fissure is foreshortened anteriorly. Olfactory bulbs and tracts are sometimes present. Complete or partial agenesis of the corpus callosum may be present. Facial distortion may be absent or subtle. Trigonocephaly and cleft lip and palate have been described, and severe mental retardation is usually present. Neuroimaging techniques confirm the diagnosis.

## NEURONAL MIGRATION DISORDERS

Neuronal migration disorders (NMDs) are perhaps the most common form of CNS malformations, yet they remain poorly understood and difficult to classify. A relatively simple division into disorders of cell proliferation and cell migration provides a framework for understanding these disorders, although substantial overlap occurs. Many other conditions are related to disturbances in neuronal organization, synaptogenesis, programmed cell death, myelination, and gliogenesis. Alternatively, these disorders have been divided into two major groups: (1) abnormal cytogenesis and histiogenesis in the first half of gestation, which includes disorders of neuronal proliferation and migration, and (2) abnormal growth and differentiation in the second half of gestation, which is more typically associated with destructive events to the developing nervous system (Evrard *et al.* 1989a).

The terms *neuronal migration disorders, neuronal heterotopias*, and *cortical dysplasias* are frequently and confusingly used interchangeably (Norman *et al.* 1995). Until better correlations between clinical, neuroimaging, and neuropathologic studies are obtained, clarification of the differences between these entities will remain elusive (Raymond *et al.* 1995; Barkovich & Kuzniecky 1996; Battaglia *et al.* 1996; Iannetti *et al.* 1996; Preul *et al.* 1997). As used here, the term *neuronal migrational disorders* refers to diffuse or generalized aberrant migrations of normally structured neurons, whereas the term *neuronal heterotopias* refers to abnormal collections of gray matter, usually lacking any type of cortical lamination that may be subependymal, subcortical, or leptomeningeal. Cortical dysplasias, in contrast, consist of abnormally structured neurons that are characterized by marked neuronal and glial cytologic abnormalities with marked disruption of the normal cortical layering and architecture. Table 13.5 lists some of the CNS malformations or associated syndromes and diseases that have been associated with the presence of neuronal migration disorders, heterotopias, or cortical dysplasias.

### DISORDERS OF NEURONAL PROLIFERATION

#### Megalencephaly

Megalencephaly is a disorder of neuronal proliferation in which the brain weight and size are greater than two standard deviations above the mean. Associated with this cell and volume proliferation is the presence of neuronal heterotopias and other neuronal migration abnormalities. Megalencephaly occurs in a wide variety of clinical disorders and syndromes, may be bilateral or unilateral, and is associated with an enormous spectrum of motor, cognitive (Sandler *et al.* 1997), and behavioral symptoms including autism (Bailey *et al.* 1993). Table 13.6 presents a list of disorders associated with a large head size (macrocephaly), and some of these conditions are related to a large brain size (megalencephaly). Of interest is a recently described syndrome with infantile onset of megalencephaly and a severe cerebral leukoencephalopathy in children who were initially normal or near normal but who developed progressive ataxia and spasticity with preserved intellect (van der Knaap *et al.* 1995). Also of interest is the recent demonstration in patients with hemimegalencephaly of the abnormal expression of the neural cell adhesion molecule LICAM in the brains of children with hemimegalencephaly (Tsuru *et al.* 1997).

#### Microcephaly

Microcephaly is present when the head circumference is greater than two standard deviations below the mean for gestational or chronologic age (whichever is appropriate) and gender. The circumference and volume of the skull are abnormally decreased because of inadequate growth and development of the brain.

In general, below-average intelligence is associated with the presence of microcephaly (Nelson & Deutschberger 1970; Dolk 1991). Nevertheless, a head circumference two to three standard deviations below the mean is not inevitably linked with intellectual retardation: 7.5% of a large group of microcephalic children had normal intelligence (Martin 1970; Sells 1977).

Disruption of cellular induction, multiplication, growth, or migration during the first 4 months of gestation is the

**Table 13.5 Diseases associated with neuronal migration disorders and heterotopias**

| | |
|---|---|
| **CNS malformation syndromes** | **Syndromes** |
| Cerebellar dysgenesis | Arthrogryposis multiplex congenita |
| Arnold–Chiari II malformation | Coffin–Siris |
| CRASH syndrome | Congenital muscular dystrophy |
| Dandy–Walker syndrome | Cornelia de Lange's syndrome |
| Hemimegalencephaly | Duchenne's muscular dystrophy |
| Hydrocephalus | Hypomelanosis of Ito |
| Lissencephaly | Incontinentia pigmenti |
| Pachygyria-macrogyria | Linear nevus sebaceus |
| Schizencephaly | Meckel–Gruber |
| **Chromosomal/genetic disorders** | Myotonic dystrophy |
| Trisomy 9, 13, 18, 21 | Neurofibromatosis |
| Deletion 4p | Orofaciodigital |
| **Metabolic disorders** | Potter's |
| GM2 gangliosidoses | Smith–Lemli–Opitz |
| Hurler syndrome | Tuberous sclerosis |
| Menkes' disease | **Teratogens** |
| Mitochondrial disorders (e.g., Leigh syndrome) | Carbon monoxide |
| Neonatal adrenoleukodystrophy | Fetal alcohol syndrome |
| Nonketotic hyperglycinemia | Maternal isotretinoic acid |
| Organic acidurias (glutaric aciduria type 2) | Mercury poisoning |
| Peroxisomal bifunctional enzyme defect | |
| Zellweger (peroxisomal disorder) | |

*Source*: From OMIM (2000); Norman *et al.* (1995); Volpe (1995).

presumed cause of familial microcephaly. During pregnancy, maternal, fetal, and environmental factors may cause microcephaly. Many cases of microcephaly are sporadic, and no underlying cause is identifiable (Cohen *et al.* 1996). Pathologic conditions that retard brain growth after birth and during the first year or two of life also may lead to microcephaly. Microcephaly may also be associated with other brain malformations or heterotopic brain growth. Microcephaly can usually but not uniformly be diagnosed by second trimester fetal ultrasonography (Bromley *et al.* 1994). MRI demonstrates additional abnormalities in approximately 90% of patients (Sugimoto *et al.* 1993).

The term *radial microbrain* (micrencephaly vera) refers to an abnormally small brain that has a normal gyral pattern, normal cortical thickness, and normal cortical lamination but the number of cortical neurons is only 30% of normal (Evrard *et al.* 1989a, 1992). A decrease in the number of radial neuronal–glial units accounts for the development of this disorder. Patients with this developmental abnormality have severe developmental retardation and profound microcephaly.

## Genetic and malformation syndromes with microcephaly

Genetic counseling in individual families with microcephaly may be very difficult and is also discussed on p. 241, Chapter 14.

**Familial microcephaly** is an autosomal-recessive, autosomal-dominant, X-linked, or polygenic disorder (McKusick 1994; Gross Tsur *et al.* 1995; Volpe 2000). The exceedingly small cerebrum contrasts with the normal cerebellum. Accompanying aberrations of cellular migration include agenesis of the corpus callosum, agyria, disrupted cortical lamination, gray matter heterotopias, macrogyria, polymicrogyria, and schizencephaly. Examination reveals obvious microcephaly, a narrow forehead, and a flat occiput. The face and ears may be of disproportionate normal size. Intellectual retardation is usually profound, and hyperactivity may dominate the patient's behavior. Visual impairment is common, and subtle-to-mild spasticity is often present. Epilepsy occurs in one-third of patients. There is a 6% risk of a family having a second microcephalic child. In families with a known pattern of inheritance, the recurrence risk may be 25–50%.

## Maternal/prenatal disorders with microcephaly

The developing nervous system is highly vulnerable to infections, including toxoplasmosis, rubella, cytomegalovirus, herpes simplex, and group B coxsackievirus, many of which can cause microcephaly (see Chapters 31 and 32). Microcephaly has also been reported in infants of women exposed to ionizing radiation from the atomic bomb or radium implantation in the cervix during the first trimester (Wood *et al.* 1967; Dekaban 1968; Sever 1995).

**Table 13.6 Etiology of macrocephaly**

| |
|---|
| **Congenital** |
| Achondroplasia |
| Benign familial |
| Cranioskeletal dysplasia |
| Craniosynostosis |
| External hydrocephalus |
| Hydranencephaly |
| Hydrocephalus |
| Megalencephaly |
| Cerebral gigantism |
| Familial |
| Autosomal-dominant or autosomal-recessive |
| Neurocutaneous syndromes |
| Porencephaly |
| **Degenerative** |
| Alexander's disease |
| Canavan's spongy degeneration |
| **Infectious** |
| Abscess |
| Subdural empyema or effusion |
| **Metabolic** |
| Generalized gangliosidosis, Gm 1 |
| Maple syrup urine disease |
| Metachromatic leukodystrophy |
| Mucopolysaccharidoses |
| Osteopetrosis |
| Rickets |
| Tay–Sachs disease |
| **Toxic** |
| Lead, vitamin A, tetracycline |
| Pseudotumor cerebri |
| **Traumatic** |
| Leptomeningeal cyst |
| Subdural hematoma or hygroma |

Maternal metabolic disorders that coexist with pregnancy, such as diabetes mellitus, uremia, and undiagnosed or inadequately treated phenylketonuria (Levy *et al.* 1996; Rouse *et al.* 1997), have been associated with neonatal microcephaly (Lenke & Levy 1982). Malnutrition, hypertension, and placental insufficiency may result in microcephaly and intrauterine growth retardation. Maternal carbon monoxide poisoning results in offspring with microcephaly, polymicrogyria, mental retardation, seizures, and occasionally hydrocephalus (Longo 1977).

Maternal alcoholism during pregnancy has also been linked with microcephaly as part of the fetal alcohol syndrome (Ouellette *et al.* 1977; Clarren & Smith 1978; Spohr *et al.* 1993; Loebstein & Koren 1997). Clinical features include growth and mental retardation, midfacial hypoplasia, short palpebral fissures, epicanthal folds, and behavioral disturbances (Rosett & Weiner, 1984). Neuropathologic findings include heterotopias, microcephaly, widespread cortical and white matter dysplasias, and defects of neuronal and glial migration (Wisniewski *et al.* 1983). Maternal cigarette smoking, as well as maternal substance abuse of cocaine and other illegal drugs, is a common cause of microcephaly (Dominguez *et al.* 1991; Loebstein & Koren, 1997).

### Postnatal disorders with microcephaly

A variety of neurologic insults to the developing nervous system in neonates and infants result in microcephaly. These insults include hypoxic–ischemic encephalopathy, intracranial hemorrhage, CNS infections, malnutrition, and inherited metabolic disorders. Pathologic findings include encephalomalacia, porencephaly, gliosis, abnormal myelination, and atrophy.

Acquired immunodeficiency syndrome in infants causes microcephaly associated with encephalopathy, delayed development, incoordination, and basal ganglia calcifications (Dickson *et al.* 1993).

Two syndromes that have gained increasing attention and that are associated with postnatal development of microcephaly are the Rett and Angelman syndromes. Dementia, ataxia, autism, and hand-wringing movements in females comprise Rett syndrome (Hagberg *et al.* 1983). Angelman syndrome (15q11–13 deletion), is associated with seizures, hypotonia, hyperreflexia, hyperkinesis, and growth failure (Fryburg *et al.* 1991; Smith *et al.* 1996). These children have an unusual facies and personality; the term *happy puppet* syndrome has been used to describe them.

Children with microcephaly display a wide variety of handicaps. Many infants have mental retardation, seizures, incoordination, movement disorders, and spasticity (Dorman 1991).

Investigation of patients with microcephaly includes evaluation for prenatal exposure to teratogens, especially alcohol, drugs, and isotretinoin (a vitamin A analog), and assessment of the family history, birth history, and associated dysmorphic conditions. Laboratory studies should include: titers for toxoplasmosis, syphilis, rubella virus, cytomegalovirus, and herpes simplex viruses; neuroimaging; evaluation of maternal and childhood metabolic disorders; and chromosome analysis.

## DISORDERS OF NEURONAL MIGRATION

### Schizencephaly

The term *schizencephaly* designates the presence of clefts in the cerebral hemispheres, which result from flawed development of the cortical mantle during cell migration in the first trimester of pregnancy (Yakovlev & Wadsworth, 1946). The clefts are almost invariably located in the area of the sylvian fissures. The fluid-filled brain cavity is covered by normal dura or a thin pia-arachnoid membrane. The gyral pattern of the neighboring gyri is abnormal. Schizencephaly is also frequently considered to be due to an encephaloclastic process associated with fetal ischemic injury in the middle cerebral artery distribution between 31 and 35 weeks gestation (Klingensmith & Cioffi-Ragan 1986). Neuroimaging techniques may demonstrate symmetric or unilateral defects in the sylvian regions (Guillen *et al.* 1995).

Controversy surrounds the use of the term *schizencephaly*, and abandonment of the term has been suggested by some neuropathologists (Norman *et al.* 1995; Friede, 1989), although it remains commonly used by radiologists. Recent studies, however, suggest that genetic factors may play a role in the development of this malformation (see p. 247). The recent publication of cases of intrauterine CMV infection in two children with schizencephaly also suggests another potential etiology for this malformation (Iannetti *et al.* 1998).

The range of clinical symptoms in children with schizencephaly is currently being reevaluated because of the availability of MRI. Children with unilateral schizencephaly are more likely to have mild or moderate impairments, whereas those with bilateral lesions usually have profound intellectual retardation, epilepsy, and generalized spasticity (Granata *et al.* 1996; Packard *et al.* 1997). Clinical findings are usually commensurate with the size of the lesion (Aniskiewicz *et al.* 1990). Children with closed-lip schizencephaly may present with hemiparesis or motor delay, whereas those with open-lip schizencephaly are more likely to present with hydrocephalus or seizures. In one recent series, 57% of patients had seizures and 91% had associated cerebral developmental anomalies including agenesis of the septum pellucidum (45%) or focal cortical dysplasia (40%) (Packard *et al.* 1997). In another series the severity of schizencephaly correlated with the severity of motor and cognitive disability but not with the severity of epilepsy (Granata *et al.* 1996).

### Focal transmural dysplasia

Focal transmural dysplasia is a newly described neuronal migration disorder in which cortical dysplasia extends from the cortex to the superolateral wall of the lateral ventricle (Barkovich *et al.* 1997). MRI findings in 18 patients demonstrated this transmural malformation. Epilepsy, developmental delay, and fixed neurologic deficits were observed. Neuropathology revealed cortical disorganization, enlarged dysplastic neurons, balloon cells, indistinct cortical gray matter–white matter junctions, and variable astrogliosis. Although the etiology of this malformation is unknown, it was suggested by Barkovich *et al.* (1997) that this malformation might be due to abnormal progenitor stem cell development.

### Porencephaly

An entity that is sometimes confused with schizencephaly is porencephaly. It results from one of two abnormal processes: in one there is disruption of normal brain tissue (see p. 355–6), and in the other a faulty induction process and aberrant neuronal migration occur (Eller & Kuller 1995a). The terms *encephaloclastic porencephaly* and *pseudoporencephaly* indicate circumscribed defects in the cerebral mantle that rarely communicate with the ventricles and that result from destruction of cerebral tissue. Survival of the developing gray matter overlying porencephalic white matter lesions is in part due to maintenance of the independent leptomeningeal and the local anastomotic circulations (Marin-Padilla 1997). In addition, functional adaptations of local interneuronal circuitry occur. It has been suggested that the sequelae of such porencephalic lesions (e.g. cerebral palsy, epilepsy) may be, in part, due to certain of these adaptive mechanisms (Marin-Padilla 1997).

Porencephaly may also be associated with seizures. Underlying hippocampal formation atrophy may be found with postoperative pathologic changes indicative of mesial temporal sclerosis (Ho *et al.* 1997).

**Encephaloclastic porencephaly** may follow severe intrauterine trauma (Viljoen 1995), and occur as a complication after amniocentesis (Eller & Kuller, 1995b) or as a complication of traumatic breech and vacuum deliveries (Odita & Hebi 1996) and after periventricular intracerebral hemorrhage with ensuing encephalomalacia in preterm infants (Pasternak *et al.* 1980). In extremely preterm infants the porencephalic lesions may involve the periphery of the brain (Cross *et al.* 1992).

**Congenital porencephaly** describes familial forms of porencephaly that are primarily autosomal-dominant disorders (Berg *et al.* 1983; Sensi *et al.* 1990; Shastri *et al.* 1993; Smit *et al.* 1984). More recently, an autosomal form of bilateral porencephaly in association with absence of the septum pellucidum and pancerebellar and vermian hypoplasia has been reported (Bonnemann *et al.* 1996).

Porencephalic cysts may be attended by an overlying encephalocele, alopecia, or other cranial defects (Yokota & Matsukado 1979). Linear sebaceous nevi and developmental failure of cerebral venous sinuses may also accompany porencephaly (Chalhub *et al.* 1975). Intracerebral cysts and porencephaly are reported in patients with the orofaciodigital syndrome type 1 (Odent *et al.* 1998).

**Clinical characteristics** of porencephaly include motor dysfunction, ranging from spastic monoparesis to hemiplegia. Supranuclear bulbar palsy is associated with bilateral lesions. Basal ganglia compromise may lead to hypotonia during the neonatal period; abnormal involuntary movements, usually athetosis, may appear during the first year of life. Delayed or impaired growth and development, epilepsy, and hydrocephalus are often present (Nixon *et al.* 1974). If the cyst dilates, the ensuing increased intracranial pressure causes progressive neurologic impairment and hydrocephalus (Tardieu *et al.* 1981).

Neuroimaging techniques, including cranial ultrasonography, reveal the cyst or cysts. In one study of 14 patients, MRI revealed porencephaly in the distribution of the middle cerebral artery in eight patients, posterior cerebral artery in three, internal carotid artery in one, and multiple vessels in two (Ho *et al.* 1997). In some patients, instilled contrast medium in conjunction with CT is necessary to determine whether the cyst communicates with the ventricular system.

A ventriculoperitoneal shunt is indicated for management of progressive enlargement of the porencephalic cyst. Furthermore, a progressive neurologic deficit may be an indication for surgical removal or shunting. In these patients, special neuroradiologic evaluation is necessary to determine the relation of the cyst to the ventricular system (Kolawole *et al.* 1987). Most patients have static neurologic deficits that require rehabilitation.

## Lissencephaly

Lissencephaly is a brain malformation manifested by a smooth cerebral surface, thickened cortical mantle, and microscopic evidence of incomplete neuronal migration (Dobyns 1989; Dobyns *et al.* 1992; Dobyns & Truwit 1995). Lissencephaly comprises the agyria–pachygyria spectrum of malformations, thus excluding polymicrogyria and other cortical dysplasias. The syndromes associated with lissencephaly are discussed on p. 244, Chapter 14.

**Type 1 lissencephaly**, or classical lissencephaly, results from abnormal neuronal migration between about 10 and 14 weeks gestation (Dobyns 1987). The brain is often small, and the ventricles are enlarged posteriorly. The corpus callosum may be small or absent. The structural pattern of the cerebral hemispheres and ventricles is distinctly immature and reminiscent of fetal brain. The superficial cellular layer resembles an immature cortex, with some separation into zones similar to layers III, V, and VI of normal cortex, although the cell population is decreased. The heterotopic neurons are separated from the superficial layer by an acellular zone, although this varies in thickness and may be absent. Gray matter heterotopias may be present in the white matter, which is much thinner than normal. Atypical forms of lissencephaly comprising agyria, pachygyria, and other changes, such as polymicrogyria, porencephaly, and intracerebral calcifications, also occur. Rare variants include lissencephaly with extreme micrencephaly (head circumference at birth of 24–28 cm; brain weight less than 100 g) and lissencephaly with cerebellar hypoplasia. Seizures are common in patients with lissencephaly, and the EEG shows various types of abnormalities (Gastaut *et al.* 1987).

The **LIS-1 gene** encodes a subunit of a brain platelet-activating factor acetylhydrolase. Recent studies have demonstrated that these gene products in the developing human brain localize to the Cajal–Retzius cells, some subplate neurons, thalamic neurons, the ventricular neuroepithelium, and, at later gestational ages, to the ependyma which suggests a potential role for these proteins in regulating neuronal migration in these structures (Clark *et al.* 1997; Isumi *et al.* 1997).

Type I lissencephaly occurs in several **associated syndromes**. Miller–Dieker syndrome (MDS) consists of severe type I lissencephaly, abnormal facial appearance, and sometimes other birth defects. The facial changes include prominent forehead, bitemporal hollowing, short nose with upturned nares, protuberant upper lip with a thin vermilion border, and a small jaw. Some patients have an unusual midline calcification in the region of the septum. Visible deletions of chromosome band 17p13.3 are observed in about half of all affected patients, whereas the remainder have submicroscopic deletions of the same region (Dobyns *et al.* 1991). Isolated lissencephaly sequence consists of type I or atypical lissencephaly and minor facial changes, such as small jaw and bitemporal hollowing.

Patients with the Norman–Roberts syndrome differ from the Miller–Dieker syndrome because they have a different facies and no evidence of a 17p13.3 deletion (Iannetti *et al.* 1993). They typically have microcephaly, bitemporal hollowing, low sloping forehead, slightly prominent occiput, widely set eyes, broad and prominent nasal bridge, and severe postnatal growth deficiency. Neurologic features include generalized spasticity, seizures, and profound developmental delay.

About 15–20% of patients with lissencephaly have submicroscopic deletions of 17p13.3 that are usually smaller than those observed in Miller–Dieker syndrome (Ledbetter *et al.* 1992). Autosomal-recessive inheritance has been observed in a few families with 'pure' isolated lissencephaly, in isolated lissencephaly with neonatal death resulting from respiratory insufficiency, and, in at least one family, with Norman–Roberts syndrome (Norman *et al.* 1976).

Non-genetic causes of type I lissencephaly include intrauterine infections such as cytomegalovirus and intrauterine perfusion failure.

### Type II lissencephaly

Type II lissencephaly is a more complex malformation than type I and consists of agyria, pachygyria, or even polymicrogyria with a pebbled surface, thickened cortex, edematous or cystic white matter, and often hydrocephalus. The cortex is severely disorganized, with no recognizable layers and widespread disruption by abnormal vascular channels and fibroglial bands. The latter often extends to the subarachnoid space, which may be partly obstructed. The white matter is poorly myelinated with large numbers of heterotopic neurons. Associated malformations include absent septum pellucidum, absent corpus callosum, vermis hypoplasia, Dandy–Walker malformation, and brainstem hypoplasia. These changes reflect a protracted process beginning as early as 6 weeks gestation and continuing as late as 24 weeks gestation (Evrard *et al.* 1989a; Dobyns *et al.* 1989). Type II lissencephaly has been observed in several syndromes, some of which have associated congenital muscular dystrophy. Walker–Warburg syndrome includes severe eye malformations and either vermian hypoplasia or Dandy–Walker malformation (Rodgers *et al.* 1994). The eye malformations may consist of microphthalmia, cataracts, Peter anomaly, congenital glaucoma, and retinal malformations, although the last malformations are the most constant.

Fukuyama congenital muscular dystrophy (see p. 713) is the least severe, although all patients are severely retarded. Eye and cerebellar malformations are minimal or absent (Yoshioka *et al.* 1994). The 'cobblestone' lissencephaly that is characteristic of type II lissencephaly has recently been reported in several families who did not have eye abnormalities or muscle disease (Dobyns *et al.* 1996b). Whether it is a related condition or a distinct entity remains undetermined at this time.

Type II lissencephaly is also seen in other conditions related to the Walker–Warburg syndrome. These include the 'muscle, eye, and brain (MEB) disease' syndrome associated with severe weakness, hypotonia with myopia, visual impairment, and abnormal eye movements and the 'cerebro-oculo-muscular syndrome' (COMS) that is similar to MEB disease (Valanne *et al.* 1994). Another rare syndrome, proliferative vasculopathy with hydranencephaly-hydrocephaly, may be related (Norman & McGillivray, 1988).

### Type III lissencephaly

A primary CNS disorder affecting neuronal survival in the brain and spinal cord in five fetuses with fetal akinesia sequence has been described in association with lissencephaly (Encha Razavi *et al.* 1996). Fetal ultrasound at 23 weeks revealed polyhydramnios and severe arthrogryposis with agenesis of the corpus callosum and vermis. Postmortem examination demonstrated lissencephaly with a hypoplastic brainstem and cystic cerebellum. An autosomal-recessive pattern of inheritance was suggested in this lethal entity.

### X-linked lissencephaly/subcortical band heterotopias

X-linked lissencephaly (XLIS) and subcortical band heterotopias (SBH) can be inherited alone or together in the same pedigree (Ross *et al.* 1997). Both conditions are associated with epilepsy and several types of neurodevelopmental disorders. Available data suggest that SBH and X-linked lissencephaly are caused by mutation of a single gene, XLIS. The brain malformation varies from classical lissencephaly, which is observed in males, to subcortical band heterotopia, which is observed primarily in females (Dobyns *et al.* 1996a). Almost all patients with SBH have been female, although several males with this condition have been reported (Dobyns *et al.* 1996a; Ono *et al.* 1997). Mutations of the gene encoding a 40 kDa protein named *doublecortin* have been reported in patients with XLIS (Gleeson *et al.* 1998). X-linked lissencephaly in association with agenesis of the corpus callosum has also been observed (Berry-Kravis & Israel, 1994).

Clinically, gestation is usually of normal duration, although many infants with lissencephaly (irrespective of the subtype) are small for gestational age and experience severe failure to thrive. Polyhydramnios is often present but is a non-specific feature. Appearance may be normal or abnormal, depending on the particular lissencephaly syndrome. For example, the facial appearance is always abnormal in children with Miller–Dieker syndrome and is usually abnormal in children with Walker–Warburg syndrome. Bitemporal hollowing and small jaw are common in all syndromes. Only a minority of children have microcephaly at birth, although virtually all become microcephalic within the first year of life. Many children with Walker–Warburg syndrome have congenital hydrocephalus and the head size is often large. Poor feeding and hypotonia are commonly observed in neonates and some have apnea. Seizures may occur during the first few days of life, but it is much more typical for them to begin later in the first year of life. Seizure types in the first year include myoclonic, tonic, and tonic–clonic. In over half the patients, seizures consist of or include infantile spasms. Other neurologic manifestations include severe or profound mental retardation, hypotonia that evolves to spastic quadriplegia, and opisthotonus. Many patients require a gastrostomy because of poor nutrition and repeated aspiration pneumonias.

CT and especially MRI reveal the smooth surface, thickened cortex, thin white matter, lack of the normal interdigitations between cortex and white matter, and enlargement of the posterior portions of the lateral ventricles (Barkovich 1995; Iannetti *et al.* 1996). Some patients also have agenesis or thinning of the corpus callosum (Fig. 13.6) (Byrd *et al.* 1988). Cerebellar malformations, especially vermian hypoplasia or Dandy–Walker malformation, are seen in Walker–Warburg syndrome. On MRI, patients with XLIS show more frontal involvement in contrast to LIS1 patients where involvement is greater in parietal and occipital regions. EEG abnormalities are common in patients with all types of lissencephalies. Hypsarrhythmia, diffuse rhythmic fast α- and β-activity, and high-voltage spike discharges or 5–7 Hz slow sharp waves or δ-waves are commonly seen (Mori *et al.* 1994).

### Recurrence risks for lissencephaly

The various clinical subtypes have different risks of recurrence in siblings. Isolated lissencephaly is causally heterogeneous. The empiric recurrence risk is 5–7% (Dobyns *et al.* 1992). The recurrence risk for Miller–Dieker syndrome depends on results of chromosome and DNA analysis; it is not inherited as an autosomal-recessive trait. The recurrence risk is 25% for isolated lissencephaly with neonatal death, Norman–Roberts syndrome, Fukuyama congenital muscular dystrophy, and Walker–Warburg syndrome. The recurrence risk for unusual types of lissencephaly, such as lissencephaly with extreme micrencephaly and lissencephaly with cerebellar hypoplasia, may be as high as 25%. The recurrence risk is 50% for brothers of males having X-linked lissencephaly with microphallus. Genetic evaluation and counseling are always indicated for families of children with lissencephaly.

### Pachygyria

Pachygyria indicates a simplified convolutional pattern with widened gyri and a decreased number of sulci; only one

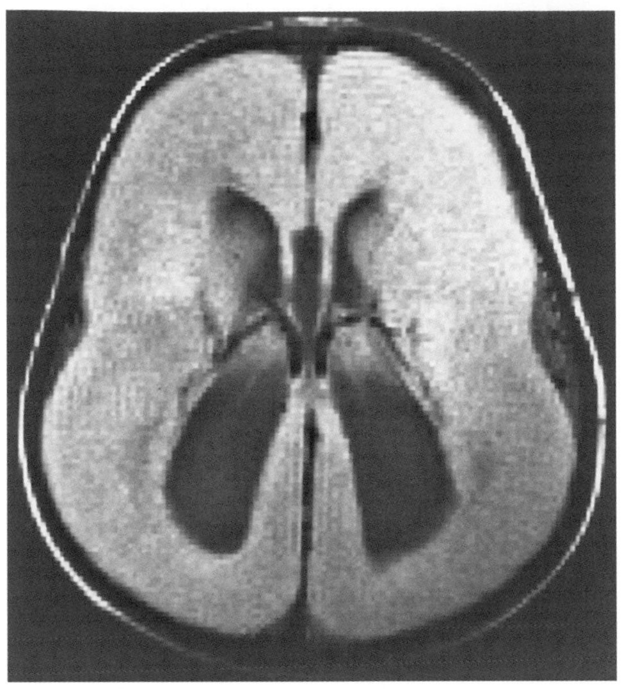
A

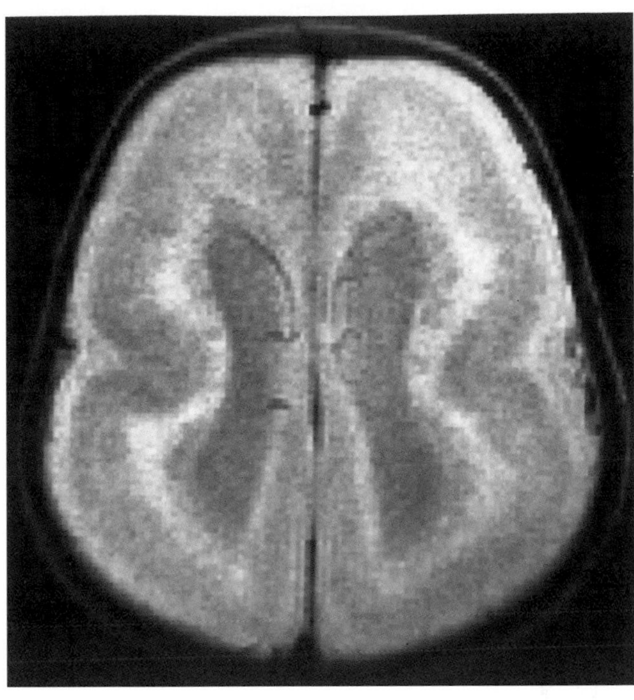
B

Figure 13.6 Lissencephaly in a 3-month-old female. (A) Smooth brain surface and dilated ventricles resulting from early arrest in neuronal migration are evident on this spin-density axial MRI scan. (B) Note the three-layer appearance from the primitive cortex peripherally, the darker matrix centrally, and the nonmigrating neurons that have proliferated in the periventricular region on a more T2-weighted image at a slightly higher level. (Courtesy Joseph R. Thompson, Department of Radiation Sciences, Loma Linda University School of Medicine, Loma Linda, CA.)

hemisphere may be involved. This disorder is caused by a defect in neuronal migration in the fourth month of gestation, and children with this disorder share many of the same clinical symptoms as children with lissencephaly (Dhellemmes *et al.* 1988). The abnormal cortical areas undergo dense gliosis and contain large, unusual neurons. Clinical findings consist of spasticity and weakness. In some patients, central rolandic and sylvian macrogyria have been associated with epilepsy, pseudobulbar palsy, and mental retardation (Kuzniecky *et al.* 1989).

## NEURONAL HETEROTOPIAS

Neuronal heterotopias are now a commonly recognized form of neuronal migration disorder (Norman *et al.* 1995; Friede 1989). Resulting from the arrested migration along radial glial elements before the fifth month of gestation, clusters of neurons can be demonstrated pathologically, and more recently by MRI. Table 13.5 also summarizes some of the more common disorders in which heterotopias have been reported. Based primarily on their locations, neuronal heterotopias have been classified into three groups: (1) periventricular; (2) subcortical white matter-diffuse laminar ('band') or focal or diffuse nodular, and (3) superficial cortical or leptomeningeal (Barkovich & Kjos 1992).

### Periventricular heterotopias

Periventricular (subependymal) heterotopias (PH) are smooth round or irregular masses of neurons that line the ventricle (Fig. 13.7). They may extend into the ventricles and are usually located in the corners or atria of the lateral ventricles or the ventrolateral regions of the temporal horns (Ball 1997). A recent series of 33 patients reported unilateral PH in 58% and bilateral lesions in 42%; 39% of patients also had unilateral focal subcortical heterotopias (Dubeau *et al.* 1995).

The causes of PH are multiple. Destructive lesions at the ependymal surface may affect proliferating or migrating neuroblasts or radial-glial processes, so that migration of intact neuroblasts does not occur (Sarnat 1995). The ependyma may be damaged by stretching during ventricular dilatation, by ventricular wall infarction, or by intrauterine infection or inflammation. Because PH and other forms of heterotopias are seen in a wide variety of genetic and metabolic conditions, it is likely that future research will clarify the mechanisms by which early neuronal migration is perturbed by environmental and other factors that allow for the development of this form of cortical dysgenesis (Kuzniecky *et al.* 1995; Crino & Eberwine 1997; Evrard *et al.* 1997).

The possibility of X-linked dominant inheritance in several kindreds with epilepsy and PH has been reported and suggests that affected females are at high risk for epilepsy

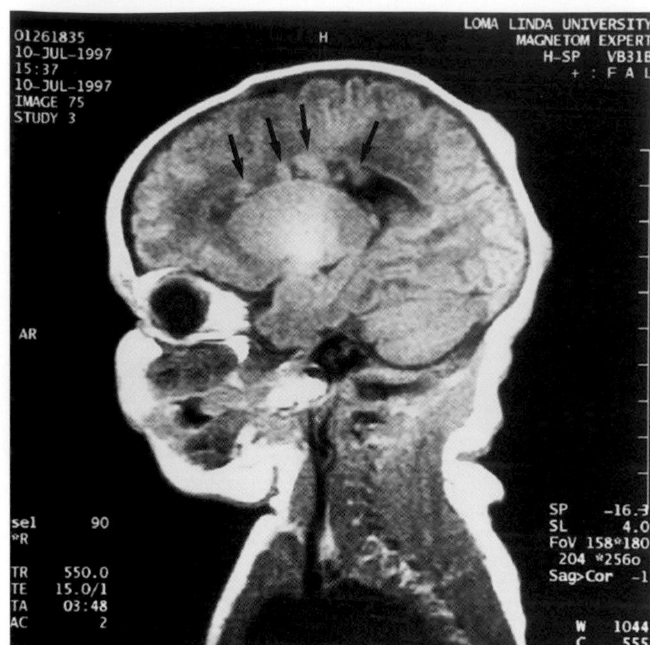


**Figure 13.7** Periventricular heterotopias in a newborn infant. This sagittal T1-weighted MRI of the brain reveals multiple nodules of ectopic gray matter versus hamartomas in the subependymal region protruding into the left lateral ventricle (black arrows). (Courtesy of Shahrokh Toranji MD, Department of Radiation Sciences, Loma Linda University School of Medicine, Loma Linda, CA.)

and that the disease may be lethal in affected males (Huttenlocher *et al.* 1994; Dubeau *et al.* 1995). Linkage to markers in distal Xq28 in patients with PH has also been reported and suggests that the PH gene may represent an important epilepsy susceptibility locus in addition to playing a key role in normal cortical development (Eksioglu *et al.* 1996). Differentiation of this form of X-linked dominant PH from tuberous sclerosis must be considered, and is based on the lack of characteristic skin lesions, more severe degrees of developmental retardation, presence of extracranial hamartomas, and different chromosomal abnormalities seen in the latter condition (DiMario *et al.* 1993; Jardine *et al.* 1996). In one kinship involving three affected sisters with PH, developmental delay, epilepsy, and dysmorphic features, including a low nasal bridge, upslanting palpebral fissures, palpebral edema, attached hypoplastic earlobes, and a thickened calvarium, were reported (Musumeci *et al.* 1996). Rectal fibrovascular polyps, urinary tract anomalies, and increased foot length were also observed.

Clinically, patients with PH may have generalized or partial complex seizures; many have no or mild clinical symptoms and normal developmental function. In one series, heterotopias were associated with unilateral or bilateral independent temporal epileptic discharges in 47% of seizure patients with subependymal lesions alone and in 61% of those who had unilateral focal subcortical heterotopias (Dubeau *et al.* 1995). Extratemporal or multifocal discharges were observed in an additional 36% of patients. Seizures may remain intractable in some patients with PH, despite temporal lobe resections suggesting a more widespread disorder with epileptogenic activity originating in or near the heterotopic tissue (Li *et al.* 1997).

### Subcortical white matter heterotopias

Heterotopias in the white matter may be classified as laminar or nodular (Friede, 1989; Barkovich 1996).

**Laminar or band heterotopias** are diffuse symmetric single or interrupted nodular bands of gray matter that are separated from the normal-appearing cortex by a thick layer of white matter (Barkovich *et al.* 1989; Palmini *et al.* 1991a; Norman *et al.* 1995). These heterotopias form symmetric ribbons of gray matter in the centrum semiovale. Patients with laminar heterotopias usually have developmental delay, neuromotor impairment, and generalized or partial complex seizures (Barkovich 1996). One form of laminar heterotopia, the 'double cortex, is associated with more severe neurologic involvement (Palmini *et al.* 1991a; Hashimoto *et al.* 1993). Affected children typically have more severe developmental delays and seizures that are difficult to control, including Lennox–Gastaut syndrome. Those patients who also have overlying cortical gyral anomalies, in association with the thickened double cortex, are also more likely to be at greater risk for developmental delay (Barkovich & Kjos 1992).

**Nodular heterotopias** are more common and consist of single or multiple nodules of gray matter, located in the subcortical white matter, that may be either focal or diffuse. They are frequently located close to the ventricular wall, lateral to the basal ganglia and thalamus or in the centrum semiovale. Microscopic examination reveals disorganized arrays of both neuronal and glial cells. These heterotopias may be seen in conjunction with other malformations such as microcephaly, agenesis of the corpus callosum, septo-optic dysplasia, and chromosomal malformations. The cerebral cortex overlying subcortical heterotopia may be thin with shallow sulci and the basal ganglia dysplastic (Barkovich 1996). Seizures and developmental delays of varying degrees are the most frequent clinical manifestations (Barkovich & Kjos 1992; Gunay & Aysun 1996). EEGs depict slow-wave background activity with spike and spike-wave complexes in the affected hemisphere (Palmini *et al.* 1991b; Barkovich 1996).

### Superficial cortical or leptomeningeal heterotopias

Superficial cortical heterotopias consist of nodular collections of glial and neuronal cells derived from layers 2 and 3 of the cortex that may herniate into the leptomeninges (Sarnat 1992). These glial neuronal heterotopias (brain warts) can be difficult to identify with MRI because they may be relatively isointense with the surrounding gray matter (Ball 1997). They can be seen in a variety of conditions including Walker–Warburg syndrome, congenital muscular dystrophy, Zellweger syndrome, Galloway–Mowat syndrome, 18p deletion, and other chromosomal disorders (Norman *et al.* 1995). They are commonly seen in association with many other severe forms of CNS malformations (e.g. microcephaly or lissencephaly), but can also occur as an isolated phenomenon.

Leptomeningeal glial–neuronal heterotopias involve ectopic collections of neurons and astrocytes that are principally located within the leptomeninges. They may have a nodular appearance but also may be present as sheets of cells overlying portions of the cortex (Norman *et al.* 1995; Volpe 2000). They are frequently seen in patients with fetal alcohol syndrome.

## AGENESIS OF THE CORPUS CALLOSUM

The corpus callosum, a forebrain commissure, originates from the primitive lamina terminalis (terminal plate). The first callosal fibers form at day 74 of gestation and formation is complete by 115 days; however, myelination continues after birth (Yakovlev & LeCours, 1967; Norman *et al.* 1995). The extent of the malformation varies from partial to complete agenesis.

Agenesis of the corpus callosum (ACC) occurs in about one to three infants per 1000 births, is usually sporadic, and may be transmitted as a sex-linked, autosomal-dominant, or autosomal-recessive trait (Castro-Gago *et al.* 1993; Lynn *et al.* 1980) (see p. 241, Chapter 14). Prenatal diagnosis of ACC can be established by 20 weeks gestation with ultrasonography (Bertino *et al.* 1988; Vergani *et al.* 1994). In about half of the reported fetal ultrasound studies, ACC is an isolated finding; in the remaining studies, other abnormalities or findings suggestive of specific syndromes are found. Male fetuses are more likely to have isolated agenesis that is considered benign.

The etiology of ACC has been associated with numerous syndromes (see Table 13.7) (Chevrie & Aicardi 1986) and several inborn errors of metabolism, including non-ketotic hyperglycinemia and fetal alcohol syndrome (Kolodny 1989; Norman *et al.* 1995). The genetically determined sex-linked type of partial agenesis of the corpus callosum is associated with seizures that are evident during the first hours of

**Table 13.7 Conditions associated with abnormal development of the corpus callosum**

| | | |
|---|---|---|
| **Associations with other organ involvement** | **Metabolic disorders** | Hypohydrotic ectodermal dysplasia |
| Asplenia, anopthalmia, coloboma | Carbohydrate-deficient glycoprotein syndrome | Jeune's thoracic asphyxiating dystrophy |
| Blepharophimosis, coloboma, hearing loss | | Kallmann |
| Congenital choanal atresia | Hurler syndrome | Marshall–Smith |
| Hirschsprung's disease | Leprechaunism (insulin receptor defect) | Meckel-Gruber |
| Median cleft face syndrome | Mitochondrial disorders (e.g., Leigh syndrome) | Microcephalic osteodysplastic primordial dwarfism |
| Morning glory syndrome | | |
| Ocular albinism | Nonketoic hyperglycinemia | Muscle, eye, and brain disease |
| Osseous lesions | Organic acidurias (3-OH-isobutyric aciduria) | Neu-Laxova |
| | Pyruvate decarboxylase deficiency | Neurofibromatosis |
| **CNS malformation syndromes** | Zellweger (peroxisomal disorder) | Norman–Roberts |
| Arachnoid cysts | | Oculo-cerebro-cutaneous |
| Arnold–Chiari II malformation | **Syndromes** | Oral-facial-digital |
| Cerebellar dysgenesis | Acrocallosal | Pena–Shokeir II |
| CRASH syndrome | Adams-Oliver | Proteus |
| Dandy–Walker syndrome | Aicardi | 'Reverse' Shapiro |
| Hydrocephalus | Andermann | Rubinstein-Taybi |
| Interhemispheric cyst | Apert | Seckel |
| Intraventricular lipomas | Baller-Gerold | Shapiro |
| Lissencephaly | Basal cell nevus | Shprintzen–Goldberg |
| | Cerebrofaciothoracic dysplasia | Smith–Lemli-Opitz |
| **Chromosomal/genetic disorders** | Coffin-Siris | Thanatophoric dwarfism |
| Aneuploidies (45, X; 47, XXY) | Cranioectodermal dysplasia | Tuberous sclerosis |
| Autosomal recessive | Di George | Walker–Warburg |
| Pseudotrisomy 13 | Ectodermal dysplasia | Whistling face |
| Trisomy 8, 11q-, 13, 16, 18 | Edward's micro-ophthalmia | |
| X-linked recessive | Frontonasal dysplasia and polydactyly | **Teratogens** |
| | Fryns | Fetal alcohol syndrome |
| | Fukuyama congenital muscular dystrophy | Maternal valproate use |
| | Goldenhar | Maternal phenylketonuria |

*Source*: From OMIM (1998); Norman *et al.* (1995), Ball (1997).

life, with subsequent profound developmental retardation (Menkes *et al.* 1964). In females, Aicardi syndrome, a sex-linked dominant condition, is associated with ACC, infantile spasms, intellectual retardation, vertebral anomalies, and chorioretinal lacunae (Fig. 13.8) (Chevrie & Aicardi 1986). The condition is probably lethal in males. Gray matter heterotopias are common. Hypsarrhythmia and burst suppression are often visualized by EEG.

ACC is also seen in association with many of the major CNS malformations. An unusual association with intraventricular lipomas (Vade & Horowitz 1992) or intracranial arachnoid cysts (Pascual-Castroviejo 1991a) is recognized, but most commonly ACC occurs in patients with lissencephaly, Dandy–Walker syndrome, and Arnold–Chiari II malformations. Of interest is the recent discovery that X-linked hydrocephalus, MASA syndrome (macrocephaly, adducted thumbs, spasticity, ACC), and certain forms of X-linked spastic paraplegia and agenesis of corpus callosum are now known to be due to mutations in the gene for the neural cell adhesion molecule L1CAM (Serville *et al.* 1992; Yamasaki *et al.* 1997). These syndromes have been reclassified as CRASH syndrome, an acronym for *c*orpus callosum hypoplasia, *r*etardation, *a*dducted *t*humbs, *s*pasticity, and *h*ydrocephalus (Fransen *et al.* 1995). L1CAM is a transmembrane glycoprotein that is mainly expressed on neurons and Schwann cells and participates in the regulation of axon outgrowth (Fransen *et al.* 1997). Mutations of the L1 gene (chromosome Xq28) are responsible for a wide spectrum of neurologic abnormalities and mental retardation.

An association between certain anti-epileptic drugs, particularly valproic acid, and various neural tube or midline defects including ACC has also been suggested (Lindhout *et al.* 1992).

Chromosomal disorders particularly trisomies 8, 13, and 18 and pseudotrisomy 13 syndrome are also associated with ACC (Lurie *et al.* 1995). Rare associations with monosomy 11q and other deletions have also been reported (Hustinx *et al.* 1993). ACC can also be seen in patients with Hirschsprung's disease (Sayed & al-Alaiyan 1996), asplenia (Devriendt *et al.* 1997), and an unusual disorder associated with mental retardation and osseous lesions (Kozlowski & Ouvrier 1993).

Other syndromes associated with ACC include the following: (1) the Meckel–Gruber syndrome, which is an autosomal-recessive disorder with principal features of renal dysplasia, polydactyly, holoprosencephaly, occipital exencephalocele, and other CNS malformations (Ahdab-Barmada & Claassen 1990); (2) Andermann syndrome, which is also an autosomal-recessive disorder described primarily in individuals from certain regions of Canada and associated with a peripheral sensorimotor neuropathy, mental retardation, and various dysmorphic features (Gurtubay *et al.* 1997); and (3) the acrocallosal syndrome (ACS), which is an autosomal-recessive disorder first reported by Schinzel in 1979 and characterized by the association of craniofacial anomalies, total or partial ACC, seizures, preaxial polysyndactyly, 'hallux duplex' of both feet, mental retardation, and, in some patients, diabetes insipidus (Gelman-Kohan *et al.* 1991; Fryns *et al.* 1997). In some patients, inverted tandem duplication of chromosome band 12p11.2-p13.3 has been observed (Pfeiffer *et al.* 1992).

Rare cases of frontonasal dysplasia (Toriello *et al.* 1986) and Fryns syndrome may be associated with ACC (Ayme *et al.* 1989). Patients with Fryns syndrome usually die in the neonatal period because of the presence of multiple congenital anomalies, including diaphragmatic defects, lung hypoplasia, cleft lip and palate, cardiac septal defects and aortic arch anomalies, renal cysts, urinary tract malformations, hypoplastic genitalia, and distal limb hypoplasia. Various forms of the orofaciodigital syndrome may also be associated with ACC (Leao *et al.* 1995).

An unusual condition with ACC is Shapiro syndrome, which is associated with spontaneous periodic hypothermia (Shapiro *et al.* 1969). Variants of this syndrome have been reported with abnormalities of water metabolism (i.e. polydipsia, polyuria, and hyponatremia) not associated with endocrine dysfunction (Mooradian *et al.* 1984) or with episodic hyperhidrosis and hypothermia (LeWitt *et al.* 1983). During attacks, patients are described as confused, withdrawn, lethargic, or ataxic. More recently a 'reverse' Shapiro syndrome has been reported (Hirayama *et al.* 1994). These patients have periodic hyperthermia rather than hypothermia. The existence of Shapiro syndrome, however,

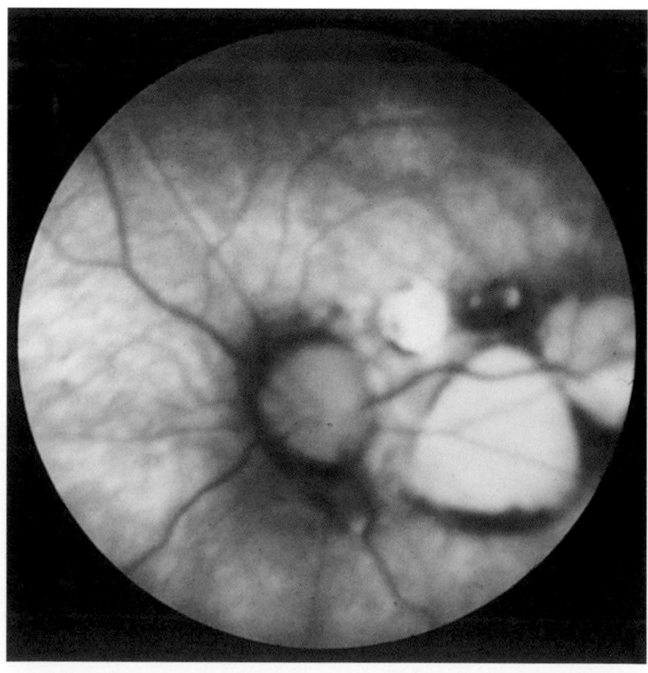

**Figure 13.8** Aicardi syndrome. This fundus photograph depicts the retinal lacunae characteristic of the syndrome. (Courtesy of the Division of Pediatric Neurology, University of Minnesota Medical School, Minneapolis, MN.)

has been questioned (Norman *et al.* 1995). Because many of the patients first present in adulthood, the relation to the congenital malformation of ACC seems unlikely.

Pathologic findings in ACC are various. The lateral ventricles are shifted laterally, with the resultant formation of a large, midline interhemispheric subarachnoid space. The foramina of Monro are malformed and elongated to reach the lateral ventricles, and the third ventricle is enlarged, its roof extending dorsally (Friede 1989; Sarnat 1992). Accompanying abnormalities may include heterotopias, microgyria, abnormal cerebral fissures, porencephalic cysts, and hydrocephalus. The sulci over the medial surface of the hemisphere may manifest an unusual radial pattern. Failure of decussation causes the fiber tracts to form large ipsilateral bundles of Probst. More profound pathologic deviations from normal have been typical of either the X-linked hereditary type or Aicardi syndrome (Fig. 13.8).

Clinically, the extent and nature of neurologic compromise result from the congenital absence of the corpus callosum and the associated brain abnormalities. Absence of the corpus callosum may be accompanied by mild or subtle clinical manifestations (Parrish *et al.* 1979). Normal intelligence is not unusual. Mild compromise of skills requiring matching of visual patterns and crossed tactile localization has been described. Severe compromise may be present, including intellectual retardation, epilepsy, failure to thrive, spasticity, and hydrocephalus; these findings are particularly likely to occur in children with extensive malformations (Lacey 1985).

Patients with agenesis of the corpus callosum often have asynchrony of sleep spindles, and hemispheric electrical activity may appear to be independent of the other side (Lynn *et al.* 1980). Neuroimaging techniques document the unique pattern resulting from the abnormal space between the lateral ventricles and the upward displacement and enlargement of the third ventricle (see Fig. 6.19).

### Wide or persistent cavum septum pellucidum

Persistence of the cavum septum pellucidum is believed to be a variant of normal. Recent studies suggest that children who have this finding may have subtle forms of cerebral dysgenesis and are at risk for a variety of neurodevelopmental disorders, although this has been disputed (Schaefer *et al.* 1996).

## CEREBELLAR MALFORMATIONS

Malformations of the cerebellum and vermis may be categorized as related to agenesis, hypoplasia, or hyperplasia. These classifications are descriptive and are likely to undergo substantial revision as the genetic regulation of posterior fossa structures and its relation to malformations or disease processes are increasingly understood. Associated conditions that can be seen with cerebellar and vermian malformations are listed in Table 13.8.

**Table 13.8 Conditions associated with abnormal cerebellar development**

| | | |
|---|---|---|
| **Associations with other organ involvement** | Porencephaly | **Syndromes** |
| Congenital hepatic fibrosis | Posterior fossa cyst | CHARGE association |
| Congenital hip dislocation | Rhombencephalosynapsis | COACH |
| Congenital lymphedema | Spinal dysraphism | Cornelia de Lange's |
| Hirschsprung's disease | Tectocerebellar dysraphia | Dekaban |
| Hypogonadotropic hypogonadism | Werdnig-Hoffmann disease | Down syndrome |
| Immunodeficiency syndromes | | Fukuyama congenital muscular dystrophy |
| Optic coloboma | **Chromosomal/genetic disorders** | Fryns |
| Progressive pancytopenia | Autosomal dominant | Hoyeraal-Hreidarsson |
| Tapeto-retinal degeneration | Autosomal recessive | Marinesco-Sjogren |
| | Down syndrome | Meckel-Gruber |
| **CNS/PNS malformation syndromes** | Chromosome 5 deletion (Cri-du-chat) | Menkes |
| Arrhinencephaly | Trisomy 9, 13, 10, 18 | Neu-Laxova |
| Arnold-Chiari II malformation | X-linked | Neurocutaneous melanosis |
| Cranial meningocele | | Oral-facial-digital (type II, type VI) |
| CRASH syndrome | **Metabolic disorders** | Otopalatal-digital |
| Dandy-Walker | Carbohydrate-deficient glycoprotein | Ritscher-Schinzel (3C) |
| Hydrocephalus | syndrome | Walker-Warburg |
| Joubert | Mitochondrial disorders | Whistling face |
| Lissencephaly/pachygyria | Muscle phosphofructokinase deficiency | |
| Microcephaly | | **Teratogens** |
| Occipital meningomyelocele | | Fetal alcohol syndrome |
| Pontocerebellar hypoplasia | | Maternal isotretinoin use |

*Source*: From OMIM (2000); Norman *et al.* (1995); Ball (1997).

## AGENESIS

Isolated agenesis of the cerebellum is distinctly uncommon and usually associated with motor deficits (Hamilton & Grafe 1994; Glickstein 1994). The dentate nuclei, vermis, and cerebellar peduncles are poorly developed (Macchi & Bentivoglio 1987). This condition and related conditions are diagnosed more frequently since the advent of modern neuroimaging techniques (Adamsbaum *et al.* 1994). Cerebellar agenesis has been associated with chromosomal defects, such as trisomies 13 and 18. Cerebellar agenesis has been described in association with a variety of CNS malformations and syndromes. It can occur with arrhinecephaly (Leech *et al.* 1997).

In contrast to complete agenesis of the cerebellum, hypoplasia of varying degrees occurs more commonly (deSouza *et al.* 1994; Shevell & Majnemer 1996). Cerebellar hypoplasia can occur in the majority of the conditions listed in Table 13.8. It may also occur sporadically or be inherited as a familial (X-linked) trait (al Shahwan *et al.* 1995). Cerebellar hypoplasia has also been detected in patients with mitochondrial respiratory chain disorders (Lincke *et al.* 1996). Findings on examination include mild-to-moderate developmental disability, microcephaly, typical 'cerebellar' findings, and impaired fine motor skills.

Unilateral cerebellar defects are more common than bilateral hemispheric agenesis or hypoplasia and are usually asymptomatic (Boltshauser *et al.* 1996). Hemiagenesis is accompanied by poor development of the red nucleus, contralateral inferior olive, and ipsilateral brachium conjunctivum. Presenting signs may include delayed motor development, contralateral torticollis, unusual head nodding, and ataxia.

Recent studies have found that mice lacking the Math1 gene fail to form granule cells and are born with a cerebellum that is devoid of an external germinal layer (Ben Arie *et al.* 1997). Math1, the mouse homolog of the Drosophila gene atonal, encodes a basic helix-loop-helix transcription factor that is specifically expressed in the precursors of the external germinal layer. Since the granule cells are the predominant neurons in the cerebellum, these findings suggest one potential mechanism for the pathogenesis of malformations involving the cerebellum.

### Pontocerebellar hypoplasia

Pontocerebellar hypoplasia (PCH) is distinct from disorders associated with cerebellar hypoplasia because the ventral pons is affected (Barth 1993; Malandrini *et al.* 1997). Barth has described the following two variants: (1) PCH-1, which is associated with a form of spinal anterior horn degeneration similar to Werdnig–Hoffmann disease; and (2) PCH-2, which is associated with an early-onset choreiform, and dystonic movement disorder that is often severe. PCH-1 presents in the neonatal period with respiratory insufficiency, frequent congenital contractures, and a combination of central and peripheral motor signs; patients usually die before the age of 1 year. PCH-2 is likely an autosomal-recessive disorder. Patients do not have spinal anterior horn pathology but do have microcephaly and severely impaired mental and motor development and are likely to die during childhood (Barth *et al.* 1995).

### Tectocerebellar dysraphia

Tectocerebellar dysraphia (TCD) is an extremely rare condition in which both the cerebellar hemispheres and brainstem tectum are hypoplastic (Hori 1994; Demaerel *et al.* 1995). Occipital encephaloceles are also common and some relation to rhombencephalosynapsis in which the cerebellar hemispheres are fused has been proposed.

## AGENESIS OF THE VERMIS

Agenesis of the vermis is usually partial but may be complete. In partial agenesis the posterior vermis is absent, which is consistent with its embryologic development; the anterior part of the vermis is formed before the posterior area. In cases of complete vermain agenesis the insult occurs earlier than in partial agenesis.

Clinically, agenesis of the vermis may be asymptomatic. Neurologic findings result from abnormalities in cerebellar hemispheres, nuclei, and associated brainstem pathways. Neurologic features include hypotonia in infants and incoordination, tremor, and truncal ataxia in children. Delayed fine and gross motor milestones, nystagmus, and decreased deep tendon reflexes also occur. Mild neurologic symptoms may improve with maturation. Agenesis of the vermis may be an associated finding with myelomeningocele, cranial meningoceles, agenesis of the corpus callosum, heterotopias, HPE, and other conditions listed in Table 13.8 (Schaefer *et al.* 1996). Vermian agenesis can also occur with fusion of the cerebellar hemispheres (rhombencephalosynapsis) and on rare occasions cerebral hemispheric fusion may also be present (Aydingoz *et al.* 1997; Sergi *et al.* 1997; Romanengo *et al.* 1997). Vermian agenesis may also be inherited as an autosomal-dominant (Rivier & Echenne 1992) or X-linked disorder (Illarioshkin *et al.* 1996).

Cerebellar hypoplasia or vermian agenesis can be detected using fetal ultrasound, usually by the end of the first trimester or early in the second trimester (van Zalen-Sprock *et al.* 1996). Findings of isolated vermian agenesis without evidence of a Dandy–Walker malformation are usually but not universally indicative of a good prognosis (Keogan *et al.* 1994). Diagnosis of vermian agenesis or the Dandy–Walker syndrome should not be made before 18 weeks gestation, because the development of the cerebellar vermis may be incomplete at that time (Bromley *et al.* 1994).

### Joubert syndrome

Joubert syndrome is an autosomal-recessive form of agenesis of the cerebellar vermis (Joubert *et al.* 1969; King *et al.* 1984; Saraiva & Baraitser 1992; Maria *et al.* 1997). It consists of episodic hyperpnea and apnea, disorders of ocular movement, ataxia, hypotonia, and mental retardation. The respiratory abnormality worsens with stimulation and improves with maturation. Abnormal respiration with episodic tachypnea and apnea can occur in several other syndromes (e.g. Rett, Mohr, or Dandy–Walker), but these usually present later in childhood (Boltshauser *et al.* 1987). Joubert syndrome has been classified into two subtypes by some investigators with the differentiating feature being the absence (type A) or presence (type B) of retinal dystrophy (Saraiva & Baraitser 1992).

The retinal dystrophy has been previously classified as a variant of Leber's congenital amaurosis (Lambert *et al.* 1989). The retinal dystrophy is always present in those patients in whom renal cysts occur. Also present are abnormalities of smooth pursuit; pendular, torsional, optokinetic, or other forms of nystagmus; or oculomotor apraxia. Vestibulo-ocular reflexes are usually intact, but smooth pursuit movements are impaired. Congenital hepatic fibrosis has also been reported in some patients, usually in association with congenital medullary cystic renal disease (Lewis *et al.* 1994). The renal cysts are multiple, small, and cortical, and affected kidneys also have interstitial chronic inflammation and fibrosis.

Neuroimaging techniques reveal an enlarged fourth ventricle and interpeduncular fossa, dilated cisterna magna, thickened superior cerebellar peduncles, and varying degrees of vermian hypoplasia (Fig. 13.9) (Kendall *et al.* 1990; Maria *et al.* 1997). As a result of midbrain, vermian, and superior cerebellar peduncle abnormalities, axial neuroimaging reveals a unique 'molar tooth' appearance of these structures (Maria *et al.* 1997). Also reported with MRI are thinned optic tracts, enlarged temporal horns in the absence of hydrocephalus, high signal of the cerebral periventricular white matter, abnormal signal in the decussation of the superior cerebellar peduncles, and abnormal embryonic vessels associated with the dysplastic folia of the cerebellar hemispheres (Sener 1995).

Joubert syndrome with retinal dystrophy and renal cysts may represent a variant of the carbohydrate-deficient glycoprotein syndrome (Hagberg *et al.* 1993; Jensen *et al.* 1995). Others have suggested that Joubert syndrome is a member of a spectrum of congenital malformation syndromes involving the CNS, eye, liver, and kidneys (Lewis *et al.* 1994; Silverstein *et al.* 1997). Joubert syndrome should also be differentiated from the COACH syndrome, which consists of *c*erebellar vermis hypo/aplasia, *o*ligophrenia, *a*taxia, *c*oloboma, and *h*epatic fibrosis (Gentile *et al.* 1996).

Several other syndromes with vermian agenesis need to be differentiated from Joubert syndrome. The Ritscher–Schinzel syndrome or 3C (craniocerebello-cardiac) syndrome is another condition with vermian agenesis or hypoplasia that is associated with cardiac and cranial defects (Kosaki *et al.* 1997). Cardiac lesions include endocardial cushion or conotruncal defects. Speech, and to a lesser extent motor, delays are the major developmental disabilities and postnatal growth deficiencies are common. Characteristic

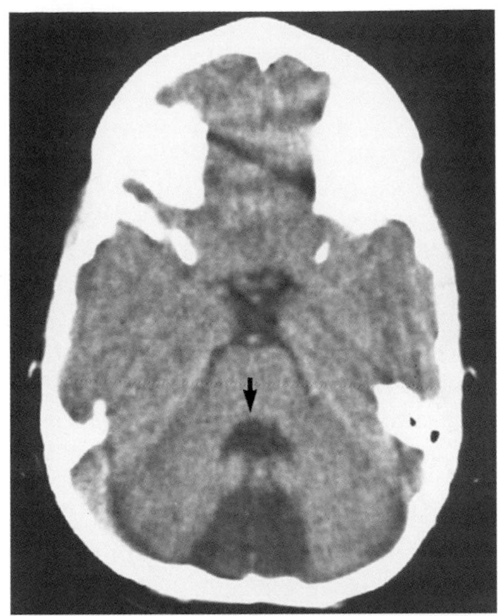
A

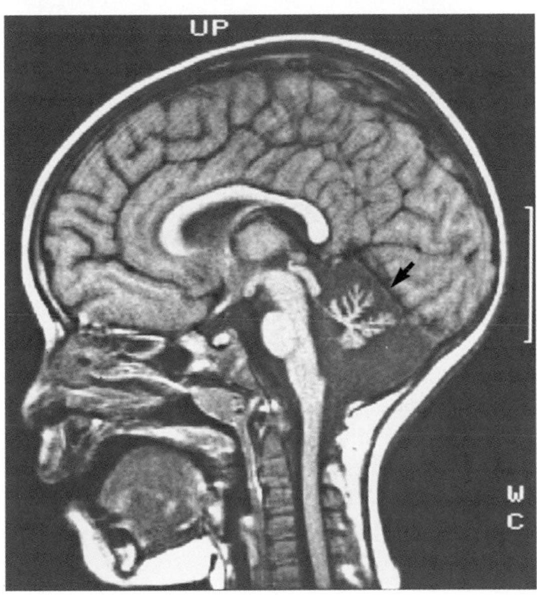

B

Figure 13.9 Cerebellar vermian hypoplasia in a 3-year-old male. (A) Moderate fourth ventricle dilatation (arrow) and large cisterna magna with little intervening vermian tissue seen on this axial CT scan. (B) Midsagittal T1-weighted MRI revealing leaflike small cerebellar vermis (arrow) surrounded by CSF. (Courtesy Joseph R. Thompson, Department of Radiation Sciences, Loma Linda University School of Medicine, Loma Linda, CA.)

dysmorphic features of this disorder are present, as well as coloboma, cleft palate, bifid uvula, short neck, syndactyly, and hypoplasia of the nails. Also, patients with CHARGE association (*c*oloboma of the eye, *h*eart defect, *a*tresia of the choana, *r*etarded growth and development, *g*enital hypoplasia, and *e*ar anomalies or deafness) may have intermittent hyperpnea and cerebellar hypoplasia, and thus need to be distinguished from patients with Joubert syndrome (Menenzes & Coker 1990).

Recent studies suggest that Joubert syndrome and other forms of vermian agenesis may result from a specific gene defect (Maria *et al.* 1997). Several members of the PAX family of genes (PAX2, PAX5, PAX8) contribute to mid-hindbrain formation (Hatten & Heintz 1995). The EN family of genes also encode for cerebellar development, and targeted disruption of certain of these genes results in abnormalities of cerebellar development (Maria *et al.* 1997). Although EN gene family members are regulated by the WNT1 gene, mutations in WNT1 in a series of Joubert syndrome patients were not detected (Pellegrino *et al.* 1997).

Other recent investigations have identified the nephronophthisis (NPH) gene complex as potentially causing Joubert syndrome (Hildebrandt *et al.* 1998). In the autosomal-recessive form of Joubert syndrome (type A), homozygous deletions have been described as causative in more than 80% of patients. In type B Joubert syndrome, different combinations of the extrarenal symptoms with the NPH gene occur. Homozygous deletions of the NPH1 region in type B Joubert syndrome patients have not been found.

A recent study reported on the follow-up of 19 children with Joubert syndrome (Steinlin *et al.* 1997). Three children who died before 3 years of age demonstrated marked respiratory dysfunction and profound development delay. The remaining children had variable motor development; walking was typically achieved between 2 and 10 years of age. Developmental testing found that four children had profound delays, nine were mild to moderately delayed, and the rest were untestable. Renal involvement was present in four children. It was also observed that ophthalmologic and renal involvement could develop over several years and required periodic monitoring. Normal intelligence despite multiple handicaps has been noted by other observers (Ziegler *et al.* 1990). Several children with Joubert syndrome showing autistic behavior have been described (Holroyd *et al.* 1991).

## CEREBELLAR HYPERPLASIA

Unilateral cerebellar enlargement has been reported in some patients with hemimegalencephaly (Sener 1997b). Ipsilateral brainstem enlargement also is present. The term *total hemimegalencephaly* has been suggested to differentiate it from unilateral megalencephaly in which just the cerebral hemispheres are involved. Hemi-enlargement of the cerebellum has also been recognized in several disorders associated with somatic hemihypertrophy, including Beckwith syndrome, Russell–Silver syndrome, and Klippel–Trenaunay–Weber syndrome (Bodensteiner *et al.* 1997).

Macrocerebellum, consisting of diffusely enlarged bilateral cerebellar hemispheres, has been reported in four children with developmental delay, hypotonia, preserved reflexes, delayed or abnormal maturation of the visual system, oculomotor apraxia, and delayed cerebral myelination (Bodensteiner *et al.* 1997). The diagnosis was established by MRI volumetric determinations and differentiated from the Lhermitte–Duclos syndrome in which there is diffuse hamartomatous enlargement of the cerebellum.

## MACRO CISTERNA MAGNA

The cisterna magna comprises the subarachnoid space posterior to the inferior half of the cerebellum. It may appear prominent as a normal variant. About 1% of children will have an enlarged cisterna magna as determined by neuroimaging studies. A recent review of a group of pediatric patients with macro cisterna magna has suggested that they are at greater risk for neurodevelopmental impairment including incoordination, ataxia, hypotonia, oculomotor abnormalities, and seizures (Schaefer *et al.* 1994).

## DANDY–WALKER SYNDROME

The Dandy–Walker syndrome (DWS) consists of a malformation of the fourth ventricle and cerebellum and occurs in approximately 1 in 30 000 live births. The recurrence risk is low (1–5%) when DWS is not associated with a mendelian disorder (see p. 240, Chapter 14). The malformation is most likely due to a developmental cerebellar defect that originates before embryologic differentiation of the foramina of the fourth ventricle (Golden *et al.* 1987; Norman *et al.* 1995). The cystic transformation of the fourth ventricle and attendant hydrocephalus have been ascribed to atresia of the foramina of the fourth ventricle, the foramen of Magendie, and the lateral paired foramina of Luschka (Epstein and Johanson, 1987). Postmortem studies often reveal intact foramina (Hart *et al.* 1972). The massive cystic formation may originate from compromised absorption of ventricular fluid and subsequent increased pressure because of failure of the normal perforation of the superior coverings of the third and fourth ventricles (Gardner, 1977).

### Pathologic findings

The fourth ventricle is grossly misshapen and is a large, ependymal-lined cyst that extends into the spinal canal (Norman *et al.* 1995; Pascual-Castroviejo *et al.* 1991b). The cerebellar hemispheres are rudimentary and displaced superiorly, and the posterior vermis is hypoplastic or absent. Rostral fluid-containing spaces, including the aqueduct of Sylvius, third ventricle, and lateral ventricles, are grossly enlarged. The posterior fossa is enlarged with upward displacement of the lateral sinuses, tentorium, and torcular.

Numerous brain abnormalities accompany the Dandy–Walker malformation, including agenesis of the corpus callosum, polymicrogyria, agyria, gray matter heterotopias, aqueductal stenosis, Klippel–Feil syndrome, microcephaly, posterior fossa lymphomas, hamartomas of the infundibulum, hemimegalencephaly, and syringomyelia (Hart *et al.* 1972; Parikh *et al.* 1994). Other non-neural associated abnormalities include polydactyly, syndactyly, cleft palate, polycystic kidneys, and abnormal lumbar vertebrae.

Chitayat *et al.* (1994) have summarized the various single gene disorders, chromosomal aberrations, teratogen-induced conditions, and other disorders that are sporadic or of undetermined inheritance associated with the Dandy–Walker malformation. Among the syndromes associated with DWS are the Marden–Walker syndrome (Ozkinay *et al.* 1995), Fryns syndrome (Ayme *et al.* 1989; Riela *et al.* 1995), Neu-Laxova syndrome (Shapiro *et al.* 1992), molybdenum cofactor deficiency (Pintos Morell *et al.* 1995), Coffin-Siris syndrome (Norman *et al.* 1995), and neurocutaneous melanosis (Kadonaga *et al.* 1992).

## Clinical characteristics

Clinical manifestations are often evident during infancy. Delayed motor development, hydrocephalus, nystagmus, spasticity, titubation, and apnea are common features. The posterior portion of the head is enlarged, and a flattened protuberance is present in the inferior occipital area (Tal *et al.* 1980). Difficulties in older children and adults may be manifestations of increased intracranial pressure and ataxia (Maria *et al.* 1987). In a retrospective long-term follow-up study of 20 patients with DWS surgically treated, normal cerebellar function was seen in 50% of patients and intellectual function was normal in 45% (Gerszten & Albright 1995). There was no correlation between cerebellar size and intellectual development or cerebellar function. There was also no correlation between the type of shunt and the subsequent cerebellar size.

An uncommon but well-recognized occurrence in patients with Dandy–Walker malformation is sudden unexpected death that may occur without uncal or tonsillar herniation (Elterman *et al.* 1995). Vascular compromise of the posterior fossa circulation secondary to local increases in intracranial pressure may be a factor.

Cranial ultrasonography accurately defines the posterior fossa cyst and hydrocephalus. Lateral plain radiographs may prove diagnostic; the posterior fossa is enlarged, with superior placement of the torcular herophili and lateral sinus grooves. CT, MRI, or cranial ultrasonography best demonstrates the characteristic pattern of hydrocephalus and cystic enlargement of the fourth ventricle (Fig. 13.10). Prenatal sonographic features include ventriculomegaly and concurrent non-CNS anomalies in about half the patients (Estroff *et al.* 1992; Bromley *et al.* 1994).

Familial forms of DWS have been described with autosomal-recessive or X-linked-recessive inheritance. DWS or cerebellar hypoplasia may be associated with maternal exposure to isotretinoin in the first trimester and can be detected prenatally (Nyberg *et al.* 1988).

The presence of an arachnoid cyst may prove confounding because clinical findings may be similar (Arai & Sato 1991). This condition must be distinguished from

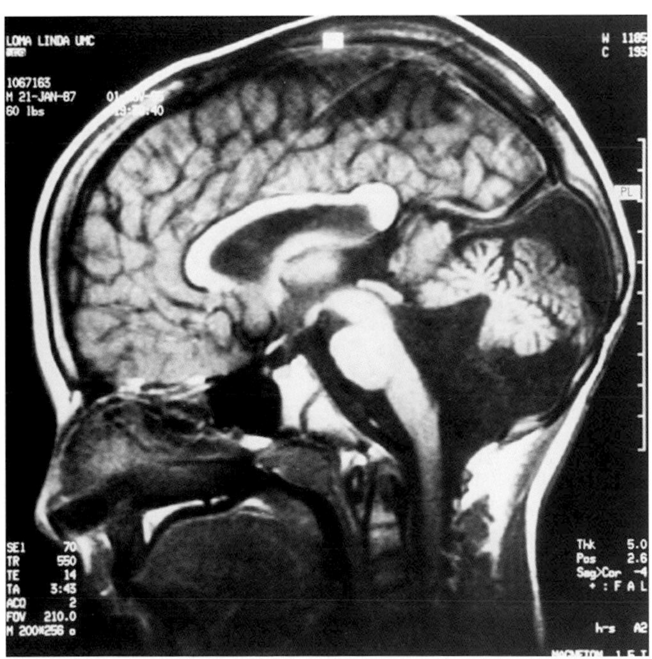


Figure 13.10 Large 2-cm posterior fossa arachnoid cyst in an 8-year-old male status after cystoperitoneal shunting is seen on a T2-weighted axial MRI image. Also present is a large fourth ventricle that interconnects with this cyst and that also distorts cerebellum. (Courtesy of Shahrokh Toranji MD, Department of Radiation Sciences, Loma Linda University School of Medicine, Loma Linda, CA.)

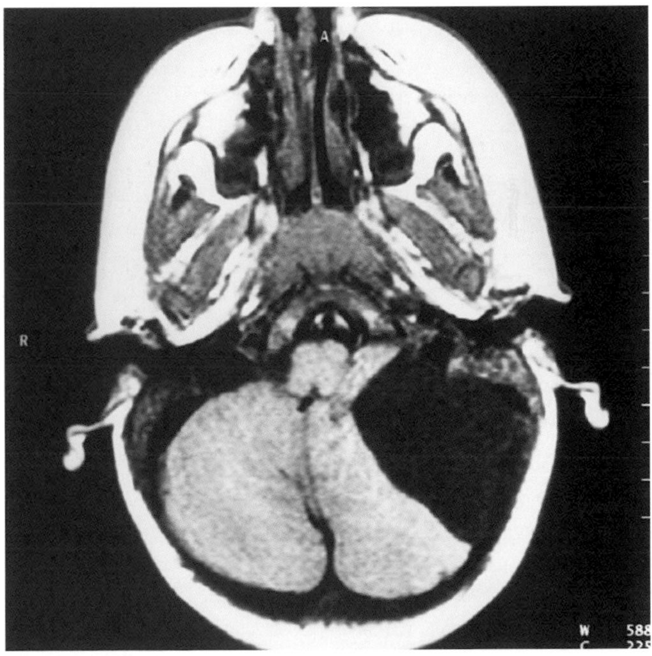

Figure 13.11 Posterior fossa arachnoid cyst in a 3-year-old male presenting with seizures. T1-weighted axial image of the posterior fossa demonstrates a sharply marginated cystic lesion of the left aspect of the posterior cranial fossa compressing and deforming the left cerebellar hemisphere and mildly compressing and displacing the fourth ventricle to the right. (Courtesy of Shahrokh Toranji MD, Department of Radiation Sciences, Loma Linda University School of Medicine, Loma Linda, CA.)

DWS (Haller *et al.* 1971; Menezes *et al.* 1980). Neuroimaging techniques reveal a normal-sized fourth ventricle that is displaced anteriorly by the arachnoid cyst (Fig. 13.11) (Rock *et al.* 1986). If necessary, metrizamide CT will demonstrate whether the cyst communicates with the ventricular system.

### Management

A shunt from the ventricles, cyst, or both has replaced removal of the cyst wall as the primary treatment for Dandy–Walker or posterior fossa cysts (Kalidasan *et al.* 1995). Surgery may be indicated when there is occipital bossing, distortion, or obliteration of CSF cisterns of the posterior fossa, compression and deformity of the brain surrounding the cyst, disturbed CSF circulation, or a non-communicating cyst (Arai & Sato, 1991; Domingo & Peter, 1996). When the ventricles and cyst communicate, a cystoperitoneal shunt may suffice (Sawayal & McLaurin, 1981).

## INTRACRANIAL ARACHNOID CYSTS

Intracranial arachnoid cysts are benign, non-genetic development cysts that contain spinal fluid and occur within the arachnoid membrane (Rengachary & Watanabe 1981; Pascual-Castroviejo *et al.* 1991a). The mechanism of formation during embryogenesis is uncertain (Naidich *et al.* 1985/86). The cysts occur in proximity to arachnoid cisterns, most often in the sylvian fissure (Table 13.9). Arachnoid cysts occur most often in males and in patients with Marfan syndrome. Common neurologic features are headache, seizures, hydrocephalus, focal enlargement of the skull, and signs and symptoms of elevated intracranial pressure and developmental delay, as well as specific signs or symptoms resulting from neural compression. Some arachnoid cysts remain asymptomatic (Mason *et al.* 1997). Progressive enlargement and intracystic or subdural hemorrhage are potential complications. Suprasellar arachnoid cysts may produce neuroendocrine dysfunction, hydrocephalus, and optic nerve compression. Posterior fossa cysts are now more frequently recognized with the use of MRI and CT and frequently require surgical treatment (Domingo & Peter 1996).

**Table 13.9 Distribution of arachnoid cysts**

| Location | Percentage |
|---|---|
| Sylvian fissure | 49 |
| Cerebellopontine angle | 11 |
| Quadrigeminal area | 10 |
| Vermian area and sellar-suprasellar area | 9 |
| Interhemispheric fissure | 5 |
| Cerebral convexity | 4 |
| Clival area | 3 |

*Source*: Modified from Rengachary & Watanabe (1981).

In a recent series of 61 children with arachnoid cysts, about 53% of cases were diagnosed before age 1 year, 42% were supratentorial, and 46% infratentorial (Pascual-Castroviejo *et al.* 1991a). Macrocephaly was the presenting symptom in 72% and associated features included the following: cranial asymmetry in 39%, aqueductal stenosis in 16%, and agenesis of the corpus callosum in 13%. Developmental delay was a common finding and many of the patients with larger cysts required either cystoperitoneal shunting or cyst fenestration.

Skull radiographs may suggest the diagnosis; CT or MRI is the definitive diagnostic procedure (Weiner *et al.* 1987). Injection of contrast medium into the cyst to document communication with the ventricular system is seldom necessary.

### Management

When symptoms warrant, surgical intervention to decompress the cyst, including shunting procedures, is required (Harsh *et al.* 1986; Raffel and McComb, 1988; Pascual-Castroviejo *et al.* 1991a). Arachnoid cysts may occur with or without hydrocephalus. The success rate of fenestration is higher in those patients without hydrocephalus (i.e. 73% required no additional treatment) compared with hydrocephalus patients (32%) (Fewel *et al.* 1996). About 12% of patients treated with fenestration alone may require a cystoperitoneal shunt. In general, cyst fenestration should be the primary procedure in patients without hydrocephalus. If hydrocephalus is present, cyst fenestration is still recommended, but a ventriculoperitoneal shunt should be placed if hydrocephalus is marked or after fenestration if the hydrocephalus is progressive (Fewel *et al.* 1996).

# POSTNEURONAL MIGRATION DEFECTS

## HYDROCEPHALUS

The diagnosis, clinical features, management and prognosis of fetal and neonatal hydrocephalus are discussed in detail in Section XI of this book.

### Aqueductal stenosis

Aqueductal stenosis leads to a form of non-communicating hydrocephalus. Partial or complete obstruction of the aqueduct of Sylvius is associated with congenital structural malformations, hemorrhage, infection, neoplasms, and vascular malformations. Concomitant occlusion of the subarachnoid space may occur. Specific pathologic types of aqueductal stenosis, including congenital narrowing, aqueductal forking, septum formation, and aqueductal gliosis, are difficult to differentiate clinically (Drachman & Richardson 1961). The inflammatory process subsequent to neonatal meningitis and intraventricular hemorrhage can cause aqueductal gliosis. Hereditary aqueductal stenosis is transmitted as an X-linked recessive trait (Edwards 1961). Rare cases of autosomal-recessive inheritance are also reported (Castro Gago *et al.* 1996).

Aqueductal stenosis may accompany Arnold–Chiari malformations, myelomeningocele, and neurofibromatosis. Aqueductal stenosis may also be secondary to an existing communicating hydrocephalus (Nugent *et al.* 1979).

In experimental animals, vitamin A excess, mumps encephalitis, and other viruses cause aqueductal gliosis with associated aqueductal stenosis and hydrocephalus (Volpe 2000). In humans, mumps encephalitis has been associated with acquired aqueductal stenosis and hydrocephalus after a latent period of 3 months to 4 years (Spataro *et al.* 1976). The pathogenesis in experimental animals and humans may be the propensity for selective infection of ependymal cells by the mumps virus (Volpe 2000).

Patients with congenital aqueductal stenosis are hydrocephalic at birth. Cranial ultrasonography demonstrates enlarged lateral and third ventricles with a normal or small fourth ventricle. Other neuroimaging techniques may detect tumor, vascular malformation, and associated congenital anomalies.

Remarkably, some patients with congenital and even early acquired aqueductal stenosis are asymptomatic until later childhood or early adult life; some remain free of symptoms. When they become apparent, manifestations include findings consistent with chronic increased intracranial pressure, such as an enlarged head, headache, seizures, gait disturbance, decreased visual acuity, dementia, and occasionally CSF rhinorrhea (Little *et al.* 1975).

Hypothalamic–pituitary disturbance may occur, including precocious or delayed puberty, impotence, short stature, obesity, hypothyroidism, temperature instability, diabetes insipidus, and amenorrhea. Abnormalities of growth hormone, antidiuretic hormone, thyroid stimulating hormone, gonadotropins, and gonadotropin-releasing hormone have been documented (Fiedler & Krieger 1975; Hier & Wiehl, 1977). Treatment is similar to that for progressive hydrocephalus. After shunting procedures, patients with hypothalamic-pituitary disturbance often improve.

## HYDRANENCEPHALY

Hydranencephaly is a devastating CNS malformation consisting of near complete absence of the cerebral hemispheres. A variety of destructive or developmental abnormalities occurring after the fourth month of gestation may lead to hydranencephaly (Halsey *et al.* 1971; Evrard *et al.* 1989a). Animal models of hydranencephaly have demonstrated that different intrauterine viruses (Flanagan & Johnson 1995) or vascular occlusion (Wintour *et al.* 1996) can cause this malformation. Intrauterine CMV and toxoplasmosis have also been reported to cause hydranencephaly (Kubo *et al.* 1994).

### Pathologic findings

The cranium is intact and therefore does not suggest anencephaly. Only small portions of the frontal, temporal, and occipital cortex are identifiable. A well formed and somewhat thickened sac consists of an outer leptomeningeal layer and a rudimentary representation of the cerebral cortex; no suggestion of normal ventricular configuration or ependymal lining can be delineated. The optic nerves are attenuated. The brainstem is also involved, as evidenced by underdeveloped cerebellar peduncles, pons, and medulla.

Compromise of blood flow within the fetal internal carotid arteries, toxoplasmosis or CMV may be the basis of the extensive CNS malformation (Vogel & McClenahan 1952; Altschuler 1973). Hydranencephaly has also been reported as a result of maternal cocaine use (Rais-Bahrami & Naqvi 1990) and in association with a younger maternal age (Lubinsky 1997). Fetal ultrasound can be used for diagnosis (Agrawal *et al.* 1996).

At least four cases have been reported of hydranencephaly in association with a proliferative vasculopathy that is believed to occur in the first trimester (Harding *et al.* 1995). It has been suggested that this is an autosomal-recessive disorder that differs from encephaloclastic forms of hydranencephaly.

Hydranencephaly may develop in neonates and older infants after widespread cerebral infarction associated with extensive meningitis, intracerebral hemorrhage, and ischemia (Lindenberg & Swanson 1967). Hydranencephaly has been reported in association with 13q22 deletion (Gershoni-Baruch *et al.* 1996).

### Clinical characteristics

Neonates may appear normal in the perinatal period. The head circumference is usually within normal limits. After a few weeks, abnormal neurologic findings become apparent, including spasticity, myoclonic seizures, and an enlarged head circumference from hydrocephalus.

Cranial ultrasonography readily demonstrates this malformation (Fig. 13.12A). Transillumination of the skull is startling because the islands of tissue, sagittal sinus, and meningeal blood vessels are quite visible. Islands of preserved cortical tissue are seen as small opacities. Other neuroimaging techniques provide detailed documentation of the extent of the malformation (Fig. 13.12B) and may be required to distinguish severe hydrocephalus or severe subdural effusions from hydranencephaly. EEG reveals suppressed or absent activity corresponding to the loss of brain tissue. Other EEG abnormalities have been described in hydranencephalic infants with Lennox–Gastaut syndrome (Velasco *et al.* 1997). Somatosensory evoked response studies usually demonstrate an absent cortical response (Tayama *et al.* 1992).

Although an infant may occasionally survive for one or two years, most die before one year of age. Ventriculoperitoneal shunting may be necessary in selected patients with associated progressive hydrocephalus.

## POLYMICROGYRIA

Cytoarchitectonic analysis of the microgyric layers and their continuity with the layers of normal cortex allow some

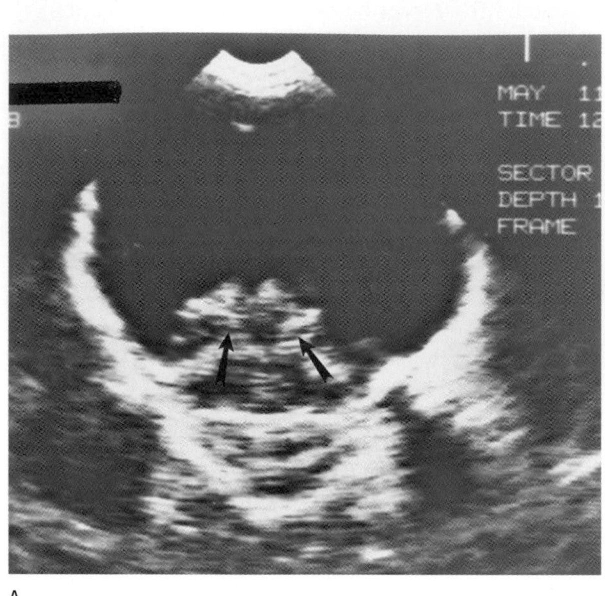


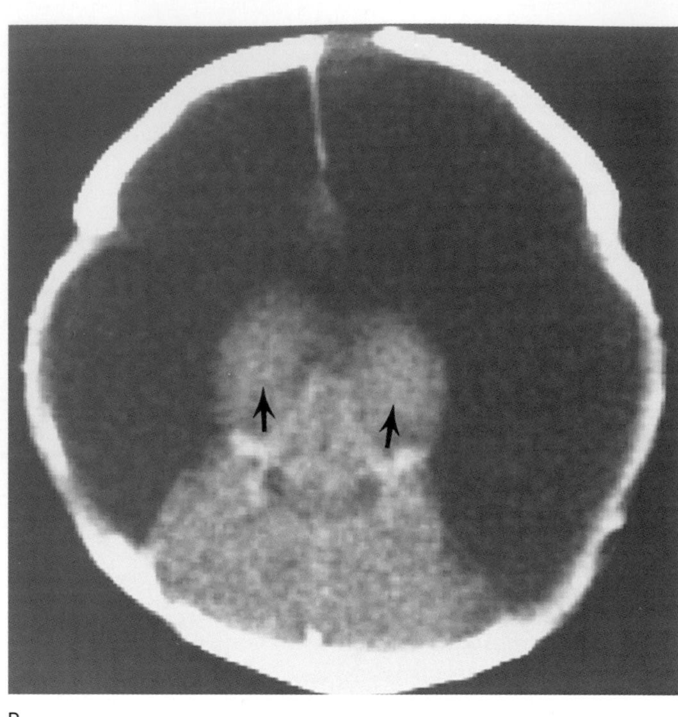

A B

Figure 13.12 Hydranencephaly in a 1-day-old female. (A) CSF-filled cranial cavity with posterior fossa and diencephalic structures (arrows) depicted on coronal, transbregmatic cranial sonogram. (B) Axial CT scan demonstrating CSF-filled supratentorial compartment except for thalamic nuclei (arrows) and small residuum of medial right occipital lobe tissue. (Courtesy Joseph R. Thompson, Department of Radiation Sciences, Loma Linda University School of Medicine, Loma Linda, CA.)

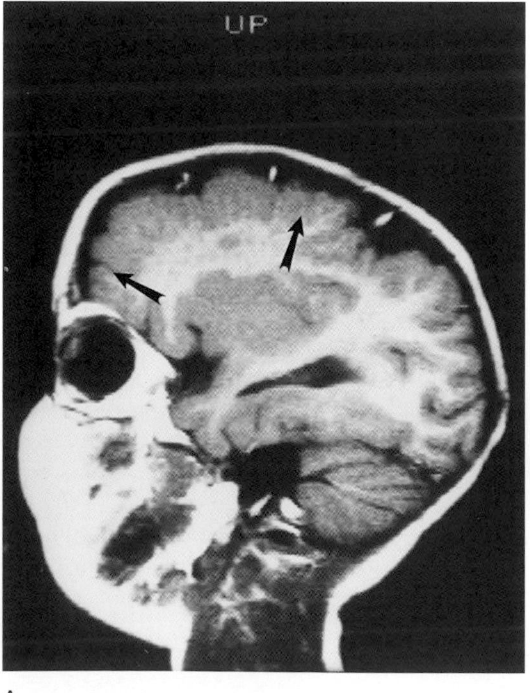


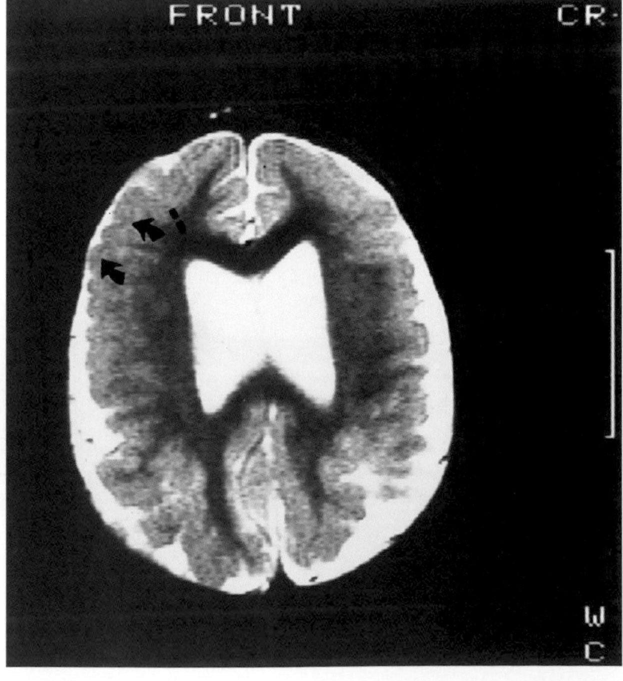


A B

Figure 13.13 Polymicrogyria. (A) T1-weighted spin-echo sagittal view demonstrating irregular, closely spaced small frontal gyri (arrows). Note normal occipital lobe gyri for comparison. (B) T2-weighted spin-echo axial view at level of body of lateral ventricles. Note closely spaced, small gyri of right frontal lobe (arrows). Note normal occipital lobe gyri for comparison.

understanding of the mechanism that underlies microgyria formation (Richman *et al.* 1974; Evrard *et al.* 1989a). The superficial and deep cellular layers of microgyri appear as normal cortical layers II (the most superficial layer), III, IV, and VI. The defect in microgyria is in the middle cortical layer, which has a reduced cellular population. Because the last cells to migrate form the superficial cortex, the presence of a normal superficial cortical layer documents normal neuronal migration. Microgyria, which most likely results from a postmigratory encephaloclastic injury presumably resulting from perfusion failure, produces laminar destruction of the middle layers of the cerebral cortex rather than an arrest of neuronal migration (Fig. 13.13).

Polymicrogyria may be caused by intrauterine hypoxia or ischemia (Evrard *et al.* 1989a), maternal cytomegalic inclusion disease or toxoplasmosis (Crome & France, 1959; Iannetti *et al.* 1998), maternal carbon monoxide poisoning (Ginsberg & Myers, 1978), or an associated finding with the type II Arnold–Chiari malformation, lissencephaly, schizencephaly, and other CNS malformations. Selected groups of patients have been reported in whom polymicrogyria has been detected with MRI in bilateral perisylvian regions (Gropman *et al.* 1997), parasagittal parieto-occipital regions (Guerrini *et al.* 1997), occipital cortex (Kuzniecky *et al.* 1997), and in the cerebellum (Sasaki *et al.* 1997):

## Key Points

- Serious malformations occur in up to 3% of newborns. These frequently involve the nervous system and in more than 60% of infants the etiology can not be determined. Increasingly genetic, teratogenic and infectious etiologies are identified as the cause of these disorders.
- Spina bifida in conjunction with myelomeningocele and hydrocephalus remains common (about 4.6 cases/10 000 births) with the evaluation and management of such infants requiring a multidisciplinary approach.
- Subtle forms of the Arnold–Chiari malformation should be considered in children who present with unexplained recurrent headaches, ataxia, neck pain, or swallowing difficulties.
- Holoprosencephaly, due to failure of the embryonic forebrain to separate, is associated with severe developmental delay, spastic quadriplegia, seizures and failure to thrive.
- Neuronal migrational disorders, neuronal heterotopias and cortical dysplasias are increasingly recognized as the cause of epilepsy syndromes and disorders of cognition based on neuroimaging or neuropathology of tissue taken at the time of epilepsy surgery. Classification of these disorders remains elusive and will depend on correlating genetic, clinical and imaging abnormalities.
- Schizencephaly is associated with the presence of clefts in the cerebral hemispheres. Children with bilateral schizencephaly are likely to have severe neurologic impairments whereas those with unilateral schizencephaly are more likely to have mild or moderate disabilities.
- Lissencephaly, characterized by a brain with a smooth cerebral surface, thickened cortical mantle and incomplete neuronal migration, is usually associated with severe developmental delay and epilepsy. Several forms have been recognized. Type I lissencephaly is most frequently associated with the Miller–Dieker syndrome (17p13.3 deletion) with affected infants having a characteristic facial appearance. Type I lissencephaly may also be seen with the Norman–Roberts syndrome. These patients have a different facial appearance and do not have the same chromosomal deletion. Type II lissencephaly is associated with a cobblestone, pebbled brain surface, thickened cortex, edematous cystic white matter and often hydrocephalus. It has been seen with congenital muscular dystrophy and the Walker–Warburg syndrome. X-linked lissencephaly and subcortical band heterotopias are both caused by mutation of a single gene, XLIS that encodes a 40 kDa protein, *Doublecortin.* Almost all patients with subcortical band heterotopias are female. Both conditions are associated with epilepsy and developmental delay.
- Agenesis of the corpus callosum (1–3/1000 births) is a relatively common nervous system malformation and is seen in association with a wide variety of other brain malformations and syndromes. Clinical symptoms and findings cover a wide spectrum of involvement.
- Cerebellar agenesis or hypoplasia frequently occurs in conjunction with other nervous system malformations as well as in association with mitochondrial disorders. Agenesis of the vermis is most commonly recognized in patients diagnosed with Joubert syndrome that presents as an autosomal recessive disorder in the neonatal period with episodic hyperpnea and apnea, disorders of ocular movement, retinal dystrophy, ataxia, hypotonia, and developmental delay. The majority of patients who survive with Joubert syndrome have significant long-term neurologic impairment.
- The Dandy–Walker syndrome (1/30 000 births) includes cystic dilation of the fourth ventricle with hypoplasia and superior displacement of the cerebellum. Hydrocephalus, delayed development, nystagmus, and spasticity are common. The majority of patients require shunting and most patients have serious long-term cognitive and cerebellar dysfunction.
- Intracranial arachnoid cysts may be benign but can cause a variety of neurologic symptoms depending on their location, size and whether they create a mass effect. Surgical decompression of symptomatic patients is indicated. Cysts occur equally in supratentorial and infratentorial compartments; sometimes the cysts are seen in conjunction with hydrocephalus.
- Aqueductal stenosis is a common cause of hydrocephalus and frequently occurs in conjunction with other nervous system malformations. It may be inherited as an X-linked recessive disorder.

## REFERENCES


Adamsbaum C, Moreau V, Bulteau C *et al.* (1994) Vermian ageneis without posterior fossa cyst. *Pediatr Radiol* 24: 543.

Agrawal P K, Agrawal U & Agrawal N K (1996) Prenatal sonographic diagnosis of hydranencephaly. *J Indian Med Assoc* 94: 322.

Ahdab-Barmada M & Claassen D (1990) A distinctive triad of malformations of the central nervous system in the Meckel-Gruber syndrome. *J Neuropathol Exp Neurol* 49: 610.

Al Shahwan S A, Bruyn G W & al Deeb S M (1995) Non-progressive familial congenital cerebellar hypoplasia. *J Neurol Sci* 128: 77.

Alman B A, Bhandari M & Wright J G (1996) Function of dislocated hips in children with lower level spina bifida. *J Bone Joint Surg* 78B: 294.

Altschuler G (1973) Toxoplasmosis as a cause of hydrocephaly. *Am J Dis Child* 125: 251.

Amer Ta & el-Shmam O M (1997) Chiari malformation type I: a new MRI classification. *Magn Reson Imaging* 15: 397.

✪ Anderson D J (1997) Cellular and molecular biology of neural crest cell lineage determination. *Trends Genet* 13: 276.

Anderson F M (1975) Occult spinal dysraphism: a series of 73 cases. *Pediatrics* 55: 826.

Anderson N G, Jordan S, MacFarlane M R *et al.* (1994) Diastematomyelia: diagnosis by prenatal sonography. *Am J Roentgenol* 163: 911.

✪ Aniskiewicz A S, Frumkin N L, Brady D E *et al.* (1990) Magnetic resonance imaging and neurobehavioral correlates in schizencephaly. *Arch Neurol* 74: 911.

✪ Arai H & Sato K (1990) Posterior fossa cysts: clinical, neuroradiological and surgical features. *Childs Nerv Syst* 7: 156.

Archer C R, Horenstein S & Sundaram M (1977) The Chiari malformation presenting in adult life. *J Chronic Dis* 30: 369.

✪ Aronyk K E (1993) The history and classification of hydrocephalus. *Neurosurg Clin N Am* 4: 599.

Ashwal S, Peabody J L, Schneider S *et al.* (1990) Anencephaly: clinical determination of brain death and neuropathologic studies. *Pediatr Neurol* 6: 233.

Aydingoz U, Cila A & Aktan G (1997) Rhombencephalosynapsis associated with hand anomalies. *Br J Radiol* 70: 764.

Ayme S, Julian C, Gambarelli D *et al.* (1989) Fryns syndrome: report on 8 new cases. *Clin Genet* 35: 191.

Bailey A, Luthert P, Bolton P *et al.* (1993) Autism and megalencephaly. *Lancet* 341: 1225.

Balci S, Onol B, Ercal M D *et al.* (1993) Autosomal recessive alobar holoprosencephaly with cyclops in three female sibs: prenatal ultrasonographic diagnosis at 18th week. *Clin Dysmorphol* 2: 165.

✪ Ball W S Jr. (1997) *Pediatric neuroradiology.* New York, NY: Lippincott-Raven Publishers.

✪ Barkovich A J (1995) *Pediatric neuroimaging*, 2nd edn. New York, NY: Raven Press,

✪ Barkovich A J (1996) Subcortical heterotopia: a distinct clinicoradiologic entity. *AJNR Am J Neuroradiol* 17: 1315.

Barkovich A J, Jackson D E Jr & Boyer R S (1989) Band heterotopias: a newly recognized neuronal migration anomaly. *Radiology* 171: 455.

Barkovich A J & Kjos B O (1992) Gray matter heterotopias: MR characteristics and correlation with developmental and neurologic manifestations. *Radiology* 182: 493.

Barkovich A J, Kuzniecky R I, Bollen A W *et al.* (1997) Focal transmantle dysplasia: a specific malformation of cortical development. *Neurology* 49: 1148.

✪ Barkovich A J & Kuzniecky R I (1996) Neuroimaging of focal malformations of cortical development. *J Clin Neurophysiol* 13: 481.

Barth P G (1993) Pontocerebellar hypoplasias. An overview of a group of inherited neurodegenerative disorders with fetal onset. *Brain Dev* 15: 411.

Barth P G, Blennow G, Lenard H G *et al.* (1995) The syndrome of autosomal recessive pontocerebellar hypoplasia, microcephaly, and extrapyramidal dyskinesia (pontocerebellar hypoplasia type 2): compiled data from 10 pedigrees. *Neurology* 45: 311.

Battaglia G, Arcelli P, Granata T *et al.* (1996) Neuronal migration disorders and epilepsy: a morphological analysis of three surgically treated patients. *Epilepsy Res* 26: 49.

✪ Becker L E & Hinton D R (1995) Pathogenesis of craniosynostosis. *Pediatr Neurosurg* 22: 104.

Belman A L, Diamond G, Dickson D *et al.* (1988) Pediatric acquired immunodeficiency syndrome: neurologic syndromes. *Am J Dis Child* 142: 29.

Ben Arie N, Bellen H J, Armstrong D L *et al.* (1997) Math1 is essential for genesis of cerebellar granule neurons. *Nature* 390: 169.

Berg R A, Aleck K A & Kaplan A M (1983) Familial porencephaly. *Arch Neurol* 40: 567.

Berry-Kravis E & Israel J (1994) X-linked pachygyria and agenesis of the corpus callosum evidence for an X-chromosome lissencephaly locus. *Ann Neurol* 36: 229–233.

Bertino R E, Nyberg D A, Cyr D R *et al.* (1988) Prenatal diagnosis of agenesis of the corpus callosum. *J Ultrasound Med* 7: 251.

Biglan A W (1990) Ophthalmologic complications of meningomyelocele: a longitudinal study. *Trans Am Ophthalmol Soc* 89: 389.

Bindal A K, Storrs B B & McLone D G (1991) Occipital meningoceles in patients with the Dandy–Walker syndrome. *J Neurosurg* 28: 844.

Bodensteiner J B, Schaefer G B, Keller G M *et al.* (1997) Macrocerebellum: neuroimaging and clinical features of a newly recognized condition. *J Child Neurol* 12: 365.

Boemers T M, Soorani Lunsing I J, de Jong T P *et al.* (1996) Urological problems after surgical treatment of scoliosis in children with myelomeningocele. *J Urol* 155: 1066.

Boltshauser E, Lange B & Dumermuth G (1987) Differential diagnosis of syndromes with abnormal respiration (tachypnea-apnea). *Brain Dev* 9: 462.

Boltshauser E, Steinlin M, Martin E *et al.* (1996) Unilateral cerebellar aplasia. *Neuropediatrics* 27: 50.

Bonnemann C G & Meinecke P (1996) Bilateral porencephaly, cerebellar hypoplasia, and internal malformations: two siblings representing a probably new autosomal recessive entity. *Am J Med Genet* 63: 428.

Botkin J R (1988) Anencephalic infants as organ donors. *Pediatrics* 82: 250.

Bradford D S, Heithoff K B & Cohen M (1991) Intraspinal abnormalities and congenital spine deformities: a radiographic and MRI study. *J Pediatr Orthop* 11: 36.

Breningstall G N, Marker S M & Tubman D E (1992) Hydrosyringomyelia and diastematomyelia detected by MRI in myelomeningocele. *Pediatr Neurol* 8: 267.

Brennand D M, Jehanli A M, Wood P J *et al.* (1998) Raised levels of maternal serum secretory acetylcholinesterase may be indicative of fetal neural tube defects in early pregnancy. *Acta Obstet Gynecol Scand* 77: 8.

Brock D J H, Scrimgeour J B & Nelson M N (1975) Amniotic fluid alpha-fetoprotein measurements in the early prenatal diagnosis of central nervous system disorders. *Clin Genet* 7: 163.

Bromley B & Benacerraf B R (1995) Difficulties in the prenatal diagnosis of microcephaly. *J Ultrasound Med* 14: 303.

Bromley B, Nadel A S, Pauker S *et al.* (1994) Closure of the cerebellar vermis: evaluation with second trimester US. *Radiology* 193: 761.

Brooks B S, El-Gammal T, Hartlage P *et al.* (1981) Myelography of sacral agenesis. *AJNR Am J Neuroradiol* 2: 319.

Buckton K E, O'Riordan M L, Ratcliffe S *et al.* (1980) AG-band study of chromosomes in liveborn infants. *Ann Hum Genet* 43: 227.

Buyse G, Verpoorten C, Vereecken R *et al.* (1995) Treatment of neurogenic bladder dysfunction in infants and children with neurospinal dysraphism with clean intermittent (self) catheterization and optimized intravesical oxybutynin hydrochloride therapy. *Eur J Pediatr Surg* 1[5 Suppl]: 31.

✪ Byers P H (1993) Osteogenesis imperfecta. In: Royce P M, Steinmann B, eds. *Connective tissue and its heritable disorders: molecular, genetic, and medical aspects.* New York: Wiley-Liss.

Byrd S E, Bohan T P, Osborn R E *et al.* (1988) The CT and MR evaluation of lissencephaly. *AJNR Am J Neuroradial* 9: 923.

✪ Byrd S E, Darling C F & McLone D G (1991) Developmental disorders of the pediatric spine. *Radiol Clin North Am* 29: 711.

Cai C & Oakes W J (1997) Hindbrain herniation syndromes: the Chiari malformations (I and II). *Semin Pediatr Neurol* 4: 156.

Carter C O (1976) Genetics of common single malformations. *Br Med Bull* 25: 52.

✪ Casey A T, Kimmings E J, Kleinlugtebeld A D *et al.* (1997) The long-term outlook for hydrocephalus in childhood. A ten-year cohort study of 155 patients. *Pediatr Neurosurg* 27: 63.

Castro-Gago M, Alonso A & Eiris Punal J (1996) Autosomal recessive hydrocephalus with aqueductal stenosis. *Childs Nerv Syst* 12: 188.

Castro-Gago M, Rodriguez Nunez A, Eiris J *et al.* (1993) Familial agenesis of the corpus callosum: a new form. *Arch Fr Pediatr* 50: 327.

Catalans L W & Sever J L (1971) The role of viruses as causes of congenital defects. *Ann Rev Microbiol* 25: 255.

Caviness V S (1976) The Chiari malformations of the posterior fossa and their relation to hydrocephalus. *Dev Med Child Neurol* 18: 103.

Chalhub E G, Volpe J J, Gado M H (1975) Linear nevus sebaceous syndrome associated with porencephaly and non-functioning major cerebral venous sinuses. *Neurology* 25: 857.

Chambers G K, Cochrane D D, Irwin B *et al.* (1996) Assessment of the appropriateness of services provided by a multidisciplinary meningomyelocele clinic. *Pediatr Neurosurg* 24: 92.

Chan A, Robertson E F, Haan E A *et al.* (1995) The sensitivity of ultrasound and serum alpha-fetoprotein in population-based antenatal screening for neural tube defects. South Australia 1986–1991. *Br J Obstet Gynaecol* 102: 370.

Chapman P H, Swearingen B & Caviness V S (1989) Subtorcular occipital encephaloceles: anatomical considerations relevant to operative management. *J Neurosurg* 71: 375.

Charney E G B, Rorke L B, Sutton L N *et al.* (1987)

Management of Chiari II complications in infants with myelomeningocele. *J Pediatr* 111: 364.

Chatkupt S, Speer M C, Ding Y *et al.* (1994) Linkage analysis of a candidate locus (HLA) in autosomal dominant sacral defect with anterior meningocele. *J Med Genet* 52: 1.

Chen J, Chang S, Duncan S A *et al.* (1996) Disruption of the MacMARCKS gene prevents cranial neural tube closure and results in anencephaly. *Proc Natl Acad Sci USA* 93: 6275.

Chevrie J J & Aicardi J (1986) The Aicardi syndrome. In: Pedley T, Meldrum B, eds. *Recent advances in epilepsy.* Edinburgh: Churchill Livingstone, 1986.

Chitayat D, Moore L, Del Bigio M R *et al.* (1994) Familial Dandy-Walker malformation associated with macrocephaly, facial anomalies, developmental delay, and brain stem dysgenesis: prenatal diagnosis and postnatal outcome in brothers. A new syndrome? *Am J Med Genet* 52: 406.

Clark G D, Mizuguchi M, Antalffy B *et al.* (1997) Predominant localization of the LIS family of gene products to Cajal–Retzius cells and ventricular neuroepithelium in the developing human cortex. *J Neuropathol Exp Neurol* 56: 1044.

Clarren S K & Smith D W (1978) The fetal alcohol syndrome. *N Engl J Med* 298: 1063.

Cohen M M & Lemire R J (1982) Syndromes with cephaloceles. *Teratology* 25: 161.

Cohen T, Zeitune M, McGillivray B C *et al.* (1996) Segregation analysis of microcephaly. *Am J Med Genet* 65: 226.

Colgan M T (1981) The child with spina bifida: role of the pediatrician. *Am J Dis Child* 135: 854.

Copp A J, Brook F A, Estibeiro J P *et al.* (1990) The embryonic development of mammalian neural tube defects. *Prog Neurobiol* 35: 363.

✪ Cowan W M (1992) Development of the nervous system. In: Asbury A K, McKhann G M, McDonald W I, eds. *Diseases of the nervous system, clinical neurobiology.* Philadelphia: W B Saunders.

Crino P B & Eberwine J (1997) Cellular and molecular basis of cerebral dysgenesis. *J Neurosci Res* 50: 907.

Crome L K & France N E (1959) Microgyria and cytomegalic inclusion disease in infancy. *J Clin Pathol* 12: 427.

Cross J H, Harrison C J, Preston P R *et al.* (1992) Postnatal encephaloclastic porencephaly – a new lesion? *Arch Dis Child* 67: 307.

Davidoff A M, Thompson C V, Grimm J M *et al.* (1991) Occult spinal dysraphism in patients with anal agenesis. *J Pediatr Surg* 26: 1001.

de Carvalho Neto J, Dias L S & Gabrieli A P (1996) Congenital talipes equinovarus in spina bifida: treatment and results. *J Pediatr Orthop* 16: 782.

Dekaban A S (1968) Abnormalities in children exposed to X-radiation during various stages of gestation: tentative time table of radiation injury to the human fetus. Part 1. *J Nucl Med* 9: 471.

Demaerel P, Kendall B E, Wilms G *et al.* (1995) Uncommon posterior cranial fossa anomalies: MRI with clinical correlation. *Neuroradiology* 37: 72.

DeMyer W (1971) Classification of cerebral malformations. *Birth Defects* 7: 78.

DeMyer W (1975) Median facial malformations and their implication for brain malformation. *Birth Defects* 11: 155.

Deng C, Bedford M, Li C *et al.* (1997) Fibroblast growth factor receptor-1 (FGFR-1) is essential for normal neural tube and limb development. *Dev Biol* 185: 42.

De Souza N, Chaudhuri R, Bingham J *et al.* (1994) MRI in cerebellar hypoplasia. *Neuroradiology* 36: 148.

Devriendt K, Naulaers G, Matthijs G *et al.* (1997) Agenesis of corpus callosum and anophthalmia in the asplenia syndrome. A recognizable association? *Ann Genet* 40: 14.

De Zegher F, Devlieger H & De Cock P (1992) Alternating diabetes insipidus and inappropriate antidiuresis in holoprosencephaly: relationship to intracranial pressure. *J Pediatr* 120: 161.

Dhellemmes C, Girard S, Dulac O *et al.* (1988) Agyria-pachygyria and Miller-Dieker syndrome: clinical, genetic and chromosome studies. *Hum Genet* 79: 163.

✪ Dias M S & Pang D (1995) Split cord malformations. *Neurosurg Clin N Am* 6: 339.

Dickson D W, Llena J F, Nelson S J *et al.* (1993) Central nervous system pathology in pediatric AIDS. *Ann NY Acad Sci* 693: 93.

DiMario F J Jr, Cobb R J, Ramsby G R *et al.* (1993) Familial band heretotopias simulating tuberous sclerosis. *Neurology* 43: 1424.

✪ Dobyns W B (1987) Developmental aspects of lissencephaly and the lissencephaly syndromes. In: Gilbert E F, Opitz J M, eds. *Genetic aspects of developmental pathology.* New York NY: Alan R Liss. For the March of Dimes Birth Defects Foundation, Birth Defects: Original Article Series 23: p. 225.

Dobyns W B (1989) The neurogenetics of lissencephaly. *Neurol Clin* 7: 89.

✪ Dobyns W B & Truwit C L (1995) Lissencephaly and other malformations of cortical development: 1995 update. *Neuropediatrics* 26: 132.

Dobyns W B, Curry C J R & Hoyme H E *et al.* (1991) Clinical and molecular diagnosis of Miller-Dieker syndrome. *Am J Med Genet* 48: 584.

Dobyns W B, Elias E R, Newlin A C *et al.* (1992) Causal heterogeneity in isolated lissencephaly. *Neurology* 42: 1375.

Dobyns W B, Pagon R A, Armstrong D *et al.* (1989) Diagnostic criteria for Walker–Warburg syndrome. *Am J Med Genet* 32: 195.

Dobyns W B, Patton M A, Stratton R F *et al.* (1996b) Cobblestone lissencephaly with normal eyes and muscle. *Neuropediatrics* 27: 70.

Dobyns W B, Andermann E, Andermann F *et al.* (1996a) X-linked malformations of neuronal migration. *Neurology* 47: 331.

Docherty T B, Herbaut A G & Sedgwick E M (1987) Brainstem auditory evoked potential abnormalities in myelomeningocele in the older child. *J Neurol Neurosurg Psychiatry* 50: 1318.

Dolk H (1991) The predictive value of microcephaly during the first year of life for mental retardation at seven years. *Dev Med Child Neurol* 33: 974.

Domingo Z & Peter J (1996) Midline developmental abnormalities of the posterior fossa: correlation of classification with outcome. *Pediatr Neurosurg* 24: 111.

Dominquez R, Vila-Coro A A, Slopis J M *et al.* (1991) Brain and ocular abnormalities in infants with *in utero* exposure to cocaine and other street drugs. *Am J Dis Child* 145: 688.

Dorman C (1991) Microcephaly and intelligence. *Dev Med Child Neurol* 33: 267.

Drachman D A & Richardson E P (1961) Aqueductal narrowing, congenital and acquired: a critical review of the histologic criteria. *Arch Neurol* 5: 552.

✪ Dubeau F, Tampieri D, Lee N *et al.* (1995) Periventricular and subcortical nodular heterotopia. A study of 33 patients. *Brain* 118: 1273.

✪ Dyste G N, Menezes A H, VanGilder J C *et al.* (1989) Symptomatic Chiari malformations. An analysis of presentation, management, and long-term outcome. *J Neurosurg* 71: 159.

Edwards J H (1961) The syndrome of sex-linked hydrocephalus. *Arch Dis Child* 36: 486.

✪ Eksioglu Y Z, Scheffer I E, Cardenas P *et al.* (1996) Periventricular heterotopia: an X-linked dominant epilepsy locus causing aberrant cerebral cortical development. *Neuron* 16: 77.

Elias D L, kawamoto H K Jr & Wilson L F (1992) Holoprosencephaly and midline facial anomalies: redefining classification and management. *Plast Reconstr Surg* 90: 951.

Eller K M & Kuller J A (1995a) Fetal porencephaly: a review of etiology, diagnosis, and prognosis. *Obstet Gynecol Surv* 50: 684.

Eller K M & Kuller J A (1995b) Porencephaly secondary to fetal trauma during amniocentesis. *Obstet Gynecol* 85: 865.

Ellyn B, Khatir A H & Singh S P (1980) Hypothalamic-pituitary functions in patients with transsphenoidal encephalocele and midfacial anomalies. *J Clin Endocrinol Metab* 51: 854.

Elterman R D, Bodensteiner J B & Barnard J J (1995) Sudden unexpected death in patients with Dandy-Walker malformation. *J Child Neurol* 10: 382.

Encha Razavi F, Larroche J C, Roume J *et al.* (1996) Lethal familial fetal akinesia sequence (FAS) with distinct neuropathological pattern: type III lissencephaly syndrome. *Am J Med Genet* 62: 16.

Epstein D J, Vogan K J, Trasler D G *et al.* (1993) A mutation within intron 3 of the Pax-3 gene produces aberrantly spliced mRNA transcripts in the splotch (Sp) mouse mutant. *Proc Natl Acad Sci USA* 90: 532–6.

✪ Epstein M H & Johanson C E (1987) The Dandy-Walker syndrome. In: Myrianthopoulos N C, ed. *Handbook of clinical neurology.* Amsterdam: Elsevier Science.

✪ Estin D & Cohen A R (1995) Caudal agenesis and associated caudal spinal cord malformations. *Neurosurg Clin N Am* 6: 377.

Estroff J A, Scott M R & Benacerraf B R (1992) Dandy–Walker variant: prenatal sonographic features and clinical outcome. *Radiology* 185: 755.

Evrard P, de Saint-Georges P, Kadhim H J *et al.* (1989a) Pathology of prenatal encephalopathies. In: Evrard P, Minkowski A, eds. *Child neurology and developmental disabilities.* Baltimore MD: Paul H. Brookes.

Evrard P, Kadhim H J, de Saint-Georges P *et al.* (1989b) Abnormal development and destructive processes of the human brain during the second half of gestation. In: Evrard P, Minkowski A, eds. *Developmental neurobiology.* Nestle Nutrition Workshop Series, vol 12. New York NY: Raven Press.

✪ Evrard P, Marret S & Gressens P (1997) Environmental and genetic determinants of neural migration and postmigratory survival. *Acta Paediatr* 422 [Suppl]: 20.

✪ Evrard P, Miladi N, Bonnier C *et al.* (1992) Normal and abnormal development of the brain. In: Rapin I, Segalowitz S J, eds. *Handbook of neuropsychology*, vol 6, *Child psychology.* Amsterdam: Biomedical Division, Elsevier Science.

✪ Fewel M E, Levy M L & McComb J G (1996) Surgical treatment of 95 children with 102 intracranial arachnoid cysts. *Pediatr Neurosurg* 25: 165.

Fiedler R & Krieger D T (1975) Endocrine disturbances in patients with congenital aqueductal stenosis. *Acta Endocrinol* 80: 1.

Fitz C R (1994) Holoprosencephaly and septo-optic dysplasia. *Neuroimaging Clin N Am* 4: 263.

Flanagan M & Johnson S J (1995) The effects of vaccination of Merino ewes with an attenuated Australian bluetongue virus serotype 23 at different stages of gestation. *Aust Vet J* 72: 455.

Freeman J M (1985) *Prenatal and perinatal factors associated with brain disorders.* NIH Publication No. 85–1149. Washington, DC: National Institute of Child Health and Development.

✪ Friede R L (1989) *Developmental neuropathology.* New York NY: Springer-Verlag.

Fryburg J S, Breg W R & Lindgren V (1991) Diagnosis of Angelman syndrome in infants. *Am J Med Genet* 38: 58.

Fransen E, Van Camp G, Vits L *et al.* (1997) L1-associated diseases: clinical geneticists divide, molecular geneticists unite. *Hum Mol Genet* 6: 1625.

French B N (1983) The embryology of spinal dysraphism. *Clin Neurosurg* 30: 295.

Friede R L (1989) *Developmental neuropathology.* New York NY: Springer-Verlag.

Fryns J P Devriendt K & Legius E (1997) Polysyndactyly and trigonocephaly with partial agenesis of corpus callosum: an example of the variable clinical spectrum of the acrocallosal syndrome? *Clin Dysmorphol* 6: 285.

Gardner W J (1977) Hemodynamic factors in Dandy–Walker and Arnold–Chiari malformations. *Childs Brain* 3: 200.

Gastaut H, Pinsard N, Raybaud C *et al.* (1987) Lissencephaly (agyriapachygyria): clinical findings and serial EEG studies. *Dev Med Child Neurol* 29: 167.

Gelman-Kohan Z, Antonelli J, Ankori-Cohen H *et al.* (1991) Further delineation of the acrocallosal syndrome. *Eur J Pediatr* 150: 797.

Gentile M, Di Carlo A, Susca F *et al.* (1996) COACH syndrome: report of two brothers with congenital hepatic fibrosis, cerebellar vermis hypoplasia, oligophrenia, ataxia, and mental retardation. *Am J Med Genet* 64: 514.

George T M & McLone D G (1995) Mechanisms of mutant genes in spina bifida: a review of implications from animal models. *Pediatr Neurosurg* 23: 236.

Gershoni-Baruch R & Zekaria D (1996) Deletion (13)(q22) with multiple congenital anomalies, hydranencephaly and penoscrotal transposition. *Clin Dysmorphol* 5: 289.

Gerszten P C & Albright A L (1995) Relationship between cerebellar appearance and function in children with Dandy-Walker syndrome. *Pediatr Neurosurg* 23: 86.

Gilbert J N, Jones K L, Rorke L B *et al.* (1986) Central nervous system anomalies associated with meningomyelocele, hydrocephalus, and the Arnold–Chiari malformation: reappraisal of theories regarding the pathogenesis of posterior neural tube closure defects. *Neurosurgery* 18: 559.

Ginsberg M D & Myers R E (1978) Fetal brain injury after maternal carbon monoxide intoxication. *Neurology* 26: 15.

✪ Gleeson J G, Allen K M, Fox J W *et al.* (1998) Doublecortin, a brain-specific gene mutated in human X-linked lissencephaly and double cortex syndrome, encodes a putative signaling protein. *Cell* 92: 63.

Glickstein M (1994) Cerebellar agenesis. *Brain* 117: 1209.

Golden J A & Chernoff G F (1995) Multiple sites of anterior neural tube closure in humans: evidence from anterior neural tube defects (anencephaly). *Pediatrics* 95: 506.

✪ Golden J A, Rorke L B & Bruce D A (1987) Dandy–Walker syndrome and associated anomalies. *Pediatr Neurosci* 13: 38.

Goldstein R B & Filly R A (1988) Prenatal diagnosis of anencephaly: spectrum of sonographic appearances and distinction from the amniotic band syndrome. *Am J Radiol* 151: 547.

Gowen L C, Johnson B L, Latour A M *et al.* (1996) Bracal deficiency results in early embryonic lethality characterized by neuroepithelial abnormalities. *Nat Genet* 12: 19.

✪ Granata T, Battaglia G, D'Incerti L *et al.* (1996) Schizencephaly: neuroradiologic and epileptologic findings. *Epilepsia* 37: 1185.

Gropman A L, Barkovich A J, Vezina L G *et al.* (1997) Pediatric congenital bilateral perisylvian syndrome: clinical and MRI features in 12 patients. *Neuropediatrics* 28: 198.

Gross Tsur V, Joseph A, Blinder G *et al.* (1995) Familial microcephaly with severe neurological deficits: a description of five affected siblings. *Clin Genet* 47: 33.

Guerrini R, Dubeau F, Dulac O *et al.* (1997) Bilateral parasagittal parietooccipital polymicrogyria and epilepsy. *Ann Neurol* 41: 65.

Guillen D, Pascual Castroviejo I, Lopez Martin V *et al.* (1995) Neuronal migration disorders: clinical-radiological radiological correlation. *Rev Neurol* 23: 43.

Gunay M & Aysun S (1996) Neuronal migration disorders presenting with mild clinical symptoms. *Pediatr Neurol* 14: 153.

Gundry C R & Heithoff K B (1994) Imaging evaluation of patients with spinal deformity. *Orthop Clin North Am* 25: 247.

Gurtubay I G, Yoldi M E, Carrera B *et al.* (1997) Andermann syndrome: presentation of a case. *Rev Neurol* 25: 1087.

✪ Hagberg B, Aicardi J, Dias K *et al.* (1983) A progressive syndrome of autism, dementia, ataxia, and loss of purposeful hand use in girls: Rett's syndrome: report of 35 cases. *Ann Neurol* 14: 471.

✪ Hagberg B A, Blennow G, Kristiansson B & Stibler H (1993) Carbohydrate-deficient glycoprotein syndromes: peculiar group of new disorders. *Pediatr Neurol* 9: 255.

Haller J S, Wolpert S M, Rabe E F *et al.* (1971) Cystic lesions of the posterior fossa in infants: a comparison of the clinical, radiological, and pathological findings in Dandy-Walker syndrome in extra-axial cysts. *Neurology* 21: 494.

Halsey J H Jr, Allen N & Chamberlin H R (1971) The morphogenesis of hydranencephaly. *J Neurol Sci* 12: 187.

Hamilton R L & Grafe M R (1994) Complete absence of the cerebellum: a report of two cases. *Acta Neuropathol Berl* 88: 258.

Harding B N, Ramani P & Thurley P (1995) The familial syndrome of proliferative vasculopathy and hydranencephaly-hydrocephaly: immunocytochemical and ultrastructural evidence for endothelial proliferation. *Neuropathol Appl Neurobiol* 21: 61.

Harley E H (1991) Pediatric congenital nasal masses. *Ear Nose Throat J* 70: 28.

Harsh G R, Edwards M S B & Wilson C B (1986) Intracranial arachnoid cysts in children. *J Neurosurg* 64: 835.

Hart M N, Malamud N & Ellis W G (1972) The Dandy–Walker syndrome, a clinicopathological study based on 28 cases. *Neurology* 22: 771.

Hashimoto R, Seki T, Takuma Y *et al.* (1993) The 'double cortex' syndrome on MRI. *Brain Dev* 15: 57.

Hatten M E & Heintz N (1995) Mechanisms of neural patterning and specification in the developing cerebellum. *Ann Rev Neurosci* 18: 385.

Hemphill M, Freeman J M, Martinez C R *et al.* (1982) A new, treatable source of recurrent meningitis: basioccipital meningocele. *Pediatrics* 70: 941.

Hier D B & Wiehl A C (1977) Chronic hydrocephalus associated with short stature and growth hormone deficiency. *Ann Neurol* 2: 246.

Hildebrandt F, Nothwang H G, Vossmerbaumer U *et al.* (1998) Lack of large, homozygous deletions of the nephronophthisis 1 region in Joubert syndrome type B. APN Study Group. Arbeitsgemeinschaft fur Padiatrische nephrologie. *Pediatr Nephrol* 12: 16.

Hirayama K, Hoshino Y, Kumashiro H *et al.* (1994) Reverse Shapiro's syndrome. A case of agenesis of corpus callosum associated with periodic hyperthermia. *Arch Neurol* 51: 494.

Ho S S, Kuzniecky R I, Gilliam F *et al.* (1997) Congenital porencephaly and hippocampal sclerosis. Clinical features and epileptic spectrum. *Neurology* 49: 1382.

Hockley A D, Goldin J H & Wake M J (1990) Management of anterior encephalocele. *Childs Nerv Syst* 6: 444.

Hol F A, Geurds M P, Chatkupt S *et al.* (1996) PAX genes and human neural tube defects: an amino acid substitution in PAX1 in a patient with spina bifida. *J Med Genet* 33: 655.

Hol F A, Hamel B C, Geurds M P *et al.* (1995) A frameshift mutation in the gene for PAX3 in a girl with spina bifida and mild signs of Waardenburg syndrome. *J Med Genet* 32: 52.

Holmes L B (1974) Inborn errors of morphogenesis: a review of localized hereditary malformations. *N Engl J Med* 291: 763.

Holmes L B (1994) Spina bifida: anticonvulsants and other maternal influences. *Ciba Found Symp* 181: 232.

Holmes L B, Driscoll S G & Atkins L (1976) Etiologic heterogenicity of neural tube defects. *N Engl J Med* 294: 365.

Holroyd S, Reiss A L & Bryan R N (1991) Autistic features in Joubert syndrome: a genetic disorder with agenesis of the cerebellar vermis. *Biol Psychiatry* 29: 287.

Hori A (1994) Tectocerebellar dysraphia with posterior encephalocele (Friede): report of the youngest case. Reappraisal of the condition uniting Cleland–Chiari (Arnold–Chiari) and Dandy–Walker syndromes. *Clin Neuropathol* 13: 216.

Hustinx R, Verloes A, Grattagliano B *et al.* (1993) Monosomy 11q: report of two familial cases and review of the literature. *Am J Med Genet* 47: 312.

✪ Huttenlocher P R, Taravath S & Mojtahedi S (1994) Periventricular heterotopia and epilepsy. *Neurology* 44: 51.

Iannetti P, Nigro G, Spalice A *et al.* (1998) Cytomegalovirus infection and schizencephaly: case reports. *Ann Neurol* 43: 123.

Iannetti P, Schwartz C E, Dietz Band J *et al.* (1993) Norman-Roberts syndrome: clinical and molecular studies. *Am J Med Genet* 47: 95.

✪ Iannetti P, Spalice A, Atzei G *et al.* (1996) Neuronal migrational disorders in children with epilepsy: MRI, interictal SPECT and EEG comparisons. *Brain Dev* 18: 269.

Illarioshkin S N, Tanaka H, Markova E D *et al.* (1996) X-linked nonprogressive congenital cerebellar hypoplasia: clinical description and mapping to chromosome Xq. *Ann Neurol* 40: 75.

Isada N B, Qureshi F, Jacques S M *et al.* (1993) Meroanencephaly: pathology and prenatal diagnosis. *Fetal Diagn Ther* 8: 423.

Iskandar B J, Oakes W J, McLaughlin C *et al.* (1994) Terminal syringohydromyelia and occult spinal dysraphism (see comments). *J Neurosurg* 81: 513.

Isumi H, Takashima S, Kakita A *et al.* (1997) Expression of the LIS-1 gene product in brain anomalies with a migration disorder. *Pediatr Neurol* 16: 42.

Jansen J, Taudorf K, Pedersen H *et al.* (1991) Upper extremity function in spina bifida. *Childs Nerv Syst* 7: 67.

Jardine P E, Clarke M A & Super M (1996) Familial bilateral periventricular nodular heterotopia mimics tuberous sclerosis. *Arch Dis Child* 74: 244.

Jensen P R, Hansen F J & Skovby F (1995) Cerebellar hypoplasia in children with the carbohydrate-deficient glycoprotein syndrome. *Neuroradiology* 37: 328.

Johnson S P, Sebire N J, Snijders R J *et al.* (1997) Ultrasound screening for anencephaly at 10–14 weeks of gestation. *Ultrasound Obstet Gynecol* 9: 14.

Joubert M, Eisenring J J, Robb J P *et al.* (1998) Familial agenesis of the cerebellar vermis. *Neurology* 19: 813.

Kadonaga J N, Barkovich A J, Edwards M S *et al.* (1992) Neurocutaneous melanosis in association with the Dandy-Walker complex. *Pediatr Dermatol* 9: 37.

✪ Kalidasan V, Carroll T, Allcutt D *et al.* (1995) The Dandy-Walker syndrome – a 10-year experience of its management and outcome. *Eur J Pediatr Surg* 1[Suppl.]: 16.

Kallen A J (1994) Maternal carbamazepine and infant spina bifida. *Reprod Toxicol* 8: 203.

Kalter H (1993) Case reports of malformations associated with maternal diabetes: history and critique. *Clin Genet* 43: 174.

Karol L A (1995) Orthopedic management in myelomeningocele. *Neurosurg Clin N Am* 6: 259.

Kendall B, Kingsley D, Lambert S R *et al.* (1990) Joubert syndrome: a clinico-radiological study. *Neuroradiology* 31: 502.

Keogan M T, DeAtkine A B & Hertzberg B S (1994) Cerebellar vermian defects: antenatal sonographic appearance and clinical significance. *J Ultrasound Med* 13: 607.

King M D, Dudgeon J & Stephenson J B P (1984) Joubert's syndrome with retinal dysplasia: neonatal tachypnea as due to a genetic brain-eye malformation. *Arch Dis Child* 59: 709.

Klingensmith W C 3rd, Cioffi-Ragan D T (1986) Schizencephaly. Diagnosis and progression *in utero*. *Radiology* 159: 617.

Knobloch W H & Layer J M (1971) Retinal detachment and encephalocele. *J Pediatr Ophthalmol* 8: 181.

Kolawole T M, Patel J J & Mahdi A H (1987) Porencephaly: computed tomography (CT) scan findings. *Comput Radiol* 11: 53.

Kolodny E H (1989) Agenesis of the corpus callosum: a marker for inherited metabolic disease? *Neurology* 39: 847.

Konz K R, Chia J K, Kurup V P *et al.* (1995) Comparison of latex hypersensitivity among patients with neurologic defects. *J Allergy Clin Immunol* 95: 950.

Korsvik H E & Keller M S (1992) Sonography of occult dysraphism in neonates and infants with MR imaging correlation. *Radiographics* 12: 297.

Kosaki K, Curry C J, Roeder E *et al.* (1997) Ritscher–Schinzel (3C) syndrome: documentation of the phenotype. *Am J Med Genet* 68: 421.

Kothari M J & Bauer S B (1997) Urodynamic and neurophysiologic evaluation of patients with diastematomyelia. *J Child Neurol* 12: 97.

Kozlowski K & Ouvrier R A (1993) Agenesis of the corpus callosum with mental retardation and osseous lesions. *Am J Med Genet* 48: 6.

Kubo S, Kishino T, Satake N *et al.* (1994) A neonatal case of hydranencephaly caused by atheromatous plaque obstruction of aortic arch: possible association with a congenital cytomegalovirus infection? *J Perinatol* 14: 483.

Kurauchi O, Ohno Y, Mizutani S *et al.* (1995) Longitudinal monitoring of fetal behavior in twins when one is anencephalic. *Obstet Gynecol* 86: 672.

Kurent J E & Sever J L (1973) Perinatal infections and epidemiology of anencephaly and spina bifida. *Teratology* 8: 359.

✪ Kuzniecky R, Andermann F, Tampieri D *et al.* (1989) Bilateral central macrogyria: epilepsy, pseudobulbar palsy, and mental retardation – a recognizable neuronal migration disorder. *Ann Neurol* 25: 547.

Kuzniecky R, Gilliam F & Faught E (1995) Discordant occurrence of cerebral unilateral heterotopia and epilepsy in monozygotic twins. *Epilepsia* 36: 1155.

Kuzniecky R, Gilliam F & Morawetz R (1997) Occipital lobe developmental malformations and epilepsy: clinical spectrum, treatment, and outcome. *Epilepsia* 38: 175.

✪ Lacey D J (1985) Agenesis of the corpus callosum: clinical features in 40 children. *Am J Dis Child* 139: 653.

Lambert S R, Kriss A, Gresty M *et al.* (1989) Joubert syndrome. *Arch Ophthalmol* 107: 709.

Lammer E J, Chen D T, Hoar R M *et al.* (1985) Retinoic acid embryopathy. *N Engl J Med* 313: 837.

Lary J M & Edmonds L D (1996) Prevalence of spina bifida at birth – United States, 1983–1990: a comparison of two surveillance systems. *MMWR CDC Surveill Summ* 45: 15.

Laurence K M (1964) The natural history of spina bifida cystica. *Arch Dis Child* 39: 41.

Layde P M, Edmonds L D & Erickson J D (1980) Maternal fever and neural tube defects. *Teratology* 21: 105.

Leao M J & Ribeiro Silva M L (1995) Orofaciodigital syndrome type I in a patient with severe CNS defects. *Pediatr Neurol* 13: 247.

Ledbetter S A, Kuwano A, Dobyns W B *et al.* (1992) Microdeletions of chromosome 17p13 as a cause of isolated lissencephaly. *Am J Hum Genet* 50: 182.

Leech R W, Johnson S H & Brumback R A (1997) Agenesis of cerebellum associated with arrhinencephaly. *Clin Neuropathol* 16: 90.

✪ Leech R W, Shuman R M (1986) Holoprosencephaly and related midline cerebral anomalies: a review. *J Child Neurol* 1: 3.

Lemire R J (1987) Anencephaly. In: Myrianthopoulos NC, ed. *Handbook of clinical neurology.* Amsterdam: Elsevier Science.

✪ Lemire R J, Beckwith J B & Warkany J (1978) *Anencephaly.* New York, NY: Raven Press.

Lemire R J, Beckwith J B & Shepard T H (1972) Iniencephaly and anencephaly with spinal retroflexion. A comparative study of eight human specimens. *Teratology* 6: 27–36.

✪ Lemire R J, Loeser J D, Leech R W *et al.* (1975) *Normal and abnormal development of the human nervous system.* New York, NY: Harper & Row.

Lendahl U (1997) Gene regulation in the formation of the central nervous system. *Acta Paediatr Suppl* 422: 8.

Lenke R R & Levy H L (1982) Maternal phenylketonuria: results of dietary therapy. *Am J Obstet Gynecol* 142: 548.

Levitt P, Barbe M F & Eagleson K L (1997) Patterning and specification of the cerebral cortex. *Ann Rev Neurosci* 20: 1.

Levy H L, Lobbregt D, Barnes P D *et al.* (1996) Maternal phenylketonuria: magnetic resonance imaging of the brain in offspring. *J Pediatr* 128: 770.

Lewis S M, Roberts E A, Marcon M A *et al.* (1994) Joubert syndrome with congenital hepatic fibrosis: an entity in the spectrum of oculo-encephalo-hepato-renal disorders. *Am J Med Genet* 52: 419.

LeWitt P A, Newman R P, Greenberg H S *et al.* (1983) Episodic hyperhidrosis, hypothermia, and agenesis of corpus callosum. *Neurology* 33: 1122.

Limb C J & Holmes L B (1994) Anencephaly: changes in prenatal detection and birth status, 1972 through 1990. *Am J Obstet Gynecol* 170: 1333.

Lincke C R, van den Bogert C, Nijtmans L G *et al.* (1996) Cerebellar hypoplasia in respiratory chain dysfunction. *Neuropediatrics* 27: 216.

Lindenberg R & Swanson P D (1967) Infantile hydranencephaly – a report of five cases of both cerebral hemispheres in infancy. *Brain* 90: 839.

Lindhout D, Omtzigt J G & Cornel M C (1992) Spectrum of neural-tube defects in 34 infants prenatally exposed to antiepileptic drugs. *Neurology* 42: 111.

Liptak G S, Bloss J W, Briskin H *et al.* (1988) The management of children with spinal dysraphism. *J Child Neurol* 3: 3.

Little J R, Houser O W, MacCarty C S (1975) Clinical manifestations of aqueductal stenosis in adults. *J Neurosurg* 43: 546.

Liu D P, Burrowes D M, Qureshi M N (1997a) Cyclopia: craniofacial appearance on MR and three-dimensional CT. *AJNR Am J Neuroradiol* 18: 543.

✪ Locke M D & Sarwark J F (1996) Orthopedic aspects of myelodysplasia in children. *Curr Opin Pediatr* 8: 65.

Loebstein R & Koren G (1997) Pregnancy outcome and neurodevelopment of children exposed *in utero* to psychoactive drugs: the Motherisk experience. *J Psychiatry Neurosci* 22: 192.

Longo L D (1977) The biological effects of carbon monoxide on the pregnant woman, fetus and newborn infant. *Am J Obstet Gynecol* 129: 69.

Lorber J (1971) Results of treatment of myelomeningocele: an analysis of 524 unselected cases with special reference to possible selection for treatment. *Dev Med Child Neurol* 13: 279.

Lubinsky M S (1997) Association of prenatal vascular disruptions with decreased maternal age. *Am J Med Genet* 69: 237.

Lurie I W, Ilyina H G, Gurevich D B *et al.* (1995) Trisomy 2p: analysis of unusual phenotypic findings. *Am J Med Genet* 55: 229.

Luyendijk W & Treffers P D (1992) The smile in anencephalic infants. *Clin Neurol Neurosurg* 94: S113.

Lynch S A, Bond P M, Copp A J *et al.* (1995) A gene for autosomal dominant sacral agenesis maps to the holoprosencephaly region at 7q36. *Nat Genet* 11: 93.

Lynn R B, Buchanan D C, Fenichel G M *et al.* (1980) Agenesis of the corpus callosum. *Arch Neurol* 37: 444.

Macchi G & Bentivoglio M (1987) Agenesis or hypoplasia of cerebellar structures. In: Myrianthopoulos NC, ed. *Handbook of clinical neurology.* Amsterdam: Elsevier Science.

✪ McLone D G & La Marca F (1997) The tethered spinal cord: diagnosis, significance, and management. *Semin Pediatr Neurol* 4: 192.

Malandrini A, Palmeri S, Villanova M *et al.* (1997) A syndrome of autosomal recessive pontocerebellar hypoplasia with white matter abnormalities and protracted course in two brothers. *Brain Dev* 19: 209.

✪ Maria B L, Hoang K B, Tusa R J *et al.* (1997) 'Joubert syndrome' revisited: key ocular motor signs with magnetic resonance imaging correlation. *J Child Neurol* 12: 423.

Maria B L, Zinreich S J, Carson B C *et al.* (1987) Dandy-Walker syndrome revisited. *Pediatr Neurosci* 13: 45.

✪ Marin-Padilla M (1991) Embryology and pathology of axial skeletal and neural dysraphic disorders. *Can J Neurol Sci* 18: 153.

✪ Marin-Padilla M (1997) Developmental neuropathology and impact of perinatal brain damage. II: White matter lesions of the neocortex. *J Neuropathol Exp Neurol* 56: 219.

Marsh D O, Myers G J, Clarkson T W *et al.* (1980) Fetal methylmercury poisoning: clinical and toxicological data on 9 cases. *Ann Neurol* 7: 343.

Martin H (1970) Microcephaly and mental retardation. *Am J Dis Child* 119: 128.

Martinez Lage J F, Poza M, Sola J *et al.* (1996) The child with a cephalocele: etiology, neuroimaging, and outcome. *Childs Nerv Syst* 12: 540.

✪ Mason T B 2nd, Chiriboga C A, Feldstein N A *et al.* (1997) Intracranial arachnoid cyst in a developmentally normal infant: case report and literature review. *Pediatr Neurol* 16: 59.

McComb J G (1997) Spinal and cranial neural tube defects. *Semin Pediatr Neurol* 4: 156.

McDonald C M (1995) Rehabilitation of children with spinal dysraphism. *Neurosurg Clin N Am* 6: 393.

McEnery G, Borzyskowski M, Cox T C *et al.* (1992) The spinal cord in neurologically stable spina bifida: a clinical and MRI study. *Dev Med Child Neurol* 34: 342.

McKusick V A (1994) *Mendelian inheritance in man: a catalog of human genes and genetic disorders*, 11th edn. Baltimore: Johns Hopkins University Press.

McLone D G & La Marca F (1994) The tethered spinal cord: diagnosis, significance, and not prepattern. *Development* 120: 2271.

McLone D G & La Marca F (1997) The tethered spinal cord: diagnosis, significance, and management. *Semin Pediatr Neurol* 473: 192–208.

Mealey J Jr, Dzentis A J & Hockey A A (1970) The prognosis of encephaloceles. *J Neurosurg* 32: 209.

✪ Medical Task Force on Anencephaly (1990) The infant with anencephaly. *N Engl J Med* 322: 669.

Meizner I, Levy A, Katz M *et al.* (1992) Iniencephaly: a case report. *J Reprod Med* 37: 885.

Melnick M & Myrianthopoulous N C (1987) Studies in neural tube defects. II. Pathologic findings in a prospectively collected series of anencephalics. *Am J Med Genet* 26: 783.

Menenzes M, Coker S B (1990) CHARGE and Joubert syndromes: are they a single disorder? *Pediatr Neurol* 6: 428.

Menezes A H, Bell W E & Perret G E (1980) Arachnoid cysts in children. *Arch Neurol* 55: 457.

Menkes J H, Philippart M & Clark D B (1964) Hereditary partial agenesis of the corpus callosum. *Arch Neurol* 11: 198.

Miller A, Guille J T & Bowen J R (1993) Evaluation and treatment of diastematomyelia. *J Bone Joint Surg* 75A: 1308.

Miller E, Hare J W, Cloherty J P *et al.* (1981) Elevated maternal hemoglobin Alc in early pregnancy and major congenital anomalies in infants of diabetic mothers. *N Engl J Med* 304: 1331.

Miller P, Smith D W & Shepard T H (1978) Maternal hyperthermia as a possible cause of anencephaly. *Lancet* 1: 519.

Mize R R & Erzurumlu R S (1996) Neural development and plasticity. *Progress in brain research.* Vol. 108. New York: Elsevier.

Mizuguchi M, Maekawa S & Kamoshita S (1994) Distribution of leptomeningeal glioneuronal heterotopia in alobar holoprosencephaly. *Arch Neurol* 51: 951.

Mooradian A D, Morley G K, McGeachie R *et al.* (1984) Spontaneous periodic hypothermia. *Neurology* 34: 79.

Mori K, Hashimoto T, Tayama M *et al.* (1994) Serial EEG and sleep polygraphic studies on lissencephaly (agyria-pachygyria). *Brain Dev* 16: 365.

Musumeci S A, Ferri R, Elia M *et al.* (1996) A new family with periventricular nodular heterotopia and peculiar dysmorphic features. A probable X-linked dominant trait. *Arch Neurol* 54: 61.

Naidich T P, McLone D G & Radkowski M A (1985/86) Intracranial arachnoid cysts. *Pediatr Neurosci* 12: 112.

Nakamura K, Hanabusa M & Okamoto N (1972) A classification of the anencephalic brain. *Teratology* 6: 115.

Nelson K B & Deutschberger J (1970) Head size at one year as a predictor of four-year I.Q. *Dev Med Child Neurol* 12: 487.

Nishikawa M, Sakamoto H, Hakuba A *et al.* (1997) Pathogenesis of Chiari malformation: a morphometric study of the posterior cranial fossa. *J Neurosurg* 86: 40.

Nixon G W, Johns R E Jr & Myers F F (1974) Congenital porencephaly. *Pediatrics* 54: 43.

Norman M G, Roberts M, Sirois J *et al.* (1976) Lissencephaly. *Can J Neurol Sci* 3: 39.

Norman M G & McGillivray B (1988) Fetal neuropathology of proliferative vasculopathy and hydranencephaly-hydrocephaly with multiple limb pterygia. *Pediatr Neurosci* 14: 301.

✪ Norman M G, McGillivray B C, Kalousek D K *et al.* (1995) *Congenital malformations of the brain.* New York: Oxford University Press.

Nugent F R, Al-Mefty O & Chou S (1979) Communicating hydrocephalus as a cause of aqueductal stenosis. *J Neurosurg* 51: 812.

Nyberg D A, Cyr D R, Mack L A *et al.* (1988) The Dandy–Walker malformation prenatal sonographic diagnosis and its clinical significance. *J Ultrasound Med* 7: 87.

Odent S, Le Marec B, Toutain A *et al.* (1998) Central nervous system malformations and early end-stage renal disease in oro-facio-digital syndrome type I: a review. *Am J Med Genet* 75: 389.

Odita J C & Hebi S (1996) CT and MRI characteristics of intracranial hemorrhage complicating breech and vacuum delivery. *Pediatr Radiol* 26: 782.

Ohnuma K, Imaizumi K, Masuno M *et al.* (1997) Magnetic resonance imaging abnormalities of the brain in Goldberg–Shprintzen syndrome. *Am J Med Genet* 73: 230.

Oi S, Matsumoto S (1992) A proposed grading and scoring system for spina bifida: Spina Bifida Neurological Scale (SBNS). *Childs Nerv Syst* 8: 337.

OMIM 98. Online Mendelian Inheritence in Man. http://www.ncbi.nlm.nih.gov/Omim

✪ O'Neill O R, Piatt J H Jr, Mitchell P *et al.* (1995) Agenesis and dysgenesis of the sacrum: neurosurgical implications. *Pediatr Neurosurg* 22: 20.

Ono J, Mano T, Andermann E *et al.* (1997) Band heterotopia or double cortex in a male: bridging structures suggest abnormality of the radial glial guide system. *Neurology* 48: 1701.

Osaka K, Matsumoto S & Tanimura T (1978) Myeloschisis in early human embryos. *Childs Brain* 4: 347.

Ouellette E M, Rosett H L, Rosman N P *et al.* (1977) Adverse effects on offspring of maternal alcohol abuse during pregnancy. *N Engl J Med* 297: 528.

Ozkinay F, Ozyurek A R, Bakiler A R *et al.* (1995) A case of Marden–Walker syndrome with Dandy–Walker malformation. *Clin Genet* 47: 221.

✪ Packard A M, Miller V S & Delgado M R (1997) Schizencephaly: correlations of clinical and radiologic features. *Neurology* 48: 1427.

✪ Palmini A, Andermann F, Aicardi J *et al.* (1991a) Diffuse cortical dysplasia, or the double cortex syndrome: the clinical and epileptic spectrum in 10 patients. *Neurology* 41: 1656.

✪ Palmini A, Andermann F, Olivier A *et al.* (1991b) Focal neuronal migration disorders and intractable partial epilepsy: results of surgical treatment. *Ann Neurol* 30: 750.

Pang D (1992) Split cord malformation. Part II. Clinical syndrome. *Neurosurgery* 31: 481.

Papasozomenos S & Roessman U (1981) Respiratory distress and Arnold–Chiari malformation. *Neurology* 31: 97.

Parikh J R, Mak K & Shalay K M (1994) Unilateral megalencephaly in association with Dandy–Walker complex. *Can Assoc Radiol J* 45: 394.

✪ Park T S (1992) Spinal dysraphism. *Contemporary issues in neurological surgery.* Boston, MA: Blackwell Scientific Publications.

Parrish M L, Roessmann U & Levinsohn M W (1979) Agenesis of the corpus callosum: a study of the frequency of associated malformations. *Ann Neurol* 6: 349.

✪ Pascual-Castroviejo I, Roche M C, Martinez Bermejo A *et al.* (1991a) Primary intracranial arachnoidal cysts: a study of 67 childhood cases. *Child Nerv Syst* 7: 257.

✪ Pascual-Castroviejo I, Velez A, Pascual-Pascual S I *et al.* (1991b) Dandy-Walker malformation: analysis of 38 cases. *Child Nerv Syst* 7: 88.

Pasternak J F, Mantovani J F & Volpe J J (1980) Porencephaly from periventricular intracerebral hemorrhage in a premature infant. *Am J Dis Child* 134: 673.

Payne J, Shibasaki F & Mercola M (1997) Spina bifida occulta in homozygous Patch mouse embryos. *Dev Dyn* 209: 105.

Peabody J, Emery J & Ashwal S (1989) Experience with anencephalic infants as prospective organ donors. *N Engl J Med* 321: 344.

Pellegrino J E, Lensch M W, Muenke M *et al.* (1997) Clinical and molecular analysis in Joubert syndrome. *Am J Med Genet* 72: 59.

Pensler J M, Giese S & Charrow J (1993) Surgical treatment of patients with lobar holoprosencephaly: a personal note. *J Craniofac Surg* 4: 2.

Petersen M C, Wolraich M, Sherbondy A *et al.* (1995) Abnormalities in control of ventilation in newborn infants with myelomeningocele. *J Pediatr* 126: 1011.

Pfeiffer R A, Legat G & Trautmann U (1992) Acrocallosal syndrome in a child with de novo inverted tandem duplication of 12p11.2-p13.3. *Ann Genet* 35: 41.

Pintos Morell G, Naranjo M A, Artigas M *et al.* (1995) Molybdenum cofactor deficiency associated with Dandy–Walker malformation. *J Inherit Metab Dis* 18: 86.

Preul M C, Leblanc R, Cendes F *et al.* (1997) Function and organization in dysgenic cortex. Case report. *J Neurosurg* 87: 113.

Raffel C & McComb J G (1988) To shunt or to fenestrate: which is the best treatment for arachnoid cysts in pediatric patients? *Neurosurgery* 23: 338.

Rais-Bahrami K & Naqvi M (1990) Hydranencephaly and maternal cocaine use: a case report. *Clin Pediatr Phila* 29: 729.

Raymond A A, Fish D R, Sisodiya S M *et al.* (1995) Abnormalities of gyration, heterotopias, tuberous sclerosis, focal cortical dysplasia, microdysgenesis, dysembryoplastic neuroepithelial tumour and dysgenesis of the archicortex in epilepsy. Clinical, EEG and neuroimaging features in 100 adult patients. *Brain* 118: 629.

Reid C B & Walsh C A (1996) Early development of the cerebral cortex. In: Mize R R, Erzurumlu R S eds. *Neural development and plasticity. Progress in brain research,* Vol 108. New York: Elsevier; 17–30.

Rengachary S S & Watanabe I (1981) Ultrastructure and pathogenesis of intracranial cysts. *J Neuropathol Exp Neurol* 40: 61.

Renwick J H (1972) Hypothesis: anencephaly and spina bifida are usually preventable by avoidance of a specific but unidentified substance present in certain potato tubers. *Br J Prev Soc Med* 26: 67.

Richman D P, Stewart R M & Caviness V S Jr (1974) Cerebral microgyria in a 27-week fetus: an architectonic and topographic analysis. *J Neuropathol Exp Neurol* 33: 374.

Riela A R, Thomas I T, Gonzalez A R *et al.* (1995) Fryns syndrome: neurologic findings in a survivor. *J Child Neurol* 10: 110.

Rivier F & Echenne B (1992) Dominantly inherited hypoplasia of the vermis. *Neuropediatrics* 23: 206.

Rock J P, Zimmerman R, Bello W O *et al.* (1996) Arachnoid cysts of the posterior fossa. *Neurosurgery* 18: 176.

Rodgers B L, Vanner L V, Pai G S *et al.* (1994) Walker–Warburg syndrome: report of three affected sibs. *Am J Med Genet* 49: 198.

Roessler E, Belloni E, Gaudenz K *et al.* (1996) Mutations in the human Sonic Hedgehog gene cause holoprosencephaly. *Nat Genet* 14: 357.

Romanengo M, Tortori Donati P & Di Rocco M (1997) Rhombencephalosynapsis with facial anomalies and probable autosomal recessive inheritance: a case report. *Clin Genet* 52: 184.

Rosett H L & Weiner L (1984) Alcohol and the fetus: a clinical perspective. New York: Oxford University Press.

Ross M E, Allen K M, Srivastava A K *et al.* (1997) Linkage and physical mapping of X-linked lissencephaly/SBH (XLIS): a gene causing neuronal migration defects in human brain. *Hum Mol Genet* 6: 555.

Rothman K J, Moore L L, Singer M R *et al.* (1995) Teratogenicity of high vitamin A intake. *N Engl J Med* 333: 1369.

Rouse B, Azen C, Koch R *et al.* (1997) Maternal Phenylketonuria Collaborative Study (MPKUCS) offspring: facial anomalies, malformations, and early neurological sequelae. *Am J Med Genet* 69: 89.

Rubenstein D, Cajade-Law A G & Youngman V (1996) The development of the corpus callosum in semilobar and lobar holoprosencephaly. *Pediatr Radiol* 26: 839.

Sabbagha R E, Sheikh Z, Tamura R K *et al.* (1985) Predictive value, sensitivity and specificity of ultrasonic targeted imaging for fetal anomalies in gravid women at high risk for birth defects. *Am J Obstet Gynecol* 152: 822.

Sakamoto H, Hukuba A, Fujitani K *et al.* (1991) Surgical treatment of the retethered spinal cord after repair of lipomyelomeningocele. *J Neurosurg* 74: 709.

Sandler A D, Knudsen M W, Brown T T *et al.* (1997) Neurodevelopmental dysfunction among non-referred children with idiopathic megalencephaly. *J Pediatr* 131: 320.

Saraiva J M & Baraitser M (1992) Joubert syndrome: a review [see comments]. *Am J Med Genet* 43: 726.

✪ Sarnat H (1992) *Cerebral dysgenesis. Embryology and clinical expression.* New York: Oxford University Press.

Sarnat H B (1995) Ependymal reactions to injury. A review. *J Neuropathol Exp Neurol* 54: 1.

Sasaki M, Ehara S & Watabe T (1997) Cerebellar polymicrogyria. *AJNR Am J Neuroradiol* 18: 394.

Sawaya R & McLaurin R L (1981) Dandy–Walker syndrome. *J Neurosurg* 55: 89.

Sayed M & al-Alaiyan S (1996) Agenesis of corpus callosum, hypertrophic pyloric stenosis and Hirschsprung disease: coincidence or common etiology? *Neuropediatrics* 27: 204.

✪ Schaefer G B, Sheth R D & Bodensteiner J B (1994) Cerebral dysgenesis. An overview. *Neurologic Clin* 12: 773–88.

✪ Schaefer G B, Thompson J N, Bodensteiner J B *et al.* (1996) Hypoplasia of the cerebellar vermis in neurogenetic syndromes. *Ann Neurol* 39: 382.

Schardein J L (1985) *Chemically induced birth defects*, vol. 2. Drug and chemical toxicology series. New York, NY: Marcel Dekker

Scherrer C C, Hammer F, Schinzel A *et al.* (1992) Brain stem and cervical cord dysraphic lesions in iniencephaly. *Pediatr Pathol* 12: 469.

Schneidau T, Franco I, Zebold K & Kaplan W (1995) Selective sacral rhizotomy for the management of neurogenic bladders in spina bifida patients: long-term followup. *J Urol* 154: 766.

Schinzel A (1979) Postaxial polydactyly, hallux duplication, absence of the corpus callosum, macrencephaly and severe mental retardation: a new syndrome? *Helv Paediatr Acta* 34: 141–6.

Scholler Gyure M, Nesselaar C, van Wieringen H *et al.* (1996) Treatment of defecation disorders by colonic enemas in children with spina bifida. *Eur J Pediatr Surg* 1 (Suppl. 6): 32.

Schrander-Stumpel C, Schrander J, Fryns J P *et al.* (1988) Caudal deficiency sequence in 7q terminal deletion. *Am J Med Genet* 30: 757.

Schull W J (1997) Brain damage among individuals exposed prenatally to ionizing radiation: a 1993 review. *Stem Cells* 15(suppl. 2): 129.

Seller M J, Singer J D, Coltart T M *et al.* (1974) Maternal serum alpha-fetoprotein levels and prenatal diagnosis of neural-tube defects. *Lancet* 1: 428.

Sells C J (1977) Microcephaly in a normal school population. *Pediatrics* 59: 262.

Sener R N (1995) MR imaging of Joubert's syndrome. *Comput Med Imaging Graph* 19: 481.

Sener R N (1997) MR demonstration of cerebral hemimegalencephaly associated with cerebellar involvement (total hemimegalencephaly). *Comput Med Imaging Graph* 21: 201.

Sensi A, Cerruti S, Calzolari E *et al.* (1990) Familial porencephaly. *Clin Genet* 38: 396.

Sepulveda W, Kyle P M, Hassan J *et al.* (1997) Prenatal diagnosis of diastematomyelia: case reports and review of the literature. *Prenat Diagn* 17: 161.

Sergi C, Hentze S, Sohn C *et al.* (1997) Telencephalosynapsis (synencephaly) and rhombencephalosynapsis with posterior fossa ventriculocele ('Dandy–Walker cyst'): an unusual aberrant syngenetic complex. *Brain Dev* 19: 426.

Serville F, Lyonnet S, Pelet A *et al.* (1992) X-linked hydrocephalus: clinical heterogeneity at a single gene locus. *Eur J Pediatr* 151: 515.

Sever L E (1995) Looking for causes of neural tube defects: where does the environment fit in? *Environ Health Perspect* 103(Suppl. 6): 165.

Shah K N, Rajadhyaksha S, Shah V S *et al.* (1992) EEG recognition of holoprosencephaly and Aicardi syndrome. *Indian J Pediatr* 59: 103.

Shapiro I, Borochowitz Z, Degani S *et al.* (1992) Neu-Laxova syndrome: prenatal ultrasonographic diagnosis, clinical and pathological studies, and new manifestations. *Am J Med Genet* 43: 602.

Shapiro W R, Williams G H & Plum F (1969) Spontaneous recurrent hypothermia accompanying agenesis of the corpus callosum. *Brain* 92: 423.

Shastri N J, Bharani S A, Modi U J *et al.* (1997) Familial porencephaly. *Indian J Pediatr* 60: 459.

Shevell M I & Majnemer A (1996) Clinical features of developmental disability associated with cerebellar hypoplasia. *Pediatr Neurol* 15: 224.

Shewmon D A, Capron A M, Peacock W J *et al.* (1989) The use of anencephalic infants as organ sources. *JAMA* 261: 1773.

Shiota K (1982) Neural tube defects and maternal hyperthermia in early pregnancy: epidemiology in a human embryo population. *Am J Med Genet* 12: 281.

Silverstein D M, Zacharowicz L, Edelman M *et al.* (1997) Joubert syndrome associated with multicystic kidney disease and hepatic fibrosis. *Pediatr Nephrol* 11: 746.

Smit L M, Barth P G, Valk J *et al.* (1984) Familial porencephalic white matter disease in two generations. *Brain Dev* 6: 54.

Smith A, Wiles C, Haan E *et al.* (1996) Clinical features in 27 patients with Angelman syndrome resulting from DNA deletion. *J Med Genet* (Feb): 107.

Spataro R F, Lin S R, Horner F A *et al.* (1976) Aqueductal stenosis and hydrocephalus: rare sequelae of mumps virus infection. *Neuroradiology* 12: 11.

Spohr H L, Willms J & Steinhausen H C (1993) Prenatal alcohol exposure and long-term developmental consequences. *Lancet* 341: 907.

Spranger J, Benirschke K, Hall J G *et al.* (1982) Errors of morphogenesis: concepts and terms. *J Pediatr* 100: 160.

Steinbok P & Cochrane D D (1991) The nature of congenital posterior cervical or cervicothoracic midline cutaneous mass lesions: report of eight cases. *J Neurosurg* 75: 206.

Steinbok P (1995) Dysraphic lesions of the cervical spinal cord. *Neurosurg Clin N Am* 6: 367.

Steinlin M, Schmid M, Landau K *et al.* (1997) Follow-up in children with Joubert syndrome. *Neuropediatrics* 28: 204.

✪ Stone A R (1995) Neurourologic evaluation and urologic management of spinal dysraphism. *Neurosurg Clin N Am* 6: 269.

Sugimoto T, Yasuhara A, Nishida N *et al.* (1993) MRI of the head in the evaluation of microcephaly. *Neuropediatrics* 24: 4.

Takahashi S, Miyamoto A, Oki J *et al.* (1995) Alobar holoprosencephaly with diabetes insipidus and neuronal migration disorder. *Pediatr Neurol* 13: 175.

Tal Y, Freigang B, Dunn H G *et al.* (1980) Dandy-Walker syndrome: analysis of 21 cases. *Dev Med Child Neurol* 22: 189.

Talwar D, Baldwin M A & Horbatt C I (1995) Epilepsy in children with meningomyelocele. *Pediatr Neurol* 13: 29.

Tardieu M, Evrard P & Lyon G (1981) Progressive expanding congenital porencephalies: a treatable cause of progressive encephalopathy. *Pediatrics* 68: 198.

Tayama M, Hashimoto T, Mori K *et al.* (1992) Electrophysiological study on hydranencephaly. *Brain Dev* 14: 185.

Toriello H V, Radecki L L, Sharda J *et al.* (1986) Frontonasal 'dysplasia', cerebral anomalies, and polydactyly: report of a new syndrome and discussion from a developmental field perspective. *Am J Med Genet Suppl* 2: 89.

Towfighi J & Housman C (1991) Spinal cord abnormalities in caudal regression syndrome. *Acta Neuropathol Berl* 81: 458.

Tsuru A, Mizuguchi M, Uyemura K *et al.* (1997) Immunohistochemical expression of cell adhesion molecule L1 in hemimeganencephaly. *Pediatr Neurol* 16: 45.

Vade A & Horowitz S W (1992) Agenesis of corpus callosum and intraventricular lipomas. *Pediatr Neurol* 8: 307.

Valanne L, Pihko H, Katevuo K *et al.* (1994) MRI of the brain in muscle-eye-brain (MEB) disease. *Neuroradiology* 36: 473.

Van Allen M I (1996) Multisite neural tube closure in humans. *Birth Defects Orig Artic Ser* 30: 203–25.

Van Allen M I, Kalousek D K & Chernoff G F (1993) Evidence for multi-site closure of the neural tube in humans. *Am J Med Genet* 47: 723.

van der Knaap M S, Barth P G, Stroink H *et al.* (1995) Leukoencephalopathy with swelling and a discrepantly mild clinical course in eight children. *Ann Neurol* 37: 324.

Van Zalen-Sprock R M, van Vugt J M & van Geijn H P (1996) First-trimester sonographic detetion of neurodevelopmental abnormalities in some single-gene disorders. *Prenat Diagn* 16: 199.

Vare A M & Bansal P C (1971) Anencephaly. An anatomical study of 41 anencephalic infants. *Indian J Pediatr* 38: 301.

Velasco M, Velasco F, Gardea G *et al.* (1997) Polygraphic characterization of the sleep-epilepsy patterns in a hydranencephalic child with severe generalized seizures of the Lennox-Gastaut syndrome. *Arch Med Res* 28: 297.

Venes J L, Black K L & Latack J T (1986) Preoperative evaluation and surgical management of the Chiari II malformation. *J Neurosurg* 64: 363.

Vergani P, Ghidini A, Strobelt N *et al.* (1994) Prognostic indicators in the prenatal diagnosis of agenesis of corpus callosum. *Am J Obstet Gynecol* 170: 753.

Viljoen D L (1995) Porencephaly and transverse limb defects following severe maternal trauma in early pregnancy. *Clin Dysmorphol* 4: 75.

Vogel F S & McClenahan J L (1952) Anomalies of major cerebral arteries associated with malformations of the brain, with special reference to the pathogenesis of anencephaly. *Am J Pathol* 28: 701.

✪ Volpe J J (2000) *Neurology of the newborn.* 4th edition Philadelphia, PA: WB Saunders.

Walters J, Ashwal S & Masek T (1997) Anencephaly: where do we now stand? *Semin Neurol* 17: 249.

Weiner S N, Pearlstein A E & Eiber A (1987) MR imaging of intracranial arachnoid cysts. *J Comput Assist Tomogr* 11: 236.

✪ Welch K & Winston K R (1987) Spina bifida. In: Myrianthopoulos N C, ed. *Handbook of clinical neurology.* Amsterdam: Elsevier Science.

Wininger S J & Donnenfeld A E (1994) Syndromes identified in fetuses with prenatally diagnosed cephaloceles. *Prenat Diagn* 14: 839.

Wintour E M, Lewitt M, McFarlane A *et al.* (1996) Experimental hydranencephaly in the ovine fetus. *Acta Neuropathol (Berl)* 91: 537.

Wisniewski K, Bambska M, Sher J H *et al.* (1983) A clinical neuropathological study of the fetal alcohol syndrome. *Neuropediatrics* 14: 197.

Wood J W, Johnson K G & Omori Y (1967) *In utero* exposure to the Hiroshima atomic bomb: an evaluation of head size and mental retardation twenty years later. *Pediatrics* 39: 385.

Wu M, Chen D F, Sasaoka T *et al.* (1996) Neural tube defects and abnormal brain development in F52-deficient mice. *Proc Natl Acad Sci USA* 93: 2110.

Yakovlev P I & LeCours A R (1967) The myelogenetic cycles of regional maturation of the brain. In: Minkowski A, ed. *Regional development of the brain in early life.* Oxford: Blackwell Scientific.

Yakovlev P I, Wadsworth R C (1946) Schizencephalies: a study of the congenital clefts in the cerebral mantle. *J Neuropathol Exp Neurol* 5: 116.

Yamasaki M, Thompson P & Lemmon V (1997) CRASH syndrome: mutations in L1CAM correlate with severity of the disease. *Neuropediatrics* 28: 175.

Yokota A & Matsukado Y (1979) Congenital midline porencephaly: a new brain malformation associated with scalp anomaly. *Childs Brain* 5: 380.

Yoshioka M & Kuroki S (1994) Clinical spectrum and genetic studies of Fukuyama congenital muscular dystrophy. *Am J Med Genet* 53: 245.

Younus M & Coode P E (1986) Nasal glioma and encephalocele: two separate entities: report of two cases. *J Neurosurg* 64: 516.

Zhao Q, Behringer R & de Crombrugghe B (1996) Prenatal folic acid treatment suppresses acrania and meroanencephaly in mice mutant for the Cart1 homeobox gene. *Nat Genet* 13: 275.

Ziegler A L, Deonna T & Calame A (1990) Hidden intelligence of a multiply handicapped child with Joubert syndrome. *Dev Med Child Neurol* 32: 261.

# Chapter 14 Genetics of neurodevelopmental anomalies

M. Suri and I. D. Young

## INTRODUCTION

Congenital abnormalities of the CNS are common and make a major contribution to severe disability both in childhood and in adult life. They can present before birth, in the neonatal period, or in later childhood, and can occur in isolation or as one feature of a large number of complex multiple abnormality syndromes. Their recognition is important not only for the management of the child in whom the anomaly is identified, but also because of the potential genetic implications for other family members.

There is increasing evidence that genetic factors play a major role in the etiology of many CNS malformations and associated multiple malformation syndromes. This evidence stems from several sources. First, there is the burgeoning literature on syndrome recognition and delineation which has culminated in the development of computerized resources such as the London Dysmorphology and Neurogenetics Databases (Winter & Baraitser 1999). Second, there is the added evidence provided by increasingly sophisticated neuroimaging, and finally there is the information gained from the staggering progress achieved in molecular biology over the last five years which has resulted in the isolation and characterization of many crucially important neurodevelopmental genes.

Together these developments, occurring in parallel, have provided much greater understanding of the role of genetics in malformations such as holoprosencephaly, lissencephaly, and neural tube defects. By utilizing this new information in conjunction with the results of traditional empiric risk family studies it is usually possible to give parents and other relevant family members a reasonable indication of risks to future children, together with details of the availability of specific DNA-based prenatal diagnostic options. Relevant developments shall be considered in this chapter in the context of specific malformations.

## NEURAL TUBE DEFECTS (NTDs) (see also p. 200)

This term embraces several relatively common malformations including anencephaly, iniencephaly, encephalocele, meningocele, and myelomeningocele. These arise as a consequence of impaired closure and subsequent canalization of the ectodermal neural tube. Primary neurulation, the process whereby the neural plate folds to form the neural tube, occurs between 18 and 28 days after fertilization. Secondary neurulation, involving canalization and differentiation of the closed neural tube, takes place between 4 and 8 weeks post fertilization. Most NTDs are thought to be caused by an error in primary neurulation, although there is a school of thought that reopening of a closed neural tube may be a contributory factor (Norman *et al.* 1995).

Whatever the precise embryologic mechanism there is general agreement that most cases of isolated non-syndromal anencephaly and spina bifida are caused by a 'multifactorial' interaction of genetic susceptibility with environmental factors. The precise nature of most of these factors is unknown. However, recent studies in mice indicate that certain developmental gene families, most notably those genes containing a paired box (*PAX*) domain, play an important role (Helwig *et al.* 1995). In humans it has been shown that specific mutations in the methylenetetrahydrofolate reductase (MTHFR) gene are risk factors for NTDs and in particular homozygosity for the common 677(C/T) mutation in both mother and child conveys a sevenfold increased risk (van der Put *et al.* 1998). Known environmental contributory factors include poor socio-economic status, maternal insulin dependent diabetes mellitus and valproate teratogenicity.

Despite extensive research in this field it is not yet possible to utilize molecular analysis to determine family risks which are still based on the results of empiric family studies. Average risk figures that are suitable for counseling purposes are summarized in Table 14.1. Ideally locally derived contemporary risks should be used but these are rarely available. The importance of offering high dose (4–5 mg daily) periconceptional folic acid supplementation to prospective mothers of 'high' risk pregnancies cannot be overemphasized. This has been shown to convey a 70–80% reduction in risk (MRC Vitamin Study Research Group 1991). It is important to remember that spinal dysraphism, embracing abnormalities such as cord tethering, diastematomyelia, and intradural lipoma, also convey multifactorial recurrence risks for open NTDs so that folic acid supplementation should be offered to relevant female relatives.

NTDs also occur in several single-gene disorders and syndromes, as summarized in Table 14.2. It is particularly important that these are recognized, as the recurrence risk will usually be much greater than for an isolated NTD. Furthermore, syndromal NTDs will almost certainly not be susceptible to periconceptional folic acid prophylaxis. There is evidence that isolated anencephaly can occasionally show autosomal recessive inheritance, particularly in the Iranian Jewish population (Zlotogora 1995), and there have been a few reports of pedigrees consistent with X-linked recessive

**Table 14.1 Multifactorial recurrence risks for NTDs**

| Affected relative | Risk (%) |
|---|---|
| First degree (50% of genes shared) | |
| One sibling | 4 |
| Two siblings | 10 |
| One parent | 4 |
| One parent and one sibling | 10 |
| Second degree (25% of genes shared) | |
| One uncle or aunt | 1–2 |
| One nephew or niece | 1–2 |
| One half sibling | 1–2 |
| Two second degree relatives | 4 |
| Third degree (12.5% of genes shared) | |
| One first cousin | 0.5–1 |
| Two first cousins | 1–2 |
| Three or more first cousins | 4 |

*Example*: A woman who has a sister with spina bifida is planning a pregnancy. This baby will have an aunt with a NTD. Thus the risk that the baby will be affected, without folic acid prophylaxis, equals 1–2%.

transmission of non-syndromal NTDs (Baraitser & Burn 1984). However, the vast majority of isolated non-syndromal NTDs are thought to be multifactorial in etiology and to convey multifactorial recurrence risks as already outlined (Table 14.1).

NTDs also occur in several chromosome abnormalities such as trisomy 13, trisomy 18 and the 22q11 deletion syndrome (Nickel & Magenis 1996). Hence when assessing any child with an NTD for the purpose of genetic counseling, due consideration should be given to chromosome analysis in the evaluation protocol (Table 14.3). Finally NTDs can also occur in the amniotic band syndrome when rupture of the amnion has occurred before 45 days gestation (Higginbottom *et al.* 1979) and in the 'Schisis Association', this being the term used to account for the tendency of NTDs, oral clefts, omphaloceles, and diaphragmatic herniae to occur together more often than would be expected by chance (Czeizel 1981). The incidence of schisis-type malformations in siblings in Czeizel's original series was seven out of 190 (3.7%).

## HYDROCEPHALUS (see also p. 226 and p. 739)

Congenital hydrocephalus is a relatively common anomaly with an incidence approaching 1 in 1000 births (Blackburn & Fineman 1994). The causes are numerous and include environmental factors such as trauma and infection together with the well recognized association with NTDs. Hydrocephalus also occurs in many chromosome abnormalities, such as triploidy and trisomy 13, and features in a large number of multiple malformation syndromes the more common of which are listed in Table 14.4.

The recurrence risk for isolated non-syndromal ('uncomplicated') hydrocephalus is relatively low, with family study derived sibling recurrence risks of between 1 and 4% (Burton 1979; Adams *et al.* 1982; Varadi *et al.* 1988). It has been noted that the recurrence risk for male siblings of a male proband tends to be higher (i.e. 4%) than for female siblings of a female proband (1–2%), and it is now well recognized that a small proportion of all cases of hydrocephalus show X-linked inheritance. Most, if not all, of these X-linked cases are now known to be caused by mutations in the *LICAM* gene which is located at Xq28 (Rosenthal *et al.* 1992).

*LICAM* encodes a neuronal cell adhesion molecule, known as L1, which is involved in neuronal migration and axonal extension. Mutations in *LICAM* can result in three different phenotypes, i.e. X-linked hydrocephalus, the MASA syndrome

**Table 14.2 Single-gene disorders in which NTDs may occur**

| Disorder | Inheritance | MIM no. | Features |
|---|---|---|---|
| Craniotelencephalic dysplasia | AR | 218670 | Craniosynostosis, frontal encephalocele, hydrocephalus |
| Cryptophthalmos syndrome | AR | 219000 | Cryptophthalmos, occipital encephalocele, renal agenesis syndactyly |
| Frontofacionasal dysplasia | AR | 229400 | Eyelid coloboma, facial clefting, frontal encephalocele |
| Knobloch's syndrome | AR | 267750 | Myopia, occipital encephalocele |
| Meckel's syndrome | AR | 249000 | Occipital encephalocele, polycystic kidneys, polydactyly |
| Roberts syndrome | AR | 268300 | Cleft lip/palate, frontal encephalocele, hypertelorism, phocomelia |
| Sacral agenesis (Currarino triad) | AD | 176450 | Anorectal malformation, anterior meningocele, partial sacral agenesis |
| Spondylocostal dysplasia (Jarcho–Levin syndrome) | AR | 277300 | Multiple rib and vertebral abnormalities |
| Walker–Warburg syndrome | AR | 236670 | Encephalocele, hydrocephalus, lissencephaly, retinal dysplasia |

*Key*: AD, autosomal dominant; AR, autosomal recessive; MIM, Mendelian inheritance in man (McKusick 1998).

**Table 14.3 Genetic assessment of NTDs**

| | |
|---|---|
| • Family history | Pedigree data to include all first, second and third degree relatives, relevant terminations of pregnancy, stillbirths, and neonatal deaths |
| • Pregnancy history | Maternal illness, e.g. IDDM<br>Drug exposure – especially valproate |
| • Examination | Other congenital malformations and/or dysmorphic features |
| • Investigations | Chromosome analysis, to include 22q FISH, if other abnormalities noted |

Key: IDDM, insulin dependent diabetes mellitus.

(M = Mental retardation, A = Aphasia, S = Shuffling gait, A = Adducted thumbs), and complicated spastic paraplegia type 1. Males with X-linked hydrocephalus show severe retardation in association with flexed adducted thumbs (Fig. 14.1) and other CNS malformations, most notably aqueduct stenosis and bilateral absence of the pyramids. This latter finding is a particularly useful discriminatory diagnostic feature (Kenwrick *et al.* 1996). Carrier females sometimes show mild learning difficulties (Halliday *et al.* 1986).

Mutation analysis for *LICAM* is now available on a limited basis. When a mutation is identified genetic counseling on the basis of X-linked inheritance is relatively straightforward. At present, screening techniques can only identify approximately 80–90% of all mutations, so that failure to identify a mutation in *LICAM* does not exclude a diagnosis of X-linked hydrocephalus. Consequently, if the clinical and pathologic features are typical it would be unwise to counsel on the basis of a low recurrence risk even if mutation analysis is negative.

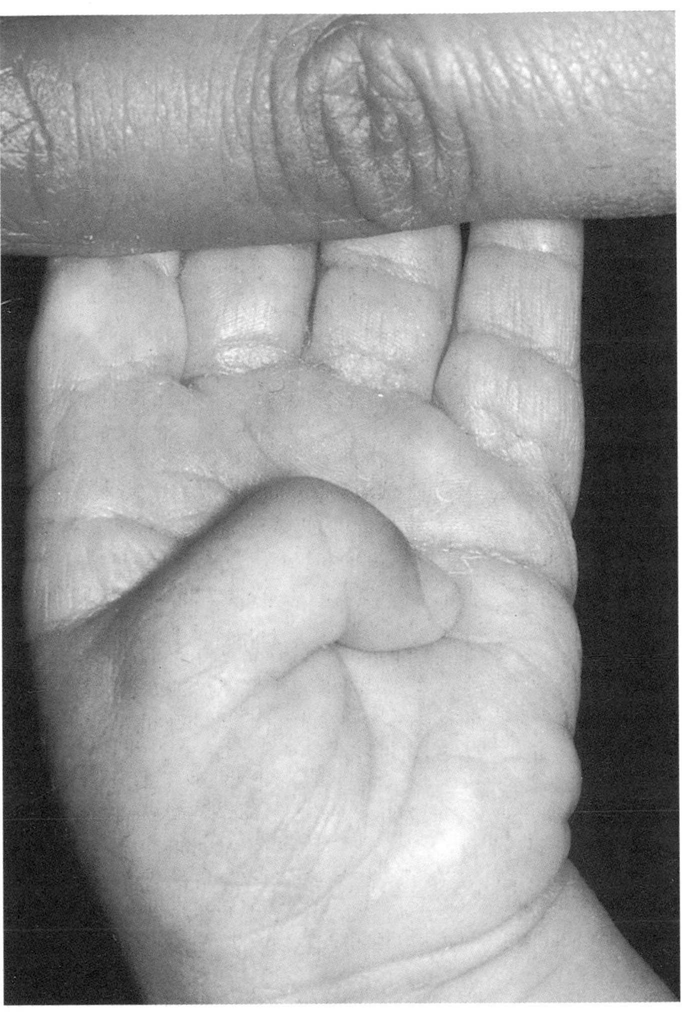

Figure 14.1 The hand of a child with X-linked hydrocephalus showing a clasped adducted thumb.

**Table 14.4 Malformation syndromes in which hydrocephalus is a characteristic feature**

| Syndrome | Inheritance | MIM no. | Associated features |
|---|---|---|---|
| Aase–Smith | AD | 147800 | Arthrogryposis, cleft palate, congenital heart defect |
| Apert | AD | 101200 | Craniosynostosis, syndactyly |
| FG | XR | 305450 | Agenesis of corpus callosum, hypotonia, imperforate anus |
| Hydrocephaly/VATER association | NK | 192350 | VATER spectrum |
| Hydrolethalus | AR | 236680 | Micrognathia, microphthalmia, polydactyly |
| Linear sebaceous nevus | NK | 163200 | Hyperpigmentation, nevus sebaceous, seizures |
| Osteopetrosis (severe congenital form) | AR | 259700 | Cranial nerve and marrow compression, dense bones |
| Thanatophoric dysplasia | AD | 187600 | Craniosynostosis, short limbs, small chest |
| Walker–Warburg | AR | 236670 | Encephalocele, lissencephaly, retinal dysplasia |

*Key*: AD, autosomal dominant; AR, autosomal recessive; XR, X-linked recessive; NK, not known; VATER, *v*ertebral, *a*nal, *t*racheo-*e*sophageal and *r*adial/*r*enal abnormalities; MIM, Mendelian inheritance in man (McKusick 1998).

## HYDRANENCEPHALY AND PORENCEPHALY

Hydranencephaly is characterized by complete or almost complete absence of the cerebral hemispheres in the presence of intact meninges and a relatively normal skull. Most cases represent sporadic events within a family and are thought to be the consequence of a destructive process such as infection or an intrauterine vascular accident. Thus usually the recurrence risk for siblings is very low. However genetic counseling is complicated by the reports of a condition known as encephaloclastic proliferative vasculopathy which shows autosomal recessive inheritance (Fowler *et al.* 1972; Harper & Hockey 1983; Moeschler & Marin Padilla 1989). In this rare disorder there is abnormal focal vascularization of the cortical mantle by proliferating tufts of blood vessels which exert a disruptive effect through hemorrhagic necrosis. The existence of this rare entity emphasizes the importance and value of detailed neuropathologic assessment. Although hydranencephaly is not often seen in children with multiple malformation syndromes, it has been reported in two male siblings in association with hypoplastic kidneys and 2/3 toe syndactyly (Bendon *et al.* 1987).

Porencephaly refers to a fluid-filled cavity in the brain which is separated from the ventricular system and subarachnoid space (p. 214). As with hydranencephaly, most cases are sporadic and are probably caused by a destructive process such as infection, hemorrhage or vascular occlusion. However, just as with hydranencephaly, counseling is complicated by several reports of familial porencephaly, often involving multiple generation transmission of hemiplegia with or without convulsions (Berg *et al.* 1983; Smit *et al.* 1984; Zonana *et al.* 1986). Debus *et al.* (1998) have reported that 16 out of 24 children with porencephalic cysts seen over a 10-year period had an apparent genetic risk factor for thrombophilia, such as heterozygous factor V Leiden deficiency or protein C deficiency (p. 395). At present it is difficult to know how best to interpret the significance of these findings, as heterozygous factor V Leiden deficiency is relatively common in the general population. However, this report does raise the possibility that a proportion of cases of familial porencephaly could be caused by a hereditary tendency to thrombophilia.

## DANDY–WALKER MALFORMATION (DWM) (see also p. 224)

In this developmental abnormality, partial or complete absence of the cerebellar vermis is associated with cystic dilatation of the fourth ventricle, elevation of the tentorium and transverse sinuses, and the early onset of hydrocephalus. This condition shows marked etiological heterogeneity (Chitayat *et al.* 1994). Approximately 50% of cases diagnosed prenatally are caused by a chromosome abnormality (Nyberg *et al.* 1991), such as one of the viable autosomal trisomy syndromes (i.e. trisomy 8, 9, 13, 18, and 21), triploidy, or more subtle imbalance such as 2q, 3q, and 6p deletion or 8p, 8q, and 17q duplication. Known environmental causal agents include prenatal exposure to infection such as cytomegalovirus and rubella and to drugs such as warfarin and valproic acid. A DWM is a recognized finding in a large number of multiple malformation syndromes, the most commonly encountered of which are listed in Table 14.5. Murray *et al.* (1985) noted that in 23 of 113 reviewed cases of DWM there was another midline abnormality such as a cleft lip or palate, congenital heart defect or neural tube defect. They proposed that in these situations the recurrence risk quoted should be that appropriate for the other malformation, i.e. usually around 2–5%.

When a DWM occurs in isolation the recurrence risk is low. Pooling the results from two studies gives a risk of 1% for siblings (Burton 1979; Murray *et al.* 1985). However, it was noted that 3 out of 44 of the siblings of the index cases in one of these series had another midline defect, an observation which emphasizes the importance of offering

**Table 14.5 Syndromes featuring a Dandy–Walker malformation**

| Syndrome | MIM no. | Inheritance | Features |
|---|---|---|---|
| Aase–Smith | 147800 | AD | Arthrogryposis, cleft palate, congenital heart defect |
| Aicardi | 304050 | XD | Chorioretinitis, infantile spasms |
| Cerebro-oculo-muscular | 236670 | AR | Congenital muscular dystrophy, encephalocele, lissencephaly |
| Fryns | 229850 | AR | Corneal clouding, diaphragmatic hernia, small nails |
| Hydrolethalus | 236680 | AR | Hydrocephalus, polydactyly |
| Joubert | 213300 | AR | Cerebellar vermis agenesis, episodic tachypnea, polydactyly, retinopathy |
| Meckel–Gruber | 249900 | AR | Encephalocele, polycystic kidneys, polydactyly |
| Oculo-cerebro-cutaneous | 164180 | NK | Microphthalmia, orbital cysts, periorbital skin tags |
| Oro-facial-digital type I | 311200 | XD | Cleft lip, oral frenulae, polydactyly, syndactyly |
| Smith–Lemli–Opitz types I and II | 268670, 270400 | AR | Genital anomaly, microcephaly, ptosis, syndactyly |
| Walker–Warburg | 236670 | AR | Encephalocele, hydrocephalus, lissencephaly, retinal dysplasia |

*Key*: AD, autosomal dominant; AR, autosomal recessive; XD, X-linked dominant; NK, not known; MIM, Mendelian inheritance in man (McKusick 1998).

detailed prenatal ultrasound monitoring in subsequent pregnancies.

## AGENESIS OF THE CORPUS CALLOSUM (ACC) (see also p. 219)

Of all the cerebral malformations discussed in this chapter, ACC almost certainly demonstrates the greatest etiological heterogeneity with numerous reported chromosomal, single-gene, syndromal, and environmental causes (Dobyns 1996). Hence counseling with regard to prognosis and recurrence risk is rarely straightforward, particularly when the abnormality is detected prenatally. The difficulty of interpreting the significance of isolated ACC is illustrated by its occasional discovery in an individual of normal intelligence, and when ACC is detected prenatally as an isolated abnormality it is associated with a probability of around 85% for normal development. However, in the presence of other abnormalities the long-term outlook for normal intellectual development is poor (Gupta & Lilford 1995).

ACC has been observed in a very large number of chromosome abnormalities (Dobyns 1996). This suggests that either many genes are involved in the development of the corpus callosum, in keeping with the 'reductionist' interpretation of the effects of chromosome imbalance, or that the corpus callosum is particularly sensitive to any disturbance in the meticulously orchestrated cascade of events which determine normal development. Chromosome abnormalities in which ACC commonly occurs include the 4p- (Wolf-Hirschhorn) syndrome, duplication 8p and 11q, and trisomy 13 and 18. The long list of other rarer chromosome abnormalities in which ACC has been reported emphasizes the importance of detailed chromosome analysis in all cases.

The London Dysmorphology Database (Winter & Baraitser 1999) lists 175 non-chromosomal syndromes in which ACC has been described. Many of these show single-gene inheritance as indicated in Table 14.6. Although some of these disorders have been mapped to particular chromosome regions, the relevant genes have been isolated in only a few instances. Notable examples include the X-linked α-thalassemia/mental retardation (ATR-X) syndrome (Gibbons *et al.* 1995), which is caused by mutations in the *XH2* gene at Xq13, and the MASA syndrome which is caused by mutations in *LICAM* as discussed above in the section on hydrocephalus.

When present in isolation, ACC is generally stated to convey a low (<5%) recurrence risk for siblings and offspring, although the present authors are not aware of any specific family studies that have been undertaken to confirm this. Counseling is complicated by several reports of multiple family members being affected with ACC, or with ACC as part of an apparently 'private' unique syndrome (e.g. da Silva 1988). Hence the genetic evaluation of every child with ACC should involve not only detailed chromosome analysis, as previously discussed, but also a full family history and thorough examination for other developmental and/or neurologic abnormalities.

## MICROCEPHALY (see also p. 211)

This constitutes a difficult and relatively common problem in genetic counseling, particularly if microcephaly is defined as a head circumference greater than 2 standard deviations (SD) below the mean for age and sex, as this will embrace almost 2.5% of the general population. However around only 10% of such individuals will show significant mental retardation in contrast to almost 50% of the 0.15% of the population ascertained if a stricter diagnostic criterion of >3 SD below the population mean is applied (Dolk 1991).

Microcephaly has numerous causes, both environmental and genetic and in many cases it can be very difficult to establish a precise diagnosis. Known environmental causes include intrauterine infection and exposure to various agents including radiation, alcohol, and high circulating levels of maternal phenylalanine. Genetic causes can be considered under the categories of chromosomal, syndromal and isolated.

**Table 14.6 Single-gene disorders in which agenesis of the corpus callosum is a common finding**

| Disorder | Inheritance | MIM no. | Features |
|---|---|---|---|
| Acrocallosal syndrome | AR | 200990 | Mental retardation, pre and postaxial polydactyly |
| Aicardi syndrome | XD | 304050 | Chorioretinitis, infantile spasms |
| α-thalassemia/mental retardation | XR | 301040 | Genital anomalies, hypotonia, mental retardation |
| Andermann syndrome | AR | 218000 | Mental retardation, peripheral neuropathy |
| FG syndrome | XR | 305450 | Anal stenosis, hypotonia, macrocephaly |
| MASA syndrome | XR | 308840 | Adducted thumbs, shuffling gait, speech delay |
| Septo-optic dysplasia | NK | 182230 | Hypopituitarism, optic nerve hypoplasia |
| Toriello–Carey syndrome | AR | 217980 | Cardiac and laryngeal abnormalities, Pierre-Robin anomaly |
| Walker–Warburg syndrome | AR | 236670 | Encephalocele, hydrocephalus, lissencephaly, retinal dysplasia |
| Zellweger syndrome | AR | 214100 | Camptodactyly, high forehead, hypotonia, stippled epiphyses |

*Key*: AR, autosomal recessive; XR, X-linked recessive; XD, X-linked dominant; NK, not known (dominant and recessive inheritance reported); MIM, Mendelian inheritance in man (McKusick 1998).

**Table 14.7 Genetic assessment of microcephaly**

| | |
|---|---|
| • History | Family history, ? parental consanguinity |
| | Pregnancy exposure to teratogens |
| | Possible pre, peri or postnatal asphyxia |
| | OFC at birth |
| • Examination | General for dysmorphic features |
| | Neurologic and ophthalmologic |
| • Parents | Maternal and paternal OFC |
| | Maternal phenylketonuria |
| • Investigations | Chromosome analysis |
| | Congenital infection screen |
| | Metabolic screen |
| | Neuroimaging to include cranial CT and/or MRI |

OFC, occipitofrontal circumference.

*Chromosomal.* Almost any degree of autosomal imbalance will have severe neurodevelopmental consequences often in association with microcephaly, so that chromosome analysis is an essential step in the investigation of any microcephalic infant (Table 14.7). If a strong suspicion of a chromosome abnormality persists despite a normal chromosome result, then consideration should be given to more detailed chromosome analysis using a technique such as multiple subtelomeric fluorescent in-situ hybridization (FISH) (Flint *et al.* 1995).

*Syndromal.* The 1999 edition of the London Dysmorphology Database (Winter & Baraitser 1999) identifies 457 syndromes in which microcephaly has been described. Some of the more commonly encountered examples are listed in Table 14.8. To this list should be added several other relatively rare disorders in which microcephaly occurs in association with ocular and/or other neurologic abnormalities (Table 14.9) (Baraitser 1997).

*Isolated* ('Simple' or 'true'). Non-syndromal microcephaly can show both autosomal dominant and autosomal recessive inheritance. In the autosomal dominant form (or forms) intellectual impairment is usually mild and may be absent (Rossi *et al.* 1987; Merlob *et al.* 1988). In classical autosomal recessive 'pure' microcephaly characteristic features are a sloping forehead, relatively large ears, micrognathia, and an amiable extrovert personality. It is probable that several different loci exist for autosomal recessive microcephaly, one of which has recently been localized to chromosome 8p22-pter by autozygosity mapping (Jackson *et al.* 1998).

Estimates of the recurrence risk for unexplained non-syndromal microcephaly vary from 1 in 8 to 1 in 5 and if the parents are consanguineous then a figure of 1 in 4 should probably be quoted (Tolmie *et al.* 1987). These empirical risks indicate that at least half of the unexplained non-syndromal cases result from autosomal recessive inheritance. The same applies when microcephaly is associated with symmetrical spastic paraplegia (Bundey 1992).

## HOLOPROSENCEPHALY (HPE) (see also p. 212)

This is a severe malformation that is caused by a failure of cleavage of the embryonic forebrain or prosencephalon (Cohen & Sulik 1992). In normal development, the prosencephalon divides transversely into the telencephalon and the diencephalon. The telencephalon divides in the sagittal plane to form the cerebral hemispheres and the olfactory tracts and bulbs. The paired thalamic and subthalamic nuclei, the optic chiasm and optic nerves, and the unpaired pineal gland and neurohypophysis develop from the diencephalon. In HPE there is failure of cleavage of both the telencephalon and diencephalon. The pathologic features of HPE include an undivided or partially divided cerebral hemisphere, usually with absent olfactory bulbs (arhinencephaly), absent or hypoplastic corpus callosum, and fused thalami.

**Table 14.8 Dysmorphic syndromes in which microcephaly is a characteristic feature**

| Syndrome | Inheritance | MIM no. | Associated features |
|---|---|---|---|
| Angelman | –[a] | 105830 | Ataxia, convulsions, inappropriate laughter |
| Bloom | AR | 210900 | Chromosome breakage, leukemia, photosensitivity |
| Cerebro-oculo-skeletal (COFS) | AR | 214150 | Arthrogryposis, cataracts, microphthalmia |
| Cockayne | AR | 216400 | Deafness, DNA repair defect, photosensitivity, premature aging |
| Cornelia de Lange | NK | 122470 | Hirsutism, micromelia, short stature, synophrys |
| Fetal alcohol | – | – | Congenital heart defects, short palpebral fissures, smooth philtrum |
| Meckel | AR | 249000 | Occipital encephalocele, polycystic kidneys, polydactyly |
| Roberts | AR | 268300 | Cleft lip/palate, chromosome puffing, phocomelia |
| Rubinstein–Taybi | AD | 180849 | Beaked nose, broad thumbs, downward sloping palpebral fissures |
| Seckel | AR | 210600 | Prominent nose, receding forehead, short stature |
| Smith–Lemli–Opitz types I and II | AR | 268670, 270400 | Hypospadias, ptosis, syndactyly<br>Raised 7-dehydrocholesterol in blood |

[a]Can be caused by chromosome-15 microdeletion, paternal uniparental disomy for chromosome-15, or dominantly inherited imprinting mutation.
*Key*: AD, autosomal dominant; AR, autosomal recessive; NK, not known (usually sporadic); MIM, Mendelian inheritance in man (McKusick 1998).

**Table 14.9 Neurologic and ophthalmologic syndromes with microcephaly**

| Syndrome and features | Inheritance | MIM no. |
|---|---|---|
| Aicardi–Goutieres: calcification of basal ganglia, CSF lymphocytosis | AR | 225750 |
| Jarmas: microphthalmia and retinal folds | AD | 180060 |
| Microcephaly with chorioretinopathy | AD, | 156590 |
| | AR | 251270 |
| Microcephaly with intracranial calcification (pseudo-TORCH syndrome) | AR | 600158 |
| Microcephaly with spastic quadriplegia | AR | 251280 |
| and severe retardation | XR | 311400 |

*Key*: AD, Autosomal dominant; AR, autosomal recessive; XR, X-linked recessive; MIM, Mendelian inheritance in man (McKusick 1998).

Pathologically, HPE is usually divided into three types. The most severe form is alobar HPE in which there is no separation of the cerebral hemispheres and there is a single cerebral ventricle (holoventricle). In semi-lobar HPE there is some division of the cerebral hemispheres with the inter-hemispheric fissure present posteriorly. In lobar HPE the cerebral hemispheres are almost completely separated with well-developed lateral ventricles. However, there is usually some degree of fusion of the frontal lobes, thalami, and corpora striata. Septo-optic dysplasia and arhinencephaly (absence of olfactory tracts and bulbs) are thought to represent the mild end of the HPE spectrum.

Holoprosencephaly is seen in about 1 in 250 conceptuses (Matsunaga & Shiota 1977). However, the prevalence at birth varies from 0.48 to 1.2 per 10 000 live births (Croen *et al.* 1996; Olsen *et al.* 1997)

HPE is an etiologically heterogeneous disorder. Genetic causes of HPE can be discussed under the categories of chromosomal, syndromal and isolated (non-syndromal).

*Chromosomal.* About 30–40% of all affected individuals with HPE have an underlying chromosomal abnormality (Croen *et al.* 1996; Whiteford & Tolmie 1996). This is usually a chromosome 13 abnormality such as trisomy 13, deletion or duplication of 13q, or ring 13. About 70% of patients with trisomy 13 have HPE (Taylor 1968). Other chromosomal abnormalities consistently associated with HPE include del(2p), dup(3p), del(7q), del(21q), and triploidy (Cohen & Sulik 1992). Thus chromosome analysis is strongly indicated in all children with this condition.

*Syndromal.* Holoprosencephaly can also be a component of multiple malformation syndromes. The 1999 edition of the London Dysmorphology Database (Winter & Baraitser 1999) lists 72 syndromes in which HPE has been described. Table 14.10 lists some of the more commonly seen syndromes with HPE.

*Isolated (Non-syndromal).* This can be inherited in a

**Table 14.10 Malformation syndromes in which holoprosencephaly is a characteristic feature**

| Syndrome | Inheritance | MIM no. | Associated features |
|---|---|---|---|
| Meckel | AR | 249000 | Encephalocele, polycystic kidneys, polydactyly |
| Oro-facial-digital type VI (Varadi-Papp) | AR | 277170 | Bifid 3rd metacarpal, cleft lip/palate, lingual nodules, MR, polydactyly |
| Pallister–Hall | AD | 146510 | Anal atresia, hypopituitarism, hypothalamic hamartoblastoma, polydactyly |
| Pseudotrisomy 13 | AR | 264480 | Congenital heart disease, cryptorchidism, microphthalmia, polydactyly |
| Smith–Lemli–Opitz type II | AR | 268670 | 2/3 toe syndactyly, congenital heart disease, male pseudohermaphroditism, polydactyly, raised levels of 7-dehydrocholesterol in tissues |
| Velocardiofacial | 22q11.2 microdeletion | 192430 | Congenital heart disease, cleft palate or velopharyngeal insufficiency, facial dysmorphism, learning problems, long fingers, short stature |

*Key*: AD, autosomal dominant; AR, autosomal recessive; MR, mental retardation; MIM – Mendelian inheritance in man (McKusick 1998).

Mendelian fashion. Familial non-syndromal HPE is usually inherited in an autosomal dominant manner, but autosomal recessive inheritance has also been described. In autosomal dominant HPE families, the transmitting parent is either clinically normal or may have subtle craniofacial malformations with normal brain imaging (Muenke *et al.* 1994). These 'microsigns' or 'microforms' include anosmia or hyposmia, microcephaly, hypotelorism, iris coloboma, congenital nasal pyriform aperture stenosis, single central maxillary incisor, absent or abnormal midline maxillary frenulum, and cleft palate.

As mentioned above, the autosomal dominant form of non-syndromal HPE can show marked intrafamilial variability as well as non-penetrance. The penetrance of autosomal dominant non-syndromal HPE is estimated to be about 70% (Cohen 1989). Four genes have so far been identified for autosomal dominant non-syndromal HPE. These are the Sonic Hedgehog (*SHH*) gene on 7q36 (Roessler *et al.* 1996), *ZIC2* on 13q32 (Brown *et al.* 1998) and *SIX3* on 2p21 (Wallis *et al.* 1999). Mutations in *SHH* are seen in about 14–23% of familial cases and in 0.5–10% of sporadic cases of non-syndromal HPE (Roessler *et al.* 1997, Odent *et al.* 1999). Mutations in *ZIC2* and *SIX3* are seen in very few familial and sporadic cases of non-syndromal HPE (Brown *et al.* 1998, Wallis *et al.* 1999). A fourth gene for autosomal dominant HPE has been recently identified. This is the *TGIF* gene on 18p11.3 (Gripp *et al.* 2000).

An approach to genetic counseling of parents of a child/fetus with HPE is shown in Fig. 14.2.

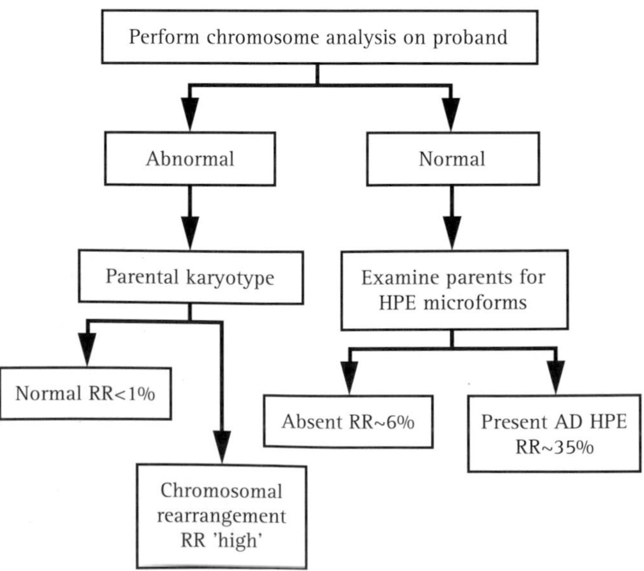


**Figure 14.2** Genetic counseling in holoprosencephaly (HPE). RR: recurrence risk.

## LISSENCEPHALY (AGYRIA–PACHYGYRIA SPECTRUM) (see also p. 213)

Lissencephaly is a severe CNS malformation in which the surface of the brain is smooth, with either complete absence of gyri and sulci (agyria) or only a few broad gyri and a few shallow sulci (pachygyria) (Barkovich *et al.* 1992). Lissencephaly results from migrational arrest of primitive neurons between 12 and 16 weeks gestation. There are two main pathologic types of lissencephaly: Classical (Type I) and Cobblestone (Type II) (Dobyns & Truwit 1995).

### CLASSICAL (TYPE I) LISSENCEPHALY

In this malformation the cerebral cortex has only 4 layers instead of the usual 6 layers (Barkovich *et al.* 1992). The surface of the brain is smooth with absent or very few sulci. Neuroradiologic findings in classical lissencephaly include agyria or pachygyria and a thick cerebral cortex with a 'figure of eight' appearance of the cortex on horizontal CT/MRI cuts due to a shallow sylvian fissure. Additional findings include a thin cortical white matter layer, dilated posterior horns of the lateral ventricles (colpocephaly), and hypoplastic corpus callosum. The cerebellum is usually normal in classical lissencephaly. When classical lissencephaly is an isolated abnormality, the phenotype is called isolated lissencephaly sequence (ILS). The clinical features of ILS are microcephaly, severe developmental delay, seizures, mild facial dysmorphism (bitemporal narrowing, short nose, thin upper lip and micrognathia), and cryptorchidism (Pilz & Quarrell 1996). About 76% of sporadic patients with ILS have a mutation in either the *LIS1* gene on 17p13.3 or the *XLIS* gene on Xq22.3–q23 (Pilz *et al.* 1998). *LIS1* codes for the β-subunit of platelet activating factor acetylhydrolase, brain isoform lb, and the gene is also called PAFAH1B1 (Hattori *et al.* 1994). *XLIS* encodes a protein called doublecortin and the gene is also called *DCX* (des Portes *et al.* 1998; Gleeson *et al.* 1998). Mutations in *LIS1* are associated with ILS in both sexes, but mutations in *XLIS* only cause ILS in males. The phenotype of an *XLIS* mutation in females is subcortical band heterotopias (SBH). This is explained by the phenomenon of random X-inactivation (Lyonization) in females. The developing cortex in females with an *XLIS* mutation has two populations of primitive neurons. The neurons in which the X-chromosome with the normal *XLIS* gene is active migrate normally to the cortex. The neurons in which the X-chromosome with the *XLIS* mutation is active do not migrate normally, and come to lie in a subcortical location, giving rise to the subcortical ribbon of gray matter seen in SBH (Fig. 14.3). Subcortical band heterotopias are rarely seen in males. Pilz *et al.* (1999) have recently identified mutations in the *LIS1* gene in 1 out of 11 males and mutations in *DCX* (*XLIS*) in 2 out of 11 males with SBH or mixed pachygyria-SBH. Subcortical band heterotopias in males could also be the result of somatic mosaicism for *LIS1* or *DCX* mutations (Gleeson *et al.* 1998, Pilz *et al.* 1999).

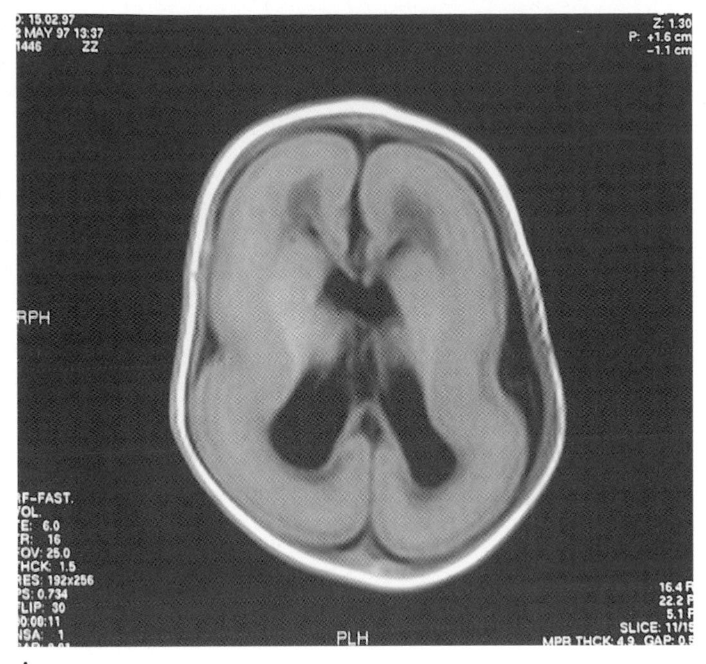


A

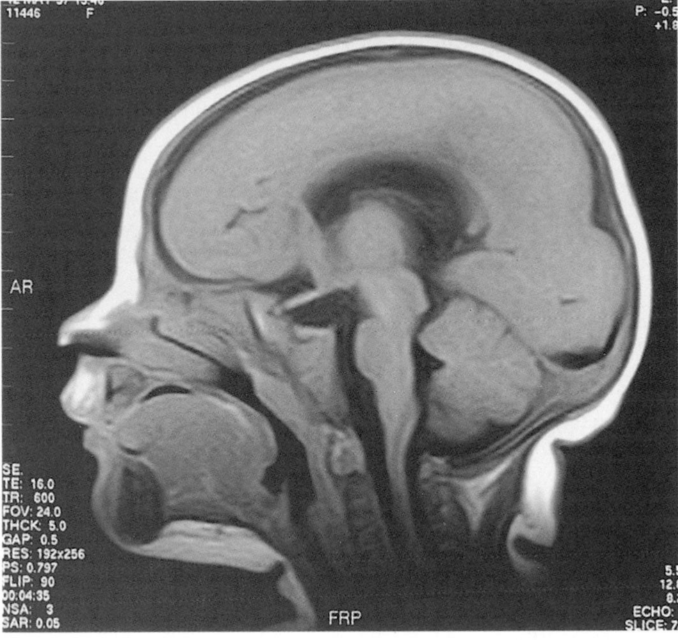


B

C

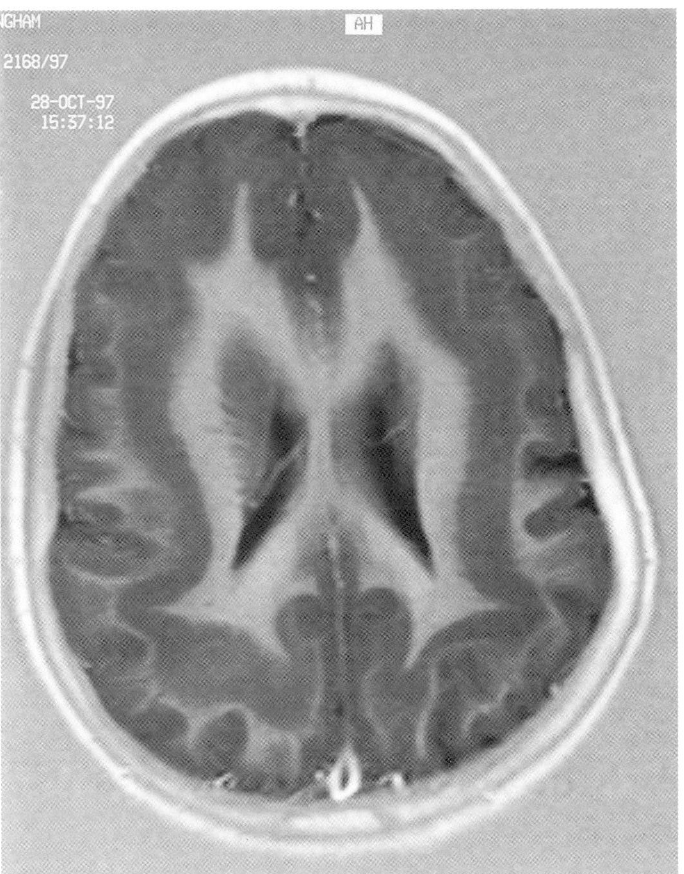


D

Figure 14.3 (A,B) MRI scans in a boy with X-linked lissencephaly and (C,D) his carrier sister. (Photographs kindly provided by Dr Tim Jaspan, University Hospital, Nottingham.)

**Table 14.11 Malformation syndromes with lissencephaly**

| Syndrome | Inheritance | MIM no./ Reference | Features |
|---|---|---|---|
| *Classical lissencephaly* | | | |
| Miller–Dieker | 17p 13.3 microdeletion | 247200 | Prominent forehead, vertical furrowing of forehead on crying |
| X-linked lissencephaly/SBH | XR | 300067 | Classical lissencephaly in hemizygous males, SBH in heterozygous females |
| Norman–Roberts | AR | 257320 | Severe microcephaly (OFC <30 cm), prominent nasal root |
| Barth microlissencephaly (radial microbrain) | AR | Barth *et al.* 1982 | Extreme microcephaly (OFC <28 cm), severe cerebellar hypoplasia, neonatal death |
| *Cobblestone lissencephaly* | | | |
| Walker–Warburg (HARD±E) | AR | 236670 | Congenital muscular dystrophy or myopathy, retinal abnormalities and/or anterior chamber dysgenesis (more severe eye abnormalities than Finnish muscle-eye-brain disease), encephalocele |
| Finnish muscle-eye-brain disease | AR | 253280 | Congenital muscular dystrophy, retinal hypoplasia, high myopia |
| Fukuyama muscular dystrophy | AR | 253800 | Severe progressive congenital muscular dystrophy, joint contractures, elevated CK, MR |
| Craniotelencephalic dysplasia | AR | 218670 | Anterior midline encephalocele, multiple craniosynostosis, bilateral microphthalmia and severe optic nerve hypoplasia |

*Key*: AR, autosomal recessive; HARD±E, hydrocephalus, agyria, retinal dysplasia ± encephalocele; OFC, occipitofrontal circumference; MIM, Mendelian inheritance in man (McKusick 1998); SBH, subcortical band heterotopia; XR, X-Linked recessive.

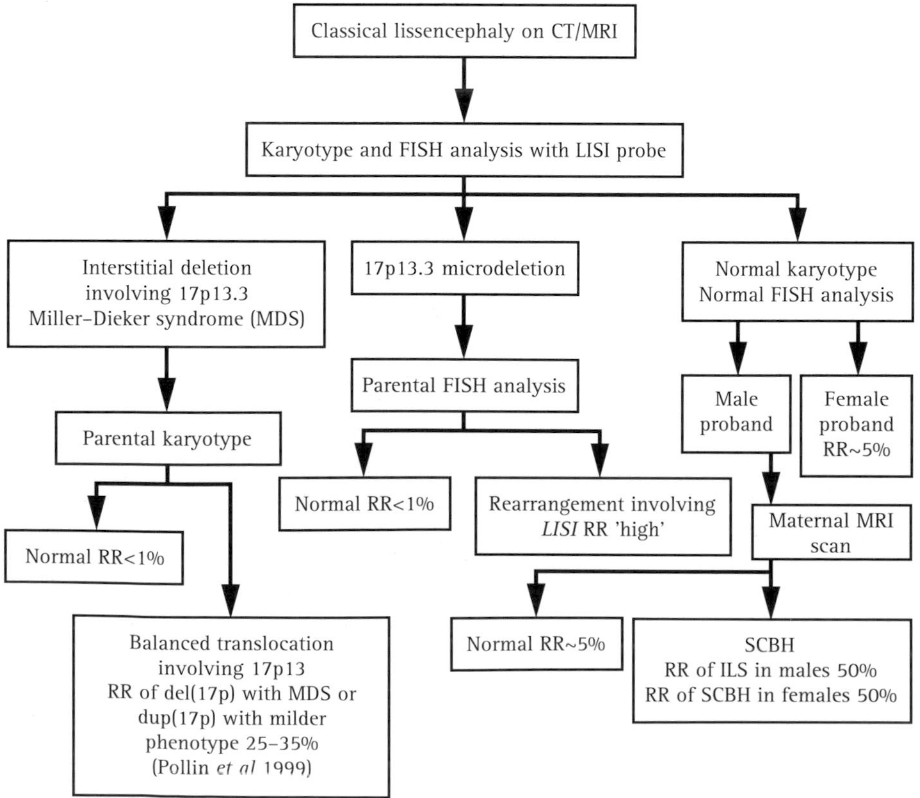


**Figure 14.4** Genetic counseling in classical lissencephaly. ILS: isolated lissencephaly, RR: recurrence risk, SCBH: subcortical band heterotropia.

Syndromal forms of classical lissencephaly are indicated in Table 14.11. An approach to counseling parents of children with classical lissencephaly is shown in Fig. 14.4.

## COBBLESTONE (TYPE II) LISSENCEPHALY

The pathologic features of this form of lissencephaly include an unlayered and severely disorganized cerebral and cerebellar cortex with neuronal and glial ectopia in the leptomeninges (Barkovich *et al.* 1992; Dobyns & Truwit 1995). The latter give the surface of the brain a cobblestone or verrucous appearance. In addition, the surface of the brain is agyric or pachygyric. Neuroradiologic features of cobblestone lissencephaly include agyria or pachygyria, a thinner cerebral cortex than in classical lissencephaly, hydrocephalus, and hypoplastic or absent corpus callosum and septum pellucidum. Posterior fossa abnormalities seen in cobblestone lissencephaly include a small cerebellum, hypoplastic vermis, Dandy–Walker malformation, and occipital encephalocele. The cerebral and cerebellar abnormalities on both CT and MRI scans help to differentiate cobblestone from classical lissencephaly. Cobblestone lissencephaly can be an isolated malformation but is usually a feature of a multiple malformation syndrome (Table 14.11). Isolated cobblestone lissencephaly is an autosomal recessive disorder (Dobyns *et al.* 1996). All syndromes with cobblestone lissencephaly are also inherited in an autosomal recessive manner with a 25% (1 in 4) sibling recurrence risk.

## SCHIZENCEPHALY (see also p. 213)

Schizencephaly is a rare congenital abnormality of the cerebral cortex that is characterized by a full thickness cleft of one or both cerebral hemispheres. The full thickness cortical clefts are characterized by a pial-ependymal seam, which is an infolding of cortical gray matter into the ventricle. This results in the fusion of the cortical pia and ventricular ependyma within the cleft. The cortical clefts in schizencephaly are lined with gray matter and the adjacent cortex often shows polymicrogyria (Norman *et al.* 1995). The most frequent sites of schizencephaly are along the primary cerebral fissures, usually the sylvian fissure. Barkovich *et al.* (1996) have classified schizencephaly as a malformation of cortical development that results from abnormal cortical organization. However, schizencephaly can also result from a disruptive process before neuronal migration is complete, i.e. about 20 weeks gestation (Norman *et al.* 1995). Neuroradiologically, schizencephaly can be of two types: 'closed-lip' (Type I) and 'open-lip' (Type II) (Barkovich *et al.* 1992). In closed-lip schizencephaly the edges of the cortical cleft appear fused. In open-lip schizencephaly the edges of the cortical cleft are well separated. This results in a large full thickness fluid-filled cortical cleft that is lined with polymicrogyric gray matter.

Although schizencephaly is usually a sporadic abnormality, siblings with schizencephaly have been reported (Robinson 1991; Hosley *et al.* 1992; Hilburger *et al.* 1993). Brunelli *et al.* (1996) found de-novo dominant mutations in the homeobox gene *EMX2* on 10q26.1 in 7 out of 8 sporadic patients with open-lip schizencephaly. Faiella *et al.* (1997) reported 10 additional patients with schizencephaly, 6 of whom were found to be heterozygous for new dominant mutations in the *EMX2* gene. These included two brothers with bilateral open-lip schizencephaly who were found to have the same 3′ splice site mutation in position 1 of exon 2. Neither parent carried this mutation. This suggests that one of the parents was a gonadal mosaic for this mutation. Faiella *et al.* (1997) also identified *EMX2* mutations in 3 out of 6 patients with unilateral closed-lip schizencephaly. The previously reported sibling recurrences of schizencephaly could therefore be the result of gonadal mosaicism for an autosomal dominant *EMX2* mutation rather than representative of autosomal recessive inheritance of schizencephaly. However, until further genes are identified for schizencephaly and gonadal mosaicism for an *EMX2* mutation is documented in additional families, parents with a single affected child with unilateral schizencephaly should be given a 1% (1 in 100) recurrence risk for this condition. Parents with a single affected child with bilateral schizencephaly should be given a 10% (1 in 10) recurrence risk (Baraitser 1997).

## CEREBELLAR HYPOPLASIA (see also p. 221)

The cerebellum develops from the alar plate of the rhombencephalon at about 28–44 days postconception (Altman *et al.* 1992). The first part of the cerebellum to form is the flocculonodular lobe. The next part of the cerebellum to develop is the vermis followed by the anterior and posterior cerebellar hemispheres. Cerebellar hypoplasia may affect only the vermis, only the hemispheres, or both. Hypoplasia of the cerebellar vermis is more frequently seen than hypoplasia of the cerebellar hemispheres or hypoplasia of the entire cerebellum. At birth, the cerebellum is normally relatively small compared with the cerebral hemispheres, and this can give the impression of cerebellar hypoplasia (Norman *et al.* 1995).

Cerebellar hypoplasia is a characteristic feature of several genetic syndromes (Table 14.12). Cerebellar hypoplasia (with or without cerebellar atrophy) can also be a feature of metabolic disorders such as Tay–Sachs disease, adenylosuccinase deficiency, and carbohydrate deficient glycoconjugate syndrome Type I (Friede 1964; Steinlin *et al.* 1998). Almost all of these disorders are inherited in an autosomal recessive manner. Children with cerebellar hypoplasia usually present with congenital ataxia or ataxic cerebral palsy (Steinlin 1998). In these children, every effort must be made to try and identify the cause of the cerebellar hypoplasia (Table 14.13). If no cause is identified for the cerebellar hypoplasia the parents should be counselled a recurrence risk of at least 10% (1 in 10). Consanguineous parents should be given a 25% (1 in 4) recurrence risk.

**Table 14.12 Malformation syndromes with cerebellar hypoplasia**

| Syndrome | Inheritance | MIM no./ Reference | Associated features |
|---|---|---|---|
| 3C (Cranio-cerebello-cardiac/Ritscher-Schinzel) | AR | 220210 | Cerebellar vermis hypoplasia, iris/retinal coloboma, congenital heart disease, mental retardation |
| COACH (cerebellar vermis aplasia/hypoplasia, oligophrenia, congenital ataxia, coloboma and hepatic fibrosis) | AR | 216360 | Cerebellar vermis hypoplasia, choroidal coloboma, hepatosplenomegaly, periportal fibrosis, mental retardation |
| Dekaban–Arimas | AR | 243910 | Cerebellar vermis hypoplasia, congenital retinal blindness, polycystic kidneys |
| Gillespie | AR | 206700 | Hypoplasia of cerebellar hemispheres or vermis, aniridia, mental retardation |
| Joubert | AR | 213300 | Cerebellar vermis hypoplasia, severe neonatal hypotonia, episodic hyperpnea, saccadic abnormality, 'molar-tooth' anomaly of midbrain, retinal dystrophy, renal cysts |
| Oro-facio-digital type VI (Varadi–Papp) | AR | 220220 | Cerebellar vermis aplasia or hypoplasia, cleft lip/palate, multiple oral frenulae, synpolydactyly, mental retardation |
| Pontocerebellar hypoplasia type 1 | AR | Barth 1993 | Hypoplasia of cerebellar hemispheres and pons, spinal anterior horn degeneration, early death |
| Pontocerebellar hypoplasia type 2 | AR | 277470 | Hypoplasia of cerebellar hemispheres and pons, microcephaly, chorea/dystonia, epilepsy, severe mental retardation |
| Carbohydrate-deficient glycoconjugate type I | AR | 212065 | Hypoplasia of cerebellar hemispheres and pons, failure to thrive, liver dysfunction, pericardial effusion, microcephaly, epilepsy, mental retardation, stroke-like episodes, inversion of nipples, abnormal fat distribution |

*Key*: AR, Autosomal recessive; Mendelian inheritance in man (McKusick 1998).

**Table 14.13 Genetic assessment of cerebellar hypoplasia**

| | |
|---|---|
| • History | Family history of congenital ataxia or ataxic cerebral palsy, parental consanguinity, exposure to teratogens (anticonvulsants, retinoic acid, methylmercury), abnormal breathing patterns as a neonate, neonatal ventilation, swallowing difficulties, jaundice, pericardial effusion, stroke-like episodes, abnormal movements |
| • Examination | Head circumference, facial dysmorphism, oral frenulae, synpolydactyly, abnormal fat distribution, inversion of nipples, abnormal saccades, retinal dystrophy, neurological findings |
| • Investigations | Chromosome analysis<br>Congenital infection screen<br>Cranial CT/MRI scan<br>Electroretinogram and visual evoked potentials<br>EMG and nerve conduction studies<br>Muscle biopsy<br>Renal ultrasound scan<br>Metabolic investigations: urine succinyladenosine levels, serum transferrin isoforms, white cell hexosaminidase A assay |

## Key Points

- Genetic factors make a major etiological contribution to most CNS malformations.
- Isolated 'non-syndromal' neural tube defects (NTDs) show multifactorial inheritance with the methylenetetrahydrofolate reductase gene being the most important susceptibility locus identified to date. NTDs also occur in chromosomal abnormalities, such as trisomy 18, and single-gene disorders, such as Meckel's syndrome.
- Isolated hydrocephalus conveys a low empiric recurrence risk for siblings of 1–4%. X-linked hydrocephalus is associated with aqueduct stenosis and is caused by mutations in the *L1CAM* gene which encodes a neuronal cell adhesion molecule.
- Most cases of hydranencephaly and porencephaly are sporadic although there have been a few reports of affected sib pairs.
- Approximately 50% of cases of Dandy–Walker malformation (DWM) diagnosed prenatally are associated with a chromosome abnormality. A non-syndromal DWM conveys a sibling recurrence risk of less than 5%.
- Agenesis of the corpus callosum shows striking etiological heterogeneity. When present as an isolated finding the recurrence risk for siblings is low.
- Microcephaly can be caused by both genetic and environmental factors. Unexplained non-syndromal microcephaly conveys a sibling recurrence risk of at least 1 in 8.
- Holoprosencephaly can be chromosomal, e.g. trisomy 13, or can be a component of a large number of single-gene multiple malformation syndromes. Several genes have been identified which can cause isolated holoprosencephaly showing autosomal dominant inheritance with reduced penetrance.
- Isolated classical (type I) lissencephaly is usually caused by a mutation in either the *LIS1* gene on chromosome 17 or the *XLIS* (doublecortin) gene on Xq22.3. Both type I and type II ('cobblestone') lissencephaly can occur in association with other abnormalities in several multiple malformation syndromes.
- Schizencephaly usually represents a sporadic event with many cases resulting from new dominant mutations in the homeobox gene *EMX2*.
- Cerebellar hypoplasia is a feature of several inherited dysmorphic and metabolic syndromes. In isolation the sibling recurrence risk is at least 1 in 10.

## REFERENCES


Adams C, Johnston W P & Nevin N C (1982) Family study of congenital hydrocephalus. *Dev Med Child Neurol* 24: 493–498.

✪ Altman N R, Naidich T P & Braffman B H (1992) Posterior fossa malformations. *AJNR Am J Neuroradiol* 13: 691–724.

Baraitser M & Burn J (1984) Neural tube defects as an X-linked condition. *Am J Med Genet* 17: 383–385.

✪ Baraitser M (1997) *The genetics of neurological disorders*, 3rd edn. Oxford: Oxford University Press.

Barkovich A J, Gressens P & Evrard P (1992) Formation, maturation and disorders of brain neocortex. *AJNR Am J Neuroradiol* 13: 423–446.

Barkovich A J, Kuzniecky R I, Dobyns W B *et al.* (1996) A classification scheme for malformations of cortical development. *Neuropediatrics* 27: 59–63.

Barth P G (1993) Pontocerebellar hypoplasias. An overview of a group of disorders with fetal onset. *Brain Dev* 15: 411–422.

Barth P G, Mullaart R, Stam F C, Sloaff J L (1982) Famalial lissencephaly with extreme neopallial hypoplasia. *Brain Development* 4: 145–151.

Bendon R W, Siddiqi T, de Courten-Myers G & Dignan P (1987) Recurrent developmental anomalies: 1. syndrome of hydranencephaly with renal aplastic dysplasia. 2. polyvalvular development heart defect. *Am J Med Genet Suppl* 3: 357–365.

Berg R A, Aleck K A & Kaplan A M (1983) Familial porencephaly. *Arch Neurol* 40: 567–569.

Blackburn B L & Fineman R M (1994) Epidemiology of congenital hydrocephalus in Utah, 1940–1979: report of an iatrogenically related 'epidemic'. *Am J Med Genet* 52: 123–129.

Brown S A, Warburton D, Brown L Y *et al.* (1998) Holoprosencephaly due to mutations in ZIC2, a homologue of Drosophila odd-paired. *Nat Genet* 20: 180–183.

Brunelli S, Faiella A, Capra V *et al.* (1996) Germline mutations in the homeobox gene EMX2 in patients with severe schizencephaly. *Nat Genet* 12: 94–96.

Bundey S (1992) *Genetics and neurology*, 2nd edn. Edinburgh: Churchill Livingstone.

Burton B K (1979) Recurrence risks for congenital hydrocephalus. *Clin Genet* 16: 47–53.

Chitayat D, Moore L & Del Bigio M R (1994) Familial Dandy–Walker malformation associated with macrocephaly, facial anomalies, developmental delay, and brain stem dysgenesis. *American J Med Genet* 52: 406–415.

Cohen M M Jr (1989) Perspectives on holoprosencephaly: Part I. Epidemiology, genetics and syndromology. *Teratology* 40: 211–235.

✪ Cohen M M Jr & Sulik K K (1992) Perpectives on holoprosencephaly: Part II. Central nervous system, craniofacial anatomy, syndrome commentary, diagnostic approach and experimental studies. *J Craniofacial Genet Dev Biol* 12: 196–244.

Croen L A, Shaw G M & Lammer E J (1996) Holoprosencephaly: epidemiologic and clinical characteristics of a California population. *Am J Med Genet* 64: 465–472.

Czeizel A (1981) Schisis Association. *Am J Med Genet* 10: 25–35.

Da Silva E (1988) Callosal defect, microcephaly, severe mental retardation and other anomalies in three sibs. *Am J Med Genet* 29: 837–843.

Debus O, Koch H G, Kurlemann G *et al.* (1998) Factor V Leiden and genetic defects of thrombophilia in childhood porencephaly. *Arch Dis Child* 78: F121–F124.

Des Portes V, Pinard J M, Billuart P *et al.* (1998) A novel CNS gene required for neuronal migration and involved in X-linked subcortical laminar heterotopia and lissencephaly syndrome. *Cell* 92: 51–61.

Dobyns W B (1996) Absence makes the search grow longer. *Am J Hum Genet* 58: 7–16.

Dobyns W B, Patton M A, Stratton R F *et al.* (1996) Cobblestone lissencephaly with normal eyes and muscle. *Neuropediatrics* 27: 70–75.

✪ Dobyns W B & Truwit C L (1995) Lissencephaly and other malformations of cortical development: 1995 update. *Neuropediatrics* 26: 132–147.

Dolk H (1991) The predictive value of microcephaly during the first year of life for mental retardation at seven years. *Dev Med Child Neurol* 33: 974–983.

Faiella A, Brunelli S, Granata T *et al.* (1997) A number of schizencephaly patients including 2 brothers are heterozygous for germline mutations in the homeobox gene EMX2. *Eur J Hum Genet* 5: 186–190.

Flint J, Wilkie A O M, Buckle V J *et al.* (1995) The detection of subtelomeric chromosomal rearrangements in idiopathic mental retardation. *Nat Genet* 9: 132–139.

Fowler M, Dow R, White T A & Green C H (1972) Congenital hydrocephalus–hydrencephaly in five siblings, with autopsy studies: a new disease. *Dev Med Child Neurol* 14: 173–188.

Friede R L (1964) Arrested cerebellar development: a type of cerebellar degeneration in amaurotic idiocy. *J Neurol Neurosurg Psychiatry* 27: 41–45.

Gibbons R J, Picketts D J, Villard L & Higgs D R (1995) Mutations in a putative global transcriptional regulator cause X-linked mental retardation with alpha-thalassaemia (ATR-X syndrome). *Cell* 80: 837–845.

Gleeson J G, Allen K M, Fox J W *et al.* (1998) Doublecortin, a brain-specific gene mutated in human X-linked lissencephaly and double cortex syndrome encodes a putative signaling protein. *Cell* 92: 63–72.

Gripp K W, Wotton D, Edwards M C *et al.* (2000) Mutations in TGIF cause holoprosencephaly and link NODAL signalling to human neural axis determination. *Nat Genet* 25: 205–208.

Gupta J K & Lilford R J (1995) Assessment and management

of fetal agenesis of the corpus callosum. *Prenat Diagn* 15: 301–312.

Halliday J, Chow C W, Wallace D & Danks D M (1986) X-linked hydrocephalus: a survey of a 20 year period in Victoria, Australia. *J Med Genet* 23: 23–31.

Harper C & Hockey A (1983) Proliferative vasculopathy and a hydranencephalic-hydrocephalic syndrome: a neuropathological study of two siblings. *Dev Med Child Neurol* 25: 232–239.

Hattori M, Adachi H, Tsujimoto M *et al.* (1994) Miller–Dieker lissencephaly gene encodes a subunit of brain platelet-activating factor acetylhydrolase. *Nature* 370: 216–218.

Helwig U, Imai K, Schmahl W *et al.* (1995) Interaction between undulated and Patch leads to an extreme form of spina bifida in double-mutant mice. *Nat Genet* 11: 60–63.

Higginbottom M C, Jones K L, Hall B D & Smith D W (1979) The amniotic band disruption complex: timing of amniotic rupture and variable spectra of consequent defects. *J Pediatr* 95: 544–549.

Hilburger A C, Willis J K, Bouldin E & Henderson-Tilton A (1993) Familial schizencephaly. *Brain Dev* 15: 234–236.

Hosley M A, Abroms I F & Ragland R L (1992) Schizencephaly: case report of familial incidence. *Pediatr Neurol* 8: 148–150.

Jackson A P, McHale D P, Campbell D A *et al.* (1998) Primary autosomal recessive microcephaly (MCPH1) maps to chromosome 8p22-pter. *Am J Hum Genet* 63: 541–546.

Kenwrick S, Jouet M & Donnai D (1996) X-linked hydrocephalus and MASA syndrome. *J Med Genet* 33: 59–65.

Matsunaga E & Shiota K (1977) Holoprosencephaly in human embryos: epidemiologic study of 150 cases. *Teratology* 16: 261–272.

✪ McKusick V A (1998) *Mendelian inheritance in man. A catalog of human genes and genetic disorders*, 12th edn. Baltimore, MD: Johns Hopkins University Press.

Merlob P, Steier D & Reisner S H (1988) Autosomal dominant isolated ('uncomplicated') microcephaly. *J Med Genet* 25: 750–753.

Moeschler J B & Marin-Padilla M (1989) Autosomal recessive encephaloclastic proliferative vasculopathy (hydrocephaly/hydranencephaly). *Am J Hum Genet* 45: A55.

MRC Vitamin Study Research Group (1991) Prevention of neural tube defects: results of the medical research council vitamin study. *Lancet* 338: 131–137.

Muenke M, Gurrieri F, Bay C *et al.* (1994) Linkage of a human malformation, familial holoprosencephaly to chromosome 7 and evidence for genetic heterogeneity. *Proc Natl Acad Sci USA* 91: 8102–8106.

Murray J C, Johnson J A & Bird T D (1985) Dandy–Walker malformation: etiologic heterogeneity and empiric recurrence risks. *Clin Genet* 28: 272–283.

Nickel R E & Magenis R E (1996) Neural tube defects and deletions of 22q11. *Am J Med Genet* 66: 25–27.

✪ Norman M G, McGillivray B C, Karlousek D K *et al.* (1995) *Congenital malformations of the brain.* New York: Oxford University Press.

Nyberg D A, Mahony B S, Hegge F N *et al.* (1991) Enlarged cisterna magna and Dandy–Walker malformation: factors associated with chromosome abnormalities. *Obstet Gynecol* 77: 436–442.

Odent S, Attie-Bitach T, Blayau M *et al.* (1999) Expression of the Sonic Hedgehog (SHH) gene during early human development and phenotypic expression of new mutations causing holoprosencephaly. *Hum Mol Genet* 8: 1683–1689.

Olsen C L, Hughes J P, Youngblood L G & Sharpe-Stimac M (1997) Epidemiology of holoprosencephaly and phenotypic characteristics of affected children: New York State, 1984–1989. *Am J Med Genet* 73: 217–226.

Pilz D T, Kuc J, Matsumoto N *et al.* (1999) Subcortical band heterotopia in rare affected males can be caused by missense mutations in DCX (XLIS) or LIS1. *Hum Mol Genet* 8: 1757–1760.

Pilz D T, Matsumoto N, Minnerath S *et al.* (1998) LIS1 and XLIS (DCX) mutations cause most lissencephaly, but different patterns of malformation. *Hum Mol Genet* 7: 2029–2037.

Pilz D T & Quarrell O W J (1996) Syndromes with lissencephaly. *J Med Genet* 33: 319–323.

Pollin T I, Dobyns W B, Crowe C A *et al.* (1999) Risk of abnormal pregnancy outcome in carriers of balanced reciprocal translocations involving the Miller–Dieker syndrome (MDS) critical region in chromosome 17p13.3. *Am J Med Genet* 85: 369–375.

Robinson R O (1991) Familial schizencephaly. *Dev Med Child Neurol* 33: 1010–1014.

Roessler E, Belloni E, Gaudenz K *et al.* (1996) Mutations in the human Sonic Hedgehog gene cause holoprosencephaly. *Nat Genet* 14: 357–360.

Roessler E, Belloni E, Gaudenz K *et al.* (1997) Mutations in the C-terminal domain of Sonic Hedgehog cause holoprosencephaly. *Hum Mol Genet* 6: 1847–1853.

Rosenthal A, Jouet M & Kenwrick S (1992) Aberrant splicing of neural cell adhesion molecular L1 mRNA in a family with X-linked hydrocephalus. *Nat Genet* 2: 107–112.

Rossi L N, Candini G, Scarlatti G (1987) Autosomal dominant microcephaly without mental retardation. *Am J Dis Child* 141: 655–659.

Smit L M E, Barth P G, Valk J & Nijiokiktjien C (1984) Familial porencephalic white matter disease in two generations. *Brain Dev* 6: 54–58.

Steinlin M (1998) Non-progressive congenital ataxia. *Brain Dev* 20: 199–208.

Steinlin M, Blaser S, Boltshauser E (1998) Cerebellar involvement in metabolic disorders: a pattern-recognition approach. *Neuroradiology* 40: 347–354.

Taylor A I (1968) Autosomal trisomy syndromes: a detailed study of 27 cases of Edwards' syndrome and 27 cases of Patau's syndrome. *J Med Genet* 5: 227–252.

Tolmie J L, McNay M, Stephenson J B P *et al.* (1987) Microcephaly: genetic counselling and antenatal diagnosis after the birth of an affected child. *Am J Med Genet* 27: 583–594.

Van der Put N M J, Gabreëls F, Stevens E M B *et al.* (1998) A second common mutation in the methylenetetrahydrofolate reductase gene: an additional risk factor for neural-tube defects? *Am J Hum Genet* 62: 1044–1051.

Váradi V, Tóth Z, Török O, Papp Z 1988. Heterogeneity and recurrence risk for congenital hydrocephalus (ventriculomegaly): a prospective study. *American Journal of Medical Genetics* 30: 305–310.

Wallis D E, Roessler E, Hehr U *et al.* (1999) Mutations in the homeodomain of the human SIX3 gene cause holoprosencephaly. *Nat Genet* 22: 196–198.

Whiteford M L & Tolmie J L (1996) Holoprosencephaly in the West of Scotland 1975–1994. *J Med Genet* 33: 578–584.

Winter R M & Baraitser M (1999) *The London dysmorphology database.* Oxford: Oxford University Press.

Zlotogora J (1995) Major gene is responsible for anencephaly among Iranian Jews. *Am J Med Genet* 56: 87–89.

Zonana J, Adornato B T, Glass S T & Webb M J (1986) Familial porencephaly and congenital hemiplegia. *J Pediatr* 109: 671–674.

# Chapter 15 Functional teratogenic effects of chemicals on the developing brain

D. F. Swaab and K. Boer

## NEUROTERATOLOGY

The conviction that the mammalian fetus is sufficiently protected against exogenous chemical factors lost support with the discovery that teratogenic effects can be produced in experimental animals by deficiencies of, for example, vitamin A (Hale 1933), vitamin $B_2$ (Warkany & Scharffenberger 1943) or by using specific chemicals such as trypan blue (Gillman *et al.* 1948). Since then, disasters have made it clear that such teratogenic effects may also occur in man. The dramatic teratogenic effect of thalidomide in man (McBride 1961; Lenz 1962) has sharply focussed attention on the possible dangers of certain medicines for the developing fetus. The observation that organic mercury compounds that were dumped into the environment by a factory engaged in the production of acetaldehyde caused Minamata's disease in Japan in 1953 (Annau 1988) has clearly shown that industrial and environmental chemicals too can be teratogenic for humans. One of the striking aspects of this outbreak of mercury poisoning was that asymptomatic women gave birth to severely mentally retarded children with a 40% smaller brain mass than that of non-affected babies. In the meantime, it has become clear that a number of prenatally occurring, irreversible defects of the CNS, such as anencephaly, spina bifida, and encephalocele, may be due to teratogenic effects of exogenous chemicals (International Clearinghouse for Birth Defects Monitoring Systems 1991).

The association between anticonvulsant drugs and congenital malformations, such as facial clefts and heart defects, has been recognized since the 1970s. Phenytoin and phenobarbitone, particularly if used together, are regarded as having serious teratogenic potential. There have been observations suggesting that the risk of congenital malformations of anti-epileptic drugs might be due to induction of folate deficiency and that the risk may be reduced by folic acid supplements (Biale & Lewenthal 1984; Steegers-Theunissen *et al.* 1993). More recently, a 10–20-fold increased risk has been reported for neural tube defects in association with valproic acid and carbamazepine exposure. Following a warning based upon animal experiments, Gomez (1980) reported on a child with a lumbosacral meningocele after first-trimester valproate exposure. Subsequently, Robert & Guibaud (1982) and others (Koch *et al.* 1983; Mastroiacovo *et al.* 1983; Robert & Rosa 1983; Lindhout & Meinardi 1984) supported the teratogenic potential of valproic acid in causing lumbosacral neural tube defects. Soon thereafter, spina bifida cases were also reported in relation to carbamazepine exposure (Rosa 1983, Lindhout & Meinardi 1984). Neural tube defects can be induced experimentally by hypervitaminosis A (Peters *et al.* 1979). On the other hand, it has been hypothesized that the occurrence of neural tube defects in human pregnancy are related to vitamin deficiency and that appropriate administration of vitamins, i.e. folic acid, will diminish the risk of occurrence (Smithells *et al.* 1980; Lipsett & Fletcher 1983; Oakley *et al.* 1983; Smithells 1983, 1992; Centers for Disease Control 1992). In the first follow-up study on *in vitro* fertilization, ovulation stimulation being one stage in the process, an increased risk of neural tube defects has been reported (Cornel 1989, 1990). Also clomiphene citrate used for ovulation induction has been associated with an increased risk of neural tube defects, but a meta-analysis showed that any such increase seems likely to be less than twofold, and there may be none (Greenland & Ackerman, 1995).

The fetal alcohol syndrome (Jones *et al.* 1976) is now recognized as an important cause of congenital malformations and neurologic handicaps. Its main features are facial dysmorphology, prenatal and postnatal growth deficiency, and neurologic impairments including mental retardation. Because it is not known if there is a threshold for alcohol intake, total abstinence from alcohol during pregnancy should be recommended.

It will be clear from the examples mentioned earlier that a balanced chemical environment is of the utmost importance for the fetus with regard to a normal structural development of its nervous system.

## FUNCTIONAL TERATOLOGY

Probably because of the thalidomide tragedy, our awareness of the dangers of drug ingestion has cautioned us against the indiscriminate use of medicines, mainly during the initial stage of pregnancy. However, even medicines that do not cause any gross morphologic malformations may cause microscopic defects or alter the intricate structure or chemical composition of fetal brain tissue, also during the second or third trimester of pregnancy, to such an extent that permanent behavioral deviations may develop later. The latter field, which is known as 'functional or behavioral teratology' (Vorhees 1989), is the main subject of this chapter. A surprisingly high proportion of pregnant women take medicines: in The Netherlands some 86% of pregnant women take medicines, including vitamins and iron supplementation (De Jong-van den Berg *et al.* 1991); whereas in a prospective study in the UK, 35% of the pregnant women took drugs (Rubin *et al.* 1986). Another study showed that in Hungary 91% of the pregnant women took medicines (70% if vitamins, iron, and calcium supplements are excluded) (Czeizel 1989). An estimated 10–15% of infants born in urban America today are exposed to cocaine *in utero* (Kosofsky *et al.* 1994). Most of these drugs and medicines are of the type that easily cross the placenta. They readily reach the fetal brain since the blood–brain barrier at this stage of development is not capable of preventing their passage. The same holds for cigarette smoking and for addictive compounds taken by the mother, e.g. heroin, morphine, methadone, alcohol, marijuana.

There are several reasons why functional neuroteratological effects of medicines were not recognized until recently, the most important one being that chemical compounds do not generally give rise to a typical syndrome in the child that can easily be recognized by the clinician as being specific to a particular compound taken by the mother during pregnancy. 'Functional teratology' is rather expressed much later in life by cognitive disturbances, mental retardation, reproductive or motor defects, disturbed language development, or sleep disturbances. This, and the long time interval between the use of medicines and the functional disturbances, often make it difficult to establish the relationship with intrauterine sequelae of chemicals.

## CHEMICALS AFFECTING BRAIN DEVELOPMENT

Many different chemicals might affect the developing brain. In fact, all those neuroactive compounds that are of importance for adult brain function appear to be involved in brain development as well (Swaab 1980). At present this principle has been established for sex hormones, corticosteroids, thyroid hormones, and neurotransmitters. Substances which alter the balance of any of these endogenous neuroactive compounds during the vulnerable periods in ontogeny, such as addictive compounds, are therefore capable of altering brain development in a permanent way. Even the use of aspirin by the mother was suspected to cause intelligence quotient (IQ) and attention deficits in the child (Pytkowicz Streissguth *et al.* 1987; but see also Klebanoff & Berendes 1988). Environmental aspects might be of importance as well. Although organic solvent mixtures cause a delay in the brain development of the rat (Stoltenberg-Didinger *et al.* 1990), a clinical study did not indicate that *in utero* exposure to relatively low levels of organic solvent can be associated with an adverse neurodevelopmental outcome (Eskenazi *et al.* 1988). Prenatal exposure to polychlorinated biphenyls (PCBs) leads to poorer short-term memory functioning (Jacobson *et al.* 1990) and lower psychomotor scores at 6 or 12 months of age (Gladen *et al.* 1988), although the latter effects were no longer visible at the later follow-up at 3, 4, or 5 years of age (Gladen & Rogan 1991). Low-level exposure to lead during early childhood is inversely associated with neuropsychological development throughout the first 7 years of life (Annau 1988; Bellinger *et al.* 1991; Baghurst *et al.* 1992).

### SEX HORMONES

In the rat, sex hormones act during the perinatal period by affecting maturation of the brain, both structurally and functionally, inducing in this way a sexual differentiation of the brain. For example, a sexual dimorphism that is evident by light microscopy occurs in the size of a part of the sexually dimorphic nucleus of the preoptic area (SDN-POA), which is determined in the rat by the levels of testosterone present around the time of birth (Gorski *et al.* 1978; Jacobson *et al.* 1980). The SDN-POA has also been found by us in the human brain. The volume of this nucleus is 2.5 times as large in men as it is in women and contains 2.2 times as many cells (Swaab & Fliers 1985; Swaab *et al.* 1992). Structural sex differences have now been described in a number of hypothalamic nuclei and adjacent brain areas (Swaab & Hofman 1995; Zhou *et al.* 1995). In addition, differences have been observed in the human hypothalamus in relation to sexual orientation (Swaab & Hofman, 1990) and gender, i.e. the feeling of being male or female (Zhou *et al.* 1995). Sex hormones coming from the fetus itself probably constitute in normal development the biological basis for sex-related brain and behavioral differences. It is therefore a matter of considerable concern that progestogens, estrogens and/or combinations thereof have frequently been prescribed to pregnant women (Reinisch & Karow 1977; Czeizel 1989), in the mistaken belief that they would prevent impending miscarriages. In the USA, 1–4.5 million pregnant women used diethylstilbestrol (DES) from 1945 until 1971. It was taken off the market to prevent miscarriage, allegedly attributable to a carcinogenic effect on the cervix and vagina in female offspring (Herbst *et al.* 1981), although randomized placebo-controlled studies almost 20 years earlier showed the inefficacy of the drug or, rather, its adverse effect on pregnancy outcome (Dieckmann *et al.* 1953). Not only are these drugs ineffective in sustaining pregnancy (Goldstein *et al.* 1989), they also increase the risk of clear cell adenocarcinoma of the vagina and the cervix among the exposed daughters to 1 per 1000 (Herbst & Anderson 1990) and anatomical malformations of the inner genital tract to more than 50% (Bibbo *et al.* 1977). In addition, a high percentage (25–33%) of infertility and possible interference with sexual function were found following intrauterine exposure to estrogens (Beral & Colwell 1981; Stenchever *et al.* 1981; Senekjian *et al.* 1988). Also, DES prenatal exposure in males has been shown to increase incidence of epididymal cysts, hypotrophic testes, and capsular induration of the testes (Bibbo *et al.* 1977). Experiments in mice show that DES exposure delays the onset of Müllerian duct development, leading to persistence of Müllerian duct remnants (Visser *et al.* 1998). There is some evidence that the risk of testicular cancer is increased by prenatal DES administration (Vessey 1989). 4,4′-

diaminostilbene-2,2′ disulfonic acid (DAS) is an intermediate in the manufacture of fluorescent whitening agents and structurally similar to the synthetic estrogen diethylstilbestrol (DES). Duration of employment in DAS production appeared negatively related to the workers' testosterone levels (Grajewski *et al.* 1996).

The use of sex hormone-related compounds during pregnancy also entails a real possibility of inducing personality disorders in the offspring.

Children exposed to estrogen have been found between 4 and 21 years of age to be generally less self-confident, less sensitive, and more dependent and group oriented than normal children (Reinisch & Karow 1977). Prenatal administration of estrogen and progesterone in boys has been reported to influence noticeably certain aspects of postnatal psychosexual development (i.e. 'masculinity', 'aggressiveness', and athletic abilities) (Yalom *et al.* 1973; Reinisch 1981; Meyer-Bahlburg *et al.* 1988). Other studies show that DES daughters have an increased incidence of bisexuality and homosexuality (Ehrhardt *et al.* 1985; Meyer-Bahlburg *et al.*, 1995). A study of Kester *et al.* (1980) showed a more masculine boyhood in DES sons, whereas exposure to progesterone in early pregnancy yielded a more feminine boyhood. A long-term follow-up study of a large group of boys and girls who had been exposed to medroxyprogesterone acetate *in utero* more than 15 years before could not demonstrate effects on intellectual development (Jaffe *et al.* 1988) or sex-dimorphic behavior (Jaffe *et al.* 1989). Prenatal exposure to phenytoin or phenobarbital went together with a remarkably high rate of trans-sexualism (Dessens *et al.* 1999), indicating that these anticonvulsive compounds interfere with sexual differentiation of the brain, possibly leading to female brain structures in a male brain in male-to-female transsexuals (Zhou *et al.* 1995).

It is worth mentioning that sexual differentiation of the brain is not only affected by sex hormones. Similar developmental effects affecting sexual differentiation have been described with drugs related to serotonin, noradrenaline (see later) and dopamine (Hull *et al.* 1984), and nicotine (Lichtensteiger & Schlumpf 1985), alcohol (McGivern *et al.* 1984), cimetidine (Anand & van Thiel 1982; McGivern 1987; but see also Walker *et al.* 1987), morphine (Vathy *et al.* 1983), barbiturates (Reinisch & Sanders 1982), and maternal stress (Dörner 1979; Ellis *et al.* 1988). When pregnant rats are exposed to stress, the SDN-POA of the male offspring becomes permanently smaller, i.e. of female size (Anderson *et al.* 1985). There is currently increasing concern about the possible impact of environmental compounds with hormone-like action on human development such as isomers of DDT and PCBs (Sharpe *et al.* 1996) and hormone-like compounds in meat from husbandry animals (Andersson & Skakkebaek, 1999). Consequently, all types of neuroactive compounds might affect sexual differentiation of the brain. This is another characteristic of the functional teratology of chemical compounds that makes this field hard to study; different compounds, when given during development, may lead to similar aspects of functional sequelae in later life.

## CORTICOSTEROIDS

Corticosteroids are used during pregnancy, for example in cases of allergic reactions, and to promote fetal lung development in cases of imminent parturition. Indeed, meta-analysis of randomized controlled trials demonstrated prenatal corticosteroid treatment to be of benefit in nearly all conditions in which the neonate is born before 34 weeks of gestation. Corticosteroid treatment dramatically reduces the risk of respiratory distress, bronchopulmonary dysplasia (De Zegher *et al.* 1992), periventricular hemorrhage, necrotizing enterocolitis and the resulting neonatal mortality (Crowley 1989). A reason for serious concern was that animal experiments indicated that exposure to corticosteroids can retard brain development and affect behavior in later life (Balázs *et al.* 1975; Taeusch 1975; Sobel 1978; Dahlof *et al.* 1980; Johnson *et al.* 1981). Marton *et al.* (1979) found retardation of psychomotor development, which persisted at least up to 2 years of life, in prematurely born children who had been exposed to corticosteroids. A follow-up study of the neurologic, physical and psychologic development of 10–12-year-old children exposed to corticosteroids once antenatally did not reveal any disturbances (Schmand *et al.* 1990; Smolders-de Haas *et al.* 1990; Dessens *et al.* 2000). However, multiple courses of corticosteroids to promote lung maturation might not be improving outcome and were recently shown in a post-hoc analysis to be accompanied by a lower birth weight, as was found in sheep, mice, and rabbits (Banks *et al.* 1999) and a smaller head circumference in human newborns (French *et al.* 1999).

## THYROID HORMONES

Thyroid hormones are essential for adequate brain development. Although thyroxine does not readily pass the placenta, low maternal free thyroxine concentrations at 12 weeks of pregnancy appeared a significant risk factor for impaired psychomotor development (Pop *et al.* 1999). In cases where hereditary congenital hypothyroidism (De Vijlder 2001, personal communication) or goiter (De Vijlder *et al.* 2000a,b) are diagnosed during pregnancy, prenatal treatment with thyroxine may be beneficial to prevent a delay in brain development, as was shown in the rat (Morreale de Escobar *et al.* 1989; Calvo *et al.* 1992). It is presumed that the reduction in brain size as a result of anti-epileptic drug use is mediated by reduced thyroid hormone levels (Kaneko *et al.* 1987).

Thyroid hormones have been injected directly into the amniotic fluid to enhance fetal lung maturation (Mashiach *et al.* 1978). Although it is known from animal experiments that such treatment may hamper brain development (Balázs 1979), no differences in neurologic or psychomotor development were detected in the treated children at the age of 5–6 years as compared with their controls (Barkai *et al.* 1988).

## NEUROTRANSMITTERS

Research indicates also that the presence of neurotransmitters, which can be subdivided into the groups acetylcholine, biogenic amines, amino acids, and peptides, are essential for normal brain development. Administration of neurotransmitters or compounds affecting their metabolism may therefore induce disturbed brain development.

### Acetylcholine

Pyridostigmine (an acetylcholinesterase inhibitor), when administered to neonatal rats, induced premature puberty and increased male sexuality in both sexes of the offspring (Hinz *et al.* 1978). Nicotine (an acetylcholine receptor agonist) enhanced cell death in the rat fetal brainstem (Kraus *et al.* 1981), while neonatal administration of chlorisodamine (a nicotine receptor blocker) prevented the normal postnatal increase in volume and cell number of the mouse superior cervical ganglion (Black & Green 1974). This might be one of the mechanisms by which smoking in the pregnant mother may have a permanent effect on brain development and school performance of the child (Butler & Goldstein 1973; Abel 1980; Sexton *et al.* 1990; Makin *et al.* 1991).

### Biogenic amines

Apart from the serotonin reuptake blocker chlorimipramine and the α-adrenergic agonist clonidine (Mirmiran *et al.* 1985; Mirmiran & de Boer 1988) (see below), there are many examples of medicines which, if used during pregnancy, impair normal brain development by upsetting the balance of the monoamines and/or influencing the sensitivity of the receptors. In animal experiments, reserpine (used as an antihypertensive drug as well as a tranquillizer) decreases the monoamine levels in the brain and has been shown to induce permanent brain and behavioral changes in offspring. These include reduced formation of neurons, hyperactivity, and increased susceptibility to audiogenic seizures. Amphetamine, which increases the release of catecholamines in the brain, is not only used as a dieting aid but is also given to children in cases of enuresis nocturna or attention deficit–hyperactivity disorder. Offspring of pregnant rats treated with such drugs show behavioral changes, most notably an inability in adulthood to adapt to new surroundings. α-Methyldopa (a false transmitter precursor for noradrenaline) and propranolol (a β-adrenergic blocker), when taken by the pregnant mother, result in a reduced head circumference in the human neonate. The use of neuroleptics such as chlorpromazine (a dopamine antagonist) during pregnancy has been reported to lead to extrapyramidal disturbances in the newborn child; while in animal experiments it impaired learning ability (for references on this section, see Swaab & Mirmiran 1984). *p*-Chlorophenylalanine, which blocks serotonin synthesis, affects cell division in regions of the posterior diencephalon known to become innervated by serotonergic fibers (Lauder *et al.* 1983; Lauder & Krebs 1984a,b). Barbiturates, which also stimulate dopamine receptors (Yanai & Feigenbaum 1981), are commonly used as hypnotics, sedatives, anticonvulsants, and in the past for the prevention of neonatal jaundice. In the large collaborative perinatal project, barbiturates were recorded to be used by 25% of the pregnant women in the USA (Reinisch & Sanders 1982). They may induce a withdrawal syndrome lasting as long as 3 months (Thornburg & Moore 1976). β-Mimetics, such as ritodrine, which are used frequently to prevent preterm delivery, may lead to less good school performance of the children later on in life (Hadders-Algra *et al.* 1986; Huisjes *et al.* 1986; Huisjes 1988). This observation has become more significant because of the apparent inefficacy of ritodrine to postpone preterm labor by more than 2 days (King *et al.* 1988; Canadian Preterm Labour Investigators Group 1992).

### Amino acids

Many compounds influencing amino acid transmitters are used during pregnancy and postnatal development. Prenatal or early postnatal treatment of rats with the frequently used tranquillizer diazepam (which acts upon the γ-aminobutyric acid (GABA)-benzodiazepine receptor complex) produces long-lasting effects on brain enzymes and behavioral disturbances such as hyperactivity, lack of acoustic startle reflexes, and sleep disturbances (Fonseca *et al.* 1976; Jakoubek 1978; Kellog *et al.* 1980; Livezey *et al.* 1985). It also reduces choline uptake in the male rat frontal cortex (Grimm 1984), induces a permanent decrease in noradrenaline level, turnover and release in the hypothalamus (Simmons *et al.* 1984; Kellogg & Retell 1986), and a permanently lower level of diazepam binding sites (Livezey *et al.* 1985). Diphenylhydantoin, administered to the pregnant rat, caused increased levels of GABA in adulthood (Vorhees 1985). Diazepam administration during pregnancy in humans results in low Apgar scores, depressed respiration and impaired suckling (Patrick *et al.* 1972; Cree *et al.* 1973). Long-term follow-up studies of such children are lacking, but regular use of large doses of benzodiazepines established in the first trimester of pregnancy can result in a child with craniofacial abnormalities, sometimes including microcephaly, having delayed motor development and mental retardation (Laegreid 1990).

### Peptides

Little is known about the possible long-term effects on brain development of this relatively recently discovered group of neurotransmitters and neuromodulators. They were originally thought to be simply hormones produced by the hypothalamus but later appeared to have important central effects as well (for reviews, see Swaab 1982; Boer & Swaab 1985).

Oxytocin is routinely used in obstetrics but may cause fetal distress, including a rise in core temperature and possibly retarded motor and speech development. Observations in the rat revealed a long-term decrease in water metabolism following administration of oxytocin to the developing rat (for references, see Boer & Swaab 1983). In addition, the use of oxytocin in inducing labor was related to a higher incidence of sudden infant death syndrome (Einspieler & Kenner 1985). Vasotocin administered to kittens induced delayed eye-opening and brain lipid content while locomotion was diminished and periods of active sleep were enhanced (Goldstein 1984). Vasopressin, which may permanently alter osmoregulation following perinatal administration and may also affect proliferation of brain cells (Boer & Swaab 1983; Boer *et al.* 1984; Boer 1993), and also its analogs, have been given to mentally retarded children (Waggoner *et al.* 1978; Anderson *et al.* 1979; Eisenberg *et al.* 1984a,b), and for the treatment of enuresis nocturna (Steener *et al.* 1986). DDAVP has been given to children following brain trauma (Wit *et al.* 1986). There are several studies showing that vasopressin may affect later blood pressure regulation, learning and memory (cf. Boer 1992). Children exposed to such compounds should consequently be followed-up for possible long-term sequelae caused by the peptide treatment in development. One of the problems of such a long-term follow-up is, however, that not enough experimental studies have been undertaken to direct the clinicians' attention to those functions that might be disturbed due to the administration of neuropeptides.

Postnatal treatment with thyrotrophin-releasing hormone (TRH) increased rat hypothalamic weight and impaired T-maze learning (Stratton *et al.* 1976). In combination with betamethasone, prenatal TRH administration accelerated somatosensory evoked potential (SEP)-assessed neural maturation (De Zegher *et al.* 1992). However, in a randomized trial in pregnant women, antenatal administration of TRH was associated with small, consistent deficits in major milestone achievements at 12 months of age (Crowther *et al.* 1997). Corticotrophin-releasing factor (CRF) accelerated eye-opening, enhanced rearing in an open field, and impaired body temperature regulation. Substance P increased pain perception and induced upregulation of its receptors (Handelmann *et al.* 1984), while neonatal exposure to a high level of ACTH 4–10 impaired adult learning behavior (McGivern *et al.* 1986).

Opioids and compounds influencing this system have strong effects on brain development. Methadone exposure of developing rats caused, for example, a delay in reflex development, eye-opening, somatic and brain growth, a regional alteration of catecholamines, hyperactivity, increased emotionality, learning disabilities, and dysfunction of thermoregulation and nociception. In children whose mothers had been exposed to opioids, abstinence symptoms were found, a high rate of mortality, sleep disturbances, delays in the sensorimotor development, retardation in somatic growth, smaller head circumference, delays in walking, problems in visual and auditory systems, aberrations in neuro-ontogeny, reduced alertness, poor attention spans, hyperactivity, learning disabilities, and social problems (Zagon & McLaughlin 1984). Naloxone, an opiate antagonist, is administered clinically to normalize the fetal heart rate (Goodlin 1981). Animal experiments have implicated naloxone as the cause of a permanent impairment of sensitivity to thermal stimuli (Sandman *et al.* 1979) and of maze learning ability (Vorhees 1981). β-Endorphin, used during delivery as an analgesic (Oyama *et al.* 1980), induces similar disturbances in the rat (Sandman *et al.* 1979). This treatment causes a reduced β-endorphin immunocytochemical staining in various brain regions (Moldow *et al.* 1981).

## ADDICTIVE COMPOUNDS

The use of addictive compounds during pregnancy is an increasing problem. Not only do 50% of Dutch women continue to smoke during pregnancy (De Jonge *et al.* 1982) and do between 28% and 62% of pregnant teenagers smoke (Albrecht *et al.* 1992), the use of marijuana, cocaine, and heroin during pregnancy is considerable as well (Sherwood *et al.* 1999). A survey done in Florida showed that 15% of the pregnant women used alcohol or drugs (Chasnoff *et al.* 1990). These compounds may also cause permanent functional sequelae in later life of the children exposed *in utero* (Table 15.1). The use of opiates, marijuana, alcohol, cigarettes, or cocaine is associated with premature labor (Stone *et al.* 1971; Kaminski *et al.* 1981; Berkowitz *et al.* 1982; Fried *et al.* 1984; Chasnoff *et al.* 1987; MacGregor *et al.* 1987) and affect motor development at the age of 2 and attention at the age of 6 in exposed children (Arendt *et al.* 1999; Leech *et al.* 1999).

### Opiates

Hard drug addiction of the mother may lead to prematurity, toxemia, breech birth, or precipitate labor. In addition, over 70% of these neonates show clinically recognizable withdrawal symptoms (Stone *et al.* 1971). Drug dependent women who have used combinations of methadone, heroin, cocaine, and other drugs during pregnancy frequently have preterm labor and a child with a smaller head circumference who functions worse neurologically and shows difficulties with early language development (Van Baar 1991). Newborns exposed to methadone *in utero*, with or without concomitant heroin, display more rapid eye movement (REM) sleep and less quiet sleep than control infants, while babies fetally exposed to opiates have a lower organization of sleep states (Dinges *et al.* 1980) and are at risk for mild psychomotor development impairment (Bunikowski *et al.* 1998).

Methadone use during pregnancy was in some studies found to be related to disturbed motor functioning (Marcus *et al.* 1982), whereas in other research no long-term developmental sequelae were found that could be directly associated with methadone exposure (Kaltenbach & Finnegan 1984). Intriguing as well as worrying is the study of Jacobson *et al.* (1990), who looked into the birth records of opiate addicts and their non-addicted siblings. It appeared that opiates or barbiturates given to the mother for pain

**Table 15.1 Functional teratology in the child during pregnancy by exposure of the mother to addictive compounds**

| Nature of disturbance | Cause | References |
|---|---|---|
| Prematurity | Heroin, hard drugs | Van Baar (1991), Stone *et al.* (1971) |
| | Alcohol | Berkowitz *et al.* (1982), Kaminski *et al.* (1981) |
| | Marijuana | Fried *et al.* (1984) |
| | Cigarette smoking | Berkowitz *et al.* (1982) |
| | Cocaine, crack | Chasnoff *et al.* (1985, 1987), MacGregor *et al.* (1987), Cherukiri *et al.* (1988) |
| Disturbed labour | Marijuana | Greenland *et al.* (1982) |
| | Cocaine | Chasnoff *et al.* (1985, 1987), Hadeed & Siegel (1989) |
| Decreased head size | Cocaine, smoking | Kosofsky *et al.* (1994), Fried & O'Connell (1987) |
| Cognitive disturbances | Smoking | Butler & Goldstein (1973), Naeye & Peters (1984), Fried *et al.* (1992) |
| | Alcohol | Jones *et al.* (1976), Clarren *et al.* (1978), Iosub *et al.* (1981), Gusella & Fried (1984), Fried & Watkinson (1988) |
| | Marijuana | Fried & Watkinson (1988), O'Connell & Fried (1991), Fried *et al.* (1992) |
| Motor disturbances | Methadone | Marcus *et al.* (1982) |
| | Smoking | Abel (1980), Naeye & Peters (1984), Gusella & Fried (1984) |
| | Marijuana | Nahas & Frick (1986) |
| | Angel dust (PCP) | Golden *et al.* (1980) |
| | Hard drugs, cocaine | Van Baar (1991), Kosofsky *et al.* (1994) |
| | Alcohol | Iosub *et al.* (1981), Gusella & Fried (1984) |
| Speech and language problems | Alcohol | Iosub *et al.* (1981), Gusella & Fried (1984) |
| | Hard drugs, cocaine | Van Baar (1991), Kosofsky *et al.* (1994) |
| Sleep disturbances | Methadone, heroin, opiates | Dinges *et al.* (1980) |
| | Alcohol, marijuana | Scher *et al.* (1988) |
| Elevated blood pressure | Maternal smoking | Beratis *et al.* (1996) |
| Reading, mathematics, general abilities, hyperactivity, attention deficits | Maternal smoking | Fried *et al.* (1992), Butler & Goldstein (1973), Naeye & Peters (1984), Fried & Watkinson (1988), Mankin *et al.* (1991) |
| Impulsive behavior | Marijhuana | O'Connell and Fried (1991), Fried *et al.* (1992) |
| | Cocaine | Richardson *et al.* (1996) |
| | Alcohol | Fried *et al.* (1992) |
| Conduct disorders, violent criminal outcomes, attention deficit, hyperactivity disorder | Smoking | Wakschlag *et al.* (1997), Rantakallio *et al.* (1992), Brennan *et al.* (1999), Milberger *et al.* (1996) |

relief during delivery between 10 and 0.5 hours before the time of birth increased the risk of the child becoming an addict in later life.

## Cocaine

Cocaine-using women have a higher rate of fetal loss (Richardson & Day 1991; Ness *et al.* 1999), precipitous labor, abruptio placentae, fetal monitor abnormalities, fetal meconium staining, and microcephaly (Chasnoff *et al.* 1987; Gingras *et al.* 1992). Disturbed labor may be the first sign of the child's CNS being affected, as the fetus usually plays an active role in the process of birth (Swaab *et al.* 1977). Fetal assessment of behavioral state development by ultrasonography in 20 cocaine-exposed fetuses predicted abnormal neonatal behavior (Hume *et al.* 1989). Autopsies of fetuses exposed to maternal cocaine use revealed hemorrhages involving the germinal matrix (Kapur *et al.* 1991). Exposure in the third trimester is associated with cerebral arterial infarction (see p. 393). Moreover, children of cocaine-using mothers show a decrease in response to environmental stimuli and are more reactive in general and more responsive to auditory stimuli (Anday *et al.* 1989) and often have transient abnormal EEGs in the first week of life showing CNS irritability, thought to be caused by changes in neurotransmitter availability (Doberczak *et al.* 1988). Indeed, an increased catecholamine activity was demonstrated in a study on cocaine-exposed newborns between 24 and 48 hours of age (Mirochnick *et al.* 1997). Children prenatally exposed to cocaine showed deficits in their ability to sustain attention on a computerized vigilance task (Richardson *et al.* 1996). In another study, no neurobehavioral effects of prenatal cocaine exposure were found in the NBAS test of the newborn 2–3 days after birth, but at 3 weeks of age a significant dose relation was found towards a poorer state regulation and greater excitability (Tronick *et al.* 1996).

An increased rate of sudden infant death syndrome in children of cocaine mothers was reported (Chasnoff *et al.* 1987) and disputed (Bauchner *et al.* 1988).

## Smoking

Smoking of the pregnant mother is associated with an increased risk of prenatal mortality and sudden infant death syndrome. In addition, children of women who were smoking during pregnancy have a smaller head circumference at birth (Fried & O'Connell 1987), are shorter, lag behind as far as memory tasks, reading, mathematics, and general abilities are concerned, and show hyperactivity (Butler & Goldstein 1973; Naeye & Peters 1984; Fried & Watkinson 1988; Fried *et al.* 1992). The performance of children of passive smokers was, in most aspects, found to be between that of children of the active smoking and the non-smoking group (Makin *et al.* 1991). Maternal smoking during pregnancy is, in addition, a risk factor for conduct disorder and criminal outcome in male offspring (Wakschlag *et al.* 1997; Brennan *et al.* 1999; Rantakallio *et al.* 1992), for attention deficit hyperactivity disorder (Milberger *et al.* 1996, 1997) and for more psychiatric disturbances (Fergusson *et al.* 1998). Neonates and infants of mothers who smoked during pregnancy have an elevation of blood pressure that is related to the number of cigarettes smoked per day (Beratis *et al.* 1996). Infants born to marijuana users exhibit more meconium staining and a longer duration of labor (Greenland *et al.* 1982), show disturbed sleep at age 3 years (Dahl *et al.* 1995) and show behavioral alterations at school age (O'Connell & Fried 1991).

The babies of mothers using marijuana have tremors, startles, and altered visual responsiveness, but these symptoms attenuate after 30 days (Fried 1982). However, at 72 months of age a deficit in sustained attention was found in such children (Fried *et al.*, 1992).

## Alcohol (see also p. 813)

The fetal alcohol syndrome (FAS) leads to an excess of stillbirths (Kaminski *et al.* 1981), an increased risk of renal agenesis or hypoplasia (Moor *et al.* 1997), deficits in academic skills in 5–6-year-old children (Coles *et al.* 1991), and in the ability to sustain attention (Brown *et al.* 1991), mental retardation, speech problems, and hyperactivity in the offspring (Clarren *et al.* 1978, Iosub *et al.* 1981). Children of 27 months of age showed decreased impulsive responses (Fried *et al.* 1992). Neuropathological observations suggest that ethanol produces disorderly neuronal and glial migration resulting in heterotopias, and leads to microcephaly, hydrocephaly, and agenesis of the corpus callosum and anterior commissure. When a pregnant woman had consumed 100–500 ml ethanol per day, 4–7 days per week, 100% of the embryos or fetuses had abnormal brain morphology, especially in the formation of the lateral ventricle walls and the cortical laminae (Konovalov *et al.* 1997). It is therefore remarkable that FAS effects were not, or hardly, seen in the children of women who had reduced their heavy alcohol consumption after the first trimester as opposed to the group that kept drinking heavily throughout pregnancy. This observation is of clinical importance (Rosett *et al.* 1978; Autti-Ramo *et al.* 1992), and illustrates the importance of discerning alcohol use in pregnant women. The continuing danger of alcohol consumption for brain development in late pregnancy is also shown by experiments in rat. Alcohol exposure from postnatal days 4–9, comparable to human third trimester exposure, induced significant brain growth deficits, even relative to body growth (Maier *et al.* 1997). In the absence of the physical features of FAS no adverse effect of prenatal alcohol exposure on cognition or sustained attention performance at the age of almost 5 years was found in a prospective study on 245 children (Greene *et al.* 1991; Body *et al.* 1991), while Mattson *et al.* found that the presence and degree of IQ deficits (1998) and other neuropsychological deficits (1997) following heavy alcohol exposure in man are not related to the physical features of FAS. In another prospective and blinded study of 38 prenatally exposed infants, EEG abnormalities at the postconceptional age of 40 weeks during REM sleep were related to subsequent motor development and during quiet sleep to mental development even in the absence of the FAS (Ioffe & Chernick 1990). In the non-human primate, weekly binge drinking as early in pregnancy as the first 6 weeks appeared as dangerous for normal behavioral and physical development as was binge drinking throughout pregnancy (Clarren *et al.* 1992). Binge drinking in the human during the period prior to the recognition of pregnancy appeared to be significantly and inversely correlated with IQ, academic achievement, classroom behavior and attention/vigilance (Sampson *et al.* 1989). It is of considerable interest that children exposed to benzodiazepines *in utero* have dysmorphic features and central nervous abnormalities resembling those of the FAS (Laegreid *et al.* 1990a,b).

It is remarkable that a decreased risk of the respiratory distress syndrome was found to be associated with maternal alcohol ingestion (Ioffe & Chernick 1987), suggesting that alcohol enhances maturation of the fetal lungs, the more so since an earlier study reported a lower 1 minute Apgar score of the child and a higher incidence of respiratory distress syndrome following treatment of pregnant women with ethanol in order to prevent premature labor (Zervoudakis *et al.* 1980).

Long-term follow-up studies of children born to alcohol consuming pregnant women showed that at 10 years of age they were still significantly smaller in weight, height, head circumference, and skinfold thickness (Day *et al.* 1999). Prenatal alcohol exposure affected length and head circumference constant over time, but growth in weight in particular between birth and 8 months (Geva *et al.* 1993; Sampson *et al.* 1994). From the large prospective study of Streissguth *et al.* (1994) it appeared that dose-dependent effects of prenatal alcohol exposure on neurobehavioral functions like attention and arithmetic, are still apparent at 14 years of age with the number of drinks per occasion as the strongest predictor.

Of even more concern may be that prenatal alcohol exposure appeared more predictive of alcohol use at the age of 14 years than was family history of alcohol problems (Baer *et al.* 1998) and may produce increased risk for later nicotine, alcohol, and drug dependence (Yates *et al.* 1998).

### OTHER AGENTS

Maternal caffeine intake was initially found to be associated with lower birth weight and smaller head circumference of the infant (Watkinson & Fried 1985), but in a large prospective cohort of 500 children, prenatal caffeine exposure was not associated with height, weight and head circumference at birth and with IQ and attention at the age of 7 years (Barr & Streissguth 1991).

In a case history of a neonate, phencyclidinè (PCP, 'angel dust') use of the mother was reported to cause respiratory depression, lethargy, floppiness, distinctive coarse flapping tremors, nystagmus, continuously roving eye movements, inability to track visually, and persistently poor food intake (Golden *et al.* 1980). However, observations of larger groups of such children, including long-term follow-up studies, are still lacking.

## ACTION OF CHEMICALS ON THE DEVELOPING BRAIN

Drugs taken by the pregnant mother may impair the developing child's brain in different ways.

### INDIRECT ACTION

This refers to an action primarily outside the brain, as in the case of aspirin which, when taken by the pregnant mother, may result in a higher incidence of intracranial bleeding and perinatal mortality (Collins 1981; Rumack *et al.* 1981). Another action of this kind is the alcohol-induced impairment of umbilical circulation, producing hypoxia and acidosis in the fetus (Mukherjee & Hodgen 1982). Alcohol exposure *in utero* affects both the pituitary–thyroid and adrenocortical system of the fetus (Rose *et al.* 1981). Prenatal exposure to barbiturates might also influence brain development indirectly, by altering liver metabolism of sex hormones (Reinisch & Sanders 1982). In animal studies, barbiturates have been shown to impair reproductive function and maze learning ability of the offspring (Middaugh *et al.* 1975; Clemens *et al.* 1979; Gupta *et al.* 1980). The demasculinization of the male rat offspring, prenatally exposed to barbiturates, was concomitant with a decreased synthesis of testosterone and decreased levels of testosterone in plasma and brain in adulthood (Gupta *et al.* 1980). Also in the human, prenatal exposure to barbiturates (for the prevention of neonatal jaundice in the Lesbos prenatal phenobarbital trial) had long-term effects on the offspring. At the age of 5–7 years the boys were taller, had a lower mean testicular volume and scored higher in the Wechsler Intelligence Scale for Children (Yaffe & Dorn 1990). No differences were seen in plasma testosterone levels, but the corticosteroid levels were significantly lower in the exposed than in the control group. In addition, psychomotor retardation caused by antiepileptic drugs might be mediated by reduced thyroid hormone levels (Kaneko *et al.* 1987).

### DIRECT ACTION

Drugs may affect brain development by interacting directly with the formation of the neuronal and glial network, e.g. by affecting cell division, cell death, cell migration, or the formation of neurites, synapses, and receptors. Most, if not all, medicines appear to affect several of these processes.

Cell division is reported to be slowed down by a number of medicines, both *in vivo* and *in vitro*. Barbiturates were found to cause a 30% reduction in the number of cerebellar Purkinje cells and a 15% reduction in hippocampal pyramidal cells. Other compounds that have similar deleterious effects include corticosteroids, chlorpromazine, alcohol, reserpine, thyroid hormones, and sex hormones (for references, see Swaab & Mirmiran 1984). Indirect evidence for decreased brain cell division is provided by the smaller head circumferences in children measured at birth following treatment with sex hormones (H. J. Huisjes 1984, personal communication), with α-methyldopa or propranolol, and diphenylhydantoin, or by the use of alcohol during human pregnancy (for references, see Swaab & Mirmiran 1984). In addition, babies of epileptic women were observed to have a smaller head circumference, suggesting an effect on cell division. This effect has been interpreted as the result of an interaction between the effect of the disease and anticonvulsant drug use (Mastroiacovo *et al.* 1988).

Cell death is augmented by nicotine (Kraus *et al.* 1981), accelerated by alcohol exposure prior to birth in the rat (Yanai 1981), and delayed by morphine in the chick embryo (Meriney *et al.* 1985).

Cell migration may be disturbed by alcohol (Jones *et al.* 1976), anticonvulsants (Trice & Ambler 1985), benzodiazepines, and monosodium glutamate (Marani *et al.* 1982). Children exposed *in utero* to benzodiazepines have dysmorphic characteristics resembling those of the fetal alcohol syndrome and distortion of neuronal migration with concomitant heterotopias (Laegreid *et al.* 1989).

The formation of neurites and synapses is known to be affected by sex hormones, corticosteroids, morphine, methadone, anticonvulsive agents, and by alcohol (for references, see Swaab & Mirmiran 1984). Prenatal nicotine exposure in rat induced a decreased stimulation of *c-fos* by hypoxia, thus potentially compromising repair of cell damage hypoxic periods (Trauth *et al.* 1999).

Receptors may also be permanently altered by neuroactive compounds given during development (Mirmiran *et al.* 1988, Gorter *et al.* 1990). Haloperidol, which blocks dopamine receptors, induced in this way a permanent decrease in the number of dopamine receptors in the striatum (Rosengarten & Friedhoff 1979). L-Dopa, which increases dopamine synthesis, permanently increased receptor density (Friedhoff *et al.* 1977). Prenatal morphine exposure in the rat increases the adult number and affinity of spinal cord opiate receptors (Kirby 1984), while prenatal exposure to diazepam results in enduring reductions in diazepam-binding sites in the rat thalamus (Livezey *et al.* 1985).

## BEHAVIOURAL ACTIONS

This mechanism involves effects of medicines on spontaneous behavioral states, namely wakefulness, quiet sleep, and REM sleep. In a study at our institute in which the long-term effect of REM sleep ('active' sleep, AS) deprivation on brain and behavior development was studied, experimental suppression of AS during early postnatal life by means of clomipramine or clonidine in rats revealed a clear-cut reduction of cortical size, a higher level of open field activity, deficient masculine sexual behavior, and disturbed sleep patterns in adulthood (Mirmiran *et al.* 1981, 1983a; Swaab & Mirmiran 1984; De Boer *et al.* 1989). These results, and those of others using different pharmacological as well as non-pharmacological approaches, argue in favor of AS as a mediating factor for normal brain maturation (Mitler 1971; Juvanes & Nowaczyk 1975; Saucier & Astick 1975), in which, of course, several mechanisms as discussed before may be involved. The specific reduction of cortical weight, together with decreased protein content, in the absence of any significant change in cell number, was highly reminiscent of the picture seen in rats reared under sensorially impoverished conditions (Rozenzweig & Bennett 1978). Furthermore, concomitant AS deprivation by means of clonidine neutralizes the effect that environmental enrichment normally exerts upon cortical growth (Mirmiran & Uylings 1983). Another intriguing finding is that prolonged AS deprivation by means of clonidine, even prior to the period of enrichment rearing, interferes with the expected extra brain growth (Mirmiran *et al.* 1983b). Apparently, cortical mechanisms underlying 'plasticity' in later life can be adversely affected by the absence of AS and/or noradrenaline disturbances in early development. Such a phenomenon may implicate abnormal sleep patterns as a potential contributory factor to learning deficiencies in humans as well. The drugs used in the AS deprivation studies, namely clomipramine (Anafranil) and clonidine (Catapresan), are also used in clinical practice (for treating depression, hypertension, migraine, nocturnal enuresis, sleep apnea, opiate withdrawal, minimal brain dysfunction, etc.). A follow-up study examined the effects of prenatal clonidine treatment of hypertensive mothers on the development of children who are now 6–8 years of age. In the exposed group compared with non-treated hypertensives, an excess of sleep disturbances was found (Huisjes *et al.* 1986), indicating that animal experiments in the field of functional teratology might give useful clues on the functions that have to be examined in children by means of long-term follow-up studies.

## MALE-MEDIATED ACTION

A neglected option is that of possible male-mediated drug effects. It is a relatively new concept that chemical exposure of male animals affects their progeny. Neonatal survival and birth weight of male rats treated with morphine sulfate, caffeine or methadone decrease markedly. In addition, adverse effects on progeny have been reported following drug administration – i.e. lead, morphine, thalidomide, caffeine, and ethanol – to males prior to mating. Systematic and convincing human studies of this topic are currently lacking, but even the authors of older studies were concerned about the relationship between increased spontaneous abortions, stillbirth, neonatal mortality and reduced family size and the professional exposure of men to excessive amounts of lead. More recently, an increased level of spontaneous abortions and congenital anomalies was found among the children of male dentists and anesthetists exposed to volatile anesthetics. In addition, an increased incidence of low birth weight infants as well as increased neonatal mortality and congenital anomalies in these infants were found among the progeny of cigarette smoking fathers (for a review, see Soyka & Joffe 1980). Increased risk of childhood cancer was not only associated with smoking by the mother during the first trimester of pregnancy, but also with smoking by the father (John *et al.* 1991). Passive smoking also affects the performance of children (Makin *et al.* 1991).

More research on the possibility that drug exposure of the father causes functional teratology is urgently needed. Abel (1991) observed a change in the immobility response of the offspring of male rats that had consumed alcohol for 7 months during the forced swimming test.

## CLINICAL AWARENESS AND FUTURE RESEARCH

It is both surprising and a source of concern how few systematic follow-up studies appear to have been carried out on the possible long-lasting functional consequences of treatments during human pregnancy. A wide variety of chemical compounds having comparable effects upon monoamine systems and/or AS, as described above, are currently in clinical use (cf. Swaab & Mirmiran 1984) and many consequently cause functional deficits. Effects of chemicals administered during development might even be carried over to following generations (Friedler 1974), possibly by affecting automodulation of genes (Campbell & Zimmerman 1982).

It is important to point out that almost all drugs used during gestation easily cross the placenta, and their level in the fetus (especially in the brain) may even be higher than in the maternal circulation (Mirkin & Singh 1976). In addition, humans are often more sensitive than animals to teratogenicity of drugs (Council on Environmental Quality 1981). One report does demonstrate a prolonged disturbance of sleep in babies born from heroin-addicted mothers (Davis & Glass 1980). Similar sleep disturbances might be responsible for the smaller head circumferences in boys, up to 4 years of age, born to mothers treated with α-methyldopa during late gestation (Moar *et al.* 1978; Ounsted *et al.* 1980). A problem is that long-term follow-up without a strong indication from animal experiments of what behavior or function has to be studied in later life will most probably fail to find disturbances. The sleep disturbances found in children where the mother used clonidine during pregnancy (Huisjes *et al.* 1986) indicated that animal experimental studies might give an indication of the right functions to study in human follow-up studies. This means that systematic search for functional teratological effects of chemicals should be encouraged.

The direct and indirect effects of a variety of clinically used drugs upon the development of the brain have been discussed here. Taken together, the literature on this subject points to a potential health hazard, not only during the first trimester of pregnancy but also throughout the entire period of gestation, and during lactation (Jason 1991; Mennella & Beauchamp 1991). The possibility that similar mechanisms are still present in later development cannot be excluded at present. Obstetricians, neonatologists, and pediatricians should, therefore, be aware that the immediate beneficial effects of many drugs may be offset by the induction of long-term or even permanent behavioral and psychological defects within the children's developing brains. This is a relevant consideration, e.g. in cases involving children suffering from attention-deficit hyperactivity disorder, who are often subjected to extremely high doses of imipramine or amphetamine-like drugs (for a review, see Gross & Wilson 1974), even though improvement often occurs eventually in the absence of any medication whatsoever. The same point can be made, of course, for the treatment of nocturnal enuresis by means of antidepressants or vasopressin. It is an unfortunate commentary at the present time that the mothers themselves are often more aware of the potential dangers inherent in the use of medicines during pregnancy than are the physicians who prescribe them. Since various publications indicate the functional developmental effects of anesthetics (Chalon *et al.* 1981; Blair *et al.* 1984; Koëter & Rodier 1986, Rodier & Koëter 1986, Rodier *et al.* 1986), it should be a point of concern not only for operations on pregnant mothers but also for pregnant staff in operating and recovery rooms. We suggest that the investigation of the link between experimental and clinical medicine in this area, namely the question of functional teratological sequelae of medications administered during early development, ought to be encouraged (Swaab 1985; Swaab & Mirmiran 1985). For those diseases that have to be treated during pregnancy and the first years of life it is of the utmost importance to select, in the future, only those compounds which combine high therapeutic potencies with low functional teratological side-effects.

## ACKNOWLEDGMENT

We are grateful to Ms W. T. P. Verweij for her secretarial help.

### Key Points

- Brain development is only partly genetically programmed
- Functional activity of brain circuits and epigenetic factors that influence this activity such as hormones and neurotransmitters determine brain development to a major degree
- This makes brain development a process that is very vulnerable to the action of medicines taken during pregnancy, drugs, chemicals that influence neurotransmitter metabolism and maternal stress
- Such factors may induce microscopic changes in the fetal brain structure and chemical composition and in this way cause permanent behavioral disorders. These alterations do not give rise to a typical syndrome but are expressed much later in life, e.g. as delayed motor or speech development, cognitive disturbances, effects on sexual orientation, gender identity or reproduction or psychiatric disorders
- This field is known as functional or behavioral teratology
- The long interval between the exposure of the fetus to chemicals and the functional disturbances, and the fact that different compounds may lead to similar functional disorders make it difficult to establish functional teratological effects in humans

## REFERENCES

Abel E (1980) Smoking during pregnancy: a review of effects on growth and development of offspring. *Hum Biol* 52: 593–625.

Abel E (1991) Alcohol consumption does not affect fathers but does affect their offspring in the forced swimming test. *Pharmacol Toxicol* 68: 68–69.

Albrecht S A, Cornelius M D, Braxter B *et al.* (1999) An assessment of nicotine dependence among pregnant adolescents. *J Subst Abuse Treat* 16: 337–344.

Anand S & van Thiel D H (1982) Prenatal and neonatal exposure to cimetidine results in gonadal and sexual dysfunction in adult males. *Science* 218: 493–494.

Anday E K, Cohen M E, Kelley N E & Leitner D S (1989) Effect of *in utero* cocaine exposure on startle and its modification. *Dev Pharmacol Ther* 12: 137–145.

Anderson D K, Rhees R W & Fleming D E (1985) Effects of prenatal stress on differentiation of the sexually dimorphic nucleus of the preoptic area (SDN-POA) of the rat brain. *Brain Res* 332: 113–118.

Anderson L T, David R, Bennet K & Dancis J (1979) Passive avoidance teaming in Lesch–Nyhan disease: effect of l-desamino-8-arginine vasopressin. *Life Sci* 24: 905–910.

Andersson A-M & Skakkebaek N E (1999) Exposure to

exogenous estrogens in food: possible impact on human development and health. *Eur J Endocrinol* 140: 477–485.

Annau Z (1988) Organometals and brain development. *Prog Brain Res* 73: 295–303.

Arendt R, Angelopoulos J, Salvator A & Singer L (1999) Motor development of cocaine-exposed children at age two years. *Pediatrics* 103: 86–92.

Autti-Ramo I, Korkman M, Hilakivi-Clarke L *et al.* (1992) Mental development of 2-year-old children exposed to alcohol *in utero*. *J Pediatrics* 120: 740–746.

Baer J S, Barr H M, Bookstein F L *et al.* (1998) Prenatal alcohol exposure and family history of alcoholism in the etiology of adolescent alcohol problems. *J Stud Alcohol* 59(5): 533–43.

Baghurst P A, McMichael A J, Wigg N R *et al.* (1992) Environmental exposure to lead and children's intelligence at the age of seven years. *N Engl J Med* 327: 1279–1284.

Balázs R (1979) Cerebellum: certain features of its development and biochemistry. *Prog Brain Res* 51: 357–372.

✪ Balázs R, Patel A J & Hajos F (1975) Factors affecting the biochemical maturation of the brain: effects of hormones during early life. *Psychoneuroendocrinology* 1: 25–36.

Banks B A, Cnaan A, Morgan M A *et al.* (1999) Multiple courses of antenatal corticosteroids and outcome of premature neonates. North American Thyrotropin-Releasing Hormone Study Group. *Am J Obstet Gynecol* 181: 709–717.

Barkai G, Zarfin Y, Ben-Harari M *et al.* (1988) *In utero* thyroxine therapy for the induction of fetal lung maturity: long term effects. *J Perinat Med* 16: 145–148.

Barr H M & Streissguth A P (1991) Caffeine use during pregnancy and child outcome: a 7-year prospective study. *Neurotoxicol Teratol* 13: 441–448.

Bauchner H, Zuckerman B, McClain M *et al.* (1988) Risk of sudden infant death syndrome among infants with *in utero* exposure to cocaine. *J Pediatrics* 113: 831–834.

✪ Bellinger D, Sloman J, Leviton A *et al.* (1991) Low-level lead exposure and children's cognitive function in the preschool years. *Pediatrics* 87: 219–227.

Beral V & Colwell L (1981) Randomized trial of high doses of stilboestrol and ethisterone therapy in pregnancy: long-term follow-up of the children. *J Epidemiol Commun Health* 35: 155–160.

✪ Beratis N G, Panagoulias D & Varvarigou A (1996) Increased blood pressure in neonates and infants whose mothers smoked during pregnancy. *J Pediatrics* 128: 806–812.

Berkowitz G S, Holford T R & Berkowitz R L (1982) Effects of cigarette smoking, alcohol, coffee and tea consumption on preterm delivery. *Early Hum Dev* 7: 239–250.

Biale Y & Lewenthal H (1984) Effect of folic acid supplementation on congenital malformations due to anticonvulsive drugs. *Eur J Obstet Biol* 18: 211–216.

Bibbo M, Gill W B, Azizi F *et al.* (1977) Follow-up study of male and female offspring of DES-exposed mothers. *Obstet Gynecol* 49: 1–8.

Black I B & Geen S C (1974) Inhibition of the biochemical and morphological maturation of adrenergic neurons by nicotinic receptor blockade. *J Neurochem* 22: 301–306.

Blair V W, Hollenbeck A R, Smith R F & Scanlon J W (1984) Neonatal preference for visual patterns: modification by prenatal anesthetic exposure? *Dev Med Child Neurol* 26: 476–483.

Boer G J (1992) Neuropeptides: a new class of transmitters, a new class of functional teratogens. In: Fujii T & Boer G J (eds) *Functional neuroteratology of short-term exposure to drugs*. Tokyo: Teikyo University Press; pp. 73–85.

Boer G J (1993) Vasopressin and oxytocin receptors and the developing brain. In: Zagon I S & McLaughlin P J (eds) *Receptors and brain development*. Chapman & Hall, London: pp. 225–248.

Boer G J & Swaab D F (1983) Long-term effects on brain and behavior of early treatments with neuropeptides. In: Zbinden G, Cuomo G, Racagni B & Weiss B (eds) Application of behavioral pharmacology in toxicology. New York: Raven Press; pp. 251–263.

Boer G J & Swaab D F (1985) Neuropeptide effects on brain development to be expected from behavioral teratology. *Peptides* 6(suppl 2): 21–28.

Boer G J, Kragten R, Kruisbrink J & Swaab D F (1984) Vasopressin fails to restore postnatally the stunted brain development in the Brattleboro rat, but affects water metabolism permanently. *Neurobehavioral Toxicology and Teratology* 6: 103–109.

Boyd T A, Ernhart C B, Greene T H, Sokol R J & Martier S 1991 Prenatal alcohol exposure and sustained attention in the pre-school years. *Neurotoxicol Teratol* 13(1): 49–55.

✪ Brennan P A, Grekin E R & Mednick S A (1999) Maternal smoking during pregnancy and adult male criminal outcomes. *Arch Gen Psychiatry* 56: 215–219.

Brown R T, Coles C D, Smith I E, Platzman K A, Silverstein J, Erickson S & Falek A (1991) Effects of prenatal alcohol exposure at school age. II. Attention and behavior. *Neurotoxicol Teratol* 13: 369–376.

Bunikowski R, Grimmer I, Heiser A, Metze B, Schafer A & Obladen M 1998 Neurodevelopmental outcome after prenatal exposure to opiates. *Eur J Pediatr* 157: 724–730.

✪ Butler N R & Goldstein H (1973) Smoking in pregnancy and subsequent child development. *BMJ* iv: 573–575.

Calvo R, Obregón M J, Escobar del Rey F *et al.* (1992) The rat placenta and the transfer of thyroid hormones from the mother to the fetus. Effects of maternal thyroid status. *Endocrinology* 131: 357–365.

Campbell J H & Zimmerman E G (1982) Automodulation of genes: a proposed mechanism for persisting effects of drugs and hormones in mammals. *Neurobehav Toxicol Teratol* 4: 435–439.

Canadian Preterm Labour Investigators Group (1992) Treatment of preterm labor with the beta-adrenergic agonist ritodrine. *N Engl J Med* 327: 308–312.

Centers for Disease Control (1992) Recommendations for the use of folic acid to reduce the number of cases of spina bifida and other neural tube defects. *MMWR Morbid Mortal Wkly Rep* 41: 1–7.

Chalon J, Tang Ch-K, Ramanathan S *et al.* (1981) Exposure to halothane and enflurane affects learning function of murine progeny. *Anesthes Analges* 60: 794–797.

Chasnoff I J, Burns K A & Burns W J (1987) Cocaine use in pregnancy: perinatal morbidity and mortality. *Neurotoxicol Teratology* 9: 291–293.

Chasnoff I J, Burns W J, Schnoll S H & Burns K A (1985) Cocaine use in pregnancy. *N Engl J Med* 313: 666–669.

Chasnoff I J, Landress H J & Barrett M E (1990) The prevalence of illicit-drug or alcohol use during pregnancy and discrepancies in mandatory reporting in Pinellas county, Florida. *N Engl J Med* 322: 1202–1206.

Cherukiri R, Minkoff H, Feldman J *et al.* (1988) A cohort study of alkaloidal cocaine ('crack') in pregnancy. *Obstet Gynecol* 72: 147–151.

✪ Clarren S K, Alvord E C Jr, Sumi S M *et al.* (1978) Brain malformations related to prenatal exposure to ethanol. *J Pediatrics* 92: 64–67.

Clarren S K, Astley S J, Gunderson V M & Spellman D (1992) Cognitive and behavioral deficits in nonhuman primates associated with very early embryonic binge exposures to ethanol. *J Pediatrics* 121: 789–796.

Clemens L G, Popham T V & Rupport P H (1979) Neonatal treatment of hamsters with barbiturates alters adult sexual behavior. *Dev Psychobiol* 12: 49–59.

Colangelo W & James D G (1982) The fetal alcohol syndrome: a review and assessment of the syndrome and its neurological sequelae. *Prog Neurobiol* 19: 271–314.

Coles C D, Brown R T, Smith I E *et al.* (1991) Effects of prenatal alcohol exposure at school age. I. Physical and cognitive development. *Neurotoxicol Teratol* 13: 357–367.

Collins E (1981) Maternal and fetal effects of acetaminophen and salicylates in pregnancy. *Obstet Gynecol* 58 (Suppl 578): 62S.

Cornel M C, ten Kate L P, te Meerman G J (1990) Association between ovulation stimulation, *in vitro* fertilisation and neural tube defects? *Teratology* 42: 201–203.

Cornel M C, ten Kate L P, te Meerman G J (1989) Ovulation induction, in vitro fertilisation and neural tube defects. *Lancet* 2: 1530.

Council on Environmental Quality (1981) Chemical hazards to human reproduction. Washington, DC: Government Printing Office.

Cree J R, Meyer S & Halley D M (1973 Diazepam in metabolism and effect on the clinical condition and thermogenesis of the new-born. *BMJ* iv: 251–255.

Crowley P (1989) Promoting pulmonary maturity. In: Chalmers I, Enkin M & Keirse M J N C (eds) *Effective care in pregnancy and childbirth*. Oxford: Oxford University Press; pp. 746–764.

Crowther C A, Hiller J E, Haslam R R & Robinson J S (1997) Australian Collaborative Trial of Antenatal Thyrotropin-Releasing Hormone: adverse effects at 12-month follow-up. ACTOBAT Study Group. *Pediatrics* Mar; 99(3): 311–317.

Czeizel A (1989) Drug use during pregnancy in Hungary. *Acta Medica Hungarica* 46: 53–62.

Dahl R E, Scher M S, Williamson D E *et al.* (1995) A longitudinal study of prenatal marijuana use. Effects on sleep and arousal at age 3 years. *Arch Pediatr Adolesc Med* 149: 145–150.

Dahlof L G, Larsson K & Hard E (1980) Sexual differentiation and adult sexual behavior of male offspring of mothers treated with corticosteroids during pregnancy. *Neurosci Lett* 5(Suppl): 128.

Davis M M & Glass P (1980) Fetal exposure to narcotics: neonatal sleep as a measure of nervous system disturbances. *Science* 209: 619–621.

Day N L, Zuo Y, Richardson G A, Goldschmidt L, Larkby C A & Cornelius M D (1999) Prenatal alcohol use and offspring size at 10 years of age. *Alcohol Clin Exp Res* 23(5): 863–9.

De Boer S, Mirmiran M, van Haaren F, Louwerse A & van de Poll N E (1989) Neurobehavioral teratogenic effects of clomipramine and alpha-methyldopa. *Neurotoxicol Teratol* 11: 77–84.

De Jonge G A & van der Klaauw M M (1982) De frequentie van roken voor, tijdens en na de zwangerschap. *Nederlands Tijdschrift Geneeskunde* 34: 1537–1543.

De Jong-van den Berg L T W, van den Nerg P B, Haaijer-Ruskamp F M *et al.* (1991) Investigating drug use in pregnancy. Methodological problems and perspectives. *Pharmacol Weekblad* 13: 32–38.

Dessens A B, Cohen-Kettenis P T, Mellenbergh G J, van de Poll N, Koppe J G, Boer K (1999) Prenatal exposure to anticonvulsants and psychosexual development. *Arch Sex Behav* 28: 31–44.

Dessens A B, Smolders-de Haas H, Koppe J G (2000) Twenty-year follow-up of antenatal corticosteroid treatment. *Pediatrics* 105: 1–7.

De Vijlder J J M & Vulsma T (2000a) Metabolic disorders causing hyperthyroidism. In: Werner & Ingbar's *The Thyroid. A Fundamental and Clinical Text.* 8th edition. Chapter 54. Eds. L E Braverman & R D Utiger.

De Vijlder J J M & Vulsma T (2000b) Genetic defects in Thyroid Hormone Synthesis and Action: Defects in Thyroid Hormone Synthesis. In: *Endocrinology*, 4th edition. Chapter 113. Eds. L J de Groot & J L Jameson.

De Zegher F, de Vries L, Pierrat V *et al.* (1992) Effect of prenatal betamethasone/thyrotropin releasing hormone treatment on somatosensory evoked potentials in preterm newborns. *Pediatr Res* 32: 212–214.

Dieckmann W J, Davis M E, Rynkiewicz L M & Pottinger R E (1953) Does the administration of diethylstilboestrol during pregnancy have therapeutic value? *Am J Obstet Gynecol* 66: 1062–1075.

✪ Dinges D F, Davis M M & Glass P (1980) Fetal exposure to narcotics: neonatal sleep as a measure of nervous system disturbance. *Science* 209: 619–621.

✪ Dittmann R W, Kappes M E & Kappes M H (1992) Sexual behavior in adolescent and adult females with congenital adrenal hyperplasia. *Psychoneuroendocrinology* 17: 153–170.

Doberczak T M, Shanzer S, Senie R T & Kandall S R (1988) Neonatal neurologic and electroencephalographic effects of intrauterine cocaine exposure. *J Pediatr* 113: 354–358.

Dörner G (1979) Psychoneuroendocrine aspects of brain development and reproduction. In: Zichella L, Pancheri P (eds) *Psychoneuroendocrinology in reproduction: an interdisciplinary approach.* Amsterdam: Elsevier, pp. 43–54.

Dwyer T, Ponsonby A L & Couper D (1999) Tobacco smoke exposure at one month of age and subsequent risk of SIDS – a prospective study. *Am J Epidemiol* 149(7): 593–602.

✪ Ehrhardt A A, Meyer-Bahlburg H F L, Rosen L R *et al.* (1985) Sexual orientation after prenatal exposure to exogenous estrogen. *Arch Sex Behav* 14: 57–75.

Einspieler C & Kenner T (1985) A possible relation between oxytocin for induction of labor and sudden infant death syndrome. *N Engl J Med* 313: 1660.

Eisenberg J, Chazan-Gologorsky S, Hattab J & Belmaker R H (1984a) A controlled trial of vasopressin treatment of childhood learning disorder. *Biol Psychiatry* 19: 1137–1141.

Eisenberg J, Hamburger-Bar R & Belmaker R H (1984b) The effect of vasopressin treatment on learning in Down's syndrome. *J Neural Transmiss* 60: 143–147.

✪ Ellis L, Ames M A, Peckham W & Burk D (1988) Sexual orientation of human offspring may be altered by severe maternal stress during pregnancy. *J Sex Res* 25: 152–157.

Eskenazi B, Gaylord L, Brachen M B & Brown D (1988) *In utero* exposure to organic solvents and human neurodevelopment. *Dev Med Child Neurol* 30: 492–501.

Fergusson D M, Woodward L J, Horwood L J (1998) Maternal smoking during pregnancy and psychiatric adjustment in late adolescence. *Arch Gen Psychiatry* 55: 721–727.

Fonseca N M, Sell A B & Cartini E A (1976) Differential behavioral responses of male and female adult rats treated with five psychotropic drugs in the neonatal state. *Psychopharmacology* 46: 263–268.

Fried P A (1982) Marihuana use by pregnant women and effects on offspring: an update. *Neurobehav Toxicol Teratol* 4: 451–454.

✪ Fried P A & O'Connell C M (1987) A comparison of the effects of prenatal exposure to tobacco, alcohol, cannabis and caffeine on birth size and subsequent growth. *Neurotoxicol Teratol* 9: 79–85.

Fried P A & Watkinson B (1988) 12- and 24-month neurobehavioral follow-up of children prenatally exposed to marihuana, cigarettes and alcohol. *Neurotoxicol Teratol* 10: 305–313.

✪ Fried P A, Watkinson B & Gray R (1992) A follow-up study of attentional behavior in 6-year-old children exposed prenatally to marihuana, cigarettes, and alcohol. *Neurotoxicol Teratol* 14: 299–311.

Fried P A, Watkinson B & Willan A (1984) Marijuana use during pregnancy and decreased length of gestation. *Am J Obstet Gynecol* 150: 23–27.

Friedhoff A J, Bonnet K A & Rosengarten H (1977) Reversal of two manifestations of dopamine receptor supersensitivity by administration of L-dopa. *Res Commun Chem Pathol Pharmacol* 16: 411–423.

Friedler G (1974) Long-term effects of opiates. In: Dancis J & Hwang J C (eds) *Perinatal pharmacology: problems and priorities.* Raven Press; New York: pp. 207–219.

Geva D, Goldschmidt L, Stoffer D & Day N L (1993) A longitudinal analysis of the effect of prenatal alcohol exposure on growth. *Alcohol Clin Exp Res* 17(6): 1124–1129.

Gillman J, Gilbert C, Gillman T & Spence I (1948) A preliminary report on hydrocephalus, spina bifida and other congenital anomalies in the rat produced by trypan blue. *S African J Med Sci* 13: 47.

✪ Gingras J L, Weese-Mayer D E, Hume R F Jr & O'Donnell K J (1992) Cocaine and development: mechanisms of fetal toxicity and neonatal consequences of prenatal cocaine exposure. *Early Hum Dev* 31: 1–24.

Gladen B C & Rogan W J (1991) Effects of perinatal polychlorinated biphenyls and dichlorodiphenyl dichloroethene on later development. *J Pediatr* 119: 58–63.

Gladen B C, Rogan W J, Hardy P *et al.* (1988) Development after exposure to polychlorinated biphenyls and dichlorodiphenyl dichloroethene transplacentally and through human milk. *J Pediatr* 113: 991–995.

Golden N L, Sokol R J & Rubin I L (1980) Angel dust: possible effects on the fetus. *Pediatrics* 65: 18–20.

Goldstein P A, Sacks H S & Chalmers T C (1989) Hormone administration for the maintenance of pregnancy. In: Chalmers I, Enkin M & Keirse M J N C (eds) *Effective care in pregnancy and childbirth.* Oxford: Oxford University Press; pp. 612–623.

Goldstein R (1984) The involvement of arginine vasotocin in the maturation of the kitten brain. *Peptides* 5: 25–28.

Gomez M R (1980) Possible teratogenicity of valproic acid. *J Pediatr* 98: 508–509.

Goodlin R C (1981) Naloxone and its possible relationship to fetal endorphin levels and fetal distress. *Am J Obstet Gynecol* 136: 16–19.

Gorski R A, Gordon J H, Shryne J E & Southam A M (1978) Evidence for a morphological sex difference within the medial preoptic area of the rat brain. *Brain Res* 148: 333–346.

Gorter J A, Kamphuis W, Huisman E *et al.* (1990) Neonatal clonidine treatment results in long-lasting changes in noradrenaline sensitivity and kindling epileptogenesis. *Brain Res* 535: 62–66.

Grajewski B, Whelan E A, Schnorr T M *et al.* (1996) Evaluation of reproductive function among men occupationally exposed to a stilbene derivative. I. Hormonal and physical status. *Am J Ind Med* 29: 49–57.

Greene T, Ernhart C B, Ager J *et al.* (1991) Prenatal alcohol exposure and cognitive development in the preschool years. *Neurotoxicol Teratol* 13: 57–68.

Greenland S, Staisch K J, Brown N & Gross S J (1982) The effects of marijuana use during pregnancy. I. A preliminary epidemiologic study. *Am J Obstet Gynecol* 143: 408–413.

Greenland S & Ackerman D L (1995) Clomiphene citrate and neural tube defects: a pooled analysis of controlled epidemiologic studies and recommendations for future studies. *Fertil Steril* Nov; 64: 936–41.

Grimm V E (1984) A review of diazepam and other benzodiazepines in pregnancy. In: Yanai J (ed) *Neurobehavioral teratology.* Amsterdam: Elsevier; pp. 153–162.

Gross M B & Wilson W C (1974) *Minimal brain dysfunction.* New York, NY: Brunnet/Mazel.

Gupta C, Sonawane B R, Yaffe S J & Shapiro B H (1980) Phenobarbital exposure *in utero*: alternations in female reproductive function in rats. *Science* 208: 508–510.

Gusella J L & Fried P A (1984) Effects of maternal social drinking and smoking on offspring at 13 months. *Neurobehav Toxicol Teratology* 6: 13–17.

Hadders-Algra M, Touwen B C L, Huisjes H *et al.* (1986) Long-term follow-up of children prenatally exposed to ritodrine. *Br J Obstet* 93: 156–161.

Hadeed A J & Siegel S R (1989) Maternal cocaine use during pregnancy: effect on the newborn infant. *Pediatrics* 84: 205–210.

Hale F 1933 Pigs born without eyeballs. *J Heredity* 25: 105.

Handelmann G E, Selsky J H & Helke C J (1984) Substance P administration to neonatal rats increases adult sensitivity to substance P. *Physiol Behav* 33: 297–300.

✪ Herbst A L & Anderson D (1990) Clear cell adenocarcinoma of the vagina and cervix secondary to intrauterine exposure to diethylstilbestrol. *Sem Surg Oncol* 6: 343–346.

Herbst A L, Hubby M M, Azizi F & Makii M M (1981) Reproductive and gynecologic surgical experience in diethylstilbestrol-exposed daughters. *Am J Obstet Gynecol* 141: 1019–1028.

Hinz G, Döcke F & Dörner G (1978) Long-term changes of sexual function in rats treated neonatally with psychotropic drugs. In: Dörner G, Kawakami M (eds) *Hormones and brain development.* Elsevier; Amsterdam: pp. 121–127.

Huisjes H J (1988) Problems in studying functional teratogenicity in man. *Prog Brain Res* 73: 51–58.

Huisjes H J, Hadders-Algra M & Touwer B C L (1986) Is clonidine a behavioural teratogen in the human? *Early Hum Dev* 14: 43–48.

Hull E M, Nishita J K, Bitran D & Dalterio S (1984) Perinatal dopamine-related drugs demasculinize rats. *Science* 224: 1011–1013.

Hume R F Jr, O'Donnell K J, Stanger C L *et al.* (1989) *In utero* cocaine exposure: observations of fetal behavioral state may predict neonatal outcome. *Am J Obstet Gynecol* 161: 685–690.

International Clearinghouse for Birth Defects Monitoring Systems (1991) *Congenital Malformations Worldwide. A report from the International Clearinghouse for Birth Defects Monitoring Systems.* Amsterdam: Elsevier.

Ioffe S & Chernick V (1987) Maternal alcohol ingestion and the incidence of respiratory distress syndrome. *Am J Obstet Gynecol* 156: 1231–1235.

Ioffe S & Chernick V (1990) Prediction of subsequent motor and mental retardation in newborn infants exposed to alcohol *in utero* by computerized EEG analysis. *Neuropediatrics* 21: 11–17.

✪ Iosub S, Fuchs M, Bingol N & Gromisch D S (1981) Fetal alcohol syndrome revisited. *Pediatrics* 68: 475–479.

Jacobson B, Nyberg K, Grönblaeth L *et al.* (1990) Opiate addiction in adult offspring through possible imprinting after obstetric treatment. *BMJ* 301: 1067–1070.

Jacobson C D, Shryne J E, Shapiro F & Gorski R A (1980) Ontogeny of the sexually dimorphic nucleus of the preoptic area. *J Comp Neurol* 193: 541–548.

Jacobson J L, Jacobson S W & Humphrey H E B (1990) Effects of *in utero* exposure to polychlorinated biphenyls and related contaminants on cognitive functioning in young children. *J Pediatr* 116: 38–45.

Jaffe B, Harlap S, Baras M *et al.* (1988) Long-term effects of MPA on human progeny: intellectual development. *Contraception* 37: 607–619.

Jaffe B, Shye D, Harlap S *et al.* (1989) Aggression, physical activity levels and sex role identity in teenagers exposed *in utero* to MPA. *Contraception* 40: 351–363.

Jakoubek B (1978) The effect of ACTH and/or tranquillizers on the development of brain macromolecular metabolism. In: Dörner G & Kawakarni M (eds) *Hormones and brain development.* Amsterdam: Elsevier; pp. 259–264.

Jason J (1991) Breast feeding in 1991. *N Engl J Med* 325: 1036–1038.

John E M, Savitz D A & Sandler D P (1991) Prenatal exposure to parents' smoking and childhood cancer. *Am J Epidemiol* 133: 123–132.

Johnson J W C, Mitzner W, Beck J C *et al.* (1981) Long-term effects of betamethasone on fetal development. *Am J Obstet Gynecol* 141: 1053–1064.

Jones K L, Smith D W & Hanson J W (1976) The fetal alcohol syndrome: clinical delineation. *Ann N Y Acad Sci* 273: 130–137.

Juvanes P & Nowaczyk T (1975) Effects of early postnatal $\alpha$-methyl-dopa treatment on behavior in the rat. *Psychopharmacologia* 42: 95–97.

Kaltenbach K & Finnegan L P (1984) Developmental outcome of children born to methadone maintained women: a review of longitudinal studies. *Neurobehav Toxicol Teratol* 6: 271–275.

Kaminski M, Franc M, Lebouvier M *et al.* (1981) Moderate alcohol use and pregnancy outcome. *Neurobehav Toxicol Teratol* 3: 173–181.

Kaneko S, Hirano T, Muramatsu E & Nomura Y (1987) Fetal and neonatal effects of antiepileptic drugs – the physical and psychomotor developments in the offspring of epileptic parents. In: Fujii T, Adams P M (eds) *Functional teratogenesis.* Tokyo: Teikyo University Press; pp. 205–215.

Kapur R P, Shaw C M & Shepard T H (1991) Brain hemorrhages in cocaine-exposed human fetuses. *Teratology* 44: 11–18.

Kellogg C K & Retell T M (1986) Release of [$^3$H]norepinephrine; alteration by early developmental exposure to diazepam. *Brain Res* 366: 137–144.

Kellogg C, Tervo D, Ison J *et al.* (1980) Prenatal exposure to diazepam alters behavioral development in rats. *Science* 207: 205–207.

Kester P, Green R, Finch S J & Williams K (1980) Prenatal 'female hormone' administration and psychosexual development in human males. *Psychoneuroendocrinology* 5: 269–285.

King J F, Grant A M, Keirse M J N C & Chalmers I (1988) Beta-mimetics in preterm labour: an overview of the randomized controlled trials. *Br J Obstet Gynaecol* 95: 211–222.

Kirby M L (1984) Alterations in fetal and adult responsiveness to opiates following various schedules of prenatal morphine exposure. In: Yanai J (ed) *Neurobehavioral teratology.* Amsterdam: Elsevier; pp. 235–248.

Klebanoff M A & Berendes H W (1988) Aspirin exposure during the first 20 weeks of gestation and IQ at four years of age. *Teratology* 37(3): 249–255.

Koch S, Göpfert-Geyer E, Jäger-Roman E *et al.* (1983) Antiepileptkia während der Schwangerschaft. Eine prospective studie über Schwangerschaftsverlauf, Fehlbildungen und kindliche Entwicklung. *Deutsche Medizinische Wochenschrift* 108: 250–257.

Koëter H B W M & Rodier P M (1986) Behavioral effects in mice exposed to nitrous oxide or halothane: prenatal vs. postnatal exposure. *Neurobehav Toxicol Teratol* 8: 189–194.

Konovalov H V, Kovetsky N S, Bobryshev Y V & Ashwell K W (1997) Disorders of brain development in the progeny of mothers who used alcohol during pregnancy. *Early Hum Dev* 48(1–2): 153–166.

Kosofsky B E, Wilkins A S, Gressens P & Evrard P (1994) Transplacental cocaine exposure: a mouse model demonstrating neuronanatomic and behavioral abnormalities. *J Child Neurol* 9: 234–241.

Kraus H F, Campbell G A, Fowler A C & Farber J P (1981) Maternal nicotine administration and fetal brain stem damage: a rat model with implications for sudden infant death syndrome. *Am J Obstet Gynecol* 140: 743–746.

Laegreid L, Olegard R, Conradi N, Hagberg G, Wahlstrom J, Abrahamsson L (1990a) Congenital malformations and maternal consumption of benzodiazepines: a case-control study. *Dev Med Child Neurol* 32: 432–441.

Laegreid L (1990b) Clinical observations in children after prenatal benzodiazepine exposure. *Dev Pharmacol Ther* 15: 186–188.

Laegreid L, Olegärd R., Walström J & Conradi N (1989) Teratogenic effects of benzodiazepine use during pregnancy. *J Pediatr* 114: 126–131.

Lancaster P A L (1987) Congenital malformations after *in vitro* fertilisation. *Lancet* ii: 1392–1393.

Lauder J M & Krebs H (1984a) Neurotransmitters in development as possible substrates for drugs of use and abuse. In: Yanai J (ed) *Neurobehavioral teratology.* Amsterdam: Elsevier; pp. 289–314.

Lauder J M & Krebs H (1984b) Humoral influences on brain development. *Adv Cell Neurobiol* 5: 3–50.

Lauder J M, Wallace J A, Wilkie M B *et al.* (1983) Roles for serotonin in neurogenesis. *Monographs in Neural Sciences* 9: 3–10.

Leech S L, Richardson G A, Goldschmidt L & Day N L (1999) Prenatal substance exposure. Effects on attention and impulsivity of 6-year-olds. *Neurotoxicol Teratol* 21: 109–118.

Lenz W (1962) Thalidomide and congenital abnormalities. *Lancet* i: 45.

Lichtensteiger W & Schlumpf M (1985) Prenatal nicotine affects fetal testosterone and sexual dimorphism of saccharin preference. *Pharmacology, Biochem Behav* 23: 439–444.

Lindhout D & Meinardi H (1984) Spina bifida and *in utero* exposure to valproate. *Lancet* ii: 396.

Lipsett M & Fletcher J C (1983) Do vitamins prevent neural tube defects (and can we find out ethically)? *The Hastings Center Report*: Aug.

Livezey G T, Radulovacki M, Isaac L & Marczynski T J (1985) Prenatal exposure to diazepam results in enduring reductions in brain receptors and deep slow wave sleep. *Brain Res* 334: 361–365.

MacGregor S N, Keith L G, Chasnoff I J *et al.* (1987) Cocaine use during pregnancy: adverse perinatal outcome. *Am J Obstet Gynecol* 157: 686–690.

Maier S E, Chen W J, Miller J A & West J R (1997) Fetal alcohol exposure and temporal vulnerability regional differences in alcohol-induced microencephaly as a function of the timing of binge-like alcohol exposure during rat brain development. *Alcohol Clin Exp Res* 21(8): 1418–1428.

✪ Makin J, Fried P A & Watkinson B 1991 A comparison of active and passive smoking during pregnancy: long-term effects. *Neurotoxicol Teratol* 13: 5–12.

Marani E, Rietveld W J & Boon M E (1982) Monosodium glutamate accelerates migration of hypothalamic perikarya at puberty. *Histochemistry* 75: 145–150.

✪ Marcus J, Hans S L & Jeruchimowicz J R (1982) Differential motor and state functioning in newborns of women on methadone. *Neurobehav Toxicol Teratol* 4: 459–462.

Marton I S, Gati I, Nemenyi M, Szondy M (1979) Psychomotor development and cord endocrine parameters of premature newborns exposed to steroid *in utero.* In: Zichella L, Pancheri P, editors. *Psychoneuroendocrinology in reproduction, an interdisciplinary approach.* Elsevier, Amsterdam 509–514.

Mashiach S, Barkai G, Sack J *et al.* (1978) Enhancement of fetal lung maturity by intra-amniotic administration of thyroid hormone. *Am J Obstet Gynecol* 130: 289–293.

Mastroiacovo P, Bertollini R & Licata D, the Italian Multicentric Registry of Birth Defects, Epilepsy Study Group (1988) Fetal growth in the offspring of epileptic women: results of an Italian multicentric cohort study. *Acta Neurologica Scand* 78: 110–114.

Mattson S N, Riley E P, Gramling L *et al.* (1997) Heavy prenatal alcohol exposure with or without physical features of fetal alcohol syndrome leads to IQ deficits. *J Pediatr* 131(5): 718–721.

Mattson S N, Riley E P, Gramling L. *et al.* (1998) Neuropsychological comparison of alcohol-exposed children with or without physical features of fetal alcohol syndrome. *Neuropsychology* 12(1): 146–53.

McBride W G (1961) Thalidomide or congenital abnormalities. *Lancet* ii: 1358.

McGivern R F (1987) Influence of prenatal exposure to cimetidine and alcohol on selected morphological parameters of sexual differentiation: a preliminary report. *Neurotoxicol Teratol* 9: 23–26.

McGivern R F, Clancy A N, Hill M A & Noble E P (1984) Prenatal alcohol exposure alters adult expression of sexually dimorphic behavior in the rat. *Science* 224: 896–898.

McGivern R F, Rose G, Berka C, Clancy A N, Beckwith B E (1987) Neonatal exposure to a high level of ACTH(4–10) impairs adult learning performance. *Pharmacol Biochem Behav* 27: 133–142.

Mennella J A & Beauchamp G K (1991) The transfer of alcohol to human milk. *N Engl J Med* 325: 981–985.

Meriney S D, Gray D B & Pilar G (1985) Morphine-induced delay of normal cell death in the avian ciliary ganglion. *Science* 228: 1451–1452.

✪ Meyer-Bahlburg H F, Feldman J F, Cohen P & Ehrhardt A A (1988) Perinatal factors in the development of gender-related play behavior: sex hormones versus pregnancy complications. *Psychiatry* 51: 260–271.

Middaugh L D, Santos C A & Zemp J W (1975) Effects of phenobarbital given to pregnant mice on behavior of mature offspring. *Dev Psychobiol* 8: 305–313.

Milberger S, Biederman J, Faraone S V *et al.* (1996) Is maternal smoking during pregnancy a risk factor for attention deficit hyperactivity disorder in children? *Am J Psychiatry* 153: 1138–1142.

Milberger S, Biederman J, Faraone S V, Chen L, Jones J (1997) Further evidence of an association between attention-deficit/hyperactivity disorder and cigarette smoking. Findings from a high-risk sample of siblings. *Am J Addict* 6: 205–217.

Mirkin B L & Singh S (1976) Placental transfer of pharmacologically active molecules. In: Mirkin B L (ed) *Perinatal pharmacology and therapeutics.* New York: Academic Press; pp. 1–69.

Mirmiran M & Uylings H B M (1983) The environmental enrichment effect upon cortical growth is neutralized by concomitant pharmacological suppression of active sleep in female rats. *Brain Res* 261: 331–334.

Mirmiran M & de Boer S (1988) Long-term effects of chemicals on developing brain and behavior. In: Kolb Meyer V (ed) *Teratogens. Chemicals which cause birth defects.* Amsterdam: Elsevier; pp. 271–314.

Mirmiran M, van de Poll N E, Corner M A *et al.* (1981) Suppression of active sleep by chronic treatment with chorimipramine during postnatal development: effects upon adult sleep and behavior in the rat. *Brain Res* 204: 129–146.

Mirmiran M, Scholtens J, van de Poll N E *et al.* (1983a) Effects of experimental suppression of active (REM) sleep during early development upon adult brain and behavior. *Dev Brain Res* 7: 277–286.

Mirmiran M, Uylings H B M & Corner M A (1983b) Pharmacological suppression of REM sleep prior to weaning counteracts the effectiveness of subsequent environmental enrichment on cortical growth in rats. *Dev Brain Res* 7: 102–105.

Mirmiran M, Brenner E, van der Gugten J & Swaab D F (1985) Neurochemical and electrophysiological disturbances mediate developmental behavioral alterations produced by medicines. *Neurobehav Toxicol Teratol* 7: 677–683.

Mirmiran M, Feenstra M G P, Dijcks F A *et al.* (1988) Functional deprivation of noradrenaline neurotransmission: effects of clonidine on brain development. *Prog Brain Res* 73: 159–172.

Mirochnick M, Meyer J, Frank D A *et al.* (1997) Elevated plasma norepinephrine after *in utero* exposure to cocaine and marijuana. *Pediatrics* 99: 555–559.

Mitler M (1971) Some developmental observations on the effects of prolonged deprivation of low voltage fast wave sleep in the deer mouse. *Dev Psychobiol* 4: 293–311.

✪ Moar V A, Jefferies M A, Mutch L M M *et al.* (1978) Neonatal head circumference and the treatment of maternal hypertension. *Br J Obstet Gynaecol* 85: 933–937.

Moldow R L, Kastin A J, Hollander C S *et al.* (1981) Brain beta-endorphin-like immunoreactivity in adult rats given beta-endorphin neonatally. *Brain Res Bull* 7: 638–686.

Moore C A, Khoury M J & Liu Y (1997) Does light-to-moderate alcohol consumption during pregnancy increase the risk for renal anomalies among offspring? *Pediatrics* 99(4): E11.

Morreale de Escobar G, Obregón M J, Ruiz de Oña & Escobar del Rey F (1989) Comparison of maternal to fetal transfer of 3,5,3′-triiodothyronine versus thyroxine in rats, as assessed from 3,5,3′-triiodothyronine levels in fetal tissues. *Acta Endocrinol (Copenhagen)* 120: 20–30.

Mukherjee A B & Hodgen G D (1982) Maternal ethanol exposure induces transient impairment of umbilical circulation and fetal hypoxia in monkeys. *Science* 218: 700–702.

✪ Naeye R L & Peters E C (1984) Mental development of children whose mothers smoked during pregnancy. *Am J Obstet Gynecol* 64: 601–607.

Nahas G & Frick H C (1986) Developmental effects of cannabis. *Neurotoxicology* 7: 381–396.

Ness R B, Grisso J A, Hirschinger N *et al.* (1999) Cocaine and tobacco use and the risk of spontaneous abortion. [Comment] *N Engl J Med* 340: 380–381.

✪ O'Connell C M & Fried P A (1991) Prenatal exposure to cannabis: a preliminary report of postnatal consequences in school-age children. *Neurotoxicol Teratol* 13: 631–639.

Oakley G P, Adams M J & James L M (1983) Vitamins and neural tube defects. *Lancet* ii: 798–799.

Ounsted M K, Moar V A, Good F J & Redman G W G (1980) Hypertension during pregnancy with and without specific treatment: the development of the children at the age of four years. *Br J Obstet Gynaecol* 87: 19–24.

Oyama T, Matsuki A, Taneichi T *et al.* (1980) Beta-endorphin in obstetric analgesia. *Am J Gynecol* 137: 613–616.

Patrick M J, Tilstone W J & Reavey P (1972) Diazepam and breast feeding. *Lancet* i: 542.

Peters P W J, Dormans J A M A & Geelen J A G (1979) Light microscopic and ultrastructural observations in advanced stages of induced exencephaly and spinal bifida. *Teratology* 19: 183–196.

✪ Pop V J, Kuijpens J L, van Baar A L *et al.* (1999) Low maternal free thyroxine concentrations during early pregnancy are associated with impaired psychomotor development in infancy. *Clin Endocrinol* 50(2): 149–155.

Pytkowicz Streissguth A, Treder R P, Barr H M *et al.* (1987) Aspirin and acetaminophen use by pregnant women and subsequent child IQ and attention decrements. *Teratology* 35: 211–219.

Rantakallio P, Läärä E, Isohanni M & Moilanen I (1992) Maternal smoking during pregnancy and delinquency of the offspring: an association without causation? *Int J Epidemiol* 21: 1106–1113.

✪ Reinisch J M (1981) Prenatal exposure to synthetic progestins increases potential for aggression in humans. *Science* 211: 1171–1173.

Reinisch J M & Karow W G (1977) Prenatal exposure to synthetic progestins and estrogens: effects on human development. *Arch Sex Behav* 6: 257–288.

Reinisch J M & Sanders S A (1982) Early barbiturate exposure: the brain, sexually dimorphic behavior and learning. *Neurosci Biobehav Rev* 6: 311–319.

✪ Richardson G A, Conroy M L & Day N L (1996) Prenatal cocaine exposure: effects on the development of school-age children. *Neurotoxicol Teratol* 18: 627–634.

Richardson G A & Day N L (1991) Maternal and neonatal effects of moderate cocaine use during pregnancy. *Neurotoxicol Teratol* 13: 455–460.

Robert E & Guibaud P (1982) Maternal valproic acid and congenital neural tube defects. *Lancet* ii: 937.

Robert E & Rosa F (1983) Valproic acid and birth defects. *Lancet* ii: 1142.

Rodier P M & Koëter H B W M (1986) General activity from weaning to maturity in mice exposed to halothane or nitrous oxide. *Neurobehav Toxicol Teratol* 8: 195–199.

Rodier P M, Aschner M, Lewis L S & Koëter H B W M (1986) Cell proliferation in developing brain after brief exposure to nitrous oxide or halothane. *Anesthesiology* 64: 680–687.

Rosa F (1983) Pregnancy outcome with maternal carbamazepine exposure. Food and Drug Administration ADR Highlights, document 1983-ADR No 11. US Food and Drug Administration, Rockville, MD.

Rose J C, Meis P J & Castro M I (1981) Alcohol and fetal endocrine function. *Neurobehav Toxicol Teratol* 3: 105–110.

Rosengarten H & Friedhoff A J (1979) Enduring changes in dopamine receptor cells of pups from drug administration to pregnant and nursing rats. *Science* 203: 1133–1135.

Rosenzweig M R & Bennett E L (1978) Experimental influences in brain anatomy and brain chemistry in rodents. In: Gottlieb G (ed) *Studies on the development of behavior and the nervous system.* New York: Academic Press; vol. 4; pp. 289–327.

✪ Rosett H L, Ouellette E M, Weiner L & Owens E (1978) Therapy of heavy drinking during pregnancy. *Obstet Gynecol* 51: 41–46.

Rubin P C, Craig G F, Gavin K & Sumner D (1986) Prospective survey of use of therapeutic drugs, alcohol, and cigarettes during pregnancy. *BMJ* 292: 81–83.

Rumack C M, Guggenheim M A, Rumack B H *et al.* (1981) Neonatal intracranial hemorrhage and maternal use of aspirin. *Obstet Gynecol* 58: 52S–56S.

Sampson P D, Streissguth A P, Barr H M & Bookstein F L (1989) Neurobehavioral effects of prenatal alcohol: part II. Partial least squares analysis. *Neurotoxicol Teratol* 11: 477–491.

Sampson P D, Bookstein F L, Barr H M & Streissguth A P (1994) Prenatal alcohol exposure, birthweight, and measures of child size from birth to age 14 years. *Am J Public Health* 84(9): 1421–1428.

Sandman C A, McGivern R F, Berka C *et al.* (1979) Neonatal administration of beta-endorphin produces 'chronic' insensitivity to thermal stimuli. *Life Sci* 25: 1755–1760.

Saucier D & Astick L (1975) Effets de l'alpha-methyl-dopa sur le sommeil du chat nouveau-né. Evolution comportementale au cours du Ier mois postnatal. *Psychopharmacologia* 42: 299–303.

Scher M S, Richardson G A, Coble P A *et al.* (1988) The effects of prenatal alcohol and marijuana exposure: disturbances in neonatal sleep cycling and arousal. *Pediatr Res* 24: 101–105.

Schmand B, Neuvel J, Smolders-de Haas H *et al.* (1990) Psychological development of children who were treated antenatally with corticosteroids to prevent respiratory distress syndrome. *Pediatrics* 86: 58–64.

Senekjian E K, Potkul R K, Frey K & Herbst A L (1988) Infertility among daughters either exposed or not exposed to diethylstilbestrol. *Am J Obstet Gynecol* 158: 493–498.

Sexton M, Fox N L & Hebel J R (1990) Prenatal exposure to tobacco: II. Effects on cognitive functioning at age three. *Int J Epidemiol* 19: 72–77.

Sharpe R M, Majdic G, Fisher J *et al.* (1996) Sexual differentiation of the male and fertility in adulthood: potential interference by environmental hormonal mimics. *Frontiers Endocrinol* 20: 181–193.

Sherwood R A, Keating J, Kavvadia V *et al.* (1999) Substance misuse in early pregnancy and relationship to fetal outcome. *Eur J Pediatr* 158: 488–492.

Simmons R D, Kellogg C K & Miller R K (1984) Prenatal diazepam exposure in rats: long-lasting, receptor-mediated effects on hypothalamic norepinephrine-containing neurons. *Brain Res* 293: 73–83.

Smithells R W (1983) Prevention of neural tube effects by vitamin supplement. In: Dobbing J (ed) *Prevention of spina bifida and other neural tube defects.* London: Academic Press; pp. 53–63.

Smithells R W (1992) Vitamins and neural-tube defects. In: Eskes T K A B (ed) *Pathogenesis and prevention.* Bussum: Medicom Europe; pp. 102–120.

Smithells R W, Sheppard S & Schorals C J (1980) Possible prevention of neural tube defects by periconceptional vitamin supplementation. *Lancet* i: 339–340.

Smolders-de Haas H, Neuvel J & Schmand B (1990) Physical development and medical history of children who were treated antenatally with corticosteroids to prevent respiratory distress syndrome: a 10- to 12-year follow-up. *Pediatrics* 86: 65–70.

Sobel E H (1978) Effects of neonatal stunting on the development of rats: early and late effects of neonatal cortisone on physical growth and skeletal maturation. *Pediatr Res* 12: 945–947.

Soyka L F & Joffe J M (1980) Male mediated drug effects on offspring. In: Schwarz R H & Yaffe S J (eds) *Drug and chemical risks to the fetus and newborn.* New York: Alan R Liss; pp. 49–66.

Steegers-Theunissen R P M, Smithells R W & Eskes T K A B (1993) Update of new risk factors and prevention of neural-tube defects. *Obstet Gynaecol Surv* 203: 45–54.

Steener H, Dittmann R W, Steen S & Commentz J C (1986) DDAVP (desmopressin) treatment in primary enuresis nocturna. *Acta Endocrinologica* (Suppl) 274: 108.

Stenchever M A, Williamson R A, Leonard J *et al.* (1981) Possible relationship between *in utero* diethylstilbestrol exposure and male fertility. *Am J Obstet Gynecol* 140: 186–193.

Stick S M, Burton P R, Gurrin L *et al.* (1996) Effects of maternal smoking during pregnancy and a family history of asthma on respiratory function in newborn infants. *Lancet* 348: 1060–1064.

Stoltenberg-Didinger G, Altenkirch H & Wagner M (1990) Neurotoxicity of organic solvent mixtures: embryotoxicity and fetotoxicity. *Neurotoxicol Teratol* 12: 585–589.

Stone M L, Slaerno L K, Green M & Zelson C (1971) Narcotic addiction in pregnancy. *Am J Obstet Gynecol* 109: 716–723.

Stratton L O, Gibson C A, Kolar K G & Kastin A J (1976) Neonatal treatment with TRH affects development, learning and emotionality in the rat. *Pharmacol Biochem Behavior* 5(Suppl 1): 65–67.

Streissguth A P, Barr H M, Sampson P D & Bookstein F L (1994) Prenatal alcohol and offspring development: the first fourteen years. *Drug Alcohol Depend* 36(2): 89–99.

Swaab D F (1980) Neuropeptides and brain development: a working hypothesis. In: Di Benedetta C, Balázs R, Gombos G & Procellati P (eds) *A multidisciplinary approach to brain development.* (Proceedings of the International Meeting, Selva di Fasano). Amsterdam: Elsevier/North Holland; pp. 181–196.

Swaab D F (1982) Neuropeptides: their distribution and function in the brain. *Prog Brain Res* 55: 97–122.

Swaab D F (1985) Influence of fetal and neonatal environment on physical, psychological and intellectual development: workshop summary. In: Marois M (ed) *Prevention of physical and mental congenital defects. B. Epidemiology, early detection and therapy, and environmental factors.* New York: Alan R Liss; pp. 463–467.

Swaab D F & Mirmiran M (1984) Possible mechanisms underlying the teratogenic effects of medicines on the developing brain. In: Yanai J (ed) *Neurobehavioral teratology.* Amsterdam: Elsevier; pp. 55–71.

Swaab D F & Fliers E (1985) A sexually dimorphic nucleus in the human brain. *Science* 228: 1112–1115.

Swaab D F & Mirmiran M M (1985) The influence of chemicals and environment on brain development: 'behavioral teratology'. In: Marois M (ed) *Prevention of physical and mental congenital defects. B. Epidemiology, early detection and therapy, and environmental factors.* New York: Alan R Liss; pp. 447–451.

✪ Swaab D F & Hofman M A (1990) An enlarged suprachiasmatic nucleus in homosexual men. *Brain Research* 537: 141–148.

Swaab D F & Hofman M A (1995) Sexual differentiation of the human hypothalamus in relation to gender and sexual orientation. *Trends Neurosci* 18: 264–269.

Swaab D F, Boer K & Honnebier W J (1977) The influence of the fetal hypothalamus and pituitary on the onset and course of parturition. In: Knight J, O'Connor M (eds) *The fetus and birth.* Amsterdam: Elsevier; pp. 379–400.

Swaab D F, Gooren L J G & Hofman M A (1992) The human hypothalamus in relation to gender and sexual orientation. *Prog Brain Res* 93: 205–219.

Swaab D F, Zhou J N, Fodor M & Hofman M A (1997) Sexual differentiation of the human brain. *Biomed Rev* 7: 17–32.

Taeusch H W (1975) Glucocorticoid prophylaxis for respiratory distress syndrome: a review of potential toxicity. *J Pediatr* 87: 617–623.

Thornburg J E & Moore K E (1976) Pharmacologically induced modifications of behavioral and chemical development. In: Mirkin B L (ed) *Perinatal pharmacology and therapeutics.* New York: Academic Press; pp. 269–354.

Trauth J A, Seidler F J, McCook E C & Slotkin T A (1999) Persistent *c-fos* induction by nicotine in developing rat brain regions: interaction with hypoxia. *Pediatr Res* 45(1): 38–45.

Trice J E & Ambler M (1985) Multiple cerebral defects in an infant exposed *in utero* to anticonvulsants. *Arch Pathol Lab Med* 109: 521–523.

Tronick E Z, Frank D A & Cabral H (1996) Late dose-response effects of prenatal cocaine exposure on newborn neurobehavioral performance. *Pediatrics* 98: 76–83.

Van Baar A (1991) *The development of infants of drug dependent mothers.* Amsterdam: Swets & Zeitlinger.

Vathy I U, Etgen A M, Rabii J & Barfield R J (1983) Effects of prenatal exposure to morphine sulfate on reproductive function of female rats. *Pharmacol Biochem Behav* 19: 777–780.

Vessey M P (1989) *Epidemiological studies of the effects of diethylstilboestrol.* IARC Scientific Publications 96: 335–348.

Visser J A, McLuskey A, Verhoef-Post M *et al.* (1998) Effect of prenatal exposure to diethylstilbestrol on Mullerian duct development in fetal male mice. *Endocrinology* 139: 4244–4251.

Vorhees C V (1981) Effects of prenatal naloxone exposure on postnatal behavioral development of rats. *Neurobehav Toxicol Teratol* 3: 295–301.

Vorhees C V (1985) Fetal anticonvulsant syndrome in rats: effects on postnatal behavior and brain amino acid content. *Neurobehav Toxicol Teratol* 7: 471–482.

Vorhees C V (1989) Behavioral teratology: what's not in a name: a reply to Cattabeni and Abbracchio. *Neurotoxicol Teratol* 11: 325–327.

Waggoner R W, Sionim A E & Armstrong S H (1978) Improved psychological status of children under DDAVP therapy for central diabetes insipidus. *Am J Psychiatry* 135: 361–362.

✪ Wakschlag L S, Lahey B B, Loeber R *et al.* (1997) Maternal smoking during pregnancy and the risk of conduct disorder in boys. *Arch Gen Psychiatry* 54: 670–676.

Walker T F, Bott J H & Bond B C (1987) Cimetidine does not demasculinize male rat offspring exposed *in utero.* *Fundamental and Applied Toxicology* 8: 188–197.

Warkany J & Scharffenberger E (1943) Congenital malformations induced in rats by nutritional deficiency. V. Effects of a purified diet lacking riboflavin. *Society for Experimental Biology and Medicine* 54: 92.

Watkinson B & Fried P A (1985) Maternal caffeine use before, during and after pregnancy and effects upon offspring. *Neurobehav Toxicol Teratol* 7: 9–17.

Wit J M, Human R, Jolies J *et al.* (1986) Effect of desglycinamide-arginine vasopressine (DGAVP) on cognitive functions in children with memory disorders. In: *Neuropeptides and brain function* (May 28–30, Utrecht, The Netherlands) [Abstr.]

Yaffe S J & Dorn L D (1990) Effects of prenatal treatment with phenobarbital. *Devel Pharmacol Ther* 15: 215–223.

Yalom I D, Green R & Fisk N (1973) Prenatal exposure to female hormones. Effect on psychosexual development in boys. *Arch Gen Psychiatry* 28: 554–561.

Yanai J (1981) Comparison of early barbiturate and ethanol effects on the CNS. *Subst Alcohol Actions Misuse* 2: 79–91.

Yanai J & Feigenbaum J J (1981) Lessened sensitivity to apomorphine induced hypothermia following prenatal exposure to phenobarbital. *IRCS Med Sci* 9: 965.

Yates W R, Cadoret R J, Troughton E P *et al.* (1998) Effect of fetal alcohol exposure on adult symptoms of nicotine, alcohol, and drug dependence. *Alcohol Clin Exp Res* 22: 914–920.

Zagon I S & McLaughlin P J (1984) An overview of the neurobehavioral sequelae of perinatal opioid exposure. In: Yanai J (ed) *Neurobehavioral teratology.* Amsterdam: Elsevier; pp. 197–234.

Zervoudakis I A, Krauss A, Fuchs F & Wilson K H (1980) Infants of mothers treated with ethanol for premature labor. *Am J Obstet Gynecol* 137: 713–718.

✪ Zhou J N, Hofman M A, Gooren L J G & Swaab D F (1995) A sex difference in the human brain and its relation to transsexuality. *Nature* 378: 68–70.

# Chapter 16

# Antenatal screening for neurologic disorders

H. Cuckle and J. Murray

## INTRODUCTION

This chapter describes current and best practice in antenatal screening for common congenital abnormalities, which affect the nervous system and present either at birth or through early developmental delay. Structural, chromosomal and genetic disorders are considered separately, as the type of abnormality determines the screening modality employed. Our central focus is on biochemical and DNA tests, as ultrasound scanning is discussed in detail elsewhere in this volume.

Antenatal screening aims to identify those at high enough risk of a specific congenital abnormality to justify the cost and hazards of prenatal diagnosis. Screening for a specific disorder is best organized in the framework of a complete program. This involves the provision of information, tests, counseling, prenatal diagnosis, and termination of affected pregnancies.

The efficiency of a screening program is determined by the discriminatory power: detection rate (proportion of affected pregnancies with positive results), false-positive rate (proportion of unaffected pregnancies with positive results), positive predictive value (risk of being affected if the result is positive), and negative predictive value (risk if negative). The practicality of the program is dependent on the acceptability of the test and cost.

## STRUCTURAL ABNORMALITIES

Biochemical screening for anencephaly and spina bifida was first introduced in the 1970s using maternal serum α-fetoprotein (AFP). Acceptability is high and in England and Wales, AFP screening, together with routine ultrasound anomaly scanning, has contributed to a dramatic fall in birth prevalence: from 4 per 1000 births before screening began to 0.1 per 1000 in 1997, the latest official statistics available. Other structural abnormalities are often incidentally identified through AFP screening but most do not have a strong neurologic component. However, ultrasound screening detects a large proportion of the rarer closed neural tube defects and other CNS abnormalities missed by AFP screening.

### MATERNAL SERUM AFP

As AFP levels in the fetus are 50 000 fold higher than in the mother, minimal leakage through an open cranial or spinal lesion will raise the maternal level. The large multicenter UK Collaborative AFP Study examined levels in nearly 300 affected and almost 20 000 unaffected pregnancies (Wald & Cuckle 1977). To allow for the rapid increase in levels with gestation and large interlaboratory differences, results were expressed as multiples of the normal gestation specific median (MoM) for the laboratory concerned. Discriminatory power was highest at 16–18 weeks gestation when, on average, the AFP level was 6.4 MoM in anencephaly and 3.8 MoM in the five-sixths of spina bifidas with open lesions; closed cases had normal levels.

Table 16.1 shows the discriminatory power predicted from a Gaussian model with the widely used 2.5 MoM cut-off. At 17 weeks most anencephalics are detected but less than two-thirds of spina bifidas, if the MoM is calculated using gestation based on menstrual dates. However, if ultrasound biparietal diameter (BPD) dating is used, spina bifida detection will increase to three-quarters. Ultrasound dating is beneficial as it reduces the contribution of gestational errors to MoM variability. Also, because the BPD is reduced on average in spina bifida by the equivalent of about two

**Table 16.1 Maternal serum AFP screening: proportion with positive results (≥2.5 MoM) according to pregnancy outcome, gestational age and dating method**

| Outcome | Gestational age (weeks)[a] | | |
|---|---|---|---|
| | 15 | 17 | 19 |
| Anencephaly | 74 | 89 | 89 |
| **Gestation by dates** | | | |
| Open spina bifida | 57 | 72 | 54 |
| Closed spina bifida | 2.5 | 2.5 | 2.5 |
| All spina bifida | 48 | 60 | 45 |
| Unaffected | 2.5 | 2.5 | 2.5 |
| **Gestation by BPD** | | | |
| Open spina bifida | 73 | 85 | 81 |
| Closed spina bifida | 25 | 25 | 25 |
| All spina bifida | 65 | 72 | 72 |
| Unaffected | 1.9 | 1.9 | 1.9 |

[a]Estimated from Gaussian frequency distributions with parameters in Wald and colleagues (1992) derived from the UK Collaborative AFP Study (Wald & Cuckle 1977).
BPD, biparietal diameter.

weeks gestation, this systematic gestational underestimation results in large MoM increases. Even in a country with an incidence of only 1 per 1000 the expected positive predictive value is 1 in 25.

## REFINEMENTS

The concentration of AFP in maternal blood is negatively correlated with maternal weight. This is presumed to be due to the fetus producing a fixed mass of AFP, which is then concentrated in varying volumes of body tissues. Published formulae are available to calculate the expected MoM value for a given weight. Dividing the observed MoM by this expected value adjusts for weight and ultimately leads to a small increase in discriminatory power.

Whilst prevalence is low in Afro-Caribbeans, women of this origin have AFP levels on average about 15% higher than Caucasians. In order to avoid a disproportionate number of false positive results, special allowances have to be made. Conversely, women with insulin dependent diabetes are at increased risk but their AFP levels are reduced by about 20% on average. A simple method of allowing for these two factors is to reduce or increase the MoM by 15% or 20% respectively or adjusting the cut-off accordingly.

In twins, the average maternal serum AFP level is about double that seen for normal singletons. In discordantly affected twin pregnancies the discriminatory power of screening is low, since the AFP from the normal co-twin tends to mask the elevation from the affected one. It is not uncommon for twins to be discovered when an ultrasound scan is performed because of raised AFP. This is often taken to be an explanation for the positive result and no further action taken. However, if the level is extremely elevated, say above 5.0 MoM, the spina bifida risk remains high.

## ULTRASOUND SCREENING (see also Chapters 17 and 18)

The discriminatory power of the ultrasound anomaly scan, usually performed at 18–20 weeks gestation, appears to be higher than for AFP screening. Anencephaly is nearly always detected and the combined results from eight prospective studies of anomaly scanning, including 95 spina bifidas and over 100 000 unaffected pregnancies yielded an 83% detection rate with no reported false positives (Cuckle & Thornton 1995). Another approach which is cheaper than anomaly scanning is to visualize the fetal skull and the brain when carrying out an earlier dating scan. In spina bifida there is a tendency for the frontal bones to be scalloped or there may be absence or curvature of the cerebellum. The combined results from six retrospective studies, mainly based on examination of photographs or scans carried out when the presence of abnormality had been established, together with six prospective studies of high risk pregnancies, yielded a detection rate over 90%. The false positive rate for cerebellar anomalies was negligible (Cuckle & Thornton 1995).

## CHROMOSOMAL DISORDERS

Second trimester biochemical screening for Down's syndrome was first proposed in the early 1980s. Introduction into routine practice has been slower than screening for anencephaly and spina bifida. In England and Wales there was no marked effect of screening on the birth prevalence until the 1990s; but by 1997 the prevalence was 1 per 1000 compared with the 1.6 per 1000 expected given the maternal age distribution (Mutton *et al.* 1998). The advent of first trimester screening, in which biochemical and ultrasound markers are combined, has resulted in a substantial increase in discriminatory power. Some Down's syndrome screening programs have now been extended to include Edwards' syndrome.

## SECOND TRIMESTER SERUM MARKERS

Many analytes have been shown to be increased or decreased on average in the serum of women with affected pregnancies but four are in widespread use. They are human chorionic gonadotrophin (hCG), the free β-subunit of hCG, AFP, and unconjugated estriol ($uE_3$): in Down's syndrome pregnancies the average level is 2.02, 2.30, 0.73, and 0.73 MoM respectively, based on meta-analysis of 47 published series (Cuckle 1995). Multi-marker test combinations are the norm using hCG or free β-hCG, and AFP, with or without $uE_3$. There has been recent interest in using inhibin A as an additional marker: based on a meta-analysis of 11 studies (Renier *et al.* 1998; Lam & Tang 1999), the average value is 1.84 MoM.

Several markers have also been discovered in maternal urine. The β-core fragment is the major metabolic product of hCG in maternal urine and second trimester levels are increased on average in affected pregnancies to a greater extent than maternal serum hCG and free β-hCG. To date there have been nine published series including a total of 364 cases and the overall average value is 3.75 MoM (Cuckle *et al.* 1999). Regardless of this, however, urinary β-core hCG is still not a suitable replacement for maternal serum hCG. First, the standard deviation of the urine marker is very wide, partly because only a random urine sample is available, and as a result discriminatory power is no better than in serum. Second, there is significant heterogeneity between the published studies, so the overall average value may be misleading. This is possibly due to differences in assay method, study design and the integrity of urine samples during transport and storage.

The statistically optimal way of interpreting an individual's marker profile is to estimate the risk of Down's syndrome from the maternal age and the MoMs; this is then compared with a fixed cut-off risk. Individual risks are calculated from a multivariate Gaussian model fitted to the overlapping frequency distributions of marker levels in affected and unaffected pregnancies.

The same statistical modeling technique can be used to

**Table 16.2 Second trimester Down's syndrome screening: predicted detection rate (DR) and false-positive rate (FPR) according to marker combination**

| Combination | DR for 5% FPR | Cut-off risk (at term) | | | | | |
|---|---|---|---|---|---|---|---|
| | | 1 in 200 | | 1 in 250 | | 1 in 300 | |
| | | DR | FPR | DR | FPR | DR | FPR |
| hCG and $uE_3$ | 56.6 | 55.0 | 4.5 | 59.0 | 5.9 | 62.3 | 7.2 |
| hCG and AFP | 59.3 | 58.0 | 4.6 | 62.0 | 6.0 | 65.0 | 7.3 |
| hCG, AFP, and $uE_3$ | 62.7 | 60.3 | 4.2 | 63.9 | 5.5 | 66.7 | 6.6 |
| hCG, AFP, $uE_3$ and inhibin | 68.9 | 66.0 | 4.0 | 69.2 | 5.1 | 71.4 | 6.0 |
| free β-hCG and $uE_3$ | 60.7 | 58.0 | 4.2 | 61.7 | 5.4 | 64.7 | 6.5 |
| free β-hCG and AFP | 62.9 | 61.3 | 4.5 | 65.0 | 5.7 | 68.2 | 7.0 |
| free β-hCG, AFP, and $uE_3$ | 66.6 | 63.5 | 4.1 | 67.0 | 5.2 | 69.8 | 6.3 |
| free β-hCG, AFP, $uE_3$, and inhibin | 72.1 | 69.2 | 4.0 | 72.1 | 5.0 | 74.4 | 6.0 |

*Source*: Based on affected parameters in Cuckle (1995) and Lam & Tang (1996), unaffected parameters from 18 000 women screened at 14–19 weeks gestation in Leeds and assuming the maternal age distribution for England and Wales in 1993–97 (Office of Population Census and Surveys, 1995–1999).
*Key*: AFP, α-fetoprotein; hCG, human chorionic gonadotrophin; $uE_3$, unconjugated estriol.

predict the outcome of a screening program (Royston & Thompson 1992). Table 16.2 shows the predicted discriminatory power. So far the detailed results of 21 large prospective studies have been published and the combined results confirm the model predictions of discriminatory power. The precise screening protocol differed between studies: all used hCG or free β-hCG together with $uE_3$ (one), AFP (seven) or both (13); most screened all women but five were restricted to those under 35 or 38; and there were 13 different risk cut-offs. Table 16.3 summarizes the combined performance and, for comparison, what would be predicted from the protocols used. Prospective studies tend to exaggerate the detection rate as non-viable true-positives are terminated, whereas the corresponding non-viable true-negatives are not discovered. Even taking account of this non-viability bias, the observed performance was at least as good as the prediction. The prospective studies also demonstrate the acceptability of screening: overall there was an 80% uptake rate and of those with screen positive results, 79% accepted invasive prenatal diagnosis.

**Table 16.3 Second trimester Down's syndrome screening: observed and predicted discriminatory power in 21 large prospective studies[a]**

| | Observed | Predicted[b] |
|---|---|---|
| Detection rate | 67% | 66% |
| False-positive rate | 4.5% | 4.6% |
| Positive predictive value | 1 in 47 | 1 in 50 |
| Negative predictive value | 1 in 2000 | 1 in 2000 |

[a]A total of 353 000 women were screened including 514 with Down's syndrome (17 studies reviewed in one paper (Cuckle 1996) and four have been published more recently (Ben 1998; Lam *et al.* 1998; Christiansen *et al.* 1999; Ward *et al.* 1999).

[b]The predicted results are based on the screening protocol in each study when applied to the maternal age distribution for England and Wales in 1993–97 (Office of Population Censuses and Surveys 1995–1999). Non-viability bias was allowed for by increasing the expected number of detected cases assuming a fetal loss rate of one-quarter (Cuckle 1999).

## FIRST TRIMESTER MARKERS

At present, most centers perform serum screening for Down's syndrome at 15–19 weeks gestation so that the same sample can be used in AFP screening. Moving to the first trimester has the obvious advantage of providing reassurance earlier in pregnancy and also where necessary, allowing for a less traumatic therapeutic abortion which would be performed before fetal movements were felt. The only disadvantage is that spina bifida detection would require either a separate AFP test after 15 weeks or reliance on the ultrasound anomaly scan at 18–20 weeks.

Three of the established second trimester markers are of value in early pregnancy, namely free β-hCG, AFP and $uE_3$; in the first trimester hCG is a much poorer marker than free β-hCG. In addition another placental product, pregnancy associated plasma protein A (PAPP-A), has consistently yielded reduced levels on average in first trimester Down's syndrome pregnancies, although the reduction is greatest in the early first trimester. Based on a meta-analysis of 44 published series, the average levels in affected pregnancies of free β-hCG, AFP and $uE_3$ are 1.98, 0.79 and 0.74 MoM, respectively; the average for PAPP-A are 0.35, 0.40 and 0.62 MoM at 6–8, 9–11 and 12–14 weeks, respectively (Cuckle & Van Lith 1999).

Several second trimester ultrasound markers have been reported but they have low discriminatory power. In contrast nuchal translucency (NT) is a highly predictive first trimester ultrasound marker. Early studies reported the NT in millimeters rather than in gestation standardized terms, resulting

**Table 16.4 First trimester Down's syndrome screening: predicted detection rate (DR) and false-positive rate (FPR) according to marker combination**

| Combination | DR for 5% FPR | Cut-off risk (at term) | | | | | |
|---|---|---|---|---|---|---|---|
| | | 1 in 200 | | 1 in 250 | | 1 in 300 | |
| | | DR | FPR | DR | FPR | DR | FPR |
| hCG and $uE_3$ | 56.6 | 55.0 | 4.5 | 59.0 | 5.9 | 62.3 | 7.2 |
| hCG and AFP | 59.3 | 58.0 | 4.6 | 62.0 | 6.0 | 65.0 | 7.3 |
| hCG, AFP, and $uE_3$ | 62.7 | 60.3 | 4.2 | 63.9 | 5.5 | 66.7 | 6.6 |
| free β-hCG and $uE_3$ | 61.0 | 59.3 | 4.5 | 63.0 | 5.7 | 65.9 | 6.9 |
| free β-hCG and AFP | 63.2 | 62.6 | 4.8 | 66.3 | 6.1 | 69.4 | 7.4 |
| free β-hCG, AFP, and $uE_3$ | 66.8 | 64.7 | 4.3 | 68.2 | 5.5 | 70.9 | 6.6 |

Source: Based on Down's syndrome parameters in Cuckle & Thornton (1995) and unaffected parameters from 18 000 women screened at 14–19 weeks gestation in Leeds, UK and assuming the maternal age distribution for England and Wales in 1993–97 (Office of Population Censuses and Surveys 1993–1997)

in lack of comparability between centers. This has now been overcome with more recent studies expressing results in MoMs. The most reliable information on the average NT in affected pregnancies is from the massive multicenter prospective intervention study organized by the Fetal Medicine Foundation. Unlike the other studies it is based on routine scanning among low risk women in non-specialist units. Among the first 326 Down's syndrome pregnancies in the study, the median NT was 2.27 MoM. Because of non-viability bias, which is even stronger in the first trimester than the second, the observed distribution of NT values is positively skewed. A 'potentially viable' subset, comprising all third trimester survivors, together with a random sample comprising half of those terminated in the first trimester and two-thirds terminated in the second, had a median of 2.02 MoM (Nicolaides *et al.* 1998).

The predicted performance of serum screening at 9–11 weeks, with and without NT determination at 11–13 weeks, is shown in Table 16.4. A Gaussian model was used with serum parameters from the meta-analysis and NT parameters from the above potential viable subset. The estimated detection rate for a 5% recall rate using PAPP-A and free β-hCG is similar to two or three marker second trimester screening. The addition of further serum markers yielded an increase comparable with inhibin A in the second trimester. NT alone had a predicted detection rate of the same magnitude and the addition of serum markers increased this to a maximum of 88%.

Among almost 100 000 completed singleton pregnancies screened in the Fetal Medicine Foundation study, the recall rate was 8% and the observed detection rate was 82% (Snijders *et al.* 1998). To allow for non-viability bias the authors made a further estimate of the detection rate by comparing the observed number of Down's syndrome births in the screened population with the number expected from the maternal age distribution. This yielded a detection rate of 78%, which is similar to the rate of 77% predicted for an 8% recall rate using the above model.

## REFINEMENTS

All the serum markers used in both the first and second trimester are negatively correlated with maternal weight. As with AFP screening it is standard practice to use weight-adjusted MoMs and benefit from a small increase in discriminatory power.

Maternal serum screening has a poorer performance in twins than in singleton pregnancies, thus even with four second trimester markers the predicted detection rate for a 5% recall rate is only 47% (Cuckle 1998). Since the NT distribution does not differ materially in singleton and twin pregnancies, first trimester screening is the method of choice.

In Edwards' syndrome the average maternal serum hCG or free β-hCG, AFP, and $uE_3$ are approximately 0.30, 0.65, and 0.45 MoM respectively. Some centers have extended the second trimester Down's syndrome screening test to routinely test for Edwards' syndrome. On the basis of published parameters using a 1 in 50 cut-off risk the predicted detection rate is 45% and the false-positive rate under 0.1%. On average PAPP-A and NT levels are similar to those in Down's syndrome, so that first trimester screening with four serum markers and NT yields a 54% predicted detection rate. Other disorders are not formally screened for, but triploidy and Turner's syndrome, which have their own marker profiles, are sometimes detected through screening.

## GENETIC DISORDERS

Whilst several neurologic disorders have a genetic origin, most are not suitable for population based screening.

Duchenne and Becker muscular dystrophy are relatively common Mendelian X-linked disorders, but new mutations and genetic heterogeneity precludes DNA testing to detect carrier mothers outside affected families. For example, in Duchenne muscular dystrophy about one-third of cases arise from a new mutation, and whilst two-thirds of those with a carrier mother have a deletion its location and size are highly variable. Tay–Sachs disease is the only Mendelian disorder for which routine antenatal screening has high discriminatory power. However, because only one in 250 000 births in the general population are affected, screening is limited to Ashkenazi Jews where the prevalence is 1 in 2500.

A number of neurologic abnormalities are now known to have a non-Mendelian genetic form of inheritance due to hereditarily unstable DNA. In myotonic dystrophy, mutations in the myotonin protein kinase gene on chromosome 19 cause hyper-expansion of a trinucleotide repeat sequence. Moderate expansion of the sequence, termed a premutation (PM), in the mother is associated with a high risk of further expansion to a full mutation (FM) when passed on to the infant. Antenatal screening for PM carriers might be feasible but the disorder is rare with a birth prevalence of 1 in 8000. A greater barrier to screening is the fact that some of the carriers may be mildly affected themselves or may manifest it at a later date. Thus antenatal screening would lead to inadvertent diagnosis of some individuals with no clinical benefit and possible psychological harm. Another disorder caused by hereditarily unstable DNA is fragile X syndrome. This is more common than myotonic dystrophy, with a birth prevalence of 1 in 4000 males and 1 in 8000 females; and carriers are clinically unaffected. Antenatal screening for fragile X syndrome is being carried out in some centers.

## TAY–SACHS' DISEASE (p. 628)

This is caused by deficient activity of β-hexosaminidase (Hex A) and in 1985 the gene for the α-subunit of the enzyme was cloned. To date more than 70 disease-causing mutations have been identified in the gene. Among Ashkenazi Jews there are just three mutations accounting for about 97% of carriers.

Before the discovery of the gene, carriers could only be identified by blood β-hexosaminidase testing. However this is technically difficult during pregnancy and the biochemical test does not identify carriers with certainty. In a study of 1364 samples tested by both biochemical and DNA methods, no mutations were found in all 43, with biochemically inconclusive results and 15 of the 67 with positive screening results (De Marchi *et al.* 1996).

In Israel a very high proportion of Ashkenazi carriers have been identified through testing outside pregnancy. In North America, community based screening schemes began in the early 1970s and have been reasonably successful; for example in Montreal the uptake rate has been estimated to be 70% (Mitchell *et al.* 1993). There is also an international program, which offers prenuptual testing specifically targeted at those of Orthodox religious persuasion (Kabak *et al.* 1993). But in most countries there is neither a concerted population based screening program nor the offer of antenatal screening to identify carrier couples. Antenatal DNA screening of Ashkenazi Jewish couples would have a 94% detection rate and a false-positive rate of about 0.1%; the positive predictive value is 1 in 4.

## FRAGILE X SYNDROME (p. 808)

The condition is caused by a mutation in a gene on the X chromosome that is characterized by a trinucleotide (cytosine-guanine-guanine) repeat sequence in the 5′ untranslated region. The sequence is polymorphic such that, in the general population, the number of repeats ranges from five to 54. Amplification of this sequence caused by mutation can result in a PM with 55–199 repeats or a FM with more than 200. The PM is asymptomatic but in carrier females confers a high risk of hyperexpansion to a FM in her offspring. Males with FM always have the clinical phenotype, unlike females, only half of whom are affected.

Screening for FMs and PMs would be most relevant to females of reproductive age. On the basis of predictions from statistical modeling the discriminatory power would be high. The predicted detection rate would approach 100% with a false-positive rate of 0.4% (Murray *et al.* 1997). Those with a FM will have a 1 in 3 chance of an affected infant and for carriers of a PM the risk is about 1 in 25.

As with other genetic disorders there are two alternatives to antenatal screening, namely active cascade testing in affected families and general population preconceptional screening. Cascade testing involves the identification of an index case, followed by systematic testing of those relatives calculated to be at high risk of having a mutation. Whilst of immeasurable benefit to the family, as a sole approach this method is unlikely to have a large impact on birth prevalence. On the basis of a model in which testing was extended to third degree relatives, only 12% of couples at high risk would be detected (Wildhagen *et al.* 1999). Other problems with this approach include the intrinsic difficulties associated with diagnosing the index case and its reliance on general family dynamics.

Preconceptional screening would be ideal as it informs couples prior to embarking on pregnancy. They would then have the option of abstaining from pregnancy, seeking prenatal diagnosis and if acceptable selective termination of pregnancy or undergoing assisted conception following preimplantation genetic diagnosis. However, in the absence of an organized infrastructure for preconceptional screening, this method is likely to prove difficult to administer. Antenatal screening offers a more practical approach as it could be carried out alongside Down's syndrome screening.

Testing can be done on mouthwash or blood samples, and is best carried out by a combination of the polymerase chain reaction (PCR) and Southern blotting. PCR is a relatively cheap, fast and reliable method by which normal alleles and smaller PMs can be accurately measured. Southern blotting is more time-consuming and expensive but is necessary for detecting larger PMs and FMs, which fail to amplify using PCR. It is also essential for differentiating between females

**Table 16.5 Fragile X syndrome screening: practical experience in four studies***

| Study | Women screened | FMs | | PMs | | Prenatal diagnoses | FM pregnancies | |
|---|---|---|---|---|---|---|---|---|
| | | No. | Rate (1 in) | No. | Rate (1 in) | | No. | Terminated |
| Finland[a] | 1738 | 0 | >1700 | 6 | 290 | 6 (100%) | 2 | 0 (0%) |
| Israel I[b] | 9459 | 4 | 2400 | 124 | 76 | 111 (90%) | 9 | 9 (100%) |
| Israel II[c] | 10587 | NS | NS | 138 | 77 | 110 (80%) | NS | NS |
| Israel III[d] | 9830 | 4 | 2500 | 118 | 83 | 118 (100%) | NS | NS |

*All studies used a cut-off of 52 repeats to define a PM except Finland, which used 60 repeats. In the Israel I study, 7 carriers had twin or repeat pregnancies, therefore uptake of prenatal diagnosis was based on 134 pregnancies.
[a]Ryynanen *et al.* (1999); [b]Pesso *et al.* (2000); [c]Falik-Zaccai *et al.* (1999); [d]Drasinover *et al.* (1999).
NS, not specified.

with homozygous (same repeat size) normal alleles and those with larger PMs or FMs, which produce similar PCR results. The most efficient testing strategy is to carry out PCR initially on all samples and Southern blotting on the approximately 30% with ambiguous PCR results. The same techniques can be applied to prenatal diagnostic samples. A major drawback with prenatal diagnosis is the inability to predict the phenotype of female fetuses with a FM, when only half of them will have fragile X syndrome. The decision to terminate a pregnancy in such circumstances is difficult. One option is to restrict screening to those with *a priori* evidence of a male fetus, based on ultrasound or DNA amplification of Y chromosome sequences in maternal blood. This uncertainty is likely to be a major hindrance to general population screening studies.

The preliminary results from five large scale population-based antenatal screening programs have now been reported (see Table 16.5). Information on the uptake of screening was only available for the Finnish study, where it was 85%, whereas all studies reported the uptake of prenatal diagnosis in the carriers and the overall rate was 87%. Only two of the studies have reported the outcome of pregnancy for cases where a fetal FM was found. Nine of the 11 were terminated, all 4 males and 5 of 7 females. These are too few data to draw conclusions about the acceptability of termination in such circumstances. However, the results of prenatal diagnosis performed because of a family history of fragile X syndrome suggest that it is acceptable. Murray and colleagues (1997) reviewed seven studies which reported the outcome of 60 prenatally diagnosed FM pregnancies. In total 43 (72%) were terminated; 16 (89%) of the 18 males and 27 (64%) of 42 females.

## INFORMING CHOICE

A fundamental component of any screening program is its ability to inform choice. In order for this to happen health professionals must provide women with sufficient information to enable them to make an informed decision. This information should be non-directive, allowing decision making to occur without undue pressure from the health professional. There are two methods by which informed decision making can be facilitated: information aids and decision aids. Information aids aim to assist women to access information whilst decision aids provide support during the process of decision making. Patient leaflets and structured decision trees are examples of each type of aid. In Britain a Working Party of The Royal College of Obstetrician and Gynaecologists (RCOG) has recommended that prior to Down's syndrome screening, all women should be informed about the condition, the likelihood of detection and the meaning and consequences of (true and false) negative and positive results (Royal College of Obstetricians and Gynaecologists 1993).

In most maternity units, face to face counseling and leaflets are the methods by which this information is imparted. However, there is mounting evidence that this approach is unsatisfactory. First the length of counseling sessions is restricted due to limited resources and as such only minimal time is devoted to imparting screening information. Second there is an apparent apathy towards screening amongst many health professionals with the consequence that they lack the knowledge to discuss basic aspects of screening (Khalid *et al.* 1994; Sadler 1997). Finally, in the UK many leaflets currently in circulation do not meet basic RCOG recommendations, which are essential if informed decision making is to be attempted (Murray *et al.* 2001). Overall therefore, the quality of information giving about antenatal Down's syndrome screening needs to be re-evaluated and improved. Whilst this presents a challenge to the antenatal clinic, it is not insurmountable.

In the UK many maternity units now recognize the need for improvement and have put in place a dedicated Screening Co-ordinator whose role includes the production and maintenance of up-to-date high quality patient literature and the education of health professionals involved in screening. Its effect on women's knowledge and informed decision making is yet to be judged. Innovative methods by which women can be informed about screening have also been suggested, including the use of videos, touch screen information systems within the antenatal clinic and internet sources. The former two have already been piloted and shown to increase knowledge and reduce anxiety respectively (Graham *et al.* 2000; Hewison *et al.* 2000).

In addition, in Britain a general health 24-hour national telephone helpline, NHS Direct, has now been established. Information-giving specific to antenatal screening could be incorporated into such a service. Finally, the NHS Executive has recently set up the Centre for High Quality Information, which aims to provide support and guidance in the production of patient information.

The concentrated efforts to promote informed decision making in antenatal screening are timely given the ever-increasing number of conditions that could potentially be tested for during pregnancy. It could be argued that until the problems experienced in Down's syndrome are overcome, other antenatal screening programs should not be instigated. However, with the bringing of these qualitative issues to the forefront, now may be an appropriate time to consider other options.

### Key Points

- Maternal serum AFP screening at 17 weeks gestation has a detection rate of 89% for anencephaly and 72% for spina bifida with a 1.9% false-positive rate.
- Ultrasound anomaly screening at 18–20 weeks has a higher detection rate with a substantially lower false-positive rate.
- Multiple marker serum screening for Down's syndrome in the second trimester has a detection rate of 67% for a 5% false-positive rate.
- Combined serum and ultrasound screening in the first trimester has an 88% detection rate for a 5% false-positive rate.
- DNA screening for Tay-Sachs disease among Ashkenazi Jewish couples has a 94% detection rate with a 0.1% false-positive rate.
- DNA screening for fragile X syndrome has a detection rate approaching 100% with a 0.4% false-positive rate.
- All forms of antenatal screening have a high uptake rate. Improved information aids and decision aids are needed to help couples make informed choices about screening.

## REFERENCES


Benn P A (1998) Preliminary evidence for associations between second-trimester human chorionic gonadotropin and unconjugated oestriol levels with pregnancy outcome in Down syndrome pregnancies. *Prenat Diagn* 18: 319–324.

Christiansen M, Lund Petersen P, Premin M *et al.* (1999) Maternal serum screening for congenital malformations and Down syndrome in Sønderjyllands county. Eight years of experience. *Ugeskr Læger* 161: 6938–6934.

Cuckle H S (1995) Improved parameters for risk estimation in Down's syndrome screening. *Prenat Diagn* 15: 1057–1065.

Cuckle H (1996) Established markers in second trimester maternal serum. *Early Human Development* 47(Suppl): 27–29.

Cuckle H (1998) Down's syndrome screening in twins. *J Med Screen* 5: 3–4.

Cuckle H (1999) Down syndrome fetal loss rate in early pregnancy. *Prenat Diagn* 19: 1175–1180.

Cuckle H S & van Lith J M M (1999) Appropriate biochemical parameters in first trimester screening for Down's syndrome. *Prenat Diagn* 19: 505–512.

Cuckle H S & Thornton J G (1995) Antenatal diagnosis and management of neural tube defects. In: Levene M I & Lilford R J, eds. *Fetal and Neonatal Neurology and Neurosurgery*. London: Churchill Livingstone 295–309.

Cuckle H S, Canick J A & Kellner L H (1999) Collaborative study of maternal urine β-core human chorionic gonadotropin screening for Down's syndrome. *Prenat Diagn* 19: 911–917.

DeMarchi J M, Caskey C T & Richards C S (1996) Population-specific screening by mutation analysis for diseases frequent in Ashkenazi Jews. *Hum Mutat* 8: 116–125.

Drasinover V, Ehrlich S, Magal N *et al.* (1999) Increased transmission of the premutated allele compared to the normal allele in female carriers of the fragile X syndrome. *Am J Hum Genet* 65(Suppl): 256.

Falik-Zaccai T C, Shackhak E, Borochowitz Z *et al.* (1999) Fragile X syndrome: population carrier screening and implication for prenatal diagnosis. *Am J Hum Genet* 65(Suppl): 1181.

Graham W, Smith P, Kamal A *et al.* (2000) Randomised controlled trial comparing the effectiveness of touch screen system with leaflet for providing women with information on prenatal tests. *BMJ* 320: 155–160.

Hewison J, Cuckle H, Baillie C *et al.* (2000) Use of videotapes for viewing at home in informed choice in Down's syndrome screening: a randomised trial. *Prenat Diagn* In Press.

Kaback M, Lim-Steele J, Dabholkar D *et al.* (1993) Tay–Sachs disease – carrier screening, prenatal diagnosis and the molecular era. An international perspective, 1970 to 1993. The International TSD Data Collection Network. *JAMA* 270: 2307–2315.

Khalid L, Price S M & Barrow M (1994) The attitudes of midwives to maternal serum screening for Down's syndrome. *Public Health* 108: 131–136.

Lam Y H & Tang M H Y (1999) Second-trimester maternal serum inhibin-A screening for fetal Down's syndrome in Asian women. *Prenat Diagn* 19: 463–467.

Lam Y H, Ghosh A, Tang M H Y *et al.* (1998) Second-trimester maternal serum alpha-fetoprotein and human chorionic gonadotropin screening for Down's syndrome in Hong Kong. *Prenat Diagn* 18: 585–589.

Mitchell J, Scriver C R, Clow C L & Kaplan F (1993) What do young people think and do when the option of cystic fibrosis carrier testing is available. *J Med Genet* 30: 538–542.

Murray J, Cuckle H, Sehmi I *et al.* (2001) Quality of written information used in Down's syndrome screening. *Prenat Diagn* In Press.

Murray J, Cuckle H, Taylor G & Hewison J (1997) Screening for fragile X syndrome; information for health planners. *Health Technology Assessment* 1(4): 1–69.

Mutton D, Ide R G, Alberman E (1998) Trends in prenatal screening for and diagnosis of Down's syndrome: England and Wales, 1989–97. *BMJ* 317: 922–923.

Nicolaides K H, Snijders R J M & Cuckle H S (1998) Correct estimation of parameters for ultrasound nuchal translucency screening. *Prenat Diagn* 18: 519–521.

Office of Population Censuses and Surveys. *Series FM1, Birth Statistics* 1995–99; Vols 22–26.

Pesso R, Berkenstadt M, Cuckle H *et al.* (2000) Screening for fragile X syndrome in women of reproductive age. *Prenat Diagn* 20: 611–614.

Renier M A, Vereecken A, van Herck E *et al.* (1998) Second trimester maternal dimeric inhibin-A in the multiple-marker screening test for Down's syndrome. *Human Reproduction* 13(3): 744–748.

Royal College of Obstetricians and Gynaecologists. *Report on the RCOG Working Group on biochemical markers and the detection of Down's syndrome*. London: RCOG Press.

Royston P & Thompson S G (1992) Model-based screening by risk with application to Down's syndrome. *Stats in Med* 11: 257–268.

Ryynanen M, Heinonen S, Makkonen M (1999) Feasibility and acceptance of screening for fragile X mutations in low risk pregnancies. *Eur J Hum Genet* 7: 212–216.

Sadler M (1997) Serum screening for Down's syndrome: how much do health professionals know? *Br J Obstet Gynaecol* 104: 176–179.

Snijders R J M, Noble P, Sebire N *et al.* (1998) UK multi-centre project on assessment of risk of trisomy 21 by maternal age and fetal nuchal-translucency thickness at 10–14 weeks of gestation. *Lancet* 352: 343–346.

Wald N J & Cuckle H (1977) Maternal serum alpha-fetoprotein measurement in antenatal screening for anencephaly and spina bifida in early pregnancy. Report of the UK Collaborative Study on alpha-fetoprotein in relation to neural-tube defects. *Lancet* i: 1323–1332.

Wald N J, Cuckle H S, Densem J W *et al.* (1992) Maternal serum screening for Down's syndrome: the effect of routine ultrasound scan determination of gestational age and adjustment for maternal weight. *Br J Obstet Gynaecol* 99: 144–149.

Ward P A, Wilson H & Wood P L (1999) The outcome of five years' implementation of maternal serum screening for Down's syndrome comparing actual age risks and mode of delivery. *J Obstet Gynaecol* 19(3): 257–261.

Wildhagen M F, Van Os T A M & Polder J J (1999) Efficacy of cascade testing for fragile X syndrome. *J Med Screening* 6: 70–76.

# Chapter 17 Antenatal assessment of CNS anomalies, including neural tube defects using abdominal ultrasound

K. D. Kalache and L. S. Chitty

## INTRODUCTION

In this chapter we describe the abnormalities of the CNS amenable to prenatal diagnosis using transabdominal ultrasound in the second and third trimesters of pregnancy. We give brief details of the etiology of abnormalities and describe the sonographic findings and prenatal management in detail. Relatively little detail regarding prognosis and long-term outcome is given, as this will be covered elsewhere in this book. However, it is important to remember that the population we see prenatally may differ from that which presents clinically to our pediatric colleagues. The spectrum of abnormalities is very broad, from the very severe, which frequently result in perinatal death (anencephaly, holoprosencephaly, hydranencephaly, etc.), to those with minor variants which may represent the one end of the spectrum of normality (mild ventriculomegaly, etc.) and will not present clinically in the postnatal period.

## MIDLINE ANOMALIES

### HOLOPROSENCEPHALY (see p. 210)

Holoprosencephaly describes a spectrum of abnormalities involving the brain and face, resulting from incomplete development and division of the embryonic forebrain or prosencephalon during early development. Since the olfactory tracts are always absent, the term arhinencephaly was originally used. Holoprosencephaly is divided into three categories depending on the degree of separation of the cerebral hemisphere: alobar, semilobar, and lobar. The most severe form is alobar holoprosencephaly where there is complete failure of separation of the forebrain into the right and left hemispheres, resulting in a single ventricle with fusion of the thalami and absence of the corpus callosum, falx cerebri, 3rd ventricle, optic tract and olfactory bulbs. Partial cleavage results in semilobar holoprosencephaly where there is some degree of separation of the anterior cerebral hemispheres, with variable degrees of fusion of the thalami and absence of the olfactory bulbs and corpus callosum. The mildest form is lobar holoprosencephaly, where there is a well-developed interhemispheric fissure with variable degrees of fusion of the lateral ventricles and frontal horns. Here the abnormality may be confined to absence of the corpus callosum and fusion of the lateral ventricles.

The prevalence of holoprosencephaly is about 1.2 per 10 000 births. The incidence is probably higher in early pregnancy because of a high intrauterine lethality. Holoprosencephaly is very heterogeneous. It can be associated with chromosome abnormalities, particularly trisomy 13 (Lehman *et al.* 1995). It may also be found in association with a variety of monogenic disorders such as Meckel–Gruber and Smith–Lemni–Opitz syndromes. Monogenic holoprosencephaly with both autosomal recessive and dominant modes of inheritance have been described. The autosomal dominant form shows very variable penetrance within a family, such that only subtle signs such as a single central incisor or reduced head circumference indicating a mildly affected parent can be seen with a severely affected child. Recent molecular genetic studies have shown that there are at least four potential loci for holoprosencephaly (Roessler *et al.* 1996; Peebles 1998; Golden 1999). Environmental teratogens, including ionizing radiation and certain alkaloids, have also been implicated in holoprosencephaly. An increased incidence of holoprosencephaly has been reported in diabetic mothers (Barr *et al.* 1983), as well as in gestational diabetes (Martinez *et al.* 1998).

In alobar and semilobar holoprosencephaly there is a single sickle-shaped ventricle occupying the anterior part of the head (Fig. 17.1A). There is complete or partial absence of the midline echo with a thin rim of cortex anteriorly, and the fused thalami posteriorly are often very prominent. The major differential diagnoses are hydranencephaly and large porencephalic cysts which may result in loss of the midline echo but the thalami are not usually fused in either case. Severe hydrocephalus may also be confused with holoprosencephaly, but in the former the midline echo is present and the thalami may be separated by the dilated 3rd ventricle. The presence of facial abnormalities may also be a clue to the underlying holoprosencephaly. These include cyclopia (single median orbit with a proboscis above the orbit) (Fig. 17.1B), ethmocephaly (hypotelorism with a proboscis in between) (Fig. 17.1C), cerebrocephaly (hypotelorism with a normally placed nose but with a single nostril), and a median or bilateral cleft lip and/or palate with hypotelorism (Fig. 17.1D). Alobar holoprosencephaly can occur without any significant facial signs. Microcephaly is a frequent finding in holoprosencephaly.

Antenatal diagnosis of lobar holoprosencephaly is difficult but has been reported, as it typically presents with some degree of enlargement of the lateral ventricles, absence of a septum pellucidum cavum, and a degree of fusion of the frontal horns, which, in the coronal view, will have a flat square roof (Nyberg *et al.* 1987; Pilu *et al.* 1987).

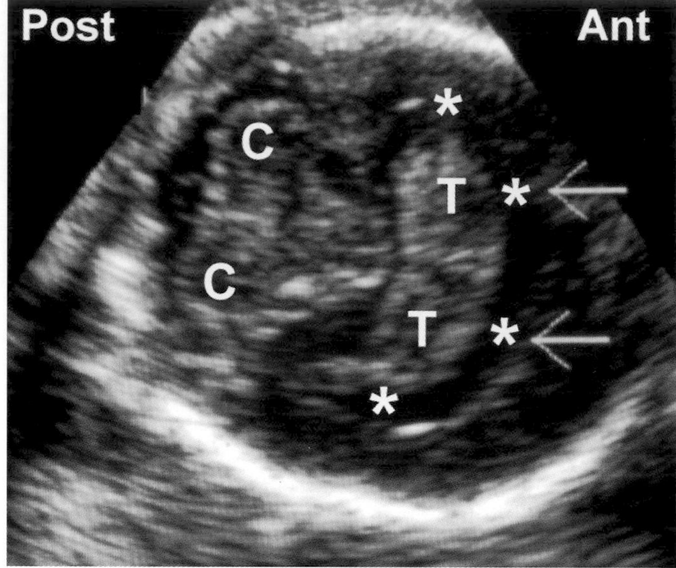

A

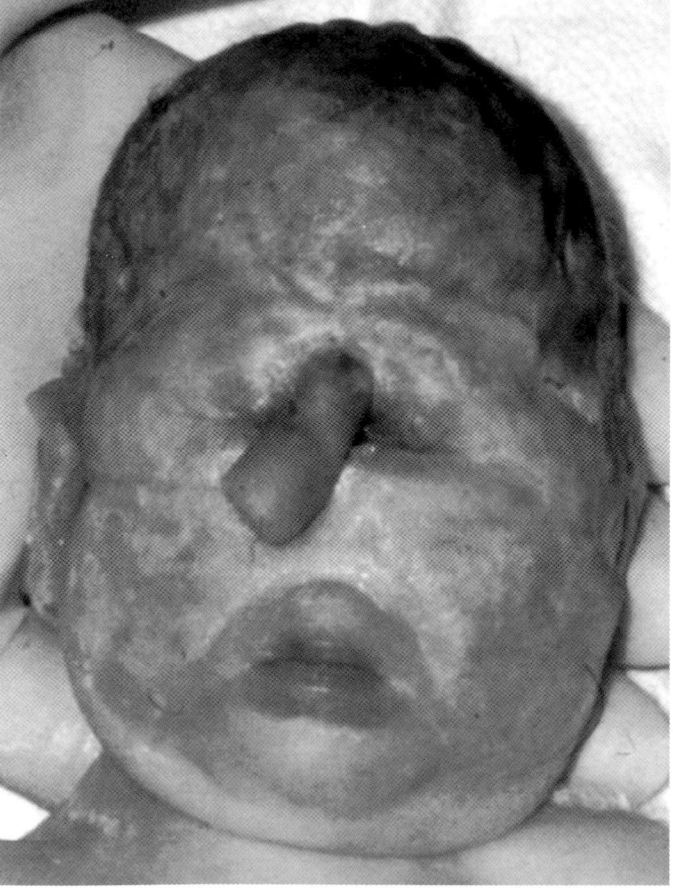
B

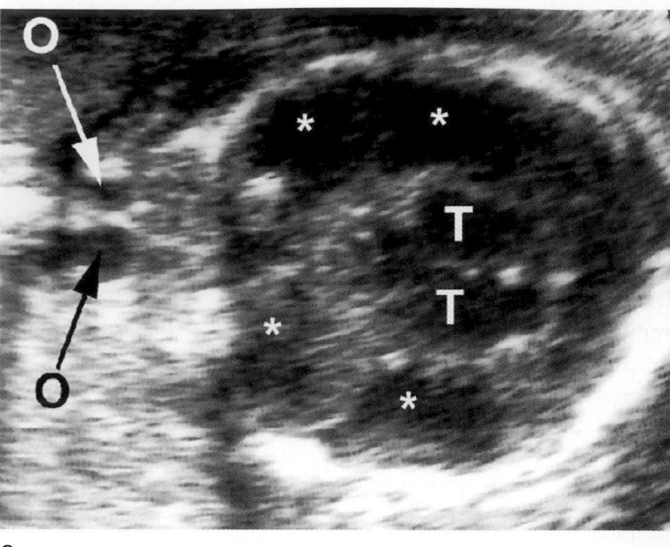

C

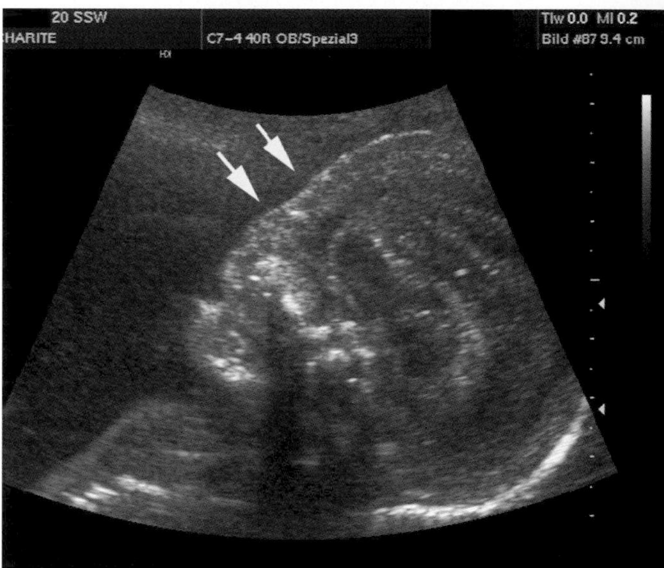

D

**Figure 17.1 Holoprosencephaly.** (A) Axial view demonstrating alobar holoprosencephaly. There is a single sickle shaped ventricle occupying the anterior part of the head (*). Note the anterior crescent-like shaped cortex rim (arrows). The thalami are fused and very prominent, T, and the cerebellum, C, is clearly seen. (B) Facial abnormalities associated with holoprosencephaly. Cyclopia with single fused orbits and proboscis above it. (C) Axial view through the orbits, O, demonstrating hypotelorism (arrows). The large thalami, T, are fused within a monoventricle (*). (D) Sagittal view in a fetus with holoprosencephaly and median cleft lip/palate. There is a an extremely flattened facial profile, as consequence of absence of the nose (arrows).

The diagnosis of holoprosencephaly should prompt a detailed anomaly scan to detect any extracranial abnormalities that may be indicative of an underlying genetic syndrome or aneuploidy. The face should be carefully examined and orbital diameters measured. Karytotyping should be discussed. Alobar and semilobar holoprosencephaly are associated with a very poor prognosis and termination of pregnancy is a reasonable option in these cases. The prognosis for lobar holoprosencephaly is uncertain but mental retardation and other neurologic sequelae are reported. If postnatal pathologic examination confirms the presence of isolated holoprosencephaly with a normal karyotype, both parents should be examined closely to look for mild features that may be associated with incomplete penetrance, and blood should be taken to look for cryptic translocations and deletions in the regions associated with holoprosencephaly. In sporadic cases of holoprosencephaly, where there is no evidence of a chromosomal or genetic abnormality, there is an empiric recurrence risk of 6% (Roach *et al.* 1975). If the findings are consistent with autosomal dominant holoprosencephaly, the overall risk for some form of abnormality in a subsequent pregnancy is 29–35%, although the severity ranges in magnitude from the severe alobar form of holoprosencephaly to an isolated single maxillary incisor (Cohen 1989).

## AGENESIS OF THE CORPUS CALLOSUM (see p. 219)

Agenesis of the corpus callosum has a heterogeneous etiology and may be associated with chromosomal abnormalities (including trisomy 18 and 13), a large number of genetic syndromes inherited in an autosomal recessive or X-linked fashion, or teratogens as in fetal alcohol syndrome and maternal ingestion of sodium valproate and cocaine.

The corpus callosum develops later than most other CNS structures, between 12 and 17 weeks of gestation. As it develops from anterior to posterior, agenesis of the corpus callosum can be partial, depending on the gestation of the insult. Sonographic diagnosis of agenesis of the corpus callosum is difficult. Many fetuses with this abnormality have a normal second trimester scan with the sonographic signs only developing later in the 3rd trimester (Bennett *et al.* 1996). The corpus callosum is not usually visible in the standard axial view of the brain, but complete agenesis of the corpus callosum may be suspected in the presence of a number of typical indirect signs. These include:

1. The sonographic appearance of three parallel lines in the midline, the lateral ones representing the medial borders of the separated hemispheres, and the middle one the falx cerebri (Fig. 17.2A). This is a result of increased separation of the hemispheres and a prominent intrahemispheric fissure secondary to absence of the main nerve fibers crossing the midline. The frontal horns are of normal size but are usually more separated than normal (Fig. 17.2B).
2. The atria and the occipital horns often show mild to moderate dilatation (Fig. 17.2A).
3. The lateral ventricles often have a teardrop shape (Fig. 17.2B).
4. The cavum septum pellucidum is absent and the 3rd ventricle may be enlarged and is usually displaced upwards (Fig. 17.2C).

A clear view of the corpus callosum can usually be obtained in the mid-sagittal plane. In a normal fetus, color Doppler will demonstrate the presence of the pericallosal artery, which is characterized by a semicircular vessel running along the superior surface of the corpus callosum (Fig. 17.2D). In agenesis of the corpus callosum the 3rd ventricle may be enlarged and is usually displaced upwards (Fig. 17.2E). Branches of the anterior cerebral artery are seen ascending linearly with a radiate arrangement and the typical pattern of the pericallosal artery is absent.

There is a high incidence of other associated intracranial abnormalities, the most common being the Dandy–Walker malformation (Pilu *et al.* 1993). Intracranial lipomas are also frequently associated with agenesis of the corpus callosum and this should be suspected when a highly echogenic mass is seen in the midline (Bork *et al.* 1996). There is also a high incidence of extracerebral malformations and a detailed anomaly scan is mandatory. Karyotyping should be offered in view of the high association with aneuploidy (Comstock *et al.* 1985; Pilu *et al.* 1993; Gupta & Lilford 1995). In the presence of aneuploidy or other abnormalities, intracranial or extracranial, the prognosis is poor and discussion of termination of pregnancy is reasonable. Counseling in isolated agenesis of the corpus callosum is difficult as the prognosis is uncertain, with most studies reporting around an 85% chance of a normal developmental outcome (Vergani *et al.* 1994; Gupta & Lilford 1995; Moutard *et al.* 1998). However, before viability it is often difficult to confirm the absence of other intracerebral abnormalities that may increase the likelihood of a poor outcome (Vergani *et al.* 1994). Furthermore, some genetic syndromes, where agenesis of the corpus callosum is the major feature, may not have any other sonographically identifiable manifestations, e.g. Aicardi syndrome.

## DANDY–WALKER SYNDROME (see p. 224)

The term Dandy–Walker syndrome defines a spectrum of disorders resulting from varying degrees of vermian agenesis and has an estimated incidence of about 1 in 30 000 births. When the agenesis is complete and there is an enlarged 4th ventricle the anomaly is called Dandy–Walker malformation (Fig. 17.3A). A partial vermian agenesis (generally of the inferior portion) without dilatation of the cisterna magna is called Dandy–Walker variant (Fig. 17.3B). Mega-cisterna refers to a condition in which the cisterna magna is enlarged without cerebellar dysgenesis.

Dandy-Walker syndrome has a heterogeneous etiology and can be associated with many chromosomal abnormalities, including trisomies 9, 13, 18 and 21, triploidy, 45,X, 6p-, and with single gene disorders such as Meckel–Gruber (Yapar *et al.* 1996), Walker–Warburg (Vohra *et al.* 1993) and Joubert syndromes (Murray *et al.* 1985). An X-linked recessive inheritance pattern has also been suggested in some families with isolated Dandy–Walker syndrome (Cowles *et al.* 1993).

The presence of Dandy–Walker malformation can be suspected *in utero* by sonographic demonstration of characteristic morphologic changes, which include:

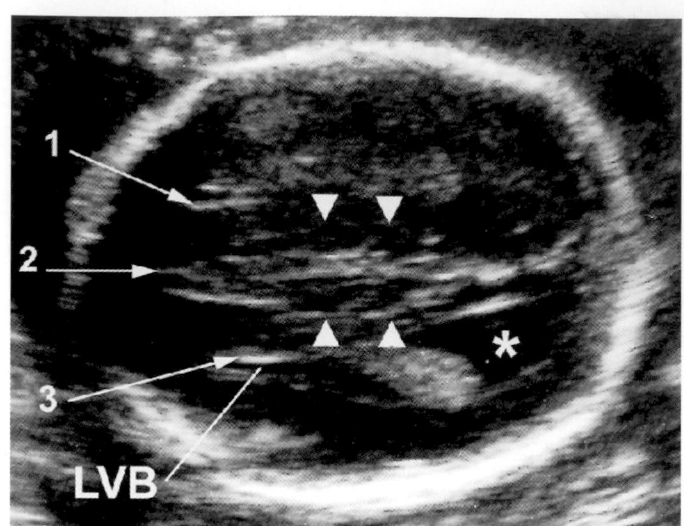
1
2
3
LVB
A

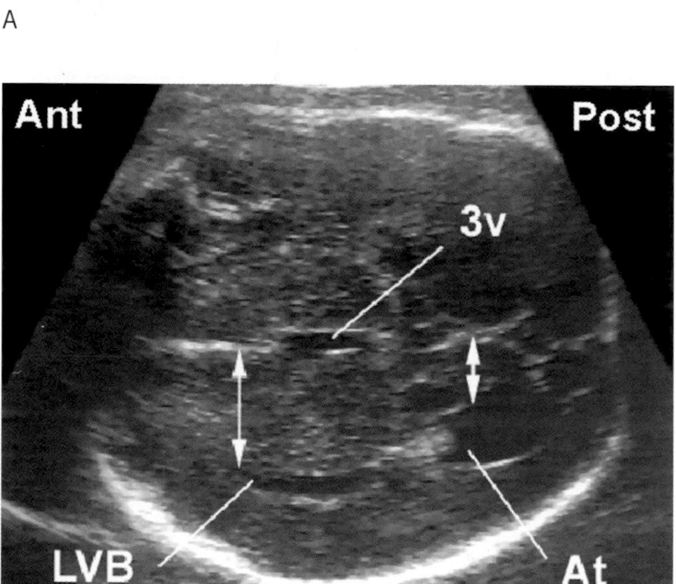
Ant
Post
3v
LVB
At
B

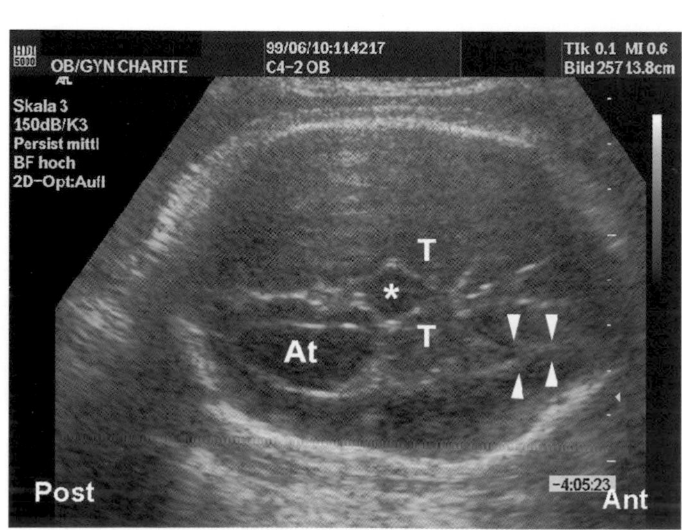
OB/GYN CHARITE
99/06/10:114217
C4-2 OB
TIk 0.1 MI 0.6
Bild 257 13.8cm
Skala 3
150dB/K3
Persist mittl
BF hoch
2D-Opt:Aufl
T
T
At
Post
-4:05:23
Ant
C

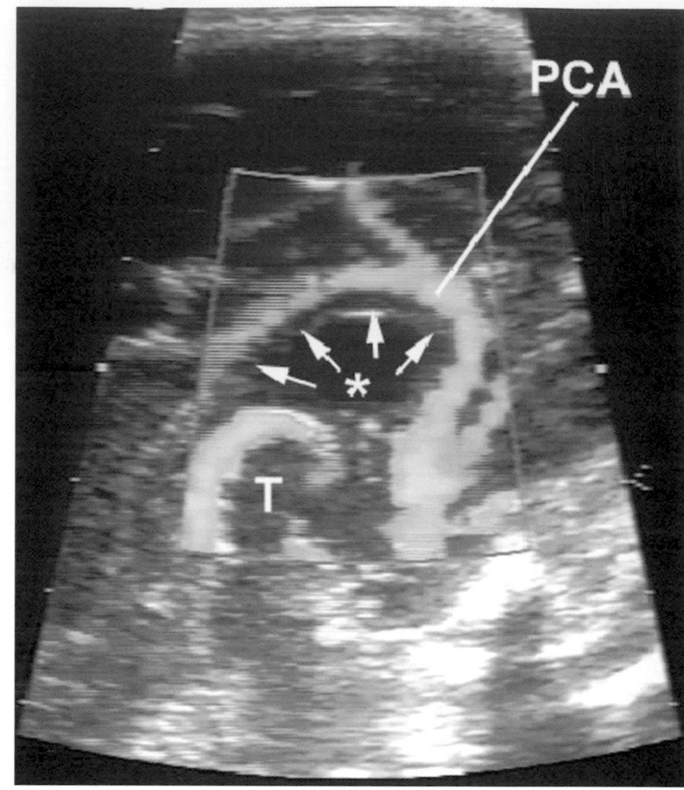
PCA
T
D

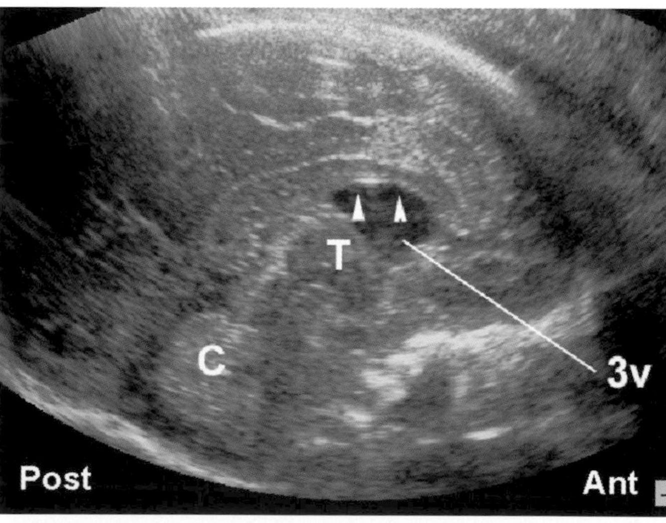
T
C
3v
Post
Ant
E

1. enlargement of the 4th ventricle,
2. separation of the cerebellar hemispheres with communication between the cisterna magna and the 4th ventricle,
3. variable degrees of ventriculomegaly.

The enlargement of the 4th ventricle is often so dramatic that the posterior fossa is occupied by a large hypoechoic area (Fig. 17.3A). In such cases the cerebellar hemispheres are widely separated and compressed against the tentorium. Ventricular dilatation mainly affects the 4th ventricle, whose over-distension also involves the aqueduct and 3rd ventricle. The incidence of ventriculomegaly associated with prenatally diagnosed Dandy–Walker malformation varies between 50 and 75% (Pilu *et al.* 1986b; Russ *et al.* 1989; Nyberg *et al.* 1988).

Dandy–Walker variant can occur in partial inferior vermian agenesis (Fig. 17.3B), but this diagnosis should not, however, be made before 18 weeks gestation because the development of the cerebellar vermis may be incomplete at that time (Russ *et al.* 1989; Bromley *et al.* 1994).

In a normal fetus, the size of the cisterna magna may vary considerably. An enlarged cisterna magna (mega cisterna magna) should be suspected when the antero-posterior diameter is greater than 10 mm (Nyberg *et al.* 1988), even then the pathologic implications are unclear.

The main differential diagnosis is an arachnoid cyst. However, unlike a Dandy–Walker malformation, this lesion usually causes a mass effect, but instead of the cystic mass separating the cerebellar hemispheres it displaces the hemispheres *en bloc*. A further differential diagnosis of a Dandy–Walker malformation includes an enlarged cisterna magna caused by communicating hydrocephalus or cerebellar hypoplasia. The latter may also be associated with karyotypic abnormalities, specifically trisomy 18 (Hill *et al.* 1991). Incorrect scanning of the fetal posterior fossa may falsely create the appearance of a dilated cisterna magna, as a result of scanning in a plane inferior to or angled more coronally than the routine axial plane.

An overall mortality rate of 12–50% has been reported in fetuses with Dandy–Walker syndrome (Nyberg *et al.* 1988). However, the prognosis for survivors is uncertain, ranging from normal development to severe disability. Prenatal recognition of this anomaly should prompt a detailed examination of the fetus to look for other abnormalities that may indicate an underlying genetic syndrome or aneuploidy, or other intracerebral abnormalities, as these will all alter the prognosis. Karyotyping should be offered. In cases with isolated Dandy–Walker syndrome, consultation with a pediatric neurologist may be helpful. Termination of pregnancy when detected before viability is an option in view of the variable outcome in isolated cases. It has been reported that the Dandy–Walker variant is a less severe anomaly than the classic Dandy–Walker malformation (Keogan *et al.* 1994). Other studies have reported that the overall guarded prognosis is similar for fetuses with Dandy–Walker malformations and Dandy–Walker variant and that the latter have a higher prevalence of karyotypic abnormalities (Nyberg *et al.* 1988). Fetuses with an antenatal diagnosis of Dandy–Walker syndrome detected before 21 weeks' gestational age tend to have worse prognosis than fetuses with a later prenatal diagnosis of the same defect (Ulm *et al.* 1997). In the absence of a recognizable syndrome, the empiric recurrence risk is around 5% (Murray *et al.* 1985).

## HYDRANENCEPHALY (see p. 225)

Hydranencephaly is defined as complete or almost complete destruction of the fetal cortex and basal ganglia. The cerebral hemispheres are replaced by cerebrospinal fluid. The thalami are usually preserved and the cerebellum has been reported as normal, small or occasionally absent. The loss of the cerebral tissue corresponds to the distribution of the anterior middle cerebral arteries and it is thought that a transient vascular insult is responsible for this condition (Russel *et al.* 1984). Other suggested etiologies include cytomegalovirus, herpes simplex virus, and maternal smoking.

On sonographic examination the head circumference is usually normal or small for gestational age. The cranial vault is fluid-filled with no cerebral cortex evident (Fig. 17.4A). A midline separation resulting from an intact falx may be seen. The thalami are usually evident with a mid-

**Figure 17.2 Agenesis of the corpus callosum.** (A) Axial view at 24 weeks. Absence of the main nerve fibers crossing the midline results in a prominent intrahemispheric fissure (arrows). Note the three parallel lines in the midline, the lateral ones (1 and 3) representing the medial borders of the separated hemispheres and the middle one (2), the falx cerebri. The occipital horns are mildly dilated (*). (B) Axial view in agenesis of the corpus callosum. The third ventricle, 3V, is mildly enlarged as a result of its upward displacement. Note the increased separation of the anterior hemispheres, the teardrop shape of the lateral ventricles and the absence of the cavum septum pellucidum. LVB, lateral ventricle body; At, atrium. (C) Axial view in agenesis of the corpus callosum. The third ventricle (*) is elevated and markedly dilated. The cavum septum pellucidum is absent. The occipital horn of the lateral ventricle, At, is larger (colpocephaly) than the anterior hemispheres (arrows). T, thalamus. (D) (see also color plate section) Mid-sagittal view in a normal fetus. Color Doppler shows the presence of the pericallosal artery, PCA, which is characterized by a semicircular vessel running along the superior surface of the hypoechoic corpus callosum (arrows). *, Cavum septum pellucidum; T, thalamus. (E) Mid-sagittal view in a fetus with corpus callosum agenesis. There is an upward displacement (arrows) of the 3rd ventricle (3v). T, thalamus; C, cerebellum.

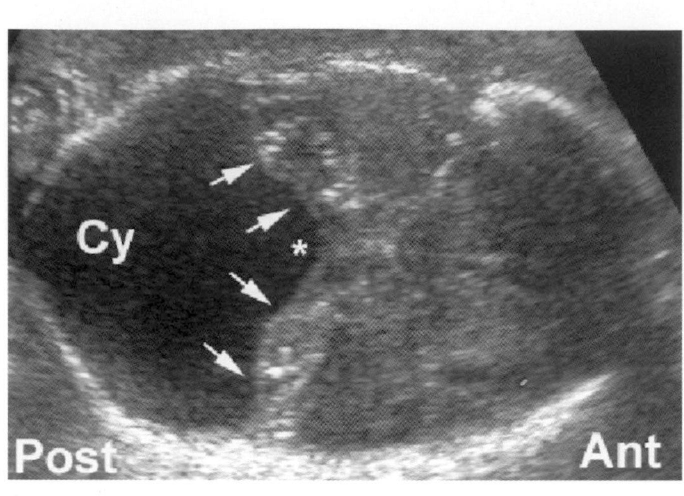


A

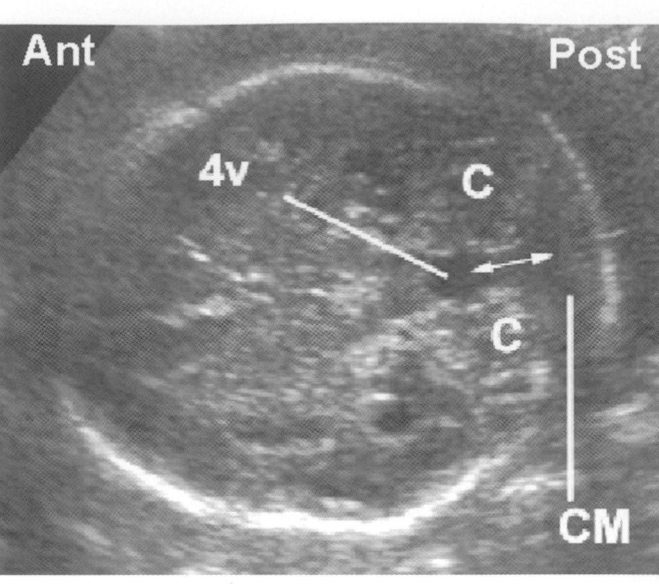


B

**Figure 17.3 Dandy–Walker syndrome.** (A) Axial view in Dandy–Walker malformation. The cisterna magna (Cy) is markedly dilated and communicates with the area of the 4th ventricle (*). The cerebellar hemispheres are separated due to the absence of the vermis (arrows). (B) Axial view in Dandy–Walker variant. There is a communication between the 4th ventricle (4v) and the cisterna magna (CM) through a defect in the cerebellar vermis (arrow). Note that the cisterna magna is not enlarged and that the cerebellar hemispheres (C) are not separated.

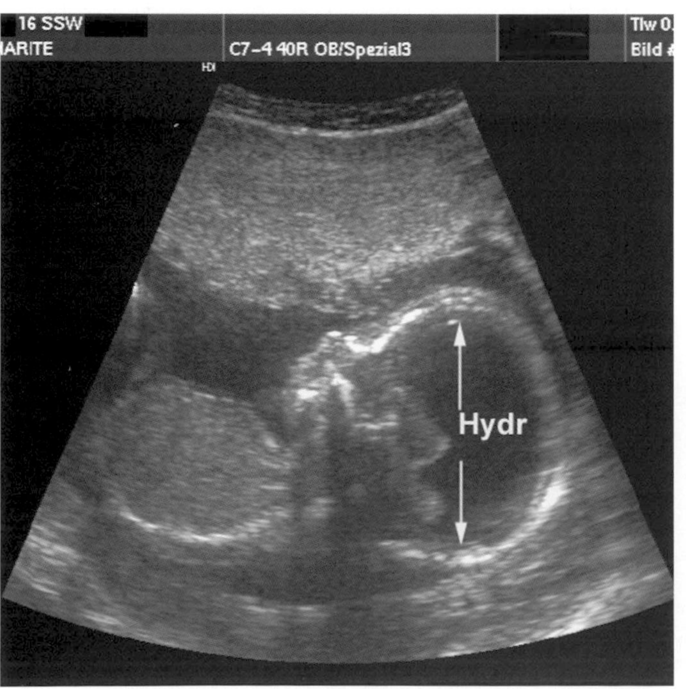


A

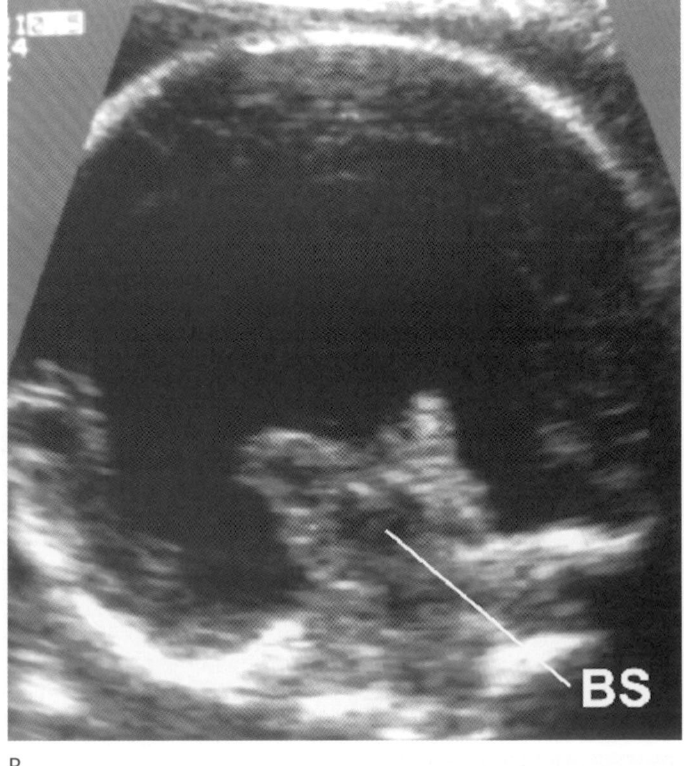


B

**Figure 17.4 Hydranencephaly.** (A) Mid-sagittal view in hydranencephaly at 16 weeks gestation. The cerebral cortex is absent with preservation of the brain stem. (B) Coronal view in hydranencephaly in the third trimester. Note that the intracranial cavity is entirely filled with fluid; however, the brain stem (BS) is still present.

line separation (Fig. 17.4B); the 3rd ventricle, choroid plexus, and cerebellum may also be seen. The main differential diagnoses include severe hydrocephalus and alobar holoprosencephaly. Absence of a midline echo, fused thalami, and facial abnormalities will indicate the presence of holoprosencephaly, whilst a dilated 3rd ventricle would suggest a diagnosis of severe hydrocephalus rather than hydranencephaly.

The sonographic evolution of hydranencephaly has been reported following intracranial hemorrhage (Edmondson *et al.* 1992). The findings are of a bright, hyperechoic mass consistent with a diagnosis of an intracranial hemorrhage. With time the echodense mass becomes more sonolucent as hydranencephaly develops. Polyhydramnios is also a common feature.

The prognosis is poor and the pregnancy usually ends in a perinatal death. However, survival for up to a year has been reported, with all infants being severely handicapped. In view of the poor prognosis, termination of pregnancy is a reasonable option. Recurrence is rare unless associated with alloimune thrombocytopenia.

## INTRACRANIAL HEMORRHAGE (see also Chapter 21)

This results from bleeding into the fetal brain and may occur spontaneously or in association with a variety of maternal or fetal conditions. The most frequent etiology is fetal alloimmune thrombocytopenia caused by maternal sensitization to fetal platelet antigens. The most commonly involved and the most clinically severe platelet antigen in caucasians being HPA-1a (Kuhn *et al.* 1992). In view of this association maternal blood should be taken to screen for anti-platelet antibodies. If positive there is a high risk of recurrence of fetal intracranial hemorrhage in subsequent pregnancies. However, the finding of antibody positivity in the mother does not guarantee that the fetus will be antigen positive, as the father may be heterozygous for the corresponding antigen. If the father is homozygous, cordocentesis should be performed to determine fetal platelet count followed by platelet transfusion to prevent fetal exsanguination after removal of the needle and intravenous administration of immune globulin to the mother for the rest of the pregnancy or/and further platelet transfusions. Delivery at 37 weeks by cesarean section is recommended.

Other etiologies include infection, congenital vascular defects, maternal drug ingestion (warfarin, cocaine), epilepsy, trauma, cholestasis of pregnancy, and other conditions that will result in fetal thrombocytopenia (thrombocytopenia absent radius syndrome, fetal congenital factor-X and factor-V deficiencies). Twin–twin transfusion with the demise of a co-twin, feto-maternal hemorrhage and hypoxic–ischemia due to maternal complications of pregnancy such as pre-eclampsia and a ruptured placenta, and episodes triggering fluctuations in blood pressure have also been implicated in the etiology of *in utero* intracranial hemorrhage.

The early signs of intracranial hemorrhage consist of irregular hyperechoic lesions in the brain parenchyma or ventricular system, which distort the normal intracranial structures (Fig. 17.5A). The echodense mass may start to

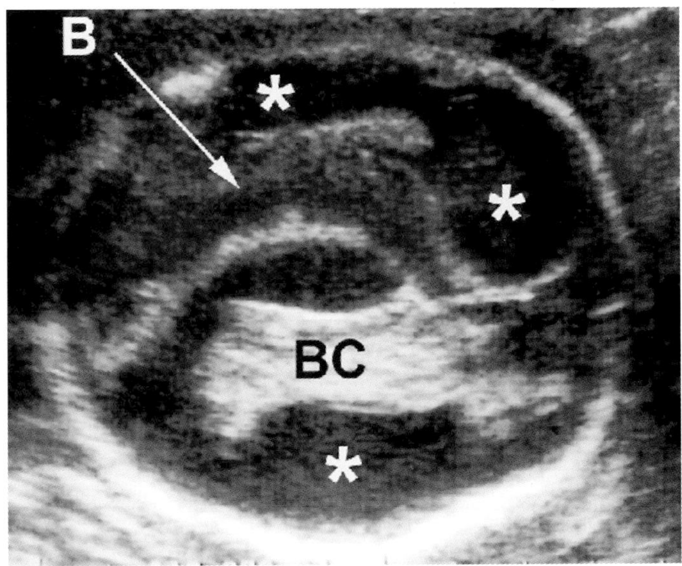


A

B

**Figure 17.5 Intracranial hemorrhage.** (A) Axial view in a fetus at 29 weeks with earlier intracranial hemorrhage. There is an irregular hyperechoic lesion corresponding to a blood clot, BC. The brain parenchyma, B, and ventricular system (*) is completely distorted. (B) Axial view in a fetus at 28 weeks gestation with earlier intracranial hemorrhage. There is severe hydrocephaly with both the hemispheres being replaced by fluid. There is only a thin rim of cerebral cortex visible (arrows).

liquify centrally and become more sonolucent. Hydrocephalus is a common association with intracranial hemorrhage. Evolution to porencephalic cyst when the lesion connects with the ventricles or hydranencephaly following extensive hemorrhage can result. The appearances of an irregular area of mixed echogenicity may be confused with a tumor. Periventricular hemorrhage has been reported *in utero* (Achiron *et al.* 1993). The initial appearances are of echogenic areas surrounding the ventricles which gradually evolve to sonolucent areas and the development of porencephalic cysts. Hemorrhage in other areas of the brain present similarly with an initial echodense mass that gradually evolves to become sonolucent. The prognosis will depend upon the extent and site of the hemorrhage. Where sequelae such as gross hydrocephalus, hydranencephaly, severe degrees of porencephaly or microcephaly results the prognosis will be extremely poor (Fig. 17.5B) (Vergani *et al.* 1996). Maternal blood should be taken to screen for antiplatelet antibodies and maternal infection, and a history of medication or recreational drug use should be sought. In the case of extensive lesions prior to viability, termination of pregnancy is a reasonable option. Periventricular and subdural hemorrhage have been reported with good outcome (Gunn *et al.* 1985; Hannigan *et al.* 1985) although fetal death may also result (Demir *et al.* 1989).

## PORENCEPHALY (see p. 214)

A porencephalic cyst is a cavity within the cerebral hemisphere filled with cerebrospinal fluid that communicates with the subarachnoid space (external), the ventricular system (internal), neither, or both. It results from an ischemic, hemorrhagic or infective event or trauma in the second or third trimester. It has been reported following inadvertent penetration of the fetal skull during amniocentesis (Eller & Kuller 1995).

In porencephaly the head is normal or large with a fluid filled cystic lesion of variable size (but usually large) that communicates with the lateral ventricle. It does not produce a mass effect but is often associated with unilateral ventriculomegaly. The main differential diagnoses include arachnoid and interhemispheric cysts. The prognosis will depend on the extent and site of the lesion. As the sonographic findings do not usually present until after viability, expectant management is usually followed. Recurrence risk is usually low unless associated with fetal alloimmune thrombocytopenia.

## SCHIZENCEPHALY (see p. 213)

Schizencephaly is a rare congenital anomaly resulting from abnormal neuronal migration causing clefts in the cerebral hemispheres. The incidence is unknown. The clefts may be unilateral or bilateral and symmetrical and extend outwards towards the skull. Intelligence may be normal with unilateral fused clefts, but patients with large bilateral clefts invariably have developmental delay (Miller *et al.* 1985). Suggested etiological factors include ischemia, fetal hypotension, recreational drugs or infection in the first trimester.

Only cases of schizencephaly with large clefts have been detected prenatally (Komarniski *et al.* 1990). Other intracerebral findings such as ventriculomegaly, agenesis of the corpus callosum and microcephaly may be a clue to underlying schizencephaly. Discussion with a neuroradiologist may help define the diagnosis in this rare condition. Prognosis is almost certainly poor in cases of schizencephaly which present prenatally, particularly if the clefts are bilateral.

## MICROCEPHALY (see p. 211)

Microcephaly is defined as a small head (<3 standard deviations below the mean for sex and age). It is usually associated with a small brain and developmental delay, although familial microcephaly with normal intelligence can occur. The incidence of microcephaly at birth ranges from 1 in 6250 to 1 in 8500, and the etiology is heterogeneous. It may be due to a neuronal proliferation disorder (Van der Knaap & Valk 1988), environmental factors such as infection or fetal alcohol syndrome, or external compression due to craniosynostosis. Microcephaly is a recognized feature of about 500 genetic syndromes (Winter & Baraitser 2000). Recurrence risks will depend on the underlying etiology but it is estimated that between 20 and 35% of idiopathic microcephaly is genetic with an autosomal recessive inheritance pattern.

The sonographic diagnosis of microcephaly should be based on measurement of the head circumference rather than relying on the biparietal diameter. This is because the biparietal diameter can be a reflection of head shape rather than absolute size (Altman & Chitty 1997). It is also important to consider the head circumference in relation to other body parameters (Fig. 17.6A), which, if all are small, may imply either incorrect dating of the pregnancy or intrauterine growth retardation. Chervenak and coworkers found in a prospective study that microcephaly could be diagnosed reliably when the occipital–frontal diameter was <4 standard deviations (SD) of the predicted mean, the head circumference <5 SD, the ratio of the head circumference to abdominal circumference <3 SD and that of the femur length : head circumference >3 SD (Chervenak *et al.* 1987).

Unless there is gross microcephaly present it is important to obtain serial ultrasound scans to determine the trend of head growth in order to establish the diagnosis. In many cases, microcephaly is not evident until the third trimester. This is particularly of relevance when considering diagnosis in women at high risk of a recurrence. These women should be advised that serial scanning will be necessary in order to establish the diagnosis, which may not become apparent until late in pregnancy, or even after birth.

Microcephaly may be a result of congenital infection, in which case intracerebral calcification may be evident. An abnormal head shape is typical for external compression due

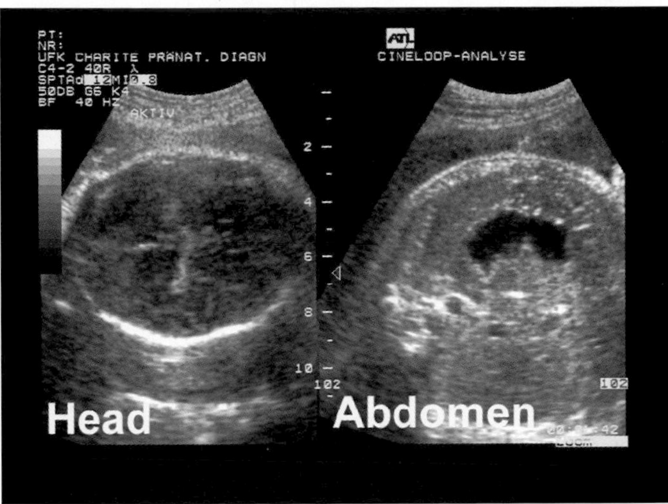


A

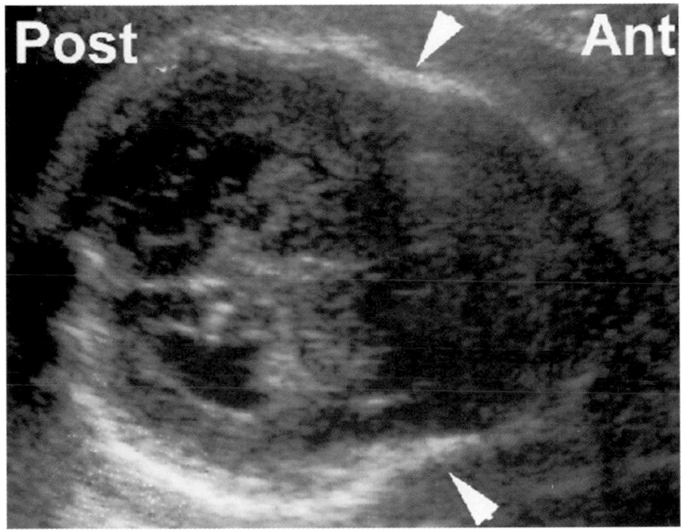


B

Figure 17.6 Microcephaly. (A) Severe microcephaly in a fetus with CMV infection as demonstrated by the small head circumference compared with the abdominal circumference. (B) Axial view in a fetus with microcephaly due to external compression (arrows) in craniosynostosis. The fetus also has mild ventriculomegaly

to craniosynostosis (Fig. 17.6B). Other associated intracranial anomalies include: lissencephaly, porencephaly, holoprosencephaly, agenesis of the corpus callosum, and ventriculomegaly, where this is secondary to brain atrophy. In view of this a detailed examination of the brain is mandatory when microcephaly is identified prenatally. As microcephaly is also a recognized feature of a number of chromosomal abnormalities and genetic syndromes, detailed sonographic examination of the fetus is required and karyotyping should be offered.

## MEGALENCEPHALY/MACROCEPHALY

Megalencephaly/macrocephaly is defined as an abnormally large head with a circumference of >2 SD above the mean. This is an uncommon abnormality with the most frequent etiology being benign familial megalencephaly. It may also occur as part of a number of genetic syndromes. In some cases, such as Beckwith–Wiedemann syndrome, there is generalized macrosomia, whereas in others, for example, achondroplasia, there is a relative macrocephaly. The head may also be enlarged secondary to an intracerebral lesion such as a tumor or obstructive hydrocephalus.

The diagnosis of megalencephaly can be made following the demonstration of a large fetal head, with the circumference lying above the 95th percentile. A detailed examination of the intracranial anatomy should be performed to rule out intracerebral lesions and other malformations. If other fetal measurements (abdominal circumference and femur length) also lie above the 95th percentile, the gestation should be confirmed, and if this is correct the diagnosis of generalized macrosomia is more likely and signs of relevant genetic syndromes should be sought. The diagnosis of benign familial megalencephaly can only be made when other fetal measurements lie within the normal range and there is a family history of large heads. One report has shown that this may not detected be until the third trimester (DeRosa *et al.* 1989).

Unilateral megalencephaly, hypertrophy of one hemisphere, can be detected *in utero*. This is often associated with ipsilateral ventricular dilatation and distortion of the midline echo. There may also be hemihypertrophy of the body and other intracranial structures such as the cerebellum and brainstem. This is usually associated with a poor outcome, unlike benign familial megalencephaly.

## INTRACRANIAL TUMOURS (see Chapter 46)

Intracranial tumours developing *in utero* are very rare. They are most commonly supratentorial (Di Rocco *et al.* 1991), with teratomas occurring more frequently than astrocytomas, craniopharyngomas and hemangioblastomas (Schlembach *et al.* 1999).

The sonographic appearance of a teratoma is that of an irregular mixed cystic and solid mass, often with areas of calcification. They usually grow rapidly, distorting the brain anatomy (Fig. 17.7). Hydrocephalus due to ventricular obstruction is common and the head circumference may be large. Polyhydramnios and high output cardiac failure have been reported (Sherer *et al.* 1993). Gliomas appear as echogenic unilateral tumors displacing the falx to the contralateral side. The sonographic appearance of choroid plexus papilloma is that of a large highly echogenic mass within the lateral ventricle associated with communicating hydrocephalus. Lipomas are well-defined echogenic masses, usually located in the midline and frequently associated with agenesis of the corpus callosum. The overall prognosis for

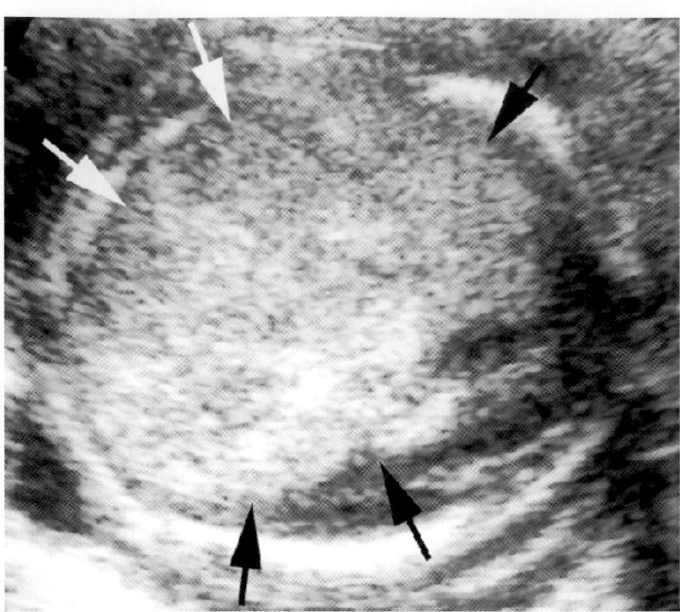

**Figure 17.7 Intracranial tumors.** Axial view in a fetus with an intracranial tumor. The mass grew rapidly over a 4-week period to fill entirely the intracranial cavity by 24 weeks. The mass was found to be a teratoma.

lipomas is good while all other intracranial tumors usually have a poor prognosis (Schlembach *et al.* 1999).

## HYDROCEPHALUS, VENTRICULOMEGALY

Both terms hydrocephalus and ventriculomegaly refer to an enlargement of the lateral ventricles due to an increase of cerebrospinal fluid, which may or may not be associated with dilatation of the 3rd and 4th ventricles (Fig. 17.8A). In general, ventriculomegaly is used to describe a more mild degree of dilatation which is usually confined to the lateral ventricles, but this can progress to frank hydrocephaly, which is one of the most common congenital anomalies, with an incidence of 0.5–3 per 1000 births.

Cerebrospinal fluid is formed mainly at the level of the choroid plexus and flows from the lateral ventricles to the 3rd ventricle and then via the cerebral aqueduct of Sylvius to the 4th ventricle. At this level, it passes through the median aperture of Magendie and then through the lateral aperture of Luschka inside the subarachnoid space. The fluid is then reabsorbed by the arachnoid granulations that are mainly distributed along the superior sagittal sinus. Hydrocephalus may be due to an obstruction (obstructive hydrocephalus) between sites of production and absorption of cerebrospinal fluid, and may be subdivided into communicating and non-communicating types. In the former, the site of obstruction is extraventricular (e.g. Arnold–Chiari malformation due to neural tube defect, encephalocele, lissencephaly) whereas in the latter, the obstruction is intraventricular (e.g., aqueduct stenosis either X-linked or idiopathic, infection including cytomegalovirus, toxoplasmosis and herpes simplex, Dandy–Walker malformation, intracranial tumors, agenesis of the corpus callosum, arachnoid cysts, aneurysm of the vein of Galen). Obstructive hydrocephalus may be associated with an increase in head circumference, whilst in the non-obstructive type, which is often secondary to primary pathology of white matter, the circumference may be normal or small. Very rarely non-obstructive hydrocephalus may be due to overproduction or reduced absorption of cerebrospinal fluid. The former condition has been observed in choroid plexus papilloma (Pilu *et al.* 1986; Anderson *et al.* 1995), and the latter in congenital absence of arachnoid granulation (Gutierrez *et al.* 1975). Hydrocephalus may be associated with a number of genetically determined syndromes and aneuploidy, although the latter is more commonly found in mild ventriculomegaly (Schlembach *et al.* 1999).

Prenatal diagnosis of fetal hydrocephalus may be difficult. In early gestation the lateral cerebral ventricles are relatively large, making the detection of pathologic dilatation difficult unless it is gross. Furthermore, in many cases ventricular dilatation does not occur until late in pregnancy, after the routine second trimester anomaly scan. Several quantitative and qualitative methods to assess the lateral ventricle have been described. The traditional method relies on measurement of the ratio of the distance from the midline echoes of the outer lateral ventricular margin to the cerebral hemispheric width. This ratio is around 90% at 15 weeks, falls to approximately 33% at 25 weeks and remains unchanged until term (Jeanty *et al.* 1981). Since the inner borders of the lateral ventricle can be accurately identified, normal ventricular size may also be verified using the largest width of the lateral ventricle in the cerebral hemisphere distal from the transducer in an axial plane at the level of the cavum septum pellucidum (Fig. 17.8B) (Pretorius *et al.* 1986; Cardoza *et al.* 1988). This measurement is normally below 10 mm and changes little from 14 to 38 weeks (Alagappan *et al.* 1994; Reece & Goldstein 1997). When screening an unselected population any measurement greater than 10 mm should be considered as potentially pathologic, but confirmation of dilatation in cases with borderline ventriculomegaly (10–12 mm) by rescanning after a week or two is essential, as dilatation may resolve spontaneously.

The most important qualitative method for assessing the lateral ventricle is the morphology of the choroid plexus, which should normally fill the atrium, but in the presence of ventriculomegaly, separation from the medial ventricular wall occurs (Fig 17.8B) (Cordoza *et al.* 1988). A separation of 3 mm or greater between the choroid plexus and the medial ventricular wall is reported to be associated with an increased risk of an abnormal outcome (Hertzberg *et al.* 1994). Ventriculomegaly may also be identified in the parasagittal plane (Fig. 17.8C). Dilatation of the 3rd ventricle, which should not normally be visible, is also a useful diagnostic aid. These qualitative parameters are

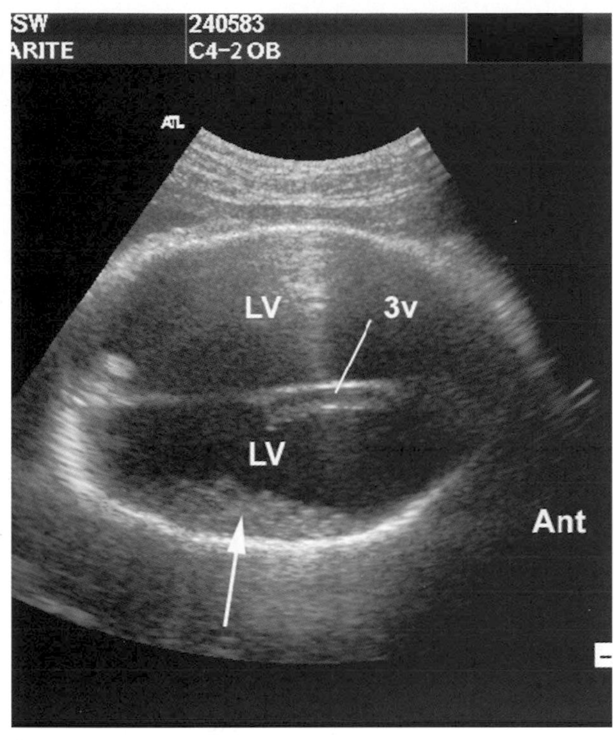


A

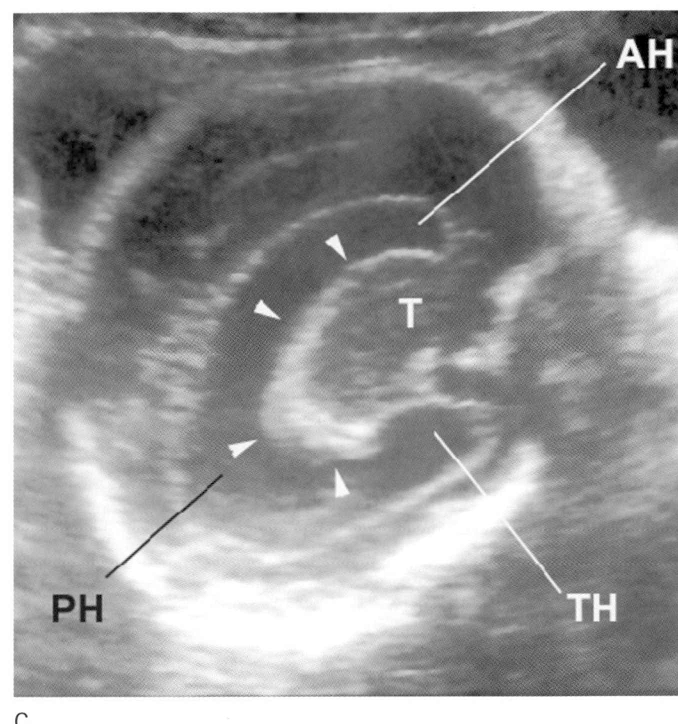


C

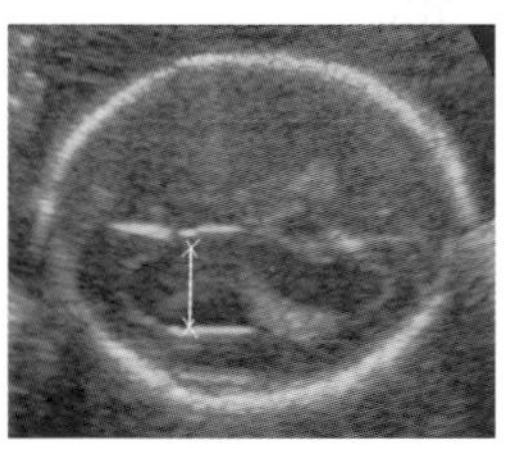

B

**Figure 17.8 Hydrocephalus.** (A) Axial view in a fetus with severe hydrocephalus at 28 weeks gestation. The lateral ventricles (LV) are enlarged; but there is still a thin rim of cerebral mantle within the distal ventricle (arrow). Note that the 3rd ventricle (3v) is enlarged, a typical feature in hydrocephalus compared with hydranencephaly. (B) Axial view in mild ventriculomegaly. The widest distance from the inner border to the outer border of the lateral ventricle (X) is measured and indicates mild dilatation. Note that there is a gap between the medial border of the lateral ventricle and the choroid plexus, which is displaced anteriorly. (C) Parasagittal view in mild ventriculomegaly. The choroid plexus (arrows) is thin and separated from the medial border of the lateral ventricle. AH, anterior horn; PH, posterior horn; TH, temporal horn; T, thalamus.

particularly useful in fetuses with borderline (10–12 mm) atrial measurements (Hilpert *et al.* 1995).

In view of the late presentation of hydrocephalus, in cases with a known increased risk, serial scanning into the third trimester is recommended. Even then a normal scan does not preclude a recurrence, as hydrocephalus can develop postnatally in some genetically determined cases. Most cases of hydrocephalus and ventriculomegaly are bilateral, but unilateral hydrocephalus has also been described (Lipitz *et al.* 1998).

Detection of ventriculomegaly or hydrocephalus should prompt a detailed scan in view of the fact that other intracranial and extracranial anomalies occur in up to 70–80% of cases. The brain and spinal cord should be examined carefully to exclude associated pathologies, and markers of aneuploidy excluded. Valat and coworkers found that the most frequent associated anomaly was a myelomeningocele (36%) followed by agenesis of the corpus callosum (11%) (Valat *et al.* 1998). Karyotyping should be discussed in all cases, but particularly when there are associated abnormalities or in the presence of mild ventriculomegaly (Goldstein *et al.* 1990; Nicolaides *et al.* 1990; Bromley *et al.* 1991). Maternal blood should be screened for infection, as should any fetal sample if an invasive procedure is done. Dommergues and coworkers showed recently that fetal serum interferon-α (IFN-α), a cytokine produced by leukocytes as a response to viral infection, was found to be detected significantly more often in the cases of ventriculomegaly with unexplained pathogenesis (Dommergues *et al.* 1996). The detection of IFN-α is suggestive of viral infection in fetuses with otherwise unexplained ventriculomegaly, and underscores the need for more extensive viral screening in such cases.

Accurate assessment of prognosis is difficult in the presence of hydrocephalus, as the literature reports predominantly selected populations, and many parents will opt to interrupt the pregnancy given an early diagnosis. Prognosis in later onset hydrocephalus will depend on the underlying etiology, but may be reasonable. In cases with early onset, severe hydrocephalus, associated abnormalities, or where aneuploidy or fetal infection is confirmed, termination of pregnancy is a reasonable option, as there is a significant risk of a poor outcome. In cases of unknown etiology, serial scanning is recommended as ventriculomegaly may often improve. Even in cases with persistent dilatation, the outcome can be good. Fetuses with this condition are reported to have around a 70% survival with normal development in 50% (Gupta *et al.* 1994).

The prognosis is better in fetuses with isolated mild ventriculomegaly (lateral ventricle width 10–15 mm), most of whom (around 85%) survive with normal development (Gupta *et al.* 1994). In cases where ventriculomegaly is associated with a normal or reduced head circumference the prognosis may be worse, as these findings imply association with white matter dysplasia.

## CHOROID PLEXUS CYSTS

Choroid plexus cysts are defined as fluid-filled space-occupying lesions present within the choroid plexus in the lateral cerebral ventricles. The precise etiology is unclear but it has been suggested that they are the result of normal epithelial folds that fill with cerebrospinal fluid and cellular debris.

The incidence of choroid plexus cysts is about 1%, but varies according to definition used and population studied (Snijders *et al.* 1994; Chitty *et al.* 1998). Whilst most fetal choroid plexus cysts resolve by around 26 weeks gestation, some persist until birth. Several studies have reported an association of choroid plexus cysts with aneuploidy, predominantly trisomy 18 where they may be present in about 30–50% of affected fetuses (Nyberg *et al.* 1993; Snijders *et al.* 1994; Gratton *et al.* 1996). The precise association with aneuploidy is difficult to define as many studies report data from populations at increased risk. However, it seems clear that when found in association with other structural abnormalities or sonographic markers of aneuploidy, or where there are other risk factors such as advanced maternal age or abnormal maternal serum biochemistry, the association with aneuploidy is increased (Snijders 1996; Chitty *et al.* 1998; Sullivan *et al.* 1999).

The normal choroid plexus has a uniform echogenic appearance. Choroid plexus cysts are usually detected on routine second trimester scan between 15 and 25 weeks of gestation when measuring the biparietal diameter, a standard measurement obtained during most fetal ultrasound examinations. They appear as round or oval sonolucent areas, clearly contrasting with the bright choroid plexus (Fig. 17.9A). They may be unilateral or bilateral, multiple or single, and vary in size from a few millimeters to large lesions measuring more than 2 cm. In a transverse plane, the proximal choroid plexus may be not visualized due to reverberation from the calvarium (Fig. 17.9B). Examination in the coronal or parasagittal plane is needed to confirm or exclude presence in the proximal hemisphere (Fig. 17.9C). When choroid plexus cysts are large they may be mistaken for ventriculomegaly (Fig. 17.9D).

Almost all choroid plexus cysts will regress by the end of the second trimester, whether or not they are associated with aneuploidy. In the absence of aneuploidy, the prognosis is good. Infant and childhood developmental follow-up of 76 children with choroid plexus cysts diagnosed prenatally showed that all of them were found to be developmentally normal (Digiovanni *et al.* 1997).

The finding of choroid plexus cysts should stimulate a detailed search for other markers of aneuploidy or structural abnormalities (Fig. 17.9E). Maternal serum screening results should be reviewed, and the level of β-hCG examined in particular as this may be low in the presence of trisomy 18. In the presence of other sonographic findings, abnormal serum biochemistry or advanced maternal age (>35 years) karyotyping should be discussed. In younger women, with no other risk factors, there is considerable debate as to what defines appropriate management after the identification of choroid plexus cysts. In general, the finding increases the prior risk slightly, but the procedural related fetal loss will often be greater than the risk of aneuploidy (Snijders 1996; Chitty *et al.* 1998).

## ARACHNOID CYSTS

Arachnoid cysts are space-occupying lesions containing cerebral spinal fluid, which are located either within the arachnoid (arachnoid cysts) or in the subarachnoid space (subarachnoid cysts). They may be midline, unilateral, bilateral, or multiple and are usually supratentorial. They can be congenital or acquired as a result of cerebral spinal fluid accumulation following hemorrhage, infection, or trauma.

The sonographic appearance of an arachnoid cyst is of a thin-walled, well-circumscribed sonolucent mass which can be uni- or multi-locular. When located on the peripheral

**Figure 17.9 Choroid plexus cysts.** (A) Axial view in bilateral choroid plexus cysts (arrows). The cysts (c) appear as sonolucent areas clearly contrasting with the bright choroid plexus. (B) Axial view in a fetus with bilateral choroid plexus cysts (c) showing that the proximal choroid plexus may not be visualized due to reverberation from the calvarium (arrows). (C) The same fetus with the proximal hemisphere now visualized showing the presence of a large choroid plexus cyst. (D) Axial view in a fetus with large choroid plexus cysts (arrows) which occupy most of the ventricle and could be mistaken for ventriculomegaly. (E) Mid-sagittal view in the same fetus showing the presence of two cysts (arrows) within the contralateral choroid plexus. Note the flat profile. The fetus was found to have trisomy 18.

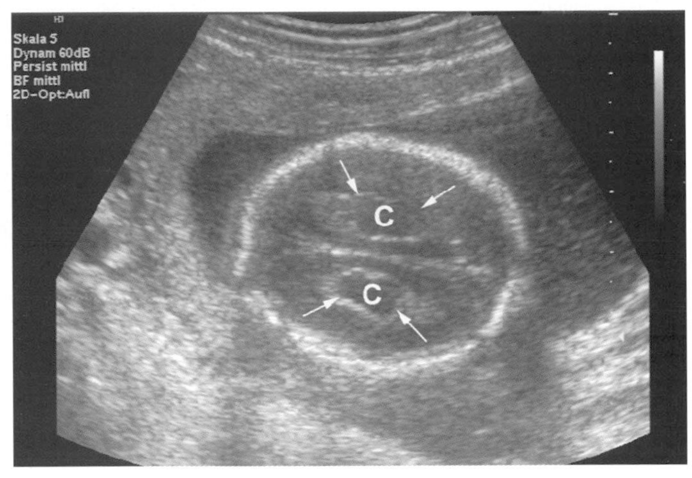
Skala 5
Dynam 60dB
Persist mittl
BF mittl
2D-Opt:Aufl
C
C

A

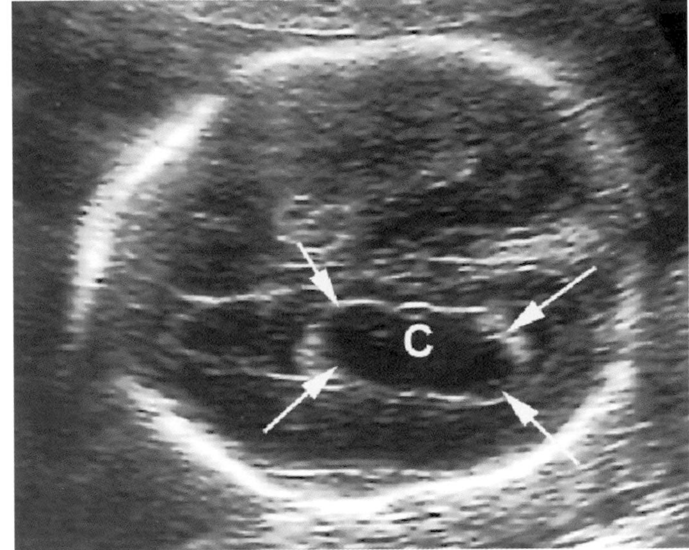
C

D

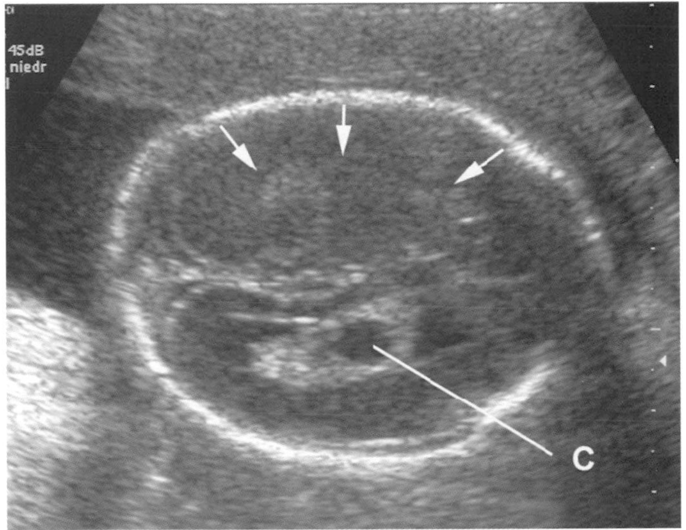
45dB
niedr
C

B

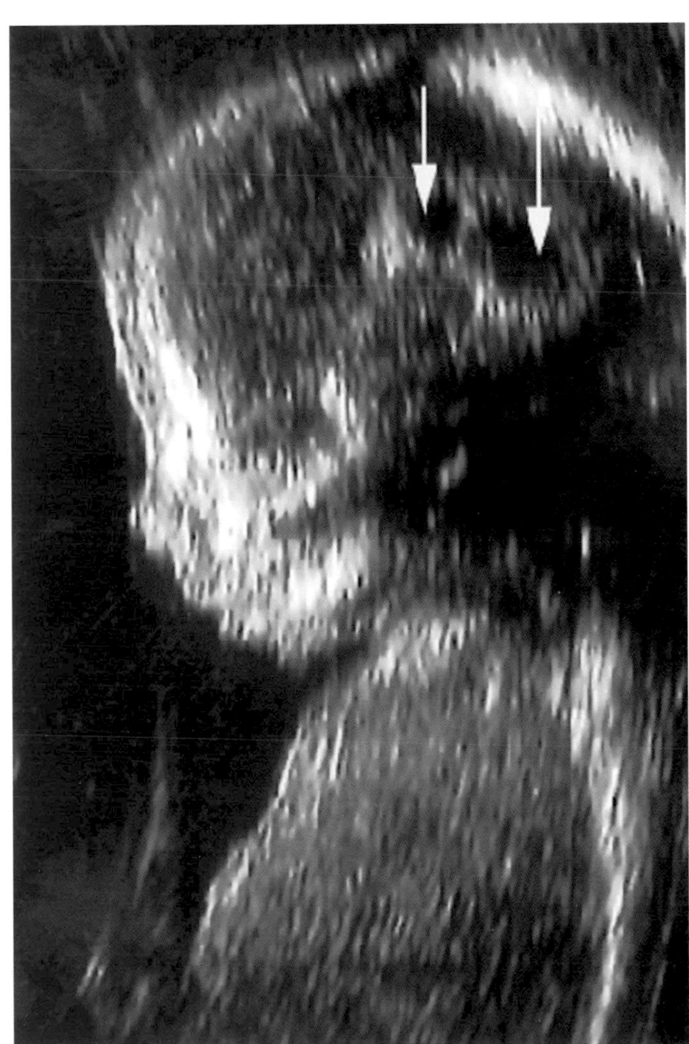

E

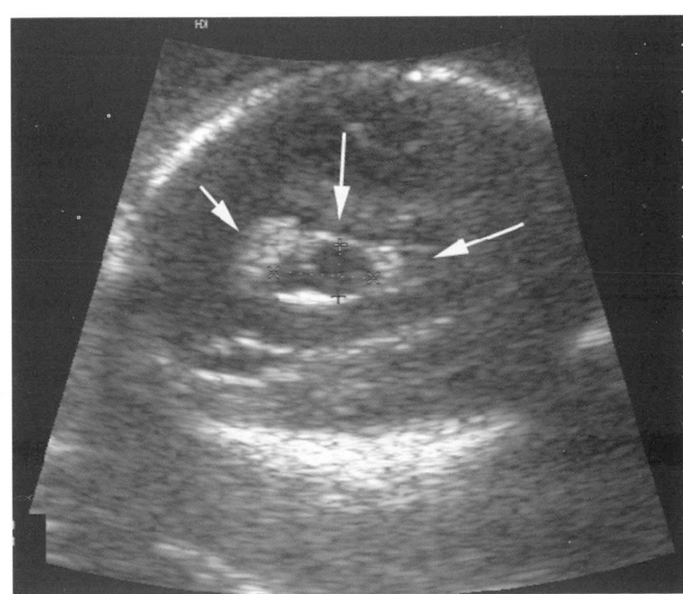

C

aspect of the brain they may be confused with a porencephalic cyst or tumor. However, unlike porencephalic cysts, they do not communicate with the ventricular system and tumors are usually located within the brain substance and are of mixed echogenicity, whereas peripheral arachnoid cysts lie between the skull and the brain surface. When in the midline, an arachnoid cyst may be confused with agenesis of the corpus callosum or an arterio-venous malformation (Fig. 17.10A,B). Less frequently, they are located in the infratentorial compartment (Fig. 17.10C), when they must be distinguished from a Dandy–Walker malformation by identifying the 4th ventricle and cerebellar vermis. Hydrocephalus may be present due to the mass effect from a large arachnoid cyst (Hassan *et al.* 1996).

Arachnoid cysts are usually isolated lesions and may occasionally be associated with other CNS malformations or extracranial abnormalities. Thus detailed sonography of the brain and the rest of the fetal anatomy is required. The outcome for the neonate is largely dependent on the location of the cysts. In spite of the large dimensions that can be reached, the clinical manifestations of arachnoid cysts may remain subtle, and between 60 and 80% of children are asymptomatic (Lena *et al.* 1995; Caldarelli & Di 1996; Bannister *et al.* 1999).

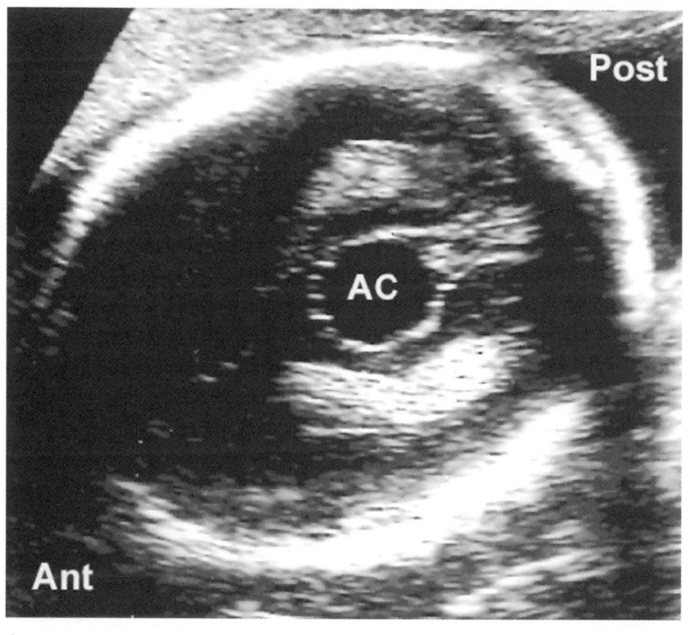


A

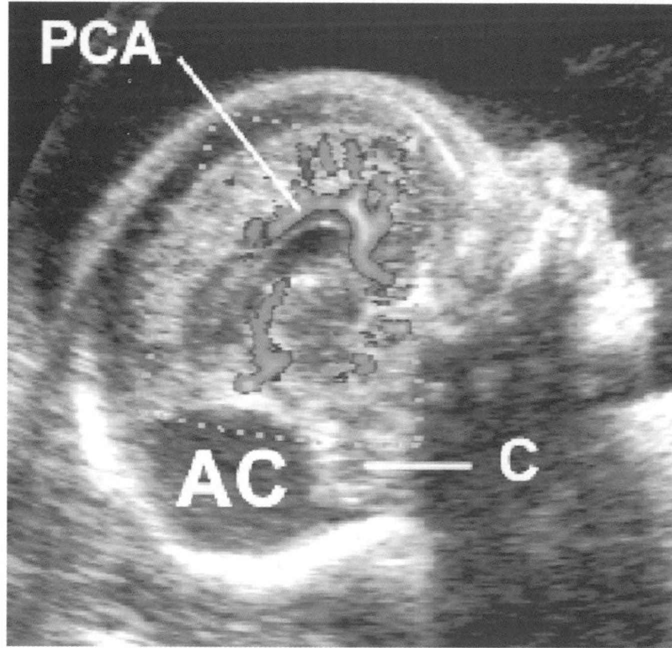


C

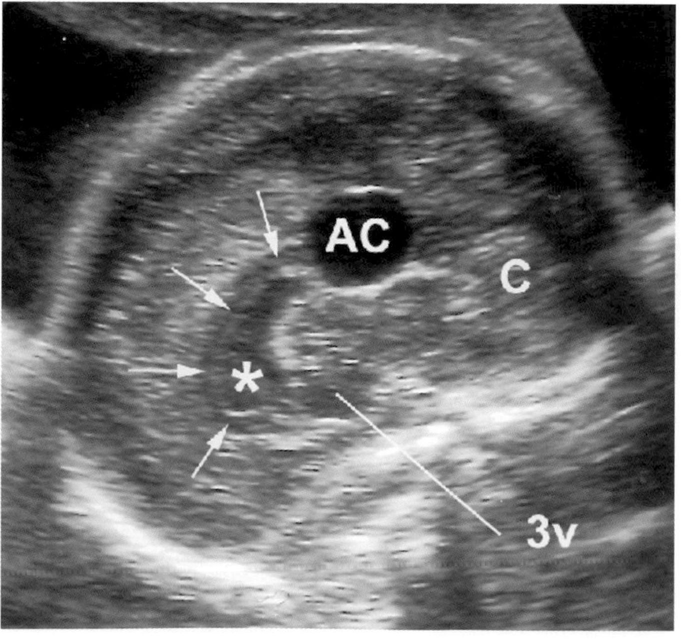


B

**Figure 17.10 Arachnoid cysts.** (A) Axial view in a fetus with a midline arachnoid cyst, AC. The cyst may be confused with a dilated 3rd ventricle as seen in agenesis of the corpus callosum. (B) Mid-sagittal view in the same fetus showing that the cyst is situated above the cerebellum, C, in the supratentorial compartment. The 3rd ventricle (3v), the cavum septum pellucidum (*) and the hypoechoic corpus callosum (arrows) are clearly visualized. (C) Mid-sagittal view in a fetus with an intratentorial archnoid cyst. In this case the cerebellum was seen above the cyst which was situated at the base of the brain. Note the normal course of the pericallosal artery, PCA, as visualized by power Doppler (see also color plate section).

## ARTERIO-VENOUS MALFORMATION (see Chapter 46)

Intracerebral arterio-venous malformations are rare, complex malformations resulting from direct arterio-venous fistulas between one or more cerebral arteries and the cerebral venous system, without intervening capillaries. In the fetus most involve the vein of Galen (Dau *et al.* 1992), although two have been reported in the frontal region (Comstock & Kirk 1991; Lee *et al.* 1994).

The sonographic appearance is of a large oval or tubular non-pulsatile sonolucent area in the midline, which may extend posteriorly to the bony cranium (Fig. 17.11A). The lesion is often surrounded by an area of increased echogenicity representing the dilated feeding vessels. Color Doppler may help to define the diagnosis by demonstrating turbulent flow within the structure (Fig. 17.11B). The lateral cerebral ventricles are usually normal, but ventriculomegaly may result, either from compression or compromise of the cerebral perfusion by diversion of blood from the brain tissue to the malformation (the so-called 'steal' phenomenon). Macrocephaly can also result. Other sonographic manifestations include enlargement of the superior vena cava, ascending aorta, and vessels leading to the head and neck. There may also be severe cardiovascular compromise manifesting as cardiomegaly, hepatomegaly, and hydrops, often with polyhydramnios. In almost all cases reported, arterio-venous malformations have presented after 30 weeks gestation (Comstock & Kirk 1991), with only a few cases being diagnosed in the second trimester (Ordorica *et al.* 1990; Ballester *et al.* 1994; Lee *et al.* 1994).

Following identification of an intracranial lesion suggestive of an arterio-venous malformation, color Doppler studies are indicated to confirm the diagnosis. As these lesions usually present late in pregnancy, expectant management should be observed with regular scanning to detect early signs of cardiac compromise. Poor prognostic

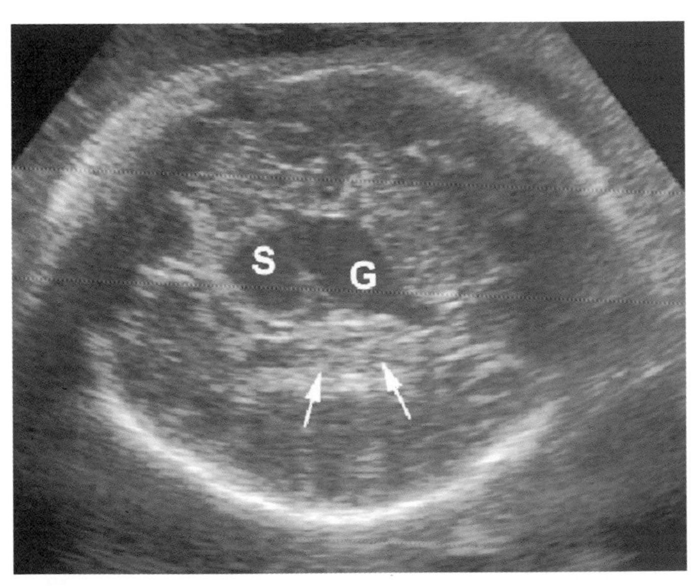


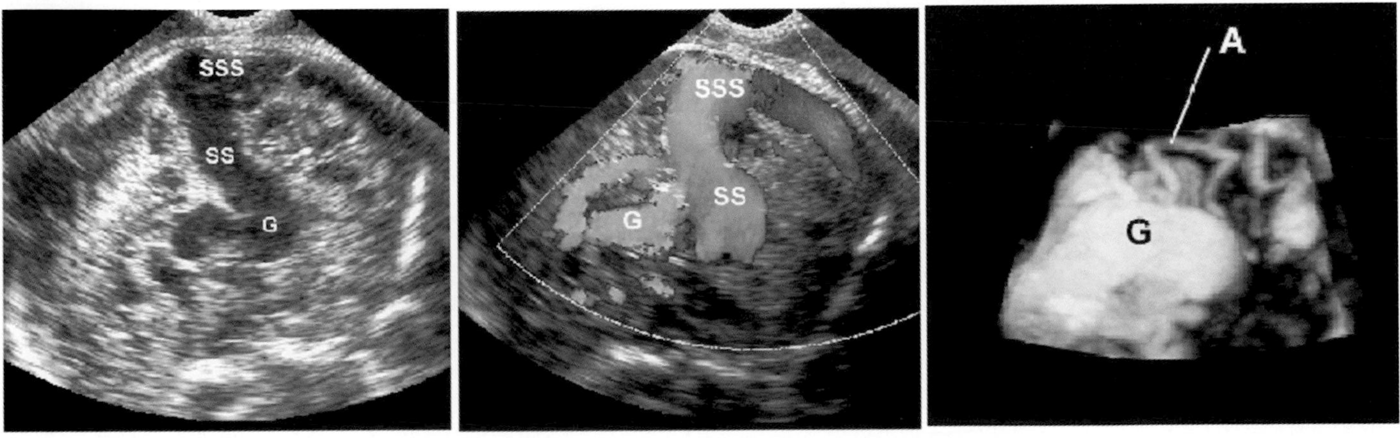


**Figure 17.11 Arterio-venous malformation.** (A) Axial view in a fetus with an arterio-venous malformation, showing the typical appearance of a vein of Galen aneurysm. There is a large tubular sonolucent area in the midline, G, which extends posteriorly, S. The lesion is often surrounded by an area of increased echogenicity representing the dilated feeding vessels (arrows). (B) Coronal section in the same fetus showing the dilated vein of Galen, G, which joins the inferior sagittal sinus, SS, which then forms the straight sinus sagittalis, SSS. (C) Same view as in (B) demonstrating confirmation by using color Doppler to show turbulent flow within the sonolucent area (see also color plate section. (D) 3-D power Doppler of the arterio-venous malformation in the same fetus. The dilated vein of Galen, G, is visualized together with the feeding artery, A.

signs are reported to include five or more feeding vessels, retrograde aortic flow and cardiomegaly (Yuval *et al.* 1997). Most studies report a very poor prognosis with early lethality if signs of severe heart failure (hydrops, cardiomegaly, etc.) are present. However, Rodesch and coworkers emphasize the high survival rate, even in the presence of cardiac failure at birth (Rodesch *et al.* 1994). They analyzed a series of 18 cases detected by ultrasound during the third trimester of pregnancy, in which 16 neonates presented with cardiac manifestations as the first clinical sign. Whilst four died shortly after birth, 12 were stabilized using medical management and subsequently underwent embolization of the arterio-venous malformation. Of those treated, 67% had a normal neurologic outcome.

## NEURAL TUBE DEFECTS (see Chapter 13)

### ANENCEPHALY AND EXENCEPHALY

Anencephaly is the absence of the cranial vault (acrania) and most parts of the brain. Cerebral hemispheres and midbrain are usually completely absent, leaving remnants of the forebrain and a generally well-formed medulla. It may be partial (meroacrania) or complete (holoacrania). In exencephaly, the brain is present but is not covered by the vault of the skull, and is therefore exposed to the amniotic fluid. There is now increasing evidence to support the theory that exencephaly is the forerunner of anencephaly with the exposed brain in exencephaly disintegrating secondary to exposure to the amniotic fluid, thus resulting in anencephaly (Timor *et al.* 1996).

Anencephaly was the first fetal malformation to be detected using transabdominal ultrasonography in a fetus of 17 weeks gestation (Campbell *et al.* 1972). In the second and third trimester the sonographic diagnosis of anencephaly is based on the symmetrical absence of the dome of the cranial vault (calvarium) (Fig. 17.12A). Variable degrees of disintegrating brain tissue may be seen. In a coronal view, facial features can be seen with the orbits clearly visible with nothing above them. The prominent, bulging eyes give the anencephalic fetus typical 'frog facies' (Fig. 17.12B). In a sagittal view, the face can be identified with normal lips and chin but the absence of the calvarium above the orbital ridge is clearly seen (Fig. 17.12A). The neck is usually short and spinal defects occur in around 50% of anencephalic fetuses. The association of limb, abdominal wall, and spinal defects in association with anencephaly suggest the limb–body-wall complex. Polyhydramnios is often a feature in the third trimester. The main differential diagnoses to be considered include severe microcephaly, where the bones of the skull may be difficult to locate but are present, and an extensive encephalocele which may have a very small ossified cranial vault. In skeletal dysplasias associated with severe degrees of hypomineralization (osteogenesis imperfecta, hypophosphatasia, and achondrogenesis type I) the skull vault may not be mineralized but the brain is present and is usually well seen because of lack of ossification of the cranial bones.

Anencephaly is uniformly lethal and termination of pregnancy should be discussed. Recurrence risk following one

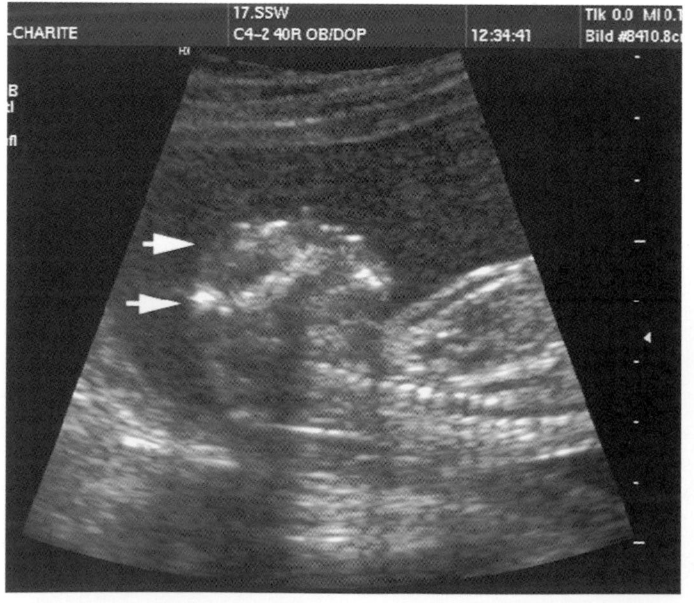


A

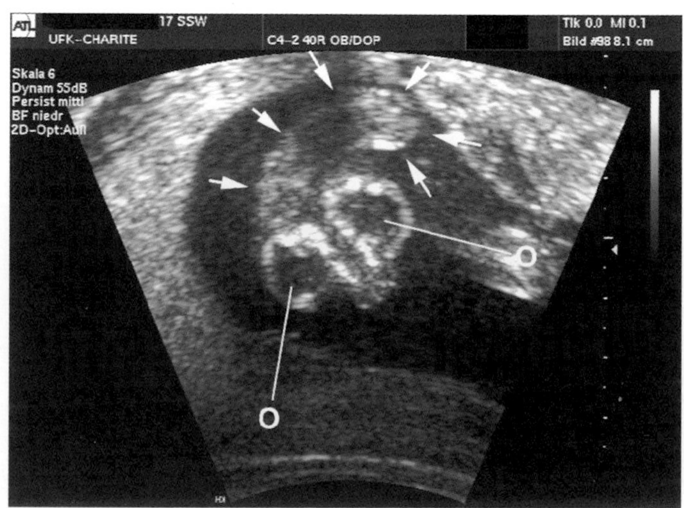


B

**Figure 17.12 Anencephaly and exencephaly.** (A) Parasagittal view in an anencephalic fetus showing the absence of the cranial vault (arrows). (B) Coronal section in a fetus with anencephaly (arrows). The prominent, bulging orbits (O) give the fetus typical 'frog facies'.

neural tube defect is around 3%, and this can be halved by taking periconceptual folic acid (Wald 1994). It is important to exclude amniotic bands as an etiology of the anencephaly, as recurrence risk in this situation is extremely small and will not be influenced by folic acid. This diagnosis usually has to await postnatal examination, unless there are obvious bands seen *in utero*.

## INIENCEPHALY

Iniencephaly is a complex malformation, consisting of exencephaly but with the bony defects restricted to the occipital region of the skull, partial or total absence of the cervical and thoracic vertebrae, rachichisis of the cervical and thoracic spine, together with fixed retroflexion of the head. There are two types: apertus (with) and clausus (without) an associated encephalocele. Other intracranial and extracranial anomalies, including hydrocephalus, holoprosencephaly, diaphragmatic hernia, urinary tract anomalies, cleft lip and palate, omphalocele and talipes, occur commonly in fetuses with iniencephaly (David & Nixon 1976).

Iniencephaly is suggested when a marked kyphoscoliosis of the spine is seen in association with fixed retroflexion of the head. An occipital encephalocele may be identifiable together with spina bifida in the cervical and thoracic area. Detailed examination of the rest of the fetus should be performed in view of the high association with extracranial abnormalities. However, as the condition is uniformly lethal, the finding of other malformations will not alter management. This is an anomaly that is readily detectable in the second trimester of pregnancy, and termination of pregnancy is a reasonable option. In the third trimester polyhydramnios may be a feature.

## CEPHALOCELE AND ENCEPHALOCELE

Cephaloceles are defined as a herniation of intracranial contents through a bony defect in the skull. Herniation of the meninges alone is termed meningocele and if there is brain tissue present as well, encephalocele. When the cerebellum is herniated as part of the cephalocele this is the Chiari type III deformity. Cephaloceles are subdivided into occipital, parietal and frontal types according to the location of the bony defect. The occurrence of the different types reflects geographic variation. They characteristically arise in the midline, with 75% of encephaloceles in the western population occurring in the occipital area followed by 13% in the frontal, with midline and parietal lesions accounting for only 12% of lesions (Chervenak *et al.* 1984). Occipital encephaloceles usually occur as an isolated lesion but may occur as part of a chromosomal (Wininger & Donnenfeld 1984) or genetic (Winter & Baraitser 2000) syndrome. The most common genetic syndrome found is the Meckel–Gruber syndrome, an autosomal recessive condition associated with bilateral enlarged cystic kidneys, polydactyly, and occasionally cardiac defects (Nyberg *et al.* 1990). Encephaloceles may also result from a disruption in the formation of the fetal skull as in amniotic band syndrome. In this situation they may be multiple or located asymmetrically.

Sonographic signs consist of a sac-like protrusion that may be irregular in outline extending from the head, most commonly in the occipital area, but it can be seen in the frontal or parietal regions. The size of the cephalocele may range from a mass exceeding the size of a cranial vault (Fig. 17.13A) to a few millimeters (Fig. 17.13B). The mass is covered by a membrane and when sonolucent represents herniation of the meninges alone (Fig. 17.13C). The diagnosis of an encephalocele is suggested when the contents of the sac are heterogeneous (Fig. 17.13A). The diagnosis of a cephalocele can only be made with certainty if a skull defect is identified with continuity between the contents of the extruded sac and intracranial structures. Identification of the bony defect can be difficult. With an encephalocele there can be distortion of the remaining intracranial contents and the lemon sign (characteristically associated with spina bifida) occurs in approximately 25% of cases. Microcephaly may be a feature if the encephalocele is large. In the absence of identification of a skull defect the main differential diagnoses include a cystic hygroma, cervical myelomeningocele, hemangioma, or epidermal cyst of the skull. Nasal teratomas and dacryocystoceles must be distinguished from anterior encephaloceles (Fig. 17.13C).

In view of the association with aneuploidy and other genetic syndromes, a detailed examination of the fetus is required and karyotyping should be offered. Prognosis depends on the location, size, content of the lesion, and presence or absence of other malformations. In isolated cephaloceles reported mortality is around 40% and there can be a significant incidence of intellectual and neurologic handicap in survivors. However, this may reflect bias in reporting as the pediatric literature does not support this apparent poor prognosis. Good prognostic signs include absence of brain tissue from the sac and an anterior location, but when present with other defects prognosis is poor. (Brown & Sheridan 1992). The empiric recurrence risk for an isolated occipital encephalocele is around 3%. When occurring as part of a genetic syndrome, the recurrence risk will be that of the syndrome.

## SPINA BIFIDA

Spina bifida results from non-fusion of the vertebral arch surrounding the spinal cord and is associated with exposure or protrusion of the spinal contents through the bony defect. When covered by skin it is called spina bifida occulta (closed spina bifida) which is more common than spina bifida aperta (open spina bifida) where there is no skin covering. If the sac only contains dura, arachnoid, and cerebro-spinal fluid it is termed a meningocele, whereas if there is also nervous tissue it is a myelomeningocele. The term rachichisis defines a widely patent dorsal opening of the spine with or without residual spinal cord. Myelomeningocele is the second most

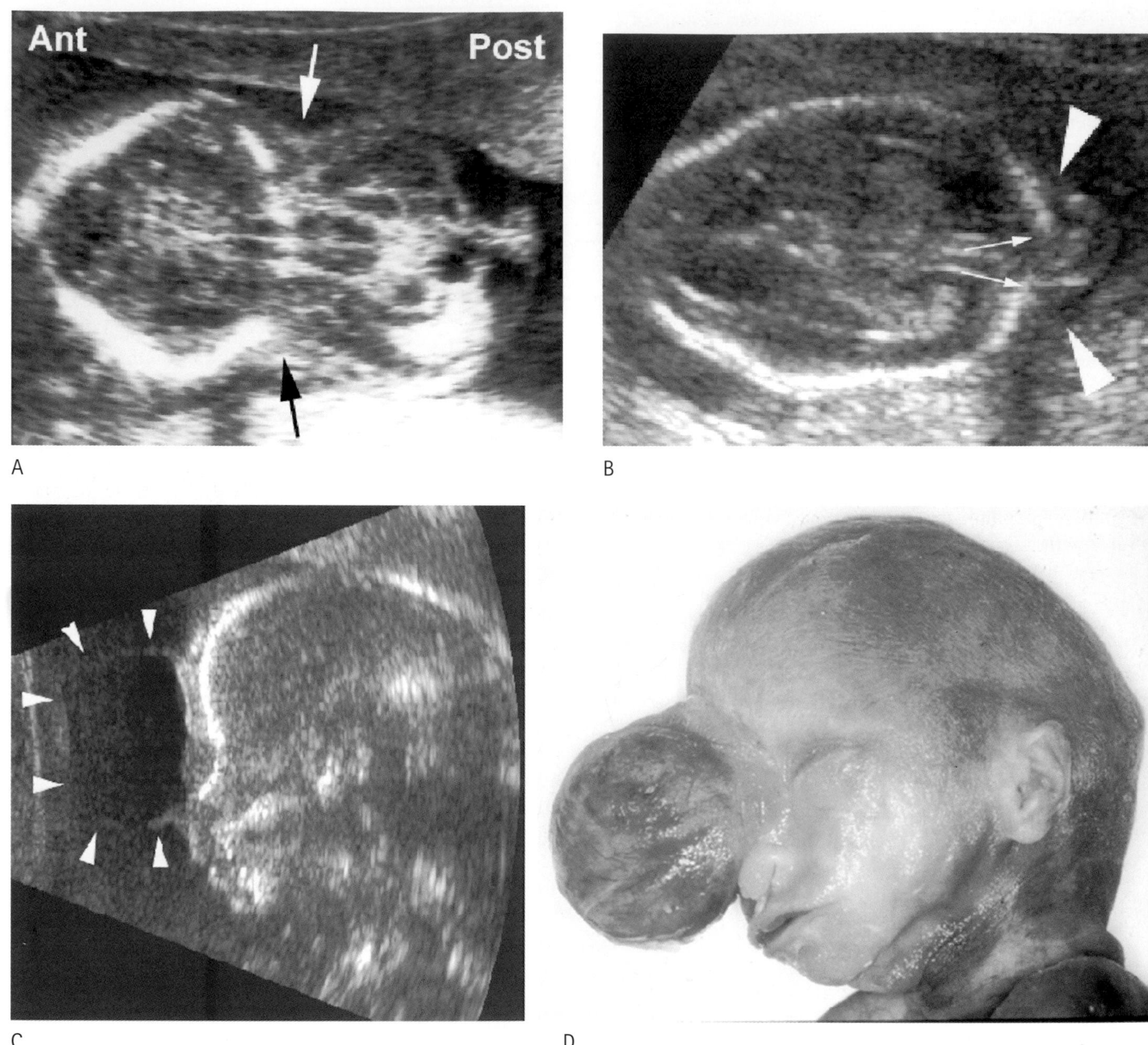


Figure 17.13 **Encephalocele.** (A) Axial view in a fetus at 22 weeks with a large occipital encephalocele (arrows). There is distortion of the remaining intracranial structures with marked microcephaly. Note the heterogeneous contents of the sac, which represents brain tissue. (B) Transversal view in a fetus with a small posterior encephalocele. There is a clear defect of the calvarium (small arrows) through which a small sac has herniated. (C) Mid-sagittal view in a fetus with a large anterior cephalocele. The sonolucent mass is covered by a membrane and there is no herniation of brain tissue. (D) Postmortem view of the same fetus.

common open neural tube defect, and as with other neural tube defects shows considerable geographic variation.

Spina bifida most commonly occurs as an isolated abnormality or with hydrocephalus, or abnormalities such as talipes that are secondary to the presence of the spina bifida. However, it is also seen as part of some chromosomal syndromes (Kennedy *et al.* 1998) or genetic syndromes. Environmental factors are also important, with an increased incidence seen in epileptic women, particularly those who are taking sodium valproate or carbamazepine during pregnancy.

The fetal spine can be examined in the sagittal, axial, and coronal planes from late in the first trimester onwards. The recognition of spinal defects requires a systematic examination of each neural arch from the cervical to the sacral region. On transverse section, the open spine has a U-shape

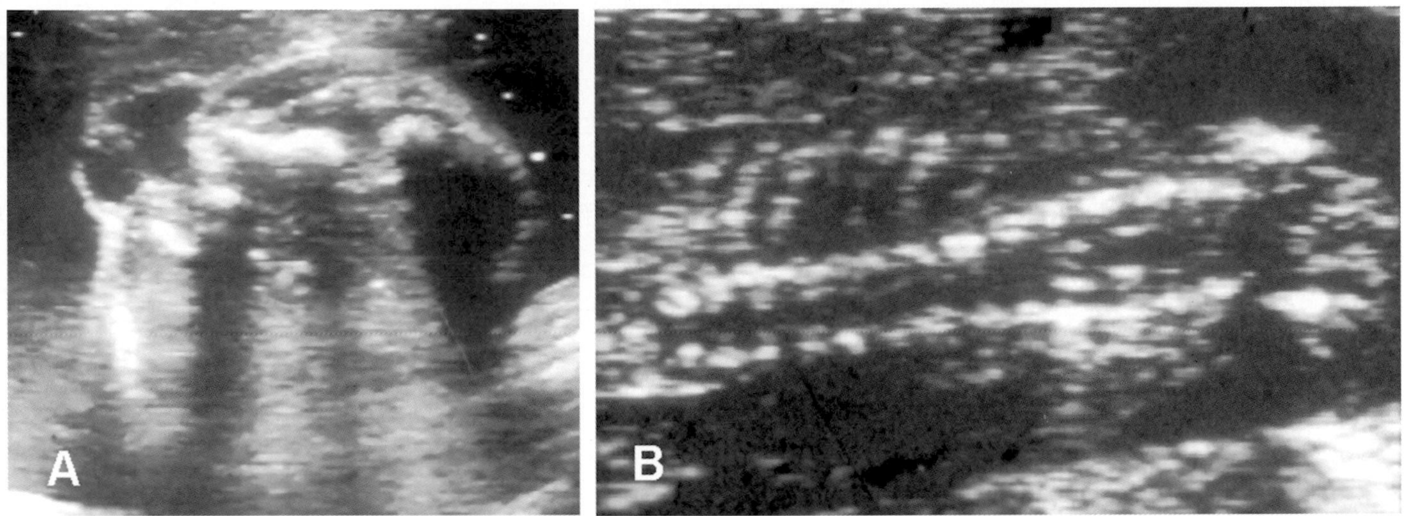


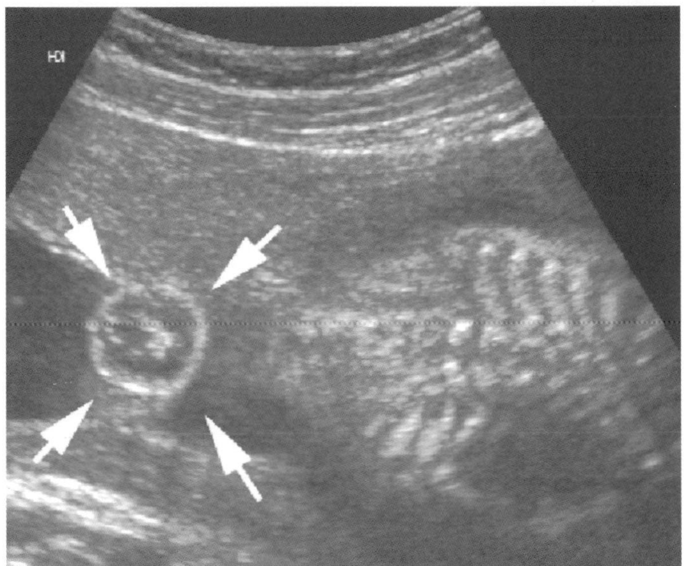

C

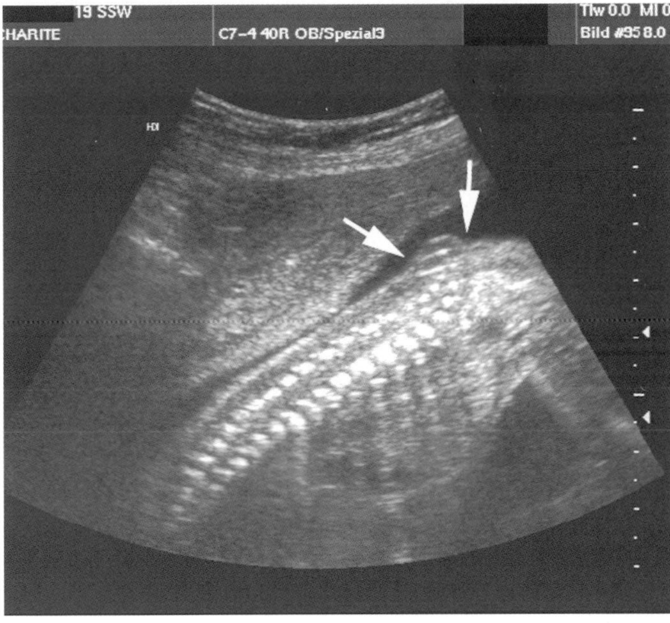


D

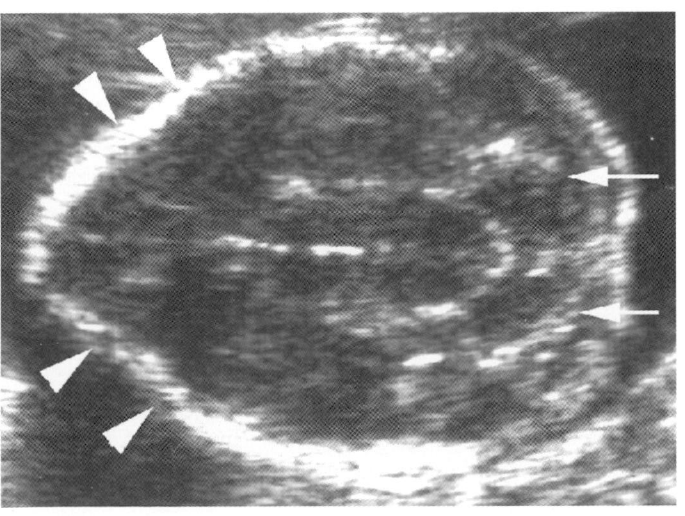

E

**Figure 17.14 Spina bifida.** (A) Axial section of the spine in fetus with spina bifida. The open spine has a typical U-shape with overlying meningocele. (B) Coronal section in the same fetus showing the divergent configuration of the affected segment of spine. (C) The presence of a meningocele or myelomeningocele (arrows) may be recognized in a frontal plane just posterior to the plane of the spine. (D) Sagittal view of the spine in a fetus with spina bifida. There is a small cystic extension from the posterior aspect of the spine (arrows). (E) Transversal view through the cerebellum in a fetus with spina bifida at 20 weeks gestation. The two typical indirect signs of this malformation are shown. The 'lemon sign' (arrowheads) refers to a loss of the convex outward shape of the frontal bones. The 'banana sign' (small arrows) refers to the banana-shaped appearance of the cerebellum, which is due to its downward displacement into the foramen magnum.

(Fig. 17.14A). However, it is the cleft in the soft tissues that is recognized more easily than the bony defect itself, such that closed lesions are relatively rarely detected *in utero*. On a coronal section, the affected bony segment shows a divergent configuration which replaces the typical parallel lines of the normal vertebral arches (Fig. 17.14B). In the presence of a meningocele or myelomeningocele the defect, overlying skin and tissues may be seen as a cystic extension from the posterior aspect of the spine (Fig. 17.14C). In the sagittal plane the defect, overlying skin and tissues may be seen (Fig. 17.14D). The presence of neural tissue within the sac indicates the presence of a myelomeningocele. However, sonography cannot reliably distinguish between meningocele and myelomeningocele.

There are several cranial features associated with spina bifida. In the second trimester fetuses with open spina bifida tend to have a disproportionately smaller biparietal diameter for the gestational age (Wald *et al.* 1980) and varying degrees of ventriculomegaly occur in almost all fetuses by the third trimester, but only in about 70% of cases in the second trimester. In 1986, Nicolaides and coworkers reported the lemon and banana signs (Fig. 17.14E), which have been a significant aid to the prenatal sonographic diagnosis of spina bifida (Nicolaides *et al.* 1986). The lemon sign refers to a loss of the convex outward shape of the frontal bones with mild flattening. It is present in virtually all fetuses with spina bifida between 16 and 24 weeks gestation, but is a less reliable marker after 24 weeks gestation when it is only present in 30–50% of cases (Nyberg *et al.* 1988; Penso *et al.* 1987; Thiagarajan *et al.* 1990). In the majority of cases of spina bifida, the cerebellum is either not detectable sonographically or has a banana-shaped appearance. Downward displacement of the cerebellum into the foramen magnum causing the Arnold–Chiari type II malformation occurs in almost all cases of thoraco-lumbar and lumbar-sacral myelomeningoceles. With the inferior displacement of the medulla and fourth ventricle into the upper cervical canal, the cerebellum becomes compressed and is flattened at the indentation of the level of the vermis. This abnormal shape may be seen from 14 weeks onwards (Blumenfeld *et al.* 1993). Cerebellar abnormalities are present in 95% of fetuses irrespective of gestation. However, the cerebellar abnormality seen most commonly before 24 weeks gestation is the banana sign (72%) whereas in later pregnancy the cerebellum is more often absent (81%) (Van den Hof *et al.* 1990).

The recognition of the lemon and banana signs has considerably enhanced the prenatal sonographic diagnosis and screening for spina bifida in both low and high risk populations. Examination of the low lumbar sacral region of the spine can be difficult in the second trimester and lesions in this area can be readily missed. However, the head is more readily visualized and identification of the intracranial signs associated with spina bifida should stimulate a detailed sonographic examination of the spine. This has resulted in a significantly increased detection rate of spina bifida using ultrasound alone in the second trimester (Chitty 1995).

Following the identification of spina bifida, detailed examination of the fetus should be performed both to look for other signs that may indicate an associated chromosomal or genetic syndrome, and also to look for evidence of neurologic damage such as talipes or a dilated renal tract. Karyotyping should be offered when other abnormalities are detected or other risk factors such as raised maternal age are present. In a recent analysis of 200 fetuses with neural tube defects, 6.5% had chromosomal abnormalities (Kennedy *et al.* 1998). However, the absence of associated sonographic abnormalities was not necessarily predictive of a normal karyotype, with 2.4% of fetuses in this category having a chromosomal abnormality. Conversely, 72% of fetuses with additional findings on ultrasound had normal chromosomes. When classified according to the site of the neural tube defect, 2.3% of anencephalics, 7.1% of encephaloceles, and 10.2% of myelomeningoceles had an abnormal karyotype.

A sonographic estimation of the level of the lesion may be a useful aid to counseling. The following landmarks may be helpful in assessing the level of involvement. In the second trimester, the last sacral ossification center is S4 and in the third trimester it is S5. T12 can be localized by identifying the last ribs, alternatively the site of the lesion can be estimated by counting upwards from the tip of the sacrum. One study has reported an accurate sonographic estimation of the level of the spinal defect to within one spinal segment in 79% of cases (Kollias *et al.* 1992). However, ultrasound has not proved to be particularly accurate in terms of predicting postnatal function. In general, the prognosis is worse the higher and the larger the lesion, and in the presence of associated abnormalities (Lorber 1971). Normal fetal lower limb movements and an intact urinary tract appear to have little prognostic value, nor does the extent of the intracerebral lesion appear to be predictive of the severity of outcome (Lorber 1971). Low sacral lesions may have a good outcome associated with normal mobility but are almost always associated with incontinence. Spina bifida occulta will usually be asymptomatic, but is rarely diagnosed prenatally.

## CONCLUSION

With advances in ultrasound technology a wide range of CNS abnormalities are now amenable to prenatal diagnosis. Other modalities such as magnetic resonance imaging may be helpful in defining the underlying pathology, but we lack data on the natural history and long-term outcome for many prenatally diagnosed abnormalities. Thus prenatal counseling of parents whose fetus has an unexpected CNS abnormality may be very difficult.

**Key Points**

- Advances in ultrasound technology have increased the potential to diagnose a wide range of central nervous system structural abnormalities
- When an abnormality is identified it is important that there is a detailed search for any additional abnormalities in the rest of the fetus since their presence markedly alters prognosis
- In some circumstances the use of other imaging modalities, such as MRI, may contribute to the diagnosis
- An incomplete understanding of natural history and lack of long-term follow-up makes prenatal counseling challenging and, when possible, the help of pediatricians and geneticists may prove invaluable

## REFERENCES


Achiron R, Pinchas O H, Reichman B *et al.* (1993) Fetal intracranial haemorrhage: clinical significance of *in utero* ultrasonographic diagnosis [see comments]. *Br J Obstet Gynaecol* 100(11): 995–999.

Alagappan R, Browning P D, Laorr A & McGahan J P (1994) Distal lateral ventricular atrium: reevaluation of normal range. *Radiology* 193(2): 405–408.

Altman D G & Chitty L S (1997) New charts for ultrasound dating of pregnancy. *Ultrasound Obstet Gynecol* 10(3): 174–191.

Anderson D R, Falcone S, Bruce J H *et al.* (1995) Radiologic-pathologic correlation. Congenital choroid plexus papillomas. *Am J Neuroradiol* 16(10): 2072–2076.

Ballester M J, Raga F, Serra S V & Bonilla M F (1994) Early prenatal diagnosis of an ominous aneurysm of the vein of Galen by color Doppler ultrasound. *Acta Obstet Gynecol Scand* 73(7): 592–595.

Bannister C M, Russell S A, Rimmer S & Mowle D H (1999) Fetal arachnoid cysts: their site, progress, prognosis and differential diagnosis. *Eur J Pediatr Surg* 9(Suppl 1): 27–28.

Barr M, Hanson J W, Currey K *et al.* (1983) Holoprosencephaly in infants of diabetic mothers. *J Pediatr* 102(4): 565–568.

Bennett G L, Bromley B & Benacerraf B R (1996) Agenesis of the corpus callosum: prenatal detection usually is not possible before 22 weeks of gestation. *Radiology* 199(2): 447–450.

Blumenfeld Z, Siegler E & Bronshtein M (1993) The early diagnosis of neural tube defects. *Prenat Diagn* 13(9): 863–871.

Bork M D, Smeltzer J S, Egan J F *et al.* (1996) Prenatal diagnosis of intracranial lipoma associated with agenesis of the corpus callosum. *Obstet Gynecol* 87(5 Pt 2): 845–848.

Bromley B, Frigoletto-FD J & Benacerraf B R (1991) Mild fetal lateral cerebral ventriculomegaly: clinical course and outcome. *Am J Obstet Gynecol* 164(3): 863–867.

Bromley B, Nadel A S, Pauker S *et al.* (1994) Closure of the cerebellar vermis: evaluation with second trimester US. *Radiology* 193(3): 761–763.

Brown M S & Sheridan P M (1992) Outlook for the child with a cephalocele. *Pediatrics* 90(6): 914–919.

Caldarelli M & Di R C (1996) Surgical options in the treatment of interhemispheric arachnoid cysts. *Surg Neurol* 46(3): 212–221.

Campbell S, Johnstone F D, Holt E M & May P (1972) Anencephaly: early ultrasonic diagnosis and active management. *Lancet* 2(7789): 1226–1227.

Cardoza J D, Filly R A & Podrasky A E (1988) The dangling choroid plexus: a sonographic observation of value in excluding ventriculomegaly. *Am J Roentgenol* 151(4): 767–770.

Cardoza J D, Goldstein R B & Filly R A (1988) Exclusion of fetal ventriculomegaly with a single measurement: the width of the lateral ventricular atrium. *Radiology* 169(3): 711–714.

Chervenak F A, Isaacson G, Mahoney M J *et al.* (1984) Diagnosis and management of fetal cephalocele. *Obstet Gynecol* 64(1): 86–91.

Chervenak F A, Rosenberg J, Brightman R C *et al.* (1987) A prospective study of the accuracy of ultrasound in predicting fetal microcephaly. *Obstet Gynecol* 69(6): 908–910.

Chitty L S (1995) Ultrasound screening for fetal abnormalities. *Prenat Diagn* 15(13): 1241–1257.

Chitty L S, Chudleigh P, Wright E *et al.* (1998) The significance of choroid plexus cysts in an unselected population: results of a multicenter study. *Ultrasound Obstet Gynecol* 12(6): 391–397.

Cohen-M M J (1989) Perspectives on holoprosencephaly: Part I. Epidemiology, genetics, and syndromology. *Teratology* 40(3): 211–235.

Comstock C H & Kirk J S (1991) Arteriovenous malformations. Locations and evolution in the fetal brain. *J Ultrasound Med* 10(7): 361–365.

Comstock C H, Culp D, Gonzalez J & Boal D B (1985) Agenesis of the corpus callosum in the fetus: its evolution and significance. *J Ultrasound Med* 4(11): 613–616.

Cowles T, Furman P & Wilkins I (1993) Prenatal diagnosis of Dandy–Walker malformation in a family displaying X-linked inheritance. *Prenat Diagn* 13(2): 87–91.

Dan U, Shalev E, Greif M & Weiner E (1992) Prenatal diagnosis of fetal brain arteriovenous malformation: the use of color Doppler imaging. *J Clin Ultrasound* 20(2): 149–151.

David T J & Nixon A (1976) Congenital malformations associated with anencephaly and iniencephaly. *J Med Genet* 13(4): 263–265.

Demir R H, Gleicher N & Myers S A (1989) Atraumatic antepartum subdural hematoma causing fetal death [see comments]. *Am Obstet Gynecol* 160(3): 619–620.

DeRosa R, Lenke R R, Kurczynski T W *et al.* (1989) *In utero* diagnosis of benign fetal macrocephaly. *Am J Obstet Gynecol* 161(3): 690–692.

Di Rocco C, Iannelli A & Ceddia A (1991) Intracranial tumors of the first year of life. A cooperative survey of the 1986–1987 Education Committee of the ISPN. *Child Nerv Syst* 7(3): 150–153.

Digiovanni L M, Quinlan M P & Verp M S (1997) Choroid plexus cysts: infants and early childhood developmental outcome. *Obstet Gynecol* 90(2): 191–194.

Dommergues M, Mahieu C D, Fallet B C *et al.* (1996) Fetal serum interferon-alpha suggests viral infection as the aetiology of unexplained lateral cerebral ventriculomegaly. *Prenat Diagn* 16(10): 883–892.

Edmondson S R, Hallak M, Carpenter R J J & Cotton D B (1992) Evolution of hydranencephaly following intracerebral hemorrhage. *Obstet Gynecol* 79(5 Pt 2): 870–871.

Eller K M & Kuller J A (1995) Porencephaly secondary to fetal trauma during amniocentesis. *Obstet Gynecol* 85(5 Pt 2): 865–867.

Golden J A (1999) Towards a greater understanding of the pathogenesis of holoprosencephaly. *Brain Dev* 21(8): 513–521.

Goldstein I, Reece E A, Pilu G L & Hobbins J C (1990) Sonographic evaluation of the normal developmental anatomy of fetal cerebral ventricles. IV: The posterior horn. *Am J Perinatol* 7(1): 79–83.

Gratton R J, Hogge W A & Aston C E (1996) Choroid plexus cysts and trisomy 18: risk modification based on maternal age and multiple-marker screening. *Am J Obstet Gynecol* 175(6): 1493–1497.

Gunn T R, Mok P M & Becroft D M (1985) Subdural hemorrhage *in utero. Pediatrics* 76(4): 605–610.

Gupta J K & Lilford R J (1995) Assessment and management of fetal agenesis of the corpus callosum. *Prenat Diagn* 15(4): 301–312.

Gupta J K, Bryce F C & Lilford R J (1994) Management of apparently isolated fetal ventriculomegaly. *Obstet Gynecol Surv* 49(10): 716–721.

Gutierrez Y, Friede R L & Kaliney W J (1975) Agenesis of arachnoid granulations and its relationship to communicating hydrocephalus. *J Neurosurg* 43(5): 553–538.

Hanigan W C, Ali M B, Cusack T J *et al.* (1985) Diagnosis of subdural hemorrhage *in utero*. Case report. *J Neurosurg* 63(6): 977–979.

Hassan J, Sepulveda W, Teixeira J & Cox P M (1996) Glioependymal and arachnoid cysts: unusual causes of early ventriculomegaly *in utero. Prenat Diagn* 16(8): 729–733.

Hertzberg B S, Lile R, Foosaner D E *et al.* (1994) Choroid plexus–ventricular wall separation in fetuses with normal-sized cerebral ventricles at sonography: postnatal outcome. *Am J Roentgenol* 163(2): 405–410.

Hill L M, Martin J G, Fries J & Hixson J (1991) The role of the transcerebellar view in the detection of fetal central nervous system anomaly. *Am J Obstet Gynecol* 164(5 Pt 1): 1220–1224.

Hilpert P L, Hall B E & Kurtz A B (1995) The atria of the fetal lateral ventricles: a sonographic study of normal atrial size and choroid plexus volume. *Am J Roentgenol* 164(3): 731–734.

Jeanty P, Dramaix W M, Delbeke D *et al.* (1981) Ultrasonic evaluation of fetal ventricular growth. *Neuroradiology* 21(3): 127–131.

Kennedy D, Chitayat D, Winsor E J *et al.* (1998) Prenatally diagnosed neural tube defects: ultrasound, chromosome, and autopsy or postnatal findings in 212 cases. *Am J Med Genet* 77(4): 317–321.

Keogan M T, DeAtkine A B & Hertzberg B S (1994) Cerebellar vermian defects: antenatal sonographic appearance and clinical significance. *J Ultrasound Med* 13(8): 607–611.

Kollias S S, Goldstein R B, Cogen P H & Filly R A (1992)

Prenatally detected myelomeningoceles: sonographic accuracy in estimation of the spinal level. *Radiology* 185(1): 109–112.

Komarniski C A, Cyr D R, Mack L A & Weinberger E (1990) Prenatal diagnosis of schizencephaly. *J Ultrasound Med* 9(5): 305–307.

Kuhn M J, Couch S M, Binstadt D H *et al.* (1992) Prenatal recognition of central nervous system complications of alloimmune thrombocytopenia. *Comput Med Imaging Graph* 16(2): 137–142.

Lee W, Kirk J S, Pryde P *et al.* (1994) Atypical presentation of fetal arteriovenous malformation. *J Ultrasound Med* 13(8): 645–647.

Lehman C D, Nyberg D A, Winter T C *et al.* (1995) Trisomy 13 syndrome: prenatal US findings in a review of 33 cases. *Radiology* 194(1): 217–222.

Lena G, van Calenberg F, Genitori L & Choux M (1995) Supratentorial interhemispheric cysts associated with callosal agenesis: surgical treatment and outcome in 16 children. *Child Nerv Syst* 11(10): 568–573.

Lipitz S, Yagel S, Malinger G *et al.* (1998) Outcome of fetuses with isolated borderline unilateral ventriculomegaly diagnosed at mid-gestation. *Ultrasound Obstet Gynecol* 12(1): 23–26.

Lorber J (1971) Results of treatment of myelomeningocele. An analysis of 524 unselected cases, with special reference to possible selection for treatment. *Dev Med Child Neurol* 13(3): 279–303.

Martinez F M, Bermejo E, Rodriguez P E *et al.* (1998) Epidemiological analysis of outcomes of pregnancy in gestational diabetic mothers. *Am J Med Genet* 78(2): 140–145.

Miller G M, Stears J C, Guggenheim M A & Wilkening G N (1984) Schizencephaly: a clinical and CT study. *Neurology* 34(8): 997–1001.

Moutard M L, Lewin F, Baron J M (1998) Pronostic des agenesies isolees du corps calleux. [Prognosis of isolated agenesis of the corpus callosum] Club Francophone de Medecine Foetale. *Neurochirurgie* 44(1 Suppl): 96–98.

Murray J C, Johnson J A & Bird T D (1985) Dandy-Walker malformation: etiologic heterogeneity and empiric recurrence risks. *Clin Genet* 28(4): 272–283.

Nicolaides K H, Campbell S, Gabbe S G & Guidetti R (1986) Ultrasound screening for spina bifida: cranial and cerebellar signs. *Lancet* 2(8498): 72–74.

Nicolaides K H, Berry S, Snijders R J *et al.* (1990) Fetal lateral cerebral ventriculomegaly: associated malformations and chromosomal defects. *Fetal Diagn Ther* 5(1): 5–14.

Nyberg D A, Mack L A, Bronstein A *et al.* (1987) Holoprosencephaly: prenatal sonographic diagnosis. *Am J Roentgenol* 149(5): 1051–1058.

Nyberg D A, Mack L A, Hirsch J & Mahony B S (1988) Abnormalities of fetal cranial contour in sonographic detection of spina bifida: evaluation of the 'lemon' sign. *Radiology* 167(2): 387–392.

Nyberg D A, Cyr D R, Mack L A *et al.* (1988) The Dandy-Walker malformation prenatal sonographic diagnosis and its clinical significance. *J Ultrasound Med* 7(2): 65–71.

Nyberg D A, Hallesy D, Mahony B S *et al.* (1990) Meckel-Gruber syndrome. Importance of prenatal diagnosis. *J Ultrasound Med* 9(12): 691–696.

Nyberg D A, Kramer D, Resta R G *et al.* (1993) Prenatal sonographic findings of trisomy 18: review of 47 cases. *J Ultrasound Med* 12(2): 103–113.

Ordorica S A, Marks F, Frieden F J *et al.* (1990) Aneurysm of the vein of Galen: a new cause for Ballantyne syndrome. *Am J Obstet Gynecol* 162(5): 1166–1167.

Peebles D M (1998) Holoprosencephaly. *Prenat Diagn* 18(5): 477–480.

Penso C, Redline R W & Benacerraf B R (1987) A sonographic sign which predicts which fetuses with hydrocephalus have an associated neural tube defect. *J Ultrasound Med* 6(6): 307–311.

Pilu G, De Palma L, Romero R *et al.* (1986a) The fetal subarachnoid cisterns: an ultrasound study with report of a case of congenital communicating hydrocephalus. *J Ultrasound Med* 5(7): 365–372.

Pilu G, Romero R, De Palma L *et al.* (1986b) Antenatal diagnosis and obstetric management of Dandy-Walker syndrome. *J Reprod Med* 31(11): 1017–1022.

Pilu G, Romero R, Rizzo N *et al.* (1987) Criteria for the prenatal diagnosis of holoprosencephaly. *Am J Perinatol* 4(1): 41–49.

Pilu G, Sandri F, Perolo A *et al.* (1993) Sonography of fetal agenesis of the corpus callosum: a survey of 35 cases. *Ultrasound Obstet Gynecol* 3: 318–329.

Pretorius D H, Russ P D, Rumack C M & Manco J M (1986) Diagnosis of brain neuropathology *in utero*. *Neuroradiology* 28(5–6): 386–397.

Reece E A & Goldstein I (1997) Early prenatal diagnosis of hydrocephalus. *Am J Perinatol* 14(2): 69–73.

Roach E, Demyer W, Conneally P M *et al.* (1975) Holoprosencephaly: birth data, genetic and demographic analyses of 30 families. *Birth Defects Orig Artic Ser* 11(2): 294–313.

Rodesch G, Hui F, Alvarez H *et al.* (1994) Prognosis of antenatally diagnosed vein of Galen aneurysmal malformations. *Child Nerv Syst* 10(2): 79–83.

Roessler E, Belloni E, Gaudenz K *et al.* (1996) Mutations in the human Sonic Hedgehog gene cause holoprosencephaly. *Nat Genet* 14(3): 357–360.

Russ P D, Pretorius D H & Johnson M J (1989) Dandy-Walker syndrome: a review of fifteen cases evaluated by prenatal sonography. *Am J Obstet Gynecol* 161(2): 401–406.

Russell L J, Weaver D D, Bull M J & Weinbaum M (1984) *In utero* brain destruction resulting in collapse of the fetal skull, microcephaly, scalp rugae, and neurologic impairment: the fetal brain disruption sequence. *Am Med Genet* 17(2): 509–521.

Schlembach D, Bornemann A, Rupprecht T & Beinder E (1999) Fetal intracranial tumors detected by ultrasound: a report of two cases and review of the literature. *Ultrasound Obstet Gynecol* 14(6): 407–418.

Sherer D M, Abramowicz J S, Eggers P C *et al.* (1993) Prenatal ultrasonographic diagnosis of intracranial teratoma and massive craniomegaly with associated high-output cardiac failure. *Am J Obstet Gynecol* 168(1 Pt 1): 97–99.

Snijders R J (1996) Isolated choroid plexus cysts: should we offer karyotyping?. *Ultrasound Obstet Gynecol* 8(4): 223–224.

Snijders R J, Shawa L & Nicolaides K H (1994) Fetal choroid plexus cysts and trisomy 18: assessment of risk based on ultrasound findings and maternal age. *Prenat Diagn* 14(12): 1119–1127.

Sullivan A, Giudice T, Vavelidis F & Thiagarajah S (1999) Choroid plexus cysts: is biochemical testing a valuable adjunct to targeted ultrasonography? *Am J Obstet Gynecol* 181(2): 260–265.

Thiagarajah S, Henke J, Hogge W A *et al.* (1990) Early diagnosis of spina bifida: the value of cranial ultrasound markers. *Obstet Gynecol* 76(1): 54–57.

Timor T I, Greenebaum E, Monteagudo A & Baxi L (1996) Exencephaly-anencephaly sequence: proof by ultrasound imaging and amniotic fluid cytology. *J Matern Fetal Med* 5(4): 182–185.

Ulm B, Ulm M R, Deutinger J & Bernaschek G (1997) Dandy-Walker malformation diagnosed before 21 weeks of gestation: associated malformations and chromosomal abnormalities. *Ultrasound Obstet Gynecol* 10(3): 167–170.

Valat A S, Dehouck M B, Dufour P *et al.* (1998) Ventriculomegalie cerebrale foetale. Etiologie et devenir, a propos de 141 observations. [Fetal cerebral ventriculomegaly. Etiology and outcome, report of 141 cases] *J Gynecol Obstet Biol Reprod Paris* 27(8): 782–789.

Van den Hof M C, Nicolaides K H, Campbell J & Campbell S (1990) Evaluation of the lemon and banana signs in one hundred thirty fetuses with open spina bifida. *Am J Obstet Gynecol* 162(2): 322–327.

van der Knaap M S & Valk J (1988) Classification of congenital abnormalities of the CNS. *Am J Neuroradiol* 9(2): 315–326.

Vergani P, Ghidini A, Strobelt N *et al.* (1994) Prognostic indicators in the prenatal diagnosis of agenesis of corpus callosum. *Am J Obstet Gynecol* 170(3): 753–758.

Vergani P, Strobelt N, Locatelli A *et al.* (1996) Clinical significance of fetal intracranial hemorrhage. *Am Obstet Gynecol* 175(3 Pt 1): 536–543.

Vohra N, Ghidini A, Alvarez M & Lockwood C (1993) Walker-Warburg syndrome: prenatal ultrasound findings. *Prenat Diagn* 13(7): 575–579.

Wald N J (1994) Folic acid and neural tube defects: the current evidence and implications for prevention. *Ciba Found Symp* 181: 192–208.

Wald N, Cuckle H, Boreham J & Stirrat G (1980) Small biparietal diameter of fetuses with spina bifida: implications for antenatal screening. *Br J Obstet Gynaecol* 87(3): 219–221.

Wininger S J & Donnenfeld A E (1994) Syndromes identified in fetuses with prenatally diagnosed cephaloceles. *Prenat Diagn* 14(9): 839–843.

Winter R M & Baraitser M (2000) *London Dysmorphology Database*. Oxford: Oxford University Press.

Yapar E G, Ekici E, Dogan M & Gokmen O (1996) Meckel-Gruber syndrome concomitant with Dandy-Walker malformation: prenatal sonographic diagnosis in two cases. *Clin Dysmorphol* 5(4): 357–362.

Yuval Y, Lerner A, Lipitz S *et al.* (1997) Prenatal diagnosis of vein of Galen aneurysmal malformation: report of two cases with proposal for prognostic indices. *Prenat Diagn* 17(10): 972–977.

# Chapter 18 Transvaginal fetal neuroscan

I. E. Timor-Tritsch and A. Monteagudo

## INTRODUCTION

The fetal CNS, and more precisely the fetal brain, is in constant development from its incipient and early stages throughout the gestation, and even after birth. It is therefore extremely important to understand the developmental changes of the brain that occur during the intrauterine life, since the sonographic appearance changes almost every month during gestation. All organs, other than the brain, assume their final sonographic appearance early in gestation; the only change that takes place in these organ systems is that they increase in size. As opposed to other organs and organ systems, the brain is the only fetal organ that changes its sonographic appearance throughout gestation.

Given that the sonographic differences occurring from week to week are subtle, and as these small differences may be visible only if high quality sonographic pictures are examined, we naturally turn to the high frequency ultrasound transducers to be able to document the fine anatomy of the fetal brain. It is known that the highest frequency transducers are those employed and utilized in the transvaginal ultrasound probes. This is the reason that the highest quality ultrasound pictures produced are those obtained by the high frequency transvaginal transducers. It is a well-known fact that the early pregnancy up to 12–14 weeks is best examined utilizing these aforementioned high frequency probes. Our approach has always been that utilizing the high frequency transvaginal probe (even later in pregnancy) will enable us to obtain high quality and high resolution images of the fetal brain.

In this chapter we will deal with technique of fetal neuroscan in general and more precisely using the transvaginal ultrasound technique, as well as the multiplanar imaging obtained by two-dimensional (2-D) and neuro 3-D ultrasound scanning techniques. Several examples of the normal and abnormal fetal neuroscan obtained by 2-D and 3-D ultrasound will also be presented.

## EQUIPMENT AND TECHNIQUE

The functioning of the available transducers as far as fetal neuroscan is concerned is limited by physical factors. Factors to consider are the size of the fetal brain and the available surface or the 'window' through which the transducer can achieve the best image, the fetal position and presentation, and last but not least, the thickness of the abdominal wall. Therefore it is easy to understand that several kinds of different transducers having a variety of frequencies and frequency ranges are used in order to obtain the best possible images. As imaging the fetal brain depends on the penetration of the sound wave through the tissues, it is clear that the progressive thickening of the fetal skull during gestation will determine in a significant way the types of ultrasound probes employed for the examination. The basic two kinds of ultrasound probes for fetal brain imaging, the transabdominal and transvaginal ultrasound probes, were tried during the last one or two decades. The *transabdominal probes* employ lower transducer frequencies whilst the *transvaginal probes* use higher ultrasound frequencies for the examination itself. During the first half of the pregnancy, high frequency transvaginal probes are usually used for scanning. The reasons for this are as follows: at earlier gestation the fetal skull is relatively thin containing less deposited calcium, and the entire body of the relatively small fetus can be easily scanned through the vaginal route. Therefore it sounds logical that during this time period high frequency probes can be used. This is also the reason that at this time transvaginal probes are the first-line transducer probes employed regardless of fetal position and presentation. If the fetus continues to present with the vertex we can employ the transvaginal ultrasound scanning approach anytime in pregnancy. If, however, the fetal head cannot be reached any more using the transvaginal route, transabdominal probes have to be used. Transvaginal ultrasound probes typically operate frequencies of 5–9 MHz, while the transabdominal probes frequencies of 3.5–7 MHz. However, at higher gestational ages the lower frequencies have to be used in order to penetrate the progressively thickening skull bones.

It should be remembered that even at the very end of the pregnancy or during the neonatal period, fetuses or the neonates can be easily scanned through the still-open anterior fontanelle. This is how neonatologists and pediatric neurologists obtain their information regarding the neonatal brain.

Transvaginal scanning, as with transfontanelle scanning of the neonatologist, obtains clinically useful brain images through the anterior fontanelle. The sections that can be obtained by scanning through this acoustic window are the median and paramedian, as well as (rotating the transducer) the coronal and the oblique sections. The tremendous advantage of transvaginal scanning of the prenatal brain is that the scanning planes obtained are identical to those obtained by the neonatal brain scan and are therefore readily comparable. The most frequent consultants to the perinatologist in the event of brain malformations are the pediatric neurosurgeons and neurologists. By presenting them with scans that are similar to those used by them in the neonatal period an immediate understanding of the location, extent and identity of the lesion in the fetal brain can be achieved.

The basic difference between the transabdominal scan and the transvaginal scan, other than the issue of the transducer frequency and picture resolution, is the direction of the scanning approach. Using transabdominal scanning, we usually scan through the temporal bone and obtain axial images of the fetal brain. If the circumstances are favorable we may obtain even a second plane – usually the coronal plane using transabdominal probes. However, adding the additional scanning route (i.e. the transvaginal route) we can obtain sagittal as well as coronal planes of the fetal brain. It is unusual to obtain axial sections using the transvaginal ultrasound probe. It should therefore be well understood that 2-D transabdominal and transvaginal techniques complement each other in obtaining all three classical planes. The 3-D volume scan of the fetal brain will circumvent some of the problems mentioned here.

As far as the actual scanning technique is concerned, the transabdominal technique is well known and is used in all laboratories by sonographers and sonologists, and will not be considered further here. More emphasis will be placed on a detailed discussion of the transvaginal sonographic examination of the fetal brain which is slowly gaining its well deserved place among the scanning options for fetuses. As said before, classically the transvaginal neuroscan relies upon the experience gained from the transfontanelle examination of the neonatal brain (Babcock *et al.* 1980; Ben-Ora *et al.* 1980; Dewbury & Aluwihare 1980; Johnson & Rumack 1980; Grant *et al.* 1981; Edwards *et al.* 1981; Slovis & Kuhns 1981; Naidich *et al.* 1986; Richardson & Grant 1986). The use of TV ultrasound technique for neuroscan was introduced in the early 1990s (Timor-Tritsch *et al.* 1988; Kushnir *et al.* 1989; Warren *et al.* 1989; Timor-Tritsch *et al.* 1990, 1991; Monteagudo *et al.* 1991a,b, 1993; Timor-Tritsch & Monteagudo 1991; Achiron & Achiron 1991; Malinger & Zakut 1993; Blaas *et al.* 1994, 1995a,b; Timor-Tritsch & Monteagudo 1996; Monteagudo & Timor-Tritsch 1997).

The technique of TV neuroscan is relatively simple. Before describing the technique we would like to emphasize the fact that there is absolutely no difference in the technique of TV fontanelle fetal neuroscan between the 2-D or the 3-D scanning methods. The probe is prepared as usual for TV scanning. The tip of the probe is well covered by a plastic sheet, a clean condom, or inserted in one digit of a surgical rubber glove. The patient is placed in the supine position and the probe is slowly advanced into the vagina to reach the anterior cervical lip. We suggest that before anything else is imaged a sagittal picture and a measurement of the cervix should be obtained for later reference. The patient's bladder should be empty in order to enable the transvaginal probe to come closer to the fetal head. The objective is to place the tip (the foot print) of the transvaginal probe opposite the anterior fontanelle. This can be obtained by twisting, turning and tilting the vaginal probe until the best image is obtained, while the abdominally placed second hand of the operator is stabilizing the fetal head or maneuvering it into the desired position for the clearest ultrasound picture.

It should be emphasized that, if a scan is required to rule out brain anomaly in a fetus in breech presentation, one should strongly consider performing an external version in order to turn the fetus into vertex presentation. This is, in most instances, easily obtained as in the late first or early second trimester, or even sometimes later, there is enough fluid to be able to perform the external version, thereby obtaining important and very clear pictures of the brain.

We place importance on the fact that the TV transducer should be an end-firing type that will enable symmetrical pictures on both sides of the scanning axis; in other words the scanning axis in the straight axis of the entirely straight probe will be identical. The use of a non end-firing or out-of-axis vaginal probe can cause the scanning of a perfectly symmetrical image of the brain to become extremely cumbersome, because the probe has to be constantly twisted and tilted into the right position, and the operator will be confused by the position of the probe and the exact location of certain structures in the brain.

## SCANNING PLANES

As mentioned before, the classical transabdominal scanning of the fetal brain may only yield the axial and coronal images. It is extremely difficult to obtain the sagittal planes. When we refer to the above-mentioned planes we mean the classical coronal, sagittal and axial planes. Using computed tomography or magnetic resonance imaging all consecutive sections are parallel to each other. However, using transvaginal fetal neuroscans it is impossible to obtain all the 'classical' planes. By performing the transvaginal fetal neuroscan with the footprint of the probe touching the anterior fontanelle it is possible to obtain tilted or slanted sections of the fetal brain in the coronal and sagittal planes. Only the median and one of the coronal sections will conform to the classical definitions of these planes. Luckily these planes are not only similar but they are also identical to those obtained by the neonatal transfontanelle imaging of the fetal brain (Ben-Ora *et al.* 1980; Dewbury & Aluwihare 1980; Cohen & Ziprkowski 1991; Grant & Richardson 1994). These similarities between the neonatal and the fetal scanning planes and sections have a practical advantage when prenatal and neonatal brain images have to be compared or to be followed regarding the pathology detected.

We attempted to standardize the planes and sections by transvaginal fetal neurosonography using anatomic landmarks and adapting a new nomenclature for labeling them, taking into consideration the fact that the transfontanelle approach is unable to create all the desired classical and parallel to each other and anatomic sections. The first assumption using this approach was that the planes generated are not parallel with each other, and therefore, they do not comply with the definitions of the classical planes imaging of the fetal head. We also assumed that some of the classical planes defined in the Nomina Anatomica (1989) have to be clarified in order to understand the new proposed planes.

The classical planes consist of the sagittal and coronal (two vertical planes), and the axial (a horizontal plane). In the coronal plane all sections from the occiput (posterior) to the forehead (anterior) are parallel to each other. The coronal planes can also be called frontal planes. In the sagittal planes there are differences in terminology of the specific planes. The 'mid sagittal plane' is called the *median plane.* On each of the two sides of the median are right and left sagittal planes. There can be multiple such right and left planes, but the term 'parasagittal' is incorrect.

Considering the planes described by us using the transvaginal probe diverge in a fan-shaped fashion from a central point (the anterior fontanelle), it is therefore incorrect to talk about 'sagittal' and 'coronal' planes in the classical sense. As said before, only one section is considered as the classical 'coronal' plane and only one section is considered the classical sagittal plane (the median plane) and the rest are oblique planes.

Toward a better understanding of this, a new nomenclature was proposed (Timor-Tritsch & Monteagudo 1996). To define each of these newly proposed sections a number of landmarks and anatomic structures were defined. The combination and clustering of these specific and well defined landmark structures enabled the exact description of every single plane. The landmark and anatomic structures taken into consideration were: the orbit, the meninges (the falx and the tentorium), ventricles and their connections (the lateral, third and fourth ventricles), the interhemispheric foramina, the choroid plexus, and the telachoroidea, midbrain structures such the corpus callosum, the head of the caudate nucleus, the thalamus and the cavum septi pellucidi, the cerebellum with its hemispheres, and the vermis.

## THE NEWLY PROPOSED PLANES

The *coronal planes* (Fig. 18.1A) are subdivided into three groups.

The **frontal group** consists of two sections. (a) In *Frontal-1*, which is also termed 'steerhead' configuration, the structures seen are the orbits and some facial structures. The homogenous brain tissue without the tip of the anterior horn of the lateral ventricles is also depicted; however, if the scanning is performed before the 16th postmenstrual week, the tips of the anterial horns are still visible using this section. (b) In *Frontal-2*; the structures seen are the orbits and the tip of the anterial horns as well as the falx.

The **middle group** consists of three sections. (a) In *Mid-coronal-1*, the structures seen are the lateral ventricles, the body of the lateral ventricles, the cavum septi pellucidi, corpus callosum, and the head of the caudate nucleus. (b) In *Mid-coronal-2*, the structures seen are the lateral ventricles with the choroid plexus entering into the third ventricle through the foramina interventricularis (Monro); the corpus callosum; and the thalamus. (c) In *Mid-coronal-3*, the structures seen are the lateral ventricles (atrium) with their choroid plexus, the corpus callosum, and the thalamus.

The **occipital group** has two subgroups: (a) *Occipital-1*, where the structures seen are the lateral ventricles (posterior horns), cerebellar hemispheres, the vermis, and at times the fourth ventricle; (b) *Occipital-2*, where the structures seen are the cerebellar hemispheres, the cerebellar vermis, the tentorium, and the cisterna magna. At times, depending on the angle, the tips of the pointed posterior horns can still be detected.

The *sagittal planes* (Fig. 18.1B) are subdivided into the following groups.

The *Median* (previously termed 'midsagittal'; as said before, only one median section is possible). The structures are: the entire corpus callosum (before the 18th to the 20th week, only parts of this can be seen); the cavum septi pellucidi; the head of the caudate nucleus; the thalamus; the tela choroidea; midbrain structures such as the corpora quadrigemina, the vermis, the tectum, the cisterna magna, and the 4th ventricle.

Right and left *Oblique-1* (previously called 'para-sagittal'). The structures are the anterior horn, atrium, and posterior horn of the lateral ventricles with the choroid plexus 'hugging' the thalami. Note: the inferior horns should not be visible through these sections since they are lateral to this plane.

Right and left *Oblique-2*. The structures contain mostly homogenous texture of the brain tissue with a horizontally oriented gaping lateral sulcus in the shape of a letter 'V' turned 90° on its side. The upper arm of the 'V' arises from the temporal lobe and is called parietal operculum. The lower arm of the 'V' is the temporal operculum. These two structures enclose an area called the insula. Toward term the insula is progressively 'buried' into the depth through the two closing opercula.

We felt that only very slight deviation from the classical anatomical planes were made and believe that this adjustment was clinically justified. The 'coronal' planes can effectively be used even in early pregnancies such as at 16–17th postmenstrual weeks to demonstrate the anatomy at that age (Fig. 18.2).

We feel that because of the simplicity and the logic behind it, this systematic method of describing the fetal brain scan by transvaginal sonography has helped us in better defining the normal and abnormal fetal brain. We once again would like to stress that it emulates the neonatal scanning of our pediatric neurologist and neurosurgeon colleagues. Even

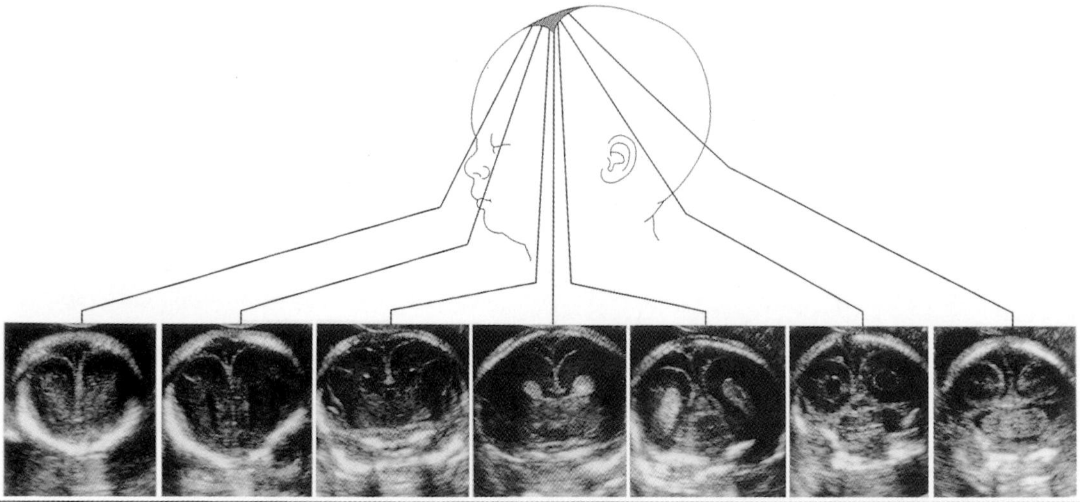

| Anatomical Structures | | FRONTAL 1 | FRONTAL 2 | MID-CORONAL 1 | MID-CORONAL 2 | MID-CORONAL 3 | OCCIPITAL 1 | OCCIPITAL 2 |
|---|---|---|---|---|---|---|---|---|
| Skull | | | Orbit | | | | | |
| Ventricles & Connections | Lateral | Only at <16 w | Anterior Horn | Body | Body<br>Choroid Plexus | Atrium<br>(Choroid Plexus) | Posterior Horn | |
| | Interventricular foramina | | | | With choroid plexus | | | |
| | Third | | | | (Virtual space) Tela choroidea | | | |
| Cavum septi pellucidi | | | | Cavum Septi Pellucidi | (Cavum Septi Pellucidi) | | | |
| Midbrain | Corpus Callosum | | | Genu | Trunk | Splenium | | |
| | Head of Caudate Nucleus | | | Caudate Nucleus | | | | |
| | Thalamus | | | | Thalamus | (Thalamus) | | |
| Cerebellum | Hemisphere | | | | | | Hemispheres | (Hemispheres) |
| | Vermis | | | | | | | Vermis |
| | 4th Ventr. | | | | | | 4th Ventricle (at times) | |
| Meninges | Falx | F | A | L | X | | | |
| | Tentorium | | | | | | Tentorium | (Tentorium) |
| Cisterna Magna | | | | | | | | Cisterna Magna |

A

Figure 18.1 The newly proposed planes and sections by transvaginal sonography. (A) Pictorial table of the different structures seen on the seven 'quasi-coronal' planes seen by 2D transvaginal sonography. The cluster of structures in any of the planes is unique only to that particular plane. (Reproduced with permission from Timor-Tritsch *et al.* 1996).

after the introduction of the 3-D fetal neuroscan (which is expected to be slow) the 2-D fetal neuroscan using the above classification will be easy to use.

## ASPECTS OF TRANSVAGINAL FETAL SCAN

**The posterior fossa.** The posterior coronal sections, such as the Mid-coronal-3, Occipital-1, and Occipital-2, provide a sufficiently good evaluation of the posterior fossa. However, at times it is feasible to scrutinize the same area using semi-axial, or even a sagittal plane. When the tip of the transvaginal transducer is closer to the posterior fontanelle it is possible to obtain a clear scan of the posterior fossa. If the scans are performed at or around the 14th to 16th postmenstrual weeks, one should be aware of the still incompletely formed vermis and that the 4th ventricle is clearly communicating through the widely open median aperture with the cerebellopeduncular cistern (cisterna magna) (Fig. 18.3A).

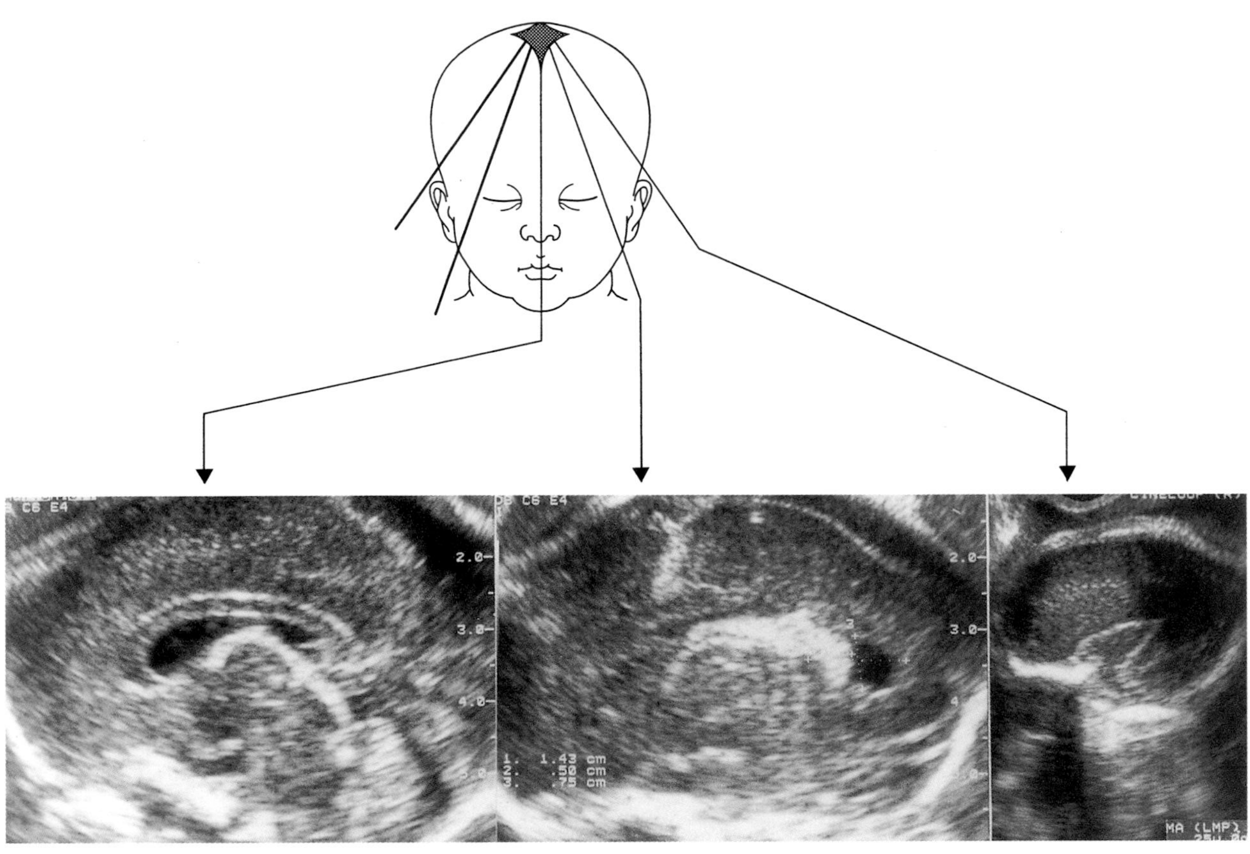

| MEDIAN | OBLIQUE-1 | OBLIQUE-2 |
|---|---|---|
| Corpus callosum | Lateral ventricle | Insula |
| Cavum septi pellucidi | Anterior horn | Parietal operculum |
| Caudate nucleus | Posterior horn | Temporal operculum |
| Thalamus | Atrium | Lateral sulcus |
| Tela choroidea | Choroid plexus | |
| Tectum | Thalami | |
| Corpora quadrigemina | | |
| Vermis | | |
| 4th ventricle | | |
| Cisterna magna | | |

B

**Figure 18.1** The newly proposed planes and sections by transvaginal sonography. (B) The different structures seen on the 'quasi-sagittal' planes obtained by 2-D transvaginal sonography. Here too, the group of structures in each plane is unique only to the plane in question. (Reproduced with permission from Timor-Tritsch *et al.* 1996.)

On the Occipital-2 section at times it is possible to detect not only the cerebellar hemisphere and the vermis, but also the surrounding fluid-filled cisterns above, lateral, and below the cerebellum itself (Fig. 18.3B).

From an occipital viewpoint in the sagittal plane it is possible to view the cerebellum, cerebellopeduncular cistern (cisterna magna), the medulla, and even the spinal cord (Fig. 18.3C). One should be aware of the fine linear echoes of the arachnoid which are sometimes visualized in the cerebellopeduncular cistern. These are normal and should not be confused with pathology. The cortex of the cerebellum is hyperechoic due to the fine invaginations of the pia mater into the cerebellar gyri and sulci, which densely cover the surface of the cerebellum. The vermis is particularly hyperechoic and easy to recognize by transvaginal sonography.

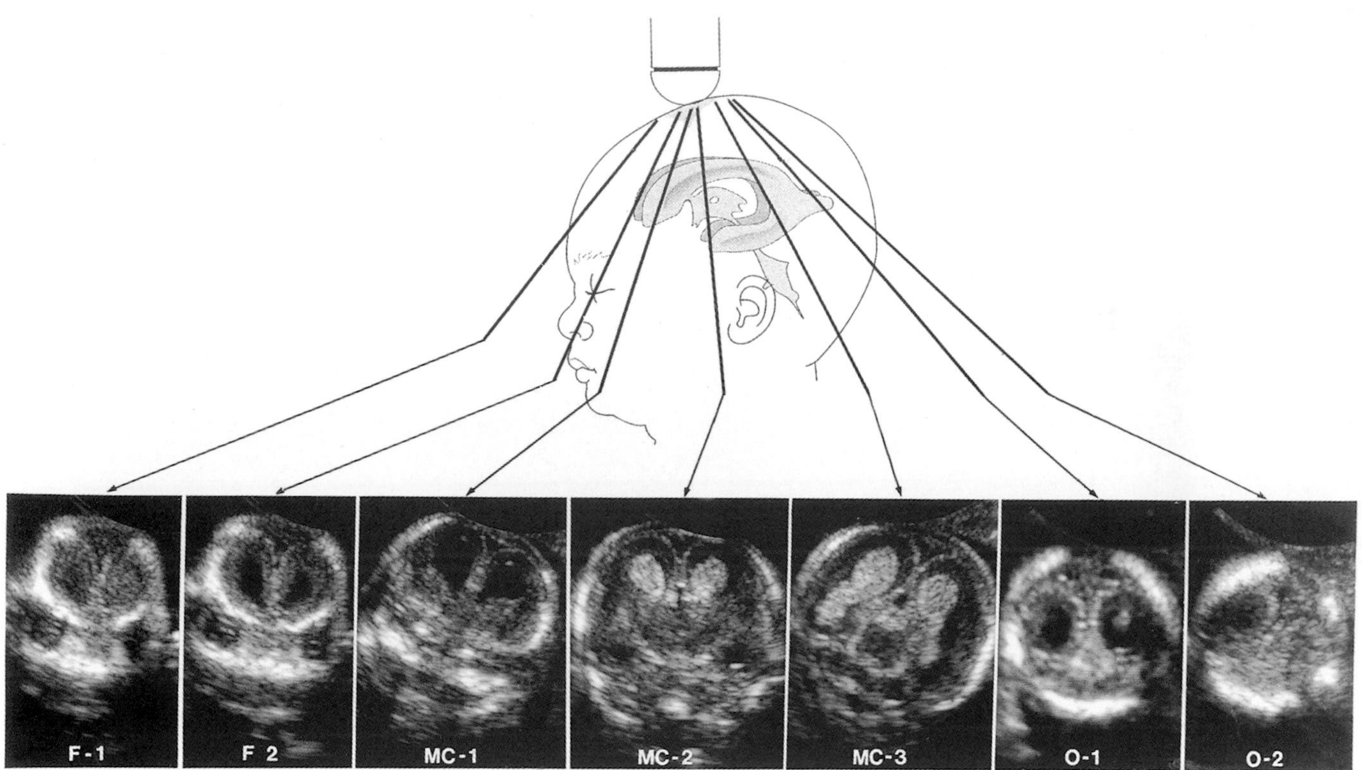


**Figure 18.2** The seven fan-shaped 'quasi-coronal' planes emanating from the anterior fontanelle imaged by 2-D transvaginal sonography at 16 postmenstrual weeks. F-1, Frontal-1; F-2, Frontal-2; MC-1, Midcoronal-1; MC-2, Midcoronal-2; MC-3, Midcoronal-3, O-1, Occipital-1; O-2, Occipital-2.

**The corpus callosum and midbrain structures.** The most representative plane to study the midbrain is the median plane. The most obvious and one of the more important structures appearing on this plane is the corpus callosum (Fig. 18.4). It starts to form at around 12 weeks and completes its anterior-to-posterior development around 20–22 weeks. The cavum septi pellucidi found under the corpus callosum and the pericallosal artery (discussed later) is seen above and following it closely (Fig. 18.4B). The thalami, caudate nuclei, 4th ventricle, and the medulla are the other structures that are also seen along the median plane. During the second and the early third trimester of pregnancy, the cavum septi pellucidi is divided into two distinct areas. The anterior is the cavum septi itself, its posterior extension is called the cavum vergae (Fig. 18.4A). The cavum vergae diminishes in size and almost disappears close to term. This is the most important scanning plane to evaluate the presence or absence of the corpus callosum. Three structures develop in close relation to each other: the corpus callosum, the pericallosal artery, and the cavum vergae. The above-mentioned midbrain structures can also be studied on the consecutive mid-coronal planes, which should be used as a control of the image obtained by the median plane.

The cavum septi pellucidi and cavum vergae are not part of the ventricular systems, as they do not have connections with the lateral ventricle.

**The ventricular system** consists of the two symmetrically positioned C-shaped lateral ventricles connecting with the 3rd ventricle in the midline through the interventricular foramina (Monroe). The CNS fluid drains into the 4th ventricle through the aqueduct and then through the median and lateral aperture into the cerebellopeduncular cistern (cisterna magna). The cerebrospinal fluid (CSF) produced by the bilaterally placed choroid plexuses situated in the atrium of the lateral ventricles is drained through these successive and previously mentioned structures into the cisterna magna and from there it is dispersed throughout the surface of the hemispheres.

As far as the individual components of the lateral ventricle are concerned, there are three horns that can be quite easily detected by transvaginal sonography: the anterior, posterior, and inferior horns. These are sometimes referred to as the frontal, occipital, and temporal horns, respectively. All three horns are relatively large at 12–14 weeks postmenstrual and their relative size compared to the rest of the brain gradually diminishes as term approaches. Clinically, the size of the lateral ventricular atrium is

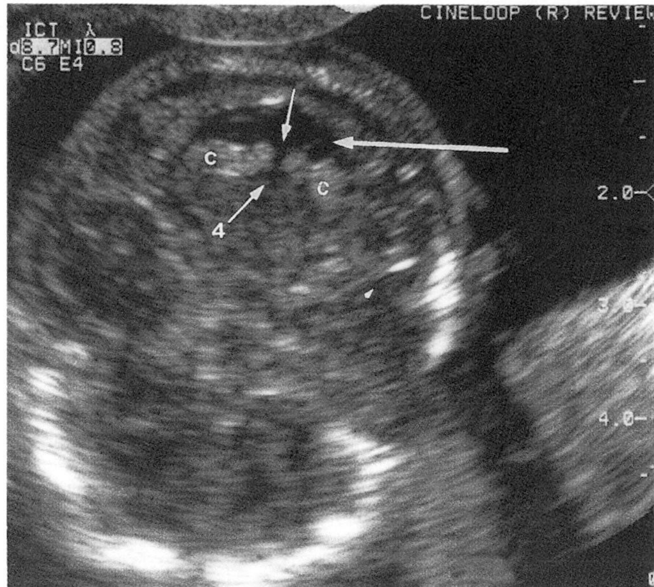

A

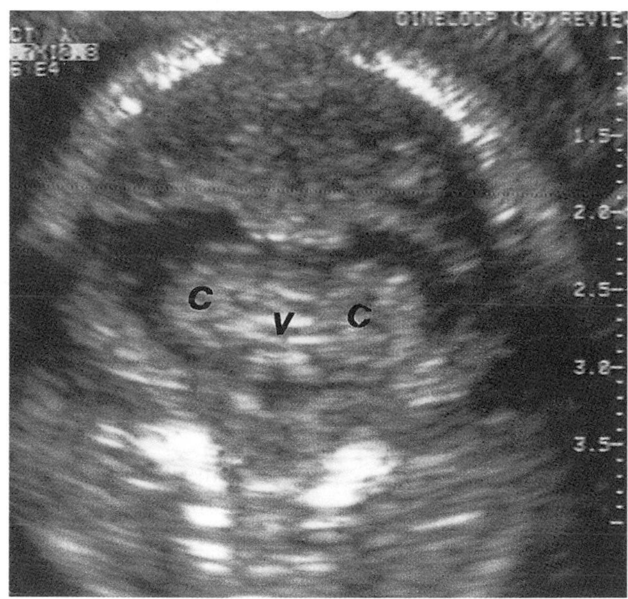


B

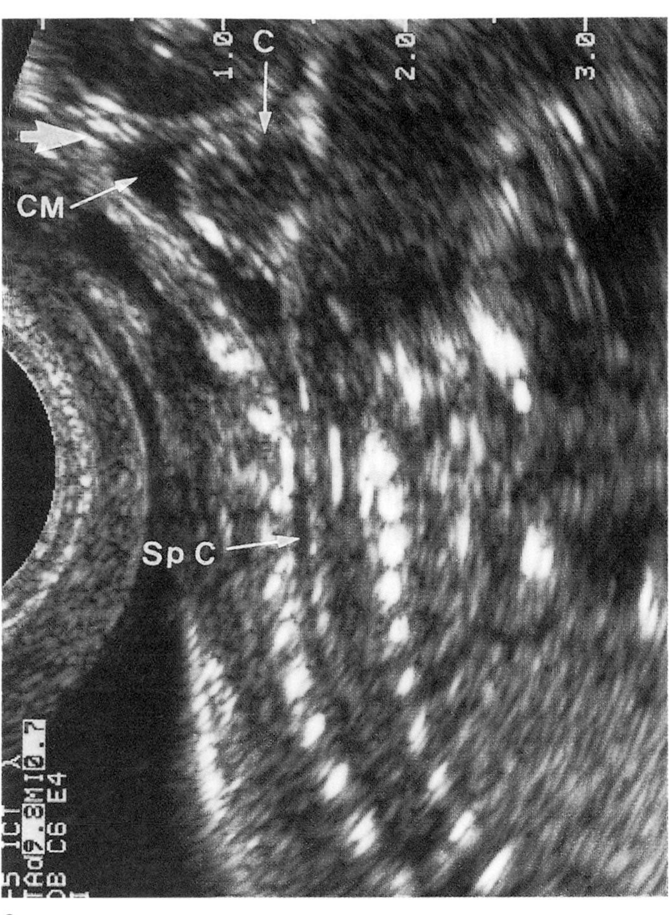


C

Figure 18.3 The posterior fossa at 16 postmenstrual weeks. (A) From an occipital viewpoint this low axial section demonstrates that the median aperture (Magendie) marked by two small opposing arrows is wide open and communicates with the 4th ventricle. The two hemispheres of the cerebellum, c, are also seen. The vermis, which is still not fully formed at this age, is not seen on this low axial section. (B) This posterior coronal (O-2) section of the brain demonstrates the echogenic vermis, v, connecting the two hemispheres of the cerebellum, c, as well as the surrounding cisterns. The cistern above the cerebellum is the cisterna ambiens. (C) A median section from an occipital approach depicts the tentorium (solid white arrow), the cisterna magna, CM, and the spinal canal, SpC, as well as the cerebellum, C.

measured as an indication of ventricular size. If the width of the lateral ventricle increases above 10 mm (four times the standard deviation of the normal) it should trigger a suspicion of true ventriculomegaly (Cardoza *et al.* 1988).

The dilatation of the posterior horn, also called colpocephaly, is probably the most sensitive indicator of ventricular dilatation. Using the transvaginal imaging method it is easy to measure the posterior horn using published nomograms (Monteagudo *et al.* 1993, 1994).

The inferior horn extends laterally into the temporal lobe. After 16 weeks in a normal fetal brain, using the Oblique-1 sections obtained by transvaginal sonography, the size of this horn remains stationary while the rest of the brain is growing. Later, after 24 weeks, it is hard to measure or detect it. If on the Oblique-1 section using 2-D ultrasound or on the three horn view obtained by 3-D transvaginal sonography the inferior horns are clearly seen, ventriculomegaly should be seriously suspected. Figure 18.5 illustrates a case of ventriculomegaly in a fetus with aqueductal stenosis.

The 3rd ventricle is rarely imaged in the second and third

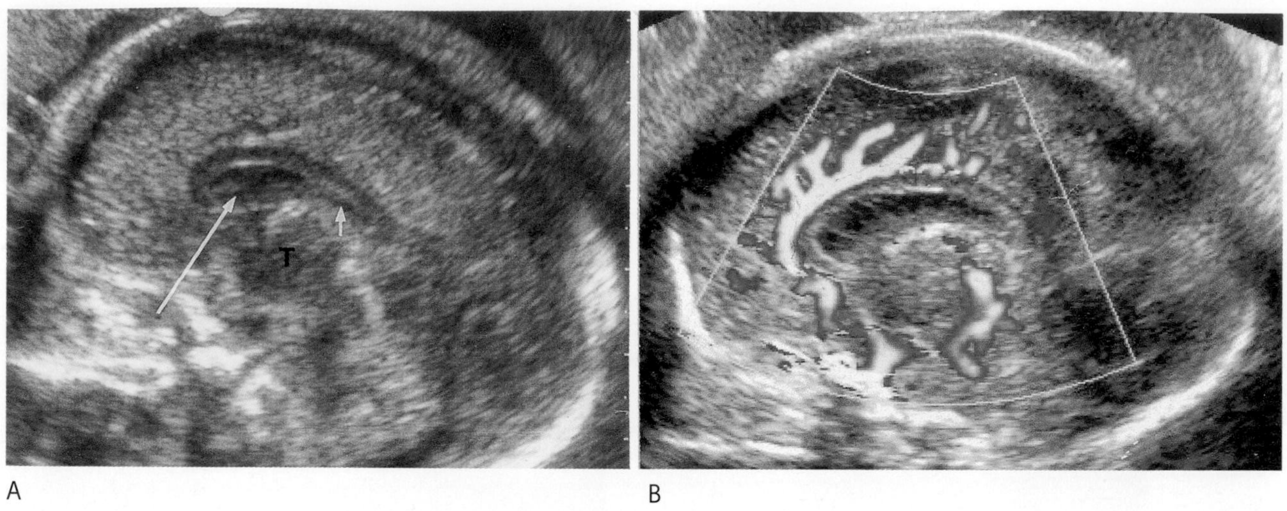


Figure 18.4 The corpus callosum at 23 postmenstrual weeks. (A) Median section demonstrating the C-shaped corpus callosum. Under it the anterior cavum septi pellucidi (long arrow) and cavum vergae (short arrow) are seen. T, thalamus. (B) Power Doppler study of the pericallosal artery above the corpus callosum.

trimesters. Any dilation of the 3rd ventricle above 5 mm using the Mid-coronal-2 section should trigger a detailed fetal neuroscan to examine the lateral ventricular system.

The 4th ventricle, seen on the median plane, usually appears as a sonolucent triangle at the level of the cerebellum.

**The choroid plexus** is found in the two lateral, the 3rd, and 4th ventricles. However, the best place to evaluate is the atrium of the lateral ventricles using the Midcoronal-3 (Fig. 18.2 – MC-2 and MC-3) and/or the Oblique-1 (Fig. 18.1B) scanning planes. Sonographically it appears as a cotton-like structure with irregular borders filling the available space of the lateral ventricles. It is richly supplied by capillaries. If it becomes thin and dangling it is considered to be a sensitive marker of ventriculomegaly (Fig. 18.5). At times sonography may detect cystic structures within the choroid plexus (see below).

**The cerebral cortex.** Information about the cerebral cortex can best be collected by transvaginal sonography. Disregarding the advances of 3-D ultrasound, it is clear that ultrasonography is able to scan only flat surfaces; therefore, the lateral and the superior surfaces of the hemispheres cannot be imaged using the standard planes. This leaves us with the flat medial surface of the cerebral hemispheres, which can be depicted using the median section to image the major gyri and sulci along the falx cerebri. Based on pathologic and developmental studies it was shown that the cerebral hemispheres are still smooth at around the 22nd postmenstrual week. By the 24th postmenstrual week the cingulate sulcus is detectable (Figure 18.6A). The biggest increase in the number and in the depth of the sulci takes place between 28 and 30 weeks postmenstrually. Using transvaginal ultrasonography we studied the development of the cingulate sulcus as well as the parieto-occipital fissure in normal fetuses from the 14th postmenstrual week to term and came to the conclusion that the developmental maturation of the normal fetal brain follows a predictable timetable and that the maturation can be followed by this technique. Typically, two or three sections of the fetal brain can be looked at to study the sulci and gyri at or after the 28th postmenstrual week. In addition to the previously mentioned median plane the other two cross-sectional planes on which sulci and gyri can be seen are the Mid-coronal-1 and -2 (Fig. 18.6B). On these sections the interhemispheric fissure, the falx and the budding of the cingulate sulcus and later, in gestation, its branches can be seen (Monteagudo & Timor-Tritsch 1997). All the above-mentioned cortical structures are detectable using this technique and may be the markers of developmental problems of the brain surface.

## THREE-DIMENSIONAL (3-D) ULTRASOUND OF THE FETAL BRAIN

Recent developments in the field of 3-D ultrasound have enabled us to expand our sonographic evaluation of the fetal brain. Replacing 2-D transvaginal or 2-D transabdominal ultrasound probes by the 3-D probes we can enhance the diagnostic abilities of the fetal neuroscan.

Using the volume acquisition mode of the 3-D ultrasound machine it is possible to obtain and simultaneously display images of the volume scan in all three planes (i.e. coronal, sagittal, and axial planes) of the fetal brain. We can see on the monitor at the same time not only the three images perpendicular to each other, but we can scroll the planes moving them back and forth, side to side, up and down, thus enabling free movement or 'navigation' within the volume. This special form of fetal neuroscan which displays 3-D planes simultaneously is called multiplanar imaging. As the

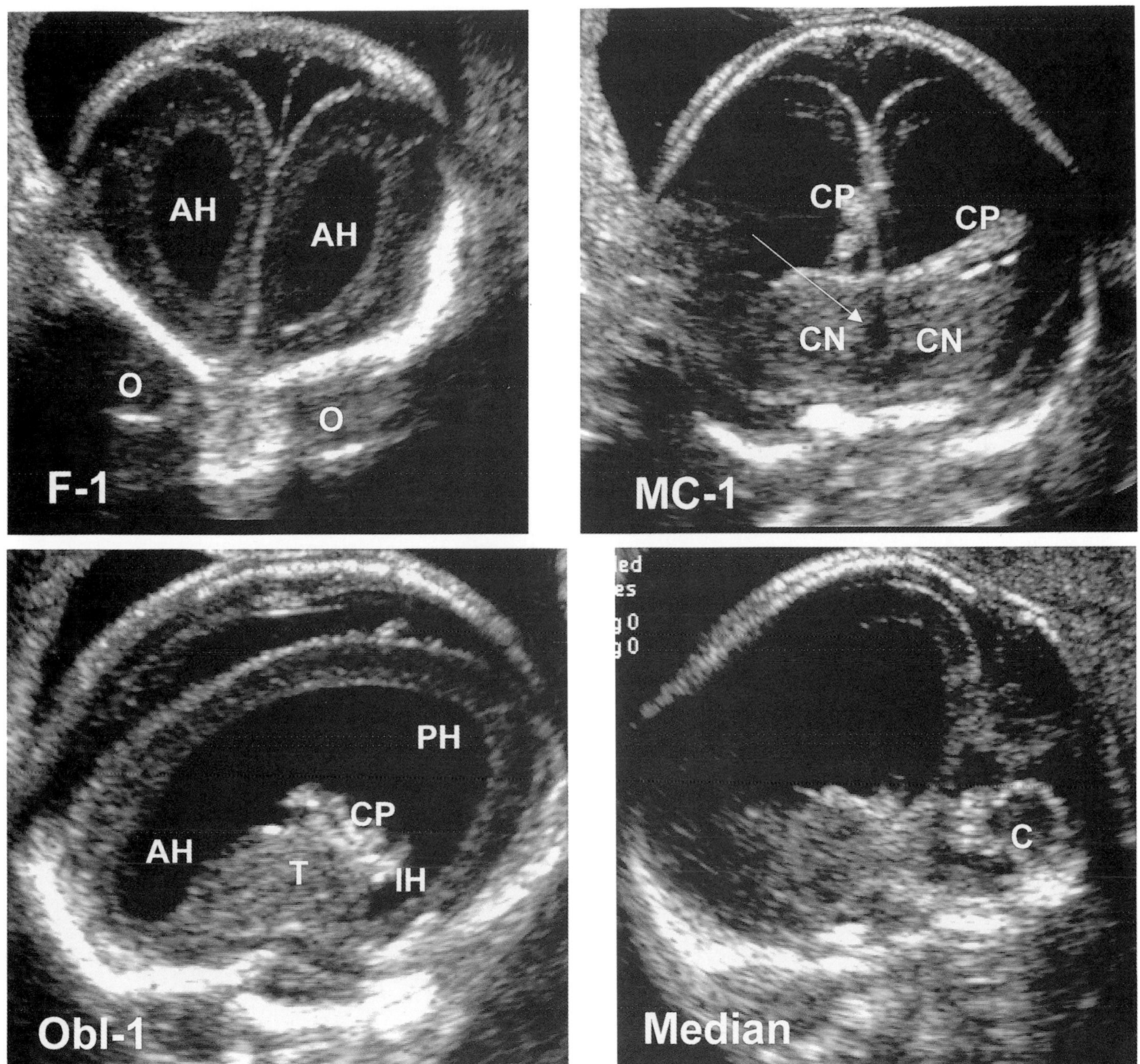


Figure 18.5 Aqueductal stenosis with hydrocephalus at 24 postmenstrual weeks. F-1, Frontal-1 section; MC-1, Midcoronal-1 section. Note the dangling choroid plexus (CP) The arrow points to the third ventricle. Obl-1, oblique-1 section (AH, anterior horn; CN, caudate nucleus; IH, inferior horn; O, orbits; T, thalamus). Median section (C, cerebellum).

the three planes are at right angles to each other this display method is also referred to as the orthogonal display. Several ultrasound machines make this display method available to clinicians.

The front-end of a 3-D ultrasound machine, of course, is the transducer. In most transducers the crystal array is mechanically moved, thus the successive sections within the volume are acquired at precise time intervals. This enables measurement within the volume itself, as the exact distances between the planes are known.

## THE 3-D FETAL NEUROSCAN TECHNIQUE

We are familiar with the Medison 3-D Voluson 530 digital ultrasound system, and therefore present our experience and results from operating this equipment.

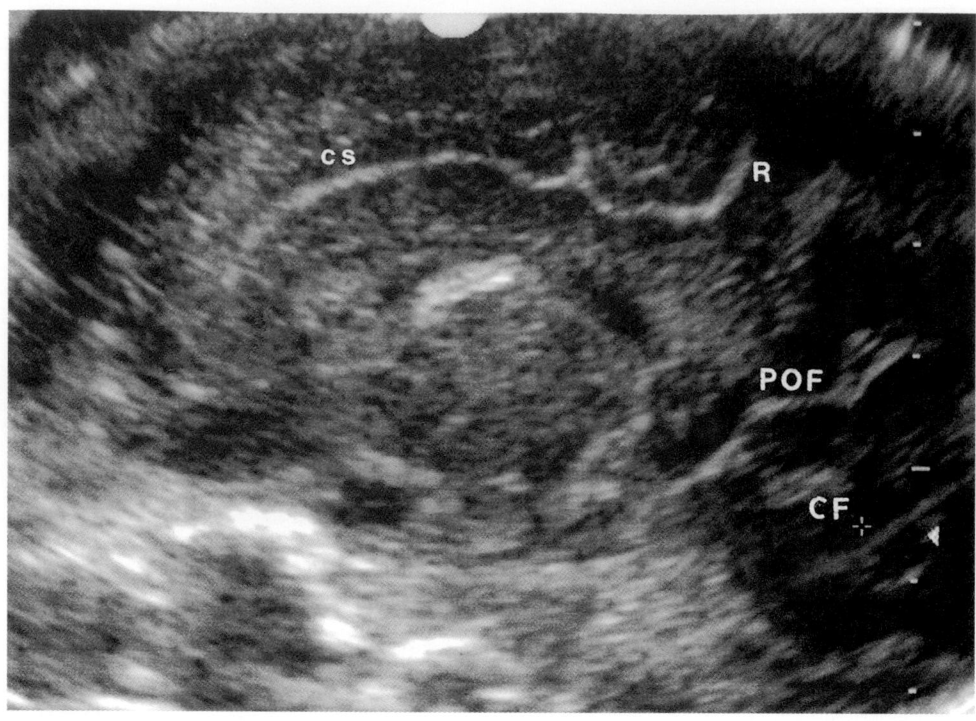


A

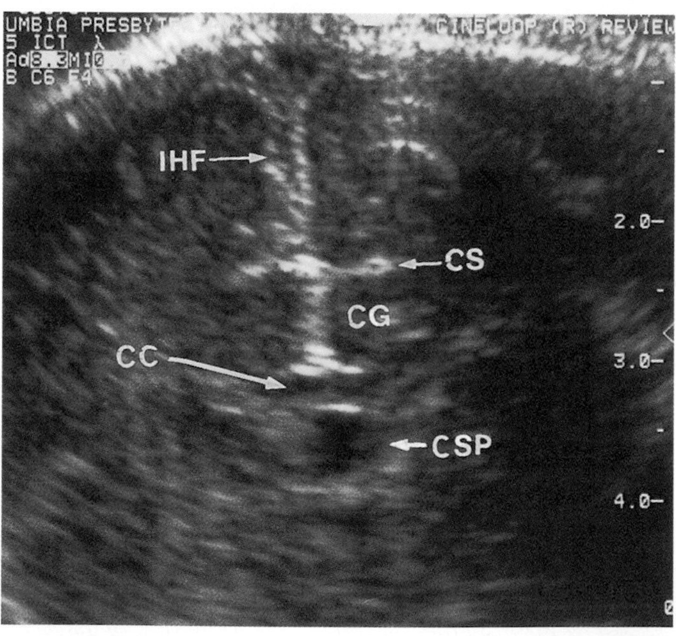


B

Figure 18.6 Gyri and sulci. (A) At 32 postmenstrual weeks a median section by transvaginal sonography shows the main sulci and fissures of the fetal brain on the medial aspect of the hemisphere (CS, callosal sulcus with its upward turning branch=R; POF, parieto-occipital fissure; CF, calcarine fissure). (B) A Midcoronal-2 section at 32 postmenstrual weeks demonstrates the interhemispheric fissure (IHF), the callosal sulcus (CS), the callosal gyrus (CG), the corpus callosum (CC) and the cavum septi pellucidi (CSP).

After identification of the fetal position and the anterior fontanelle, the 3-D volume acquisition can be started. The transvaginal probe is then used to select the region of interest. If needed, the fetal head can be gently manipulated by the examiner's free hand placed on the abdomen. A pie-shaped volume indicator region is placed to include the region of interest in both the *x* and *y* planes (Fig. 18.7). One of the three available scanning speeds is then activated. The slower the scanning speed the more information is stored. The changing plane of interest is in the 'active box' which can be recognized by its rectangular frame. As said before, by convention Box 'A' contains the coronal plane, and if 'active' this is the one that will be showing the different sections from anterior to posterior. One can move the

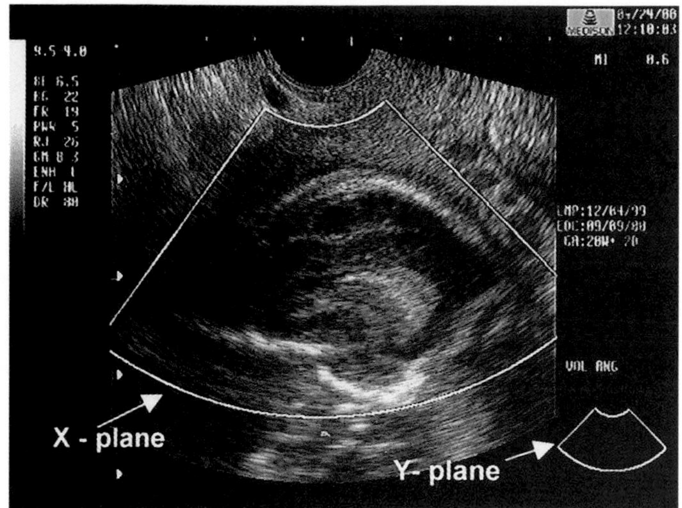


**Figure 18.7** Setting the outside boundaries to start the 3-D volume scan of the fetal brain by transvaginal sonography. The X area is placed in the sagittal plane while the Y-area is in the coronal plane. Both can be of variable size and depth.

coronal scanning plane visible in Box 'B' and then follow the appropriate coronal planes in Box 'A' (Figure 18.8A–C). The same process can then be repeated by placing the active box on the sagittal image (Box 'B') and change the sagittal planes that are indicated in Box 'A', moving them to the right and left. Finally, if the active box is transferred to Box 'C' one can examine the subsequent and successive axial planes by moving the level of horizontal plane seen in Boxes 'A' and 'B' toward the basis of the skull or toward the top of the head.

It is sometimes important to examine the anterior, posterior, and inferior horns on the same image. This is possible by tilting the volume seen in Box 'A' to the right or left and then placing the scanning planes across all three horns at the same time. We call this important viewing plane the three-horn view (3HV) (Timor-Tritsch *et al.* 2000a). On the 3HV very subtle changes in size and shape during a progressively developing ventriculomegaly can be observed (see Fig. 18.9). Using 2-D transvaginal ultrasonography we published measurements of the anterior, posterior, and inferior horns in the sagittal as well as coronal planes (Timor-Tritsch *et al.* 2000b). These measurements can be used for the 3HV. An example of obtaining the 3HV in a pathologic case with agenesis of the corpus callosum (ACC) can be seen in Fig. 18.9.

The main differences between the 2-D and 3-D fetal neuroscan studies are the following:

- Using 2-D transfontanelle fetal neuroscan, axial sections cannot be seen. This plane, however, becomes available using the 3-D technique.
- In the case of the conventional 2-D transvaginal transfontanelle neurosonography the 'sagittal' and the 'coronal' planes are radiating from the footprint of the probe placed on the fontanelle. In the case of 3-D multiplanar imaging the scanning planes are always parallel to each other.
- Using the 2-D technique the operator has to recreate the 3-D image in his or her brain and then try to pinpoint the location and the exact nature of the pathology. Using 3-D ultrasound, the marker dot enables the observer navigating within the volume to pinpoint the pathology, its extent, and the effect on adjacent structures.
- Using 3-D multiplanar imaging, pathology can be easily conveyed to the pediatric neurologist or neurosurgeon, who understands of the pathology better and faster, and can provide a more focussed plan for the postnatal management and can counsel the patient regarding the pathology.

The advantages of the 3-D fetal neuroscan are as follows:

1. It allows the observer to view the structure simultaneously in the coronal, sagittal, and axial planes.
2. As mentioned before, scrolling within the volume in any direction is possible.
3. By placing the point of intersection of three planes and creating a recognizable point (marker dot), it is possible to pinpoint structures which are then seen in the three selected planes at the same time.
4. The volume and the images can be stored for future evaluation.
5. The stored volume can be sent over networks to specialists anywhere for evaluation. The recipients can then further manipulate the volume as they desire.
6. Offline patient education and counseling are easy, using the views and, at times, the surface rendering mode.
7. During consultation with pediatric neurologists and neurosurgeons, pathology can be conveyed easier using the technique described above.
8. Another useful feature of 3-D ultrasound is the use of power angio or the color Doppler mode. In selected cases one can follow a blood vessel, and the exact course of the vessel can be ascertained or if it is missing the diagnosis can be established.

There are very few limitations of 3-D ultrasound of the fetal brain. One of them was already mentioned: the fact that the fetus may assume a breech presentation where an external version is not possible. Another limitation may be frequent fetal motion creating artifacts; however, waiting for the right time for a short pause in fetal motility can overcome this problem. The largest obstacle, as far as we are concerned, for the widespread use of 3-D imaging of the fetal brain is lack of equipment, operator inexperience, and lack of knowledge regarding the scanning procedure. These can be overcome by becoming familiar with the equipment, the right technique, and the pertinent literature.

To conclude we feel that the 3-D transvaginal sonography can effectively be used to examine the fetal brain. The

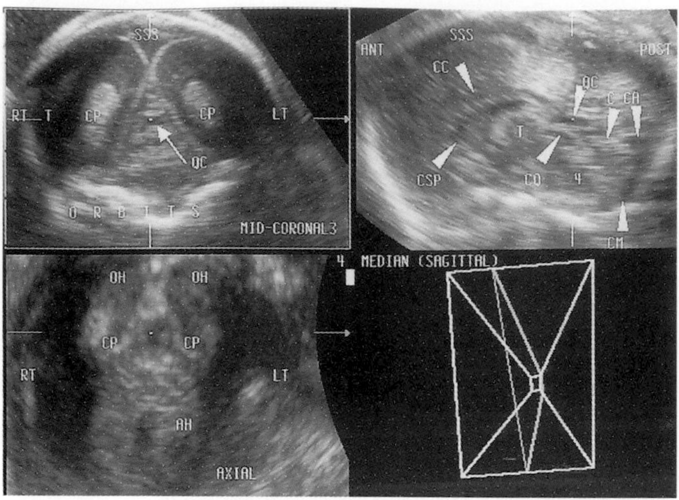


A

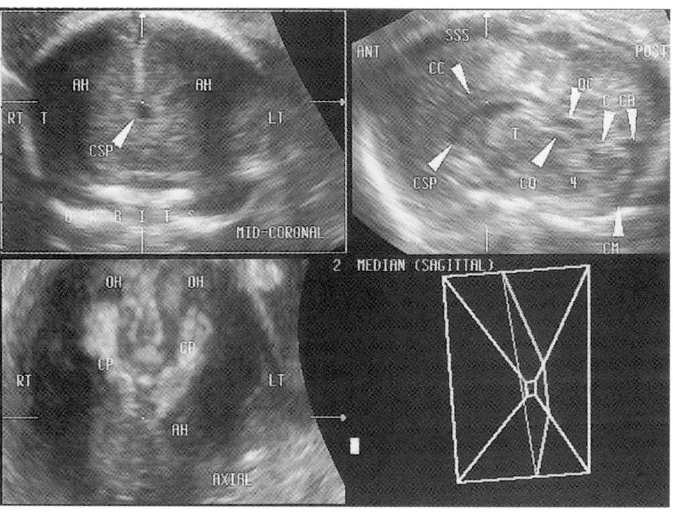


B

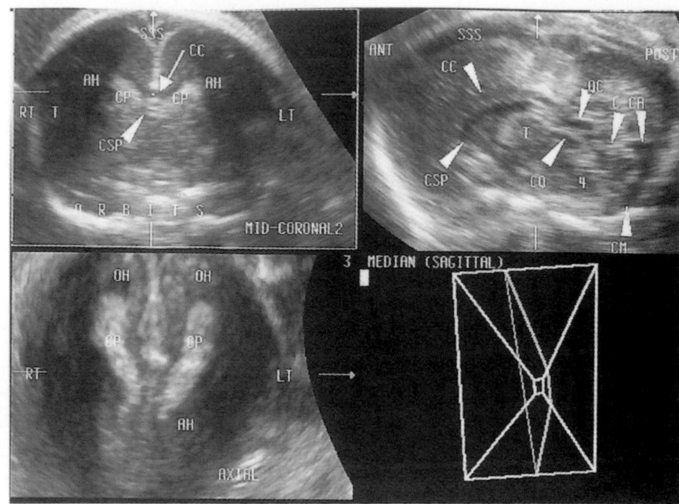


C

**Figure 18.8** The orthogonal displays of the volume scan at 22 postmenstrual weeks. The upper left box is box 'A', the upper right is box 'B', the lower left is box 'C'. In the lower right box the shape of the volume and the plane used in box 'B' is displayed. By our own choice box 'A' displays coronal sections, box 'B' contains the sagittal sections and box 'C' the axial or horizontal section. (A) Box 'A' is the active box (i.e. that image changes as the plane indicated by the white lines in box 'B' which can be moved in the anterior (frontal) or posterior (occipital) directions. In this picture box 'A' contains an anterior midcoronal section. (B) Here in Box 'B' the white line of the coronal plane was moved somewhat posteriorly resulting in a picture of the choroid plexus and the corpus callosum (cross section) in box 'A'. (C) The plane of the coronal section in box 'B' was moved further in the occipital direction therefore in box 'A' the entire choroid plexus is seen (much alike section Mid-coronal-3 by 2-D transvaginal sonography). AH, anterior horns; C, cerebellum; CA, cisterna ambiens; CC, corpus callosum; CM, cisterna magna; CP, choroid plexus; CQ, corpora quadrigemina; CSP, cavium septi pellucidi; OH, posterior horns; 4, fourth ventricle; SSS, superior sagittal sinus; T, thalamus).

possibility given to the examiner to view simultaneously and then review the brain volume in all scanning planes, by navigating or scrolling within the volume using the marker dot is clinically feasible and important. The tremendous advantage of applying 3-D technology fetal neuroscanning is that the information within the 3-D volume can be reviewed over and over again, the disk containing the volume can be mailed or sent over electronic media to a distant expert, and it can be used for teaching. Furthermore, comparison with neonatal ultrasound, MRI, or CT studies or pathology specimens can be more currently obtained. We are confident that 3-D fetal neuroscanning will find its way to the daily scanning routine of the imaging specialist.

## SELECTED FETAL NEUROPATHOLOGY USING TRANSVAGINAL TRANSFONTANELLE SCANNING

If any part of the fetal brain deviates from its normal sonographic appearance one is dealing with malformations of the CNS. These may be a result of pathologic development or they may be acquired during gestation (e.g. infection). Regardless of the cause they are called congenital brain anomalies. In order to properly diagnose such anomalies the sonographer or the sonologist has to be familiar with the developmental stages of the fetal brain. We cannot stress enough the fact that some structures may be normal early in pregnancy, however, if they are found later on they may represent pathologic development. The fetal brain is the

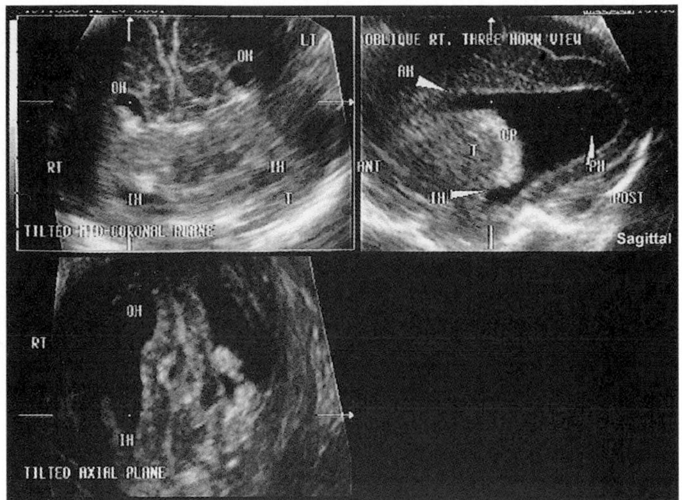


**Figure 18.9** Partial agenesis of the corpus callosum at 20 postmenstrual weeks by 3-D transvaginal sonography. Box 'A' shows the widely displaced lateral ventricles (OH) and the interhemispheric fissure connecting with the upward displaced third ventricle. Box 'B' is a picture of the right 3 HV obtained by slightly tilting the volume counter clockwise and across the line of the small white arrow in Box 'A'. Box 'C' is the horizontal section across the lateral ventricles with the typical colpocephaly (dilatation of the posterior horns) and the teardrop shaped lateral ventricle. (AH, anterior horn; IH, inferior horn; OH, posterior horn; T, thalamus).

only organ that undergoes tremendous anatomic changes throughout gestation.

Following this, some of the anomalies detectable by transvaginal sonography will be presented. It is beyond the scope of this chapter to list and show all the fetal CNS anomalies. However, the images presented here will enable the reader to understand the principle of the scanning methods and their advantages.

*NEURAL TUBE DEFECTS (NTDs)* (see Chapter 13). Considering the incidence of NTDs in the world is 2–3 per 1000 births it is important to recognize them at the earliest possible stage. Fig. 18.10 illustrates a fetus with anencephaly and rachyschysis detected at 18 weeks and 5 days gestation by transvaginal sonography. We would like to point out that it is possible to detect the exencephaly–anencephaly sequence as early as 9 to 10 weeks gestation by carefully scanning the fetal head. The head shape in the coronal, sagittal as well as in the axial planes are part of the diagnosis at these early gestational ages. We strengthened the theory of Bronshtein *et al.* (1999) who believed that the anencephaly results from the rubbing-off of exposed brain tissue, by observing the progressively diminishing amount of brain tissue in cases of exencephaly and by detecting free-floating neural cells. It is therefore felt that the exposed brain tissue is disintegrating and diminishing as gestation progresses (Timor-Tritsch *et al.* 1996; Greenbaum *et al.* 1997).

*CHOROID PLEXUS CYSTS* (see p. 286) These are fluid-filled cystic lesions in the choroid plexus and have an approximate incidence of 1% of all pregnancies. They are usually benign and disappear about the 24th postmenstrual week. An ongoing debate is reflected in the literature as to whether they are indeed markers of chromosomal anomalies. They can be detected as early as the 11th–12th week of gestation. Fig. 18.11 depicts bilateral cysts on the Midcoronal-2 section.

*VENTRICULOMEGALY AND HYDROCEPHALY* (see p. 284) These two terms are used interchangeably; however, ventriculo-

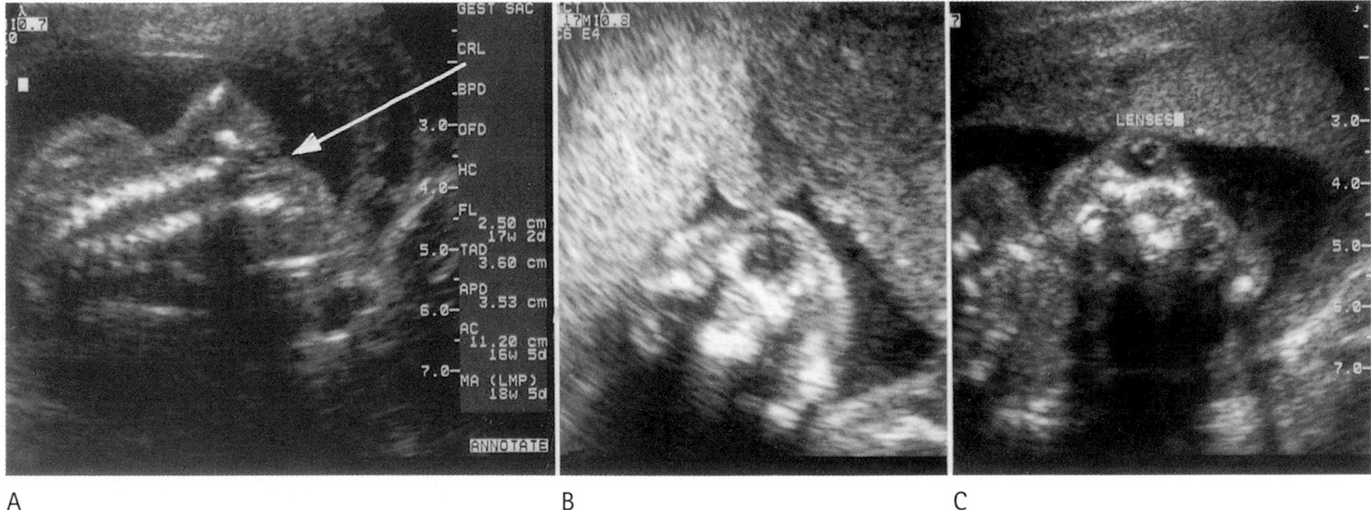


**Figure 18.10** Anencephaly and upper spinal rachyschysis at 18 postmenstrual weeks by transvaginal sonography. (A) The arrow points to the open upper spine; (B) sagittal section of the face and base of skull; (C) coronal section of the head.

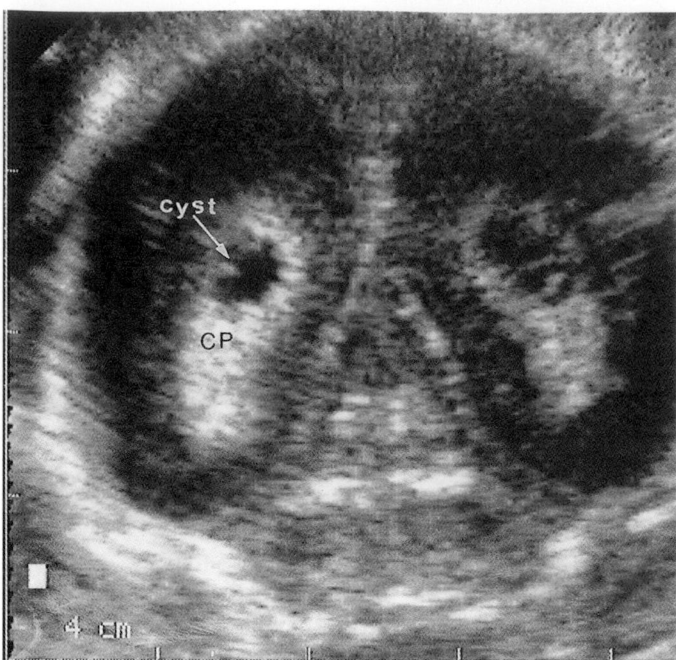


**Figure 18.11** Mid-coronal-3 section obtained by transvaginal sonography at 16 postmenstrual weeks depicting the bilateral choroid plexus cysts (CP, choroid plexus) and the infratentorial cerebellar hemispheres.

megaly is a denotation of the lateral ventricles when there is normal CNS fluid pressure present. As opposed to this, hydrocephaly is more than ventriculomegaly, since in this case there is an increased pressure of CFS fluid, causing increasing fetal head size and thinning of the brain tissue. Usually hydrocephaly is divided into non-communicating (Fig. 18.5) and communicating types. The diagnosis of hydrocephaly or ventriculomegaly is relatively simple, as there are relatively large fluid-filled spaces which can be detected easily even by transabdominal fetal neuroscan.

The size of the ventricular system can be evaluated subjectively and objectively. There are several ways to assess the size of the ventricles subjectively or qualitatively using transvaginal sonography: (a) relying on *indirect signs* such as the thickness of the cortical mantle, detection of the inferior horn (which should normally not be seen on an Oblique-1 section!), the shape and the mobility of the choroid plexus (if thin and dangling it signifies ventricular dilatation; (b) the *gestalt approach*, defined as relying on the observers experience in judging the appearance of the ventricular system; (c) looking at the third ventricle on Mid-coronal-1 or 2 sections. Anytime this ventricle is seen (usually it is slit-like!) attention to the entire ventricular system should be given.

As shown earlier the three horn views are instrumental sections that provide valuable information about the extent of this pathology. The objective assessment of ventricular size is based upon the published measurements of different parts of the lateral and the third ventricles or their ratios. These measurements are based upon TAS (Pretorius *et al.* 1986; Cardoza *et al.* 1988) or transvaginal sonography (Monteagudo *et al.* 1993, 1994).

Transvaginal sonographic evaluation of the ventricular system seems to be of high specificity in detecting mild ventriculomegaly as well as asymmetric ventriculomegaly. Their implications are well documented in the literature (Mahony *et al.* 1988; Bromley *et al.* 1991; Achiron *et al.* 1993). Using such an apparently sensitive and specific scanning route, one has to still remember that the most important prognostic factors in the outcome of prenatally detected hydrocephaly are: associated chromosomal anomalies, the amount of residual brain tissue around the ventricles, and the presence or absence of any other anomaly.

*HOLOPROSENCEPHALY* (see p. 210 and 275) At birth its incidence is 1 per 1600 births, however, at earlier scans (in the late first and early second trimester) the sonologist will encounter this anomaly more frequently (Matsunaga & Shiota 1977).

Two of the more frequent forms: alobar and semilobar types are relatively easily diagnosed any time an exhaustive fetal neuroscan is performed. Absence of the inter-hemispheric fissure (total or pential), non-disjunction of the thalami, no corpus callosum, and cavum septi pellucidi and several facial anomalies (cyclops, proboscis, median clefts, etc.) are the most frequent, but not the only features.

The lobar type has more subtle features. At times the only signs are clustered around the corpus callosum, cavum septi pellucidi, and the 3rd ventricle. The box-shaped cavity in the midbrain, below the corpus callosum without the two lateral

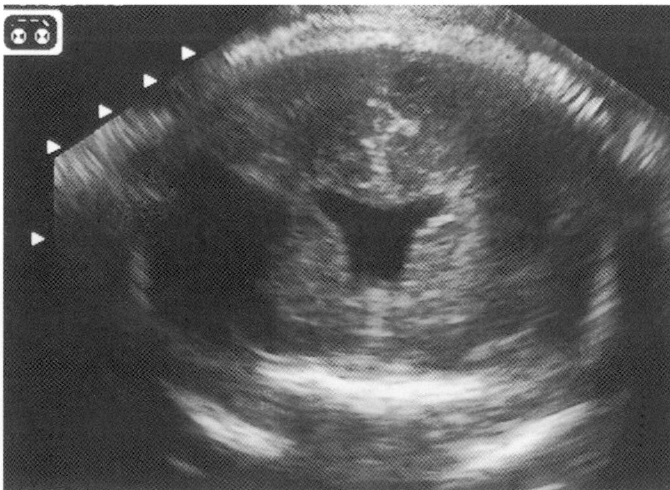

**Figure 18.12** Lobar holoprosencephaly. Typical shape of the third ventricle and the cavum septi pellucid on the Mid-coronal-1 section. The box-shaped sonolucent structure is created by the missing lateral walls of the cavum septi pellucidi (see the normal configuration on the same plane of Fig. 18.15, MC-1).

walls of the septum pellucidum give rise to the suggestion of lobar holoprosencephaly (Fig. 18.12) and its closest differential diagnosis: septo-optic displasia (Pilu *et al.* 1996). At times the final diagnosis is made after birth.

*AGENESIS OF THE CORPUS CALLOSUM* (see also Chapter 13) Our aim here is to demonstrate the diagnosis of total and/or partial agenesis of the corpus callosum (TACC, PACC). The use of transvaginal sonography seems to us indispensable to make or rule out this diagnosis in a reliable and straightforward manner (Fig. 8.13). Indeed some of the indirect diagnostic features of ACC such as the teardrop-shaped lateral ventricles on the axial section; the widely displaced upward pointing anterior horns, the upward displaced 3rd ventricle connecting in an unobstructed way with the interhemispheric fissure on coronal sections can be seen using transabdominal sonography. However, these are indirect signs. The direct observation of the presence or absence (or partial absence) of this structure is only possible using the median plane. As pointed out earlier transabdominal sonography can rarely provide this plane.

Owing to the sporadic use of transvaginal sonography many sonologists and sonographers using only transabdominal sonography diagnose and report the associated and more obvious hydrocephaly and miss the real diagnosis (i.e. ACC or PACC). This was our impression during the last five or six years looking at cases referred to us for a second opinion for hydrocephaly or ventriculomegaly. A

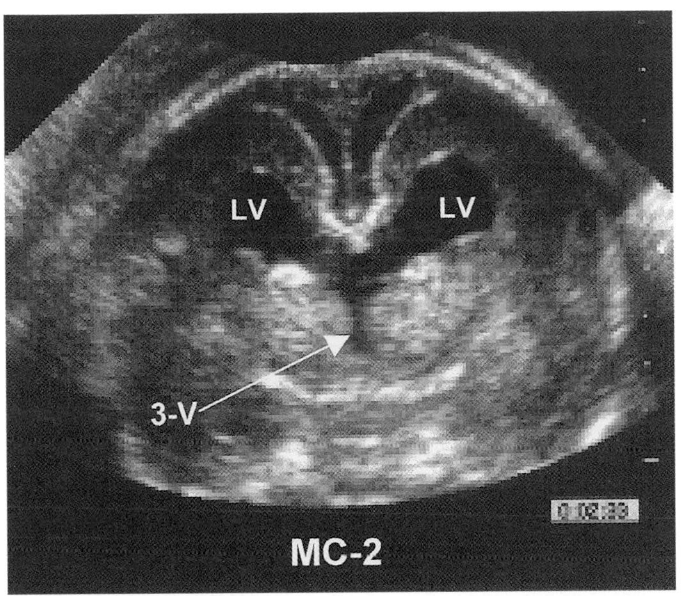


A

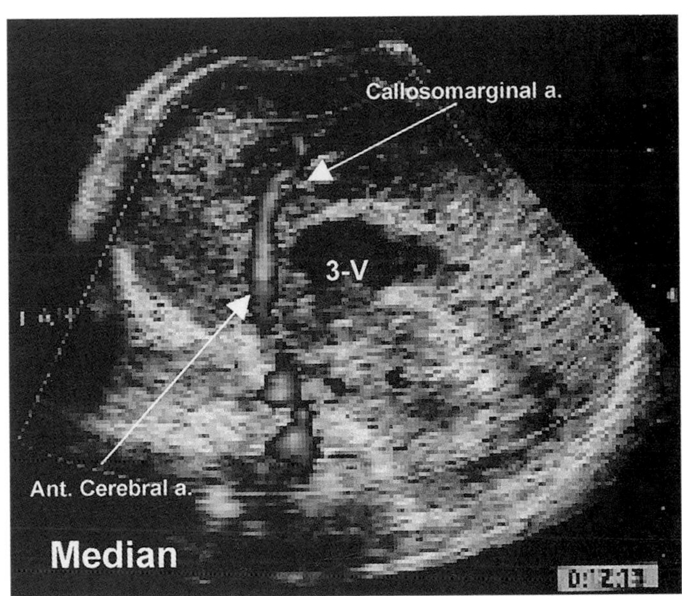


C

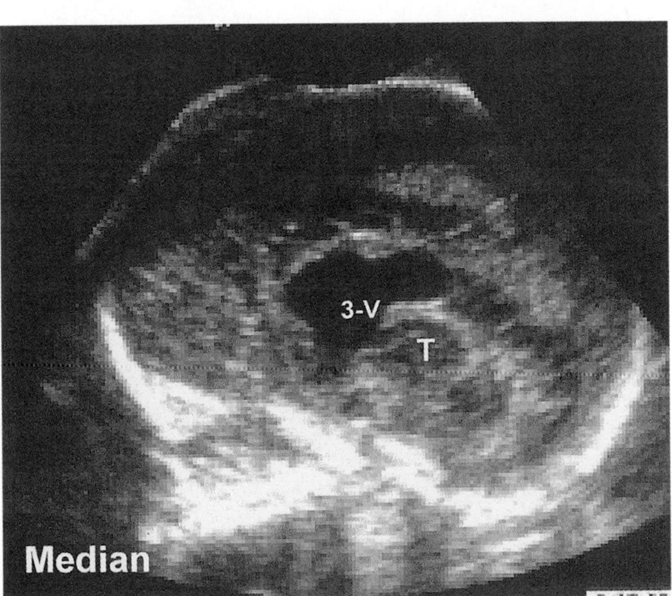


B

Figure 18.13 Total agenesis of the corpus callosum at 23 postmenstrual weeks. (A) MC-2, Mid-coronal-2 section with the 3rd ventricle (3-V) communicating with the lateral ventricles (LV) without the presence of the corpus callosum or the cavum septi pellucidi. The two median sections (B, C) and practically the same showing the upward displaced 3rd ventricle above the thalamus (T), however part (C) is a power Doppler image of the anterior cerebral and the callosomarginal arteries without the presence of the pericallosal artery.

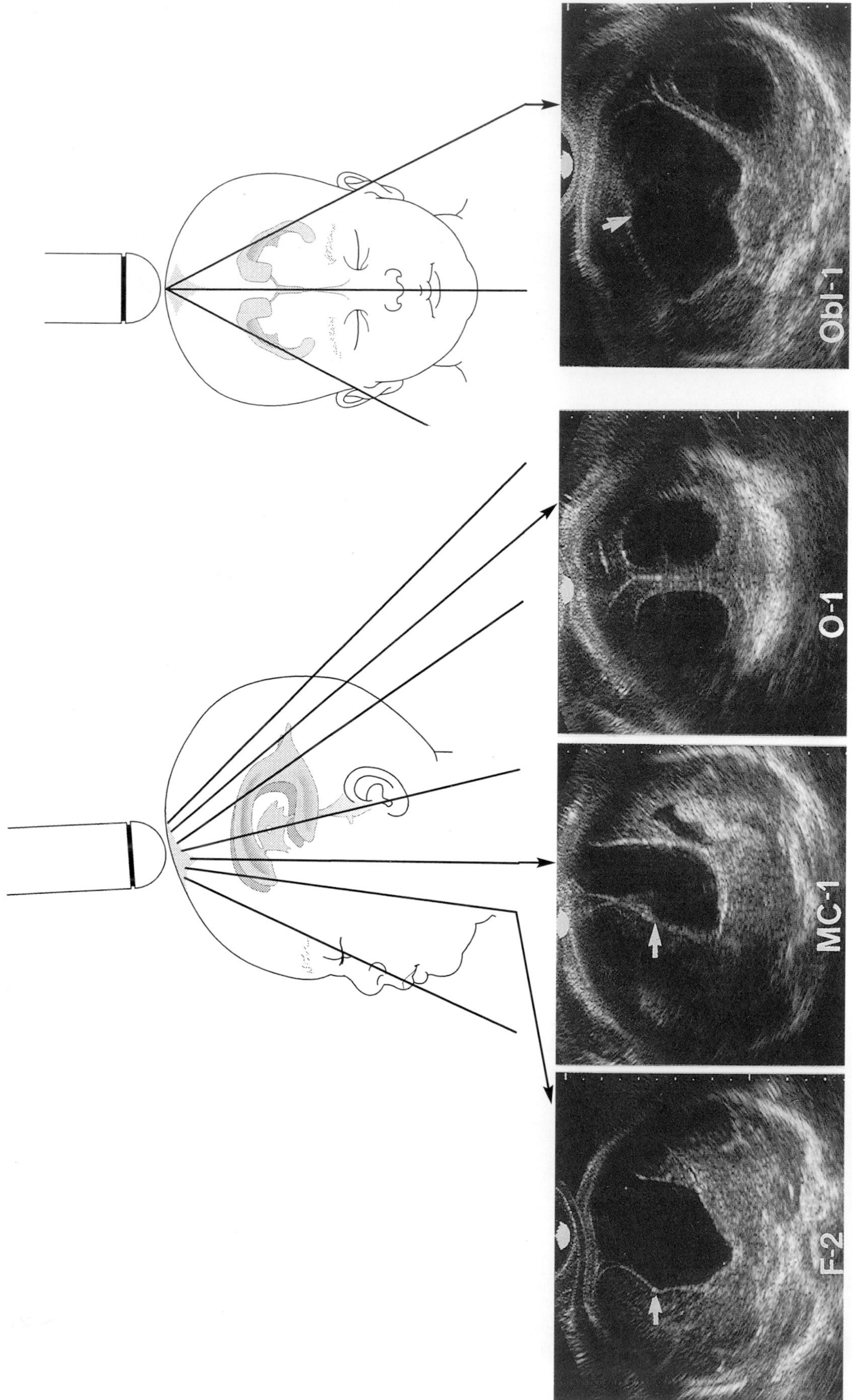


**Figure 18.14** Arachnoid cysts at 23 postmenstrual weeks. The cyst is marked by arrows. It originates probably from the area of the quadrigeminal plate. The cyst extends anteriorly and is seen on Frontal-2 (F-2) section. On the Mid-coronal-1 (MC-1) section, it is clear that the cyst is predominantly on the left side of the mid-line (the falx is displaced to the right). There was already sufficient pressure on the aqueduct to cause ventriculomegaly (note the dilatation of the posterior horn on the O-1 section). The Oblique-1 (Obl-1) section demonstrates the extent of the cyst anteriorly and posteriorly.

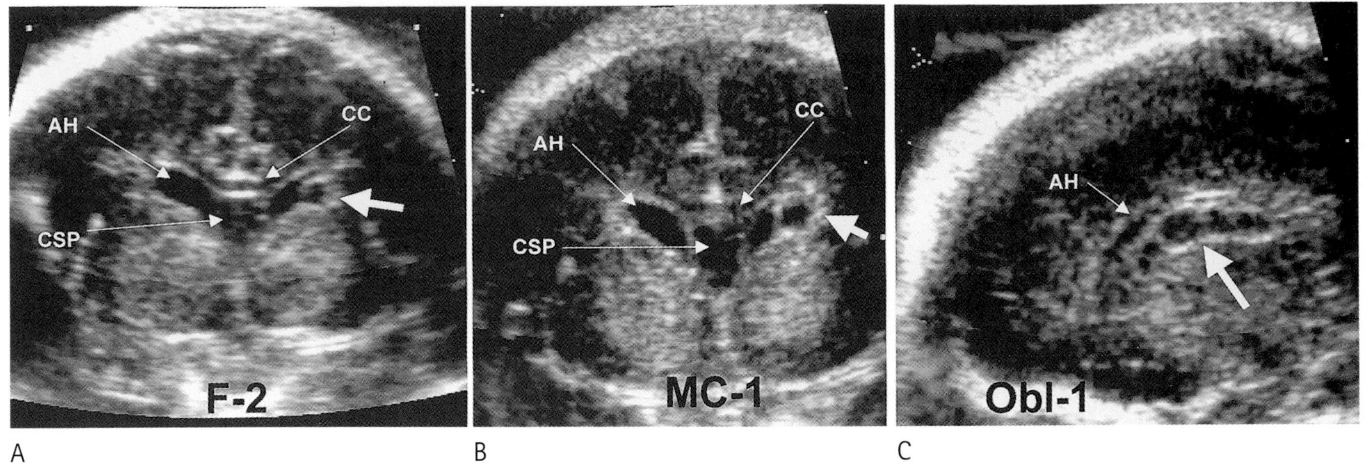


**Figure 18.15** Periventricular leukomalacia in a fetus at 28 postmenstrual weeks in a twin pregnancy. (A) Frontal-2 (F-2) section with the large arrow pointing at the lesion. (B) Mid-coronal-1 (MC-1) section; the large arrow points to the lesion. (C) Oblique-1 (Obl-1) section with the lesion highlighted with the large arrow. AH, anterior horn; CC, corpus callosum; CSP, cavum septi pellucidi.

large number of these in fact were diagnosed as ACC or PACC!

*ARACHNOID CYSTS* (see p. 286) These are CSF filled spaces which do not connect with the ventricles or the cava. They are space occupying lesions with all the effects of such lesions; however, histologically they are benign. They appear as sonolucent, thin-walled structures. Most common are left sided lesions and 10% are located in the quadrigeminal cistern (Fig. 18.14). Five to ten percent are in the posterior fossa and about 10% of them are in potentially dangerous areas (e.g. the suprasellar cistern). By exerting pressure on the flow of the CSF they may cause bilateral hydrocephaly (e.g. pressure on the interventricular foramen). If they are located on the convexity of the brain, the outcome is usually good (Hudgins *et al.* 1988).

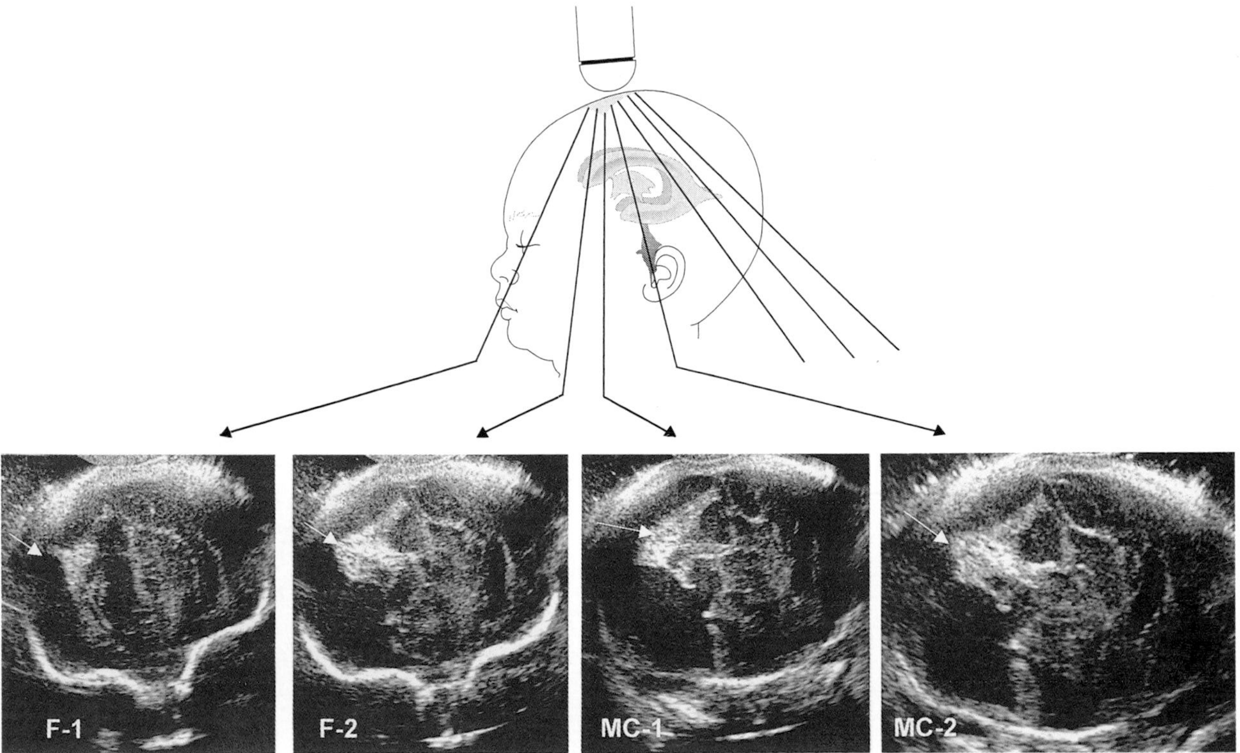

*PERIVENTRICULAR LEUKOMALACIA* (see Chapters 21 and 22) As the name implies the lesion is located in the white matter around or close to the lateral ventricles. It is believed that the relatively poorly visualized areas between two arterial supplies ('water shed areas') are affected by changes in the blood supply, resulting in this pathology (Fig. 18.15).

*INTRACRANIAL HEMORRHAGE* (Chapter 21) This rarely occurs *in utero*; however, if it occurs it is caused among other things by hypoxemia, congenital vascular anomalies, clotting defects, drugs, thrombosis of the umbilical cord or its entanglement.

One can detect fresh clots by their hyperechoic appearance within the parenchyma or in the ventricles. Sites of long standing clots may disintegrate and become porencephalic cysts (Fig. 18.16).

The neurodevelopmental long term outcome of fetuses diagnosed with intracranial hemorrhages is related to the severity and the location of the hemorrhage.

**Key Points**

- Fetal neuroscan, using transvaginal sonography in particular can detect the overwhelming majority of structural anomalies of the CNS. Its strength is that it can detect the anomalies that are developing early in gestation.
- It is important to stress that knowledge of the 'developmental timetable' of the fetal brain is essential to correct assessment of the normal and the abnormal fetal CNS. In addition, it is necessary to operate high resolution ultrasound machines by skillfully trained sonographers and sonologists.
- Three-dimensional fetal neuroscan is a promising tool which undoubtedly will be of pivotal importance in the future.

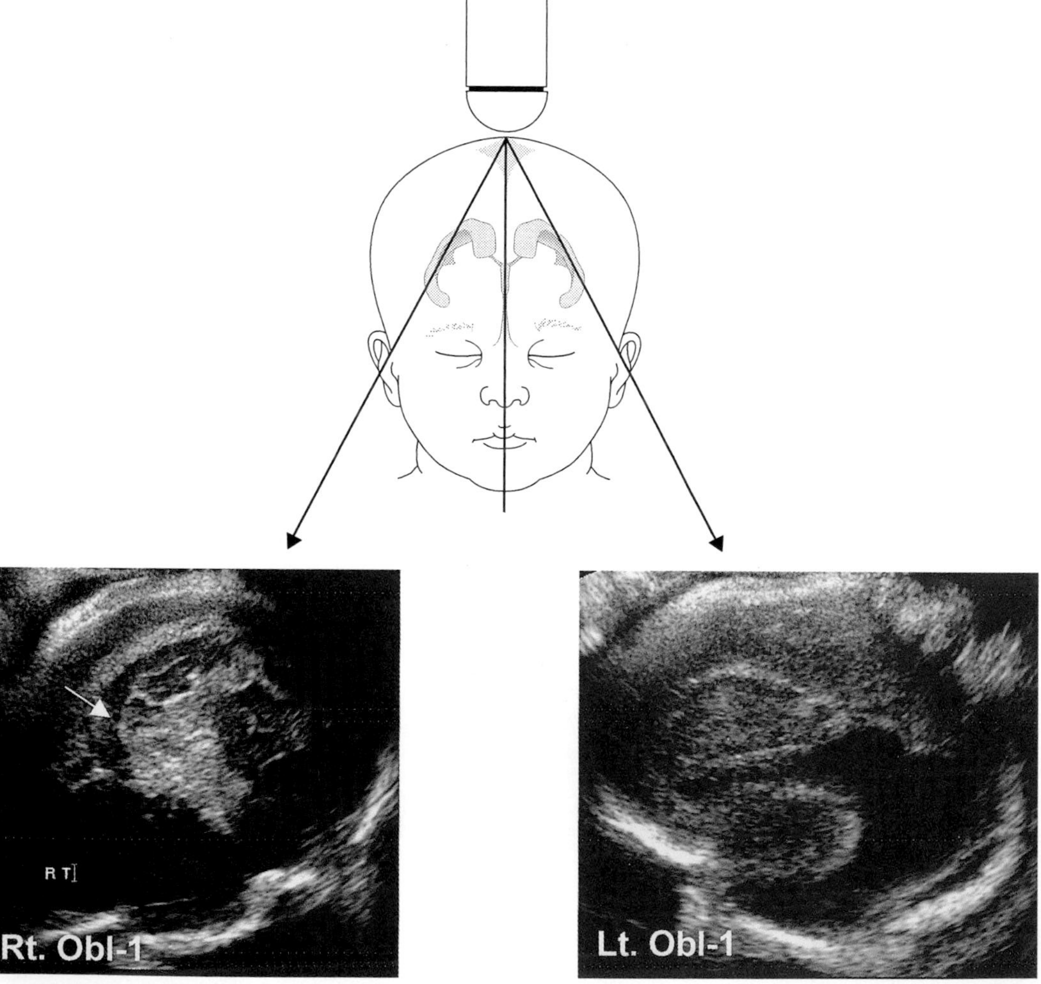


B

**Figure 18.16** Intraparenchymal bleeding, mostly in the right hemisphere, marked by the arrow. The right hemisphere is almost totally destroyed with excessive lateral ventriculomegaly. The left lateral ventricle is dilated however to a somewhat lesser degree (A) Four successive coronal sections: F-1=Frontal-1 (F-1) section, F-2–Frontal-2 (F-2) section, MC-1=Mid-coronal-1 (MC-1) section, MC-2–Mid coronal-2 (MC-2) section. (B) The right and left oblique-1 sections.

## REFERENCES


Achiron R & Achiron A (1991) Transvaginal ultrasonic assessment of the early fetal brain. *Ultrasound Obstet Gynecol* 1: 336–344.

Achiron R, Schimmel M, Achiron A *et al.* (1993) Fetal mild idiopathic lateral ventriculomegaly: Is there a correlation with fetal trisomy? *Ultrasound Obstet Gynecol* 3: 89–92.

Babcock D S, Han B K, LeQuesne G W (1980) B-mode gray scale ultrasound of the head in the newborn and young infant. *AJR Am J Radiol* 134: 457–468.

Ben-Ora A, Eddy L, Hatch G *et al.* (1980) The anterior fontanelle as an acoustic window to the neonatal ventricular system. *J Clin Ultrasound* 8: 65–67.

Blass H G, Eik-Nes S H, Kiserud T *et al.* (1994) Early development of the forebrain and midbrain: a longitudinal ultrasound study from 7 to 12 postmenstrual weeks of gestation. *Ultrasound Obstet Gynecol* 4: 183–192.

Blaas H G, Eik-Nes S H, Kiserud T *et al.* (1995a) Early development of the hindbrain: a longitudinal ultrasound study from 7 to 12 weeks of gestation. *Ultrasound Obstet Gynecol* 5: 151–160.

Blaas H G, Eik-Nes S H, Kiserud T *et al.* (1995b) Three-dimenstional imaging of the brain cavities in human embryos. *Ultrasound Obstet Gynecol* 5: 228–232.

Bromley B, Frigoletto F D & Benacerraf B R (1991) Mild fetal lateral cerebral ventriculomegaly: clinical course and outcome. *Am J Obstet Gynecol* 164: 863–867.

Bronshtein M & Ornoy A (1991) Acrania: anencephaly resulting from secondary degeneration of a closed neural tube: two cases in the same family. *J Clin Ultrasound* 19: 230–234.

Cardoza I D, Goldstein R B & Filly R A (1988) Exclusion of fetal ventriculomegaly with a single measurement of the width of the lateral ventricular atrium. *Radiology* 169: 711–714.

Cohen H L & Ziprkowski M (1991) New diagnostic insight in pediatric neurosonography. *Diagn Imag* 13: 142–146.

Dewbury K C, Aluwihare A P R (1980) The anterior fontanelle as an ultrasound window for study of the brain: a preliminary report. *Br J Radiol* 53: 81–84.

Edwards M K, Brown D L, Muller J *et al.* (1981) Cribside neurosonography: real-time sonography for intracranial investigation of the neonate. *AJR Am J Radiol* 136: 271–276.

Grant E & Richardson J (1994) Infant and neonatal neurosonography technique and normal anatomy. In: Taveras J (ed.) *Radiology diagnosis–imaging–intervention*, vol 3. Philadelphia PA: Lippincott; pp. 1–7.

Grant E G, Schellinger D, Borts F T *et al.* (1981) Real-time sonography of the neonatal and infant head. *AJR Am J Radiol* 136: 265–270.

Greenebaum E, Mansakhani M M, Heller D S & Timor-Tritsch I E (1997) Open neural tube defects: immunocyto-chemical demonstration of neuroepithelial cells in amniotic fluid. *Diagn Cytopathol* 16(2): 143–144.

Hudgins R J, Edwards M S B, Goldstein R *et al.* (1988) Natural history of fetal ventriculomegaly. *Pediatrics* 82: 692–697.

Johnson M L, Rumack C M (1980) Ultrasonic evaluation of the neonatal brain. *Radiol Clin North Am* 18: 117–131.

Kushnir U, Shalev J, Bronshtein M *et al.* (1989) Fetal intracranial anatomy in the first trimester of pregnancy: transvaginal ultrasonographic evaluation. *Neuroradiology* 31: 222–225.

Mahony B S, Nyberg D A, Hirsch J H *et al.* (1988) Mild idiopathic lateral cerebral ventricular dilatation *in utero*: sonographic evaluation. *Radiology* 169: 715–721.

Malinger G & Zakut H (1993) The corpus callosum: normal fetal development as shown by transvaginal sonography. *AJR Am J Radiol* 161: 1041–1043.

Matsunaga E & Shiota Y (1977) Holoprosencephaly in human embryos: epidemiological studies of 150 cases. *Teratology* 16: 261.

Monteagudo A & Timor-Tritsch I E (1997) Development of fetal gyri, sulci and fissures: a transvaginal sonographic study. *Ultrasound Obstet Gynecol* 9: 222–228.

Monteagudo A, Reuss M L & Timor-Tritsch I E (1991a) Imaging the fetal brain in the second and third trimesters using transvaginal sonography. *Obstet Gynecol* 77: 27–32.

Monteagudo A, Timor-Tritsch I E, Reuss M L *et al.* (1991b) Transvaginal sonography of the second and third trimester fetal brain. In: Timor-Tritsch I E, Rottern S (eds) *Transvaginal sonography*, 2nd edn. New York, NY: Chapman & Hall; 393–425.

Monteagudo A, Timor-Tritsch I E & Moomjy M (1994) *In utero* detection of ventriculomegaly during the second and third trimesters by transvaginal sonography. *Ultrasound Obstet Gynecol* 4: 193–198.

Monteagudo A, Timor-Tritsch I E & Moomjy M (1993) Nomograms of the fetal lateral ventricles using transvaginal sonography. *J Ultrasound Med* 5: 265–269.

Naidich T P, Yousefzadeh D K & Gusnard D A (1986) Sonography of the normal neonatal head. Supratentorial structures: state of the art imaging. *Neuroradiology* 28: 408–427.

Nomina anatomica, 6th edn. (1989). Authorized by the 12th International Congress of Anatomists, London, 1985. Edinburgh: Churchill Livingstone.

Pilu G, Perolo A & David C (1996) Midline anomalies of the brain. In: Timor-Tritsch I E, Monteagudo A & Cohen H L (eds) *Ultrasonography of the prenatal and neonatal brain.* Stamford, CT: Appleton & Lange; 241–258.

Pretorius D H, Drose J A & Manco-Johnson M L (1986) Fetal lateral ventricular ratio determination during the second-trimester. *J Ultrasound Med* 5: 121–124.

Richardson D J & Grant E G (1986) Scanning techniques and normal anatomy. In: Grant GE (ed). *Neurosonography of the preterm neonate.* New York, NY: Springer-Verlarg; pp. 1–24.

Slovis T L, Kuhns L R (1981) Real-time sonography of the brain through the anterior fontanelle. *AJR* 136: 277–286.

Timor-Tritsch I E & Monteagudo A (1991) Transvaginal sonographic evaluation of the fetal central nervous system. *Obstet Gynecol Clin North Am* 18: 713–748.

Timor-Tritsch I E & Monteagudo A (1996) Transvaginal fetal neurosonography: standardization of the planes and sections by anatomic landmarks. *Ultrasound Obstet Gynecol* 8: 42–47.

Timor-Tritsch I E, Farine D & Rosen M G (1988) A close look at early embryonic development with the high-frequency transvaginal transducer. *Am J Obstet Gynecol* 159: 676–681.

Timor-Tritsch I E, Peisner D B & Raju S (1990) Sonoembryology: an organ-oriented approach using a high-frequency vaginal probe. *J Clin Ultrasound* 18: 286–298.

Timor-Tritsch I E, Monteagudo A & Warren W B (1991) Transvaginal ultrasonographic definition of the central nervous system in the first and early second trimesters. *Am J Obstet Gynecol* 164: 747–753.

Timor-Tritsch I E, Blumenfeld Z, Rottem S (1991) Sonoembryology. In: Timor-Tritsch I E, Rottem S (eds) *Transvaginal sonography*, 2nd edn. New York, NY: Chapman & Hall; p. 241.

Timor-Tritsch I E, Greenebaum E, Monteagudo A & Baxi L (1996) The exencephaly-anencephaly sequence: proof by ultrasound imaging and amniotic fluid cytology. *Matern Fet Med* 5: 182–185.

Timor-Tritsch I E, Monteagudo A & Mayberry P (2000a) 3-D ultrasound evaluation of the fetal brain: the three horn view. *Ultrasound Obstet Gynecol* 16: 302–306.

Timor-Tritsch I E, Monteagudo A & Mayberry P (2000b) Three dimensional transvaginal neurosonography of the fetal brain: navigating in the volume scan. *Ultrasound Obstet Gynecol* 16: 307–313.

Warren WB, Timor-Tritsch I E, Peisner D B *et al.* (1989) Dating the early pregnancy by sequential appearance of embryonic structures. *Am J Obstet Gynecol* 161: 747–753.

Chapter 19

# Epidemiology and prevention of NTDs

N. C. Nevin

## INTRODUCTION

Neural tube defects (NTDs) constitute a major public health problem in terms of mortality, morbidity, social cost and human suffering. Before considering the epidemiology of NTDs, it is necessary to define the disorders encompassed by the term. Anencephalus affects the structures derived from or associated with the cephalic end of the neural tube. Other NTDs that occur at the cephalic end of the neural tube include herniation of brain tissue, through a defect in the skull – for example, cranial meningocele, cranium bifidum and encephalocele. Most infants are stillborn and liveborn infants survive for a short period of time, usually a few days. Spina bifida is a term describing a variety of lesions due to midline separation of the vertebrae. Most spina bifida lesions are dorsal but ventral lesions also occur. 'Open' spina bifida describes a lesion where there is exposure of neural tissues, an open spinal canal and without skin cover. If skin cover is complete, the lesion is usually cystic (spina bifida/cystica). Craniorachischisis is a combination of anencephalus with exposure of spinal cord. Spina bifida occulta describes defects in the vertebrae covered with normal skin. It may not be obvious clinically but sometimes the overlying skin may be dimpled, pigmented, have an abnormal tuft of hair or hemangioma. Radiology of the spine will reveal the underlying bony defect in the vertebrae. The management of NTDs is discussed in Chapter 45.

## EMBRYOLOGY AND PATHOGENESIS OF NTDs

The brain and spinal cord are formed from the neural tube which is developed from the dorsal folding of the neural plate. The evidence favors primary non-closure as the most likely mechanism in the formation of NTDs. The neural plate folds dorsally commencing to fuse in the thoracic region at the six somite stage. Closure proceeds in cranial and caudal directions and is completed at 23–26 days. Recently, it has been suggested that closure of the neural plate is not a continuous sequence but may involve five separate sites of closure along the length of the neural tube (Van Allen *et al.* 1993). The lower sacral and spinal cord is formed not by closure of the neural tube but by another mechanism (neuralation). There is a condensation of mesenchymal cells arising from the primitive streak followed by canalization. Some authors have suggested that NTDs can be classified as: upper NTDs including anencephalus and spina bifida above the level of T11/T12; and lower NTDs, due to neuralation defects, below level of T11/T12 (Torillo & Higgins 1985; Seller 1990).

## EPIDEMIOLOGY OF NTDs

A fundamental criterion in studying the epidemiology of congenital abnormalities is the use of standardized definitions. The European Registration of Congenital Abnormalities and Twins (EUROCAT) has developed standard definitions of NTDs (De Wals *et al.* 1984), together with an illustrated guide to the recognition of malformations of the CNS (Nevin & Weatherall, 1983). The standardization of definitions of NTDs enables accurate comparisons to be made between various countries and centers. Thus it is possible to compare variations of prevalence of NTDs with time and place. Prevalence is defined as the number of infants and/or fetuses born per annum.

The region that has been investigated most is the British Isles where many surveys have been based on multiple sources of ascertainment. The highest prevalence rates at birth for NTDs reported in a community are 4.2 per 1000 for anencephalus and 4.5 per 1000 for spina bifida in Belfast in 1964–1968 (Elwood & Nevin, 1973). Fig. 19.1 shows the changing prevalence of anencephalus in one British city from 1936–65. During 1974–79, lower prevalence rates were

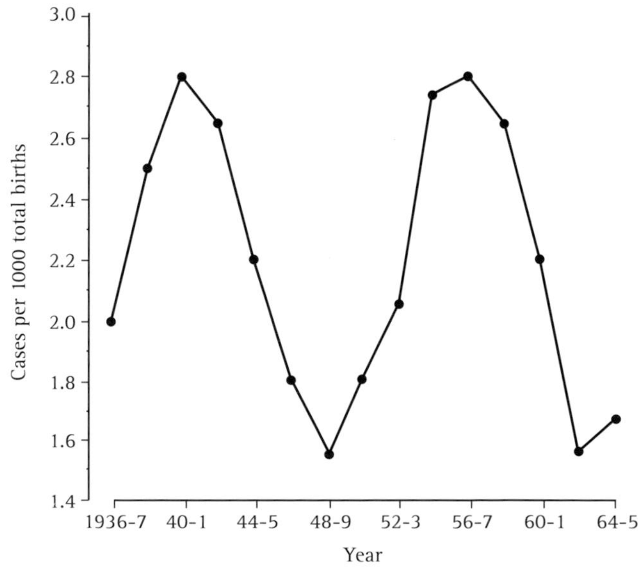


**Figure 19.1** Anencephaly prevalence rates in Birmingham, 1936–1965 (data from MacMahon *et al.* 1951, Leck 1966).

recorded; the combined rates were 6.3 per 1000 for Northern Ireland, 4.5 per 1000 for Scotland and 2.5 per 1000 for England and Wales. Prevalence rates have continued to decline over the past two decades. The geographic variation of NTDs is striking. The highest rates are found in NW Europe especially among the peoples of Ireland, Scotland, and South Wales. The EUROCAT Working Group (1991) recorded data on NTDs from six registers for congenital malformations in the British Isles (1980–86). The prevalence rates in this study included abortions as well as NTDs at birth. The prevalence rates were two to three times higher than those in eight similar registers in continental Europe. Prevalence rates for anencephalus were consistently lower than those for spina bifida. Penrose (1957) first drew attention to the general trend of a decrease in the prevalence of NTDs from west to east across Europe. Prior to 1980, few reports of prevalence rates for NTDs from Europe were available. Data are now much more extensive. Prevalence rates for NTDs are generally lower than those of the British Isles, ranging from 0.4 per 1000 births (Finland) to 1.6 per 1000 births (Hungary). The EUROCAT Working Group (1991) reported prevalence rates of NTDs in eight European registries and six British Isles registries. The rates for anencephalus (1980–88) in the eight European centers ranged from 0.3 to 0.7 per 1000 births and the rates for spina bifida were similar compared with prevalence rates of 0.9 to 1.5 for anencephalus and 1.4 to 1.8 for spina bifida in the six British Isles registries.

In the 1960s and 1970s, prevalence rates in North America and Canada were higher on the east coast and lower on the west coast. Both spina bifida and anencephalus showed a similar geographic variation. In the USA, high prevalence rates were observed in NE for both spina bifida and hydrocephalus in the 1960s and 1970s but later data did not show this geographic pattern.

The British Isles remains a relatively high-risk region, and within the British Isles the highest rates are seen in Northern Ireland, the Republic of Ireland, and in Scotland. However, recent data show prevalence rates for NTDs between 3 and 6 per 1000 births, in contrast to figures of between 6 and 10 some three decades ago (Elwood *et al.* 1992). In Quebec, Canada the prevalence rate of NTDs has been reduced by a factor of 3 during the last three decades (De Wals *et al.* 1999). The decrease in prevalence rates for NTDs has been influenced by prenatal recognition but it is clear that this is not the sole explanation and that there has been a considerable natural decline. The decrease in the prevalence of NTDs preceded any significant impact from prenatal diagnosis. Rosano *et al.* (1999) examined time trends of NTD prevalence rates from 1987 to 1996 in relation to the primary prevention policies for folic acid supplementation strategies in Atlanta (USA), England, Wales, Hungary, and Japan. They concluded that there is no evidence that up to the middle of 1996, any change in time trend was attributable to the introduction of national folate supplementation policies.

## IMPACT OF PRENATAL DIAGNOSIS

Prenatal diagnosis of NTDs is carried out by ultrasound examination (see Chapters 17 and 18) and measurement of serum α-fetoprotein (AFP) in maternal serum or in amniotic fluid (see Chapter 16). The widespread use of prenatal diagnosis for NTDs has made epidemiologic studies more difficult. True NTD prevalence rates are impossible to obtain, as there is no statutory requirement to document the presence or nature of an abnormality in the fetus of a pregnancy which has been terminated. Cuckle & Wald (1987) pointed out that the birth prevalence of anencephaly and spina bifida declined by 80% from 3.15 to 0.6 per 1000 births between 1964–72 and 1985. Over the same period notified terminations of pregnancy with a suspected NTD rose from less than 1% to 56%. They estimated prenatal diagnosis accounted for 31% of the decline in the prevalence rate of NTDs. Scotland had one of the first and most intensive population screening programmes for NTDs. From 1974 to mid-1980s, the proportion of anencephalus diagnosed prenatally with subsequent selective abortion rose to over 80% for both Glasgow and the whole of Scotland. Similarly, for spina bifida, the proportion detected prenatally reached 50–60% (Stone *et al.* 1988). The EUROCAT Working Group (1991) had as one of its aims, to evaluate the impact of prenatal diagnosis in terms of frequency and timing of termination of pregnancy. The study involved a total of 3113 cases of NTDs in 20 regions. In 11 centers the impact of prenatal diagnosis on prevalence at birth could be evaluated. In all centers, anencephaly was more frequently diagnosed prenatally and aborted than spina bifida, and prenatal diagnosis of anencephaly was made earlier during the pregnancy. In 6 of the 11 centers registering induced abortions, terminations were performed in at least 80% of total cases of anencephaly and in at least 40% of total cases of spina bifida. There was considerable regional variation in the impact of prenatal diagnosis and pregnancy termination linked to different policies and practices of prenatal screening. The impact of prenatal diagnosis and subsequent termination of pregnancy on the prevalence rates of NTDs in the USA has not been well established. Assessment of this impact on prevalence rates is crucial to the use of surveillance data to monitor trends in the occurrence of NTDs and the effectiveness of intervention strategies for these defects. Cragan *et al.* (1995) presented data from birth defects surveillance systems in six states over different time periods. Among all the pregnancies ascertained in which an infant or fetus had anencephaly or spina bifida, the percentages that were electively terminated ranged from 9% to 42%. In each system, pregnancies associated with anencephaly were terminated more frequently than those associated with spina bifida. The conclusion was that the impact of prenatal diagnosis and subsequent termination of pregnancy on the prevalence rates at birth of NTDs varied among geographic areas and populations. More recently, Forrester & Merz (2000) reached a similar conclusion using the data in the

Hawaii Birth Defects Program, where 74% of NTDs were diagnosed prenatally and 48% were terminated. It is important that all future epidemiologic studies of NTDs must incorporate pregnancies diagnosed prenatally and terminated, in order to monitor trends accurately and to establish the effectiveness of intervention strategies.

## PRIMARY PREVENTION OF NTDs

Some features of the epidemiology of NTDs are consistent with a genetic component in their etiology. First, the concordance rates for NTDs are significantly higher in monozygotic twin pairs than in dizygotic twin pairs, indicating a probable genetic component. Second, the increased risk among siblings, the offspring of parents with spina bifida and among half siblings is also consistent with a genetic component. An important issue in elucidating the possible role of genetic factors is whether NTDs are etiologically homogeneous. Some genetic heterogenicity of NTDs is established by the observation that anencephalus, spina bifida, or encephalocele may occur as a component of certain syndromes, with a Mendelian mode of inheritance, for example, Meckel's syndrome or in association with chromosomal anomalies, for example trisomy 18 (Edward's syndrome). As the majority of NTDs do not appear to have a monogenic mode of inheritance or a chromosomal anomaly, yet appear to have a genetic component, investigators have considered etiologies involving both genetic and environmental components. There are two major types: the multifactorial model and models involving major gene effects on susceptibility to environmental factors. In the multifactorial model, it is assumed that many independent genetic loci and environmental factors contribute small effects to a quantitative phenotype. In the major gene models, susceptibility to environmental factors varies according to one or more genetic loci (Little & Nevin, 1992). With the multifactorial model, the occurrence of NTDs depends on the additive effects of several abnormal genes and environmental factors. Accumulation of these aberrant genetic and environmental factors can be tolerated by the fetus to a point (the 'threshold') beyond which there is a risk of an NTD. Carter (1976) concluded that 'little is yet known about the mechanisms by which the genetic predisposition acts or the environmental factors involved'.

Among the factors that have been suggested as possibly contributing to the etiology of NTDs is maternal nutrition. Undoubtedly, good maternal nutrition is important in normal embryonic and fetal development. Warkany & Nelson (1941) found that nutritional deficiency in pregnancy, notably vitamin deficiency, could result in congenital malformations in the offspring. The mean blood levels of serum folate, red cell folate, white cell vitamin C, and riboflavin values were lower in mothers who gave birth to infants with NTDs than in control mothers (Smithells *et al.* 1976, 1980, 1983; Wild *et al.* 1986). In Scotland, a similar study demonstrated red cell folate levels were lower in mothers who had an infant with a NTD than controls (Yates *et al.* 1987). The possible role of folic acid deficiency in the etiology of NTDs prompted intervention studies using vitamin supplementation for women at increased risk of an infant with a NTD. These studies assessed the protective effect of vitamin supplementation in terms of the recurrence rate of NTDs in mothers who had had one or more affected children, and whose expected recurrence risk was up to 5% (Nevin and Johnston, 1980). A multicenter non-randomized prospective trial of periconceptional vitamin supplementation (pregnavite forte F) in the prevention of NTDs showed that of infants or fetuses born to fully supplemented mothers, the recurrence rate of a NTD was 0.6% compared with 5.0% in the infants and fetuses of unsupplemented mothers (Smithells *et al.* 1980). Subsequently, more detailed and extended reports confirmed the protective effect.

In 1983 the UK Medical Research Council initiated a randomized trial of prevention of recurrence of NTDs. Those eligible were women who had had a previous pregnancy affected by a NTD. The design of the trial assessed four supplementation regimes: (1) folic acid and minerals; (2) folic acid, other vitamins and minerals; (3) minerals only, and (4) other vitamins and minerals. Folic acid was given as 4 mg daily. A total of 1817 women had been randomized in 17 centers in the UK and 16 other countries. Half the women took folic acid and half did not. The results of the trial were very clear. There were six recurrences in 593 pregnancy outcomes in women receiving folic acid, a rate of 1.0% compared with 21 recurrences in 602 informative pregnancies in women not receiving folic acid, a rate of 3.5%. These results confirmed a protective effect of folic acid of 72%. An immediate consequence was that dietary supplementation with folic acid should be offered to all women who have had a previous pregnancy affected with a NTD (MRC Vitamin Study Group 1991). The recommended daily dose of folic acid was 5 mg for all those who had a previous affected pregnancy and who may become pregnant. The folic acid supplements should be continued to the twelfth week of pregnancy. Over 95% of pregnancies resulting in a baby with NTDs were first occurrences. It is recommended that folic acid (0.4 mg) should be given to all women planning a pregnancy.

## HOW DOES FOLIC ACID PREVENT NTDs

About 60–70% NTDs during fetal development can be prevented by periconceptional supplementation of diet with folic acid. Recently, attention has been directed to the genetic component of NTDs. There is increasing evidence that the role of the folate in NTDs is not one of simple dietary deficiency. The first genetic risk factor for NTDs identified at a molecular level is a C677T (alanine to valine) polymorphism in the gene encoding for the folate dependent enzyme, 5,10-methylenetetrahydrofolate reductase (MTHFR). Individuals who are homozygous for the mutation have a thermolabile enzyme with relatively low levels of MTHFR activity (Van der Put *et al.* 1998). The genotypes and folic acid status were assessed in 56 patients with spina bifida, 62 mothers of patients, 97 children without NTDs and 90 mothers of the controls. Of these, 20% of spina bifida patients and 18% of their mothers were homozygous for MTHFR polymorphism compared with 11% control children and 11% control mothers. The results indicate that the mutant genotype conferred an increased risk for NTDs. The risk was further increased if the mother and child had the same genotype and was greater when the mutant genotype was also associated with a low folate status (Christensen *et al.*, 1999). A polymorphism in methionine synthase reductase (MTRR), the enzyme that activates cobalamin dependent synthase, A66G, increases NTD risk when cobalamin (vitamin B12) status is low or where the MTHFR mutant phenotype is present (Wilson *et al.* 1999).

## SUMMARY

In the past three decades, there has been substantial progress in the epidemiology, in the control of NTDs by prenatal diagnosis and in understanding their etiology. The most important development in etiology has been the recognition that periconceptional folic acid supplementation greatly reduces the rates of recurrence of NTDs. Many aspects of the biology of NTD are as yet unexplained. More research on the identification of the genetic components will lead to a greater understanding of the genetic-nutrient interaction in the causation of NTDs.

### Key Points

- There is a strong geographical variation in prevalence of NTD from west to east across Europe
- Contemporary prevalence of NTD rates is not possible due to unrecorded reasons for termination of pregnancy
- In the UK there has been an 80% decline in the prevalence of NTD in a 20-year period, with only 30% of this due to prenatal diagnosis
- Periconceptual folic acid (5 mg od) reduces risk of NTD by approximately 70% in women with one or more affected pregnancies
- In all pregnancies, periconceptual folic acid (0.4 mg od) prevents 60–70% of cases of NTD
- Predisposition to NTD appears to be predominately due to a polymorphism coding for the enzyme methionine synthase reductase

## REFERENCES


Carter C O (1976) Genetics of common single malformations. *Br Med Bull* 32: 21–26.

Christensen B, Arbour L, Tran P *et al.* (1999) Genetic polymorphisms in methylenetetrahydrofolate reductase and methionine synthase, folate levels in red blood cells and risk of neural tube defects. *Am J Med Genet* 84: 151–157.

Cragan J D, Roberts H E, Edmonds L D *et al.* (1995) Surveillance for anencephaly and spina bifida and the impact of prenatal diagnosis – United States, 1985–1994. *Morbid Mortal Wkly Rep CFC Surveillance Summary* 44: 1–13.

Cuckle H & Wald N (1987) The impact of screening for neural tube defects in England and Wales. *Prenat Diagn* 7: 91–99.

De Wals P, Mastroiacova P, Weatherall J A C & Lechat M F (1984) EUROCAT Guide for the registration of congenital anomalies: 1 Department of Epidemiology, Catholic University of Louvain, Brussels.

De Wals P, Trochet C & Pinsonneault L (1999) Prevalence of neural tube defects in the province of Quebec (1992). *Can J Public Health*, Jul–Aug, 237–239.

Elwood J M, Little J & Elwood J H (eds.) (1992) *Epidemiology and control of neural tube defects.* Oxford Medical Publications, pp. 101–106.

Elwood J H & Nevin N C (1973) Factors associated with anencephalus and spina bifida in Belfast. *Br J Prevent Soc Med* 27: 73–80.

EUROCAT Working Group (1991) Prevalence of neural tube defects in 20 regions of Europe and the impact of prenatal diagnosis, 1980–1986. *J Epidemiol Commun Health* 45: 52–58.

Forrester M B & Merz R D (2000) Prenatal diagnosis and elective termination of neural tube defects in Hawaii, 1986–1997. *Fetal Diagn Ther* 15: 146–151.

Leck I (1966) Changes in the incidence of neural tube defects. *Lancet* ii: 791–792.

Little J & Nevin N C (1992) Genetic models. In: Elwood J M, Little J & Elwood J H (eds.) *Epidemiology and control of neural tube defects.* Oxford: Oxford University Press; Ch 17; pp. 677–710.

MacMahon B, Record R G & McKeown T (1951) Secular changes in the incidence of malformations in the central nervous system. *Br J Prevent Soc Med* 5: 254–258.

Medical Research Council Vitamin Study Group (1991) Prevention of Neural Tube Defects: Results of the Medical Research Council Vitamin Study. *The Lancet* 238: 131–137.

Nevin N C & Johnston W P (1980) A family study of spina bifida and anencephalus in Belfast, Northern Ireland (1964–1968). *J Med Genet* 17: 203–211.

Nevin N C & Weatherall J A C (1983) *Illustrated guide to malformations of the central nervous system at birth.* Edinburgh: Commission of the European Communities Churchill Livingstone.

Penrose L S (1957) Genetics of anencephaly. *J Ment Def Res* 1: 4–15.

Rosano A, Smithells D, Cacciani L *et al.* (1999) Time trends in neural tube defects prevalence in relation to preventive strategies: an international study. *J Epidemiol Commun Health* 53: 630–635.

Seller M J (1990) Neural tube defects: are neuralation and canalization forms causally distinct? *Am J Med Genet* 35: 394–396.

Smithells R W, Shepperd S & Schorah C J (1976) Vitamin deficiencies and neural tube defects. *Arch Dis Child* 51: 944–950.

Smithells R W, Shepperd S, Schorah C J *et al.* (1980) Possible prevention of neural tube defects by periconceptional vitamin supplementation. *Lancet* i: 339–340.

Smithells R W, Nevin N C, Seller M J *et al.* (1983) Further experience of vitamin supplementation for prevention of neural tube defect recurrences. *Lancet* i: 1027–1031.

Stone D H, Smalls M J, Rosenberg K & Womersley J (1988) Screening for congenital neural tube defects in a high risk area: an epidemiological perspective. *J Epidemiol Commun Health* 42: 271–273.

Toriello H V & Higgins J V (1985) Possible causal heterogeneity in spina bifida cystica. *Am J Med Genet* 21: 13–20.

Van Allen M I, Kalousek D K, Cheenoff G F *et al.* (1993) Evidence for multi-site closure of neural tube in humans. *Am J Med Genet* 47: 723–743.

Van der Put N M, Gabreels F, Stevens E M *et al.* (1998) A second common mutation in methylenetetrahydrofolate reductase gene: an additional risk factor for neural tube defects? *Am J Hum Genet* 62: 1044–1051.

Warkany J & Nelson R C (1941) Skeletal abnormalities in the offspring of rats reared on deficient diets. *Anat Rec* 79: 83–100.

Wild J, Read A P, Sheppard S *et al.* (1986) Recurrent neural tube defects, risk factors and vitamins. *Arch Dis Child* 61: 440–444.

Wilson A, Platt R, Wu Q *et al.* (1999) A common variant in methionine synthase reductase combined with low cobalamin (vitamin B12) increases risk for spina bifida. *Mol Genet Metab* 67: 317–323.

Yates J R W, Ferguson-Smith M A, Shenkin A & Guzman-Rodriguez R *et al.* (1987) Is disordered folate metabolism the basis for the genetic predisposition neural tube defects? *Clin Genet* 31: 279–287.

# Section IV
# Hemorrhagic and ischemic lesions

# Chapter 20

# Fetal cerebral pathology of hypoxic–ischemic origin

W. Squier

## INTRODUCTION

This chapter describes and illustrates the nature of the damage that may result from hypoxic–ischemic injury to the human brain throughout its development from the earliest weeks of gestation until the first months of postnatal life. The developing brain is particularly vulnerable to a wide variety of insults that may cause structural damage. Hypoxic–ischemic injury is one of the commonest causes of damage to the developing brain, with the possibility of subsequent serious neurologic impairment. Long-term neurologic disability affects some 4 per 1000 full-term infants, and comprises motor and cognitive disorders as well as epilepsy and visual disorders. The clinical spectrum resulting from such damage is often described within the term 'cerebral palsy' (see Chapter 44). The pattern of damage is influenced by a number of factors including the developmental age at the time of the brain injury, the precise nature and severity of the insult, and the underlying metabolic state of the fetus. Recent experimental work has begun to define some of the underlying cellular mechanisms which account for changing vulnerability of different brain areas during development (see also Chapter 23).

## TERMINOLOGY

**Hypoxia** is defined as inadequate supply of oxygen to a tissue and/or its utilization. It may be due to reduced oxygenation of the blood reaching the tissue (hypoxic hypoxia), slowing of blood flow (stagnant hypoxia), inability to transport oxygen due to reduced hemoglobin, or inability to utilize oxygen as, for example, in mitochondrial disease.

Experimentally induced hypoxia alone does not produce brain damage. In the most extreme hypoxic conditions cardiovascular collapse leads to a fall in blood pressure which causes cerebral damage.

**Ischemia** means the reduction of blood flow to a tissue, and its effects result from deprivation of metabolic substrates including oxygen, glucose, and lactate, and failure to remove toxic metabolites such as carbon dioxide and lactic acid. Ischemia is a potent cause of brain damage, whether focal, as in obstruction of an artery, or generalized as, for example, in hypotension.

**Asphyxia** is the result of failure of blood flow, with reduction of oxygen and accumulation of carbon dioxide, together with metabolic acidosis (see p. 410).

In practice these terms are often used interchangeably owing to the difficulty of establishing the precise nature of an insult, particularly in the fetus, and also of estimating the relative contribution each might have made to damage. Hypoxic–ischemic injury (HII) or asphyxia are currently the preferred terms.

## PATHOGENESIS

Many other agents are capable of damaging the developing brain. These include infections, metabolic disease, toxins, and thyroid hormone deficiency (Blair 1996). Some have characteristic hallmarks that are identifiable by brain imaging or pathology: for example, fetal infection tends to cause widespread calcification and may involve other organs such as eye, skin, and liver. However, there may be no specific identifying features and there is a danger that fetal brain damage may be wrongly attributed to HII in the absence of any other recognizable cause. This not only leads to overestimation of the importance of HII, but also may limit the search for other, perhaps preventable, causes.

One such particular example has been recognized in recent years. Epidemiologic studies have demonstrated an association between materno-fetal infections and white matter lesions (Dammann & Leviton 1997) and intraventricular hemorrhage in the neonatal brain (see Chapters 21 and 22). Increased levels of cytokines and tumor necrosis factor have been identified in the amniotic fluid of fetuses with white matter damage (Yoon 1997). Although HII alone may cause proinflammatory cytokine release within the brain, these findings have caused us to question the traditional belief that white matter lesions result solely from ischemia. Materno-fetal infections may be important and their recognition may have implications for the prevention of fetal brain damage.

The pathogenesis of white matter injury in the immature brain is multifactorial and is discussed fully on p. 375.

## FETAL CIRCULATORY INSULTS

There is now a considerable literature on events in pregnancy that lead to circulatory disturbance of the fetus and cause neuropathology. Table 20.1 lists the recognized causes of fetal HII that have been reported to damage the brain.

### Maternal medical conditions

Chronic medical conditions such as anemia or hypertension in the mother are unlikely to cause acute brain injury in the fetus, but an acute exacerbation in the maternal condition

**Table 20.1 Recognized causes of fetal brain injury**

| Event | Gestational age (weeks) | Brain injury (Ref.) |
|---|---|---|
| Maternal causes | | |
| Cardiorespiratory arrest | 22 | Hippocampal infarct (Galloway & Roessmann 1986) |
| Severe respiratory failure | 16–20 | Neuronal migration disorder (Stewart *et al.* 1975) |
| Seizures | 15–26 | MCLE (Rizzuto & Martin 1967) |
| | 24 | Fetal intraventricular hemorrhage (Minkoff *et al.* 1985) |
| Anaphylaxis (bee sting) | 22 | MCLE (Erasmus *et al.* 1982) |
| Carbon monoxide poisoning | 24 | MCLE (Beaudoing *et al.* 1969) |
| Butane gas inhalation | 30 | MCLE (Larroche 1986), |
| | 22 | Brainstem and cerebellar necrosis (Gosseye *et al.* 1982) |
| Cocaine abuse | | See Chapters 15 and 22 |
| Maternal trauma | | See text |
| Fetal causes | | |
| Multiple pregnancy | | See p. 379 |
| Low velocity car accident | | See text |
| Fetal arrhythmia | | See text |
| Non-immune hydrops | | Larroche 1995 |

MCLE, multicystic encephalomalacia.

may damage the fetal brain. Examples of this include a severe episode of asthma or status epilepticus, rendering the mother acutely and severely hypoxic. Severe maternal hypoxia as results from gas poisoning may also damage the fetal brain.

### Maternal trauma

Maternal trauma in pregnancy is relatively common and may affect the fetus directly or indirectly. Damage to the fetal brain as a result of direct trauma from a penetrating injury is well reported (Larroche 1995). Serious systemic injury to the mother as may be caused by a road traffic accident or gunshot wound may lead to maternal (and fetal) hypotension which may cause damage to the developing brain (Sidky *et al.* 1991). Injury to the fetal brain has been described, including cerebral artery infarction (Coignet *et al.* 1979), multicystic encephalomalacia (MCLE) (Ferrer & Navaro 1978) and hydranencephaly (Fowler *et al.* 1971; Larroche 1986, 1995).

### Cocaine abuse

Cocaine is widely used as a recreational drug of abuse in some parts of the world. It is a powerful vasoactive compound and if used during pregnancy has been shown to cause cerebral malformations following exposure in the first half of pregnancy, and cerebral artery infarction should exposure occur in the second half of pregnancy. Cocaine exposure has also been reported to increase the risk of placental abruption (Dusick *et al.* 1993) with the possibility of fetal cerebral injury. This subject is discussed in more detail in Chapter 15.

### Multifetal gestation

It is well recognized that multifetal gestation confers a significantly increased risk of brain injury to each fetus. This risk is increased in monozygotic twins, particularly where there is death of one twin *in utero*. This is discussed in more detail in Chapter 22.

### Fetal arrhythmia

Fetal supraventricular tachycardia is reported to cause brain damage due to cerebral hypoperfusion secondary to the impaired cardiac output (Sonesson *et al.* 1996). Cerebral lesions include cerebral artery infarction and periventricular leukomalacia. Severe or prolonged cases of fetal tachycardia may cause non-immune hydrops and if the tachycardia is episodic or brief, may be missed on fetal assessment. Non-immune hydrops is recognized to be associated with brain injury (Larroche 1995) and fetal tachycardia may be a more important cause than previously recognized.

### Road traffic accidents without physical injury to the mother

It is now well recognized that low velocity car accidents can cause fetal injury where the mother is not significantly injured. In a low velocity car accident, there will be rapid deceleration from a speed of approximately 30 mph (50 km/h) to stop within a very short distance. This causes major deceleration forces on the fetoplacental unit. If the mother is wearing a sash type of safety restraint, then the force on the placenta is great as deceleration occurs within a few centimeters. This shearing force may cause incomplete placental abruption which if non-fatal to the fetus may cause significant fetal hemodynamic changes with transient underperfusion of the cerebral circulation.

Larroche (1986) has described three cases of motor vehicle accidents where the mother was not seriously hurt, but the fetus sustained brain injury. In another case a woman at 27 weeks gestation was involved in a 35 mph/(55 km/h) crash and was not injured but her fetus suffered very severe brain damage (Fries & Hankins 1989). An Australian study reported a series of motor vehicle accidents involving 27 pregnancies, some with little or no maternal injury in which the fetus sustained extensive injury (Peperell *et al.* 1977). Agran *et al.* (1987) described nine car accidents in pregnancy with severe outcome to the fetus. In an animal study, in which pregnant primates were subjected to rapid deceleration forces, Myers (1975) proposed an alternative explanation for the fetal brain injury mediated through maternal stress.

## CELLULAR RESPONSES TO HYPOXIC–ISCHEMIC INSULT

The mechanisms and pathophysiologic effects of hypoxic–ischemic insult are discussed in detail in Chapter 23. Aspects of this which apply to pathologic effects on the brain are described in detail here.

Following a hypoxic–ischemic insult, individual cells in the brain undergo a series of reactive changes; some cells die, some react to limit damage and others produce 'scar' tissue. Once neurons die they cannot be replaced and tissue repair is by gliosis. These cellular reactions contribute to the final pattern of damage. The speed and intensity of cellular responses varies with gestational age. Their clinical significance lies in the fact that some may be identified many years after injury on brain images and may permit assessment of the timing, and possibly the nature, of the initial injury. These clinically relevant cellular reactions are outlined below.

### CELL DEATH

There are several pathways leading to death of a cell. Recent *in vitro* and *in vivo* studies have led to descriptions of a multitude of mechanisms of cell death, some overlapping. The distinction of different forms of neuronal death has become increasingly difficult. The two currently best described forms of cell death are **necrosis** and **apoptosis**. Necrosis is passive cell death caused by a severe insult, leading to rapid failure of metabolism. The integrity of the cell membrane is lost and it becomes permeable to ions such as calcium which flood into the cell.

The histologic appearances are of cell swelling, with intense bright red appearance of the cytoplasm in hematoxylin and eosin stained sections (Fig. 20.1). The nuclear membrane disappears and the nuclear chromatin lyses into an indistinct network. Necrotic cells release their contents and provoke a local inflammatory response. Necrosis has been described as cell murder induced by external agents.

Apoptosis, in contrast, is considered to be cell suicide. This form of cell death may be triggered by external agents which set in motion a cascade of intracellular enzyme mediated events, some requiring gene activation and expression, which terminate in breakdown of nuclear DNA into regular fragments. The histological characteristics of apoptosis include cell shrinkage with the nucleus becoming small, rounded and intensely basophilic in hematoxylin and eosin stained sections. Finally, the nucleus breaks up into several rounded fragments (Fig. 20.1). Apoptotic cells are rapidly phagocytosed and do not induce an inflammatory response.

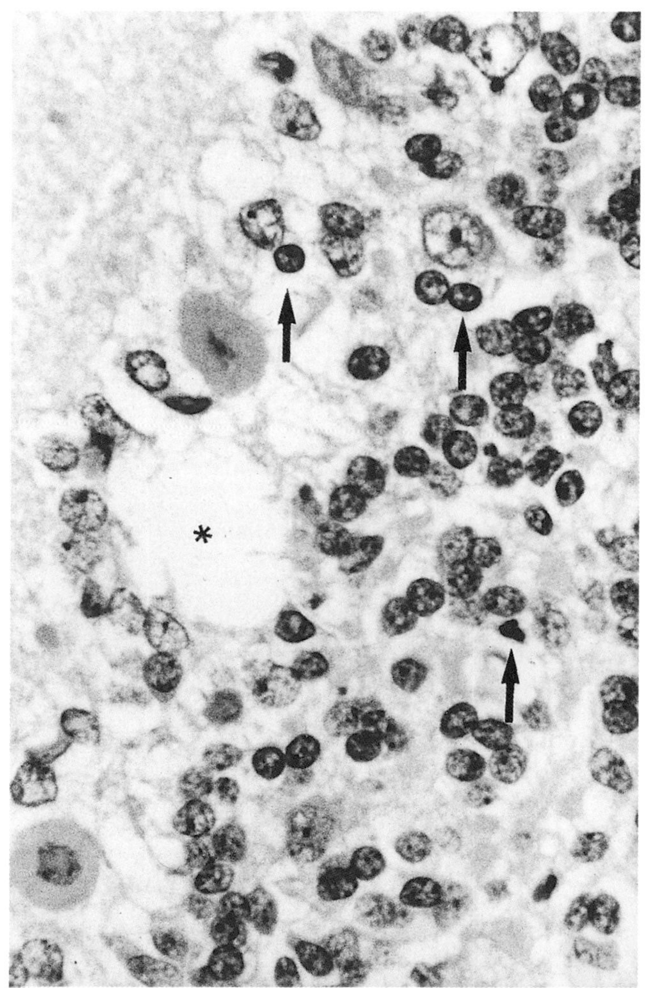

Figure 20.1 Necrosis and apoptosis. High power micrograph of cerebellar cortex 48 hours after a hypoxic–ischemic episode. One Purkinje cell has already been lost leaving an empty space (*). Two remaining Purkinje cells show changes characteristic of necrosis, that is, lysis of nuclear chromatin with uniform eosinophilia of the cytoplasm. By contrast, several cells of the underlying granular layer show rounding of the nuclei and condensation of chromatin indicating early apoptosis (arrows).

Apoptosis is thought to be the mechanism of 'programmed cell death'. This is the process by which cell populations are culled during brain development. There is a 50% over-production of cells during brain development, some forming transient structures of relevance only in brain formation, others are cells that fail to make appropriate connections.

Several factors may influence whether cells die by necrosis or apoptosis. The severity of insult is significant. Necrosis tends to occur in more severe injuries; for example, the core of an ischemic area of brain exhibits large numbers of necrotic cells while the partially perfused penumbra at the edge exhibits apoptosis. Maturity is an important factor as immature neurons die by apoptosis and necrosis, while mature differentiated neurons favor necrosis (Yue *et al.* 1997).

The most important clinical significance of the two forms of cell death is that apoptosis is an energy dependent process which takes time to complete and thus may be amenable to therapeutic intervention. It has already been shown that hypothermia shortly after HII can reduce the proportion of apoptotic cells while having no effect on necrosis (see p. 515).

## GLIOSIS

The brain's cell population includes the neurons and a number of supporting cells, including glial cells (astrocytes and oligodendroglia), microglia, and ependyma. The astrocytes play an important role in maintaining the blood–brain barrier and nurture the neurons. Oligodendroglia provide the myelin sheath around axons, which enhances the speed and efficiency of impulse transmission. Microglia are the resident phagocyte population of the brain and ependyma is the epithelial lining of the ventricular system.

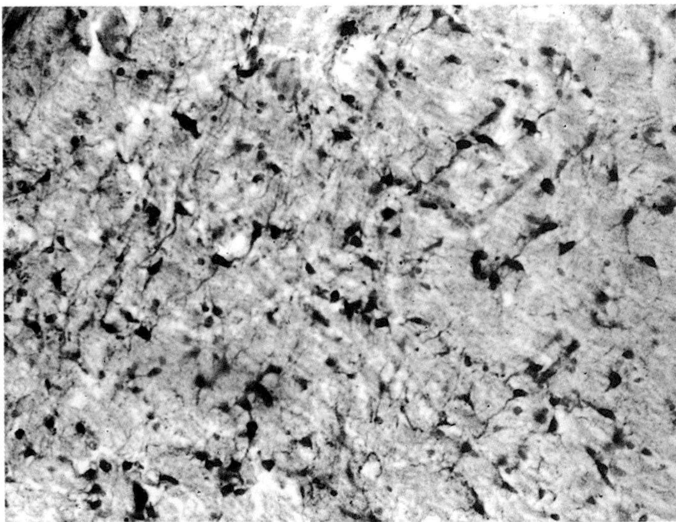

**Figure 20.2** Reactive gliosis. Reactive gliosis adjacent to an area of trauma in a fetal brain at 19 weeks gestation. The dark reactive glial cells are stained with antibodies against glial fibrillary acidic protein.

Following injury the astrocytes react by increasing in size and number. They develop extensive fibrillary processes which replace small areas of damaged tissue. Astrocytes are identified in the fetal brain from 7 weeks of gestation and are capable of generating a vigorous response by 19 weeks as illustrated in Fig. 20.2. Astrocytic gliosis can be identified by its characteristic signal change on MR scans many years after injury (Fig. 22.11).

## CAPILLARY REACTION

The endothelial cells which form the walls of blood capillaries are highly metabolically active and susceptible to HII. They react by increasing in size and thickness within 2–3 days of injury and by 5–7 days proliferate to produce new vessels. This allows increased capillary blood flow which may contribute to sparing of tissues in the penumbra of infarction. Capillary dilatation after HII is mediated by nitric oxide and blocking this action results in extension of damage.

Capillary proliferation and the resulting enhanced blood flow can be identified on brain scans. It is responsible for the phenomenon of 'cortical highlighting' which is recognized in MRI scans about 1 week after an asphyxial episode (see Fig. 6.14).

## PHAGOCYTOSIS

The brain's macrophage population, the microglia, respond to HII by enlarging and proliferating. A microglial response in the inner border of the hippocampal dentate gyrus is an established marker of previous HII in infants under 9 months of age (Del Bigio & Becker 1994). In severe injury additional macrophages are enlisted from the circulation. Macrophages engulf dead tissue and remove it via the blood vessels. Within 2–3 days of injury large macrophages are seen with distended cytoplasm containing cellular debris. Macrophages contribute to the conversion of necrotic tissue into cystic cavities. This is a process that takes a minimum of about 8–10 days. Visualization of cysts on brain scans is strong evidence for the elapse of a period of at least 1 week since injury (Fig. 22.6). Macrophages may also take up red cells in areas of hemorrhage and may persist in the tissues for many years. After this time intracytoplasmic red cells are no longer seen, but evidence of their previous existence is demonstrated by the presence of iron pigment in the cytoplasm of macrophages or free in the tissues. This is a helpful histologic pointer to hemorrhagic etiology of damage many years later.

## MINERALIZATION

Minerals are readily deposited in areas of damaged tissue in the immature brain. Focal infarcts are often rimmed by mineralized remnants of nerve cells, axons, and phagocytes. In hypoxic damage to the deep nuclei, dead nerve cells remain as mineralized ghosts and may persist for years later

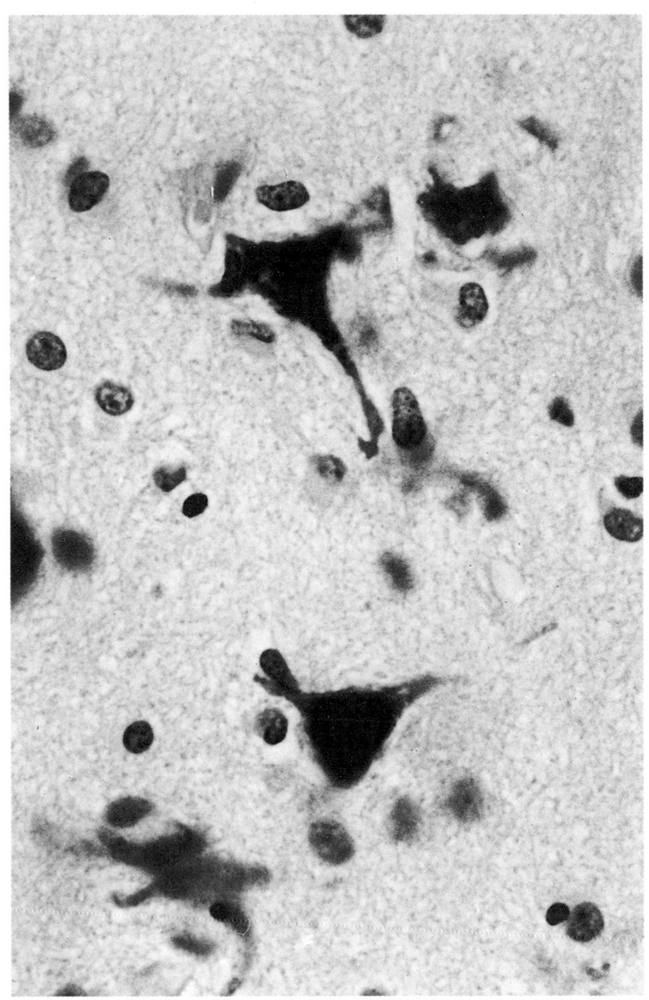

Figure 20.3 Mineralization. Thalamic neurons which have become mineralized following severe HII at birth. This child survived for 6 months.

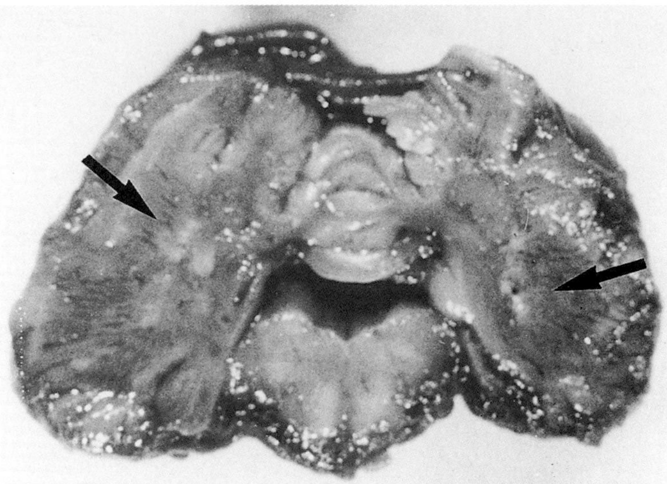

Figure 20.4 Mineralization – viral infection. Slice through the hindbrain of a neonate who died following intrauterine cytomegalovirus infection. Note dense foci of calcification in the deep cerebellar tissue (arrows).

(Fig. 20.3). Mineralization also accompanies viral infections of the brain. In this case the mineral is deposited widely throughout the brain tissue (Fig. 20.4) or as a dense periventricular band. Cerebral mineralization is readily identified in CT scans.

## FACTORS THAT INFLUENCE PATHOLOGIC OUTCOME

Many factors influence the final pathologic outcome following HII. Of primary importance is the age of the fetus at the time of insult, which is discussed in detail elsewhere in this book. The fetal factors that influence patterns of brain damage are related both to the developmental state of the brain and to the general metabolic state of the fetus. Within the brain, regional vulnerability to damage is related to changing anatomy of the blood supply and intrinsic vulnerability of specific cells.

### FETAL CEREBRAL BLOOD SUPPLY

The major blood vessels supplying the fetal brain are derived from superficial and deep sources. These vessels are radially arranged with few lateral anastomoses in the immature cortex. In ischemic conditions, cells between the radial vessels are more easily damaged, with preservation of columns of cells adjacent to perforating vessels. This is an unusual but characteristic pattern in the immature cortex (Vannucci & Vanucci 1997). Watershed zones between the superficial and deep vessels have also been considered responsible for the distribution of the white matter ischemic lesions of periventricular leukomalacia. This concept is controversial but it has been shown that the density of small vessels of the deep white matter shows a transient decrease between 28 and 36 weeks of gestation (Miyawaki 1998), corresponding to peak incidence of periventricular leukomalacia.

### INTRINSIC CELLULAR FACTORS

Different cell types within a single brain area may show profoundly different responses to an episode of sub-lethal ischemia. For example, in the immature cerebellar cortex, Purkinje cells undergo necrosis and the less mature granule cells undergo apoptosis (Yue *et al.* 1997) following HII (Fig. 20.1). The least mature cells of the inner dentate gyrus of the hippocampus are the most susceptible to HII (Del Bigio & Becker 1994).

These differences are thought to be related to the development of specific neurotransmitter systems, and acquisition of calcium binding proteins and anti-apoptotic factors. The development of aerobic respiration, as manifest by expression of mitochondrial oxidative enzyme systems, confers some resistance to HII.

### GENERAL FETAL FACTORS

General fetal factors including the metabolic state also influence response to HII. Temperature has been shown to mitigate the effects of HII in the neonatal pig (Edwards *et al.* 1995). Blood sugar is significant, and in contrast to the adult brain (Vanucci & Vanucci 1997) hyperglycemia reduces the extent of HII in the immature brain.

Intrauterine growth retardation is associated with an increased risk of prenatal white matter disease. This may be due to associated chronic acidosis or to the effects of redistribution of blood supply away from the cerebral hemispheres (Pasternak & Gorey 1998). Chronic hypoxia in the developing rat brain results in reduction of white matter volume (Ment *et al.* 1998).

### FACTORS RELATED TO THE INSULT

The severity, duration and pattern (i.e. single or repeated) of the insult bears a relationship to outcome. Acute sub-total asphyxia is particularly damaging to the brainstem nuclei and basal ganglia producing a characteristic pattern (Pasternak & Gorey 1998) sometimes referred to as 'cardiac arrest encephalopathy'. This is seen in immature infants at all stages but rarely in adults.

Chronic and less severe insults allow time for redistribution of the blood supply. Blood is diverted to the brain, heart, and adrenals. Within the brain there may be further redistribution to spare vital centers of the brainstem, thus exposing the hemispheres to relative ischemia (Pasternak & Gorey 1998).

The effect of HII may also depend on whether an insult is single or repeated. In the fetal sheep model single insults damaged the cortex while repeated insults led to infarction of the deep cerebral nuclei (Mallard *et al.* 1993), and see Chapter 23.

## PATTERNS OF DAMAGE FOLLOWING HII

The following section describes age-dependent patterns of damage seen after HII. These patterns are generally related to the developmental stage at insult, but, as noted above, other factors may operate to modify the pathology, its severity, and extent.

Brain development begins in the first days after conception and continues into adult life. In the first half of gestation the major brain structures are formed. During the second half the brain undergoes enormous growth and differentiation.

Insults occurring in the early months of brain development are likely to interrupt the normal processes of development and to induce malformations. A structure will be malformed only if it is injured before or during its period of formation. Identification of malformations can therefore be informative when attempting to pinpoint the timing of an insult to the developing brain.

In order to appreciate the nature of such patterns it is helpful to review briefly the basic stages of normal brain development. This is discussed in detail in Chapters 2 and 3.

### BRAIN DEVELOPMENT

The main structures of the brain are formed during the gestational period 0–20 weeks. The cerebral hemispheres develop as lateral pouches from the anterior neural tube. The neural tube is a simple structure lined by ependyma. Beneath this is the germinal layer, where all cells of the nervous system are generated. The germinal layer initially lines the entire neural tube but later is confined to collections of cells underlying the ependyma of the lateral ventricles, being most prominent close to the head of the caudate nucleus anteriorly and posteriorly in the medial wall of the occipital horn, close to the trigone.

The germinal matrix is responsible for generation of neurons in the first 20 weeks of gestation, and subsequently is the source of glial cells. It persists until about 36 weeks of intrauterine life. A further significance of the germinal matrix is as a potential source of hemorrhage. It consists of tightly packed, highly metabolically active, dividing cells. The blood supply is derived from a network of thin-walled capillaries. These capillaries are vulnerable to fluctuations in blood pressure in the premature infant before 36 weeks of gestation and are the primary source of intraventricular hemorrhage in this group of infants.

The brain grows by proliferation of cells which migrate from the germinal matrix to their definitive adult structures in the mature brain. All nerve cells migrate: in the human brain this takes place between 6 and 23 weeks of gestation. Neuronal migration in the cerebral hemispheres takes place with the assistance of glial cells which form radial 'guide wires' by extending long processes between the ventricular germinal zone and the brain surface where the cortex will develop. Neurons which have undergone their final mitotic division migrate along these glial guides to the cortical plate. This involves complex interaction between neuron, glial cell, and extracellular matrix proteins.

Further migration pathways are involved in development of the hindbrain. A mass of germinal tissue collects close to the lateral angles of the 4th ventricle in the rhombic hip. From here cells migrate along several pathways: some cells migrate dorsally to form the cerebellar hemispheres, others migrate either through, or over the surface of the brainstem to form the brainstem nuclei.

The importance of the stage of neuronal migration is that it occurs within a fairly precisely identified time period. Migration to the human cerebral cortex has not been identified after 23 weeks of gestation. It can be disrupted by a number of insults, including ischemia. The result of such interference is that neurons fail to reach their proper destination and form heterotopic collections of cells.

Once neurons have reached the cerebral cortex they begin to make synaptic contacts with one another; electrical activity is detected from 10–11 weeks of gestation. Neurons that fail to make successful synaptic contacts are eliminated by programmed cell death. Immature neurons are all similar in appearance in the early cortex; they only take on their characteristic morphologic appearances towards term.

## DAMAGE IN EARLY GESTATION: 0–28 WEEKS

Severe damage in the first weeks of gestation leads to gross malformations that are not compatible with life. Less severe insults may cause major malformations, for example spina bifida, encephaloceles, holoprosencephaly and agenesis of the corpus callosum.

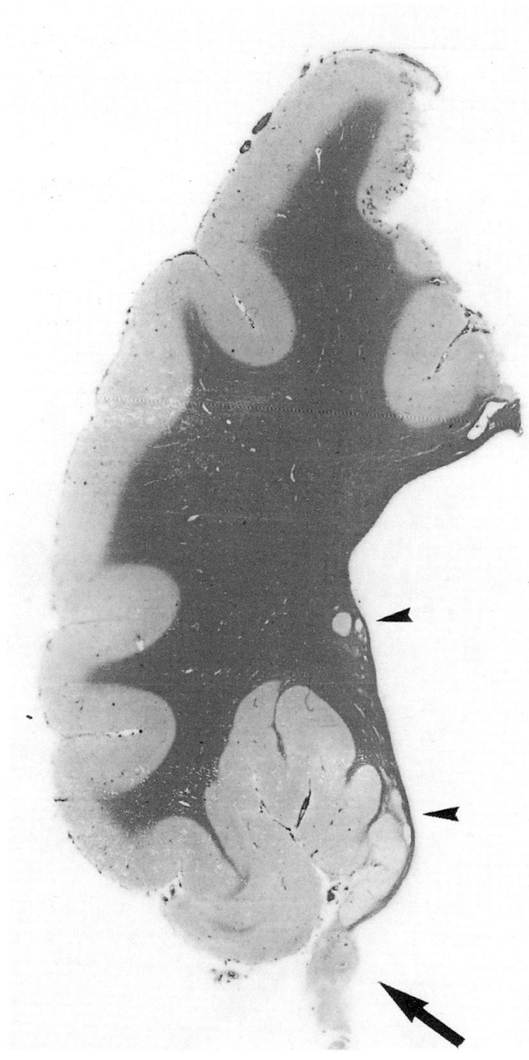

**Figure 20.5** Cortical dysplasia and heterotopia. Section of hemispherectomy specimen removed at 7 years for severe epilepsy and stained to show myelin (dark). There is an area of cortical dysplasia adjacent to a focus of cortical damage which occurred following trauma at 17 weeks of gestation (arrow). There are small heterotopic nodules in the immediately underlying white matter (arrowheads).

### The cerebral cortex: laminar necrosis

Focal ischemia of the cerebral cortex may cause necrosis; rarely this is seen in a laminar pattern similar to that described in the adult cortex. The reason for selective destruction of particular cortical layers at this stage is unknown.

### Porencephaly (see also p. 214)

If an area of cortex is completely destroyed, the necrotic tissues will be resorbed, resulting in formation of a **porencephalic cyst**. Tissues bordering on an infarct in the incompletely ischemic penumbra may suffer lesser degrees of damage, and in these areas disruption of the cortex can result in cortical dysplasia, polymicrogyria, and subcortical heterotopia (Fig. 20.5). The presence of these malformations adjacent to a porencephalic cyst are evidence of its origin in early gestation.

### Polymicrogyria (see also p. 215)

Polymicrogyria may result from ischemia, and the sporadic forms are often seen in the distribution of supply of a single cerebral artery, particularly the middle cerebral artery. When polymicrogyria is seen as a result of a known insult this always occurs before 28 weeks of gestation (Barth 1987). It may also occur in some genetically determined conditions and infections.

The macroscopic appearance of polymicrogyria is of a cortex with gyri that are too small and too numerous (Fig. 20.6). Histologically a variety of patterns are described, but essentially there is usually fusion of the outer surfaces of adjacent gyri. The underlying band of neurons may form a sweeping festoon or may be divided into irregular groups.

### Heterotopia (see also p. 217)

Groups of neurons may fail to achieve their final destination if an insult occurs during their period of migration. Neurons may be found close to the ventricular wall or in the subcortical zone. The cortex overlying neuronal heterotopias is often also dysplastic (Fig. 20.5). Focal damage to the glial limiting membrane of the cortex results in over migration of neurons into the pial membrane to form leptomeningeal heterotopia. Heterotopias resulting from an insult are evidence that the insult occurred prior to the end of neuronal migration, that is, before 23 weeks.

Periventricular nodular heterotopia and subcortical band heterotopia are genetically determined disorders resulting from mutations of the X chromosome.

### Basal ganglia

Damage to the basal ganglia has been considered characteristic of the term infant but recent studies have shown that severe HII can cause infarction of the deep cerebral nuclei at

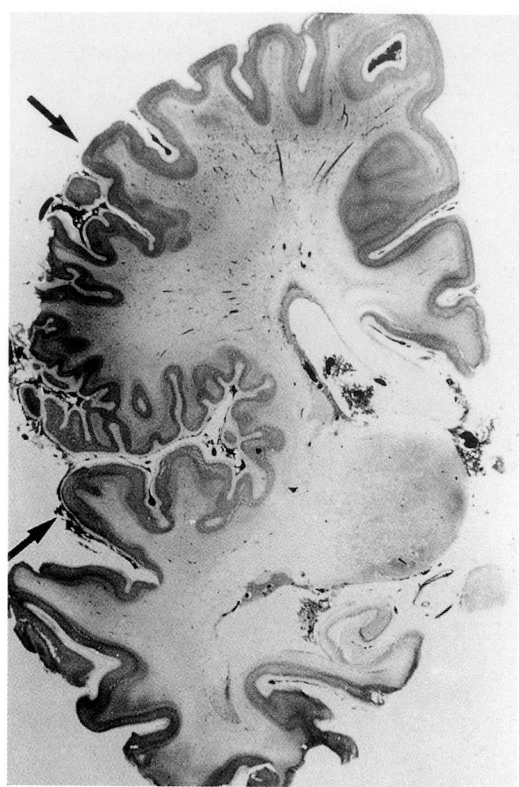

Figure 20.6 Polymicrogyria. Coronal section of the brain of a child who died at 9 years with polymicrogyria in the cortex of the Sylvian fissure (between arrows).

any stage, even as early as 24 weeks of gestation (Cohen & Roessmann 1994).

### Brainstem

The brainstem nuclei develop and mature very early in gestation. Infarction of the brainstem has been described as early as 8 weeks and may present at birth as Moebius syndrome. The damaged area is atrophic and often calcified with large proliferated blood vessels.

## DAMAGE IN MID-GESTATION: 24–36 WEEKS

In this period the two most frequent outcomes following HII are damage to the white matter, and germinal matrix hemorrhage and its sequelae. Following generation and migration of neurons the germinal matrix produces glial cell precursors which migrate out into the hemispheres where they nurture and support neurons and myelinate axons. Glial cells derived from a common precursor stem cell differentiate into astrocytes and oligodendrocytes. Astrocytes contribute to the metabolic support of neurons and form the reactive scar tissue of the brain. The oligodendroglia migrate into the white matter and wrap a membraneous sheath around axons, increasing speed and efficiency of impulse transmission. Myelination begins in the cerebral hemispheres at about 11 weeks of gestation and continues in the subcortical fibers until the third decade of adult life.

Between 24 and 36 weeks oligodendroglial migration and activity are very high and these cells appear to be particularly vulnerable to HII. Some of this damage may be mediated by excitotoxic mechanisms following ischemic axonal rupture with release of excitotoxic neurotransmitters (Kinney & Back 1998).

HII is probably responsible for a high proportion of white matter damage. Its distribution with predilection for deep periventricular areas is thought to be the result of the anatomy of the blood supply of the developing brain; this zone has been considered a watershed zone and thus particularly vulnerable to reductions in blood flow. Recent epidemiologic and clinical studies have questioned this etiological argument and there is convincing evidence that much fetal white matter disease is associated with materno-fetal infections and mediated by mechanisms associated with inflammation, particularly elevated levels of cytokines (Dammann & Leviton 1997). Thus the etiology of premature white matter disease is uncertain. Further it should be remembered that many other conditions including metabolic, toxic and infections may lead to destruction of fetal white matter (Blair 1996). This is discussed in detail in Chapter 22.

White matter disease in the premature brain may appear in a number of patterns, focal or diffuse, which are related to nature and severity of the insult.

### Periventricular leukomalacia (see also Chapter 22)

This term describes white matter pathology involving extensive areas of the deep white matter, and includes a spectrum of damage from mild diffuse gliosis to frank focal infarction (Fig. 20.7). The classical appearance is of multiple small infarcts in the deep white matter, characteristically located close to the frontal horns and the occipital horns of the lateral ventricles (Fig. 20.8). The infarcts appear as yellow spots macroscopically, due to mineral deposition in the surrounding tissue, and they may become centrally cystic. Between focal infarcts the white matter is diffusely gliotic.

Larger cystic infarcts may persist or fuse with the ventricle; smaller cysts collapse and are replaced with glial tissue. Loss of white matter and its shrinkage with subsequent gliosis contribute to overall reduction in volume and ventriculomegaly. The enlarged ventricles have squared-off frontal horns and the corpus callosum is thin (Fig. 20.9).

In some cases there is diffuse white matter gliosis without development of focal cysts. This is sometimes termed 'telencephalic leukoencephalopathy'. Diffuse white matter damage is seen in a considerable proportion of stillborn and neonatal brains at post-mortem.

### Multicystic leukoencephalopathy (see also p. 478)

Occasionally the white matter is so severely damaged that it is reduced to a mass of large cystic spaces, which may be predominantly subcortical or periventricular or both. There

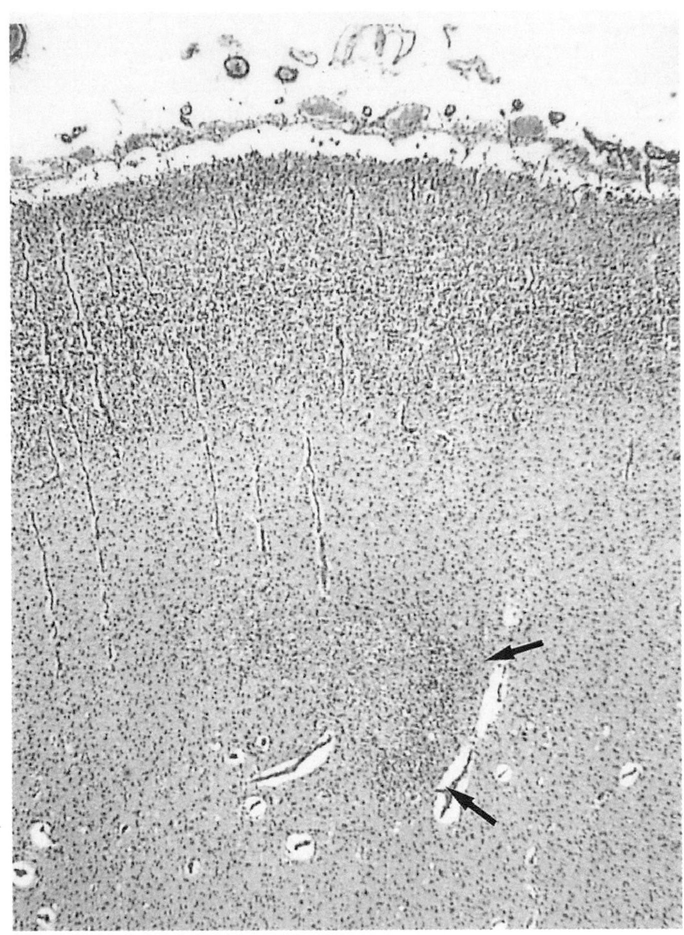

Figure 20.7 Periventricular leukomalacia. Developing periventricular leukomalacia at 30 weeks gestation. There is a focus of increased cellularity (arrows) indicating an early gliotic lesion. Note the prominent radial blood vessels at this gestational age.

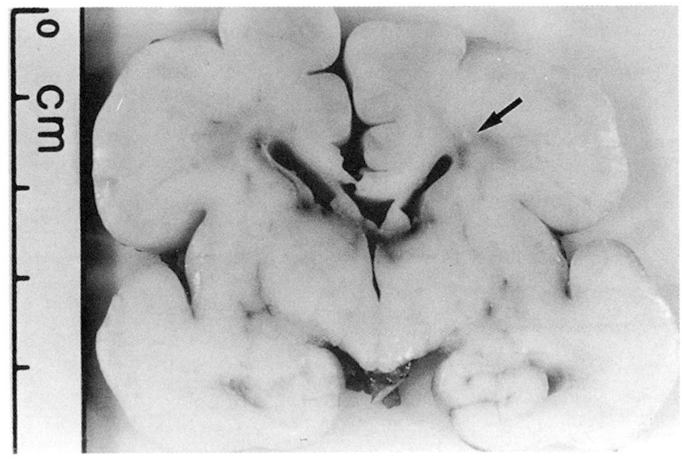


Figure 20.8 Periventricular leukomalacia. Coronal slice of an immature brain at 28 weeks gestation showing a tiny cyst (arrow) in the deep white matter adjacent to the lateral ventricles.

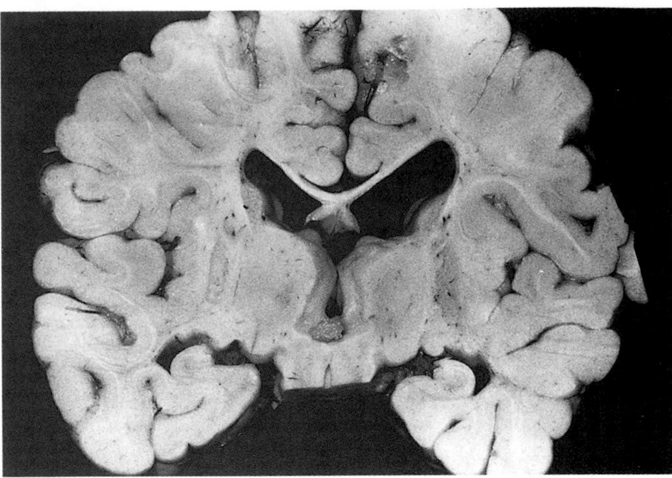

Figure 20.9 Periventricular leukomalacia. Coronal slice of the brain of a child who died at 7 months with a history of cerebral palsy. Note the reduction in white matter volume, thin corpus callosum and large, square lateral ventricles. The cortex is well preserved.

are many examples reported in the literature. The infants are usually damaged between 30 and 44 weeks of gestation and have suffered acute and severe interruption of fetal blood supply (Larroche 1986). Examples include infants of mothers who have suffered bee-sting anaphylaxis with hypotensive shock, or been involved in road traffic accidents, or had severe hemorrhage with hypovolemia.

Much of the white matter is replaced by large cysts with extensive gliosis between them (Fig. 20.10). The overlying cortex retains some aspects of its original gyral pattern but is severely or completely depleted of neurons and consists

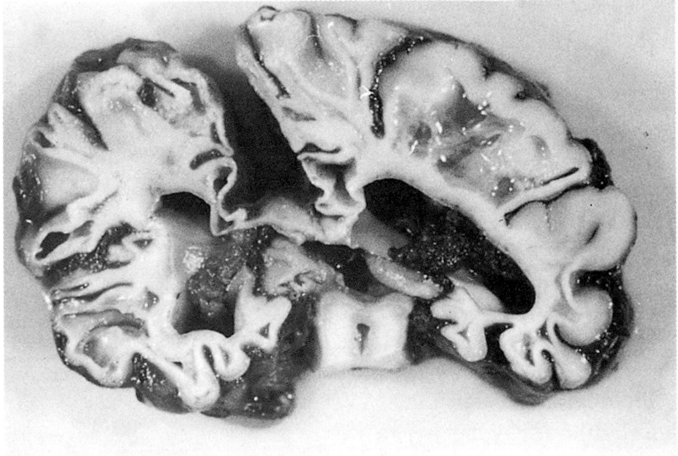

Figure 20.10 Multicystic leukoencephalopathy. Coronal slice of the brain of an infant who survived for 10 weeks following severe asphyxia at birth. Multiple large cysts replace most of the white matter of the cerebral hemispheres. The overlying cortex is thin and the lateral ventricles are dilated.

largely of glial cells. The basal ganglia and brainstem are usually also damaged, firm, and gliotic.

**Germinal matrix hemorrhage** (see also Chapter 21)
Germinal matrix hemorrhage and its sequelae are common in the premature infant. As noted above, as long as the germinal matrix persists its delicate vascular network is a potential source of bleeding. Germinal matrix hemorrhage typically occurs in infants under 36 weeks of gestation and is most frequent in very young premature babies of less than 24 weeks. Hemorrhage is most frequent in the first 2 days after birth and is associated with low cerebral blood flow. Autoregulation of cerebral blood flow is impaired in the sick neonate, and the cerebral circulation is passive and vulnerable to fluctuations in systemic blood pressure.

Germinal matrix hemorrhages may be single or multiple; unilateral or bilateral. The most frequent site is overlying the head of the caudate nucleus, particularly in older infants. Hemorrhage in the wall of the posterior horn of the lateral ventricles is common in younger babies (Fig. 20.11).

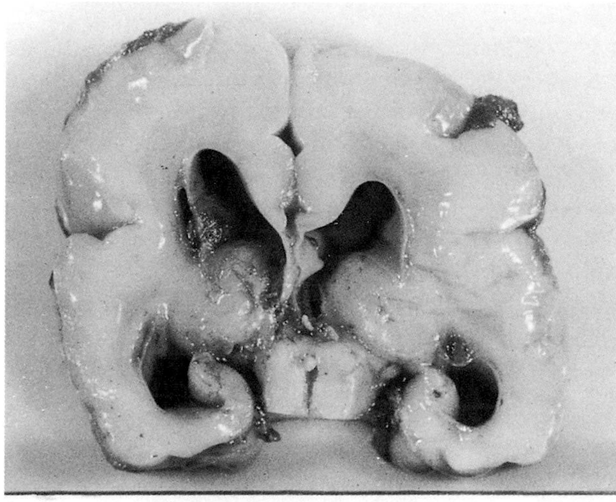

Figure 20.11 Germinal matrix hemorrhage. There is a small linear hemorrhage in the germinal matrix adjacent to the left lateral ventricle.

**Intraventricular hemorrhage** (see also Chapter 21)
Rupture of hemorrhage into the ventricular system has serious short and long term consequences. Blood entering the ventricular system passes with the cerebrospinal fluid (CSF) into the lateral and 3rd ventricles, through the narrow mid-brain aqueduct and into the 4th ventricle. It leaves the ventricular system through the foramina of Lushka and Magendie to enter the basal cisterns and from there is taken with the CSF flow over the surface of the brain to drain back into the sagittal sinus.

In the short term, blood in the ventricular system may clot and obstruct the flow of CSF, causing acute hydrocephalus. Blood has an irritant effect on the lining of the ventricular system and causes shedding of the ependyma with reactive glial proliferation (Fig. 20.12). This proliferative reaction can itself cause narrowing of parts of the ventricular system and obstruction of CSF flow, causing hydrocephalus of more chronic onset (Fig. 20.13). This most frequently occurs in the mid-brain aqueduct, the exit foramina of the 4th ventricle and the arachnoid granulations of the sagittal sinus where CSF resorption is impaired.

If the mid-brain aqueduct is stenosed the lateral and 3rd ventricles dilate. When the exit foramina of the 4th ventricle are obstructed hydrocephalus involves the entire ventricular system and the aqueduct is widened and rounded. If CSF resorption at the arachnoid villi is impaired the CSF

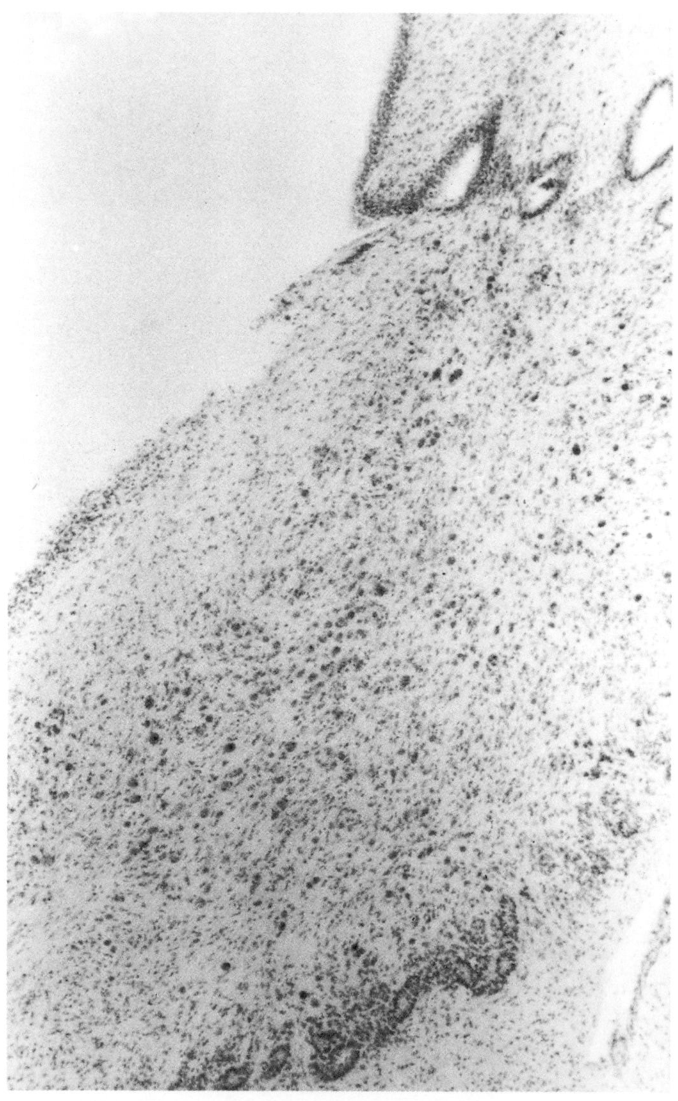

Figure 20.12 Post-hemorrhagic ependymal gliosis. Wall of the 4th ventricle showing a cushion of glial cells growing through damaged ependyma which is forming a row of tubules or rosettes in reaction to injury. The many dark cells in the gliotic tissue are macrophages containing hemosiderin.

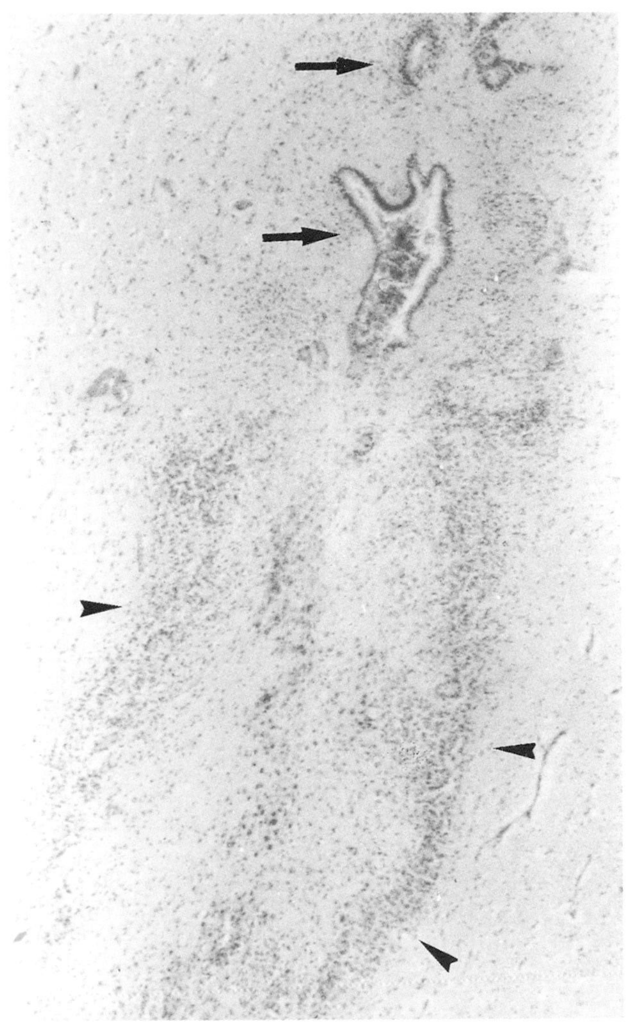

Figure 20.13 Post-hemorrhagic aqueduct stenosis. Sections of the mid-brain aqueduct in the brain of an infant with severe post-hemorrhagic hydrocephalus. The aqueduct is narrowed to a series of tiny channels (arrows) but the original size is indicated by a band of reactive ependymal and glial cells (arrowheads).

spaces over the surface of the brain are increased as well as those within the brain causing 'communicating hydrocephalus'.

### Parenchymal hemorrhagic infarction (see p. 341)

A particularly serious consequence of germinal matrix hemorrhage is development of parenchymal hemorrhagic infarction in the white matter adjacent to the bleed. This occurs in about 15% of cases of germinal matrix hemorrhage (Volpe 1989) and is associated with a high incidence of cerebral palsy. Infarction appears to result from venous stasis. The infarcted zone extends out into the parenchyma adjacent to the germinal matrix bleed (Fig. 20.14). Histology of a hemorrhagic infarct in the early stages shows numerous macrophages continuing phagocytosed red cells in the area, many flanking blood vessels. These cells are very prominent as reduced venous drainage hinders their normal clearance.

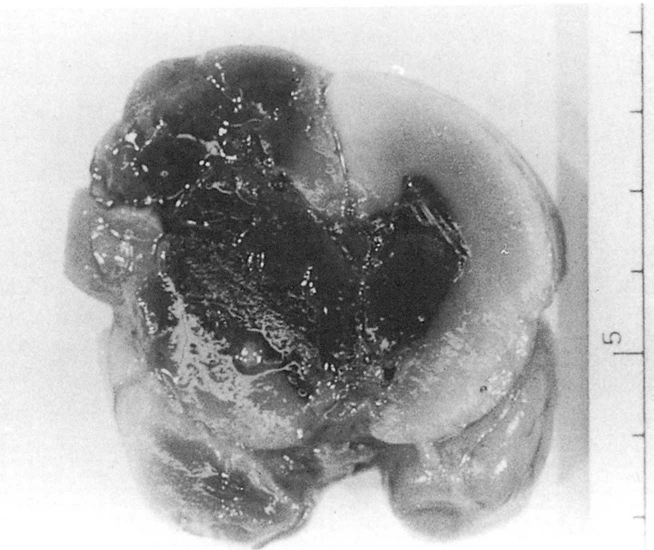


Figure 20.14 Parenchymal hemorrhagic infarction. Coronal slice of a 24 week fetal brain shows bilateral intraventricular hemorrhage with parenchymal hemorrhagic infarction adjacent to the hemorrhage on the left side.

The mechanisms of hemorrhagic infarction are unclear. It is possible that blood clot causes mechanical obstruction of draining veins or that free blood in the tissues causes vasospasm. There may be some contribution from the asphyxial damage which initially precipitated germinal matrix hemorrhage.

The infarcted tissue is eventually resorbed leaving a cystic cavity which becomes continuous with the ventricular cavity and causes irregular, unilateral dilatation. The lesion is almost always unilateral (Volpe 1989) which assists in its distinction from PVL.

## DAMAGE IN LATE-GESTATION: 36 WEEKS TO TERM

As the brain approaches maturity the pathologic results of HII become more similar to those seen in the adult brain, in that the gray matter becomes vulnerable to damage. However, certain patterns are virtually specific to the infant brain.

Documented patterns of damage following HII in the term brain involve specific areas of the cortex, the deep gray nuclei, the hippocampus, brainstem, and posterior limb of the internal capsule (Barkovitch 1992; Rutherford *et al.* 1998) (Figs 20.15 and 20.16).

### The cerebral cortex

The cerebral cortex is frequently damaged in the term infant exposed to HII. The patterns of cortical damage are multiple

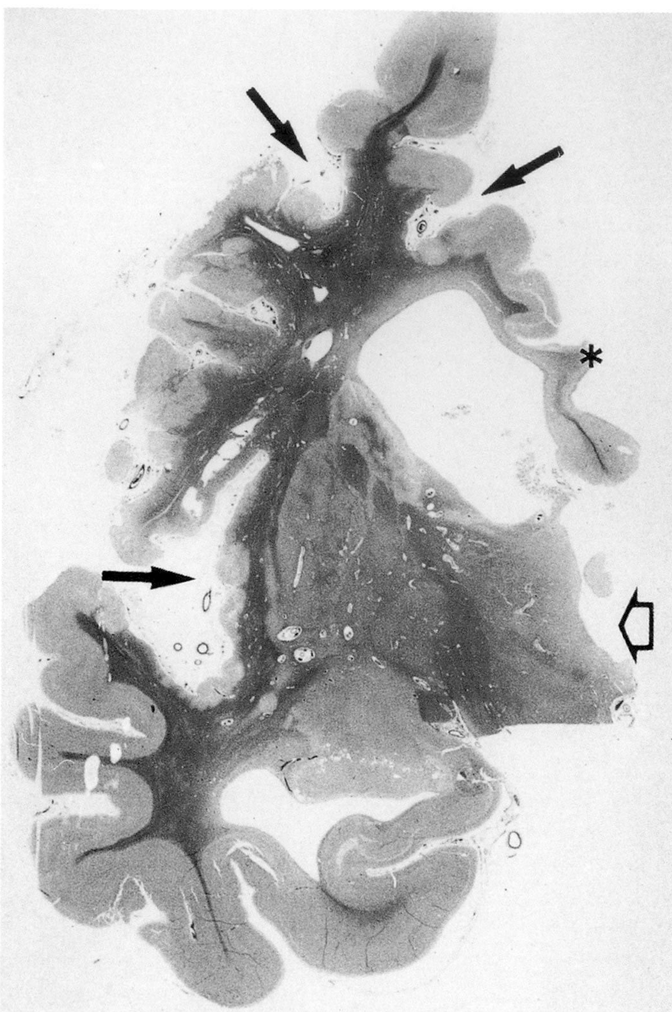


Figure 20.15 Old HII. Coronal section of a cerebral hemisphere of a child who died at 7 months of age. The section is stained to show myelin which is dark. Note the small volume of white matter and thin corpus callosum (*). The lateral ventricle is large and square. The 3rd ventricle is dilated due to atrophy of the thalamus (open arrow). There are multiple areas of ulegyria (arrows) where the cortex of the deep parts of sulci has been more severely damaged than the cortex in adjacent gyral crests.

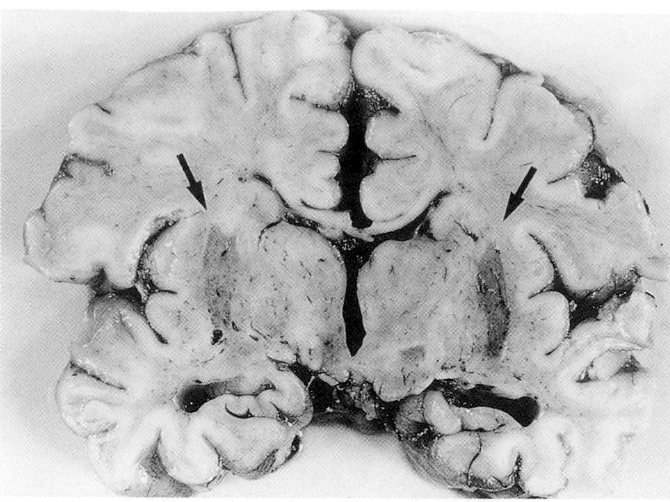

Figure 20.16 HII at term. Coronal slice of the brain of an infant who suffered severe asphyxia at birth at 41 weeks and 3 days and survived for 2 weeks. There is severe edema. The ventricles are compressed and the cortex appears a prominent white band. There is discoloration of the putamina bilaterally (arrows) due to recent infarction and reactive capillary proliferation.

and complex and depend on extrinsic factors, such as vascular anatomy as well as intrinsic factors at a cellular level within particular regions of the cortex. Involvement of the anterior cerebrum, particularly the territory of supply of the internal carotid arteries is common. This may be due to altered blood flow patterns after prolonged fetal asphyxia. An alternative hypothesis is that acute brain swelling in asphyxia causes compression of the internal carotid arteries as they enter the skull.

Damage in the cortical watershed areas is also common. The watershed areas are the terminal zones between the main cerebral arteries, where the blood supply is most tenuous if blood flow falls. In the infant brain this involves the dorsal parasagittal cortex and the inferolateral areas of the parieto-occipital lobes.

The capillary supply to the developing cerebral cortex is very simple and consists of vessels that pass in at right angles from the superficial meningeal vessels. The intracortical capillaries have few lateral anastamoses. If flow is reduced, the cells closest to capillaries are spared but intervening tissue is lost. This results in columnar cortical necrosis which is not seen in the older brain. Following long term survival the residual pericapillary cells are seen as rounded masses in glial scar tissue.

Vulnerability of the perirolandic cortex has been demonstrated in MRI studies of asphyxiated infants (Barkovich 1992). This strip of cortex is the source of the corticospinal tracts which are actively myelinating at this stage. It has been suggested that the metabolic demands of myelination increase vulnerability to HII.

### Ulegyria

Another pattern of cortical damage that is characteristic of the term infant is ulegyria. The term describes preferential necrosis of the depths of sulci with sparing of gyral crests (Fig. 20.17). It has been suggested that this pattern results from the relative infrequency of capillaries in sulcal depths. Ulegyria is only rarely seen following asphyxia in adults. Selective cortical damage in deep cerebellar folia is seen in Fig. 20.18.

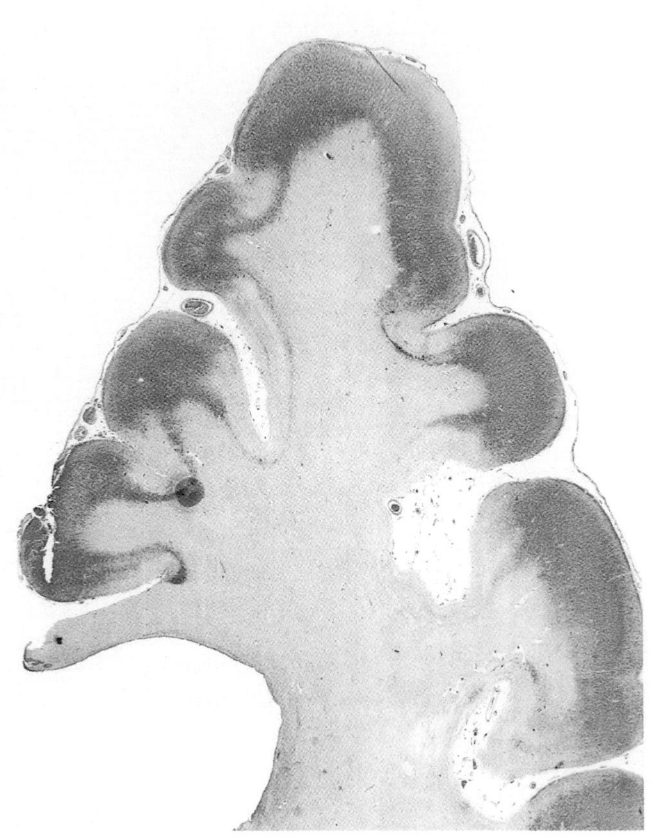

Figure 20.17 Ulegyria. This section of the frontal lobe is stained with antibodies against a neuronal marker MAP-2. Note selective loss of neurons from the depths of sulci and neuronal preservation in the gyral crests.

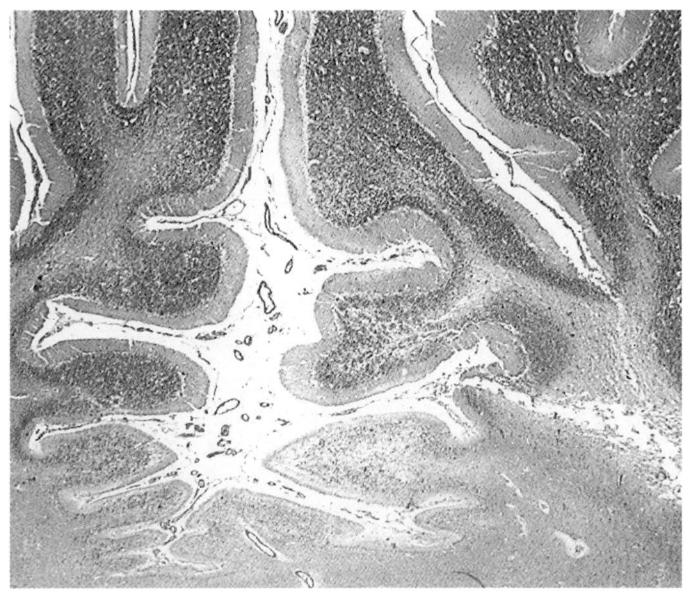

Figure 20.18 Selective cortical atrophy. Section of cerebellar cortex of an infant who suffered HII. There is preferential loss of neurons and cortical atrophy in the deeper folia which are pale and shrunken.

### Basal ganglia

Damage to the thalamus and basal ganglia may be seen after sufficiently severe HII at any gestational age, frequently associated with cortical damage. The ventrolateral nucleus of the thalamus and posterior putamen are often involved (Fig. 20.16).

Infants who survive ischemic damage to the basal ganglia show atrophy of these nuclei with widening of the 3rd ventricle. In infants who suffer acute near-total asphyxia, selective damage to the deep nuclei with complete or relative sparing of the cortex and white matter is described (Pasternak & Gorey 1998). Histologic examination often shows gliosis with mineralization of remaining neurons.

'Status marmoratous' or 'marbling' of the thalamus results from aberrant myelination of glial fibers in the damaged thalamus. The glial fibers result from earlier asphyxial damage. Marbling is only seen after 6 months of age when the thalamic white matter is normally myelinated. Further, shrinkage of the thalamus due to the ischemic neuronal loss in early life leads to closer packing of normal myelinated fibers which further contributes to the increased myelin in the structure. Status marmoratus is visible on MRI scans.

## DAMAGE OCCURRING AT ANY AGE

Some injuries occur irrespective of gestational age. Obstruction of a cerebral artery will lead to total necrosis of tissue in the area of supply at any age: this is the basis of many examples of porencephaly and probably of some cases of schizencephaly. The age at which this occurs may be suggested if malformed tissues are identified in the borders of the infarct.

### Brainstem necrosis 'cardiac arrest encephalopathy'

A highly specific pattern of necrosis of the nuclei of the brainstem occurs following a period of total ischemia to the brain; sometimes termed 'cardiac arrest encephalopathy'. This phenomenon is seen throughout gestation and at term but is only rarely seen in adults.

There is symmetrical necrosis of the nuclei of the brainstem from medulla through the mid-brain and extending up to the basal ganglia (Fig. 20.19). Infants with this form of damage have an extremely poor prognosis (Pasternak & Gorey 1998).

### Arterial infarction (see p. 393)

Infarction in the territory of a single cerebral artery is not uncommon in the infant brain. The middle cerebral arteries are most frequently involved; the left more than the right. The clinical outcome is very variable, most infants do extremely well but a few have motor disabilities and epilepsy. MRI scans of populations of neonates suggest that many cases occur at birth and often without any clinical signs or symptoms (Bouza *et al.* 1994); however, histologic examination of specimens from a series of children with

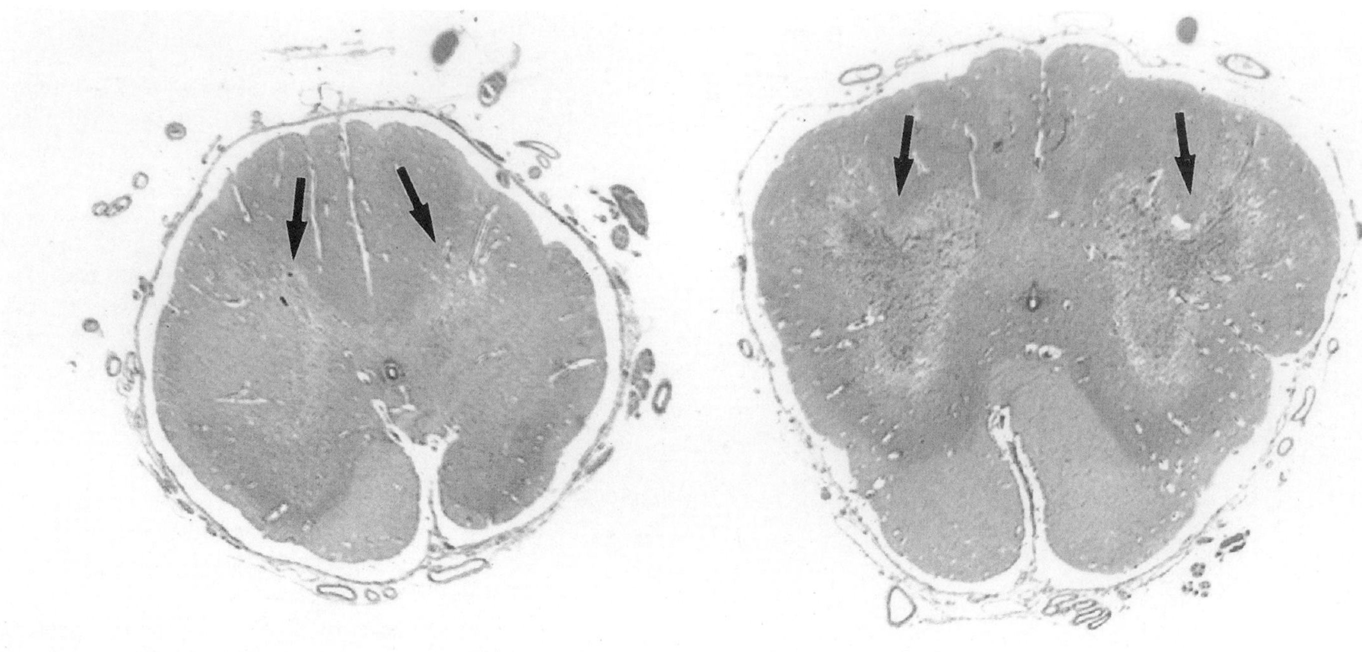

**Figure 20.19** Brainstem necrosis. This 28 weeks premature infant suffered a severe HII 20 days before death. These brainstem sections show symmetrical necrosis (arrows).

severe epilepsy has shown that approximately half of these cases had infarcts before 28 weeks of gestation.

### Schizencephaly (see also p. 213)

This is the term applied to a complete slit-like lesion of the cerebral mantle extending from the meninges to the ventricular wall. Originally, it was described as a malformation and in some cases genetic linkage has been described. Full thickness infarction of an area of the brain wall may cause similar appearances if the resulting cystic space collapses with apposition of the walls.

### Hydranencephaly (see also p. 227)

This describes the brain that has had extensive infarction of most of both of the two hemispheres, leaving them as thin-walled, fluid-filled cysts. The membrane consists of remnants of meninges and glial tissue. The damage usually involves the territory of supply of the internal carotid arteries with sparing of inferior temporal lobes, occipital lobes, and the hindbrain.

## HYPOGLYCEMIA

While the purpose of this chapter is to describe the effects of HII on the developing brain, it is appropriate to mention the role of hypoglycemia, which has a complex interaction with HII in the immature brain. In contrast to the adult, hypoglycemia compounds the damage caused by HII (Vannucci & Vannucci 1997).

Cases where there has been pure hypoglycemia at birth are not common and very few have had post-mortem examinations. Findings in these cases and in experimental studies show that the damage due to hypoglycemia differs in distribution from that caused by HII. More recent imaging studies using MRI and SPECT (Chiu *et al.* 1998; Traill *et al.* 1998) have demonstrated a marked predilection for the posterior parts of the cerebral hemispheres, causing atrophy of cortex and underlying white matter. This is unlike the damage due to HII and it is important to distinguish these patterns of injury.

### Key Points

- Circulatory disturbances may damage the fetal brain secondary to maternal medical conditions, maternal trauma or cocaine abuse
- Fetal conditions such as cardiac arrhythmia and road traffic accidents may damage the brain
- The pattern of brain injury in a fetus depends on the gestational age at which the insult occurs
- Neuronal migration disorders may occur as the result of insults occurring in the developing brain in the first 23 weeks of gestation

## REFERENCES


Agran P F, Dunkle D E, Winn D G & Kent D (1987) Fetal death in motor vehicle accidents. *Ann Emerg Med* 16: 1355–1358.

Barkovitch A J (1992) MR and CT evaluation of profound neonatal and infantile asphyxia. *AJNR Am J Neuroradiol* 13: 959–972.

✪ Barth P G (1987) Disorders of neuronal migration. *Le Journal Canadien Des Sciences Neurologiques* 14: 1: 1–16.

Beaudoing A, Gachon J, Butin L P *et al.* (1969) Les consequences foetales de l'intoxication oxycarbonnee de la mere. *Pediatrie* 2: 539–553.

✪ Blair E (1996) Obstetric antecedents of cerebral palsy. *Fetal Matern Med Revi* 8: 199–215.

Bouza H & Dubowitz L M *et al.* (1994) Late magnetic resonance imaging and clinical findings in neonates with unilateral lesions on cranial ultrasound. *Dev Med Child Neurol* 36: 951–964.

Chiu N, Huang C & Chang Y *et al.* (1998) Technetium-99m-HMPAO brain SPECT in neonates with hypoglycemic encephalopathy. *J Nucl Med* 39(10): 1711–1713.

Cohen M & Roessman U (1994) *In utero* brain damage: relationship of gestational age to pathological consequences. *Dev Med Child Neurol* 36: 263–270.

Coignet J, Palix C, Tommasi C *et al.* (1979) Apport de la sonographie dans la souffrance du nouveau-ne. *Pediatrie* 34: 787–797.

✪ Dammann O & Leviton A (1997) Maternal intrauterine infection, cytokines, and brain damage in the preterm newborn. *Pediatr Res* 42(1): 1–8.

Del Bigio M R & Becker L E (1994) Microglial aggregation in the dentate gyrus: a marker of mild hypoxic-ischaemic brain insult in human infants. *Neuropath App Neurobiol* 20: 144–151.

Dusick A M, Covert R F, Schreiber M D *et al.* (1993) Risk of intracranial hemorrhage and other adverse outcomes after cocaine exposure in a cohort of 323 very low birth weight infants. *J Pediatr* 122: 438–445.

Edwards A D, Yue X, Squier M V *et al.* (1995) Specific inhibition of apoptosis after cerebral hypoxia-ischaemia by moderate post-insult hypothermia. *Biochem Biophys Res Commun* 217: 1193–1199.

Erasmus C, Blackwood W & Wilson J (1982) Infantile multicystic encephalomalacia after maternal bee sting anaphylaxis during pregnancy. *Arch Dis Child* 57: 785–787.

Ferrer I & Navarro C (1978) Multicystic encephalomalacia of infancy. *J Neurol Sci* 38: 179–189.

Fowler M, Brown C & Cabrera K F (1971) Hydranencephaly in a baby after an aircraft accident to the mother: case report and autopsy. *Pathology* 3: 21–30.

Fries M H & Hankins G D (1989) Motor vehicle accident associated with minimal maternal trauma but subsequent fetal demise. *Ann Emerg Med* 18: 301–304.

Galloway P G & Roessmann U (1986) Neuronal karynorrhexis in Sommer's sector in a 22 week stillborn. *Acta Neuropathol* 70: 343–344.

Gosseye S, Golaire M C & Larroche J-C (1982) Cerebral, renal and splenic lesions due to fetal anoxia and their relationship to malformations. *Dev Med Child Neurol* 24: 510–518.

Kinney H C & Back S A (1998) Human oligodendroglial development: relationship to periventricular leukomalacia. *Semin Pediatr Neurol* 5(3) Sep: 180–189.

✪ Larroche J-C (1986) Fetal encephalopathies of circulatory origin. *Biol Neonate* 50: 61–74.

Larroche J-C (1995) Fetal cerebral pathology of circulatory origin. In: *Fetal and neonatal neurology and neurosurgery*, 2nd edn. Levene M I, Lilford R J (eds) Edinburgh: Churchill Livingstone, pp. 321–334.

✪ Mallard E C, Williams C E, Gunn A J *et al.* (1993) Frequent episodes of brief ischemia sensitize the fetal sheep brain to neuronal loss and induce striatal injury. *Research* 33; 1: 61–65.

Ment L R, Schwartz M, Makuch R W *et al.* (1998) Association of chronic sublethal hypoxia with ventriculomegaly in the developing rat brain. *Dev Brain Res* 111: 197–203.

Minkoff H, Schaffer R M, Delke I *et al.* (1985) Diagnosis of intracranial hemorrhage *in utero* after a maternal seizure. *Obstet Gynecol* 65: 22S–24S.

Miyawaki T, Matsui K, Takashima S (1998) Developmental characteristics of vessel density in the human fetal and infant brains. *Early Hum Dev* 53: 65–72.

Myers R E (1975) Maternal psychological stress and fetal asphyxia: a study in the monkey. *Am J Obstet Gynecol* 122: 47–59.

✪ Pasternak J F & Gorey M T (1998). The syndrome of acute near-total intrauterine asphyxia in the term infant. *Pediatr Neurol* 18: 391–398.

Pepperell R J, Rubinstein E & MacIsaac I A (1977) Motor-car accidents during pregnancy. *Med J Austr* 1: 203–205.

Rizzuto N & Martin L (1967) Le probleme de l'encephalopathie foetale kystique survenant au cours du deuxieme tiers de la grossesse. *Biologia Neonatorum* 11: 115–127.

✪ Rutherford M A, Pennock J M, Counsell S J *et al.* (1998) Abnormal magnetic resonance signal in the internal capsule predicts poor neurodevelopmental outcome in infants with hypoxic-ischemic encephalopathy. *Pediatrics* 102(2): 323–328.

Sidky I H, Daikoku N H & Gopal J (1991) Insignificant blunt maternal trauma with lethal fetal outcome: a case report. *Maryland Med J* 40: 1083–1085.

Sonesson S-E, Winberg P, Lidegran M & Westgren M (1996) Foetal supraventricular tachycardia and cerebral complications. *Acta Paediatr* 85: 1249–1252.

Stewart R M, Richman D P & Caviness V S (1975) Lissencephaly and pachygyria. An architectonic and topographical analysis. *Acta Neuropathol* 31: 1–12.

Traill Z, Squier M & Anslow P (1998) Brain imaging in neonatal hypoglycaemia. *Arch Dis Child Fetal Neonat Edn* 79: F145–F147.

✪ Vannucci R C & Vannucci S J (1997) A model of perinatal hypoxic-ischaemic brain damage. *Ann N Y Acad Sci* 835: 234–249.

Volpe J J (1989) Current concepts of brain injury in the premature infant. *AJR* 153: 243–251.

Yoon B H, Romero R, Yang S H *et al.* (1996) Interleukin-6 concentrations in umbilical cord plasma are elevated in neonates with white matter lesions associated with periventricular leukomalacia. *Am J Obstet Gynecol* 174(5): 1433–1440.

✪ Yue X, Mehmet J, Penrice J *et al.* (1997) Apoptosis and necrosis in the newborn piglet brain following transient cerebral hypoxia-ischaemia. *Neuropathol App Neurobiol* 23: 16–25.

# Chapter 21 Neonatal intracranial hemorrhage

M. I. Levene and L. S. de Vries

## INTRODUCTION

Hemorrhages involving the neonatal brain are among the most frequent and important conditions affecting the newborn. Intracerebral hemorrhage is more common in the neonatal period than at any other time, but there is a wide spectrum of hemorrhagic lesions, with differing etiologies and varying prognostic significance. Table 21.1 lists the types of hemorrhage reported in the newborn brain and each will be discussed separately.

With the introduction of modern imaging techniques in the late 1970s, intracranial hemorrhage could be studied in living infants and information on its pathogenesis and outcome in surviving children assessed. Recent studies describe an incidence of intracranial hemorrhage in asymptomatic healthy full-term infants of 3.5–5% (Heibel *et al.* 1993; Mercuri *et al.* 1998). Before that, information could only be obtained from autopsy material which would bias the findings towards the more severe degrees of hemorrhage. Despite the obvious limitations of post-mortem studies, a definite trend can be observed over the last 60 years. In 1938, Craig analyzed 126 post-mortem examinations in which intracranial hemorrhage was discovered and found subdural hematoma to be common, occurring in almost half of the cases. A similar assessment 40 years later from Hammersmith Hospital, UK autopsies during the years 1978–79 showed a considerable decline in the proportion of subdural hemorrhages, with a corresponding marked increase in the percentage of germinal matrix hemorrhage–intraventricular hemorrhage (GMH–IVH) (Levene *et al.* 1985). This is due to a marked reduction in the number of fatal subdural hemorrhages associated with more careful obstetric management of the second stage of labor and the relative increase in cases of GMH–IVH associated with longer survival of very premature infants supported by neonatal intensive care who are most at risk of GMH–IVH. This is now the most frequent and important cause of intracranial hemorrhage in neonatal medicine.

**Table 21.1 Localization and site of origin of various types of intracranial hemorrhage**

| Type of hemorrhage | Site of origin |
|---|---|
| Subdural | – |
| Subarachnoid | Primary |
| | Secondary to intraventricular hemorrhage |
| | Subarachnoid hematoma |
| Intraventricular | Germinal matrix |
| | Choroid plexus |
| | Cerebral parenchyma |
| Intraparenchymal | Periventricular white matter |
| | Thalamus |
| | Arteriovenous malformation |
| Intracerebellar | – |

## GERMINAL MATRIX HEMORRHAGE AND INTRAVENTRICULAR HEMORRHAGE

The terminology used to describe hemorrhage in and around the lateral ventricles is confusing and lacks a clear consensus view. Intraventricular hemorrhage is an imprecise term used to describe bleeding within the ventricular cavities but arising from any site. It may be impossible to distinguish on ultrasound examination the presence of liquid phase blood in the lateral ventricle. Consequently, the distinction between unruptured GMH and IVH can often not be made confidently by this imaging technique alone. The generic term 'periventricular hemorrhage' is also widely used to refer to hemorrhage originating in the germinal matrix, often with involvement of the lateral ventricles and on occasions extending into the periventricular white matter. It is now clear that hemorrhage occurring *de novo* in the periventricular white matter, without germinal matrix bleeding, also occurs not infrequently, and this condition might be referred to more accurately as periventricular hemorrhage. For these semantic reasons we have chosen to use the term 'germinal matrix hemorrhage–intraventricular hemorrhage' (GMH–IVH) to refer to a common form of intracranial hemorrhage usually seen in premature infants. Throughout this section the term 'GMH–IVH' is used in a general sense to describe the condition that other authors have described by a variety of terms but which we believe to refer to the same condition. There is now growing evidence that a proportion of hemorrhagic lesions in the cerebral parenchyma have quite a different pathophysiologic basis from GMH–IVH and are ischemic in origin. This is discussed in detail in Chapter 22.

### PATHOLOGY

Kowitz (1914) was the first to publish a report of IVH in the neonate and included 128 cases, but Ruckensteiner & Zollner

(1929) were the first to recognize that, in premature infants, blood in the ventricles commonly occurred as the result of hemorrhage within the subependymal germinal matrix. The subependymal germinal matrix is a transient structure and is initially the site of vigorous neuroblast and glioblast mitotic activity. When cell division is complete and after the majority of the neurons have completed their migration, the relative size of the periventricular germinal matrix progressively decreases, but a conspicuous mass of cells persist over the head and body of the caudate nucleus until 33–34 weeks of gestation. Residual matrix tissue persists in the roof of the temporal horn and in the external wall of the occipital horn. These glial precursors develop into oligodendrocytes and astrocytes and migrate all over the cerebrum.

The arterial supply of the germinal matrix is from the recurrent artery of Heubner (a branch of the anterior cerebral artery), as well as terminal branches of the lateral striate arteries. These vessels divide to give the germinal matrix a rich bed of vascular afferents. Takashima & Tanaka (1978) have suggested that the germinal matrix represents a border zone between the striate and thalamic arteries and as such is particularly vulnerable to infarction (see below). Venous drainage of the germinal matrix is via many small veins into the terminal vein. These are joined anteriorly at the level of the foramen of Monro by the septal, choroidal, and thalamostriate veins just before the terminal vein turns sharply back on itself (Takashima & Tanaka 1978). The terminal vein drains into the internal cerebral vein and then into the vein of Galen.

The site of GMH depends on the maturity of the infant. In the least mature infants (24–28 weeks), Hambleton & Wigglesworth (1976) found GMH to be larger and occur most frequently over the body of the caudate nucleus, and in more mature infants the lesion was seen over the head of the caudate nucleus.

Although some disagreement still exists concerning the vascular origin of GMH, the predominant view at present is that hemorrhage arises from the thin walled veins (Grontoft 1953; Cole *et al.* 1974; Nakamura *et al.* 1990; Moody *et al.* 1994; Ghazi-Birry *et al.* 1997). In a large number of cases examined histologically, blood from the GMH was seen tunneling along the perivenous space of a germinal matrix vein leading to compression of patent veins and secondary rupture of smaller connecting venous tributaries (Ghazi-Birry *et al.* 1997). This in turn causes venous stasis, increased venous pressure and reduced perfusion pressure through this part of the brain.

Hambleton & Wigglesworth (1976), using post-mortem injection techniques, failed to show evidence of rupture of either veins or arteries, but reported hemorrhage to occur as the result of disruption of the capillary bed.

The immature veins are vulnerable to rupture as the result of under-developed basal lamina, incomplete glial support, and poor matrix support. Ment *et al.* (1995) have suggested that the immaturity is transient. They showed that the germinal matrix vessels change significantly over the first four days of life to greater continuity of the basement membrane, and by 10 days after birth the length and number of tight junctions had increased and the number of supporting cells surrounding the germinal matrix vessels

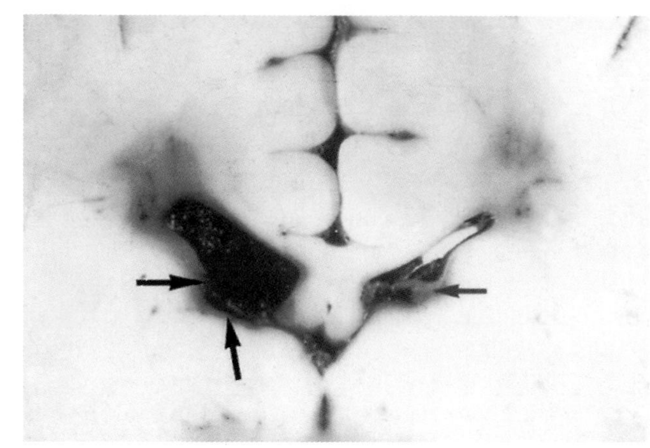

A

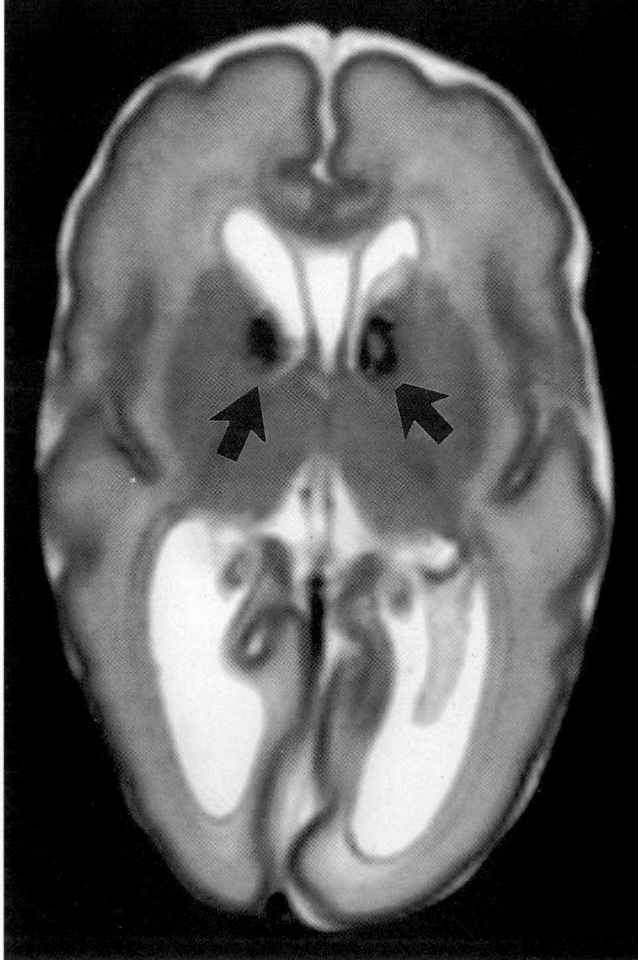

B

Figure 21.1 (A) Bilateral GMH (arrowed) with rupture into the left lateral ventricle, which is filled with clot. (B) Appearances on T2-weighted MR axial scan (GMH arrowed).

had risen. This rapid maturation, presumably as a result of early birth, accounts for the frequency of GMH in the first few days of life.

In 80 per cent of cases of GMH, blood ruptures through the ependyma into the lateral ventricles, causing IVH. GMH is bilateral in half of affected brains, with a slight left-sided preponderance (Donn & Bowerman 1985). In bilateral lesions the hemorrhages are usually asymmetrical (Fig. 21.1). Bleeding sites may be multiple and in some cases develop in the roof of the temporal horn and posteriorly in the germinal matrix of the external wall of the lateral ventricle. Bleeding may also extend into the caudate nucleus and other adjacent structures. Blood may also extend into the ventricle from primary bleeding of the tela choroidea and from the choroid plexus.

## Parenchymal hemorrhage

Parenchymal hemorrhage occurs in approximately 15% of infants with GMH–IVH and is usually unilateral and does not involve the cortical mantle. If the baby survives the lesion, a large porencephalic cavity may develop (see p. 356).

It has been thought in the past that parenchymal hemorrhage was due to direct extension of hemorrhage into the periventricular white matter, but this has now been discounted as a likely explanation for its development. Bleeding into an area of previously compromised periventricular white matter occurs as a result of periventricular leukomalacia (PVL) which may be confused with primary parenchymal hemorrhage. PVL is described in detail in the next chapter but is usually a symmetrical condition compared with the very asymmetrical appearance of parenchymal hemorrhage.

The cause of parenchymal hemorrhage is now thought to be due to venous infarction. The deep periventricular white matter is served by a fan-shaped leash of short and long medullary veins which flow vertically into subependymal veins (Takashima & Tanaka 1978, Takashima *et al.* 1986), and this is illustrated in Fig. 21.2. A careful pathologic study of infants dying with periventricular intraparenchymal cerebral hemorrhage showed that the ependyma remained intact, indicating that direct spread from the lateral ventricle could not have occurred (Gould *et al.* 1987). These authors suggested that clot in the germinal matrix causes obstruction to the terminal vein with reduction in cerebral perfusion in the white matter drained by these veins. There is evidence for this mechanism from pathologic specimens (Pape & Wigglesworth 1979), and an example is shown in Fig. 21.3. Histology showed that the hemorrhage is mainly perivascular and radiates outwards from the angle of the lateral ventricle, closely following the distribution of the medullary veins draining the white matter. Marked ischemic injury was not found (Gould *et al.* 1987). Low cerebral blood flow in the periventricular region has been shown by positron emission tomography to occur on the side of GMH–IVH, which is most likely to reflect the low perfusion seen in venous infarction (Volpe *et al.* 1983).

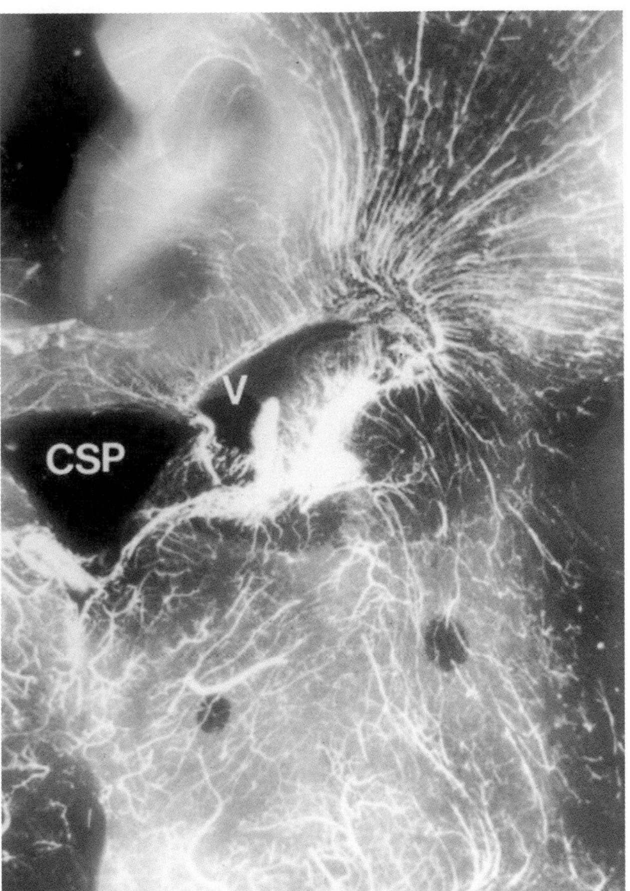


**Figure 21.2** Microvenography showing the fan-shaped leash of veins in the deep periventricular white matter of a neonate of 28 weeks of gestation. V, ventricle; CSP, cavum septi pellucidi. (Reproduced with permission from Elsevier Science, from Takashima *et al.* 1986.)

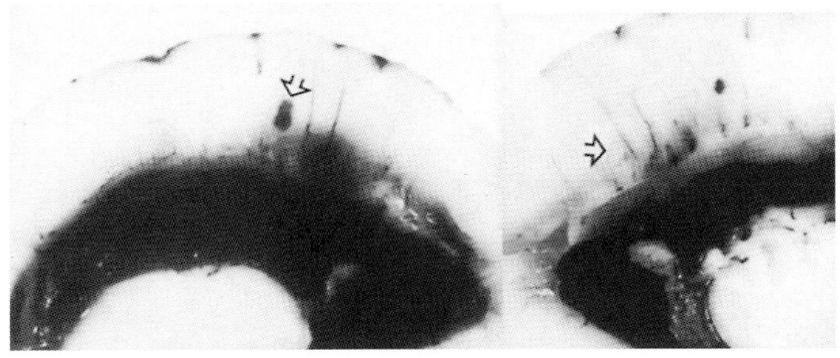

**Figure 21.3** Close-up of the two hemispheres from an infant of 30 weeks of gestation showing distention of both lateral ventricles with clot. There is congestion of the veins draining the deep periventricular white matter. Note also the white spots of periventricular leukomalacia (arrowed) and the secondary bleeding into the necrotic tissue.

Venous infarction has also been reported to occur following intraventricular clot formation (Pape & Wigglesworth 1979). We have reported ultrasound evidence for

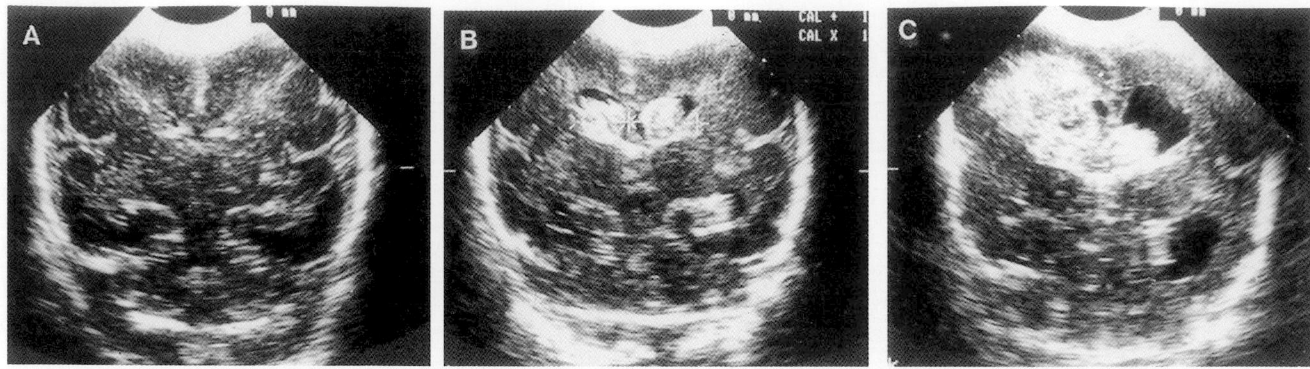


**Figure 21.4** Evolution of GMH–IVH in an infant born at 27 weeks. (A) Normal scan on day 1. (B) Large bilateral intraventricular hemorrhage on day 2. (C) Right-sided parenchymal involvement on day 3.

extension of GMH–IVH in 15% of infants with this form of hemorrhage over a period of up to 48 hours (Levene & de Vries 1984). The initial lesion is one of distention of the ventricle with clot, and subsequently extension of echodensity into the periventricular white matter occurs (Fig. 21.4).

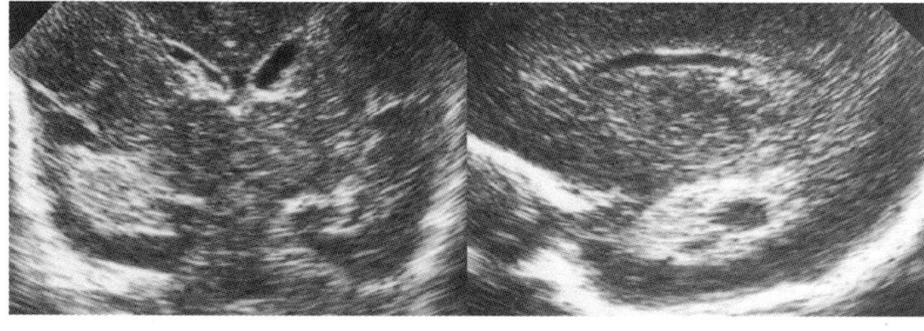

A

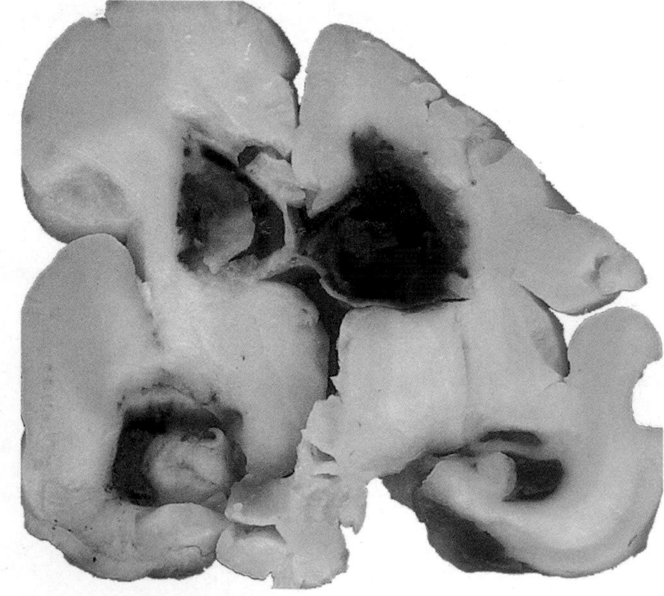

B

**Figure 21.5** Focal temporal lobe infarction secondary to GMH seen on ultrasound coronal scan (left) and parasagittal scan (right). (With permission of Dr P. Govaert.)

A recent report (Govaert *et al.* 1999) suggests that a discrete unilateral haemorrhagic lesion in the temporal lobe (Fig. 21.5) or around the atrium of very premature infants is secondary to venous infarction of either the inferior ventricular vein or the lateral atrial veins. These lesions are suggested to occur as a result of GMH causing obstruction to these veins with eventual venous infarction.

It has been suggested that blood within the lateral ventricle liberates vasoactive compounds that induce local arterial spasm within the periventricular arteries to produce ischemia with subsequent infarction (Stutchfield & Cooke 1989). The time-scale for the evolution of this lesion will be similar to that of venous infarction (White *et al.* 1975; Edvinsson *et al.* 1986). Stutchfield & Cooke (1989) found that 45% of premature infants with ultrasound evidence of parenchymal infarction had cerebrospinal fluid (CSF) potassium concentrations above 2 SD from the mean.

Blood in the ventricular system may remain in the liquid phase, but when it is present in large amounts clots develop. In severe cases a cast of clot involving the lateral, third and fourth ventricular system forms and, if the infant survives, ventricular dilatation is almost inevitable (see Chapter 43). Alternatively, multiple small clots may develop which are suspended in the liquid phase of the intraventricular blood, and these may also cause obstruction to CSF drainage. Blood commonly collects in the subarachnoid spaces of the posterior fossa and may extend into the basal cistern.

## INCIDENCE

Although prenatal hemorrhage is well documented (see Chapter 20) it occurs rarely and GMH–IVH is essentially a postnatal event. The incidence of GMH–IVH is directly related to the maturity of the infant, and for infants weighing below 1500 g (approximating to 30 weeks of gestation) the current incidence is about 30–40%, although some centers report significantly lower figures (Allan *et al.* 1997). The incidence of hemorrhage increases with reducing gestational age below 30 weeks (see Fig. 21.6) and conversely becomes progressively less common with

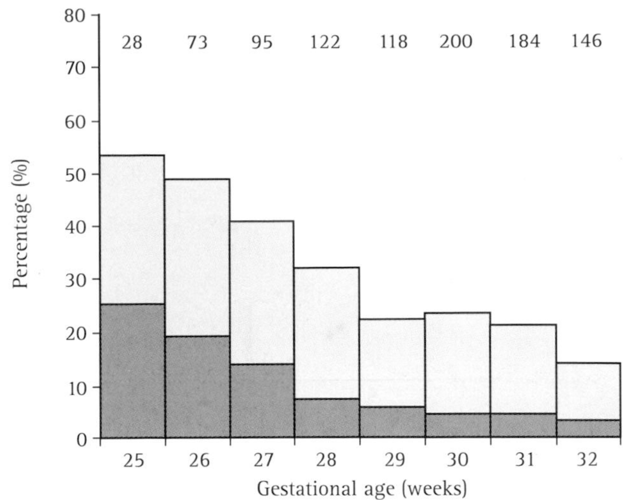


Figure 21.6 Incidence of GMH–IVH in extremely premature infants by gestational age from Wilhelmina Children's Hospital, Utrecht (1994–96). The number at the top of each column refers to the number of infants in each group, shaded areas represent proportion with parenchymal hemorrhage.

advancing gestational age. Intraparenchymal hemorrhage was reported in the 1990s to be relatively uncommon with an average incidence of 5% (range 2–11%) (Batton *et al.* 1994; Cooke 1994; Rademaker *et al.* 1994; Claris *et al.* 1996; Allan *et al.* 1997).

In the last decade, with the introduction of high uptake of antenatal corticosteroids and surfactant therapy, the incidence of GMH–IVH appears to be falling. In the USA the incidence of GMH–IVH was 9% in 1990–93 compared with 23% in 1982–85 (Allan *et al.* 1994). The decline in incidence is particularly marked for intraparenchymal lesions (Allan *et al.* 1994, Cooke 1994, Cooke 1999).

### Incidence in mature infants

The true incidence in infants of 35 weeks of gestation and above is difficult to derive as most infants born at this maturity are healthy and are not referred to neonatal units for intensive care or intracranial scanning. Those that are referred are clearly highly selected, and the incidence of GMH–IVH in this group will not be representative of the whole population. Although GMH–IVH is uncommon in mature infants it is well documented (Cartwright *et al.* 1979, Palma *et al.* 1979, Mitchell & O'Tuama 1980, Scher *et al.* 1982, Fenichel *et al.* 1984). By 35–36 weeks, involution of the subependymal germinal matrix is almost complete and bleeding in this area is uncommon. The overall incidence of GMH–IVH diagnosed by ultrasound is 2–5% of an unselected, asymptomatic group of full-term infants (Hayden *et al.* 1985; Heibel *et al.* 1993; Mercuri *et al.* 1998). It was bilateral in approximately one-half of cases (Hayden *et al.* 1985) and in a group of 1000 unselected low-risk full-term infants approximately 1% had associated IVH (Heibel *et al.* 1993). IVH due to choroid plexus hemorrhage (see below) accounted for a further 1%.

Mature infants described in isolated case reports are likely to be symptomatic for the attending clinicians to perform scans, and it is not surprising that in these infants the majority of lesions are extensive and some involve the cerebral parenchyma. Asphyxia may precede the hemorrhage in mature infants, but this is not invariable, and often there are no obvious risk factors. IVH in full-term infants has been reported to be due to choroid plexus or tela choroidea hemorrhage, vascular malformations or extension of parenchymal hemorrhagic infarcts, and these are all discussed on p. 360. Thalamic hemorrhage (see p. 361) is reported to be the commonest cause of IVH in full-term infants who present with acute onset of hemorrhage up to 1 month of age (Roland *et al.* 1990). Other causes in mature babies include blunt abdominal trauma (Wehberg *et al.* 1992), and following aspiration of an intraventricular reservoir (Moghal *et al.* 1992). The prognosis for a group of infants presenting at term with *symptomatic* IVH was mixed (Jocelyn & Casiro 1992). One-half were apparently normal at a mean age of 36 months, but one-third had severe handicaps. In general, extensive IVH occurring in full-term infants is very unusual.

## TIMING OF THE BLEED

As discussed above, GMH–IVH is generally a condition that occurs after birth. Initially, the age at onset of hemorrhage was inferred from autopsy material and reflected a bias towards the most severe cases. Indirect methods designed to time the onset of GMH–IVH have depended on analysis of the proportion of radioactively labeled red cells (Tsiantos *et al.* 1974) or the proportion of mature erythrocytes in the intracerebral clot found at autopsy (Emerson *et al.* 1977). These studies suggested that most bleeds occurred within the first 48 hours after birth.

The introduction of real-time ultrasound allowed frequent scanning of high-risk infants to accurately time the onset of GMH–IVH. Approximately 90% of these hemorrhages occur in the first week of life (Bejar *et al.* 1980; de Crespigny *et al.* 1982; Levene *et al.* 1982; Thorburn *et al.* 1982; Dolfin *et al.* 1983; Szymonowicz & Yu 1984a; Ment *et al.* 1984a) and the majority within the first 3 days of life. Approximately half of all cases of GMH–IVH occur in the first 24 hours of life (Dolfin *et al.* 1983; Beverley *et al.* 1984a; McDonald *et al.* 1984b, Perlman & Volpe 1986).

Very early hemorrhage has been described. Anderson *et al.* (1988) reported a group of infants with established GMH–IVH by 1 hour after birth, and infants with very early hemorrhage (<12 hours) have been considered to be an etiologically distinct group (Leviton *et al.* 1988). Others have reported 19–27% of infants with GMH–IVH developed very early lesions, less than 12 hours from birth (Leviton *et al.* 1991b, Ment *et al.* 1992). Factors in labor may be particularly important in the development of these early lesions (see below).

Late-onset GMH–IVH is not uncommon, and in one study 15% of very low birth weight infants developed hemorrhage after 2 weeks of life (Trounce *et al.* 1986). Hecht *et al.* (1983) reported 17 infants with late onset of hemorrhage after 1 week of age, and all but two were confined to the region of the germinal matrix. Late onset GMH–IVH beyond the first week of life is reported to occur in the caudothalamic groove and be associated with the development of chronic lung disease (Smets *et al.* 1997), but the pathophysiology of these lesions is unclear. If late GMH–IVH occurs, it is usually benign with little likelihood of serious adverse outcome.

Repeated ultrasound scans have shown that in 10–20% of infants, progression in the initial size of the GMH–IVH occurs over 24–48 hours, and this is illustrated in Fig. 21.4 (Shankaran *et al.* 1982; Levene & de Vries 1984; Rademaker *et al.* 1994). Venous infarction is probably the most common mechanism by which this happens, and this is discussed on p. 341.

## ETIOLOGY

GMH–IVH is a condition of prematurity related to rupture of small vessels within the germinal matrix, and is most likely to occur in babies with respiratory distress syndrome (RDS). Many other factors have been described in the etiology of the condition, but in many studies the timing of the hemorrhage has not been established and, consequently, the cause and effect of hemorrhage may become confused. The most useful studies are those that have accurately timed the onset of GMH–IVH and analyzed risk factors only up until the time of hemorrhage. The following represents those risk factors that have been consistently reported to be important.

### Prenatal factors

It has been suggested that early onset GMH–IVH before 12 hours of age represents a group of babies in whom prenatal factors are particularly important in the development of the condition (Anderson *et al.* 1988; Leviton *et al.* 1988).

Although prenatal factors are not a major factor in the etiology of GMH–IVH, they are increasingly recognized as being important in some cases. In a small group of babies known to have prenatal onset of parenchymal hemorrhage, pre-eclampsia, HELLP (Hemolysis, Elevated Liver enzymes, Low Platelets), fetal heart decelerations on the cardiotocograph and absent end-diastolic flow have all been described (de Vries *et al.* 1998a).

A number of reports have shown that maternal pre-eclampsia is associated with a significantly reduced risk of GMH–IVH (Kuban *et al.* 1992; Developmental Epidemiology Network Investigators 1998), even for large lesions (Shankaran *et al.* 1996). Further analysis suggests that this effect may not be direct but reflects the more mature nature of babies born to mothers with pregnancy induced hypertension (Developmental Epidemiology Network Investigators 1998). Others have suggested that markers of a chronic hypoxic intrauterine environment may increase the risk of GMH–IVH. In particular, elevated uric acid as a marker of previous hypoxic-ischemic exposure (Perlman & Risser 1998) and total nucleated red blood cell count on day 1 of $>2.0 \times 10^9$/l (Green *et al.* 1995). Other protective factors for severe GMH–IVH include female sex and African-American maternal race (Shankaran *et al.* 1996).

A full course of antenatal corticosteroids is a very important factor in reducing the risk of GMH–IVH (Shankaran *et al.* 1996), but it is not clear whether this is due to a direct effect on the brain or mediated through reduction in the severity of lung disease (see p. 349). Use of β-sympathomimetic tocolysis has been suggested to double the risk of GMH–IVH developing in the infant (Groome *et al.* 1992), although this has not been reported by others (Levene *et al.* 1982; Leviton *et al.* 1991a; Anderson *et al.* 1992).

Prenatal factors shown to increase the risk of GMH–IVH include histologic signs of amniotic infection (Developmental Epidemiology Network Investigators 1998) and this probably has its effect through cytokine release (see p 376). Heavy maternal smoking may also be a factor for increasing risk of smaller hemorrhages (Spinillo *et al.* 1995).

### Intrapartum factors

In studies of monitoring in labor, the fetuses that subsequently developed severe GMH–IVH with parenchymal involvement, there were significantly increased numbers of abnormal fetal heart rate patterns, although the numbers reported were small (Strauss *et al.* 1985) or possibly the result of earlier fetal insult (de Vries *et al.* 1998b). Others have shown no predictive benefit from cardiotocography in labor (Levene *et al.* 1982; Beverley *et al.* 1984a; Tejani *et al.* 1984).

No report has found that cord blood gases predict the overall risk of GMH–IVH (Beverley & Chance 1984; Beverley *et al.* 1984a; Tejani *et al.* 1984; Tejani & Verma 1989; Ment *et al.* 1992), but a low cord pH (<7.2) was a predictive factor for early onset GMH (Leviton *et al.* 1991a). Low Apgar scores have been correlated with the development of hemorrhage (Beverley *et al.* 1984a; Strauss *et al.* 1985; Tejani & Verma 1989; Ment *et al.* 1992; D'Souza *et al.* 1995). The majority of reports find no such association (Levene *et al.* 1982; Thorburn *et al.* 1982; de Crespigny & Robinson 1983; Beverley & Chance 1984; Hawgood *et al.* 1984; Leviton *et al.* 1991a). Szymonowicz *et al.* (1984b) have found that severe facial bruising, a feature of birth trauma, was a strong predictor of infants likely to develop more severe forms of hemorrhage.

Condition at birth appeared to be associated with early onset GMH–IVH (Leviton *et al.* 1991a), and exposure of the fetus to the active phase of labor (defined as commencing when the cervix reached 4 cm dilatation) also increased the risk of more severe hemorrhage (Anderson *et al.* 1992). The importance of method of delivery on the development of

GMH–IVH is controversial. Vaginal delivery and vertex delivery were considered to be important independent variables in the development of early hemorrhage (Ment *et al.* 1992), but another five well-conducted studies have found no significant difference in the incidence of GMH–IVH between infants born vaginally and those presenting either by the breech or vertex (Levene *et al.* 1982; de Crespigny & Robinson 1983; Bada *et al.* 1984; Tejani *et al.* 1984; Strauss *et al.* 1985).

Most reports do not find that elective Cesarean section, when the woman is not in labor, protects the infant from developing GMH–IVH (Levene *et al.* 1982; Bada *et al.* 1984; Strauss *et al.* 1985; Morales *et al.* 1989; Malloy *et al.* 1991). Another study found Cesarean section to lower the incidence of GMH–IVH compared with vaginal delivery, but neither reduced the severity of hemorrhage, nor reduced the mortality rate (de Crespigny & Robinson 1983). A protective effect of Cesarean section has been claimed by others (Thorburn *et al.* 1982; Tejani *et al.* 1984; Leviton *et al.* 1991b), but in the former study the majority of infants delivered by section was significantly more mature, thus reducing the likelihood of GMH–IVH occurring. There is no good evidence that Cesarean section protects the premature infant against GMH–IVH. Breech delivery is associated with higher risk of large GMH–IVH, but this effect is lost in multivariate analysis (Shakaran *et al.* 1996).

It has been suggested that infants born outside a perinatal center and transported in have a higher incidence of GMH–IVH (Clark *et al.* 1981; Levene *et al.* 1982; Hawgood *et al.* 1984). The transported infants are highly selected, as those who are in good condition at birth may not be referred, thus biasing the group towards those with more severe illness and who are more likely to have intracerebral hemorrhage. Clark *et al.* (1981) studied a group of very low birth weight infants in a geographically well-defined area. All infants born outside the perinatal center were referred in and there was no selection on the basis of severity of illness. Only 29% of the inborn infants had GMH–IVH compared with 79% of those outborn.

### Lung disease and its complications

Respiratory distress syndrome (RDS) is the most consistently recognized risk factor predisposing to GMH–IVH in premature infants. The association between massive intracranial hemorrhage (many of which were GMH–IVH in origin) and the presence of RDS was first made by Harrison *et al.* (1968). They attributed the hemorrhage to severe hypoxia consequent on the lung disease. Subsequently, the association has been confirmed by other groups (Cooke 1981; Levene *et al.* 1982; Thorburn *et al.* 1982; Perlman *et al.* 1983; Szymonowicz *et al.* 1984b; D'Souza *et al.* 1995), but there is probably not a causal relationship between RDS and hemorrhage. Infants with severe RDS require mechanical ventilation and are subject to complications associated with this form of treatment. It has been suggested that hypercapnia, pneumothorax, and the fluctuating pattern of systemic blood pressure cause GMH–IVH, and these are discussed below.

Hypercapnia occurs commonly as a complication of severe RDS and is a potent vasodilator of newborn intracerebral arterioles (Archer *et al.* 1986). This is thought to be an important factor in the development of GMH. A number of studies have reported hypercapnia to be an independent factor in the evolution of GMH–IVH (Dykes *et al.* 1980; Cooke 1981; Levene *et al.* 1982; Szymonowicz *et al.* 1984b; Wallin *et al.* 1990). Levene *et al.* (1982) found that 81% of low birth weight infants who had both hypercapnia ($PaCO_2$ > 6 kPa) and severe acidosis (pH < 7.1) developed GMH–IVH, and more than half of these infants had moderate or severe degrees of hemorrhage.

Metabolic acidosis has also been reported to be an important independent variable in the development of GMH–IVH (Cooke 1981; Levene *et al.* 1982; Hawgood *et al.* 1984), although others have not confirmed this (Thorburn *et al.* 1982). In the older literature infusion of sodium bicarbonate to treat metabolic acidosis has been claimed to be an important cause of GMH–IVH (Simmons *et al.* 1974; Anderson *et al.* 1976; Wigglesworth *et al.* 1976). The rapid or large infusion of a hypertonic base induces osmotic gradients between blood and brain, causing cerebral shrinkage and subsequent hemorrhage. It has been calculated that an infusion of 10 ml of molar concentration sodium bicarbonate over less than 4 hours will produce such a gradient (Finberg 1977). Subsequent prospective studies also suggested that rapid infusion of hyperosmolar sodium bicarbonate was associated with a significantly increased incidence of GMH–IVH (Papile *et al.* 1978; Hawgood *et al.* 1984). Dykes *et al.* (1980) found that administration of sodium bicarbonate after the first day of life was also a significant risk factor in the development of GMH–IVH. A controlled study of bicarbonate infusion in high-risk premature infants could not confirm this as a cause of GMH–IVH (Corbet *et al.* 1977). These studies did not account for the timing of the hemorrhage, and confusion between cause and effect is possible. There are no recent reports suggesting that sodium bicarbonate infusion is an important risk factor prior to the onset of GMH–IVH, but dosage of this agent is now considerably less than previously reported. Unless large volumes of sodium bicarbonate or other hyperosmolar solutions are used these substances are unlikely to produce GMH–IVH by a direct effect.

Pneumothorax has frequently been reported to cause or be an important factor in the development of GMH–IVH (Dykes *et al.* 1980; Lipscomb *et al.* 1981; Peabody 1981; Hill *et al.* 1982; Thorburn *et al.* 1982; Szymonowicz *et al.* 1984a,b; Wallin *et al.* 1990), although a number of other equally careful studies have failed to substantiate this association (Cooke *et al.* 1981; Levene *et al.* 1982). In a prospective study, GMH–IVH was usually found to have developed within 6 hours of the clinical diagnosis of pneumothorax (Hill *et al.* 1982). In each infant in whom blood pressure was measured, there was an increase in diastolic pressure and a fall in pH at the time of pneumothorax. Hill *et al.* (1982)

suggest that GMH–IVH occurs as the direct result of the increase in blood pressure consequent on the development of pneumothorax.

High frequency ventilation (HFV) has been reported to be associated with an increased risk of intracranial hemorrhage (HiFO Study Group 1993; Wiswell *et al.* 1996). A meta-analysis of nine studies comparing HFV with conventional ventilation showed no excess of GMH–IVH or more severe forms of IVH (Clark *et al.* 1996) and more recent Cochrane reviews show that high frequency jet or oscillation ventilation as elective treatment is not associated with an excess of GMH–IVH (Bhuta & Henderson-Smart 1999a; Henderson-Smart *et al.* 1999). In a review of rescue high-frequency oscillatory ventilation versus conventional ventilation in preterm infants there was an increase in IVH of any grade compared with conventional ventilation (RR* 1.77; CI* 1.06, 2.96) and that there is a strong trend towards more severe forms of IVH (Bhuta & Henderson-Smart 1999b).

### Cardiovascular factors

It is generally thought that ill premature infants cannot regulate their CBF constant in the presence of changes in systemic blood pressure and, consequently, extremes of CBF predispose to either ischemia or hemorrhage in the vulnerable germinal matrix (Lou *et al.* 1979; Pape & Wigglesworth 1979). A number of studies have attempted to relate loss of autoregulation to the development of hemorrhage (Milligan 1980; Ment *et al.* 1981; Ahmann *et al.* 1983), but all have major methodologic problems and do not prove the hypothesis.

Acute changes in blood pressure due to rapid infusions of blood or plasma and leading to GMH–IVH have been reported (Dykes *et al.* 1980; Milligan 1980; McDonald *et al.* 1984b, Hawgood *et al.* 1984), but it is of considerable interest that most studies that have assessed the relationship between blood pressure and GMH–IVH have shown a strong relationship between periods of hypotension and the development of hemorrhage (Miall-Allen *et al.* 1987; Watkins *et al.* 1989), with occasional exceptions (D'Souza *et al.* 1995). Mehrabani *et al.* (1991) found that hypotension associated with pneumothorax increased the risk of more severe GMH–IVH by almost ten times compared with infants who had pneumothorax without hypotension. The explanation for this association may be that hypotension causes infarction of the germinal matrix as originally suggested by Towbin (1968). An alternative explanation is that hypotension causes a resetting of the vascular tone within the germinal matrix, and when the blood pressure increases to a more normal level (not necessarily hypertensive) GMH occurs. To support this, a Japanese group (Funato *et al.* 1992) continuously scanned a group of infants at risk of GMH–IVH. They accurately timed the onset of hemorrhage in four cases, and in all four an increase of blood pressure was noted at the time of the hemorrhage compared with the lower blood pressure prior to the bleed. They suggest that GMH–IVH is due to a reperfusion injury. In support of this, Goddard-Finegold *et al.* (1982) produced GMH–IVH in an animal model by rapid volume expansion in puppies that had been previously rendered hypotensive. This did not occur following infusion in untreated normotensive animals.

It has been reported that GMH–IVH occurs mainly in infants who are ventilated and show an unstable pattern of blood pressure characterized by rapid beat-to-beat fluctuations (Perlman *et al.* 1983; Van Bel *et al.* 1987). Perlman *et al.* (1983) suggested that the fluctuating blood pressure pattern led to similar changes in CBF which caused rupture of the germinal matrix vessels. In contrast, Miall-Allen *et al.* (1989) in a similar study assessed the coefficient of variation in systolic blood pressure prior to the onset of GMH–IVH and found that the percentage of time when this was greater than 5% was significantly higher in those infants who did not develop hemorrhage. They did not see the very large beat-to-beat variations reported by Perlman *et al.* (1983). The risk of GMH–IVH may be related to the propagation of this blood pressure variability to the brain through an open ductus arteriosus (Mullaart *et al.* 1994).

It has been observed that another important and common cause of sudden marked changes in systolic pressure is the handling of the infant (Perry *et al.* 1990), but there was no correlation between attempts at reducing these responses and the subsequent development of GMH–IVH. In support of this, no differences in the incidence of GMH–IVH was found in a controlled study of premature babies who had a 'reduced manipulation' protocol compared with the standard 'frequent handling' management (Bada *et al.* 1990).

The role of increased intracerebral venous pressure has also been suggested to be an important cause of GMH–IVH (Reynolds *et al.* 1979). Little is known of the relationship between RDS and venous pressure, but anatomical evidence exists for severe venous stasis in the right atrium, jugular veins, and deep venous system of Galen in neonatal respiratory disease. Increased intracranial venous pressure observed during the course of mechanical ventilation has been reported by Vert *et al.* (1975), and others have also reported increased pressure in the right atrium (Perlman & Volpe 1986) and major changes in perfusion pressure due to fluctuating venous pressure (Perlman & Volpe 1987). Toubas *et al.* (1978) have described an increase in central venous pressure in hypothermic experimental animals.

It has been reported that infants with patent ductus arteriosus (PDA) are at increased risk of developing GMH–IVH due to hemodynamic disturbances associated with the ductal shunt (Perlman *et al.* 1981; Martin *et al.* 1982). Additionally, once the ductus has been surgically ligated there is a sudden increase in systemic blood pressure (Marshall *et al.* 1982) which may cause GMH. Other studies have shown no correlation between GMH–IVH and PDA (Ment *et al.* 1984a) or acute onset or extension of an existing GMH–IVH lesion after surgical ligation of the ductus (Strange *et al.* 1985). A careful hemodynamic study of Doppler assessment of the

* RR, relative risk; OR, odds ratio; CI, confidence interval.

ductal patency has suggested that larger PDA diameter and higher right ventricular output are significantly associated with the risk of subsequently developing a severe GMH–IVH (Evans & Kluckow 1996).

It is most likely that cardiovascular hemodynamic instability is a key risk factor for the development of GMH–IVH and it is the constellation of critical changes in CBF mediated by interaction between the baby's spontaneous respiratory activity and the ventilator via a PDA which is the critical factor in the development of hemorrhage of this type.

### Extravascular pressure

The brain loses extracellular fluid over the first few days of life, and it has been suggested that shrinkage predisposes to vessel rupture due to a lower tissue hydrostatic pressure and an acute increase between intra- and extravascular pressure gradients (DeCourten & Rabinowicz 1981). Others have shown that prevention of postnatal water loss from the brain by prolactin injection prevents intracerebral hemorrhage (Coulter *et al.* 1985). A high serum sodium concentration (>145 mmol/l), as a marker of reduced extravascular volume, was correlated with the development of GMH–IVH, but no significant association could be found (Lupton *et al.* 1990).

### Coagulation defects

It has been postulated by a variety of researchers that after capillary rupture has occurred, bleeding is more likely to continue in the presence of coagulation disturbances (Chessels & Wigglesworth 1972; Foley & McNicol 1977; Setzer *et al.* 1982; Thorburn *et al.* 1982; Beverley *et al.* 1984b; McDonald *et al.* 1984a). Few studies have examined clotting before the onset of hemorrhage, and results are conflicting. Beverley *et al.* (1984b) found no significant differences at birth in a variety of coagulation studies in infants who later developed GMH–IVH, but at 48 hours of age there were significant differences in activated partial thromboplastin time and the activity of some clotting factors between the non-hemorrhage and GMH–IVH groups, but they could not show a relationship between the timing of GMH–IVH and the severity of coagulopathy. Conversely, McDonald *et al.* (1984a) found a significant association between coagulopathy in the first few hours of life and subsequent GMH–IVH or extension of intracranial hemorrhage. The use of heparin to maintain patency of intravascular catheters is an equivocal risk factor. A fourfold increased risk has been reported from a retrospective study (Lesko *et al.* 1986), but a more recent randomized control study has shown no increased risk (Chang *et al.* 1997).

Indomethacin, a potent prostaglandin synthetase inhibitor, is used widely in premature infants to close a PDA and has been suggested to be a risk factor for GMH. Corazza *et al.* (1984) found that indomethacin significantly prolonged the bleeding time within 2 hours of its administration, but they and others (Maher *et al.* 1985) could find no convincing link between indomethacin administration and the initiation or maximal size of hemorrhage. More recently indomethacin has been convincingly shown to reduce the risk of GMH–IVH (see p. 350).

### Other factors

Flush solutions containing benzyl alcohol as a preservative have been suggested to cause GMH–IVH (Menon *et al.* 1984, Hiller *et al.* 1986), and withdrawal of benzyl alcohol from clinical use was associated with a considerable reduction in the number of infants with moderate or severe hemorrhage (Jardine & Rogers 1989). Clearly, iatrogenic causes of GMH–IVH must always be suspected, as new treatments are commonly introduced into neonatal medicine in an uncontrolled manner. Placing an umbilical artery catheter at the level of $T_6$–$T_{11}$ (a high position) has been suggested to cause retrograde flow in the cerebral circulation, and in a retrospective study, placement of the catheter in the high position compared with the low ($L_3$–$L_5$) was significantly associated both with the development of GMH–IVH and its severity (Schick *et al.* 1989).

Vigorous and frequent physiotherapy has been described to be the cause of a particular type of intracranial hemorrhage that may be confused with GMH–IVH in extremely premature infants (Harding *et al.* 1998). In survivors this lesion leads to encephaloclastic porencephaly. Its origin is thought to be hemorrhagic infarction and is similar pathologically to the findings seen in older infants with shaking injuries as a result of non-accidental injury caused by shearing of bridging vessels over the brain surface.

### A unifying hypothesis

GMH–IVH may occur when the structural integrity of the vessel wall is compromised and then ruptures following subsequent changes in intravascular pressure or blood flow. An additional hypothetical factor may be alterations in extravascular pressure. Various factors may be associated with acute changes in intravascular pressure which can be either respiratory or cardiovascular in origin. Respiratory risk factors include mechanical ventilation and pneumothorax which induce vasodilatation secondary to hypercapnia. The most important cardiovascular factors are those that cause a change in CBF, and hypotensive infants may be most vulnerable once the blood pressure is restored. The changes in blood pressure and consequently in blood flow through the germinal matrix are most likely to occur in the presence of hypercapnia and hypoxia, as these factors maximally dilate the cerebral arterioles. Prostaglandins play an important role in the vascular tone of the germinal matrix vessels, and factors may act at this level to predispose the infant to changes in local blood flow and rupture of compromised vessels. Once rupture has occurred, coagulopathy will exacerbate bleeding, which may then become more extensive and rupture into the lateral ventricles. Further impaired flow as the result of venous congestion (p. 340) occurs in the periventricular white matter, leading to venous infarction. This mechanism is summarized in Figure 21.7.

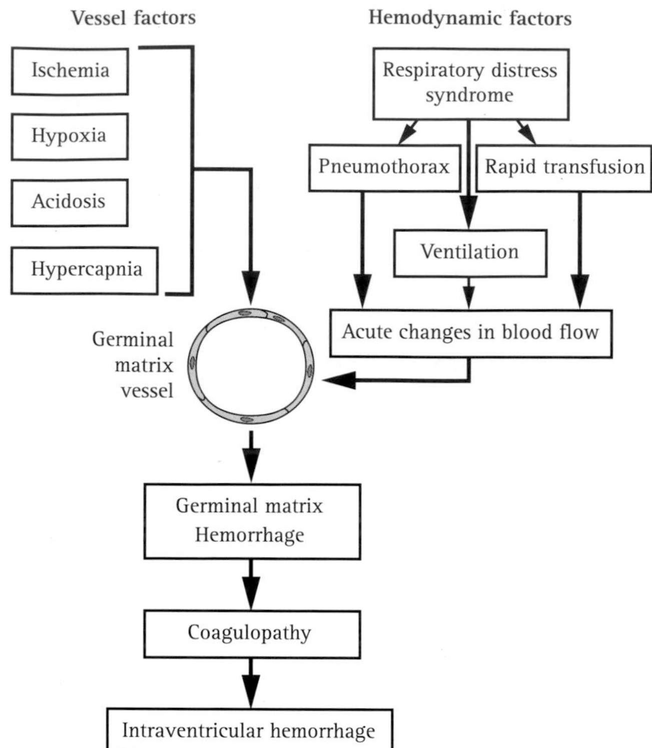


Figure 21.7 A model for the development of GMH and IVH which is dependent on both vessel and hemodynamic factors.

## DIAGNOSIS

### Clinical

This is discussed in detail in Chapter 6, and will be summarized briefly here. Before the introduction of scanning techniques, GMH–IVH was thought to be a devastating condition with obvious clinical signs. Volpe (1977) described two clinical manifestations: a rapidly evolving catastrophic deterioration and, less commonly, a slower saltatory course. Lazzara *et al.* (1978) reported the main physical signs associated with GMH–IVH diagnosed by computerized tomography (CT) to include a tense fontanelle and either increase or decrease in spontaneous activity. In another study, decerebrate posturing was seen in one-half of infants who were shown to have GMH–IVH on CT scans, but clonic seizures were seen equally frequently in the group of infants without hemorrhage (Krishnamoorthy *et al.* 1977).

With the introduction of routine scanning techniques it was recognized that the majority of infants with GMH–IVH showed no overt symptoms. Burstein *et al.* (1979) reported that the frequency of 'silent' hemorrhage was as high as 68% in a group of very low birth weight infants.

Comprehensive neurologic assessment methods have shown that a variety of clinical signs correlate with the presence of GMH–IVH, including impaired visual tracking, abnormal popliteal angle, later development of roving eye movements, decrease in tone, and poor motility (Dubowitz *et al.* 1981). Others have also found infants with GMH–IVH to have increased tone in the lower limbs (particularly popliteal angle) and hypotonia of the neck (particularly flexor muscles) and upper limb girdle muscles. In addition, those with GMH–IVH had brisker tendon reflexes and clonus of the ankle (Stewart *et al.* 1983a).

Clinical assessment at full-term in prematurely born infants is useful in predicting outcome and has been shown to be a better predictor of poor outcome than neonatal ultrasound abnormalities (Dubowitz *et al.* 1984). Of the 62 infants considered normal at 40 weeks, 91% were assessed as normal at 1 year. Abnormal movement patterns associated with intracranial pathology are discussed in detail in Chapter 8.

### Imaging (see also Chapter 6)

CT was first used to diagnose GMH–IVH in 1976 (Pevsner *et al.* 1976) but is inappropriate for routine clinical use. In 1979, ultrasound was shown to be a sensitive method for diagnosing GMH–IVH and has now become widely used as a convenient and safe method for detecting this condition. More recently the role of magnetic resonance imaging (MRI) has been explored in the diagnosis of intracranial hemorrhage and this technique may be able to time accurately the onset of these lesions (Keeney *et al.* 1991, Zuerrer *et al.* 1991). The role of these three techniques in diagnosing hemorrhage, is fully discussed in Chapter 6.

### Electroencephalography (see also Chapter 11)

Cukier *et al.* (1972) first described a specific EEG abnormality associated with GMH–IVH. This was referred to as a positive Rolandic sharp wave, and the association has been confirmed subsequently by other workers (Blume & Dreyfus-Brisac 1982). Unfortunately, this abnormality appears not to be sensitive for uncomplicated GMH–IVH (Watanabe *et al.* 1983; Clancy *et al.* 1984), nor specific (Lombroso 1982). Positive Rolandic sharp waves have also been reported in periventricular leukomalacia (Lombroso 1982; Marret *et al.* 1986), and this particular EEG pattern is common when GMH–IVH is associated with severe leukomalacia. Therefore, the EEG may not be a useful method for diagnosing GMH–IVH alone but may be of value in prognosis because of frequently associated parenchymal lesions. The role of this technique is fully discussed in Chapter 11.

## PREVENTION OF GMH–IVH

There is a large body of data investigating the role of vitamins and drugs in the prevention of GMH–IVH (Table 21.2) and a few studies have shown convincing data that GMH–IVH can be prevented when treatment is given either prenatally or postnatally. Figures 21.8 and 21.9 summarize this data where up-to-date systematic reviews are available.

**Table 21.2 Agents evaluated in preventing GMH–IVH.**

| Postnatal administration | Antenatal administration |
|---|---|
| *Ethamsylate | *Corticosteroids |
| *Factor XIII concentrate | *Phenobarbitone |
| *Fresh frozen plasma | *Vitamin K |
| *Indomethacin | |
| *Pancuronium | |
| *Phenobarbitone | |
| Surfactant | |
| Tranexamic acid | |
| *Vitamin A | |
| *Vitamin E | |

*These have been shown on at least one randomized control study to significantly reduce the risk of hemorrhage. See the text for a detailed discussion.

## Antenatal drug interventions

*ANTENATAL CORTICOSTEROIDS* (Fig. 21.8) To date 18 randomized controlled trials involving over 3700 babies have evaluated the role of corticosteroids in improving perinatal outcome when given antenatally to women in premature labor. A systematic review (Crowley 1999) of all these trials has shown that corticosteroid administration is associated with a significant reduction in the risk of intraventricular hemorrhage diagnosed by ultrasound (OR 0.48; CI 0.32, 0.72). There is also a strong trend towards improving long-term neurologic outcome in survivors (OR 0.62; CI 0.36, 1.08). It is not known whether the steroids reduce the incidence of GMH–IVH through the reduction in risk and severity of respiratory distress syndrome, stabilization of blood pressure, or whether there is a direct cerebral protective effect. Studies of postnatal rescue corticosteroid administration to premature babies with severe lung disease within 96 hours of birth have shown no reduction in the risk of severe IVH.

*ANTENATAL PHENOBARBITONE* (Fig. 21.8) To date there have been 8 trials involving over 1600 babies of phenobarbitone given to mothers in preterm labor to prevent GMH–IVH and these have been systematically reviewed (Crowther & Henderson-Smart 1999a). When all 8 studies were compared there was a significant reduction in the rate of GMH–IVH of all grades of severity (RR 0.75; CI 0.65, 0.88) and in more severe grades of IVH (RR 0.49; CI 0.32, 0.74). There were few data on outcome of survivors, but no difference in the incidence of adverse outcome was found when the children between 18 and 36 months of age were assessed.

The methodological quality of some of these reports was questioned (Crowther & Henderson-Smart 1999a). Some studies failed to randomize, others did not have a placebo arm, and the rates of exclusion of many of these studies was high. When these studies were excluded, the protective effect of antenatally administered phenobarbitone disappeared. Therefore the benefit of antenatal phenobarbitone in preventing disability has not been proven and if only high-quality randomized controlled trials are considered, there is no evidence that antenatally administered phenobarbitone has any effect.

*ANTENATAL MAGNESIUM SULFATE* There have been a number of retrospective reports of magnesium sulfate given either to terminate preterm labor or used as treatment for

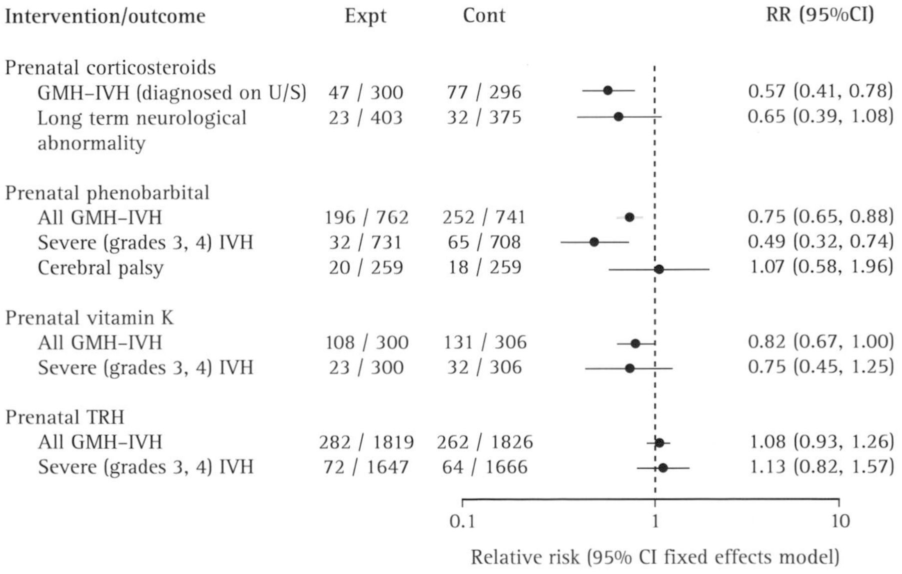

| Intervention/outcome | Expt | Cont | RR (95%CI) |
|---|---|---|---|
| Prenatal corticosteroids | | | |
| GMH–IVH (diagnosed on U/S) | 47 / 300 | 77 / 296 | 0.57 (0.41, 0.78) |
| Long term neurological abnormality | 23 / 403 | 32 / 375 | 0.65 (0.39, 1.08) |
| Prenatal phenobarbital | | | |
| All GMH–IVH | 196 / 762 | 252 / 741 | 0.75 (0.65, 0.88) |
| Severe (grades 3, 4) IVH | 32 / 731 | 65 / 708 | 0.49 (0.32, 0.74) |
| Cerebral palsy | 20 / 259 | 18 / 259 | 1.07 (0.58, 1.96) |
| Prenatal vitamin K | | | |
| All GMH–IVH | 108 / 300 | 131 / 306 | 0.82 (0.67, 1.00) |
| Severe (grades 3, 4) IVH | 23 / 300 | 32 / 306 | 0.75 (0.45, 1.25) |
| Prenatal TRH | | | |
| All GMH–IVH | 282 / 1819 | 262 / 1826 | 1.08 (0.93, 1.26) |
| Severe (grades 3, 4) IVH | 72 / 1647 | 64 / 1666 | 1.13 (0.82, 1.57) |

0.1 1 10

Relative risk (95% CI fixed effects model)

**Figure 21.8** Results of systematic reviews of prenatal drug interventions to prevent GMH–IVH or disability.

maternal hypertension in protecting the fetus against the subsequent development of cerebral palsy (Nelson & Grether 1995, Schendel *et al.* 1996). The precise mechanism by which neuroprotection is apparently conferred is unknown, but a number of studies have investigated whether antenatal magnesium sulfate treatment reduces the incidence of GMH–IVH. In retrospective observational studies, the evidence that magnesium sulfate prevents GMH–IVH is equivocal, but a recent study of 799 babies with birthweight ≤ 1 kg showed that it had no protective effect for the more severe types of IVH (Kimberlin *et al.* 1998).

A systematic review of randomized controlled trials of magnesium sulfate in women in preterm labor described only two, both of poor quality. There was no difference in GMH–IVH in the only trial that reported neurologic complications in the newborn (Crowther & Moore 1999). It has been suggested that when magnesium sulfate is used in conjunction with indomethacin to suppress preterm labor there is a significant excess of babies who develop severe IVH compared with the babies of mothers given magnesium sulfate alone (Iannucci *et al.* 1996). There has also been a report that antenatal magnesium sulfate may increase neonatal mortality (Mittendorf *et al.* 1997), although this is disputed and further prospective studies are still on-going.

A recent retrospective study has suggested that premature infants exposed to antenatal magnesium sulfate were found to have a reduced risk of cystic PVL (FineSmith *et al.* 1997), but there are no other studies to substantiate this.

*ANTENATAL VITAMIN K* (Fig. 21.8) A recent systemic review has compared 5 randomized studies involving 420 women to evaluate the role of vitamin K in the prevention of GMH–IVH, given to women in labor or very likely to deliver a premature infant (Crowther & Henderson-Smart 1999b). The rationale for giving vitamin K is to reduce the tendency to coagulopathy in the immature infant, which is probably an important factor in the subsequent development of hemorrhage. Despite initial enthusiasm for this therapy, the effects appear to be marginal. Antenatal vitamin K was associated with a strong, but non-significant trend towards reduction in the overall rate of GMH–IVH (RR 0.82; CI 0.67–1.00) as well as a somewhat less strong reduction in the more severe types of IVH (RR 0.75; CI 0.45, 1.25). Unfortunately, only one of these 5 studies was rated as of acceptable quality by the reviewers and this study showed a non-significant trend towards protection against GMH–IVH. Follow-up of babies enrolled into these studies was very poor and no differences were seen.

*THYROTROPIN-RELEASING HORMONE* (Fig. 21.8) Thyroid hormone has been postulated as an important factor in maturation of the developing lung and the immature CNS. Administration of thyrotropin-releasing hormone (TRH) together with corticosteroids to mothers in, or at high risk of, premature labor has been evaluated in its outcome on GMH–IVH. To date 11 trials have been published involving over 4500 women. In a systematic review of these studies (Crowther *et al.* 1999) there was no difference in the incidence of either any GMH–IVH or of severe IVH between the two groups. Information on the outcome of survivors was available for only one of these studies (ACTOBAT 1995) and there was an increased incidence of motor delay (RR 1.31; CI 1.09–1.56), motor impairment (RR 1.51; CI 1.01, 2.24), and social delay (RR 1.25; CI 1.03–1.51) in the TRH treated group. This is a worrying finding and suggests that TRH may have a negative effect on early brain development.

## Postnatal drug interventions

*POSTNATAL PHENOBARBITONE* This was the first agent claimed to prevent GMH–IVH. Donn *et al.* (1981) gave two loading doses of 10 mg/kg intravenously 12 hours apart and adjusted the maintenance dose to achieve a serum level of 20–30 µg/ml by the third day of life. GMH–IVH occurred in only 4 of the 30 (13%) infants in the phenobarbitone group compared with 14 of the 30 (47%) control infants ($p = 0.01$). They reported their results again after studying a total of 105 babies and continued to show an impressive reduction in the incidence of GMH–IVH in the treated group (Donn *et al.* 1982). This study was not performed blind and the neonatal staff knew which infants received the drug. Since this original report a further 7 randomized control studies have been published on phenobarbitone given postnatally and the development of GMH–IVH (Morgan *et al.* 1982; Whitelaw *et al.* 1983; Bedard *et al.* 1984; Porter *et al.* 1985; Kuban *et al.* 1986; Anwar *et al.* 1986; Ruth *et al.* 1988). Some of these studies were not conducted blind (Anwar *et al.* 1986; Ruth *et al.* 1988). The loading dose varied between 20 and 30 mg/kg, and all the studies achieved serum phenobarbitone levels within the therapeutic anticonvulsant range. Whitelaw *et al.* (1983) reported that in spontaneously breathing infants the loading dose of phenobarbitone was associated with a high incidence of respiratory failure within hours of giving the drug.

Horbar (1992) has reported the results of a meta-analysis on these 8 studies and concluded that there is no evidence that phenobarbitone reduces the incidence or severity of GMH–IVH compared with controls.

There have been only 2 follow-up reports of infants from these phenobarbitone studies. There were no differences at 18 months in neurologic items (Krishnamoorthy *et al.* 1990) or in neurodevelopmental impairment at a mean age of 27 months (Ruth *et al.* 1988). In conclusion, there is no evidence that postnatally administered phenobarbitone has any benefit in the prevention of GMH–IVH.

*POSTNATAL INDOMETHACIN* (Fig. 21.9) Indomethacin is a potent prostaglandin synthetase inhibitor and inactivates prostaglandin and other prostaglandin-like compounds. In an animal study, Ment *et al.* (1983) found in puppies that indomethacin significantly reduced the incidence of GMH–IVH induced by a hypotension/hypertension technique. The

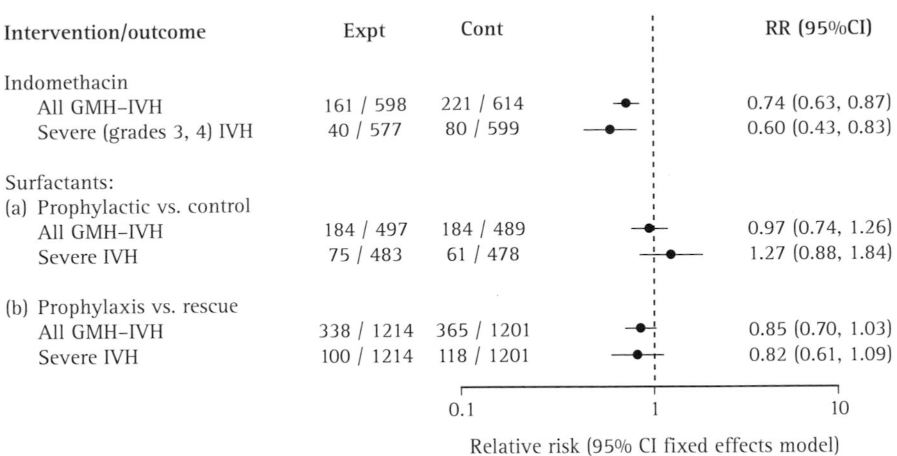

Intervention/outcome
Expt
Cont
RR (95%CI)
Indomethacin
All GMH–IVH
161 / 598
221 / 614
0.74 (0.63, 0.87)
Severe (grades 3, 4) IVH
40 / 577
80 / 599
0.60 (0.43, 0.83)
Surfactants:
(a) Prophylactic vs. control
All GMH–IVH
184 / 497
184 / 489
0.97 (0.74, 1.26)
Severe IVH
75 / 483
61 / 478
1.27 (0.88, 1.84)
(b) Prophylaxis vs. rescue
All GMH–IVH
338 / 1214
365 / 1201
0.85 (0.70, 1.03)
Severe IVH
100 / 1214
118 / 1201
0.82 (0.61, 1.09)
0.1
1
10
Relative risk (95% CI fixed effects model)


**Figure 21.9** Results of systematic reviews of postnatal interventions to prevent GMH–IVH.

pretreated puppies had significantly fewer fluctuations in blood pressure, and indomethacin appeared to ameliorate lability of blood pressure. This same group has subsequently shown in a series of randomized controlled studies that indomethacin significantly reduces the incidence of GMH–IVH in premature infants (Ment *et al.* 1985b, 1988, 1994). These studies randomized 431 infants to receive indomethacin (0.1 mg/kg IV at 6 and 12 postnatal hours and every 24 hours for two more doses or placebo. The mechanism of action is unclear but may involve free-radical scavenging effect or inhibition of active calcium transport in vascular smooth muscle.

Fowlie (1999) has reported a systematic review of 15 randomized controlled studies using prophylactic indomethacin in premature infants (≤1750 g). The incidence of GMH–IVH of all grades was significantly reduced in indomethacin treated groups (RR 0.74; CI 0.63, 0.87). When only more severe degrees of hemorrhage were reported (Papille grade 3 and 4) this effect was still present (RR 0.60; CI 0.43, 0.83).

Two of these studies reported neurodevelopmental outcome of study babies (Bandstra *et al.* 1988; Ment *et al.* 1994). Both showed a trend towards less severe disability in the indomethacin group. One study showed that there was a significant improvement in Stanford–Binet IQ scores at 36 months when both maternal education and infant birth weight were controlled for ($p = 0.044$) (Ment *et al.* 1996). There were no significant differences for the incidence of cerebral palsy between the two groups. The systematic review showed a trend towards an increased incidence of necrotizing enterocolitis in the indomethacin group.

The evidence supports the suggestion that indomethacin treatment within 24 hours of birth reduces the risk of GMH–IVH in very low birth weight infants and may reduce disability, although this remains unproven at the present time.

*POSTNATAL ETHAMSYLATE* As GMH–IVH occurs by capillary bleeding from the germinal matrix, Morgan *et al.* (1981) suggested that ethamsylate, a drug known to reduce capillary bleeding, may prevent this form of hemorrhage. They enrolled 70 very low birth weight infants in a double-blind controlled study using 0.1 mg/kg of drug or placebo. There was a significantly reduced incidence of GMH–IVH in ethamsylate treated infants, but the frequency of larger bleeds was no different between the two groups. They subsequently enrolled more infants (not in a randomized manner) and reported that there was a reduction in neurologic abnormalities at follow-up, as well as a reduction in the number of ventriculoperitoneal shunts needed to treat posthemorrhagic hydrocephalus (Cooke & Morgan 1984). It has been suggested that as well as the platelet effect, ethamsylate reduces the synthesis of prostaglandins (Ment *et al.* 1984b), which may protect the germinal matrix from rapid fluctuations in CBF.

A multicenter trial assessing the effect of ethamsylate in the prevention of GMH–IVH (Benson *et al.* 1986) has also suggested that ethamsylate has a protective effect in both reducing the incidence of IVH and limiting the size of the eventual lesion. A total of 330 very low birth weight infants were enrolled, and only 18.5% of the treated group developed IVH or parenchymal hemorrhage compared with 29.8% of the controls. There was no difference in mortality between the two groups. The surviving infants in this study were followed-up to the age of 2.5 years, and those who received ethamsylate appear to have had significantly higher cognitive scores on Griffiths assessment than the placebo group. There were no significant differences in disability between the two groups (R. W. I. Cooke, personal communication). Subsequently, a smaller randomized controlled study has also shown a significant reduction in overall GMH–IVH as well as in more severe hemorrhage (Chen 1993).

*POSTNATAL VITAMIN E* Chiswick *et al.* (1983) from Manchester, UK have claimed that early treatment with vitamin E protects against IVH in premature infants. They attempted to distinguish, by ultrasound scanning, ruptured from unruptured GMH, and on this basis showed an apparent protective effect of vitamin E on the frequency of GMH–IVH. However, when the combined incidences of both GMHs and IVHs were compared there was no difference in the incidence of GMH–IVH between the two groups. It is not possible using ultrasound to make the distinction, Chiswick *et al.* claim, but they subsequently reported the results of a larger prospective randomized trial (Sinha *et al.* 1987). Unfortunately, this study was not carried out in a blind manner, but they found that both inborn and outborn babies pretreated with vitamin E had a lower incidence of IVH and parenchymal hemorrhage.

Two further studies have suggested that vitamin E has an effect in protecting against GMH–IVH (Speer *et al.* 1984; Fish *et al.* 1990). In a randomized control study of intramuscular vitamin E in neonates of birth weight 1 kg or less, this agent was shown to significantly reduce the incidence of any type of intracranial hemorrhage as well as severe hemorrhage only in the group of infants with a birth weight of 750 g and below (Fish *et al.* 1990). There appeared to be no complications of treatment in this study. Another study of infants weighing less than 1 kg at birth (Phelps 1984) showed that 14 of 43 infants pretreated with vitamin E developed severe hemorrhage compared with only 4 of 42 given placebo.

In an overview of 4 vitamin E studies that assessed its effect on GMH–IVH, Law *et al.* (1990) concluded that 'vitamin E supplementation might not prevent neurological disability [as the result of GMH–IVH], and at best it would do so in no more than 2.5 per cent of all treated infants'.

It is suggested that vitamin E stabilizes endothelial membranes, thus limiting the extent of hemorrhage (Chiswick *et al.* 1983; Speer *et al.* 1984). Alternatively, prevention of mitochondrial damage by its activity in scavenging oxygen free-radicals has been proposed as its main mechanism of action (Ment 1985a). In addition, it has been shown that superoxide dismutase (a powerful oxygen free-radical scavenger) reduces the incidence of periventricular hemorrhage in an animal model (Ment *et al.* 1985a).

Evidence has accumulated in the USA suggesting that a particular form of parenteral vitamin E (E-Ferol) causes thrombocytopenia, renal dysfunction, and cholestatic liver failure (Bove *et al.* 1985). It is not clear whether this is a direct effect of the vitamin preparation or occurs as a result of the vehicle in which the drug is administered. In view of the potential hazards of this agent and doubt as to its efficacy in preventing GMH–IVH, we cannot recommend it for routine use in premature infants.

*POSTNATAL PANCURONIUM* Pancuronium, a non-depolarizing neuromuscular blocker, has also been shown to prevent GMH–IVH in premature infants with marked beat-to-beat fluctuations in blood pressure (Perlman *et al.* 1985). This pattern occurs in infants who actively expire against a positive-pressure inspiratory breath of the mechanical ventilator. Perlman *et al.* (1985) recognized a group of infants with the fluctuating blood pressure pattern, and paralyzed a randomly selected proportion of them. GMH–IVH developed in all ten spontaneously breathing infants, but only 5 of 14 given pancuronium developed hemorrhage, and in 4 of the 5 GMH–IVH developed after the paralysis had worn off. On closer examination of their data only 20 of the 166 (12%) infants they studied actually developed GMH–IVH, an incidence well below that reported previously by Volpe in a population of very low birth weight infants (Tarby & Volpe 1982). This must raise the question of how representative of high-risk infants was their cohort.

Two previous studies of pancuronium failed to show any significant reduction in the incidence of GMH–IVH (Pollitzer *et al.* 1981; Greenhough *et al.* 1984). Further information must be obtained on the safety and efficacy of neuromuscular blockade in the prevention of GMH–IVH before it becomes routinely accepted.

*POSTNATAL PLASMA EXPANSION* Beverley *et al.* (1985) reported a reduction in the incidence of GMH–IVH from 41 to 14% by means of early infusion of 10 ml/kg of fresh frozen plasma (FFP) on admission to the neonatal unit and then again at 48 hours from birth. This was highly statistically significant ($p = 0.022$). The mechanism by which FFP prevents hemorrhage is unclear. They did not find that it reduced the frequency of clotting abnormalities in these infants, but did not report blood pressure data. It is possible that the reduction in incidence of severe GMH–IVH was related to the prevention of cerebral ischemia due to the effects of the FFP stabilizing the cerebral circulation.

More recently, a much larger study (Northern Neonatal Nursing Initiative Trial Group, 1996) involving 776 babies compared early administration of 20 ml/kg fresh frozen plasma (FFP) with 20 ml/kg of a gelatin based plasma substitute (Gelofusin) and a control group with no bolus infusion. There was no difference in mortality or in IVH diagnosed at autopsy (ultrasound data was not reported). There was no difference in the number of disabled children alive at two years after birth (100% follow-up).

*POSTNATAL VITAMIN A* Low levels of vitamin A have been reported in a group of very low birth weight babies who sustained severe intracranial bleeding (Papagaroufalis *et al.* 1988). Vitamin A has a role in the integrity of vascular endothelium, and this may be important in the pathogenesis of GMH–IVH. This group organized a randomized control study to supplement a group of very immature infants with either intramuscular vitamin A (5000 IU within 12 hours and then 3750 IU daily) or placebo (Papagaroufalis *et al.* 1991). There was a significant reduction in severe GMH–IVH in the vitamin A group and a trend towards reduction in all grades of hemorrhage.

*POSTNATAL FACTOR XIII CONCENTRATE* Premature infants with intracranial hemorrhage have been shown to have a markedly reduced platelet count, and low fibrinogen and factor XIII activity (Shirahata *et al.* 1990). Shirahata *et al.* gave factor XIII concentrate within 6 hours of birth to a group of premature infants at risk of GMH–IVH and found a significant reduction in the incidence of hemorrhage in the group treated with factor XIII compared with controls.

*POSTNATAL TRANEXAMIC ACID* Another drug that reduces fibrinolytic activity of the germinal matrix is tranexamic acid, and this has also been assessed for its ability to prevent GMH–IVH. In a double-blind controlled study of 100 very low birth weight infants, no reduction in either the incidence or severity of hemorrhage was found (Hensey *et al.* 1984).

*EXOGENOUS SURFACTANT* (Fig. 21.9) Exogenous surfactant is a very effective agent in reducing mortality in premature infants with RDS. A number of studies have evaluated the role of surfactant in the prevention of GMH–IVH. A systematic review (Soll 1999) of prophylactic use of both synthetic and natural surfactants found no evidence that surfactant reduces the risk of GMH–IVH (any grade), or severe IVH, or the development of subsequent cerebral palsy. A second systematic review (Soll & Morley 1999) of prophylactic surfactant versus selective use in premature infants showed a strong trend towards prophylactic use, reducing the risk of all GMH–IVH (OR 0.85, CI 0.70, 1.03) and severe IVH (OR 0.82, CI 0.61, 1.09).

The effects of rapid instillation of surfactant into the trachea on cerebral function and blood pressure have been examined. A short period of electrocerebral depression was reported lasting less than 10 minutes after instillation of the surfactant (Hellstrom-Westas *et al.* 1992). The effect of surfactant on blood pressure has also been reported. A transient fall in mean arterial blood pressure of 6 mmHg (Cowan *et al.* 1991) and 9.3 mmHg (Hellstrom-Westas *et al.* 1992) immediately after giving the surfactant may be an important factor in the EEG changes and the later development of GMH–IVH.

*GENERAL METHODS* It has been noted that hypercapnia vasodilates cerebral arterioles and together with failure of autoregulation may predispose to GMH. Lou *et al.* (1982) have retrospectively analyzed the $PaCO_2$ values following elective intubation and resuscitation in a group of very premature infants. They suggested that hyperventilation might re-establish autoregulation in these babies and consequently prevent GMH–IVH. No infant developed hemorrhage whose early $PaCO_2$ was less than 25 mmHg, and hemorrhage tended to occur in the infants with the highest $PaCO_2$ levels measured in the first hour. All the infants with early GMH–IVH were born vaginally. The authors claim that the severity of the infant's lung disease was not the reason for the differences in $PaCO_2$ and the reduced incidence of GMH–IVH. These results must be treated with caution in view of the retrospective and uncontrolled nature of this study and the demonstration that hypocapnia is an important factor in the development of cystic PVL (p. 380).

Two controlled studies have been conducted to compare the neonatal outcome for elective versus selective Cesarean section in the very premature baby (Zlatnik 1993). The results for reduction of the risk of intracranial pathology were contradictory, but taken together these studies were small and no significant effect was reported.

A group in Melbourne (Szymonowicz *et al.* 1986) has attempted to modify early neonatal management in order to reduce the incidence of GMH–IVH in infants with a birth weight below 1250 g. They achieved significant improvement in measurements of pH, body temperature and blood pressure measured on admission to the neonatal unit, and subsequently found significantly lower $PaCO_2$ tensions and higher blood pressure measurements. Infants treated by these methods had a 36% incidence of GMH–IVH compared with a 60% incidence in infants of the same birth weight treated by less aggressive means in a previous period. This was a highly significant reduction in the incidence of hemorrhage ($p<0.001$). They claim that changes in neonatal management may account for an apparent reduction in the incidence of GMH–IVH in drug studies, particularly if these are not performed blind.

Handling of small, sick infants is known to be associated with large swings in systemic blood pressure (see p. 347). Bada *et al.* (1990) have attempted to assess whether a protocol of reduced manipulation of these babies reduces the incidence of GMH–IVH. There were no statistically significant differences between the standard management group and the reduced handling group. The differences in intervention time in the two groups were only significant for the first 48 hours, and even on the first day of life when the differences were greatest this amounted to an average of 2.4 hours.

## PROGNOSIS

Determining the prognosis in infants who had sustained GMH–IVH is confused due to other confounding variables. GMH–IVH occurs in prematurely born infants, and it is known that very low birth weight infants have significantly lower scores of cognitive ability and motor adaptation than infants born at full-term. In a subgroup of very low birth weight babies without any evidence of brain pathology following repeated ultrasound examinations, in the newborn period, when compared with full-term control infants, they show significantly more clumsiness and lower IQ scores (Levene *et al.* 1992). Clearly the effect of very premature birth has its own long-term effects on brain function, quite apart from the effect of GMH–IVH. In addition to premature birth, other confounding variables include the general effects of severe prematurity on the developing, specific pathology such as periventricular leukomalacia (see Ch. 22) and later effects of socioeconomic class (Vohr & Ment 1996).

### Mortality

Death in extremely premature infants may be due to a variety of causes including lung disease, sepsis, necrotizing enterocolitis, and brain hemorrhage. At autopsy, cerebral hemorrhage may be found, but this may not be the primary cause of death, and deciding what single insult killed the infant may be impossible. In general, it appears that the more severe the degree of hemorrhage, the higher is the mortality (Thorburn *et al.* 1981; Shankaran *et al.* 1982; Smith *et al.* 1983). Hemorrhage confined to the region of the germinal matrix does not increase the risk of death, but intraparenchymal involvement has a high mortality. Approximately one-half (Martin *et al.* 1984; Ahmann *et al.* 1983; de Vries *et al.* 1998b) to three-quarters (Thorburn *et al.* 1981; Trounce *et al.* 1986) of infants with intraparenchymal lesions die, although the staff and parental attitudes towards large IVH may influence the survival statistics.

### Neurodevelopmental outcome

Early studies reporting outcome are biased towards those cases with the most obvious clinical presentation as it was only those who had CT scans performed (Krishnamoorthy *et al.* 1979; Kosmetatos *et al.* 1980). Studies in which all very premature infants had regular ultrasound scans provide more accurate follow-up data. There appears to be little increased risk of handicap in infants with grade I hemorrhage confined to the region of the germinal matrix, compared with similar infants without GMH–IVH (Shankaran *et al.* 1982; Papile *et al.* 1983; Stewart *et al.* 1983b). Some authors have also suggested that moderate hemorrhage (clot in the lateral ventricles with no parenchymal extension) does not significantly increase the risk of adverse outcome compared with mild GMH–IVH (Papile *et al.* 1983; Stewart *et al.* 1983b; Dubowitz *et al.* 1984). However, others have suggested a definite trend between the size of GMH–IVH and incidence of severe disability (Catto-Smith *et al.* 1985). The latter authors report that two-thirds of infants with this form of hemorrhage had major disability, an incidence higher than most other follow-up studies. In summary, the prognosis for infants with uncomplicated GMH–IVH (no parenchymal extension or ventricular dilatation) is very likely to be good with respect to these infants not developing cerebral palsy.

Studies relating the severity of GMH–IVH to outcome in school-age children agree that providing hemorrhage does not extend into the cerebral parenchyma and there is no significant ventricular dilatation the outcome is no different from infants born of the same degree of prematurity but without evidence of GMH–IVH (Lowe & Papile 1990; Levene *et al.* 1992; Vohr *et al.* 1992). At 5 years of age, 60% of children with Papile grade III and IV hemorrhage were normal on neurologic assessment, and children with grade I and II GMH–IVH had no worse outcome than prematurely born children with no GMH–IVH (Vohr *et al.* 1992). Lowe & Papile (1990) found that on a battery of tests the children with previous GMH–IVH (Papile grade I and II) did not perform significantly worse on any one test, but when all tests were compared together they did perform less well than a prematurely born group without hemorrhage. Similarly, when a group of very low birth weight infants were seen at 5 years and tests of motor impairment (degree of clumsiness) performed, although the presence of GMH–IVH did not impair performance, when those infants who had 'prolonged flare' as well as GMH–IVH were considered, the 'double ultrasound abnormality' was associated with less good motor performance (Levene *et al.* 1992). Motor coordination was impaired at 5 years in very low birth weight infants to the same degree whether or not the child had IVH in the neonatal period (Vohr *et al.* 1992). There is a suggestion that language development at 3 years of age may be worse in infants with a birth weight below 1000 g if they had sustained GMH–IVH (Grunau *et al.* 1990).

The underlying etiology of parenchymal hemorrhage is discussed in the next section, but follow-up studies agree that there is a high incidence of adverse neurodevelopmental outcome whatever the cause. Major handicap ranges from 67 to 100% of infants with parenchymal involvement (Shankaran *et al.* 1982; Stewart *et al.* 1983b; Papile *et al.* 1983; Dubowitz *et al.* 1984; Catto-Smith *et al.* 1985, TeKoiste *et al.* 1985; de Vries *et al.* 1998b). McMenamin *et al.* (1984) have suggested that outcome following this form of hemorrhage is much worse in infants weighing less than 1000 g at birth compared with larger babies. Furthermore, they found that survivors of large parenchymal lesions all had more significant handicap than those surviving less extensive parenchymal involvement. The distinction between the ultrasound appearances of periventricular leukomalacia and parenchymal involvement due to venous infarction may be very difficult in the first week of life. Evolution to porencephaly or multiple cystic degeneration helps to clarify the pathology, and this is why early abnormal ultrasound appearances (those present in the first two weeks of life) are less good at predicting adverse outcome than those made later when the lesions have had time to evolve fully (Cooke 1987; Stewart *et al.* 1987; Nwaesei *et al.* 1988). MRI used to assess the degree of myelination predicts neurodevelopmental outcome at 3 years of age, but was found to be less accurate in its predictive ability than cranial ultrasound (van der Bor *et al.* 1992).

In a study of 1625 premature infants born between 1990 and 1997, de Vries *et al.* (1998b) found that 11% of survivors with large IVH (blood distending the ventricle in the acute phase and clot filling >50% of the ventricle) developed cerebral palsy compared with 67% who developed it after surviving unilateral parenchymal hemorrhage. The most common form of cerebral palsy was spastic hemiplegia, contralateral to the side of the parenchymal hemorrhage. The location of the unilateral parenchymal hemorrhage also appears to predict risk of cerebral palsy. Nine of 10 babies with parenchymal lesions in the fronto-parietal region did not develop cerebral palsy, compared with all survivors of apparent hemorrhage in the occipital region who did so (Rademaker *et al.* 1994).

### Porencephaly

The prognosis for established porencephaly is also controversial. A bad prognosis with cerebral palsy (Guzzetta *et al.* 1986; Cooke 1987) and developmental impairment (Cooke 1987) has been reported, but de Vries *et al.* (1985) suggest that the outcome in infants with porencephaly is much more benign. It is important to note that despite extensive hemorrhage and early signs of cerebral palsy, the eventual disability may be mild and the child should be able to attend a normal school (Fawer *et al.* 1983). The outcome of 16 prematurely born infants with posthemorrhagic porencephalic cavities was reviewed at a mean age of 33 months (Blackman *et al.* 1991). They found that 81% of the children had cerebral palsy, but only 19% had moderate or severe cognitive deficits. De Vries *et al.* (2000) have reported that the appearance of asymmetry of myelination in the posterior limb of the internal capsule predicts subsequent development of cerebral palsy.

## SEQUELAE OF GMH–IVH

### Metabolic complications

A number of hormonal disturbances or metabolic problems are described in association with various types of intracranial hemorrhage. Some of these are also discussed on p. 485 as they may occur as the result of birth asphyxia or other forms of intracranial pathology.

Inappropriate antidiuretic hormone secretion has been reported in a few premature infants with CT scan diagnosis of intracranial hemorrhage (Moylan *et al.* 1978). Central diabetes insipidus has also been reported in a premature infant with GMH–IVH (Adams *et al.* 1976). This was a transient condition and required short-term treatment with a vasopressin-like agent.

Hyperpyrexia following GMH–IVH is well recognized (Gomes & Weerasuriya 1975), and this is seen particularly in full-term infants and may occur following a variety of different forms of intracranial hemorrhage. Elevated body temperature may persist for weeks and may initially cause confusion with meningitis, particularly if there is a high CSF white cell count with low glucose.

### Subependymal pseudocyst

Cyst formation is a relatively common finding in the subependymal region at the head of the caudate nucleus in the newborn (Fig. 21.10). Cavitation within the germinal matrix is referred to as a pseudocyst because it is not lined by epithelium (Larroche 1972). These commonly develop after a small hemorrhage in the region of the germinal matrix and are easily recognized on ultrasound. They may develop following a variety of insults including prenatal infection with rubella or cytomegalovirus (Shaw & Alvord 1974). They may also occur as a 'normal' event if the rapidly developing germinal matrix outgrows its blood supply. In some cases the pseudocysts may be more anterior and bilateral (Rademaker *et al.* 1993), and care must be taken not to confuse them with cystic periventricular leukomalacia (see p. 383). When the pseudocyst occurs following GMH–IVH it has no prognostic significance, and if it represents the only cerebral insult the prognosis is excellent.

### Encephaloclastic porencephaly

Encephaloclastic porencephaly refers to a fluid-filled defect lying within the cerebral parenchyma and communicating with a lateral ventricle.

Porencephaly occurs relatively commonly in the perinatal brain due to a variety of insults. The pathology of porencephaly is discussed in Chapter 13 and the antenatal diagnosis and significance is discussed in Chapter 17. Porencephaly may occur as a result of intracranial hemorrhage or infarction.

Porencephaly is a common finding in premature infants at the site of a pre-existing venous infarct (see p. 341) and

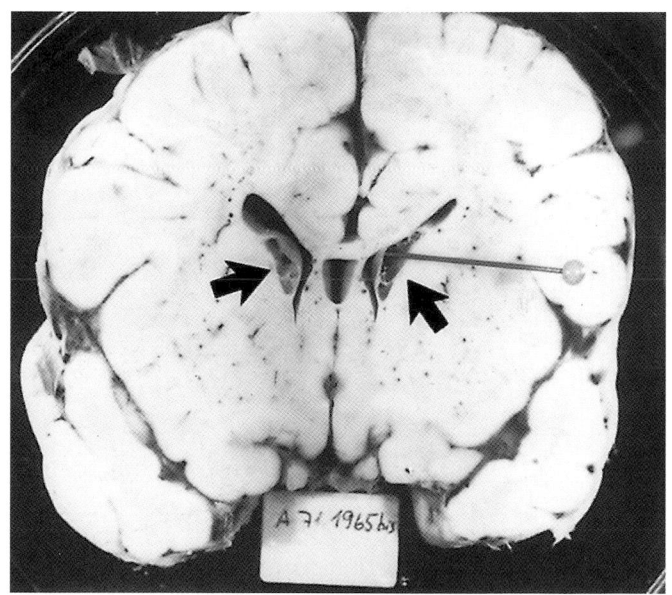

A

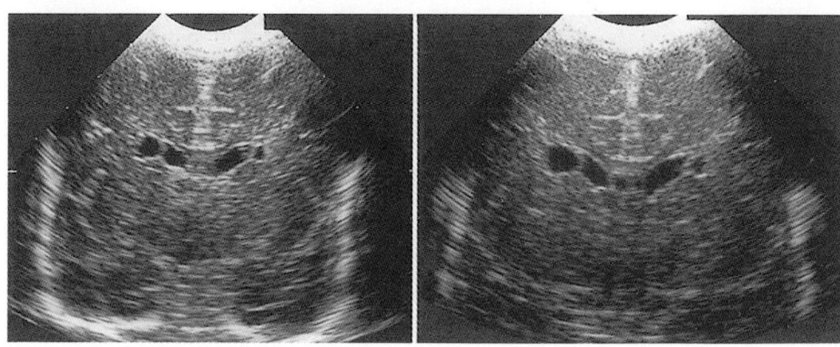

B

**Figure 21.10** (A) Bilateral subependymal pseudocysts (arrowed) in the germinal matrix. (B) Ultrasound scans showing bilateral pseudocysts.

develops in approximately two-thirds of infants with parenchymal hemorrhage or hemorrhagic infarction (Pasternak *et al.* 1980), and these can be detected by imaging techniques. The time interval between initial hemorrhage and its evolution through to porencephaly may be 6–8 weeks.

The prognosis for infants and children with porencephaly depends entirely on the underlying cause of the porencephalic lesion. Its prognosis in infants with porencephaly secondary to venous infarction is discussed on p. 355. Rarely the porencephalic cavity progressively expands, and this may cause deterioration in cerebral function (Tardieu *et al.* 1981). Although the measured CSF pressure is not elevated, ventriculoperitoneal shunting can result in remarkable improvement of focal motor deficits and intellectual development.

### Posthemorrhagic hydrocephalus

This complication occurs relatively frequently following GMH–IVH, and is discussed in detail in Chapters 43 and 44.

## SUBDURAL HEMORRHAGE

Fatal subdural hemorrhage is now rare but the incidence of this condition in surviving infants is difficult to ascertain. Various CT studies have reported subdural hemorrhage to account for 4–11% of infants with symptomatic intracranial hemorrhage (Le Blanc & O'Gorman 1980; Bergman *et al.* 1985), but it may be associated with little or no clinical signs and therefore remain clinically undiagnosed.

## ETIOLOGY

Subdural hemorrhage may be due to a number of different underlying causes, but birth trauma is the most commonly recurring factor.

### Dural tear

This was usually associated with rapid delivery of the infant's head or trauma associated with difficult instrumental delivery. The dura mater divides the brain into three compartments: the two cerebral hemispheres, and the cerebellum. The main folds are the falx cerebri and the tentorium cerebelli. The major venous sinuses are contained within these folds, and dural tears are likely to cause extensive bleeding from the adjacent sinus. Welch & Strand (1986) have suggested that some extensive subdural hemorrhages are due to arterial bleeding, which is also likely to be due to trauma.

The fetal head withstands the compressive effects of labor well if the mechanical forces are applied evenly. With passage of the head through the birth canal the head molds to a long occipito-frontal diameter. If delivery is too rapid, then the mechanical forces are less well tolerated and there will be sudden changes in head shape. This causes stretching and possibly tearing of the dura. As long-axis stretching is most common, it is the vertical part of the tentorium that is most stressed and liable to rupture (Fig. 21.11). Subdural hemorrhage in the posterior fossa usually arises from rupture of the vein of Galen, straight or lateral sinuses. The most common site of hemorrhage appears to be at the falco-tentorial junction near the incisura (Huang & Shen 1991). Tears of the falx cerebri are rare, and occasionally subdural hemorrhage is associated with sinus thrombosis (Craig 1938).

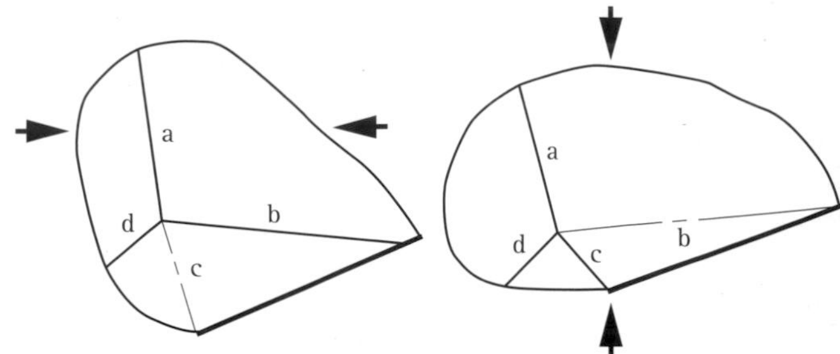


Figure 21.11 Dural tears associated with compressional stress to the neonatal head. The diagram on the left shows the effect of occipitofrontal compression with greatest strain on the vertical part of the tentorium (c). The diagram on the right shows the effect of compression between vault and base, with greatest strain on the horizontal part of the tentorium (b). Falx cerebri (a); line of junction of tentorium and falx (d). (Redrawn from Holland 1922.)

Vacuum extraction has also been associated with the development of dural tears (Hayashi *et al.* 1987; Romodanov & Brodsky 1987; Hanigan *et al.* 1990; Huang & Shen 1991; Castillo & Fordham 1995; Odita & Hebi 1996). The application of the vaccum cup to the vertex with longitudinal traction exerts vertical stresses on the tentorium with tearing and hemorrhage similar to that seen with forceps delivery. Vacuum extraction has been reported to be associated commonly with intracranial hemorrhage. Hanigan *et al.* (1990) described a distinctive pattern of hemorrhage due to vacuum extraction with extension over the superior surface of the cerebellum or inferior surface of the occipital lobe. Avrahami *et al.* (1993) scanned ten babies born by the vaccum extractor who showed no clinical signs of either trauma or asphyxia and found that all of them showed evidence of hemorrhage representing a combination of subarachnoid, intradural tentorial bleeding and small juxta-tentorial intracerebral hemorrhage, although in no cases were these bleeds thought to be severe. Other intracranial lesions including GMH–IVH, cerebellar hemorrhage and arterial infarction have also been reported as the result of vacuum extraction (Castillo & Fordham 1995). The reported prognosis from SDH due to vacuum extraction is generally good (Hayashi *et al.* 1987; Odita & Hebi 1996)

### Occipital osteodiastasis

Subdural hemorrhage may be associated with vaginal breech delivery in which there is excessive extension of the infant's neck. This causes separation of the squamous and lateral portions of the occipital bone (osteodiastasis) and direct injury to structures within the posterior cranial fossa, including the cerebellum and brainstem (Hemsath 1934; Wigglesworth & Husemeyer 1977). Exceptionally this may occur due to parietal diastasis. The prognosis is reported to be worse than in babies who have sustained subdural hemorrhage as the result of vacuum extraction (Odita & Hebi 1996).

### Bridging vein rupture

The most common cause of subdural hemorrhage is rupture of the superior cerebral bridging veins (Pape & Wigglesworth 1979). These lesions occur most commonly over the cerebral convexity (Fig. 21.12) and may be seen in association with subarachnoid hemorrhage. Convexity subdural hemorrhages may be more common in infants with coagulation disorders or those undergoing exchange transfusions (Morgan *et al.* 1983).

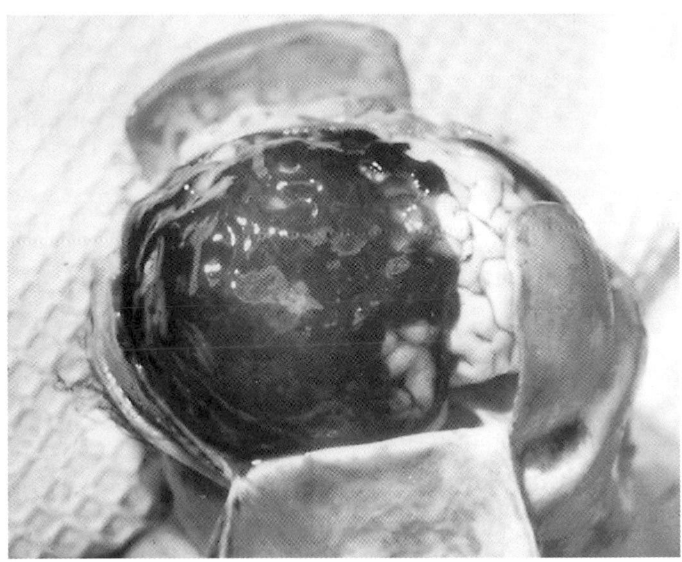

**Figure 21.12** Subdural hematoma over the right cerebral hemisphere. After reflection of the skull, thick blood clot remained over the cerebral convexity. (Reproduced, with permission, from Larroche 1984.)

### Convexity hemorrhage

The term 'convexity hemorrhage' is used because the precise origin of the bleeding is unclear and compression of the brain may occur with eventual infarction, thus making determination of the underlying lesion difficult. These lesions have also been referred to as lobar hemorrhages (Hanigan *et al.* 1995).

### Other causes

Subdural hemorrhage in infants may also be caused by shaking associated with non-accidental injury and subsequent meningitis, particularly if the latter is due to *Haemophilus influenzae*. These are, however, rarely seen in the neonatal period. A chronic subdural hemorrhage may be due to asymptomatic bleeding in the neonatal period which causes insidious symptoms some weeks or months after birth. In this case there is accumulation of fluid around the initial bleed due to an osmotic effect that creates a space occupying lesion. Determining the timing of the original bleed may be very difficult.

Rebleeding after the onset of subdural hemorrhage may occur up to four days later (Craig 1938). Rebleeding occurs as the result of resuscitation with restoration of blood pressure, or as the result of falling intracranial pressure in the few days after the original bleed.

## CLINICAL FINDINGS

These may be non-specific and depend on the severity and localization of the hemorrhage. In some cases symptoms may be delayed and only occur after a period of apparent neurologic normality (chronic subdural collection). This may be due to dural tear without damage to major vessels. More commonly, symptoms and signs are due to either raised intracranial pressure or associated asphyxial injury (Hayashi *et al.* 1987).

Massive hemorrhage may be associated with shock, coma, and rapid demise. Posterior fossa hemorrhage has been reported to produce a recognizable symptom complex (Govaert *et al.* 1990). This includes a tense fontanelle, decrease or absence of motor tone, lethargy, and reduced or absent primitive reflexes, apnea, irregular patterns of breathing, facial palsy, and skew deviation of the eyes. A fixed bradycardia and sighing respiration are particular features of posterior fossa pathology. Although seizures are commonly seen, they are not necessary for the clinical diagnosis (Govaert *et al.* 1990). Retinal hemorrhages have been reported in approximately 25% of cases (Hayashi *et al.* 1987).

Convexity subdural hemorrhage may present with generalized or multifocal seizures. Occasionally, focal neurologic signs are seen, in particular a difference in tone between the two sides. Volpe (1977) suggests that the most distinctive sign of compression is a non-reactive or sluggish pupil due to third cranial nerve compression. It is likely that most infants with mild subdural bleeding have no symptoms or signs at all.

## DIAGNOSIS

Ultrasound is not very reliable in diagnosing or excluding small subdural lesions. Large convexity hemorrhages, particularly when causing displacement of midline structures, should be detected on ultrasound examination, or the echo-free subdural effusion may be seen. Scanning through the posterior fontanelle (Maertens 1989), mastoid fontanelle (Buckley *et al.* 1997) or foramen magnum (Sudakoff *et al.* 1993) may add precision to the diagnosis of tentorial abnormalities.

CT and MRI are more sensitive techniques for detecting smaller lesions, but even with these techniques distinction between small subdural hemorrhage and normal appearance may be impossible (Ludwig *et al.* 1980). Subdural bleeding should be considered in all asphyxiated infants and, as its compressive effects are treatable, CT or MRI examination is recommended whenever this possibility is considered.

The features of subdural hemorrhage on CT scans have been described by Govaert *et al.* (1990):

1. Pericerebellar subdural hematoma. Intracerebellar hemorrhage may be present.
2. Obvious hemorrhage in or around the tentorial apex, straight sinus and behind the third ventricle. These tend to coalesce to form a triangular area with its base against the occipital bone.
3. Presence of hemorrhage between the posterior cerebral hemorrhages.

Infants with CT or MRI evidence of posterior fossa hemorrhage may have either subdural or cerebellar hemorrhage, and distinction between the two may be difficult. The two conditions appear to occur with equal frequency in the neonate (Scotti *et al.* 1981), but intracerebellar hemorrhage is more common in premature infants, and subdural hemorrhage is more likely in full-term infants (Menezes *et al.* 1983). Figure 21.13 shows an example of subdural hemorrhage due to a tentorial tear diagnosed by CT.

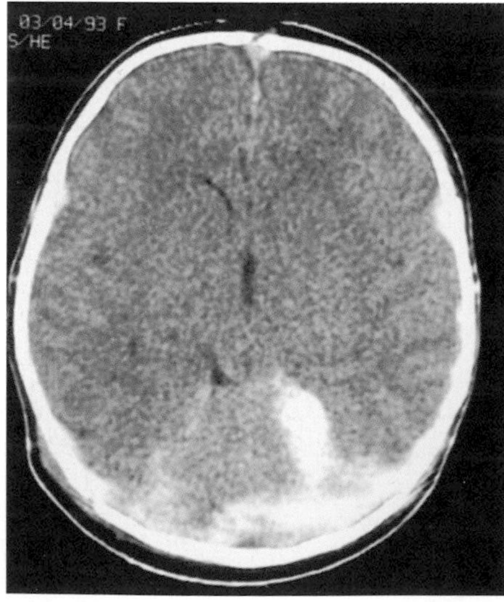


**Figure 21.13** CT scan showing subdural hemorrhage associated with a tear of the left fold of the tentorium cerebelli.

## TREATMENT

Convexity hemorrhages causing a midline shift should be decompressed by subdural tap. Craniotomy may be necessary if the collection is not accessible to needling through the fontanelle. It is, however, important to distinguish clinical signs arising from diffuse cerebral involvement as occurs in asphyxia from focal abnormalities arising from hemorrhage. Treatment directed towards a minor collection will not improve the clinical signs or eventual prognosis in the presence of more diffuse cerebral injury.

The neurosurgical management of subdural hemorrhage is controversial. Massive subdural hemorrhage in the posterior cranial fossa may require aspiration of clot at craniotomy. Definite indications for craniotomy include signs of brainstem compression and raised intracranial pressure due to developing hydrocephalus (Huang & Shen 1991). The management of less severe subdural hemorrhage is expectant. Neurosurgical management of hydrocephalus may be necessary.

## PROGNOSIS

In the most severe cases the prognosis is poor and approximately half of infants with subdural hemorrhage diagnosed by CT are neurologically abnormal at follow-up, presumably related to associated cerebral injury. More recent data reporting the outcome of less severe forms of subdural hemorrhage are more optimistic. The majority of infants with subdural hemorrhage appear to do well (Hayashi *et al.* 1987; Castillo & Fordham 1995; Odita & Hebi 1996), although those born by the breech, presumably with basal hemorrhage secondary to occipital osteodiastasis are reported to have a worse prognosis (Odita & Hebi 1996). Normal survivors have been reported following surgical evacuation of a large posterior fossa hemorrhage (Menezes *et al.* 1983).

## COMPLICATIONS

### Hydrocephalus

Hydrocephalus may develop as the result of two mechanisms following subdural hemorrhage; obstructive and resorptive (Govaert & de Vries 1997). In the former the mass effect of the hemorrhage causes acute obstruction to CSF flow, particularly at the site of the aqueduct or fourth ventricle, with symptoms or signs developing a few days after the onset of the lesion. Later, a disturbance in CSF resorption at the arachnoid granulations may cause late onset of hydrocephalus in infancy some weeks after birth.

### Secondary cerebral infarction

Govaert *et al.* (1992b) have reported a series of seven cases of cerebral artery infarction in association with intracranial hemorrhage due to tentorial tears. They postulate that arterial compression occurs as the result of one of two mechanisms. First, supratentorial intracranial hypertension causes uncal herniation with occlusion of the ipsilateral posterior cerebral artery. Second, convexity subdural hemorrhage in the posterior fossa causes compression of the ipsilateral middle cerebral artery or its branches. Prolonged arterial compression leads to cerebral infarction in the distribution of that vessel (see also Chapter 22).

## SUBARACHNOID HEMORRHAGE

Subarachnoid hemorrhage (SAH) may be primary or secondary to blood tracking through the ventricular system, usually from an IVH (see p. 340). Blood exits from the fourth ventricle through the foramina of Luscka and Magendie into the subarachnoid space. Primary hemorrhage is due to either leakage from the fine vessels of the leptomeningeal plexus, or to rupture of the larger veins within the subarachnoid space. It is quite unlike SAH seen in adults, which is a devastating condition caused by rupture of an arterial aneurysm.

Minor focal SAH is commonly seen in autopsy specimens, particularly in premature infants. These small lesions are probably clinically insignificant. It may be impossible to distinguish subpial hemorrhage microscopically from that confined to the subarachnoid space, and this distinction can only be made histologically (Friede 1972). The etiology of both conditions is probably hypoxic and develops due to oozing from veins. SAH may occur in full-term babies owing to a congenital coagulopathy, or one that is secondary to vitamin K deficiency (Chaou *et al.* 1984). The incidence of primary SAH diagnosed by CT scanning has been reported to be 7% of 118 infants of birth weight less than 1800 g (Shinnar *et al.* 1982). A large study of premature infants <2.0 kg reported the incidence of SAH diagnosed by ultrasound to be 7% (Paneth *et al.* 1994).

Larroche (1977) described 33 cases of a much more extensive form of primary SAH occurring over the cerebral convexity, often involving the temporal lobes (Figs 21.14 and 21.15) and these have also been referred to by Hanigan *et al.* (1995) as lobar hemorrhages (see p. 357). This lesion has a sharply defined border and may be very extensive, causing severe hemorrhagic necrosis to underlying cortical and subcortical structures due to a compressive effect. The convexity lesion was mainly seen in infants with bleeding disorders and particularly those having an exchange transfusion. The underlying cause of this condition is unclear but arterial occlusion cannot be excluded (see also convexity hemorrhage, p. 357).

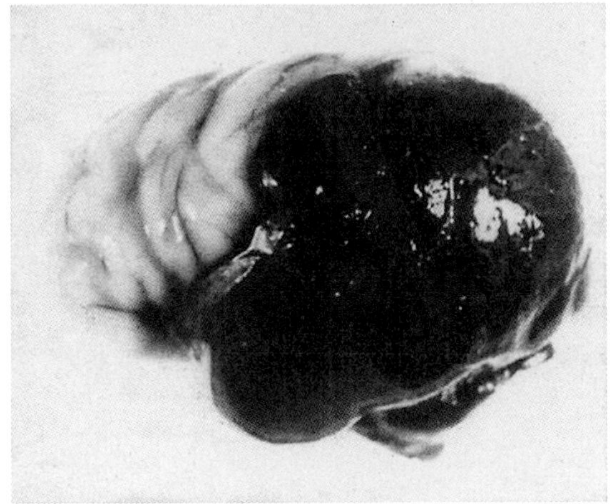

A

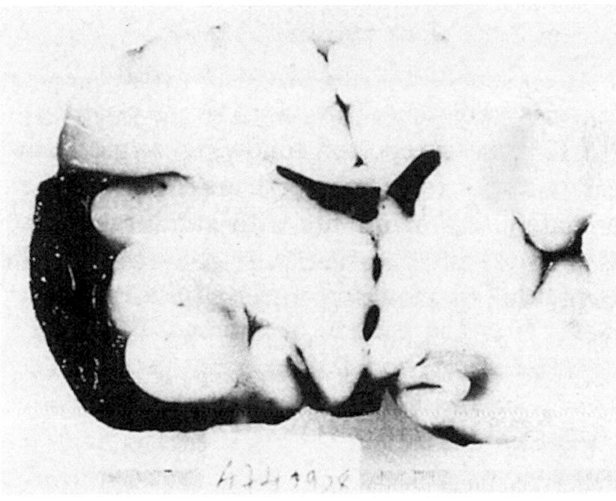

B

Figure 21.14 (A) SAH over the left temporal, parietal and occipital lobes. (B) Coronal section shows a small GMH–IVH with SAH compressing and displacing the left hemisphere. (Reproduced, with permission, from Larroche 1984).

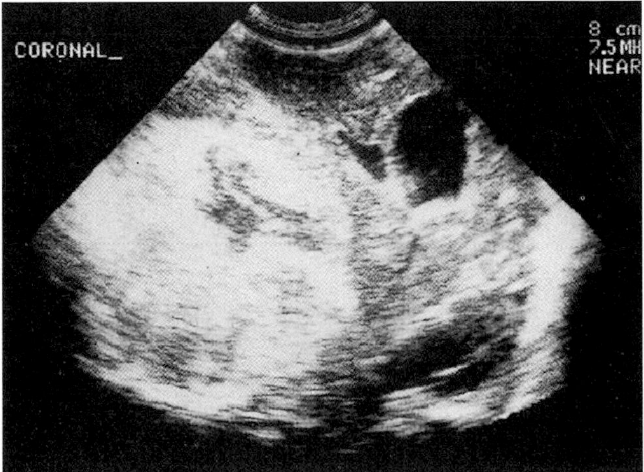


Figure 21.15 Ultrasound scan showing massive right-sided convexity hemorrhage in an infant born with severe allo-immune thromobocytopenia.

### CLINICAL FINDINGS

The majority of infants with SAH are asymptomatic. Massive convexity SAH may cause symptoms similar to large subdural hemorrhage with coma and shock. Large convexity lesions may also produce focal signs. The classical symptom associated with this type of hemorrhage is convulsion. Convulsions are usually generalized and often multifocal. The infants usually behave and feed remarkably normally between seizures. Nystagmus and apneic episodes have also been reported to be associated with SAH. Asphyxia often accompanies significant SAH, and the symptoms may be related to this more generalized abnormality.

### DIAGNOSIS

Traditionally the diagnosis has been made by lumbar puncture. A non-traumatic tap with free flow of blood-stained

CSF that does not clear in successive tubes strongly suggests the diagnosis of SAH, but this will not distinguish primary from secondary hemorrhage. Brain imaging by CT or MR is the most sensitive method for making the diagnosis, although SAH may be indistinguishable from subdural hemorrhage under certain conditions. Abnormal echogenicity in the intracerebral cisterns has been described as a sensitive ultrasound sign for SAH, but is poorly specific (Kazam *et al.* 1994).

### PROGNOSIS

The prognosis is generally thought to be good even in infants presenting with seizures (Rose & Lambroso 1970), but Fenichel *et al.* (1984) reported that only five out of ten infants with the CT diagnosis of SAH were subsequently normal. The follow-up period in these infants was short, and further information is awaited. Posthemorrhagic hydrocephalus may occur following primary SAH, but this is not common.

## CHOROID PLEXUS HEMORRHAGE

Bleeding from the choroid plexus is a common cause of IVH. Larroche (1977) has reported minor bleeding into the choroid plexus to be associated with, or to cause, IVH in 25% of cases. In another post-mortem study, Friede (1975) found choroid plexus hemorrhage in only 7% of neonatal brains. Heibel *et al.* (1993) scanned the brain of 1000 consecutively born, clinically normal full-term infants on day 3 of life and found that 1.1% of these babies had choroid plexus hemorrhage; two were confined to the choroid plexus and nine had ruptured into the lateral ventricles. The most frequent site of bleeding is into the posterior tufts at the level of the glomus. Autopsy studies emphasize that choroid plexus hemorrhage occurs most commonly in full-term infants (Donat *et al.* 1978, Lacey & Terplan 1982) and may arise following birth asphyxia.

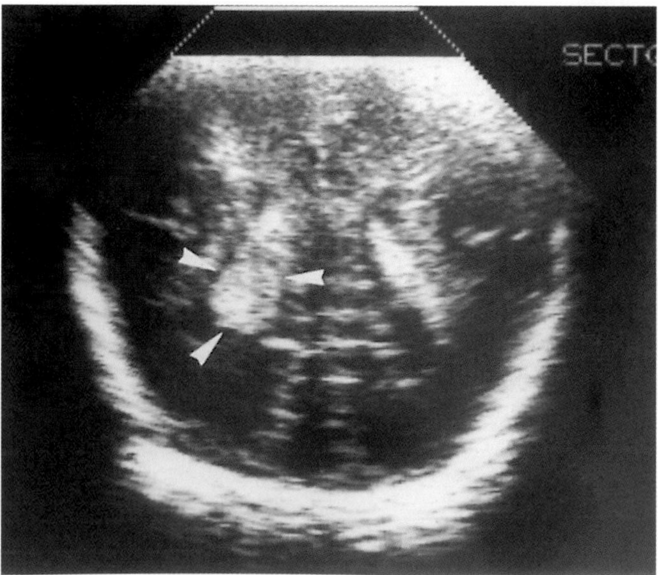


**Figure 21.16** Choroid plexus hematoma (arrows) adherent to the left choroid plexus, diagnosed on ultrasound scanning. (Reproduced, with permission, from Levene *et al.* 1985.)

### DIAGNOSIS

There are no recognized clinical features of choroid plexus hemorrhage and the diagnosis can be made by ultrasound (Fig. 21.16), CT, or MRI examination.

## INTRACEREBELLAR HEMORRHAGE

Primary hemorrhage into the cerebellum is well recognized (Fig. 21.17) and has been reported to occur in 2.5% of a high-risk preterm population (Merrill *et al.* 1998). Diffuse microscopic hemorrhages are seen in premature infants and not uncommonly in association with periventricular hemorrhage or, rarely, with meningoencephalitis (Larroche 1977). They usually arise either within the cerebellar cortex or, less commonly, in the subependymal layer of the roof of the fourth ventricle (Pape & Wigglesworth 1979). It has been suggested that bleeding into the cerebellar folia is related to poor vascularization of the cerebellar cortex (Pape & Wigglesworth 1979). Large primary cerebellar hematomata are much less common and have been diagnosed in life in both premature (Grunnet & Shields 1975; Martin *et al.* 1976; Peterson *et al.* 1984) and full-term infants (Rom *et al.* 1978; Ravenel 1979; Fishman *et al.* 1981). Massive cerebellar hemorrhage of prenatal onset has been described (Hadi *et al.* 1994). Bleeding disorders or severe rhesus isoimmunization have been reported to be common etiological factors.

Secondary hemorrhages due to occipital osteodiastasis associated with breech delivery have been described (Wigglesworth & Husemeyer 1977) or a face-mask applied by a tight-fitting band around the back of the infant's head (Pape *et al.* 1976). The tight band caused distortion of the occipital bone and probably mechanical trauma to the cerebellum with venous infarction.

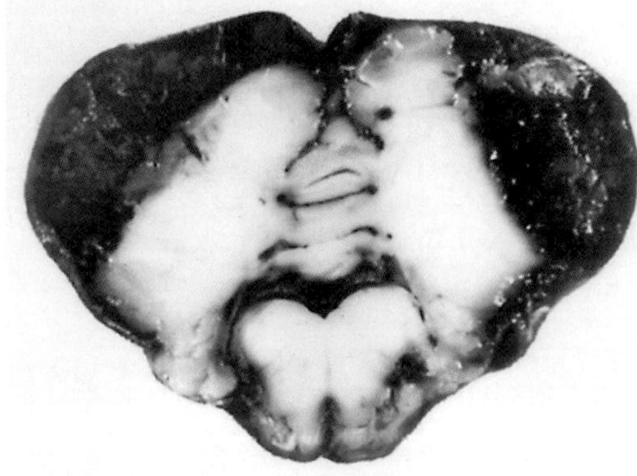

**Figure 21.17** Bilateral cerebellar hematoma in an infant born at 28 weeks of gestation.

## DIAGNOSIS

Clinical features include apnea and bradycardia, seizures, fixed bradycardia, opisthotonus, and nystagmus. These features are similar to those described for infants with subdural hemorrhage arising in the posterior cranial fossa, and these two conditions may be extremely difficult to distinguish even by imaging techniques (Scotti *et al.* 1981). Merrill *et al.* (1998) have described a clinically silent presentation in a group of premature infants with cerebellar hemorrhage.

Routine ultrasound scanning has a low detection rate for intracerebellar hemorrhage, but views through the posterior fontanelle have been reported to increase the detection rate significantly (Merrill *et al.* 1998). Diagnosis may also be made by CT or MRI examination.

## MANAGEMENT

Suboccipital craniotomy has been performed successfully in a few full-term infants (Rom *et al.* 1978; Ravenel 1979), but conservative management has also been advocated, apparently with good outcome (Fishman *et al.* 1981).

# THALAMIC HEMORRHAGE

This may be primary or due to extension of hemorrhage arising from the germinal matrix. It has been reported to be secondary to thrombosis of deep central veins (see p. 340), with hemorrhagic infarction in the thalamus and adjacent gray matter. This is most likely to occur in the most immature infants.

Primary hemorrhage into the thalamus in the newborn has been described and there may be secondary rupture into the lateral ventricle (Trounce *et al.* 1985; Roland *et al.* 1990; de Vries *et al.* 1992; Govaert *et al.* 1992a). It is almost always unilateral and has been reported less commonly in preterm infants (De Vries *et al.* 1992). Two recent cases with acute onset have been described in apparently healthy 8-week-old infants (Incorpora *et al.* 1999). The cause of this type of lesion is unknown but does not appear to be due to an arterio-venous malformation, trauma, or coagulopathy. Asphyxia is a predisposing factor in a number of unilateral cases (de Vries *et al.* 1992). Cerebral vein thrombosis has been suggested to be a cause in two cases (Govaert *et al.* 1992a), and hemorrhagic infarction in three cases (Roland *et al.* 1990). Hemorrhagic infarction of the thalamus (Fig. 21.18) may be indistinguishable macroscopically from primary hemorrhage. Very rarely, hemorrhage into the basal ganglia may occur due to microangiomata. Alonso *et al.* (1984) have reported two such cases occurring in neonates.

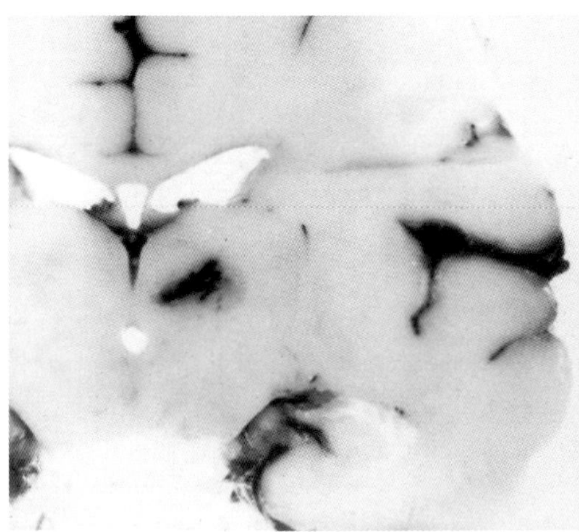

**Figure 21.18** Hemorrhagic infarction within the right thalamus in a premature infant with congenital listeriosis. SAH is also visible in the Sylvian fissure.

## DIAGNOSIS

A specific clinical syndrome associated with primary thalamic hemorrhage has been described. The condition presents usually in previously well babies at about 7–14 days with acute onset of seizures and a bulging fontanelle. In the initial report, most had dramatic eye signs, including sunsetting and eye deviation downwards and outwards to the side of the thalamic lesion. The abnormal eye posture is due to the close proximity of the hemorrhage to the frontomesencephalic pathway of the optic tract. Later reports have not confirmed these ophthalmic findings (Roland *et al.* 1990). Facial palsy, apnea, irritability, and opisthotonic posturing have also been reported in a proportion of affected infants. A minority of infants had pre-existing asphyxia (Roland *et al.* 1990; de Vries *et al.* 1992) and meningitis (Govaert *et al.* 1992a, Perlman *et al.* 1992).

Diagnosis may be confirmed by ultrasound, CT or MRI examination (Fig. 21.19). Roland *et al.* (1990) reported a minority of babies had decreased tissue attenuation adjacent to the hemorrhage on CT, suggestive of thalamic infarction. Evidence of venous thrombosis has been reported on CT (Roland *et al.* 1990) and MRI (Govaert *et al.* 1992a). Cerebral angiography is necessary to exclude microangiomata, but this is rarely indicated. Confusion has arisen between this condition and infants with the appearance of bilateral 'bright' thalamic lesions, as illustrated on p. 476 (Kotagel *et al.* 1983; Donn *et al.* 1984; Kreusser *et al.* 1984; Voit *et al.* 1985; Shen *et al.* 1986). All these cases occurred in full-term infants sustaining severe asphyxia who were profoundly neurologically abnormal from birth. Autopsy showed these cases, reported as 'bright' thalamic appearances, to be due to hemorrhagic necrosis (Kreusser *et al.* 1984). These case reports appear to be fundamentally different from the 'benign' intrathalamic hemorrhage originally reported by Trounce *et al.* (1985).

## PROGNOSIS

The infants with unilateral thalamic hemorrhage showed abnormal neurologic signs for some time. Initial reports

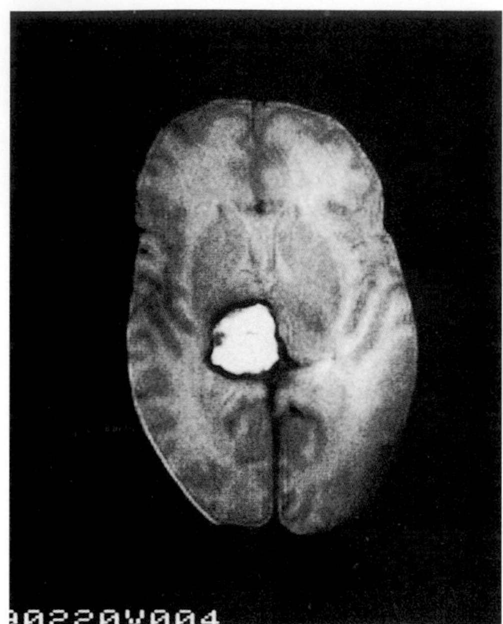


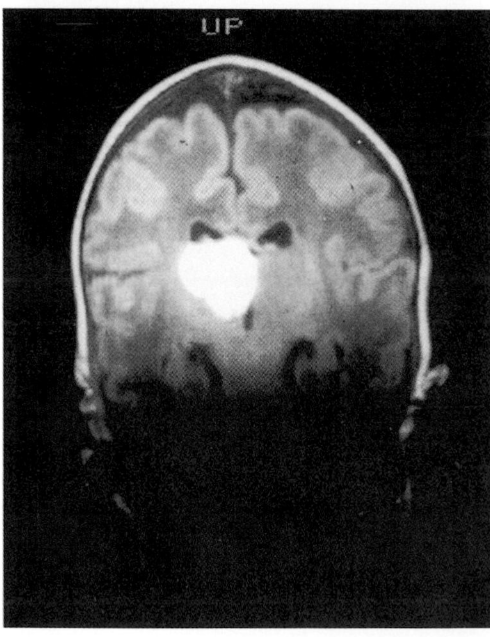


**Figure 21.19** Unilateral thalamic hemorrhage seen on MRI in a preterm infant of 34 weeks gestational age. (A) Spin echo T1, 500/15 TR/TE. (B) T2, 2500/90 TR/TE.

suggested that the majority of infants had no neurodevelopmental abnormality at 18 months, but later follow-up suggests that approximately half have moderate-to-severe neurodevelopmental sequelae (personal observation on reported cases, Roland *et al.* 1990). In contrast, all asphyxiated infants with a bilateral bright thalamic appearance are dead or severely handicapped.

## PARENCHYMAL HEMORRHAGE

The distinction between a primary hemorrhagic process extending from an intraventricular bleed and bleeding into previously ischemic periventricular tissue is difficult and is discussed in detail on p. 341. In addition, confusion between primary parenchymal hemorrhage and cerebral artery infarction may easily occur. Distinction between these two conditions is possible, and cerebral artery infarction is discussed in Chapter 22.

Most of the reported cases of primary intraparenchymal hemorrhage have been associated with fetal or neonatal coagulopathy (Bleyer & Skinner 1976; Zalneraitis *et al.* 1979; Chaou *et al.* 1984; Motohara *et al.* 1984; Whitelaw *et al.* 1984, Morales & Stroup 1985; Sadowitz & Balcom 1985; Sia *et al.* 1985; Matsuzaka *et al.* 1989; Michaud *et al.* 1991). Prenatal intracranial hemorrhage is discussed in detail in Chapter 20. The most common cause for the bleeding disorder is vitamin K deficiency (Aydinli *et al.* 1998). This occurs in solely breast-fed infants who are not given vitamin K at birth. Intracranial hemorrhage due to vitamin K deficiency is most likely to occur beyond the neonatal period and may be devastating in its severity. In one study of 11 babies with intracranial hemorrhage due to vitamin K deficiency, 75% of them suffered long-term neurodisability (Aydinli *et al.* 1998). It is now clear that a single prophylactic vitamin K injection will protect the full-term infant from significant, late intracranial hemorrhage due to vitamin K deficiency (Matsuzaka *et al.* 1989).

Other causes include isoimmune thrombocytopenia and specific clotting factor deficiency. $\alpha_1$-antitrypsin deficiency may present with intracranial hemorrhage associated with coagulation disorders (Jenkins *et al.* 1982; Hope *et al.* 1982; Payne & Hasegawa 1984; Bussel *et al.* 1997). Intraparenchymal hemorrhage has been reported following heparinization for extracorporeal membrane oxygenation therapy (Bowerman *et al.* 1985; Watson *et al.* 1990). Intracranial hemorrhage appears to be particularly common in premature infants treated with this technique (Cilley *et al.* 1986). Very rarely, parenchymal hemorrhage in infants may occur and be caused by an intracerebral tumor (Palma *et al.* 1979), or an arterio-venous malformation of the choroid plexus (Wakai *et al.* 1990), or vein of Galen aneurysm. McLellan *et al.* (1986) have reported a case of localized hematoma (Fig. 21.20) in the frontoparietal area caused by aneurysmal rupture of the middle cerebral artery. Protein C deficiency, a very rare cause of intravascular thrombosis and secondary coagulopathy, has been reported to be associated with severe intracranial hemorrhage (Voutsinas *et al.* 1991), and periventricular leukomalacia (personal case), as has transplacental transfer of an acquired factor VII:C inhibitor (Ries *et al.* 1995). Blueberry muffin lesions (cutaneous hematopoeisis in severely anemic babies) has been reported to be associated with extensive intraparenchymal hemorrhage (Smets & van Aken 1998).

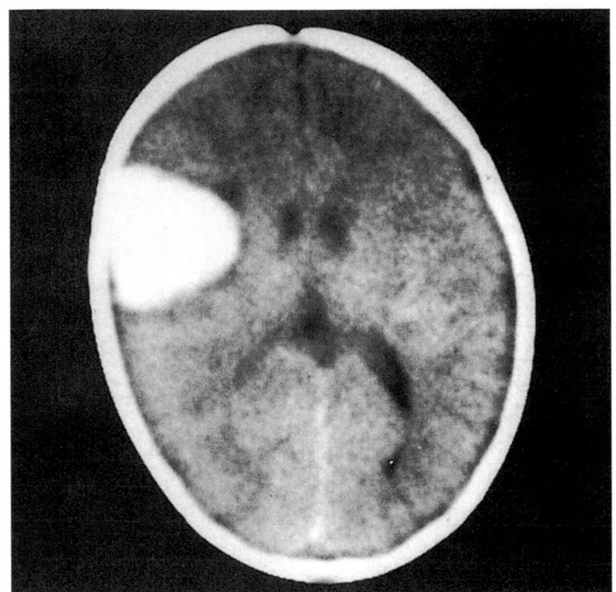

A

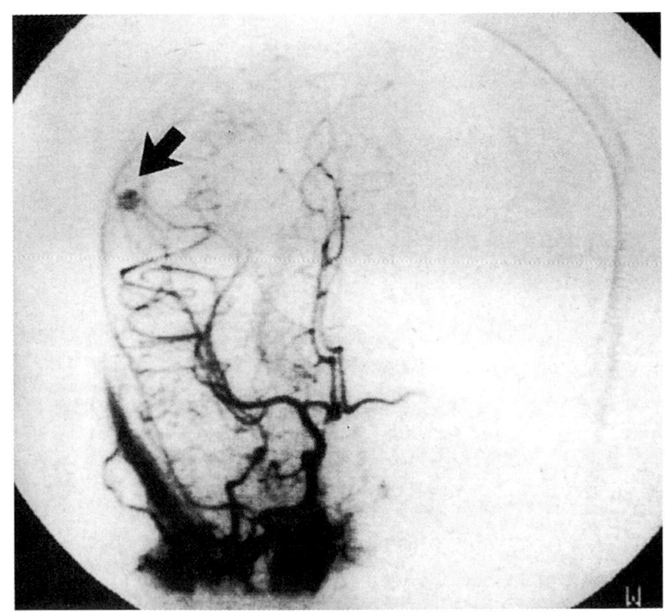

B

Figure 21.20 (A) Parenchymal hematoma in the right frontoparietal lobe seen on CT. (B) Angiography shows an arterial aneurysm (arrow) in an ascending branch of the right middle cerebral artery. (Reproduced, with permission, from McLellan *et al.* 1986.)

## DIAGNOSIS

Clinical features usually suggest a bleeding disorder, as multiple petechial hemorrhages are present on the infant's skin. The infant may only show minor neurologic disturbances including lethargy and irritability. Seizures are common. Diagnosis is confirmed by ultrasound, CT and MRI examination (Fig. 21.21).

## MANAGEMENT

Hemorrhage due to vitamin K deficiency is a preventable condition if synthetic vitamin K is given routinely to all infants at birth. Vitamin K should be given to infants with intracerebral hemorrhages, and other clotting disorders should be treated as appropriate. Platelet transfusions may be necessary in infants with severe thrombocytopenia. A history of allo-immune thrombocytopenia with intracranial hemorrhage in a sibling should alert the obstetrician to the high risk of prenatal bleeding in subsequent pregnancies. Measurement of fetal platelets with intrauterine platelet transfusion if necessary may reduce the risk of prenatal bleeding in subsequent pregnancies (Bussel *et al.* 1997). Postnatally, specific neurologic treatment is only necessary if progressive ventriculomegaly occurs.

## PROGNOSIS

From the case-reports published up to the present time it appears that approximately one-third of infants die, one-third are handicapped and one-third are subsequently neurologically normal.

# OTHER CRANIAL HEMORRHAGES

## EXTRADURAL (EPIDURAL) HEMORRHAGE

This has been very rarely reported in the neonatal literature and is usually due to trauma, often as a result of skull fracture with resultant underlying arterial bleeding. Skull fracture is rare in newborn infants owing to poor mineralization of the skull vault, but becomes progressively more common with trauma after 40 weeks of gestation. Extradural hemorrhage has been reported as the result of complicated breech delivery and difficult instrumental maneuvres. Takagi *et al.* (1978) found extradural hemorrhage to account for only 1.5% of all intracranial hemorrhages discovered at autopsy.

An extradural hemorrhage is usually associated with a cephalhematoma over the fracture. The diagnosis is best made by CT or MR scanning. The imaging features are a biconvex mass adjacent to the inner table of the skull. Early liquifaction of the clot within 24–48 hours is seen on scanning, and fluid levels within the clot may also be seen. Lam *et al.* (1991) reported six cases in full-term infants diagnosed by ultrasound and confirmed on CT examination.

Infants in whom the diagnosis is made on imaging are usually relatively well and the major symptom is seizures, but between fits the babies are not neurologically abnormal (Lam *et al.* 1991). Acute extradural hemorrhage may cause intracranial hypertension, uncal herniation and secondary infarction due to nipping of a major cerebral artery.

A large convexity extradural collection may require evacuation via a craniotomy if needle evacuation is not successful in relieving the intracranial mass effect. The

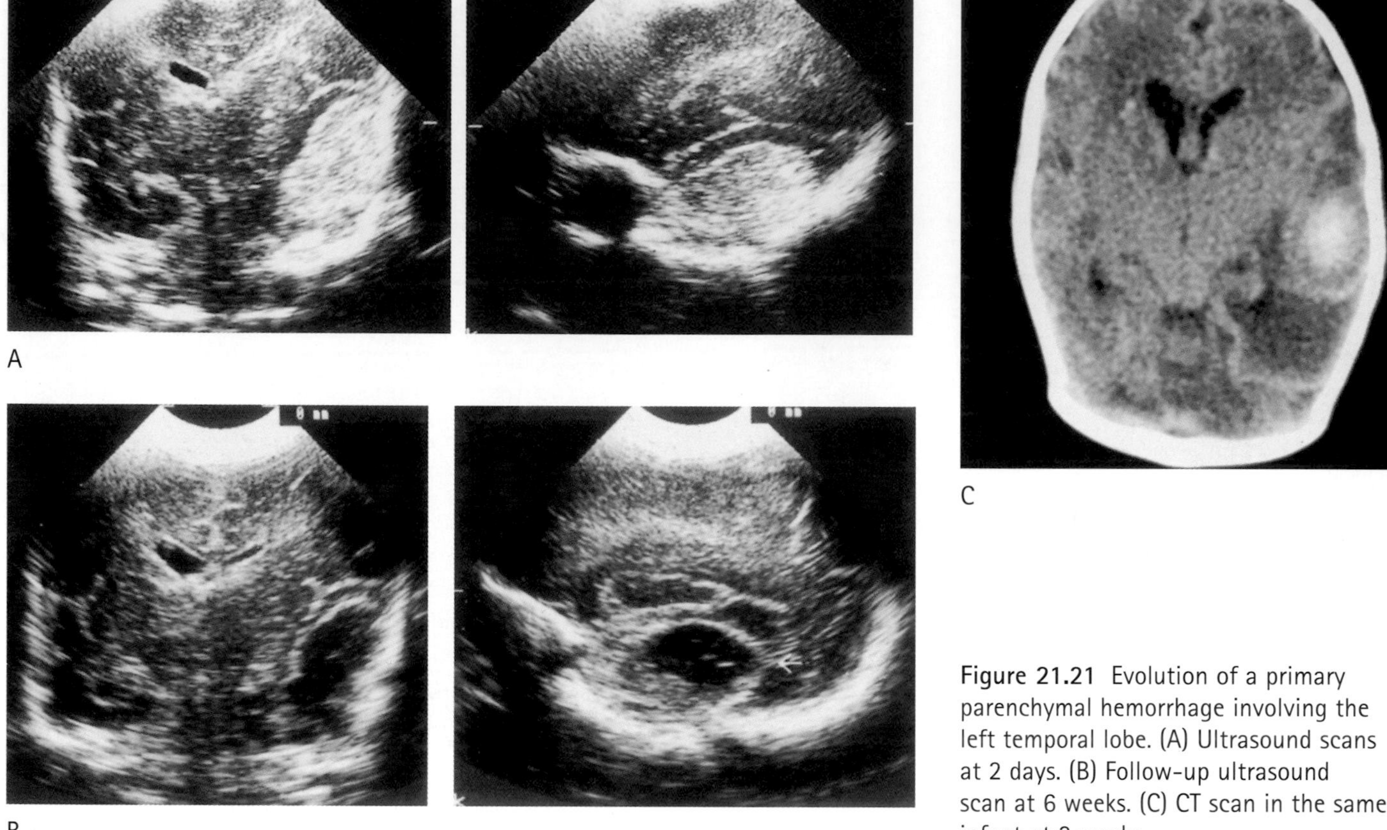

Figure 21.21 Evolution of a primary parenchymal hemorrhage involving the left temporal lobe. (A) Ultrasound scans at 2 days. (B) Follow-up ultrasound scan at 6 weeks. (C) CT scan in the same infant at 3 weeks.

prognosis is good in mild cases, but is poor in severe hemorrhage with arterial rupture.

## SUBAPONEUROTIC HEMORRHAGE

This is not an intracranial hemorrhage, but refers to bleeding over the infant's skull, but under the cranial aponeurosis (subgaleal space). It may occur spontaneously and has been reported particularly in babies of Afro-Caribbean origin and may also be associated with vitamin K deficiency, particularly in association with vacuum extraction (Ahuja *et al.* 1969) and, less commonly, hemophilia. Ng *et al.* (1995) describe an incidence of 0.8 per 1000 deliveries in a Chinese population and almost all were instrumental deliveries. They reported that vacuum extraction represented a 60-fold increase in risk for this condition.

Rapid and massive blood loss may occur into the subaponeurotic space with shock and hypotension, and this may cause severe secondary cerebral ischemia. A fluctuant 'fluid filled' swelling is present over the scalp, usually in the occipital region. It may rapidly expand as active bleeding occurs into it and become very tight and bluish in appearance. Rarely, the hemorrhage may not be obvious or not occur for up to 48 hours. The infant's hemoglobin level may fall, but in severe and acute cases the hemoglobin level remains normal as there has not been enough time for hemodilution to develop. Treatment involves careful observation and monitoring for signs of shock. Resuscitation must be undertaken early with plasma or blood. The reported mortality is 19–25% (Govaert *et al.* 1992c, Ng *et al.* 1995) and many of the babies who died had associated asphyxia, although it may be difficult to know whether the underestimated hypovolemia as a result of the hemorrhage was a major factor in the asphyxial state.

## CEPHALHEMATOMA

This refers to bleeding between the periosteum of the skull and the bone. The blood is confined by the periosteal membrane and therefore precisely overlies the affected bone. Because the bleeding is slow the hematoma may not be noticed on the first day of life and may appear to grow over the first few days. It usually remains for several weeks, and may heal leaving a raised calcified edge. It usually affects the parietal bone and may be bilateral. Rarely, the occipital bone is affected when the cephalhematoma crosses the midline. Hemorrhage is due to the skull being buffeted either by the maternal pelvis or the trauma of instrumental delivery (forceps or vacuum extractor). There is rarely an underlying extradural hemorrhage (p. 363) and skull fracture should be considered.

## CEREBRAL SINUS AND VENOUS THROMBOSIS

Thrombosis of the cerebral veins or sinuses is very rarely reported in the newborn, but as it may be confused with intracranial hemorrhage or predispose to hemorrhagic infarction it will be considered in this section. The condition is certainly more common than is reported in the literature.

### ANATOMY

The venous drainage of the brain can be considered as an internal and an external system. The external system drains the cerebral cortex and much of the white matter via the dural sinuses and external cortical veins. The internal system drains the basal ganglia, pons, and medulla via the internal cerebral veins, and vein of Galen. Thrombosis of the internal cerebral veins is thought to be less common than dural sinus thrombosis and may extend from primary dural sinus thrombosis.

### ETIOLOGY

Factors associated with the development of venous thrombosis include both local and systemic causes. Reported causes include sepsis (meningitis, septicemia, otitis media, and brain abscess), birth or postnatal trauma (particularly skull fracture) and impaired blood flow through the sinuses and veins (dehydration particularly associated with gastroenteritis and polycythemia). Impairment in venous drainage leading to sinus thrombosis may occur secondary to placement of a thin catheter in the internal jugular or subclavian veins (Gebara *et al.* 1995). We have seen a number of cases associated with systemic thrombophilic disorders such as factor V Leiden and protein C deficiency. A thrombophilia screen should be performed in all cases.

### CLINICAL FEATURES

There are no specific neurologic signs that suggest neonatal cerebral venous thrombosis, but this condition should be suspected in dehydrated infants or those with pre-existing neurologic disease if exacerbation of neurologic features occur. General signs include features of raised intracranial pressure, convulsions, hypertonia, and opisthotonus. Rivkin *et al.* (1992) have reported lethargy and unexplained seizures to be the main symptoms in a group of seven infants with cerebral venous thrombosis. We have seen this condition on MRI in asymptomatic, routinely scanned babies.

### DIAGNOSIS

Ultrasound is unlikely to diagnose thrombosis in superficial sinuses because the vessels are too close to the skull. Color flow Doppler has not been reported to reliably diagnose this condition. CT scans may suggest the diagnosis by increased density along the course of the vein of Galen and straight sinus (Eick *et al.* 1981) or a high-density thrombus in a cerebral cortical vein. CT enhancement may reveal specific abnormalities (Rao *et al.* 1981) including gyral or tentorial enhancement, and a filling defect in the straight sinus ('empty delta sign'). MRI appears to be the most sensitive method for diagnosing this condition (Fig. 21.22), and more extensive disease was recognized on MRI than suspected by CT examination (Rivkin *et al.* 1992). Venous magnetic resonance angiography may show a filling defect in the drainage system due to thrombosis formation. Associated intracranial and intraventricular hemorrhage has been reported with cerebral venous thrombosis (Ehlers & Courville 1936).

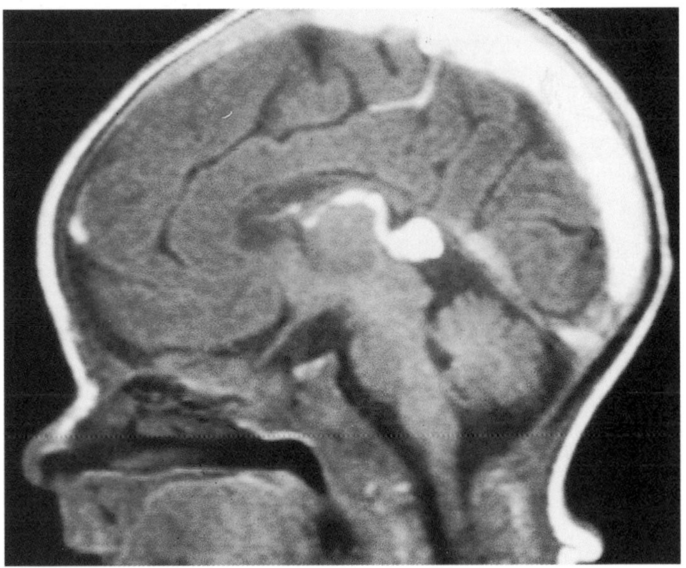

**Figure 21.22** MR scan (T1-weighted image) showing thrombosis (high signal) within the vein of Galen, straight sinus, and superior sagittal sinus.

It has been suggested that some cases of thalamic hemorrhage (see p. 361) are secondary to thrombosis of deep cerebral veins (Roland *et al.* 1990; Govaert *et al.* 1992a).

### MANAGEMENT

There are very few reports of the management of sinus vein thrombosis in the neonatal period and the most appropriate management is expectant. General management includes attention to the state of hydration and management of seizures.

The use of heparin and urokinase are very controversial. There are two reports of thrombolysis for sinus vein thrombosis using urokinase (Higashida *et al.* 1989) given systemically (1000 IU/h for 12 hours) and by local administration through a transfemoral vein catheter to close to the sagittal sinus (Gebara *et al.* 1995).

**Key Points**

- GMH–nIVH is the commonest form of intracranial hemorrhage in premature infants (30–40% of very low birthweight infants; 15% of these will involve the cerebral parenchyma).
- The most convincing drug shown to prevent GMH–IVH is antenatally administered corticosteroids and postnatal indomethacin. No drugs have been definitely shown to reduce disability.
- If the GMH–IVH does not involve the parenchyma and is not associated with ventricular dilatation the child is not at increased risk of disability compared with age matched children. The majority of those with parenchymal hemorrhage will develop cerebral palsy.
- Subarachnoid hemorrhage is common in premature infants and the prognosis is generally good.
- Cerebral sinus thrombosis is rarely diagnosed but has a relatively good prognosis. A thrombophilic tendency is often a causative factor.

## REFERENCES


Adams J M, Kenny J D, Rudolph A J (1976) Central diabetes insipidus following intraventricular hemorrhage. *J Pediatr* 88: 292–294.

Ahmann P A, Dykes F D, Lazzara A *et al.* (1983) Relationship between pressure passivity and subependymal/intraventricular hemorrhage as assessed by pulsed Doppler ultrasound. *Pediatrics* 72: 665–669.

Allan W C, Vohr B, Makuch R W *et al.* (1997) Antecedents of cerebral palsy in a multicenter trial of indomethacin for intraventricular hemorrhage. *Arch Pediatr Adolesc Med* 151: 580–585.

Alonso A, Taboada D, Alvarez J A *et al.* (1984) Spontaneous hematomas caused by microangiomatosis of the basal ganglia. *Child Brain* 11: 202–211.

Anderson G D, Bada H S, Sibai B M *et al.* (1988) The relationship between labor and route of delivery in the preterm infant. *Am J Obstet Gynecol* 158: 1382–1390.

Anderson G D, Bada H S, Shaver D C *et al.* (1992) The effect of Cesarean section on intraventricular hemorrhage in the preterm infant. *Am J Obstet Gynecol* 166: 1091–1101.

Anderson J M, Bain A D, Brown J K *et al.* (1976) Hyaline-membrane disease, alkaline buffer treatment, and cerebral intraventricular hemorrhage. *Lancet* i: 117–119.

Avrahami E, Frishman E & Minz M (1993) CT demonstration of intracranial hemorrhage in term newborn following vacuum extractor delivery. *Neuroradiology* 35: 107–108.

Aydinli N, Citak A, Caliskan C *et al.* (1998) Vitamin K deficiency – late onset intracranial hemorrhage. *Eur J Paediatr Neurol* 2: 199–203.

Bada H S, Korones S B, Anderson G D *et al.* (1984) Obstetric factors and relative risk of neonatal germinal layer/intraventricular hemorrhage. *Am J Obstet Gynecol* 148: 798–804.

Bada H S, Korones S B, Perry E H *et al.* (1990) Frequent handling in the neonatal intensive care unit and intraventricular hemorrhage. *J Pediatr* 117: 126–131.

Bandstra E S, Montalvo B M, Goldberg R N *et al.* (1988) Prophylactic indomethacin for prevention of intraventricular hemorrhage in premature infants. *Pediatrics* 82: 533–542.

Batton Daniel G, Holtrop P, DeWitte D *et al.* (1994) Current gestational age-related incidence of major intraventricular hemorrhage. *J Pediatr* 125: 623–625.

Bedard M P, Shankaran S, Slovis T L *et al.* (1984) Effect of prophylactic phenobarbital on intraventricular hemorrhage in high-risk infants. *Pediatrics* 73: 435–439.

Bejar R, Curbelo V, Coen R W (1980) Diagnosis and follow-up of intraventricular and intracerebral hemorrhages by ultrasound studies of infant's brain through the fontanelles and sutures. *Pediatrics* 66: 661–673.

✪ Benson J W T, Drayton M R, Hayward C *et al.* (1986) Multicentre trial of ethamsylate for prevention of periventricular hemorrhage in very low birthweight infants. *Lancet* ii: 1297–1300.

Bergman I, Bauer R E, Barmada M A *et al.* (1985) Intracerebral hemorrhage in the full-term neonatal infant. *Pediatrics* 75: 488–496.

Beverley D W, Chance G (1984) Cord blood gases, birth asphyxia and intraventricular hemorrhage. *Arch Dis Child* 59: 884–897.

Beverley D W, Chance G W, Inwood M J *et al.* (1984a) Intraventricular haemorrhage: timing of occurrence and relationship to perinatal events. *Br J Obstet Gynaecol* 91: 1007–1013.

Beverley D W, Chance G W, Inwood M J *et al.* (1984b) Intraventricular hemorrhage and haemostasis defects. *Arch Dis Child* 59: 444–448.

Beverley D W, Pitts-Tucker T J, Congdon P J *et al.* (1985) Prevention of intraventricular hemorrhage by fresh frozen plasma. *Arch Dis Child* 60: 710–713.

Bhuta T, Henderson-Smart D J (1999a) Elective high frequency jet ventilation versus conventional ventilation for neonatal respiratory distress syndrome in preterm infants. *Cochrane Database of Systematic Reviews.* Issue 3. Oxford: Update.

Bhuta T, Henderson-Smart D J (1999b) Rescue high frequency oscillatory ventilation versus conventional ventilation for pulmonary dysfunction in preterm infants. *Cochrane Database of Systematic Reviews.* Issue 3. Oxford: Update.

Blackman J A, McGuinness G A, Bale J F & Smith W L (1991) Large postnatally acquired porencephalic cysts: unexpected development outcomes. *J Child Neurol* 6: 58–64.

Bleyer W A & Skinner A L (1976) Fatal neonatal hemorrhage after maternal anticonvulsant therapy. *J Am Med Assoc* 235: 626–627.

Blume W T & Dreyfus-Brisac C (1982) Positive Rolandic sharp waves in neonatal EEG: types and significance. *Electroencephalog Clin Neurophysiol* 53: 227–282.

Bove K, Kosmetatos N, Wedig K E *et al.* (1985) Vasculopathic hepatotoxicity associated with E-Ferol syndrome in low-birthweight infants. *J Am Med Assoc* 254: 2422–2430.

Bowerman R A, Zwischenberger J B, Andrews A F & Bartlett R H (1985) Cranial sonography of the infant treated with extracorporeal membrane oxygenation. *Am J Roentgenol* 145: 161–166.

Buckley K M, Taylor G A, Estroff J A *et al.* (1997) Use of the mastoid fontanelle for improved sonographic visualization of the neonatal midbrain and posterior fossa. *Am J Roentgenol* 168: 1021–1025.

Burstein J, Papile L A & Burstein R (1979) Intraventricular hemorrhage in premature newborns: a prospective study with CT. *Am J Roentgenol* 132: 631–635.

Bussel J B, Zabusky M R, Berkowitz R L & McFarland J G (1997) Fetal alloimmune thrombocytopenia. *N Engl J Med* 337: 22–26.

Cartwright G W, Culbertson K, Schreiner R L & Garg B P (1979) Changes in clinical presentation of term infants with intracranial hemorrhage. *Dev Med Child Neurol* 21: 730–737.

Castillo M & Fordham L A (1995) MR of neurologically symptomatic newborns after vacuum extraction delivery. *AJNR Am J Neuroradiol* 16: 816–818.

Catto-Smith A G, Yu V Y H, Bajuk B *et al.* (1985) Effect of neonatal periventricular hemorrhage on neurodevelopmental outcome. *Arch Dis Child* 60: 8–11.

Chang G Y, Lueder F L, DiMichele D M, Radkowski M A, McWilliams L J, Jansen R D (1997) Heparin and the risk of intraventricular hemorrhage in premature infants. *J Pediatr* 131: 362–366.

Chaou W-T, Chou M-L & Eitzman D V (1984) Intracranial hemorrhage and vitamin K deficiency in early infancy. *J Pediatr* 105: 880–884.

Chen J (1993) Ethamsylate in the prevention of periventricular-intraventricular hemorrhage in premature infants. *J Formosan Med Assoc* 92: 889–893.

Chessells J M & Wigglesworth J S (1972) Coagulation studies in preterm infants with respiratory distress and intracranial hemorrhage. *Arch Dis Child* 47: 564–570.

Chiswick M L, Johnson M, Woodhall C *et al.* (1983) Protective effect of vitamin E (*dl*-alpha-tocopherol) against intraventricular hemorrhage in premature babies. *Br Med J* 287: 81–84.

Cilley R E, Zwischenberger J B, Andrews A F *et al.* (1986) Intracranial hemorrhage during extracorporeal membrane oxygenation in neonates. *Pediatrics* 78: 699–704.

Clancy R R, Tharp B R & Enzman D (1984) EEG in premature infants with intraventricular hemorrhage. *Neurology* 34: 583–590.

Claris O, Besnier S, Lapillonne A, Picaud J C & Salle B L (1996) Incidence of ischemic-hemorrhage cerebral lesions in premature infants of gestational age ≤28 weeks: a prospective ultrasound study. *Biol Neonate* 70: 29–34.

Clark C E, Clyman R I & Roth R S (1981) Risk factor analysis of intraventricular hemorrhage in low birth weight infants. *J Pediatr* 99: 625–628.

Clark R H, Dykes F D, Bachman T E & Ashurst J T (1996) Intraventricular hemorrhage and high-frequency ventilation: A meta-analysis of prospective clinical trials. *Pediatrics* 98: 1058–1061.

Cole V A, Durbin G M, Olaffson A *et al.* (1974) Pathogenesis of intraventricular hemorrhage in newborn infants. *Arch Dis Child* 49: 722–728.

Cooke R W (1981) Factors associated with periventricular hemorrhage in very low birth weight infants. *Arch Dis Child* 56: 425–431.

Cooke R W I (1987) Early and late cranial ultrasonographic appearances and outcome in very low birthweight infants. *Arch Dis Child* 62: 931–937.

Cooke R W I (1994) Survival and cerebral morbidity in preterm infants. *Lancet* 343: 1578.

✪ Cooke R W I (1999) Trends in incidence of cranial ultrasound lesions and cerebral palsy in very low birthweight infants 1982–93. *Arch Dis Child Fetal Neonat Ed* 80: F115–117.

Cooke R W I, Morgan I M & Coad N A G (1981) Pneumothorax, mechanical ventilation, and periventricular hemorrhage. *Lancet* i: 555.

Cooke R W I & Morgan M E I (1984) Prophylactic ethamsylate for periventricular hemorrhage. *Arch Dis Child* 59: 82–84.

Corazza M S, Davis R F, Merritt A *et al.* (1984) Prolonged bleeding time in preterm infants receiving indomethacin for patent ductus arteriosus. *J Pediatr* 105: 292–296.

Corbet A J, Adams J M, Kenny J D *et al.* (1977) Controlled trial of bicarbonate therapy in high-risk premature newborn infants. *J Pediatr* 91: 771–776.

Coulter D M, La Pine T R & Gooch M (1985) Treatment to prevent postnatal loss of brain water reduces the risk of intracranial hemorrhage in the beagle puppy. *Pediatric Research* 19: 1322–1326.

Cowan F, Whitelaw A, Wertheim D & Silverman M (1991) Cerebral blood flow velocity changes after rapid administration of surfactant. *Arch Dis Child* 66: 1105–1109.

✪ Craig W S (1938) Intracranial hemorrhage in the new-born. *Arch Dis Child* 13: 89–124.

✪ Crowley P (1999) Prophylactic corticosteroids for preterm delivery (Cochrane Review). In: *The Cochrane Library, Issue 2.* Oxford: Update Software.

✪ Crowther C A & Henderson-Smart D J (1999a) Phenobarbital prior to preterm birth for the prevention of neonatal periventricular hemorrhage (PVH) (Cochrane Review). In: *The Cochrane Library*, Issue 2. Oxford: Update Software.

Crowther C A & Henderson-Smart D J (1999b) Vitamin K prior to preterm birth for the prevention of periventricular hemorrhage (Cochrane Review). In: *The Cochrane Library*, Issue 2. Oxford: Update Software.

Crowther C A & Moore V (1999) Magnesium for preventing preterm birth after threatened preterm labour (Cochrane Review). In: *The Cochrane Library*, Issue 2. Oxford: Update Software.

Crowther C A, Alfirevic Z & Haslam R R (1999) Prenatal thyrotropin-releasing hormone (TRH) for preterm birth. *Cochrane Library Issue 2.* Oxford, Update Software.

Cukier F, Andre M, Monod N & Dreyfus-Brisac C (1972) Apport de l'EEG au diagnostic des hemorrhagies intra-ventriculaires du premature. *Revue Electro-encephalographie et Neurophysiologique Clinique* 2: 318–322.

D'Souza S W, Janakova H, Minors D *et al.* (1995) Blood pressure, heart rate, and skin temperature in preterm infants: associations with periventricular hemorrhage. *Arch Dis Child* 72: F162–F167.

Developmental Epidemiology Network Investigators (1998) The correlation between placental pathology and intraventricular hemorrhage in the preterm infant. *Pediatr Res* 43: 15–19.

De Crespigny L Ch & Robinson H P (1983) Can obstetricians prevent neonatal intraventricular hemorrhage? *Aust NZ J Obstet Gynaecol* 23: 146–149.

De Crespigny L, Mackay R, Muston L J *et al.* (1982) Timing of neonatal cerebroventricular hemorrhage with ultrasound. *Arch Dis Child* 57: 231–233.

De Vries L S, Dubowitz L M S & Dubowitz V (1985) Predictive value of cranial ultrasound in the newborn baby: a reappraisal. *Lancet* ii: 137–140.

De Vries L S, Smet M, Goemans N *et al.* (1992) Unilateral thalamic hemorrhage in the pre-term and full-term newborn. *Neuropediatrics* 23: 153–156.

✪ De Vries L S, Eken P, Groenendaal F *et al.* (1998a) Antenatal onset of haemorrhagic and/or ischaemic lesions in preterm infants: prevalence and associated obstetric variables. *Arch Dis Child Fetal Neonatal Edn* 78: F51–56.

De Vries L S, Rademaker K J, Groenendaal F *et al.* (1998b) Correlation between neonatal cranial ultrasound, MRI in infancy and neurodevelopmental outcome in infants with a large intraventricular hemorrhage with or without unilateral parenchymal involvement. *Neuropediatrics* 29: 180–188.

De Vries L S *et al.* (2000) *Neuropediatrics* (In press).

DeCourten G M & Rabinowicz T (1981) Intraventricular hemorrhage in premature infants: reappraisal and a new hypothesis. *Dev Med Child Neurol* 23: 389–403.

Dolfin T, Skidmore M B, Fong K W *et al.* (1983) Incidence, severity and timing of subependymal and intraventricular hemorrhages in preterm infants born in a perinatal unit as detected by serial real-time ultrasound. *Pediatrics* 71: 541–546.

Donat J F, Okazaki H, Kleinberg F & Reagan T J (1978) Intraventricular hemorrhages in full-term and premature infants. *Mayo Clinic Proceedings* 53: 437–441.

Donn S M & Bowerman R A (1985) Unilateral germinal matrix hemorrhage in the newborn. *J Ultrasound Med* 4: 251–253.

Donn S M, Roloff D W & Goldstein G W (1981) Prevention of intraventricular hemorrhage in preterm infants by phenobarbitone: a controlled trial. *Lancet* ii: 215–217.

Donn S M, Roloff D W & Goldstein G W (1982) Phenobarbitone and neonatal intraventricular hemorrhage. *Lancet* i: 1240–1241.

Donn S M, Bowerman R A, DiPietro M A & Gebarski S S (1984) Sonographic appearance of neonatal thalamic-striatal hemorrhage. *J Ultrasound Med* 3: 231–233.

Dubowitz L M S, Levene M I, Morante A *et al.* (1981) Neurologic signs in neonatal intraventricular hemorrhage: a correlation with real-time ultrasound. *J Pediatr* 99: 127–133.

Dubowitz L M S, Dubowitz V, Palmer P G *et al.* (1984) Correlation of neurologic assessment in the preterm newborn infant with outcome at one year. *J Pediatr* 105: 452–456.

Dykes F D, Lazzara A, Ahmann P *et al.* (1980) Intraventricular hemorrhage: a prospective evaluation of etiopathogenesis. *Pediatrics* 66: 42–49.

Edvinsson L, Lou H C & Tvede K (1986) On the pathogenesis of regional cerebral ischaemia in intracranial hemorrhage: a causal influence of potassium? *Pediatr Res* 20: 478–480.

Ehlers H & Courville C B (1936) Thrombosis of internal cerebral veins in infancy and childhood. *J Pediatr* 8: 600–623.

Eick J J, Miller K D, Bell K A & Tutton R H (1981) Computed tomography of deep cerebral venous thrombosis in children. *Neuroradiology* 140: 399–402.

Emerson P, Fujimura M, Howat P *et al.* (1977) Timing of intraventricular hemorrhage. *Arch Dis Child* 52: 183–187.

Evans N & Kluckow M (1996) Early ductal shunting and intraventricular hemorrhage in ventilated preterm infants. *Arch Dis Child* 75: F183–F186.

Fawer C-L, Levene M I & Dubowitz L M S (1983) Intraventricular hemorrhage in a preterm neonate: discordance between clinical course and ultrasound scan. *Neuropediatrics* 14: 242–244.

Fenichel G M, Webster D L & Wong W K T (1984) Intracranial hemorrhage in the term infant. *Arch Neurol* 41: 30–34.

Finberg L (1977) The relationship of intravenous infusions and intracranial hemorrhage – a commentary. *J Pediatr* 91: 777–778.

Fine Smith R B, Roche K, Yellin P B *et al.* (1997) Effect of magnesium sulfate on the development of cystic periventricular leukomalacia in preterm infants. *Am J Perinatol* 14: 303–307.

Fish W H, Cohen M, Franzek D *et al.* (1990) Effect of intramuscular vitamin E on mortality and intracranial hemorrhage in neonates of 1000 grams or less. *Pediatrics* 85: 578–584.

Fishman M A, Percy A K, Cheek W R & Speer M E (1981) Successful conservative management of cerebellar hematomas in term neonates. *J Pediatr* 98: 466–468.

Foley M E & McNicol G P (1977) An *in vitro* study of acidosis, platelet function, and perinatal cerebral intraventricular hemorrhage. *Lancet* i: 1230–1232.

✪ Fowlie P W (1999) Intravenous indomethacin for preventing mortality and morbidity in very low birth weight infants (Cochrane Review). In: *The Cochrane Library*, Issue 2. Oxford: Update Software.

Friede R L (1972) Subpial hemorrhage in infants. *J Neuropathol Exp Neurol* 31: 548–556.

Friede R L (1975) *Developmental neuropathology.* Vienna: Springer-Verlag.

Funato M, Tamai H, Noma K *et al.* (1992) Clinical events in association with timing of intraventricular hemorrhage in preterm infants. *J Pediatr* 121: 614–619.

Gebara B M, Goetting M G & Wang A M (1995) Dural sinus thrombosis complicating subclavian vein catheterization: treatment with local thrombolysis. *Pediatrics* 95: 138–140.

Ghazi-Birry H S, Brown W R, Moody D M, Challa V R, Block S M & Reboussin D M (1997) Human germinal matrix: Venous origin of hemorrhage and vascular characteristics. AJNR *Am J Neuroradiol* 18: 219–229.

Goddard-Finegold J, Armstrong D & Zeller R S (1982) Intraventricular hemorrhage following volume expansion after hypovolaemic hypotension in the newborn beagle. *J Pediatr* 100: 796–799.

Gomes W J & Weerasuriya N (1975) Hyperpyrexia in neonates: a sign of intraventricular hemorrhage. *Indian Pediatrics* 12: 505–507.

✪ Gould S J, Howard S, Hope P L & Reynolds E O R (1987) Periventricular intraparenchymal cerebral hemorrhage in preterm infants: the role of venous infarction. *J Pathol* 151: 197–202.

Govaert P, Calliauw L, Vanhaesebrouck P *et al.* (1990) On the management of neonatal tentorial damage. Eight case reports and a review of the literature. *Acta Neurochirurg* 106: 52–64.

Govaert P, Achten E, Vanhaesebrouck P, de Praeter C & van Damme J (1992a) Deep cerebral venous thrombosis in thalamo-ventricular hemorrhage of the term newborn. *Pediatr Radiol* 22: 123–127.

Govaert P, Vanhaesebrouck P & de Praeter C (1992b) Traumatic neonatal intracranial bleeding and stroke. *Arch Dis Child* 67: 840–845.

Govaert P, Vanhaesebrouck P, De Praeter C, Moeins K & Leroy J (1992c) Vacuum extraction, bone injury and neonatal subgaleal bleeding. *Eur J Pediatr* 151: 532–5.

Govaert P & de Vries L S (1997) *An atlas of neonatal brain sonography. Clinics in Developmental Medicine* 141–142 p. 109–126. London: Mac Keith Press.

Govaert P, Smets K, Matthys E & Oostra A (1999) Neonatal focal temporal lobe or atrial wall haemorrhagic infarction. *Arch Dis Child Fetal Neonatal En* 81: F211–F216.

Green D W, Hendon B & Mimouni F B (1995) Nucleated erythrocytes and intraventricular hemorrhage in preterm neonates. *Pediatrics* 96: 475–478.

Greenhough A, Wood S, Morley C J & Davis J A (1984) Pancuronium prevents pneumothoraces in ventilated premature babies who actively expire against positive pressure inflation. *Lancet* i: 1–3.

Grontoft O (1953) Intracerebral and meningeal hemorrhages in perinatally deceased infants. I. Intracerebral hemorrhages. *Acta Obstet Gynaecol Scand* 32: 308–324.

Groome L J, Goldenberg R L, Cliver S P *et al.* (1992) March of Dimes Multicenter Study Group 1992 Neonatal periventricular-intraventricular hemorrhage after maternal sympathomimetic tocolysis. *Am J Obstet Gynecol* 167: 873–879.

Grunau R V, Kearney S M & Whitfield M F (1990) Language development at 3 years in pre-term children of birth weight below 1000 g. *Br J Disord Commun* 25: 173–182.

Grunnet M L & Shields W O (1975) Cerebellar hemorrhage in the premature infant. *J Pediatr* 88: 605–608.

Guzzetta F, Shackelford G D, Volpe S *et al.* (1986) Periventricular intraparenchymal echodensities in the premature newborn: critical determinant of neurologic outcome. *Pediatrics* 78: 995–1006

Hadi H A, Finley J, Mallette J W & Strickland D (1994) Prenatal diagnosis of cerebellar hemorrhage: medicolegal implications. *Am J Obstet Gynecol* 170: 1392–1395.

Hambleton G & Wigglesworth J S (1976) Origin of intraventricular hemorrhage in the preterm infant. *Arch Dis Child* 51: 651–659.

Hanigan W C, Morgan A M, Stahlberg L K & Hiller J L (1990) Tentorial hemorrhage associated with vacuum extraction. *Pediatrics* 85: 534–539.

Hanigan W C, Powell F C, Palagallo G & Miller T C (1995) Lobar hemorrhages in full-term neonates. *Child Nerv Syst* 11: 276–280.

Harding J E, Miles F K I & Becroft D M (1998) Chest physiotherapy may be associated with brain damage in extremely premature infants. *Journal Pediatr* 132: 440–444.

Harrison V C, Heese H & Klein M (1968) Intracranial hemorrhage associated with hyaline membrane disease. *Arch Dis Child* 43: 116–120.

Hawgood S, Spong J & Yu V Y H (1984) Intraventricular hemorrhage: incidence and outcome in a population of very low birth weight infants. *Am J Dis Child* 138: 136–139.

Hayashi T, Hashimoto T, Fukuda S *et al.* (1987) Neonatal subdural hematoma secondary to birth injury. Clinical analysis of 48 survivors. *Child Nerv Syst* 3: 23–29.

Hecht S T, Filly R A, Callen P W & Wilson-Davis S L (1983) Intracranial hemorrhage: late onset in the preterm neonate. *Radiology* 149: 697–699.

Heibel M, Heber R, Bechinger D & Kornhuber H H (1993) Early diagnosis of perinatal cerebral lesions in apparently normal full-term newborns by ultrasound of the brain. *Neuroradiology* 35: 85–91.

Hellstrom-Westas L, Bell A H, Skov L *et al.* (1992) Cerebroelectrical depression following surfactant treatment in preterm neonates. *Pediatrics* 89: 643–647.

Hemsath F A (1934) Birth injury of the occipital bone with a report of thirty-two cases. *Am J Obstet Gynecol* 27: 194–203.

Henderson-Smart D J, Bhuta T, Cools F & Offringa M (1999) Elective high frequency oscillatory ventilation versus conventional dysfunction in preterm infants. *Cochrane Database of Systematic Reviews*, Issue 3. Oxford: Update.

Hensey O J, Morgan M E I & Cooke R W I (1984) Tranexamic acid in the prevention of periventricular hemorrhage. *Arch Dis Child* 59: 719–721.

HiFO Study Group (1993) Randomized study of high-frequency oscillatory ventilation in infants with severe respiratory distress syndrome. *J Pediatr* 122: 609–619.

Higashida R T, Helmer E & Halbach V V (1989) Direct thrombolytic therapy for superior sagittal sinus thrombosis. *Am J Roentgenol* 10: S4–S6.

Hill A, Perlman J M & Volpe J J (1982) Relationship of pneumothorax to occurrence of intraventricular hemorrhage in the premature newborn. *Pediatrics* 69: 144–149.

Hiller J L, Benda G I, Rahatzad M *et al.* (1986) Benzyl alcohol toxicity: impact on mortality and intraventricular hemorrhage among very low birthweight infants. *Pediatrics* 77: 500–506.

Holland E (1922) Cranial stress in the foetus during labour and on the effects of excessive stress on the intracranial contents. *J Obstetr Gynecol Br Empire* 29: 549–569.

Hope P L, Hall M A, Millward-Sadler G H & Normand I C S (1982) Alpha-1-antitrypsin deficiency presenting as a bleeding diathesis in the newborn. *Arch Dis Child* 57: 68–79.

Horbar J D (1992) Prevention of periventricular-intraventricular hemorrhage. In: Sinclair J C, Bracken M B (eds) *Effective care of the newborn infant.* Oxford: University Press, pp. 562–589.

Huang C C & Shen E Y (1991) Tentorial subdural hemorrhage in term newborns: ultrasonographic diagnosis and clinical correlates. *Pediatric Neurology* 7: 171–177.

Iannucci T A, Besinger R E, Fisher S G *et al.* (1996) Effect of dual tocolysis on the incidence of severe intraventricular hemorrhage among extremely low-birth-weight infants. *Am J Obstet Gynecol* 175: 1043–1046.

Incorpora G, Pavone P, Smilari P G *et al.* (1999) Late primary unilateral thalamic hemorrhage in infancy: Report of two cases. *Neuropediatrics* 30: 264–267.

Jardine D S & Rogers K (1989) Relationship of benzyl alcohol to kernicterus, intraventricular hemorrhage, and mortality in preterm infants. *Pediatrics* 83: 153–160.

Jenkins H R, Leonard J V, Kay J D S *et al.* (1982) Alpha-1-antitrypsin deficiency, bleeding diathesis, and intracranial hemorrhage. *Arch Dis Child* 57: 722–723.

Jocelyn L J & Casiro O G (1992) Neurodevelopmental outcome of term infants with intraventricular hemorrhage. *Am J Dis Child* 146: 194–197.

Kazam E, Rudelli R, Monte W *et al.* (1994) Sonographic diagnosis of cisternal subarachnoid hemorrhage in the premature infant. *AJNR Am J Neuroradiol* 15: 1009–1020.

Keeney S E, Adcock E W & McArdle C B (1991) Prospective observations of 100 high-risk neonates by high-field (1.5 tesla) magnetic resonance imaging of the central nervous system: I. Intraventricular and extracerebral lesions. *Pediatrics* 87: 421–430.

Kimberlin D E, Hauth J C, Goldenberg R L *et al.* (1998) The effect of maternal magnesium sulfate treatment on neonatal morbidity in < or = 1000-gram infants. *Am J Perinatol* 15: 635–641.

Kosmetatos N, Dinter C, Williams M L, Lourie H & Berne A S (1980) Intracranial hemorrhage in the premature: its predictive features and outcome. *Am J Dis Child* 134: 855–859.

Kotagel S, Toce S, Kotagel P & Archer C (1983) Symmetrical bithalamic and striatal hemorrhage following perinatal hypoxia in a term infant. *J Comput Assist Tomogr* 7: 353–355.

Kowitz H L (1914) Intrakranielle blutungen and Pachymeningitis Haemorrhagia chronica interna bis Neugeborensen und Sauglingen. *Virchows Archiv. A. Pathological Anatomy and Physiology* 215: 233–246.

Kreusser K L, Schmidt R E, Shackelford G D & Volpe J J (1984) Value of ultrasound for identification of acute hemorrhagic necrosis of thalamus and basal ganglia in an asphyxiated term infant. *Ann Neurol* 16: 361–363.

Krishnamoorthy K S, Fernandez R A, Momose K J *et al.* (1977) Evaluation of neonatal intracranial hemorrhage by computerized tomography. *Pediatrics* 59: 165–172.

Krishnamoorthy K S, Kuban K C K, Leviton A *et al.* (1990) Periventricular–intraventricular hemorrhage sonographic localization, phenobarbital, and motor abnormalities in low birth weight infants. *Pediatrics* 85: 1027–1033.

Kuban K C K, Leviton A, Krishnamoorthy K S *et al.* (1986) Neonatal intracranial hemorrhage and phenobarbital. *Pediatrics* 77: 443–450.

✪ Kuban K C K, Leviton A, Pagano M *et al.* (1992) Maternal toxemia is associated with reduced incidence of germinal matrix hemorrhage in premature babies. *J Child Neurol* 7: 70–76.

Lacey D J & Terplan K (1982) Intraventricular hemorrhage in full-term neonates. *Dev Med Child Neurol* 24: 332–337.

Lam A, Cruz G B & Johnson I (1991) Extradural hematoma in neonates. *J Ultrasound Med* 10: 205–209.

Larroche J-C (1972) Sub-ependymal pseudocysts in the newborn. *Biol Neonate* 21: 170–183.

Larroche J-C (1977) *Developmental pathology of the neonate.* Amsterdam: Excerpta Medica.

Larroche J-C (1984) Perinatal brain damage. In: Adams J H, Corsellis J, Duchen L W (eds) *Greenfield's neuropathology.* Edward Arnold, London pp. 451–489.

Law M R, Wijewardene K & Wald N J (1990) Is routine vitamin E administration justified in very low-birthweight infants? *Dev Med Child Neurol* 32: 442–450.

Lazzara A, Ahmann P A, Dykes T D *et al.* (1978) Clinical predictability of intraventricular hemorrhage in preterm infants. *Ann Neurol* 4: 187.

Le Blanc R & O'Gorman A M (1980) Neonatal intracranial hemorrhage: a clinical and serial computerized tomographic study. *J Neurosurg* 53: 642–651.

Lesko S M, Mitchell A A, Epstein M F *et al.* (1986) Heparin use as a risk factor for intraventricular hemorrhage in low-birth-weight infants. *N Engl J Med* 314: 1156–1160.

Levene M I & de Vries S H (1984) Extension of neonatal intraventricular hemorrhage. *Arch Dis Child* 59: 631–636.

✪ Levene M I, Fawer C-L & Lamont R F (1982) Risk factors in the development of intraventricular hemorrhage in the preterm neonate. *Arch Dis Child* 57: 410–417.

Levene M I, Williams J L & Fawer C-L (1985) Ultrasound of the infant brain. *Clin Dev Med* 92: 4.

Levene M, Dowling S, Graham M (1992) Impaired motor function (clumsiness) in 5 year old children: correlation with neonatal ultrasound scans. *Arch Dis Child* 67: 687–690.

Leviton A, Pagano M & Kuban K C K (1988) Etiologic heterogeneity of intracranial hemorrhages in preterm newborns. *Pediatr Neurol* 4: 274–278.

✪ Leviton A, Fenton T, Kuban K C & Pagano M (1991a) Labor and delivery characteristics and the risk of germinal matrix hemorrhage in low birth weight infants. *J Child Neurol* 6: 35–40.

Leviton A, Pagano M, Kuban K C K *et al.* (1991b) The epidemiology of germinal matrix hemorrhage during the first half-day of life. *Dev Med Child Neurol* 33: 138–145.

Lipscomb A P, Thorburn R J, Reynolds E O R *et al.* (1981) Pneumothorax and cerebral hemorrhage in preterm infants. *Lancet* i: 414–416.

Lombroso C T (1982) Neonatal electroencephalography. In: Niedermeyer E, daSilva F L (eds) *Electro-encephalography.* Baltimore: Urban & Schwarzenberg.

Lou H C, Lassen N A & Friis-Hansen B (1979) Is arterial hypertension crucial for the development of cerebral hemorrhage in premature infants? *Lancet* i: 1215–1217.

Lou H C, Phibbs R H, Wilson S L & Gregory G A (1982) Hyperventilation at birth may prevent early periventricular hemorrhage. *Lancet* i: 1407.

Lowe J & Papile L A (1990) Neurodevelopmental performance of very-low-birth-weight infants with mild periventricular intraventricular hemorrhage. *Am J Dis Child* 144: 1242–1245.

Ludwig B, Brand M & Brockerhoff P (1980) Postpartum CT examination of the heads of full term infants. *Neuroradiology* 20: 145–154.

Lupton B A, Roland E H, Whitfield M F & Hill A (1990) Serum sodium concentration and intravascular hemorrhage in premature infants. *Am J Dis Child* 144: 1019–1021.

Maertens P (1989) Imaging through the posterior fontanelle. *J Child Neurol* 4(suppl): S62–S67.

Maher P, Lane B, Ballard R *et al.* (1985) Does indomethacin cause extension of intracranial hemorrhages: a preliminary study. *Pediatrics* 75: 497–500.

Malloy M H, Onstad L & Wright E (1991) The effect of cesarian delivery on birth outcome in very low birth weight infants. *Obstet Gynecol* 77: 498–503.

Marret S, Parain D, Samson-Dollfus D *et al.* (1986) Positive rolandic sharp waves and periventricular leukomalacia in the newborn. *Neuropediatrics* 17: 199–202.

Marshall T A, Marshall F & Reddy P P (1982) Physiologic changes associated with ligation of the ductus arteriosus in preterm infants. *Journal of Pediatrics* 101: 749–753.

Martin C G, Snider A R, Katz S M *et al.* (1982) Abnormal cerebral blood flow patterns in preterm infants with a large patent ductus arteriosus. *Journal of Pediatrics* 101: 587–593.

Martin D J, Pape K E & Daneman A (1984) The site of neonatal periventricular hemorrhage: an important prognostic sign of mortality and morbidity. *Ann Radiol* 27: 243–246.

Martin R, Roesmann U & Fanaroff A (1976) Massive intracerebellar hemorrhage in low birth weight infants. *Journal of Pediatrics* 89: 290–292.

Matsuzaka T, Yoshinaga M, Tsuji Y *et al.* (1989) Incidence and causes of intracranial hemorrhage in infancy: a prospective surveillance study after vitamin K prophylaxis. *Brain Dev* 11: 384–388.

McDonald M M, Johnson M L & Rumack C M (1984a) Role of coagulopathy in newborn intracranial hemorrhage. *Pediatrics* 74: 26–31.

McDonald M M, Rumack C M & Johnson M L (1984b) Timing and antecedents of intracranial hemorrhage in the newborn. *Pediatrics* 74: 32–36.

McLellan N J, Prasad R & Punt J (1986) Spontaneous subhyaloid and retinal hemorrhages in an infant. *Arch Dis Child* 61: 1130–1132.

McMenamin J B, Shackelford G D & Volpe J J (1984) Outcome of neonatal intraventricular hemorrhage with periventricular echodense lesions. *Ann Neurol* 15: 285–290.

Mehrabani D, Gowen C W & Kopelman A E (1991) Association of pneumothorax and hypotension with intraventricular hemorrhage. *Arch Dis Child* 66: 48–51.

Menezes A H, Smith D E & Bell W E (1983) Posterior fossa hemorrhage in the term neonate. *Neurosurgery* 13: 452–456.

Menon P A, Thach B T, Smith C H *et al.* (1984) Benzyl alcohol toxicity in a neonatal intensive care unit: incidence, symptomatology and mortality. *Am J Perinatol* 1: 288–292.

Ment L R, Ehrenkranz R A & Lange R C (1981) Alterations in cerebral blood flow in preterm infants with intraventricular hemorrhage. *Pediatrics* 68: 763–769.

Ment L R, Stewart W B, Scott D T & Duncan C C (1983) Beagle puppy model of intraventricular hemorrhage: randomized indomethacin prevention trial. *Neurology* 33: 179–184.

Ment L R, Duncan C C, Ehrenkranz R A *et al.* (1984a) Intraventricular hemorrhage in the preterm neonate: timing and cerebral blood flow changes. *J Pediatr* 104: 419–425.

Ment L R, Stewart W B & Duncan C C (1984b) Beagle puppy model of intraventricular hemorrhage: ethamsylate studies. *Prostaglandins* 27: 245–256.

Ment L R, Stewart W B & Duncan C C (1985a) Beagle puppy model of intraventricular hemorrhage: effect of superoxide dismutase on cerebral blood flow and prostaglandins. *J Neurosurg* 62: 563–569.

Ment L R, Duncan C C, Ehrenkranz R A *et al.* (1985b) Randomized indomethacin trial for prevention of intraventricular hemorrhage in very low birthweight infants. *J Pediatr* 107: 937–943.

Ment L R, OH W & Philip A G S *et al.* (1992) Risk factors for early intraventricular hemorrhage in low birth weight infants. *J Pediatr* 121: 776–783.

Ment L R, Oh W & Ehrenkranz R A (1994) Low dose indomethacin and prevention of intraventricular hemorrhage: a multicener randomized control trial. *Pediatr* 93: 543–550.

✪ Ment L R, Vohr B, Oh W *et al.* (1996) Neurodevelopmental outcome at 36 months corrected age of preterm infants in the multicenter indomethacin intraventricular hemorrhage prevention trial. *Pediatrics* 98: 714–715.

Ment L R, Westerveld M, Makuch R, Vohr B & Allan W C (1998) Cognitive outcome at 4½ years of very low birth weight infants. *Pediatr* 102: 159–160.

✪ Mercuri E, Dubowitz L, Paterson Brown S & Cowan F (1998) Incidence of cranial ultrasound abnormalities in apparently well neonates on a postnatal ward: correlation with antenatal and perinatal factors and neurological status. *Arch Dis Child Fetal Neonatal Edn* 79: F185–F189.

Merrill J D, Piecuch R E, Fell S C *et al.* (1998) A new pattern of cerebellar hemorrhages in preterm infants. *Pediatrics* 102: E62.

Miall-Allen V M, de Vries L S & Whitelaw A G L (1987) Mean arterial blood pressure and neonatal cerebral lesions. *Arch Dis Child* 62: 1068–1069.

Michaud J L, Rivard G E & Chessex P (1991) Intracranial hemorrhage in a newborn with hemophilia following elective cesarean section. *Am J Pediatr Hematol Oncol* 13: 473–475.

Milligan D W A (1980) Failure of autoregulation and intraventricular hemorrhage in preterm infants. *Lancet* i: 896–898.

Mitchell W & O'Tuama L (1980) Cerebral intraventricular hemorrhages in infants: a widening age spectrum. *Pediatrics* 65: 35–39.

Mittendorf R, Covert R, Boman J *et al.* (1997) Is tocolytic magnesium sulphate associated with increased total paediatric mortality? *Lancet* 350: 1517.

Moghal N E, Quinn M W, Levene M I & Puntis J W L (1992) Intraventricular hemorrhage after aspiration of ventricular reservoirs. *Arch Dis Child* 67: 448–449.

Moody D M, Brown W R, Challa V R & Block S M (1994) Alkaline phosphatase histochemical staining in the study of germinal matrix hemorrhage and brain vascular morphology in a very-low-birth-weight neonate. *Pediatr Res* 35: 424–430.

Morales W J & Stroup M (1985) Intracranial hemorrhage *in utero* due to isoimmune neonatal thrombocytopenia *Obstet Gynecol* 65: 205–215.

Morales W J, O'Brien W F, Knuppel R A *et al.* (1989) The effect of mode of delivery on the risk of intraventricular hemorrhage in nondiscordant twin gestations under 1500 g. *Obstet Gynecol* 73: 107–110.

Morgan M E I, Benson J W T & Cooke R W I (1981) Ethamsylate reduces the incidence of periventricular hemorrhage in very low birth weight babies. *Lancet* ii: 830–831.

✪ Morgan M E I, Massey R F & Cooke R W I (1982) Does phenobarbitone prevent periventricular hemorrhage in very low birth weight babies? A controlled trial. *Pediatrics* 70: 186–189.

Morgan M E I, Hensey O J & Cooke R W I (1983) Convexity cerebral hemorrhage in the neonate: *in vivo* ultrasound diagnosis. *Arch Dis Child* 58: 814–818.

Motohara K, Matsukura M, Matsuda I *et al.* (1984) Severe vitamin K deficiency in breast-fed infants. *J Pediatr* 105: 943–945.

Moylan F M, Herrin J T, Krishnamoorthy K *et al.* (1978) Inappropriate antidiuretic hormone secretion in premature infants with cerebral palsy. *Am J Dis Child* 132: 399–402.

Mullaart R A, Hopman J C W, Rotteveel J J *et al.* (1994) Cerebral blood flow fluctuation in neonatal respiratory distress and periventricular hemorrhage. *Early Hum Dev* 37: 179–185.

Nakamura Y, Okudera T, Fukuda S & Hashimoto T (1990) Germinal matrix hemorrhage of venous origin in preterm neonates. *Hum Pathol* 21: 1059–1062.

Nelson K B & Grether J K (1995) Can magnesium sulfate reduce the risk of cerebral palsy in very low birthweight infants? *Paediatr* 95: 263–269.

Ng P C, Siu Y K & Lewindon P J (1995) Subaponeurotic hemorrhage in the 1990s: a 3-year suveillance. *Acta Paediatr* 84: 1065–1069.

Northern Neonatal Nursing Initiative Trial Group (1996) Randomised trial of prophylactic early fresh-frozen plasma or gelatin or glucose in preterm babies: outcome at 2 years. *Lancet* 348: 229–232.

Nwaesei C G, Allen A C & Vincer M J (1988) Effect of timing of cerebral ultrasonography on the prediction of later neurodevelopmental outcome in high-risk preterm infants. *J Pediatr* 112: 970–975.

Odita J C & Hebi S (1996) CT and MRI characteristics of intracranial hemorrhage complicating breech and vacuum delivery. *Pediatr Radiol* 26: 782–785.

Palma P A, Miner M E, Morriss F H *et al.* (1979) Intraventricular hemorrhage in the neonate born at term. *Am J Dis Child* 133: 941–944.

Paneth N, Rudelli R, Kazam E & Monte W (1994) *Brain Damage in the Preterm Infant.* Clinics in Developmental Medicine No 131. Cambridge: Cambridge, University Press.

Papagaroufalis C, Pantazatou E, Megreli Ch *et al.* (1988) Low vitamin A plasma levels (VAPL) preceding massive intracranial bleeding (MIB) in very-low-birth-weight (VLBW) neonates. *Pediatr Res* 23: 556A.

Papagaroufalis C, Megreli Ch, Hagjigeorgi Ch & Xanthou M (1991) A trial of vitamin A supplementation for the prevention of intraventricular hemorrhage in very low birth weight infants. *J Perinatal Med* 19(suppl 1): 382–387.

Pape K E, Armstrong D L & Fitzhardinge P M (1976) Central nervous system pathology associated with mask ventilation in the very low birth weight infant: a new etiology for intracerebellar hemorrhages. *Pediatrics* 58: 473–483.

✪ Pape K E & Wigglesworth J S (1979) hemorrhage, ischaemia and the perinatal brain. *Clin Dev Med* 69/70.

✪ Papile L-A, Burstein J, Burstein R *et al.* (1978) Relationship of intravenous sodium bicarbonate infusions and cerebral intraventricular hemorrhage. *J Pediatr* 93: 834–836.

Papile L-A, Munsick-Bruno G & Schaefer A (1983) Relationship of cerebral intraventricular hemorrhage and early childhood neurologic handicap. *J Pediatr* 103: 273–277.

Pasternak J F, Mantovani J F & Volpe J J (1980) Porencephaly from periventricular intracerebral hemorrhage in a premature infant. *Am J Dis Child* 134: 673–675.

Payne N R & Hasegawa D K (1984) Vitamin K deficiency in newborns. *Pediatrics* 73: 712–716.

Peabody J L (1981) Mechanical ventilation of the newborn ... good news ... bad news. *Crit Care Med* 9: 710–713.

Perlman J M & Volpe J J (1986) Are venous circulatory abnormalities important in pathogenesis of intraventricular hemorrhage in preterm infants? *Ann Neurol* 20: 434–435.

Perlman J M & Volpe J J (1987) Are venous circulatory abnormalities important in the pathogenesis of hemorrhagic and/or ischemic cerebral injury? *Pediatrics* 80: 705–711.

Perlman J M & Risser R (1998) Relationship of uric acid concentrations and severe intraventricular hemorrhage/leukomalacia in the premature infant. *J Pediatr* 132: 436–439.

Perlman J M, Hill A & Volpe J J (1981) The effect of patent ductus arteriosus on flow velocity in the anterior cerebral arteries: ductal steal in the premature newborn infant. *J Pediatr* 99: 767–771.

Perlman J M, McMenamin J B & Volpe J J (1983) Fluctuating cerebral blood flow velocity in respiratory distress syndrome: relation to the development of intraventricular hemorrhage. *N Engl J Medicine* 309: 204–209.

Perlman J M, Goodman S, Kreusser K L & Volpe J J (1985) Reduction in intraventricular hemorrhage by elimination of fluctuating cerebral blood flow velocity in preterm infants with respiratory distress syndrome. *N Engl J Med* 312: 1353–1357.

Perry E H, Bada H S & Ray J D (1990) Blood pressure increases, birth weight-dependent stability boundary, and intraventricular hemorrhage. *Pediatrics* 85: 727–732.

Peterson C M, Smith W L & Franklen E A (1984) Neonatal intracerebellar hemorrhage: detection by real-time ultrasound. *Radiology* 150: 391–392.

Peysner P H, Garcia-Bunuel R, Leeds N & Finkelstein M (1976) Subependymal and intraventricular hemorrhage in neonates: early diagnosis by computed tomography. *Radiology* 119: 111–114.

Phelps D L (1984) Vitamin E and CNS hemorrhage. *Pediatrics* 74: 1113–1114.

Pollitzer M J, Reynolds E O R, Shaw D G & Thomas R M (1981) Pancuronium during mechanical ventilation speeds recovery of the lungs of infants with hyaline membrane disease. *Lancet* i: 346–348.

Porter F L, Marshall R E, Moore J A & Miller H (1985) Effect of phenobarbital on motor activity and intraventricular hemorrhage in preterm infants with respiratory disease weighing less than 1500 grams. *Am J Perinatol* 2: 63–66.

Rademaker K J, de Vries L S & Barth P G (1993) Subependymal pseudocysts: ultrasound diagnosis and findings at follow-up. *Acta Paediatr Scand* 82: 394–399.

Rademarker K J, Groenendaal F, Jansen G H *et al.* (1994) Unilateral haemorrhagic parenchymal lesions in the preterm infant: shape, site and prognosis. *Acta Paediatr Scand* 83: 602–608.

Rao K C V G, Knipp H C & Wagner E J (1981) Computed tomographic findings in cerebral sinus and venous thrombosis. *Radiology* 140: 391–398.

Ravenel S D (1979) Posterior fossa hemorrhage in the term newborn: report of two cases. *Pediatrics* 64: 39–42.

Reynolds M L, Evans C, Reynolds E O R *et al.* (1979) Intracranial hemorrhage in the preterm sheep fetus. *Early Hum Dev* 3/2: 163–186.

Ries M, Wolfel D & Maier-Brandt B (1995) Severe intracranial hemorrhage in a newborn infant with transplacental transfer of an acquired factor VIII:C inhibitor. *J Pediatr* 127: 649–650.

Rivkin M J, Anderson M L & Kaye E M (1992) Neonatal idiopathic cerebral venous thrombosis: an unrecognized cause of transient seizures or lethargy. *Ann Neurol* 32: 51–56.

Roland E H, Flodmark O & Hill A (1990) Thalamic hemorrhage with intraventricular hemorrhage in the full-term newborn. *Pediatrics* 85: 737–742.

Rom S, Serfontein G L & Humphreys R P (1978) Intracerebellar hematoma in the neonate. *J Pediatr* 93: 486–488.

Romodanov A P & Brodsky Y S (1987) Subdural hematomas in the newborn: surgical treatment and results. *Surg Neurol* 28: 253–258.

Rose A L & Lombroso C T (1970) Neonatal seizure states: a study of clinical, pathological, and electroencephalographic features in 137 full-term babies with a long-term follow-up. *Pediatrics* 45: 404–425.

Ruckensteiner E & Zollner F (1929) Uber die Blutungen im Gebiete der Vena terminalis bei Neugeborenen. *Frankfurt Zeitschrift für Pathologie* 37: 568–578.

Ruth V, Virkola K, Paetau R & Raivio K O (1988) Early high-dose phenobarbital treatment for prevention of hypoxic-ischemic brain damage in very low birth weight infants. *J Pediatr* 112: 81–86.

Sadowitz P D & Balcom R (1985) Intrauterine intracranial hemorrhage in an infant with isoimmune thrombocytopenia. *Clin Pediatr* 24: 655–657.

Schendel D E, Berg C J, Yeargin-Allsopp M *et al.* (1996) Prenatal magnesium sulfate exposure and the risk for cerebral palsy or mental retardation among very low-birth-weight children aged 3 to 5 years. *JAMA* 276: 1805–1810.

Scher M S, Wright F S, Lockman L A & Thompson T R (1982) Intraventricular hemorrhage in the full-term neonate. *Arch Neurol* 39: 769–772.

Schick J B, Beck A L & DeSilva H N (1989) Umbilical artery catheter position and intraventricular hemorrhage. *J Perinatol* 9: 382–385.

Scotti G, Fodmark O, Harwood-Nash D C & Humphries R P (1981) Posterior fossa hemorrhages in the newborn. *J Comput Assist Tomogr* 5: 68–72

Setzer E S, Webb I B & Wassenaar J W (1982) Platelet dysfunction and coagulopathy in intraventricular hemorrhage in the premature infant. *J Pediatr* 100: 599–605.

Shankaran S, Bauer C R, Bain R *et al.* (1996) Prenatal and perinatal risk and protective factors for neonatal intracranial hemorrhage. *Arch Pediatr Adolesc Med* 150: 491–497.

Shankaran S, Slovis T L, Bedard M P & Poland R L (1982) Sonographic classification of intracranial hemorrhage: a prognostic indicator of mortality, morbidity and short-term neurologic outcome. *J Pediatr* 100: 469–475.

Shaw C-M & Alvord E C (1974) Subependymal germinolysis. *Arch Neurol* 31: 374–381.

Shen E Y, Huang C C, Chyou S C *et al.* (1986) Sonographic finding of the bright thalamus. *Arch Dis Child* 61: 1096–1099.

Shinnar S, Molteni R A, Gammon K *et al.* (1982) Intraventricular hemorrhage in the premature infant: a changing outlook. *N Engl J Med* 306: 1464–1468.

Shirahata A, Nakamura T, Shimono M, Kaneko M & Tanaka S (1990) Blood coagulation findings and the efficacy of factor XIII concentrate in premature infants with intracranial hemorrhages. *Thrombosis Res* 57: 755–763.

Sia C G, Amigo N C, Harper R G *et al.* (1985) Failure of cesarian section to prevent intracranial hemorrhage in siblings with isoimmune neonatal thrombocytopenia. *Am J Obstet Gynecol* 153: 79–81.

Simmons M A, Adcock E W, Bard H & Battaglia F C (1974) Hypernatraemia and intracranial hemorrhage in neonates. *N Engl J Med* 291: 6–10.

Sinha S, Davies J, Toner N *et al.* (1987) Vitamin E supplementation reduces the incidence of periventricular hemorrhages in very preterm babies. *Lancet* i: 466–471.

Smets K, De Kezel C & Govaert P (1997) Subependymal caudothalamic groove hyperechogenicity and neonatal chronic lung disease. *Acta Paediatrica* 86: 1370–1373.

Smets K & Van Aken S (1998) Fetomaternal hemorrhage and prenatal intracranial bleeding: two more causes of blueberry muffin baby. *Eur J Pediatr* 157: 932–934.

Smith W L, McGuinness G, Cavanaugh D & Courtney S 1983 Ultrasound screening of premature infants: longitudinal follow-up of intracranial hemorrhage. *Radiology* 147: 445–448.

✪ Soll R F & Morley C J (1999) Prophylactic versus selective use of surfactant for preventing morbidity and mortality in preterm infants (Cochrane Review). In: *The Cochrane Library*, Issue 2. Oxford: Update Software.

Speer M E, Blifeld C, Rudolph A J *et al.* (1984) Intraventricular hemorrhage and vitamin E in very low birth weight infant: evidence for efficacy of early intramuscular vitamin E administration. *Pediatrics* 74: 1107–1112.

Spinillo A, Ometto A, Stronati M *et al.* (1995) Epidemiologic association between maternal smoking during pregnancy and intracranial hemorrhage in preterm infants. *J Pediatr* 127: 473–479.

Stewart A L, Reynolds E O R & Hope P L (1987) Probability of neurodevelopmental disorders estimated from ultrasound appearance of brains of very preterm infants. *Dev Med Child Neurol* 29: 3–11.

Stewart A L, Thorburn R J, Lipscomb A P & Amiel-Tison C (1983a) Neonatal neurologic examinations of very preterm infants: comparison of results with ultrasound diagnosis of periventricular hemorrhage. *Am J Perinatol* 1: 6–11.

Stewart A L, Thorburn R J, Hope P L *et al.* (1983b) Ultrasound appearance of the brain in very preterm infants and neurodevelopmental outcome at 18 months of age. *Arch Dis Child* 58: 598–604.

Strange M J, Myers G, Kirklin J K *et al.* (1985) Surgical closure of patent ductus arteriosus does not increase the risk of intraventricular hemorrhage in the preterm infant. *J Pediatr* 107: 602–604.

Strauss A, Kirz D, Modanlou H D & Freeman R K (1985) Perinatal events and the very low-birth weight infant. *Am J Obstet Gynecol* 151: 1022–1027.

Stutchfield P R & Cooke R W I (1989) Electrolytes and glucose in cerebrospinal fluid of premature infants with intraventricular hemorrhage: role of potassium in cerebral infarction. *Arch Dis Child* 64: 470–475.

Sudakoff G S, Montazemi M & Rifkin M D (1993) The foramen magnum: the underutilized acoustic window to the posterior fossa. *J Ultrasound Med* 12: 205–210.

Szymonowicz W & Yu V Y H (1984a) Timing and evolution of periventricular hemorrhage in infants weighing 1250 g or less at birth. *Arch Dis Child* 59: 7–12.

Szymonowicz W, Yu V Y H & Wilson F E (1984b) Antecedents of periventricular hemorrhage in infants weighing 1250 g or less at birth. *Arch Dis Child* 59: 13–17.

Szymonowicz W, Yu V Y H, Walker A & Wilson F (1986) Reduction in periventricular hemorrhages in preterm infants. *Arch Dis Child* 61: 661–665.

Takagi T, Nagai R, Wakabayashi S *et al.* (1978) Extradural hemorrhage in the newborn as a result of birth trauma. *Child Brain* 4: 306–318.

Takashima S & Tanaka K (1978) Microangiography and vascular permeability of the subependymal matrix in the premature infant. *Can J Neurol Sci* 5: 45–50.

Takashima S, Mito T & Ando Y (1986) Pathogenesis of periventricular white matter hemorrhages in preterm infants. *Brain Devel* 8: 25–30.

Tarby T J & Volpe J J (1982) Intraventricular hemorrhage in the premature infant. *Pediatr Clin North Am* 29: 1077–1089.

Tardieu M, Evrard P & Lyon G (1981) Progressive expanding congenital porencephalies: a treatable cause of progressive encephalopathy. *Pediatrics* 68: 198–202.

Tejani N, Rebold B, Tuck S *et al.* (1984) Obstetric factors in the causation of early periventricular-intraventricular hemorrhage. *Obstet Gynecol* 64: 510–515.

Tejani N & Verma U L (1989) Correlation of Apgar scores and umbilical artery acid-base status to mortality and morbidity in the low birth weight neonate. *Obstet Gynecol* 73: 597–600.

TeKoiste K A, Bennett F C & Mack L A (1985) Follow-up of infants receiving cranial ultrasound for intracranial hemorrhage. *Am J Dis Child* 139: 299–303.

Thorburn R J, Lipscomb A P, Stewart A L *et al.* (1981) Prediction of death and major handicap in very preterm infants by brain ultrasound. *Lancet* i: 1119–1121.

Thorburn R J, Lipscomb A P, Stewart A L (1982) Timing and antecedents of periventricular hemorrhage and of cerebral atrophy in very preterm infants. *Early Hum Dev* 7: 221–238.

Toubas P L, Hof R P, Heymann M & Rudolph A (1978) Effects of hypothermia and rewarming on the neonatal circulation. *Archives Françaises Pediatrie* (suppl) 35: 84–92.

Towbin A (1968) Cerebral intraventricular hemorrhage and subependymal matrix infarction in the fetus and premature newborn. *Am J Pathol* 52: 121–134.

✪ Trounce J Q, Dodd K L, Fawer C-L *et al.* (1985) Primary thalamic hemorrhage in the newborn: a new clinical entity. *Lancet* i: 190–192.

Trounce J Q, Rutter N & Levene M I (1986) A prospective study of the incidence of periventricular leukomalacia and intraventricular hemorrhage in the preterm neonate. *Arch Dis Child* 61: 1196–1202.

Tsiantos A, Victorin L, Relier J P *et al.* (1974) Intracranial hemorrhage in the prematurely born infant. Timing of clots and evaluation of clinical signs and symptoms. *J Pediatr* 85: 854–859.

Van Bel F, Van de Bor M, Stijnen T *et al.* (1987) Aetiological role of cerebral blood-flow alterations in development and extension of peri-intraventricular hemorrhage. *Dev Med Child Neurol* 29: 601–614.

van der Bor M, den Ouden L, Guit G L (1992) Value of cranial ultrasound and magnetic resonance imaging in predicting neurodevelopmental outcome in preterm infants. *Pediatrics* 90: 196–199.

Vert P, Nomin P & Sibout M (1975) Intracranial venous pressure in the newborn: variations in physiological state and in neurologic and respiratory distress. In: Stern L (ed) *Intensive care in the newborn.* New York: Masson.

✪ Vohr B & Ment L R (1996) Intraventricular hemorrhage in the preterm infant. *Early Hum Dev* 44: 1–16.

Vohr B, Coll C G, Flanagan P & Oh W (1992) Effects of intraventricular hemorrhage and socioeconomic status on perceptual, cognitive, and neurologic status of low birth weight infants at 5 years of age. *J Pediatr* 121: 280–285.

Voit T, Lemburg P & Stork W (1985) NMR studies in thalamic-striatal necrosis. *Lancet* ii: 445.

Volpe J J (1977) Neonatal intracranial hemorrhage: pathophysiology, neuropathology and clinical features. *Clin Perinatol* 4: 77–102.

Volpe J J, Herscovitch P, Perlman J M & Raichle M E (1983) Positron emission tomography in the newborn: extensive impairment of regional blood flow with intraventricular hemorrhage and hemorrhagic involvement. *Pediatrics* 72: 589–601.

Voutsinas L, Gorey M T, Gould R *et al.* (1991) Venous sinus thrombosis as a cause of parenchymal and intraventricular hemorrhage in the full-term neonate. *Clin Imaging* 15: 273–275.

Wakai S, Andoh Y, Nagai M *et al.* (1990) Choroid plexus arteriovenous malformation in a full-term neonate. *Journal of Neurosurgery* 72: 127–129.

Wallin L A, Rosenfeld C R, Laptook A R *et al.* (1990) Neonatal intracranial hemorrhage: II. Risk factor analysis in an inborn population. *Early Hum Dev* 23: 129–137.

Waanabe K, Hakamada S, Kuroyanagi M *et al.* (1983) Electroencephalographic study of intraventricular hemorrhage in the preterm newborn. *Neuropaediatr* 14: 225–230.

Watkins A M C, West C R & Cooke R W I (1989) Blood pressure and cerebral haemorrhage and ischaemia in very low birthweight infants. *Early Hum Development* 19: 103–110.

Watson J W, Brown D M, Lally K P *et al.* (1990) Complications of extracorporeal membrane oxygenation in neonates. *South Med J* 83: 1262–1265.

Wehberg K, Vincent M, Garrison B *et al.* (1992) Intraventricular hemorrhage in the full-term neonate associated with abdominal compression. *Pediatrics* 89: 327–329.

Welch K & Strand R (1986) Traumatic parturitional intracranial hemorrhage. *Dev Med Child Neurol* 28: 156–164.

White R P, Hagen A A, Morgan H *et al.* (1975) Experimental study on the genesis of cerebral vasospasm. *Stroke* 6: 52–57.

Whitelaw A, Placzek M, Dubowitz L *et al.* (1983) Phenobarbitone for prevention of periventricular hemorrhage in very low birth weight infants. *Lancet* ii: 1168–1170.

Whitelaw A G, Haines M E, Bolsover W & Harris E (1984) Factor V deficiency and antenatal intraventricular hemorrhage. *Arch Dis Child* 59: 997–999.

Wigglesworth J S & Husemeyer R P (1977) Intracranial birth trauma in vaginal breech delivery: the continued importance of injury to the occipital bone. *Br J Obstet Gynaecol* 84: 684–691.

Wigglesworth J S, Keith I H, Girling D J & Slade S A (1976) Hyaline membrane disease, alkali and intraventricular hemorrhage. *Arch Dis Child* 51: 755–759.

Wiswell T E, Graziani L J, Kornhauser M S *et al.* (1996) High-frequency jet ventilation in the early management of respiratory distress syndrome is associated with a greater risk for adverse outcome. *Pediatrics* 98: 1035–1043.

Zalneraitis E L, Young R S K & Krishnamoorthy K S (1979) Intracranial hemorrhage *in utero* as a complication of isoimmune thrombocytopenia. *J Pediatr* 95: 611–614.

Zlatnik F J (1993) The Iowa premature breech trial. *Am J Perinatol* 10: 60–63.

Zuerrer M, Martin E & Boltshauser E (1991) MR imaging of intracranial hemorrhage in neonates and infants at 2.35 tesla. *Neuroradiology* 33: 223–229.

# Chapter 22 Cerebral ischemic lesions

L. S. de Vries and M. I. Levene

## INTRODUCTION

Brain ischemia occurs as the result of a variety of perinatal insults. During intrapartum asphyxia, cerebral hypoperfusion together with hypoxia produces a typical pathologic and clinical appearance which is discussed in Chapter 23. In this section we will refer to the more specific condition of cerebral ischemia associated to some extent with vascular compromise. This may develop in the watershed area between the vascular territory of two arterial beds, as occurs in a number of infants with leukomalacia, or following infarction of the whole or a branch of a major cerebral artery.

## LEUKOMALACIA

Leukomalacia literally means 'softening of the white matter' and has been recognized as a pathologic entity for longer than periventricular hemorrhage. This condition is now well recognized to be an important cause of neurodevelopmental sequelae. The etiology of leukomalacia was until recently considered to be basically ischemic, but there is now increasing data suggesting that inflammatory processes as well as increased vulnerability of oligodendroglia to oxidative stress also play an important role. Different forms of white matter disease can occur and the condition is especially more diffuse in the less mature preterm infants who are now surviving in ever increasing numbers. The diagnosis using cranial ultrasound is not very reliable in the noncystic form, but the use of neonatal MRI is now increasing and will hopefully advance our understanding of this condition.

### HISTORICAL REVIEW

Ischemic lesions in general and periventricular leukomalacia (PVL) in particular have commonly been diagnosed at autopsy, before the era of the newer imaging techniques. PVL has been known to pathologists for more than a century and was first described by Virchow in 1867, who noted yellowish-white areas in the periventricular white matter, which he associated with infection, and he named the condition 'congenital interstitial encephalitis'. Parrot (1873) reviewed the condition around the same time in a series of reports and pointed out that the problem was more common in premature infants and he therefore assumed that the immature white matter might be especially vulnerable in this age group. A major advance in understanding this condition occurred in 1962 when Banker & Larroche described the pathologic changes in 51 infants. They introduced the name 'periventricular leukomalacia' to describe their observation of the periventricular 'white spots' seen macroscopically (Fig. 22.1) and the softening (malacia) of the white matter (leukos). Perinatal anoxia was noted in the clinical history of all their cases, and they were the first to suggest that the condition was vascular in origin. Van den Bergh (1969) and De Reuck *et al.* (1972) further stressed the vascular origin of these lesions and attributed the cause to hypoperfusion of the boundary zones between ventriculofugal and ventriculopetal arteries. This hypothesis was supported by Armstrong & Norman in 1974, who showed that hemorrhages could occur as a secondary process into these ischemic lesions (Fig. 22.2). Leech & Alvord (1974) reported that the lesions could extend beyond the periventricular region into the subcortical white matter. Takashima & Tanaka (1978) performed post-mortem cerebral angiography and showed that the boundary zones between the ventriculofugal and ventriculopetal arteries were affected in the infants with PVL. Takashima *et al.* (1978) performed similar studies in more mature infants and showed a relatively avascular triangle in the white matter at the depths of the sulci. These areas corresponded well with the site of the subcortical lesions seen in

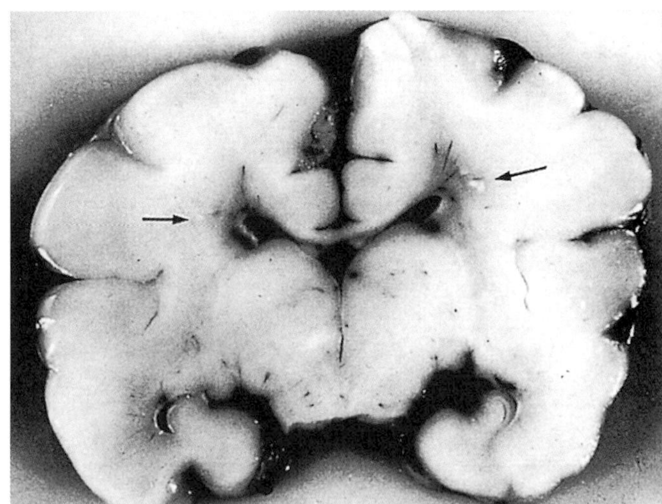

Figure 22.1 Bilateral 'white spots' (arrowed) of PVL. Histologically, glial proliferation and calcification were present. Small bilateral germinal matrix hemorrhage is also present.

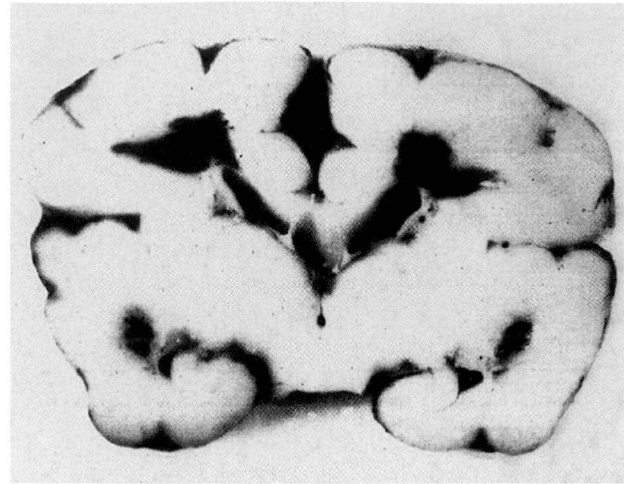

Figure 22.2 Hemorrhagic necrosis into bilateral PVL lesions.

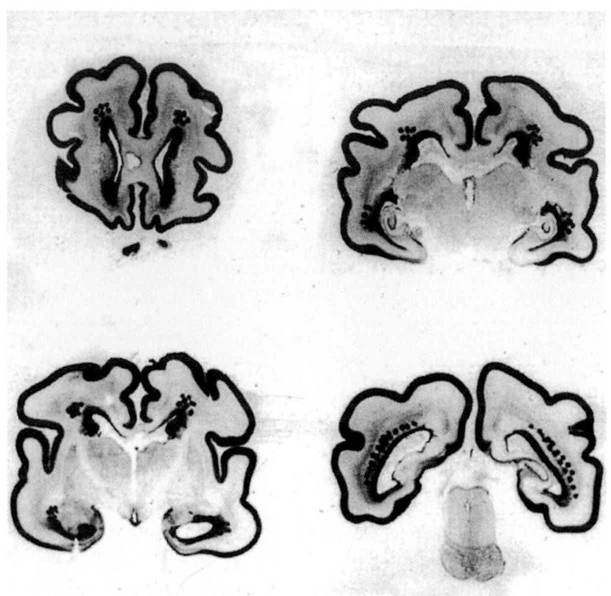

Figure 22.3 Distribution of PVL lesions. The sites of predilection of white matter lesions are superimposed on brain sections stained with cresyl violet. (Reproduced, with permission, from Larroche 1984.)

more mature infants. They therefore suggested that the distribution of these cystic lesions was related to the maturity of the vascular supply.

Kuban & Gilles (1985) and Nelson *et al.* (1991) did not support the ventriculofugal/ventriculopetal periventricular white matter vascular border zone model, as they were not able to confirm the existence of ventriculofugal arteries described by van den Bergh and De Reuck. Kuban & Gilles (1985) injected the cerebral arteries of human fetal cadavers with silicone and looked at these specimens using high-power stereomicroscopic observations of thick specimens, and were unable to visualize ventriculofugal arteries. When they examined these specimens at low magnification and without stereoscopy they were able to reproduce the results of van den Bergh, and concluded that both van den Bergh as well as De Reuck mistook transcerebral channels within the periventricular white matter, superimposed on the distal ends of striate arteries, for ventriculofugal arteries. Similar conclusions were drawn by Moody *et al.* (1990) using different techniques. They suggested that the medullary veins, which converge in a radial fashion out of the centrum semiovale towards the ventricles, were mistaken for ventriculofugal arteries, and once again questioned the ventriculofugal/ventriculopetal vascular border zone model as the basis for PVL.

During more recent years, it has become clear that hypoperfusion may play a role but other, probably more important, factors are involved, such as excitatory amino acids, the vulnerability of immature oligodendrocytes to oxidative stress, and the role of proinflammatory cytokines (see below).

## PATHOLOGY

Macroscopical examination of PVL shows a typical distribution of the periventricular lesions involving the external angle of the lateral ventricles (centrum semiovale), the corona radiata, the optic radiation (trigone and occipital horn), and the auditory radiation (temporal horn) (Fig. 22.3).

Histologic findings depend on the duration between the insult and the time of death. The earliest changes consist of coagulation necrosis, characterized by loss of architecture, and this can be found within 5–8 hours following an insult. A few days later, nuclear debris, astrocytes and macrophages are noted to fill the periphery of the necrotic area. These macrophages can remain for months or years. The center of the necrotic area may liquify, resulting in small cavities, usually not communicating with the lateral ventricles (Fig. 22.4). Calcified capillaries can sometimes be noted in the periphery of these areas. Cavitation is not always observed, and gliosis and persisting macrophages may be noted instead. Thinning of the white matter with enlargement of the lateral ventricles is present in both cases.

Owing to the prolonged survival of severely ill very low birth weight (VLBW) infants, the morphologic expression of the brain insult has changed significantly from the histology originally described by Banker & Larroche (1962). Paneth *et al.* (1990) reported autopsy findings of 22 preterm infants who died beyond 5 days of age. Of these infants, 15 had either acute or chronic white matter necrosis, but this was restricted to the periventricular white matter in only a minority of the cases. Only 3 infants had histologic findings as originally reported by Banker & Larroche in 1962. The other 12 infants either did not have the classic histologic features of PVL, or if they did, the lesions were not restricted to the periventricular white matter. They concluded that in the VLBW infant white matter necrosis need not be restricted

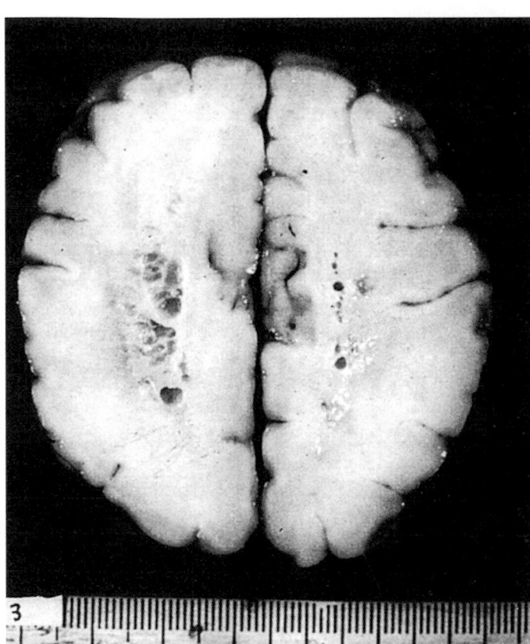

Figure 22.4 Multicystic leukomalacia. Horizontal section of brain from an infant of 29 weeks of gestation who survived for 5 weeks. (Reproduced, with permission, from Larroche 1984.)

to the periventricular region and can sometimes be histologically different from PVL as originally described.

The use of immunohistochemistry has improved our understanding of this condition considerably. Using this technique, Deguchi *et al.* (1997, 1999) showed the distribution of PVL in 85 infants (22–41 weeks gestation) to be more widespread in the most immature infants, involving the deep and intermediate white matter. It was shown that GFAP positive astrocytes were increased in the deep white matter, often also spreading to the intermediate white matter in all PVL cases. Cells positive for tumor necrosis factor-α (TNF-α) were present in 69% of PVL cases and β-amyloid precursor protein (β-APP) in 76% of cases. β-APP is a membrane spanning glycoprotein generated in the neuronal cell body that is transported to axons and accumulates in damaged axons. It can either be a marker of axonal injury, or it may be upregulated in response to brain injury. Some studies have suggested that β-APP is a growth factor and a protector against excitotoxic or ischemic insults. It is an excellent marker for foci of necrosis and can readily identify the otherwise subtle morphologic features of white matter necrosis in the immature brain. Ninety-four per cent of the infants with a gestational age below 29 weeks showed widespread distribution of PVL, whereas most of those with a gestational age greater than 34 weeks developed focal PVL.

GFAP, TNF-α or β-APP positive cells were not found in any of the controls. β-APP positive axons proved to be a useful marker for demonstrating the type of PVL. In a subsequent study they pointed out that β-APP positive cells were only seen in the *early* stages of prenatal PVL (Meng *et al.* 1997). The same group (Meng & Takashima 1999) also studied the expression of transforming growth factor-β1 in PVL, a factor considered to be synthesized in response to brain injury. This factor was observed in glial cells around necrotic foci in the white matter and was only present in the subacute stage of PVL, in those with focal stages and in the more mature infants (gestational age >32 weeks). They suggested that transforming growth factor-β1 might contribute to tissue remodeling and healing after ischemic injury.

The incidence of PVL in these pathologic studies varies between 7 and 34% (Armstrong & Norman 1974; Pape & Wigglesworth 1979), but increases to over 80% by taking only those infants who required ventilation and survived beyond the first 7 days of life (Shuman & Selednik 1980). In a more recent study, 68% of the 22 VLBW infants who survived at least 6 days were diagnosed as having some degree of white matter necrosis (Paneth *et al.* 1990).

Kuban *et al.* (1999) found a clear association of white matter disorders with intraventricular hemorrhage (IVH) and ventriculomegaly. Infants with both were at 18–29-fold greater risk of white matter damage. In this study no distinction was made between an echolucency following a unilateral parenchymal hemorrhage or bilateral echodensities characteristic of early stage PVL.

Prenatal onset of leukomalacia was also noted by pathologists when studying stillbirths or infants who died within the first few days of life. The incidence varied from 1.1% (Sims 1985) to 20% in stillbirths and 16.4% of infants who died within the first 3 days of life. Of the preterm infants, 14.3% had prenatal onset PVL which consisted of widespread necrosis (Iida 1993).

## PATHOPHYSIOLOGY

There is no generally accepted pathophysiologic mechanism to explain the development of PVL and a number of different theories exist.

### The vascular theory

The historical concept that PVL is caused by hypoperfusion is supported by only a few animal studies. Abramovicz (1964) obliterated the basilar artery and ligated one or both common carotid arteries in mature cats. Subsequently, he was able to show patchy infarcts close to the ventricular wall in the centrum semiovale.

Other groups have used dogs as animal models. Young *et al.* (1982) produced systemic hypotension either by withdrawal of blood or by injection of *E. coli* into the peritoneum, and showed a significant reduction of cerebral blood flow (CBF) in the periventricular white matter while the blood flow to the cortical and deep gray matter was preserved. Ment *et al.* (1985a) induced hemorrhagic hypotension in beagle puppies and found similar results. Yoshioka *et al.* (1992) performed bilateral carotid artery occlusion in 7 mongrel puppies and found that 6 of the 7 brains had uni- or multiloculated cysts in the periventricular white matter and significantly reduced myelination compared with controls. Using bilateral carotid artery occlusion in 5-day-old rats, Uehara *et al.* (1999) were able to induce white matter changes in 90.9% of the animals. Matsuda *et al.* (1999) induced systemic hypotension in fetal sheep by rapid withdrawal of 35% of the fetoplacental blood volume and produced periventricular white matter lesions, consisting of coagulation necrosis and/or diffuse axonal swelling in 5 out of 6 fetuses. An interesting observation was made by Ohyu *et al.* (1999) who performed repeated umbilical cord occlusion in near-term fetal sheep and subsequently detected multiple necrotic foci predominantly in the periventricular white matter.

A reduction in CBF after hypocarbia due to vasoconstriction was noted in several animal experiments (Saphiro *et al.* 1980). Reuter & Disney (1986) have shown, that there is a non-linear positive correlation between $PaCO_2$ and regional CBF in the white matter of newborn dogs.

In different types of animal experiments, the periventricular white matter has appeared to be more susceptible than other areas of the brain. Ment *et al.* (1985a) noted a regional increase in glucose utilization in the periventricular white matter and therefore assumed uncoupling between local CBF and glucose metabolism in the periventricular white matter. This uncoupling was also noted by Cavazutti & Duffy (1982), who looked at hyperemia following hypoxia. They found that the compensatory hyperemia was less pronounced in the periventricular white matter, while an extremely high rate of glycolysis was found in this area compared with other regions of the brain. Prostaglandin $E_2$, a potent vasodilator, was also carefully studied by Ment *et al.* (1985b) in beagles subjected to hypotension. The concentration of prostaglandin $E_2$ was shown to increase to a lesser extent in the periventricular white matter than in the cortex and gray matter.

## The excitotoxic theory

Animal studies suggest that hypoperfusion alone could be an oversimplification in explaining the pathophysiology of PVL, and an increasing number of these studies are looking at the role of excitatory amino acids in relation to neuronal damage (see Chapters 23 and 28). Gressens *et al.* (1999) were able to induce cystic PVL by injecting the glutaminergic analog ibotenate intracerebrally into newborn mice. By simultaneously injecting a trophic factor, vasoactive intestinal peptide (VIP), a reduction up to 87% of these excitotoxic lesions was obtained. Using the same model, this group also showed a protective effect of a glycine antagonist and NO synthase inhibitor (Marret *et al.* 1999). Meng & Takashima (1999) also suggested that exogenous transforming growth factor-β1 could have a therapeutic effect, being involved in a delayed glial response. They studied 25 neonates with PVL using immunohistochemistry and found this growth factor to be present in 16 cases, especially in the subacute stage of PVL and only in the more mature infants (greater than 32 weeks gestation). The expression was more obvious in *focal* PVL.

## The oligodendroglial theory

Following the work of Oka *et al.* (1993) who showed that cultured oligodendroglial cells were highly vulnerable to glutamate induced cell death, Back *et al.* (1998) extensively studied maturation dependent vulnerability of oligodendrocytes (OLs) to oxidative stress. They were able to develop an *in vitro* system to study two distinct OLs maturational stages: the preOL and the mature-OL, the preOL being the mitotically active premyelinating precursor to the mature myelin basic protein positive OL. They examined whether OLs display maturation dependent survival in response to cystine deprivation, the latter being a form of oxidative stress that involves depletion of intracellular glutathione. PreOLs in contrast to OLs indeed displayed increased susceptibility to death associated with free radical mediated injury, induced by glutathione depletion or exogenous reactive oxygen species. Maturation of OLs correlated with increased resistance to oxidative stress. The increased vulnerability of the preOLs to oxidative stress correlated with a greater dependence on intracellular glutathione for survival. The toxicity of glutathione depletion was prevented by glutathione replacement. Glutathione depletion caused a marked rise in reactive oxygen species, whose toxicity could be prevented by antioxidants α-tocopherol and idebenone. Increased susceptibility of preOLs to oxidative stress may be due to delayed maturational expression of genes that suppress apoptosis.

Alternatively, the death of preOLs may be regulated by a specific pathway triggered by oxidative stress that is down-regulated in mature OLs. Jelinski *et al.* (1999) used 7-day-old rats for a hypoxic–ischemic model, exposing them to 8% oxygen with temporary occlusion of the carotid arteries. Oligodendroblasts were identified using the O4 antibody. They suggest that the vulnerable glial cell type that makes a contribution to the development of PVL is the oligodendroblast, as a decrease of these cells was seen within 24 hours after the insult. Another group studied the distribution and development of ferritin-containing cells by immunohistochemistry and found that the OL was the predominant cell type. Ferritin-positive cells were present in the periventricular and subcortical white matter from 25 weeks onwards. They suggested that ferritin-positive glia were related to the process of myelination and maturation of the OL (Ozawa *et al.* 1994).

## The cytokine theory

Many recent experimental as well as human studies have provided strong evidence for a causal relationship between ascending intrauterine infection, the production of pro-inflammatory cytokines, and white matter damage (see reviews by Dammann & Leviton 1997a, 1998, 1999 and Rothwell *et al.* 1997). The first animal study suggesting the importance of infection was by Gilles *et al.* in 1976. They administered intraperitoneal *E. coli* endotoxin to neonatal kittens for 6 days and found telencephalic leukoencephalopathy at post-mortem. The severity of the lesions appeared to be related to the dose of the endotoxin. More recently, Yoon *et al.* (1997a) performed hysteroscopy in rabbits at 20–21 days of gestation and inoculated either *E. coli* ($n$=31) or saline ($n$=14), treating both groups with ampicillin-sulbactam. The rabbits were killed 5–6 days later. They noted histologic evidence of white matter damage in 12 of the *E. coli* inoculated group compared with none in the saline group ($p < 0.005$).

Levels of endotoxin measured in a clinical setting were measured by Okumura *et al.* (1999a). They were unable to show a correlation between raised endotoxin levels and the presence of PVL and, unfortunately, were unable to perform simultaneous cytokine measurements.

Many bacterial products besides endotoxin can stimulate the production of cytokines. Deguchi *et al.* (1996) and Yoon *et al.* (1997b) used immunohistochemical staining on brain sections having histologic evidence of PVL, and compared them with brain sections without leukomalacia. Expression of TNF-α and interleukin-6 was found significantly more often in brain sections that showed evidence of leukomalacia. Interleukin-6 has been reported to play a role in guiding the developing bipotential oligodendrocyte precursor cell, 0-2A, towards the astrocyte and away from the pathway leading to a mature oligodendrocyte (Kahn & de Vellis 1994). Deguchi *et al.* (1996) noted that TNF-α was mainly expressed in glial cells in the deep white matter. It is of interest that TNF-α expression was also present in the controls during the late fetal period, but later than in the leukomalacia cases. These two studies provided further support for the hypothesis that proinflammatory cytokines play a role in the genesis of PVL. Even more convincing is the study by Dommergues *et al.* (2000) who pretreated pups with interleukin 1-β, IL-6, IL-9 or TNF-α. They were able to show that the pretreated pups developed significantly larger cortical and white matter damage than controls when later exposed to the neurotoxin ibotenate. Induction of TNF-α and inducible nitric oxide synthase were, however, also detected following fetal hypoxia induced by repetitive umbilical cord occlusion (Ohyu *et al.* 1999)

Several groups have subsequently measured cytokines both in the amniotic fluid, in fetal plasma, and cord blood. TNF-α, interleukin-1 and interleukin-6 all play a role in normal pregnancy (Opsjln *et al.* 1993), but levels have been shown to be elevated in the amniotic fluid of pregnant women with chorioamnionitis (Yoon *et al.* 1997c). Baud *et al.* (1999a) were able to find an association between the amniotic fluid level of interleukin-1β and the degree of vascular extension of chorioamnionitis. TNF-α best predicted the development of severe early neonatal infection. In this study, the cytokines were unable to predict the development of PVL, but Yoon *et al.* (1997c) did show a significant relationship between raised interleukin-1β and interleukin-6 levels in the amniotic fluid with white matter lesions. Gomez *et al.* (1998) measured interleukin-6 levels in both the amniotic fluid as well as the fetal plasma in women with preterm labor and premature prolonged rupture of membranes and found interleukin-6 in fetal plasma to be significantly higher in the fetus who went on to develop severe neonatal morbidity, which also included PVL. In another study by Yoon's group interleukin-6 concentrations greater than 400 pg/ml in umbilical cord plasma were associated with a sixfold increase in white matter disease (Yoon *et al.* 1996).

## CLASSIFICATION

Unfortunately there is no agreement on classification of lesions of the brain parenchyma. Following the introduction of the term 'periventricular leukomalacia' by Banker & Larroche in 1962, many groups of pathologists have used this term, but others have identified more widespread white matter damage, consisting of hypertrophic astrocytes, amphophilic globules, necrotic foci, and acutely damaged glia which were widespread in the cerebral white matter. This condition has been referred to as 'leukoencephalopathy' (Gilles & Murphy 1969). Kuban *et al.* (1999) prefer to describe echodensities and echolucencies as one condition, even in cases with a classic unilateral parenchymal hemorrhage. Paneth (1999) proposed the term 'white matter damage.'

As the majority of papers cited in this chapter use the term periventricular leukomalacia (PVL), we also prefer to use it and will only describe 'white matter damage' when quoting papers using that term. We have been using a grading system for PVL (Table 22.1) that is now quite commonly employed by other groups (de Vries *et al.* 1992). Using a grading system is essential when comparing the different studies in this field.

**Table 22.1 Classification of periventricular and subcortical leukomalacias based on cranial ultrasound findings (de Vries *et al.* 1992)**

|  |  |
|---|---|
| • Grade I | Periventricular echodense area, present for 7 days or more |
| • Grade II | Periventricular echodense areas evolving into localized frontoparietal cysts |
| • Grade III | Periventricular echodense areas evolving into multiple cysts in the parieto-occipital white matter |
| • Grade IV | Echodense areas in the deep white matter, with evolution into multiple subcortical cysts |

## INCIDENCE

The first reports of PVL described the ultrasound findings in a small number of cases only. Recently, however, several population studies have been performed, reporting an incidence of between 2.3 and 17.8% (Levene *et al.* 1983; Sinha

**Table 22.2 Incidence of ultrasound-diagnosed extensive cystic PVL from 17 studies**

| Reference | Incidence (%) | Group selection[a] | Population |
|---|---|---|---|
| Levene *et al.* (1983) | 7.5 | <1500 g | 120 |
| Bozynski *et al.* (1985) | 5 | <1201 g | 138 |
| Weindling *et al.* (1985) | 8 | <1500 g or 34 weeks | 124 |
| Fawer *et al.* (1985a) | 4.8 | <35 weeks | 83 |
| Sinha *et al.* (1985) | 17.8 | <33 weeks | 219 |
| Calvert *et al.* (1986) | 2.3 | <1501 g | 431 |
| Trounce *et al.* (1986) | 9.5 | <1501 g | 200 |
| Graham *et al.* (1987) | 8.3 | <1501 g | 200 |
| Zorzi *et al.* (1988) | 5.2 | <33 weeks | 154 |
| Tzogalis *et al.* (1988) | 16 | <35 weeks | 81 |
| de Vries *et al.* (1988) | 3.2 | <35 weeks | 676 |
| Pidcock *et al.* (1990) | 7.9 | <33 weeks | 288 |
| Ikonen *et al.* (1992) | 10.6 | <33 weeks | 103 |
| Perlman *et al.* (1996) | 2.3 | <1750 g | 632 |
| | 3.2 | <1500 g | |
| Zupan *et al.* (1996) | 9.2 | <33 weeks | 753 |
| Spinillo *et al.* (1998) | 5.7 | <33 weeks | 349 |
| Stevenson *et al.* (1998) | 6 | <1501 g | 2771 |

[a] Birth weight or gestational age.

*et al.* 1985; Weindling *et al.* 1985a; Trounce *et al.* 1986b; Zupan *et al.* 1996; Perlman *et al.* 1996; Stevenson *et al.* 1998; Spinillo *et al.* 1998) (Table 22.2). The incidence will vary with the type of patient admitted to the intensive care unit (Larroche *et al.* 1986), the type of transducer used (5 or 7.5 MHz), the number of ultrasound examinations performed, and the definition used to describe PVL. Those authors who find a low incidence have restricted the term 'PVL' to apply to infants who developed extensive cystic lesions, while those giving a higher incidence have also included localized cystic lesions restricted to the centrum semiovale (Fawer *et al.* 1985b). Trounce *et al.* (1986b) reported a 9.5% incidence of cystic PVL. If prolonged flares were included in the PVL category, the incidence increased to 26%. The incidence of flares (echodensities seen in two planes and lasting more than 2 weeks) was found to be 12.5%. Extensive cystic lesions, both in the trigone and in the centrum semiovale, were noted in only 2.7% of all the infants. Stevenson *et al.* (1998) studied a very large inborn cohort with a birth weight <1500 g. PVL was noted in 6% of the 2771 infants who had ultrasound examinations after 2 weeks, but no distinction for cystic PVL was made. We feel that this distinction is of significance, in relation to later outcome (see below). An incidence of periventricular infarction of 48% was reported by Nwaesei *et al.* (1984), who studied those infants who died beyond 21 days of life.

## TIMING

The onset of PVL usually occurs in the perinatal period, but any severe deterioration in the condition of the infant, such as occurs with necrotizing enterocolitis or septicemia, up until 40 weeks of postmenstrual age, can still lead to this condition (Rushton *et al.* 1985; de Vries *et al.* 1986; Perlman *et al.* 1996; Zupan *et al.* 1996). Repeated ultrasound examinations beyond the first 2 weeks of life are therefore of importance (Townsend *et al.* 1999). This is in contrast to germinal matrix hemorrhage – intraventricular hemorrhage (GMH–IVH), which is known to occur rarely beyond the first week of life (Partridge *et al.* 1983, Fawer *et al.* 1984). PVL may also be due to insults occurring *in utero* (Barth 1984; Larroche 1986; Szymonowicz *et al.* 1986; Bejar *et al.* 1988, 1990; Baetmann *et al.* 1996), and this is discussed in more detail in Chapter 20. A recent study by Hayakawa *et al.* (1999) used EEG recordings within 72 hours of life to determine the time of onset in 26 infants with cystic PVL. Acute stage abnormalities were present in 14 of these infants, suggestive of a perinatal onset. The EEG was initially normal in 7 infants who were considered to have a postnatal onset, and chronic stage abnormalities were recognized in the remaining 5, suggestive of antenatal onset PVL.

## ETIOLOGY

A relatively small number of studies have been carried out to identify risk factors for leukomalacia. Early on, the risk factors identified for PVL in these studies were based on small numbers of cases and were not as uniform as those previously identified for GMH–IVH, but this has changed over the last few years. In some studies, infants with extensive cystic leukomalacia were compared with controls or infants with GMH–IVH while in others infants with prolonged flares also formed part of the PVL study group. Infants with associatated GMH–IVH were included in some studies and excluded in others, which complicated interpretation and comparison of the results.

## Prenatal factors

In contrast to GMH–IVH, prenatal risk factors have been identified by several groups.

### Multiple gestation

Bejar *et al.* (1988) identified a condition referred to as antenatal white matter necrosis in 13 out of 127 (10.3%) preterm infants with a gestational age below 36 weeks. This was defined as cystic lesions present at birth or developing during the first 3 days of life. Placental vascular anastomoses in multiple pregnancies, funisitis, and purulent amniotic fluid were identified as independent risk factors. A second study from the same group (Bejar *et al.* 1990) identified antenatal white matter necrosis in 14 out of 101 (13.8%) infants who were members of twin or triplet sets. Using logistic regression analysis, antenatal white matter necrosis was predicted by the presence of artery-to-artery or vein-to-vein anastomoses and by intrauterine fetal death of a co-twin. The incidence of antenatal white matter necrosis in infants of multiple gestation was reported to be 13.8%, and this was not significantly higher than the same condition occurring in singletons. Monochorionic infants, however, had an incidence of antenatal white matter necrosis of 30% which was significantly higher ($p < 0.005$) than the 3.3% incidence reported in singletons or dichorionic infants. Burguet *et al.* (1999) also found monochorionic twin placentation to be an important risk factor for cerebral palsy. The relation between death of a co-twin and severe neurologic sequelae has been reported previously (Szymonowicz *et al.* 1986, Rydhstrom & Ingemarsson 1993) (see Chapter 47). Multifetal pregnancy reduction was also shown to be an additional risk factor for PVL (Geva *et al.* 1998).

### Tocolysis

Baerts *et al.* (1990) reported the possible adverse role of indomethacin, used during pregnancy as a tocolytic agent. Using multivariate analysis they identified indomethacin as an independent and significant risk factor for cystic PVL ($p = 0.001$). Spinillo *et al.* (1998) found that the long term use of ritodrine increased the risk for transient echodense lesions.

### Fetal heart rate patterns

Okamura *et al.* (1997) examined fetal heart rate tracings for base line heart rate, variability, and decelerations. They also described a specific pattern, 'the flip flop' pattern, which is an oscillatory tracing pattern with increased baseline variability and tachycardia with superimposed deceleration. This 'flip flop pattern' was significantly more common in the fetuses who went on to develop cystic PVL.

### Infection

More than a decade ago, several groups noted an association between bacterial contamination or infection and antenatal white matter necrosis (Leviton & Gilles 1984; Sims *et al.* 1985; Bejar *et al.* 1988). Bejar *et al.* (1988) identified funisitis and purulent amniotic fluid as independent risk factors for antenatal white matter necrosis. Leviton & Gilles (1984) showed that 85% of infants who died with white matter lesions had a Gram-negative bacteremia. Sims *et al.* (1985) found that brain lesions of prenatal onset were associated with amnionitis and acute intrauterine infection.

Several more recent studies have looked at obstetric antecedents of PVL. Perlman *et al.* (1996) studied 632 preterm infants, each weighing 1750 g or less and identified preterm rupture of membranes and chorioamnionitis to be significant predictors of cystic PVL, using univariate analysis. Zupan *et al.* (1996) showed that 19% of the infants who had abnormal white cell count/C-reactive protein, or positive bacterial cultures, or whose mothers had signs of infection, developed PVL compared with 6% of those without these signs. Verma *et al.* (1997) studied 745 preterm infants with birth weights below 1750 g. They made a distinction between cases with preterm rupture of membranes, refractory preterm labor with intact membranes, and delivery initiated by the physician for maternal or fetal indications. They noted that the incidence and severity of both IVH as well as PVL significantly increased in both preterm rupture of membranes and preterm labor. Alexander *et al.* (1998) looked at an even larger group of preterm infants with birth weights of 1500 g or less and found that 7% of them had been exposed to chorioamnionitis. Using multiple regression analysis and adjusting for preterm rupture of membranes, a significant association was found with the development of cystic PVL (OR 3.4; 95% CI 1.6–7.3).

In several studies identifying risk factors for cerebral palsy, chorioamnionitis and prolonged rupture of membranes were found to be major predictors of cerebral palsy (Nelson & Ellenberg 1985; Grether *et al.* 1996; Murphy *et al.* 1996; O'Shea *et al.* 1998a,b; Burguet *et al.* 1999).

### Antepartum hemorrhage

Three groups identified antepartum hemorrhage as a risk factor for PVL (Sinha *et al.* 1985; Weindling *et al.* 1985a; Calvert *et al.* 1986). Other groups were unable to confirm this (Trounce *et al.* 1988; Tzogalis *et al.* 1988). Gibbs & Weindling (1994) reported placental abruption to be associated with a fourfold increased incidence of PVL and large hemorrhages; 10 out of 29 cases developed cystic PVL compared with 10% of their matched controls.

## Intrapartum factors

### Place of birth

Being outborn was identified as an independent risk factor for PVL by de Vries *et al.* (1988b) but not others (Trounce *et al.* 1988; Tzogalis *et al.* 1988). As those infants who are transported to a neonatal intensive care unit are highly selected, care should be taken to interpret data collected in a tertiary intensive care unit. Grether *et al.* (1996) found that being born in a level I facility was significantly associated with the development of cerebral palsy.

### Mode of delivery

To date, the mode of delivery has not been found to be of importance in the development of PVL. Ikonen *et al.* (1988) reported that infants who developed PVL were delivered significantly more often by the vaginal route ($p < 0.003$). Emergency Cesarean section was associated with an increased risk for PVL in one study by de Vries *et al.* 1988b who found the need for an emergency Cesarean section significantly higher in infants with extensive cystic PVL than those who developed a large GMH–IVH. Baud *et al.* (1998a) showed a significant reduction in PVL when the infant was delivered by Cesarean section in the presence of chorioamnionitis (OR 0.15; 95% CI 0.04–0.57). Hansen & Leviton (1999) found vaginal delivery to be associated with white matter disease, but only on univariate analysis; the strength of this relationship was markedly reduced on multivariate analysis when inflammation was taken into account. This suggests that vaginal delivery is only a marker for antecedent inflammation and/or infection.

### Condition at birth

Both cord blood gases as well as Apgar scores have been reported by some groups to predict the risk of developing PVL (Sinha *et al.* 1985; Weindling *et al.* 1985a; Calvert *et al.* 1986; Tzogalis *et al.* 1988; de Vries *et al.* 1988b) but not in other careful studies (Trounce *et al.* 1988; Ikonen *et al.* 1988, 1992; Perlman *et al.* 1996).

### Gestational age

Immaturity has been shown to be inversely related to the frequency and degree of GMH–IVH (Trounce *et al.* 1988). This is not a consistent finding for PVL, and it appears that the infant's brain may remain susceptible to PVL for a longer period of gestation. In some studies (Calvert *et al.* 1986; Ikonen *et al.* 1988) infants with PVL were matched with controls who had a similar gestational age, making it impossible to identify gestational age as a risk factor. It should also be taken into account that the gestational age at birth may not bear much relationship to the age at which a baby develops PVL following an acute clinical deterioration many weeks after birth (de Vries *et al.* 1986; Pelman *et al.* 1996; Zupan *et al.* 1996). No relationship between the gestational age and PVL was found by several groups (Weindling *et al.* 1985a; de Vries *et al.* 1988b; Trounce *et al.* 1988, Ikonen *et al.* 1992). Tzogalis *et al.* (1988) did find, however, that infants who developed PVL were significantly less mature than their normal controls (29.8 vs. 31.9 weeks). In a study by Ikonen *et al.* (1988), 12 infants with extensive cystic PVL were all noted to have a gestational age of 31 or 32 weeks. De Vries *et al.* (1988b) noted that infants with extensive cystic PVL were significantly more mature than infants who developed large hemorrhages (30.1 vs. 28.3 weeks) (Fig. 22.5), a finding supported by Perlman *et al.* (1996) (gestational age 29.4 weeks for PVL compared with 26.6 weeks for large GMH–IVH, $p < 0.01$). In the study by Stevenson *et al.* (1999), PVL varied between 6 and 7% for those infants weighing 500–1500 g. Bejar *et al.* (1988) found antenatal white matter necrosis to be inversely related to the birth weight, and was more frequent in infants weighing more than 1000 g (19%).

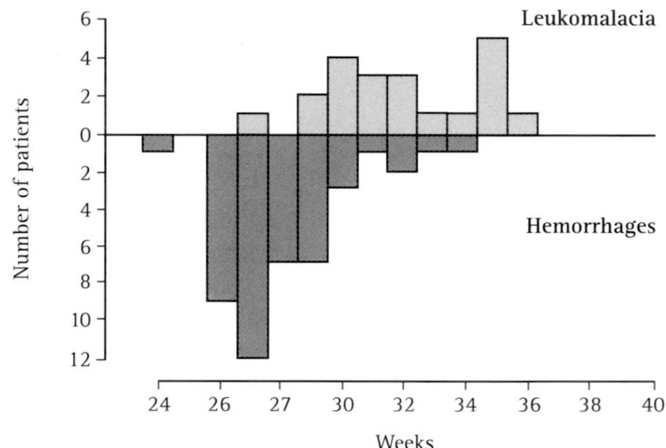


**Figure 22.5** Age in postmenstrual weeks at the onset of hemorrhagic and ischemic lesions.

## Lung disease and its complications

While respiratory distress syndrome is the most consistently recognized risk factor predisposing to GMH–IVH in preterm infants, this is not the case for PVL. Mechanical ventilation has, however, been identified by most groups to have a significant association with PVL (Sinha *et al.* 1985; Weindling *et al.* 1985a; de Vries *et al.* 1988b; Trounce *et al.* 1988). Sinha *et al.* (1990) compared babies with early onset PVL to infants with late-onset PVL (days 4–70), and noted that hyaline membrane disease was associated with the latter group, while a history of intrauterine growth restriction and recurrent apnea was more common in the early onset group. Complications associated with mechanical ventilation, such as pneumothorax, hypocarbia, and hypercapnia have all been identified as risk factors for PVL, and these are discussed below.

### Hypercapnia and hypocarbia

Hypercapnia has only been identified as a risk factor by one group (Trounce *et al.* 1988), but several studies have shown hypocarbia to be associated with cystic PVL. This was first found by Calvert *et al.* (1987) and has subsequently been confirmed by Iida *et al.* (1992) and Ikonen *et al.* (1992). In the latter study, significantly longer periods of carbon dioxide levels below 4 kPa (30 mmHg) were found in infants who developed PVL than in those that did not. In an earlier study, Ikonen *et al.* 1988, looking at a smaller number of infants with extensive cystic PVL, noted that a mean duration of carbon dioxide levels below 4 kPa (30 mmHg) was longer in the affected infants, but the results did not reach statistical significance. The mean highest pH during the first 72 hours was, however, significantly higher in infants with PVL than in controls. These findings are in agreement with earlier reports by Greisen *et al.* (1986, 1987) who noted an increase in the incidence of infants with major neurologic sequelae when trying to reduce the incidence of GMH–IVH by hyperventilating the infants.

It appears that those infants with only mild respiratory distress are especially at risk of experiencing periods of hyperventilation. With the introduction of high frequency oscillation, there has been concern about an increase in the number of cases with cystic PVL. Wiswell *et al.* (1996a) have pointed out that high frequency jet ventilation may produce substantial hypocapnia: 18 out of 52 surviving infants developed cystic PVL. Logistic regression analysis revealed that infants with cystic PVL were significantly more likely to have greater cumulative hypocarbia below a threshold of 3.3 kPa (25 mmHg) during the first day of life. In another study, Wiswell *et al.* (1996b) randomized 73 preterm infants to receive high frequency jet ventilation or conventional ventilation and found that those being treated with high frequency jet ventilation were significantly more likely to develop cystic PVL ($p = 0.022$). A recent meta-analysis was however unable to relate an increased risk of cystic-PVL with high frequency ventilation (Cools & Offringa 1999). Vannucci *et al.* (1995, 1997) studied the effect of hyper- and hypocarbia in an immature hypoxia–ischemia rat model and noted an adverse effect of hypocarbia as well as a protective effect of mild hypercarbia.

#### Pneumothorax

Several studies have identified pneumothorax as a risk factor for PVL (Sinha *et al.* 1985, Trounce *et al.* 1988, de Vries *et al.* 1988b).

### Cardiovascular factors

As PVL is considered by some to be related to hypoperfusion of the boundary zones between ventriculofugal and ventriculopetal arteries, hypotension was expected to be an important risk factor of the occurrence of PVL. No period of hypotension was documented in any of the seven cases studied by Weindling *et al.* (1985a). In the largest cohort studied so far (Trounce *et al.* 1988), systolic blood pressure data were carefully analyzed but no relation between hypotension and the development of PVL could be established. Watkins *et al.* (1989) reported that there was a strong association between hypotension and IVH but there was a lack of an association between hypotension and the occurrence of periventricular ischemic lesions. Iida *et al.* (1992) did find hypotension to be significantly related to the development of PVL in a small group of infants. It should be stressed that other factors identified as risk factors, such as septicemia, surgery, and apneic spells, may all be associated with fluctuations in blood pressure. Lou *et al.* (1979) performed radioactive xenon studies in sick preterm infants and showed a marked reduction in CBF coinciding with hypotension.

#### Patent ductus arteriosus

An association between a patent ductus arteriosus and PVL has been reported in two studies (Sinha *et al.* 1985; de Vries *et al.* 1988b). Infants with a patent ductus arteriosus may have reduced CBF as measured by Doppler ultrasound. Following administration of indomethacin, a further reduction in CBF velocity has been shown in Doppler studies (Cowan 1986; Evans *et al.* 1987), but no data have been published showing an association between postnatal treatment with indomethacin and the development of PVL.

### Hyperbilirubinemia

Trounce *et al.* (1988) first identified hyperbilirubinemia as an independent variable associated with PVL. In the same year, Ikonen *et al.* (1988) also noted that serum bilirubin levels were significantly higher in a group of 12 infants with PVL when compared with the levels of 12 matched controls. They speculated that bilirubin toxicity may play an additional role in the damage of the periventricular white matter. To further support this, they performed a second study, looking prospectively at a cohort of 103 infants with gestational age below 33 weeks. They once again were able to identify the mean levels of total serum bilirubin as a significant independent risk factor. The hyperbilirubinemia usually coincided with prolonged hypocarbia (<4 kPa), identified as the second independent risk factor. Their hypothesis was that the toxic effects of a high bilirubin concentration may be especially deleterious to brain tissue that has already been underperfused due to prolonged hypocarbia. This finding would fit in with data from van de Bor *et al.* (1989), who showed that there is an increasing prevalence of cerebral palsy in preterm infants with increasing total serum bilirubin levels. In a recent study by Graziani *et al.* (1992), however, there was no evidence to suggest that hyperbilirubinemia was causally related to cerebral palsy or periventricular cysts.

### Hypothyroxinemia

Leviton *et al.* (1999) studied 1414 preterm infants with birth weights of 1500 g or less, and were able to show that the preterm infants with a thyroxine level below 67.8 nmol/l had twice the risk of 'echolucencies' as their peers with higher thyroxine levels. The multicenter antenatal TRH study noted a trend toward more motor impairment in the TRH treated group (Crowther *et al.* 1997). Antenatal treatment, however, combined TRH with corticosteroids.

### Postnatal dexamethasone treatment

There is some concern about the (early) use of dexamethasone and its effect on neurodevelopmental outcome. Yeh *et al.* (1998) randomized 133 infants within the first 12 hours after birth and treatment was continued for 4 weeks. They showed a significant increase in neuromotor dysfunction at 2 years of age (25/63 vs. 12/70). O'Shea *et al.* (1999) showed that more infants treated with dexamethasone developed cerebral palsy (25% vs. 9%) at 1 year of age. Papile *et al.* (1998) showed poor head growth following dexamethasone treatment. Shinwell *et al.* (2000) performed a randomized multicenter study in which dexamethasone or a placebo was given within 12 hours of age and continued for 3 days. Long term follow-up on 159 infants showed a significantly higher incidence of cerebral palsy (49 compared to 15%; OR 4.62; 95% CI 2.38–8.98) in those treated with dexamethasone. Infants treated with dexamethasone had more cystic PVL but this did not reach statistical significance (22% compared with 13%). It is of interest that 22% of their cerebral palsy cases did not have any ultrasound abnormalities. Shinwell and colleagues propose the possibility of a direct neurotoxic effect of dexamethasone in the neonatal period. As the study involved 18 centers, it can not also be excluded that the standard of neonatal ultrasonography was not of the same level in all centers and that some of the infants with cystic PVL were missed.

### Pyruvate carboxylase deficiency

Brun *et al.* (1999) have suggested that this metabolic disorder can present on ultrasound scan with appearance similar to cystic PVL. They confused subependymal pseudocysts with 'frontal cystic-PVL'.

## UNIFYING HYPOTHESIS

Although PVL can still be considered an ischemic lesion, the vulnerability of the white matter to other factors also appears to play an important role. First, the increased vulnerability of the immature oligodendrocyte to glutamate was shown by Back *et al.* (1998) using cultured oligodendroglia. Second, the proinflammatory cytokines play a role, probably even before delivery. An association of raised interleukins 1 and 6 and TNF-α which has been studied in the amniotic fluid as well as in the cord blood, and white matter disease is now well established, with data coming from both animal experiments as well as from human clinical studies. Cytotoxic cytokines can, however, also be released *during* ischemia. After delivery, complications related to mechanical ventilation can occur and we are now well aware that vasoconstriction due to hypocarbia is a rather common risk factor. Care should be taken to avoid this, especially when using high frequency ventilation.

## PREVENTION

The first results about possible prevention of PVL are now being published, but their clinical utility is still very limited.

### Antenatal drug intervention

Nelson & Grether (1995) showed a reduction in cerebral palsy cases after *in utero* exposure to magnesium sulfate. Another retrospective study (FineSmith *et al.* 1997) even showed a significant reduction in the incidence of cystic PVL among 492 infants each weighing less than 1750 g. Canterino *et al.* (1999), however, were unable to show a protective effect of this drug on the development of severe ultrasound abnormalities in 918 infants with birth weights below 1750 g. There are no convincing data available at present to suggest that magnesium sulfate prevents antenatal PVL.

Antenatal steroids lead to a significant reduction in the incidence of PVL in appropriate for gestational age preterm infants delivered following preterm labor with or without ruptured membranes, but not in those with fetal growth restriction (Elimian *et al.* 1999). Baud *et al.* (1999b) showed a reduced risk of cystic PVL with antenatal administration of betamethasone, but not with dexamethasone (4.4% vs. 11%, compared with 8.4% when no corticosteroids were given at all). Betamethasone and dexamethasone differ by only one methyl group, but betamethasone has a longer half life. It has been suggested that sulfating agents present in dexamethasone may be neurotoxic. The study was, however, retrospective and uncontrolled.

Russell & Cooke (1995) randomly allocated 400 infants with gestational ages between 24 and 32 weeks to receive either allopurinol or a placebo for the first 7 days of life. They were unable to show a protective effect for the development of cystic PVL, bronchopulmonary dysplasia, or retinopathy of prematurity. Hypoxanthine levels at birth were, however, significantly higher in infants who went on to develop cystic PVL. These data are in agreement with recent findings by Perlman & Risset (1998) who found significantly higher uric acid concentrations on day 1 in those who went on to develop severe intraventricular hemorrhages or cystic PVL.

## DIAGNOSIS AND EVOLUTION OF PVL

With the use of newer imaging techniques it is now well recognized that many infants with PVL survive. Performing sequential ultrasound studies, valuable information about the timing, the evolution of the ultrasound changes, and the possible risk factors have been reported in the mid-1980s (Dolfin *et al.* 1984; Chow *et al.* 1985).

### Ultrasound

Correlation with autopsy findings has varied a lot in the literature. A high sensitivity and specificity was found by several groups (Nwaesei *et al.* 1984; Fawer *et al.* 1985a; Trounce *et al.* 1986a; de Vries *et al.* 1988a), but other groups showed a low sensitivity (Szymonowicz *et al.* 1984; Baarsma *et al.* 1987; Hope *et al.* 1988; Carson *et al.* 1990; Paneth *et al.* 1990). The data of Hope *et al.* (1988) were especially disappointing, with a sensitivity of only 28% and a specificity of 86%. There were many false negatives due to failure to detect very small areas of PVL and diffuse gliosis. In other studies, it was also noted that the main problem appears to be that not all infants with ischemic lesions detected on histology had areas of increased echogenicity on cranial ultrasound. The presence of hemorrhage into these areas increased the sensitivity of the ultrasound diagnosis. The sensitivity was very good once cystic lesions had developed during life. The frequency of the ultrasound transducers (5 vs. 7.5 MHz), the interval between serial ultrasound examinations, and the time that elapsed between the last scan and the post-mortem studies should all be taken into account when interpreting these data.

Timing the onset of the lesion can be deduced from the evolution of the ultrasound changes. Areas of increased echogenicity are usually seen within 24–48 hours following an acute clinical episode (Fig. 22.6A). This increase in echogenicity was initially thought to be due to hemorrhages occurring in the ischemic areas, following restoration of the circulation. Several authors have now shown that non-hemorrhagic infarction is also able to give this echogenic appearance (Martin *et al.* 1983; Delaporte *et al.* 1985; Trounce *et al.* 1986a). This can be confirmed at autopsy or by the use of a computerized tomography (CT) scan within a week following the lesions, or for longer by MRI.

It is assumed that severe congestion may cause this increase in echogenicity. The densities can resolve but usually persist until the dense areas break down into cystic lesions 2–4 weeks later. The cysts appear in clusters in the area of previous echogenicity. They vary in diameter

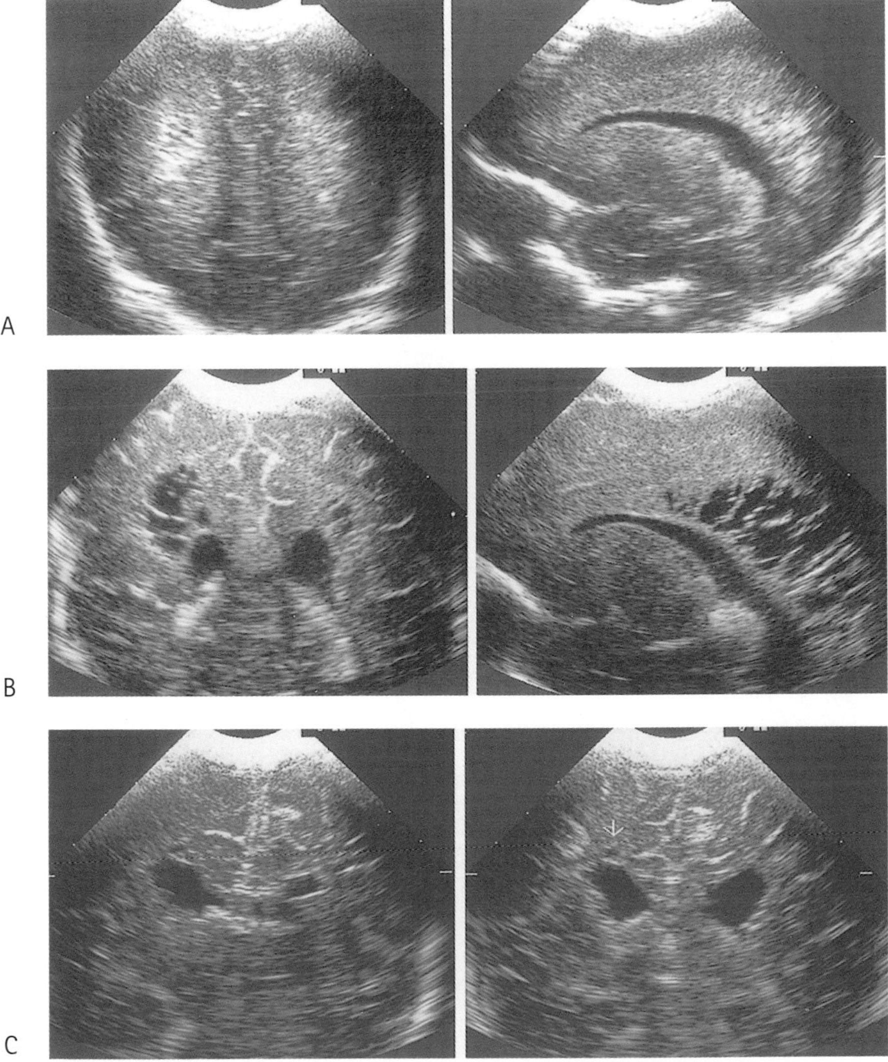


**Figure 22.6** Cranial ultrasound performed on day 10 in a preterm infant (gestational age 28 weeks; birth weight 800 g) showing increased echogenicity, more marked on the right than on the left on the coronal view (**A, left**) and the right parasagittal view (**A, right**). Same views in the same child, shown 6 weeks later (**B**), showing extensive cystic evolution. The cysts are separate from the lateral ventricles and are more extensive than would have been expected on the basis of the preceding echogenicity. At 6 months of age mild *ex vacuo* dilatation is shown as well as only one remaining cyst (arrow) (**C**).

between a few millimeters to over a centimeter and do not usually communicate with the ventricles (Fig. 22.6B). When PVL occurs together with a large intraventricular hemorrhage (IVH) and posthemorrhagic ventricular dilatation, communication of the cystic lesions with the ventricular system does occur and is referred to as pseudoventricle formation (Grant *et al.* 1986). The cysts remain for several weeks, but tend to become smaller and are usually not visible on ultrasound examination once the infant is 2–3 months old (Fig. 22.6C, Fig. 22.7). When the cysts become less apparent, dilatation of the lateral ventricles can be noted (Bozynski *et al.* 1985). The outline of the cysts may disappear completely, as was observed in a child with PVL who died at 8 months of age. Histologic examination showed gliosis, delayed myelination, and mild ventricular dilatation (Trounce *et al.* 1986a). A similar case was reported by Rodriguez *et al.* (1990) who found a linear glial scar in the area where the periventricular cysts were initially seen using ultrasound. Most reports concerning cystic PVL have described the development of cysts in the periventricular white matter. Tsuru *et al.* (1995) described the evolution of cysts in the cerebellar folia in three premature infants, and Coley & Hogan (1997) reported one preterm infant who developed cysts in the corpus callosum.

A small number of cases develop small localized cysts in the centrum semiovale (Fig. 22.8). These cysts are usually unilateral and few in number and can only be visualized with a 7.5 MHz transducer. These localized cysts were at first only noted in the fronto-parietal periventricular white matter but in recent years small and localized cysts have also been seen more posteriorly in the parieto-occipital white matter. These small cysts take longer to develop (3–4 weeks) and are only present for 1–3 weeks.

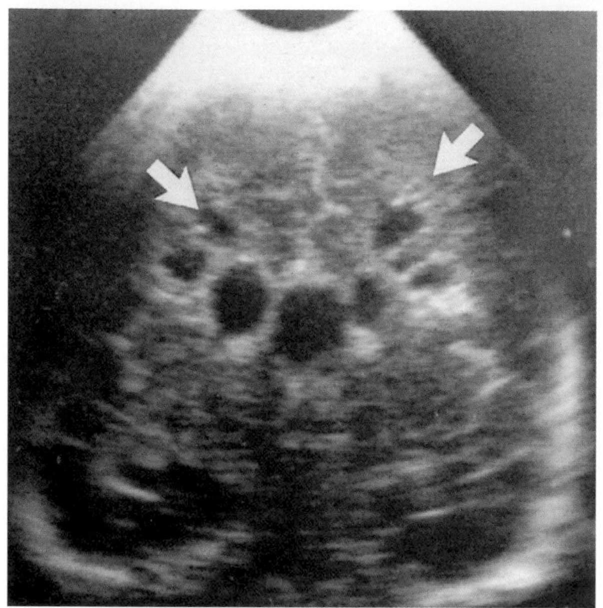

A

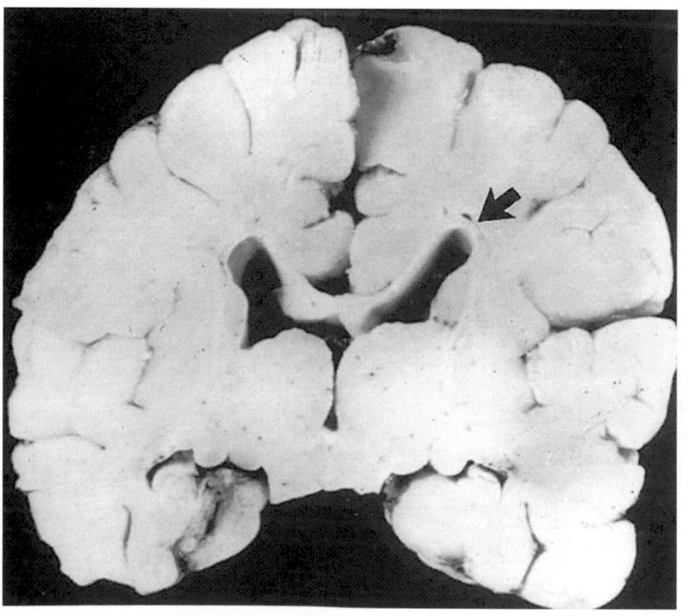

B

**Figure 22.7** Evolution of cystic PVL lesions. **(A)** Coronal ultrasound scan showing multiple echo-free cavities (arrows) in the white matter. **(B)** The infant died 3 months later, and at autopsy the brain showed collapse of the cavities, which were only just visible (arrow).

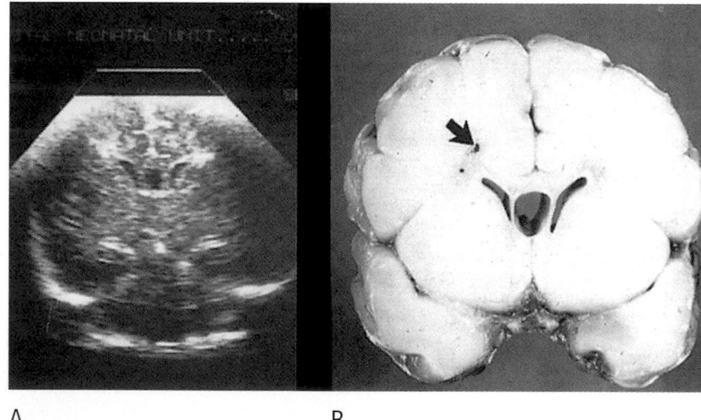

A B

**Figure 22.8** Cystic PVL. **(A)** Midcoronal ultrasound scan showing echodense areas in the periventricular white matter with small cysts on the left side. **(B)** Post-mortem correlate showing a small cyst on the left (arrowed) with discoloration and softening of the periventricular white matter on the right.

While it is relatively uncommon for a child to develop cystic lesions, many infants develop increased echogenicity at the external angle of the lateral ventricle without, or with less, apparent echogenicity around the occipital horns (McMenamin *et al.* 1984; Di Pietro *et al.* 1986; Guzzetta *et al.* 1986). Trounce *et al.* (1986b) defined the periventricular echodensities as prolonged 'flares' if they persisted for at least 14 days (Fig 22.9). Such flares subsequently resolve,

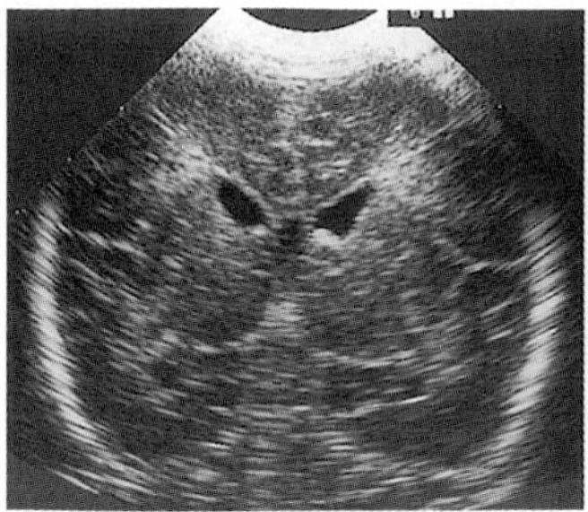
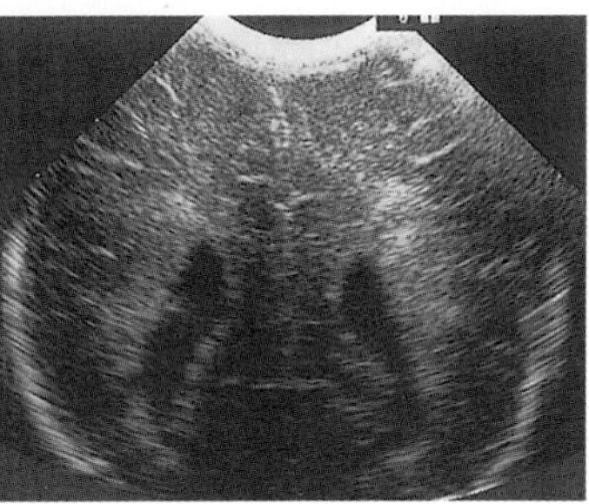

**Figure 22.9** Cranial ultrasound, coronal views, performed on day 14 in a preterm infant (gestational age 28 weeks; birth weight 1100 g). Increased echogenicity is noted, especially at the level of the external angle of the lateral ventricles.

but mild ventricular dilatation can be observed in some of these infants when they are scanned again between 6 and 9 months of age, and this can be asymmetrical where the periventricular echodensities were asymmetrical to start with. Subsequent widening of the interhemispheric fissure has also been recorded in a few infants with flares in the neonatal period, possibly indicating some degree of atrophy. In a few infants who died, gliosis has been observed at autopsy, and it is therefore likely that these flares represent a milder degree of PVL (McMenamin *et al.* 1984; Fawer *et al.* 1985a; Trounce *et al.* 1986a; de Vries *et al.* 1988a).

### Magnetic resonance imaging (see also p. 70)

The use of MRI plays an important role in the early stage of PVL, when it is still uncertain whether cysts will evolve. It has been described that many infants with areas of increased periventricular echogenicity on ultrasound show small petechial hemorrhages within a larger area of abnormal signal intensity but these can also be present in those infants without subsequent cystic evolution (Schouman-Claeys *et al.* 1993; van Wezel-Meijler *et al.* 1998). Cysts are sometimes seen at an earlier stage, with more anatomical detail and can be more numerous and extensive than seen on ultrasound (Sie *et al.* 2000). Petechial or more extensive hemorrhages within the areas recognized as 'flares' on ultrasound were present in 50% of their 50 infants studied using early MRI. Early detection of the diffuse component of PVL can possibly be detected at a very early stage using diffusion-weighted MRI. Inder *et al.* (1999a) reported one case who showed marked restriction of water diffusion on day 5 in the absence of abnormal signal on conventional MRI and without increased echogenicity on ultrasound. The infant went on to develop extensive cystic PVL. The same group was also able to show the postmigrational development of polymicrogyria by performing MRI at 31 and at 40 weeks postmenstrual age in an infant with cystic PVL (Inder *et al.* 1999b). In the infants with localized cysts, neonatal MRI tended to show more extensive changes in signal intensity throughout the periventricular white matter and MRI performed during the second year of life showed more extensive gliosis than would be expected on the basis of the few localized cysts seen in the neonatal period (de Vries *et al.* 1993).

Recent MRI studies have also shed some light on the significance of identifying transient echodensities on ultrasound. Van Wezel-Meijler *et al.* (1998) showed a strong positive correlation between presence of echodensities on ultrasound and the degree of signal change of the periventricular white matter on MRI, suggesting that echodensities on ultrasound and signal intensity changes in the periventricular white matter on MRI are due to the same lesion. Signal changes were often still present on MRI following disappearance on ultrasound and sometimes these were more extensive than the echodensities had been. In a small number of cases signal changes were seen on MRI in the absence of (previous) echodensities on ultrasound, suggesting that MRI is more sensitive than ultrasound. Follow-up of these 42 infants until 12 months corrected age (van Wezel-Meijler *et al.* 1999) showed that abnormalities found with both imaging techniques were associated with a high incidence of transient motor problems during infancy. It was of interest, however, that the degree of echogenicity had the highest predictive value, compared with duration of the echodensities and signal changes on MRI. A recent study by Maalouf *et al.* (1999) showed that a large number of infants with a gestational age below 30 weeks (22/29) have diffuse and excessive high signal intensity in the white matter (DEHSI) on T2-weighted images at term. This was commonly associated with the development of cerebral atrophy, a sign suggestive of white matter disease.

### Magnetic resonance spectroscopy (see Ch. 10)

This has been shown to be of value in predicting the importance of these early echodensities. Hamilton *et al.* (1986) showed that all infants with periventricular echodensity who had a PCr/Pi ratio below the normal range either died or developed extensive cystic lesions, while most of those with normal ratios did not develop extensive cystic lesions (page 142). Groenendaal *et al.* (1997) studied 19 infants with cystic PVL, using proton magnetic resonance spectroscopy and were able to show that this test predicted neurodevelopmental outcome (Fig. 22.10). *N*-acetyl aspartate:choline ratios significantly related to the grade of PVL and also showed a correlation with developmental quotients at 12 months or more.

### Neurophysiology

Other techniques have recently become available to aid early prediction as to the significance of these areas of increased echogenicity. Connell *et al.* (1987) used continuous 24-hour, four-channel EEG recordings and noted marked abnormalities (seizures, low amplitude) in those infants who had densities that subsequently evolved into extensive cystic lesions, while the EEG findings of those with transient periventricular densities and subsequently normal development were normal (page 167). The importance of positive Rolandic

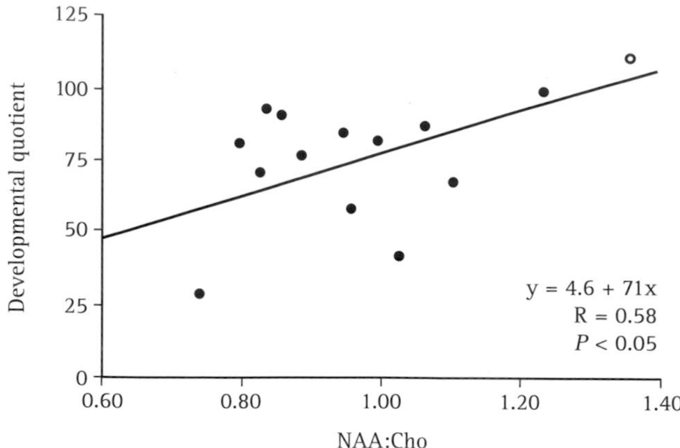


**Figure 22.10** Correlation between developmental quotients and NAA:Cho ratio in 15 preterm infants with cystic PVL, studied using proton magnetic resonance spectroscopy at 40 weeks postmenstrual age. ○, normal; ● handicap. (Reproduced with permission from *Dev Med Child Neurol* 39: 1997; Groenendaal *et al.* Fig. 3).

sharp waves has been recognized by several groups (Marret *et al.* 1992, 1997; Baud *et al.* 1998b; Okumura *et al.* 1999b). A recent retrospective study by Baud *et al.* (1998b) showed the presence of positive Rolandic sharp waves to be very specific markers of PVL. The sensitivity was, however, only 32.4% for the less mature infants (<28 weeks gestation) compared to 87.8% for those with a gestational age between 28 and 32 weeks, with a specificity of 100% and 99.8% respectively. The value of evoked responses is discussed in detail in Chapter 12. Abnormalities of both visual as well as somatosensory evoked potentials are still of limited value in the infants with PVL (de Vries *et al.* 1987; Pierrat *et al.* 1993; Ekert *et al.* 1997). Visual evoked responses and somatosensory evoked potentials performed at 40 weeks of postmenstrual age were, however, absent in infants having subcortical lesions, and EEG recordings were severely abnormal in the acute stages. Abnormalities were still present at 40 weeks in infants with subcortical leukomalacia, while abnormalities seen in the infants with PVL were only present in the acute phase, with complete recovery at 40 weeks of postmenstrual age in most infants.

## OUTCOME

In the 1980s there were many follow-up studies of infants who had developed GMH–IVH in the neonatal period (Thorburn *et al.* 1981; Catto-Smith *et al.* 1985). These studies suggested that the size of the hemorrhages and the presence of ventricular dilatation were of prognostic significance (Palmer *et al.* 1982; Stewart *et al.* 1983). Ultrasound examinations were often still performed with linear array equipment utilizing a 5 or 3.5 MHz transducer. It is therefore likely that cases of PVL were missed, or that densities seen in the acute phase were interpreted as parenchymal hemorrhages. Stewart *et al.* (1983) stressed the predictive value of cerebral atrophy, diagnosed when irregular ventricular dilatation was noted in association with normal or delayed head growth. They assumed this to be due to ischemia and cerebral infarction. De Vries *et al.* (1985a) were the first to compare the neurodevelopmental outcome of infants with a large IVH (with or without intraparenchymal involvement) with infants who developed extensive cystic PVL. At early follow-up (9–24 months) they noted that 43% of the infants with large hemorrhages were functioning at a normal level, compared with none of those with extensive cystic lesions. Only 3 of the 23 infants with large hemorrhages, who also showed associated ischemic lesions on their ultrasound scans, were severely handicapped with quadriplegia and severe mental retardation. The presence of ischemic lesions was thus of more predictive value than the size of the hemorrhage.

At present follow-up studies dealing with PVL can be divided into three main categories:

- Reports of infants with the ultrasound diagnosis of (cystic) PVL with the inherent variation in the definition of the condition.
- Populations of preterm infants in which attempts are made to identify specific ultrasound abnormalities with outcome. In these studies there are often uncertainties about both the quality of the imaging as well as the number of scans performed.
- Selection of ex-preterm infants with established spastic diplegia in whom the diagnosis of PVL is made by MRI in childhood (Fig. 22.11).

### Extensive cystic leukomalacia

*CATEGORY 1* The number of infants in the this category are usually small (Bowerman *et al.* 1984; Bozynski *et al.* 1985; Weindling *et al.* 1985b; Calvert *et al.* 1986; Rogers *et al.* 1994). Most infants developed cerebral palsy, with or without associated seizures, visual impairment, and a variable degree of mental retardation. Rogers *et al.* (1994) performed measurements of the periventricular region where the cysts were seen and found the antero-posterior extent on parasagittal view, a measurement that helped to predict the type and severity of motor and cognitive disabilities. Bilateral cystic PVL with a width of greater than 2 cm was always associated with the development of quadriplegia.

In four other studies, infants with PVL were studied and follow-up data reported. Monset-Couchard *et al.* (1988) studied 30 infants with a spectrum of cystic PVL. While 8 out of 11 infants with minor cystic lesions were normal at follow-up, all infants with severe cystic lesions had neurologic sequelae. Cases including posterior lesions or presenting solely with such lesions had a worse outcome. Fazzi *et al.* (1994) described neurodevelopmental outcome at 5–7 years in 37 infants with PVL. All infants with large cysts

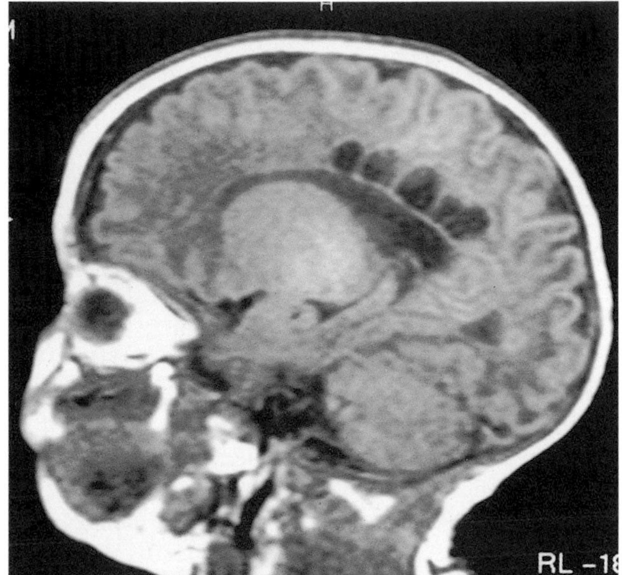


A

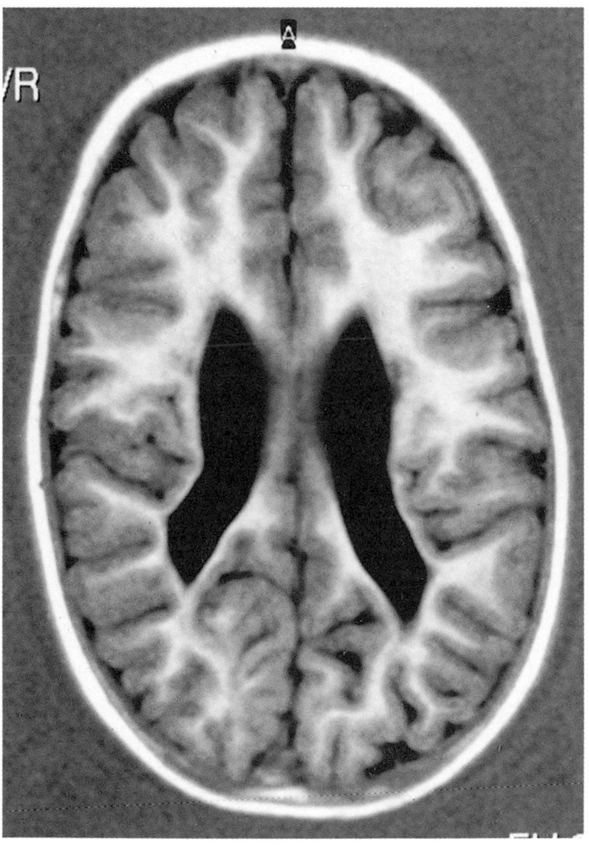


B

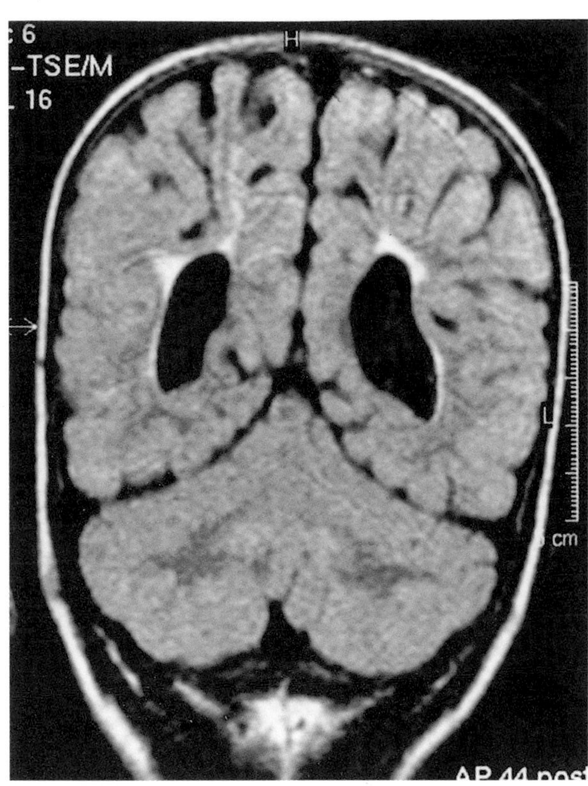


C

**Figure 22.11** MR scan at 40 weeks postmenstrual age of a child who developed extensive cystic PVL following a necrotizing enterocolitis. (**A**) A T1-weighted sequence shows multiple cysts separate from the lateral ventricle on this parasagittal view. A repeat MR scan was done at 20 months. (**B**) The inversion recovery scan at mid-ventricular level shows delay in myelination, particularly around the irregularly dilated occipital horns. (**C**) The FLAIR sequence shows moderate irregular ventricular dilatation and high signal intensity suggestive of gliosis.

(>5 mm) developed cerebral palsy, compared with 2 out of 11 with small cysts. A further 7 had mild neurologic signs. Prognosis was related to site and number of cysts. They also noted that the cognitive profiles were disharmonic, with a better verbal than performance IQ.

The study of Fujimoto *et al.* (1994b) is one of the few not to find either the size or the site of the cysts as predicting the development of cerebral palsy. They studied 24 infants (25–37 weeks gestation) with cystic-PVL, 14 with symmetrical parieto-occipital cysts, and 10 with asymmetrical cysts. Those with symmetrical cysts all developed cerebral palsy compared with 60% of those with asymmetrical cysts.

Bennett *et al.* (1990) were unable to confirm the predictive value of cystic lesions. Only 4 out of 15 (26.7%) infants with cystic PVL developed cerebral palsy compared with 4 out of

9 infants (44.4%) with severe intracranial hemorrhage. Their data may be criticized, as infants having localized cystic lesions were grouped together with infants having extensive cysts.

*CATEGORY 2* These are largely population based studies (Graziani *et al.* 1987; Graham *et al.* 1987; Zorzi *et al.* 1988; Bennett *et al.* 1990; Pidcock *et al.* 1990; Fazzi *et al.* 1992). Graham *et al.* (1987) described the correlation between ultrasound findings and neurodevelopmental outcome at 18 months in 156 survivors of a cohort of infants each weighing 1500 g or less. All infants with PVH alone or GMH–IVH confined to the lateral ventricle were normal at follow-up. The presence of cysts accurately predicted abnormal outcome (94%) and was highly specific (96%). Of the 12 infants with cerebral palsy, 10 had ultrasound evidence of PVL. No infants with cysts confined to the frontal region or the centrum semiovale developed cerebral palsy, while cysts in the occipital region were always associated with a poor outcome.

Zorzi *et al.* (1988) studied 154 preterm infants of 32 weeks or less. Of these, 24 (15.5%) had intraparenchymal cystic lesions related to intraparenchymal hemorrhage in 8 cases and to PVL in a further 16 cases. The 8 infants with one large cyst developed cerebral palsy, and a severe deficit was present in 4 of them. All infants with extensive cystic PVL developed cerebral palsy, while 1 out of 4 with localized cystic PVL and 3 out of 4 with unilateral localized cystic PVL were normal at follow-up. The site of the cystic lesions was taken into account, and cysts were present in the occipital region in the majority of the infants studied.

Pidcock *et al.* (1990) studied 127 infants of 32 weeks or less who had some degree of periventricular echodensity, classified as mild, moderate, or severe. The evolution of cysts was also taken into account and cysts were divided into three groups, depending on their size. Of the 127 infants, 26 developed cerebral palsy and all had cystic lesions. In 8 infants, moderate to severe periventricular echodensity with cysts of less than 2 mm were present, and in the other 18, cysts were over 3 mm in size. It is of interest that 19 out of 36 infants with cystic lesions did not develop cerebral palsy, and in 5 of these 19 infants cystic lesions were large. These authors explained that the absence of cerebral palsy in these infants was related to the site of the cysts, being either anterior or posterior to the caudothalamic notch, suggesting sparing of the corticospinal tracts. The absence of cerebral palsy in the presence of diffuse cysts had been previously noted by the same group in three infants (Graziani *et al.* 1987).

Pinto-Martin *et al.* (1995) published 2-year follow-up data of 777 infants each weighing 501–2000 g. They found brain lesions diagnosed by ultrasound to be powerful predictors of cerebral palsy, especially the disabling form. Parenchymal echolucencies and ventricular enlargement were the most powerful predictors in a multivariate logistic regression analysis (OR 15.4, 95% CI 7.6–31.1) but the presence of a GMH–IVH also carried a risk (OR 3.5, 95% CI 1.7–6.9). This study can however be criticized, as only 47% of their cases had an ultrasound examination beyond the first week of life and no information is given about the type of transducer used.

*CATEGORY 3* An increasing number of recent follow-up studies have selected babies on the basis of their history (preterm birth) and the type of cerebral palsy (spastic diplegia). A relation between abnormalities and sensorimotor outcome has been established, often with special attention to visuo-perceptual impairment. Koeda & Takeshita (1992) reported that the volume of the peritrigonal white matter of the parietal and occipital lobes was significantly correlated with visuo-perceptual impairment in diplegic children following preterm delivery. Goto *et al.* (1994) found thinning of the parietal and/or occipital white matter in diplegic children with visuo-spatial cognitive deficit. Ito *et al.* (1996) measured the ratio of the areas of the posterior horns to the anterior horns and found a negative correlation with visuo-perceptual ability. Fedrizzi *et al.* (1996) performed MRI in 30 children with spastic diplegia, when they were 6–14 years old. They studied the relation between the pattern of cognitive impairment and their MRI features. They noted a significant difference between verbal and performance IQ, indicating a specific failure in the visuo-spatial function, as indeed they had shown previously at 3 years of age (Fedrizzi 1993). The severity of abnormalities on MRI (ventricular dilatation, white matter reduction or involvement and thinning of the posterior part of the corpus callosum) correlated with the full scale and performance IQ but not with the verbal IQ. Several other studies (Cioni *et al.* 1997a) also found a strong correlation between the degree of MRI abnormalities and sensorimotor outcome. Melhem *et al.* (2000) showed a significant association between lateral ventricular volumes and the degree of motor and cognitive impairment. Only Yokochi *et al.* (1991) reported that neither the degree of ventricular dilatation nor the amount of white matter loss correlated with the degree of mental impairment.

The works of Marin-Padilla (1997) and Inder *et al.* (1999a) have helped to foster a better understanding of the cognitive problems that arise following damage to the white matter, by showing that destruction of axonic fibers can cause input deprivation and output isolation on the overlying gray matter, thus affecting its subsequent development. The gray matter 'survives' but is deprived of incoming inputs (corticopetal fibers) and is unable to establish connections with distant cortical regions (cortico-fugal fiber destruction). This can result in *ex vacuo* dilatation due to antero- and retrograde degeneration of damaged axis cylinders, causing a generalized reduction of white matter fibers. Inder *et al.* (1999b) used a quantitative three-dimensional volumetric MRI technique and were able to show a reduction in cortical gray matter volume at term.

Performing MRI later in infancy has led to two interesting observations. Iai *et al.* (1994) measured several ratios of the corpus callosum in 43 infants with spastic diplegia and found a significant correlation between the ratio of the thickness of the splenium to the length of the corpus callosum and the level of motor impairment. Yokochi (1997) performed MRI in 44 preterm infants with spastic cerebral palsy. All had changes on MRI compatible with PVL. In 22 of these infants, abnormalities were seen in the pulvinar (posterior part of the thalamus) and the posterior part of the internal capsule in addition to the abnormalities in the periventricular white matter. The gestational age at delivery of these infants had been significantly greater compared with those not having thalamic involvement. Mental retardation and paroxysmal ocular downward deviation were also more common in these infants.

### Transient periventricular echodensities

The outcome of infants with transient periventricular echodensities has so far been reported in only a few studies (McMenamin *et al.* 1984; de Vries *et al.* 1988c; Appleton *et al.* 1990; Levene *et al.* 1992; Ringelberg and van de Bor 1993; Fazzi *et al.* 1994). Dammann & Leviton (1997) reviewed the studies that mentioned transient densities and proposed to make a distinction between brief flares (1–6 days), intermediate flares (7–13 days) and prolonged flares (14 or more days). The exact duration of flares will, however, not always be known as this requires sequential scans after the first week of life. In the study of McMenamin *et al.* (1984), 32 infants with small intraparenchymal echodensities were studied. These were bilateral in 50% of the cases. A total of 22 infants survived, and small cysts developed in only 3 infants. In 14 of them the outcome was normal, 6 showed mild deficits, 2 moderate deficits, and none was severely handicapped. De Vries *et al.* (1988c) studied 59 infants with transient periventricular echodensities. The neurodevelopmental outcome of 53 of these infants was compared with 92 infants with normal ultrasound scans. Four of the 53 infants with periventricular echodensities developed spastic diplegia and 24 developed transient dystonia, whereas only 8 of the 92 infants with normal ultrasound scans demonstrated this finding ($p < 0.001$) (Fig. 22.12). The persistence of the echodensities was important, as it was noted that densities remaining for more than 10 days were most likely to be associated with subsequent problems. The site of the densities was also important, as both infants with densities in the trigone were noted to develop cerebral palsy. When re-examining 44 of these infants at the age of 6 years and comparing them to 62 infants with normal ultrasound scans, no differences in cognitive abilities were found between the groups, but the results of standardized motor assessment showed that performance decreased significantly with increasing duration of periventricular densities (Jongmans *et al.* 1993). Fawer *et al.* (1987) studied 24 infants with PVL, 5 of whom had densities present for more than 2 weeks without subsequent evolution into cystic lesions. Three of these infants with frontal densities were found to be normal at follow-up while the other two infants who were noted to have densities in the frontoparietal or frontoparieto-occipital white matter developed spastic diplegia. In a subsequent study by Fawer & Calame (1991), children were assessed at 5 years of age. Children with small focal PVL (tiny cysts or persistent echodensities) had lower cognitive abilities on the McCarthy scale and were noted to have more abnormal neuromotor signs and more attention deficits when compared with children giving normal scans or having isolated hemorrhage.

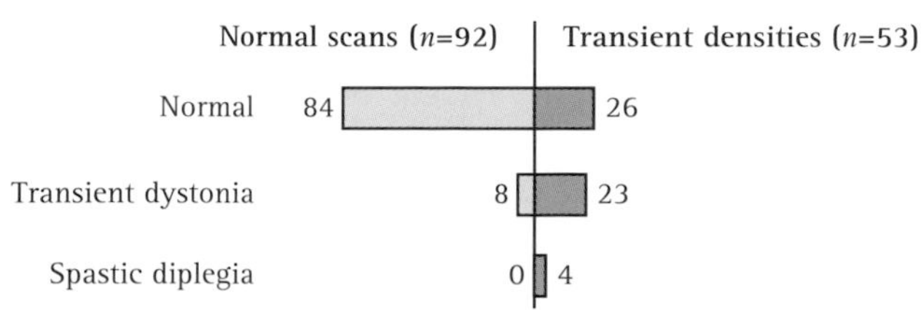


**Figure 22.12** Neurodevelopmental outcome of infants without ultrasound abnormalities and infants with transient periventricular echodensities.

Similar data were collected by Appleton *et al.* (1990), who looked at the neurodevelopmental outcome of 15 infants who had periventricular echodensities in the absence of associated IVH. At follow-up, 4 infants had neurologic abnormalities (spastic diplegia in 2 infants with densities persisting for 21 and 35 days, respectively). On the other hand, Pidcock *et al.* (1990), using a 5 or 7.5 MHz transducer, were unable to confirm this: none of their infants with mild, moderate or severe echodensities, who did not develop cystic lesions, developed cerebral palsy. In another follow-up study of VLBW infants at 5 years, the presence of transient periventricular echodensities (referred to as prolonged flare) on the neonatal scans predicted motor impairment (clumsiness), but only when GMH–IVH occurred in the same baby (Levene *et al.* 1992). In the group of infants studied by Ringelberg & van de Bor (1993) only 10 infants with flares persisting beyond the first week of life were included and 1 of these (10%) developed cerebral palsy. Fazzi *et al.* (1994) studied 12 infants with ‘prolonged flares’, which they defined as present for more than 14 days. Of these, 6 developed cerebral palsy, 4 had mild neurologic signs, and only 2 were normal. It is possible that the long duration of the flares explains the high incidence of cerebral palsy in this study. Aziz *et al.* (1995) were unable to find a distinction between the outcome of infants with transient parenchymal echodensities and those who went on to develop cysts. Their infants were scanned with a 5 or 7.5 MHz transducer and it can therefore not be excluded that some of their cystic cases, if scanned with a 5 MHz transducer, were missed. As in the previous study, 50% of their cases with transient densities developed cerebral palsy.

De Vries *et al.* (1993) reported MRI data of 15 infants with PVL, diagnosed using cranial ultrasound in the neonatal period, who all developed cerebral palsy, of whom 6 had extensive cystic PVL, and none was able to walk. Four infants had localized small cysts in the frontoparietal periventricular white matter and one of them was walking independently. Five had transient periventricular echodensities and three learned to walk at 20 and 26 months, respectively. All infants with extensive cystic PVL on neonatal ultrasound had an irregular ventricular enlargement, a decrease in peritrigonal white matter and extensive gliosis as shown by MRI. In the other two groups, gliosis was present in all, but tended to be less extensive, especially in those with transient periventricular echodensities only. Ventricular enlargement was present in only one of the five infants with transient echodensities on ultrasound. When comparing the MRI data with the initial ultrasound data, there was, in general, good agreement between neonatal ultrasound data and later changes on MRI, but in some cases extensive MRI abnormalities were seen in spite of apparently localized abnormalities on cranial ultrasound (Fig. 22.13). Van Wezel-Meijer *et al.* (1999) performed both neonatal MRI scans and repeats at 12 months corrected age in a group of infants with transient densities on ultrasound. Transient tone abnormalities during the first year were common, but none developed cerebral palsy. On the repeat MRI scan at 1 year corrected age, gliosis was noted in 10 infants. The lack of cerebral palsy cases can probably be explained by the fact that infants with severe and inhomogeneous echodensities were not eligible for this study.

A

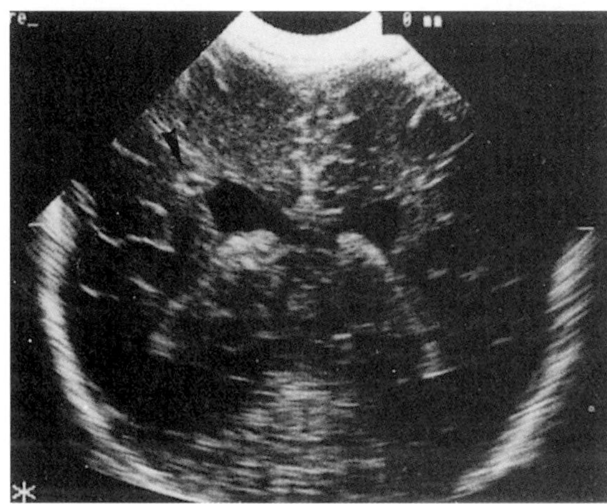

B

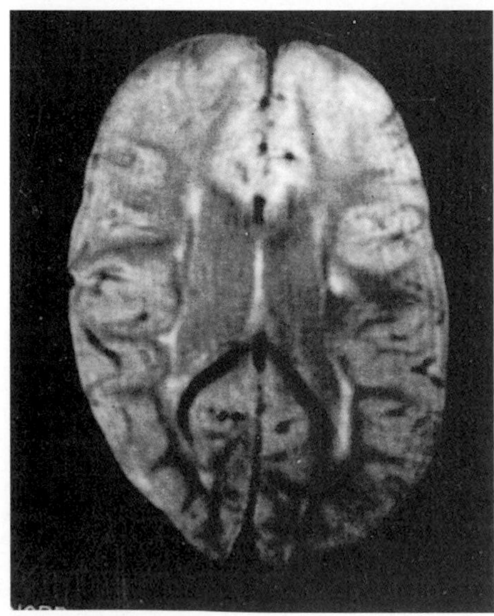

Figure 22.13 Localized cystic PVL. (A) Coronal ultrasound scan showing a localized cystic lesion on the right (arrowhead). (B) MRI scan of the same infant at 12 months of age showing on a short T2 sequence ventricular enlargement and bilateral periventricular areas of increased signal intensity suggestive of gliosis. (Reproduced, with permission, from de Vries *et al.* 1993.)

Bos *et al.* (1998) combined ultrasound data with general movement studies and noted the latter to be of better predictive value, especially when these abnormal general movements persisted for longer.

All these studies would imply that transient periventricular echodensity or non-cavitating parenchymal densities is less predictive, but they should not be disregarded as they probably represent mild PVL.

### Ventriculomegaly

Ventriculomegaly or ventricular enlargement should be mentioned as a separate entity. This finding can be seen in the absence of excessive head growth and has therefore also been referred to *ex vacuo* dilatation, related to a decrease in white matter. This phenomenon appears to be especially common in the less mature premature infants without any preceding GMH–IVH or transient echodensities. Leviton & Gilles (1996) reviewed this condition and hypothesized that this is a well recognized form of 'neonatal white matter disease'. Diffuse astrocytosis is recognized at post-mortem, poor head growth and delayed myelination on MRI is seen in survivors. They relate these findings to oligodendrocyte demise and dysfunction.

Several follow-up studies have found that ventriculomegaly is associated with a poor outcome. Whitaker *et al.* (1996) noted a poorer cognitive function at 6 years of age in those with ventriculomegaly and parenchymal involvement. Ventriculomegaly was recently identified as the most important predictor for a IQ of less than 70 (OR 19; 95% CI 4.5–80.6) by Ment *et al.* (1999). They did not find an association with PVL, but this condition had a very low incidence in their population.

### Cerebral visual impairment (see also Chapter 38)

Several groups have paid special attention to associated visual impairment (de Vries *et al.* 1985, 1987; Calvert *et al.* 1986; Scher *et al.* 1989; Gibson *et al.* 1990; Eken *et al.* 1994; Fedrizzi *et al.* 1996; Jacobsen *et al.* 1996; Cioni *et al.* 1997b). Of the 15 infants with extensive cystic PVL reported by Calvert *et al.* (1986), 8 had associated visual problems; 6 had bilateral squints, 1 was blind and 1 had severe visual impairment. Scher *et al.* (1989) reported longitudinal data on visual acuity, visual field, and motor development in 10 infants with leukomalacia, non-cystic in 9 and cystic in 1. The diagnosis was made using CT or MRI in 9 and using ultrasound in only 1. Low visual acuity was found in 2 infants, 1 with cystic lesions and in 1 with non-cystic PVL.

Reduced visual fields were also noted in 2 out of 6 infants tested at 72 weeks of age. Gibson *et al.* (1990) found that 7 of the 14 infants with cystic PVL developed squints, including 70% of those with occipital cystic lesions. In a prospective longitudinal study of 51 preterm infants, Eken *et al.* (1994) have again noted the risk of associated visual impairment in infants with cystic leukomalacia. No ultrasound abnormalities were present in 18 infants: 17 had a variety of GMH–IVH and 16 had PVL (non-cystic in 5). From 40 weeks of postmenstrual age until 18 months of age, visual acuity and visual evoked potentials were performed at regular intervals. None of the infants without ultrasound abnormalities or with GMH–IVH had impaired visual acuity beyond 3 months of corrected age. Impaired visual acuity was noted only in infants with extensive cystic PVL. Of the 11 infants with cystic lesions, acuity estimates were unrecordable or more than one octave below the tenth centile in 4 children and on the tenth centile in 3. The visual problems were especially severe in the more mature preterm infants (35–37 weeks of gestation) with cysts extending into the deep white matter. The authors stress the importance of early visual testing, as this enables us to identify infants with visual impairment at an early age. When these children were tested again at 5½ years of age, none of the 7 with cerebral visual impairment at 18 months had improved. Good correlations were found both for visual acuity as well as cognition for the whole group (van den Hout *et al.* 1998).

Cioni *et al.* (1997b) investigated visual outcome in 96 preterm infants who either had a normal ultrasound scan (18 cases) prolonged transient echodensities (34 infants) or severe cystic-PVL (44 infants). MRI was available in 12 of the cystic-PVL cases, 6 of the moderate PVL group and none of the controls. They found a high incidence of cerebral visual impairment, consisting mainly of low visual acuity, severe oculomotor disorders and reduced visual field in the infants with cystic PVL. These findings were less common in the moderate PVL group. Abnormalities of the optic radiation on MRI correlated with visual outcome (specificity 82%, sensitivity 69%). MRI abnormalities in the visual cortex were highly specific (100%) but had a very low sensitivity (15%). A very similar study was performed in 38 preterm infants by Lanzi *et al.* (1998). Cerebral visual impairment was present in 66% of these infants and once again there was a good correlation between the degree of visual impairment and abnormalities on MRI, consisting mainly of an abnormal MR signal in the optic radiation and atrophy of the calcarine cortex in the most severe cases. In 6 of the 9 blind patients optic atrophy was also noted. In an earlier study they also noted abnormalities in the lateral geniculate body in 2 of their blind cases (Uggetti *et al.* 1996).

### Subcortical leukomalacia

Leech *et al.* first reported in 1974 that white matter lesions can extend into the deep white matter. Involvement of the subcortical white matter appears to be more common in neonates with a gestational age above 34 weeks. This is supported by post-mortem angiography studies by Takashima *et al.* (1978) who showed a triangular, watershed area at the depth of the sulci in the full-term infant (Fig. 22.14). The development of extensive cystic lesions in the subcortical white matter is not at all common (Fig. 22.15)

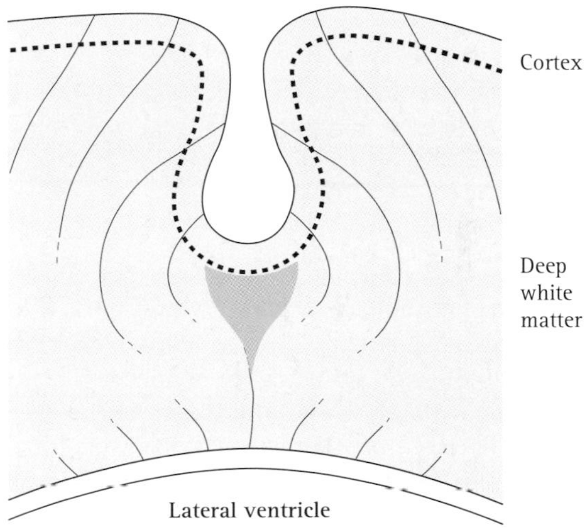


Figure 22.14 A coronal section through cortex, white matter and lateral ventricle. There is a watershed area of subcortical white matter (stippled) exposed to ischemic injury. (Redrawn from Takashima *et al.* 1978 © American Medical Society.)

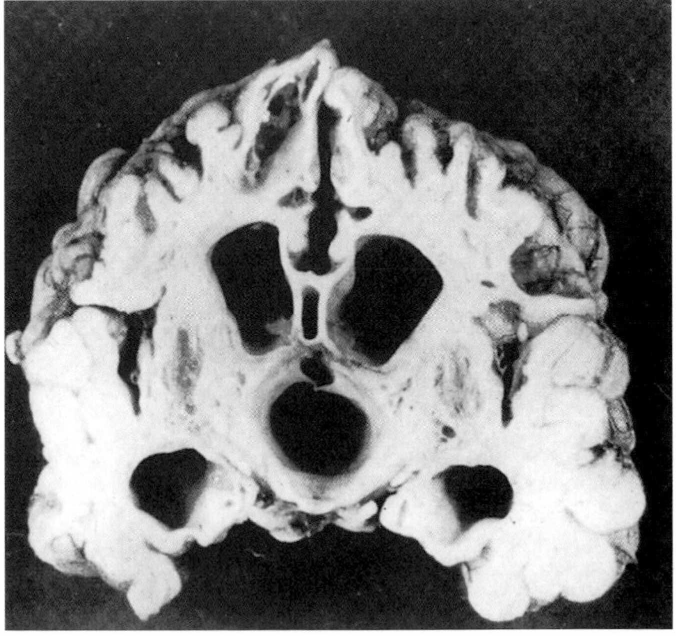

Figure 22.15 Cystic subcortical leukomalacia. There is an irregular cavity in the subcortical region on the left side.

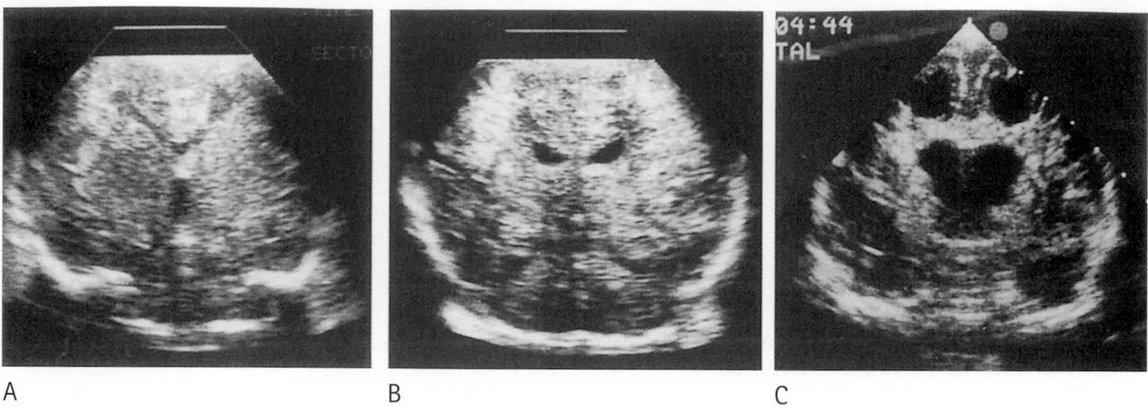


Figure 22.16 Evolution of subcortical leukomalacia on ultrasound scans. (A) Coronal scan showing a 'fuzzy' brain with slit-like ventricles. (B) Same infant 5 days later showing increased echodensity around the lateral ventricles. (C) Scan at 7 months of age showing multiple subcortical cysts and ventricular dilatation.

and in its most extensive form may be described as multicystic leukoencephalomalacia (MCLE) which is discussed on p. 478. The appearance of these cystic lesions was first shown in living infants using pneumoencephalography by Taboada *et al.* (1980), who found rounded dilated lateral and third ventricles in nine microcephalic infants. In an attempt to explain the apparent conservation of the thickness of the cerebral parenchyma they performed pneumoencephalographic studies, needling the anterior fontanelle. Using this method they were able to show separate subcortical cysts. CT scans of these infants merely showed areas of decreased attenuation and dilatation of the ventricles.

Ultrasonography can show the evolution of subcortical leukomalacia non-invasively, as was first described by Pfister-Goedeke & Boltshauser (1982). The evolution of the ultrasound changes is as follows. The cysts occur within 2–3 weeks after the insult and tend to be larger in diameter than in the infants with PVL (see Fig. 22.16). The cysts are noted to persist far beyond 40 weeks of postmenstrual age and can be recognized by ultrasonography as long as the fontanelle permits this form of examination to be performed. De Vries *et al.* (1985b, 1987) and Eken *et al.* (1994) especially noted associated visual problems in infants with extensive cystic PVL and especially in those with cysts extending into the subcortical white matter. So far, no distinction has been made between infants with lesions restricted to the periventricular white matter and infants with subcortical lesions, but as most of the studies were looking at infants with a gestational age of 32 weeks or less, the majority of the studies mentioned above would have included infants mainly with lesions in the periventricular white matter. Lutschg *et al.* (1983) reported on 8 full-term and 2 preterm infants who suffered birth asphyxia and subsequently developed subcortical leukomalacia as diagnosed by CT. All infants were hypo- or hypertonic at 3 months of age, with microcephaly in 7 and infantile spasms in 9. Trounce & Levene (1985) and de Vries *et al.* (1987) noted a marked difference between the outcome in infants with periventricular lesions and those with subcortical lesions. De Vries *et al.* (1987) noted that while eight survivors with cystic PVL all developed diplegia and a squint, quadriplegia was found in the seven survivors with cysts extending into the deep white matter. Associated problems, such as cortical blindness, microcephaly, severe mental retardation and seizures, were also commonly seen in most of the infants with subcortical lesions.

This marked difference in later outcome fitted in well with MRI findings, performed between 9 and 18 months of age. Infants with PVL showed delayed myelination, especially around the irregularly dilated occipital horns. On the short $T_2$ spin echo sequence, areas of high signal intensity, suggestive

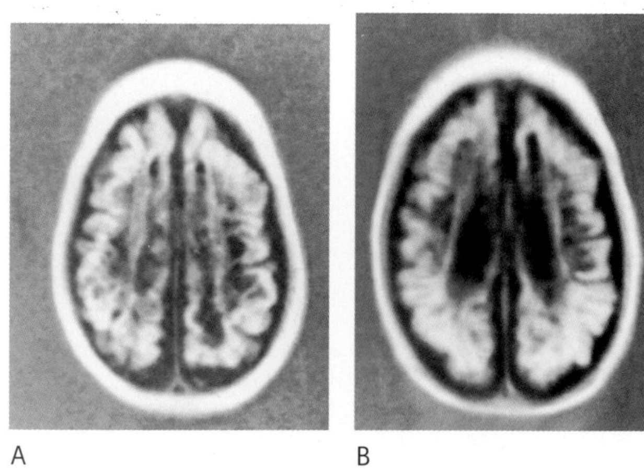


Figure 22.17 MRI scans of an infant with subcortical cystic leukomalacia (same child as illustrated in Fig. 22.10). (A) Inversion recovery at the mid-ventricular level (6 months of corrected age) showing multiple subcortical cysts. No myelination is seen. (B) Same child at 12 months at a higher level. The cysts remain visible with still no evidence of myelination.

of gliosis, were noted in areas where the cystic lesions were initially seen on cranial ultrasound (see Fig. 22.11). Subsequent scans did, however, show progression of myelination. The children with subcortical lesions, however, showed persistence of the cystic lesions and little or no myelination. There was also evidence of marked cortical atrophy, indicating that the initial lesions were much more extensive than could be visualized by ultrasonography in the neonatal period. At follow-up very little if any progression of myelination was noted (Fig. 22.17). Yokochi (1998) performed MRI in 13 children with subcortical leukomalacia and border zone infarction. Mental retardation was more marked in these cases than motor impairment, which consisted mainly of truncal swaying and ataxia.

## CEREBRAL ARTERY INFARCTION

Infarction of a major artery or a branch arising from it is now recognized in an increasing number of newborn infants. Bleeding into an infarcted area occurs relatively often and we believe that many infants previously thought to have had 'primary parenchymal hemorrhage' have in fact

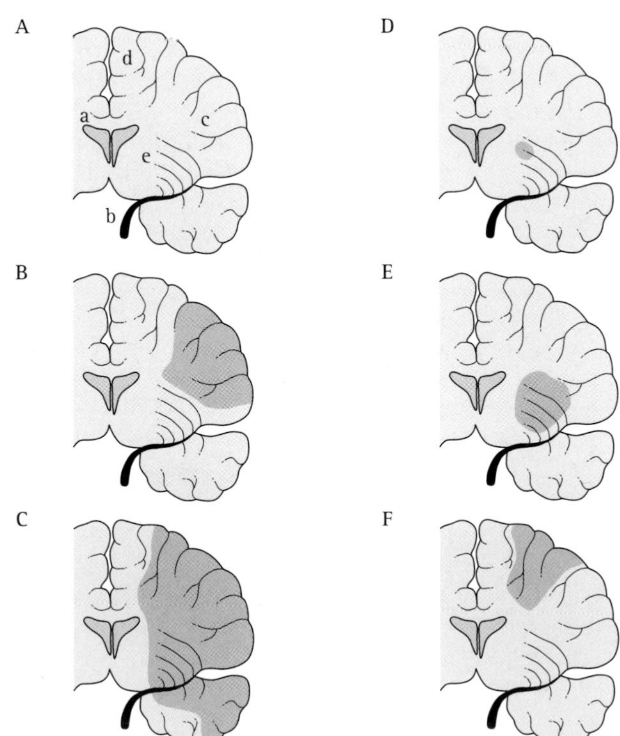


**Figure 22.18** Schematic drawing, showing (**A**) the different branches of the middle cerebral artery, with (**B**) involvement of a cortical branch; (**C**) involvement of the main branch; (**D**) involvement of one or (**E**) more lenticulostriate branches and (**F**) the boundary zone between the anterior and middle cerebral artery (Adapted from Kappelle *et al.* 1991; with permission, *Neuropediatrics* 28: 1997; de Vries *et al.*, Fig. 1 © by the Lancet Ltd).

sustained neonatal 'stroke' with secondary hemorrhage. Knowledge of this condition and use of appropriate imaging techniques should allow its differentiation.

Lesions involving the left hemisphere are three to four times more common than those of the right hemisphere. This is suggested to be due to either hemodynamic differences between right and left carotid arteries arising as the result of a patent ductus arteriosus or preferential flow of placental emboli into the left side vessels rather than the right. Middle cerebral artery infarction occurs twice as commonly as involvement of any other artery. The anterior cerebral artery is rarely recognized to be affected, but this may reflect the silent nature of symptoms related to involvement of this vessel.

Both de Vries *et al.* (1997) as well as Mercuri *et al.* (1999) used a classification according to the main artery involved. Infarcts in the territory of the middle cerebral artery were further subdivided into main branch, cortical branch, and lenticulostriate branch infarctions (Fig 22.18).

### PATHOLOGY

Cerebral infarction in the neonate has been defined as a severe disorganization or even complete disruption of both gray and white matter caused by embolic, thrombotic, or ischemic events (Barmada *et al.* 1979). Friede (1975) has reviewed the earlier pathology literature on this condition and described five cases of his own. These were all wedge shaped hemorrhagic lesions involving cortical, subcortical, and deep periventricular white matter. Friede (1975) could only positively identify these lesions as infarctive histologically.

Larroche (1977) described the pathologic appearance of cerebral artery infarction in six cases. In those infants dying in the acute stage of the condition, the hemisphere was swollen and deeply congested. There was involvement of both white matter and cortex, with secondary hemorrhagic infarction in some cases. In those infants who survived for longer, contraction of the affected area was seen with softening and multiple cystic degeneration giving a honeycomb appearance on sectioning (Fig. 22.19). The extent of the atrophic process was thought to reflect the level of arterial infarction. In some cases, infarction occurred very early in fetal life, and these brains showed extensive porencephalic cyst formation. This is discussed in more detail in Chapter 20. More recently, Aso *et al.* (1990) performed autopsies in nine cases and found that all but one of these had one or more additional lesions, such as PVL, pontosubicular necrosis, and anoxic–ischemic neuronal necrosis.

### INCIDENCE

The introduction of modern imaging techniques has confirmed the pathologist's impression that neonatal stroke occurs commonly. Over 150 cases have been reported where the diagnosis was made in life (Billard *et al.* 1982; Hill *et al.* 1983; Mannino & Trauner 1983; Mantovani & Gerber 1984; Ment *et al.* 1984; Nanni *et al.* 1984; Voorhies *et al.* 1984;

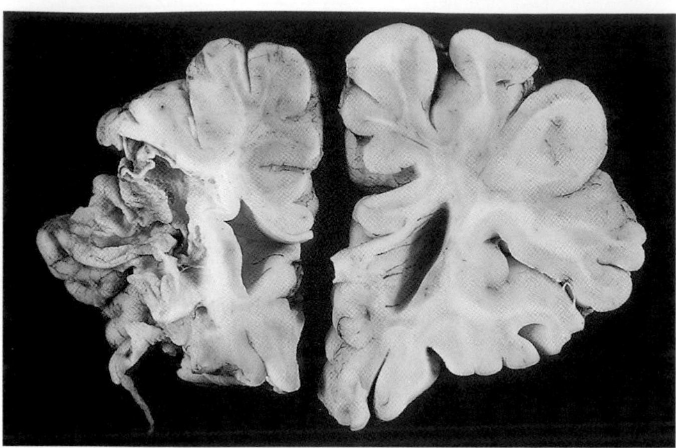

**Figure 22.19** Infarction involving cortex and white matter in the distribution of the middle cerebral artery. The infant developed following cardiac surgery and the infarction may have been due to an embolus during this procedure. (Courtesy of Dr P. Nikkels, Department of Paediatric Pathology, Utrecht.)

Clancy *et al.* 1985; Levy *et al.* 1985; Chasnoff *et al.* 1986; Trauner & Mannino 1986; Filipek *et al.* 1987; Levene 1987; Roodhooft *et al.* 1987; Wulfeck *et al.* 1991; Fujimoto *et al.* 1992; Perlman *et al.* 1994; Koelfen *et al.* 1995; Jan & Camfield 1998; de Vries *et al.* 1997; Mercuri *et al.* 1999). Data concerning the incidence are scarce and reflect the population from which the data are drawn. Barmada *et al.* (1979) reported cerebral infarction in over 5% of infants examined at *autopsy*. More recent studies have looked at newborn infants admitted to a neonatal unit with seizures and/or apneas. Lien *et al.* (1995) found a prevalence of 0.01% (1:10 000). Estan & Hope (1997) studied a 7-year cohort and reported a prevalence of 0.025% (1:4000), which is rather similar to the findings of Perlman *et al.* (1994) who found a prevalence of 0.02% (1:5000). We also estimate the incidence of 'neonatal stroke' to be 1 in 5000 full-term infants (Levene 1987). Several groups found neonatal stroke to be the second most common cause for neonatal seizures (Levy *et al.* 1985; Lien *et al.* 1995; Estan & Hope 1997). In the latter study, 49% of the infants had seizures due to hypoxic–ischemic encephalopathy and 12% due to unilateral cerebral infarction.

## TIMING OF THE INFARCTION

Neonatal stroke can occur both before, as well as in the immediate, perinatal neonatal period. Before the era of widespread use of neuroimaging techniques, it was a common belief that a prenatal stroke was more common, but at present there is little data in the literature to support this. As the infants are often well enough to go to the postnatal ward, subtle seizures, occurring during the first few days, may go unnoticed and the child may first present at 4–6 months of age with an asymmetrical grasp. Mercuri *et al.* (1995), however, showed that when the threshold to perform neonatal imaging, and in particular MRI, is low in infants with neonatal seizures, focal infarction will be identified in the majority of these infants. Using ultrasound or conventional MRI, the lesions only become apparent during the first week of life. Diffusion-weighted imaging always clearly showed the area of infarction on the initial scan. It is reported that acute diffusion-weighted changes are maximal between 1 and 5 days after the acute lesion and normalize between 1 and 2 weeks (Mercuri & Cowan 1999). These findings suggest a perinatal onset, as diffusion-weighted imaging abnormalities become less obvious within 2 weeks after the onset (Cowan *et al.* 1994).

## ETIOLOGY

Stroke in the newborn does not appear to be the same condition as seen in older children and adults. In children the most common cause of stroke is hemorrhage (either arteriovenous malformation, aneurysm, or tumor), and arterial occlusion occurs less frequently (Eeg-Olofsson & Ringheim 1983). Hemorrhagic stroke is less common in the newborn; although venous infarction due to sinus thrombosis is well recognized it is less frequently seen at autopsy than cerebral artery occlusion.

The causes of neonatal stroke fall into three groups: embolization, thrombosis, and ischemia (Mannino & Trauner 1983). Embolic causes are the most commonly reported (Barmada *et al.* 1979) and twin-to-twin transfusion as well as congenital heart disease are well recognized. Emboli arising from a patent ductus arteriosus or the placenta (Cocker *et al.* 1965) have also been reported. Temporal artery catheterization has been related to ipsilateral cerebral infarction (Bull *et al.* 1980), and disseminated intravascular coagulation and sepsis have also been associated with the development of thrombotic arterial infarction. Clancy *et al.* (1985) reported that asphyxia and polycythemia were additional important predisposing factors, and described one infant who had sustained severe and prolonged hypertension before the stroke. In a review of 24 term infants with cerebral artery infarction, none had evidence of severe acute asphyxia, but 14 had perinatal abnormalities that included abnormal CTG (continuous decelerations below 90 with slow recovery) and 11 had meconium stained liquor (Mercuri *et al.* 1999).

In some reports, infarction of watershed areas between cerebral artery vascular distributions are included with descriptions of single artery infarction (Mercuri & Cowan 1999). These watershed infarctions are most probably due to severe partial intermittent asphyxia, which is discussed in detail in Chapter 23, and are probably best considered separately from single vessel infarction.

Maternal cocaine abuse (p. 256) has also been considered to cause stroke (Chasnoff *et al.* 1986; Hoyme *et al.* 1990; Dominguez *et al.* 1991; Volpe 1992). In a study of 43 women who abused crack cocaine during pregnancy, 17% of their infants had evidence of cortical infarction (stroke) compared with only 2% of the matched control group (Heier *et al.* 1991). The teratogenic effects of cocaine are discussed in Chapter 15. Recent studies have illustrated the importance of extensive studies for an underlying coagulopathy. Especially activated protein-C resistance caused by factor V Leiden mutation, is increasingly being recognized as an underlying problem (Debus *et al.* 1998; Varelas *et al.* 1998; Thorarensen *et al.* 1997). Association with elevated maternal cardiolipin and antiphospholipid antibodies have also been occasionally reported (Silver *et al.* 1992; Akanli *et al.* 1998; de Klerk *et al.* 1997).

Adverse perinatal events were present in 11 of the 24 infants studied by Mercuri *et al.* (1999). However, none of these had a pH < 7.0 and only 5 infants had a 1 min Apgar score below 5. Other studies also did not find significant birth asphyxia among their cases (Levy *et al.* 1985; Jan *et al.* 1998; Perlman *et al.* 1994).

Although neonatal stroke is most commonly seen in full-term infants, it has also been reported in premature neonates (Barmada *et al.* 1979; de Vries *et al.* 1988d; Amato *et al.* 1990; de Vries *et al.* 1997). De Vries *et al.* (1997) have shown that middle cerebral artery infarction does occur in preterm infants, but that involvement of the main branch is less common in the preterm population, who more often present with cortical infarction or infarction of one or more lenticulostriate branches of the middle cerebral artery.

## DIAGNOSIS

Acute onset of seizures is the most common presenting feature. Billard *et al.* (1982) reported the onset of fits between 8 and 60 hours after birth in all 8 of their cases, and fits occurred in 10 out of 11 reported by Clancy *et al.* (1985). In the 16 infants studied by Mercuri *et al.* (1995), 6 presented with seizures occurring within the first 24 hours and 8 between 24 and 48 hours. In contrast, clinical seizures were only noted in 2 of the 17 preterm infants studied by de Vries *et al.* (1997). Among full-term infants presenting with seizures, cerebral infarction is recognized to be the second most common cause (Estan & Hope 1997) with hypoxic–ischemic encephalopathy being the most common one. The convulsions are usually of the focal clonic variety, but multifocal tonic or subtle seizures may all be seen. Many of the infants show no major clinical neurologic abnormality between seizures. Three of the 18 infants reported by Fujimoto *et al.* (1992) and 5 out of 16 studied by Mercuri *et al.* (1995) presented with apneas, requiring a short period of mechanical ventilation in some. In most studies, treatment with only phenobarbitone was sufficient, but among the 7 infants reported by Filipek *et al.* (1987), 5 required more than one drug to control the seizures. Infants with middle cerebral artery infarction may show asymmetry or hypotonia on early neurologic examination, but Mercuri *et al.* (1999) did not find these early neurologic abnormalities to be predictive of an adverse neurologic outcome. Infants with posterior cerebral artery infarction may develop abnormal eye signs, which later can be shown to be due to homonymous hemianopia.

### Imaging

#### Ultrasonography

Diagnosis by ultrasound is possible, but this modality is not always reliable. If hemorrhagic infarction is present the focal increased echodensity is obvious, but Hill *et al.* (1983) have reported increased echoes from non-hemorrhagic infarcted areas. Sometimes, extensive stroke may show none or relatively subtle changes on ultrasound. A wedge-shaped increase in echogenicity tends to become more apparent by the end of the first week (Fig. 22.20A). Hernanz-Schulman *et al.* (1988) noted the absence of gyral definition, absence of vascular pulsations, altered parenchymal echogenicity and territorial distribution as characteristic sonographic findings. Absence of arterial pulsations were also noted by Messer *et al.* (1991) and Perlman *et al.* (1994). Taylor (1994) however, studied 8 infants using color Doppler sonography and noted an increase in size and number of visible vessels in the periphery of the infarct, and increased mean blood flow velocity in vessels supplying or draining the infarcted areas in 4 infants. A diminished vessel size number was found in one case. Repeat studies showed the development of multiple small irregular blood vessels in the periphery of the infarct in two cases.

Although ultrasound may not always detect cerebral artery infarction in its early stages, it may be useful later when the honeycomb cystic lesions have developed. At this stage some *ex vacuo* dilatation of the ipsilateral ventricle can also be noted.

#### Computerized tomography

As the lesion extends into the cortex, its full extent can be better identified using CT or MRI (Fig. 22.20B). CT is of more value than ultrasound in establishing the diagnosis, but a normal scan within 48 hours of birth does not exclude this condition. At least two scans over 1 week are necessary before the condition can be excluded. The classic appearance is a wedge-shaped area of low attenuation with irregular margins. If bleeding occurs into the infarcted region, areas of high attenuation may be seen on CT scan examination. A mass effect may be seen due to severe edema surrounding the infarcted area. It has been reported that complete occlusion of the common or internal carotid arteries may be associated with no focal abnormalities on CT (Voorhies *et al.* 1984). The infants described in this study had all suffered very severe perinatal asphyxia and are not typical of most infants with cerebral artery infarction. Rescanning some months later shows full-thickness loss of cerebral tissue in the same distribution (Fig. 22.20C). Thalamic atrophy can also be found later during the first year and is regarded to be due to retrograde degeneration (Giroud *et al.* 1995).

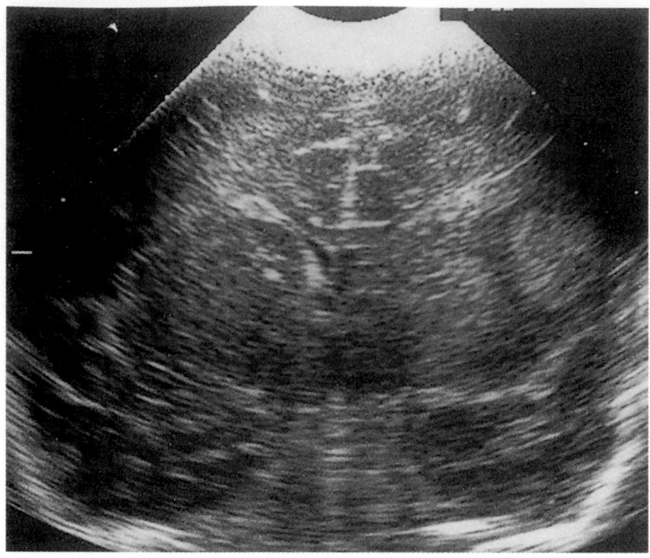

A

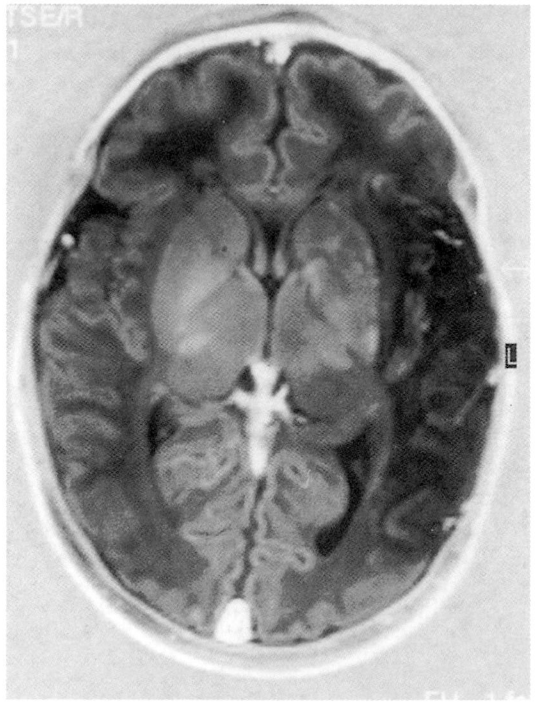

B

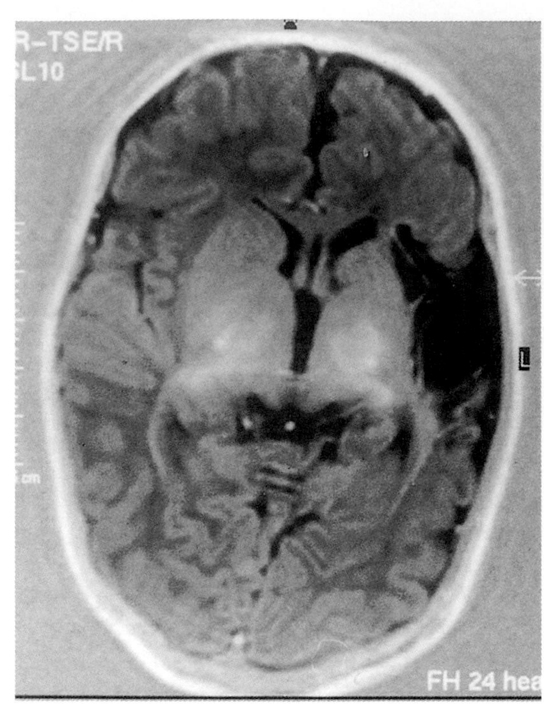

C

**Figure 22.20** Middle cerebral artery infarction in a fullterm infant. **(A)** Cranial ultrasound, coronal view, day 3, showing areas of increased echogenicity in the distribution of the main branch of the left middle cerebral artery. **(B)** MRI, IR sequence of the same infant performed on day 7, shows a large area of low signal intensity in the same region. **(C)** repeat MRI, IR sequence at 3 months of age shows cystic evolution in the affected area. Also note the absence of the normal myelination of the posterior limb on the affected side and involvement of the basal ganglia. (Reproduced, with permission, from de Vries *et al.*, *Neuropediatrics* 28: 1997; Figs 2 and 3).

### Magnetic resonance imaging

The more widespread use of MRI has been especially useful in the diagnosis of focal infarction, but some hours at least must pass before MR images can show abnormality after an acute stroke event (Mercuri & Cowan 1999). At a very early stage (24–48 hours), when CT scans or even conventional MRI may fail to detect a focal infarction, diffusion-weighted imaging does identify the lesion within hours after its onset. In diffusion-weighted MRI, image contrast depends mainly on differences in the molecular motion of water rather than changes in T1 or T2. Increases in T1 or T2 appear later and probably require the presence of vasogenic edema. Cowan *et al.* (1994) were the first to use this technique in neonatal infarction and showed that the diffusion-weighted changes were most marked on the initial scan, at a stage that the changes were not or less clearly seen on conventional MRI. Even when only conventional MR sequences are used, more anatomical detail is obtained compared with ultrasound or CT. Mercuri *et al.* (1995) reported on 16 infants with neonatal seizures who had early MRI, of whom 10 had evidence of focal infarction. Although the lesion was also identified using ultrasound in 9, MRI provided much better anatomical definition of the extent of the lesions. Focal white matter hemorrhages were found in a further 4 cases and only 2 infants presenting with seizures did not show any abnormalities on MRI. Similar data were reported by Rollins *et al.* (1994). A repeat scan can show thalamic atrophy (Giroud *et al.* 1995) and asymmetry at the level of the mesencephalon, which can be seen as early as 6 weeks after the onset (Bouza *et al.* 1994). Smith & Baumann (1991) found ipsilateral atrophy of the pons or midbrain to be strongly associated with *congenital* lesions. These changes are referred to as Wallerian degeneration due to transaxonal neuronal degeneration. Using MRI in preterm infants with unilateral thalamic echogenicities, de Vries *et al.* (1997) identified areas of focal infarction, which looked very similar to lacunar infarcts in children and adults (Fig. 22.21). These lesions occur following occlusion or spasm of one or more of the lenticulostriate branches of the middle cerebral artery.

Little data is available about focal infarction in preterm infants except for the pathologic study by Paneth *et al.* (1994), who found lesions in the thalami or basal ganglia in 17% of the post-mortem cases belonging to a cohort born in the New Jersey counties between 1984 and 1987. Performing MRI enables us to perform proton spectroscopy and MR angiography (MRA) during the same session. Groenendaal *et al.* (1995) described three infants with a middle cerebral artery and one with a posterior cerebral artery infarction. Lactate resonances were present and confined to the area of

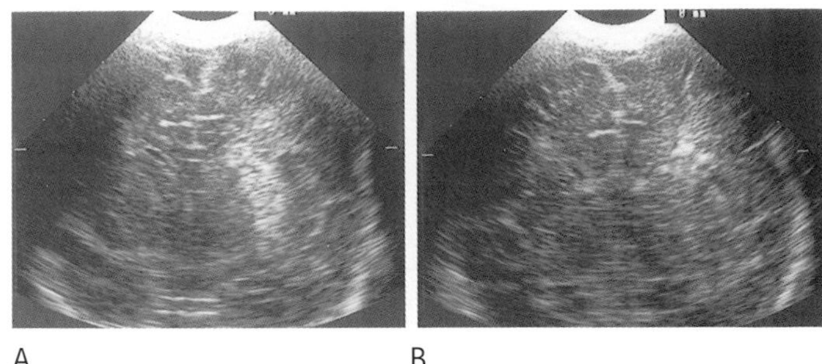

A B

**Figure 22.21** Cranial ultrasound, coronal views, showing **(A)** a giant lacunar infarction, seen as a wedge shaped echogenic area at the level of the caudate nucleus and the striate on day 1 with **(B)** associated periventricular echogenicity in a more posterior coronal view, in a monozygous twin, following the death of the co-twin at 35 weeks.

infarction in the two infants who were scanned within the first two weeks of life and in one of them lactate was still present on a repeat scan at 3 months of age. All four showed a decrease in *N*-acetyl aspartate to choline ratios in the area of infarction. MRA can sometimes show a decreased flow in the middle cerebral artery on the affected side (Fig. 22.22) which can resolve and be no longer present on a follow-up scan suggesting transient vasospasm. Koelfen *et al.* (1993)

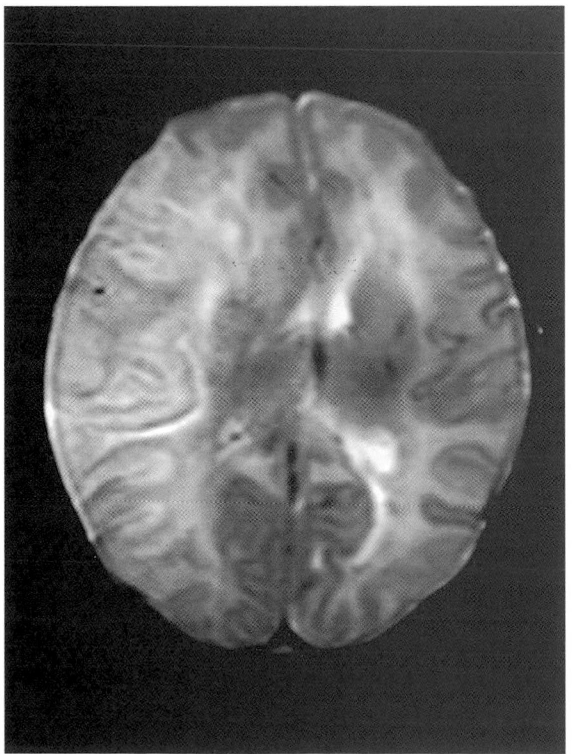

A

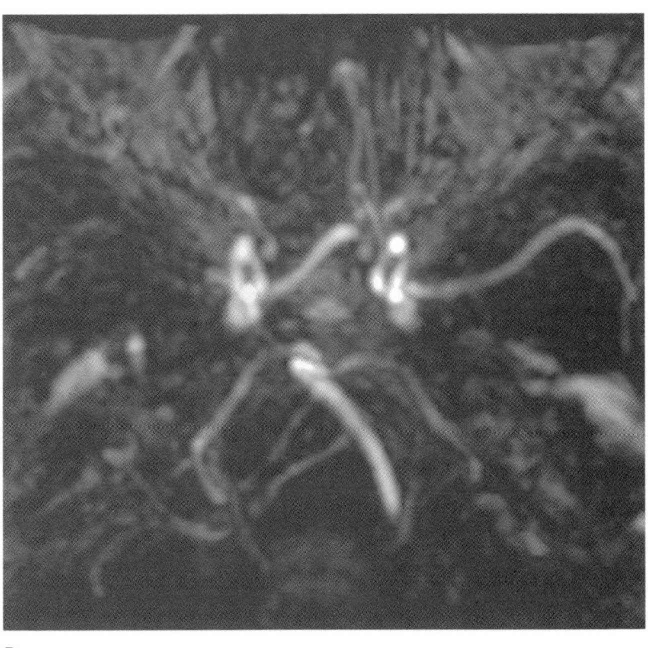

B

**Figure 22.22** Middle cerebral artery infarction in a fullterm infant. **(A)** MRI, a T2 weighted SE sequence, performed on day 7, shows increased signal intensity in the distribution of the right middle cerebral artery. **(B)** MR angiography, performed during the same examination. A difference in signal intensity is seen between the right and left middle cerebral artery, suggestive of decreased flow on the right side.

performed MRA on 8 infants with a middle cerebral artery infarct aged 1.5–8.4 years. MRA studies still showed abnormalities corresponding to the expected vascular distribution of the parenchymal lesion. MRA was normal in one case and showed a hypoplastic middle cerebral artery main stem with or without visible flow in the secondary branches in the other 7 infants.

### Radionuclide brain scanning

This is also of value in diagnosing cerebral artery infarction and is particularly useful if there is marked edema around the infarcted lesion. $\gamma$-Emitting technetium is retained only in areas of damaged blood–brain barrier and thus will delineate the area of vascular damage (Fig. 22.23). O'Brien *et al.* (1979) performed technetium scans on 85 asphyxiated full-term infants and found uptake in the region of the middle cerebral artery in 20% of cases. It has been reported that technetium brain scans may be negative in the first week following cerebral infarction (Harwood-Nash & Fitz 1976).

### Cerebral arteriography

This is a highly invasive procedure in infancy and unnecessary in most cases (Roodhooft *et al.* 1987), especially now that MRA has become more widely available. Less invasive digital intravenous angiography has been used in the diagnosis of neonatal occlusive vascular disease (Voorhies *et al.* 1984). Contrast medium is injected via an umbilical venous catheter that has been advanced to lie near the right atrium. This technique, although relatively safe, is probably not necessary, as surgical treatment to remove an embolus is not feasible.

### Electroencephalography

EEG has also been used in the diagnosis of neonatal stroke (Billard *et al.* 1982; Mantovani & Gerber 1984; Clancy *et al.* 1985; Levy *et al.* 1985; Mercuri *et al.* 1999). This investigation revealed focal abnormalities in almost all patients. These included persistent localized voltage reduction, focal slowing, sharp waves, and focal seizure activity. Mercuri *et al.* (1999) found an abnormal background pattern, even when only recorded on two channels, to be the best predictor of adverse neurologic outcome.

## PROGNOSIS

The outlook in most cases is relatively good. Spastic hemiplegia is the most important sequel, particularly following infarction of the main branch of the middle cerebral artery. Two-thirds of children with hemiplegia, however, are of normal intelligence. Homonymous hemianopia may follow posterior cerebral artery infarction. Outcome is very much dependent on the threshold to perform MRI and on the artery involved and whether the main branch is involved or only a cortical branch or one of the lenticulostriate branches. De Vries *et al.* (1997) noted that involvement of the lenticulostriate branches was more common in the preterm infants. Only 3 out of 16 infants with involvement of a cortical branch or one or more lenticulostriate branches developed cerebral palsy in contrast to all 5 survivors with main branch involvement. Govaert *et al.* (2000) recently suggested that cranial ultrasound was important in the prediction of hemiplegia. In the parasagittal view attention should be paid to involvement of the central groove, which

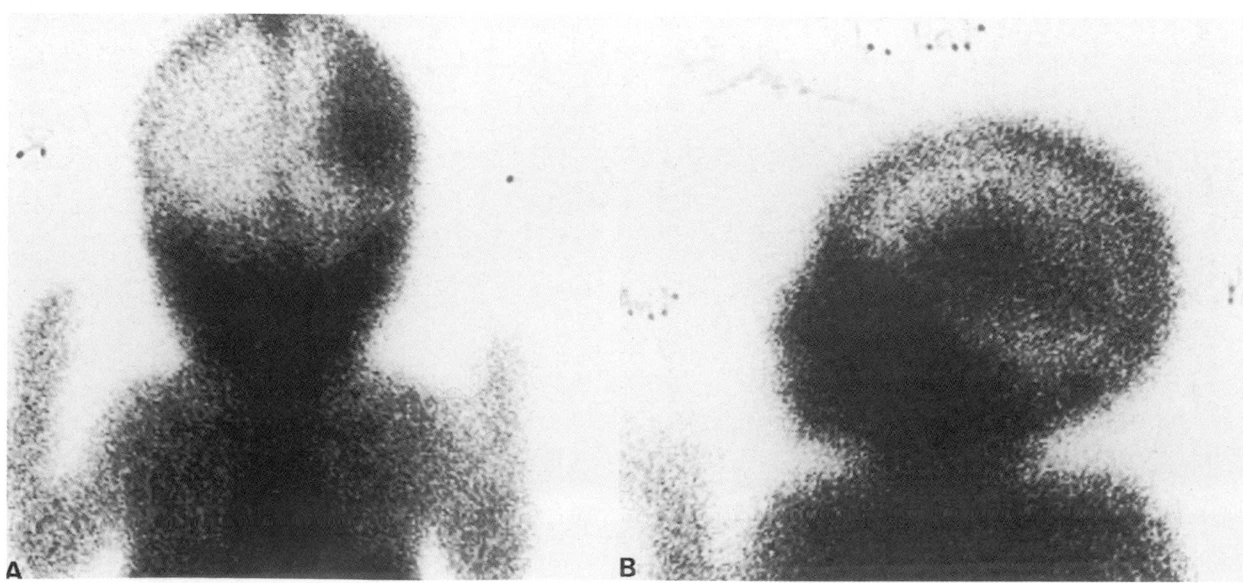


Figure 22.23 Radionuclide technetium scan of an infant with middle cerebral artery infarction. There is retention of radionuclide tracer in the region supplied by the left middle cerebral artery on (A) coronal and (B) sagittal planes.

is usually present in those with involvement of the main branch and those with involvement of the anterior trunk of the middle cerebral artery. Published follow-up data from case reports suggest that over half of all infants surviving neonatal stroke are entirely normal at 12–18 months of age. Trauner & Mannino (1986) found that 8 out of 10 infants with neonatal cerebral infarction were normal at 2–5 years. The two children in whom neurologic deficits were found were only mildly affected. In a later study, the same group (Wulfeck *et al.* 1991) reported that a hemiplegia initially noted in 11 out of 14 cases had resolved in 5 of these 11 cases by 2 years of age. A subsequent study by the same group (Trauner *et al.* 1993) noted some degree of hemiparesis in 21 of their 29 cases, but a very favorable prognosis in terms of intellectual outcome. Seizures were a common complication and occurred beyond the neonatal period in 52% of their infants.

In the study of Fujimoto *et al.* (1992) only 5 of the 28 infants (28%) developed hemiplegia and 11 of the 16 infants studied by Sran & Baumann (1988) were also making apparently normal developmental progress. In the cohort studied by Mercuri *et al.* (1999) only 5 of the 24 infants (20%) developed a hemiplegia. A further 2 had mild asymmetry and 2 had mild global delay. Only those cases with involvement of the hemisphere, basal ganglia as well the internal capsule on their first scan tended to develop a hemiplegia or an asymmetry of tone. In another report that assessed visual function, sequential studies were performed on 12 babies with focal infarction (Mercuri *et al.* 1996). A relatively high incidence of abnormalities was reported on at least one of their battery of tests.

Goodman & Graham (1996) noted that half of all children with hemiplegia have psychiatric disorders including problems with behavior, emotions, or relationships severe enough to interfere with the child's everyday life. They usually present with irritability, anxiety, and hyperactivity/inattention.

Evidence of modified organization was shown by Lewine *et al.* (1994) combining magnetoencephalography and MRI in an adult who had suffered a left-sided middle cerebral artery infarction as a neonate. Following right median nerve stimulation, activation of the left inferior temporal gyrus as well as ipsilateral right median parietal cortex was noted. Using functional MRI, more data leading to a better understanding of cortical reorganization are to be expected.

In summary and based on the estimated incidence of perinatal cerebral vascular infarction, it might be expected that this condition is the cause of the neurologic deficit in up to 20% of children with cerebral palsy (Levene 1987).

### Key Points

- PVL refers to damge of the periventricular white matter and is largely a disorder of the immature brain
- There is no generally accepted model for the pathogenesis of PVL
- Clinical risk factors for PVL include multiple gestation, chorioamnionitis, hypocarbia, hyperbilirubinemia, hypothyroxinemia and postnatal dexamethasone therapy
- Cavitating lesions seen on ultrasound imaging are highly associated with the development of cerebral palsy, visual impairment and a variable degree of learning disability
- Transient periventricular echodensity is considerably less predictive of adverse outcome, but may increase the risk of neurologic and functional impairment
- The incidence of cerebral artery infarction in the newborn is approximately 1:5000 and may occur before, during or after birth
- Important etiological factors include maternal cocaine abuse and inherited thrombophilia
- Spastic hemiplegia is the most common sequel of this condition and over 60% of affected children have normal intelligence. Homonymous hemianopia may follow posterior cerebral artery infarction

## REFERENCES


Abramovicz A (1964) The pathogenesis of perinatal brain damage and their conditions of occurrence in primates. *Adv Neurol* 27: 85–95.

Akanli L F, Trasi S S, Thuraisamy K *et al.* (1998) Neonatal middle cerebral artery infarction: association with elevated maternal anticardiolipin antibodies. *Am J Perinatol* 15: 399–402.

✪ Alexander J M, Gilstrap L C, Cox S M *et al.* (1998) Clinical chorioamnionitis and the prognosis for very low birth weight infants. *Obstet Gynecol* 91: 725–729.

Amato M, Huppi P, Herschkowitz N & Huber P (1991) Prenatal stroke suggested by intrauterine ultrasound and confirmed by magnetic resonance imaging. *Neuropediatrics* 22: 100–102.

Appleton R E, Lee R E J & Hey E N (1990) Neurodevelopmental outcome of transient neonatal intracerebral echodensities. *Arch Dis Child* 65: 27–29.

Armstrong D & Norman M G (1974) Periventricular leukomalacia in neonates: complications and sequelae. *Arch Dis Child* 49: 367–375.

Aso K, Scher M & Barmada M A (1990) Cerebral infarcts and seizures in the neonate. *J Child Neurol* 5: 224–228.

✪ Aziz K, Vickar D B, Sauve R S *et al.* (1995) Province-based study of neurologic disability of children weighing 500 through 1249 grams at birth in relation to neonatal cerebral ultrasound findings. *Pediatrics* 95: 837–844.

Baarsma R, Laurini R N, Baerts W & Okken A (1987) Reliability of sonography in non-haemorrhagic periventricular leukomalacia. *Pediatric Radiology* 17: 189–191.

✪ Back S A, Gan X, Li Y, Rosenberg P A & Volpe J J (1998) Maturation-dependent vulnerability of oligodendrocytes to oxidative stress-induced death caused by glutathione depletion. *J Neurosci* 18: 6241–6253.

✪ Baetmann M, Kahn T, Lenard H-G & Voit T (1996) Fetal CNS damage after exposure to maternal trauma during pregnancy. *Acta Paediatr* 85: 1331–1338.

Baerts W, Fetter W P F, Hop W C J *et al.* (1990) Cerebral lesions in preterm infants after tocolytic indomethacin. *Dev Med Child Neurol* 32: 910–918.

Banker B Q & Larroche J-C (1962) Periventricular leukomalacia of infancy: a form of neonatal anoxic encephalopathy. *Arch Neurol* 7: 386–410.

Barmada M A, Moossy J & Shuman R M (1979) Cerebral infarcts with arterial occlusion in neonates. *Ann Neurol* 6: 495–502.

Barth P G (1984) Prenatal clastic encephalopathies. *Clin Neurol Neurosurg* 86: 65–75.

✪ Baud O, Ville Y, Zupan V *et al.* (1998a) Are neonatal brain lesions due to intrauterine infection related to mode of delivery? *Br J Obstet Gynecol* 105: 121–124.

✪ Baud O, d'Allest A-M, Lacaze-Masmonteil T *et al.* (1998b) The early diagnosis of periventricular leukomalacia in premature infants with positive Rolandic sharp waves on serial electroencephalography. *J Pediatr* 132: 813–817.

✪ Baud O, Emilie D, Pelletier E *et al.* (1999a) Amniotic fluid concentrations of 'interleukin-1 beta, interleukin-6 and TNF-alpha in chorioamnionitis before 32 weeks of gestation: histological associations and neonatal outcome. *Br J Obstet Gynaecol* 106: 72–77.

✪ Baud O, Foix-L'Helias L, Kaminski M *et al.* (1999b) Antenatal glucocorticoid treatment and cystic periventricular leukomalacia in very premature infants *N Engl J Med* 341: 1190–1196.

Bejar R, Wozniak P, Allard M *et al.* (1988) Antenatal origin of neurologic damage in newborn infants. I. Preterm infants. *Am J Obstet Gynecol* 159: 357–363.

Bejar R, Vigliocco G, Gramajo H *et al.* (1990) Antenatal origin of neurologic damage in newborn infants. II. Multiple gestations. *Am J Obstet Gynecol* 162: 1230–1236.

Bennett F C, Silver G, Leung E J & Mack L A (1990) Periventricular echodensities detected by cranial ultrasonography: usefulness in predicting neurodevelopmental outcome in low-birth weight, preterm infants. *Pediatrics* 85: 400–404.

Billard C, Dulac O & Diebler R (1982) Ramollissement cérebral ischemique du nouveau-né: une étiologie possible des états de mal convulsifs neonatale. *Arch Françaises de Pediatrie* 39: 677–683.

✪ Bos A F, Martijn A, Okken A & Prechtl H F (1998) Quality of general movements in preterm infants with transient periventricular echodensities. *Acta Paediatrica* 87: 328–335.

✪ Bouza H, Rutherford M, Acolet D *et al.* (1994) Evolution of early hemiplegic signs in full-term infants with unilateral brain lesions in the neonatal period: a prospective study. *Neuropediatrics* 25: 201–207.

Bowerman R A, Donn S M, DiPietro M A *et al.* (1984) Periventricular leukomalacia in the preterm infant: sonographic and clinical features. *Radiology* 151: 383–388.

Bozynski M E, Nelson M N, Matalon T A S *et al.* (1985) Cavitary periventricular leukomalacia: incidence and short term outcome in infants weighing <1200 grams at birth. *Dev Med Child Neurol* 27: 572–577.

✪ Brun N, Robitaille Y, Grignon A *et al.* (1999) Pyruvate carboxylase deficiency: prenatal onset of ischemia-like brain lesions in two sibs with the acute neonatal form. *Am J Med Genet* 84: 94–101.

Bull M J, Schreiner R L, Garg B P *et al.* (1980) Neurologic complications following temporal artery catheterization. *J Pediatr* 96: 1071–1073.

✪ Burguet A, Monnet E, Pauchard J Y *et al.* (1999) Some risk factors for cerebral palsy in very premature infants: importance of premature rupture of membranes and monochorionic twin placentation. *Biol Neonate* 75: 177–186.

Calvert S A, Hoskins E M, Fong K W & Forsyth S C (1986) Periventricular leukomalacia: ultrasonic diagnosis and neurological outcome. *Acta Paediatr Scand* 75: 489–496.

Calvert S A, Hoskins E M & Fong K W (1987) Etiological factors associated with the development of periventricular leukomalacia. *Acta Paediatr Scand* 76: 254–259.

✪ Canterino J C, Verma U L, Visintainer P F *et al.* (1999) Maternal magnesium sulfate and the development of neonatal periventricular leukomalacia and intraventricular hemorrhage. *Obstet Gynecology* 93: 396–402.

Carson S C, Hertzberg B S, Bowie J D & Burger P C (1990) Value of sonography in the diagnosis of intracranial haemorrhage and periventricular leukomalacia: a postmortem study of 35 cases. *Am J Neuroradiol* 11: 677–683.

Catto-Smith A G, Yu V Y H, Bajuk B *et al.* (1985) Effect of neonatal periventricular haemorrhage on neurodevelopmental outcome. *Arch Dis Child* 60: 8–11.

Cavazutti M & Duffy T E (1982) Regulation of cerebral blood flow in normal and hypoxic newborn dogs. *Ann Neurol* 11: 247–257.

Chasnoff I J, Bussey M E, Savich R & Stack C M (1986) Perinatal cerebral infarction and maternal cocaine use. *J Pediatr* 108: 456–459.

Chow P P, Morgan J G & Taylor K J W (1985) Neonatal periventricular leukomalacia: a real-time sonographic diagnosis with CT correlation. *Am J Radiol* 145: 155–160.

✪ Cioni G, Fazzi B, Ipata A E *et al.* (1996) Correlation between cerebral visual impairment and magnetic resonance imaging in children with neonatal encephalopathy. *Dev Med Child Neurol* 38: 120–132.

✪ Cioni G, Di Paco M C, Bertucelli B *et al.* (1997a) MRI findings and sensorimotor development in infants with bilateral spastic cerebral palsy. *Brain Dev* 19: 245–253.

✪ Cioni G, Fazzi B, Coluccini M *et al.* (1997b) Cerebral visual impairment in preterm infants with periventricular leukomalacia. *Pediatr Neurol* 17: 331–338.

Clancy R, Malin S, Laraque D *et al.* (1985) Focal motor seizures heralding stroke in fullterm neonates. *Am J Dis Child* 139: 601–606.

Cocker J, George S W & Yates P O (1965) Perinatal occlusion of the middle cerebral artery. *Dev Med Child Neurol* 7: 235–243.

✪ Coley B D & Hogan M J (1997) Cystic periventricular leukomalacia of the corpus callosum. *Pediatr Radiol* 27: 583–585.

Connell J A, Oozeer R C, Regev R *et al.* (1987) Continuous 4 channel EEG monitoring in the evaluation of echodense ultrasound lesions and cystic leukomalacia. *Arch Dis Child* 62: 1019–1024.

✪ Cools F & Offringa M (1999) Meta-analysis of elective high frequency ventilation in preterm infants with respiratory distress syndrome. *Arch Dis Child* 80: F15–F20.

Cowan F (1986) Indomethacin, patent ductus arteriosus, and cerebral blood flow. *J Pediatr* 109: 341–344.

✪ Cowan F M, Pennock J M, Hanrahan J D *et al.* (1994) Early detection of cerebral infarction and hypoxic-ischemic encephalopathy in neonates using diffusion-weighted magnetic resonance imaging. *Neuropediatrics* 25: 172–175.

✪ Crowther C A, Hiller J E, Haslam R R *et al.* (1997) Australian Collaborative Trial of Antenatal Thyrotropin-Releasing Hormone: adverse effects at 12-month follow-up. ACTOBAT Study Group 99: 311–317.

✪ Dammann O & Leviton A (1997a) Maternal intrauterine infection, cytokines, and brain damage in the preterm newborn. *Pediatr Res* 42: 1–8.

✪ Dammann O & Leviton A (1997b) Duration of transient hyperechoic images of white matter in very-low-birthweight infants: a proposed classification. *Dev Med Child Neurol* 39: 2–5.

Dammann O & Leviton A (1998) Infection remote from the brain, neonatal white matter damage, and cerebral palsy in the preterm infant. *Semin Pediatr Neurol* 5: 190–201.

✪ Dammann O & Leviton A (1999) Brain damage in preterm newborns: might enhancement of developmentally regulated endogenous protection open a door for prevention? *Pediatrics* 104: 541–550.

✪ Debus O, Koch H G, Kurlemann G *et al.* (1998) Factor V Leiden and genetic defects of thrombophilia in childhood porencephaly. *Arch Dis Child* 78: F121–F124.

✪ Deguchi K, Mizuguchi M & Takashima S (1996) Immunohistochemical staining of tumor necrosis factor-alpha in neonatal leukomalacia. *Pediatr Neurol* 14: 13–14.

✪ Deguchi K, Oguchi K & Takashima S (1997) Characteristic neuropathology of leukomalacia in extremely low birth weight infants. *Paediatr Neurol* 16: 296–300.

✪ Deguchi K, Oguchi K, Matsuura N *et al.* (1999) Periventricular leukomalacia: relation to gestational age and axonal injury. *Pediatr Neurol* 20: 370–374.

✪ De Klerk O L, de Vries T W & Sinnige L G F (1997) An unusual cause of neonatal seizures in a newborn infant. *Pediatrics* 100: E8.

Delaporte B, Labrune M, Imbert M C & Dahan M (1985) Early echographic findings in non-haemorrhagic periventricular leukomalacia in the premature infant. *Pediatr Radiol* 15: 82–84.

De Reuck J, Chattha A S & Richardson E P (1972) Pathogenesis and evolution of leukomalacia in infancy. *Arch Neurol* 27: 229–236.

De Vries L S, Dubowitz L M S, Dubowitz V *et al.* (1985a) Predictive value of cranial ultrasound: a reappraisal. *Lancet* ii: 137–140.

De Vries L S & Dubowitz L M S (1985b) Cystic leukomalacia in preterm infants: site of lesion in relation to prognosis. *Lancet* ii: 1075–1076.

De Vries L S, Regev R & Dubowitz L M S (1986) Late onset cystic leukomalacia. *Arch Dis Child* 61: 298–299.

De Vries L S, Connell J C, Pennock J M *et al.* (1987) Neurological, electrophysiological and MRI abnormalities in infants with extensive cystic leukomalacia. *Neuropediatrics* 18: 61–66.

De Vries L S, Wigglesworth J S, Regev R & Dubowitz L M S (1988a) Evolution of periventricular leukomalacia during the neonatal period and infancy: correlation of imaging and postmortem findings. *Early Hum Dev* 17: 205–219.

De Vries L S, Regev R, Dubowitz L M S, Whitelaw A G M, Aber V R (1988b) Perinatal risk factors for the development of extensive cystic leukomalacia. *Am J Dis Child* 142: 732–735.

De Vries L S, Regev R, Pennock J M *et al.* (1988c) Ultrasound evolution and later outcome of infants with periventricular densities. *Early Hum Dev* 16: 225–233.

De Vries L S, Regev R, Connell J A *et al.* (1988d) Localised cerebral infarction in the premature infant: ultrasound diagnosis and correlation with CT and MRI. *Pediatrics* 81: 31–34.

De Vries L S, Eken P & Dubowitz L M S (1992) The spectrum of leukomalacia using cranial ultrasound. *Behav Brain Res* 49: 1–6.

De Vries L S, Eken P, Groenendaal F *et al.* (1993) Correlation between the degree of periventricular leukomalacia diagnosed using cranial ultrasound and MRI later in infancy in children with cerebral palsy. *Neuropediatrics* 24: 263–268.

✪ De Vries L S, Groenendaal F, Eken P *et al.* (1997) Infarcts in the vascular distribution of the middle cerebral artery in preterm and fullterm infants. *Neuropediatrics* 28: 88–96.

De Vries L S, Groenendaal F, Eken P *et al.* (1999) *Neuropediatrics* 30: 314–319.

Di Pietro M A, Brody B A & Teele R L (1986) Peritrigonal echogenic 'blush' on cranial sonography: pathologic correlates. *Am J Radiol* 146: 1067–1072.

Dolfin T, Skidmore M B, Fong K W *et al.* (1984) Diagnosis and evolution of periventricular leukomalacia: a study with real-time ultrasound. *Early Hum Dev* 9: 105–109.

Dominguez R, Vila-Coro A A, Slopis J M & Bohan T P (1991) Brain and ocular abnormalities in infants with *in utero* exposure to cocaine and other street drugs. *Am J Dis Child* 145: 688–695.

Dommergues M A, Patkai J, Renauld J C, Evrard P & Gressens P (2000) Proinflammatory cytokines and interleukin-9 exacerbate excitotoxic lesions of the newborn murine neopallium. *Ann Neurol* 47: 54–63.

Eeg-Olofsson O & Ringheim Y (1983) Stroke in children: clinical characteristics and prognosis. *Acta Paediatr Scand* 72: 391–395.

Eken P, van Nieuwenhuizen O, van der Graaf Y *et al.* (1994) Relation between neonatal cranial ultrasound abnormalities and cerebral visual impairment in infancy. *Dev Med Child Neurol* 36: 3–15.

✪ Eken P, de Vries L S, van Nieuwenhuizen O *et al.* (1996) Early predictors of cerebral visual impairment in infants with cystic leukomalacia. *Neuropediatrics* 27: 16–25.

✪ Ekert P G, Taylor M J, Keenan N K *et al.* (1997) Early somatosensory evoked potentials in preterm infants: their prognostic utility. *Biol Neonate* 71: 83–91.

✪ Elimian A, Verma U, Canterino J *et al.* (1999) Effectiveness of antenatal steroids in obstetric subgroups. *Obstet Gynecol* 93: 174–179.

✪ Estan J & Hope P (1997) Unilateral neonatal cerebral infarction in full term infants. *Arch Dis Child* 76: F88–F93.

Evans D M, Levene M I & Archer L N J (1987) The effect of indomethacin on cerebral blood-flow velocity in premature infants. *Dev Med Child Neurol* 29: 776–782.

Fawer C-L & Calame A (1991) Significance of ultrasound appearances in the neurological development and cognitive abilities of preterm infants at 5 years. *Eur J Pediatr* 150: 515–520.

Fawer C-L, Calame A & Anderegg A (1984) Real-time ultrasonography in the neonate: a systematic study of high risk infant population. *Helvet Acta Paediatr* 39: 34–45.

Fawer C-L, Calame A, Perentes E & Anderegg A (1985a) Periventricular leukomalacia: a correlation study between real-time ultrasound and autopsy findings. *Neuroradiology* 27: 292–300.

Fawer C-L, Calame A & Furrer M-T (1985b) Neurodevelopmental outcome at 12 months of age related to cerebral ultrasound appearances of high risk preterm infants. *Early Hum Dev* 11: 123–132.

Fawer C-L, Diebold P & Calame A (1987) Periventricular leukomalacia and neurodevelopmental outcome in preterm infants. *Arch Dis Child* 62: 30–36.

Fazzi E, Lanzi G, Gerardo A *et al.* (1992) Neurodevelopmental outcome in very-low-birth-weight infants with or without periventricular haemorrhage and/or leukomalacia. *Acta Paediatr* 81: 808–811.

✪ Fazzi E, Orcesi S, Caffi L *et al.* (1994) Neurodevelopmental outcome at 5–7 years in preterm infants with periventricular leukomalacia. *Neuropediatrics* 25: 134–139.

✪ Fedrizzi E, Inverno M, Botteon G *et al.* (1993) The cognitive development of children born preterm and effected by spastic diplegia. *Brain Dev* 15: 428–432.

✪ Fedrizzi E, Inverno M, Bruzzone M G *et al.* (1996) MRI features of cerebral lesions and cognitive functions in preterm spastic diplegic children. *Paediatr Neurol* 15: 207–212.

Filipek P A, Krishnamoorthy K S, Davis K R & Kuehnle K (1987) Focal cerebral infarction in the newborn: a distinct entity. *Paediatr Neurol* 3: 141–147.

✪ FineSmith R B, Roche K, Yellin P B *et al.* (1997) Effect of magnesium sulfate on the development of cystic periventricular leukomalacia in preterm infants. *Am J Perinatol* 14: 303–307.

Friede R (1975) *Developmental neuropathology.* Vienna: Springer-Verlag.

Fujimoto S, Yokochi K, Togari H *et al.* (1992) Neonatal cerebral infarction: symptoms, CT findings and prognosis. *Brain Dev* 14: 48–52.

✪ Fujimoto S, Togari H, Yamaguchi N (1994a) Hypocarbia and cystic periventricular leukomalacia in preterm infants. *Arch Dis Child* 71: F107–F110.

✪ Fujimoto S, Yamaguchi N, Togari H *et al.* (1994b) Cerebral palsy of cystic periventricular leukomalacia in low-birth-weight infants. *Acta Paediatr* 83: 397–401.

✪ Geva E, Lerner-Geva L, Stavorovsky Z *et al.* (1998) Multifetal pregnancy reduction: a possible risk factor for periventricular leukomalacia. *Fertil Steril* 69: 845–850.

✪ Gibbs J M & Weindling A M (1994) Neonatal intracranial lesions following placental abruption. *Eur J Pediatr* 153: 195–197.

Gibson N A, Fielder A R, Trounce J Q & Levene M I (1990) Ophthalmic findings in infants of very low birthweight. *Dev Med Child Neurol* 32: 7–13.

✪ Gilles F H & Murphy S F (1969) Perinatal telencephalic leucoencephalopathy. *J Neurosurg Psychiatry* 32: 404–413.

Gilles F H, Leviton A & Kerr C S (1976) Endotoxin leukoencephalopathy in the telencephalon of the newborn kitten. *J Neurol Sci* 27: 183–191.

✪ Gilles F H, Leviton A, Golden J A *et al.* (1998) Groups of histopathologic abnormalities in brains of very low birthweight infants. *J Neuropathol Exp Neurol* 57: 1026–1034.

✪ Giroud M, Fayolle H, Martin D *et al.* (1995) Late thalamic atrophy in infarction of the middle cerebral artery territory in neonates. *Child Nerv Syst* 11: 133–136.

✪ Gomez, Romero R, Ghezzi F *et al.* (1998) The fetal inflammatory response syndrome. *Am J Obstet Gynecol* 179: 194–202.

✪ Goodman R & Graham P (1996) Psychiatric problems in children with hemiplegia: cross sectional epidemiological survey. *BMJ* 312: 1065–1069.

✪ Goto M, Ota R, Iai M *et al.* (1994) MRI changes and deficits of higher brain functions in preterm diplegia. *Acta Paediatr* 83: 506–511.

Govaert P, Matthys E, Zecic A *et al.* (2000) Perinatal cortical infarction within middle cerebral artery trunks. *Arch Dis Child* 82: F59–F63.

Graham M, Levene M I, Trounce J Q & Rutter N (1987) Prediction of cerebral palsy in very low birth weight infants: prospective ultrasound study. *Lancet* ii: 593–596.

Grant E G, Schellinger D, Smith Y & Uscinkski R H (1986) Periventricular leukomalacia in combination with intraventricular hemorrhage; sonographic features and sequelae. *Am J Neuroradiol* 7: 443–447.

Graziani L J, Pasto M, Stanley C *et al.* (1987) Neonatal neurosonographic correlates of cerebral palsy in preterm infants. *Pediatrics* 78: 88–95.

Graziani L J, Mitchell D G, Kornhauser M, Pidcock F S, Merton D A, Stanley C, McKee L 1992 Neurodevelopment of preterm infants: neonatal neurosonographic and serum bilirubin studies. *Pediatrics* 89: 229–234.

✪ Graziani L J, Spitzer A R, Mitchell D G *et al.* (1992) Mechanical ventilation in preterm infants: neurosonographic and developmental studies. *Pediatrics* 90: 515–522.

Greisen G, Munck H & Lou H (1986) May hypocarbia cause ischaemic brain damage in the preterm infant? *Lancet* ii: 460.

Greisen G, Munck H & Lou H (1987) Severe hypocarbia in preterm infants and neurodevelopmental deficit. *Acta Paediatr Scand* 76: 401–404.

✪ Gressens P, Besse L & Robberecht P *et al.* (1999) Neuroprotection of the developing brain by systemic administration of vasoactive intestinal peptide derivatives. *J Pharmacol Exp Ther* 288: 1207–1213.

✪ Grether J K, Nelson K B, Emery III E S & Cummins S K (1996) Prenatal and perinatal factors and cerebral palsy in very low birth weight infants. *J Pediatr* 128: 407–414.

✪ Groenendaal F, van der Grond J, Witkamp T D & de Vries L S (1995) Magnetic resonance spectroscopic imaging in neonatal stroke. *Neuropediatrics* 26: 243–248.

✪ Groenendaal F, van der Grond J & van Haastert I (1997) Early cerebral proton MRS and neurodevelopmental outcome in infants with cystic leukomalacia. *Dev Med Child Neurol* 39: 373–379.

Guzzetta F, Shackelford G D, Volpe S *et al.* (1986) Periventricular intraparenchymal echodensities in the premature newborn: critical determinant of neurologic outcome. *Pediatrics* 78: 995–1006.

Hamilton P A, Hope P L, Cady F B *et al.* (1986) Impaired energy metabolism in brains of newborn infants with increased cerebral echodensities. *Lancet* i: 1242–1246.

Hansen A & Leviton A (1999) Labor and delivery characteristics and risks of cranial ultrasonographic abnormalities among very-low-birth-weight infants. The Developmental Epidemiology Network Investigators. *Am J Obstet Gynecol* 181: 997–1006.

Hayakawa F, Okumura A, Kato T, Kuno K & Watanabe K (1999) Determination of timing of brain injury in preterm infants with periventricular leukomalacia with serial neonatal electroencephalography. *Pediatrics* 104: 1077–1081.

Harwood-Nash D C & Fitz C R (1976) *Neuroradiology in infants and children.* St Louis, MO: CV Mosby.

Heier L A, Carpanzano C R & Mast J (1991) Maternal cocaine abuse: the spectrum of radiologic abnormalities in the neonatal CNS. *Am J Neuroradiol* 12: 951–956.

Hernanz-Schulman M, Cohen W & Genieser N B (1988) Sonography of cerebral infarction in infancy. *Am J Radiol* 150: 897–902.

Hill A, Martin D J, Danemann A & Fitz C R (1983) Focal ischaemic cerebral injury in the newborn: diagnosis by ultrasound and correlation with computed tomographic scans. *Pediatrics* 71: 790–793.

✪ Holling E E & Leviton A (1999) Characteristics of cranial ultrasound white-matter echolucencies that predict disability: a review. *Dev Med Child Neurol* 41: 136–139.

Hope P J, Gould S J, Howard S *et al.* (1988) Ultrasound diagnosis of pathologically verified lesions in the brains of very preterm infants. *Dev Med Child Neurol* 30: 457–471.

Hoyme H E, Jones K L, Dixon S D *et al.* (1990) Prenatal cocaine exposure and fetal vascular disruption. *Pediatrics* 85: 743–747.

✪ Iai M, Tanabe Y, Goto M, Sugita K & Niimi H (1994) A comparative magnetic resonance imaging study of the corpus callosum in neurologically normal children and children with spastic diplegia. *Acta Paediatr* 83: 1086–1090.

Iida K, Takashima S & Takeuchi Y (1992) Etiologies and distribution of neonatal leukomalacia. *Pediatr Neurol* 8: 205–209.

✪ Iida K (1993) Neuropathologic study of newborns with prenatal-onset leukomalacia. *Paediatr Neurol* 9: 45–48.

Ikonen R S, Kuusinen E J & Janas M O (1988) Possible etiological factors in extensive periventricular leukomalacia of preterm infants. *Acta Paediatr Scand* 77: 489–495.

Ikonen R S, Janas M O, Koivikko M J *et al.* (1992) Hyperbilirubinaemia, hypocarbia and periventricular leukomalacia in preterm infants: relationship to cerebral palsy. *Acta Paediatr Scand* 81: 802–807.

✪ Ito J, Saijo H, Araki A *et al.* (1996) Assessment of visuoperceptual disturbance in children with spastic diplegia using measurements of the lateral ventricles on cerebral MRI. *Dev Med Child Neurol* 38: 496–502.

✪ Inder T, Huppi P, Zientara G P *et al.* (1999a) Early detection of periventricular leukomalacia by diffusion-weighted magnetic resonance imaging techniques. *J Pediatr* 134: 631–634.

✪ Inder T, Huppi P, Zientara G P *et al.* (1999b) The postmigrational development of polymicrogyria documented by magnetic resonance imaging from 31 weeks' postconceptional age. *Ann Neurol* 45: 798–801.

✪ Jacobsen L, Ek U, Fernell *et al.* (1996) Visual impairment in preterm children with periventricular leukomalacia–visual, cognitive and neuropaediatric characteristics related to cerebral imaging. *Dev Med Child Neurol* 38: 724–735.

✪ Jan M M & Camfield P R (1998) Outcome of neonatal stroke in full-term infants without significant birth asphyxia. *Eur J Pediatr* 157: 846–848.

✪ Jelinski S E, Yager J Y & Juurlink B H J (1999) Preferential injury of oligo-dendroglioblasts by a short hypoxic-ischemic insult. *Brain Res* 815: 150–153.

Jongmans M, Henderson S, de Vries L S & Dubowitz L M S (1993) Duration of periventricular densities in preterm infants and neurological outcome at six years. *Arch Dis Childhood* 69: 9–13.

✪ Kahn M A & De Vellis J (1994) Regulation of an oligodendrocyte progenitor cell line by the interleukin-6 family of cytokines. *Glia* 12: 87–98.

✪ Koeda T & Takeshita K (1992) Visuo-perceptual impairment and cerebral lesions in spastic diplegia with preterm birth. *Brain Devel* 14: 239–244.

✪ Koelfen W, Freund M, Koming S *et al.* (1993) Results of parenchymal and angiographic magnetic resonance imaging and neuropsychological testing of children after stroke as neonates. *Eur J Pediatr* 152: 1030–1035.

✪ Koelfen W, Freud M & Varnholt V (1995) Neonatal stroke involving the middle cerebral artery in term infants: clinical presentation, EEG and imaging studies, and outcome. *Dev Med Child Neurol* 37: 204–212.

Kuban K C K & Gilles F H (1985) Human telencephalic angiogenesis. *Ann Neurol* 17: 539–548.

✪ Kuban K C (1998) White matter disease of prematurity, periventricular leukomalacia, and ischemic lesions. *Dev Med Child Neurol* 40: 571–573.

✪ Kuban S, Sanocka U, Leviton A *et al.* (1999) White matter disorders of prematurity: association with intraventricular hemorrhage and ventriculomegaly. *J Pediatr* 134: 539–546.

✪ Lanzi G, Fazzi E, Uggetti C *et al.* (1998) Cerebral visual impairment in periventricular leukomalacia. *Neuropediatrics* 29: 145–150.

Larroche J-C (1977) *Developmental pathology of the neonate.* Amsterdam: Excerpta Medica.

Larroche J-C (1984) Perinatal brain damage. In: Adams J H, Corsellis J A N & Duchen L W (eds) *Greenfield's neuropathology*, 4th edn. London: Edward Arnold.

Larroche J-C (1986) Fetal encephalopathies of circulatory origin. *Biol Neonate* 50: 61–74.

Larroche J-C, Bethmann O, Beadoin M & Couhard M (1986) Brain damage in the premature infant: early lesions and new aspects of sequelae. *Italian J Neurol Sciences (suppl)* 5: 43–52.

Leech R W & Alvord E C (1974) Morphologic variation in periventricular leukomalacia. *Am J Pathol* 74: 591–600.

Levene M I (1987) *Neonatal neurology.* Edinburgh: Churchill Livingstone.

Levene M I & Trounce J Q (1986) Cause of neonatal convulsions: towards more precise diagnosis. *Arch Dis Child* 61: 78–79.

Levene M I, Wigglesworth J S & Dubowitz V (1983) Hemorrhagic periventricular leukomalacia: a real-time ultrasound study. *Pediatrics* 71: 794–797.

Levene M I, Dowling S, Graham M *et al.* (1992) Impaired motor function (clumsiness) in 5 year old children: correlation with neonatal ultrasound scans. *Arch Dis Child* 67: 687–690.

Leviton A & Gilles F H (1984) Acquired perinatal leukoencephalopathy. *Ann Neurol* 16: 1–8.

Leviton A & Paneth N (1990) White matter damage in preterm newborns – an epidemiologic perspective. *Early Hum Dev* 24: 1–22.

✪ Leviton A (1993) Preterm and cerebral palsy: is tumor necrosis factor-alpha the missing link? *Dev Med Child Neurol* 35: 549–558.

✪ Leviton A & Gilles F (1996) Ventriculomegaly, delayed myelination, white matter hypoplasia, and 'periventricular' leukomalacia: how are they related? *Pediatr Neurol* 15: 127–136.

✪ Leviton A, Paneth N, Reuss M L *et al.* (1999) Hypothyroxinaemia of prematurity and the risk of cerebral white matter damage. *J Pediatr* 134: 706–711.

Levy S R, Abrams I F, Marshall P C & Rosquette E E (1985) Seizures and cerebral infarction in the full-term newborn. *Ann Neurol* 17: 366–370.

✪ Lewine J D, Stur R S, Davis L E *et al.* (1994) Cortical organization in adulthood is modified by neonatal infarct: A case study. *Radiology* 190: 93–96.

✪ Lien J M, Towers C V, Quilligan E J *et al.* (1995) Term early-onset neonatal seizures: obstetric characteristics, etiologic classifications, and perinatal care. *Obstet Gynecol* 85: 163–169.

Lou H C, Lassen N A & Friis-Hansen B (1979) Impaired autoregulation of cerebral blood flow in the distressed newborn infant. *J Pediatr* 94: 118–121.

Lutschg J, Hanggeli C & Huber P (1983) The evolution of cerebral hemispheric lesions due to pre- or perinatal asphyxia (clinical and neuroradiological correlation). *Helvet Paediatr Acta* 38: 245–254.

✪ Maalouf E F, Duggan P J, Rutherford M A *et al.* (1999) Magnetic resonance imaging of the brain in a cohort of extremely preterm infants. *J Pediatr* 135: 351–357.

McMenamin J B, Shackelford G D & Volpe J J (1984) Outcome of neonatal IVH with periventricular echodense lesions. *Ann Neurol* 15: 285–290.

Mannino F L & Trauner D A (1983) Stroke in neonates. *J Pediatr* 102: 605–610.

Mantovani J F & Gerber G J (1984) 'Idiopathic' neonatal cerebral infarction. *Am J Dis Child* 138: 359–362.

✪ Marin-Padilla M (1997) Developmental neuropathology and impact of perinatal brain damage. II: White matter lesions of the neocortex. *J Neuropathol Exp Neurol* 56: 219–235.

✪ Marret S, Parain D, Samson-Dollfus D *et al.* (1986) Positive rolandic sharp waves and periventricular leukomalacia in the newborn. *Neuropediatrics* 17: 199–202.

✪ Marret S, Parain D, Jeannot E *et al.* (1992) Positive rolandic sharp waves in the EEG of the premature newborn: a five year prospective study. *Arch Dis Child* 67: 948–951.

✪ Marret S, Mukendi R, Gadisseux J F *et al.* (1995) Effect of ibotenate on brain development: an excitotoxic mouse model of microgyria and posthypoxic-like lesions. *Neuropathol Exp Neurol* 54: 358–370.

✪ Marret S, Parain D, Ménard J F *et al.* (1997) Prognostic value of neonatal electroencephalography in premature newborns less than 33 weeks of gestational age. *Electroencephalogr Clin Neurophysiol* 102: 178–185.

✪ Marret S, Bonnier C, Raymackers J M *et al.* (1999) Glycine antagonist and NO synthase inhibitor protect the developing mouse brain against neonatal excitotoxic lesions. *Pediatr Res* 45: 337–342.

Martin D J, Hill A, Fitz C R *et al.* (1983) Hypoxic/ischaemic cerebral injury in the neonatal brain: a report of monographic features with computed tomographic correlation. *Pediatr Radiol* 13: 307–312.

Matsuda T, Okuyama K, Cho K, Hoshi N, Matsumoto Y, Kobayashi Y & Fujimoto S (1999) Induction of antenatal periventricular leukomalacia by hemorrhagic hypotension in the chronically instrumented fetal sheep. *Am J Obstet Gynecol* 181: 725–730.

Melhem E R, Hoon A H, Ferrucci J T *et al.* (2000) Periventricular leukomalacia: relationship between lateral ventricular volume on brain MR images and severity of cognitive and motor impairment. *Radiology* 214: 199–204.

✪ Meng S Z, Arai Y, Deguchi K & Takashima S (1997) Early detection of axonal and neuronal lesions in prenatal-onset periventricular leukomalacia. *Brain Dev* 19: 480–484.

✪ Meng S Z & Takashima S (1999) Expression of transforming growth factor-beta 1 in periventricular leukomalacia. *J Child Neurol* 14: 377–381.

Ment L R, Duncan C C & Ehrenkrantz R A (1984) Perinatal cerebral infarction. *Ann Neurol* 16: 559–568.

Ment L R, Stewart W B, Duncan C C *et al.* (1985a) Beagle puppy model of perinatal cerebral infarction: acute changes in cerebral blood flow and metabolism during hemorrhagic hypotension. *J Neurosurg* 63: 441–447.

Ment L R, Stewart W B, Duncan C C *et al.* (1985b) Beagle puppy model of perinatal cerebral infarction: acute changes in cerebral prostaglandins during hemorrhagic hypotension. *J Neurosurg* 63: 899–904.

✪ Ment L R, Vohr B, Allan W *et al.* (1999) The etiology and outcome of cerebral ventriculomegaly at term in very low birth weight preterm infants. *Pediatrics* 104: 243–248.

✪ Mercuri E & Cowan F (1999) Cerebral infarction in the newborn infant: review of the literature and personal experience. *Eur J Paediatr Neurol* 3: 255–63.

✪ Mercuri E, Cowan F, Rutherford M A *et al.* (1995) Ischaemic and haemorrhagic brain lesions in newborns with seizures and normal Apgar scores. *Arch Dis Child* 73: F67–F74.

✪ Mercuri E, Atkinson J, Braddick O *et al.* (1996) Visual function and perinatal focal cerebral infarction. *Arch Dis Child* 75: F76–F81.

✪ Mercuri E, Rutherford M A, Cowan F *et al.* (1999) Early prognostic indicators of outcome in infants with neonatal cerebral infarction: a clinical, electroencephalogram, and magnetic resonance imaging study. *Pediatrics* 103: 39–44.

✪ Messer J, Haddad J & Casanova R (1991) Transcranial Doppler evaluation of cerebral infarction in the neonate. *Neuropediatrics* 22: 147–151.

Monset-Couchard M, de Bethmann O, Radvyani-Bouvet M-F, Papin C, Bordarier C & Relier J P (1988) Neurodevelopmental outcome in cystic periventricular leukomalacia (CPVL) (30 cases). *Neuropediatrics* 19: 124–131.

Moody D M, Bell M A & Challa V R (1990) Anatomic features of the cerebral vascular pattern that predict vulnerability to perfusion or oxygenation deficiency. *Am J Neuroradiol* 11: 431–439.

✪ Murphy D J, Squier M V, Hope P L *et al.* (1996) Clinical associations and time of onset of cerebral white matter damage in very preterm babies. *Arch Dis Child* 75: F27–F32.

Nanni G S, Kaude J V & Reeder J D (1984) Ischemic brain infarct in a neonate: ultrasound diagnosis and follow-up. *J Clin Ultrasound* 12: 229–231.

Nelson K B & Ellenberg J H (1985) Antecedents of cerebral palsy. I. Univariate analysis of risk factors. *N Engl J Med* 315: 81–86.

Nelson M D, Gonzalez-Gomez I & Gilles F H (1991) The search for human telencephalic ventriculofugal arteries. *Am J Neuroradiol* 12: 215–222.

✪ Nelson K B & Grether J K (1995) Can magnesium sulfate reduce the risk of cerebral palsy in very low birthweight infants? *Pediatrics* 1995 Feb; 95(2): 263–269.

Nwaesei C G, Pape K E, Martin D J *et al.* (1984) Periventricular infarction diagnosed by ultrasound: a postmortem correlation. *J Pediatrics* 105: 106–110.

O'Brien M J, Ash J M & Gilday D L (1979) Radionucleide brain scanning in perinatal hypoxia. *Dev Med Child Neurol* 21: 161–168.

✪ Ohyu J, Marumo G, Ozawa H *et al.* (1999) Early axonal and glial pathology in fetal sheep brains with leukomalacia induced by repeated umbilical cord occlusion. *Brain Dev* 21: 248–252.

✪ Opsjln S L, Wathen N C, Tingulstad S *et al.* (1993) Tumor necrosis factor, interleukin-1, and interleukin-6 in normal human pregnancy. *Am J Obstet Gynecol* 169: 397–404.

✪ O'Shea T M, Klinepeter K L, Meis P J & Dillard R G (1998a) Intrauterine infection and the risk of cerebral palsy in very low-birth weight infants. *Paediatr Perinat Epidemiol* 12: 72–83.

✪ O'Shea T M, Klinepeter K L & Dillard R G (1998b) Prenatal events and the risk of cerebral palsy in very low birth weight infants. *Am J Epidemiol* 147: 362–369.

✪ O'Shea T M, Kothadia J M, Klinepeter K L *et al.* (1999) Randomized placebo-controlled trial of a 42 day tapering course of dexamethasone to reduce the duration of ventilator dependency in very low birth weight infants: outcome of study participants at 1-year adjusted age. *Pediatrics* 104: 15–21.

✪ Oka A, Belliveau M J, Rosenberg P A & Volpe J J (1993) Vulnerability of oligodendroglia to glutamate: pharmacology, mechanisms and prevention. *J Neurosci* 13: 1441–1453.

✪ Okamura M, Itakura A, Kurauchi O *et al.* (1997) Fetal heart rate patterns associated with periventricular leukomalacia. *Int J Gynecol Obstet* 56: 13–18.

✪ Okumura A, Hayakawa F, Kato T *et al.* (1999a) Correlation between the serum level of endotoxin and periventricular leukomalacia in preterm infants. *Brain Dev* 21: 378–381.

Okumura A, Hayakawa F, Kato T *et al.* (1999b) Positive Rolandic sharp waves in preterm infants with periventricular leukomalacia: their relation to background electroencephalographic abnormalities. *Neuropediatrics* 30: 278–282.

✪ Ozawa H, Nishida A, Mito T & Takashima S (1994) Development of ferritin-positive cells in cerebrum of human brain. *Pediatr Neurol* 10: 44–48.

Palmer P, Dubowitz L M S, Levene M I & Dubowitz V (1982) Developmental and neurological progress of preterm infants with intraventricular haemorrhage and ventricular dilatation. *Arch Dis Child* 57: 748–753.

Paneth N, Rudelli R, Monte W *et al.* (1990) White matter necrosis in very low birth weight infants: neuropathologic and ultrasonographic findings in infants surviving six days or longer. *J Pediatr* 116: 975–984.

✪ Paneth N, Rudelli R, Kazam E *et al.* (1994) Associated pathological lesions: cerebellar haemorrhage, pontosubicular necrosis, basal ganglia necrosis. *Clin Dev Med* 131: 163–170.

✪ Paneth N (1999) Classifying brain damage in preterm infants. *J Pediatr* 134: 527–529.

Pape K E & Wigglesworth J S (1979) Haemorrhage, ischaemia and the perinatal brain. *Clin Dev Med* 69/70.

✪ Papile L-A, Tyson J E, Stoll B J *et al.* (1998) A multicenter trial of two dexamethasone regimens in ventilator-dependent premature infants. *N Engl J Med* 333: 1112–1118.

Parrot J (1873) Etude sur la ramollisement de l'encephale chez la nouveau-né. *Arch Physiol Norm Pathol* 5: 59–73, 176–195, 283–330.

Partridge J C, Babcock D S, Steichen J J & Bokyung K H (1983) Optimal timing for diagnostic ultrasound in low birth weight infants for detection of intracranial haemorrhage and ventricular dilatation. *J Pediatr* 102: 281–287.

✪ Perlman J M, Rollins N K & Evans D (1994) Neonatal stroke: clinical characteristics and cerebral blood flow velocity measurements. *Pediatric Neurology* 11: 281–284.

✪ Perlman J M, Risser R & Broyles R S (1996) Bilateral cystic periventricular leukomalacia in the premature infant: associated risk factors. *Pediatrics* 97: 822–827.

✪ Perlman J M & Risser R (1998) Relationship of uric acid concentrations and severe intraventricular haemorrhage/leukomalacia in the premature infant. *J Pediatr* 132: 436–439.

Pfister-Goedeke L & Boltshauser E (1982) Postnatale Entwicklung einer multilokularen zystischen Enczephalopathie beim Neugeborenen. *Helvet Paediatr Acta* 37: 59–65.

Pidcock F S, Graziani L J, Stanley C *et al.* (1990) Neurosonographic features of periventricular echodensities associated with cerebral palsy in preterm infants. *J Pediatr* 116: 417–422.

Pierrat V, Eken P, Duquennoy C *et al.* (1993) Prognostic value of early somatosensory evoked potentials in neonates with cystic leukomalacia. *Dev Med Child Neurol* 35: 683–690.

✪ Pinto-Martin J, Riolo S, Cnaan A *et al.* (1995) Cranial ultrasound prediction of disabling and non-disabling cerebral palsy at age two in a low birth weight population. *Pediatrics* 95: 249–254.

Reuter J H & Disney T A (1986) Regional cerebral blood flow and cerebral metabolic rate of oxygen during hyperventilation in the newborn dog. *Pediatric Research* 20: 1102–1106.

Ringelberg J & van der Bor M (1993) Outcome of transient periventricular echodensities in preterm infants. *Neuropediatrics* 24: 269–273.

Rodriguez, Claus D, Verellen G & Lyon G (1990) Periventricular leukomalacia: ultrasonic and neuropathological correlations. *Dev Med Child Neurol* 32: 347–355.

✪ Rogers B, Msall M, Owens T *et al.* (1994) Cystic periventricular leukomalacia and type of cerebral palsy in preterm infants. *J Pediatr* 125: S1–S8.

✪ Rollins N K, Morriss M C, Evans D & Perlman J M (1994) The role of early MR in the evaluation of the term infant with seizures. *Am J Neuroradiol* 15: 239–248.

Roodhooft A M, Parizel P M, Van Acker K J *et al.* (1987) Idiopathic cerebral arterial infarction with paucity of symptoms in the full-term neonate. *Pediatrics* 80: 381–385.

✪ Rothwell N J, Loddick S A & Stroemer P (1997) Interleukins and cerebral ischaemia; *Int Rev Neurobiol* 40: 281–298.

Rushton D I, Preston P R & Durbin G M (1985) Structure and evolution of echodense lesions in the neonatal brain. *Arch Dis Child* 60: 798–808.

✪ Russell G A & Cooke R W (1995) Randomised controlled trial of allopurinol prophylaxis in very preterm infants. *Arch Dis Childh Fetal Neonatal Edn* 73: F27–F31.

✪ Rydhstrom H & Ingemarsson I (1993) Prognosis and long-term follow-up of a twin after antenatal death of the co-twin. *J Reprod Med* 38: 142–146.

Saphiro H M, Greenberg J H, Van Horn Naughton K & Reivich M (1980) Heterogeneity of local cerebral blood flow – $p_aCO_2$ sensitivity in neonatal dogs. *J App Physiol* 49: 113–118.

Scher M S, Dobson V, Carpenter N A & Guthrie R D (1989) Visual and neurological outcome of infants with periventricular leukomalacia. *Dev Med Child Neurol* 31: 353–365.

✪ Schouman-Claeys E, Henry-Feugeas M C, Roset F *et al.* (1993) Periventricular leukomalacia: correlation between MR imaging and autopsy findings during the first 2 months of life. *Radiology* 189: 59–64.

✪ Shinwell E S, Karplus M, Reich D *et al.* Early postnatal dexamethasone therapy is associated with increased incidence of cerebral palsy. Presented at the Hot topics, Ross conference meeting 1999.

Shinwell E S, Karplus M, Reich D *et al.* (2000) Early postnatal dexamethasone therapy is associated with increased incidence of cerebral palsy. *Arch Dis Child Fetal and Neonat Ed* 83: F177–186.

Shuman R M & Selednik L J (1980) Periventricular leukomalacia: a one year autopsy study. *Arch Neurol* 37: 231–235.

✪ Sie L T L, van der Knaap M S, van Wezel-Meyler G *et al.* (1997) Early magnetic resonance imaging compared to ultrasound in neonates with periventricular leukomalacia. *Neuropediatrics* 28: 350A.

Sie L T L, van der Knaap M S, van Wezel-Meyler G, Taets van Amerongen A H M, Lafeber H N & Valk J (2000) Early magnetic resonance imaging compared to ultrasound in neonates with periventricular leukomalacia. *American Journal of Neuroradiology* 21: 852–861.

✪ Silver R K, MacGregor S N, Pasternak & Neely S E (1992) Fetal stroke associated with elevated maternal anticardiolipin antibodies. *Obstetrics and Gynecology* 80: 497–499.

✪ Silver R M, Schwinzer B & McGregor J A (1993) Interleukin-6 levels in amniotic fluid in normal and abnormal pregnancies: preeclampsia, small-for-gestational-age fetus, and premature labor. *Am J Obstet Gynecol* 169: 1101–1105.

Sims M E, Beckwitt Turkel S *et al.* (1985) Brain injury and intrauterine death. *Am J Obstet Gynecol* 151: 721–723.

Sinha S K, Davies J M, Sims D G & Chiswick M L (1985) Relation between periventricular haemorrhage and ischaemic brain lesions diagnosed by ultrasound in very preterm infants. *Lancet* ii: 1154–1155.

Sinha S K, D'Souza S W, Rivlin E & Chiswick M L (1990) Ischaemic brain lesions diagnosed at birth in preterm infants: clinical events and developmental outcome. *Arch Dis Child* 65: 1017–1020.

Smith C D & Baumann R J (1991) Clinical features and magnetic resonance imaging in congenital and childhood stroke. *J Child Neurol* 6: 263–272.

✪ Spinillo A, Capuzzo E, Stronati M *et al.* (1998) Obstetric risk factors for periventricular leukomalacia among preterm infants. *Br J Obstet Gynaecol* 105: 865–871.

Sran S K & Baumann R J (1988) Outcome of neonatal strokes. *Am J Dis Child* 142: 1086–1088.

✪ Stevenson D K, Wright L L, Lemons J A *et al.* (1998) Very low birth weight outcomes of the National Institute of Child Health and Human Development Neonatal Research Network, January 1993 through December 1994. *Am J Obstet Gynecol* 179: 1632–1639.

Stewart A L, Thorburn R J, Hope P L *et al.* (1983) Ultrasound appearance of the brain in very preterm infants and neurodevelopmental outcome at 18 months of age. *Arch Dis Child* 58: 598–604.

Szymonowicz W, Yu V Y H & Wilson F E (1984) Antecedents of periventricular haemorrhage in infants weighing 1250 grams or less at birth. *Arch Dis Child* 59: 13–17.

Szymonowicz W, Preston H & Yu V Y H (1986) The surviving monozygotic twin. *Arch Dis Child* 61: 454–458.

Taboada D, Alonso A, Olague R *et al.* (1980) Radiological diagnosis of periventricular and subcortical leukomalacia. *Neuroradiology* 20: 33–41.

Takashima J & Tanaka K (1978) Development of cerebral architecture and its relationship to periventricular leukomalacia. *Arch Neurol* 35: 11–16.

Takashima J, Armstrong D & Becker L E (1978) Subcortical leukomalacia: relationship to development of the cerebral sulcus and its vascular supply. *Arch Neurol* 35: 470–472.

✪ Takashima S, Iida K & Deguchi K (1995) Periventricular leukomalacia, glial development and myelination. *Early Hum Dev* 43: 177–184.

✪ Taylor G A (1994) Alterations in regional cerebral blood flow in neonatal stroke: preliminary findings with color Doppler sonography. *Pediatr Radiol* 24: 111–115.

✪ Thorarensen O, Ryan S, Hunter J *et al.* (1997) Factor V Leiden mutation: an unrecognized cause of hemiplegic cerebral palsy, neonatal stroke and placental thrombosis. *Ann Neurol* 42: 372–375.

Thorburn R J, Lipscomb A P, Stewart A L *et al.* (1981) Prediction of death and major handicap in very preterm infants by brain ultrasound. *Lancet* i: 1119–1121.

✪ Townsend S F, Rumack C M, Thilo E H *et al.* (1999) Late neurosonographic screening is important to the diagnosis of periventricular leukomalacia and ventricular enlargement in preterm infants. *Pediatr Radiol* 29: 347–352.

Trauner D A & Mannino F L (1986) Neurodevelopmental outcome after neonatal cerebrovascular incident. *J Pediatr* 108: 459–461.

✪ Trauner D A, Chase C, Walker P & Wulfeck B (1993) Neurologic profiles of infants and children after perinatal stroke. *Pediatr Neurol* 9: 383–386.

Trounce J Q & Levene M I (1985) Diagnosis and outcome of subcortical cystic leukomalacia. *Arch Dis Child* 60: 1041–1044.

Trounce J Q, Rutter N & Levene M I (1986a) Periventricular leucomalacia and intraventricular haemorrhage in the preterm neonate. *Arch Dis Child* 61: 1196–1202.

Trounce J Q, Fagan D & Levene M I (1986b) Intraventricular haemorrhage and periventricular leukomalacia: ultrasound and autopsy correlation. *Arch Dis Child* 62: 1203–1207.

Trounce J Q, Shaw O E, Levene M I & Rutter N (1988) Clinical risk factors and periventricular leucomalacia. *Arch Disease Child* 63: 17–22.

✪ Tsuru A, Mizuguchi M & Takashima S (1995) Cystic leukomalacia in the cerebellar folia of premature infants. *Acta Neuropathologica* 90: 400–402.

Tzogalis D, Fawer C L, Wong Y & Calame A (1988) Risk factors associated with the development of peri-intraventricular haemorrhage and periventricular leukomalacia. *Helvetica Paediatrica Acta* 43: 363–376.

✪ Uehara H, Yoshioka H, Kawase S *et al.* (1999) A new model of white matter injury in neonatal rats with bilateral carotid artery occlusion. *Brain Res* 837: 213–220.

Uggetti C, Egitto M G, Fazzi E *et al.* (1996) Cerebral visual impairment in periventricular leukomalacia: MR correlation. *Am J Neuroradiol* 17: 979–985.

Van de Bor M, van Zeben-van der A T M, Verloove-Vanhoorick S P *et al.* (1989) Hyperbilirubinaemia in preterm infants and neurodevelopmental outcome at 2 years of age: results of a national collaborative survey. *Pediatrics* 83: 915–920.

Van den Bergh R (1969) The periventricular intracerebral blood supply. In: Meyer J, Lechner H & Eichhorn O (eds) *Research of the cerebral circulation.* Springfield, IL: Charles C Thomas; pp. 52–65.

✪ Van den Hout B M, Eken P, van der Linden D *et al.* (1998) Visual, cognitive and neurodevelopmental outcome at 5½ years in children with perinatal haemorrhagic–ischaemic brain lesions. *Dev Med Child Neurol* 40: 820–828.

✪ Vanhulle C, Marret S, Parain D *et al.* (1998) Convulsions neonatales focalisees et infarctus arteriel cerebral. *Arch Pediatrie* 5: 404–408.

✪ Vannucci R C, Twofighi J, Heitjan D F & Brucklacher R M (1995) Carbon dioxide protects the perinatal brain from hypoxic–ischemic damage: an experimental study in the immature rat. *Pediatrics* 95: 868–874.

✪ Vannucci R C, Brucklacher R M & Vannucci S (1997) Effect of carbon dioxide on cerebral metabolism during hypoxia-ischemia in the immature rat. *Pediatric Res* 42: 24–29.

✪ Van Wezel-Meijler G, van der Knaap M S, Sie L T L *et al.* (1998) Magnetic resonance imaging of the brain in premature infants during the neonatal period. Normal phenomena and reflection of mild ultrasound abnormalities. *Neuropediatrics* 129: 89–96.

✪ Van Wezel-Meijler G, van der Knaap M S, Oosting J *et al.* (1999) Predictive value of neonatal MRI as compared to ultrasound in premature infants with mild periventricular white matter changes. *Neuropediatrics* 30: 231–238.

✪ Varelas P N, Sleight B J, Rinder H M *et al.* (1998) Stroke in a neonate heterozygous for factor V Leiden. *Pediatr Neurol* 18: 262–264.

✪ Verma U, Tejani N, Klein S *et al.* (1997) *Am J Obstet Gynecol* 176: 275–281.

Virchow R (1867) Zur pathologishen Anatomie des Gehirns. I. Congenitale Enzephalitis und Myelitis. *Virchows Archiv* 38: 129–142.

Volpe J J (1992) Effect of cocaine use on the fetus. *N Engl J Med* 327: 399–407.

Voorhies T M, Lipper E G, Lee B C P *et al.* (1984) Occlusive vascular disease in asphyxiated newborn infants. *J Pediatr* 105: 92–96.

Watkins A M C, West C R & Cooke R W I (1989) Blood pressure and cerebral haemorrhage and ischaemia in very low birthweight infants. *Early Hum Dev* 19: 103–110.

Weindling A M, Wilkinson A R, Cook J *et al.* (1985a) Perinatal events which precede periventricular haemorrhage and leukomalacia in the newborn. *Br J Obstet Gynaecol* 92: 1218–1223.

Weindling A M, Rochefort M J, Calvert S A *et al.* (1985b) Development of cerebral palsy after sonographic detection of periventricular cysts in the newborn. *Dev Med Child Neurol* 27: 800–806.

✪ Whitaker A H, Feldman J F, Van Rossem R *et al.* (1996) Neonatal cranial ultrasound abnormalities in low birth weight infants: relation to cognitive outcomes at six years of age. *Pediatrics* 98: 719–729.

✪ Wiswell T E, Graziani L J, Kornhauser M S *et al.* (1996a) Effects of hypocarbia on the development of cystic periventricular leukomalacia in premature infants treated with high-frequency jet ventilatation. *Pediatrics* 98: 918–924.

Wiswell T E, Graziani L J, Kornhauser M S *et al.* (1996b) High-frequency jet ventilatation in the early management of respiratory distress syndrome is associated with a greater risk for adverse outcomes. *Pediatrics* 98: 1035–1043.

Wulfeck B B, Trauner D A & Tallal P A (1991) Neurologic, cognitive and linguistic features of infants after early stroke. *Paediatr Neurol* 7: 266–269.

✪ Yeh T F, Lin Y J, Huang C C *et al.* (1998) Early dexamethasone therapy in premature infants: a follow-up study. *Pediatrics* 101: e7.

✪ Yokochi K, Aiba K, Horie M *et al.* (1991) Magnetic resonance imaging in children with spastic diplegia: correlation with the severity of their motor and mental abnormality. *Dev Med Child Dev* 33: 18–25.

✪ Yokochi K (1997) Thalamic lesions revealed by MR associated with periventricular leukomalacia and clinical profiles of subjects. *Acta Paediatrica* 86: 493–496.

✪ Yokochi K (1998) Clinical profiles of subjects with subcortical leukomalacia and border zone infarction revealed by MRI. *Acta Paediatrica* 87: 879–883.

✪ Yoon B H, Romero R, Ha Yang S *et al.* (1996) Interleukin-6 concentrations in umbilical cord plasma are elevated in neonates with white matter lesions associated with periventricular leukomalacia. *Am J Obstet Gynecol* 174: 1433–1440.

✪ Yoon B H, Kim C J, Romero R *et al.* (1997a) Experimentally induced intrauterine infection causes fetal brain white matter lesions in rabbits. *Am J Obstet Gynecol* 177: 797–802.

✪ Yoon B H, Romero R, Kim C J *et al.* (1997b) High expression of tumor necrosis factor-alpha and interleukin-6 in periventricular leukomalacia. *Am J Obstet Gynecol* 177: 406–411.

✪ Yoon B H, Jun J K, Romero R *et al.* (1997c) Amniotic fluid inflammatory cytokines (interleukin-6, interleukin-1 beta and tumor necrosis factor-alpha), neonatal brain white matter lesions and cerebral palsy. *Am J Obstet Gynecol* 177: 19–26.

Yoshioka H, Goma H, Ochi M *et al.* (1992) Experimental periventricular leukomalacia in the puppy: neurology, $^{31}$P-MRS and neuropathology. *Biol Neonate* 62: 303.

Young R S K, Hernandez M J & Yagel S K (1982) Selective reduction of blood flow to white matter during hypotension in newborn dogs: a possible mechanism of periventricular leukomalacia. *Ann Neurol* 12: 445–448.

Zorzi C, Angonese I, Zaramella P *et al.* (1988) Periventricular intraparenchymal cystic lesions: critical determinant of neurodevelopmental outcome in preterm infants. *Helvet Paediatr Acta* 43: 195–202.

✪ Zupan V, Gonzalez P, Lacaze-Masmonteil T *et al.* (1996) Periventricular leukomalacia: risk factors revisited. *Dev Med Child Neurol* 38: 1061–1067.

# Section V
# Perinatal asphyxia

# Chapter 23 Pathophysiology of asphyxia

L. Bennet, J. A. Westgate, P. D. Gluckman and A. J. Gunn

## INTRODUCTION

For most of the 20th century the concept of perinatal brain damage centered around cerebral palsy and intrapartum asphyxia. It is only in the last 20 years that this view has been seriously challenged by clinical and epidemiologic studies which have demonstrated that approximately 70–90% or more of cerebral palsy is unrelated to intrapartum events (MacLennan 1999). Many term infants who subsequently develop cerebral palsy are believed to have sustained asphyxial events in mid-gestation. In some cases, prenatal injury may lead to chronically abnormal heart tracings, and impaired ability to adapt to labor which may be confounded with an acute event.

In those infants who do have evidence for an acute, perinatal event, the key link between exposure to asphyxia and subsequent neurodevelopmental impairment is the early onset of neonatal encephalopathy (MacLennan 1999). Newborns with mild encephalopathy are completely normal to follow-up, while all of those with severe (stage III) encephalopathy die or have severe handicap. In contrast, only half of those with moderate (stage II) hypoxic–ischemic encephalopathy develop handicap; however, even those who do not develop neurologic impairment are at risk of future academic failure (Robertson & Finer 1993).

At the same time it has become clear that the predictive value for cerebral palsy of various markers for potentially injurious asphyxia, such as abnormal fetal heart rate tracings, is consistently weak (Nelson *et al.* 1996). For example, more than half of babies born with severe acidosis (base deficit >16 mmol/l and pH <7.0) do not develop even mild encephalopathy, while conversely encephalopathy can still occur, although at low frequency, in association with relatively modest acidosis (Low 1997). These data contrast with the presence of (very) non-reassuring fetal heart rate tracings and severe metabolic acidosis in those infants who do develop neonatal encephalopathy (Westgate *et al.* 1999).

## CHARACTERISTICS OF PERINATAL ASPHYXIAL ENCEPHALOPATHY

Perinatal asphyxial encephalopathy has a number of distinct characteristics that limit extrapolation from studies of the neonatal or adult brain. First, the etiology of the insult is generally global, affecting the whole fetus. Thus the fetal systemic and cardiovascular responses are critical to understanding the pathogenesis of injury. Second, the insult is generally reversible, whether spontaneously or therapeutically (e.g. delivery and resuscitation) and so can be associated with an evolving pattern of cerebral dysfunction and delayed injury after the insult. Third, although the injury may be a single acute episode, it is commonly due to repeated insults. Fourth, many of the insults occur in the stable and warmer thermal environment of the uterus. Finally, the maturity of the brain has a considerable effect on how neurons and glia respond to asphyxia.

It is now understood that the fetal response to asphyxia is not stereotypical, but rather depends upon both the nature of the insult and the condition of the fetus (Fig. 23.1). In fact, it appears that the fetus is spectacularly good at defending itself against such insults, and injury occurs only in a very narrow window between intact survival and death. This chapter focusses on recent developments in our understanding of the factors that determine whether the brain is

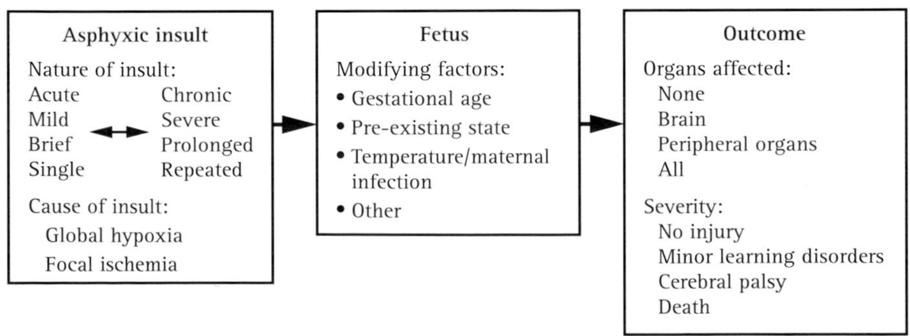


**Figure 23.1** Flow diagram of the determinants of cerebral injury after perinatal asphyxia.

damaged after an asphyxial insult. We will review the systemic adaptations of the fetus to asphyxia, the underlying cellular mechanisms of cerebral damage, and the factors modulating neuronal death.

## SYSTEMIC AND CARDIOVASCULAR ADAPTATION TO ASPHYXIA

The systemic adaptations of the fetus to whole body asphyxia are critical to outcome. Although the focus of most of the classic studies in this area was to delineate the cardiovascular and cerebrovascular responses, more recently the relationship between particular patterns of asphyxia and neural outcome has been examined. The great majority of studies of the pathophysiology of asphyxia have been performed in the chronically instrumented fetal sheep, studied *in utero*.

### ADAPTATIONS TO FETAL LIFE

The fetus is highly adapted to intrauterine conditions, which include low partial pressures of oxygen and relatively limited supply of other substrates compared with postnatal life. The fetus cannot store oxygen and is wholly dependent on a steady supply, but the fetus normally exists with a surplus of oxygen relative to its metabolic needs. This surplus provides a significant margin of safety when oxygen delivery is impaired. For the fetus hypoxia is perhaps the greatest challenge to its wellbeing *in utero* and consequently the fetus has several adaptive features, some unique to the fetus, which help it to defend itself from injury. These adaptive features include: higher blood flow to organs; left shift of the oxygen dissociation curve which increases the capacity to carry oxygen and oxygen extraction at typical oxygen tensions; the capacity to significantly reduce energy-consuming processes, greater anaerobic capacity in many tissues, and the capacity to redistribute blood flow towards essential organs away from the periphery. During hypoxia the fetus can maintain normal oxygen consumption until oxygen delivery is reduced by half. Additional structural features of the fetal circulation also augment these adaptive features including the systems of 'shunts', such as the ductus arteriosus, and preferential blood flow streaming in the inferior vena cava to avoid intermixing of oxygenated blood from the placenta and deoxygenated blood in the fetal venous system. These features ensure maximal oxygen delivery to essential organs such as the brain and heart. The preferential streaming patterns may be augmented during hypoxia to help maintain oxygen delivery to these organs.

These adaptations work sufficiently well in the majority of cases that even the concept of 'birth asphyxia' itself has been controversial. However, from recent studies where cerebral function has been monitored from birth in infants with clinical evidence of birth asphyxia, it is clear that many such children did have a precipitating episode in the immediate peripartum period, with evidence of acute evolving cerebral injury (Hellstrom Westas *et al.* 1995; Roth *et al.* 1997; Westgate *et al.* 1999). Follow-up of these children has shown a significant number to have long term cognitive or functional sequelae demonstrating that birth asphyxia is a true syndrome (Roth *et al.* 1997).

### ETIOLOGY OF ASPHYXIA

Systemic fetal asphyxia may be of fetal, placental or maternal origin. Fetal causes include decreased fetal hemoglobin (e.g. hemolysis or feto-maternal hemorrhage), cord prolapse, cord compression, cord entanglements, and true knots in the cord. Placental causes include placenta previa, vasa previa, and placental abruption. Maternal causes include systemic hypoxia (for example anemia or hemorrhage), and reduced utero-placental blood flow due to hypotension, vasospasm accompanying hypertension, and uterine hyperactivity.

Clearly, the different etiological factors lead to different patterns of asphyxia, which may be acute, chronic, or acute on the background of chronic impairment. In labor, fetal asphyxia will most commonly be brief, but frequently repeated. Perfusion of the placenta has been shown to be inversely proportional to the rise in intrauterine pressure during contractions (Janbu & Nesheim 1987). Conversely, catastrophic events such as cord prolapse or abruption will cause a single profound immediate insult. After placental abruption fetal blood loss with volume contraction further potentiates the direct effects of hypoxia on the fetus.

### HYPOXIA

The response of the fetal sheep to moderate, stable hypoxia has been extensively characterized (Giussani *et al.* 1994). Fetal isocapnic hypoxia is typically induced by reduction of maternal inspired oxygen fraction to 10%. In the late gestation fetus, this is associated with an initial transient, moderate bradycardia followed by tachycardia, and a rise in blood pressure (Fig. 23.2). There is an overall increase in combined ventricular output (CVO), and increased flow to essentially all organs (Giussani *et al.* 1994; Hanson 1997). As hypoxia becomes greater there is a rapid transition in the distribution of CVO, with further increases in blood flow to vital organs, such as the brain, heart, and adrenals, at the expense of peripheral organs which show a decrease in flow (Giusani *et al.* 1994; Jensen 1996). This phenomenon is termed 'centralization' of the circulation.

Cerebral oxygen consumption is little changed, even if arterial oxygen content falls as low as 1 mmol/l thanks to the compensating increases in both cerebral blood flow (CBF) and oxygen extraction (Parer 1998). Within the brain there is a greater increase in blood flow to the brainstem compared with the cerebrum, such that oxygen delivery is fully maintained to the brainstem, but not to the cerebrum (Jensen 1996). Nitric oxide (NO) has been shown to play a role in mediating the local increase in CBF (Hanson 1997).

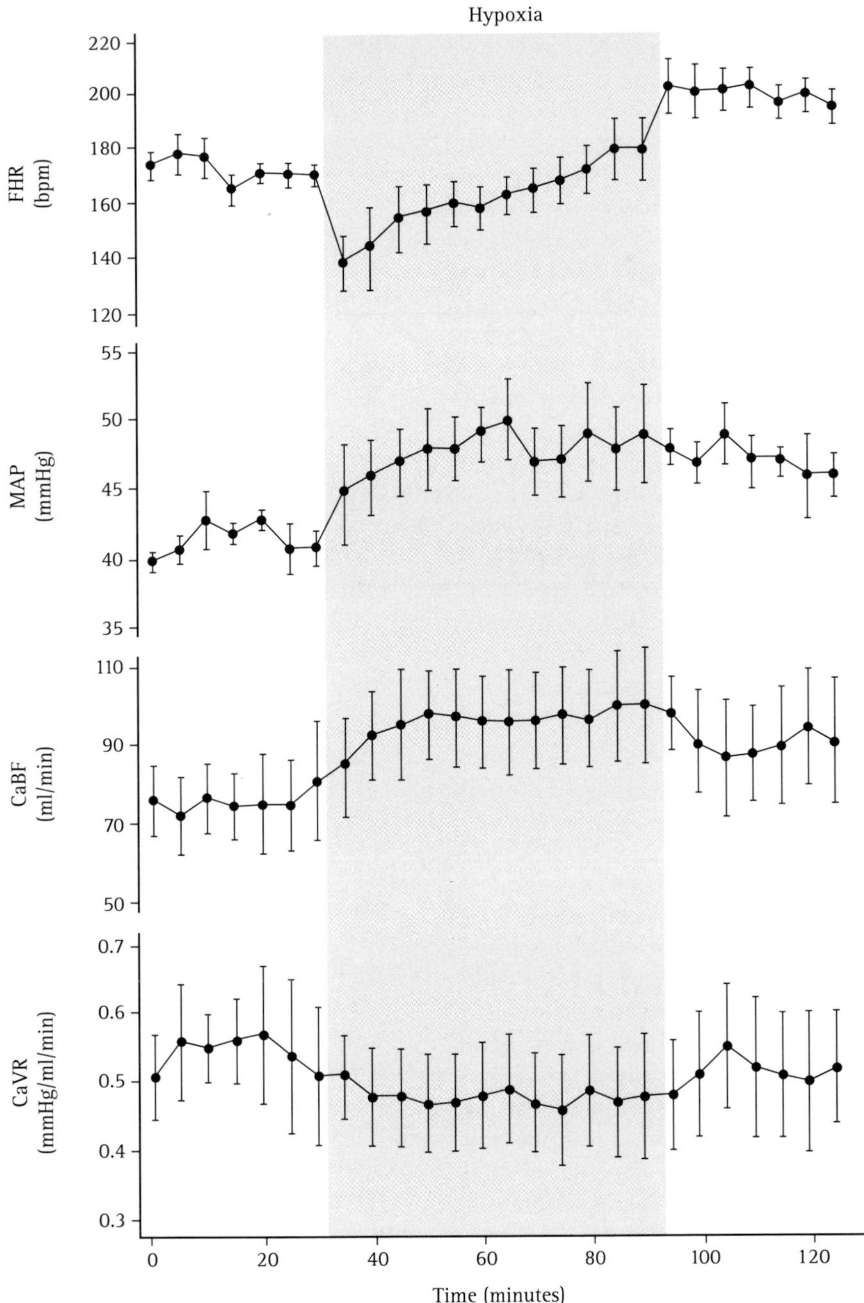


**Figure 23.2** The responses in the near-term fetal sheep to moderate isocapnic hypoxia for 60 minutes, induced by altering the maternal inspired gas mixture, showing changes in fetal heart rate (FHR), mean arterial blood pressure (MAP), carotid blood flow (CaBF), and carotid vascular resistance (CaVR). Moderate hypoxia is associated with a sustained redistribution of blood flow away from peripheral organs to essential organs such as the brain (see Giussani *et al.* 1994 for review). Data derived from Bennet *et al.* (1998).

Components of these changes in fetal heart rate (FHR) and CVO are reflexly mediated and the afferent limbs are in part mediated by muscarinic (parasympathetic) pathways, and by α-adrenergic stimulation (Giussani *et al.* 1997; Hanson 1997). The adrenergic input is derived partly from the sympathetic neural system and partly by circulating catecholamines released from the adrenal medulla. The rise in blood pressure during asphyxia is at least partly mediated by increased release of vasopressors, including the catecholamines, arginine vasopressin and angiotensin II (Giussani *et al.* 1997; Hanson 1997). There are also large adrenocorticotrophic and cortisol responses to hypoxia. Their role in the cardiovascular response to hypoxia is unclear, but cortisol has been shown to modulate the actions of other vasopressors (Tangalakis *et al.* 1992).

### Prolonged hypoxia

The effect of prolonged hypoxemia on cerebral metabolism in near-term fetal sheep has been studied during stepwise reductions of the maternal inspired oxygen concentration from 18% to 10–12% over four successive days (Richardson & Bocking 1998). Until the fetal arterial oxygen saturation was reduced to less than 30% of baseline, cerebral oxidative metabolism remained stable. At the lowest inspired oxygen concentration (with 3% $CO_2$) a progressive metabolic acidemia was induced. Initially, CBF increased, thus maintaining cerebral oxygen delivery as seen in acute studies. Eventually, when the pH fell below 7.00, cerebral oxygen consumption fell to less than 50% of control values.

If mild-to-moderate hypoxia is continued the fetus may be able to fully adapt, as measured by normalization of FHR, blood pressure, the incidence of fetal breathing, and body movements, although redistribution of blood flow is maintained (Richardson & Bocking 1998). These fetuses can improve tissue oxygen delivery to near baseline levels by increasing hemoglobin synthesis, mediated by greater erythropoietin release (Kitanaka *et al.* 1989). This is consistent with the clinical situation of 'brain sparing' in growth retardation.

### Maturational changes in responses to hypoxia

The cardiovascular response to fetal hypoxia appears to be age related. In the premature fetal sheep before 100 days (0.7) gestation, isocapnic hypoxia and hemorrhagic hypotension are not associated with hypertension, bradycardia, or peripheral vasoconstriction. Thus it has been suggested that peripheral vasomotor control starts to develop at 0.7 gestation, coincident with maturation of neurohormonal regulators and chemoreceptor function (Jensen 1996; Hanson 1997). However, when interpreting these results it is also important to consider the degree of hypoxia in relation to the much greater anaerobic capacity of the premature fetus. This is discussed below in the section on premature fetal asphyxia. It is likely that the degree of hypoxia attained in these studies did not reduce tissue oxygen availability below the critical threshold for this developmental stage.

## ASPHYXIA

Studies of asphyxia by definition involve both hypoxia and hypercapnia with metabolic acidosis. It is important to appreciate that in these studies of asphyxia a greater depth of hypoxia is typically attained than is possible using maternal inhalational hypoxia. Further, asphyxia can be induced relatively abruptly, limiting the time available for adaptation. Brief, total clamping of the uterine artery or umbilical cord leads to a rapid reduction of fetal oxygenation within a few minutes, and this is associated with massive hemodynamic changes and rapid metabolic deterioration (Parer 1998). In contrast, gradual partial occlusion induces a slow fetal metabolic deterioration without the acute fetal cardiovascular responses of bradycardia and hypertension; this is a function of the relative hypoxia attained (de Haan *et al.* 1993).

The responses to moderate asphyxia are similar to those described above for hypoxia, with redistribution of blood flow to essential organs (Parer 1998). During profound asphyxia, corresponding with a severe reduction of uterine blood flow to 25% or less and a fetal arterial oxygen content of less than 1 mmol/l, the cardiovascular responses of the normal fetus are substantially different. Bradycardia is sustained and there is a generalized vasoconstriction involving essentially all organs (Parer 1998). CBF does not increase or may even fall despite initially increased fetal blood pressure, due to significantly increased cerebral vasoconstriction. In the near-term sheep, within the brain, blood flow is preferentially redirected during asphyxia to protect structures important for survival such as the brainstem. Speculatively this redirection may maintain autonomic function at the expense of the cerebrum (Jensen 1996). Further, the reduced oxygen content limits oxygen extraction from the blood. The combination of these two factors, restricted CBF and reduced oxygen extraction, profoundly restricts cerebral oxygen consumption (Parer 1998). Partial cord compression for 90 minutes, titrated to induce severe asphyxia in near-term fetal sheep, had effects similar to those following a correspondingly severe reduction of uterine perfusion (Parer 1998; Ikeda *et al.* 1998). Both methods produced similar levels of asphyxia and cerebral injury (Ikeda *et al.* 1998).

Figure 23.3 shows the cardiovascular and cerebrovascular responses of a near-term fetus to asphyxia of rapid onset. This figure demonstrates the failure of carotid blood flow (CaBF, used as an index of CBF) to increase during asphyxia in contrast to the rise seen during hypoxia (Fig. 23.2). CaBF is instead briefly maintained around control values before falling. The failure of CBF to increase is not due to hypotension but rather is a function of a significant rise in cerebral vascular resistance as demonstrated by the increase in carotid vascular resistance (Figure 23.3) (Parer 1998; Bennet *et al.* 1998). During asphyxia blood pressure initially increases markedly but as asphyxia proceeds the fetus becomes hypotensive (Fig. 23.3). The sustained bradycardia and increased peripheral resistance in the late gestation fetus during asphyxia are mediated by chemoreflexes; a logarithmic rise in circulating catecholamine levels further augments the peripheral vasoconstriction (Hanson 1997). Hypotension is primarily related to asphyxial impairment of myocardial contractility, due to a direct inhibitory effect of profound acidosis and depletion of myocardial glycogen stores (Rosen *et al.* 1986). Once glycogen is depleted, there is rapid loss of high energy metabolites such as ATP in mitochondria (Shelley 1961). During a shorter episode, e.g. 5 min, of asphyxia, the fetus may not become hypotensive. If the

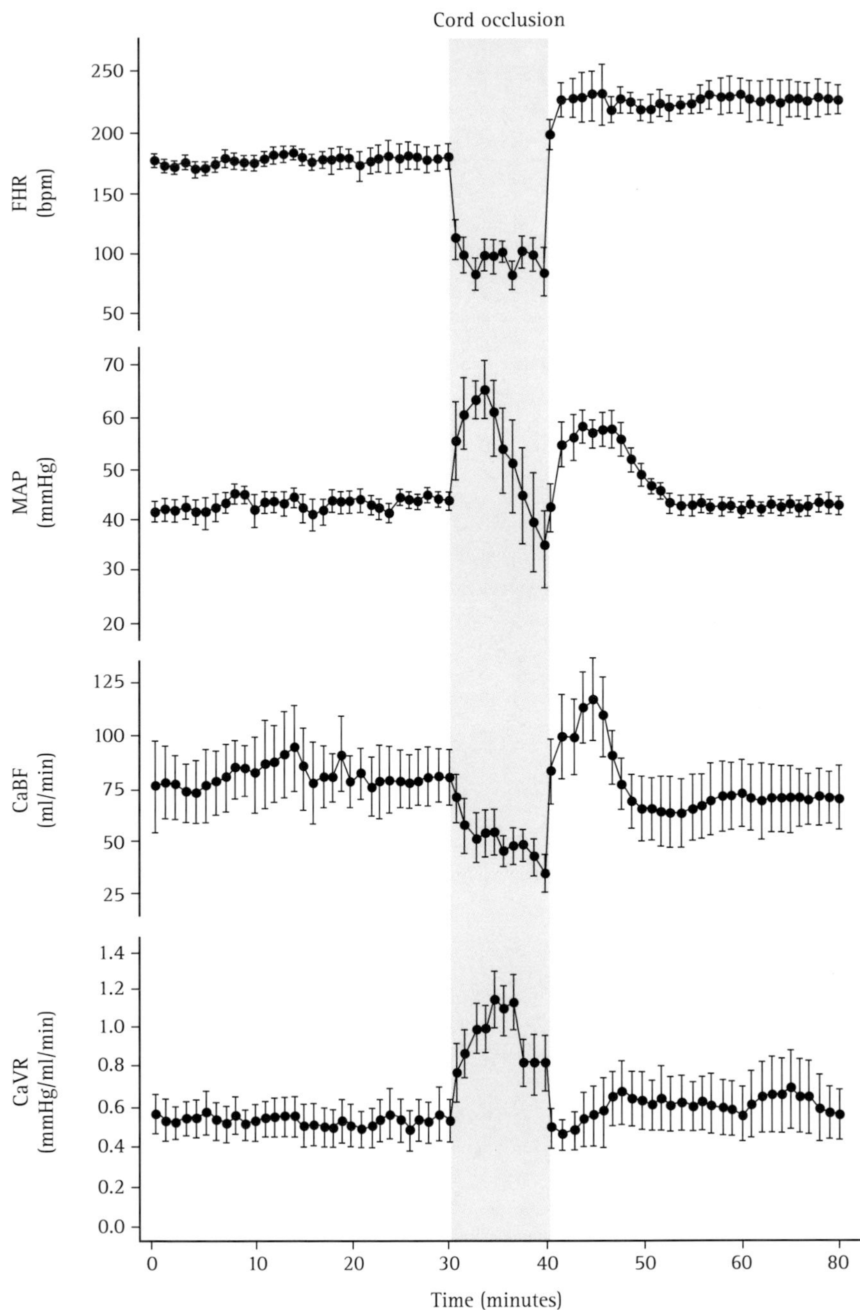


**Figure 23.3** The responses in the near-term fetal sheep to complete umbilical cord occlusion for 10 minutes. In contrast to the response to moderate hypoxia, the profound fall in fetal heart rate (FHR) is maintained throughout the occlusion. Fetal mean arterial blood pressure (MAP) was initially elevated but then fell to below normal just prior to release. Carotid blood flow (CaBF) did not increase, and this was associated with a large increase in carotid vascular resistance (CaVR). Hypotension and hypoperfusion develop in the second half of the occlusion. Data derived from Bennet *et al.* (1998).

insult is repeated before myocardial glycogen can be replenished, successive periods of asphyxia will be associated with increasing duration of hypotension.

Another possible factor leading to impaired contractility during asphyxia is myocardial injury, which has been found after severe birth asphyxia and with congenital heart disease in limited case series (Donnelly 1987). Studies in adult animals have shown that there may be a significant delay in recovery of cardiac contractility after reperfusion from brief ischemia in the absence of necrosis. This delayed recovery has been termed 'myocardial stunning', and this may contribute to progressive myocardial dysfunction and to delayed recovery of heart rate after repeated umbilical cord occlusions in the fetal lamb (Gunn *et al.* 2000).

### Progressive asphyxia

During gradually induced asphyxia, even to arterial oxygen contents of less than 1 mmol/l, fetal adaptation may be closer to that seen with hypoxia. Progressive reduction of uterine perfusion over a 3–4 h period in near-term fetal sheep, led to a mean pH <7.00, serum lactate levels > 14 mM, with a fetal mortality of 53%. Surviving animals remained normotensive and normoglycemic, and CBF was more than doubled. Interestingly however, in surviving

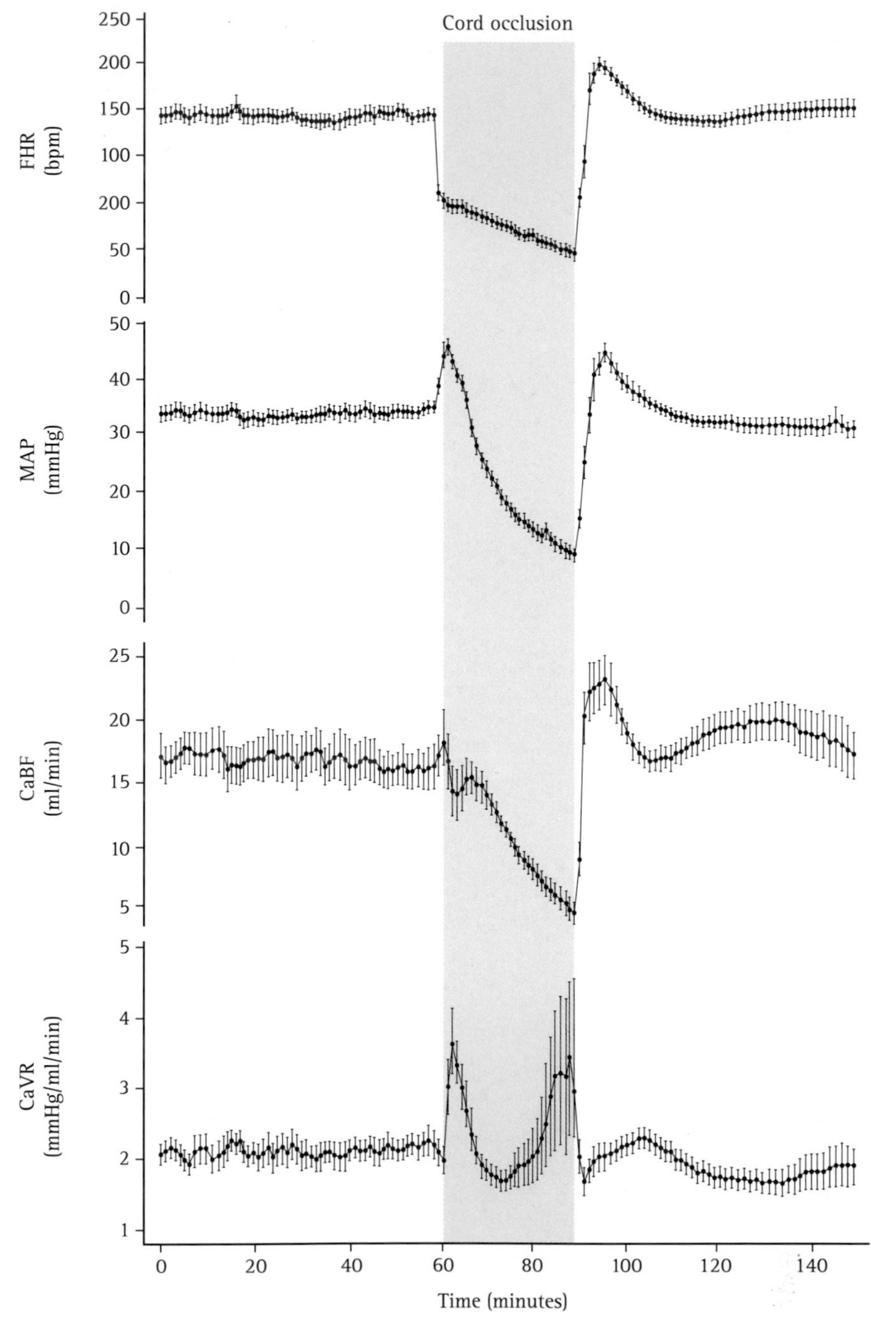


**Figure 23.4** The responses of the mid-gestation (0.6 gestation) fetal sheep to complete umbilical cord occlusion for 30 minutes, showing fetal heart rate (FHR), mean arterial blood pressure (MAP), carotid blood flow (CaBF) and carotid vascular resistance (CaVR). Contrary to early reports, the overall response of the premature fetus was similar to that of the near-term fetus, with sustained bradycardia, redistribution of blood flow away from the periphery to essential organs with initial hypertension. With continued asphyxia there was failure of adaptation with profound hypotension and hypoperfusion. The major difference with the near-term fetus (Fig. 23.3) was that the premature fetus was able to survive such a prolonged period of cord occlusion. Data derived from Bennet *et al.* (1999).

fetuses neuronal damage was limited to selective loss of the very large, metabolically active cerebellar Purkinje cells (De Haan *et al.* 1993).

## Brief repeated asphyxia

In normal human labor, uterine contractions are relatively brief (typically less than one or two minutes). Total umbilical cord occlusions have been studied in fetal lambs near term at frequencies consistent with active labor, either 1 min out of every 2.5 min or 2 min out of every 5 min, continued for many hours until fetal hypotension (<20 mmHg) occurred (de Haan *et al.* 1997a,b). There was an initial sustained rise in blood pressure during early occlusions followed after 15 min by the appearance of a biphasic pattern. This pattern was characterized by an initial rise in blood pressure at the start of each occlusion, followed by a fall. From then on a progressive fall in the nadir of fetal arterial blood pressure occurred with each occlusion.

At a pH between 7.04 and 6.85 in individual fetuses, the recovery of arterial blood pressure after each occlusion became markedly delayed. The rapid decompensation associated with this sustained hypotension was associated with delayed recovery of the fetal heart rate in only a third of cases, illustrating the poor diagnostic value of fetal heart rate monitoring to identify the compromised fetus (de Haan *et al.* 1997a). Histologic analysis demonstrated the presence of focal neuronal damage in the parasagittal cortex, the thalamus and the cerebellum, while the hippocampus and striatum were almost wholly spared (de Haan *et al.* 1997b).

## Maturational changes in fetal responses to asphyxia

The premature fetus at 90 days gestation, prior to the onset of cortical myelination, can tolerate extended periods of up to 20 minutes of umbilical cord occlusion without neuronal loss (Keunen *et al.* 1997). The very prolonged cardiac survival (up to 30 minutes, Fig. 23.4) (Bennet *et al.* 1999) corresponds with the maximal levels of cardiac glycogen that are seen at this gestation (Shelley 1961). Interestingly, while the premature fetal response to hypoxia appears to be different to that seen at term, the response during asphyxia was similar to that seen in more mature fetuses, with sustained bradycardia, accompanied by circulatory centralization, initial hypertension, then a progressive fall in pressure (Bennet *et al.* 1998, 1999). Similarly to the term fetus, there was no increase in blood flow to the brain and again this was due to a significant increase in vascular resistance rather than to hypotension (Bennet *et al.* 1999). The mechanism mediating this remains speculative. As shown in Figs 23.4 and 23.5, once blood pressure begins to fall CaBF falls in parallel. The fall in pressure is partly a function of the loss of redistribution of blood flow as seen in Fig. 23.5 with a rise in femoral blood flow. The mechanisms mediating this loss of redistribution are unknown, but are likely to relate to profound local peripheral acidosis. A similar phenomenon is also seen at term, near the end of occlusion.

In the latter half of a maximal interval of asphyxia in the preterm fetus, there is progressive failure of CVO, with a fall in both central and peripheral perfusion. This phase is much less likely to be seen for any significant duration in the term fetus, as glycogen stores in the term fetus are depleted more

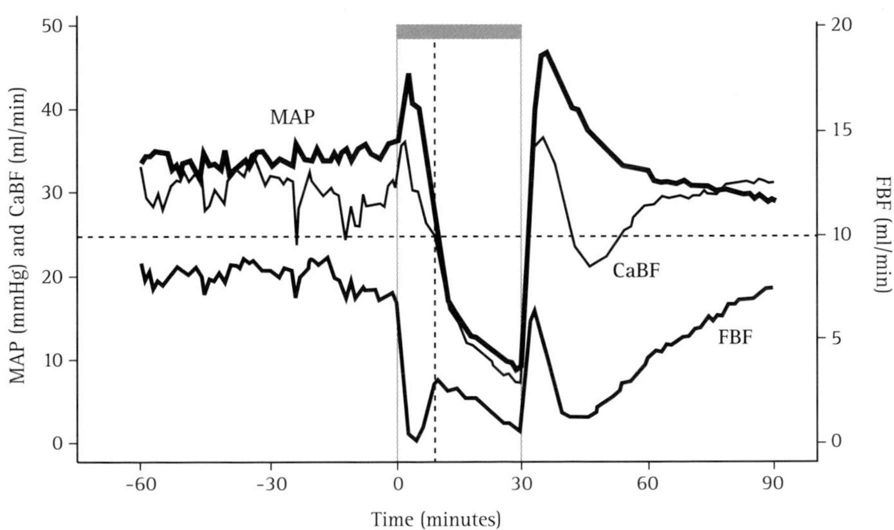


**Figure 23.5** An example of the relationship between hypotension and carotid and femoral blood flow (CaBF and FBF) during cord occlusion in a 0.6 gestation fetal sheep. The start and end of occlusion are shown by the solid lines and the bar. Note that the CaBF began to fall only when MAP was below baseline levels (shown by the dotted horizontal line), and thereafter paralleled the changes in MAP very closely. It is interesting that this also corresponded with failure of peripheral vasoconstriction (increased FBF, shown by the vertical dotted line). Similar changes are seen near-term, but with earlier onset of hypotension and hypoperfusion.

quickly. The term fetus is unable to survive such prolonged periods of sustained hypotension, and typically will recover from a maximum of 10–12 minutes of cord occlusion compared with up to 30 minutes at 0.6 gestation. As a consequence of this extended survival the premature fetus is exposed to profound and prolonged hypotension and hypoperfusion. It may be speculated that during this final phase of asphyxia in the premature fetus there is a catastrophic failure of redistribution of blood flow within the fetal brain, which places previously protected areas of the brain such as the brainstem at risk of injury (Myers 1977), consistent with clinical reports (Barkovich & Sargent 1995). Post-asphyxia, a brief period of arterial hypertension and hyperperfusion is followed by a prolonged period of hypoperfusion, despite normalization of blood pressure, with a reduction in cerebral oxygenation as measured by near-infrared spectroscopy (Fig. 23.6) (Bennet *et al.* 1999). This post-asphyxial hypoperfusion and reduced cerebral oxygenation may contribute further to cerebral injury.

## Chronic asphyxia

In addition to its potential impact on neurodevelopment (as outlined below, p. 423), chronic asphyxia may also adversely affect the ability of the fetus to adapt to acute insults (Hanson 1998). Chronic placental insufficiency leads to fetal arterial hypertension and myocardial hypertrophy, with increased umbilical artery resistance. Consistent with this, experimentally growth retarded fetuses exhibit sustained

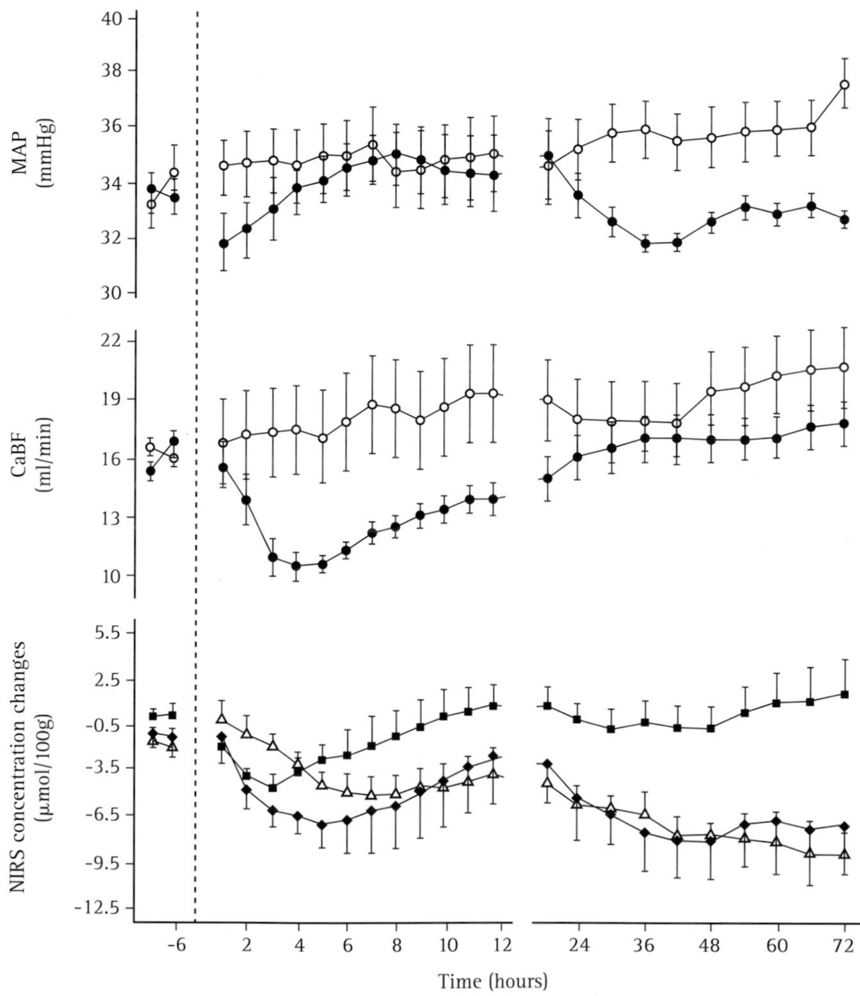


**Figure 23.6** The recovery of the near mid-gestation (0.6 gestation) fetal sheep following 30 minutes of complete umbilical cord occlusion (denoted by the heavy dashed line; for occlusion data see Fig. 23.4). In the top and middle panels, open symbols are control fetuses and closed symbols are asphyxiated fetuses. Post-asphyxia carotid blood flow (CaBF) showed a secondary fall, with a nadir after 4–6 h. This secondary change was not due to a fall in mean arterial blood pressure (MAP). The NIRS data (bottom panel) include only the asphyxia group. A similar secondary fall was seen in total cerebral hemoglobin (◆), which is the combination of oxyhemoglobin (■) and deoxyhemoglobin (△), and provides an index of total cerebral blood volume. Significantly this fall was mainly due to a significant reduction in cerebral oxyhemoglobin around 2–4 hours post-asphyxia suggesting a true impairment of cerebral perfusion. This may have contributed to the final injury. Data derived from Bennet *et al.* (1999).

elevation of plasma catecholamines, cortisol, and prostaglandin $E_2$, with a significant fall in corticotrophin, and when challenged with hypoxia have a blunted rise in plasma catecholamines. These adaptations are associated with a blunted cardiovascular response to further acute hypoxic challenges. Similar observations have been made in newborn rats exposed to chronic hypoxia *in utero*, and in the llama, a species adapted to the hypoxemia of high altitude (Hanson 1998; Richardson & Bocking 1998).

## PATHOGENESIS OF CELL DEATH

### WHAT INITIATES NEURONAL INJURY?

At the most fundamental level, injury requires a period of insufficient delivery of oxygen and substrates such as glucose (and other substances such as lactate in the fetus) such that neurons (and glia) cannot maintain homeostasis. If oxygen is reduced but substrate delivery is effectively maintained (i.e. pure or nearly pure hypoxia), the cells adapt in two ways. First, they can use anaerobic metabolism to support their production of high-energy metabolites for a time. The use of anaerobic metabolism is of course very inefficient since anaerobic glycolysis produces lactate and only 2 ATP, whereas aerobic glycolysis produces 38 ATP. Thus glucose reserves are rapidly consumed, and a metabolic acidosis develops with local and systemic consequences. Second, they can to some extent reduce non-obligatory energy consumption. This is clearly seen in neurons, where moderate hypoxia typically induces a switch to lower frequency states requiring less oxygen consumption. As an insult becomes more severe, neuronal activity will then cease completely, at a threshold above that which causes actual neuronal depolarization.

In contrast, under conditions of combined reduction of oxygen and substrate the neuron's options are much more limited, as not only is there less oxygen, but there is also much less glucose available to allow anaerobic metabolism. This may occur during either pure ischemia (reduced tissue blood flow) and even more critically during conditions of hypoxia–ischemia i.e. both reduced oxygen content, and reduced total blood flow. In the fetus, hypoxia–ischemia commonly occurs due to hypoxic cardiac compromise. Under these conditions depletion of high energy metabolites will occur much more rapidly and profoundly, while at the same time, there may actually be *less* acidosis both because there is much less glucose available to be metabolized to lactate, and because the insult is evolving more quickly.

These concepts help to explain the consistent observation, discussed later in this chapter, that most cerebral injury after acute insults occurs in association with hypotension and consequent tissue hypoperfusion or ischemia. Technically, asphyxia is defined as the combination of impaired respiratory gas exchange (i.e. hypoxia and hypercapnia) accompanied by the development of metabolic acidosis. When we think about the impact on the brain of clinical asphyxia it will be critical to keep in mind that this definition tells us much about things that can be measured relatively easily (blood gases and systemic acidosis) and essentially nothing about blood pressure or perfusion of the brain.

### CEREBRAL INJURY: AN 'EVOLVING' PROCESS

The seminal concept to emerge from both experimental and clinical studies is that brain cell death does not necessarily occur during hypoxia or ischemia (the 'primary' phase of injury), but rather they may precipitate a cascade of biochemical processes leading to delayed cell death hours or even days afterwards (the 'secondary' phase). The sequence is illustrated in Fig. 23.7. Experimental studies have demonstrated the existence of both a primary phase of energy failure during hypoxia–ischemia, a 'latent' phase during which oxidative metabolism normalizes, followed by secondary failure of oxidative metabolism in piglets (Lorek *et al.* 1994) and immature rats (Blumberg *et al.* 1997). Clinically, neural injury with no initial recovery of oxidative metabolism is seen after sufficiently severe or prolonged asphyxia (Azzopardi *et al.* 1989), but in many other cases infants show initial, transient recovery of cerebral oxidative metabolism followed by a secondary deterioration, with cerebral energy failure from 6 to 15 hours after birth (Azzopardi *et al.* 1989; Roth *et al.* 1997). In asphyxiated infants there is a close correlation between the degree of

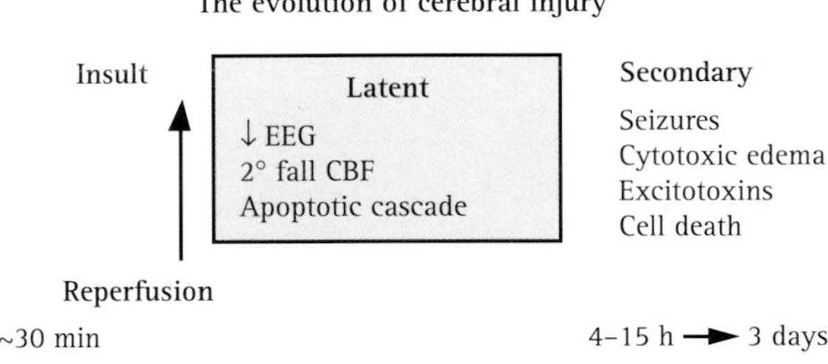


**Figure 23.7** Flow chart illustrating the relationship between the mechanisms active in the pathophysiologically defined phases of cerebral injury after a severe reversible hypoxic–ischemic insult. During the immediate *reperfusion* period, lasting approximately 30 minutes, cellular energy metabolism is restored, with resolution of the acute hypoxic depolarization and cell swelling. This is followed by a *latent* phase, with near-normal oxidative cerebral energy metabolism as shown by magnetic resonance spectroscopy, but depressed electroencephalogram (EEG) activity, and often a delayed period of reduced cerebral blood flow (CBF). The latent phase is believed to be associated with the intracellular components of the apoptotic cascade. This may be followed by *secondary* deterioration with delayed seizures and cytotoxic edema, extracellular accumulation of potential cytotoxins (such as the excitatory neurotransmitters), and 4–15 h after the asphyxia, failure of oxidative metabolism and damage. The changes in the secondary phase may take 3 days or more to resolve.

secondary energy failure and neurodevelopmental outcome at 1 and 4 years of age (Roth *et al.* 1997).

A critical aspect of these findings is that a single 'subthreshold' insult that causes either minor or no neural injury can lead to a phase of increased vulnerability to further insults. Conversely, the delayed evolution of cell death after more severe insults suggests the potential for the prevention of brain cell death by interrupting the events which lead to secondary cell death (Gunn & Gluckman 1998).

### FOCAL INSULTS

Post-asphyxial encephalopathy is typically associated with global, reversible hypoxia–ischemia. Purely focal lesions can occur in the newborn, typically in infants with no evidence of exposure to asphyxia. The evolution of injury is quite different from that seen after global insults with reperfusion. In a focal ischemic injury, such as adult stroke, there is a dense ischemic core characterized by primary cell death with pannecrosis. This core is surrounded by an ischemic 'penumbra' which has some residual blood supply. Damage extends from the core out to the penumbra over a few hours under experimental conditions. The evolution of damage in the penumbra has been associated with waves of depolarization which deplete remaining cellular energy reserves (Lipton 1999).

## PATHOPHYSIOLOGIC CORRELATES OF THE PHASES OF NEURAL INJURY

Many of the pathophysiologic events associated with evolution of injury have been characterized in a model of reversible cerebral ischemia in the chronically instrumented fetal sheep, studied *in utero* (Williams *et al.* 1991). The primary and secondary phases of injury seen in this paradigm are shown in Fig. 23.8. During carotid artery occlusion, the EEG shows an immediate loss of amplitude, becoming isoelectric after 30 seconds, and remains so until the end of occlusion. After 30 minutes of occlusion, the EEG remains suppressed for 5–9 hours. During this period of reduced neural activity, a secondary hypoperfusion develops, which reflects depressed cerebral metabolism (Gunn *et al.* 1997). The significance of this remains elusive, as this is also seen after 'threshold' insults which do not cause cell death. In the adult, the duration but not the depth of the secondary reduction in CBF has been correlated with the severity of the insult (Michenfelder & Milde 1990). The secondary phase is marked by an abrupt onset of seizure activity, with an increase in CBF (Gunn *et al.* 1997) and cytotoxic edema. The delayed seizure activity peaks rapidly at approximately 12 hours, then progressively resolves over 1–2 days. The residual EEG intensity after resolution of seizures is related to the amount of neuronal death in the underlying cortex.

The development of cytotoxic edema can be monitored using cortical impedance (Williams *et al.* 1991). This is a technique whereby the electrical resistance (impedance) to a low amplitude alternating current is measured; the impedance of a tissue rises concomitantly as cells depolarize and fluid shifts from the extracellular to the intracellular space. Thus a rise in impedance reflects cell swelling. As shown in Fig. 23.8, there is a rapid rise in impedance during ischemia, which almost completely resolves over 30–60 minutes of reperfusion. The secondary evolution of cytotoxic oedema, initiated after the onset of seizures, peaks much later and takes 2–3 days to resolve. Even if seizures are abolished by infusion of a selective glutamate antagonist, the secondary rise is only delayed (Tan *et al.* 1992), suggesting that the edema is not a direct consequence of seizures but rather primarily reflects ongoing encephalopathic processes. The timing of secondary edema is consistent with that of secondary energy failure after perinatal asphyxia, as measured by magnetic resonance spectroscopy (MRS) in the infant (Reynolds *et al.* 1991) and piglet (Lorek *et al.* 1991). Interestingly, studies in near-term fetal sheep using near infrared spectroscopy also suggest that mitochondrial failure occurs in this delayed phase (Marks *et al.* 1996).

Histologic analysis after 3 days' recovery shows that 30 minutes of ischemia causes consistent injury of the parasagittal cortex and dorsal hippocampus, with macroscopically visible laminar necrosis. Our group has shown that microscopically there is at least 75–90% neuronal death in the parasagittal cortex, with lesser loss in other areas (Gunn *et al.* 1997) and this is illustrated in Fig. 23.9. The depths of the sulci tend to show greater damage than the adjacent gyri. This pattern of injury with predominant parasagittal and sulcal injury, is a classic 'watershed' distribution which is commonly seen in asphyxiated term neonates (Volpe 1995).

### THE PRIMARY PHASE

Once the neuron's supply of high-energy metabolites such as ATP can no longer be maintained during hypoxia–ischemia, there is failure of the energy dependent mechanisms of intracellular homeostasis such as the $Na^+/K^+$ ATP-dependent pump. Neuronal depolarization occurs leading to sodium and calcium entry into cells. This in turn favors further cation and water entry, leading to cell swelling (cytotoxic edema). If sufficiently severe this may cause immediate neuronal lysis, but before this stage, the swollen neurons may still recover if hypoxia is stopped or if the osmotic environment is manipulated (*in vitro*) to prevent cell swelling (Goldberg & Choi 1993). Finally, re-uptake of excitatory amino acid neurotransmitters (EAAs) such as glutamate is also energy dependent. Thus typically, ischemia is associated with extracellular accumulation of the EAAs. Receptor mediated binding by these neurotransmitters further favors both immediate swelling, by opening receptor linked $Na^+/K^+$ channels (e.g. the α-amino-3-hydroxy-5-methyl-4-isoxazolepropionic acid, AMPA, subtype of glutamate receptor) as well as calcium entry (e.g. the *N*-methyl D-aspartate, NMDA, subtype of glutamate receptor) (Choi 1995).

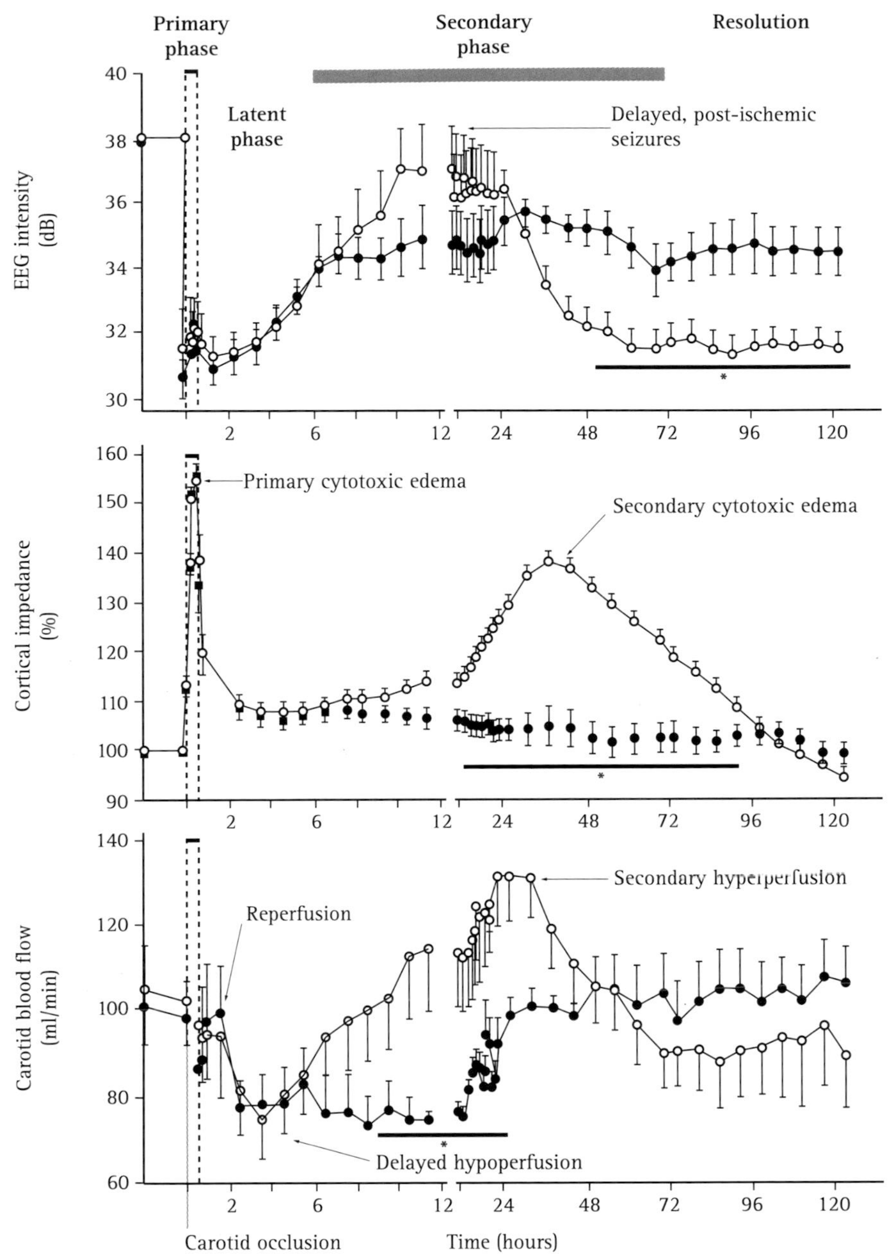


**Figure 23.8** The relationship between the phases of neural injury and changes in the fetal electroencephalogram (EEG), impedance and carotid blood flow after 30 minutes of global cerebral ischemia in the near-term fetal sheep. Impedance is a measure of cytotoxic edema in the parietal cortex. Fetuses received either sham cooling (○) or cerebral hypothermia (●) started 5.5 h after reperfusion, and continued until 72 h. The hypothermia group shows better recovery of EEG intensity after resolution of delayed seizures, and complete suppression of the secondary rise in impedance. The phase of secondary hypoperfusion is extended by hypothermia but resolves spontaneously despite continued cooling for 72 h. Data derived from Gunn *et al.* (1998). Mean ± SEM, $^*p < 0.05$.

Ionic calcium is normally actively maintained at very low concentrations in the cell (10 000-fold lower than in extracellular fluid). This gradient allows calcium to be used by the cell as an intracellular signaling mechanism. Although the rise in intracellular calcium during hypoxia does not cause immediate cell death, it can inappropriately activate enzymes and signal transduction systems that favor free radical production, kinase activities and hydroxyapatite precipitation which are all potentially damaging (Choi 1995). Oxygen free radicals are derived partially from such calcium activated enzymatic processes and partly from excess purine production, as ATP is exhausted. It is generally

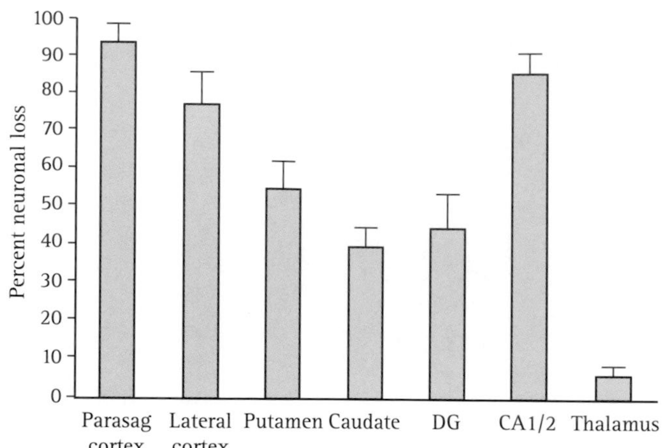


**Figure 23.9** Comparison of neuronal loss (mean ± SEM) in different brain regions 5 days after severe ischemia (bilateral carotid artery occlusion for 30 minutes) in the near-term fetal sheep. Injury is greatest in the parasagittal cortex and in the underlying dorsal horn of the hippocampus. In contrast, the granule cells of the dentate gyrus (DG) of the hippocampus and the nuclei of the striatum and thalamus (Putamen and Caudate) are relatively spared. This pattern of injury is in the classic 'watershed' distribution (see Refs Gunn *et al.* 1997, 1998).

believed that oxygen free radicals play a particular role in damaging essential cell membrane components during the immediate recovery from asphyxia (the reperfusion phase), when tissue oxygen levels abruptly recover (Fellman & Raivio 1997).

## THE DELAYED PHASE

Although neurons (and glia) may initially recover from the primary injury, processes initiated by exposure to hypoxia–ischemia may lead to cell death hours or days later. The longer and more severe the insult, generally the greater proportion of primary neural death (Beilharz *et al.* 1995). Delayed appearance of histologically defined cell death has been directly demonstrated after asphyxial brain injury from clinical and experimental studies (Gunn 2000).

### Necrosis and apoptosis

Two morphologic patterns of delayed cell death have been described: necrosis and apoptosis (Raff 1992). Necrosis is defined by loss of plasma membrane integrity associated with a random pattern of DNA degradation. Typically there is swelling of the cytoplasm and organelles, with little change initially to the nucleus. Apoptosis is defined by shrinkage of the cell, 'karyohexis', associated with specific endonuclease mediated DNA degradation. Eventually, the shrunken cell breaks into small fragments. Karyohexis is the classic microscopic picture of condensation of chromatin (i.e. a dark shrunken nucleus) with loss of the reticular formation in the cytoplasm (leading to eosinophilia on light microscopy). The active degradation of DNA by endonucleases, which cleave the chromatin at internucleosomal points, leads to fragments of fixed size, with a characteristic laddered appearance on chromatography.

By analogy with the active process of developmental loss of excess cells (including neurons) it is suggested that an apoptotic morphology reflects active cell death, involving a cascade of 'suicide' processes (Raff 1992). In contrast, necrosis is suggested to reflect biophysical damage to the cell (cell membrane instability, ion shifts, etc.), particularly lysis in the primary phase. Both are clearly described in infants dying after perinatal asphyxia (Edwards *et al.* 1997; Scott & Hegyi 1997). Apoptosis may be initiated by several intracellular pathways, but the final events involve alterations in the ratio of various intracellular factors such as Bcl (which inhibits apoptosis) and Bax which promotes apoptosis, and to activation of a family of proteases related to interleukin converting enzyme, known as caspases (Lipton 1999). The final events involve endonuclease mediated DNA fragmentation (Beilharz *et al.* 1995).

Although a greater proportion of necrotic cell death is seen with increasing severity of the primary insult (Beilharz *et al.* 1995), it has become clear that the underlying processes may not be as clearly separated as originally thought. Even slowly evolving, treatable cell death can occur by necrosis (Colbourne *et al.* 1999), and hypoxic cell death *in vitro* appears to include a combination of both apoptotic and necrotic processes, with one or the other being more prominent depending on factors such as maturity (Gottron *et al.* 1997; Porteracailliau *et al.* 1997). Furthermore, there is evidence that mitochondrial calcium overload is a critical event in both apoptotic and necrotic cell death and that 'anti-apoptotic' nuclear proteins such as Bcl can also inhibit necrotic cell death (Lipton 1999).

The concept remains an important one, considering that if neuronal and glial cell death is an active response, mediated by activation of second and third messenger events after an acute event (whether specifically due to a preset 'death program' or to less specific pathways initiated by excess free calcium, inflammatory pathways and/or cytotoxins), then it should logically be possible to interrupt these events.

### Intracellular calcium accumulation

The events promoting or sustaining delayed cell death after reperfusion are not known. Mitochondrial calcium overload during hypoxia–ischemia appears to be one of the critical steps initiating delayed death (Choi 1995), and therapeutic strategies to reduce calcium induced neuronal death are discussed in Chapter 28. Other proposed damaging factors that may also contribute include loss of trophic growth factor support and free radical release during reperfusion.

### Microglial activation

There is a close temporal association between microglial activation and the development of apoptosis, and thus this has been proposed to be a causal relationship (Lees 1993). Microglia are the macrophages resident in the brain, but other macrophages may also cross from the circulation and play a role in the activation of the neuroimmune system after asphyxial injury. Activated microglia express a number of cytotoxic cytokines such as tumor necrosis factor alpha (TNF-α) as well as the cytotoxic radicals NO and $H_2O_2$. This neuroimmune system has probably evolved as a protective response to viral and bacterial infection at the cost of retaining a potential neurotoxic role (Lees 1993).

### Seizures and excitotoxins

In the human neonate, seizure activity is a bad prognostic indicator (Hellstrom Westas *et al.* 1995). *In vivo* microdialysis after ischemia in the fetal sheep shows that both glutamate and NO are induced in the secondary phase (Tan *et al.* 1996). The elevation in extracellular glutamate is closely associated with the onset of post-asphyxial seizures, and treatment with a specific antagonist of the NMDA type of glutamate receptor potently abolishes the seizures. However, this treatment had no effect on the most severely affected region (the parasagittal cortex) and had a modest effect in more peripheral regions, suggesting that these post-ischemic seizures only have a partial role in extending the area of brain injury (Tan *et al.* 1992).

## ENDOGENOUS PROTECTIVE MECHANISMS

A number of endogenous protective responses of the brain act to limit injury. These responses include release of neuromodulators/inhibitory neurotransmitters, induction of neurotrophic factors and intracellular anti-apoptotic systems, and postnatally, spontaneous cerebral hypothermia. An illustration of the potential protective effects of endogenous cellular responses is that a single, subthreshold insult that does not cause damage may markedly increase resistance to a subsequent more severe insult. Several hours must elapse for preconditioning to be seen, and its effect then attenuates after several days, consistent with the time course of a wide range of stress gene responses to ischemia (Massa *et al.* 1996). Several of the mechanisms discussed below may be involved, including induction of anti-apoptotic genes such as Bcl-2, growth factors such as insulin-like growth factor or fibroblast growth factor, free radical scavengers, adenosine, and the heat shock proteins.

### Inhibitory neuromodulators

Ischemia and asphyxia are typically associated with a large increase in inhibitory neuromodulators such as γ-amino butyric acid (GABA), adenosine and cerebral opioids (Shuaib & Kanthan 1997). Microdialysis studies in the fetal lamb suggest that compared with postnatal studies, there is a disproportionately large release of GABA relative to that of the excitotoxins during ischemia (Tan *et al.* 1996). Interestingly, adult species such as the turtle that are very tolerant to hypoxia, also show a very elevated GABA response to anoxia (Nilsson & Lutz 1991). After reperfusion in the fetal lamb, there is a rapid fall in cerebral GABA levels (Tan *et al.* 1996), with no elevation of GABA during the secondary phase. This loss of GABA release during the secondary phase may be one contributor to the development of very intense seizures that are difficult to manage.

It has been proposed that endogenous release of these inhibitory factors may help limit cerebral injury by reducing neural activity and by providing a counter balance to the excitatory neurotransmitters, and thus that increasing cerebral inhibitory responses may be a logical treatment (Shuaib & Kanthan 1997). However, the results of many studies using this approach have been contradictory with, for example, evidence of protection both with agonists and antagonists to the adenosine receptors (Bona *et al.* 1997; Shuaib & Kanthan 1997). This is discussed in detail in Chapter 28.

### Endogenous neurotrophic factors

Cerebral injury is associated with neurotrophic activity (defined by the ability to support neuronal survival *in vitro*), which is considerably greater in the immature brain than later in life (Hughes *et al.* 1999). Studies suggest that neuronal injury is associated with rapid, transient, activity dependent expression of neurotrophins (such as nerve growth factor-β, brain derived growth factor, neurotensin 3, and activin A) in neurons, contrasting with a delayed and more persistent injury induced expression of certain growth factors (insulin-like growth factor 1 (IGF-1) and transforming growth factor beta (TGF-β) within glia (Hughes *et al.* 1999). For example, the broadly anti-apoptotic agent IGF-1 and two of its binding proteins (IGFBP-2 and IGFBP-3) are intensely induced 3–5 days after hypoxic–ischemic injury in the developing brain. The binding proteins may perhaps act to transport and target IGF-1 to particular cell types. Endogenous administration of growth factors, including IGF-1 and TGF-β, is neuroprotective (Hughes *et al.* 1999) (see p. 512).

### Cerebrovascular responses in the delayed phase

A delayed period of hyperperfusion or 'luxury perfusion' is well described after perinatal asphyxia (Ilves *et al.* 1998). There is evidence that this hyperperfusion in the delayed phase may in part protect marginally viable tissue (Abi Raad *et al.* 1999). Putatively neuroprotective agents such as the calcium antagonists which depress blood pressure, and thus impair CBF in the post-asphyxial period, may aggravate brain injury (Gunn & Gluckman 1998). Factors that may mediate the hyperperfusion phase include NO (Marks *et al.* 1996), and prostacyclin (Walton *et al.* 1997). NO is a volatile, rapidly regulated, neuromodulator that can be produced by NO synthases (NOS) in endothelial cells (eNOS), neurons (nNOS) and by neutrophils or microglia (inducible NOS, or iNOS). Citrulline, a degradation production of NO, is induced

**Table 23.1 Summary of cardiovascular and cerebrovascular adaptations to asphyxia**

- The healthy fetus has considerable aerobic and anaerobic reserves to cope with transient or mild hypoxia
- The fetal defences against hypoxia depend on the type and severity of the insult, maturation, and fetal wellbeing
- During moderate hypoxia blood flow is redirected to key organs, and flow is also redirected within the brain towards the structures important for autonomic function such as the brainstem
- During severe asphyxia of rapid onset the adaptations are similar but more extreme. Blood flow to the brain as a whole may not be increased, but appears to be maintained so long as blood pressure is normal or raised
- Progression of severe asphyxia results in failure of adaptation and progressive hypotension and hypoperfusion.

*Variable decelerations*

- Intermittent or repeated insults as seen during labor allow partial recovery and adaptation between periods of hypoxia, but eventually hypotension begins to develop during hypoxia and becomes progressively more severe
- The initial changes in the fetal heart rate during acute asphyxia are reflex mediated. Thus FHR changes during variable decelerations poorly reflect the development of fetal hypotension or acidosis
- In previously healthy fetuses, late recovery from severe variable decelerations is seen only in a subgroup of profoundly compromised fetuses

**Table 23.2 Acidosis and the pathogenesis of cell death**

- There is no intrinsic, physiologic relationship between the amount of systemic anerobic metabolism (as reflected by metabolic acidosis) and the development of neuronal injury. The crude clinical correlation between the two is simply consistent with the fact that hypoxic–ischemic damage occurs under anaerobic conditions
- Systemic acidosis during asphyxia is primarily related to peripheral vasoconstriction, acting to redistribute blood flow to essential organs. Even when a proportion of whole body anaerobic metabolism is central, so long as sufficient glucose is available to neurons to support basal energy metabolism, injury will not occur. Thus profound arterial metabolic acidosis may still accompany successful protection of the brain, with a normal outcome
- During very prolonged periods of asphyxia with ongoing lactic acidosis, very severe acidosis may compromise fetal adaptation, including blood flow redistribution and cardiac contractility, promoting hypotension and thus causing cerebral hypoxia–ischaemia
- Conversely during more acute insults, with impaired tissue perfusion, less glucose is delivered to neurons and so less lactate is produced. Thus, injury may occur despite relatively modest levels of acidosis
- Acute-on-chronic insults where there is reduced fetal metabolic reserve also have the potential to lead to injury after relatively short periods of acute asphyxia and moderate acidosis

in extracellular brain fluid in the secondary phase after ischemia, which may suggest a role for NO in delayed injury (Tan *et al.* 1996) (see p. 417).

It is vital to take into consideration the multiple roles of NO in order to interpret its effects on neural injury. The endothelial NO is a vasodilator which under physiological conditions plays an important role in the regulation of cerebral blood flow (CBF), cerebral autoregulation, blood flow–metabolism coupling and the control of platelet aggregation and adhesion (Faraci & Heistad 1998). NO has also been shown to play a role in regulating fetal CBF (Hanson 1997). Thus, it is perhaps not surprising that as most NO production derives from induction of endothelial NOS, non-specific inhibition of NO production following ischemia has been associated with increased cerebral injury, probably due to impairment of cerebral perfusion (Marks *et al.* 1996).

nNOS is $Ca^{2+}$ dependent and thus activated by intracellular calcium accumulation during ischemia, and nNOS expression in the developing brain correlates with regions of selective neuronal loss in the developing rat brain. iNOS is inducible by cytokines and released by activated macrophages in very highly concentrated killing bursts. Macrophage activation occurs in the delayed phase of injury, and thus it is a likely mediator of cytotoxicity in that phase. Selective inhibition of nNOS or iNOS is suggested to be neuroprotective (Bolanos & Almeida 1999) (see p. 509). However, much more work is required to dissect their contribution to brain damage.

**Table 23.3 Summary: the evolution of neural injury**

- Neuronal death does not necessarily occur at the time of the insult. Hypoxia–ischaemia may activate pre-existing cell death pathways, leading to evolving cell death
- The different stages of evolution of delayed cell death are reflected in characteristic pathophysiologic changes. Experimentally, successful intervention has been shown in the reperfusion and latent phases. To date no successful treatment has been shown with therapy delayed until after the onset of secondary deterioration.
- During recovery from a mild 'threshold' insult, the fetus may be more vulnerable to any further insult or to environmental factors such as hyperthermia or impaired cardiovascular function.

## Acidosis: friend or foe?

The systemic acidosis caused by asphyxia is both associated with and can exacerbate fetal compromise, for example by impairing cardiac contractility. The direct effect on neural injury, however, is complex. *In vitro*, acidosis limits both hypoxic and excitotoxic neuronal injury in hippocampal neurons (Giffard *et al.* 1990; Tombaugh 1994). It is a striking observation that in experimental studies in the fetal sheep, the dorsal horn of the hippocampus is very vulnerable to short periods of dense ischemia or asphyxia, but has been reported to be spared after both brief repeated asphyxia and prolonged partial asphyxia (de Haan *et al.* 1997b). Consistent with the hypothesis that local acidosis may actually protect this region, a very profound acidosis developed during brief repeated cord occlusions (pH 6.83 ± 0.03) (de Haan *et al.* 1997b), whereas there was only a mild metabolic acidosis after 10 minutes of umbilical cord occlusion with severe selective loss in the cornu ammonis fields of the hippocampus (5 minutes after reperfusion the mean pH was >7.10) (Mallard *et al.* 1992).

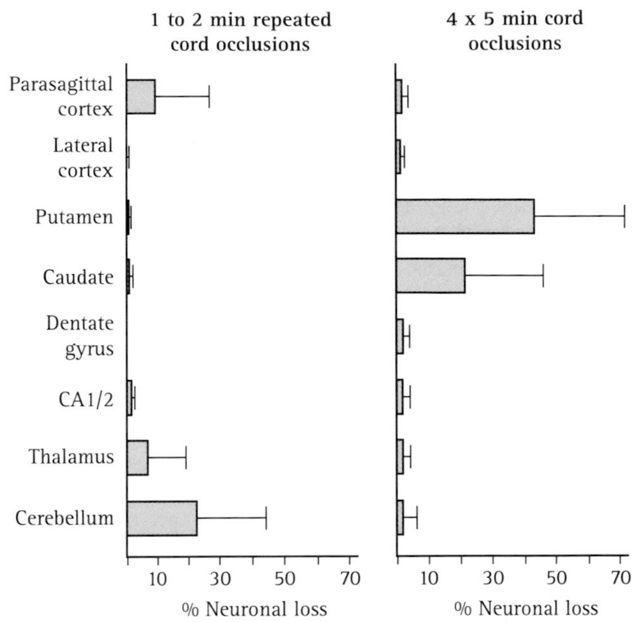


**Figure 23.10** The distribution of neuronal loss assessed after 3 days recovery from two different patterns of prenatal asphyxia in near-term fetal sheep. The left panel shows the effects of brief (1 or 2 min) cord occlusions repeated at frequencies consistent with established labor. Occlusions were terminated after a variable time, when the fetal blood pressure fell below 20 mmHg for two successive occlusions. This insult led to damage in the watershed regions of the parasagittal cortex and cerebellum (de Haan *et al.* 1997b). The right hand panel shows the effect of five minute episodes of cord occlusion, repeated four times, at intervals of 30 minutes. This paradigm is associated with selective neuronal loss in the putamen and caudate nucleus, which are nuclei of the striatum. CA 1/2 and the dentate gyrus are regions of the hippocampus. Mean ± SD. Data derived from de Haan *et al.* (1997c).

# PATHOPHYSIOLOGIC DETERMINANTS OF ASPHYXIAL INJURY

Recent studies using well defined experimental paradigms of asphyxia in the near-term fetal sheep have explored the relationship between the distribution of neuronal damage and the type of insult. These studies suggest that the key factor precipitating and localizing injury is local cerebral hypoperfusion due to hypotension. In addition, a number of factors modify the impact of asphyxia on the brain, including the pattern of repetition of insults as well as fetal factors such as gestational age, pre-existing metabolic state, and cerebral temperature (see Fig. 23.1).

## HYPOTENSION AND THE 'WATERSHED' DISTRIBUTION OF NEURONAL LOSS

The development of hypotension appears to be the critical factor precipitating neural injury after acute insults. This is readily understood as reduced perfusion will reduce the supply of glucose for anerobic metabolism, compounding the reduction of oxygen delivery and concentration. The real life importance of hypotension is supported by both the pattern of neural damage, and the correlation of injury with arterial blood pressure across multiple paradigms.

The close relationship between changes in CaBF and blood pressure during asphyxia is shown by Figs 23.3–23.5. In these fetuses, mean arterial blood pressure (MAP) initially rose with intense peripheral vasoconstriction. At this time CaBF was maintained. As cord occlusion was continued MAP eventually fell, probably as a function of impaired cardiac contractility and failure of peripheral redistribution. When MAP fell below baseline, carotid blood flow fell in parallel. It appeared that there was a small window during which flow was maintained as pressure was falling (Fig. 23.5), suggesting that autoregulation was intact. This is consistent with the normal relatively narrow range of fetal cerebrovasculature autoregulation (Parer 1998).

In the term fetus, neural injury has been commonly reported in areas such as the parasagittal cortex, the dorsal horn of the hippocampus, and the cerebellar neocortex after a range of insults including pure ischemia, prolonged single complete umbilical cord occlusion, and prolonged partial asphyxia and repeated brief cord occlusion (Figs 23.9, left panel and 23.10) (de Haan 1993, 1997b; Gunn *et al.* 1992, 1997; Mallard *et al.* 1992). These areas are 'watershed' zones within the borders between major cerebral arteries, where perfusion pressure is least, and, clinically, lesions in these areas in adults and children are typically seen after systemic hypotension (Torrik 1984).

Some data suggest that limited or localized white or gray matter injury may occur even when significant hypotension is not seen (de Haan *et al.* 1983; Ikeda *et al.* 1998), particularly when hypoxia is very prolonged (Rees *et al.* 1998). Clearly there may have been some relative hypoperfusion in these studies. Nevertheless, there is a strong correlation between either the depth or duration of hypotension and the amount of neuronal loss within individual studies of acute asphyxia (Gunn *et al.* 1992; de Haan *et al.* 1997b,c; Ikeda *et al.* 1998).

This is also seen between similar paradigms causing severe fetal acidosis that have been manipulated to either cause fetal hypotension (Gunn *et al.* 1992; Ikeda *et al.* 1998) or not (de Haan *et al.* 1993). In fetal lambs exposed to prolonged severe partial asphyxia, as judged by the degree of metabolic compromise, neuronal loss occurred only in those in whom one or more episodes of acute hypotension occurred (Ikeda *et al.* 1998). In contrast, in a similar study where an equally 'severe' insult was induced gradually and titrated to maintain normal or elevated blood pressure throughout the insult, no neuronal loss was seen outside the cerebellum (de Haan *et al.* 1993).

## PATTERN OF INJURY: REPEATED INSULTS

The one apparent exception to a general tendency to a 'watershed' distribution after global asphyxial insults near-term, is the selective neuronal loss in striatal nuclei (putamen and caudate nucleus; Fig. 23.10, right panel) which is seen when relatively prolonged periods of asphyxia or ischemia are repeated (Mallard *et al.* 1993; de Haan *et al.* 1997c). Whereas 30 minutes of continuous cerebral ischemia leads to predominantly parasagittal cortical neuronal loss, with only moderate striatal injury, when the insult was divided into three episodes of ischemia, a greater proportion of striatal injury was seen relative to cortical neuronal loss (Figs 23.9 and 23.11) (de Haan *et al.* 1997c). Intriguingly, significant striatal involvement was also seen after prolonged partial asphyxia in which distinct episodes of bradycardia and hypotension occurred (Gunn *et al.* 1992).

It is thus likely that the pathogenesis of striatal involvement in the near-term fetus is related to the precise timing of the relatively prolonged episodes of asphyxia and not to more severe local hypoperfusion, since the striatum is not in a watershed zone but rather within the territory of the middle cerebral artery. The vulnerability of the medium sized neurons of the striatum to this type of insult may be related to a greater release of glutamate into the striatal extracellular space after repeated insults compared with a single insult of the same cumulative duration. Consistent with this, immunohistochemical techniques have shown that inhibitory striatal neurons were primarily affected (Mallard *et al.* 1995).

## PREMATURE BRAIN INJURY: THE EFFECT OF MATURATION

Surprisingly little work has been done to resolve the effect of maturation on sensitivity to injury. This is of critical importance, for two reasons. First, in recent years improvements in

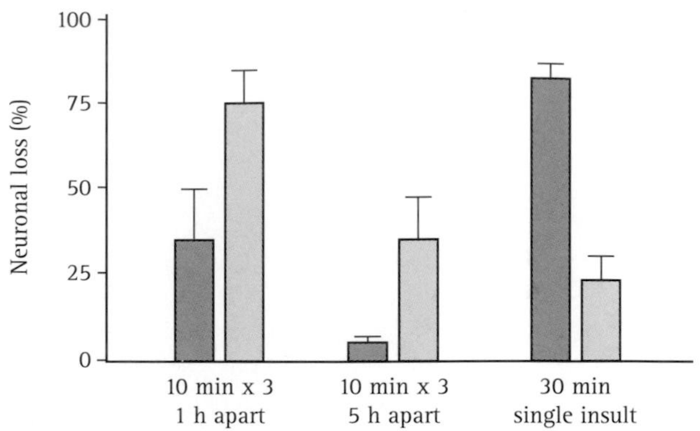


Figure 23.11 The effects of different intervals between insults on the distribution of cerebral damage after ischemia in the near-term fetal sheep. Cerebral ischemia was induced by carotid occlusion for 10 minutes and repeated three times, at intervals of either 1 h or 5 h, compared with a single continuous episode of 30 minutes occlusion. The divided insults were associated with a preponderance of striatal injury, whereas a single episode of 30 minutes of carotid occlusion was associated with severe cortical neuronal loss. Increasing the interval to 5 h nearly completely abolished cortical injury, but was still associated with significant neuronal loss in the striatum. Light bars are results for striatum and dark bars are those for parasagittal cortex. Data derived from Mallard *et al.* (1993).

obstetric and pediatric management have resulted in significantly increased survival of preterm infants from 24 weeks of gestation, with an associated increase in later handicap (Kiely & Susser 1992). Second, many infants may sustain neural injuries well before birth, including a significant number of infants with cerebral palsy (Stanley 1992) (see also Chapters 20 and 44). The characteristic patterns of cerebral injury in the preterm fetus differ from those seen at term or after birth. Key features include preferential injury of subcortical structures and white matter.

### Cortical susceptibility

Clinical imaging data suggest that profound asphyxia before 32 weeks gestation is associated with injury to subcortical structures, particularly the diencephalon (including the thalamus), basal ganglia and brainstem (Barkovich & Sargent 1995). This is consistent with the patterns observed in infants with cerebral palsy of prenatal origin who show predominantly diencephalic lesions, variably associated with PVL, cortical or subcortical lesions and ventricular dilatation (Volpe 1995). Similarly, in fetal sheep at 0.65 to 0.7 gestation (96 to 102 days), a maturation comparable to the 28 week gestation human fetus, 30 minutes of cerebral ischemia induced by reversible carotid occlusion, led to the development of subcortical infarction involving the deeper layers (V and VI) of the cortex, and underlying white matter tracts

(Reddy *et al.* 1998). In contrast, the same insult in the near-term fetal sheep leads to neuronal loss which is greatest in the superficial layers (II, III and IV) of the cortex.

This difference is consistent with the stages of anatomical maturation. As neurons migrate into the cortex during development, the deeper layers are populated first and thus mature first, while the superficial layers include immature, migrating neurons which are less metabolically active and are still using primarily anaerobic pathways (Hansen 1977). Another factor may be progressive maturation of the neuronal glutamate receptors during and after migration (Gressens *et al.* 1996). This is an area requiring considerably greater attention.

### Pathogenesis of white matter injury

In the very low birth weight infant the distinctive white matter lesion, periventricular leukomalacia (PVL) is the major pathologic associate of later developmental handicap. Key factors that have been identified include vascular development, the intrinsic vulnerability of the oligodendrocyte to neurotoxic factors, and exposure to maternal/chorionic membrane infection. PVL classically occurs in areas that represent arterial end zones or border zones (Perlman 1998). Prolonged hypoperfusion due to hypotension or associated with hypocapnia potentially exposes these areas to greater ischemia as discussed above.

The immaturity of oligodendrocyte precursors is clearly critical, as the period of greatest risk for PVL is before myelination has begun, at a time when oligodendrocyte precursors are actively proliferating and differentiating. Such actively differentiating cells have an increased metabolic demand and are sensitive to substrate limitation. It has been suggested that developing oligodendroglia are very sensitive to the excitatory neurotransmitter glutamate and to free radical toxicity because of a developmental lack of antioxidant enzymes to mediate oxidative stress (Rivkin *et al.* 1995).

Finally, compelling evidence has recently linked prenatal inflammation or infection to later cerebral palsy (Nelson *et al.* 1998). Exposure to maternal or placental infection is associated both with increased risk of preterm birth and also with brain lesions predictive of cerebral palsy (Dammann & Leviton 1997). It is likely that the effect of infection is mediated by systemic inflammation since fetal plasma interleukin levels including interleukins 1, 8, 9, TNF-$\alpha$ and the interferons, are strongly and independently associated with PVL (Dammann & Leviton 1997; Nelson *et al.* 1998) (see also Chapter 22).

### Intraventricular hemorrhage (IVH) and white matter injury

The pathogenesis of these disorders is discussed in detail in Chapters 21 and 22. IVH with extension in to the periventricular regions is also associated with adverse outcome. The white matter injury appears to be a venous infarction with hemorrhage occurring as a secondary phenomenon. Further, there is evidence of prolonged loss of cerebrovascular autoregulation post-asphyxia which may leave the fetal brain vulnerable to factors causing fluctuations in blood pressure and thus CBF; this is proposed to be a key mechanism in the pathogenesis of IVH. Other factors that may contribute to IVH include the fragility of immature germinal matrix capillaries, deficient vascular support, and a limited vasodilatory capacity impairing perfusion during asphyxia. In this regard, the antenatal administration of glucocorticoids has been associated with a significant reduction in the sonographic incidence of severe IVH and the associated white matter involvement (p. 349).

## PRE-EXISTING METABOLIC STATUS AND CHRONIC HYPOXIA

While the original studies of factors influencing the degree and distribution of brain injury, primarily by Myers (Myers 1977), focussed on metabolic status, the issue remains controversial. It has been suggested, for example, that hyperglycemia is protective against hypoxia–ischemia in the infant rat (Vannucci *et al.* 1997) but not in the piglet (LeBlanc *et al.* 1993). The extreme differences between these neonatal species in the degree of neural maturation and activity of cerebral glucose transporters may underlie the different outcomes (Vannucci *et al.* 1997). The most common metabolic disturbance to the fetus is intrauterine growth retardation associated with placental dysfunction. Although there is reasonable clinical information that this condition is usually associated with a greater risk of brain injury, recent studies have suggested a greatly reduced rate of encephalopathy in affected patients over time (Westgate *et al.* 1999). This would suggest that the apparently increased sensitivity to injury is mostly due to reduced aerobic reserves, leading to early onset of systemic compromise during labor.

Neural maturation is markedly altered in intrauterine growth retardation with some aspects delayed and others advanced (Cook *et al.* 1988; Stanley *et al.* 1989). This is likely to influence the response to asphyxia but also to introduce a confounding independent effect on neural development. Severe growth retardation has been associated with altered neurotransmitter expression, reduced cerebral myelination, altered synaptogenesis and smaller brain size (Kramer *et al.* 1990). The effect of the timing and severity of placental restriction has been examined in a range of studies in fetal sheep (Rees *et al.* 1998). Chronic mild growth retardation due to peri-conceptual placental restriction was associated with delayed formation of neuronal connections in the hippocampus, cerebellum, and visual cortex, but did not alter neuronal migration or numbers. In contrast, in studies in the near mid-gestation fetus, hypoxia induced by a variety of methods was associated with a reduction in numbers of Purkinje cells in the cerebellum and delayed development of neural processes. With more severe hypoxia the cortex and hippocampus were also affected and there

**Table 23.4 Summary of the determinants of acute asphyxial neural injury**

- Cerebral perfusion is linearly compromised by hypotension during asphyxia. The combination of reduced perfusion with hypoxia (i.e. hypoxia–ischemia) not only further reduces the amount of oxygen delivered to the brain but also compounds this by reducing the supply of glucose for anaerobic metabolism. This commonly leads to a 'watershed' distribution of injury
- Increased spacing between relatively prolonged episodes of ischemia or asphyxia is associated with a relative increase in striatal injury
- The brain matures from rostral to caudal. Thus, in the premature brain the cortex is relatively immature, particularly in the superficial layers, and is less susceptible to hypoxic–ischemic injury than subcortical white matter and structures
- The dominant neuropathologic correlate of handicap in surviving premature infants is the distinctive white matter lesion, PVL, which occurs before oligodendrocyte maturation, and is strongly associated with evidence of maternal infection, with a fetal systemic inflammatory response, and with exposure to asphyxia (p. 423)
- Environmental conditions during recovery from asphyxia can critically affect outcome. Experimentally, moderate cerebral hypothermia initiated in the latent phase and continued until resolution of secondary changes can dramatically reduce neural injury

was reduced subcortical myelination. The cerebellum develops later in gestation than the hippocampus, and thus appears to be more susceptible to the effects of hypoxia (Rees *et al.* 1998).

## CEREBRAL TEMPERATURE

There is now good evidence from a range of species and paradigms that small, clinically relevant changes in post-ischemic cerebral temperature can critically modulate encephalopathic processes that are initiated during hypoxia–ischemic insults, and which extend into the secondary phase of neuronal loss (Gunn 2000). Conversely, prolonged mild hyperthermia during the secondary phase increases injury. The role of therapeutic hypothermia in neonatal brain protection is discussed on p. 515.

While asphyxia may not be preventable, experimental data make it clear that cerebral injury is an evolving process, which can be modified by numerous external factors such as blood pressure management, infection, and temperature. This means that the opportunity exists to provide effective treatment for asphyxia. However, considerable research still needs to be done to refine our understanding of the mechanisms of injury and to develop appropriate therapeutic strategies for different clinical situations, including the very premature infant.

## ACKNOWLEDGMENTS

The authors' work reported in this review has been supported by National Institutes of Health grant RO-1 HD32752, and by grants from the Health Research Council of New Zealand, Lottery Health Board of New Zealand, and the Auckland Medical Research Foundation.

**Key Points**

- Acute onset of asphyxia is associated with bradycardia, increased systemic blood pressure, but no increase in cerebral blood flow (CBF)
- Progressive asphyxia is associated with a doubling of CBF with no hypotension
- In the primary phase of asphyxial neuronal injury, depolarization occurs leading to $Na^{+}$ and $Ca^{++}$ entry with cell swelling (cytotoxic edema) and extracellular accumulation of excitatory amino acid neurotransmitters
- In the delayed phase, neuronal necrosis and/or apoptosis occurs as the result of a number of intraneuronal biochemical events

## REFERENCES

Abi Raad R, Tan W K, Bennet L *et al.* (1999) Role of the cerebrovascular and metabolic responses in the delayed phases of injury after transient cerebral ischemia in fetal sheep. *Stroke* 30: 2735–2742.

Azzopardi D, Wyatt J S, Cady E B *et al.* (1989) Prognosis of newborn infants with hypoxic-ischemic brain injury assessed by phosphorus magnetic resonance spectroscopy. *Pediatr Res* 25: 445–451.

Barkovich A J & Sargent S K (1995) Profound asphyxia in the premature infant: imaging findings. *AJNR Am J Neuroradiol* 16: 1837–1846.

Beilharz E J, Williams C E, Dragunow M *et al.* (1995) Mechanisms of delayed cell death following hypoxic-ischemic injury in the immature rat: evidence for apoptosis during selective neuronal loss. *Brain Res* 29: 1–14.

Bennet L, Peebles D M, Edwards A D, Rios A & Hanson M A (1998) The cerebral hemodynamic response to asphyxia and hypoxia in the near-term fetal sheep as measured by near-infrared spectroscopy. *Pediatr Res* 44: 951–957.

Bennet L, Rossenrode S, Gunning M I *et al.* (1999) The cardiovascular and cerebrovascular responses of the immature fetal sheep to acute umbilical cord occlusion. *J Physiol (Lond)* 517: 247–257.

Blumberg R M, Cady E B, Wigglesworth J S *et al.* (1997) Relation between delayed impairment of cerebral energy metabolism and infarction following transient focal hypoxia-ischaemia in the developing brain. *Exp Brain Res* 113: 130–137.

Bolanos J P & Almeida A (1999) Roles of nitric oxide in brain hypoxia–ischemia. *Biochim Biophys Acta* 1411: 415–436.

Bona E, Aden U, Gilland E *et al.* (1997) Neonatal cerebral hypoxia-ischemia – the effect of adenosine receptor antagonists. *Neuropharmacology* 36: 1327–1338.

Choi D W (1995) Calcium: still center-stage in hypoxic–ischemic neuronal death. *Trends Neurosc* 18: 58–60.

Colbourne F, Sutherland G R & Auer R N (1999) Electron microscopic evidence against apoptosis as the mechanism of neuronal death in global ischemia. *J Neurosci* 19: 4200–4210.

Cook C J, Gluckman P D, Williams C E & Bennet L (1988) Precocial neural function in the growth retarded fetal lamb. *Pediatr Res* 24: 600–605.

Dammann O & Leviton A (1997) Maternal intrauterine infection, cytokines, and brain damage in the preterm newborn. *Pediatr Res* 42: 1–8.

de Haan H H, Van Reempts J L, Vles J S, de Haan J & Hasaart T H (1993) Effects of asphyxia on the fetal lamb brain. *Am J Obstet Gynecol* 169: 1493–1501

de Haan H H, Gunn A J & Gluckman P D (1997a) Fetal heart rate changes do not reflect cardiovascular deterioration during brief repeated umbilical cord occlusions in near-term fetal lambs. *Am J Obstet Gynecol* 176: 8–17.

de Haan H H, Gunn A J, Williams C E & Gluckman P D (1997b) Brief repeated umbilical cord occlusions cause sustained cytotoxic cerebral edema and focal infarcts in near-term fetal lambs. *Pediatr Res* 41: 96–104.

de Haan H H, Gunn A J, Williams C E *et al.* (1997c) Magnesium sulfate therapy during asphyxia in near-term fetal lambs does not compromise the fetus but does not reduce cerebral injury. *Am J Obstet Gynecol* 176: 18–27.

Donnelly W H (1987) Ischemic myocardial necrosis and papillary muscle dysfunction in infants and children. *Am J Cardiovasc Pathol* 1: 173–188.

Edwards A D, Cox P, Hope P L *et al.* (1997) Apoptosis in the brains of infants suffering intrauterine cerebral injury. *Pediatr Res* 42: 684–689.

Faraci F M & Heistad D D (1998) Regulation of the cerebral circulation: role of endothelium and potassium channels. *Physiol Rev* 78: 53–97.

Fellman V & Raivio K O (1997) Reperfusion injury as the mechanism of brain damage after perinatal asphyxia. *Pediatr Res* 41: 599–606.

Giffard R G, Monyer H, Christine C W & Choi D W (1990) Acidosis reduces NMDA receptor activation, glutamate neurotoxicity, and oxygen-glucose deprivation neuronal injury in cortical cultures. *Brain Res* 506: 339–342.

Giussani D A, Spencer J A D & Hanson M A (1994) Fetal cardiovascular reflex responses to hypoxaemia. *Fetal and Maternal Medicine Review* 6: 17–37.

Goldberg M P & Choi D W (1993) Combined oxygen and glucose deprivation in cortical cell culture – calcium-dependent and calcium-independent mechanisms of neuronal injury. *J Neurosci* 13: 3510–3524.

Gottron F J, Ying H S & Choi D W (1997) Caspase inhibition selectively reduces the apoptotic component of oxygen-glucose deprivation-induced cortical neuronal cell death. *Mol Cell Neurosci* 9: 159–169.

Gressens P, Marret S & Evrard P (1996) Developmental spectrum of the excitotoxic cascade induced by ibotenate: a model of hypoxic insults in fetuses and neonates. *Neuropathol Appl Neurobiol* 22: 498–502.

Gunn A J (2000) Cerebral hypothermia for the prevention of neural injury after perinatal asphyxia. *Curr Opin Paediatr* 12: 111–115.

Gunn A J & Gluckman P D (1998) Pharmacologic strategies for the prevention of perinatal brain damage. *Semin Perinatol* 3: 87–101.

Gunn A J, Parer J T, Mallard E C *et al.* (1992) Cerebral histological and electrophysiological changes after asphyxia in fetal sheep. *Pediatr Res* 31: 486–491.

Gunn A J, Gunn T R, de Haan H H *et al.* (1997) Dramatic neuronal rescue with prolonged selective head cooling after ischemia in fetal lambs. *J Clin Invest* 99: 248–256.

Gunn A J, Gunn T R, Gunning M I *et al.* (1998) Neuroprotection with prolonged head cooling started before postischemic seizures in fetal sheep. *Pediatrics* 102: 1098–1106.

Gunn A J, Maxwell L, de Haan H H *et al.* (2000) Delayed hypotension and sub-endocardial injury after repeated umbilical cord occlusion in near-term fetal lambs. *Am J Obstet Gynecol* 183: 1564–1572.

Hansen A (1977) Extracellular potassium concentration in juvenile and adult rat brain cortex during anoxia. *Acta Physiol Scand* 99: 412–420.

Hanson M A (1997) Do we now understand the control of the fetal circulation? *Eur J Obstet Gynecol Reprod Biol* 75: 55–61.

Hanson M A (1998) Role of chemoreceptors in effects of chronic hypoxia. *Comparative Biochem Physiol A Mol Integr Physiol* 119: 695–703.

Hellstrom Westas L, Rosen I & Svenningsen N W (1995) Predictive value of early continuous amplitude integrated EEG recordings on outcome after severe birth asphyxia in full term infants. *Arch Dis Child Fetal Neonat Edn* 72: F34–F38.

Hughes P E, Alexi T, Walton M *et al.* (1999) Activity and injury-dependent expression of inducible transcription factors, growth factors and apoptosis-related genes within the central nervous system. *Prog Neurobiol* 57: 421–450.

Ikeda T, Murata Y, Quilligan E J, Choi B H, Parer J T, Doi S & Park S D (1998) Physiologic and histologic changes in near-term fetal lambs exposed to asphyxia by partial umbilical cord occlusion. *Am J Obstet Gynecol* 178: 24–32.

Ilves P, Talvik R & Talvik T (1998) Changes in Doppler ultrasonography in asphyxiated term infants with hypoxic-ischaemic encephalopathy. *Acta Paediatr Scand* 87: 680–684.

Janbu T & Nesheim B I (1987) Uterine artery blood velocities during contractions in pregnancy and labour related to intrauterine pressure. *Br J Obstet Gynaecol* 94: 1150–1155.

Jensen A (1996) The brain of the asphyxiated fetus – basic research. *Eur J Obstet Gynecol Reprod* 65: 19–24.

Keunen H, Blanco C E, Van Reempts J L & Hasaart T H (1997) Absence of neuronal damage after umbilical cord occlusion of 10, 15, and 20 minutes in midgestation fetal sheep. *Am J Obstet Gynecol* 176: 515–520.

Kiely J L & Susser M (1992) Preterm birth, intrauterine growth retardation and perinatal mortality. *Am J Public Health* 82: 343–344.

Kitanaka T, Alonso J G, Gilbert R D, Siu B L, Clemons G K & Longo L D (1989) Fetal responses to long-term hypoxemia in sheep. *Am J Physiol* 256: R1348–54.

Kramer M S, Olivier M, McLean F H *et al.* (1990) Impact of intrauterine growth retardation and body proportionality on fetal and neonatal outcome. *Pediatrics* 86: 707–713.

LeBlanc M H, Huang M, Vig V *et al.* (1993) Glucose affects the severity of hypoxic-ischemic brain injury in newborn pigs. *Stroke* 24: 1055–1062.

Lees G J (1993) The possible contribution of microglia and macrophages to delayed neuronal death after ischemia. *J Neurol Sci* 114: 119–122.

Lipton P (1999) Ischemic cell death in brain neurons. *Physiol Rev* 79: 1431–1568.

Lorek A, Takei Y, Cady E B *et al.* (1994) Delayed ('secondary') cerebral energy failure after acute hypoxia-ischemia in the newborn piglet: continuous 48-hour studies by phosphorus magnetic resonance spectroscopy. *Pediatr Res* 36: 699–706.

Low J A (1997) Intrapartum fetal asphyxia: definition, diagnosis, and classification. *Am J Obset Gynecol* 176: 957–959.

MacLennan A, The International Cerebral Palsy Task Force, Gunn A J, Bennet L & Westgate J A (1999) A template for defining a causal relation between acute intrapartum events and cerebral palsy: international consensus statement. *BMJ* 319: 1054–1059.

Mallard E C, Gunn A J, Williams C E *et al.* (1992) Transient umbilical cord occlusion causes hippocampal damage in the fetal sheep. *Am J Obstet Gynecol* 167: 1423–1430.

Mallard E C, Williams C E, Gunn A J *et al.* (1993) Frequent episodes of brief ischemia sensitize the fetal sheep brain to neuronal loss and induce striatal injury. *Pediatr Res* 33: 61–65.

Mallard E C, Waldvogel H J, Williams C E *et al.* (1995) Repeated asphyxia causes loss of striatal projection neurons in the fetal sheep brain. *Neuroscience* 65: 827–836.

Marks K A, Mallard E C, Roberts I *et al.* (1996) Nitric oxide synthase inhibition attenuates delayed vasodilation and increases injury following cerebral ischemia in fetal sheep. *Pediatr Res* 40: 185–191.

Massa S M, Swanson R A & Sharp F R (1996) The stress gene response in brain. *Cerebrovasc Brain Metab Rev* 8: 95–158.

Michenfelder J D & Milde J H (1990) Postischemic canine cerebral blood flow appears to be determined by cerebral metabolic needs. *J Cereb Blood Flow Metab* 10: 71–76.

Myers R E (1977) Experimental models of perinatal brain damage: relevance to human pathology. In: Gluck L (ed). *Intrauterine asphyxia and the developing fetal brain.* Chicago, IL: Year Book Medical; pp. 37–97.

Nelson K B, Dambrosia J M, Ting T Y & Grether J K (1996) Uncertain value of electronic fetal monitoring in predicting cerebral palsy. *N Engl J Med* 334: 613–618.

Nelson K B, Dambrosia J M, Grether J K & Phillips T M (1998) Neonatal cytokines and coagulation factors in children with cerebral palsy. *Ann Neurol* 44: 665–675.

Nilsson G E & Lutz P L (1991) Release of inhibitory neurotransmitters in response to anoxia in turtle brain. *Am J Physiol* 261: R32–R37.

Parer J T (1998) Effects of fetal asphyxia on brain cell structure and function: limits of tolerance. *Comp Biochem Physiol A Mol Integr Physiol* 119: 711–716.

Perlman J M (1998) White matter injury in the preterm infant: an important determination of abnormal neurodevelopment outcome. *Early Hum Dev* 53: 99–120.

Porteracailliau C, Price D L & Martin L J (1997) Excitotoxic neuronal death in the immature brain is an apoptosis-necrosis morphological continuum. *J Comp Neurol* 378: 70–87.

Raff M C (1992) Social controls on cell survival and cell death. *Nature* 356: 397–400.

Reddy K, Mallard C, Guan J *et al.* (1998) Maturational change in the cortical response to hypoperfusion injury in the fetal sheep. *Pediatr Res* 43: 674–682.

Rees S, Mallard C, Breen S *et al.* (1998) Fetal brain injury following prolonged hypoxemia and placental insufficiency: a review. *Comp Biochemi Physiol A, Mol Integr Physiol* 119: 653–660.

Reynolds E O, McCormick D C, Roth S C *et al.* (1991) New non-invasive methods for the investigation of cerebral oxidative metabolism and haemodynamics in newborn infants. *Ann Med* 23: 681–686.

Richardson B S & Bocking A D (1998) Metabolic and circulatory adaptations to chronic hypoxia in the fetus. *Comp Biochem Physiol A Mol Integr Physiol* 119: 717–723.

Rivkin M J, Flax J, Mozell R *et al.* (1995) Oligodendroglial development in human fetal cerebrum. *Ann Neurol* 38: 92–101.

Robertson C M & Finer N N (1993) Long-term follow-up of term neonates with perinatal asphyxia. *Clin Perinatol* 20: 483–500.

Rosen K G, Hrbek A, Karlsson K & Kjellmer I (1986) Fetal cerebral, cardiovascular and metabolic reactions to intermittent occlusion of ovine maternal placental blood flow. *Acta Physiol Scand* 126: 209–216.

Roth S C, Baudin J, Cady E *et al.* (1997) Relation of deranged neonatal cerebral oxidative metabolism with neurodevelopmental outcome and head circumference at 4 years. *Dev Med Child Neurol* 39: 718–725.

Scott R J & Hegyi L (1997) Cell death in perinatal hypoxic-ischaemic brain injury. *Neuropathol Appl Neurobiol* 23: 307–314.

Shelley H J (1961) Glycogen reserves and their changes at birth and in anoxia. *Br Med Bull* 17: 137–143.

Shuaib A & Kanthan R (1997) Amplification of inhibitory mechanisms in cerebral ischemia: an alternative approach to neuronal protection. *Histol Histopathol* 12: 185–194.

Stanley F J (1992) Survival and cerebral palsy in low birthweight infants: implications for perinatal care. *Paediatr Perinat Epidemiol* 6: 298–310.

Stanley O, Fleming P & Morgan M (1989) Abnormal development of visual function following intrauterine growth retardation. *Early Hum Dev* 19: 87–101.

Tan W K M, Williams C E, Gunn A J *et al.* (1992) Suppression of postischemic epileptiform activity with MK-801 improves neural outcome in fetal sheep. *Ann Neurol* 32: 677–682.

Tan W K M, Williams C E, During M J *et al.* (1996) Accumulation of cytotoxins during the development of seizures and edema after hypoxic-ischemic injury in late gestation fetal sheep. *Pediatr Res* 39: 791–797.

Tangalakis K, Lumbers E R, Moritz K M, Towstoless M K & Wintour E M (1992) Effect of cortisol on blood pressure and vascular reactivity in the ovine fetus. *Exp Physiol* 77: 709–717.

Tombaugh G C (1994) Mild acidosis delays hypoxic spreading depression and improves neuronal recovery in hippocampal slices. *J Neurosci* 14: 5635–5643.

Torvik A (1984) The pathogenesis of watershed infarcts in the brain. *Stroke* 15: 221–223.

Vannucci S J, Maher F & Simpson I A (1997) Glucose transporter proteins in brain: delivery of glucose to neurons and glia. *Glia* 21: 2–21.

Volpe J J (1995) Hypoxic-ischemic encephalopathy: neuropathology and pathogenesis. In: WB Saunders (ed). *Neurology of the Newborn*, 3rd edn. Philadelphia, PA: WB Saunders Company; pp. 279–313.

Walton M, Sirimanne E, Williams C *et al.* (1997) Prostaglandin H synthase-2 and cytosolic phospholipase A(2) in the hypoxic-ischemic brain – role in neuronal death or survival. *Mol Brain Res* 50: 165–170.

Westgate J A, Gunn A J & Gunn T R (1999) Antecedents of neonatal encephalopathy with fetal acidaemia at term. *Br J Obstet Gynaecol* 106: 774–782.

Williams C E, Gunn A J & Gluckman P D (1991) The time course of intracellular edema and epileptiform activity following prenatal cerebral ischemia in sheep. *Stroke* 22: 516–521.

# Chapter 24 Antenatal prediction of asphyxia

K. A. Sorem and M. L. Druzin

## INTRODUCTION

Perinatal asphyxia is a hypoxic–ischemic insult that may occur antepartum, intrapartum, or after birth. Historically, perinatal asphyxia was thought to be associated with brain damage and cerebral palsy (Little 1862), yet it is unlikely to be the cause of cerebral palsy unless the asphyxial insult is near lethal (Winkler *et al.* 1999). Recent analysis of cerebral palsy and birth asphyxia indicates that only 10% of cases of cerebral palsy (1–2 per 10 000) were associated with birth asphyxia (Nelson & Ellenberg 1968). Conversely, 2% of newborns have 'asphyxial exposure', and the majority of these recover without neurologic sequelae (Low 1993). Nevertheless, asphyxial brain injury remains a significant cause of perinatal morbidity and mortality, and identification of the fetus at risk for asphyxia remains a clinical challenge.

## DEFINITION OF PERINATAL ASPHYXIA

A task force of the World Federation of Neurology Group has defined asphyxia as a condition of impaired gas exchange which, if it persists, leads to progressive hypercapnea and hypoxemia (Box & Nelson 1993). Fetal asphyxia occurs as a result of absent or insufficient placental blood flow due to acute or chronic events. These include umbilical cord occlusion, altered placental gas exchange (placental abruption, insufficiency or previa), inadequate perfusion of the maternal side of the placenta (maternal hypotension, vasospasm, or abnormal contractions), and impaired maternal oxygenation (severe anemia, cardiac or pulmonary disease). Newborn asphyxia may result from cardio-respiratory complications after delivery, including respiratory distress syndrome, apnea, and birth trauma. Hypoxic ischemia is defined as tissue damage resulting from inadequate oxygen and substrate delivery. If blood flow and oxygenation are restored, the tissue damage is minimal; however, with prolonged asphyxia irreversible cell loss may occur.

The terms 'perinatal asphyxia' and 'hypoxic–ischemic injury' imply a specific cause and effect which may be difficult to determine clinically. Therefore, specific criteria for the definition of perinatal asphyxia have been suggested by The American College of Obstetricians and Gynecologists (ACOG), which states that 'in assessing a possible link between perinatal asphyxia and neurologic deficit in an individual patient, the following criteria must be present before a plausible link can be made: (1) profound umbilical artery metabolic or mixed acidemia (pH <7.00), (2) persistence of an Apgar score of 0–3 for longer than 5 minutes, (3) neonatal neurologic sequelae, (4) multi-organ system dysfunction, e.g. cardiovascular, gastrointestinal, hematologic, pulmonary or renal' (AMCOG 1992).

Complete assessment of the neonate at risk for neurologic sequelae includes evaluation of CNS dysfunction, including seizures, abnormal respiration, altered activity states (such as hyperalertness or somnolence), impaired reflexes (such as suck and gag), abnormal ocular responses, or a bulging anterior fontanelle. Additionally, abnormal EEGs may be observed in newborns with hypoxic–ischemic encephalopathy. Clinical features of neonatal hypoxic–ischemic encephalopathy are shown in Table 24.1 (Carter *et al.* 1993). Although multiple organ systems may be affected by hypoxic–ischemic injury, including cardiovascular, respiratory, renal, metabolic, gastrointestinal and hematologic, only CNS involvement has residual sequelae at long term follow-up (Shankaran *et al.* 1991). One clinical classification of intrapartum fetal asphyxia described by Low is shown in Table 24.2.

## PATHOPHYSIOLOGY OF PERINATAL ASPHYXIA

Hypoxic–ischemic damage begins during the injury (impaired placental exchange) and extends into the period of

**Table 24.1 Clinical features of neonatal hypoxic–ischemic encephalopathy**

| Time after birth (hours) | Clinical features |
|---|---|
| 12–24 | Hyperalertness; hyper-excitability; seizures; apnea; jitteriness; weakness. |
| 24–72 | Obtundation or coma; ataxic respirations with respiratory arrest; abnormal oculomotor reflexes; impaired papillary response; intracranial hemorrhage (premature neonates) with subsequent deterioration. |
| >72 | Persistent stupor; abnormal or absent sucking, swallowing, and gag reflexes; generalized hypotonia; weakness. |

*Source*: Modified from Volpe JJ (1987) Hypoxic ischemic encephalopathy: clinical aspects. In: *Neurology of the newborn*, 2nd edn. Philadelphia, PA: WB Saunders; p. 236, with permission.

**Table 24.2 Classification of intrapartum fetal asphyxia**

| Asphyxia | Metabolic acidosis at delivery | Encephalopathy | Cardiovascular, respiratory, or renal complication |
|---|---|---|---|
| Mild | + | ± | ± |
| Moderate | + | ++ | ± |
| Severe | + | +++ | +++ |

*Source*: Modified from Low JA (1997) Intrapartum fetal asphyxia: definition, diagnosis, and classification. *Am J Obstet Gynecol* 176: 957–959, with permission.

resuscitation or reperfusion. At the biochemical level, cellular injury within the CNS initiates a cascade of molecular events which leads to accumulation of excitatory amino acids, increased intracellular calcium, and increased free radical production (Delivoria-Papadapoulos & Mishra 1998). Oxidative metabolism is replaced by anaerobic metabolism, resulting in the accumulation of nicotinamide-adenine dinucleotide (NADH), flavin-adenine dinucleotide (FADH), and lactic acid. ATP is depleted as glycolysis fails to keep up with cellular demands, and transcellular ionic pumps fail, leading to the disruption of sodium, chloride, calcium, and cellular water. Cytotoxic edema evolves. Free fatty acids accumulate as membrane phospholipids break down and undergo peroxidation by oxygen free-radicals. Glutamate is generated from axon terminals, along with nitric oxide, both of which may be directly toxic to adjacent neuronal cells. Cell death may follow due to the effects of acidosis, energy failure, and lipid peroxidation (Vanucci & Perlman 1997; Vanucci & Palmer 1997). Furthermore, depletion of growth factors and inflammatory cells may lead to extensive cellular damage within the CNS (Gluckman & Williams 1992).

Following prolonged hypoxic–ischemic injury, some cells within the CNS may not recover function, resulting in regional or global infarction. In adults and experimental animals, the therapeutic window of intervention and recovery is longer than that of the fetus and newborn because the process of cellular destruction is much more rapid in the perinatal period (Vanucci & Palmer 1997). In the human fetus and neonate, the therapeutic window is estimated to be less than 2 hours (Vanucci & Perlman 1997).

Infant laboratory primates subjected to hypoxic–ischemic injury demonstrate distinct patterns of CNS damage, depending on the nature of the asphyxial insult. Brief total asphyxia damages subcortical nuclei in the thalamus and brainstem, whereas prolonged partial asphyxia damages cerebral white matter, beginning in parasagittal areas (Meyers 1975). Pasternak reported a study of 11 term human infants who sustained an acute near total intrauterine asphyxia and demonstrated a similar pattern of brain damage, depending on the magnitude and timing of the hypoxic–ischemic insult. On postnatal MRI, acute near total asphyxia appeared to damage the thalamus, brainstem, and basal ganglia, presumably because of the relatively high

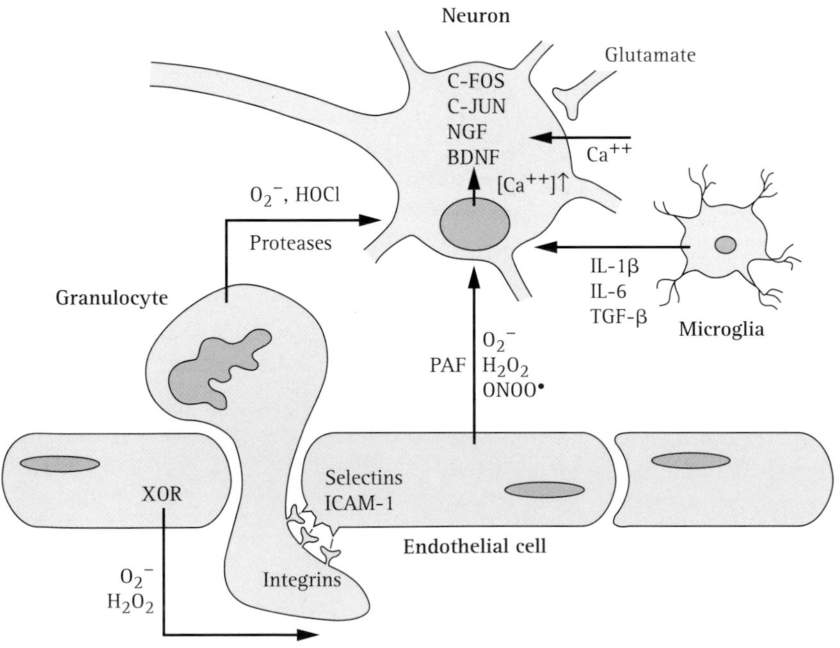


**Figure 24.1** Reperfusion injury and neuronal damage following hypoxic insult. Reactive oxygen metabolites generated by endothelial and parenchymal cells lead to cell necrosis and end organ damage. NGF, nerve growth factor; BDNF, brain derived neurotrophic factor; TGF, transforming growth factor; PAF, platelet-activating factor; ONOO•, peroxynitrite. (From Fellman V & Raivio K (1997) Reperfusion injury as the mechanism of brain damage after perinatal asphyxia. *Pediatr Res* 41: 600, with permission.)

basal metabolic rate, whereas subacute partial asphyxia led to damage primarily in the cerebral hemispheres due to shunting of blood to the brainstem and cerebellum (Pasternak & Gorey 1998).

After brief episodes of asphyxia, restoration of blood flow may lead to re-oxygenation and end organ survival. However, reperfusion of ischemic brain tissue after a severe insult may deliver harmful reactive oxygen metabolites causing further tissue damage. In addition to damaging the cell directly, reactive oxygen metabolites delivered by reperfusion also promote the expression of adhesion molecules on endothelial or parenchymal cells. This leads to accumulation of neutrophils that cause necrosis of cortical brain cells or delayed neuronal death through apoptosis. Pathologic evidence of cellular damage includes cell shrinkage, membrane blebbing, chromatin concentration, and DNA fragmentation (Tominaga *et al.* 1993). Therefore, it appears that cell damage occurs during both the ischemic and reperfusion phase of an asphyxial insult (Fellman & Raivio 1991).

After a severe asphyxial event, neonates often enter a phase of neurologic depression characterized by suppressed EEG and abnormal activity level. Oxygen free-radicals may induce prolonged cerebral hypoperfusion, reducing cerebral metabolism, protein synthesis, and electrical activity (Leffler *et al.* 1989). Post-asphyxial seizures in the neonate lasting more than 30 minutes are associated with poor neurologic outcome and cerebral infarction (Mellits *et al.* 1982; Williams *et al.* 1992). Seizures that are primarily multifocal clonic type may add additional insult to the injured brain by increasing metabolic demands on cortical cells.

## FETAL RESPONSE TO ASPHYXIA (see also Chapter 23)

A fetal asphyxial insult may vary from hypoxia (decreased oxygenation) to anoxia (absent oxygenation). The fetus may not tolerate complete anoxia for more than 10 minutes, and survivors of complete total cord occlusion generally show multiple cerebral lesions, primarily in the brain stem. Through physiologic compensatory mechanisms, experimental fetal sheep have been shown to be capable of surviving an 80% decrease in cerebral oxygen uptake (Field *et al.* 1991), indicating that the healthy fetus may tolerate even extreme hypoxia. During a hypoxic event, blood flow is reduced to the pulmonary, renal and splanchnic areas with preferential perfusion of the heart, brain, and adrenal glands (Peters *et al.* 1979). Within the brain, hypoxia leads to preferential blood flow to the brain stem, with decreased blood flow to white matter and the cerebral cortex.

One fetal response to hypoxia, bradycardia, results from chemoreceptor stimulation of the vagus nerve. Increased sympathetic activity and peripheral vasoconstriction increase fetal blood pressure and maintain bradycardia (Hanson 1988). In addition to CNS regulation of fetal heart rate via sympathetic and parasympathetic neurons, catecholamines released from the adrenal glands directly depress the myocardium, leading to late cardiac decelerations observed on fetal heart rate monitoring. Although anaerobic glycolysis and the accumulation of pyruvate and lactate lead ultimately to metabolic acidosis, brain injury appears to be associated more strongly with fetal hypotension than with the degree of hypoxia or acidosis (Mallard *et al.* 1992; De Haan *et al.* 1997). Loss of fetal heart rate variability may accompany fetal hypoxia (Paul *et al.* 1975) as well as other conditions that indicate CNS depression, such as drug exposure and structural CNS anomalies. In a 10-year study of antepartum fetal heart rate monitoring, Ayodeji & Kuhn reported that 19% of fetuses with 'critical reserve patterns' (late decelerations and loss of variability) had major structural malformations, suggesting that some fetuses may have inappropriate responses to hypoxia based on pre-existing CNS abnormalities (Ayodeji & Kuhn 1986). Genetics may also influence the fetal response to asphyxia, as demonstrated in animal models, which show that factors that mediate the response to induced hypoxia are genetically determined (Labudova *et al.* 1999).

Changes in fetal activity include decreased gross body movements and cessation of fetal breathing (Vintzileos *et al.* 1991). Koos *et al.* demonstrated in studies on fetal sheep that decreases in fetal breathing movements are evident after a decrease in fetal $PO_2$ of 6 mmHg (Koos *et al.* 1987). This effect appears to be gestational age-dependent, with immature fetuses exhibiting less hypoxic inhibition than fetuses close to term. The biochemical mechanisms of the hypoxic inhibition of fetal breathing movements may result from changing brain stem concentrations of adenosine, which may be mediated by local levels of prostaglandin $E_2$ (Kitterman *et al.* 1983). Both the severity and duration of hypoxia contribute to the effect on fetal breathing movements, as well as to the decreased eye movements and gross body movements observed with hypoxemia.

## MARKERS FOR PERINATAL ASPHYXIA

Fetal meconium in the amniotic fluid is a relatively common finding in labor, occurring in 18% of deliveries. Although meconium may indicate that fetal stress has occurred, it does not predict neurologic impairment in the normal term fetus (Nelson & Ellenberg 1984). Prior to the widespread use of electronic fetal monitoring, the Collaborative Perinatal Study (1966) reported that 64% of the cases of amniotic fluid meconium were attributable to chorioamnionitis and only 0.2% to recognized intrapartum hypoxemic disorders (Anonymous 1966). Katz & Bowes suggest that among some fetuses with asphyxial exposure, it is the underlying asphyxia, rather than the observed meconium that is responsible for the pulmonary pathology (Katz & Bowes 1992). However, the phenomenon of meconium aspiration syndrome in neonates born by Cesarean section in the absence of known adverse antepartum or intrapartum events indicates that meconium may also have direct effects on pulmonary vasculature. *In vitro* studies have demonstrated that macrophages may transport meconium directly from the amniotic fluid into the umbilical cord (Altschuler *et al.* 1992), where it stimulates the release of vasoconstrictors within the placenta and fetus. Whether the vasoconstrictive effect of meconium contributes to damage within vulnerable cerebral vessels is speculative. In one study of 43 children with spastic quadriplegia, staining of the amniotic fluid was the only identified risk factor for cerebral palsy. Although all of the children had neuroimaging studies which identified lesions consistent with the type of severe brain damage produced by hypoxic ischemia, not all of the newborns had abnormal umbilical artery pH or elevated base deficit (Naeye 1995).

Apgar scores, long used to quantify clinical depression in the first minutes of life (Apgar 1953), reflect several variables including gestational age, muscular disorders, CNS abnormalities, cardiorespiratory problems, and maternal medication, in addition to antepartum or intrapartum hypoxia. Whereas moderately and briefly low Apgar scores are not related to subsequent neurologic outcome, severely low, late and very late Apgar scores are much better predictors of cerebral palsy. A 10-min Apgar score of 3 or less indicates persistent hypoperfusion or hypoxia and is associated with a 16.7% risk of cerebral palsy (Freeman & Nelson 1988). A score of 3 or less at 20 min post delivery is associated with a 59% mortality rate and cerebral palsy in 57% of survivors (Nelson & Ellenberg 1981).

Evaluation of the acid–base status of the fetus and neonate has improved identification of newborns at risk for neurologic complications associated with antepartum or intrapartum asphyxia. The normal umbilical artery pH for term newborns is 7.2 (SD ± 0.08) and the mean base deficit is 8.3 mmol/l (SD ± 4.0 mmol/l) (Skyes & Johnson 1982), indicating that all newborns respond to the relative hypoxia of labor with a mixed metabolic and respiratory acidosis. This is not surprising, given the repetitive interruption of uteroplacental blood flow occurring with uterine contractions. In the normal term fetus with an intact CNS these episodes of intermittent hypoxia are well tolerated. The level of fetal acidemia that is considered pathologic or associated with increased morbidity and mortality is controversial. Umbilical artery pH less than 7.0 has been reported as an indicator of a neonate at increased risk for neurologic abnormalities (Hauth 1996), and ACOG has included an umbilical artery pH of 7.00 as a cut-off for clinically relevant acidemia in its definition of perinatal asphyxia. In a study of 3506 newborns, 87 of whom had pH less than 7.00, Goldaber suggests that the level of pathologic fetal acidemia is even lower (Goldaber *et al.* 1991). Factors such as prematurity, fetal growth restriction, infection, hypertension, collagen vascular diseases, and prolonged pregnancy may all contribute to both a decreased tolerance to labor and a diminished fetal response.

Interpretation of umbilical artery blood gases requires examination of the $PO_2$, $PCO_2$ and bicarbonate, as well as the base deficit. According to Low, a base deficit of greater than 12 to 16 (occurring in 0.5% and 2% of newborns, respectively) represents the threshold for significant metabolic acidosis (Low 1997). Others have proposed the threshold as 15 mmol/l, with a compensatory calculation for severe hypercarbia ($PCO_2$ greater than 66 mmHg), indicating a mixed respiratory and metabolic acidosis (Goldaber *et al.* 1991). Kruger *et al.* has reported a threshold of 4.8 mmol/l for clinically significant lactate levels in fetal scalp blood, correlating with an increased risk of hypoxic–ischemic encephalopathy (Kruger *et al.* 1999). All of these measurements, however, reflect a cumulative fetal response and do not indicate the timing or duration of the asphyxial exposure. As with Apgar scores, only extremely abnormal values of pH and base deficit are associated with abnormal neurologic outcome, as 80% of infants with umbilical cord pH less than 7.0 at birth will have normal neurologic development (Goodwin *et al.* 1992).

Other markers for hypoxemia and asphyxia, such as neonatal lymphocyte count, nucleated red blood cells (NRBC), and urinary lactate to creatinine ratios have been investigated for their utility in determining the timing of an asphyxial event. In 1941, Anderson reported that chorionic capillaries within the placentas of fetuses with intrauterine asphyxia had an increase in NRBCs (Anderson 1941). Phelan and Korst subsequently observed that a NRBC count greater than 10 per 100 white blood cells was significantly higher in infants who were neurologically impaired as a result of hypoxic ischemia (Phelan *et al.* 1995; Korst *et al.* 1996). In one study of 46 neurologically impaired infants, lower NRBC counts were observed in intrapartum asphyxial events closer to the birth than those with presumed asphyxial events more remote from delivery. Infants whose identified hypoxemic events were uterine ruptures had lower numbers of NRBCs than those whose asphyxial exposures were described by abnormal fetal heart rate tracings (non-reactive EFM tracings or tachycardia) (Phelan *et al.* 1995). In Naeye's study of 16 neonates with hypoxic–ischemic encephalopathy, lymphocyte counts of greater than 10 000/mm$^3$ were significantly higher than those observed in control groups consisting of infants with low Apgar scores and without cerebral palsy. Elevated lymphocyte counts in the affected neonates were also observed compared with infants with cerebral palsy from developmental delays unrelated to antepartum and intrapartum events (Naeye & Localio 1995). In a recent report of 40 newborns with asphyxial exposure and 58 control infants, Huang *et al.* reported a significantly elevated urinary lactate to creatinine ratio in infants with hypoxic exposure who developed encephalopathy (16.75), compared with both normal infants (0.09) and infants with asphyxial exposure who did not develop encephalopathy (0.19) (Huang *et al.* 1999).

Because of the high number of false positive rates of any abnormal findings on fetal heart rate monitoring, and the impossibility of excluding antenatal causes, the exact timing of subcatastrophic asphyxial events in studies such as these cannot be determined, limiting the precision of the NRBCs and elevated neonatal lymphocytes as markers for perinatal asphyxia. Because of advances in potential therapies for infants exposed to hypoxic–ischemic events (Palmer & Vannucci 1993), recognition of neonates at risk and understanding the timing of the insult remain critical clinical research goals.

## NEUROIMAGING AND PERINATAL HYPOXIC–ISCHEMIC BRAIN INJURY (see also Chapter 6)

Later evidence for hypoxic–ischemic brain injury in the neonate is available from a variety of imaging modalities, including computed tomography (CT), single photon emission computed tomography (SPECT), magnetic resonance imaging (MRI), positron emission tomography (PET) and cranial sonography. Although one case of *in utero* fetal cerebral intra-parenchymal ischemia diagnosed by MRI has been reported in a severely growth restricted fetus (Sibong *et al.* 1998), this technique has not been utilized clinically for antepartum fetal detection of hypoxic–ischemic brain injury. The antenatal MRI finding in this case report was described as subtentorial frontoparietal intraparenchymal heterogeneous lesion with cerebral edema, and the follow-up autopsy showed significant hemispheric white matter lesions.

In term infants with neuroimaging abnormalities following asphyxial events, the ischemic injury results in diffuse infarctions in the parasagittal cortex and parieto-occipital cortex. Thromboembolic multifocal infarcts, thalamic, and basal ganglia infarcts and middle cerebral artery infarcts may also be observed. In one study of 11 infants who suffered acute near-total intrauterine asphyxia, imaging studies reported a consistent pattern of injury in the subcortical brain nuclei with relative sparing of the white matter. Seven of the 11 infants with hypoxic ischemic encephalopathy and this pattern of brain injury had good cognitive outcomes; however, long-term neurologic deficits included spastic quadriplegia, mild cerebral palsy, deafness, and behavioural abnormalities and dystonia. Although 10 of the 11 patients did not have significant multiorgan system failure, the one infant who died in the neonatal period had evidence of hepatic abnormality (Pasternak & Gorey 1998). Another study of 20 term infants with moderate-to-severe hypoxic–ischemic encephalopathy, decreased tissue attenuation in the central gray matter (thalami and basal ganglia) was observed in the absence of cortical changes. This pattern of injury indicated an extremely poor prognosis, with 35% of infants expiring in the neonatal period and the remaining survivors all affected with neurologic abnormalities including spastic quadriplegia, microcephaly, and seizures (Roland *et al.* 1998).

In preterm infants with hypoxic–ischemic encephalopathy, brain injuries usually result from hemorrhage, either in the vascular subependymal areas, within the cerebral ventricles, or within the parenchyma. Infrequently, the periventricular white matter region is affected bilaterally and periventricular leukomalacia (PVL) results. The specific pattern of perinatal CNS damage in the preterm infant is demonstrated primarily in the deep strata of the cerebellum, germinal tissue, periventricular white matter and basal ganglia, in contrast to mainly cortical damage in the term infant. This distinction is influenced by three gestational age-dependent factors: (1) presence or absence of germinal matrix tissue, (2) the underlying process of CNS organogenesis, and (3) the degree of development of neurovasculature (Towbin 1986). Neurodevelopmental prognoses among preterm infants with asphyxial exposure and abnormal neuroimaging studies vary widely, with factors such as infection and developmental immaturity contributing to possible CNS damage from asphyxial exposure.

Neuropathologic studies confirm the findings of neuroimaging and have shown that both the gray matter and the white matter of the brain may undergo necrosis as a result of lethal hypoxic ischemia. In one post-mortem study of 120 perinatal deaths attributed to perinatal asphyxia, CNS necrosis was observed in 16 infants, including lesions that occurred in the antepartum period as well as intrapartum (Low *et al.* 1989). In the first half of pregnancy, ischemic CNS insults may lead to porencephalic cysts, multicystic encephalomalacia, and hydrancephaly. In this study of term infants, two infants with antenatal hypoxic ischemia had evidence of PVL. In five infants remote from term, the hypoxic–ischemic insult occurred in the 12-hour period before the onset of labor, presumably due to antepartum hemorrhage. The pattern of CNS pathology in this group showed neuronal necrosis of the cerebral cortex, and the inferior olive and dorsal nucleus of the vagus nerve of the brain stem, large germinal matrix hemorrhage, and intraventricular hemorrhage. The four neonates in the intrapartum asphyxia group delivered with clinical evidence of asphyxia as well as abnormal pH and acid–base status. The observed neuropathology in the intrapartum asphyxia group included extensive neuronal necrosis of the basal ganglia and thalamus, with limited necrosis in the cerebellar cortex and brain stem.

In summary, establishing the temporal relationship between an asphyxial event and the associated findings on neuroimaging and neuropathology is difficult and imprecise. Term and preterm infants exhibit different patterns of brain injury after asphyxial events, and the pattern associated with asphyxial injury remote from delivery may occasionally be distinct. Neonates who expire of sudden cardiorespiratory failure as a result of catastrophic asphyxia may not demonstrate any neuropathologic findings because of rapid demise. Furthermore, as mentioned earlier, findings consistent with an acute intrapartum event do not rule out preexisting subclinical subacute lesions that may enhance fetal susceptibility to the intermittent hypoxia of normal and abnormal labors.

## ANTEPARTUM ASPHYXIA

In the United States, perinatal mortality, which includes late fetal deaths (after 28 weeks) as well as early neonatal deaths (less than 6 days of life), has been declining steadily since 1965, reaching 8.7 per 1000 in 1991 (US Department of Health and Human Services 1995). Antepartum deaths may be due to a variety of causes including congenital malformations, pregnancy complications and infection, as well as to chronic or acute hypoxic ischemia. Of the 70–90% of fetal deaths that occur prior to the onset of labor, approximately one-third are due to hypoxia (Lammer *et al.* 1989). In contrast, intrapartum fetal deaths are primarily asphyxial, in some cases due to severe hypoxia or anoxia, and in some cases due to abnormal fetal response.

Reducing the rate of lethal antepartum asphyxia remains a difficult clinical task, not only because of the unpredictable nature of the underlying causes but also because of the relatively long period of time over which it may occur (Grant & Elborne 1989). Identifying subcatastrophic hypoxial insults that may lead to long-term neurologic morbidity is yet more complex. One strategy to reduce antepartum fetal deaths is to identify pregnancies that are at increased risk for decreased uteroplacental blood flow, such as those complicated by hypertension, collagen vascular diseases and diabetes, and to subject these patients to a schedule of antepartum evaluation or testing. Fetuses at risk for antenatal acute and chronic asphyxia, including those with intrauterine fetal growth restriction (Soothill *et al.* 1987) and prolonged pregnancy, may also benefit from antepartum surveillance.

**Table 24.3 Indications for antepartum fetal testing**

| | |
|---|---|
| • Asthma | • Polyhydramnios |
| • Abnormal fetal heart tones | • Poor obstetric history |
| • Cardiac disease | • Prolonged pregnancy |
| • Cholestasis of pregnancy | • Preeclampsia |
| • Chronic hypertension | • Preterm labor |
| • Collagen vascular disease | • Preterm premature rupture of membranes |
| • Congenital anomalies | • Prior stillbirth |
| • Decreased fetal movement | • Renal disease |
| • Diabetes | • Rh disease (isoimmunization) |
| • Fetal growth restriction | • Sickle cell disease |
| • Intrauterine procedure | • Substance abuse |
| • Multiple gestation | • Third trimester bleeding |
| • Oligohydramnios | • Thyroid disease |
| • Placenta previa | |

## ANTEPARTUM FETAL TESTING

Fetal well-being is currently evaluated using several antepartum tests including the non-stress test, contraction stress test, ultrasonographic evaluation of the fetal biophysical state, and fetal Doppler. Of the tests that involve observations of fetal heart rate by cardiotocography, the non-stress test is the most widely used. The use of the non-stress test evolved from observations of fetal heart tracings in labor as well as in experimental animal models. Whereas late decelerations and loss of variability on electronic fetal monitoring (EFM) have been linked with fetal acidosis (Murata *et al.* 1982), accelerations of the fetal heart in response to fetal activity, contractions, or external stimulation, have been associated with adequate fetal oxygenation and neurologic response. To produce a normal (reactive) fetal heart rate tracing on EFM, the fetal heart must demonstrate intact electrical conduction pathways involving myocardial, neurologic and hormonal receptors as well as intact sympathetic and parasympathetic reflexes and normal myocardial contractility (Dalton *et al.* 1983).

The normal fetal heart baseline is between 110 and 160 bpm. The healthy term fetus demonstrates an average of 34 heart rate accelerations per hour, averaging 20 to 25 bpm above baseline and lasting up to 40 seconds (Patrick *et al.* 1984). At term, fetal heart rate accelerations are associated with fetal movement more than 85% of the time and more than 90% of fetal body movements are accompanied by accelerations. The association of fetal heart rate accelerations and fetal movement increases with advancing gestational age, representing neurologic maturation and integration of reflex responses and autonomic tone.

The most common cause for absent fetal heart rate accelerations is fetal sleep, although other factors such as maternal narcotics, CNS depressants, maternal smoking, or β-blockers may reduce fetal heart rate variability as well (Keegan *et al.* 1979; Phelan 1979; Margulis *et al.* 1984). Episodes of low fetal movement associated with diminished fetal heart rate variability indicate a quiet fetal sleep cycle, and may last from 20 to 120 minutes in the term fetus. Active sleep cycles in the fetus occur throughout most of a 24-hour day and involve increased fetal breathing, increased fetal heart rate variability, rapid eye movements, and occasional body movements. Brief periods of 'wakefulness' occur approximately 15–20% of the day and are associated with increased gross body movements, and maximal fetal heart rate variability.

### NON-STRESS TEST

The non-stress test (NST) is usually performed in an outpatient setting, with the patient in a reclining chair or bed with left lateral tilt to avoid supine hypotension. The fetal heart rate is monitored using the Doppler ultrasound transducer, and the tocodynamometer is used to detect uterine contractions. During the test the patient reports fetal activity, although the record of these fetal movements does not affect the interpretation of the test. As with intrapartum fetal monitoring, acute fetal hypoxemia in the antepartum period may cause profound decreases in fetal movement and heart rate accelerations. Chronic hypoxia, however, may yield a more gradual decline in fetal function and response as compensatory circulatory shunting occurs.

Guidelines for interpretation of fetal heart rate (FHR) monitoring have been developed by the Research Planning Workshop for the National Institute of Child Health and Human Development (1996) (Anonymous 1997). These guidelines apply to interpretation of antepartum as well as intrapartum EFM. First, any patterns of the fetal heart rate are reported as baseline, periodic, or episodic. Second, the following five components of fetal heart rate patterns must be described qualitatively and quantitatively: (1) baseline rate, (2) baseline variability, (3) presence of accelerations, (4) periodic or episodic decelerations and (5) changes or trends in fetal heart rate patterns over time. An acceleration of the fetal heart rate is defined as a visually abrupt increase in the FHR above baseline. The peak is to be greater than or equal to 15 bpm over the baseline and lasting 15 seconds or more. Prior to 32 weeks gestation, accelerations are defined as 10 bpm over baseline for duration of 10 seconds or greater. The most widely applied definition of a normal or reactive non-stress test involves two accelerations meeting the above criteria in a 20-minute period.

On initial testing, 85% of NSTs will be reactive and 15% will be non-reactive (Lavery 1982). The NST is most predictive when it is normal or reactive. A reactive NST has been associated with a perinatal mortality of approximately 5 per 1000 (Phelan 1981). Although the rate of perinatal demise after a non-reactive NST is considerably higher, up to 40 per 1000, this group contains a large number of false positive tests, as high as 75–90% (Lavery 1982). The majority of fetuses with a non-reactive NST will not suffer death or morbidity following the test; however, follow-up testing is generally indicated, either by prolonged NST, contraction stress test, or biophysical profile.

Vibroacoustic stimulation (VAS) has been used to stimulate the fetus that may be in a quiet sleep state. The artificial larynx, which generates a sound pressure of 82 dB measured at 1 meter of air, is the most commonly used device (Gagnon *et al.* 1989). VAS has been shown to increase the mean duration of heart rate accelerations, the mean amplitude of accelerations and total time spent in accelerations. FHR variability and gross body movements are also increased. Using VAS in the setting of non-reactive NSTs, the incidence of non-reactivity is reduced from 14 to 9%, and the time spent in testing is reduced. In one study by Druzin *et al.*, the incidence of non-reactive NSTs in fetuses after 26 weeks was significantly decreased with the use of VAS (Druzin *et al.* 1989), obviating the need for further testing to follow-up a non-reactive test.

Significant bradycardia, defined as a fetal heart rate of less than 90 bpm or a fall in the fetal baseline more than 40 bpm (Druzin *et al.* 1981; ACOG 1984), has been observed in 1–2% of all NSTs. Bradycardia on NST has been associated with increased perinatal morbidity and mortality, including intrauterine fetal demise, structural malformations, and fetal growth restriction (Bourgeois *et al.* 1984; Druzin 1989). Moreover, the incidence of abnormal intrapartum FHR tracing and subsequent Cesarean delivery is higher in those with bradycardia on antepartum heart tracing on NST compared with those who have reactive NSTs without significant bradycardia. Although a non-reactive NST is also associated with an abnormal intrapartum FHR tracing and increased intervention rate, the positive predictive value of the tracing with bradycardia leading to Cesarean delivery is higher (Dashow & Read 1984). Because perinatal mortality rates may be as high as 25% in fetuses with spontaneous significant bradycardias, delivery is generally indicated for the term fetus, but management of the preterm fetus may be more complex. Presence or absence of variability in the setting of significant bradycardia may not be helpful in distinguishing fetuses at increased risk for perinatal hypoxia. Corticosteroid administration and conservative management may follow assessment of the amniotic fluid index and targeted ultrasound for fetal anomalies, with continuous fetal monitoring for the early preterm fetus.

In high-risk pregnancies, increasing the interval of testing to twice per week can reduce the false negative rate of the NST. Boehm *et al.* reported an overall decrease in the fetal death rate from 6.1/1000 to 1.9/1000 when twice weekly testing was used (Boehm *et al.* 1986). Because the fetal death rate is increased in pregnancies with diabetes, hypertension, and fetal growth restriction, these pregnancies should be monitored with twice weekly NSTs. The incidence of fetal death following a normal NST in prolonged pregnancies is not significantly increased over the general tested pregnant population (2.7/1000) (Barss *et al.* 1981); however, the risk–benefit ratio of intervention on behalf of the term mature fetus may favor induction of labor in some cases.

## CONTRACTION STRESS TEST

The contraction stress test (CST), also known as the oxytocin challenge test, was the first antepartum test used for fetal surveillance. When contractions produce decreased blood flow in the intervillous spaces of the placenta, varying degrees of hypoxia may lead to signs of stress in the fetus. On FHR monitoring, the fetus with diminished placental respiratory reserve may respond to the stress of contractions with late decelerations. Interpretation of the presence or absence of late decelerations and the pattern of decelerations form the basis for interpretation of the CST.

Prior to the test, which is generally performed on a labor and delivery suite or specialized antepartum testing unit, maternal blood pressure is monitored periodically while uterine contractions and FHR are recorded using external monitors. Oxytocin is administered by intravenous infusion, beginning at 0.5 mU/min. The infusion is doubled every 15 minutes until three contractions in 10 minutes are achieved. After the CST is achieved, FHR monitoring should continue until contractions cease. As an alternative to oxytocin infusion, the nipple stimulation test may be used. Using self-nipple massage, over 85% of patients can achieve adequate uterine contractions for evaluation (Oki *et al.* 1987) with no difference in the incidence of positive and negative tests compared with the CST. Absolute contraindications to the CST include premature preterm rupture of the membranes, third trimester bleeding, and cervical incompetence. Relative contraindications include preterm labor, polyhydramnios, prior Cesarean section, and multiple gestation.

Interpretation of the CST follows the definitions described by Freeman (1975). A positive (abnormal) test is defined as a 10-minute segment of the FHR tracing which includes at least three contractions, each followed by late decelerations. A negative (normal) test is one with no late decelerations after three uterine contractions. A CST with negative windows and occasional late decelerations is read as suspicious, and equivocal describes the tracing with occasional late decelerations and no negative window. A CST with both negative and positive windows is interpreted as positive. A suspicious or equivocal CST should be repeated in 24 hours, and most of these tests will become negative. Bruce *et al.* observed that 5 of 67 patients with initial CSTs read as suspicious were subsequently positive (Bruce *et al.* 1978).

Although a negative CST has been consistently associated with a good outcome (perinatal mortality less than 1/1000 within 1 week of the test), the relatively high false positive rate (up to 30%) limits the utility of the test (Evertson *et al.* 1978; Freeman *et al.* 1982). Furthermore, Druzin *et al.* reported that a non-reactive NST with a negative contraction stress test did not have the same predictive accuracy as the reactive NST (Druzin *et al.* 1980). Overall, the rate of perinatal death following a positive CST is elevated at 7–15%. Although a positive CST is an indication for delivery, it is not necessarily an indication for Cesarean section, as labor may proceed safely with continuous FHR monitoring. The positive CST had been associated not only with an increased incidence of fetal death, but also with an increased incidence of perinatal morbidity as detected by low 5-minute Apgar scores, fetal growth restriction, and meconium stained amniotic fluid, intrapartum fetal distress, and neonatal depression.

No prospective randomized trials with sufficient numbers of risk-matched gravidas have been reported for either the CST or the NST. Evaluation of the current literature shows a wide range of testing standards and thresholds yielding a yet wider range of test sensitivity, specificity, and positive predictive values. Because the positive predictive value depends on the incidence of fetal compromise in a given population, the application of these tests to low-risk patients will decrease the performance of the test. For both the NST and the CST the specificity is relatively high (>90%), with sensitivities of 45–55%. Most evaluations of the CST use perinatal mortality as a primary outcome measure with few conclusions regarding the impact of abnormal tests on perinatal morbidity and neurologic outcome. Because of the low sensitivity of these tests (i.e. high number of false positives), additional fetal testing may be performed prior to intervention (delivery), especially when the fetus is known or suspected to be immature.

## BIOPHYSICAL PROFILE

Fetal hypoxemia has been shown to alter biophysical activities such as fetal breathing and movement, as well as tone and heart rate patterns. Fetal biophysical profile (BPP) scoring was therefore developed using dynamic ultrasound examination to assess the well-being of the fetus. Ultrasound examination of the fetus is also used to detect abnormalities of amniotic fluid, fetal size, placental location, and umbilical cord insertion site. Fetal biophysical responses to asphyxia include both acute and chronic responses. The acute fetal response to hypoxia includes changes in CNS regulated activities, such as breathing and movement. Chronic responses to decreased oxygenation include low levels of amniotic fluid and restricted fetal growth.

The BPP method as described by Manning *et al.* uses real time ultrasound for scored evaluation of fetal breathing movements, fetal tone, gross body movements, and amniotic fluid volume (Manning *et al.* 1985). A NST may follow the ultrasound examination of the fetus. The longitudinal scan plane is used to view the fetus with simultaneous evaluation of upper and lower extremities, as well as the fetal thorax. The test continues for 30 minutes or until all the parameters have been observed. Two points are scored for each of the above variables for a maximum score of 8 out of 8. If the NST is generally performed if one of more of the other four variables is abnormal, two points are scored for a reactive NST, and the total for a normal test is then scored as 10 out of 10. All of the components are assumed to be of equal significance, and therefore are each assigned two points. In one analysis of 342 abnormal tests, Manning demonstrated that the distribution of score variables is almost equal among possible combinations (Manning *et al.* 1990).

According to Vintzileos, fetal biophysical activities that appear earliest in fetal development are the last to disappear with fetal hypoxia (Vintzileos *et al.* 1983). The fetal tone center in the cortex begins to function at approximately 8 weeks. Fetal tone, therefore, would be the last parameter to be lost with deteriorating fetal condition. The fetal movement center, which functions at approximately 9 weeks, would be more sensitive than fetal tone. Fetal breathing, which develops at approximately 20 weeks, may be lost sooner than movement and tone. Finally, fetal heart rate reactivity, which relies on development of the posterior thalamus and medulla as well as intact CNS reflexes, may not reliably appear until the late third trimester (>28 weeks). Using this hypothesis, the BPP may be used to evaluate the preterm fetus in which FHR reactivity has not been established.

Like the reactive NST, a normal BPP is highly predictive of a non-asphyxiated fetus with intact CNS responses. In one prospective blinded study of 216 high-risk pregnancies, Manning found no perinatal deaths when all five variables of the test were normal (Manning *et al.* 1980). However, unlike the NST, several aspects of fetal response are evaluated using the BPP, and the resulting proportion of normal

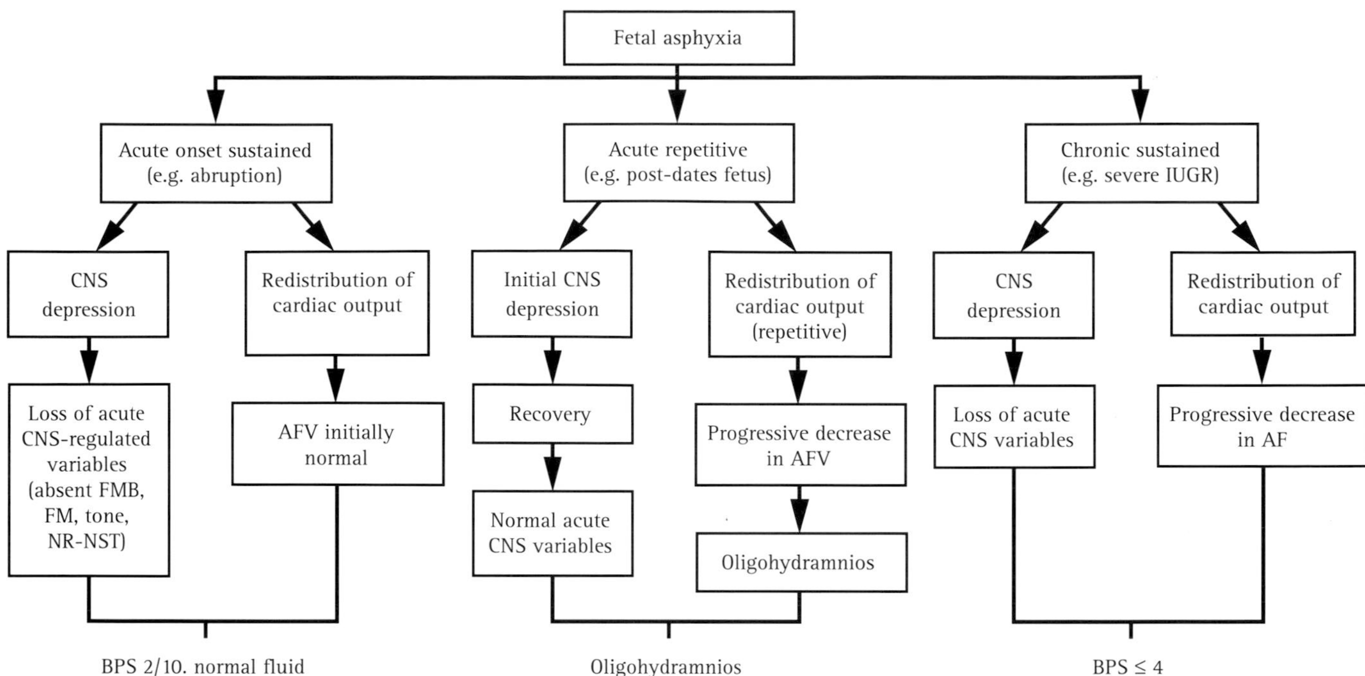


**Figure 24.2** Schematic representation of the mechanisms by which the fetal response to hypoxic insult may affect the biophysical score. The fetal responses may vary with acute versus chronic hypoxia and will be affected by the duration, severity, rate of onset, and repetitive frequency of the insult. CNS, central nervous system; IUGR, intrauterine growth restriction; FBM, fetal breathing movements; FM, fetal movement; NR-NST, non-reactive non-stress test; AFV, amniotic fluid volume; BPS, biophysical profile score. (From Tsang HH & Manning FA, Biophysical profile scoring. In: Druzin ML, ed. *Antepartum fetal assessment.* Boston, MA: Blackwell Scientific; p. 33, with permission.)

**Table 24.4 Biophysical profile scoring and interpretation**

| Biophysical variable | Normal (score=2) | Abnormal (score=0) |
|---|---|---|
| Fetal breathing movements | At least one episode of fetal breathing movement of at least 30 seconds duration in 30 minutes | Absent fetal breathing or no episode of greater than 30 seconds in 30 minutes |
| Gross body movements | At least three discrete body or limb movements in 30 minutes | Two or fewer body or limb movements in 30 minutes |
| Fetal tone | At least one episode of active extension with return to flexion of fetal limbs or trunk, includes opening and closing the hand | Either slow extension with return to partial flexion, or movement of the limb in full extension or no fetal movement |
| Reactive non-stress test | At least two episodes of fetal heart rate acceleration of greater than or equal to 15 bpm and of at least 15 seconds duration associated with fetal movement in 30 minutes | Less than two episodes of acceleration of fetal heart rate greater than or equal to 15 bpm, and of at least 15 seconds in duration associated with fetal movement in 30 minutes |
| Amniotic fluid volume | At least one pocket of amniotic fluid that measures 2 cm by 2 cm in two perpendicular planes | Either no amniotic fluid pocket or a pocket less than 2 cm in two perpendicular planes |

*Source*: From Tsang HH & Manning FA, Biophysical profile scoring. In: Druzin ML, ed. *Antepartum fetal assessment.* Boston, MA: Blackwell Scientific; p. 33, with permission.

tests is higher (97.5%). A false negative rate of the BPP is also lower than that of the NST alone (2–5/1000). Similar to the NST, the use of vibroacoustic stimulation of the fetus with an abnormal or equivocal BPP has been shown to improve the biophysical score without decreasing the false negative rate (Inglis *et al.* 1993). Moreover, the scoring system for the BPP (see Table 23.4) may reveal a spectrum of fetal asphyxial response. Good obstetric management mandates interpretation of the individual components as well as consideration of obstetric factors, such as gestational age, underlying fetal and maternal disease, maternal drug exposure, and prematurity. According to a summary of data in eight studies of BPP for fetal evaluation, involving 23 780 patients and 54 337 tests, the overall corrected perinatal mortality of the BPP was calculated at 0.726/1000 (Manning 1992).

To evaluate the effect of fetal assessment by BPP on the risk of perinatal morbidity, Manning evaluated the incidence of cerebral palsy in fetuses that were evaluated by BPP compared with those who were not. In a retrospective study of 84 947 live births over a 5-year period, the overall incidence of cerebral palsy was 3.68/1000. The incidence of cerebral palsy in 26 290 referred high risk patients who had antenatal testing with BPP was 1.33/1000 live births compared with 4.74/1000 in 58 657 untested patients (Manning *et al.* 1998). In another study examining the relationship between abnormal BPP and cerebral palsy, Manning reported that the fetuses with abnormal BPP were more likely to develop fetal distress in labor (88.8%), acidosis (77.7%), and neonatal seizures (88.8%). Antenatal asphyxia as predicted based on BPP appears to be associated with cerebral damage in 29.6% of cases (Manning *et al.* 1997).

A combined strategy of nonstress testing, evaluation of amniotic fluid index (AFI), biophysical profile, umbilical velocimetry and contraction stress testing may be used in

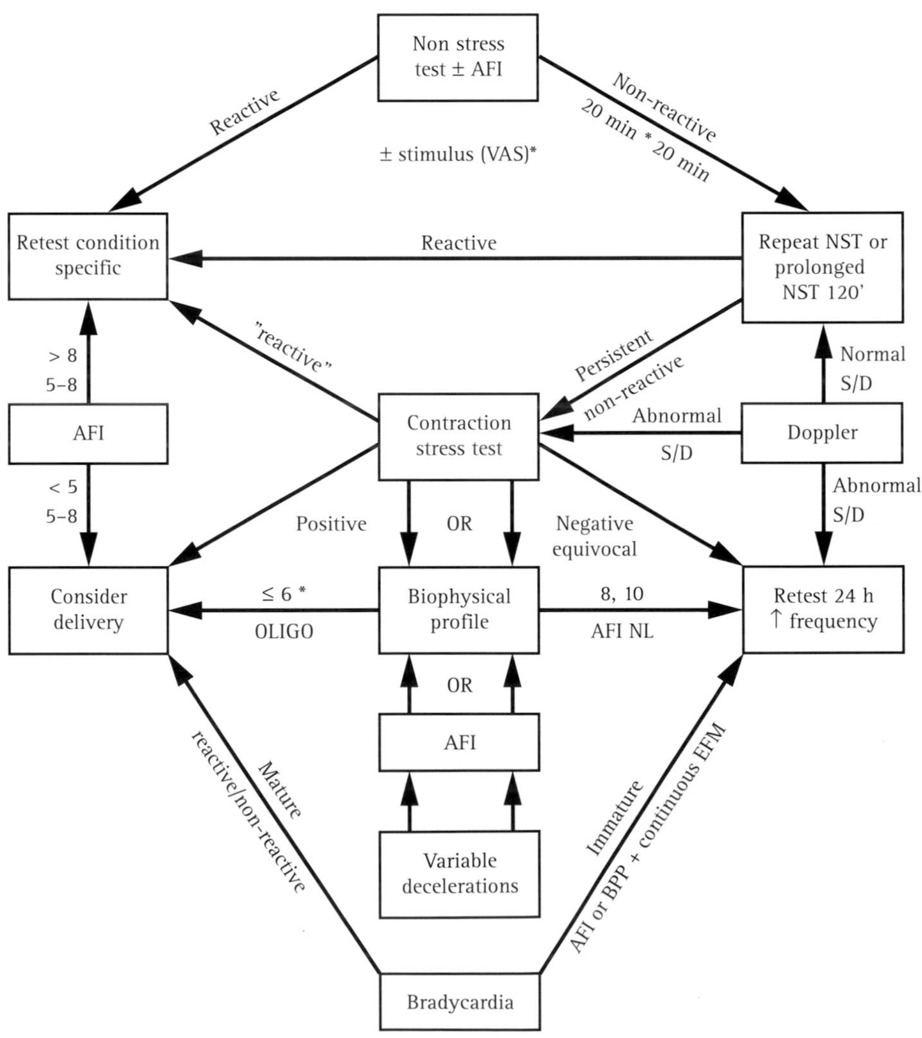


**Figure 24.3** Fetal antepartum testing scheme. The most commonly used antepartum test is the non-stress test (NST). Depending on abnormalities of testing, other follow-up tests may be indicated. AFI, amniotic fluid index; VAS, vibroacoustic stimulation; BPP, biophysical profile; S/D; systolic to diastolic ratio.

the antepartum assessment of the fetus at risk for hypoxic stress. One general algorithm for fetal evaluation in the antepartum testing unit at Stanford University is represented in Fig. 24.3. The specific indication for testing, the gestational age, and other compounding maternal and fetal factors may influence the testing interval as well as the combined number of tests required to raise the suspicion of fetal jeopardy to the point of delivery. When abnormal antepartum testing indicates the need for delivery, this may be accomplished by either the vaginal or abdominal route, depending on the fetal response to the stress of labor and other obstetric indications.

## DOPPLER VELOCIMETRY OF THE UMBILICAL VESSELS (see also Chapter 9)

Because of the need for better antenatal tests to reduce unnecessary intervention in pregnancies with false positive tests, umbilical artery Doppler velocimetry has been widely investigated. The principle upon which Doppler testing of the fetus may be useful relies on an incomplete understanding of the physiology of uteroplacental blood flow. Continuous wave Doppler systems generate flow velocity waveforms that reflect the distribution and intensity of the Doppler frequency shifts over time. Provided the angle of insonation and the transmitted frequency of the ultrasound beam are constant, these frequency shifts are proportional to changes in flow velocity within the umbilical vessels.

Clinically, the most commonly used fetal Doppler evaluation is reported as the ratio of the peak systolic velocity waveform to the nadir at diastole. The greater the diastolic flow, the lower the ratio. As the peripheral resistance increases, the diastolic flow falls, resulting in an elevated *S*/*D* ratio. At various gestational ages the fetal circulation demonstrates characteristic Doppler waveforms. In the first trimester of pregnancy, the uterine artery has high pulsatility and consequently generates a Doppler waveform with reduced diastolic flow (elevated *S*/*D* ratio). This pattern results from elevated downstream resistance in the uterine vessels. As resistance in the placental vessels drops in the second trimester from growth of small muscular arteries in the tertiary stem villi of the placenta, diastolic flow increases, and the *S*/*D* ratio decreases. This pattern of decreasing pulsatility and increasing diastolic flow continues throughout normal gestation. By 30 weeks gestation, the *S*/*D* ratio in the umbilical artery should be less than 3.0. Absent or reverse diastolic flow reflects an abnormally elevated level of fetal peripheral resistance that may indicate fetal jeopardy.

Other methods of reporting fetal arterial Doppler waveforms include the pulsatility index and the resistance index. The pulsatility index is calculated as the systolic minus the diastolic values divided by the mean of the velocity waveform profile ($S - D$/mean). The resistance index (Pourcelot ratio) is expressed as $S - D/S$. These indices may be useful when there is absent or reversed end diastolic flow.

Several studies have suggested that umbilical artery Doppler provides a reasonable estimation of umbilical cord blood flow. Decreases in the *S*/*D* ratio, therefore, reflect placental abnormalities in flow and resistance, rather than hypoxia or asphyxia *per se*. Using a sheep model, Trudinger *et al.* embolized the umbilical placental circulation with microspheres each day for nine days and observed the resulting Doppler waveforms (Trudinger *et al.* 1987). The umbilical *S*/*D* ratio increased steadily with increasing vascular resistance in the placental bed. However, umbilical blood flow did not fall significantly until the placental resistance was maximal. Morrow & Ritchie used a similar model of progressive embolization and likewise observed a progressive increase in the *S*/*D* ratio, followed by absent end diastolic flow, then reversed diastolic flow (Morrow & Ritchie 1989). In this study, increasing the blood viscosity 100% by increasing the fetal hematocrit had minimal effect on the *S*/*D* ratio, indicating that umbilical blood flow, not necessarily hypoxia, induced abnormal Doppler waveforms in the umbilical artery. Because decreased umbilical artery flow may not produce hypoxemia in the well compensated fetus, abnormal Doppler velocimetry neither reliably predicts antenatal hypoxic–ischemic conditions nor demonstrates chronic asphyxia.

In assessing placental function and umbilical blood flow, Doppler velocimetry has been investigated as an antenatal predictor of fetal condition. In one study by Devoe *et al.*, Doppler velocimetry was used along with NST and amniotic fluid evaluation to determine the predictive value in predicting poor perinatal outcome as determined by fetal distress in labor, low 5-minute Apgar scores, neonatal acidosis and perinatal mortality (Devoe *et al.* 1990). The overall perinatal mortality using all three techniques was 2.1 per 1000. Although each method had a specificity of approximately 90%, sensitivities for the NST and Doppler velocimetry were 69% and 21%, respectively. The positive predictive value of all three tests combined in predicting abnormal outcome was 100%. In a meta-analysis of 12 randomized controlled trials of Doppler velocimetry in high risk pregnancies, Alfirevic and colleagues detected a significant decrease in perinatal deaths and Cesarean deliveries for fetal distress among pregnancies in which Doppler velocimetry was used for antenatal surveillance (Alfirevic & Nielson 1995).

Although Doppler velocimetry has not been shown to be predictive of poor pregnancy outcome in low risk pregnancies (Mason *et al.* 1993), this antenatal test performs better in pregnancies at risk for intrauterine growth restriction, including hypertension and collagen vascular diseases. An elevation of the *S*/*D* ratio may precede the identification of fetal growth restriction, and may be more predictive of neonatal morbidity than the NST alone (Trudinger *et al.* 1986). Because the absence of diastolic flow in pregnancies complicated by fetal growth restriction has been associated with increased perinatal mortality, these fetuses may require either intense on-going fetal surveillance or delivery.

Abnormal Doppler velocimetry appears to be associated with abnormal fetal conditions including aneuploidy (Martinex-Crespo *et al.* 1996), and major structural malformations (Tannirandorn *et al.* 1993), indicating a possible need for a combination of antenatal tests in evaluating the well-being of these high risk fetuses.

## INTRAPARTUM FETAL ASSESSMENT

Controversy exists over the role of intrapartum fetal heart rate monitoring for the prediction and prevention of hypoxic–ischemic brain damage, with emphasis on cerebral palsy. Perinatal brain injury is a recognized cause of some cases of severe neurologic deficit and cerebral palsy, with approximately 10% attributable to intrapartum hypoxic ischemic events (Nelson & Ellenberg 1986). Efforts to reduce the number of fetuses with severe intrapartum asphyxia and those with hypoxic–ischemic brain injury in the era of widespread use of fetal heart rate monitoring have been disappointing. Although intrapartum mortality has decreased with fetal heart rate monitoring since the 1970s and significant improvements in perinatal and neonatal care have evolved, the incidence of cerebral palsy has remained unchanged (1–2/1000). Despite an extremely low overall incidence of cerebral palsy due to hypoxic–ischemic brain injury (1–2/10 000), the pediatric, obstetric, and medicolegal interest in the topic remains high.

In a review article addressing the association of intrapartum hypoxic–ischemic cerebral injury with cerebral palsy, Perlman suggests four possible explanations for the stability of the incidence of cerebral palsy: (1) most cases of brain injury associated with cerebral palsy are not related to perinatal events; (2) improved survival of very premature infants who are at greatest risk of developing hemorrhagic ischemic brain injury and cerebral palsy; (3) limitations of current markers of perinatal stress to identify those infants who are at greatest risk of developing hypoxic–ischemic brain injury because of intrapartum asphyxia; (4) lack of effective postnatal interventions to reduce brain injury in neonates with hypoxic–ischemic encephalopathy (Perlman 1997).

Although it is clear that intrapartum fetal asphyxia of sufficient degree and duration will cause fetal death and neurologic morbidity in some survivors, it is not clear whether or not the use of electronic fetal monitoring (EFM) in labor can prevent asphyxial brain injuries. Randomized clinical trials of EFM versus intermittent auscultation have failed to demonstrate a clear improvement in neonatal neurologic outcome. Thacker *et al.* reviewed 12 published clinical trials with 58 855 pregnancies from 10 centers worldwide and concluded that the significant differences in outcome with the use of EFM included a reduction in intrapartum asphyxia, a decrease in neonatal seizures, and an increase in operative vaginal and abdominal deliveries (Thacker *et al.* 1995). Because of the slight contribution of intrapartum asphyxia to the rate of cerebral palsy, an impact of EFM on the rate of cerebral palsy would not be expected, even with the large number of patients evaluated. Nelson *et al.* reviewed FHR tracings in 78 of 95 infants identified with cerebral palsy in California. Although decreased variability was associated with cerebral palsy, the false positive rate was extremely high (Nelson *et al.* 1996).

Several other studies that have retrospectively examined intrapartum FHR tracings of asphyxiated infants have highlighted the difficulty of using EFM as a predictor of hypoxic–ischemic brain injury in labor. Ahn evaluated FHR tracings of 300 neurologically impaired infants, 24 of whom had normal intrapartum FHR patterns. Intrapartum reactivity appeared to be evident in brain damaged infants only in cases of asphyxial events preceding labor (54%) or with postnatal injury (46%) (Ahn *et al.* 1998). In one matched case control study of 71 term infants with intrapartum asphyxia defined as umbilical arterial blood base deficit of greater that 16 mmol/l, Low *et al.* evaluated FHR tracings for evidence of abnormal intrapartum patterns. They found that the pattern of minimal-to-absent variability and late and prolonged decelerations to be most strongly associated with moderate-to-severe intrapartum asphyxia (Low *et al.* 1999). Because most abnormal intrapartum patterns are not specific for asphyxia and the positive predictive value of these findings is very low, the potential for unnecessary intervention in labor is high when abnormal FHR patterns are observed by the clinician. Low and others have concluded that intrapartum detection of asphyxia is possible but difficult, and that the window of opportunity to intervene is small.

In 1996, guidelines for interpretation of FHR were developed by the Research Planning Workshop for the National Institute of Child Health and Human Development in order to standardize the definitions of normal and abnormal FHR patterns for intrapartum as well as antenatal surveillance. Nevertheless, no consensus was established regarding which FHR pattern or patterns constitute fetal distress, or what clinical responses are appropriate. Even the term 'fetal distress' to describe a potentially hypoxic fetus is controversial, with ACOG favoring the term 'non-reassuring fetal status.' Given the wide range of fetal responses to hypoxic injury and the lack of consensus on whether or not neurologic damage results from a 'continuum of reproductive casualty' (Goodwin 1999), interpretation of FHR patterns will remain possible but difficult.

Despite its disappointing performance in clinical trials, EFM is used for intrapartum fetal assessment in over 75% of all labors in the United States. Additional tests of fetal well-being in labor, such as fetal scalp blood sampling and vibroacoustic stimulation, are also used to reduce the number of false positive interpretations of FHR patterns that could lead to unnecessary interventions. Intelligent computer systems for interpretation of EFM continue to show promise, as do continuous intrapartum pH, $PO_2$ and $sPO_2$ monitoring. None of the techniques for continuous fetal biochemical monitoring is in clinical use because of technical problems and the difficulties with continuing the measurements of these parameters throughout labor.

Fetal pulse oximetry has the potential to provide continuous meaningful data regarding the state of fetal oxygenation in labor, and the results of a large multicenter clinical trial are now pending. One of the many technical challenges in the development of fetal oximetry has been continuous placement of the probe against the fetal cheek throughout labor, including the second stage when fetal blood flow shifts may be significant. Both Dildy *et al.* (1993) and Luttkus *et al.* (1995) reported that a reliable signal is obtained only 50% of the time in labor. Moreover, the accuracy of measurement of fetal $O_2$ which has a mean $O_2$ saturation of approximately 58% (Dildy *et al.* 1993), may be unstable at relatively low and clinically critical values. Other difficulties with continuous fetal oximetry include variations in measurements due to variables such as meconium, fetal and maternal movement, caput formation and thick, curly hair (Dildy *et al.* 1997). Nevertheless, technological improvements in fetal pulse oximetry hold continuing promise for reducing the Cesarean section rate for nonreassuring fetal status, as well as for improving the detection of severe hypoxic–ischemic insult in labor.

## SUMMARY

Overall, significant advances in obstetric and neonatal care, along with improvements in the antenatal prediction and prevention of fetal asphyxia, have led to the observed decline in perinatal morbidity and mortality over the last half-century. Ultrasound techniques have allowed clinicians to observe fetal anatomy, biophysical status, the intrauterine environment, and fetal response to stress. The etiologies of fetal/neonatal brain disorders are diverse and associated with intrapartum events in only a small minority of cases. The detection and prevention of neurologic damage, therefore, remain a continual challenge. Early identification of risk factors for neurologic sequelae as well as advancements in understanding neonatal response to hypoxia have been crucial to the development of strategies to limit further injury.

Identification and timely delivery of the fetus exposed to hypoxic stress may improve the neurologic outcomes in some cases. However, this strategy could lead to avoidable complications of prematurity if the diagnosis of hypoxia is in error. Intrapartum management of fetuses based on electronic fetal monitoring remains imperfect. A lower threshold for operative delivery, as a strategy for reducing hypoxic ischemic neurologic injury, will not be effective unless the diagnostic accuracy of tests for impending fetal neurologic injury improves.

### Key Points

- Perinatal asphyxia is a hypoxic ischemic insult that may occur antepartum, intrapartum or after birth.
- Perinatal asphyxia was thought to be associated with brain damage and cerebral palsy, yet it is unlikely to be the cause for cerebral palsy unless the severity of the asphyxial insult is nearly lethal.
- Recent analysis of cerebral palsy and birth asphyxia indicates that only 10% of cases of cerebral palsy (1–2 per 10 000) were associated with birth asphyxia.
- Fetal asphyxia occurs as a result of absent or insufficient placental blood flow due to acute or chronic events.
- The terms 'perinatal asphyxia' and 'hypoxic ischemic injury' imply a specific cause and effect which may be difficult to determine clinically.
- Hypoxic ischemic damage begins during the injury (impaired placental exchange) and extends into the period of resuscitation or reperfusion.
- Although meconium may indicate that fetal stress has occurred, it does not predict fetal neurological impairment.
- Later evidence for hypoxic ischemic brain injury in the neonate is available from variety of imaging modalities, including computed tomography (CT), single photon emission computed tomography (SPECT), magnetic resonance imaging (MRI), positron emission tomography (PET) and cranial sonography.
- Fetal well being is currently evaluated using several antepartum tests including the nonstress test, contraction stress test, ultrasonographic evaluation of the fetal biophysical state, and fetal Doppler.
- Significant advances in obstetrical and neonatal care along with improvements in the antenatal prediction and prevention of fetal asphyxia, have led to the observed decline in perinatal morbidity and mortality over the last half-century.

## REFERENCES


ACOG (1994) *Antepartum fetal surveillance.* American College of Obstetricians and Gynecologists Technical Bulletin 188, January 1994.

Ahn M O, Korst L M & Phelan J P (1998) Normal fetal heart rate pattern in the brain damaged infant: A failure of intrapartum fetal monitoring. *J Mat Fetal Invest* 8: 58–60.

Alfirevic Z & Nielson J P (1995) Doppler ultrasonography in high-risk pregnancies: systematic review with meta-analysis. *Am J Obstet Gynecol* 172: 1379–1387.

Altschuler G, Arizawa M & Molnar-Nadasdy G (1992) Meconium induced umbilical cord vascular necrosis and ulceration. A potential link between placenta and poor pregnancy outcome. *Obstet Gynecol* 79: 760–766.

AMCOG (1992) *Fetal and neonatal injury.* American College of Obstetricians and Gynecologists Technical Bulletin 163.

Anderson G W (1941) Studies on the nucleated red blood cell count in the chronic capillaries and cord blood of various ages of pregnancy. *Am J Obstet Gynecol* 42: 1–12.

Anonymous (1966) *The collaborative study on cerebral palsy, mental retardation and other neurological and sensory disorders of infancy and childhood manual.* Bethesda, MD: Public Health Service.

Anonymous (1997) *Electronic fetal heart rate monitoring: research guidelines for interpretation.* National Institute of Health Research Planning Workshop. *Am J Obstet Gynecol* 177: 1385–1390.

Apgar V (1953) A proposal for a new method of evaluation of the newborn infant. *Current Res Anesth Analg* 32: 260–267.

Ayodeji O & Kuhn R (1986) Abnormal antepartum cardiotocography and major fetal abnormalities. *Aust NZ J Obstet Gynaecol* 26: 120–123.

Barss V A, Frigoletto F D & Diamond F (1981) Stillbirth after nonstress testing. *Obstet Gynecol* 65: 541–544.

Bax M & Nelson K B (1993) Birth asphyxia: a statement. *Dev Med Child Neurol* 35: 1022–1024.

Boehm F H, Salyer S, Shah D M *et al.* (1986) Improved outcome of twice-weekly nonstress testing. *Obstet Gynecol* 67: 566–570.

Bourgeois F J, Thiagarajah S & Harbert G M (1984) The significance of fetal heart rate decelerations during nonstress testing. *Am J Obstet Gynecol* 150: 213–216.

Bruce S L, Petrie R H & Yeh S Y (1978) The suspicious contraction stress test. *Obstet Gynecol* 51: 415–418.

Carter B S, Haverkamp A D & Merenstein G B (1993) The definition of acute perinatal asphyxia. *Clin Perinatol* 20: 287–304.

Dalton K J, Dawes G S & Patrick J E (1983) The autonomic nervous system and fetal heart rate variability. *Am J Obstet Gynecol* 146: 456–462.

Dashow E E & Read J A (1984) Significant fetal bradycardia during antepartum fetal heart rate testing. *Am J Obstet Gynecol* 148: 187–190.

De Haan H H, Gunn A J & Gluckman P D (1997) Fetal heart rate changes do not reflect cardiovascular deterioration during brief repeated umbilical cord occlusions in near-term fetal lambs. *Am J Obstet Gynecol* 176: 8–17.

Delivoria-Papadapoulos M & Mishra O P (1998) Mechanisms of cerebral injury in perinatal asphyxia and strategies for prevention. *J Pediatr* 132: S30–S34.

Devoe L D, Gardner P, Dear C *et al.* (1990) The diagnostic value of concurrent nonstress testing, amniotic fluid measurement, and doppler velocimetry in screening a general high-risk population. *Am J Obstet Gynecol* 163: 1040–1047.

Dildy G A, Clark S L & Garite T J *et al.* (1999) Current status of the multicenter randomized clinical trial on fetal oxygen saturation monitoring in the United States. *Eur J Obstet Gynecol Reprod Biol* 72: S43–S50.

Dildy G A, Clark S L & Louks C A (1993) Preliminary experience with intrapartum fetal pulse oximetry in humans. *Obstet Gynecol* 81: 630–635.

Druzin M L (1989) Fetal bradycardia during antepartum testing. *J Reprod Med* 34: 47–51.

Druzin M L, Edersheim T G & Hutson J M *et al.* (1989) The effect of vibroacoustic stimulation on the nonstress test at gestational ages of thirty two weeks or less. *Am J Obstet Gynecol* 166: 1476–1478.

Druzin M L, Gratacos J & Keegan K *et al.* (1981) Antepartum fetal heart rate testing VII. The significance of bradycardia. *Am J Obstet Gynecol* 139: 194–198.

Druzin M L, Gratacos J & Paul R H (1980) Antepartum fetal heart rate testing: predictive reliability of 'normal' tests in the prevention of antepartum death. *Am J Obstet Gynecol* 137: 746–747.

Evertson L R, Gauthier R J & Collea J L (1978) Fetal demise following negative contraction stress test. *Obstet Gynecol* 51: 671–673.

Fellman V & Raivio K (1991) Reperfusion injury as the mechanism of brain damage after perinatal asphyxia. *Pediatr Res* 41: 599–606.

Field D R, Parer J T, Baker B W *et al.* (1991) Fetal heart rate variability and cerebral oxygen consumption in fetal sheep during asphyxia. *Eur J Obstet Gynecol Reprod Biol* 42: 145–153.

Freeman J M & Nelson K (1988) Intrapartum asphyxia and cerebral palsy. *Pediatrics* 82: 240–249.

Freeman R K (1975) The use of the oxytocin challenge test for antepartum clinical evaluation of uteroplacental respiratory function. *Am J Obstet Gynecol* 121: 481–489.

Freeman R, Anderson G & Dorchester W (1982) A prospective multi-institutional study of antepartum fetal heart rate monitoring. I. Risk of perinatal mortality according to antepartum fetal heart rate results. *Am J Obstet Gynecol* 143: 771–777.

Gagnon, Foreman J & Hunse C, *et al.* (1989) Effects of low frequency vibration on human term fetuses. *Am J Obstet Gynecol* 161: 1479–1485.

Gluckman P D & Williams C E (1992) When and why do brain cells die? *Dev Med Child Neurol* 34: 1010–1014.

Goldaber K G, Gilstrap L C & Leveno K J *et al.* (1991) Pathologic fetal acidemia. *Obstet Gynecol* 78: 1103–1107.

Goodwin T M (1999) Clinical implications of perinatal depression. *Obstet Gynecol Clin* 26: 711–723.

Goodwin T M, Belai I & Hernandez P *et al.* (1992) Asphyxial complications in the term newborn with severe umbilical acidemia. *Am J Obstet Gynecol* 167: 1506–1512.

Grant A & Elbourne D (1989) Fetal movement counting to assess fetal well being. In: Chalmers I, Enkin M & Keirse MJNC, eds. *Effective Care in Pregnancy and Childbirth.* Oxford: Oxford University Press; 440.

Hanson M A (1988) The importance of baro- and chemoreflexes in the control of the fetal cardiovascular system. *J Dev Physiol* 10: 491–511.

Hauth J C (1996) Fetal monitoring: Utility and interpretation of umbilical cord gases and fetal blood sampling. In: *Acute Perinatal Asphyxia in Term Infants.* Bethesda, MD: National Institutes of Health; pp. 63–72.

Huang, C-C, Wang S-T, Chang Y-C *et al.* (1999) Measurement of urinary lactate: creatinine ratio for the early identification of newborn infants at risk for hypoxic-ischemic encephalopathy. *N Engl J Med* 341: 328–335.

Inglis S R, Druzin M L, Wagner W E & Kogut E (1993) The use of vibroacoustic stimulation during the abnormal or equivocal biophysical profile. *Obstet Gynecol* 82: 371–374.

Katz V L & Bowes W A Jr (1992) Meconium aspiration syndrome: reflections on a murky subject. *Am J Obstet Gynecol* 166: 171–183.

Keegan K, Paul R & Broussard P *et al.* (1979) Antepartum fetal heart rate testing. III. The effect of phenobarbitol on the nonstress test. *Am J Obstet Gynecol* 133: 579–582.

Kitterman J A, Liggins G C, Fewell J E *et al.* (1983) Inhibition of breathing movements in fetal sheep by prostaglandins. *J Appl Physiol* 54: 687–692.

Koos B J, Matsuda K & Power G G (1987) Fetal breathing, sleep state, and cardiovascular responses to graded hypoxia in sheep. *J Appl Physiol* 62: 1033–1039.

Korst L M, Phelan J P, Ahn M O & Martina G I (1996) Nucleated red blood cells: an update on the marker for fetal asphyxia. *Am J Obstet Gynecol* 175: 843–846.

Kruger K, Hallberg B & Blennow M *et al.* (1999) Predictive value of fetal scalp blood lactate concentrations and pH as markers of neurologic disability. *Am J Obstet Gynecol* 181: 1072–1078.

Labudova O, Schuller E & Yeghiazarjan *et al.* (1999) Genes involved in the pathophysiology of perinatal asphyxia. *Life Sciences* 64: 1831–1838.

Lammer E J, Brown L E, Anderka M T & Guyer B (1989) Classification and analysis of fetal deaths in Massachusetts. *JAMA* 261: 1757–1762.

Lavery J P (1982) Nonstress fetal heart rate testing. *Clin Obstet Gynecol* 25: 689–705.

Leffler C W, Busija D W & Mirro R *et al.* (1989) The effects of ischemia on brain blood flow and oxygen consumption in newborn pigs. *Am J Physiol* 257: H1917–H1926.

Little W J (1862) On the influence of abnormal parturition, difficult labors, premature birth, and asphyxia neonatorum on the mental and physical condition of the child, especially in relation to deformities. *Trans Obstet Soc Lond* 2: 293.

Low J (1997) Intrapartum fetal asphyxia: definition, diagnosis and classification. *Am J Obstet Gynecol* 176: 957–959.

Low J A (1993) The relationship of asphyxia in the mature fetus to long-term neurologic function. *Clin Obstet Gynecol* 36: 82–90.

Low J A, Robertson D M & Simpson L L (1989) Temporal relationship of neuropathologic conditions caused by perinatal asphyxia. *Am J Obstet Gynecol* 160: 608–614.

Low J A, Victory R & Derrick J (1999) Predictive value of electronic fetal monitoring for intrapartum asphyxia with metabolic acidosis. *Obstet Gynecol* 93: 285–291.

Luttkus A, Fengler T W & Friedman W *et al.* (1995) Continuous monitoring of fetal oxygen saturation by pulse oximetry. *Obstet Gynecol* 85: 183–186.

Mallard E C, Gunn A J & Williams E C *et al.* (1992) Umbilical cord occlusion causes cerebral damage in the fetal sheep. *Am J Obstet Gynecol* 167: 1423–1430.

Manning F A (1992) Biophysical profile scoring. In: Nijhuis J, ed. Fetal Behavior. New York: Oxford University Press; p. 241.

Manning F A, Platt L D, Sipos L (1980) Antepartum fetal evaluation: development of a fetal biophysical profile. *Am J Obstet Gynecol* 136: 787–795.

Manning F A, Morrison I, Lange I R *et al.* (1985) Fetal assessment based on fetal biophysical profile scoring: Experience in 12 620 referred high-risk pregnancies. *Am J Obstet Gynecol* 151: 343–350.

Manning F A, Bondagji N, Harman C R *et al.* (1997) Fetal assessment based on the fetal biophysical score: Relationship of last BPS to subsequent cerebral palsy. *Journal de Gynecologie, Obstetrique et Biologie de la Reproduction.* 26: 720–729.

Manning F A, Bondagji N, Harman C R *et al.* (1998) *Am J Obstet Gynecol* 178: 696–706.

Manning F A, Morrison I R, Harman C R & Menticoglou S M (1990) The abnormal biophysical profile: analysis of distribution of abnormal variables. *Am J Obstet Gynecol* 162: 918–927.

Margulis E, Binder D, Cohen A *et al.* (1984) The effect of propranolol on the nonstress test. *Am J Obstet Gynecol* 148: 340–341.

Martinex-Crespo J M, Comas C & Ojuel H *et al.* (1996) Umbilical artery pulsatility index in early pregnancies with chromosomal anomalies. *Br J Obstet Gynaecol* 103: 330–334.

Mason G C, Lilford R J, Porter J & Tyrell S (1993) Randomized comparison of routine versus highly selective use of doppler ultrasound in low risk pregnancies. *Br J Obstet Gynaecol* 100: 130–133.

Mellits E, Holden K & Freeman J (1982) Neonatal seizures: II. A multivariate analysis of factors associated with outcome. *Pediatrics* 70: 177–185.

Meyers R E (1975) Four patterns of perinatal brain damage and their conditions of occurrence in primates. *Adv Neurol* 10: 223–234.

Morrow R & Ritchie K (1989) Doppler ultrasound velocimetry and its role in obstetrics. *Clin Perinatol* 16: 771–778.

Murata Y, Martin C B, Ikenoue T *et al.* (1982) Fetal heart rate accelerations and late decelerations during the course of intrauterine death in chronically catheterized Rhesus monkeys. *Am J Obstet Gynecol* 144: 218–223.

Naeye R (1995) Can meconium in the amniotic fluid injure the fetal brain? *Obstet Gynecol* 86: 720–724.

Naeye R L & Localio A R (1995) Determining the time before birth when ischemia and hypoxemia initiated cerebral palsy. *Obstet Gynecol* 86: 713–719.

Nelson K B & Ellenberg J H (1981) Apgar scores as predictors of chronic neurologic disability. *Pediatrics* 68: 36–64.

Nelson K B & Ellenberg J H (1984) Obstetric complications as risk factors for cerebral or seizure disorders. *JAMA* 251: 1843–1848.

Nelson K B & Ellenberg J H (1986) Antecedents of cerebral palsy. Multivariate analysis of risk. *N Engl J Med* 315: 81–86.

Nelson K B, Dambrosia J M, Ting T Y & Grether J K (1996) Uncertain value of fetal heart monitoring in predicting cerebral palsy. *N Engl J Med* 334: 613–618.

Oki E Y, Keegan K A, Freeman R D & Dorchester W (1987) The breast-stimulated contraction stress test. *J Reprod Med* 32: 919–923.

Palmer C & Vannucci R C (1995) Potential new therapies for perinatal cerebral hypoxia–ischemia. *Clinics in Perinatology* 20: 411–432.

Pasternak J F & Gorey M T (1998) The syndrome of acute near total intrauterine asphyxia in the term infant. *Pediatr Neurol* 18: 391–398.

Patrick J, Carmichael L, Chess L & Staples C (1984) Acceleration of the human fetal heart at 38 to 40 weeks gestational age. *Am J Obstet Gynecol* 148: 35–41.

Paul R H, Suidan A K & Yeh S *et al.* (1975) Clinical fetal monitoring: VII. The evaluation of and significance of intrapartum baseline FHR variability. *Am J Obstet Gynecol* 123: 206–210.

Peeters L L, Sheldon R D & Jones M D *et al.* (1979) Blood flow to fetal organs as a function of arterial oxygen content. *Am J Obstet Gynecol* 135: 637–646.

Perlman J M (1997) Intrapartum hypoxic ischemic cerebral brain injury and subsequent cerebral palsy: medicolegal issues. *Pediatrics* 99: 851–859.

Phelan J P (1979) Diminished fetal reactivity with smoking. *Am J Obstet Gynecol* 136: 230–233.

Phelan J (1981) The nonstress test: a review of 3000 tests. *Am J Obstet Gynecol* 139: 7–10.

Phelan J P, Ahn M O, Korst L M & Martin G I (1995) Nucleated red blood cells: a marker for fetal asphyxia? *Am J Obstet Gynecol* 173: 1380–1384.

Roland E H, Poskitt K, Rodrigues E *et al.* (1998) Perinatal hypoxic ischemic injury: clinical features and neuroimaging. *Ann Neurol* 44: 161–166.

Shankaran S, Woldt E, Koepke T *et al.* (1991) Acute neonatal morbidity and long-term central nervous system sequelae of perinatal asphyxia in term infants. *Early Hum Dev* 25: 135–148.

Sibony O, Stempfle N, Luton D *et al.* (1998) *In utero* fetal cerebral intraparenchymal ischemia diagnosed by nuclear magnetic resonance. *Dev Med Child Neurol* 40: 122–123.

Skyes G S & Johnson P (1982) Do Apgar scores indicate asphyxia? *Lancet* 1: 494–496.

Soothill P W, Nicolaides K H & Campbell S (1987) Perinatal asphyxia, hyperlacticaemia, hypoglycemia, and ethyroblastosis in growth retarded fetuses. *BMJ* 294: 1051–1053.

Tannirandorn Y, Witoonpanich P & Phaosavasdi S (1993) Doppler umbilical artery flow velocity waveforms in pregnancies complicated by major fetal malformations. *J Med Assoc Thai* 76: 494–500.

Thacker S B, Stroup D F & Peterson H B (1995) Efficacy and safety of intrapartum fetal monitoring. An update. *Obstet Gynecol* 86: 613–620.

Tominaga T, Kure S, Narisawa K & Yoshimoto T (1993) Endonuclease activation following focal ischemic injury in the rat brain. *Brain Res* 608: 21–26.

Towbin A (1986) Obstetric malpractice litigation: The pathologist's view. *Am J Obstet Gynecol* 155: 927–935.

Trudinger B J, Cook C M & Jones L *et al.* (1986) A comparison of fetal heart rate monitoring and umbilical artery waveforms in the recognition of fetal compromise. *Br J Obstet Gynaecol* 93: 171–175.

Trudinger B J, Stevens D, Connelly A *et al.* (1987) Umbilical artery flow velocity waveforms and placental resistance: The effects of embolization of the umbilical circulation. *Am J Obstet Gynecol* 157: 1443–1448.

US Department of Health and Human Services (1995) *Childbirth USA '94*. Washington, DC: US Government Printing Office.

Vannucci R C & Palmer C (1997) Hypoxic ischemic encephalopathy: pathogenesis and neuropathology. In: Farnoff A A & Martin R J, eds. *Neonatal and Perinatal Medicine*. Philadelphia, PA: Mosby-Yearbook; pp. 856–877.

Vannucci R C & Perlman J M (1997) Interventions for perinatal hypoxic ischemic encephalopathy. *Pediatrics* 100: 1004–1014.

Vintzileos A M, Campbell W A, Ingardia C J & Nochimson D J (1983) The fetal biophysical profile and its predictive value. *Obstet Gynecol* 62: 271–278.

Vintzileos A M, Fleming A D & Scorza W E *et al.* (1991) Relationship between fetal biophysical profile and umbilical cord gas values. *Am J Obstet Gynecol* 165: 707–713.

Williams C E, Gunn A J & Mallard E C *et al.* (1992) Outcome after ischemia in the developing sheep brain: an electroencephalographic and histological study. *Ann Neurol* 31: 14–21.

Winkler C L, Hanth J C, Tucker J M *et al.* (1991) Neonatal complications at term as related to the degree of umbilical artery acidemia. *Am J Obstet Gynecol* 164: 637–641.

Chapter 25

# Intrapartum monitoring for asphyxia

D. A. Miller

## FETAL HEART RATE AUSCULTATION

Auscultation of the fetal heart, described as early as the 17th century in Le Goust's 'Humani Foetus Historia' (Philippeaux 1879), was first reported in Western medical literature by Mayor (1818). In 1822, Le Jumeau reported his observations of the fetal heart sounds using Laennec's stethoscope and proposed that auscultation of the fetal heart could be useful in confirming pregnancy, diagnosing multiple pregnancy, determining fetal position, and judging the state of fetal health or disease by changes in strength and frequency of the heart tones (Le Jumeau 1822). Later, Kennedy (1833), Schwartz (1870), Winckel (1893) and others described fetal heart rate (FHR) changes associated with umbilical cord compression, head compression, and fetal distress. Kilian (1849) and Winckel (1893), proposed indications for forceps delivery based upon FHR abnormalities such as tachycardia, bradycardia, 'irregularity', and 'impurity of tone'. Schwartz (1870) and Seitz (1903) speculated upon the relationship between FHR changes and fetal oxygenation. Remarkably, these observations were made using only the stethoscope (mediate auscultation), or the ear of the examiner placed directly upon the maternal abdomen (immediate auscultation). It was not until 1917 that Hillis described the modified stethoscope known today as the DeLee–Hillis fetoscope (Hillis 1917; DeLee 1922).

## ELECTRONIC FETAL MONITORING

In 1906, Cremer recorded the first fetal electrocardiograph (ECG). Placing one electrode on the maternal abdomen above the fundus and another in the vagina, he observed small fetal electrical impulses among the higher voltage maternal signals (Cremer 1906). Despite technological improvements, the quality of abdominal fetal ECG tracings remains unreliable, and the clinical usefulness of the technique is limited.

The concept of direct application of the ECG electrode to the fetus *in utero* was introduced in the 1950s (Smyth 1953; Sureau 1956; Kaplan & Toyama 1958), with results clearly superior to those obtained abdominally. During the 1960s, Hon (1966) in the USA, Caldeyro-Barcia *et al.* (1966) in Uruguay and Hammacher (1967) in Germany pioneered the development of electronic monitoring. The first practical clinical electronic fetal monitor became available in the USA in 1968, and throughout the 1970s fetal monitoring became increasingly incorporated into obstetric management. By 1978, more than half of all labors were monitored electronically (Williams & Hawes 1979). The National Center for Health Statistics reported that EFM was used in 83% of all births in the USA in 1997 (National Center for Health Statistics 1999).

## FETAL ASPHYXIA

The objective of electronic fetal monitoring (EFM) is to identify the fetus in distress so that measures might be taken in time to avert permanent damage or death. The term 'fetal distress' although commonly used, remains poorly defined. It has been described as 'a condition in which fetal physiology is so altered as to make death or permanent injury a probability within a relatively short period of time' (Kirschbaum 1969). Some investigators have based the definition on FHR abnormalities (Haverkamp *et al.* 1979; Haesslin & Niswander 1980), and others on abnormal fetal blood gas values or low Apgar scores. Most agree that the term denotes some degree of disruption of normal fetal oxygenation, ranging from hypoxia to asphyxia. Hypoxia is defined as the reduction of oxygen supply to tissues below physiologic levels. Asphyxia, derived from the Greek word meaning 'a stopping of the pulse', is defined by Webster's as 'a lack of oxygen or excess carbon dioxide that is usually caused by interruption of breathing' (Webster's 1985). The World Federation of Neurology Group defined asphyxia as a condition of impaired gas exchange which, if it persists, leads to progressive hypoxemia and hypercapnia (Bax & Melson 1993). Low *et al.* defined asphyxia as a combination of hypoxia, hypercapnia, and metabolic acidosis (Low *et al.* 1997). Historically, the clinical diagnosis of birth asphyxia has been based upon a variety of findings, including meconium passage, abnormal FHR patterns, low Apgar scores, abnormal blood gases, and neonatal neurologic abnormalities. When present together, these findings are highly suggestive of a birth-related asphyxial insult. Isolated abnormal findings, however, correlate poorly with birth asphyxia and subsequent neurologic impairment. Gilstrap *et al.* (1989) recommended that the diagnosis of birth asphyxia be reserved for infants who are severely depressed (5-min Apgar < 3) and acidotic (pH < 7.00) at birth, require resuscitation, and have seizures in the first day of life. The ACOG Committee on Obstetrics, Maternal and Fetal Medicine (1991) stated that:

> A neonate who has had severe hypoxia close to delivery that is severe enough to result in hypoxic encephalopathy will show other evidence of hypoxic damage including all of the following: (1) a profound umbilical artery metabolic or mixed acidemia (pH < 7.00), (2) persistence of an Apgar score of 0–3 for longer than 5 minutes, (3) neonatal neurologic sequelae, e.g. seizures, coma, hypotonia, and (4) multiorgan system dysfunction, e.g. cardiovascular, gastrointestinal, hematologic, pulmonary, or renal.

The Committee further opined 'the term birth asphyxia is imprecise and should not be used' (ACOG 1991). However, the terminology is entrenched and continues to generate confusion and debate.

## ASPHYXIA AT THE CELLULAR LEVEL

At the cellular level, asphyxia triggers a cascade of events, including membrane depolarization, disruption of normal energy metabolism, altered release and re-uptake of neurotransmitters, ion shifts, protease activation, free-radical production and phospholipid degradation (Johnson 1993). Profound and prolonged asphyxia may lead to cell death, and eventually, death of the organism. Levels of asphyxia that are sublethal to the organism, however, may result in clinical evidence of cellular dysfunction. Clinical manifestations of asphyxial myocardial injury include conduction abnormalities, myocardial dysfunction, and congestive heart failure. Manifestations of asphyxia in the gastrointestinal tract include hypoxic–ischemic mucosal injury, stress ulcers, hepatic injury and necrotizing enterocolitis. In the lungs, sequelae include meconium aspiration, persistent pulmonary hypertension, impaired surfactant production, and respiratory distress syndrome. Asphyxial renal injury may lead to renal insufficiency or acute renal failure. Hematologic manifestations include thrombocytopenia, neutropenia, and disseminated intravascular coagulation. In the CNS, impaired neuronal water regulatory mechanisms and disruption of the blood–brain barrier may lead to cerebral edema and neuronal necrosis. Resultant disruption of normal membrane depolarization, neurotransmission and receptor stimulation may lead to seizures and respiratory depression. One of the most publicized consequences of fetal asphyxia is cerebral palsy (see Chapter 47).

## ASPHYXIA AND FHR ABNORMALITIES

As early as the 19th century, researchers using auscultation recognized that certain FHR patterns were associated with poor perinatal outcome. Kennedy (1833) related Bodson's description of fetal distress in association with a FHR pattern exhibiting 'slowness of its return when a contraction is passing on'. Schwartz (1838) recommended frequent counting of the fetal heart tones in labor, and implicated 'asphyxic intoxication' as a cause of alterations in their 'individual normal frequency'. Referring to Schwartz's description of the relationship between FHR decelerations and uterine contractions, Gültekin-Zootzmann (1975) noted that 'in those cases in which the heart sounds returned slowly to their earlier rhythm, or when the attenuations persisted or deteriorated during the pauses, the result would be a weak, moribund or dead fetus'. Seitz (1903) described three progressively ominous stages of FHR deceleration. He attributed the first two stages to irritation and paralysis of the vagal centers, and the third to paralysis of all extracardiac nerve centers, concluding that it was possible to detect early signs of compromise before the fetus was actually in danger. The introduction of EFM and fetal scalp blood sampling in the 1960s provided additional tools for evaluating the fetus. Hon and Quilligan (1967) proposed a system for classification of FHR decelerations, and Kubli *et al.* (1969) demonstrated the relationship between the type and severity of FHR deceleration and the fetal scalp pH. They reported that fetuses with no decelerations, early decelerations or mild variable decelerations had average scalp pH values >7.29, while those with severe variable or late decelerations had pH values <7.15. Many investigators have demonstrated the importance of FHR variability as a marker of fetal well-being (Hon & Lee 1963; Paul *et al.* 1975; Hammacher *et al.* 1968; Martin 1982). Clark *et al.* (1984) reported that FHR accelerations of 15 bpm for 15 seconds in response to fetal scalp stimulation predicted a scalp pH >7.19. Smith (1986) reported a similar relationship between fetal scalp pH and the FHR response to vibroacoustic stimulation, with an artificial larynx applied to the maternal abdomen over the fetal head for <3 seconds. All 30 fetuses exhibiting FHR accelerations in response to this stimulus had scalp pH values >7.25. The work of these and many other investigators has helped to clarify the complex relationship between fetal biochemistry and the neurologic regulation of FHR.

## ELECTRONIC FETAL MONITORING vs. TRADITIONAL AUSCULTATION

With EFM rapidly replacing the traditional practice of intermittent intrapartum FHR auscultation, a series of non-randomized studies in the mid-1970s reported significantly lower perinatal mortality rates in electronically monitored patients (Chan *et al.* 1973; Kelly & Kulkani 1973; Edington *et al.* 1975; Koh *et al.* 1975; Shenker *et al.* 1975; Tutera & Newman 1975; Lee & Baggish 1976; Amato 1977; Paul *et al.* 1977; Johnstone *et al.* 1978; Hamilton *et al.* 1978). These studies were not randomized and employed non-concurrent controls. Critics have cited rapidly improving neonatal care and falling perinatal mortality rates as possible sources of bias. MacDonald & Grant (1987) pointed out that, over the time period of these studies, hospitals not using EFM experienced rates of improvement in perinatal outcome similar to those seen in hospitals that were using EFM. Despite the inevitable shortcomings of non-randomized trials, these studies had the effect of validating the use of EFM.

In 1976, the first of a series of randomized, controlled trials was published, comparing EFM to intermittent auscultation of the FHR during labor. To date, there have been nine such studies; five in high-risk populations (Renou *et al.* 1976; Haverkamp *et al.* 1976, 1979; Luthy *et al.* 1987; Vintzileos *et al.* 1993), two in low-risk populations (Kelso *et al.* 1978; Wood *et al.* 1981), and two in combined low- and high-risk populations (MacDonald *et al.* 1985; Neldam *et al.* 1986). These trials are summarized in Table 25.1.

## RANDOMIZED CONTROLLED TRIALS OF EFM vs. AUSCULTATION

In 1976, Haverkamp and associates in Denver, reported the first prospective, randomized study of 483 high-risk obstetric patients, comparing electronic fetal monitoring with intermittent FHR auscultation in labor (Haverkamp *et al.* 1976). A point-rating system (Goodwin *et al.* 1969) was used to assess risk status. In the EFM group, a scalp electrode was placed as soon as possible. Auscultation in the control group was performed every 15 minutes in the first stage of labor and every 5 minutes in the second stage, for 30 seconds after uterine contractions. Electronic monitoring was employed in both groups, but was blinded in the control group. In the EFM group, FHR patterns were evaluated using the criteria of Kubli *et al.* (1969). In patients with late decelerations or severe variable decelerations that persisted after 15 minutes of corrective measures (oxygen, positional changes, correction of hypotension), delivery was effected. Fetal distress in the control group was diagnosed by the presence of bradycardia to 100 bpm after three or more consecutive contractions. Delivery was accomplished if fetal distress was not relieved within 15 minutes. There were no significant differences in outcome between the EFM and control groups as measured by perinatal mortality, Apgar scores, cord blood pH values, neurological signs in the neonate, or neonatal nursery morbidity. The monitored group, however, had significantly higher incidences of Cesarean section overall (16.5% vs. 6.8%), and Cesarean section for fetal distress (7.4% vs. 1.2%). Questions have been raised concerning the comparability of the two groups. For instance, review of the monitor tracings revealed a higher incidence of abnormal FHR patterns early in labor in the study group. Furthermore, the study group had a higher incidence of maternal post-partum infectious morbidity (13.2% vs. 4.6%) which was not explained by the increased rate of Cesarean birth. These findings suggest that the study group may have represented a higher risk population than did the control group, and that effective randomization was not achieved.

The second study, by Renou *et al.* (1976) in Melbourne, Australia randomized 350 high-risk patients into EFM and auscultation groups. High-risk patients were defined as those with a poor obstetric history, a medical or obstetric complication, an abnormal FHR detected by auscultation, or meconium in the amniotic fluid. Continuous EFM was performed in the study group, and scalp pH was measured if the FHR tracing were judged to be abnormal. Abnormalities were defined as a slowing of the FHR in relation to the contraction cycle, a baseline FHR less than 100 bpm, or loss of normal beat-to-beat variability (Renou & Wood 1974). The protocol for auscultation in the control group was not reported. Criteria for obstetric intervention were not specified in either group. There were no significant differences between the groups with respect to perinatal mortality, Apgar scores, or maternal or neonatal infection. Patients in the monitored group, however, had significantly higher cord blood pH values and significantly lower incidences of admission to the neonatal intensive care unit (NICU), neonatal neurologic signs and/or symptoms, and neonatally diagnosed brain damage (not further defined). The Cesarean section rate was significantly higher in the monitored group than in the control group (22.3% vs. 13.7%); however, the indications for intervention were not specified, making this

**Table 25.1 Prospective randomized clinical trials of EFM vs. intermittent FHR auscultation**

| First authors | Year | *N* (total) | Risk status | Perinatal mortality | Neonatal neurologic signs | Cesarean section rate |
|---|---|---|---|---|---|---|
| Haverkamp | 1976 | 483 | High | 0 | 0 | ↑ |
| Renou | 1976 | 350 | High | 0 | ↓ | ↑ |
| Kelso | 1978 | 504 | Low | 0 | 0 | ↑ |
| Haverkamp | 1979 | 690 | High | 0 | 0 | ↑ |
| Wood | 1981 | 989 | Low | 0 | 0 | 0 |
| MacDonald | 1985 | 12 964 | Combined | 0 | ↓ | 0 |
| Neldam | 1986 | 969 | Combined | 0 | 0 | 0 |
| Luthy | 1987 | 246 | High (PTL) | 0 | 0 | 0 |
| Vintzileos | 1993 | 1428 | High | ↓ | 0 | 0 |

0 = No difference
↓ = Lower in EFM group
↑ = Higher in EFM group

difference difficult to interpret. The authors commented that the difference in Cesarean section rates was not statistically significant after removal of six patients in the monitored group who had had a previous Cesarean birth. The rationale for removing these patients on the basis of their previous operations was unclear since, presumably, the initial decision had been made to allow them a trial of labor. The rates of Cesarean section for fetal distress were not reported.

Kelso *et al.* (1978) in Sheffield, UK published the first randomized, controlled trial comparing EFM and intermittent auscultation in 504 low-risk patients. High-risk patients were excluded according to listed criteria, including multiple gestation, breech presentation, hypertension and diabetes, among other medical and obstetric complications. Continuous EFM was employed in study patients, with a fetal scalp electrode placed as early as possible. Auscultation in the control group was performed for 1 minute at least every 15 minutes, during and immediately following a contraction. Cross-over was not permitted, and scalp pH determination was not utilized. The dip area (Shelley & Tipton 1971) was used as a measure of fetal distress in the EFM group; however, criteria for intervention were not specified. In the control group, a FHR higher than 160 bpm or lower than 120 bpm was considered indicative of fetal distress. There were no significant differences between the groups with respect to perinatal mortality, low Apgar scores, cord blood pH values, NICU admissions or lengths of stay, neonatal or maternal infections, or abnormal neonatal neurologic findings. The only significant difference between the groups was an increase in the incidence of Cesarean birth in the monitored group (9.5% vs. 4.4%). There was no statistical difference, however, in the incidence of Cesarean section for fetal distress (EFM 1.6%, control 1.2%).

In 1979, Haverkamp and associates published a second randomized, controlled trial in high-risk patients which was similar in design to the first, but included additional measures of infant status as well as the option to perform fetal scalp pH determination during labor (Haverkamp *et al.* 1979). Blinded EFM in the control group was not performed in this trial. A total of 690 high-risk patients were randomized into three groups. In the first group, fetal assessment during labor was accomplished by intermittent auscultation. The second group had continuous EFM alone, and the third group had continuous EFM with the option to measure scalp blood pH as needed. Risk assessment guidelines, auscultation protocols, and criteria for the diagnosis of fetal distress were the same as in their previous study. Among the three groups, no significant differences were found in perinatal mortality, Apgar scores, cord blood pH values, maternal or neonatal infectious morbidity, NICU admissions or neonatal neurologic abnormalities. A significant increase in the incidence of Cesarean birth was demonstrated in the group with EFM alone (EFM alone – 18%, EFM with the option to scalp sample – 11%, auscultation – 6%). The option to perform scalp sampling resulted in an intermediate Cesarean section rate that was not significantly different from either of the other groups. When analyzed together, electronically monitored patients had a significantly higher incidence of Cesarean section for fetal distress than did controls (5.2% vs. 0.43%).

The fifth trial was published by Wood *et al.* (1981) in Melbourne, Australia. A total of 989 low-risk patients (890 at one hospital and 99 at another) were randomized to receive EFM or intermittent auscultation. High-risk pregnancies were excluded, based upon listed criteria including previous preterm delivery, meconium stained amniotic fluid, fetal tachycardia or bradycardia, maternal renal disease, hypertension, diabetes, and other medical and obstetric complications. Monitored patients had placement of a fetal scalp electrode as early as possible. The protocol for auscultated patients was not described. Scalp pH measurements were made as needed. Fetal distress was diagnosed as in the previous studies by Renou and colleagues (Renou & Wood 1974; Renou *et al.* 1976). The criteria for operative intervention were not specified. No significant differences between the groups were seen in perinatal mortality, Apgar scores, cord blood pH values, NICU admissions, or neonatal neurologic abnormalities. In this study, the Cesarean section rates were not significantly different between the groups (4% in the monitored group and 2% in the auscultated group), although the overall rate of operative intervention (including forceps) was significantly higher in the monitored group. Rates of Cesarean section for fetal distress were not reported. It should be noted that the randomization process was compromised at the hospital that undertook the larger study, requiring subsequent data manipulation.

MacDonald *et al.* (1985), in Dublin and Oxford, published a randomized, controlled trial comparing EFM with intermittent FHR auscultation in 12 964 pregnancies. It was the first study to calculate prospectively the sample size needed to demonstrate statistically significant differences between the groups. Prior to initiation of the study, estimates were made of the anticipated frequencies of intra-partum stillbirths, neonatal deaths, neonatal seizures in survivors and other severe abnormal neurologic characteristics. They calculated that 13 000 patients would be needed to demonstrate a 50% reduction in the combined incidence of intra-partum stillbirths, neonatal deaths and neonatal seizures in survivors (power 75%, $p < 0.05$). A trial of that size would have a 50% chance of detecting a 50% reduction in the rate of seizures, alone. Risk status was determined according to listed criteria, and 22.5% of the study participants were identified as high risk. Amniotomy was performed within 1 hour of admission in all patients, and those with either no fluid or moderate to dense meconium were excluded from participation in the study. In the EFM group, a fetal scalp electrode was applied as early as possible, and scalp pH measurements were used as needed. Criteria for evaluation of the FHR tracings were similar to those of Kubli *et al.* (1969). Suspicious or ominous tracings were those with marked tachycardia or bradycardia, moderate tachycardia or bradycardia with decreased variability, absent-minimal variability, late decelerations, moderate-to-severe variable decelerations, and other difficult-to-interpret patterns. In the first stage of labor, scalp pH was determined if such patterns persisted for at least 10 minutes. A scalp pH <7.20 was an indication for delivery. If the fetal scalp pH was between 7.20 and 7.25 with persistent suspicious or ominous FHR patterns, or <7.20 regardless of the FHR pattern, delivery was accomplished. If the scalp pH was >7.25, but the tracing remained suspicious or ominous, the scalp pH was repeated within 30 to 60 minutes. In the second stage of labor, delivery was effected if FHR abnormalities persisted for at least 10 minutes. In the control group, FHR auscultation was performed every 15 minutes for 60 seconds in the first stage of labor, and between each contraction during the second stage. If the FHR was <100 bpm or >160 bpm during three contractions and could not be corrected with conservative measures, a scalp pH was measured and managed as above, or delivery was expedited, depending on the stage of labor. Blood sampling also was performed at unspecified intervals in the control group when labor exceeded 8 hours. There were no significant differences between the groups in perinatal mortality, low Apgar scores, neonatal trauma, resuscitation requirement, NICU admissions or infectious morbidity. Among the 28 perinatal deaths, asphyxia was considered to be the primary cause in 7 cases in each group. There were significantly more cases of neonatal seizures and persistent neurologic abnormalitics (>1 week) in the control group; however, no differences with respect to neurologic abnormality remained at 1-year and 4-year follow-up (3 cases in each group). Labor was significantly shorter in the EFM group, and analgesia (meperidine) was required less often. Twice as many fetuses with low scalp pH (<7.20) were identified in the EFM group, and scalp sampling was used more frequently (EFM 4.4%, control 3.5%). The Cesarean section rate in the EFM group (2.4%) was not significantly different from the auscultated group (2.2%). Overall rates of operative delivery were higher in the EFM group (10.6% vs. 8.5%) due to an increased incidence of forceps delivery (8.2% vs. 6.3%). Rates of Cesarean section for fetal distress were not significantly different (EFM 0.4%, control 0.2%). In the control group, the allocated method of auscultation was used throughout labor in 97.7%. The remaining 2.3% crossed over and underwent EFM secondary to prolonged labor (1.3%), meconium (0.2%), FHR abnormality (0.4%), and other reasons (0.4%). In patients randomized to EFM, only 80.7% used it throughout labor.

The overall frequency of seizures in the 22.5% who were classified as high risk was 4.3/1000. This was significantly higher than in the low-risk group (2.6/1000). The incidence of seizures in surviving neonates was the same in both groups (2.3/1000). Electronic monitoring did not reduce the seizure incidence to a greater extent in high-risk patients than in low-risk patients. In this study, the largest to date, EFM was associated with no increase in maternal morbidity.

Neldam and associates (1986) in Copenhagen, Denmark, reported a randomized, controlled trial of EFM vs. intermittent auscultation in 969 combined low- and high-risk patients. The study excluded women with pregestational diabetes mellitus. In the EFM group, monitoring was initiated when patients no longer desired to ambulate. A scalp electrode was placed as soon as possible, thereafter. In the control group, fetal heart tones were auscultated twice an hour for at least 15 seconds at cervical dilatation <5 cm, every 15 minutes from 5 cm until the second stage of labor, and for 30 seconds after each contraction or at least every five minutes during the second stage. Scalp pH sampling was optional, and was performed only five times (EFM 3, control 2). In the EFM group, intervention was considered if FHR abnormalities remained unresolved after 15 minutes of corrective measures. These abnormalities included bradycardia <120 bpm, tachycardia >160 bpm, late decelerations, variable decelerations (not further specified), silent FHR pattern (beat-to-beat variability <5 bpm), and saltatory pattern (variability >25 bpm). Intervention was considered in the control group if the FHR was <100 bpm following three or more consecutive contractions. No statistical differences were detected between the groups with respect to perinatal mortality, low Apgar scores, seizures, NICU admissions or lengths of stay. Significantly more pathological FHR patterns were detected in the EFM group; however, there was no difference in the incidence of Cesarean delivery between the groups.

The eighth study, by Luthy *et al.* (1987) in Seattle and Vancouver compared EFM and auscultation in 246 high-risk patients with preterm labor. Inclusion criteria were preterm labor, singleton gestation, cephalic presentation, estimated gestational age 26–32 weeks and estimated fetal weight 700–1750 g. Patients with preterm premature rupture of the membranes were not excluded. In the EFM group, external monitoring was used until advanced cervical dilatation (7 cm), at which time amniotomy was performed and a scalp electrode was placed. In those with ruptured membranes, a scalp electrode was placed once delivery was inevitable. Ominous FHR patterns were those with persistent late decelerations with at least three successive contractions in the absence of correctable cause, FHR >180 bpm with total loss of variability persisting more than 15 minutes, FHR <100 bpm for more than 3 minutes, or severe variable decelerations persisting for more than 30 minutes. An ominous FHR pattern lasting for more than 30 minutes, or a scalp pH of <7.20 was an indication for delivery. In the control group, auscultation was performed for at least 30 seconds, at least every 15 minutes in the first stage of labor, and at least every 5 minutes in the second stage. Ominous patterns were those with FHR <100 bpm for more than 30 seconds after three or more consecutive contractions, baseline FHR >180 bpm for more than 15 minutes, or <100 bpm for more than 60 seconds. Scalp pH was used as clinically indicated in both groups. Fetal scalp pH <7.20 or ominous FHR patterns in the absence of a correctable cause were considered indications for delivery. The groups did not differ with respect to the use of tocolytics, corticosteroids, oxytocin, or regional anesthesia. There were no differences in perinatal mortality, low Apgar scores, cord pH values, neonatal seizures, respiratory distress syndrome, or intracranial hemorrhage. Cesarean section rates were similar (EFM 15.6%, controls 15.2%). There was no difference in the incidence of Cesarean section for fetal distress (EFM 8.2%, controls 5.6%).

The most recent randomized trial, published by Vintzileos *et al.* (1993), was conducted in Athens, Greece, and compared EFM and intermittent auscultation in 1428 patients in a population with high baseline perinatal mortality rates of 20.4–22.6 per 1000. The relatively high incidence of the outcome measure to be studied (perinatal death) markedly improved the likelihood of detecting a statistically significant effect of EFM. Using an average incidence of 21 perinatal deaths per 1000, they prospectively calculated that a sample of 2210 patients would have an 80% chance of detecting a 67% reduction in perinatal mortality at the 0.05 level of significance. Reviews were conducted every 3 months, and the study was ended after the third review in light of a statistically significant five-fold decrease in perinatal mortality in the EFM group. The study included women with singleton living fetuses with estimated gestational ages greater than 26 weeks. Fetuses with known congenital or chromosomal anomalies were excluded. In the EFM group, external monitoring was used as long as satisfactory tracings were obtained. Scalp electrodes were placed as needed. In the control group, FHR auscultation was performed every 15 minutes during the first stage of labor, and every 5 minutes during the second stage. The FHR was counted during contractions and for at least 30 seconds immediately afterward. Non-reassuring patterns in the EFM group included late decelerations, prolonged decelerations <80 bpm for >2 minutes, severe variables <70 bpm for >60 seconds, variable decelerations with a rising baseline and loss of variability, tachycardia with decreased variability (<5 bpm), persistent decreased variability or a sinusoidal pattern. In the auscultated group, non-reassuring patterns included a FHR <100 bpm during and immediately after a contraction, a persistent FHR <100 bpm or >160 bpm. Scalp sampling was not used in either group, and cross-over was not permitted. In both groups, if non-reassuring FHR patterns failed to resolve after 20 minutes of conservative measures, delivery was accomplished. There were significantly fewer perinatal deaths in the EFM group than in the controls (2.6/1000 vs. 13/1000). Furthermore, there were no hypoxia-related perinatal deaths in the EFM group, whereas 6 such deaths occurred in the auscultated group (0.9%). This difference was statistically significant. The groups did not differ significantly with respect to low Apgar scores, NICU admissions or lengths of stay, ventilator requirements, neonatal hypoxic–ischemic encephalopathy, intraventricular hemorrhage, seizures, hypotonia, necrotizing enterocolitis or respiratory distress syndrome. Although the incidence of Cesarean section for fetal distress was significantly higher in the EFM group (5.3% vs. 2.3%), the overall incidence of Cesarean birth was not significantly different between the EFM and control groups (9.5% vs. 8.6%).

## POTENTIAL BENEFITS OF ELECTRONIC FETAL MONITORING

When EFM was introduced in the 1960s, proponents anticipated marked reductions in perinatal mortality and neonatal neurologic injury. Regarding the former, eight out of nine randomized clinical trials conducted over the last 20 years have failed to detect a statistically significant difference in perinatal mortality between EFM and intermittent FHR auscultation (Table 25.1). However, it is crucial to point out that many non-randomized trials (Chan *et al.* 1973; Kelly & Kulkani 1973; Edington *et al.* 1975; Koh *et al.* 1975; Shenker *et al.* 1975; Tutera & Newman 1975; Lee & Baggish 1976; Amato 1977; Paul *et al.* 1977; Johnstone *et al.* 1978; Hamilton *et al.* 1978) demonstrated significant reductions in intra-partum death rates when electronic monitoring was introduced, and only one of the nine randomized trials (Vintzileos *et al.* 1993) had sufficient statistical power to demonstrate a reduction in perinatal death. In that trial, electronically monitored patients had a statistically significant five-fold improvement in perinatal mortality compared to those followed in labor with intermittent auscultation. In comparison to the high perinatal mortality rates (20.4–22.6/1000) in the study by Vintzileos *et al.* (1993), MacDonald *et al.* (1985) calculated the combined anticipated frequencies of intra-partum stillbirths and neonatal deaths in his population to be 3 per 1000. In such a population, a study with an 80% likelihood of detecting a 50% reduction in perinatal mortality ($p < 0.05$), would require more than 33 000 patients (Fleiss 1981). The total number of patients in all nine studies, combined, was 18 623. A recent meta-analysis of the nine published randomized trials by Vintzileos *et al.* (1995a) reported a significantly lower incidence of perinatal mortality due to fetal hypoxia in monitored patients. Subsequent meta-analysis by Thacker & Stroup (1999) did not support this conclusion. Vintzileos *et al.* (1995b) further reported that electronic monitoring was superior to intermittent auscultation in detecting fetal acidemia at birth in 1419 patients who had umbilical cord blood acid–base measurements at delivery.

With respect to neonatal neurologic injury, the problem of sample size was the same. Seven of the nine trials (Haverkamp *et al.* 1976, 1979; Luthy *et al.* 1987; Vintzileos *et al.* 1993; Kelso *et al.* 1978; Wood *et al.* 1981) showed no benefit of EFM (Table 25.1). Two trials (Renou *et al.* 1976; MacDonald *et al.* 1985) reported fewer neonatal seizures in the EFM groups. Electronic monitoring was associated with a lower incidence of seizures in the meta-analysis by Thacker & Stroup (1999), but not in the meta-analysis by Vintzileos *et al.* (1995a) The only study to examine long-term neurodevelopment (MacDonald *et al.* 1985; Grant *et al.* 1989) found no difference between the groups in the incidence of neurologic abnormality at 1 or 4 years of age.

Assuming that the school-age incidence of cerebral palsy is approximately 2 per 1000, and that approximately 10% of cerebral palsy is attributable to birth asphyxia, the anticipated incidence of asphyxia-related cerebral palsy is roughly 0.2 per 1000. A study large enough to detect a 50% reduction in the incidence of asphyxia-related cerebral palsy (power 80%, $p < 0.05$) would require more than 500 000 patients (Fleiss 1981). It is not surprising that the randomized trials to date have been unable to detect a statistically significant reduction in cerebral palsy with the use of EFM.

No randomized trials have investigated possible associations between specific FHR patterns and long-term neurologic outcome. However, Nelson *et al.* (1996) reported a population-based study of the association of cerebral palsy with specific intra-partum FHR patterns. Multiple late decelerations (OR 3.9; 95% CI, 1.7 to 9.3), and decreased beat-to-beat variability (OR 2.7; 95% CI, 1.1 to 5.8) were associated with an increased risk of cerebral palsy. The risk persisted after correction for multiple other risk factors. Because of the low prevalence of the outcome in question, the false-positive rate of these FHR abnormalities for predicting cerebral palsy was 99.8%.

## POTENTIAL RISKS OF ELECTRONIC FETAL MONITORING

Early concerns regarding the potential for maternal or neonatal infections in electronically monitored patients have proven to be unfounded. Only one study (Haverkamp *et al.* 1976) demonstrated an increased risk of maternal infectious morbidity in patients randomized to EFM. These results are difficult to interpret in light of the fact that fetal scalp electrodes were used in both the EFM and control groups (FHR tracings were recorded in the control group, but clinicians did not have access to them). The largest randomized trial to date (MacDonald *et al.* 1985) revealed no increased infectious morbidity in electronically monitored patients. Current evidence does not support an association between EFM and increased infectious morbidity.

Meta-analyses of the randomized trials of EFM versus auscultation identify a higher risk of operative intervention in the monitored group compared with controls (Vintzileos *et al.* 1995a; Thacker & Stroup 1999). Data from the most recent randomized trials, however, suggest that the effect of EFM on Cesarean section rates is minimal. While four early randomized trials (Haverkamp *et al.* 1976, 1979; Renou *et al.* 1976; Kelso *et al.* 1978) reported significantly more Cesarean deliveries in electronically monitored patients, the five most recent studies (Wood *et al.* 1981; Neldane *et al.* 1986; Luthy *et al.* 1987; MacDonald *et al.* 1985; Vintzileos *et al.* 1993) have shown no such difference. Moreover, as the use of EFM in the USA has increased to include 83% of all births, fetal distress was identified as a complication of labor in only 3.6% of births in the USA in 1997 (National Center for Health Statistics 1999) and the incidence of Cesarean section for fetal distress has increased by only 1.5% since 1974 (from 0.4% in 1974 to 1.9% in 1977) (Rosen 1981; National Center for Health Statistics 1999). This increase reflects less than 10% of the total rise in the rate of Cesarean births. Since the introduction of EFM, nearly 30 years of research and clinical experience have refined the interpretation of FHR patterns. Additional tools such as fetal scalp pH determination, fetal scalp stimulation, and vibroacoustic stimulation help to confirm fetal well-being in the presence of non-reassuring tracings that may previously have prompted operative intervention. Continued improvement in our understanding of the capabilities and limitations of EFM should lead to fewer unnecessary Cesarean sections.

Despite the lack of consensus on many points, EFM has been shown to be at least as effective in identifying fetal compromise as is frequent FHR auscultation with intensive, one-on-one nursing. While this level of individualized nursing care may be available in some settings, most delivery units will find the personnel requirements to be impractical and cost prohibitive.

## OTHER METHODS OF FETAL MONITORING

One of the major shortcomings of EFM is a high rate of false-positive results. Even the most ominous patterns are associated with evidence of newborn compromise in no more than 50–65% of cases (Tejani *et al.* 1975; Banta & Thacker 1979; Clarke *et al.* 1984). This has led to exploration of alternative methods of evaluating fetal status.

### INTRAPARTUM FETAL SCALP pH DETERMINATION (see also Chapter 26)

Intermittent sampling of scalp blood for pH determination was described in the 1960s and studied extensively in the 1970s. However, its use has been limited by many factors, including the requirements for cervical dilation and membrane rupture, technical difficulty of the procedure, the need for serial pH determinations and uncertainty regarding interpretation and application of results. Moreover, a recent review from a large obstetric center revealed no changes in the rates of fetal distress, Cesarean section for fetal distress, low Apgar scores, meconium aspiration or perinatal asphyxia when scalp pH sampling was eliminated from clinical practice Goodwin *et al.* (1994).

The applicability of continuous intrapartum monitoring of fetal scalp pH was explored in the 1970s (Stam *et al.* 1976; Sturbois *et al.* 1977; Bloch 1978; Lauersen *et al.* 1979). Lauersen *et al.* (1979) reported 76.9–87% correlation between the readings of a continuous fetal scalp tissue pH electrode and intermittent fetal scalp pH determinations. The technique was considered to be clinically useful in 65% of the 40 patients studied. Complications included inflammation at the electrode site in one case and breakage of the electrode during application in another, with retention of a fragment of the electrode in the fetal scalp. The authors reported good correlation between the continuous pH readings and the immediate neonatal outcome. Others have reported no correlation between pH values and outcome (Small *et al.* 1989). Inconsistent correlation with outcome and technical obstacles have limited the usefulness of this technique. Investigators exploring the potential of transcutaneous $PO_2$ (Huch *et al.* 1980; Willcourt & Queenan 1981; Aarnoudse *et al.* 1985) and $PCO_2$ (Bergmans *et al.* 1993) monitoring have encountered similar limitations.

## COMPUTER ANALYSIS OF FHR

Subjective interpretation of FHR tracings by visual analysis is hampered by inconsistency and imprecision. In attempt to overcome this limitation, Dawes and others derived a system of numeric analysis of FHR (Dawes 1991). Computer analysis of intrapartum FHR records has been reported to be more precise than visual assessment (Pello *et al.* 1991; Dawes *et al.* 1992). However, intrapartum computer analysis has not been shown to improve prediction of neonatal outcome. Keith *et al.* reported the results of a multicenter trial of an intelligent computer system using clinical data in addition to FHR data (Keith *et al.* 1995). In 50 cases analyzed, the system's performance was indistinguishable from that of 17 expert clinicians. The authors reported that the system was highly consistent, recommended no unnecessary intervention, and performed better than all but two of the experts.

## FETAL PULSE OXYMETRY

Intrapartum reflectance fetal pulse oxymetry is a modification of transmission pulse oxymetry that indirectly measures the oxygen saturation of hemoglobin in fetal blood (Dildy *et al.* 1996a). An intrauterine sensor provides continuous assessment of fetal oxygen saturation as long as it maintains contact with fetal skin. Sensors have been reported to obtain reliable signals 45–60% of the time (Dildy *et al.* 1993). In fetal sheep, normal aerobic metabolism is maintained at oxygen saturations above 30% (Oesburg *et al.* 1992; Nijland *et al.* 1995). Below that level, metabolic acidosis may develop. Dildy *et al.* (1994) reported a multicenter experience with 291 human subjects. A wide range of $SpO_2$ values was noted, however, during the second stage of labor, an $SpO_2$ value of 33% was 2 standard deviations below the mean, consistent with the lower limit of normal in animal studies. In 122 patients, Seelbach-Gobel *et al.* (1994) reported than an $SpO_2$ less than 30% for greater than 10 minutes predicted a postpartum pH <7.2 in more than 50% of cases. Dildy *et al.* (1996b) later reported on 1101 paired umbilical artery and vein specimens. An umbilical arterial blood $SaO_2$ >30% was associated with an umbilical arterial blood pH <7.13 in only 1% of cases, while an umbilical arterial blood $SaO_2$ < 30% was associated with an umbilical arterial blood pH <7.13 in 8.6% of cases.

A German multicenter study (Kuhnert *et al.* 1998) including 46 fetuses validated the critical threshold $SpO_2$ of 30% and concluded that $SpO_2$ values below this level for more than 10 minutes correlated with decreased intrapartum scalp pH and decreased postpartum cord blood pH values. Intrapartum fetal oxygen saturation monitoring is an evolving technology that may prove a useful clinical assessment of fetal status. Studies have demonstrated the potential of this modality to predict fetal acid–base status, however, further investigation is needed to assess the impact of oxygen saturation monitoring on perinatal outcome.

# MANAGEMENT OF INTRAPARTUM FETAL DISTRESS

Timely diagnosis and appropriate management of intrapartum fetal distress remain among the most challenging tasks facing the obstetrician. During the intrapartum period, uterine contractions subject the fetus and the uteroplacental exchange unit to intermittent episodes of diminished maternal blood flow. These brief interruptions in oxygen delivery are usually well tolerated by the healthy fetus; however, repetitive or prolonged hypoxic stress may overwhelm the fetal compensatory mechanisms and lead to acidosis and asphyxia. In such cases, the fetus will usually exhibit FHR patterns indicative of stress or distress. Clear understanding of the pathophysiology of these patterns is essential in order to optimize fetal outcome and minimize unnecessary operative deliveries.

The National Institute of Child Health and Human Development published guidelines in 1997 for interpretation of FHR monitoring and standardization of nomenclature (Anonymous 1997). Interpretation of the FHR tracing is based upon: (1) the baseline FHR, (2) variability in the FHR, and (3) periodic and/or episodic patterns classified according to their temporal relationship to uterine contractions.

## BASELINE FETAL HEART RATE

The normal FHR baseline ranges from 110 to 160 bpm. It is commonly closer to 160 bpm in early pregnancy, declining as gestational age advances. Likewise, the FHR may gradually decrease during the course of labor. In general, a FHR baseline below 110 bpm is termed bradycardia, and a rate in excess of 160 bpm is termed tachycardia. Abnormalities in the FHR baseline may have very different causes and consequences. It is important, therefore, to characterize the underlying etiology as accurately as possible and to institute appropriate therapy at the earliest possible time.

## BRADYCARDIA

Bradycardia is defined as an abnormally low baseline FHR (<110 bpm), and must be differentiated from the abrupt FHR changes characteristic of decelerations. Although FHR decelerations are very common, true fetal bradycardia is not. A bradycardic FHR baseline between 100 bpm and 110 bpm in association with otherwise reassuring FHR patterns most likely represents a normal variant. Rarely, fetal bradycardia may be seen in association with maternal β-blocker therapy, hypothermia, hypoglycemia, hypothyroidism, or fetal cardiac conduction defects (i.e. congenital atrio-ventricular block).

Documentation of fetal heart block should prompt a search for structural fetal cardiac abnormalities, which are present in 20% of cases. Other possible causes of heart block include viral infections (i.e. cytomegalovirus) and maternal systemic lupus erythematosis with anti-Ro (SSA) antibodies. Most congenital causes of fetal bradycardia do not present as acute changes in the FHR and rarely require emergency intervention. Any abrupt decline in the FHR below 110 bpm more likely represents a deceleration than a change in the baseline, and should be considered pathologic until proven otherwise.

## TACHYCARDIA

Fetal tachycardia has many possible etiologies. It may result from decreased vagal and/or increased sympathetic outflow, associated with fever, infection, fetal anemia, or fetal hypoxia. Other possible causes include maternal hyperthyroidism, sympathomimetic medications (ritodrine, terbutaline), parasympatholytic medications (atropine, phenothiazines), and fetal cardiac arrhythmias. The underlying etiology should be identified and treated, when possible.

The source of any maternal fever must be aggressively sought. Specifically, intra-amniotic infection must be excluded. The diagnosis of chorioamnionitis requires intrapartum antibiotic therapy. Possible causative medications should be discontinued, and maternal hyperthyroidism should be excluded. Fetal cardiac arrhythmias may require ultrasonographic evaluation to rule out structural lesions and cardiac failure. Anti-arrhythmic therapy may be instituted if deemed necessary. Although tachycardia alone does not necessarily indicate fetal distress, it is commonly seen in association with other FHR patterns suggestive of hypoxia, including loss of variability and repetitive late decelerations. In such cases, consideration should be given to fetal scalp pH determination or delivery.

## SINUSOIDAL PATTERN

The sinusoidal FHR pattern is an uncommon FHR baseline abnormality. The pattern presents as a smooth sine wave with an amplitude of 5–15 bpm and a frequency of 2–5 cycles/min. Variability is decreased, and accelerations are absent. Although the pathophysiologic mechanism is not known, this pattern classically is associated with fetal hypoxia secondary to severe fetal anemia. It may also occur in association with amnionitis (Gleicher *et al.* 1980), fetal sepsis, or administration of narcotic analgesics. A persistent sinusoidal pattern that is not attributable to medications is a concerning finding. Labor should be allowed to continue only in the presence of a normal fetal scalp pH or other FHR evidence of fetal well-being.

## FETAL HEART RATE VARIABILITY

Variability in the FHR results from the interaction of the sympathetic and parasympathetic arms of the fetal autonomic nervous system. Modulation of vagal tone occurs in response to blood pressure changes detected by aortic arch baroreceptors. Oxygen and carbon dioxide fluctuations, detected by chemoreceptors, similarly affect vagal outflow. Continual adjustments in vagal tone are manifested in the FHR tracing as 'short-term' ('beat-to-beat') variability superimposed upon broader, cyclical (3–5 cycles/min) 'long-term' variability. In clinical use, the term 'FHR variability' refers to a composite of the two (Fig. 25.1). Moderate FHR variability (6–25 bpm) reflects a normally oxygenated, non-acidotic vagal connection between the fetal CNS and the cardiac conduction system. Normal variability is a well-document predictor of fetal well-being (Hon & Lee 1963; Krebs *et al.* 1979; Hammacher *et al.* 1968; Paul *et al.* 1975; Martin 1982). Marked variability (>25 bpm), or 'saltatory' FHR pattern, is uncommon and most often represents an exuberant autonomic response of a normal fetus. On occasion, it may reflect increased catecholamine release in the early stages of fetal hypoxia. Careful evaluation of the associated FHR findings should help to clarify such cases. Decreased variability (0–5 bpm) most often reflects decreased fetal CNS activity associated with a fetal sleep state. However, fetal anomalies, medications (analgesics, magnesium sulfate, benzodiazepines, phenothiazines), and fetal acidosis can lead to decreased variability. Huey *et al.* (1979) reported significantly less FHR variability at scalp pH values less than 7.20 than at values above 7.20. Persistently decreased variability in a non-anomalous fetus (not attributable to medications or fetal sleep state) is a concerning sign, particularly when associated with other FHR patterns

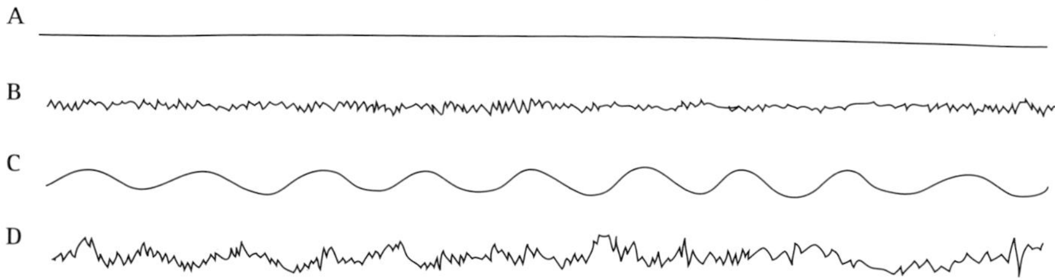


**Figure 25.1** Fetal heart rate variability. (A) Short-term variability is absent, long-term variability is absent – abnormal. (B) Short-term variability present, long-term variability absent – abnormal. (C) Short-term variability is absent, long-term variability is present – abnormal. (D) Short-term variability is present, long-term variability is present – normal.

suggestive of fetal hypoxia or acidosis. In such cases, demonstration of fetal well-being is desirable in order to allow labor to continue. Reassurance may be obtained by several different means, including fetal scalp pH determination. A fetal scalp pH >7.25 provides evidence of a non-acidotic fetus. In the presence of a persistently non-reassuring FHR tracing, however, the pH determination should be repeated every 30–60 minutes. A scalp pH of 7.20–7.25 is suspicious, and should be repeated within 30–60 minutes, regardless of other FHR findings. A scalp pH < 7.20, when confirmed, is an indication for delivery. A more practical and less invasive approach employs fetal scalp stimulation or vibroacoustic stimulation. Frequently, these stimuli will provoke FHR accelerations and improve FHR variability, providing reassurance that the fetus is not acidotic. If reassurance cannot be obtained, delivery should be considered.

## PERIODIC AND EPISODIC PATTERNS

The FHR baseline frequently is interrupted by accelerations and/or decelerations in rate. Patterns that occur sporadically are termed 'episodic patterns'. Those that occur with periodicity (with uterine contractions) are referred to as 'periodic patterns'. Examples of episodic patterns are FHR accelerations and variable decelerations not associated with contractions. Examples of periodic patterns include late decelerations, early decelerations and variable decelerations that occur with uterine contractions. Episodic and periodic patterns have important clinical implications.

### Accelerations

Accelerations in FHR occur in association with fetal movement, probably as a result of increased catecholamine release and decreased vagal stimulation of the heart (Fig. 25.2). Starting at approximately 30–32 weeks gestation, they normally occur during the fetal wake state at a rate of 15–20 per hour. The occurrence of at least two qualifying FHR accelerations (15 bpm for 15 seconds) in a period of 10 to 20 minutes constitutes a 'reactive' FHR pattern. The presence of a reactive FHR pattern is a reassuring finding, reflecting a normally oxygenated, non-acidotic CNS–cardiac axis. The persistent absence of spontaneous accelerations, on the other hand, is abnormal and may reflect fetal compromise. A non-reactive FHR tracing must be interpreted carefully in the context of the clinical presentation and other FHR characteristics. During labor, the frequency and amplitude of FHR accelerations may be diminished by fetal sleep state, common medications (narcotics, $MgSO_4$), or fetal acidosis. In the absence of spontaneous accelerations, fetal scalp stimulation or vibroacoustic stimulation often provoke fetal movement and FHR accelerations. Such accelerations are associated with normal scalp pH values (Clark *et al.* 1984; Smith *et al.* 1986; Irion *et al.* 1996; Spencer 1991). If these measures fail to provoke FHR accelerations, and if other FHR characteristics are non-reassuring, consideration should be given to fetal scalp pH determination and/or delivery.

### Decelerations

Decelerations in the FHR most commonly are encountered during the intrapartum period. They are divided into three categories, early, variable, and late, based upon the temporal relationship to the onset of a uterine contraction (Fig. 25.3).

#### Early decelerations

Early decelerations are uniform, shallow dips in the FHR (rarely below 100 bpm) that start when a contraction starts and end when the contraction ends. They probably result from fetal head compression and reflex augmentation of vagal tone. Perinatal outcome is not adversely affected by these decelerations, and they are considered clinically benign.

#### Variable decelerations

Variable decelerations result from umbilical cord compression and have a variable temporal relationship to uterine contractions. Initially, umbilical vein compression decreases fetal venous return and causes reflex FHR elevation ('shoulder'). Subsequent umbilical arterial compression dramatically increases fetal peripheral resistance and produces a rapid-onset baroreceptor-mediated slowing of the heart rate. Maximum vagal tone may result in a junctional or idioventricular escape rhythm which appears as a relatively stable rate of 60–70 bpm. As the cord is decompressed, this sequence of events occurs in reverse. Isolated variable decelerations usually have little clinical significance. Repetitive severe variable decelerations, however, may not allow sufficient fetal recovery, resulting in persistent hypoxemia, hypercapnia and respiratory acidosis. Prolonged tissue hypoperfusion may lead to metabolic acidosis and, ultimately, fetal death. In animal models, Clapp *et al.* (1988) reported that frequent episodes of hypoxemic stress, produced by umbilical cord occlusion over a period of hours, produced fetal injury even in the absence of acidosis.

When repetitive, severe variable decelerations are present, prolapse of the umbilical cord must be excluded.

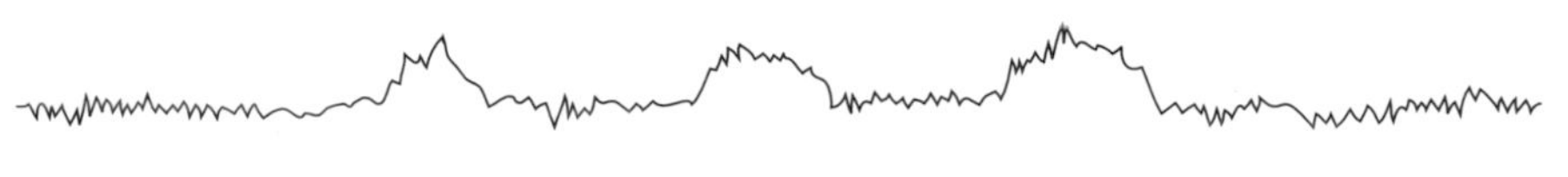

Figure 25.2 Fetal heart rate accelerations.

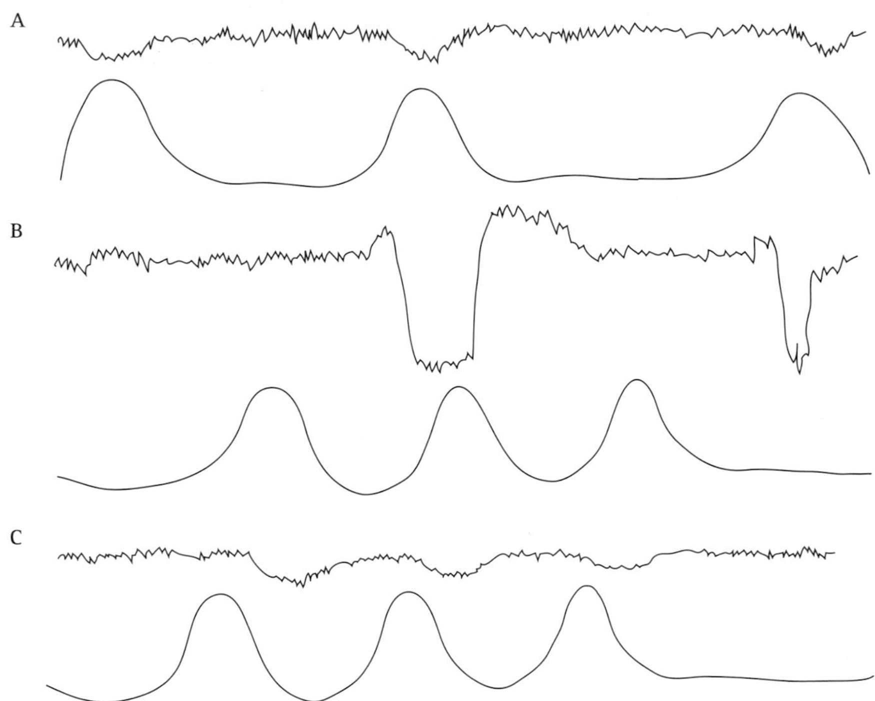


**Figure 25.3** Fetal heart rate declerations: (A) early; (B) variable; (C) late.

Maternal positional changes may relieve cord compression. Uterine hypertonus or tachysystole may be relieved by discontinuing oxytocin, administering uterine relaxants, or both. Intrapartum amnioinfusion is a procedure by which fluid is infused through an intrauterine catheter into the amniotic cavity in attempt to restore the amniotic fluid volume to normal. The goals of the procedure are: (1) to relieve the intermittent umbilical cord compression that results in variable FHR decelerations and transient fetal hypoxemia, and (2) to dilute thick meconium in attempt to prevent meconium aspiration syndrome. The benefits of amnioinfusion are well documented (Miyazaki & Nevarez 1985; MacGregor *et al.* 1991; Strong *et al.* 1990; Chauhan *et al.* 1992; Nageotte *et al.* 1985, 1991; Owen *et al.* 1990; Wu 1989; Hofmeyr 1996a,b; Spong *et al.* 1994; Lo & Rogers 1993; Schrimmer *et al.* 1991; Mahomed *et al.* 1998; Macri *et al.* 1992). Intrapartum amnioinfusion has been shown to reduce significantly the incidence of thick meconium, intrapartum variable FHR decelerations, low umbilical artery pH values, low Apgar scores, meconium aspiration, and meconium aspiration syndrome. Randomized trials of the effect of amnioinfusion on repetitive variable decelerations and Cesarean section for fetal distress are summarized in Figs 25.4 and 25.5 (Miyazaki & Nevarez 1985; MacGregor *et al.* 1991; Strong *et al.* 1990; Chauhan *et al.* 1992; Nageotte *et al.* 1985, 1991; Owen *et al.* 1990; Wu 1989; Hofmeyr 1996a,b). Repetitive severe variable decelerations that persist despite the above measures must be evaluated in the context of the associated FHR patterns. In the absence of reassuring FHR findings, delivery should be expedited.

Occasionally, variable decelerations fail to return promptly to baseline, and may more accurately be termed 'prolonged decelerations'. Prolonged decelerations usually result from cord compression (cord prolapse, tight nuchal cord), or other acute interruption of uteroplacental transfer of oxygen (tetanic contraction, uterine rupture, maternal hypotension, maternal apnea, placental abruption). Umbilical cord prolapse must be excluded. Maternal positional changes and/or manual elevation of the fetal head may relieve cord compression, if present. Documentation of separate maternal and fetal heart rates is necessary. Heart block may be ruled-out by ultrasound confirmation of identical atrial and ventricular rates. Acute maternal hypotension (i.e. epidural anesthesia) may respond to positional changes, fluids and ephedrine, if necessary. Tetanic uterine contractions often are relieved by discontinuing oxytocin, however, uterine relaxants ($MgSO_4$, terbutaline) occasionally are required. Oxygen is administered to the mother by face mask. If the above measures fail to result in resolution of the prolonged deceleration, rapid delivery is indicated.

### Late deceleration

Late decelerations reflect inadequate uteroplacental transfer of oxygen during uterine contractions. Typically, they are uniform decelerations that start after the onset of a contraction and end after the contraction ends. During uterine contractions, disruption of maternal uteroplacental perfu-

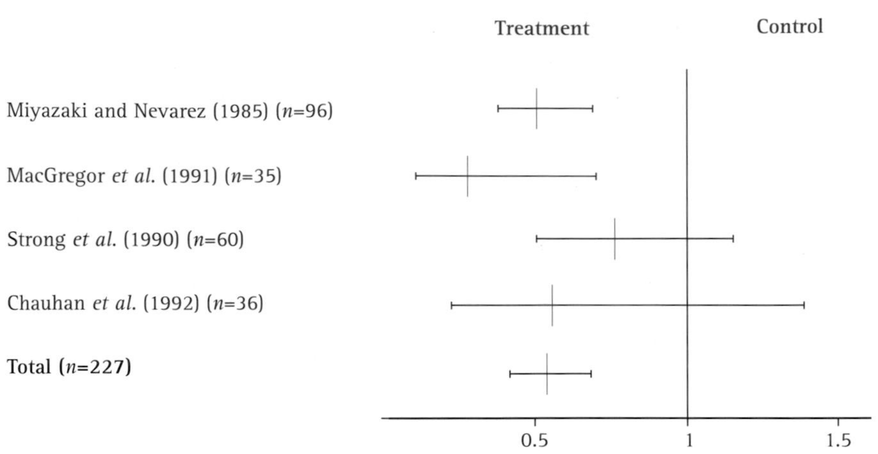


**Figure 25.4** Results of randomized trials of amnioinfusion for the treatment of persistent variable decelerations.

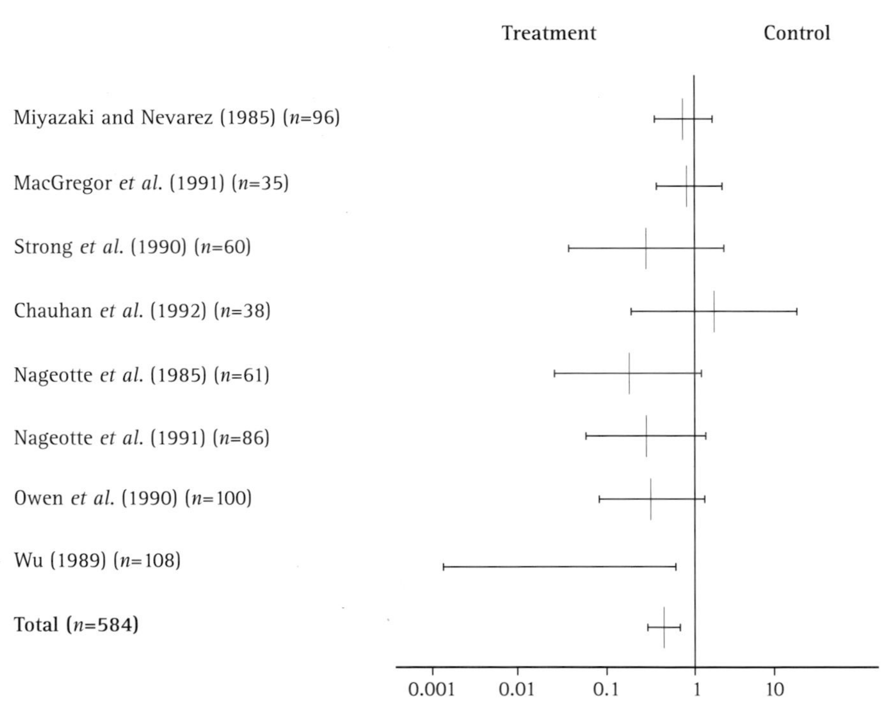


**Figure 25.5** Results of randomized trials of the effect of amnioinfusion on the incidence of Cesarean section for fetal distress.

sion causes a decline in fetal $PO_2$. When the fetal $PO_2$ falls below a critical threshold, a complex chemoreceptor- and baroreceptor-mediated reflex is initiated. Centralization of blood volume (favoring perfusion of the brain, heart and adrenals) occurs via vasoconstriction in the vascular beds of the limbs and gut. The resulting increase in peripheral resistance provokes a reflex deceleration in the FHR. Isolated late decelerations within an otherwise normal tracing usually have little clinical significance. However, continuing hypoxic stress, as evidenced by repetitive late decelerations, may lead to metabolic acidosis, asphyxia, and eventually fetal death. The goal in treating late decelerations is to improve uteroplacental perfusion and oxygen delivery to the fetus. Usual measures include: (1) left lateral decubitus position, to improve maternal venous return and cardiac output; (2) face mask $O_2$; (3) intravenous fluid bolus of 250–500 ml of crystalloid to restore the maternal intravascular volume and improve cardiac output, and (4) discontinuation of oxytocin. In the presence of late decelerations with decreased FHR variability, reassurance of fetal well-being is imperative in order to justify continuation of labor. A normal fetal scalp pH (>7.25), or an acceleratory FHR response to fetal scalp or vibroacoustic stimulation provides reassurance that acidosis is not present. A pattern of repetitive late decelerations without such reassurance suggests fetal distress and is an indication for delivery.

## CONCLUSION

Dramatic changes in intrapartum management have taken place over the last two decades, highlighted by the rapid proliferation of electronic fetal monitoring (EFM), the decline in maternal and perinatal mortality, and the rising utilization of Cesarean section. Many widely held beliefs have been challenged. Large case-control studies have demonstrated the limited contribution of 'birth asphyxia' to the incidence of cerebral palsy. Randomized trials have dampened some of the early enthusiasm regarding the potential benefits of EFM. Nevertheless, the objective of intrapartum management remains the same: to optimize the outcome for both mother and fetus by (1) preventing intrapartum fetal asphyxia and possible long-term sequelae, and (2) avoiding unnecessary operative deliveries. To that end, the most effective resource available to the obstetrician is a thorough understanding of the FHR patterns associated with normal and abnormal fetal physiologic states.

### Key Points

- The objective of electronic fetal monitoring (EFM) is to identify the fetus in distress so that measures might be taken in time to avert permanent damage or death.
- The term 'fetal distress' although commonly used, remains poorly defined.
- Despite the lack of consensus on many points, EFM has been shown to be at least as effective in identifying fetal compromise as is frequent FHR auscultation with intensive, one-on-one nursing. While this level of individualized nursing care may be available in some settings, most delivery units will find the personnel requirements to be impractical and cost prohibitive.
- One of the major shortcomings of EFM is a high rate of false-positive results.
- Other methods of fetal monitoring include: sampling of scalp blood for pH determination, computer analysis of FHR, and fetal pulse oxymetry.
- Timely diagnosis and appropriate management of intrapartum fetal distress remain among the most challenging tasks facing the obstetrician.
- Interpretation of the FHR tracing is based upon: the baseline FHR, variability in the FHR, and periodic and/or episodic patterns classified according to their temporal relationship to uterine contractions.
- Changes in intrapartum management have taken place over the last two decades, highlighted by the rapid proliferation of electronic fetal monitoring, the decline in maternal and perinatal mortality, and the rising utilization of Cesarean section.
- The objective of intrapartum management is to optimize the outcome for both mother and fetus by (1) preventing intrapartum fetal asphyxia and possible long-term sequelae, and (2) avoiding unnecessary operative deliveries.
- To achieve this goal the most effective resource available to the obstetrician is a thorough understanding of the FHR patterns associated with normal and abnormal fetal physiologic states.

## REFERENCES


Aarnoudse J G, Huisjes H J, Gordon H *et al.* (1985) Fetal subcutaneous scalp $PO_2$ and abnormal heart rate during labor. *Am J Obstet Gynecol* 153:565–566.

ACOG (1991) Committee on Obstetrics, Maternal and Fetal Medicine of the American College of Obstetrics. *Utility of umbilical cord blood acid–base assessment.* ACOG Committee Opinion No. 91, February 1991.

Amato J L (1977) Fetal monitoring in a community hospital: a statistical analysis. *Obstet Gynecol* 50:269–274.

Anonymous (1997) Electronic fetal heart rate monitoring: research guidelines for interpretation. National Institute of Child Health and Human Development Research Planning Workshop. *Am J Obstet Gynecol* 177(6):1385–1390.

Banta H D & Thacker S B (1979) *Costs and benefits to electronic fetal monitoring: a review of the literature.* Rockville, MD: National Center for Health Services Research; 1979. Report No.: DHEW-PHS-79-3245.

Bax M & Melson K B (1993) Birth asphyxia: a statement. *Dev Med Child Neurol* 35:1022–1024.

Bergmans M G M, van Geijn H P, Weber T *et al.* (1993) Fetal transcutaneous $PCO_2$ measurements during labor. *Eur J Obstet Gynecol* 51:1–7.

Bloch B (1978) Measurement of fetal scalp pH by continuous-recording scalp electrode and correlation with capillary blood pH. *S Afr Med J* 54:448–450.

Caldeyro-Barcia R, Mendez-Bauer C, Posiero J J *et al.* (1966) Control of the human fetal heart rate during labor. In: Cassels D E (ed.) *The heart and circulation of the newborn and infant.* New York, NY: Grune & Stratton; 7–36.

Chan W H, Paul R H & Toews J (1973) Intrapartum fetal monitoring: maternal and fetal morbidity and perinatal mortality. *Obstet Gynecol* 41:7–13.

Chauhan S P, Rutherford S E, Hess L W & Morrison J C (1992) Prophylactic intrapartum amnioinfusion for patients with oligohydramnios. A prospective randomized study. *J Reprod Med* 37:817.

Clapp J F, Peress N S, Wesley M & Mann L I (1988) Brain damage after intermittent partial cord occlusion in the chronically instrumented fetal lamb. *Am J Obstet Gynecol* 159:504–509.

Clark S L, Gimovsky M L & Miller F C (1984) The scalp stimulation test: a clinical alternative to fetal scalp blood sampling. *Am J Obstet Gynecol* 148:274–277.

Cremer M V (1906) Ueber die Direckte Ableitung der Aktionsstrome des Menchlichen Herzens vom Oesophagus und ueber das Elektrokardiogramm des Fetus. *Munch Med Wochenschr* 53:811.

Dawes G S (1991) Computerised analysis of the fetal heart rate. *Eur J Obstet Gynecol Reprod Biol* 42(Suppl):S5–S8.

Dawes G S, Moulden M, Sheil O & Redman C W G (1992) Approximate entropy, a statistic of regularity, applied to fetal heart rate data before and during labor. *Obstet Gynecol* 80:763–768.

DeLee J B (1922) Ein nues stethoskopf fur die Geburtshilfe besonders geeignet. *Zentralbl Gynaekol* 46:1688.

Dildy G A, Clark S L & Loucks C A (1993) Preliminary experience with intrapartum fetal pulse oximetry in humans. *Obstet Gynecol* 81:630–635.

Dildy G A, van den Berg P P, Katz M *et al.* (1994) Intrapartum fetal pulse oximetry: fetal oxygen saturation trends during labor and relation to delivery outcome. *Am J Obstet Gynecol* 171:679–684.

Dildy G A, Clark S L, Loucks C A (1996a) Intrapartum fetal pulse oximetry: Past, present, and future *Am J Obstet Gynecol* 175(1):1–9.

Dildy G A, Thorp J A, Yeast J D & Clark S L (1996b) The relationship between oxygen saturation and pH in umbilical blood: implications for intrapartum fetal oxygen saturation monitoring. *Am J Obstet Gynecol* 175(3 Pt 1):682–687.

Edington P T, Sibanda J & Beard R W (1975) Influence on clinical practice of routine intra-partum fetal monitoring. *BMJ* 3:341–343.

Fleiss O O (1981) *Statistical methods for rates and proportions*, 2nd edn. Chichester: John Wiley; pp. 38 45.

Gültekin-Zootzmann B (1975) The history of monitoring the human fetus. *J Perinat Med* 3:135–144.

Gilstrap L C, Leveno K J, Burris J *et al.* (1989) Diagnosis of birth asphyxia on the basis of fetal pH, Apgar score, and newborn cerebral dysfunction. *Am J Obstet Gynecol* 161:825–830.

Gleicher H, Runowicz C & Brown B (1980) Sinusoidal fetal heart rate patterns in association with amnionitis. *Obstet Gynecol* 56:109.

Goodwin J W, Dunne J T & Thomas R W (1969) Antepartum identification of the fetus at risk. *Can Med Assoc J* 101:458.

Goodwin T M, Milner-Masterson L & Paul R H (1994) Elimination of fetal scalp blood sampling on a large clinical service. *Obstet Gynecol* 83(6):971–974.

Grant A, O'Brien N, Joy M, Hennessy E & MacDonald D (1989) Cerebral palsy among children born during the Dublin randomized trial of intrapartum monitoring. *Lancet* 2:1233–6.

Haesslein H C & Niswander K R (1980) Fetal distress in term pregnancies. *Am J Obstet Gynecol* 137:245–253.

Hamilton L A, Gottschalk W, Vidyasagar D *et al.* (1978) Effects of monitoring on perinates. *Int J Gynaecol Obstet* 15:483–490.

Hammacher K (1967) The diagnosis of fetal distress with an electronic fetal heart monitor. In: Horsky J & Stembera Z K (ed.) *Intrauterine dangers to the fetus.* Amsterdam: Excerpta Medica.

Hammacher K, Huter K A, Bokelmann J & Werners P H (1968) Foetal heart frequency and perinatal condition of the foetus and newborn. *Gynaecologia* 166:439–460.

Haverkamp A D, Thompson H E, McFee J G & Cetrullo C (1976) The evaluation of continuous fetal heart rate monitoring in high-risk pregnancy. *Am J Obstet Gynecol* 125:310–320.

Haverkamp A D, Orleans M, Langendoerfer S *et al.* (1979) A controlled trial of the differential effects of intrapartum fetal monitoring. *Am J Obstet Gynecol* 134:399–408.

Hillis D S (1917) Attachment for the stethoscope. *JAMA* 68:910.

Hofmeyr G J (1996) Amnioinfusion for intrapartum umbilical cord compression (potential or diagnosed by electronic fetal heart rate monitoring). In: Enkin M W, Keirse M J N C, Renfrew M J & Neilson J P (eds.) *The Cochrane Database of Systematic Reviews: Pregnancy and Childbirth Module.* The Cochrane Collaboration; Issue 3. Oxford: Update Software.

Hofmeyr G J (1996) Amnioinfusion for meconium-stained liquor in labour. In: Enkin M W, Keirse M J N C, Renfrew M J, Neilson J P (eds.) *The Cochrane Database of Systematic Reviews: Pregnancy and Childbirth Module.* The Cochrane Collaboration; Issue 3. Oxford: Update Software.

Hon E H (1966) The human fetal circulation in normal labor. In: Cassels D E (ed.) *The heart and circulation of the newborn and infant.* New York NY: Grune & Stratton; 37–52.

Hon E H & Lee S T (1963) The electronic evaluation of the fetal heart rate. VIII. Patterns preceding fetal death: further observations. *Am J Obstet Gynecol* 87:814–826.

Hon E H, Quilligan E J (1967) The classification of fetal heart rate. *Conn Med* 31:779.

Huch A, Huch R, Schneider H & Peabody J (1980) Experience with transcutaneous $PO_2$ (tc$PO_2$) monitoring of mother, fetus and newborn. *J Perinat Med* 8:51–72.

Huey J R Jr, Paul R H, Hadjiev A A *et al.* (1979) Fetal heart rate variability: an approach to automated assessment. *Am J Obstet Gynecol* 134(6):691–695.

Irion O, Stuckelberger P, Moutquin J M *et al.* (1996) Is intrapartum vibratory acoustic stimulation a valid alternative to fetal scalp pH determination? *Br J Obstet Gynaecol* 103:642–647.

Johnson M V (1993) Cellular alterations associated with perinatal asphyxia. *Clin Invest Med* 16(2):122–132.

Johnstone F D, Campbell D M & Hughes G J (1978) Antenatal care: has continuous intrapartum monitoring made any impact on fetal outcome? *Lancet* 1:1298–1300.

Kaplan S & Toyama S (1958) Fetal electrocardiography: utilizing abdominal and intrauterine leads. *Obstet Gynecol* 11:391.

Keith R D F, Beckly S, Garibaldi J M *et al.* (1995) A multicentre comparative study of 17 experts and an intelligent computer system for managing labour using the cardiotocogram. *Br J Obstet Gynaecol* 102(9):688–700.

Kelly V C & Kulkarni D (1973) Experiences with fetal monitoring in a community hospital. *Obstet Gynecol* 41:818–824.

Kelso I M, Parsons R J, Lawrence G F *et al.* (1978) An assessment of continuous fetal heart rate monitoring in labor: a randomized trial. *Am J Obstet Gynecol* 131:526–532.

Kennedy E (1833) *Observations of Obstetrical Auscultation.* Dublin: Hodges & Smith.

Kilian (1849) quoted by Jaggard W W (1888). In: Hirst B C (ed.) *A system of obstetrics.* Philadelphia, PA: Lea Broth.

Kirschbaum T H (1969) Editorial: Diagnosis of fetal distress. *Obstet Gynecol.* 34:721–8.

Koh K S, Greves D, Yung S *et al.* (1975) Experience with fetal monitoring in a university teaching hospital. *Can Med Assoc J* 112:455–462.

Krebs H B, Petres R E, Dunn L J *et al.* (1979) Intrapartum fetal heart rate monitoring. 1. Classification and prognosis of fetal heart rate patterns. *Am J Obstet Gynecol* 133:762–772.

Kubli F W, Hon E H, Khazin A F & Takemura H (1969) Observations on heart rate and pH in the human fetus during labor. *Am J Obstet Gynecol* 104:1190–1206.

Kuhnert M, Seelbach-Goebel G & Butterwegge M (1998) Predictive agreement between the fetal arterial oxygen saturation and fetal scalp pH: results of the German multicenter study. *Am J Obstet Gynecol* 178(2):330–335.

Lauersen N H, Miller F C & Paul R H (1979) Continuous intrapartum monitoring of fetal scalp pH. *Am J Obstet Gynecol* 133:44–50.

Le Jumeau J A (de Kergaradec) (1822) Mémoire sur l'Auscultation appliquée à l'Etude de la Grossesse ou Recherches sur deux nouveaux signes propres à faire reconnaître plusieurs circonstances de l'Etat de Gestation; lu à l'Académie royale de médecine, dans sa séance générale du 26 décembre 1821. Paris, 1822.

Lee W K & Baggish M S (1976) The effect of unselected intrapartum fetal monitoring. *Obstet Gynecol* 47:516–520.

Lo K W & Rogers M (1993) A controlled trial of amnioinfusion: the prevention of meconium aspiration in labour. *Aust NZ J Obstet Gynaecol* 33:51–54.

Low J A, Lindsay B G & Derrick E J (1997) Threshold of metabolic acidosis associated with newborn complications. *Am J Obstetr Gynecol* 177:1391–1394.

Luthy D A, Kirkwood K S, van Belle G *et al.* (1987) A randomized trial of electronic fetal monitoring in preterm labor. *Obstet Gynecol* 69:687–695.

MacDonald D, Grant A, Sheridan-Pereira M *et al.* (1985) The Dublin randomized controlled trial of intrapartum fetal heart rate monitoring. *Am J Obstet Gynecol* 152:524–539.

MacDonald D, Grant A. Fetal surveillance in labour – the present position. Bonnar J, ed. *Recent advances in obstetrics and gynaecology,* vol. 15. London: Churchill Livingstone; pp. 83–100.

MacGregor S N, Banzhaf W C, Silver R K & Depp R (1991) A prospective randomized evaluation of intrapartum amnioinfusion. *J Reprod Med* 36:69.

Macri C J, Schrimmer D B, Leung A *et al.* (1992) Prophylactic amnioinfusion improves outcome of pregnancy complicated by thick meconium and oligohydramnios. *Am J Obstet Gynecol* 167:117.

Mahomed K, Mulambo T, Woelk G *et al.* (1998) The Collaborative Randomised Amnioinfusion for Meconium Project (CRAMP): 2. Zimbabwe. *Br J Obstet Gynaecol* 105(3):309–313.

Martin C B (1982) Physiology and clinical use of fethal heart rate variability. *Clin Perinatol* 9:339–352.

Mayor H (1818) Biblioth Univ. de Genève, Nov 9, quoted by Thomas H (1935) *Classical contributions to obstetrics and gynecology.* Springfield, Illinois: Charles C Thomas.

Miyazaki F S & Nevarez F (1985) Saline amnioinfusion for relief of repetitive variable decelerations: a prospective randomized study. *Am J Obstet Gynecol* 153:301–306.

Nageotte M P, Bertucci L, Towers C V, Lagrew D L & Modanlou H (1991) Prophylactic amnioinfusion in pregnancies complicated by oligohydramnios: a prospective study. *Obstet Gynecol* 77:677.

Nageotte M P, Freeman R K, Garite T J & Dorchester W (1985) Prophylactic intrapartum amnioinfusion in patients with preterm premature rupture of membranes. *Am J Obstet Gynecol* 153:557.

National Center for Health Statistics, Vol. 47, No. 18, April 29, 1999.

Neldam S, Osler M, Hansen P K *et al.* (1986) Intrapartum fetal heart rate monitoring in a combined low- and high-risk population: a controlled clinical trial. *Eur J Obstet Gynecol Reprod Biol* 23:1–11.

Nelson, Karin B, Dambrosia, James M, Ting, Tricia Y, Grether & Judith K (1996) Uncertain value of electronic fetal monitoring in predicting cerebral palsy. *N Engl J Med* 334(10) 7:613–618.

Nijland R, Jongsma H W, Nijhuis J G *et al.* (1995) Arterial oxygen saturation in relation to metabolic acidosis in fetal lambs. *Am J Obstet Gynecol* 172:810–819.

Oeseburg B, Ringnalda B E M, Crevels J *et al.* (1992) Fetal oxygenation in chronic maternal hypoxia: what's critical? *Adv Exp Med Biol* 317:499–502.

Owen J, Henson B V & Hauth J C (1990) A prospective randomized study of saline solution amnioinfusion. *Am J Obstet Gynecol* 162:1146–9.

Paul R H, Huey J R & Yaeger C F (1977) Clinical fetal monitoring – its effect on cesarean section rate and perinatal mortality: five-year trends. *Postgrad Med* 61:160–164.

Paul R H, Suidan A K, Yeh S & Hon E H (1975) The evaluation and significance of intrapartum baseline FHR variability. *Am J Obstet Gynecol* 123:206–210.

Pello L C, Rosevear B M, Dawes G S *et al.* (1991) Computerized fetal heart rate analysis in labor. *Obstet Gynecol* 78:602–610.

Philippeaux (1879) Notice biographique et bibliographique sur Philippe Le Goust. *Archives de tocologie des maladies des femmes, Paris* 6:304.

Renou P & Wood C (1974) Interpretation of the continuous fetal heart rate record. *Clin Obstet Gynaecol* 1:191–215.

Renou P, Chang A, Anderson I & Wood C (1976) Controlled trial of fetal intensive care. *Am J Obstet Gynecol* 126:470–476.

Rosen M G (Chairman) (1981) *Consensus Task Force on Cesarean Childbirth.* National Institutes of Health

Publication No. 82-2067, Washington DC, US Dept of Health and Human Services; October 1981; pp. 49, 125, 275.

Schrimmer D B, Macri C J & Paul R H (1991) Prophylactic amnioinfusion as a treatment for oligohydramnios in laboring patients: a prospective, randomized trial. *Am J Obstet Gynecol* 165:972–975.

Schwartz H (1838) *Die vorzeitgen Athembewegungen.* Leipzig 1838.

Schwartz H (1870) *Arch Gynaekol* 1:361.

Seelbach-Gobel B, Butterwegge M, Kuhnert M & Heupel M (1994) Fetal reflectance pulse oximetry *sub partu.* Experiences – prognostic significance and consequences – goals. *Zeitschr Geburtshilfe Perinatol* 198:67–71.

Seitz L (1903) *Die fetalen Herztone unter der Geburt.* Munchen: Habil-Schrift.

Shelley T, Tipton R H (1971) Dip Area: A quantitative measure of fetal heart rate patterns. *J Obstet Gynecol Br Commonw* 78:694–701.

Shenker L, Post R C & Seiler J S (1975) Routine electronic monitoring of fetal heart rate and uterine activity during labor. *Obstet Gynecol* 46:185–189.

Small M L, Beall M, Platt L D *et al.* (1989) Continuous tissue pH monitoring in the term fetus. *Am J Obstet Gynecol* 161(2):323–329.

Smith C V, Nquyen H N, Phelan J P & Paul R H (1986) Intrapartum assessment of fetal well-being: a comparison of fetal acoustic stimulation with acid–base determinations. *Am J Obstet Gynecol* 155:726–728.

Smyth C N (1953) *Lancet* 2:1124.

Spencer J A (1991) Predictive value of a fetal heart rate acceleration at the time of fetal blood sampling in labour. *J Perinat Med* 19(3):207–215.

Spong C Y, Ogundipe O A & Ross M G (1994) Prophylactic amnioinfusion for meconium-stained amniotic fluid. *Am J Obstet Gynecol* 171:931–935.

Stamm O, Latscha U, Janecek P & Campana A (1976) Development of a special electrode for continuous subcutaneous pH measurement in the infant scalp. *Am J Obstet Gynecol* 124:193–195.

Strong T H Jr, Hetzler G, Sarno A P & Paul R H (1990) Prophylactic intrapartum amnioinfusion: a randomized clinical trial. *Am J Obstet Gynecol* 162:1374–1375.

Sturbois G, Uzan S, Rotten D *et al.* (1977) Continuous subcutaneous pH measurement in human fetuses: correlations with scalp and umbilical blood pH. *Am J Obstet Gynecol* 128:901–903.

Sureau C L (1956) Recherches electrocardiographiques foetal au cours de la gestation et du travail: premiers resultal d'une nouvelle technique d'enregistrement par electrodes endouterines. *Gynecol Obstet* 55:21.

Tejani N, Mann L, Bhakthavathsalan A *et al.* (1975) Correlation of fetal heart rate-uterine contraction patterns and fetal scalp blood pH. *Obstet Gynecol* 46:392–396.

Thacker S B & Stroup D F (1999) Continuous electronic heart rate monitoring versus intermittent auscultation for assessment during labor (Cochrane Review). In: *The Cochrane Library,* vol. 3 (Oxford: Update Software.

Tutera G & Newman R L (1975) Fetal monitoring: its effect on the perinatal mortality and caesarean section rates and its complications. *Am J Obstet Gynecol* 122:750–754.

Vintzileos A M, Antsaklis A, Varvarigos I *et al.* (1993) A randomized trial of intrapartum electronic fetal heart rate monitoring versus intermittent auscultation. *Obstet Gynecol* 81:899–907.

Vintzileos A M, Nochimson D J & Guzman E R (1995a) Intrapartum electronic fetal heart rate monitoring versus intermittent auscultation: a meta-analysis. *Obstet Gynecol* 85:149–155.

Vintzileos A M, Nochimson D J, Antsaklis A, Varvarigos I, Guzman E R & Knuppel R A (1995b) Comparison of intrapartum electronic fetal heart rate monitoring versus intermittent auscultation in detecting fetal acidemia at birth. *Am J Obstet Gynecol* 173:1021–4.

*Webster's ninth new collegiate dictionary* (1985) Springfield, Mass: Merriam-Webster, Inc.

Willcourt R & Queenan J T (1981) Fetal scalp blood sampling and transcutaneous $PO_2$. *Clin Perinatol* 8:87–99.

Williams R L & Hawes W E (1979) Cesarean section, fetal monitoring and perinatal mortality in California. *Am J Public Health* 69:864.

Winckel F (1893) *Lehrbuch der Geburtshilfe.* Leipzig: Veit.

Wood C, Renou P, Oats J *et al.* (1981) A controlled trial of fetal heart rate monitoring in a low-risk obstetric population. *Am J Obstet Gynecol* 141:527–534.

Wu B T (1989) Intrapartum amnio-infusion in patients with oligohydramnios. *Chyng Hua Fu Chan Ko Tsa Chih* 24:2.

Chapter 26

# Prediction of asphyxia with fetal gas analysis

S. De la Fuente and P. Soothill

## INTRODUCTION

The word 'asphyxia' etymologically comes from the Greek word for 'pulse-less', which we equate to 'death', and so in our view, the general usage of this term is so poorly defined as to be useless. It is used to mean a sick baby at birth, which, for many years, has been recognized as being associated with long-term neurological lesions in infants (Little 1862). Major recent advances in obstetric and neonatal care have led to greater expectations by doctors and patients for excellent pregnancy, delivery and newborn outcomes. Perinatal mortality has fallen so substantially that reducing preventable neurological handicap has now become the priority; consequently, death is no longer an adequate end-point with which to assess obstetric care.

Despite the widely recognized association between poor condition at birth and long-term damage, the diagnosis of asphyxia has been confused not only because of the lack of an adequate definition but also because there is no simple direct linear relationship between the severity of asphyxia and the amount of damage that results. Further confounding factors include the duration and frequency of the asphyxial events and the gestational age at which they occur. Moreover, animal studies, which have attempted to describe the effects of 'chronic asphyxia', have tended to study hypoxia over several hours rather than the more clinically relevant time period, which is weeks. Finally, the inevitable lack of experimental studies in humans has led to notorious differences of opinion in interpreting the relationship between cause and effect of asphyxia and neurological handicaps.

The complexity described above is reflected in the consensus reached for the clinical definition of fetal asphyxia. This requires three criteria to be met: a lack of oxygen in the blood, an abnormal acid–base status and a pathophysiological effect on the neonate. By these criteria, at least 2% of all neonates experience asphyxia during labor and delivery, and some of them are damaged as a result (Low 1997). However, in many of these cases, the damage will have occurred before the labor started (e.g. as a result of chronic placental dysfunction), and it has become increasingly clear that this has often been under-recognized due to the difficulty in obtaining objective criteria of measurement.

In this chapter, we will review the methods of assessing fetal blood gases and acid–base status and evaluate them as predictors of 'asphyxia', whilst clearly distinguishing between acute and chronic disease.

## DEFINITIONS

### HYPOXIA, ACIDOSIS, ASPHYXIA AND HYPOXIC ISCHEMIC ENCEPHALOPATHY

The World Federation of Neurology Group defined **asphyxia** as 'a condition of impaired gas exchange leading, if it persists, to progressive hypoxemia and hypercapnia' (Bax & Nelson 1993). Significant hypoxemia in the fetus is usually followed by metabolic acidosis, so some authors feel that any definition must also include this aspect to meet the pathophysiological process (Low 1997). For the word asphyxia to have any meaning other than hypoxia and/or acidosis, the reader should consider its links to clinical consequences, and so in addition to blood gas and acid–base balance analysis, pathological effects shortly after birth may be considered. Central nervous system, cardiac, respiratory and renal complications are usually associated with severe asphyxia and can be readily identified. The neurological features are often described as hypoxic–ischemic encephalopathy (HIE) which is a common disease of the newborn and has a strong association with chronic disability in childhood (Sarnat & Sarnat 1976). In neonatal medicine, this term has come to replace the diagnosis of birth asphyxia.

Although HIE is helpful in neonatal medicine, because it includes postnatal information, the term cannot be used prospectively in fetal medicine, and the word 'asphyxia' is often taken to be synonymous with fetal hypoxia and/or acidosis (Soothill *et al.* 1989). However, these measurements should be interpreted only as a very rough identifier of a group at high risk for asphyxia at birth rather than being diagnostic.

$PO_2$ and $PCO_2$ are terms that refer to the partial pressure of a gas. They can be defined as the tension required to maintain the same amount of a gas dissolved in the water phase of plasma, which, under normal conditions, is not greater than 2% of the total oxygen contained in the blood.

**Hypoxemia** means a decreased oxygen content in blood and can be produced either because of reduced $PO_2$ or reduced hemoglobin concentration (Soothill *et al.* 1989). **Hypoxia** refers to reduced use of oxygen by the tissues. This can be caused either by impaired supply from hypoxemia, impaired blood flow or reduced uptake of oxygen by the tissues (e.g. metabolism failure from cyanide poisoning). A low $PO_2$ should be defined as a partial pressure of oxygen more than 2 standard deviations (2SD) below the normal mean for gestational age in the blood, and before labor, this measurement is relatively simple to define, because gestational age-dependent charts are available (Nicolaides *et al.* 1989; Soothill *et al.* 1986). After the onset of delivery, it is not always clear what range should apply because the 'normal' values are changed by the duration of labor, the use of anesthetics and the mode of delivery.

**Acidosis** refers to a high hydrogen ion concentration in the tissues. While fetal tissue pH is relatively stable, its measurement is not realistically possible. **Acidemia** refers to a high $H^+$ ion concentration in the blood, which can be easily measured, and it usually reflects the levels in the tissues. In adults, acidemia is defined as a pH of 7.35 or less in arterial blood. In the fetus, the cut-off values to define acidemia are less clear and are dependent on the site of blood sampling. Traditionally, the definition was a pH of less than 7.20 for fetal scalp blood or 2SDs below the mean (pH 7.10–7.18) in the umbilical artery after delivery (Gilstrap 1998). However, this approach is still not clear because to produce complications in the newborn, in the absence of other problems such as trauma or sepsis, umbilical arterial acidosis must be more severe. The American College of Obstetricians and Gynecologists has recommended considering a pH less than 7.00 as pathological or severely acidemic in the umbilical artery at birth. pH values less than 6.61 in the umbilical arterial blood have been described as probably incompatible with life (Belai *et al.* 1998). Before delivery, interpretation is simpler because normal reference ranges for fetal gases have been established throughout the pregnancy by cordocentesis (Nicolaides *et al.* 1989).

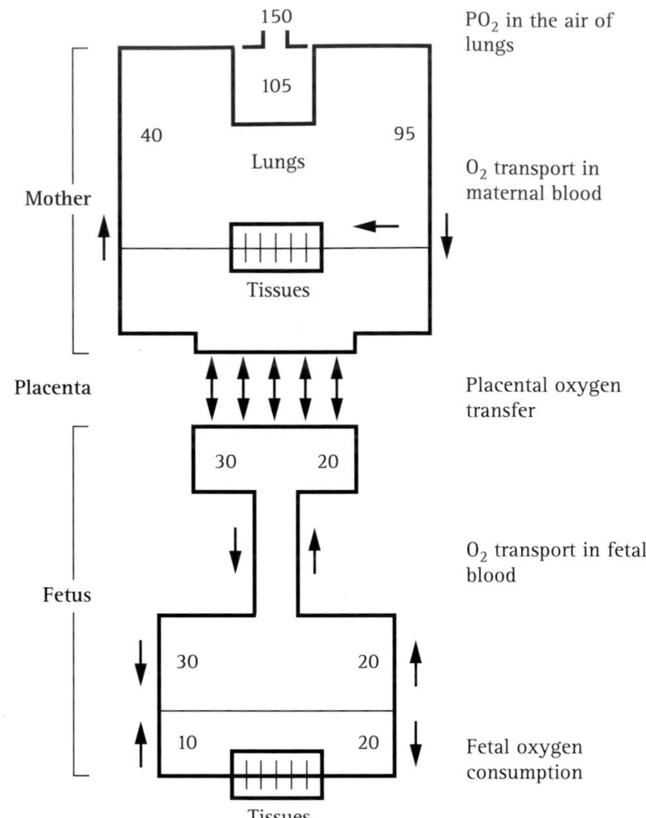


Figure 26.1 Oxygen gradient between the maternal lungs and the fetal tissues. Modified from Towell (1976).

## NORMAL OXYGEN DELIVERY TO THE FETUS

### OXYGEN CARRIAGE IN THE BLOOD

As shown in Fig. 26.1, gases are transported from the mother to the fetus and vice versa by a double circulatory system through the placenta. Oxygen diffuses down a decreasing gradient of partial pressure from air in the lungs ($PO_2$ 150 mmHg), pulmonary capillary vessels (105 mmHg), arterial blood (95 mmHg), placental vessels (30–40 mmHg), umbilical venous fetal blood (20–30 mmHg) to finally equilibrate $PO_2$ with the fetal tissues at a $PO_2$ of around 10–20 mmHg in a term fetus (Towell 1976).

Despite the low $PO_2$ levels, fetal blood has a high oxygen content due to both the high affinity of fetal haemoglobin and its high concentration; the latter increases in a linear fashion from the second trimester throughout pregnancy (Nicolaides *et al.* 1988). Not only is the blood oxygen content quite high, but normally, the organs, especially the heart and brain, are well perfused because of the high fetal cardiac output. Indeed, when under stress, there are physiological compensatory mechanisms including blood redistribution and a further increase in fetal oxygen extraction (see later). For all of these reasons, oxygen delivery to some organs per gram of tissue is actually greater in the fetus than to the same organ in the adult.

The flow of oxygen to the tissues is known as oxygen delivery, which is the product of the volume of blood flow to a tissue and its oxygen content. The latter is dependent on the hemoglobin concentration and oxygen saturation. The ability of hemoglobin to carry oxygen varies in different physiological conditions and is affected by the hemoglobin oxygen affinity. This property correlates the amount of oxygen bound to hemoglobin for a given $PO_2$ in a sigmoid curve known as the hemoglobin dissociation curve (Fig. 26.2). The oxygen saturation is the percentage of hemoglobin that is oxygenated and accounts for about 98% of the total oxygen in blood. The affinity for oxygen is dependent on the type of hemoglobin and fetal hemoglobin has a greater affinity for oxygen than the adult type, so its curve is shifted to the left. This means that at the same $PO_2$, fetal hemoglobin will be more saturated than adult. This is described by the *P*50, which is the partial pressure of oxygen at which the hemoglobin is 50% saturated; for fetal hemoglobin, this level is 21 mmHg, whereas for the adult, it is 27 mmHg. Due to this property, at the levels of $PO_2$ in the fetus, 13 ml of oxygen are carried by 100 ml of blood. This is very similar to the 15 ml per 100 ml carried by the maternal blood, and so the fetus is not hypoxemic despite the lower $PO_2$ (Willcourt 1987). It is therefore not surprising

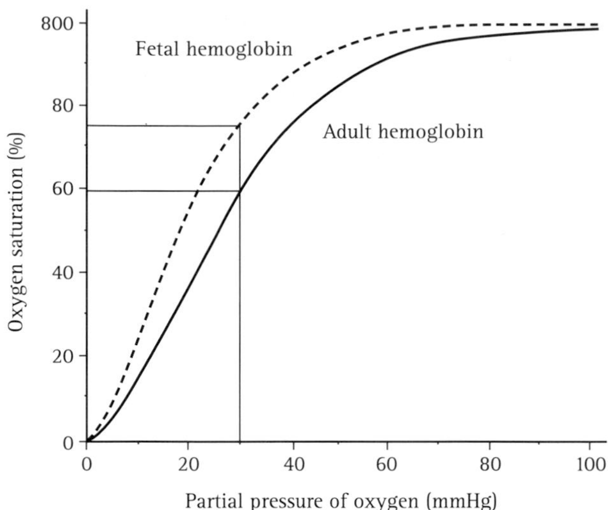


**Figure 26.2** $PO_2$ dissociation curve of adult and fetal hemoglobin.

that the saturation of fetal hemoglobin is on average about 60% in the umbilical vein at term (Bozzetti *et al.* 1987; McNamara *et al.* 1982; Richardson *et al.* 1998).

In the fetus, the hemoglobin dissociation curve can be affected by pH and perhaps temperature. By increasing temperature or decreasing pH the hemoglobin molecule becomes less bound to oxygen, and the dissociation curve is shifted to the right. 2,3-Diphosphoglycerate (2,3-DPG), a product of glycolysis, causes a right shift of the adult dissociation curve, but it has little effect with fetal hemoglobin (Soothill *et al.* 1988).

At term, the uterine blood flow is 1200 ml/min with a $PO_2$ of about 95 mmHg. It leaves the uterine veins with a $PO_2$ of about 40 mmHg, and this difference is due to fetal, uterine and placental oxygen extraction. Fetal oxygen extraction is the ratio between fetal oxygen consumption and oxygen delivery, and it also can be expressed in mathematical terms as:

$$\text{Oxygen extraction} = (CvO_2 - CaO_2)/CvO_2,$$

where Cv and Ca represent the venous and arterial oxygen content, respectively.

Using cord blood gases from normal vaginal deliveries and Cesarean sections (CS) at term, Rurak estimated that, at a fetal umbilical artery $PaO_2$ of 20 mmHg, the human fetus extracts about 47% of the available oxygen (Rurak *et al.* 1987). Because the umbilical artery flow, estimated from Doppler studies, is about 120 ml/min/kg fetus (Gill *et al.* 1984) and the venous–arterial oxygen difference is 6–7 vol/100 ml, it has been calculated that the fetus consumes at term roughly 20–30 ml of oxygen per minute. This changes during the pregnancy, and the umbilical arterial $PO_2$ falls significantly with gestational age (Soothill *et al.* 1986), suggesting an increased fractional oxygen extraction in the human fetus as the gestation progresses (Richardson *et al.* 1998). Oxygen extraction has been found to be increased under some conditions where oxygen delivery is reduced, such as cord compression or CS after labor (Richardson *et al.* 1998).

## CIRCULATION

When the oxygenated blood comes back to the fetus from the placenta through the umbilical vein, it enters the fetal liver where it joins the umbilical segment of the left portal vein (Callen 1994). This vessel, before reaching the main portal stem, divides into small branches supplying the hepatic parenchyma and a thin muscular vein, the ductus venosus. The majority of blood goes through the liver to the inferior vena cava, but a proportion (which can vary) will bypass this organ through the ductus. Color Doppler studies have shown two streams, the left and the right, and these have been seen to extend into the inferior vena cava before the right atrium (Kiserud *et al.* 1992). The right stream carries the less oxygenated blood from the liver and the inferior part of the body to the right atrium and ventricle. The left pathway transports the more oxygenated blood directly from the placenta through the ductus venosus to the left atrium. This differential flow is facilitated by the Eustachian valve and septum primum, which conduct the blood through the foramen ovale to the left chambers.

From the left ventricle, the blood goes to the aortic arch and through the neck vessels to the brain. Soon after the division of the vessels to the head and neck, the aortic arch joins the ductus arteriosus, which shunts blood from the pulmonary artery into the aorta, and so a mixture of oxygenated and deoxygenated blood is distributed to the rest of the fetal body. Finally the umbilical arteries, which arise from the internal iliac arteries, reach the placenta and complete the circulatory cycle.

## NORMAL GAS EXCHANGE ACROSS THE PLACENTA – DIFFUSION vs. PERFUSION LIMITATION

Fetal vessels in the placenta are distributed into 15–20 cotyledons. Here, the vessels divide to form the villous tree, which is bathed by maternal blood in the intervillous space. The human placenta is consequently classified as the hemochorial type and feto-maternal exchange occurs across the syncytial-vascular membrane in an area that varies from 4 to 14 $m^2$ (Sadler 1995). Comparing the placenta with the lung, it appears to be a less efficient organ, because despite their similar weight, the oxygen transfer rate at term is about 24 ml of oxygen per minute, which is about 10–20 times less than the oxygen exchanged by the lungs (Longo 1981).

The circulation of the fetal blood in the villi permits the exchange of gases by diffusion, favored by the high partial pressure gradients between the maternal and fetal blood flow. The exchange is restricted by diffusion of the molecules across the membrane but also by the blood flow in both fetal and maternal compartments (Longo 1981). In other words, if the blood flow is slow enough, and if the membrane is sufficiently permeable to $O_2$, maternal and fetal blood could exit the exchanger with similar $pO_2$ values.

### FETAL RESPIRATION

Normal respiration in fetal cells requires oxygen and glucose to produce energy. Glucose is transformed into pyruvate in the cytoplasm from where it enters into the mitochondria and is metabolized by the Krebs cycle. As a consequence, carbon dioxide and high-energy electrons are produced, which are carried by NADH and $FADH_2$ into a complex system of electron carriers in the mitochondrial inner membrane (respiratory chain). Here, they combine with molecular oxygen to produce water in a series of redox reactions that lead to a net production of 36 molecules of ATP at the end of the cycle.

## IMPAIRED OXYGEN DELIVERY TO THE FETUS

Under conditions of abnormally low oxygen levels, the process of metabolizing glucose occurs in a less efficient way than when there is ample oxygen. Pyruvate cannot enter the Krebs cycle to be oxidated but is instead transformed into lactate by accepting $H^+$ from NADH. The overall net energy production of the process is only two molecules of ATP compared with 36 released by the aerobic pathway. With anaerobic respiration, the fetal cells can continue to work for a while but at the expense of increasing the $H^+$ ion concentration in the cytoplasm and subsequently in the blood. When the oxygen supply is restored, the accumulated lactate is converted back to pyruvate, and NADH hydrogen is transferred to the flavoprotein cytochrome chain.

When placental gas exchange is significantly impaired (at any step of the oxygen transport pathway) and the compensatory mechanisms have become insufficient, the fetus develops hypoxemia. Also, progressive hypercapnia will occur, and so respiratory acidosis will be developed. This is reflected in an umbilical artery $PCO_2$ of 75 mmHg or more at birth (Low 1994) with a correspondingly low pH. Such a respiratory acidosis can occur in a variety of clinical conditions, such as in a sudden decrease of placental or umbilical perfusion or maternal hypoventilation. If the situation persists, anaerobic metabolism will eventually lead to metabolic acidosis where base will be consumed (buffer base <30 mmol/l), the umbilical artery base deficit may fall to as low as 12–16 mmol/l, and the pH will decrease.

By strict definition, respiratory acidosis occurs when there is an increased $PCO_2$ with a low pH but a normal bicarbonate ($HCO_3^-$) and metabolic acidosis is a low pH with a normal $PCO_2$ but decreased $HCO_3^-$. Mixed acidosis is when there is an increased $PCO_2$ as well as a decreased $HCO_3$. In severe respiratory acidosis, $HCO_3^-$ will be increased by 1 mEq/l for each 10 mmHg increased $PCO_2$, but it is important to realize that $HCO_3$ is not measured in blood by most blood gas machines but calculated from the $PCO_2$ and pH measurements.

Chronic fetal hypoxemia from placental dysfunction leads to hypoxia, hypercapnia, hyperlacticemia and acidosis, and so mixed respiratory and metabolic acidosis (Nicolaides *et al.* 1989). Such a mixed chronic acidemia in SGA fetuses has been shown to be associated with somewhat reduced subsequent neurodevelopment (Soothill *et al.* 1995). In contrast, a short-term, acute, mixed acidosis can be severe, and no abnormal outcome would be expected, provided the fetus was well before this event. These factors make the distinction between respiratory and metabolic acidosis no longer useful, and the terms chronic or acute acidosis are preferred, (Bobrow & Soothill 1999).

In studies by cordocentesis in normal pregnancies, the umbilical vein lactate concentration was higher than in the artery towards the end of pregnancy, suggesting that the normoxemic human fetus consumes lactate of placental origin (Soothill *et al.* 1986). In anemic human fetuses, it has been possible to study the arteriovenous lactate difference, and it has been shown that the placenta clears lactate from

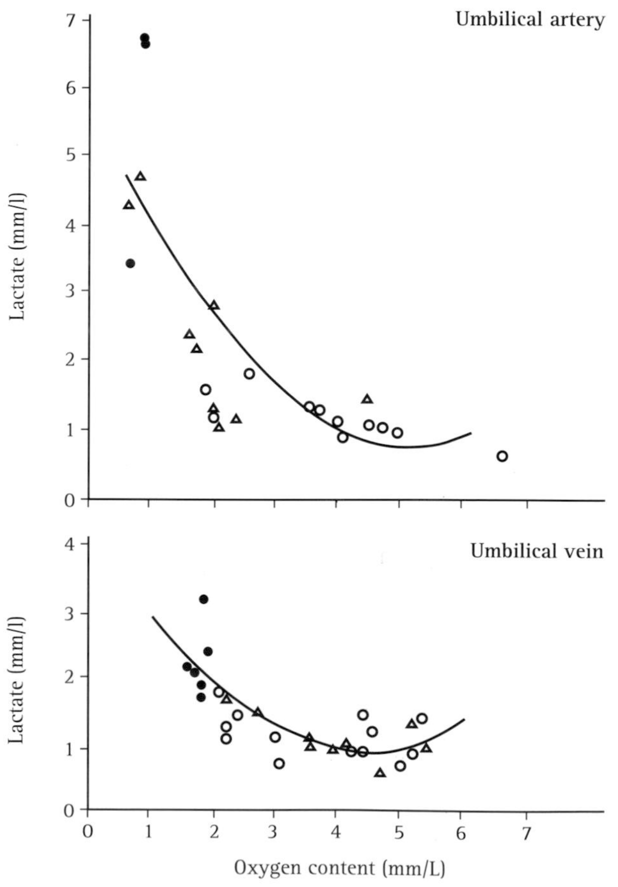


**Figure 26.3** Relationship between fetal plasma lactate concentration to blood oxygen content in 32 rhesus-affected pregnancies. Adapted from Soothill *et al.* (1987a). Open circles indicate the values before transfusion, open triangles indicate the values from subsequent transfusions, and solid circles indicate values from hydropic fetuses.

the fetal circulation as a result of transfer to the mother or metabolism. As shown in Fig. 26.3, the placental capacity to clear lactate is exceeded when anemia is severe, and as a consequence, the lactate venous concentration rises (Soothill *et al.* 1987a) (see later). Also, in hypoxic SGA fetuses, lactic acid is increased (Soothill *et al.* 1987b), probably due to reduced oxidative metabolism, and here, the origin of lactate seems to be fetal (Nicoloides *et al.* 1989). Therefore, it has been suggested that the placenta can repay a fetal oxygen debt, which is analogous to the liver repaying such a deficiency for the muscles in the heavily exercising adults.

## ASPHYXIA

The predictive value of cord blood acidemia at birth for poor subsequent neonatal outcome, particularly brain damage, is very weak (Ruth & Raivio 1988; Fee *et al.* 1990). Although this may be partly explained by variation between individuals, it is clear that the mechanism leading to asphyxia, the gestational age at which it occurred as well as its severity and duration are all important elements when determining the predictive value of blood gases for prognosis. Furthermore, not only is the prediction of damage in a population weak, but the severity of damage in an individual patient depends on many other factors, such as the previous metabolic and cardiovascular states and the repetition or pattern of any previous hypoxic insults.

Asphyxial events, either 'acute' or 'chronic', can have different causes, characteristics and consequences. Therefore, the way to distinguish acute from chronic is not only based on duration, and a time cut-off, but also the nature of the disease and its cause. However, in general events lasting hours are classified as acute and those acting over weeks, chronic (Bobrow & Soothill 1999). This fundamental distinction has not been adequately appreciated in the past, especially when counselling the parents of children asphyxiated at birth, and so these different groups are described separately in the rest of this section.

### ACUTE ASPHYXIA

#### Pathophysiology (see also Chapter 23)

Acute asphyxia is usually followed by a number of changes in the fetal circulation mediated by the autonomic nervous system (Jensen & Lang 1992). The initial response is an increase in the systemic blood pressure due to a rapid and profound vasoconstriction and consequently a decrease in the blood flow to peripheral organs (Jensen *et al.* 1987). Although the total umbilical blood flow is maintained, in hypoxia, the proportion of blood passing through the ductus venosus to the inferior vena cava is increased, thereby reducing the oxygen delivery to the liver (Rudolph 1983; Paulick *et al.* 1990).

A redistribution process tends to facilitate delivery of the most oxygenated blood to the heart, brain and adrenal glands at the expense of the lungs, kidneys, gastrointestinal tract and carcass (Peeters *et al.* 1979; Bocking *et al.* 1988; Ball *et al.* 1994a,b). Blood flow to the heart and brain is maintained overall, but redistribution occurs within the brain, favoring the brainstem at the expense of cerebrum and choroid plexuses. Also, a good blood supply to the adrenals seems to be vital for fetal sheep survival, and vasodilatation leads to almost a doubling of oxygen delivery in hypoxia (Jensen *et al.* 1987). The redistribution responses do not occur in medically sympathectomized fetal sheep (Jensen & Lang 1992), and so seem to be mediated by a chemoreflex (Jensen & Hanson 1995) and possibly modulated by endogenous opioids (Espinoza *et al.* 1989).

During acute hypoxia, cerebral and myocardial oxidative metabolism are maintained due to an increased blood flow, increased cerebral oxygen extraction and decreased myocardial work (Richardson 1989; Low *et al.* 1994). Fetal oxygen consumption is maintained by increased oxygen extraction when fetal oxygen delivery is mildly or moderately reduced for as long as 24 h. With a more severe episode of hypoxia, where oxygen delivery is reduced to over 50%, these mechanisms become inefficient and decompensation occurs. The fetus develops severe metabolic acidosis, hypotension, and variable degrees of damage influenced by individual levels of tolerance (Ball *et al.* 1994a).

#### Causes

Oxygen delivery to the uterus can be acutely affected by many conditions that result in maternal hypotension, impairment of utero-placental blood supply, placental abruption or obstruction of umbilical blood flow. Very severe maternal hypotension can be caused by many conditions such as massive maternal hemorrhage, an exaggerated response to hypotensive drugs or after epidural anesthesia. The latter can occur due to the loss of sympathetic tone in the legs, which leads to vasodilatation when epidural or spinal anesthesia is undertaken without adequate intravascular volume preload. Hypertonic uterine contractions can cause a reduction of the maternal blood supply due to a high intrauterine pressure and high tension in the uterine wall, which is crossed by branches of the uterine artery to reach the placenta. Placental abruption occurs when the placenta is partly or completely detached from the uterine wall, so losing part or all the gas exchange surface. This is usually a sudden phenomenon, which occurs more frequently in some obstetric conditions such as pre-eclamsia. Finally, cord compression can also interrupt fetal gas exchange. This can be intermittent with uterine contractions in labor, when the umbilical cord is around the neck or in oligohydramnios, but also sustained as seen in true knots or cord prolapse.

#### Diagnosis with blood gases

The blood gas and acid–base state have been used to assess fetal well-being during labor or following birth. The American College of Obstetricians and Gynecologists has stated that a plausible link between perinatal asphyxia and a subsequent neurological deficit cannot be made unless the umbilical artery pH is less than 7.00, accompanied by both a significant metabolic component as well as an abnormal newborn course (American College of Obstetricians and Gynecologists 1992). An abnormal newborn course refers to persistently low Apgar scores (e.g. 0–3 for longer than 5 min), signs of newborn encephalopathy and other organ compromises such as in the cardiovascular, respiratory and renal systems.

Due to the heterogeneity of factors related to the nature and severity of the exposure to asphyxia, it is still not possible to predict the occurrence or extent of damage in an individual fetus (Parer 1998). As mentioned above, acidosis does not predict neurologic dysfunction (Ruth & Raivio 1988; Fee *et al.* 1990), and also a very wide range of acid–base values are found in babies with a normal condition, as indicated by Apgar scores (Helwig *et al.* 1996). At present, the long-term outcome is better predicted by classifying the severity of the intrapartum asphyxia combined with consideration of the short-term neonatal events rather than blood gases alone (Low 1997).

Although it is not possible to predict asphyxia at birth or its future consequences with fetal blood gases only, normal results may help to exclude intrapartum hypoxia as a cause of brain damage (Winkler *et al.* 1991). However, it has to be considered that a fetus could have been damaged by an earlier acute asphyxial event that was corrected before labor started such that the blood gases at delivery would not necessarily be abnormal. In the same way, gas analysis can be affected by attempting to improve the condition of an asphyxiated fetus during labor with the use of maternal oxygen therapy or tocolysis (Tejani *et al.* 1983; Burke *et al.* 1989; McNamara *et al.* 1993).

### Scalp blood gases

Cardiotocography (CTG) is a good tool for detecting fetal acidosis, but the specificity of a non-reassuring test is poor, giving an unacceptably high false positive rate. One study reported a 99.8% false positive rate in a group of 155 636 children over 2500 g and estimated that according to CTG criteria, 2324 non-beneficial CS would have been done to avoid one child with cerebral palsy (Nelson *et al.* 1996).

Intrapartum scalp blood samples to improve fetal assessment in the presence of ominous CTG patterns have been effective in reducing the increased intervention rate (Zalar & Quilligan 1979; Ayromlooli & Garfinkel 1980; Young *et al.* 1980; Katz *et al.* 1981), but the technique is only possible after cervical dilatation and rupture of the membranes. After a small incision in the scalp, a capillary blood sample can be obtained for testing. It provides only a single 'snapshot' of fetal acid/base status and so gives no information about the previous fetal condition or the trend of change. There are some devices for continuous tissue pH measurement (Small *et al.* 1989), but more recently, the trend has been to replace these with non-invasive techniques. A scalp blood pH between 7.24 and 7.20 is considered borderline and less than 7.2 as acidotic (Bretscher & Saling 1967). It is important to keep in mind that scalp blood pH may be influenced by the maternal acid–base status and perhaps caput succedaneum (O'Connor *et al.* 1979).

Although scalp sampling has been very useful for many years, there are some concerns about the technique. It is relatively invasive and so could increase the transmission rate of infectious diseases such as HIV. The necessity of repeated sampling and the technical difficulties involved in obtaining adequate samples can be a problem. The equipment used is relatively expensive and may be required infrequently. Also, the poor correlation between pH and predictable neurologic consequences in the child has led some to rely on fetal heart-rate monitoring and propose that scalp pH sampling should be removed from standards of care (Perkins 1997).

### Optical spectroscopy

In the last few years, there has been a trend towards non-invasive devices to continuously monitor fetal oxygenation, especially of the brain. Optical spectroscopy is a technique that estimates blood oxygen saturation based on the different absorption properties of oxyhemoglobin and deoxyhemoglobin to red and near infra-red light (Benaron *et al.* 1995). This wavelength can penetrate through the fetal skull and brain, from where it is scattered in a constant way. Differences detected in diffused or transmitted light intensity can be attributed to the different absorption coefficient of oxygenated to deoxygenated hemoglobin (Kurth *et al.* 1993; Benaron *et al.* 1995). There are two optical spectroscopy-based techniques to monitor fetal hemoglobin oxygen saturation in labor, cerebral optical spectroscopy and fetal pulse oximetry. Cerebral optical spectroscopy uses a transmission device, with light-emitting diodes and a photo-detector positioned on opposite sides of the vascular bed. This allows the measurement of light absorption of the entire cerebral vascular bed, which is mainly venous blood (Wahr *et al.* 1996).

Pulse oximetry was introduced to medicine in the late 1970s, and thereafter, it has been used in several medical disciplines such as anesthetics, adult and neonatal intensive care. It uses a reflectance system, where the light-emitting diode and photo-detector are positioned adjacent to one another, on the same skin surface, with a pulsed signal to detect changes in the pulsatile arterial bed. A recent validation of the technique in human fetuses has included comparisons with umbilical vein oxygen saturation and cord blood pH at birth (McNamara *et al.* 1992). An oxygen saturation of less than 30% is a useful threshold to define a risk of fetal acidosis (Carbonne *et al.* 1997; Goffinet *et al.* 1997; East *et al.* 1997; Kuhnert *et al.*, 1993), but acidosis follows only when a low oxygen saturation is maintained for long periods. In one study of 400 labors, the fetal pH fell by 0.02 pH units/10 min, while the fetal saturation was less or equal 30%. Acidosis was never found when the saturation was under 30% for less than 10 min in a previously non-acidemic fetus (Seelbach-Gobel *et al.* 1999).

Currently, the optical devices are being used in association with CTG and fetal scalp blood analysis, but in view of the problems with both mentioned above, the role of the non-invasive oximetry techniques may increase in the future. Randomized trials comparing CTG and fetal scalp sampling with CTG and pulse oximetry are being considered, but to the knowledge of the authors, none has been reported at the time of writing.

### Cord blood gases

Blood samples can be easily obtained from the umbilical artery and vein after delivery from a section of the cord clamped before the neonate takes a first breath. This is a very useful technique to assess retrospectively the condition of the fetus, and its results can give a valuable guide to immediate neonatal care. Cord blood gases have helped us to understand many aspects of the pathophysiology and incidence of asphyxia at birth and to evaluate both our management of labor and the efficacy of new methods of fetal assessment (Gordon & Johnson 1985). However, unless acidemia is severe its correlation with neurologic dysfunction is quite poor (see above).

Attempts to improve the prediction of asphyxia include determination of the origin of acidosis (maternal or fetal) to distinguish between respiratory and metabolic acidosis (Ingemarsson & Arulkumaran 1986; Goodwin *et al.* 1992; Low *et al.* 1994) and to assess differences in arteriovenous pH, $PCO_2$ and $PO_2$ (Westgate *et al.* 1994; Belai *et al.* 1998). Since the duration of the insult is usually not known, Low has theorized that the umbilical arterio-venous buffer base difference may help, because it varies inversely with the duration of the acute asphyxia (<6 mmol/l indicating long-term and > 6 mmol/l short-term). A small arterial–venous difference is also expected in placental dysfunction (Low *et al.* 1994).

It is very important that appropriate normal ranges are used to interpret cord blood pH. Often, a low normal pH is interpreted as abnormal – some published values are shown in Table 1. Even when these ranges are used, values below the normal range (–2 SD) are usually associated with a normal outcome.

## CHRONIC ASPHYXIA

### Pathophysiology (see also Chapter 23)

The animal models of chronic asphyxia do not completely resemble human placental dysfunction, so care must be taken when trying to use these data to understand the process in the human fetus (Soothill *et al.* 1989). Also, animal experiments described as 'chronic' have often referred to hours or, at most, days of study, so the results may be more relevant to acute rather than chronic asphyxia in humans. However, some data are available, and in the sheep fetus, when hypoxia is prolonged over several days, oxygen consumption is no longer sustained and starts to fall with diminishing oxygen delivery (Anderson *et al.* 1986). With chronic oxygen restriction over several days, redistribution of blood flow to vital organs becomes less pronounced than with acute asphyxia (Richardson *et al.* 1998). A considerable reduction in oxygen consumption can be tolerated because of adaptive mechanisms such as reduced fetal activity and a lowered metabolic rate: therefore, the growth-retarded fetus can become less active (Richardson *et al.* 1998). In the human, the hypoxemic small-for-gestational-age (SGA) fetus further compensates by increasing oxygen transport in the blood by increasing the manufacture of hemoglobin (Soothill *et al.* 1987a) as a result of increased plasma erythropoietin (Snijders *et al.* 1993).

Fetal growth retardation has been induced experimentally in several species using maternal under-nutrition, chronic hypoxia, prolonged reduction in uterine blood flow, reduction in placental size, and endocrine alterations. A sheep model, using the pre-conceptual removal of endometrial caruncles, has been able to produce fetal growth retardation by reducing placental size. The study showed that the fetuses were chronically starved, hypoxemic, polycythemic, and hypoglycemic (Robinson *et al.* 1979), so mimicking the findings in human chronic placental dysfunction.

Severe fetal anemia can also reduce fetal oxygen content and cause acidemia when the hemoglobin concentration has

**Table 26.1 Normal pH values for umbilical artery at birth (vaginal delivery vs. CS)**

| Authors | Vaginal delivery Mean ±SD | –2 SD | Cesarean section Mean ±SD |
|---|---|---|---|
| Helwig *et al.* (1996) | 7.26 ± 0.08 | 7.10 | – |
| Ruth & Raivio (1988) | 7.29 ± 0.07 | 7.15 | 7.31 ± 0.03 |
| Loh *et al.* (1998) | 7.21 ± 0.08 | 7.05 | 7.22 ± 0.07 |
| Yeomans *et al.* (1985) | 7.28 ± 0.05 | 7.18 | – |
| Yoon and Kim (1994) | 7.24 ± 0.07 | 7.10 | No labor 7.27 ± 0.05<br>Labor 7.26 ± 0.05 |

The lower limit of normal (–2SD) is shown for normal vaginal deliveries.

dropped to about one-third of the normal value for the gestational age (4–6 g/dl) with an oxygen content below 2 mmol/l (Soothill *et al.* 1987a) (Fig. 3). The fetus reacts by increasing the blood-flow velocity and redistributing oxygen delivery in favor of the most vital organs (Fumia *et al.* 1984), as in placental insufficiency, thus leading to a decrease in pH and $HCO_3$ and an increase in umbilical artery lactate concentration. The terminal state of fetal hydrops is interpreted as the inability of the fetus to sustain the increased cardiac output in hypoxic conditions (Soothill *et al.* 1987c).

## Causes

### Maternal

Sustained reduction in fetal oxygen availability throughout the pregnancy can occur as a consequence of severe maternal disease causing maternal hypoxemia, including cardiac and respiratory diseases. However, in order to produce significant fetal effects, the maternal disease may be sufficiently severe to produce infertility. Other maternal diseases, particularly those affecting the uteroplacental vascular bed (pre-eclampsia, connective tissue diseases, diabetes, chronic hypertension) may reduce fetal oxygenation. In general, maternal anemia does not affect fetal oxygenation, because the determining factor for placental oxygen transfer is the $PO_2$ difference, which is not affected by maternal anemia. Since maternal oxygen supply to the placenta is usually maintained by increased maternal blood flow and the fetal hemoglobin concentration is normal (Soothill 1994), the fetal blood oxygen content will be normal. This has been confirmed in animal studies when chronically anemic pregnant ewes have shown that the fetus is not hypoxemic or acidemic (Mostello *et al.* 1991).

### Placental

Variable grades of hypoxemia and metabolic acidosis may occur in placental dysfunction (Pardi *et al.* 1987; Soothill *et al.* 1987b). The most established cause is when the normal cytotrophoblast invasion of the distal segments of the spiral arteries during the late first and early second trimester is incomplete (Pijnenborg *et al.* 1980). This process has been shown to occur incompletely in women who develop pre-eclampsia and when there is fetal growth restriction probably due to an abnormal interaction between trophoblast and the spinal arteries (Khong *et al.* 1986), which leads to a dysfunctional placenta. Others have postulated that the origin of fetal hypoxia in these SGA fetuses is due to a failure of oxygen transport from the intervillous space to the umbilical vein. If this were so, the intervillous $PO_2$ would be very close to maternal arterial $PO_2$. This 'chronic intra-placental hyperoxia' may be the cause of a reaction in the trophoblast and the villous core responsible for the impairment of oxygen transport (Kingdom & Kaufmann 1997).

Whatever the site of the problem, many other abnormal nutrient and hormonal findings also occur in SGA fetuses and probably relate to impaired placental function. These results have been reviewed previously, and they are beyond the scope of this chapter (Soothill *et al.* 1992a; Soothill 1994).

### Fetal

Diseases of the fetus can occasionally lead to hypoxia and also acidosis, particularly severe fetal anemia (Soothill *et al.* 1987c) as a result of hemolysis (Rhesus immunization), infections (Parvovirus B-19), feto-maternal hemorrhage or hemoglobinopathies (alpha-thalassemia major). Structural heart abnormalities can produce abnormal organ perfusion due to reduced cardiac output. This is also seen in some fetal cardiac arrhythmias, especially in congenital heart block or supraventricular tachycardia, where the high heart rate prevents a normal filling of the main cardiac chambers, consequently reducing the ventricular ejection volume. Finally, another cause of abnormal gases in the fetus is cardiac failure due to a hyperdynamic circulation resulting from intra (hemangioma, arterio-venous malformation) or extra-fetal shunts (twin-to-twin transfusion, TRAP sequence, placental and cord arteriovenous malformations).

## Diagnosis with blood gases

In contrast to acute asphyxia, in which acidemia is caused by acute changes in a previously healthy child, with rapidly changing blood-gas results, in chronic situations, fetal blood gases are more representative of the fetal condition and reflect better the underlining pathology. In these situations, hypoxemia is usually sustained and almost always progressive. When acidemia has developed, a cause–effect relationship with neurological damage seems more likely (Soothill *et al.* 1992b).

Cordocentesis allows fetal blood to be obtained directly from cord vessels during pregnancy from about 18 weeks onwards. Initially, the procedure was done with fetoscopic guidance (Rodeck & Campbell 1978), but more recently, it was simplified to ultrasound guidance (Daffos *et al.* 1983). The needle is directed under ultrasound control to the vessels at about 1 cm from the placental insertion of the cord, ideally targeting the vein. This is the safest place to sample, and the procedure-related risk of pregnancy loss is no higher than 2% as long as a free loop of the cord is avoided. Nevertheless, on some rare occasions, the sample has to be obtained from the right ventricle of the fetal heart or the intrahepatic portion of the umbilical vein, but fetal paralysis or analgesia might be considered in these cases (Montemagno & Soothill 1997). Due to the difference in the gas composition, it is important to identify the vessel sampled as artery or vein to accurately establish the fetal acid–base status. In this sense, perhaps cardiac samples would not be ideal since this blood does not exactly match with 'arterial' or 'venous' composition, because it is incompletely mixed (foramen ovale, ductus arteriosus).

Fetal blood sampling has shown that severe acidosis can occur in non-laboring high-risk fetuses (Nicolaides *et al.* 1986). Normal reference ranges of umbilical venous and arterial blood $PO_2$, $PCO_2$, pH and lactate have been obtained for appropriate gestational age fetuses (Soothill *et al.* 1986; Nicolaides *et al.* 1989); see Table 2.

**Table 26.2 Blood gases, pH and lactate in 208 AGA and 196 SGA fetuses obtained by cordocentesis at 18–38 weeks gestation**

| Parameter | AGA fetuses Mean ± SD | SGA fetuses Mean ± SD |
|---|---|---|
| U artery $PO_2$ | 28.0 ± 4.2 | 20.8 ± 8.0 |
| U vein $PO_2$ | 42.7 ± 7.4 | 31.5 ± 10.0 |
| U artery $PCO_2$ | 35.0 ± 2.0 | 47.3 ± 10.1 |
| U vein $PCO_2$ | 34.9 ± 3.8 | 41.0 ± 9.9 |
| U artery pH | 7.37 ± 0.03 | 7.32 ± 0.07 |
| U vein pH | 7.41 ± 0.03 | 7.35 ± 0.08 |

Only figures for 25 weeks are shown. Since the normal values change with gestational age, the figures shown must not be used to assess results at any gestational age other than 25 weeks. *Source*: Nicolaides *et al.* (1989).

The demonstration of chronic intrauterine hypoxia and acidosis in some growth-retarded fetuses (Soothill *et al.* 1987b) has led some to attempt maternal oxygen therapy, aimed at improving fetal blood gases, while waiting for fetal viability (Nicolaides *et al.* 1987). Although this led to an increased fetal $PO_2$ and improved Doppler flow patterns, no improvements were seen in fetal weight (Battaglia *et al.* 1992) or fetal oxygen consumption (Harding *et al.* 1992). Furthermore, artificial supplements of oxygen and nutrients in theory could be harmful (Harding *et al.* 1992), making this therapy difficult to recommend. Therefore, at present, no *in utero* treatment is possible, and the prognosis depends on the gestational age at which chronic hypoxia and acidosis develop.

Even chronically severely acidotic fetuses may survive and appear well if they can be delivered above 32 weeks gestation, although they might be damaged by chronic oxygen deficiency (Soothill 1994). The mode of delivery in these babies is almost always by CS, because they have achieved a point where placental function is so poor that there is no margin of safety or fetal reserve to withstand even the uterine contractions of normal labor.

A very important advance was when it was shown that hypoxic fetuses can be identified by the non-invasive test of Doppler. Indeed, some have claimed that after knowing the Doppler study results, fetal blood gases have little further value in predicting perinatal death (Nicolini *et al.* 1990). Nevertheless, there is some evidence that infants who were chronically acidemic as fetuses may have lower developmental quotients (Soothill *et al.* 1992b), and although this does not establish acidemia as necessarily causative, it appears that this is quite likely. It has been hypothesized that if the fetuses with placental dysfunction are delivered when they are hypoxemic, but before they become acidemic, neurological damage might be avoided (Soothill 1994).

## Other methods

Nowadays, the only direct clinical method to identify chronic fetal acidemia is cordocentesis, but because it is not free of risk, its use has been limited. Indirect methods to search for chronic asphyxia have been developed, such as CTG and biophysical profile score (BPS), but these are ineffective because of a high false positive rate (Low *et al.* 1986) and a weak association with neonatal morbidity (Soothill *et al.* 1993) and because they do not usually become abnormal until a pre-terminal stage (Ribbert *et al.* 1993).

Currently, Doppler ultrasound is the only non-invasive method that is able to predict with acceptable specificity the existence of chronic asphyxia in the fetus (Nicolaides *et al.* 1988) by detecting the hemodynamic changes that occur in response to fetal hypoxemia and acidemia. Studies in pregnancies with growth-retarded fetuses have shown that altered fetal gases at cordocentesis are associated with an increased impedance to flow in umbilical arteries, descending thoracic aorta, and decreased impedance in common carotids and cerebral arteries (Bilardo *et al.* 1990). Umbilical artery pulsatility index (PI) progressively increases as chronic hypoxemia develops, and the end diastolic flow (EDF) often becomes absent or reversed when acidemia is present (Steiner *et al.* 1995). In advanced acidemia, venous Doppler flow also becomes abnormal, probably reflecting myocardial failure due to hypoxia and ischemia (Hecher *et al.* 1995; Rizzo *et al.* 1995).

When abnormal umbilical arterial Doppler results are obtained in a fetus with normal anatomy, it is possible to classify these SGA fetuses as growth-restricted as a consequence of dysfunctional placenta. This diagnosis makes an active management approach essential. Alternatively, normal Dopplers with a SGA fetus at the end of the pregnancy virtually exclude placental insufficiency as causing the small fetal size. These babies can be regarded merely as SGA (Holmes & Soothill 1999). It appears that the obstetric management of these cases does not need to be any different from the normal population (Soothill *et al.* 1999). Nevertheless, screening with umbilical artery Dopplers in a low-risk population has proven to be of limited value (Beattie & Dornan 1989), and at the moment, it is only recommended if the fetus is small for the date. Although antenatal estimation of the fetal weight is possible by ultrasound, it has an error of 10–15% (Chauhan *et al.* 1998), but this varies with the use of different formulae and is increased at both ends of the Gaussian distribution. We opted to use the measurement of the abdominal circumference and classify the fetus as SGA if this is below 2SD for the gestation.

## CONCLUSIONS

Asphyxia is a poor term, which everyone involved in the care of newborns and fetuses should now try to avoid. The word is probably best replaced with 'acidemia', but this has to be used with a very clear understanding of the difference between acute and chronic as described above. The title of this chapter therefore becomes something of a self fulfilling prophecy, but certainly, normal blood gases can be extremely useful in excluding acidosis as a cause of brain damage.

When looked at from the view of a doctor caring for a child with brain damage, obstetric data may give an indication of whether chronic acidosis is likely to have been the cause. The first is the birth weight. If this was less than 2 SD for the gestational age, a chronic *in utero* cause of the brain damage becomes much more likely. This opinion would be supported by oligohydramnios on ultrasound scan but above all by an abnormal umbilical artery Doppler assessment. If the Dopplers were abnormal (umbilical artery PI > 2SD) in a baby with a birth weight less than 2SD, then chronic placental insufficiency is almost certain (Bobrow & Soothill 1999) and so should be seriously considered as the cause of any brain damage.

Normal blood gases make previous chronic acidosis very unlikely. Acidosis at birth is very common and, when acute, is very rarely a cause of brain damage. Acidosis at birth in a baby with the other features of chronic placental insufficiency is important and may be a valuable predictor of outcome.

### Key Points

- The terms asphyxia, hypoxemia, acidosis and acidemia are often used in a confusing and sometimes interchangeable way, which leads to confusion and misunderstanding
- Asphyxia is defined as a condition of impaired gas exchange, which if persistent, will lead to progressive hypoxemia and hypercapnia – about 2% of neonates are born with the condition
- The effect of asphyxia on the individual neonate is variable and difficult to predict. Outcome depends on the severity of the asphyxia, its duration, the gestational age at which it occurred, and the mechanisms that led to its development
- It is important to distinguish between acute (hours) and chronic (weeks) asphyxia as the mechanisms and effects are different.
- Less than 20% of cerebral palsy may be the result of events which occur in labour or delivery
- Fetal scalp blood sampling remains the standard technique to assess acid/base status in labour although other techniques, such as pulse oximetry are being evaluated as direct estimates of oxygen status

## REFERENCES


✪ American College of Obstetricians and Gynecologists (1992) Fetal and neonatal neurologic injury. Washington, DC: *American College of Obstetricians and Gynecologists*, ACOG technical bulletin no. 163.

Anderson D F, Parks C M & Faber J J (1986) Fetal $O_2$ consumption in sheep during controlled long-term reductions in umbilical blood flow. *Am J Physiol* 250: H1037–H1042.

Ayromlooli J & Garfinkel R (1980) Impact of fetal scalp blood pH on the incidence of caesarean section performed for fetal distress. *Int J Gynaecol Obstet* 17: 391–392.

Ball R H, Espinoza M I, Parer J T *et al.* (1994a) Regional blood flow in asphyxiated fetuses with seizures. *Am J Obstet Gynecol* 170: 156–161.

Ball R H, Parer J T, Caldwell L E *et al.* (1994b) Regional blood flow and metabolism in ovine fetuses during severe cord occlusion. *Am J Obstet Gynecol* 171: 1549–1555.

Battaglia C, Artini P G, D'Ambrogio G *et al.* (1992) Maternal hyperoxygenation in the treatment of intrauterine growth retardation. *Am J Obstet Gynecol* 167:430–435.

Bax M & Nelson K B (1993) Birth asphyxia: a statement. *Dev Med Child Neurol* 35: 1002–1004.

Beattie R B & Dornan J C (1989) Antenatal screening for intrauterine growth retardation with umbilical artery Doppler ultrasonography. *BMJ* 298(6674):631–635.

Belai Y, Goodwin T M, Durand M *et al.* (1998) Umbilical arteriovenous $pO_2$ and $pCO_2$ differences and neonatal morbidity in term infants with severe acidosis. *Am J Obstet Gynecol* 178:13–19.

Benaron D A, Kurth C D, Steven J M *et al.* (1995) Transcranial optical path length in infants by near-infrared phase-shift spectroscopy. *J Clin Monit* 11:109–117.

Bilardo C M, Nicolaides K H & Campbell S (1990) Doppler measurements of fetal and uteroplacental circulations: relationship with umbilical venous blood gases measured at cordocentesis. *Am J Obstet Gynecol* 162:115–120.

Bobrow C S, Soothill P W (1999) Causes and consequences of fetal acidosis. *Arch Dis Child Fetal Neonatal* 80:F246–F249.

Bocking A D, Ganong R, White S E *et al.* (1988) Circulatory response to prolonged hypoxemia in fetal sheep. *Am J Obstet Gynecol* 159:1418–1424.

Bozzetti P, Buscaglia M, Cetin I *et al.* (1987) Respiratory gases, acid-base balance and lactate concentrations of the midterm human fetus. *Biol Neonate* 52:188–197.

Bretscher J & Saling E (1967) pH values in the human fetus during labor. *Am J Obstet Gynecol* 97:906–911.

Burke M S, Porreco R P, Day D *et al.* (1989) In trauterine resuscitation with tocolysis. An alternate month clinical trial. *J Perinatol* 9:296–300.

Callen P W (1994) Ultrasound evaluation of normal fetal anatomy. In: Callen P W (ed.) *Ultrasonography in obstetrics and gynecology*. Philadelphia, PA: WB Saunders 2nd edn, pp. 144–188.

Carbonne B, Langer B, Goffinet F *et al.* (1997) Multicenter study on the clinical value of fetal pulse oximetry. II. Compared predictive values of pulse oximetry and fetal blood analysis. The French Study Group on Fetal Pulse Oximetry. *Am J Obstet Gynecol* 177: 593–598.

Chauhan S P, Charania S F, McLaren R A *et al.* (1998) Ultrasonographic estimate of birth weight at 24 to 34 weeks: a multicenter study. *Am J Obstet Gynecol* 179:909–916.

Daffos F, Capella-Pavlovsky M & Forestier F (1983) Fetal blood sampling via the umbilical cord using a needle guided by ultrasound. Report of 66 cases. *Prenat Diagn* 3:271–277.

East C E, Dunster K R, Colditz P B *et al.* (1997) Fetal oxygen saturation monitoring in labour: an analysis of 118 cases. *Aust NZJ Obstet Gynaecol* 37:397–401.

Espinoza M, Riquelme R, Germain A M *et al.* (1989) Role of endogenous opioids in the cardiovascular responses to asphyxia in fetal sheep. *Am J Physiol* 256:R1063–1068.

Fee S C, Malee K, Deddish R *et al.* (1990) Severe acidosis and subsequent neurologic status. *Am J Obstet Gynecol* 162:802–86.

Fumia F D, Edelstone D I & Holzman I R (1984) Blood flow and oxygen delivery to fetal organs as functions of fetal hematocrit. *Am J Obstet Gynecol* 150:274–282.

Gill R W, Kossoff G, Warren P S *et al.* (1984) Umbilical venous flow in normal and complicated pregnancy. *Ultrasound Med Biol* 10:349–363.

Gilstrap L C (1998) In: Creasy R & Resnik R (eds.) *Maternal-fetal medicine* Philadelphia, PA: Saunders. *Chapter 22*, 4th edn, pp. 331–339.

Goffinet F, Langer B, Carbonne B *et al.* (1997) Multicenter study on the clinical value of fetal pulse oximetry. I. Methodologic evaluation. The French Study Group on Fetal Pulse Oximetry. *Am J Obstet Gynecol* 177:1238–1246.

Goodwin T M, Belai I, Hernandez P *et al.* (1992) Asphyxial complications in the term newborn with severe umbilical acidemia. *Am J Obstet Gynecol* 167:1506–1512.

Gordon A & Johnson J W (1985) Value of umbilical blood acid–base studies in fetal assessment. *J Reprod Med* 30:329–336.

Harding J E, Owens J A & Robinson J S (1992) Should we try to supplement the growth retarded fetus? A cautionary tale. *Br J Obstet Gynaecol* 99:707–709.

Hecher K, Campbell S, Doyle P *et al.* (1995) Assessment of fetal compromise by Doppler ultrasound investigation of the fetal circulation. Arterial, intracardiac, and venous blood flow velocity studies. *Circulation* 91:129–138.

Helwig J T, Parer J T, Kilpatrick S J *et al.* (1996) Umbilical cord blood acid-base state: what is normal? *Am J Obstet Gynecol* 174:1807–1812.

Holmes R & Soothill P W (1999) Small fetuses with normal Dopplers are appropriately grown with normal pregnancy outcome. Presented at BMFMS 1999. *J Obstet Gynaecol* 19:S23.

Ingemarsson I & Arulkumaran S (1986) Fetal acid–base balance in low-risk patients in labour. *Am J Obstet Gynecol* 155:66–69.

Jensen A, Lang U (1992) Foetal circulatory responses to arrest of uterine blood flow in sheep: effects of chemical sympathectomy. *J Dev Physiol* 17:75–86.

Jensen A & Hanson M A (1995) Circulatory responses to acute asphyxia in intact and chemodenervated fetal sheep near term. *Reprod Fertil Dev* 7:1351–1359.

Jensen A, Hohmann M, Kunzel W (1987) Dynamic changes in organ blood flow and oxygen consumption during acute asphyxia in fetal sheep. *J Dev Physiol* 9:543–559.

Katz M, Meizner I, Mazor M *et al.* (1981) Fetal heart rate patterns and scalp blood pH as predictors of fetal distress. *Isr J Med Sci* 17:260–265.

Khong T Y, De Wolf F, Robertson W B *et al.* (1986) Inadequate maternal vascular response to placentation in pregnancies complicated by pre-eclampsia and by small-for-gestational age infants. *Br J Obstet Gynaecol* 93:1049–1059.

Kingdom J C & Kaufmann P (1997) Oxygen and placental villous development: origins of fetal hypoxia. *Placenta* 18:613–621, 623–66.

Kiserud T, Eik-Ness S H, Hellevik L R *et al.* (1992) Ductus venosus: a longitudinal Doppler velocimetric study of the human fetus. *J Matern Fetal Invest* 2:5–11.

Kuhnert M, Seelbach-Goebel B, Butterwegge M (1998) Predictive agreement between the fetal arterial oxygen saturation and fetal scalp pH: results of the German multicenter study. *Am J Obstet Gynecol* 178:330–335.

Kurth C D, Steven J M, Benaron D *et al.* (1993) Near-infrared monitoring of the cerebral circulation. *J Clin Monit* 9:163–170.

Little W J (1862) On the influence of abnormal parturition, difficult labour, premature birth and asphyxia neonatorum on the mental and physical condition of the child, especially in relation to deformities. *Trans London Obstet Soc* 3:293–325.

Loh S F, Woodworth A & Yeo G S (1998) Umbilical cord blood gas analysis at delivery. *Singapore Med J* 39:151–155.

Longo L D (1981) The interrelations of maternal–fetal transfer and placental blood flow. In: Young M, Boyd RDH, Longo L D *et al.* (1981) (eds.) *Placental transfer methods and interpretations.* Placenta Supplement 2. Philadelphia, PA: WB Saunders pp. 45–64.

Low J A (1997) Intrapartum fetal asphyxia: Definition, diagnosis, and classification. *Am J Obstet Gynecol* 176:957–959.

Low J A, McGrath M J, Marshall S J *et al.* (1986) The relationship between antepartum fetal heart rate, intrapartum fetal heart rate, and fetal acid-base status. *Am J Obstet Gynecol* 154:769–776.

Low J A, Panagiotopoulos C & Derrick E J (1994) Newborn complications after intrapartum asphyxia with metabolic acidosis in the term fetus. *Am J Obstet Gynecol* 170:1081–1087.

McNamara H, Chung D C, Lilford R *et al.* (1992) Do fetal pulse oximetry readings at delivery correlate with cord blood oxygenation and acidaemia? *Br J Obstet Gynaecol* 99:735–738.

McNamara H, Johnson N & Lilford R (1993) The effect on fetal arteriolar oxygen saturation resulting from giving oxygen to the mother measured by pulse oximetry. *Br J Obstet Gynecol* 100:446–449.

Montemagno R & Soothill P W (1997) Invasive procedures. In Fisk N and Moise K (eds.) *Fetal therapy, invasive and transplacental.* Cambridge: Cambridge University Press, pp 9–26.

Mostello D, Chalk C, Khoury J *et al.* (1991) Chronic anemia in pregnant ewes: maternal and fetal effects. *Am J Physiol* 261:R1075–R1083.

✪ Nelson K B, Dambrosia J M, Ting T Y *et al.* (1996) Uncertain values of electronic fetal monitoring in predicting cerebral palsy. *N Engl J Med* 334:613–618.

Nicolaides K H, Soothill P W, Rodeck C H *et al.* (1986) Ultrasound-guided sampling of umbilical cord and placental blood to assess fetal wellbeing. *Lancet* 1:1065–1067.

Nicolaides K H, Campbell S, Bradley R J *et al.* (1987) Maternal oxygen therapy for intrauterine growth retardation. *Lancet* 1:942–945.

Nicolaides K H, Bilardo C M, Soothill P W *et al.* (1988) Absence of end diastolic frequencies in umbilical artery: a sign of fetal hypoxia and acidosis. *Br Med J* 297:1026–1027.

Nicolaides K H, Soothill P W, Clewell W H *et al.* (1988) Fetal haemoglobin measurement in the assessment of red cell isoimmunisation. *The Lancet* 1 (8594):1073–1075.

✪ Nicolaides K H, Economides D L & Soothill P W (1989) Blood gases, pH and lactate in appropriate- and small-for-gestational-age fetuses. *Am J Obstet Gynecol* 161:996–1001.

Nicolini U, Nicolaidis P, Fisk N M *et al.* (1990) Limited role of fetal blood sampling in prediction of outcome in intrauterine growth retardation. *Lancet* 336:768–772.

O'Connor M C, Hytten F E & Zanelli G D (1979) Is the fetus 'scalped' in labour? *Lancet* 2:947–949.

Pardi G, Buscaglia M, Ferrazzi E *et al.* (1987) Cord sampling for the evaluation of oxygenation and acid–base balance in growth-retarded human fetuses. *Am J Obstet Gynecol* 157:1221–1228.

Parer J T (1998) Effects of fetal asphyxia on brain cell structure and function: limits of tolerance. *Comp Biochem Physiol A Mol Integr Physiol* 119:711–716.

Paulick R P, Meyers R L, Rudolph C D *et al.* (1990) Venous responses to hypoxemia in the fetal lamb. *J Dev Physiol* 14:81–88.

Peeters L L H, Sheldon R E, Jones M D (1974) *et al.* Blood flow to fetal organs as a function of arterial oxygen content. *Am J Obstet Gynecol* 135:637–646.

Perkins R P (1997) Requiem for a heavyweight: the demise of scalp blood pH sampling. *J Matern Fetal Med* 6:298–300.

Pijnenborg R, Dixon G, Robertson W B *et al.* (1980) Trophoblastic invasion of human decidua from 8 to 18 weeks of pregnancy. *Placenta* 1:3–19.

✪ Ribbert L S, Visser G H, Mulder E J *et al.* (1993) Changes with time in fetal heart rate variation, movement incidences and haemodynamics in intrauterine growth retarded fetuses: a longitudinal approach to the assessment of fetal well being. *Early Hum Dev* 31:195–208.

Richardson B S (1989) Fetal adaptive responses to asphyxia. *Clin Perinatol* 16: 595–611.

Richardson B, Nodwell A, Webster K *et al.* (1998) Fetal oxygen saturation and fractional extraction at birth and the relationship to measures of acidosis. *Am J Obstet Gynecol* 178:572–579.

Rizzo G, Capponi A, Arduini D *et al.* (1995) The value of fetal arterial, cardiac and venous flows in predicting pH and blood gases measured in umbilical blood at cordocentesis in growth retarded fetuses. *Br J Obstet Gynaecol* 102:963–969.

Robinson J S, Kingston E J, Jones C T *et al.* (1979) Studies on experimental growth retardation in sheep. The effect of removal of a endometrial caruncles on fetal size and metabolism. *J Dev Physiol* 1:379–398.

Rodeck C H & Campbell S (1978) Sampling pure fetal blood by fetoscopy in second trimester of pregnancy. *Br Med J* 2:728–730.

Rudolph A M (1983) Hepatic and ductus venosus blood flows during fetal life. *Hepatology* 3:254–258.

Rurak D, Selke P, Fisher M *et al.* (1987) Fetal oxygen extraction: Comparison of the human and sheep. *Am J Obstet Gynecol* 156:360–366.

✪ Ruth V J, Raivio K O (1988) Perinatal brain damage: predictive value of metabolic acidosis and the Apgar score *BMJ* 297:24–27.

Sadler T W (1995) Fetal membranes and placenta. In: Sadler T W (ed.) *Medical Embryology* Baltimore, MD: Williams & Wilkins, 7th edn, pp. 101–121.

Sarnat H B & Sarnat M S (1976) Neonatal encephalopathy following fetal distress. *Arch Neurol* 33:696–705.

Seelbach-Gobel B, Heupel M, Kuhnert M *et al.* (1999) The prediction of fetal acidosis by means of intrapartum fetal pulse oximetry. *Am J Obstet Gynecol* 180:73–81.

Small M I, Beall M, Platt L D *et al.* (1989) Continuous tissue pH monitoring in the term fetus. *Am J Obstet Gynecol* 161:323–329.

Snijders R J, Abbas A, Melby O *et al.* (1993) Fetal plasma erythropoietin concentration in severe growth retardation. *Am J Obstet Gynecol* 168:615–619.

Soothill P W (1994) Diagnosis of intrauterine growth retardation and its fetal and perinatal consequences. *Acta Paediatr Suppl* 399:55–59.

Soothill P W, Nicolaides K H, Rodeck C H *et al.* (1986) Effects of gestational age on fetal and intervillous blood gas and acid–base values in human pregnancy. *Fetal Ther* 1:168–175.

Soothill P W, Nicolaides K H, Rodeck C H *et al.* (1987a) Relationship of fetal haemoglobin and oxygen content to lactate concentration in Rh isoimmunized pregnancies. *Obstet Gynecol* 69:268–271.

✪ Soothill P W, Nicolaides K H, Campbell S (1987b) Prenatal asphyxia, hyperlacticaemia, hypoglycaemia, and erythroblastosis in growth retarded fetuses. *BMJ* (*Clin Res Ed*) 294:1051–1053.

Soothill P W, Nicolaides K H & Rodeck C H (1987c) Effect of anaemia on fetal acid–base status. *Br J Obstet Gynaecol* 94:880–883.

Soothill P W, Lestas A N, Nicolaides K H *et al.* (1988) 2,3-Diphosphoglicerate in normal, anaemic and transfused human fetuses. *Clin Sci* 1988; 74:527–530.

Soothill P W, Nicolaides K H & Rodeck C H (1989) Fetal blood gas and acid–base parameters. In Rodeck C H (ed.) *Fetal medicine/I.* Oxford: Blackwell Scientific, pp 57–89.

Soothill P W, Ajayi R A & Nicolaides K N (1992a) Fetal biochemistry in growth retardation. *Early Hum Dev* 29:91–97.

Soothill P W, Ajayi R A, Campbell S *et al.* (1992b) Relationship between fetal acidaemia at cordocentesis and subsequent neurodevelopment. *Ultrasound Obstet Gynecol* 2:80–83.

Soothill P W, Ajayi R A, Campbell S *et al.* (1993) Prediction of morbidity in small and normally grown fetuses by fetal heart rate variability, biophysical profile score and umbilical artery Doppler studies. *Br J Obstet Gynaecol* 100:742–745.

✪ Soothill P W, Ajayi R A, Campbell S *et al.* (1995) Fetal oxygenation at cordocentesis, maternal smoking and childhood neuro-development. *Eur J Obstet Gynecol Reprod Biol* 59:21–24.

Soothill P W, Bobrow C S & Holmes R (1999) Small for gestational age is not a diagnosis. *Ultrasound Obstet Gynecol* 13:225–228.

Steiner H, Staudach A, Spitzer D *et al.* (1995) Growth deficient fetuses with absent or reversed umbilical artery end-diastolic flow are metabolically compromised. *Early Hum Dev* 41:1–9.

Tejani N A, Verma U L, Chatterjee S *et al.* (1983) Terbutaline in the management of acute intrapartum fetal acidosis. *J Reprod Med* 28:857–861.

Towell M E (1976) Fetal respiratory physiology. In: Goodwin J W, Godden J O, Chance G W (eds) *Perinatal medicine.* Toronto: Longman Canada pp. 171–186.

Wahr J A, Tremper K K, Samra S *et al.* (1996) Near-infrared spectroscopy: theory and applications. *J Cardiothorac Vasc Anesth* 10:406–418.

Westgate J, Garibaldi J M & Greene K R (1994) Umbilical cord blood gas analysis at delivery: a time for quality data. *Br J Obstet Gynaecol* 101:1054–1063.

Willcourt R F (1987) Fetal blood gases and pH: current application. In Studd J (ed.) *Progress in Obstetric and Gynecology*, Vol. 6. Edinburgh: Churchill Livingstone; pp. 155–174.

Winkler C L, Hauth J C, Tucker J M *et al.* (1991) Neonatal complications at term as related to the degree of umbilical artery acidaemia. *Am J Obstet Gynecol* 164:637–641.

✪ Yeomans E R, Hauth J C, Gilstrap L C 3rd *et al.* (1985) Umbilical cord pH, $PCO_2$, and bicarbonate following uncomplicated term vaginal deliveries. *Am J Obstet Gynecol* 151:798–800.

Yoon B H & Kim S W (1994) The effect of labor on the normal values of umbilical blood acid-base status. *Acta Obstet Gynecol Scand* 73: 555–561.

Young D C, Gray J H, Luther E R *et al.* (1980) Fetal scalp blood pH sampling: Its value in an active obstetric unit. *Am J Obstet Gynecol* 136:276–281.

✪ Zalar R W & Quilligan E J (1979) The influence of scalp sampling on the caesarean section rate for fetal distress. *Am J Obstet Gynecol* 135:239–246.

# Chapter 27 The asphyxiated newborn infant

M. I. Levene

## INTRODUCTION

In the developed world, birth asphyxia is arguably the most common cause of perinatally acquired severe brain injury in full-term infants. It is a tragedy for a normally developed fetus to sustain cerebral injury during the last hours of prenatal life and then to survive for many more years with a major disability.

For pediatricians, birth asphyxia remains a frustrating condition to treat as prevention of the condition is outside their control, and there have been few or no improvements in clinical management in the last 20 years. The antenatal and intrapartum aspects of detection and prevention are discussed in Chapters 24, 25 and 26. Potentially effective new brain protection therapy for birth asphyxia is discussed in Chapter 28.

## DEFINITION

Apnea at birth is a relatively common feature, particularly in premature infants. This may cause the Apgar score to be depressed and require the infant to be resuscitated. There may be little evidence that the baby has suffered the hypoxic–ischemic pathophysiological insult inherent in the term 'birth asphyxia'. Because of the fundamental differences in the definition and neuropathological sequelae of asphyxia between preterm and full-term infants, this chapter only discusses perinatal asphyxia with reference to the mature infant. The neuropathological insults seen in premature infants are predominantly hemorrhagic or ischemic, and intrapartum events only rarely precipitate these conditions. They are discussed in detail in Section IV.

The term asphyxia refers to impairment of placental or pulmonary gas exchange resulting in hypoxemia, hypercapnia and acidosis. 'Birth asphyxia' is widely used as a clinical diagnosis, but there is little consensus as to what is meant by it. Hypoxic–ischemic insult better describes the patho-physiology of intrapartum asphyxia and stresses the two major components of the condition. Hypoxia on its own is well tolerated by the immature brain, providing that minimum quantities of metabolic substrate (mainly glucose) are delivered to the brain. Cerebral ischemia is not well tolerated, and pure ischemic lesions may occur as the result of sudden hypovolemia. The cerebral lesions that develop following an episode of intense ischemia are different to those seen when hypoxia and ischemia act together, as occurs as the result of intrapartum asphyxia. Pure ischemic lesions in premature and full-term infants are discussed in Chapter 22.

The fetus is well adapted to the rigors of labor, and these protective mechanisms are discussed in the previous chapter. Severe hypoxic–ischemic insult may overwhelm these adaptive mechanisms and cause the vital organs to be compromised. The determinants of whether the insult is severe enough to cause dysfunction are its intensity and duration. An intense insult such as cord prolapse or massive placental abruption causes the fetus to be rapidly compromised, whereas a less intense insult such as intermittent placental insufficiency associated with hypertonic uterine contractions will need a longer duration to have a similarly severe effect on the fetus. It is often not possible to know clinically either the degree of intensity or the duration of the intrapartum insult.

## THE 'ASPHYXIA SYNDROME'

There is no universally accepted clinical definition of asphyxia, and all the following features are used as possible markers of the condition; indeed, a recent statement on this condition recommended that the term 'birth asphyxia' should not be used (Bax & Nelson 1993). There are many conditions in medicine that cannot be diagnosed accurately with a blood test or radiological procedure. In these cases, a careful clinical history, together with exclusion of alternative diagnoses, usually suffices to make the diagnosis. There is no test to diagnose birth asphyxia, and it is necessary to adopt a similar approach to that for the diagnosis of migraine or epilepsy. This will involve considering asphyxia as a syndrome, or collection of features, with the exclusion of alternative conditions (Levene 1995). To adopt this approach, it is necessary for three aspects to be considered:

1. assessment of diagnostic criteria
2. exclusion of alternative possible diagnoses
3. consideration of results from contributory diagnostic tests.

Each of these is considered below.

### Assessment of diagnostic criteria

None of the features listed below on their own are diagnostic, but the more that are present, so the more likely it is that asphyxia has occurred. The presence of four out of six items should make the diagnosis of moderate probability, providing that the exclusion criteria are met, and five or six out of six gives a good probability of the diagnosis being generally accepted.

The most common time for a baby to be acutely asphyxiated is at the end of labor, with birth releasing the fetus from a hostile intrauterine environment. In these cases, there is likely to be evidence of increasing fetal distress, poor adaptation to birth and hypoxic–ischemic encephalopathy with evidence of transient impairment in other organ systems. Less commonly, a severe asphyxial event may occur several hours or even days prior to delivery such as prolonged, but reversible, uterine hypertonus due to excess pharmacological stimulation or transient severe maternal hypotension. Under these conditions, the baby may not show fetal distress immediately prior to birth, as cardiovascular recovery from the acute event has occurred, and the baby may be born in relatively good condition. The baby may, nevertheless, show signs of HIE, although the sequence may be altered (e.g. very early convulsions) by the interval between insult and delivery.

Nucleated red blood cells (NRBCs) in the peripheral blood film have been suggested to be a marker of asphyxia (see p. 430). Asphyxiated full-term infants had a significantly higher NRBC count than non-asphyxiated babies of the same gestational age (Phelan *et al.* 1995). There was no statistically significant difference in the numbers of asphyxiated babies with evidence of a more prolonged asphyxial insult as opposed to a terminal severe asphyxial event. Babies thought to have a long-standing asphyxial event had NRBCs present beyond 80 h from birth compared with babies who had sustained a more acute asphyxial event.

### Fetal distress

Fetal asphyxia during labor occurs as the result of placental compromise or, rarely, umbilical cord compression. These conditions affect the entire fetus, and methods to detect fetal distress usually monitor the effects of these insults on the cardiovascular system. Chapter 25 discusses these methods. There is no clinically reliable method for assessing central nervous system function during labor, and evidence of fetal distress does not necessarily indicate that the fetal brain has been compromised. Intrapartum fetal monitoring is not good at distinguishing fetal stress (a normal reaction to the rigors of labor) from fetal distress. Consequently, abnormalities on a cardiotocograph (CTG) are relatively poorly sensitive to intrapartum asphyxia (high number of false positives). The CTG is, however, more likely to be a relatively specific test as a normal CTG probably indicates that the fetus is not suffering from acute intrapartum asphyxia at the time that the CTG is being registered.

### Passage of meconium

Meconium is passed prior to delivery in 10–20% of full-term infants. Heavy contamination of the amniotic fluid has been suggested to be a feature of fetal distress (Meis *et al.* 1978). The passage of meconium is, however, a very weak marker of those babies likely to sustain irreversible cerebral injury as the result of intrapartum asphyxia. Nelson & Ellenberg (1984) reported that only 0.4% of infants weighing more than 2500 g who had meconium-stained liquor were later found to have cerebral palsy.

### Metabolic acidosis

Anaerobic metabolism is a normal physiological response during episodes of hypoxemia with generation of lactic acid. Fetal acidosis may be measured by scalp blood pH or by the base deficit, which better reflects the metabolic component of a low pH. The severity of the metabolic acidosis may reflect either the duration or the intensity of the asphyxial event, but metabolic acidosis does not correlate with those infants who later are shown to have sustained neurological deficit (see Chapter 26). Although fetal acidosis is widely taken to be pH $<7.20$, a more reliable value indicating the possibility of neurological compromise is $\leq 7.05$ or $\leq 7.0$.

### Maladaptation at birth

This refers to the baby who is born in a less than optimal condition, and this can be measured as a low Apgar score or delay in establishing spontaneous respiration. Maladaptation is most likely to occur in preterm infants and does not imply that the baby has suffered a significant hypoxic–ischemic event immediately prior to birth.

Virginia Apgar first described the scoring system which now bears her name (Apgar 1953) and proposed that it should be assessed 1 min after birth. Later, Drage *et al.* (1964) recommended reassessment 5 min after birth. This system is effective for describing the infant's condition shortly after birth but relates poorly to preceding events and is a very weak predictor of those infants who are later identified as having neurodevelopmental deficits caused by perinatal asphyxia (see p. 494). The Apgar score may be influenced by non-asphyxial factors such as prematurity and maternal drug (opiate) depression. Nevertheless, depression of the Apgar score has been widely used in diagnosing perinatal asphyxia, and a score of 3 or less at 5 min is often taken as indicating severe asphyxial insult (Nelson & Ellenberg 1981; Ergander *et al.* 1983).

Donald (1959) defined 'asphyxia neonatorum' as failure to establish spontaneous ventilation at birth, but there may be many causes for this, including depression of ventilation due to drugs, trauma, and, rarely, neuromuscular disorders affecting the onset of spontaneous breathing. Delay in spontaneous respiratory activity is not a good predictor of neurological disability (Ergander *et al.* 1983).

Attempts have been made to identify babies at high risk of neonatal seizures on the basis of very early neonatal markers. Poor condition, as measured by the combination of three factors at birth (Apgar score of $\leq 5$ at 5 min, the need for intubation and a cord blood pH of $\leq 7.00$), has been reported to increase the risk of neonatal seizures (and presumably disability) 340-fold (Perlman & Risser 1996).

### Hypoxic–ischemic encephalopathy

Disturbances in the neurological behavior of the infant following birth may be a sensitive indicator of significant cerebral asphyxial insult. Hypoxic–ischemic encephalopathy (HIE) is a term used to describe a consistent pattern of neurological signs that progress in a regular manner. The clinical features of HIE are described on p. 478. HIE is not the only cause of encephalopathy in the newborn period (Nelson & Leviton 1991), and alternative causes must be considered and excluded before HIE can be reliably used as a feature of neurological deficit. In particular, neonatal convulsions alone with clinical interseizure normality are not a feature of HIE, nor is the baby who shows an unchanging pattern of neurological abnormalities in the newborn period. It has been suggested that in the majority of cases, 'neonatal encephalopathy' in full-term babies may not be due to intrapartum events, but may originate in the antepartum period (Adamson *et al.* 1995).

It is likely that intrapartum asphyxia severe enough to cause neurodevelopmental handicap will be associated with clinical neurological dysfunction, and if no abnormalities occur, the infant appears to be at little risk. Unfortunately, HIE must be a retrospective diagnosis and does not appear to correlate well with the Apgar scores (Levene *et al.* 1986).

### Multiorgan involvement

Severe asphyxia may cause disturbance in a number of organ systems other than the brain (see p. 484). The kidneys and myocardium are particularly vulnerable, but gastrointestinal, endocrine and lung complications may also occur. Evidence of acute and transient compromise to more than one organ suggests that an acute asphyxial event in labor was the common pathway by which these organs were affected. Recently, series of cases have been described of babies who developed HIE with the later development of cerebral palsy and who had no, or only a minor, multiorgan system dysfunction (Pasternak & Gorey 1998, Phelan *et al.* 1998). In most of these cases, intrapartum asphyxia was documented to be of short duration (mean 32 min) and was severe and unexpected such as occurs with uterine rupture and cord prolapse (Phelan *et al.* 1998).

## Exclusion of alternative possible diagnoses

All the individual features of 'asphyxia' discussed above may occur as the result of alternative causes. Failure to establish spontaneous respirations immediately after birth may be due to maternal opiate administration or, more rarely, neuromuscular disorders. Later-onset encephalopathy may be due to a number of conditions, which can be relatively easily excluded (Table 27.1). Hypoglycemia occurs more commonly in asphyxiated infants and may not be severe enough to cause encephalopathy. Severe and persistent hypoglycemia suggests that the abnormal neurological behavior is more likely to be due to hypoglycemia rather than it being an associated factor.

**Table 27.1 Exclusion criteria in consideration of the birth asphyxia syndrome**

| |
|---|
| Meningitis |
| Cerebral hemorrhage |
| Perinatal stroke |
| Brain malformation |
| Dysmorphic or chromosomal conditions |
| Inborn errors of metabolism |
| Severe hypoglycemia |

Routine lumbar puncture, brain imaging, biochemical screening (urine and blood) for inborn errors of metabolism and careful examination for subtle dysmorphic features should be a part of the assessment of all infants in whom the diagnosis of asphyxia is suspected.

## Contributory diagnostic tests

There are three important diagnostic tests that help to determine whether acute asphyxial insult has occurred prior to delivery; EEG, imaging and Doppler assessment. Each of these is discussed in detail below. An hypoxic–ischemic event usually causes a consistent abnormality in these tests, and this may change with time from the insult. These diagnostic tests may also help with prognosis.

Secondary microcephaly is an important sign of acute cerebral injury. If the occipitofrontal head circumference was in the normal range at birth, with rapid slowing in head (brain) growth after birth, then this is an important indicator that an insult had occurred around the time of birth. It is not possible to define the cause of the insult, and its timing may have been several days or even weeks prior to delivery. Accurate serial head-circumference measurements are simple and important assessments of cerebral injury.

# INCIDENCE

The incidence of birth asphyxia in full-term infants has been variously reported from the USA, Sweden and Britain to be between 1.8 and 9.0 cases per 1000 deliveries (Brown *et al.* 1974; MacDonald *et al.* 1980; Finer *et al.* 1981; Nelson & Ellenberg 1981; Ergander *et al.* 1983; Levene *et al.* 1985a; Thornberg *et al.* 1995a). The incidence of low Apgar scores in babies with birth weights of less than 1500 g is 15-fold higher than infants weighing over 3000 g (Palme-Kilander 1992). In two studies, asphyxia was defined as an Apgar score of 3 or less at 5 min (Nelson & Ellenberg 1981; Ergander *et al.* 1983), and another included all infants who required intermittent positive-pressure ventilation for more than 1 min (MacDonald *et al.* 1980). In a cohort of all babies born in Sweden in 1985, 1.6 per 1000 live-born infants did not breathe spontaneously within 20 min of delivery (Palmer-Kilander 1992). In another more recent Swedish study, 6.9 per 1000 live-born term babies had an Apgar score <7 at 5 min (Thornberg *et al.* 1995a).

Three studies reported the incidence of HIE. Brown *et al.* (1974) found that 5.9 per 1000 full-term deliveries showed clinical signs due to intrapartum asphyxia, and in Leicester, we reported an incidence of 6.0 per 1000 inborn infants (Levene *et al.* 1985a). Moderate and severe HIE occurred in 1.1 and 1.0 per 1000 infants, respectively. One-quarter of the infants with HIE born in Leicester showed intrauterine growth retardation, which is comparable to the 29% reported by Finer *et al.* (1981). A third study of births in Sweden reported 'birth asphyxia with HIE' to occur in 1.8 per 1000 of term births from 1985 to 1991 (Thornberg *et al.* 1995a). Intrauterine growth retardation was six times more common in the asphyxiated than the control group.

The incidence of perinatal asphyxia is much more common in the developing world than in developed countries. The World Health Organization estimates that nearly 4 million newborn infants suffer moderate or severe asphyxia with 'at least 800 000 dying and an equal number developing sequelae such as epilepsy, mental retardation, cerebral palsy and learning disabilities' (World Health Organization 1991). In India, the incidence of death due to birth asphyxia in mature infants was estimated to be 10 per 1000 (Costello & Manandhar 1994). In Nigeria, the incidence of HIE is reported to be 26.5 per 1000 livebirths (Airedale 1991), some four to five times higher than in Britain and the USA. There is a trend towards a higher prevalence of asphyxia in Africa than Asia (Ellis & Manandhar 1999).

In the West, there appears to have been a reduction in the incidence of asphyxia in full-term infants over recent years. In the USA, infant mortality (all birth weights) due to intrauterine hypoxia and birth asphyxia has fallen from 253 per 1000 births in 1970 to 39 per 1000 by 1981 (Wegman 1984). The incidence of infants with convulsions apparently due to severe asphyxia, born in Montreal in Canada, and weighing more than 2500 g at birth fell from 1.8 per 1000 in 1960 to 0.7 per 1000 in 1978–1980 (Cyr *et al.* 1984). Figures from Paris (Amiel-Tison 1979) have shown a dramatic fall in the incidence of mild and moderate encephalopathy in full-term infants over a 4-year period. In 1974, the incidence of this condition was 18.9 per 1000, and for the years 1976–1978, it had fallen to 3.9 per 1000. There was, however, no change in the proportion of infants who were stillborn due to intrapartum asphyxia or who had the most severe form of encephalopathy. Two cohorts of full-term infants born in England in 1976–1980 and 1984–1988 showed that there had been a decline in the incidence of HIE from 7.7 per 1000 to 4.6 per 1000 in the intervening 4-year period (Hull & Dodd 1992).

## PATHOLOGY

Consistent pathological features associated with birth asphyxia have been recognized since the 19th century. Ulegyria or gyral scarring was first described by Bressler (1899), and status marmoratus or état marbre involving the basal ganglia was reported by Anton (1893). Despite these observations, no single distinct or uniform pathological appearance is recognized following severe hypoxic–ischemic injury. The brain may be globally affected with extensive swelling and necrosis, or pathological lesions may be more focal and discrete. These heterogeneous and clinically unpredictable appearances are related to the variety of pathophysiological insults to which the fetus is exposed. The majority of pathological lesions seen in the brain following asphyxia have been explained either as ischemic injury based on a vascular etiology or as the vulnerability of certain regions of the brain to metabolic injury.

The major factors affecting the development of particular pathological lesions include:

1. Developmental age at which the insult occurs. Insults in the first half of pregnancy will lead to disruption of neuronal migration and pachygyria (p. 329). Involvement of the white matter occurs commonly in immature infants (periventricular leukomalacia) and often in conjunction with periventricular hemorrhage. This condition, together with subcortical leukomalacia, is discussed in detail in Chapter 22, and this section will deal mainly with neuronal necrosis, which is commonly seen in full-term infants following asphyxia.
2. The appearance of the asphyxiated brain depends on the duration between the onset of the insult and the age at which it is examined. Within hours of the insult, the brain may appear grossly normal. In the first 48 h, histological examination may be unremarkable, but later, acidophilic staining of the cytoplasm with pyknosis or nuclear fragmentation is seen (Pape & Wigglesworth 1979). Electron microscopy reveals a diffuse change involving both vascular endothelium and neurons. Hemorrhage may be present on removing the brain from the skull. Subdural bleeding due to tentorial tears may be seen, and subarachnoid hemorrhage is particularly common.
3. Duration of the insult. This is discussed in detail in Chapter 23. A very short, but intense, insult may cause a different pattern of cerebral injury than a more protracted partial intermittent form of asphyxial compromise. Animal studies have shown that episodes of partial asphyxia produce lesions predominantly in cortical and subcortical structures. Acute and total asphyxia produced a totally different type of injury involving thalamus, brainstem and spinal cord structures (Myers 1972). Cerebral edema did not occur following acute asphyxia. When episodes of total asphyxia are superimposed upon episodes of partial asphyxia, mixed lesions may develop.
4. Partial intermittent asphyxia has also been produced in animal studies by a variety of means, but in all, there has been maintenance of some blood flow despite very low oxygen concentrations. In these studies, brain injury affects primarily the cerebral cortex with severe brain swelling. The distribution of injury is described

mainly in areas of brain between two arterial supplies: the so-called watershed distribution. Deeper structures in the brain are either spared or significantly less badly affected. Human post-mortem studies have shown a similar distribution of lesions, and imaging studies on surviving children have supported these findings.

## Cerebral edema

Within 24–48 h, gross swelling with marked flattening and widening of the gyri and obliteration of the sulci may occur. The brain at this time is soft and very friable. In some cases, cerebral herniation may have occurred with grooving of the uncus and partial cerebellar displacement through the foramen magnum, but this is infrequent. On cutting the brain, the ventricles are slit-like, and little cerebrospinal fluid drains out. Protrusion of the infundibulum into the interpeduncular cistern may occur (Larroche 1984).

Brain swelling and intracranial hypertension do not occur in all severely asphyxiated full-term infants (Pryse-Davies & Beard 1973; Levene *et al.* 1987), and the factors involved in their development are not clear. Klatzo (1967) has classified brain edema into two types: cytotoxic and vasogenic. In vasogenic edema, there is an increase in leakiness of the blood–brain barrier, allowing entry of serum proteins into the cerebral parenchyma. The resulting increase in intracerebral osmotic pressure leads to the accumulation of fluid within the extracellular compartment of the brain. Cytotoxic edema is due to the failure of cellular membrane pumps with entry of $Na^+$ and swelling of the cells (see above). Cytotoxic edema probably occurs earlier and in response to the initial hypoxic–ischemic insult and may affect the gray matter in preference to the white matter (Klatzo 1985). Later, and in response to a less clearly defined insult, the blood–brain barrier opens to proteins. The swollen brain seen at autopsy probably results predominantly from vasogenic edema, and this does not reach a maximum effect until 48 h after birth (Anderson & Belton 1974). In a fetal lamb model, vasogenic edema did not appear to be a significant feature following hypoxic–ischaemic insult, at least in the first 24 h (Tweed *et al.* 1981).

## Injury to gray matter

It is rare for isolated lesions to occur in only one area of the brain, and multiple or focal sites of involvement are usual, but for the sake of clarity, neuropathological features will be described under separate subheadings.

### Cortex

In the acute stages following asphyxia, the cerebral cortex may appear normal, but within a week or two, it may become fluctuant to touch and occasionally cystic. On a cut section, the cortex may show a gray–brown discoloration (Larroche 1984). Ulegyria, a macroscopic appearance of gyral sclerosis with widening of the sulci, is seen in some infants who have survived the asphyxial event by months or years (Fig. 27.1). This is probably a watershed insult (see

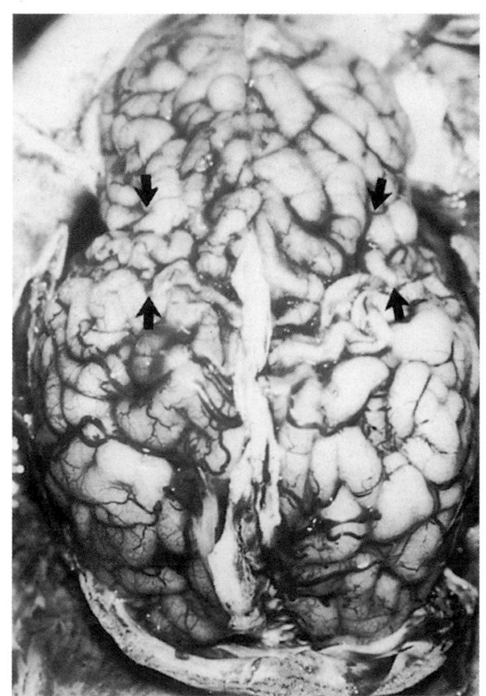

A

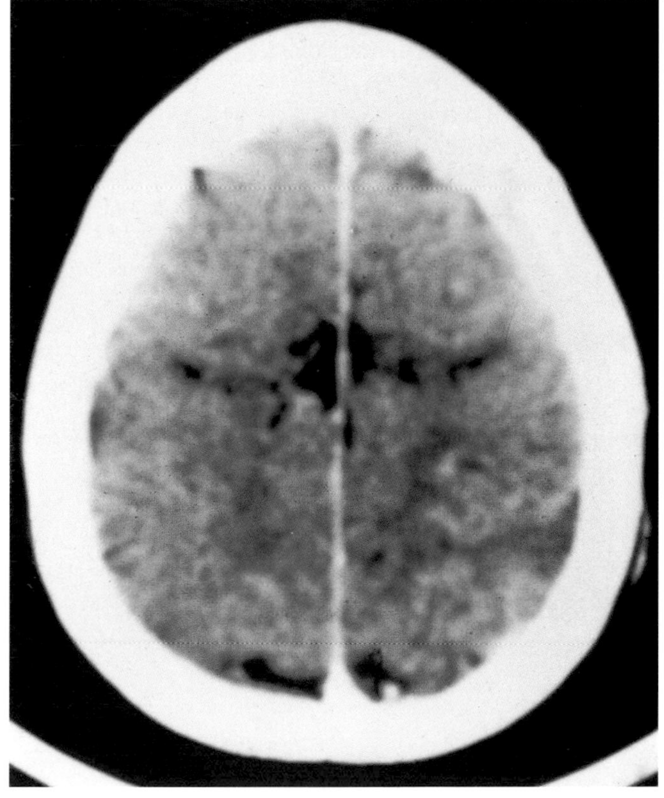

B

**Figure 27.1** Ulegyria. (A) There is sclerosis and cortical atrophy of the brain in the region between the anterior and middle cerebral arteries (arrows). (B) Computerized tomography scan showing areas of low attenuation representing ulegyria in the central corticosubcortical area.

below). Microscopically, cortical involvement may be focal or diffuse and may preferentially involve certain cortical layers, notably III and V, with II being well preserved (Larroche 1984). This may be due to relative differences in metabolic rate (Farkas-Bargeton & Diebler 1978). The hippocampus is particularly vulnerable to hypoxic insult, and partial or total destruction of pyramid cells within this area is almost invariable following significant cerebral asphyxic injury (Larroche 1977). Other particularly vulnerable areas include the pre- and postcentral gyri and the visual cortex around the calcarine fissure.

## Parasagittal injury

Progressive periods of asphyxial insult cause increased neuronal loss as the duration of insult lengthens (Williams *et al.* 1992), but the cerebrum is not uniformly affected. Severe asphyxia in mature fetal sheep produces selective damage in the regions of the parasagittal cortex and striatum (Gunn *et al.* 1992). Volpe (1977) has drawn particular attention to the parasagittal injury seen in full-term asphyxiated infants. Cortical necrosis occurring at the junction between the territories of the anterior, middle and posterior cerebral arteries has been produced experimentally in animals (Brierley *et al.* 1969) and recognized at autopsy in the brains of children (Adams *et al.* 1966). These authors have related this boundary zone injury to hypotension affecting the region between major arterial distribution. Similar lesions (Fig. 27.2) have been produced in fetal monkeys by inducing maternal hypotension for 1–5 h (Brann & Myers 1975).

This lesion has been diagnosed during life by means of technetium brain scans (Volpe & Pasternak 1977) or positron emission tomography (Volpe *et al.* 1985). Seventeen infants with evidence of significant postasphyxial encephalopathy were studied within the first 5 days. There was a consistent, symmetrical decrease in CBF of up to 50% to the parasagittal regions that was more marked posteriorly than anteriorly.

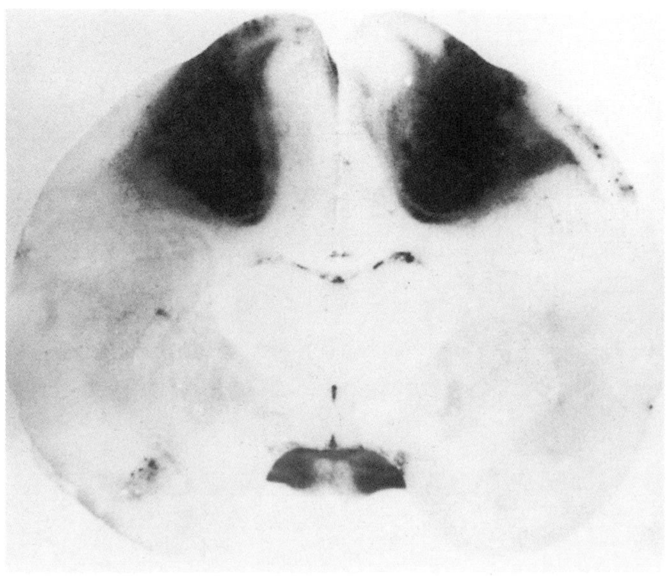

Figure 27.2 Parasagittal injury. Coronal section through a fetal monkey brain showing an asphyxial injury similar to the parasagittal watershed lesion. Reproduced, with permission, from Brann & Myers (1975).

## Subcortical structures

The region immediately below the cortical ribbon is particularly vulnerable to the effects of perinatal asphyxia due to the temporary vascular watershed exposed in full-term infants. Cortical and subcortical structures at the depths of sulci are particularly likely to develop infarction (Fig. 27.3) and may evolve to subcortical leukomalacia (see p. 391) or multiple cystic encephalomalacia.

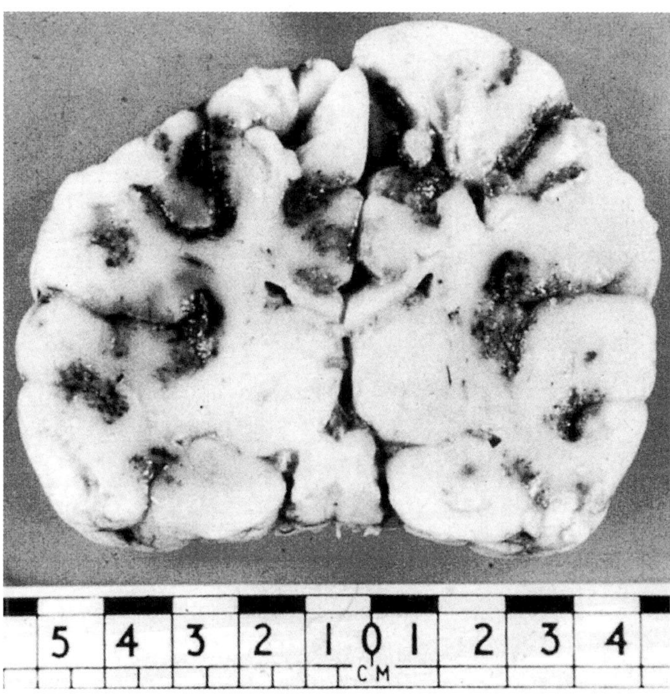


Figure 27.3 Deep cortical and subcortical hemorrhagic necrosis. The depths of the sulci are most severely involved.

Barth *et al.* (1984) have described a pattern of injury that occurs as the result of asphyxia in the central corticosubcortical area (Figs 27.1B and 27.4). This is the primary motor and sensory cortical areas. The distribution of this injury cannot be explained on the basis of a watershed distribution, and it is thought that infarction occurs as a result of the increased metabolic rate of these neurons during asphyxia. This lesion gives a typical appearance on computerized tomography (CT) (Barth *et al.* 1984).

## Basal ganglia

Status marmoratus is the classical neuropathological lesion affecting the basal ganglia and is seen only in infants who survive the asphyxia by many months. This is a visible marble-like appearance of the thalamus and basal ganglia

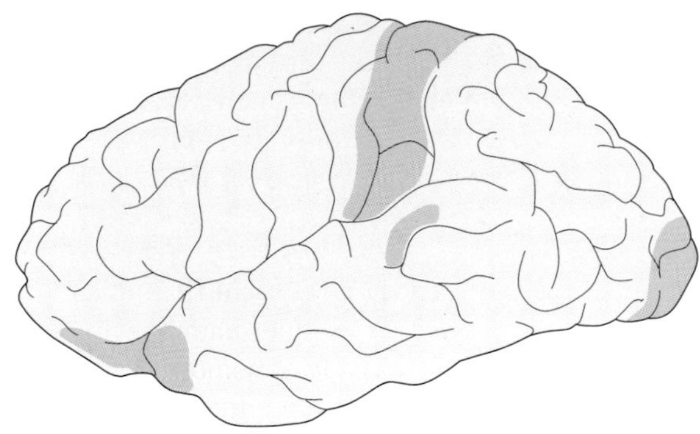

Figure 27.4 Distribution of vulnerable cortical and subcortical injury. (Redrawn, with permission, from Barth *et al.* (1984) © Masson Editeur).

and is due to abnormal myelination. Rorke (1982) states that this is a rare condition and is uncommonly seen even in infants who survive for many years after severe asphyxial insults. Rorke found lesions confined to the basal ganglia in only 3% of perinatal autopsies, but these lesions were relatively commonly seen together with more extensive cerebral injury. The majority of infants with selective damage to the thalamus had frank infarction with or without hemorrhage. Cystic infarction is also seen, and in some cases has been related to maternal drug addiction (Rorke 1982). Lesions apparent in the thalamus usually indicate more extensive involvement throughout the central nervous system.

Hemorrhage or hemorrhagic infarction involving the basal ganglia is seen frequently following birth asphyxia in full-term infants (Fig. 27.5). A consistent abnormality involving the thalamus and basal ganglia has been reported in surviving severely asphyxiated newborn infants (Kotagel *et al.* 1983; Morimoto *et al.* 1985) and is especially associated with acute, near total intrauterine asphyxia at the end of labor (Pasternak & Gorey 1998). These lesions have been recognized on ultrasound, CT and magnetic resonance imaging (MRI) (Voit *et al.* 1987; Barkovich 1992; Eken *et al.* 1994; Pasternak & Gorey 1998). Autopsy correlation suggests that this may be due to capillary proliferation and microcalcification. This may reflect evolving status marmoratus, and when these appearances are seen, the prognosis is very poor. They should not be confused with a unilateral thalamic hemorrhage (see p. 361). Scanning these children at a later stage may reveal symmetrical bi-thalamic calcification (Colamaria *et al.* 1988), and this also appears to be a good marker of previous severe asphyxial injury (Fig. 27.6). MR scans in infancy may show characteristic abnormalities of the basal ganglia (Fig. 27.7).

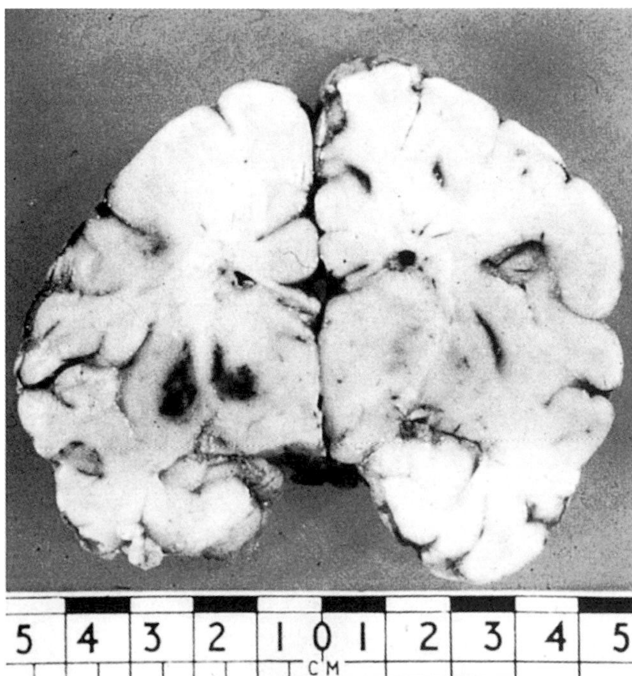


Figure 27.5 Hemorrhagic infarction of the left basal ganglion. Both the lentiform nucleus and lateral thalamus are involved, with the white matter or the internal capsule being spared.

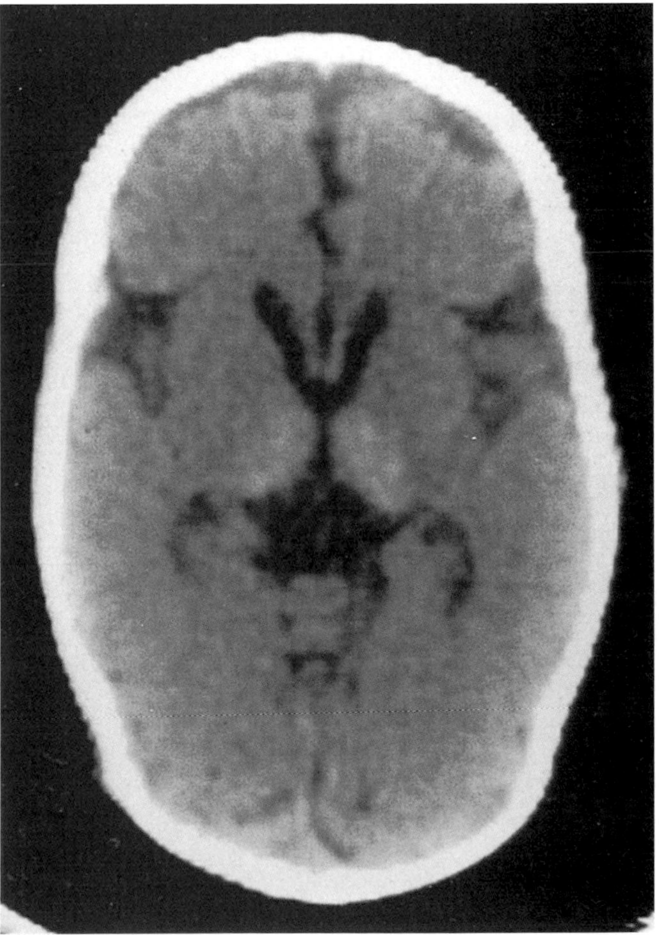

Figure 27.6 Bright thalami seen on a CT scan in an infant who had suffered from severe birth asphyxia some months earlier. The high attenuation was due to calcification. Note also the generalized cerebral atrophy.

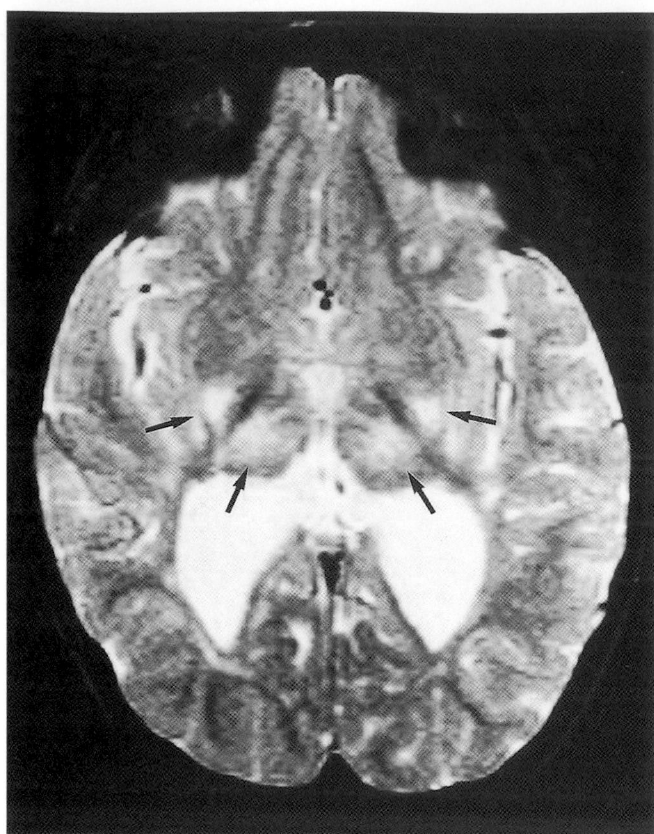

Figure 27.7 Axial MR scan showing abnormal T2 signal in the thalami and the lentiform nuclei (arrows) in a 2-year-old child with a dystonic form of cerebral palsy.

### Brainstem

Injuries to the brainstem are usually associated with concomitant lesions to the basal ganglia, as mentioned above. The most vulnerable structure is the inferior colliculus, probably due to its high metabolic rate, but the reticular formation, lateral geniculate bodies and pontine nuclei may also be involved. Leech & Alvord (1977) found evidence of brainstem lesions in 15 out of 16 (93%) brains that they examined. Lesions from the diencephalon, through the midbrain, pons, medulla and cord, have been described in some infants (Schneider *et al.* 1975). Lesions are rarely evident on macroscopic examination. Brainstem injury also involving the basal ganglia has been reported to be associated with abnormal eye movements, facial diplegia and poor sucking reflex in a surviving child (Roland *et al.* 1988).

### Cerebellum

The cerebellum is more resistant to the effects of asphyxia than the cerebrum, and pathological involvement following perinatal asphyxia has been reported infrequently. The dentate nuclei, Purkinje cells, and internal granular layers appear to be most vulnerable. Interestingly, the external granular layer is usually normal (Larroche 1977). Bilateral lesions may occur in the watershed region between the two superior and inferior cerebellar arteries (Friede 1975). Occipital diastasis may cause local trauma to the cerebellum and is described in Chapter 21. One-third of infants found at post-mortem to have obvious brain swelling showed cerebellar herniation (Pryse-Davies & Beard 1973).

### Spinal cord

Lesions within the cord are rarely obvious on macroscopic examination, but evidence of asphyxial injury is present microscopically. The gracile and cuneate nuclei, nuclei of the medulla oblongata, and the anterior horn cells are particularly vulnerable. Trauma to the spinal cord may be associated with intrapartum asphyxia (see Chapter 40).

### Multicystic leukoencephalopathy (MCLE)

This is a rare, but well-recognized, form of pathology that is seen as the end result of severe hypoxic–ischemic insult. MCLE occurs in mature babies and is very rarely reported to occur below 35 weeks of gestational age. Multiple areas of cavitation form a honeycomb appearance in the cortex and subcortical white matter. The gyral shape is usually not distorted and is maintained by the molecular layer and leptomeninges. Cavitation is most common in the distribution of the carotid arterial supply (frontal, parietal and temporal lobes), and the occipital region is severely involved less commonly. The brainstem and cerebellum are spared. Imaging studies (Keeney *et al.* 1991) have shown a similar distribution of cavities to autopsy studies (Fig. 27.8).

The babies have usually sustained clear evidence of intrapartum asphyxial insult, although the type of insult is variable. Acute compromise such as placental abruption, more sustained partial intermittent asphyxia, and severe fetomaternal hemorrhage have all been implicated in its causation. MCLE has also been reported as the result of very severe insults in the neonatal period including cardiovascular collapse and meningitis (Frigieri *et al.* 1996). The babies show markedly abnormal neurological behavior with grade III (severe) encephalopathy.

It is not clear what the underlying pathophysiology is that results in MCLE, and its evolution is unpredictable. Two explanations have been advanced. In the first, it is suggested that severe edema and the high water content of the immature brain cause a further impairment of cerebral blood flow (Friede 1975). We have anecdotally recognized clinical evidence of severe brain swelling preceeding the development of extensive cavitation in a number of cases. An alternative hypothesis is that it is due to intense vasospasm in the distribution of the carotid vasculature rather than the vertebrobasilar vessels that are devoid of sympathetic innervation (Sheth *et al.* 1995). This accounts for the distribution of the cavitation.

## CLINICAL FEATURES

Mature infants exposed to a period of asphyxia usually show a definite and predictable sequence of neurological

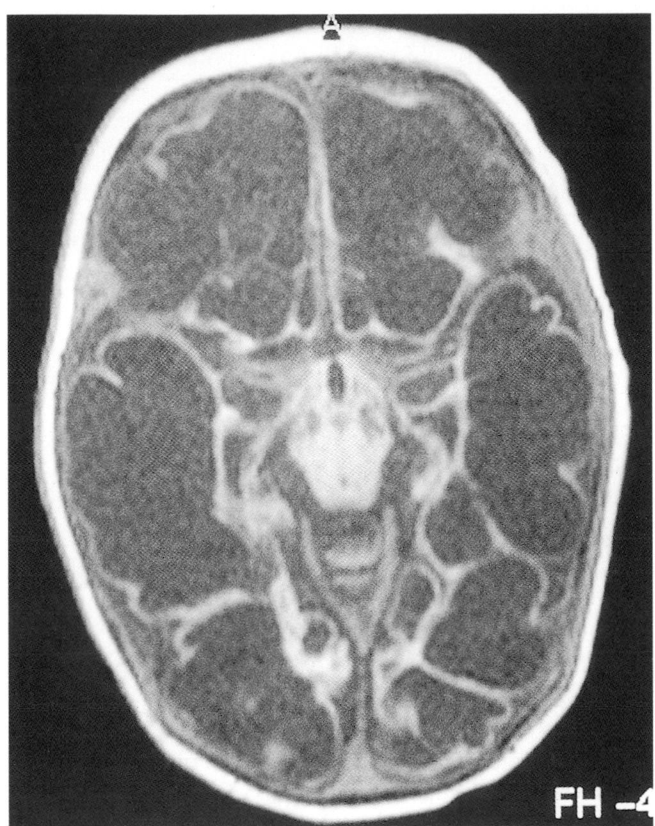


Figure 27.8 Multicystic leukoencephalopathy. Axial MR T1 weighted image showing extensive cavitation with destruction of most of the cerebral tissue in this section.

symptoms and signs. The relationship between an acute hypoxic–ischemic event and the sequence of abnormal signs has been described in infants who have sustained 'near-miss sudden infant death syndrome' and who had previously been normal. A number of these babies showed a consistent progression of signs, including an initial period of near normality followed by seizures, deterioration in conscious level and deepening coma (Constantinou *et al.* 1989). This sequence is very similar to that seen in severely asphyxiated infants. Premature babies may also show a similar sequence of neurological abnormalities (Niijima & Levene 1989), but this is uncommon, and HIE is only reliably seen in the full-term neonate.

The severity and progression of symptoms depend on the intensity of the hypoxic–ischemic event. The reason for the regular progression is not clear but certainly reflects pathophysiological changes in terms of CBF, cerebral metabolism and increase in brain swelling. Some of the clinical features, such as differential tone between upper and lower limbs, can be explained on the basis of parasagittal vascular injury. Chapter 8 details the clinical assessment and the features seen in infants with birth asphyxia. In this section, discussion is confined to the progression and clinical grading of HIE.

Sarnat & Sarnat (1976) were the first to devise a method to describe the progression of symptoms in asphyxiated full-term infants and combined it together with EEG activity. The clinical stages are shown in Table 27.2. Subsequently, a number of methods based on the Sarnat scheme have been described that can be used to refer to the maximum level of

**Table 27.2 Clinical grading system for post-asphyxial encephalopathy (Sarnat & Sarnat 1976 © American Medical Society)**

| | Mild (1) | Moderate (2) | Severe (3) |
|---|---|---|---|
| Level of consciousness | Hyperalert | Lethargic | Stuporose |
| Neuromuscular control | | | |
| Muscle tone | Normal | Mild hypotonia | Flaccid |
| Posture | Mild distal flexion | Strong distal flexion | Intermittent decerebration |
| Stretch reflexes | Overactive | Overactive | Decreased or absent |
| Segmental myoclonus | Present | Present | Absent |
| Complex reflexes | | | |
| Suck | Weak | Weak or absent | Absent |
| Moro | Strong: low threshold | Weak: incomplete; high threshold | Absent |
| Oculovestibular | Normal | Overactive | Weak or absent |
| Tonic neck | Slight | Strong | Absent |
| Autonomic function | Generalized sympathetic | Generalized parasympathetic | Both systems depressed |
| Pupils | Mydriasis | Miosis | Variable; often unequal; poor light reflex |
| Heart rate | Tachycardia | Bradycardia | Variable |
| Bronchial and salivary secretions | Sparse | Profuse | Variable |
| Gastrointestinal motility | Normal or decreased | Increased; diarrhoea | Variable |
| Seizures | None | Common; focal or multifocal | Uncommon (excluding decerebration) |

neurological abnormality in mature infants (Amiel-Tison 1979; Finer *et al.* 1981; Fenichel 1983; Levene *et al.* 1985a; Amiel-Tison & Ellison 1986). All these methods utilize a three-point grading system referring to mild, moderate and severe abnormality.

### Mild encephalopathy

These infants show no alteration in conscious level but appear to be 'hyperalert'. They spend more time in an awake and restless state, often with staring eyes. They show excessive response to stimulation and are jittery with spontaneous or exaggerated Moro reflexes. The infant's passive limb tone is normal, but there is usually some mild increase on assessment of active tone. When held in a sitting position, some head lag is noticeable, but the tone in the neck extensors is relatively increased compared with the flexers. Limb reflexes are normal or slightly increased, but sustained ankle clonus may be elicitable. Clinically apparent seizures do not occur. The sucking reflex is often weak, and the infants need encouragement to complete feeds. Sarnat & Sarnat (1976) found the duration of mild encephalopathy to range between 1.5 and 18 h, but we allow up to 48 h for complete recovery to occur (Levene *et al.* 1985a). Amiel-Tison & Ellison (1986) allow up to 7 days for complete recovery in mild encephalopathy.

### Moderate encephalopathy

The main features of this condition are seizures and lethargy with a reduction in spontaneous movements. These infants are slower to react to stimuli, and their responses may be incomplete. A somewhat higher threshold is usually necessary before a reaction is seen. The infants lie in a more hypotonic posture with abducted arms and legs. A consistent feature is differential tone between upper and lower limbs. The arms show much less spontaneous movement and are relatively hypotonic compared with the legs (Volpe & Pasternak 1977). Tendon jerks are exaggerated and the Moro reflex incomplete. Autonomic function is largely parasympathetic with relative bradycardia and constricted pupils. The sucking reflex is poor and feeding incomplete; tube feeding is usually necessary. Onset of convulsions is most common after 12 h from birth but may be seen earlier. They may be subtle or fragmentary and relatively easy to control pharmacologically. Sarnat & Sarnat (1976) found that these infants showed abnormal behavior for a mean of 4.7 days. Complete recovery (if it occurs) may take several weeks, but some improvement is usually seen by the end of the first week.

### Severe encephalopathy

These infants are comatose with severe hypotonia and usually require respiratory support from birth. They are profoundly hypotonic with no spontaneous movements. Seizures are frequent and may be prolonged. The most severely asphyxiated infants of this group may have no seizure activity associated with an isoelectric EEG. Tendon jerks and primitive reflexes are usually absent. The infants have no suck reflex but may show abnormal sucking-like seizure movements. Pupils are fixed and dilated or react only sluggishly to light. Infants who die due to asphyxia all have severe encephalopathy. With recovery, the infants may show a progression from hypotonia to extensor hypertonicity (Brown *et al.* 1974). Some infants can recover fully, but this may take up to 6 weeks.

Both moderate and severe encephalopathy follow a progression of clinical signs. In the first few hours, the infant may breathe spontaneously and show increasing tone and movement activity. Seizures initially appear to be subtle and then become more overt and last for a longer time with progression of the encephalopathy. The infant later becomes more hypotonic and enters a period of stabilization, although seizures may continue to be a problem. Subsequently, signs of clinical recovery occur in some infants. Others show changes in their pattern of neurological abnormality predictive of severe neurodevelopmental sequelae.

The timing and distribution of abnormal neurological signs may correlate with the type of asphyxial insult and the distribution of ensuing brain injury. Infants in whom HIE developed after severe acute asphyxial insult and who were shown to have permanent brain impairment tended to have earlier seizure onset (mean 6.6 h) compared with a mean onset of 11.1 h in infants with evidence of a more protracted aspyhxial insult (Ahn *et al.* 1998). Specific patterns of abnormal neurological signs have been reported in babies with differing distribution of anatomical brain lesions due to asphyxia. Full-term infants with predominantly basal ganglia involvement on MR imaging are reported to show persistent and diffuse neurological abnormalities compared with those who sustain injury mainly in the white matter who show a different clinical pattern with improved sucking reflex and less severe abnormalities in tone (Mercuri *et al.* 1999).

## INVESTIGATIONS

The diagnosis of birth asphyxia is usually made on clinical criteria. Evidence for intrapartum compromise such as fetal bradycardia, passage of meconium, CTG abnormalities, low Apgar scores, or delay in establishing respiration will alert the clinician to the condition, and the subsequent evolution of clinical signs and symptoms is usually sufficient to make a firm diagnosis of HIE. Some infants present late to the clinician, and information on intrapartum events may be absent or incomplete. Investigations may be necessary to elucidate the cause of the neurological abnormalities or to monitor an asphyxiated infant who receives neuromuscular paralysis to facilitate mechanical ventilation. It is important to consider alternative causes for encephalopathy in every baby thought to have been asphyxiated. Meningitis is the most common treatable condition that may cause similar symptoms to HIE. Lumbar puncture should be performed in all infants who are encephalopathic. Asphyxia and neonatal meningitis may occur in the same infants.

A further important role for investigative techniques is to provide prognostic information in the acute stages of HIE. This is further discussed in the section on outcome.

### Imaging

Imaging techniques such as ultrasound, CT and MRI have been used to study the neonatal brain following birth asphyxia. Details of these techniques together with examples of pathology are discussed in Chapter 6.

The commonly described pathological conditions affecting the brain of mature infants have been recognized by means of imaging techniques. These abnormalities are described on p. 71.

Cerebral edema is recognized on ultrasound imaging as a generalized increase in echodensity throughout the brain, loss of normal anatomical landmarks, and slit-like ventricles after 24 h of life (Babcock & Ball 1983; Martin *et al.* 1983; Skeffington & Pearse 1983; Williams 1983). The CT appearance of cerebral edema includes extensive areas of low attenuation, which appears to be related to the severity of the asphyxial insult (for examples, see p. 72). Moderate or severe involvement affecting white matter or cortex occurs in approximately 40% of asphyxiated full-term infants examined by CT (Flodmark *et al.* 1980; Magilner & Wertheimer 1980; Schrumpf *et al.* 1980; Fitzhardinge *et al.* 1981; Finer *et al.* 1983; Adsett *et al.* 1985; Lipp-Zwahlen *et al.* 1985a). This represents a high-risk group of infants who were selected for scanning in view of the severity of their neurological involvement. Signs of brain swelling on an MR scan were seen in almost all infants scanned within 5 days of life with HIE and disappeared rapidly after this time (Rutherford *et al.* 1995). Abnormalities include small extracerebral space, loss of the Sylvian fissures, narrowing of the interhemispheric fissure and slit-like anterior horns of the lateral ventricles.

The basal ganglia show a variety of abnormalities following birth asphyxia, including echodensity confined to the region of the basal ganglia (Levene *et al.* 1985b; Shen *et al.* 1986). This latter condition (see p. 476) has been reported only rarely and has been assumed to be due to edema, but Shen *et al.* (1986) report that the increase in echoes persists for over 6 months in some cases; this is far too long to be due to edema. CT and MRI have shown local lesions apparently confined to the thalamus (Shewman *et al.* 1981; Morimoto *et al.* 1985; Voit *et al.* 1985; Rutherford *et al.* 1995) (see Figs 27.6 and 27.7). These appearances may be due to infarction, edema, calcification or hemorrhage (Kotagel *et al.* 1983). Shewman *et al.* (1981) have reported that the high-attenuation thalamic lesions show considerable enhancement on infusion of radiopaque dye, suggesting that they are due to postischemic hypervascularity. The distinction between the bilateral thalamic density and thalamic hemorrhage is discussed in detail on p. 477.

Asphyxiated infants show a high incidence of intracranial hemorrhage diagnosed by various imaging techniques. Their incidence ranges from 19 to 73% of at-risk infants (Flodmark *et al.* 1980; Magilner & Wertheimer 1980; Fitzhardinge *et al.* 1981; Gerard *et al.* 1981; Finer *et al.* 1983; Adsett *et al.* 1985; Lipp-Zwahlen *et al.* 1985a). Analysis of cumulative data gives an overall risk of hemorrhage of approximately 30% in infants showing clinical evidence of significant asphyxia. More than half of the lesions are due to subarachnoid hemorrhage.

Infarction of a major cerebral artery occurs relatively commonly in asphyxiated babies (Voorhies *et al.* 1983) and should be apparent on brain imaging. This condition is discussed fully in Chapter 23. Imaging detects an abnormality in the distribution of the affected vessel. Ultrasound may be a useful screening test for this condition, but infarction of a major cerebral artery may occur in the presence of a normal ultrasound scan, so that it is important to perform CT or MR scans on all full-term infants in whom cerebral artery infarction is suspected. Clinical suspicion should be aroused by focal convulsions or the presence of asymmetrical neurological signs. The tissue supplied by the infarcted vessel usually becomes necrotic and is replaced by a porencephalic cyst, again seen in the vascular distribution of the affected vessel. This is a useful marker in the older child with this particular lesion.

Cortical abnormality is seen on ultrasound imaging only if a very high frequency (10-MHz transducer) is routinely used. These changes occur between 48 and 72 h (Eken *et al.* 1994) and correlate with laminar necrosis on histology. Cortical/subcortical changes are well recognized also on MR imaging and may represent a breakdown of deep white matter (Rutherford *et al.* 1995).

Multicystic leukomalacia, involving the periventricular region, and subcortical leukomalacia (see p. 391) have also been diagnosed by ultrasound following severe birth asphyxia (Babcock & Ball 1983; Martin *et al.* 1983; Levene *et al.* 1985b; Trounce & Levene 1985; Frigieri *et al.* 1996).

In practice, all infants with moderate or severe post-asphyxial encephalopathy should have a routine ultrasound scan performed within 48 h of birth. Clinically significant and treatable lesions should be suspected by this technique, particularly if a midline shift is present. A convexity subdural or subarachnoid hemorrhage will require CT or MR scanning to delineate its precise position and its response to treatment if this is undertaken (Fig. 27.9).

MR imaging shows a changing pattern of abnormalities after an hypoxic–ischemic insult (Martin & Barkovich 1995). The precise sequence depends on the type of asphyxial insult and the region of brain most compromised. In the first 2–3 days, a low signal on T1-weighted images and a high signal on T2-weighted images are seen. In acute total asphyxia, signal changes may be particularly present in the lentiform nucleus as well as other parts of the basal ganglia and along the corticospinal tracts. Following severe partial intermittent asphyxia, the abnormal signal may be

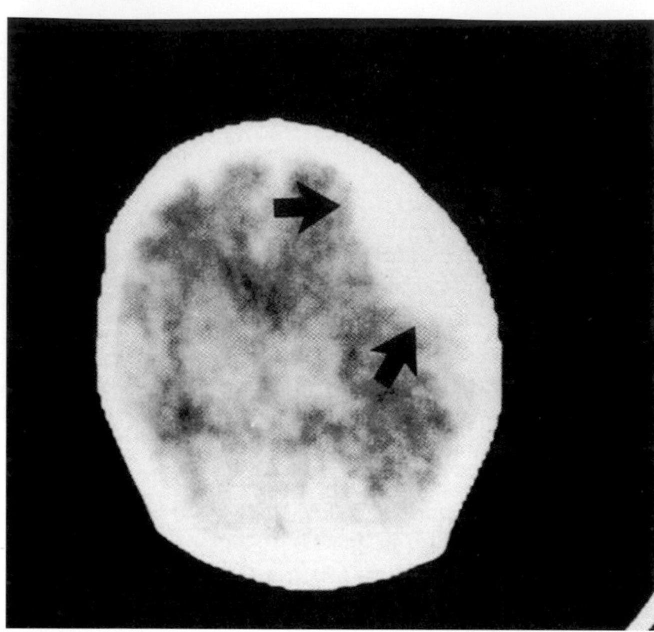

Figure 27.9 CT scan showing convexity left-sided hemorrhage (arrowed) present in a severely asphyxiated infant. Note the midline shift and extensive areas of low attenuation.

particularly obvious in the vascular boundary zones. By 4–5 days, T1 shortening becomes evident in the abnormal area and, at about 7 days, becomes most pronounced and may persist for 4 weeks or more. A low signal on T2-weighted images slowly develops over the first month and may persist for 2–3 months. In babies with the most severe form of asphyxia, MR abnormalities tend to occur in areas of developing or established myelination (Martin & Barkovich 1995).

Two earlier MR markers of post-asphyxial injury are loss of T1-weighted signal from the posterior limb of the internal capsule and abnormal high T1-weighted signal in the deep portions of the pre- and postcentral gyri. Early diffusion weighted imaging appears to be more sensitive to damage than conventional MR imaging (Cowan *et al.* 1994).

## Measurement of intracranial pressure

Cerebral edema may occur as the result of hypoxic–ischemic insult and leads to intracranial hypertension in some cases. Direct assessment of intracranial pressure by means of a subarachnoid catheter has shown that only 50% of asphyxiated infants actually develop intracranial hypertension, and monitoring may not significantly alter the outcome in the majority of infants (Levene *et al.* 1987).

Attempts have been made to measure intracranial pressure (ICP) both directly and indirectly across the anterior fontanelle. The latter has the obvious advantage of being non-invasive but may also be less accurate. Unfortunately, indirect transfontanelle methods are unreliable and inaccurate.

### Direct methods

Doubts about the accuracy of indirect methods have prompted a number of attempts at invasive measurement of ICP in infants. Goitein & Amit (1982) described placement through the fontanelle of a 22-gauge Quick-Cath into the subdural space, and found no complications associated with this technique. Levene & Evans (1983) used a fine subarachnoid catheter inserted percutaneously to monitor ICP and have used this successfully in over 30 infants without complications associated with the technique. McWilliam & Stephenson (1984) published a method for monitoring ICP directly from the anterior horn of the lateral ventricle. To date, this has not been described in the neonate.

Methods to measure ICP directly using devices inserted into the skull are more accurate and reliable, and all appear to be remarkably safe in clinical practice.

### Normal ICP

Normal ICP in full-term infants is derived from indirect measurement using transfontanellar devices and is probably inaccurate and unreliable. For obvious reasons, there are no data from direct measurement techniques in normal babies. Kaiser & Whitelaw (1987) have reported normal lumbar cerebrospinal fluid pressure to range from 0 to 5.5 mmHg measured at lumbar puncture. In practice, I estimate normal ICP in mature normal neonates to be <6 mmHg.

### Cerebral perfusion pressure

This concept has been used in adults and children to describe the resistance to cerebral perfusion due to elevations in ICP. Cerebral perfusion pressure (CPP) is calculated by subtracting ICP from the mean arterial blood pressure (MAP):

$$\text{CPP} = \text{MAP} - \text{ICP}.$$

In essence, the driving force of blood through the cerebral arterioles will be reduced by increments in ICP if the MAP remains unchanged.

A critically low CPP has been associated with poor outcome in adults (Rowan *et al.* 1972) and infants (Raju *et al.* 1983). The normal range for CPP in infants has been prone to the same methodological problems inherent in the measurement of ICP.

## Electrodiagnostic tests

These methods include electroencephalography and evoked responses and are discussed in detail in Chapters 11 and 12. They are important investigations that help to strengthen the clinical diagnosis of birth asphyxia.

Polygraphic electroencephalography is a widely available technique applicable to the newborn infant. This technique has been shown to be a good prognostic indicator following birth asphyxia (Watanabe *et al.* 1980; Takeuchi & Watanabe 1989), but it requires considerable skill and experience in the interpretation of the tracings. It is limited to short recordings lasting only minutes in time. For this reason, methods to continuously monitor cerebral electrical activity have been developed. Continuous EEG or cerebral function monitoring have a twofold role in asphyxiated infants. Firstly, they may provide useful prognostic information (see p. 497), and secondly, they may aid the diagnosis of seizures. These methods are also of value in prognosis following HIE, and this is also discussed in Chapter 11.

### Doppler assessment

Consistent changes in Doppler signals from major cerebral arteries following birth asphyxia have been described (Levene *et al.* 1989), and these changes occur in a particular sequence (p. 132). Doppler ultrasound has also been shown to be a useful prognostic indicator following birth asphyxia (Levene *et al.* 1989), and this is discussed on p. 497. Doppler ultrasound has not been shown to have a role in the acute management of birth asphyxia.

### Biochemical methods

As indicated in the section on the pathophysiology of birth asphyxia, a cascade of biochemical reactions occur during and after an asphyxial event, and so, changes in biochemical markers are potentially useful methods for monitoring the progress of the condition. Table 27.3 lists the biochemical markers reported in the literature to assess the diagnosis or progress of an asphyxial insult. These methods focus on changes in the body or brain's energy states, hormonal response or markers of brain-based proteins usually accessible only at lumbar puncture.

The problem with many of these markers is that they assess total body effects of asphyxia rather than just those affecting the brain. It is suggested that as the blood–brain barrier in neonates is less functionally competent, aerobically derived enzymes may cross more readily into the systemic circulation, thus enabling cerebral pathology to be monitored reliably on blood specimens than in older patients. Recent studies have assessed these markers in CSF that reflect the brain condition more closely. The main purpose of these biochemical markers is in the prediction of outcome, and this is discussed on p. 497.

#### Energy metabolism

Anaerobic metabolism, a precursor of asphyxia, causes both respiratory and metabolic acidosis with fall in blood pH and increase in lactate. Acidosis has been proposed as a marker of duration and/or severity of hypoxic–ischemic insult. Cord-blood pH varies depending on whether on artery or vein is sampled; the pH of arterial blood is normally lower than venous blood. Severe cord-blood acidosis (arterial pH <7.05) occurs in about 2.5% of unselected full-term infants (Westgate 1993), but few of these babies show major signs of 'asphyxia'. In one study, 61% of all babies with a pH <7.00 did not require admission to a neonatal unit (Goldaber *et al.* 1991), and in another study, only 22% of babies with a similar degree of cord-blood acidosis developed seizures (Perlman & Risser 1996). A normal arterial cord-blood level may be useful in suggesting that anaerobic metabolism had not occurred immediately prior to delivery.

In an acidotic fetus, the size of the difference may indicate whether the acidosis has occurred acutely or not. Chronic anaerobic metabolism will produce a smaller difference as the placenta will have had time to equilibrate the difference. A large difference suggests acute onset of acidosis. Low *et al.* (1993) found a significantly poorer neurodevelopmental outcome in babies with metabolic acidosis who had a narrow

**Table 27.3 Biochemical markers reported to be used in the diagnosis of birth asphyxia and/or prediction of outcome following a hypoxic–ischemic event**

| Energy metabolism | Hormones | Brain derived proteins |
|---|---|---|
| Fetal blood pH | Vasopressin | Aspartate/glutamate |
| Cord blood pH (A–V) difference | Erythropoeitin | GFAP |
| Cord blood $PCO_2$ (A–V) difference | Noradrenaline | Myelin basic protein |
| Buffer base | Insulin | BDNF |
| Lactate (blood, brain) | Prolactin | Nestin |
| Urinary lactate/pyruvate ratio | Growth hormone | |
| Lactate/pyruvate ratio | Catecholamines | |
| Lactate dehydrogenase and isoenzymes | ACTH | Brain enzymes |
| Hydroxybutyrate dehydrogenase | Endorphins | Creatine kinase (CK-BB) |
| Hypoxanthine (blood, CSF) | Somatostatin | Neuron specific enolase |
| Cyclic AMP | Aldosterone | |
| Adenosine | | |
| Uric acid/creatinine ratio | | Cytokines |
| | | TNFα |
| | | IL-1β |
| | | IL-6 |

A–V difference compared with those with similar metabolic acidosis, but a large A–V difference.

Lactate production as the result of anaerobic metabolism is an important component of metabolic acidosis detected at birth. Intracerebral lactic acid accumulation may be responsible for the development of cerebral edema, but it is suggested that there is poor correlation between blood lactic acidemia and intracerebral levels. Recently, elevated lactate, as expressed by a high urinary lactate:creatinine ratio, has been shown to correlate well with short-term complications of asphyxia including HIE (Huang *et al.* 1999). Acidemia as the result of fetal compromise usually resolves spontaneously (Farkas *et al.* 1995), but lactate levels in brain white and gray matter remain elevated for a considerably longer time after resolution of systemic blood lactate levels (Thoresen *et al.* 1998). $^{1}$H MRS has shown that high levels of intracerebral lactate occur shortly after acute asphyxia in full-term human neonates (Leth *et al.* 1996; Groenendaal *et al.* 1994; Hanrahan *et al.* 1996; Penrice *et al.* 1996) and that high levels or prolonged detection of lactate predict bad outcome.

The energy state within the brain can be assessed in a number of ways, both directly and indirectly. The high-energy molecule ATP is necessary for normal cellular function, and this can be directly assessed by measuring the PCr/$P_i$ ratio using $^{31}$P MRS (Ch. 10). Wyatt *et al.* (1989) produced a series of phosphorus spectra from asphyxiated babies and showed that there is a delayed deterioration in the brain energy state suggestive of a slowly progressive disruption of oxidative phosphorylation in brain tissue (Figs 10.3 and 27.10). In the hours after a severe hypoxic–ischemic insult, the PCr/$P_i$ ratio falls, indicating a continuing degradation of high-energy substrate to inorganic phosphorus. This degradation in ATP is associated with a poor outcome (Lorek *et al.* 1994; Martin *et al.* 1996; Roth *et al.* 1997). It is, however, unlikely that MRS will ever be available as a routine technique for monitoring cerebral function following birth asphyxia, but it provides invaluable insight into the pathophysiology of this condition.

During hypoxia, ATP is degraded to AMP and thence to hypoxanthine (Hx). This is discussed in detail on p. 143. Cyclic AMP is synthesized in mitochondria from ATP and has been shown to be very low in CSF samples in term asphyxiated infants, and these have been shown to have a very poor outcome (Pourcyrous *et al.* 1999). Saugstad (1975) suggested that Hx is a sensitive and specific measure of energy state following perinatal asphyxia. Various studies have shown there to be a wide overlap between Hx in normal control and asphyxiated fetuses (O'Connor *et al.* 1981). In a study of cord-blood Hx measurements, Thiringer (1983) found a poor correlation between Hx and low Apgar scores, but abnormal clinical findings correlated better. Hx is not a specific measure of cerebral energy breakdown but reflects whole-body changes. The liver and brain appear to contribute most to total Hx following severe fetal hypoxia,

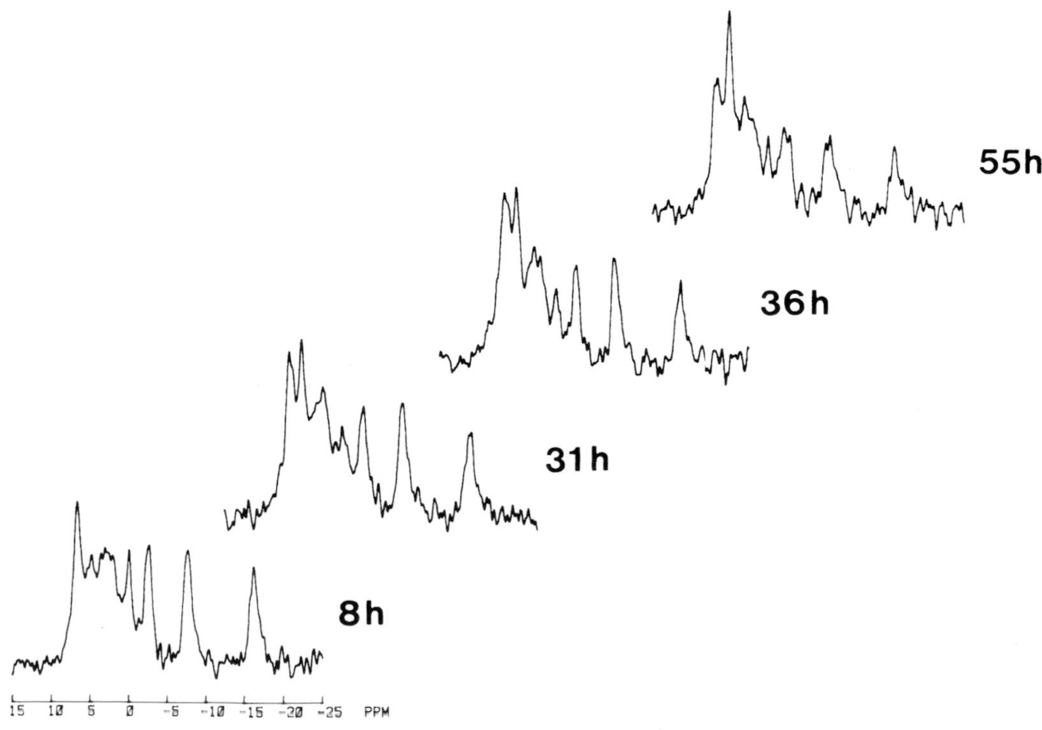


Figure 27.10 A series of MRS phosphorus spectra from a severely asphyxiated full-term infant scanned at varying times from birth (ages indicated in hours) showing a progressive deterioration of the PCr/$P_i$ ratio with time. Reproduced, with permission, from Wyatt *et al.* (1989).

and consequently, Hx is of little value in the prediction of neurological outcome.

### Brain enzymes

Creatine kinase (CK) is derived from brain, heart and skeletal muscle in response to tissue injury. Attempts have been made to separate the three isoenzymes chemically in order to study changes in the brain-derived enzyme (CK-BB) following asphyxia. Worley *et al.* (1985) have shown CK-BB to be derived from both neurons and astrocytes. A variety of methods, including electrophoretic separation (Cuestas 1980; Walsh *et al.* 1982) and radioimmunoassay (Thompson *et al.* 1980; Worley *et al.* 1985), have been used to measure CK-BB. These methods, particularly electrophoresis, have been criticized because they do not separate the various component CK-BB accurately from cardiac enzyme CK-MB (Hoo & Goedde 1982). Apparent measurements of CK-BB can be badly contaminated by CK-MB, thus rendering results unreliable.

Studies have shown that low levels of CK-BB predict a subsequent normal outcome reasonably well, and significantly elevated levels found during the first 12 h of life predict a later neurological abnormality in a relatively high proportion of asphyxiated newborn infants (Walsh *et al.* 1982; Fernandez *et al.* 1987). Others could not, however, find any correlation between the levels of CK-BB isoenzyme in cord blood and depressed Apgar scores or cord-blood pH (Amato *et al.* 1986; Ruth 1989). In addition, there was no correlation between CK-BB activity and developmental quotient at 2 years (Ruth 1989). The role of the CK-BB isoenzyme in quantifying cerebral injury is not clear. Certainly, earlier techniques have failed to separate accurately the various isoenzymes.

Lactate and hydroxybutyrate dehydrogenase (LDH and HBDH) have been used as indicators of neurological damage in asphyxiated newborn infants. Isoenzyme studies have suggested that LDH originated from neuronal tissue, but studies have not suggested that blood enzyme levels are good discriminators of at-risk infants (Hall *et al.* 1980). Elevated levels of LDH and its isoenzymes LDH2 and LDH3 in CSF have been suggested to be better predictors of death and disability (Dalens *et al.* 1981; Fernandez *et al.* 1986).

Neuron-specific enolase (NSE) is released into both CSF and serum following damage to the brain. Studies have shown that babies with HIE have higher levels of NSE than controls and that those with the most severe grades of HIE had the highest NSE levels in CSF (Thornberg *et al.* 1995b). Infants who died or sustained motor deficit as the result of asphyxial insult were found to have the highest levels of NSE in CSF (Garcia-Alix *et al.* 1994).

### Brain-derived proteins

A number of brain-derived proteins have been found to be elevated in the CSF of neonates who have sustained an hypoxic–ischemic insult. These include glial fibrillary acidic protein (GFAP), a structural protein of intermediate filaments in astroglia (Blennow *et al.* 1995), myelin basic protein (Garcia-Alix *et al.* 1994), brain-derived neurotrophic factor (BDNF) (Korhonen *et al.* 1998), and nestin, an intermediate filament protein derived from reactive astrocytes (Grigelioniene *et al.* 1996).

The CSF concentration of the excitatory neurotransmitter amino acids, glutamate and aspartate, have been shown to increase by over 250% in asphyxiated infants (Hagberg *et al.* 1993). The highest increase was reported in the infants with the most severe forms of HIE.

### Hormones

Asphyxia is a potent stimulator of a wide endocrine response. There is a massive catecholamine release in response to birth, and this is even greater in asphyxia (Largercrantz *et al.* 1992). Inappropriately high insulin levels are reported in a group of asphyxiated babies, and these babies were reported to have a worse outcome (Davis *et al.* 1999). Elevated growth hormone and depressed prolactin values have been reported in asphyxiated neonates (Varvarigou *et al.* 1996), and this may reflect pituitary compromise. Hypoxia is also known to stimulate release of arginine vasopressin from the pituitary, and high levels of vasopressin have been found in the cord plasma of asphyxiated babies (De Vane & Porter 1980), but this did not correlate with neurodevelopmental outcome at 2 years (Ruth *et al.* 1988).

Erythropoietin (Epo) is produced by the fetal kidney within a few hours of a hypoxic insult. In a group of infants with apparent acute asphyxia, those infants with definite adverse outcome had significantly higher cord blood Epo levels than asphyxiated controls without abnormal outcome (Ruth *et al.* 1988). Epo deserves further attention as a sensitive biochemical marker of intrapartum hypoxia, but it is not a specific marker of a cerebral injury. Excess nucleated red blood cells in peripheral blood may occur as a result of abnormal Epo production and may be a marker of chronic hypoxia (p. 472).

### Cytokines

Cytokines are a group of chemical messengers with both pro- and anti-inflammatory actions and are released as the result of tissue injury. A number of specific cytokines including TNF$\alpha$, IL-1$\beta$, IL-6, and IL-8 have been shown to be elevated in the CSF of asphyxiated babies compared with controls (Martin-Ancel *et al.* 1997; Oygur *et al.* 1998; Savman *et al.* 1998). The magnitude of response to IL-6 has also been shown to correlate with neurodevelopmental outcome (Martin-Ancel *et al.* 1997; Savman *et al.* 1998).

## COMPLICATIONS

During the acute hypoxic–ischemic insult, changes occur in the distribution of blood flow in order to preserve circulation to the most vital organs, as described in Chapter 23. In summary, blood flow to the brain, heart, and adrenals increases in inverse proportion to the arterial oxygen content and at the expense of blood flow to the kidneys, liver and gastrointestinal tract. This accounts for the increased vulnerability of some organs to acute asphyxial events, and anticipation of complications is important in the appropriate management of such infants.

## Kidney

Asphyxia in fetal or newborn animals causes a marked reduction in renal blood flow (Rudolph 1969) with a significant increase in the vascular resistance of the kidney (Alward *et al.* 1978), and renal failure is a relatively common complication of severe hypoxic–ischemic insult (Dauber *et al.* 1976). Renal failure may also occur due to myoglobinuria following tissue breakdown in asphyxiated infants (Kojima *et al.* 1985). Doppler studies of renal hemodynamics after birth asphyxia have shown an increase in apparent renal vascular resistance (Akinbi *et al.* 1994) and a reduction in renal systolic flow velocity, which predicts the development of acute renal failure (Luciano *et al.* 1998).

The incidence of renal impairment, as defined by oliguria, following birth asphyxia has been reported to vary between 23 and 55% (Perlman & Tack 1988; Fernandez *et al.* 1989). Acute renal failure (defined as a plasma creatinine level >130 μmol/l for at least 2 consecutive days) was reported in 19% of a group of asphyxiated infants born at 34 weeks of gestational age and above (Roberts *et al.* 1990). There was a relatively poor concordance in these studies between renal impairment and HIE. A more sophisticated assessment of renal tubular function has shown that urinary concentrations of *N*-acetyl-glucosaminidase (NAG) was significantly higher in a group of full-term asphyxiated neonates compared to controls (Willis *et al.* 1997). There was also a significant increase in urinary NAG excretion with increasing severity of perinatal asphyxia, as indicated by the HIE grade.

## Gastrointestinal tract

Asphyxiated babies have been shown to be more likely to have abnormalities in intestinal motility with intolerance of enteral feeds (Berseth & McCoy 1992). Necrotizing enterocolitis (NEC) is the major complication affecting the bowel in asphyxiated infants, although this is rare amongst cohorts of full-term asphyxiated infants (Perlman *et al.* 1989). Fitzhardinge (1977) reported one-third of infants with NEC to have suffered asphyxia before its onset. Although NEC is much more common in premature infants, it is also described following asphyxia in full-term infants (Goldberg *et al.* 1983). Abnormal liver function tests are also described in asphyxiated infants (Goldberg *et al.* 1983; Zanardo *et al.* 1985). Asphyxiated infants also show an apparent increase in resistance of mesenteric vessels (Akinbi *et al.* 1994), which may predispose them to post-asphyxial bowel problems.

## Cardiovascular system

### Cardiac output

Compromise of myocardial contractility may reduce cardiac output due to decreased stroke volume with subsequent systemic hypotension. In extreme cases, cardiogenic shock and heart failure may occur (Burnard & James 1961; Cabal *et al.* 1980). Acute cardiac dilatation associated with asphyxia may cause functional tricuspid atresia, further impairing cardiac function (Bucciarelli *et al.* 1977). In a group of infants with low Apgar scores and acidosis (pH <7.10), their blood pressure, cardiac output, and stroke volume were found to be lower than a similar, but non-acidotic, group. Myocardial dysfunction detected by Doppler ultrasound studies has been reported in 28–50% of asphyxiated infants (Perlman *et al.* 1989; van Bel & Walther 1990; Bennhagen *et al.* 1998). Dopamine is valuable in increasing blood pressure in asphyxiated infants (Di Sessa *et al.* 1981) by its inotropic effect, which improves cardiac output and stroke volume (Walther *et al.* 1985).

### Myocardial infarction

Ischemic necrosis of the papillary muscle following severe birth asphyxia has been found in a high proportion of autopsy specimens (Donnelly *et al.* 1980; De Sa & Donnelly 1984). Evidence for myocardial ischemia is often present on ECG assessment (Daga *et al.* 1983; Primhak *et al.* 1985).

## Lung

Meconium aspiration is a common accompaniment of HIE. Hypoxia induces fetal gasping during labor as well as passage of meconium, and meconium aspiration occurs before the infant is born. Pulmonary hypertension is a common complication of meconium aspiration, and the ensuing systemic hypoxemia may further compromise cerebral function. Pulmonary hypertension has been reported to be a specific complication of birth asphyxia and may be severe (Perlman *et al.* 1989). It has been suggested that in some asphyxiated infants, the pulmonary hypertension may be due to pulmonary embolism (Arnold *et al.* 1985).

The breathing pattern of asphyxiated full-term infants shows a variety of abnormal patterns compared with controls. There are more apneic periods and longer duration of apneic episodes when they occurred. The duration of time spent in periodic breathing was also prolonged (Sasidharan 1992).

## Metabolism

A variety of metabolic problems may arise in asphyxiated infants, including hyponatremia, hypoglycemia, hypocalcemia, metabolic acidosis, and hyperammonemia. Hyponatremia may occur due to fluid retention as a result of renal compromise or due to inappropriate antidiuretic hormone secretion (IADHS). Perinatal asphyxia causes high levels of circulating ADH (Daniel *et al.* 1978; Speer *et al.* 1984), and fluid retention occurs as a result of this (see above). IADHS is recognized by the combination of dilute plasma and concentrated urine.

Transient hyperammonemia, in association with severe perinatal asphyxia, has been described (Goldberg *et al.* 1979). Some of the clinical features seen in these infants and thought to be due to asphyxia, including hyperthermia, hypertension and lack of beat-to-beat variability, may have been caused by the hyperammonemia. The reason for the transient elevation in serum ammonia levels is not known.

### Hematological complications

Disseminated intravascular coagulation (DIC) occurs commonly following intrapartum asphyxia (Chessels & Wigglesworth 1970; Chadd *et al.* 1971; Anderson *et al.* 1974; Suzuki & Morishita 1998). Bleeding due to DIC may cause severe secondary complications including intracranial hemorrhage. Anderson *et al.* (1974) could find no evidence that DIC was associated with significant intracerebral thrombus deposition.

In a group of asphyxiated babies, there was a marked abnormality in a number of variables suggestive of DIC (Suzuki & Morishita 1998). These included significantly low levels of factor XIII, and elevated thrombin–antithrombin (TAT) complexes, D-dimer, fibrin and fibrinogen degradation products (FDP), and soluble fibrin monomer complexes (SFMC).

## MANAGEMENT

The immediate management of birth asphyxia is directed first towards rapid and efficient resuscitation and then stabilization of the infant's condition. Asphyxia may compromise the functions of a variety of immature organ systems (see p. 485), and anticipation of such complications with appropriate management is essential. The management of the asphyxiated infant must be considered in relation to general systemic complications as well as directing therapy towards the brain. Brain-oriented management (Chapter 28) is misplaced if complications such as systemic hypotension are unrecognized or inadequately treated. Severely asphyxiated infants must be treated in the same manner as the very-low-birth-weight infant, with adequate monitoring and the provision of cerebrally oriented intensive care, should this be necessary.

### RESUSCITATION

Dawes (1968) has described the sequence of events that occur during experimental asphyxia of fetal rhesus monkeys. Immediately following the asphyxial insult, there is an episode of regular small-volume breaths followed by a fall in the heart rate and cessation of breathing. This is termed primary apnea, and the animal looks cyanosed as a result of these changes. With no intervention, the period of primary apnea lasts for up to a minute and is followed by spontaneous gasping, which is maintained for a further 4–5 min before a second period of apnea develops. If resuscitation is not undertaken at the stage of secondary apnea, then the animal will die. This sequence of events is similar to those that have been observed to occur in the human newborn. These stages are summarized in Fig. 27.11.

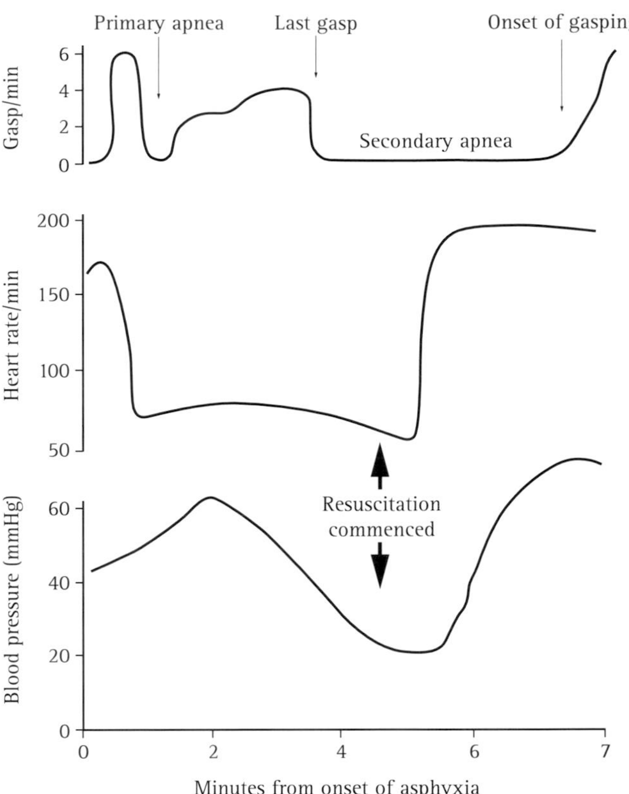


Figure 27.11 Physiological effects of acute asphyxia and the response to resuscitation. Redrawn, with permission, from Dawes (1968).

The need for resuscitation can be anticipated in many cases, and risk factors are listed in Table 27.4. Despite this, in a national Swedish survey, 19% of all babies who required resuscitation were not anticipated prior to delivery (Palme-Kilander 1992).

| Table 27.4 Factors indicating a significantly increased risk that an infant may need resuscitation at birth |
|---|
| Prematurity |
| Diagnosis of fetal distress |
| Heavy meconium staining of the liquor |
| Fetal acidosis (pH < 7.2) measured from a scalp sample |
| Known major congenital malformation |
| Twins |
| Any delivery under general anesthesia |
| Mid-cavity or rotational forceps |
| Rhesus disease |
| Significant antepartum hemorrhage |

### Immediate measures

At birth, the newborn baby's condition should be rapidly assessed and priority given to three major aspects of resuscitation in the following order:

1. Airway. Establish a safe and secure airway.
2. Breathing. Establish adequate and appropriate ventilation.
3. Circulation. Ensure that the heart rate and cardiac output is appropriate.

This section is not intended to act as a guide to resuscitation methods, but it is most important that all professional personnel working in an environment where it is planned to deliver babies must be trained and regularly retrained in appropriate resuscitation techniques. All equipment must be regularly checked to ensure that it is in working order. It has been shown in China that the introduction of neonatal resuscitation program guidelines developed by the American Academy of Pediatrics and the American Heart Association produced a threefold reduction in perinatal mortality (Zhu *et al.* 1997).

Babies who fail to rapidly adapt to birth by establishing spontaneous breathing and become pink should be quickly dried and transferred to a resuscitation trolley. The type of resuscitation depends on the infant's degree of depression. This can be summarized as:

1. Apneic with a heart rate above 100 beats per minute (bpm). This represents primary apnea, and the infant requires little more than vigorous cutaneous stimulation and oxygen blown across his or her nostrils.
2. Apneic with a heart rate below 100 bpm. This may represent the stage of secondary apnea. Suction of the mouth and nares should be applied followed by inflation of the lungs by means of a bag and a tight-fitting face-mask. The heart rate should pick up, and the color should improve. The baby will then usually rapidly develop spontaneous respirations. Some babies may be apneic because their mothers have recently been given an opiate for pain relief. Naloxone is a specific opiate antagonist and should be given (0.1 mg/kg by deep intramuscular injection) if the mother has received opiates within 4 h of delivery.
3. Pesistent failure to breathe and/or persistent bradycardia. The baby should be intubated and given intermittent positive-pressure ventilation (IPPV).
4. Persistent bradycardia or asystole. IPPV and cardiac massage should be rapidly started. Vascular access should be quickly established, and intravenous drugs such as adrenaline and calcium gluconate should be given. Adrenaline appears to be as effective if given down the endotracheal tube.

It has been the practice in many delivery rooms to resuscitate babies with 100% oxygen. This has recently been questioned as leading to a number of potential risks including reduction of cerebral blood flow (Lundstrom *et al.* 1995) and excessive free-radical release (Saugstad 1998). A large, randomized control trial of the effects of newborn resuscitation with room air compared to 100% oxygen has shown that babies who received room-air resuscitation had fewer postnatal problems than those who received 100% oxygen, although none of the differences were statistically significant (Saugstad *et al.* 1998). In particular, mortality in the first 7 days, overall neonatal mortality, and death from moderate or severe HIE were all less in the room air group. There appears to be little justification for routinely resuscitating asphyxiated newborn babies in high oxygen concentrations.

It is important during resuscitation to prevent cold stress and unnecessary utilization of oxygen to maintain body temperature. Every effort should be made to prevent the baby from becoming cold during resuscitation. The future role of therapeutic hypothermia is discussed on p. 515.

It is usually unnecessary to correct metabolic acidosis as a routine procedure during resuscitation. If the baby has a good circulation and adequate ventilation, then he or she should be able to correct his or her own metabolic acidosis. Early assessment of arterial pH is helpful as a baseline, and a further measure should be made 1 h later. If correction has not occurred by the second measure, then the careful use of sodium bicarbonate solution may be necessary. The routine use of albumin in neonatal resuscitation is controversial, but there is no evidence that this practice is beneficial for the baby and may be associated with additional myocardial compromise (Roberton 1997).

The role of intravenous glucose during resuscitation is discussed on p. 489.

## SYSTEMIC MANAGEMENT

### Respiratory support

Following immediate resuscitation, respiratory support may be necessary for comatose infants with severe encephalopathy and those with coincident lung disease, of which meconium aspiration is the most common. Infants with frequent and prolonged convulsions may also need to be supported by mechanical ventilation, and this may become necessary as a result of their anticonvulsant management. Careful assessment of arterial blood gas estimates is necessary to provide appropriate support. Spontaneously breathing infants should be electively intubated and ventilated if they develop hypercapnia due to depression of respiratory drive or lung disease [$P\text{aCO}_2 > 7$ kPa (53 mmHg)]. The fear of inducing respiratory arrest by adequate dosage of anticonvulsants is irrational. The effects of prolonged or frequent seizures make the need to treat this complication adequately essential (see Chapter 37). If fear of the infant requiring mechanical ventilation is a factor in avoiding adequate anticonvulsant therapy, then the infant should be referred to a center where this can be safely and rapidly undertaken. Hypoxia should also be avoided, and although there are no clear guidelines, the $P\text{aCO}_2$ should be maintained in the range of 10–12 kPa (75–90 mmHg) in mature infants.

Hyperventilation in the management of suspected cerebral oedema is discussed on p. 491.

### Fluids

Fluid restriction is widely used in the management of asphyxiated infants to prevent brain swelling, but the evidence that fluid intake contributes to cerebral edema is lacking. The baby should be given only the volume of fluid necessary to keep him or her just adequately hydrated. This requires at least daily measurement of serum osmolality and urinary concentration (specific gravity), aiming to maintain the serum osmolality in the region of 290 mOsm/l and the urinary specific gravity at 1010.

Fluid restriction may be important in asphyxiated infants who have complications such as inappropriate antidiuretic hormone (ADH) secretion and renal compromise. Inappropriate ADH secretion is suspected by demonstrating dilute plasma and concentrated urine. The fluid intake should be restricted until the serum osmolality and serum sodium levels return to normal.

Oliguria due to renal compromise is managed by maintenance of careful fluid balance. Daily measurement of plasma creatinine levels is a sensitive method of assessing renal function. Assessment of the state of hydration in severely oliguric patients is facilitated by measurement of central venous pressure. Acute renal failure is best managed conservatively.

### Blood pressure

Hypotension occurs frequently in severely asphyxiated infants, and continuous monitoring of arterial blood pressure is essential (Diprose *et al.* 1986). Plasma is often ineffective in restoring normotension, and dopamine (5–15 μg/kg/min) or dobutamine (2.5–15.0 μg/kg/min) is usually necessary to raise the blood pressure into the normal range. Care must be taken with albumin therapy for hypotension as this may put an additional volume load on an already compromised myocardium.

### Hemostasis

Disturbances in blood clotting are most commonly due to disseminated intravascular coagulation. Management is supportive, and there is no place for systemic heparinization. The infant should receive additional vitamin K and may require either fresh frozen plasma for replacement of clotting factors or platelet transfusions, or both. Regular hematological checks of clotting function should be performed in all infants with severe birth asphyxia.

### Infection

A high index of suspicion for infection must be maintained in all ill infants. Routine use of antibiotics cannot be recommended and should be used only for clinical indications or suspected infection. Early neonatal meningitis may present clinically in a manner similar to birth asphyxia, and if there is any doubt, a lumbar puncture must be performed.

## STANDARD BRAIN-ORIENTED MANAGEMENT

Traditionally, the standard management of the asphyxiated infant has been directed towards achieving a stable condition, adequate treatment of seizures and preventing or controlling cerebral edema. Increased awareness of subtle fits or asymptomatic electroconvulsive seizure activity in infants given neuromuscular relaxing agents has led to a wider use of continuous EEG monitoring (see p. 175). Adequate control of seizures is essential, and this is discussed in Ch. 37.

When analysing the effect of drugs in hypoxic–ischemic injury, the pathogenesis of the injury must be considered in relation to the pharmacological action of the drug. Following perinatal asphyxia, both the primary and the secondary cerebral insults may vary in severity, and, although interdependent, they may not necessarily be sequential. Ideally, in order to predict the likelihood of acute intracerebral sequelae, it is necessary to know for how long the fetus or infant has suffered significant cerebral underperfusion and whether there was a period of complete anoxia (cardiac arrest). Once resuscitation has been achieved, further variables include whether or not cerebral hypoperfusion (the 'no reflow phenomenon') has developed and whether intracranial hypertension intervened to impede cerebral perfusion further. The measurement of cerebral blood flow is fundamental to understanding these events, but this is not possible in the routine management of the asphyxiated newborn infant (see Chapter 10). Uncertainty concerning the duration of intrapartum asphyxia is common in the clinical setting, and this makes assessment and management of birth asphyxia largely empirical.

### Glucose

The decision as to whether or not to give asphyxiated infants glucose remains unresolved. The deleterious effects of high levels of glucose on asphyxial cerebral injury in the adolescent or mature animal have been reviewed by Myers *et al.* (1983). This has been extended by some to the fetus and newborn, but the evidence to support this is very limited.

More recent data have shown conclusively that there is a fundamental difference in the way the immature and mature brain responds to glucose infusion. The immature brain appears to be protected by elevated blood glucose levels immediately prior to asphyxia compared with animals that were not exposed to additional glucose (Vannucci & Mujsce 1992). The evidence that administration of glucose after asphyxia in immature animals is beneficial remains controversial. Hattori & Wasterlain (1990) have shown that glucose treatment following hypoxic–ischemic insult in 7-day-old rat pups protects against neuropathological damage compared to controls. Another study also using 7-day-old rat pups found that treatment with glucose immediately after hypoxic–ischemic insult caused more severe neuronal damage than in animals exposed to a similar insult without glucose infusion (Sheldon *et al.* 1992).

It is clear that hypoglycemia following asphyxia must be avoided. In the human situation, it is not possible to give clear advice about the use of additional glucose following a severe asphyxial event, and we must await a controlled study in the context of birth asphyxia.

## Anticonvulsants

It has not been shown that convulsions following birth asphyxia cause additional direct cerebral injury, although these data are difficult to acquire. The fits may only reflect existing neuronal compromise, and therefore, multiple anticonvulsant therapy to suppress all convulsive activity (either clinically observed or electrophysiologically evident) may not be justified. It is inappropriate to not treat infants with postasphyxial convulsions, particularly when frequent or lasting more than a few minutes. In my view, it is not necessary to abolish all convulsions, but treatment should be instituted for frequent (three or more convulsions per hour) or prolonged convulsions (any fit or electroconvulsive episode lasting more than 1 min).

The management of neonatal convulsions is considered in detail in Chapter 37.

### Barbiturates

This group of drugs has multiple actions on the central nervous system and is still the mainstay of brain-oriented management of the asphyxiated newborn infant. The cerebral effects of barbiturates are listed here, but these effects are dose-related and may be specific to one type of barbiturate only.

1. reduction in cerebral metabolic rate; thiopentone reduces this by up to 50% (Michenfelder 1974)
2. depression of cerebral function, including suppression of the EEG to the point at which it becomes isoelectric
3. reduction in cerebral blood flow due to an increase in cerebral vascular resistance (Pierce *et al.* 1962; Hanson *et al.* 1975)
4. anticonvulsant effects
5. reduction of cerebral edema (Simeone *et al.* 1979) in part related to reduction in cerebral blood flow
6. oxygen free radical consumption (Flamm *et al.* 1978)
7. biochemical modification of the cell, including stabilization of lysosomal membranes, reduction in intracellular calcium concentrations and modified neurotransmitter release (Steen & Michenfelder 1980).

The benefit of barbiturates in the management of hypoxic–ischemic injury has been demonstrated in human and animal studies but only when the drug was given before the asphyxial event (Campbell *et al.* 1968; Cockburn *et al.* 1969; Goodlin & Lloyd 1970). There have been a number of randomized clinical trials assessing the cerebral protective effects of a barbiturate (phenobarbitone or thiopentone) in neonates following birth asphyxia. There were no significant differences in outcome, but 14 of the 17 infants given thiopentone treatment required inotropic support for hypotension compared with only seven of 15 controls (Goldberg *et al.* 1986). Eyre & Wilkinson (1986) have reported the use of thiopentone in six severely asphyxiated neonates. The dosage was sufficient to produce an isoelectric EEG. In two infants, the infusion was stopped because of hypotension, and in all six, the outcome was death or severe handicap.

More recently, a randomized (none blinded) controlled study of phenobarbitone (40 mg/kg over 1 h) prior to the onset of seizures in 20 severely asphyxiated babies showed that the outcome at 3 years was significantly better than in a similar group of babies where phenobarbitone was only given after onset of seizures (Hall *et al.* 1998). However, a meta-analysis of barbiturate treatment in asphyxia did not show an overall beneficial effect when all the studies were considered together (Evans & Levene 1998).

In a paper entitled 'brain-orientated intensive care', Svenningsen *et al.* (1982) recommended the routine use of phenobarbitone within an hour of delivery in all severely asphyxiated infants. Using this as well as other methods, they claim to have reduced the mortality and incidence of neurodevelopmental handicap. It seems unlikely that the effect of phenobarbitone in the dosage used (10 mg/kg) would have any significant protective effect on the brain. It is more likely that these authors, by paying more careful attention to all aspects of the care of asphyxiated infants, have thereby improved the outlook.

Phenobarbitone is the first-line anticonvulsant (20 mg/kg loading dose followed by 3 mg/kg 12-hourly). The dosage of phenobarbitone should be carefully monitored in asphyxiated infants as toxicity may easily occur. Gal *et al.* (1984) have shown that asphyxiated neonates require about half the maintenance dose compared with non-asphyxiated infants to achieve a similar plasma concentration.

### Other anticonvulsants

If frequent or prolonged convulsions continue, then a second half loading dose of phenobarbitone can be given (10 mg/kg). Clonazepam is used as a second-line anticonvulsant (100 μg/kg loading dose) followed by an intermittent dosage regimen every 24 h. Phenytoin is also widely used to treat post-asphyxial convulsions, but is contraindicated with lignocaine (see below). A loading dose of 20 mg/kg may be used to achieve control of frequent seizures, but maintenance therapy is difficult to control.

More recently, two other anticonvulsants have been used to treat asphyxiated newborn infants; midazolam (0.05 mg/kg as a loading dose followed by 0.15 mg/kg/h) and lignocaine (lidocaine) (2 mg/kg as a loading dose followed by 6 mg/kg/h). There may be synergism between these drugs, and they may be a useful combination in babies with refractory seizures. The potentially cardiotoxic effects of lignocaine are rarely seen, but are more common if phenytoin has been given prior to the infusion of lignocaine having been started.

Anticonvulsants can be stopped once the infant is thought to be neurologically normal on clinical examination.

## Cerebral edema

There is some dispute as to the role of cerebral edema in contributing to acute cerebral injury following asphyxia. Brann & Myers (1975) have shown evidence of cerebral edema both macroscopically and microscopically within 2 h of severe asphyxia in a fetal monkey. In our experience, the median time for severe intracranial hypertension (intracranial pressure >15 mmHg) to develop in the human neonate following asphyxia is 26 h (unpublished data). These data are not of course incompatible, but the implication that early cerebral edema has a role in the primary pathogenesis of brain injury following intrapartum hypoxic–ischemic injury is unsubstantiated. Cerebral edema severe enough to cause secondary cerebral hypoperfusion is a potential complication of asphyxia, and adequate treatment of intracranial hypertension will not *per se* prevent brain injury. Levene *et al.* (1987) have analyzed the results of monitoring and treating raised intracranial pressure in full-term asphyxiated infants. In less than 10% of the babies studied, could intervention to control intracranial hypertension have had any significant beneficial effect on outcome.

There is no evidence that the routine monitoring of intracranial pressure and appropriate management makes any improvement in outcome.

### Corticosteroids

The role of steroids in the management of asphyxia is controversial, with few data available for either newborn humans or experimental animals. Studies on 5-day-old rats, whose brains at that age are at a comparable state of development to the full-term human brain, showed that treatment with dexamethasone before asphyxiation resulted in less severe cerebral effects than in untreated animals (Adlard & De Souza 1976). The use of steroids following neonatal asphyxia was ineffective in treating or preventing cerebral edema (De Souza & Dobbing 1973).

It has been suggested that dexamethasone has its main benefit in treating vasogenic edema and is less effective in cytotoxic edema (Yamaguchi *et al.* 1976), but in clinical practice, both types of brain swelling probably occur together. Corticosteroids have their major role in the treatment of focal cerebral edema associated with tumor or abscess, neither of which bears a close resemblance to the generalized brain swelling that occurs following perinatal asphyxia. In addition, there is a body of evidence on the adverse effects of steroids on the developing brain even when used over a short period of time (Weichsel 1977). Fitzhardinge *et al.* (1974) found measurable differences in neurological function of children who had received hydrocortisone only in the first 24 h of life, compared with untreated controls. Levene & Evans (1985) found no improvement in cerebral perfusion pressure within 6 h of giving dexamethasone. There is no good evidence for the beneficial effect of using steroids after a hypoxic–ischemic insult in the newborn, and their use is not recommended.

### Hyperventilation

There is a predictable relationship between $PaCO_2$, and cerebral blood flow. Increasing carbon dioxide tension induces cerebral arteriolar vasodilatation with increase in cerebral blood flow and vice versa (see Fig. 27.12). In adults, for every 0.13 kPa (1 mmHg) change in $PaCO_2$, there is approximately a 3% change in cerebral blood flow over the physiological range for $PaCO_2$ (Bruce 1984). This proportional change diminishes for levels of $PaCO_2$ below 2.7 kPa (20 mmHg). Following perinatal asphyxia, the arteriolar response may be less sensitive to changes in $PaCO_2$, and in some, there may be a paradoxical increase in cerebral blood flow with controlled hyperventilation (Sankaran 1984). Cerebral ischemia is an important component of the pathophysiology of postasphyxial injury in cerebral hypoperfusion, and it is possible that severe hyperventilation may exacerbate impaired reperfusion to the compromised brain. This is strongly implicated in PVL in premature infants (p. 380).

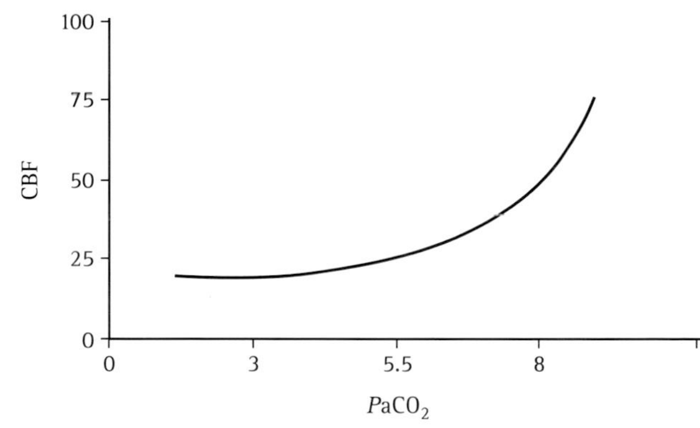


**Figure 27.12** Relationship between $PaCO_2$ and cerebral blood flow (CBF). Redrawn from Bruce (1984).

There have been no clinical trials of hyperventilation in asphyxiated newborn infants. In practice, we attempt to maintain the $PaCO_2$ in asphyxiated infants who are mechanically ventilated at about 4.5 kPa (34 mmHg). A high positive end-expiratory pressure (PEEP) level is likely to produce a higher $PaCO_2$ (Stewart *et al.* 1981), and PEEP should be kept as low as possible in asphyxiated infants who are mechanically ventilated. Hyperventilation should be avoided.

### Osmotic agents

A variety of agents, including mannitol, glycerol, and urea, have been used to shrink the swollen neonatal brain. These agents act by inducing a higher osmotic pressure across the blood–brain barrier, thereby causing intracerebral shrinkage. A theoretical hazard is the entry of the osmotic agent into the brain through the damaged blood–brain barrier, causing a rebound effect of brain swelling. In a neonatal animal model, mannitol significantly reduced the brain water content when given immediately after an asphyxial event (Mujsce *et al.* 1988), but it did not reduce the severity or distribution of brain damage in treated versus untreated animals. Mannitol is the only osmotic agent where published data exist on its use in the newborn. Marchal *et al.* (1974) in an uncontrolled study gave mannitol to 225 babies with the diagnosis of asphyxia, although the precise indications for treatment varied. Early treatment was defined as mannitol infusion (1 g/kg) before the baby was 2 h of age. There were significantly fewer deaths ($p = 0.005$), and the survivors had a better neurological outcome ($p = 0.014$) in the early treatment group compared with those treated after 2 h. A fall in intracranial pressure and an improvement in cerebral perfusion pressure was found on each occasion when mannitol (1 g/kg over 20 min) was infused intravenously in a group of severely asphyxiated babies (Levene & Evans 1985). This appears to be the only agent which is of proven value in treating intracranial hypertension in the asphyxiated newborn. Despite the reduction in ICP in many babies, our follow-up data did not suggest that this made any difference to long-term outcome.

### Barbiturates

As mentioned above, barbiturates increase cerebral vascular resistance, thereby reducing cerebral blood flow, and it is this action that contributes to the lowering of intracranial pressure in the swollen brain. It is unlikely that this will improve cerebral perfusion pressure.

## OUTCOME

Prediction of outcome in asphyxiated infants is of obvious importance for the parents, as they will ask 'will my baby be handicapped?' An accurate and honest answer may be available from the results of good follow-up studies. Another important aspect of predicting outcome is the question of when it is appropriate to abandon resuscitative efforts or withdraw intensive care in infants likely to be severely handicapped. The answers to these questions are beginning to emerge, but a critical review of the assessment methods is necessary, and this is discussed in detail below. A major problem in the evaluation of follow-up studies is the failure to distinguish whether the data refer to full-term babies only or a mixture of mature and immature infants. In addition, the problem of defining what is asphyxia influences outcome statistics. For the purpose of this review, only reports from full-term infants will be considered, and the outcome from different assessment techniques will be discussed separately. The utility of any test can be evaluated from its sensitivity, specificity and positive predictive value. Sensitivity refers to the percentage of handicapped infants detected by the test, and specificity is the percentage of normal infants detected by a normal test. Positive predictive value is the proportion of times a positive test predicts adverse outcome. To evaluate any assessment of outcome, all these variables should be considered. Wherever it has been possible to calculate these figures, they are given in the text.

There is some evidence that the prognosis following intrapartum asphyxia has improved over recent years (Finer *et al.* 1983). A Swedish study reported that 50% of infants surviving asphyxia between 1973 and 1976 had significant neurodevelopmental sequelae, in contrast to a 17% incidence of handicap in those born between 1976 and 1979 (Svenningsen *et al.* 1982). Svenningsen *et al.* related the improved outcome to the introduction of brain-oriented intensive care, but there has been no single therapeutic innovation that has improved the outcome for asphyxiated babies over recent years.

Few data are available for the outcome of asphyxiated term babies born in developing countries. One recent study from Kathmandu in Nepal reports that the overall risk of death or major disability at 1 year of age in a group of term babies with signs of neonatal encephalopathy was 62% compared with only 4% of normal controls (Ellis *et al.* 1999). This is considerably higher than in the developed world. The relative risk of impairment in survivors of grade I neonatal encephalopathy was 5.3 (95% CI 0.9, 30), and for grade II neonatal encephalopathy, 32.1 (95% CI 7.9, 131).

## MORTALITY

The mortality rate of live-born asphyxiated infants depends on the severity of the insult and the intensity of treatment. If asphyxia is defined by depression of the Apgar score, then mortality increases inversely to gestational age and birth weight. MacDonald *et al.* (1980) report an overall mortality of 46% in severely asphyxiated infants of all gestational ages, and the presence of intrauterine growth retardation, respiratory distress syndrome, and hypothermia were all associated with a significantly higher risk of death. In another study, over half of the infants died, if born with an Apgar score of 0 at birth, or delay in establishing respiration until 20 min after birth (Scott 1976). In the well-known study of Nelson & Ellenberg (1981) over 40 000 infants had an accurate assessment of the Apgar score. Those with a birth weight below 2500 g with severe depression of the Apgar score at 15 and 20 min had approximately a 90% chance of dying, but this was considerably less in infants weighing more than 2500 g (Table 27.5).

Delay in establishing spontaneous respiration also seems to predict the risk of death. Steiner & Nelligan (1975) have shown that infants who have not established regular breathing 30 min after return of the heartbeat subsequently have a very poor outcome. They suggest that resuscitation under these circumstances should not be continued for longer than this time. By contrast, a Swedish study found that 25% of babies who had not breathed spontaneously by 20 min were without significant handicap (Ergander *et al.*

**Table 27.5 Risk of death or cerebral palsy (CP) in infants with Apgar scores of 0–3 at varying times from birth**

| | Birth weight < 2500 g | | Birth weight > 2500 g | |
|---|---|---|---|---|
| Age (min) | Death in first year (%) | CP (%) | Death in first year (%) | CP (%) |
| 1 | 26 | 2 | 3 | 0.7 |
| 5 | 55 | 7 | 8 | 0.7 |
| 10 | 67 | 7 | 18 | 5 |
| 15 | 84 | 0 | 48 | 9 |
| 20 | 96 | 0 | 59 | 57 |

*Source*: Data from Nelson & Ellenberg (1981).

1983). Peliowski & Finer (1992) have reviewed the literature and report the outcome of only 35 full-term babies who did not breathe spontaneously by 30 min, and 24 (80%) died or were significantly handicapped.

### When to abandon resuscitation

1. If an infant has no cardiac output after 10 min of effective resuscitation, then treatment should be abandoned.
2. If a baby is not breathing spontaneously by 30 min, then the value of further resuscitation should be seriously questioned. Other causes for failure to breathe spontaneously should be considered, such as opiate depression and neuromuscular disorders. The final decision to abandon resuscitation should be made by the most senior neonatologist/pediatrician available.

## DISABILITY

Babies born apparently dead, but resuscitated rapidly, may subsequently be neurologically normal (Steiner & Nelligan 1975; Scott 1976; Jain *et al.* 1991). Casalaz *et al.* (1998) described 29 babies of gestational age 36 weeks and above, born with a zero 1 min Apgar score and who were successfully resuscitated. Forty-five per cent of these babies were subsequently described as normal, and a further 34% died prior to discharge from hospital. Of those who went home, only 31.5% were disabled. Disability probably depends on the duration and severity of the asphyxial insult as well as the development of cardiovascular complications.

Asphyxia has been described as having an all or none effect. The majority of very severely asphyxiated babies die, and the majority of the remainder are without major neurological deficit and are often reported as being 'normal' at follow-up. Only a very small proportion are disabled. This effect may be illusory as there are very few good long-term follow-up studies to assess the children for less severe forms of disability such as clumsiness, attention deficit disorders and learning problems.

Finer *et al.* (1983) in Canada have regularly assessed a group of full-term asphyxiated infants at 27 months, 3.5 years (Robertson & Finer 1985) and 8 years (Robertson *et al.* 1989). They showed that there is a gradation of effect on the intelligence quotient (IQ) for different degrees of severity of the asphyxial insult. At 3.5 years, the children with moderate hypoxic–ischemic encephalopathy (HIE) had a median Stanford Binet IQ of 92.3 compared with 101.5 in babies with mild HIE (Robertson & Finer 1985). At 8 years, there was a difference in IQ of 11 points between children with moderate HIE and mild HIE and 17 points between moderate HIE and an unasphyxiated control group (Robertson *et al.* 1989). Children who survived severe HIE had a median IQ of 48 at 8 years. Cognitive impairment as measured by the IQ therefore appears to represent a continuum of disability reflecting the severity of the initial asphyxial insult.

The classical disability suffered by the survivors of severe asphyxia is cerebral palsy. This may be associated with intellectual impairment, blindness and epilepsy, but the motor deficit is invariably present with these other disabilities. Mental retardation alone is not a recognized sequel to intrapartum asphyxia. Two distinct forms of cerebral palsy occur as the result of birth asphyxia at full term: spastic quadriplegia and choreoathetosis, or a combination of these two. These two patterns of motor deficit presumably reflect the regions of the brain predominately affected by the asphyxial process (see p 474).

The late onset of dystonia (including athetosis) with normal intelligence has been described many years following perinatal asphyxia (Saint Hilaire *et al.* 1991; Scott & Jankovic 1996). The mean age of onset in these studies was over 10 years, with progression over a further 7–10 years. In one study, the latency in neonates with an hypoxic–ischemic aetiology was 27.6 years (Scott & Jankovic 1996). In another study, none of the subjects were severely disabled by the dystonia (Saint Hilaire *et al.* 1991).

### Fetal assessment

#### Passage of meconium

Thick meconium present in the liquor at the onset of labor carries a sevenfold increased risk of perinatal death (MacDonald *et al.* 1985). Meconium staining of the liquor does not, however, predict the risk of subsequent disability. Ninety-nine per cent of all babies born with meconium-stained liquor do not have cerebral palsy (Freeman & Nelson 1988).

#### Acidosis

Low *et al.* (1978) defined fetal acidosis as an umbilical artery buffer base of less than 34 mmol/l, and these infants had on average a lower 1- and 5-min Apgar score than a control, non-acidotic group. However, they could find no differences in neurological outcome between the acidotic and control groups at 12 months of age. Ruth & Raivio (1988) assessed umbilical arterial acid–base values on 982 live-born (mainly full-term) infants and correlated these measurements with neurodevelopmental outcome at 12 months of age. The positive predictive value for low pH (<7.16) and high lactate (>5.4 mmol/l) with reference to abnormal outcome was only 8 and 5%, respectively. Therefore, acidosis at birth does not appear to predict adverse outcome and cannot be used as a measure of potential compromise to the fetal brain.

### Cardiotocography

Fetal condition is assessed widely by means of measuring the fetal heart rate (see Chapter 25). This can be done intermittently by means of a stethoscope or by an electronic device. Fetal distress is diagnosed on the basis of fetal tachycardia (>160 bpm) or bradycardia (<120 bpm) or decelerations in the heart rate in response to, or following, a contraction. Continuous electronic fetal heart rate monitoring and evaluation of changes in heart rate with contractions (cardiotocography) have become very widely used in recent years, but there are relatively few data on the long-term prediction of outcome.

Grant (1989) has reviewed the literature on fetal monitoring and performed meta-analyses on the published data. When electronic fetal monitoring with scalp blood sampling for fetal pH is compared with intermittent auscultation, there is no significant reduction in perinatal deaths (odds ratio 0.81, 95% CI 0.22–2.98). Cardiotocogram (CTG) monitoring increases the risk of Cesarean section fourfold compared with intermittent auscultation. When the effect of electronic fetal monitoring and scalp sampling was compared with intermittent auscultation on neonatal seizures, there was a significant reduction in the number of infants with convulsions in those fetuses continuously monitored (odds ratio 0.49, 95% CI 0.29–0.82).

There are limited data on the correlation with CTG monitoring and subsequent disability. Painter *et al.* (1978) followed up 38 full-term infants with 'ominous' fetal heart-rate patterns. These infants showed moderate to severely variable patterns with or without late decelerations. Of the 38 infants, five were neurologically abnormal at 1 year of age, and four in the group had patterns showing severe variability. Surprisingly, few of these infants had depressed Apgar scores. A subsequent report stated that none of these children were abnormal in later childhood (Paneth & Stark 1983). Ingemarrson *et al.* (1981) showed that fewer infants were born with depressed Apgar scores over three time periods following the introduction of CTG monitoring, but in the high-risk full-term pregnancies, there was no statistically significant reduction in neurological sequelae at 2 years, although there was a trend towards improvement. This study was undertaken over a period of time when many changes were introduced in both obstetric and neonatal management, and no firm conclusions on the prognostic value of abnormal CTGs can be made.

In a limited follow-up study from Dublin of electronic fetal heart rate monitoring versus intermittent auscultation, there were no differences in the number of children with cerebral palsy in the two groups (Grant *et al.* 1989).

In conclusion, CTG monitoring increases the rate of operative deliveries, but does not reduce the risk of perinatal death. There is good evidence that the number of neonatal convulsions is reduced in the group that are electronically monitored but that there is no reduction in the risk of cerebral palsy.

## Apgar scores

Depression of the Apgar score has traditionally been widely used as a method for determining asphyxia and predicting outcome. The risk of handicap following depression of the Apgar score is best estimated from the data of Nelson & Ellenberg (1981) and is shown in Table 27.5. In full-term infants, the risk only becomes significant if the Apgar score remains 0–3 at 20 min. Depression of the Apgar score to this degree at 15 min is associated with less than a 10% risk of subsequent cerebral palsy in surviving infants. In another study, 93% of infants with severely depressed Apgar scores (0 at 1 min and/or 0–3 at 5 min) were normal at follow-up (Thomson *et al.* 1977).

An overview of three studies where the outcome of full-term babies with depressed Apgar scores of 3 or less at 5 min showed that this carried an overall risk of mortality of 16% but only a 3% risk of handicap in surviving infants (Peliowski & Finer 1992). Levene *et al.* (1986) identified a group of infants at risk of handicap following intrapartum asphyxia and assessed the sensitivity of various degrees of Apgar score depression (Table 27.6). They found an Apgar score of 5 or less at 10 min to be the most sensitive predictor

**Table 27.6 Sensitivity and specificity of six different grades of Apgar depression (Levene *et al.* 1986 © by the Lancet Ltd)**

| Depression of Apgar score | *n* | Sensitivity (%) | Specificity (%) |
|---|---|---|---|
| < 3 at 1 min: > 5 by 5 min | 42 | 13 | 38 |
| < 5 at 5 min: > 5 by 10 min | 35 | 17 | 67 |
| < 3 at 5 min: > 5 by 10 min | 10 | 13 | 90 |
| < 5 at 10 min: > 5 by 20 min | 15 | 43 | 95 |
| < 3 at 10 min: > 5 by 20 min | 5 | 17 | 99 |
| < 5 at 20 min: or more | 3 | 13 | 100 |

of outcome, and this was also highly specific. Apgar scores do not reflect how long the infant suffered from intrapartum asphyxia, and this is, in most cases, a blunt instrument for predicting outcome.

### Onset of spontaneous respiration

The time to establish spontaneous respiration is used by many as an index of the severity of asphyxia. Unfortunately, factors other than hypoxic–ischemic insult may cause depression of respiration, such as the administration of maternal drugs and neuromuscular disease of the newborn. Failure to establish spontaneous respiration by 30 min carries a very high risk of handicap or death (see above). Scott (1976) reported a remarkably low risk of handicap in a group of surviving infants who had shown no spontaneous respiration by 20 min from birth. Ergander *et al.* (1983) reported that 71% of babies who had established spontaneous respiration by 20 min were normal or only had minimal handicap. In another study, almost 70% of mature infants who had required IPPV for more than 1 min were normal (Mulligan *et al.* 1980). Fysh *et al.* (1982) reported an infant who did not establish regular respiration for 25 min and who had an arterial pH of 6.6 at 1 h. This infant was entirely normal at 3 years of age, and it is interesting to note that she had neither convulsions nor any other neurological abnormality in the newborn period, supporting the contention that the severity of clinical neurological abnormality is the more important predictor of adverse outcome.

### Hypoxic–ischemic encephalopathy (HIE)

Moderate or severe encephalopathy following intrapartum asphyxia has been shown to be a more sensitive predictor of death or severe neurodevelopmental sequelae than depression of the Apgar scores (Levene *et al.* 1986). Different studies have reported an outcome related to the severity of hypoxic–ischemic encephalopathy (HIE) (Sarnat & Sarnat 1976; Finer *et al.* 1981, 1983; Low *et al.* 1985; Robertson & Finer 1985; Amiel-Tison & Ellison 1986; Levene *et al.* 1986), and these methods are discussed in Chapter 8. Although some vary slightly in their definition of the grades of encephalopathy, there is remarkable consensus when predicting adverse outcome. Results from five of these studies are shown in Table 27.7. No infant with mild HIE developed significant neurodevelopmental handicap. The one handicapped infant in the study of Levene *et al.* (1986) had congenital myopathy. The incidence of severe handicap or death in the moderate encephalopathy group varied between 15 and 27%. Robertson & Finer (1985) found all infants with severe encephalopathy to have a poor outcome, but this was not the case in the majority of studies. Surprisingly, up to 25% of infants comatose due to asphyxia, but who survived, were without any significant handicap.

Peliowski & Finer (1992) have reported a meta-analysis of five published studies reporting outcome by severity of HIE. The risk of death for babies with severe, moderate, and mild HIE is 61, 5.6, and less than 1%, respectively. In surviving infants, the risk of severe neurological handicap for severe, moderate and mild HIE is 72, 20, and less than 1%, respectively.

The duration of time that infants show clinical neurological abnormalities following asphyxia correlates well with the risk of handicap. Sarnat & Sarnat (1976) reported that a good outcome was seen in infants with moderate encephalopathy (lethargy, hypotonia and seizures) if abnormal clinical signs had disappeared within 5 days of life. In another study, only infants with neurological signs persisting for more than 6 weeks developed cerebral palsy (Scott 1976). Recovery to a normal neurological score by 7 days after birth was found by Thompson *et al.* (1997) to be a very good prognostic marker.

### Scoring systems

Various scoring systems to summarize the extent of neurological abnormalities after asphyxia have been developed (Lipper *et al.* 1986; Bao *et al.* 1993; Perlman & Risser 1996; Ekert *et al.* 1997; Thompson *et al.* 1997; Carter *et al.* 1998). Lipper *et al.*'s postasphyxial score (PAS) was assigned within the first 24 h, based on 17 items, six of which are related to tone. The optimal (maximum) score was 39, and no infants with a score of 6 or less survived without a severe handicap. The PAS correctly predicted abnormal outcome (sensitivity) at 1 year in 95% of infants and showed a specificity of 83%. Thompson *et al.* (1997) devised a score based on nine signs

**Table 27.7 Proportion of handicapped children depending on their degree of PAE (only full-term infants are included)**

| | | Proportion severely abnormal or dead (%) | | | |
|---|---|---|---|---|---|
| Reference | *n* | Mild (1) | Moderate (2) | Severe (3) | Duration of follow-up (years) |
| Sarnat & Sarnat (1976) | 21 | – | 25 | 100 | 1 |
| Finer *et al.* (1981) | 89 | 0 | 15 | 92 | 3.5 |
| Robertson & Finer (1985) | 200 | 0 | 27 | 100 | 3.5 |
| Low *et al.* (1985) | 42 | –[a] | 27 | 50 | 1 |
| Levene *et al.* (1986) | 122 | 1[b] | 25 | 75 | 2.5 (median) |

[a]Mild and moderate HIE considered together.

[b]Handicap due to congenital myopathy.

**Table 27.8 Comparison of three scoring systems for prediction of term infants at-risk of poor outcome following asphyxia**

| Author | Scoring system | Outcome variable | Sensitivity (%) | Specificity (%) | PPV (%) |
|---|---|---|---|---|---|
| Perlman & Risser (1996) | pH ≤7.00<br>Delivery room intubation<br>Apgar ≤5 at 5 min | Neonatal seizures | 80 | 98.8 | 80 |
| Ekert *et al.* (1997) | Spontaneous respiration ≥10 min<br>Onset seizures ≤4 h | HIE | 71 | 73 | 69 |
| Carter *et al.* (1998) | Score ≥6[a] | Multiorgan failure | – | – | 73 |

[a]See text for scoring system.
PPV = positive predictive value.

(two based on tone or posture) with a maximum abnormality score of 22. They showed that babies with a maximum score of >15 had a positive predictive value of 92% with sensitivity and specificity of 71 and 96% respectively. Levene *et al.* (1986) found a moderate or severe encephalopathy to have a positive predictive value for adverse outcome (handicap or death) of 96% and a specificity of 78%.

Three further systems have attempted to look at very early markers of neonatal complications that fall short of neurodevelopmental outcome (Perlman & Risser 1996). The aim of these studies was to identify a group of babies soon after birth who were at risk of permanent injury and in whom timely intervention may improve outcome (see Chapter 28). Table 27.8 shows the sensitivity, specificity and positive predictive value of these scoring systems. Caution must be exercised in interpreting the predictive value of these tests as neurodevelopmental outcome was not assessed, but rather variables that may or may not be good markers of the risk of adverse outcome.

The type of abnormal neurological signs may also predict poor outcome. Brown *et al.* (1974) recognize two clinical categories that are particularly associated with death or handicap. In the group with persistent hypotonia, only 16% were normal, and in those in whom hypotonia evolved to extensor hypertonia, only 23% were normal. Among infants with a predominant extensor type of abnormality, 56% were normal on follow-up. Apathy in the newborn period had also been reported to occur more frequently in infants with abnormal outcome, but no children were found to be severely handicapped in this group (De Souza & Richards 1978). Convulsions may predict outcome to some extent. Approximately half of the asphyxiated infants with neonatal seizures have some functional handicap (see Chapter 37).

It is clear that the severity of abnormal neurological behavior occurring after birth in infants who have suffered intrapartum asphyxia is an excellent predictor of subsequent outcome.

The pattern of abnormal neurological signs in asphyxiated babies may correlate with the distribution of brain injury. Full-term infants with predominantly basal ganglia involvement on MR imaging have persistent and diffuse neurological abnormalities compared with those who sustain injury mainly in the white matter. These latter show a different clinical pattern with an improved sucking reflex and less severe abnormalities in tone (Mercuri *et al.* 1999). Rosenbloom (1994) has described a group of severely asphyxiated babies with later development of dyskinetic (choreoathetoid) cerebral palsy to have relatively little evidence of HIE in the neonatal period presumably because of cortical sparing.

### Brain imaging

Computerized tomography (CT) is reported to be a good predictor of bad neurodevelopmental outcome in asphyxiated babies when extensive areas of hypodensity are seen in scans taken at 7–14 days after birth (Fitzhardinge *et al.* 1981; Adsett *et al.* 1985; Lipper *et al.* 1986). The sensitivity and specificity of abnormal scans (diffuse or global decrease in density) in the prediction of major handicap or subsequent death are reported to be 90–91 and 60–80%, respectively (Adsett *et al.* 1985; Lipper *et al.* 1986). In contrast, others have shown no correlation between abnormal CT scans and outcome, but these studies were performed within 7 days from birth (Finer *et al.* 1983; Lipp-Zwahlen *et al.* 1985b). In summary, CT appears to be a good predictor of subsequent outcome in asphyxiated full-term infants, but only if the scan is done after the first week of life. This limits the value of this technique in the acute management of the severely asphyxiated infant in whom withdrawal of care is considered.

More recently, MR imaging has been widely used in the early assessment of asphyxiated infants. The sequence of changes seen on MR has been described in Chapter 6. Early changes on MR that are associated with a bad outcome include abnormalities in the basal ganglia (Rutherford *et al.* 1996; Aida *et al.* 1998; Barkovich *et al.* 1998) and extensive abnormalities in the periventricular white matter (Rutherford *et al.* 1996). Cortical highlighting in the perirolandic area (Rutherford *et al.* 1996; Barkovich *et al.* 1998) is also seen in infants with a poor prognosis, but all of these usually show abnormalities in the basal ganglia as well.

The best predictor of bad outcome in MR scans taken in the first 10 days of life is abnormality of signal intensity within the posterior limb of the internal capsule (PLIC)

(Rutherford *et al.* 1998). This is best seen on IR sequences and was often associated with more extensive abnormalities within the basal ganglia. An abnormal or equivocal signal intensity within the PLIC predicted abnormal outcome with a sensitivity of 90%, specificity of 100% and positive predictive value of 100%.

Two scoring systems have been described, which rate abnormalities seen on early MR scans in term asphyxiated infants (Rutherford *et al.* 1995; Barkovich *et al.* 1998). In MR studies performed before the seventh day after birth, higher scores as the result of basal ganglia abnormalities were most highly predictive of adverse outcome at 12 months (Barkovich *et al.* 1998).

### Electroencephalography

These techniques are discussed fully in Chapter 11. The EEG abnormalities seen in mature asphyxiated infants and associated with a poor prognosis include isoelectric recordings and periodic patterns (Sarnat & Sarnat 1976; Holmes *et al.* 1982; Wertheim *et al.* 1994; Selton & Andre 1997) and persistent low-voltage states (Holmes *et al.* 1982). Holmes *et al.* (1983) have shown that some infants with a burst suppression pattern can be stimulated to produce continuous activity, and in these infants, the prognosis is better. A normal EEG in asphyxiated infants is usually associated with an excellent prognosis (Rose & Lombroso 1970; Sarnat & Sarnat 1976; Watanabe *et al.* 1980; Wertheim *et al.* 1994; Selton & Andre 1997).

Peliowski & Finer (1992) have performed a meta-analysis on four studies where early EEG assessment could be correlated with outcome in groups of asphyxiated mature neonates. Severe EEG abnormalities included burst suppression, low-voltage, or isoelectric EEGs, and moderate EEG abnormality included slow wave activity. The overall risk of death or handicap derived from these studies is 95% for a severely abnormal EEG, 64% for a moderately abnormal EEG, and 3.3% for a normal or mildly abnormal EEG. Further studies published since this meta-analysis have confirmed these findings (Wertheim *et al.* 1994; Selton & Andre 1997). Cerebral function monitoring (a single channel compressed EEG signal) is now widely used in neonates and is discussed in detail in Chapter 11. Burst suppression or paroxysmal activity has been reported to be associated with a poor outcome (Thornberg & Ekstrom-Jodal 1994), and these abnormalities may be present within 4 h of birth (Eken *et al.* 1995).

Evoked response EEGs such as visual, auditory, and somatosensory evoked potentials may also provide accurate prognostic information in asphyxia, and the role of these techniques in the prediction of outcome following birth asphyxia is discussed in Chapter 12.

### Intracranial pressure

Continuous measurement of intracranial pressure by a subarachnoid catheter gives some prognostic information (Levene *et al.* 1987). No infant with a sustained rise in intracranial pressure of 15 mmHg or more lasting for an hour or more survived without major handicap. Infants with sustained elevations in intracranial pressure above 10 mmHg generally had a worse prognosis than those without a rise to this level, but a cut-off of 10 mmHg was not as sensitive for handicap as a sustained elevation to 15 mmHg.

Interestingly, low cerebral perfusion pressure did not predict outcome as well as intracranial hypertension (Levene *et al.* 1987). This is probably because hypotension can cause a low cerebral perfusion pressure without any significant cerebral edema. The hypotension reflects cardiovascular injury with a good prognosis rather than cerebral compromise.

### Doppler assessment

The use of Doppler ulrasound to assess cerebral hemodynamics has been shown to be a useful prognostic indicator in term asphyxiated newborns (Archer *et al.* 1986; Levene *et al.* 1989; Low *et al.* 1994; Liao & Hung 1997; Ilves *et al.* 1998). The measurement of PRI (Pourcelot's resistance index; see p. 132) predicts outcome in asphyxiated full-term infants with an 86% accuracy (Archer *et al.* 1986). A low PRI (<0.55) predicted adverse outcome with a sensitivity and a specificity of 100 and 81%, respectively. In a more recent study using duplex Doppler that allows calculation of cerebral blood flow velocity (CBFV) within the anterior cerebral artery, Levene *et al.* (1989) showed that a CBFV value above 3SDs from the mean had a positive predictive value for adverse outcome (death or handicap) of 94% compared with 83% for a PRI < 0.55. The sensitivity for high CBFV was 57%, and the specificity 88%. The advantage of Doppler assessment is that abnormalities become apparent within 12–60 h after birth (Archer *et al.* 1986; Levene *et al.* 1989; Ilves *et al.* 1998).

### Magnetic resonance spectroscopy (see also Chapter 10 and p. 483)

This technique allows separation of a variety of biochemical compounds within the brain, and changes related to asphyxia have been studied in full-term newborn infants. Two techniques have been used, based on $^{31}$P and $^{1}$H proton spectroscopy. The former provides information on phosphorylated energy states within the brain. The phosphorus metabolites ATP, phosphocreatine (PCr) and inorganic phosphorus ($P_i$) can be measured, and the PCr/$P_i$ ratio has been used to assess the state of degradation of the cerebral energy state. Degradation in ATP is associated with a poor outcome (Moorcroft *et al.* 1991; Roth *et al.* 1992, 1997; Lorek *et al.* 1994; Martin *et al.* 1996) A PCr/$P_i$ ratio below the range of values from normal infants predicted an adverse outcome after asphyxia with a sensitivity and a specificity of 88 and 83%, respectively. The positive predictive value was 64% (Moorcroft *et al.* 1991). $^{1}$H proton spectroscopy has also been evaluated in a group of severely asphyxiated infants, and high levels of intracerebral lactate and low *N*-acetylaspartate (NAA) predict adverse outcome (Peden *et al.* 1993;

Groenendaal *et al.* 1994; Hanrahan *et al.* 1996; Leth *et al.* 1996; Penrice *et al.* 1996).

## NEONATAL BRAIN DEATH

The concept of brain death is now well established in children, and guidelines on diagnosis have been published in both the USA (Task Force 1987) and Britain (British Paediatric Association 1991). These criteria are compared in Table 27.9. Both documents agree that brain death cannot be diagnosed in premature infants, but there is some disagreement as to the diagnosis of brain death in the mature neonate. The British Paediatric Association document states that in infants of 37 weeks' gestation to 2 months of age, 'given the state of knowledge it is rarely possible to diagnose confidently brain stem death at this age', and in infants below 37 weeks' gestation, 'the concept of brain stem death is inappropriate for infants of this age group'. In the USA, the Special Task Force of the American Academy of Pediatrics concludes that 'in term newborns (>38 weeks' gestation), the criteria [for diagnosing brain death] are useful seven days after the neurologic insult'.

These differences revolve around the rapid developmental changes seen in the later stages of gestation and the early weeks of life. This means that there cannot be absolute reliance placed on the presence or absence of brainstem reflexes at this developmental age. Volpe (1987) describes two infants with apparent brain death including coma, absent respiration, loss of pupillary responses to light, and loss of other brainstem responses who survived. One, a 35-week-old infant, showed near-normal development at 1 year of age, and the other, a full-term infant, regained brainstem reflexes 24 h following the first examination and left hospital alive, albeit in a persistent vegetative state.

Another difference between the American and British criteria is the inclusion of laboratory data (EEG and radionuclide angiography) in the American guidelines. The natural history of the isoelectric EEG in the neonatal period is now well established in terms of predicting bad outcome, but many babies with this abnormality survive despite irreversible brain injury (see p. 497). Limited experience of radionuclide angiography in the neonatal period in confirming brain death makes its routine use questionable.

**Table 27.9 Comparison of the British and US (American Academy of Pediatrics) criteria for the diagnosis of brain death**

| Criteria | British Paediatric Association | AAP Special Task Force |
|---|---|---|
| Preconditions | Comatose and apneic<br>Clear diagnosis | Comatose and apneic<br>Clear diagnosis<br>Flaccid tone and absence of spontaneous movements |
| Exclusions | Drug, endocrine and metabolic causes excluded<br>Neuromuscular blockade has been demonstrably reversed<br>No hypothermia | Toxic and metabolic disorders excluded<br>Sedative, hypnotic and paralytic drugs excluded<br>No hypotension<br>No hypothermia |
| Absence of brainstem function | No pupillary response<br>No corneal reflex<br>No vestibulo-ocular reflex<br>(Caloric test)<br>No doll's eyes reflex<br>No motor response to pain in cranial nerve V distribution<br>No gag reflex to suction of trachea<br>Apnea persists despite a rise in $PaCO_2$ > 50 mmHg (6.6 kPa) against a background of normoxia | Absence of movement of bulbar musculature including facial and oropharyngeal muscles<br>No corneal reflex<br>No vestibulor-ocular reflex or spontaneous eye movements<br>No cough reflex<br>No smiling or rooting reflex<br>No gag reflex on suction of trachea<br>Respiratory movements absent with patient off ventilator<br>Apnea using standardized methods after other criteria met |
| Laboratory tests | Not necessary | EEG – electrocerebral silence over 30 min<br>CBF – cerebral radionuclide angiogram demonstrating arrest of carotid circulation at base of skull and absence of intracranial arterial circulation |
| Observation period | Two examinations 12–24 h apart by two separate clinicians, one of whom is a pediatrician and one not primarily involved in the child's care | Two examinations and EEGs separated by:<br>in infants 7 days to 2 months – 48 h apart<br>in infants 2–12 months – 24 h apart |

Ashwal & Schneider (1989) described the clinical course of 18 premature and full-term infants whom they felt showed the features of brain death including coma, apnea and absent brainstem reflexes. Additional information including EEG and radionuclide scanning was performed in most. Nine of the 18 infants with clinical signs of brain death had an isoelectric EEG on the first examination, and 11 of the 17 in whom radionuclide scanning was performed showed no evidence of cerebral blood flow. Serum levels of phenobarbitone greater than 25 µg/ml were thought to suppress the EEG and make this investigation unreliable. They conclude that in full-term infants, the persistence of clinical signs of brainstem death was inconsistent with survival, and in premature infants, the persistence of the signs for 3 days was inconsistent with survival off the ventilator. They also report that an isolectric EEG in the absence of factors known to suppress the EEG was associated with inevitable death if the clinical signs of brain death persisted for 24 h. Although all the babies in this study died, some survived for some time in a persistent vegetative state. This underlines the difficulty in neonates of diagnosing 'brain death' in the context of brainstem death. It is not unusual for some brainstem functions, such as respiratory activity, to persist despite the fact that the brain has been massively and irreparably damaged.

Some investigations are helpful in the evaluation of irreversible and massive cerebral injury. These include severe EEG abnormalities as described on p. 497, abnormal Doppler values (low PRI or high CBFV; see p. 133) and MRS if this is available. A sequence of changes within the anterior cerebral artery detected by Doppler ultrasound have been described as a feature of neonatal brain death. These include initially a decrease and subsequent loss of the diastolic component, followed by the appearance of retrograde flow and, finally, loss of both systolic and diastolic flow in the cerebral vessel with preservation of flow in the common carotid artery (McMenamin & Volpe 1983). In my experience, this is a very rare sequence of events and cannot be relied on to make the diagnosis of brain death in the neonatal period.

## INDICATIONS FOR WITHDRAWAL OF CARE

It is my belief that the criteria for brain death in the neonate are not helpful, and the clinical decision as to when to withdraw care should be made after full evaluation of all the laboratory information and repeated clinical assessment of the child. My practice is to assess severely asphyxiated infants with EEG (or CFM) at 6 h and to reassess EEG together with a Doppler study at the age of 24 h. If these tests at 6 and 24 h are all abnormal, the term 'irreversible brain injury', is used and the parents are advised that the prognosis is extremely poor. When speaking to the parents, the terms 'irreversible' and 'massive brain injury' are more honest than 'brain death', with its implications that the child will not survive off the mechanical ventilator. Many of these babies do breathe once disconnected from the ventilator, and this may cause considerable distress to the parents if they are not warned about this in advance.

### Key Points

- There is no single or generally agreed diagnosis of 'birth asphyxia'. The diagnosis can be assessed retrospectively by attention to seven clinical features.
- Cerebral pathology resulting from a hypoxic ischemic insult depends on gestational age of the infant when the insult occurred as well as the severity and duration of the insult.
- Access to expert and rapid resuscitation immediately after birth is essential for asphyxiated newborn infants.
- There are few proven evidence based interventions in the management of the asphyxiated newborn infant. Postnatal corticosteroid treatment and hyperventilation are potentially hazardous.
- There is no evidence that suppressing all seizure activity with anticonvulsant drugs improves the subsequent outcome of the baby.
- The best clinical predictor of adverse outcome is severity of HIE; moderate and severe HIE has a 25% and 80% risk of adverse outcome respectively.

## REFERENCES


Adams J H, Brierley J B & Connor R C R (1966) The effects of systemic hypotension upon the human brain: clinical and neuropathological observations in 11 cases. *Brain* 89:235–268.

Adamson S J, Alessandra L M, Badawi B *et al.* (1995) Predictors of neonatal encephalopathy in full term infants. *BMJ* 311:598–602.

Adlard B P F & De Souza S W (1976) Influence of asphyxia and of dexamethasone on ATP concentrations in the immature rat brain. *Biol Neonate* 24:82–88.

Adsett D B, Fitz C R & Hill A (1985) Hypoxic–ischaemic cerebral injury in the term newborn: correlation of CT findings with neurological outcome. *Dev Med Child Neurol* 27:155–160.

Ahn M O, Korst L M, Phelan J P *et al.* (1998) Does the onset of neonatal seizures correlate with the timing of fetal neurologic injury? *Clin Pediatr* 37:673–676.

Aida N, Nishimura G, Hachiya Y *et al.* (1998) MR imaging of perinatal brain damage: comparison of clinical outcome with initial and follow-up MR findings. *Am J Neuroradiol* 19:1909–1921.

Airedale A I (1991) Birth asphyxia and hypoxic–ischaemic encephalopathy: incidence and severity. *Ann Trop Paediatr* 11:331–335.

Akinbi H, Abbasi S, Hilpert P L *et al.* (1994) Gastrointestinal and renal blood flow velocity profile in neonates with birth asphyxia. *J Pediatr* 125:625–627.

Alward C T, Hook J B & Helmrath T A (1978) Effects of asphyxia on renal function in the newborn piglet. *Pediatr Res* 12:225–228.

Amato M, Gambon R C & von Muralt G (1986) Accuracy of apgar score and arterial cord-blood pH in diagnosis of perinatal brain-damage assessed by CK-BB isoenzyme measurement. *J Perinatal Med* 14:335–338.

Amiel-Tison C (1979) Birth injury as a cause of brain dysfunction in full-term newborns. In: Korobkin R & Guilleminault L (eds) *Advances in perinatal neurology.* New York: Spectrum; vol. 1.

Amiel-Tison C & Ellison P (1986) Birth asphyxia in the fullterm newborn: early assessment and outcome. *Dev Med Child Neurol* 28:671–682.

Anderson J M & Belton N R (1974) Water and electrolyte abnormalities in the human brain after severe intrapartum asphyxia. *J Neurol Neurosurg Psychiatry* 37:514–520.

Anderson J M, Brown J K & Cockburn F (1974) On the role of disseminated intravascular coagulation in the pathology of birth asphyxia. *Dev Med Child Neurol* 16:581–591.

Anton G (1893) Uber die Betheiligung der basalen Gehringaglien bei Bewegungsstorungen und insbesondere bei der Chorea; nut Demonstrationen von Gehirnschaitten. *Wiener Klinische Wochenschrift* 6:859–861.

Apgar V (1953) A proposal for a new method of evaluation of the newborn infant. *Curr Res Anesthesia Analgesia* 32:260–267.

Archer L N J, Levene M I & Evans D H (1986) Cerebral artery Doppler ultrasonography for prediction of outcome after perinatal asphyxia. *Lancet* ii:1116–1118.

Arnold J, O'Brodovich H & Whyte R *et al.* (1985) Pulmonary thromboemboli after neonatal asphyxia. *J Pediatr* 106:806–809.

Ashwal S & Schneider S (1989) Brain death in the newborn. *Pediatrics* 84:429–437.

Babcock D S & Ball W (1983) Postasphyxial encephalopathy in full-term infants: ultrasound diagnosis. *Radiology* 148:417–423.

Bao X L, Yu R J & Li Z S (1993) 20 item neonatal behavioural neurological assessment used in predicting prognosis of asphyxiated newborn. *Chin Med J* 106:211–215.

Barkovich A J (1992) M R and C T evaluation of profound neonatal and infantile asphyxia. *Am J Neuroradiol* 13:950–972.

Barkovich A J, Hajnal B L, Vigneron D *et al.* (1998) Prediction of neuromotor outcome in perinatal asphyxia: evaluation of MR scoring systems. *Am J Neuroradiol* 19:143–149.

Barth P G, Valk J & Olislagers-de Slegte R (1984) Aspect scanographique des zones corticales et sous-corticales centrales dans les paralysies cerebrales. *J Neuroradiol* 11:65–71.

Bax M & Nelson K B (1993) Birth asphyxia: a statement. *Dev Med Child Neurol* 35:1023–1024.

Bennhagen R G, Weintraub R G, Lundstrom N R *et al.* (1998) Hypoxic–ischaemic encephalopathy is associated with regional changes in cerebral blood flow velocity and alterations in cardiovascular function. *Biol Neonate* 73:275–286.

Berseth C L & McCoy H H (1992) Birth asphyxia alters neonatal intestinal motility in term neonates. *Pediatrics* 90:669–673.

Blennow M, Hagberg H & Rosengren L (1995) Glial fibrillary acidic protein in the cerebrospinal fluid: a possible indicator of prognosis in full-term asphyxiated newborn infants? *Pediatr Res* 37:260–264.

Brann A W & Myers R E (1975) Central nervous system findings in the new born monkey following severe *in utero* partial asphyxia. *Neurology* 25:327.

Bressler J (1899) Klinische und pathologisch-anatomische Beitrage zur Mikrogyrie. *Archiv für Psychiatrie* 31:566–573.

Brierley J B, Brown A W, Excell B J *et al.* (1969) Brain damage in the rhesus monkey resulting from profound arterial hypotension. 1. Its nature, distribution and general physiological correlates. *Brain Res* 13:68–100.

British Paediatric Association (1991) *Diagnosis of brain stem death in infants and children. A working party report of the British Paediatric Association.* London: British Paediatric Association.

Brown J K, Purvis R J, Forfar J O *et al.* (1974) Neurological aspects of perinatal asphyxia. *Dev Med Child Neurol* 16:567–580.

Bruce D A (1984) Effects of hyperventilation on cerebral blood flow and metabolism. *Clin Perinatol* 11:673–680.

Bucciarelli R L, Nelson R M, Egan E A *et al.* (1977) Transient tricuspid insufficiency of the newborn: a form of myocardial dysfunction in stressed newborns. *Pediatrics* 59:330–334.

Burnard E D & James L A (1961) Failure of the heart after undue asphyxia at birth. *Pediatrics* 28:545–547.

Cabal L A, Devaskar U, Siassi B *et al.* (1980) Cardiogenic shock associated with perinatal asphyxia in preterm infants. *J Pediatr* 4:705–710.

Campbell A G M, Milligin J E & Talner N S (1968) The effect of pretreatment with pentobarbital, meperdine or hyperbaric oxygen on the response to anoxia and resuscitation in newborn rabbits. *J Pediatr* 72:518–527.

Carter S, McNabb F & Merenstein G B (1998) Prospective validation of a scoring system for predicting neonatal morbidity after acute perinatal asphyxia. *J Pediatr* 132:619–623.

Casalaz D M, Marlow N & Speidel B D (1998) Outcome of resuscitation following unexpected apparent stillbirth. *Arch Dis Childhood* 78:F112–F115.

Chadd M A, Elwood P C, Gray O P *et al.* (1971) Coagulation defects in hypoxic full-term newborn infants. *Br Med J* iv:516–518.

Chernick V, Manfreda J, de Booy V *et al.* (1988) Clinical trial of naloxone in birth asphyxia. *J Pediatr* 113:519–525.

Chessells J M & Wigglesworth J S (1970) Secondary haemorrhagic disease of the newborn. *Arch Dis Childhood* 45:539–543.

Cockburn F, Daniel S S, Dawes G S *et al.* (1969) The effect of pentobarbital anesthesia on resuscitation and brain damage in fetal rhesus monkeys asphyxiated on delivery. *J Pediatr* 75:281–291.

Colamaria V, Curatolo P, Cusmai R *et al.* (1988) Symmetrical bithalamic hyperdensities in asphyxiated full-term newborns: an early indicator of status marmoratus. *Brain Dev* 10:57–59.

Constantinou J E C, Gillis J, Ouvrier R A *et al.* (1989) Hypoxic–ischaemic encephalopathy after near miss sudden infant death syndrome. *Arch Dis Childhood* 64:703–708.

Cuestas R A (1980) Creatine kinase isoenzymes in high-risk infants. *Pediatr Res* 14:935–938.

Cyr R M, Usher R H & McLean F H (1984) Changing patterns of birth asphyxia and trauma over 20 years. *Am J Obstet Gynecol* 48:490–498.

Daga S R, Prabhu P G, Chandrashekhar L *et al.* (1983) Myocardial ischaemia following birth asphyxia. *Ind Pediatr* 20:567–571.

Dalens B, Viallard J-L, Raynauld E-J *et al.* (1981) CSF levels of lactate and hydroxybutyrate dehydrogenase as indicators of neurological sequelae after neonatal brain damage. *Dev Med Child Neurol* 23:228–233.

Daniel S S, Husain M K, Milliez J *et al.* (1978) Renal response of the fetal lamb to complete occlusion of the umbilical cord. *Am J Obstet Gynecol* 131:514–519.

Dauber I M, Krauss A N, Symchych P S *et al.* (1976) Renal failure following perinatal asphyxia. *J Pediatr* 88:851–855.

Davis D J, Creery W D & Radziuk J (1999) Inappropriately high plasma insulin levels in suspected perinatal asphyxia. *Acta Paediatr* 88:76–81.

Dawes G (1968) *Fetal and neonatal physiology.* Chicago, IL: Year Book.

De Sa D J & Donnelly W H (1984) Myocardial necrosis in the newborn. *Perspec Pediatr Pathol* 8:295–311.

De Souza S W & Dobbing J (1973) Cerebral oedema in developing brain. III. Brain water and electrolytes in immature asphyxiated rats treated with dexamethasone. *Biol Neonate* 22:388–397.

De Souza S W & Richards B (1978) Neurological sequelae in newborn babies after perinatal asphyxia. *Arch Dis Childhood* 53:564–569.

De Vane G W & Porter J C (1980) An apparent stress-induced release of arginine vasopressin by human neonates. *J Clin Endocrinol Metab* 51:1412–1416.

Di Sessa T G, Leitner M, Ti C C *et al.* (1981) The cardiovascular effects of dopamine in the severely asphyxiated neonate. *J Pediatr* 99:772–776.

Diprose G K, Evans D H, Archer L N J *et al.* (1986) Dinamap fails to detect hypotension in very low birthweight infants. *Arch Dis Childhood* 61:771–773.

Donald I (1959) Birth: adaptation from intrauterine to extrauterine life. In: Holland E & Bourne A (eds) *British obstetric practice.* London: Heinemann.

Donnelly W H, Bucciarelli R L & Nelson R M (1980) Ischemic papillary muscle necrosis in stressed newborn infants. *J Pediatr* 96:295–300.

Drage J S, Kennedy C & Schwarz B K (1964) The Apgar score as an index of neonatal mortality: a report from the collaborative study of cerebral palsy. *Obstet Gynecology* 24:222–230.

Eken P, Jansen G H, Groenendaal F *et al.* (1994) Intracranial lesions in the full term infant with hypoxic ischaemic encephalopathy: ultrasound and autopsy correlation. Neuropediatrics 25:301–307.

Eken P, Toet M C, Groenendaal F *et al.* (1995) Predictive value of early neuroimaging, pulsed Doppler and neurophysiology in full term infants with hypoxio–ischaemic encephalopathy. *Arch Dis Childhood* 73:F75–F80.

Ekert, Perlman M, Steinlin M *et al.* (1997) Predicting the outcome of postasphyxial hypoxic–ischaemic encephalopathy within 4 hours of birth. *J Pediatr* 131:613–617.

Ellis M & Manandhar D (1999) Progress in perinatal asphyxia. *Semin Neonatol* 4:183–191.

Ellis M, Manandhar N, Shrestha P S *et al.* (1999) Outcome at 1 year of neonatal encephalopathy in Kathmandu, Nepal. *Dev Med Child Neurol* 41:689–695.

Ergander U, Eriksson M & Zetterstrom R (1983) Severe neonatal asphyxia: incidence and prediction of outcome in the Stockholm area. *Acta Paediatr Scand* 72:321–325.

Evans D J & Levene M I (1998) Anticonvulsants for preventing mortality and morbidity in full term newborns with perinatal asphyxia (Cochrane Review). In: *The Cochrane Library, issue 1.* Oxford: Update Software.

Eyre J A & Wilkinson A R (1986) Thiopentone-induced coma after severe birth asphyxia. *Arch Dis Childhood* 61:1084–1089.

Farkas A G, Robson S C, Kyei-Mensah A *et al.* (1995) Acid-base changes after severe birth acidaemia. *J Perinatal Med* 23:249–255.

Farkas-Bargeton E & Diebler M F (1978) A topographical study of enzyme maturation in human cerebral neocortex: a histological and biochemical study. In: Brazier M A B Petsche H (eds) *Architectonics and the cerebral cortex.* New York, NY: Raven Press.

Fenichel G M (1983) Hypoxic–ischemic encephalopathy in the newborn. *Arch Neurol* 40:261–266.

Fernandez F, Quero J Verdu A *et al.* (1986) L D H isoenzymes in CSF in the diagnosis of neonatal brain damage. *Acta Neurol Scand* 74:30–33.

Fernandez F, Verdu A, Quero J *et al.* (1987) Serum CPK-BB isoenzyme in the assessment of brain damage in asphyctic term infants. *Acta Paediatr Scand* 76:914–918.

Fernandez F, Barrio V, Guzman J *et al.* (1989) Beta-2-microglobulin in the assessment of renal function in full term newborns following perinatal asphyxia. *J Perinatal Med* 17:453–459.

Finer N N, Robertson C M, Richards R T *et al.* (1981)

Hypoxic-ischemic encephalopathy in term neonates: perinatal factors and outcome. *J Pediatr* 98:112–117.

Finer N N Robertson C M, Peters K L *et al.* (1983) Factors affecting outcome in hypoxic-ischemic encephalopathy in term infants. *Am J Dis Children* 137:21–25.

Fitzhardinge P M (1977) Complications of asphyxia and their therapy. In: Gluck L (ed) *Intrauterine asphyxia and the developing fetal brain.* Chicago, IL: Year Book.

Fitzhardinge P M, Eisen E, Lejtonyi C *et al.* (1974) Sequelae of early steroid administration to the newborn infant. *Pediatrics* 53:877–883.

Fitzhardinge P M, Flodmark O, Fitz C R *et al.* (1981) The prognostic value of computed tomography as an adjunct to assessment of the term infant with postasphyxial encephalopathy. *J Pediatr* 99:777–781.

Flamm E S, Demopoulos H B, Seligman M L *et al.* (1978) Free radicals in cerebral ischaemia. *Stroke* 9:445–447.

Flodmark O, Becker L E, Harwood-Nash D C *et al.* (1980) Correlation between computed tomography and autopsy in premature and full-term neonates that have suffered perinatal asphyxia. *Radiology* 137:93–103.

Freeman J & Nelson K (1988) Intrapartum asphyxia and cerebral palsy. *Pediatrics* 82:240–249.

Friede R L (1975) *Developmental neuropathology.* Berlin: Springer

Frigieri G, Guidi B, Costa Zaccarelli S *et al.* (1996) Multicystic encephalomalacia in term infants. *Child's Nerv Syst* 12:759–764.

Fysh W J, Turner G M & Dunn P M (1982) Neurological normality after extreme birth asphyxia: case report. *Br J Obstet Gynaecol* 89:24–26.

Gal P, Toback J, Erkan N V *et al.* (1984) The influence of asphyxia on phenobarbital dosing requirements in neonates. *Dev Pharmacol Ther* 7:145–152.

Garcia-Alix A, Cabanas F, Pellicer A *et al.* (1994) Neuron-specific enolase and myeline basic protein: relationship of cerebrospinal fluid concentrations to the neurologic condition of asphyxiated full-term infants. *Pediatrics* 93:234–240.

Gerard P, Verheggen P, Bachy *et al.* (1981) Interet de la tomodensitometrie cerebrate chez les enfants nes asphyxies. *Archives Françaises de Pediatrie* 38:591–596.

Goitein K J & Amit Y (1982) Percutaneous placement of subdural catheter for measurement of intracranial pressure in small children. *Crit Care Med* 10:46–48.

Goldaber K G, Gilstrap L C, Leveno K J *et al.* (1991) Pathological fetal acidemia. *Obstet Gynaecol* 78:1103–1107.

Goldberg R N, Cabal L A, Sinatra F R *et al.* (1979) Hyperammonemia associated with perinatal asphyxia. *Pediatrics* 64:336–341.

Goldberg R N, Thomas D W, Sinatra F R (1983) Necrotizing enterocolitis in the asphyxiated full-term infant. *Am J Perinatol* 1:40–42.

Goldberg R, Moscoso P, Bauer C *et al.* (1986) Use of barbiturate therapy in severe perinatal asphyxia: a randomized controlled trial. *J Pediatr* 109:851–856.

Goodlin R C & Lloyd D (1970) Use of drugs to protect against fetal asphyxia. American *J Obstet Gynaecol* 107:227–231.

Grant A (1989) Monitoring the fetus during labour. In: Chalmers I, Enkin M & Keirse M J N C (eds) *Effective care in pregnancy and childbirth.* Oxford: Oxford University Press; vol 2, pp. 846–882.

Grigelioniene G, Blennow M, Torok C *et al.* (1996) Cerebrospinal fluid of newborn infants contains a deglycosylated from of the intermediate filament nestin. *Pediatr Res* 1996;40:809–814.

Groenendaal F, Veenhoven R H, van der Grond J *et al.* (1994) Cerebral lactate and *N*-acetyl-aspartate/choline ratios in asphyxiated full-term neonates demonstrated *in vivo* using proton magnetic resonance spectroscopy. *Pediatr Res* 35:148–151.

Gunn A J, Parer J T, Mallard E C *et al.* (1992) Cerebral histologic and electrocorticographic changes after asphyxia in fetal sheep. *Pediatr Res* 31:486–491.

Hagberg H, Thornberg E, Blennow M *et al.* (1993) Excitatory amino acids in the cerebrospinal fluid of asphyxiated infants: relationship to hypoxic-ischemic encephalopathy. *Acta Paediatr* 82:925–929.

Hall R T, Kulkarni P B, Sheehan M B *et al.* (1980) Cerebrospinal fluid lactate dehydrogenase in infants with perinatal asphyxia. *Dev Med Child Neurol* 22:300–307.

Hall R T, Hall F K & Daily D K (1998) High-dose phenobarbital therapy in term newborn infants with severe perinatal asphyxia: A randomised, prospective study with three year follow up. *J Pediatr* 345–348.

Hanrahan J D, Sargentoni J, Azzopardi D *et al.* (1996) Cerebral metabolism within 18 hours of birth asphyxia: a proton magnetic resonance spectroscopy study. *Pediatr Res* 39:584–590.

Hanrahan J D, Cox I J, Azzopardi D *et al.* (1999) Relation between proton magnetic resonance spectroscopy within 18 hours of birth asphyxia and neurodevelopment at 1 year of age. *Dev Med Child Neurol* 41:76–82.

Hanson J. Anderson R & Sundt T (1975) Influence of cerebral vasoconstricting and vasodilating agents on blood flow in regions of cerebral ischemia. *Stroke* 6:642–648.

Hattori H & Wasterlain C G (1990) Posthypoxic glucose supplement reduces hypoxic-ischemic brain damage in the neonatal rat. *Ann Neurol* 28:122–128.

Holmes G, Rowe J, Hafford J *et al.* (1982) Prognostic value of the electroencephalogram in neonatal asphyxia. *Electroencephalog Clin Neurophysiol* 53:60–72.

Holmes G L, Rowe J & Hafford J (1983) Significance of reactive burst suppression following asphyxia in full term infants. *Clin Electroencephalog* 14:138–141.

Hoo J J & Goedde H W (1982) Determination of brain type creatine kinase for diagnosis of perinatal asphyxia – choice of method. *Pediatr Res* 16:806.

Huang C C, Wang S T, Chang Y C *et al.* (1999) Measurement of the urinary lactate:creatinine ratio for the early identification of newborn infants at risk for hypoxic-ischemic encephalopathy. *N Eng J Med* 341:328–335.

Hull J & Dodd K L (1992) Falling incidence of hypoxic-ischaemic encephalopathy in term infants. *Br J Obstet Gynaecol* 9:386–391.

Ilves P, Talvik R & Talkvik T (1998) Changes in Doppler ultrasonography in asphyxiated term infants with hypoxic-ischaemic encephalopathy. *Acta Paediatr* 87:680–684.

Ingemarsson E, Ingemarsson I & Svenningsen N W (1981) Impact of routine fetal monitoring during labor on fetal outcome with long-term follow-up. *Am J Obstet Gynecol* 141:29–38.

Jain L, Ferre C, Vidyasagar D *et al.* (1991) Cardiopulmonary resuscitation of apparently stillborn infants: survival and long-term outcome. *J Pediatr* 118:778–782.

Kaiser A M & Whitelaw A G L (1987) Noninvasive monitoring of intracranial pressure – fact or fancy? *Dev Med Child Neurol* 29:320–326.

Keeney S E, Adcock E W & McArdle C B (1991) Prospective observations of 100 high-risk neonates by high-field (1.5 Tesla) magnetic resonance imaging of the central nervous system. II. Lesions associated with hypoxic-ischemic encephalopathy. *Pediatrics* 87:431–438.

Klatzo I (1967) Neuropathological aspects of brain damage. *J Neuropathol Exp Neurol* 26:1–5.

Klatzo I (1985) Brain oedema following brain ischaemia and the influence of therapy. *Br J Anaesthesia* 57:18–22.

Kojima T, Kobayashi T, Matsuzaki S *et al.* (1985) Effects of perinatal asphyxia and myoglobinuria on development of acute neonatal renal failure. *Arch Dis Childhood* 60:908–912.

Korhonen L, Riikonen R, Nawa H *et al.* (1998) Brain derived neurotrophic factor is increased in cerebrospinal fluid of children suffering from asphyxia. *Neurosci Lett* 240:151–154.

Korst L M, Phelan J P *et al.* (1996) Nucleated red blood cells: an update on the market for fetal asphyxia. *Am J Obstet Gynaecol* 175:843–846.

Kotagel S, Toce S S, Kotagel P *et al.* (1983) Symmetric bithalamic and striatal hemorrhage following perinatal hypoxia in a term infant. *J Comput Assist Tomogr* 7:353–355.

Larroche J-C (1977) *Developmental pathology of the neonate.* Amsterdam: Excerpta Medica.

Larroche J-C (1984) Perinatal brain damage. In: Adams J H, Corsellis J A N & Duchen L W (eds) *Greenfield's neuropathology.* London: Arnold.

Lassen N A (1996) The luxury perfusion syndrome and its possible relation to acute metabolic acidosis localised within the brain. *Lancet* ii:1113–1115.

Leech R W & Alvord E C (1977) Anoxic-ischemic encephalopathy in the human neonatal period: the significance of brain stem involvement. *Arch Neurol* 34:109–113.

Leth H, Toft P B, Peitersen B *et al.* (1996) Use of brain lactate levels to predict outcome after perinatal asphyxia. *Acta Paediatr* 85:859–864.

Levene M I (1995) Birth asphyxia. In: David T J *Recent Advance In Paediatrics.* Edinburgh: Churchill Livingstone; pp. 13–27.

Levene M I & Evans D H (1983) Continuous measurement of subarachnoid pressure in the severely asphyxiated newborn. *Arch Dis Childhood* 58:1013–1015.

Levene M I & Evans D H (1985) Medical management of raised intracranial pressure after severe birth asphyxia. *Arch Dis Childhood* 60:12–16.

Levene M I, Kornberg J & Williams T H C (1985a) The incidence and severity of post-asphyxial encephalopathy in full-term infants. *Early Human Dev* 11:21–28.

Levene M I, Williams J L & Fawer C-L (1985b) *Ultrasound of the infant brain,* No. 92. Oxford: Spastics International Medical Publications.

Levene M I, Sands C, Grindulis H *et al.* (1986) Comparison of two methods of predicting outcome in perinatal asphyxia. *Lancet* i:67–91.

Levene M I, Evans D H, Forde A *et al.* (1987) The value of intracranial pressure monitoring in asphyxiated newborn infants. *Dev Med Child Neurol* 29:311–319.

Levene M I, Fenton A C, Evans D H *et al.* (1989) Severe birth asphyxia and abnormal cerebral blood-flow velocity. *Dev Med Child Neurol* 31:427–434.

Liao H T & Hung K L (1997) Anterior cerebral artery Doppler ultrasonograpy for prediction of outcome after perinatal asphyxia. *Chung-Hua Min Kuo Hsiao Erh Ko I Hsueh Tsa Chih* 38:208–212.

Lipper E G, Voorhies T M, Ross G *et al.* (1986) Early predictors of one-year outcome for infants asphyxiated at birth. *Dev Med Child Neurol* 28:303–309.

Lipp-Zwahlen A E, Deonna T, Chrzanowski R *et al.* (1985a) Temporal evolution of hypoxic-ischaemic brain lesions in asphyxiated full-term newborns assessed by computerized tomography. *Neuroradiology* 27:138–144.

Lipp-Zwahlen A E, Deonna T, Micheli J L *et al.* (1985b) Prognostic value of neonatal C T scans in asphyxiated term babies: low density score compared with neonatal neurological signs. *Neuropediatrics* 16:209–217.

Lorek A, Takei Y, Cady E B *et al.* (1994) Delayed ('secondary') cerebral energy failure after acute hypoxia–ischemia in the newborn piglet: continuous 48-hour studies by phosphorus magnetic resonance spectroscopy. *Pediatr Res* 36:699–706.

Low J A (1993) The relationship of asphyxia in the mature fetus to long-term neurologic function. *Clin Obstet Gynecol* 36:82–90.

Low J A, Galbraith R S, Muir D *et al.* (1978) Intrapartum fetal asphyxia: a preliminary report in regard to long-term morbidity. *Am J Obstet Gynecol* 130:525–533.

Low J A, Galbraith R S, Muir D W *et al.* (1985) The relationship between perinatal hypoxia and newborn encephalopathy. *Am J Obstet Gynecol* 152:256–260.

Low J A, Galbraith R S, Raymond M J *et al.* (1994) Cerebral blood flow velocity in term newborns following intrapartum fetal asphyxia. *Acta Paediatr* 83:1012–1016.

Luciano R, Gallini F, Romagnoli C *et al.* (1998) Doppler evaluation of renal blood flow velocity as a predictive index of acute renal failure in perinatal asphyxia. *Eur J Pediatr* 157:656–660.

Lundstrom K, Pryds O & Greisen G (1995) Oxygen at birth and prolonged cerebral vasoconstriction in preterm infants. *Arch Dis Childhood* 73:F81–F84.

MacDonald D, Grant A, Sheridan-Pereira M *et al.* (1985) The Dublin randomised trial of intrapartum fetal heart monitoring. *Am J Obstet Gynecol* 152:524–539.

MacDonald H M, Mulligan J C, Allan A C *et al.* (1980) Neonatal asphyxia. 1. Relationship of obstetric and neonatal complications to neonatal mortality in 38 405 consecutive deliveries. *J Pediatr* 96:898–902.

Magilner A D & Wertheimer I S (1980) Preliminary results of a computed tomography study of neonatal brain hypoxia–ischemia. *J Comput Assist Tomogr* 4:457–463.

Marchal C, Costagliola P, Leveau Ph *et al.* (1974) Traitement de la souffrance cerebrale neonatale d'origine anoxique par le mannitol. Revue de Pédiatrie 9:581–589.

Martin D J, Hill A, Fitz C R *et al.* (1983) Hypoxic/ischemic cerebral injury in the neonatal brain. Pediatric Radiology 13:307–312.

Martin E, Buchli R, Ritter S *et al.* (1996) Diagnostic and prognostic value of cerebral $^{31}$P magnetic resonance spectroscopy in neonates with perinatal asphyxia. *Pediat Res* 40:749–748.

Martin-Ancel A, Garcia-Alix A, Pascual-Salcedo D *et al.* (1997) Interleukin-6 in the cerebrospinal fluid after perinatal asphyxia is related to early and late neurological manifestations. *Pediatrics* 100:789–791.

McMenamin J B & Volpe J J (1983) Doppler ultrasonography in the determination of neonatal brain death. *Ann Neurol* 14:302–307.

McWilliam R C & Stephenson J B P (1984) Rapid bedside technique for intracranial pressure monitoring. *Lancet* ii:73–75.

Meis P J, Hall M & Marshall J (1978) Meconium passage: a new classification for risk assessment during labor. *Am J Obstet Gynecol* 131:509.

Menke J A, Miles R, McIlhany M *et al.* (1982) The fontanelle tonometer: a noninvasive method for measurement of intracranial pressure. *J Pediatr* 100:960–963.

Mercuri E, Guzzetta A, Haataja L *et al.* (1999) Neonatal neurological examination in infants with hypoxic ischaemic encephalopathy: correlation with MRI findings. *Neuropaediatrics* 30:83–89.

Michenfelder J D (1974) The interdependency of cerebral function and metabolic effects following massive doses of thiopental in the dog. *Anesthesiology* 41:231–236.

Minns R A (1984) Intracranial pressure monitoring. *Arch Dis Childhood* 59:486–488.

Moorcroft J, Bolas N M, Ives N K *et al.* (1991) Global and depth resolved phosphorus magnetic resonance spectroscopy to predict outcome after birth asphyxia. *Arch Dis Childhood* 66:1119–1123.

Mori M, Nishizaki T & Okada Y (1992) Protective effect of adenosine on the anoxic damage of hippocampal slice. *Neuroscience* 46:301–307.

Morimoto K, Sumita Y, Kitajima H *et al.* (1985) Bilateral, asymmetrical hemorrhagic infarction of the basal ganglia and thalamus following neonatal asphyxia. *No To Shinkei* 37:133–137.

Mujsce D J, Stern D R, Vannucci R C *et al.* (1988) Mannitol therapy in perinatal hypoxic–ischemic brain damage. *Ann Neurol* 24:338.

Mulligan J C, Painter M J, O'Donoghue P A *et al.* (1980) Neonatal asphyxia. II. Neonatal mortality and long-term sequelae. *J Pediatr* 96:903–907.

Myers R E (1972) Two patterns of perinatal brain damage and their conditions of occurrence. *Am J Obstet Gynecology* 112:246–276.

Myers R E, Wagner K R, Courten-Myers G M *et al.* (1983) Brain metabolic and pathologic consequences of asphyxia. In: Milunsky A, Haddow R Alpert E (eds) *Advances in perinatal medicine.* New York, NY: Plenum, vol. 3.

Nelson K B & Ellenberg J H (1981) Apgar scores as predictors of chronic neurological disability. *Pediatrics* 68:36–44.

Nelson K B & Ellenberg J H (1984) Obstetric complications as risk factors for cerebral or seizure disorders. *JAMA* 251:1843–1848.

Nelson K B & Leviton A (1991) How much of neonatal encephalopathy is due to birth asphyxia? *Am J Dis Children* 145:1325–1331.

Niijima S & Levene M I (1989) Post-asphyxial encephalopathy in a preterm infant. *Dev Med Child Neurol* 31:395–397.

O'Connor M C, Harkness R A, Simmonds R J *et al.* (1981) The measurement of hypoxanthine, xanthine, inosine and uridine in umbilical cord blood and fetal scalp blood samples as a measure of fetal hypoxia. *Br J Obstet Gynaecol* 88:381–390.

Oygur N, Sonmez O, Saka O *et al.* (1998) Predictive value of plasma and cerebrospinal fluid tumour necrosis factor-α and interleukin-1β concentrations on outcome of full term infants with hypoxic–ischaemic encephalopathy. *Arch Dis Childhood* 79:F190–F193.

Painter M J, Depp R & O'Donogue P D (1978) Fetal heart rate patterns and development in the first year of life. *Am J Obstet Gynecol* 132:271–277.

Palme-Kilander C (1992) Methods of resuscitation in low-Apgar-score newborn infants – A national survey. *Acta Paediatr Scand* 81:739–744.

Paneth N & Stark R I (1983) Cerebral palsy and mental retardation in relation to indicators of perinatal asphyxia. *Am J Obstet Gynecol* 147:960–966.

Pape K E & Wigglesworth J S (1979) *Haemorrhage, ischaemia and the perinatal brain.* London: Spastics International.

Pasternak J F & Gorey M T (1998) The syndrome of acute near-total intrauterine asphyxia in the term infant. *Pediatr Neurol* 18:391–398.

Peden C J, Rutherford M A, Sargentoni J *et al.* (1993) Proton spectroscopy of the neonatal brain following hypoxic–ischaemic injury. *Dev Med Child Neurol* 35:502–510.

Peliowski A & Finer N N (1992) Birth asphyxia in the term infant. In: Sinclair J C, Bracken M B (eds) *Effective care of the newborn infant.* Oxford Oxford University Press, pp. 249–279.

Penrice J, Cady E B, Lorek A *et al.* (1996) Proton magnetic resonance spectroscopy of the brain in normal preterm and term infants, and early changes after perinatal hypoxia–ischemia. *Pediatr Res* 40:6.

Perlman J M & Tack E D (1988) Renal injury in the asphyxiated newborn infant: relationship to neurologic outcome. *J Pediatr* 113:875–879.

Perlman J M, Tack E D, Martin T *et al.* (1989) Acute systemic organ injury in term infants after asphyxia. *Am J Dis Childhood* 143:617–620.

Perlman J M & Risser M S (1996) Can asphyxiated infants at risk for neonatal seizures be rapidly identified by current high-risk markers? *Pediatrics* 97:456–462.

Phelan J P, Ahn M O, Korst L *et al.* (1998) Intrapartum fetal asphyxial brain injury with absent multiorgan system dysfunction. *J Maternal–Fetal Med* 7:19–22.

Phelan J P, Myoung O A, Korst L M *et al.* (1995) Nucleated red blood cells: a marker for fetal asphyxia? *Am J Obstet Gynaecol* 173:1380–1384.

Philip A G S, Long J G & Donn S M (1981) Intracranial pressure. Sequential measurements in full-term and pre-term infants. *Am J Dis Children* 135:521–524.

Pierce E C, Lambertson C J, Deutsch S *et al.* (1962) Cerebral circulation and metabolism during thiopental anesthesia and hyperventilation in man. *J Clin Invest* 41:1664–1671.

Pourcyrous M, Bada H S, Yang W *et al.* (1999) Prognostic significance of cerebrospinal fluid cyclic adenosine monophosphate in neonatal asphyxia. *J Pediatr* 134:90–96.

Primhak R A, Jedeikin R, Ellis G *et al.* (1985) Myocardial ischaemia in asphyxia neonatorum. *Acta Paediatr Scand* 74:595–600.

Pryse-Davies J & Beard R W (1973) A necropsy study of brain swelling in the newborn with special reference to cerebellar herniation. *J Pathol* 109:51–73.

Raju T N & Vidyasagar D (1982) Intracranial and cerebral perfusion pressure: methodology and clinical considerations. *Med Instrum* 16:154–156.

Raju T N, Doshi U & Vidyasagar D (1983) Low cerebral perfusion pressure: an indicator of poor prognosis in asphyxiated term infants. *Brain Dev* 5:478–482.

Roberton N R (1997) Use of albumin in neonatal resuscitation. *Eur J Pediatr* 156:428–431.

Roberts D S, Haycock G B, Dalton R N *et al.* (1990) Prediction of acute renal failure after birth asphyxia. *Arch Dis Childhood* 65:1021–1028.

Robertson C & Finer N (1985) Term infants with hypoxic–ischaemic encephalopathy: outcome at 3.5 years. *Dev Med Child Neurol* 27:473–484.

Robertson C M T, Finer N N & Grace M G A (1989) School performance of survivors of neonatal encephalopathy associated with birth asphyxia at term. *J Pediatr* 114:753–760.

Robinson R O, Rolfe P & Sutton P (1977) Non-invasive method for measuring intracranial pressure in normal newborn infants. *Dev Med Child Neurol* 19:305–308.

Roland E H, Hill A & Norman M G *et al.* (1988) Selective brainstem injury in an asphyxiated newborn. *Ann Neurol* 23:89–92.

Rorke L B (1982) *Pathology of perinatal brain injury.* New York, NY: Raven Press.

Rose A L & Lombroso C T (1970) A study of clinical, pathological and electroencephalographic features in 137 full-term babies with a long term follow up. *Pediatrics* 111:133–141.

Rosenbloom L (1994) Dyskinetic cerebral palsy and birth asphyxia. *Dev Med Child Neurol* 36:285–289.

Roth S C, Baudin J, Cady E *et al.* (1997) Relation of deranged neonatal cerebral oxidative metabolism with neurodevelopmental outcome and head circumference at 4 years. *Dev Med Child Neurol* 39:718–725.

Rowan J O, Johnston H, Harper A M *et al.* (1972) Perfusion in intracranial hypertension. In: Borck M, Dietz H (eds) *Intracranial pressure*. New York, NY: Springer.

Rudolph A M (1969) The course and distribution of the fetal circulation. In: Wolstenholme G O'Connor M J A (eds) *Foetal autonomy*. London: Churchill.

Ruth V J (1989) Prognostic value of creatine kinase BB-isoenzyme in high risk newborn infants. *Arch Dis Childhood* 64:563–568.

Ruth V J & Raivio K O (1988) Perinatal brain damage: predictive value of metabolic acidosis and the Apgar score. BMJ 297:24–27.

Ruth V, Autti-Ramo I, Granstrom M-L *et al.* (1988) Prediction of perinatal brain damage by cord plasma vasopressin, erythropoietin, and hypoxanthine values. *J Pediatr* 113:800–815.

Rutherford M A, Pennock J M, Schwieso J E *et al.* (1995) Hypoxic ischaemic encephalopathy: early magnetic resonance imaging findings and their evolution. *Neuropediatrics* 26:183–191.

Rutherford M A, Pennock J, Schwieso J *et al.* (1996) Hypoxic-ischaemic encephalopathy: early and late magnetic resonance imaging findings in relation to outcome. *Arch Dis Childhood* 75:F145–F151.

Rutherford M A, Pennock J M, Counsell S J *et al.* (1998) Abnormal magnetic resonance signal in the internal capsule predicts poor neurodevelopmental outcome in infants with hypoxic ischemic encephalopathy. Pediatrics 102:323–329.

Saint Hilaire M-H, Burke R E, Bressman S B *et al.* (1991) Delayed-onset dystonia due to perinatal or early childhood asphyxia. *Neurology* 41:216–222.

Salmon J H, Hajjar W & Bada H S (1977) The fontogram: a noninvasive intracranial pressure monitor. *Pediatrics* 60:721–725.

Sankaran K (1984) Hypoxic-ischemic encephalopathy: cerebrovascular carbon dioxide reactivity in neonates. *Am J Perinatol* 1:114–117.

Sarnat H B & Sarnat M S (1976) Neonatal encephalopathy following fetal distress. *Arch Neurol* 33:696–705.

Sasidharan P (1992) Breathing pattern abnormalities in full term asphyxiated newborn infants. *Arch Dis Childhood* 67:440–442.

Saugstad O D (1975) Hypoxanthine as a measurement of hypoxia. *Pediatr Res* 9:158–161.

Saugstad O D (1998) Resuscitation with room-air or oxygen supplementation. *Clin Perinatol* 25:741–756.

Saugstad O D, Rootwelt T & Aalen O (1998) Resuscitation of asphyxiated newborn infants with room air or oxygen: an international controlled trial: the Resair 2 study. *Pediatrics* 102.

Savman K, Blennow M, Gustafson K *et al.* (1998) Cytokine response in cerebrospinal fluid after birth asphyxia. *Pediatr Res* 43:746–751.

Schrumpf J D, Sehring S, Killpack S *et al.* (1980) Correlation of early neurologic outcome and CT findings in neonatal brain hypoxia and injury. *J Comput Assist Tomogr* 4:445–450.

Scott B L & Jankovic J (1996) Delayed-onset progressive movement disorders after static brain lesions. *Am Acad Neurol* 46:68–74.

Scott H (1976) Outcome of very severe birth asphyxia. *Arch Dis Childhood* 51:712–716.

Selton D & Andre M (1997) Prognosis of hypoxic-ischaemic encephalopathy in full term newborns – value of neonatal electroencephalography. *Neuropediatrics* 28:276–280.

Sheldon R A, Partridge C, Ferriero D M (1992) Postischemic hyperglycemia is not protective to the neonatal rat. *Pediat Res* 32:489–493.

Shen E Y, Huang C C, Chyou S C *et al.* (1986) Sonographic finding of the bright thalamus. *Arch Dis Childhood* 61:1096–1099.

Sheth R J, Bodensteiner J B, Riggs J E (1995) Differential involvement of the brain in neonatal asphyxia: a pathogenic explanation. *J Child Neurol* 10:463–466.

Shewman D A, Fine M, Masdeu J C *et al.* (1981) Postischemic hypervascularity of infancy: a stage in the evolution of ischemic brain damage with characteristic CT scan. *Ann Neurol* 9:358–365.

Simeone F A, Frazer G, Lawner P (1979) Ischemic brain oedema: comparative effects of barbiturates and hypothermia. *Stroke* 10:8–12.

Skeffington F S & Pearse R G (1983) The 'bright brain'. *Arch Dis Childhood* 58:509–511.

Speer M E, Gormon W A, Kaplan S L *et al.* (1984) Elevation of plasma concentrations of arginine vasopressin following perinatal asphyxia. *Acta Paediatr Scand* 73:610–614.

Steen P A & Michenfelder J D (1980) Mechanisms of barbiturate protection. *Anesthesiology* 53:183–190.

Steiner H & Nelligan G (1975) Perinatal cardiac arrest: quality of the survivors. *Arch Dis Childhood* 50:696–702.

Stewart A R, Finer N N & Peters K L (1981) Effects of alterations of inspiratory and expiratory pressures and inspiratory/expiratory ratios on a mean airway pressure, blood gases and intracranial pressure. *Pediatrics* 67:474–481.

Suzuki S & Morishita S (1998) Hypercoagulability and DIC in high-risk infants. *Semin Thrombosis Hemostasis* 24:463–466.

Svenningsen N W, Blennow G, Lindroth M *et al.* (1982) Brain-orientated intensive care treatment in severe neonatal asphyxia: effects of phenobarbitone protection. *Arch Dis Childhood* 57:176–183.

Takeuchi T & Watanabe K (1989) The EEG evolution and neurological prognosis of perinatal hypoxia in neonates. *Brain Dev* 11:115–120.

Task Force (1987) Guidelines for the determination of brain death in children. *Pediatrics* 80:298–300.

Thiringer K (1983) Cord plasma hypoxanthine as a measure of foetal asphyxia: comparison with clinical assessment and laboratory measures. *Acta Paediatr Scand* 72:231–237.

Thompson C M, Puterman A S, Linley L L *et al.* (1997) The value of a scoring system for hypoxic ischaemic encephalopathy in predicting neurodevelopmental outcome. *Acta Paediatr* 86:757–761.

Thompson R J, Graham J G, McQueen I N F *et al.* (1980) Radio immunoassay of brain type creatine kinase-BB isoenzyme in human tissues and in serum of patients with neurological disorders. *J Neurol Sci* 47:241–254.

Thomson A J, Searle M & Russell G (1977) Quality of survival after severe birth asphyxia. *Arch Dis Childhood* 52:620–626.

Thoresen M, Hallstrom A, Whitelaw A *et al.* (1988) Lactate and pyruvate changes in the cerebral gray and white matter during posthypoxic seizures in newborn pigs. *Pediatr Res* 44:746–754.

Thornberg E & Ekstrom-Jodal B (1994) Cerebral function monitoring: a method of predicting outcome in term neonates after severe perinatal asphyxia. *Acta Paediatr* 83:596–601.

Thornberg E, Thiringer K, Odeback A *et al.* (1995a) Birth asphyxia: incidence, clinical course and outcome in a Swedish population. *Acta Paediatr* 84:927–932.

Thornberg E, Thiringer K, Hagberg H *et al.* (1995b) Neuron specific enolase in asphyxiated newborns: association with enceophalopathy and cerebral function monitor trace. *Arch Dis Childhood* 72:F39–F42.

Trounce J Q, Levene M I (1985) The diagnosis and outcome of subcortical cystic leukomalacia. *Arch Dis Childhood* 60:1041–1044.

Tweed W A, Pash M & Doig G (1981) Cerebrovascular mechanisms in perinatal asphyxia: the role of vasogenic brain edema. *Pediatr Res* 15:44–46.

Van Bel F & Walther F J (1990) Myocardial dysfunction and cerebral blood flow velocity following birth asphyxia. *Acta Paediatrica Scandinavica* 79:756–762.

Vannucci R C & Mujsce D J (1992) Effect of glucose on perinatal hypoxic-ischemic brain damage. *Biol Neonate* 62:215–224.

Varvarigou A, Vagenakis A G, Makri M *et al.* (1996) Prolactin and growth hormone in perinatal asphyxia. *Biol Neonate* 69:76–83.

Voit T, Lemburg P, Neuen E *et al.* (1987) Damage of thalamus and basal ganglia in asphyxiated full-term neonates. *Neuropediatrics* 18:176–181.

Voit T, Lemburg P & Stork W (1985) NMR studies in thalamic-striatal necrosis. *Lancet* ii:445.

Volpe J J (1977) Observing the infant in the early hours after asphyxia. In: Gluck L (ed) *Intrauterine asphyxia and the developing fetal brain*. Chicago, IL: Year Book.

Volpe J J (1987) Brain death determination in the newborn. *Pediatrics* 80:293–297.

Volpe J J & Pasternak J F (1977) Parasagittal cerebral injury in neonatal hypoxic-ischemic encephalopathy: clinical and neuroradiologic features. *J Pediatr* 91:472–476.

Volpe J J, Herscovitch P, Perlman J M *et al.* (1985) Positron emission tomography in the asphyxiated term newborn: parasagittal impairment of cerebral blood flow. *Ann Neurol* 17:287–296.

Voorhies T M, Ehrlich M E, Frayer W *et al.* (1983) Occlusive vascular disease in perinatal cerebral hypoxia-ischemia. *Am J Perinatol* 1:1–5.

Walsh P, Jedeikin R, Ellis G *et al.* (1982) Assessment of neurologic outcome in asphyxiated term infants by use of serial CK-BB isoenzyme measurement. *J Pediatr* 101:988–992.

Walther F J, Siassi B, Ramadan N A *et al.* (1985) Cardiac output in newborn infants with transient myocardial dysfunction. *J Pediatr* 107:781–785.

Watanabe K, Miyazaki S, Hara K *et al.* (1980) Behavioural state cycles, background EEGs and prognosis of newborns with perinatal hypoxia. *Electroencephalogr Clin Neurophysiol* 49:618–625.

Wegman M E (1984) Annual summary of vital statistics – 1983. *Pediatrics* 74:981–990.

Weichsel M E (1977) The therapeutic use of glucocorticoid hormones in the perinatal period: potential neurological hazards. *Ann Neurology* 2:364–366.

Wertheim D, Mercuri E, Faundez J C *et al.* (1994) Prognostic value of continuous electroencephalographic recording in full term infants with hypoxic ischaemic encephalopathy. *Arch Dis Childhood* 71:F97–F102.

Westgate J (1993) The assessment of acid-base status at birth. DM thesis 114–143, University of Plymouth.

Williams C E, Gunn A J, Mallard C *et al.* (1992) Outcome after ischemia in the developing sheep brain: an electroencephalo-graphic and histological study. *Ann Neurol* 31:14–21.

Willis F, Summers J, Minutillo C *et al.* (1997) Indices of renal tubular function in perinatal asphyxia. *Arch Dis Childhood* 77:F57–F60.

World Health Organization (1991) Child health and development: health of the newborn. Geneva: World Health Organization.

Worley G, Lipman B, Genolb I M *et al.* (1985) Creatine kinase brain isoenzyme: relationship of cerebrospinal fluid concentration to the neurologic condition of newborns and cellular localization in the human brain. *Pediatrics* 76:15–21.

Wyatt J S, Edwards A D, Azzopardi D *et al.* (1989) Magnetic resonance and near infrared spectroscopy for investigation of perinatal hypoxic–ischaemic brain injury. *Arch Dis Childhood* 64:953–963.

Yamaguchi M, Shirakata S, Yamasaki S *et al.* (1976) Ischemic brain edema and compression brain edema. *Stroke* 7:77–83.

Zanardo V, Bondio M, Pesini G *et al.* (1985) Serum glutamic–oxaloacetic transaminase and glutamic–pyruvic transaminase activity in premature and full-term asphyxiated newborns. *Biol Neonate* 47:61–69.

Zhu X Y, Fang H Q, Zeng S P *et al.* (1997) The impact of the neonatal resuscitation programme guidelines (NRPG) on the neonatal mortality in a hospital in Zhuhai, China. *Singapore Med J* 38: 485–487.

# Chapter 28 Neuroprotection of the fetal and neonatal brain

H. Hagberg, K. Blomgren and C. Mallard

## PATHOPHYSIOLOGIC MECHANISMS (see also Chapter 23)

### INTRODUCTION

Hypoxia–ischemia induces a reduction in the supply of oxygen and substrates, which results in a shift from oxidative to anaerobic metabolism with production of lactic acid leading to intra- and extracellular acidosis. In spite of the relatively low metabolic needs of the immature brain (Duffy *et al.* 1975), anaerobic glycolysis is insufficient to meet the metabolic needs of the tissue, and a gradual decrease of tissue ATP levels will ensue. Deficient energy will lead to failure to maintain transmembrane ionic gradients, release of neuroactive compounds into the extracellular compartments and activation of lipases, proteases and endonucleases.

The hypoxic–ischemic insult itself should not be considered as the terminal event but rather as the primary event leading to brain injury delayed by hours or even days (secondary brain injury). Clinical studies involving repeated magnetic resonance studies in severely asphyxiated human neonates have demonstrated that infants maintain normal cerebral phosphate spectra some hours after resuscitation, but this phase of recovery is followed by deterioration of energy rich compounds 12–48 h after the insult reflecting a phase of secondary neuronal compromise (Azzopardi *et al.* 1989). A similar biphasic pattern of secondary energy failure has been demonstrated in piglets (Lorek *et al.* 1994) and rats (Blumberg *et al.* 1997) during reperfusion after experimental hypoxia–ischemia. The concept of secondary brain injury is important as it indicates the existence of a potential therapeutic window for neuroprotective treatment after hypoxia–ischemia, and indeed, experimental studies have shown that a variety of therapies (Tuor *et al.* 1996; Hagberg 1997) are effective when administered following an hypoxic–ischemic insult.

It is important, however, to bear in mind that the division into primary and secondary events is likely to be a simplification of the actual situation. Regions suffering from severe insults may rapidly become irreversibly injured, whereas other areas subjected to milder degrees of hypoxia–ischemia may undergo selective neuronal death with a time-course that is delayed considerably. Furthermore, regions distant from, but in synaptic contact with, the primarily affected site will become hypotrophic and functionally depressed after the insult (diaschisis phenomenon) due to the interruption of circuitry (leading to ante- and retrograde axonal degeneration) and lack of trophic influences (Johansson & Grabowski 1994), which may lead to cell death in these distant regions (Joashi *et al.* 1999). Tissue repair and compensatory mechanisms may further modulate the extent of the lesions, and the functional consequences are difficult to predict, especially in the immature brain with its great plasticity and potential for recruitment of stem cells.

### NEUROCHEMICAL MECHANISMS

During reperfusion, a complex process is started where multiple partly interrelated factors act in concert in a viscous cycle leading to secondary brain injury. All components of this cycle have not been fully elucidated, but oxygen free radicals (OFRs), excitatory amino acids (EAAs), intracellular calcium regulation, nitric oxide (NO), gene activation/apoptosis, trophic factors and the immuno-inflammatory system are implicated in the process (Fig. 28.1) (Johnston *et al.* 1995; Palmer 1995; Tuor *et al.* 1996).

#### Excitatory amino acids (EAAs)

EAAs such as glutamate are the main excitatory transmitters in the brain, but, in addition, they have been known for a long time to exert toxic effects (excitotoxicity) if applied to the nervous system (Olney & Ho 1970). There are a number of naturally occurring EAA agonists that exert excitotoxicity to humans, e.g. domoic acid (blue mussels, gulf of St Lawrence), β-oxaloamino-alanine (grass pee, Asia) and beta-methylamino-alanine (plant, Guam), which causes short- or long-lasting memory deficits, lathyrism and motor disease, respectively (Stone 1993).

EAA receptors are present on virtually all neurons. There are three ionotropic EAA receptor subclasses: the *N*-methyl-D-aspartate (NMDA), the α-amino-3-hydroxy-5-methyl-4-isoxazole-propionic acid (AMPA) and the kainate receptors that are named after their respective most selective receptor agonist. There are also metabotropic receptors that are coupled to G proteins and stimulate phosphoinositide hydrolysis or decrease cAMP formation (Fig. 28.2).

The NMDA receptor has a high permeability to sodium and calcium (Foster *et al.* 1990). It is composed of a number of subunits, including the NR1 and NR2A-D, and it has been suggested that different isoforms of the NMDA receptor complex exist in the CNS, differing in structure and functional properties (Dannhardt & Kohl 1998). There are several modulatory sites on the receptor sensitive to glutamate,

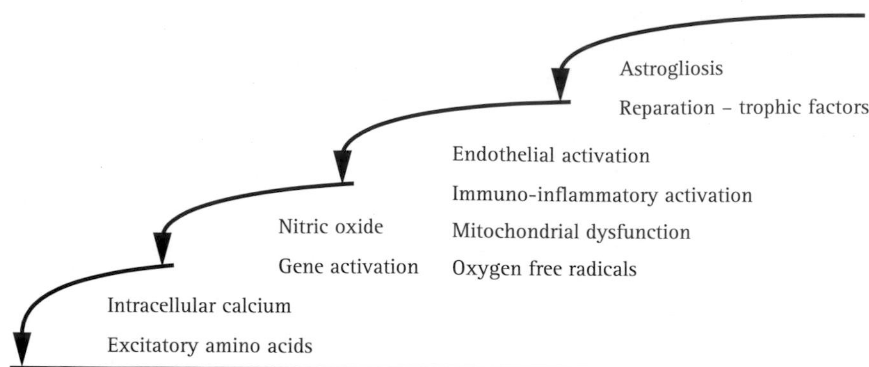


**Figure 28.1** Brain injury cascade after hypoxia–ischemia. Multiple factors are involved in the pathophysiology of perinatal brain injury. Depolarization of membranes and activation of excitatory amino acid receptors increase intracellular calcium, which induces production of nitric oxide, oxygen free radicals and mitochondrial dysfunction. During the later phases, the endothelial activation, inflammatory response, production of growth factors/astroglial reaction may be critical components.

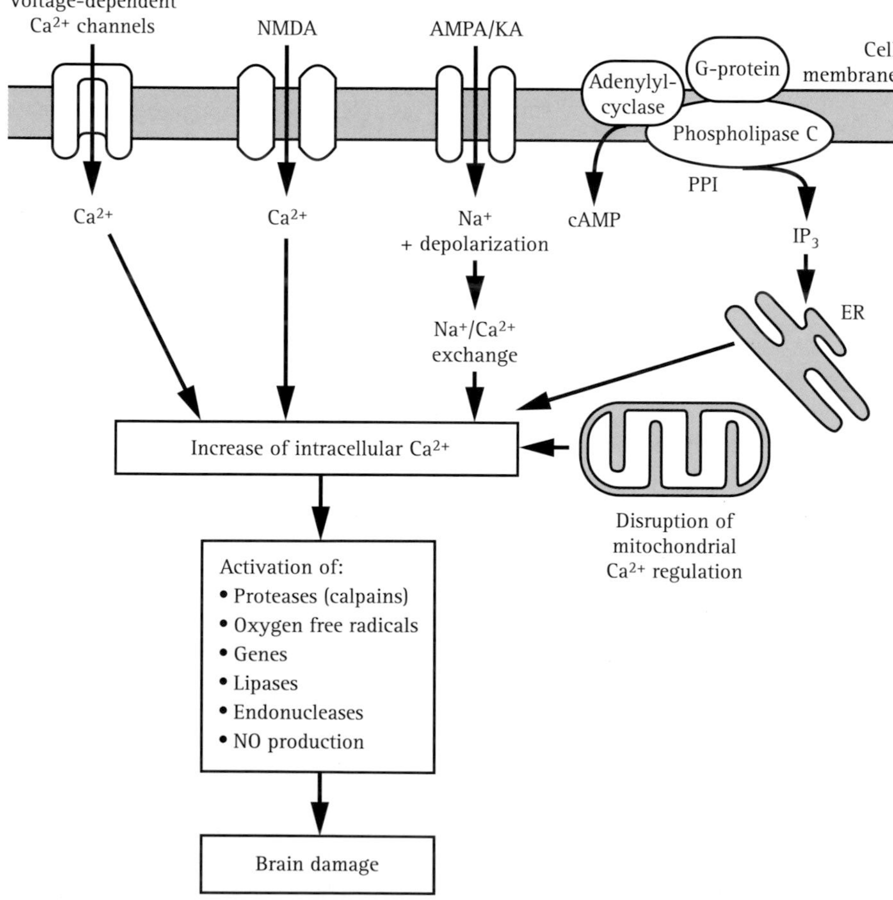


**Figure 28.2** Excitatory amino acids and intracellular calcium after hypoxia–ischemia. Activation of ionotropic receptors (NMDA, AMPA and kainate) and metabotropic receptors results in an increased concentration of intracellular calcium. Metabotropic receptor activation leads to synthesis of inosine triphosphate ($IP_3$) and mobilization of calcium from the endoplasmatic reticulum (ER). Intracellular overflow of calcium in combination with mitochondrial impairment will lead to the activation of a number of processes leading to brain damage.

glycine, $Zn^{2+}$, polyamine, spermine, the redox state, $H^+$ and ion channel sites, including that of $Mg^{2+}$ (Foster *et al.* 1990; Dannhardt & Kohl 1998).

The expression of EAA receptors is enhanced in the immature brain, which reflects the critical role of these receptors for neuronal development (McDonald & Johnston 1990). Hence, the immature brain is also markedly more vulnerable to excitotoxicity (especially NMDA) than the adult (McDonald & Johnston 1990).

Glutamate is the main 'natural' agonist candidate for excitotoxicity *in vivo*. Recent reports suggest, however, that microglia produce a peptide with NMDA receptor agonistic properties (Giulian *et al.* 1993). In addition, microglia/monocytes in the brain of humans and guinea-pigs (but not rats and mice) produce quinolinic acid in response to inflammatory neurological conditions and trauma (Heyes *et al.* 1997), which may be important considering its marked toxicity.

There is ample support for a role of EAAs in the pathophysiology of hypoxic ischemic brain injury. There is a high density of NMDA and other EAA receptors in regions vulnerable to hypoxia–ischemia (Greenamyre *et al.* 1987), and disruption of these receptors precedes the appearance of cell damage (Silverstein *et al.* 1987). Accumulation of phosphoinositides is enhanced in response to hypoxia–ischemia, implying that metabotropic receptors are also involved in the immature brain under these conditions (Chen *et al.* 1988). Extracellular concentrations of EAAs and, to some extent, glycine increase during neonatal hypoxia–ischemia (Hagberg *et al.* 1987; Andiné *et al.* 1991), followed by a secondary increase during reflow (Tan *et al.* 1996; Puka-Sundvall *et al.* 1997). Blocking NMDA receptors before or after hypoxia–ischemia reduces subsequent brain damage in most animal models (Barks & Silverstein 1992; Hagberg 1992). In immature rats, the AMPA receptor antagonist NBQX reduced brain damage moderately when given after hypoxia–ischemia (Hagberg *et al.* 1994), but another AMPA receptor antagonist (LY293558) did not provide neuroprotection in newborn pigs (LeBlanc *et al.* 1995). Treatment with voltage-dependent $Na^+$ channel blockers, acting as glutamate release inhibitors, reduce injury (Gilland *et al.* 1994), which provides additional support for the excitotoxic hypothesis of cell death in neonatal animals.

The mechanism of excitotoxicity in response to hypoxia–ischemia is unclear. Previously, accumulation of EAAs during hypoxia–ischemia was thought to lead to overactivation of EAA receptors, leading to post-synaptic overload of calcium and neuronal death. However, glutamate, asparate and cysteine levels are not as high extracellularly after hypoxia–ischemia in the immature brain (Hagberg *et al.* 1987) as in the adult brain (Hagberg *et al.* 1985) and NMDA receptor antagonists are highly efficacious even if administered several hours after the insult (Wasterlain *et al.* 1993), i.e. at the point when EAAs returned to nearly normal levels, suggesting that other mechanisms are at play (see mitochondrial dysfunction).

### Calcium

Calcium ($Ca^{2+}$) has been one of the key issues in cell injury for more than two decades (Siesjö 1986), and calcium is still considered to be important in this respect (Choi 1995). $Ca^{2+}$ ions are ubiquitous intracellular second messengers, acting as key regulators of numerous cellular functions (Miller 1987). In order to allow efficient $Ca^{2+}$-dependent signaling, the intracellular $Ca^{2+}$ concentration ($[Ca^{2+}]_{i.c.}$) is strictly regulated at a level of 100 nM, i.e. 10 000 times lower than the extracellular concentration (Miller 1991). The large electrochemical gradient is being upheld through ATP-requiring processes at the level of the cell membrane ($Na^+/Ca^{2+}$ exchange and $Na^+/K^+$-ATPase, $Ca^{2+}$-ATPase-mitochondria and endoplasmic reticulum (Miller 1991) (Fig. 28.2). After a few minutes of complete anoxia or ischemia in the adult brain, transmembrane ionic gradients cannot be maintained, and a rapid depolarization (anoxic depolarization) occurs, with a concomitant rise of $[Ca^{2+}]_{i.c.}$ (Siesjö 1986). A marked rise of $[Ca^{2+}]_{i.c.}$ may trigger a number of toxic processes like activation of calpains, apoptosis, phospholipases, endonucleases, OFR formation and NO production. According to *in vitro* studies, the rise of $[Ca^{2+}]_{i.c.}$ tends to be slower and less pronounced in immature neurons (Bickler *et al.* 1993). According to extracellular microelectrode recordings *in situ* in cerebral cortex during complete anoxia in 7-day-old rats (Hansen 1977; Puka-Sundvall *et al.* 1994), there is a protracted and variable increase of potassium and a decrease of calcium, being very different from the corresponding changes in the adult brain. It is presently unknown to what extent these extracellular changes correlate to intracellular ionic events or to the development of brain injury. Radioisotope $^{45}Ca$ accumulates to some extent in the brain tissue and calcium-dependent enzymes like calpains, and phospholipase C are activated (Chen *et al.* 1988; Blomgren *et al.* 1995), offering some indirect information in support of an increase of $[Ca^{2+}]_{i.c.}$ in the immature brain during hypoxia–ischemia.

During reflow, the $^{45}Ca$ radioactivity is initially normal, followed by a secondary accumulation in the tissue 5–72 h after HI, preferentially in regions with brain injury (Stein & Vannucci 1988). It is not known how these measurements correspond to intracellular ionic activities or whether this accumulation of $^{45}Ca$ precedes, or is a consequence of, brain injury. The calcium entry blocker flunarizine administered prior to (but not after) hypoxia–ischemia attenuated brain injury in 7-day-old rats (Silverstein *et al.* 1986), but high doses were administered, and non-specific effects of the drug make the interpretation difficult (Tuor *et al.* 1996). Nimodipine, an L-type voltage-selective calcium channel blocker, is not neuroprotective in the immature brain (Chumas *et al.* 1993).

In conclusion, calcium is held to be one of the most critical molecules in cell injury, but more specific information with regard to the immature brain is needed. The danger of increased levels of $Ca^{2+}$ has been emphasized. Recently, however, it was suggested that a decrease of cytosolic $Ca^{2+}$

was associated with cellular perturbation and an increase of apoptotic-like cell death.

### Oxygen free radicals (OFRs)

OFRs are atoms or molecules that contain one or more unpaired electrons (Halliwell 1992), which makes the free radicals react with other molecules, and subsequently, the molecular structure of lipids and proteins is impaired in the cell with devastating consequences for CNS functions (Halliwell 1992; Saugstad 1996).

There are several pathways by which OFRs are produced in the brain (Halliwell 1992; Phillis 1994; Palmer 1995). The superoxide radical ($O_2\cdot^-$) is produced by: (1) electron leakage from the electron transport chain in mitochondria; (2) oxidation of hypoxanthine to xanthine and urate by xanthine oxidase (mainly in endothelial cells), (3) degradation of free fatty acids by phospholipase $A_2$ into arachidonic acid and subsequent oxidation of arachidonic acid by cyclooxygenase and lipooxygenase, and (4) NADPH oxidase activity in macrophages, neutrophils and microglia (Palmer 1995; Akopov *et al.* 1996).

The $O_2\cdot^-$ radical has a relatively low reactivity and does not easily cross cell membranes. The scavenging enzyme superoxide dismutase converts $O_2\cdot^-$ into hydrogen peroxide ($H_2O_2$), which is not very reactive but is readily diffusable and can react with $Fe^{2+}$ ions to form hydroxyl radicals (·OH) (Fig. 28.3). The ·OH radical reacts with almost every molecule at diffusion limited speed in the presence of transition metals such as $Fe^{2+}$ ions and exerts its toxic effects on DNA and activates poly (ADP-ribose) synthetase and depletes cellular $NAD^+$ and ATP. The ·OH radical initiates lipid peroxidation, whereby polyunsaturated fatty acids are converted to peroxyl radicals in a self-perpetuating reaction that disrupts membrane function. Thiol groups on enzymes and structural proteins are oxidized with a loss of enzyme function and cytoskeletal disruption (Halliwell 1992). There are several defense systems in the brain to reduce the formation of OFRs and several pathways for their inactivation (Fig. 28.3). The $O_2\cdot^-$ radical is dismutated by superoxide dismutase (SOD) into $H_2O_2$, which is converted to water and oxygen by either of the two enzymes catalase or glutathione peroxidase. Vitamin E ($\alpha$-tocopherol) is a lipid soluble scavenger that inhibits lipid peroxidation. There are reports suggesting that scavenging systems may be less well developed in immature animals (Saugstad 1996; Tuor *et al.* 1996). Chelation of transition metals such as iron is another endogenous protective mechanisms against excessive formation of OFRs (Palmer 1995). There is evidence for increased hypoxanthine levels, free-radical formation and lipid peroxidation during reperfusion after hypoxia–ischemia in neonatal mice, newborn piglets, immature rats and fetal sheep (Hasegawa *et al.* 1993; Bågenholm *et al.* 1997, 1998). Treatment with the 21-aminosteroid tirilazad mesylate, a lipid peroxidation inhibitor, after hypoxia–ischemia in 7-day-old rats reduces brain damage (Bågenholm *et al.* 1996). Allopurinol and its

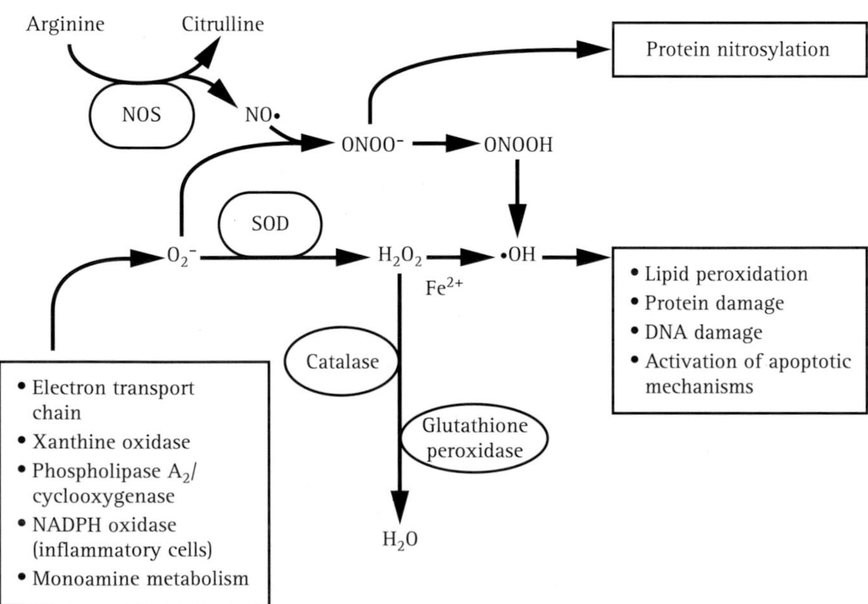


**Figure 28.3** Schematic representation of the role of oxygen free radicals and nitric oxide in brain damage. Superoxide ($O_2^-$) is formed by several reactions and nitric oxide (NO·) by conversion of arginine to citrulline by nitrous oxide synthase (NOS). Superoxide generates hydrogen peroxide ($H_2O_2$) through the action of superoxide dismutase (SOD), and the highly reactive hydroxyl adduct (·OH) is formed either via a reaction catalyzed by ferrous iron ($Fe^{2+}$) or from peroxynitrate ($ONOO^-$). Oxygen free radicals are inactivated through the combined activity of SOD, catalase and glutathione peroxidase.

metabolite oxypurinol, being inhibitors of xanthine oxidase and OFR scavengers in high concentrations, reduce brain damage when administered before or after hypoxia–ischemia (Palmer *et al.* 1993). Furthermore, the iron chelator deferoxamine attenuates hypoxic–ischemic brain damage (Palmer *et al.* 1994). All these pharmacologic agents penetrate poorly across the blood–brain barrier, and it has been suggested that OFR production is initiated in endothelial and immuno-inflammatory cells from within the vascular compartment (Palmer 1995), which is supported by the fact that pretreatment with SOD chelated to polyethylenglycol (PEG-SOD) affords acute beneficial effects in asphyxiated lambs (Rosenberg 1989) and newborn piglets (Armstead *et al.* 1992) in spite of no penetrance across the vascular wall (Matsumiya *et al.* 1991). In adult ischemia, it has been suggested that neutrophils are a major source of free-radical production in the reperfusion phase (Phillis 1994; Matsuo *et al.* 1995).

### Nitric oxide (NO)

The hypothesis that NO, a free radical, is involved in brain injury was supported by the demonstration that inhibition of NO synthesis attenuated NMDA toxicity (Dawson *et al.* 1993). Production of NO, first known as endothelium-derived relaxing factor, occurs through conversion of arginine to citrulline (Fig. 28.3) by three different nitric oxide synthases (NOS): neuronal NOS (nNOS), endothelial NOS (eNOS) and macrophage or inducible NOS (iNOS) (Jaffey & Snyder 1995). NO acts on guanylate cyclase to produce cGMP. Both eNOS and nNOS are expressed constitutively, but all types of NOS can be induced in response to a variety of stimuli. Both eNOS and nNOS are dependent upon $Ca^{2+}$ binding for activation and nNOS is activated by NMDA receptor stimulation (Jaffey & Snyder 1995). The activity of iNOS is mainly expressed in inflammatory cells and produces large amounts of NO and its activity is $Ca^{2+}$ independent (Iadecola & Ross 1997). NO is a vasodilator, but it is also a free radical and binds to iron and thiol groups of proteins including metabolic enzymes. NO· and $O_2^{\cdot-}$ react very quickly to form peroxynitrite ($ONOO^-$) (Fig. 28.3). The $ONOO^-$ radical is freely diffusible in its protonated form, oxidizes thiol groups, induces protein nitrosylation/mitochondrial impairment, and decomposes into ·OH and nitrogen dioxide (Fig. 28.3) (Craw & Beckman 1995). Early investigations on the role of NO in ischemic brain injury yielded conflicting results, and it has now become evident that the different subtypes of NOS have to be considered separately (Huang *et al.* 1994; Iadecola & Ross 1997). Studies using pharmacological methods and knock-out mice in adult rodents have demonstrated that eNOS confers protection, whereas nNOS and iNOS enhance injury in response to focal ischemia (Huang *et al.* 1994; Iadecola & Ross 1997).

It is not known whether the same mechanisms occur in the newborn brain, but the citrulline/arginine ratio increases after hypoxia–ischemia (Tan *et al.* 1996; Thoresen *et al.* 1997), indicating that NO is produced in increasing amount during reperfusion (Brock *et al.* 1995). Ferriero *et al.* (1996) demonstrated that neonatal knock-out mice for nNOS develop a smaller brain injury than wild-type mice following hypoxia–ischemia, suggesting that NO produced by nNOS exerts toxic effects, in accordance with the finding that regional expression of nNOS corresponds to regions of vulnerability in developing rats (Black *et al.* 1995). Selective lesion of cells with NOS activity prior to a hypoxic–ischemic insult decreases brain injury (Ferriero *et al.* 1995) and non-specific NOS inhibitors provide neuroprotection if administered before the insult (Trifiletti, 1992) or in the late reperfusion phase (Palmer & Roberts 1997). Other studies in fetal sheep demonstrated, however, that NOS inhibition early after hypoxia–ischemia attenuated vasodilation and increased brain injury (Marks *et al.* 1996).

In summary, the data are partly contradictory, but there is evidence to suggest that at the early stages of the insult and first hours of reperfusion, NO produced by eNOS exerts beneficial vascular effects, whereas in the later stages of reperfusion, massive amounts of NO are produced by nNOS or iNOS, which will confer predominantly neurotoxic effects.

### Activation of apoptotic mechanisms

Recent data in the adult brain indicate that at least some cells in the brain exhibit some of the features of apoptotic, rather than necrotic, cell death after hypoxia–ischemia (MacManus & Linnik 1997). It is important to point out, however, that in the immature brain, the morphology of cell death after hypoxia–ischemia or after application of excitotoxins is usually distinctly different from apoptosis as it occurs during CNS development (Ishimaru *et al.* 1999). There is however, ample support for the possibility that hypoxic–ischemic cell death shares important biochemical features with apoptotic cell death, which may be important in the context of cerebroprotection.

Necrosis is a passive response to environmental disruption characterized by swelling of cytoplasm and mitochondria, lysis of organelles, spilling of intracellular contents with triggering of inflammation and secondary breakdown of the genomic DNA into fragments of many different sizes. Apoptosis, however, is an active process by which unnecessary, damaged, or aged cells are removed. Approximately half of the population of neurons are discarded by apoptosis during brain development in the complicated process of selection, differentiation and wiring of the CNS (Sarnat 1992). The cellular contents are disposed with little or no extracellular spilling or inflammatory reaction. Apoptosis often involves activation of certain genes and synthesis of specific proteins, and therefore, the term 'programmed cell death' is sometimes used as a synonym. However, this is not fully correct because apoptosis can occur without gene transcription and translation (MacManus & Linnik 1997). In the latter stages, DNA is fragmented into 200-bp fragments corresponding to the amount of DNA associated with one histone. This can be detected as a laddered pattern on electrophoresis, or by positive *in-situ* DNA end-labeling (e.g. TUNEL-staining).

The molecular mechanisms of apoptosis are beyond the scope of this article, and several recent reviews are available (Johnson *et al.* 1995; MacManus & Linnik 1997; Kroemer *et al.* 1998). Briefly, the apoptotic process can be subdivided into four different phases: signaling, activation, commitment and execution. There are a number of factors that are able to induce apoptosis, such as loss of trophic support and release of OFR, EAAs, and NO (MacManus & Linnik 1992; Kroemer *et al.* 1998). These signals may or may not lead to activation, depending on the state of a number of modulators. The expression of proapoptotic proteins like Bax, Bad, myc, p53, or some mitochondrial factors will promote activation, whereas antiapoptotic factors like bcl-2, bcl-$X_L$, gadd45, or PCNA will counteract it. A predominance of proapoptotic modulators will lead further to commitment and execution. The entire process of activation, commitment, and execution is orchestrated by a family of cysteine proteases called caspases (Cohen 1997). There are to date at least 13 known caspases, and they all have an absolute requirement for an aspartate residue at the site of cleavage (Johnson *et al.* 1995). This is a very unusual substrate specificity, which enables the caspases to target a limited number of specific proteins, thereby disrupting essential homeostatic processes and initiating the orderly disassembly of cells. Among the known caspase substrates are actin, fodrin and lamin (leading to disassembly of the cytoskeleton and nuclear envelope), PARP (disabling DNA repair), and ICAD/DFF45 (initiating DNA fragmentation) (Enari *et al.* 1998). It has been demonstrated that caspase inhibitors can prevent cell death in many (but not all) *in vitro* systems of apoptosis (Johnson *et al.* 1995; Cohen 1997), supporting the concept of a key role for these proteases.

The concepts of apoptosis, a developmentally regulated ongoing process in the perinatal period, and necrosis are not readily separated. EAA receptor agonists that trigger necrosis in the mature brain trigger apoptosis in the neonatal brain (Portera-Cailliau *et al.* 1997). DNA fragmentation (Ferrer *et al.* 1994), and the appearance of cells with morphological signs of apoptosis can also be detected after hypoxia–ischemia in animals (Ferrer *et al.* 1994; Mehmet *et al.* 1994) and in humans (Scott & Hegyi 1997). It has been suggested that apoptosis occurs more frequently after hypoxia–ischemia in the brain of immature, than older, rats (Sidhu *et al.* 1997). Furthermore, caspase-3 activity (the key executioner of apoptosis) increases several-fold during reperfusion (3–48 h post-HI) (Cheng *et al.* 1998; Wang *et al.* 2001), paralleled by a loss of the proenzyme and an increase of the intermediate and active forms of caspase-3 (29 and 17 kDa fragments) on Western blots (Wang *et al.* 2001). These biochemical measures of caspase-3 activation occur concomitantly with the appearance of cells being immunopositive for active caspase-3 and showing signs of DNA fragmentation (Zhu *et al.* 2000). In addition, the appearance of active caspase-3 was paralleled by the detection of caspase-3-specific cleavage products of PARP and fodrin, as well as a loss of ICAD. The loss of ICAD, for example, indicates that the mechanism of caspase-3-mediated DNA fragmentation is present after hypoxia–ischemia in the immature brain (Fig. 28.4). Recently, it was shown that 7-day-old transgenic mice overexpressing Bcl-$X_L$ were

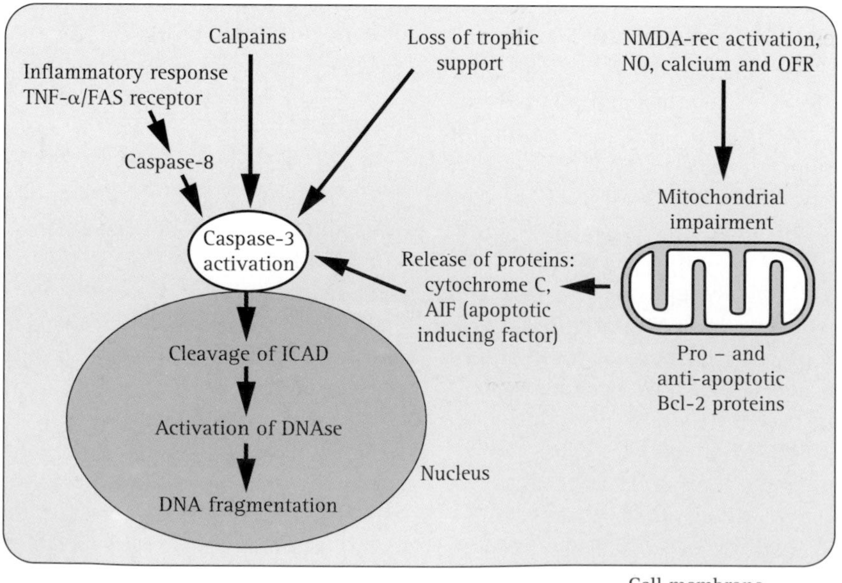


**Figure 28.4** The tentative role of caspase-3 in cell injury. Caspase-3 is activated by inflammatory factors, calpains, loss of trophic support and through the action of proteins released from mitochondria. The activation of caspase-3 leads to cleavage of inhibitory protein of caspase activated DNAase (ICAD) and, subsequently, activation of nuclear DNAse and DNA fragmentation.

resistant to hypoxic–ischemic and axotomy-induced cell death (Parsadanian *et al.* 1998) in support of the fact that anti-apoptotic proteins of the Bcl-2 family are important modulators also under these conditions. Finally, the pan-caspase inhibitor boc-aspartyl-fluoromethylketone (BAF) reduced hypoxic–ischemic brain injury markedly in the 7-day-old rat, even when treatment was started as late as 3 h following the insult (Cheng *et al.* 1998). In conclusion, there is convincing evidence that some apoptosis-like mechanisms are activated in the immature brain in response to excitotoxicity, axotomy and hypoxia–ischemia, and a critical role for caspase-3 is suggested by a number of studies.

### Calpains

Calpains, like the caspases, are cysteine proteases, but the calpains are calcium-activated, and their substrate specificity is not as strict. Calpains have been postulated to have important regulatory roles with regard to signal transduction cascades and cytoskeletal turnover (Croall & DeMartino 1991). Calpains have been implicated in the process of necrosis, and activation may impair cellular function through induction of axonal degeneration and cytoskeletal disruption (Wang & Yuen 1997). Calpains have also been suggested to play a role in apoptosis (Squier & Cohen 1997; Leist & Nicotera 1998). Both calpains and caspases were activated in cerebellar granule cell apoptosis, and cell death was inhibited by both calpain and caspase inhibitors, suggesting that both protease families were involved (Nath *et al.* 1996). Calpain inhibitors have been shown to reduce brain injury in adult models of ischemia (Bartus *et al.* 1994). The calpain activity is high in the developing brain, especially in the white matter (Croall & DeMartino 1984; Blomgren & Karlsson 1989). In immature rat brains, hypoxia–ischemia increased the calpain activity (Ostwald *et al.* 1993), and calpains were translocated to membranes, where they were activated as judged by the accumulation of calpain-specific cleavage products of α-fodrin during the early and late phases of reperfusion (Blomgren *et al.* 1995). Fodrin degradation was most pronounced in the white matter, suggesting a role in white matter injury. In addition, calpastatin, the endogenous calpain inhibitor was up-regulated in areas that remained undamaged, but degraded in areas where excessive activation of calpains and infarction occurred (Blomgren *et al.* 1999). In conclusion, calpains appear to be involved in both necrotic and apoptotic processes, particularly in the immature brain.

### Mitochondrial dysfunction

Mitochondrial respiration is depressed in the immature brain after hypoxia–ischemia (Gilland *et al.* 1998), which leads to a partly anaerobic energy production during reflow, characterized by increased glucose utilization (Blennow *et al.* 1995; Gilland *et al.* 1996) and elevated tissue lactate levels (Groenendeal *et al.* 1994; Gilland & Hagberg 1996). This early period with relatively preserved high-energy phosphates is subsequently replaced by a phase of secondary energy failure (Azzopardi *et al.* 1989; Penrice *et al.* 1997).

The factors involved in mitochondrial dysfunction are partly unknown, but there are data to suggest that increased glutamate cycling acts synergistically with secondary energy failure as the NMDA receptor fluxes more calcium into neurons when energy failure partly depolarizes neuronal membranes (Novelli *et al.* 1998). Furthermore, NMDA receptor activation may impair mitochondria by acting as a trigger of OFR and NO production, which are known to be mitochondrial toxins (Beal *et al.* 1993). This assumption is supported by the finding that NMDA receptor antagonists improve mitochondrial respiration (Gilland *et al.* 1998), attenuate hyperutilization of glucose (Gilland & Hagberg 1996), and prevent secondary energy depletion (Gilland *et al.* 1998) and brain injury after hypoxia–ischemia in immature rats. Furthermore, data in adult animals suggest that NMDA receptor stimulation activates poly-ADP-ribose polymerase (PARP) with consumption of NAD, which may lead to depletion of cellular ATP and susequent cell death, especially under conditions of mitochondrial impairment (Eliasson *et al.* 1997).

Recent data suggest that mitochondria have a key role in the control of cell death (Kroemer *et al.* 1998). Mitochondria in isolated cells exposed to stressful stimuli undergo membrane permeability transition (MPT), which involves opening of a mega-pore in the inner mitochondrial membrane (Zoratti & Szabo 1995). MPT will cause the potential and proton gradient to collapse ultimately leading to ATP depletion and cell death. Opening of the mega-pore can be prevented by the immunosuppressant cyclosporin-A, and this drug has been shown to reduce injury in the adult brain after ischemia (Uchino *et al.* 1995) and hypoglycemia (Friberg *et al.* 1998) *in vivo*. It would be anticipated that MPT leads to necrotic cell death, but disruption of the mitochondrial membrane function, including MPT and/or mitochondrial release of caspase activators (e.g. cytochrome C, apoptosis-inducing factor), is a common manifestation also of apoptosis (Golstein 1997). Furthermore, the Bcl-2 like proteins, which play key roles in apoptosis (Kroemer *et al.* 1998), including that of immature neurons (Parsadanian *et al.* 1998), appear to be attached to the interface between the inner and outer mitochondrial membranes, offering further support for mitochondria as center-stage players in the regulation of cell death (Fig. 28.4). In summary, mitochondria may play a dual role in the pathophysiology of injury after hypoxia–ischemia: firstly, deficient mitochondrial ATP production may contribute to secondary energy failure, and secondly, mitochondrial impairment may trigger apoptotic-like cell death.

### Trophic factors

There are several families of endogenously produced neurotrophic factors that are known to regulate the long-term survival and differentiation of neurons in the central nervous system (CNS). Many of these factors are also induced in the CNS after cerebral injury and afford protection against brain injury when administered either before or after the insult.

### The neurotrophin family

These include nerve growth factor (NGF), brain-derived neurotrophic factor (BDNF), neurotrophin-3 (NT-3), and neurotrophin-4/5 (NT-4/5) and are involved in the regulation of neuronal differentiation, dendritic and axonal growth and synapse formation (Barbacid 1995). The biological effects of the neurotrophins are mediated via specific receptor tyrosine kinases, so-called trk receptors. There are three high-affinity receptors, trk A, trk B and trk C, that predominantly bind NGF, BDNF, and NT-3, respectively. All neurotrophins also bind to the low-affinity receptor p75, but the exact function of this receptor is not known.

BDNF mRNA and protein are widely distributed throughout the brain, with a particularly high expression in cholinergic projection areas and the olfactory system (Yan *et al.* 1997). In comparison, the distribution of NGF and NT-3 in the brain is more limited. During development, the mRNA expression of the neurotrophins coincides with the onset of neurogenesis. The expression of NT-3 and NGF is generally high during brain development and then declines to adult levels, except for the expression in the hippocampus, which remains high in the adult (Maisonpierre *et al.* 1990). In contrast, BDNF mRNA is expressed at relatively low levels in developing brain regions and increases with maturation of these regions.

The neurotrophins and their receptors are induced following a range of insults to the brain, including seizures, kindling stimulation in the hippocampus, kainic acid injection, transient forebrain ischemia, focal ischemia, middle cerebral artery occlusion and hypoglycemia. For example, following cerebral ischemia, there is an increased mRNA expression of both BDNF and NGF in the hippocampus, while the expression of NT-3 is down-regulated (Lindvall *et al.* 1992). BDNF is also induced by seizure activity in the neonatal rat. Inhibition of the increase in BDNF results in brain injury in the hippocampus, which is not normally seen, suggesting that BDNF may act as an endogenous neuroprotector following seizures (Tandon *et al.* 1999). In neonatal rats, a single intra-cerebroventricular injection of BDNF has markedly protective properties following a hypoxic–ischemic insult. When given before the insult, BDNF protects against 90% of tissue loss, whereas when given after the ischemic episode, 50% of the tissue is saved. This protection appears to be age-related since the same procedure in 21-day-old old or adult rats only afforded moderate protection. The protection was associated with the activation of the trk B receptor since trk phosphorylation was mainly seen in the younger age group (Cheng *et al.* 1997). Similarly, an i.c.v. injection of NGF prior to, and 48 h following, a hypoxic–ischemic insult in 7-day-old rats stimulates phosphorylation of the trk A receptor and protects against cerebral damage (Holtzman *et al.* 1996).

### The insulin-like growth factors (IGFs)

IGF-I and IGF-II play important roles in the development of the nervous system in stimulating cell proliferation and differentiation (D'Ercole *et al.* 1996). Both IGF-I and IGF-II are synthesized in the brain during embryogenesis, and during brain development, the mRNA expression for IGF-I and II is particularly high in cell populations undergoing proliferation. After birth, levels gradually decline towards adult levels. IGF-I protein has been demonstrated in forebrain structures such as the neocortex, hippocampus and basal ganglia, Purkinje neurons of the cerebellum, and several brainstem nuclei. Similarly, the distribution of IGF-II protein expression is seen throughout the brain such as in myelinated tracts.

The IGFs exert their biological effects via two surface tyrosine kinase receptors: type I IGF receptors and type II IGF receptors. The type I IGF receptor is the main receptor for IGF-I, while IGF-II is recognized with lesser affinity. Studies both *in vitro* and *in vivo* suggest that the trophic effects of the IGFs are mainly mediated through the type I IGF receptor. In the blood, the IGFs are bound to carrier proteins, the IGF-binding proteins (IGFBPs). The IGFBPs have also been identified in cerebral spinal fluid (CSF), choroid plexus and astrocytes in the CNS. The exact function of the IGFBPs is not known, but it is believed that they regulate the activity of the IGFs since the IGFBPs have been shown to have both inhibitory and stimulatory effects on IGF actions. It has also been suggested that they may function as a delivery system in tissue. To date, six different IGFBPs (1–6) have been identified.

*In vitro* studies have shown that IGF-I promotes the survival and neurite extension of cortical neurons, hypothalamic cells and prevents apoptosis of cerebellar granule cells. IGF-I also appears to be very important for oligodendrocyte development and myelination of the brain, demonstrated by the small brain size and reduced myelination in transgenic mice lacking IGF.

The IGF system is clearly activated following brain injury, with increased expression of both IGF-I mRNA and IGFBPs 2,3 and 5 after hypoxic–ischemic injury in neonatal and adolescent rats (Gluckman *et al.* 1992). *In vitro* experiments have demonstrated that IGF-I protects neuronal cells from calcium-mediated hypoglycemic damage, apoptosis of cortical neurons following NMDA, and NO-mediated neurotoxicity, and inhibits apoptosis of cerebellar granule cells following low-potassium induced cell death. Furthermore, numerous studies, in both immature and adult animals, have shown that IGF-I affords cerebral protection even when administered some hours after hypoxia–ischemia (Gluckman *et al.* 1998). IGF-I can be cleaved by proteases into des-N (1–3)-IGF-I (des-IGF-I) and the N-terminal tripeptide, glycine–proline–glutamate (GPE). It has recently been shown that GPE has neuroprotective effects following hypoxic–ischemic injury in adult rats and reduces the extent of damage in the cortex and hippocampus (Guan *et al.* 1999). However, whether GPE has similar neuroprotective effects in the immature brain is still unknown. At present, it is not clear how GPE exerts its neuroprotective effects, but there is some evidence to suggest an interaction with the NMDA receptor.

The production of IGF-I appears to be, at least partially, under the regulation of growth hormone (GH). Furthermore, GH receptors (GH-R) are abundantly expressed in the rat brain in neuronal, glial and endothelial cells. It has therefore been suggested that GH may exert neuroprotective effects, similar to those shown by IGF-I. It is not known whether GH crosses the blood–brain barrier (BBB) but peripheral treatment with GH increases the amount of GH-R mRNA in the brain (Gustafson *et al.* 1999) and increases the immunoreactivity of IGF-I in CSF of injured rats (Scheepens *et al.* 1999). Moderate neuroprotection (20% reduction in injury) has been demonstrated following daily s.c. administration of GH (50 or 100 mg/kg) to 7-day-old rats following hypoxia–ischemia. In contrast, a smaller dose of GH (15 μg/g/day) did not rescue neurons from cell death following hypoxia–ischemia in 21-day-old rats.

The exact neuroprotective mechanisms of the neurotrophins and the growth factors are not known. However, several possible neuroprotective pathways have been identified downstream of the activation of the tyrosine kinase receptor (Fig. 28.5). Central to many of these pathways is the signaling through phosphatidylinositol 3-kinase (PI 3-kinase), which can result in down-regulation of apoptotic-related proteins, including BAD and caspase-3 (Singleton *et al.* 1996; Tamatani *et al.* 1998). Alternatively, neuroprotection may be mediated via the induction of NF-kB which also can inhibit apoptotic-like cell death. Further support for these theories comes from the finding that inhibition of these pathways increases apoptosis.

## Vascular and immuno-inflammatory mechanisms

Pathological processes in the brain often involve the endothelium and its interactions with circulating blood elements. Neutrophils, monocytes and platelets are activated by the endothelium, and, vice versa, immuno-inflammatory cells activate the endothelium to produce a number of humoral factors and to express adhesion molecules (Akopov *et al.* 1996). The activation of vascular/inflammatory cell components have been implicated in adult neurological diseases like multiple sclerosis, infection, amyotrophic lateral sclerosis, stroke and trauma (Kochanek & Hallenbeck 1992). These events are, however, likely to play a role also in the pathogenesis of injury in the immature brain (Palmer 1995).

### Immuno-inflammatory cells

The recruitment of myelomonocytic cells during acute inflammation is different in the brain as compared to other tissues (Lawson & Perry 1995). The CNS response to excito-

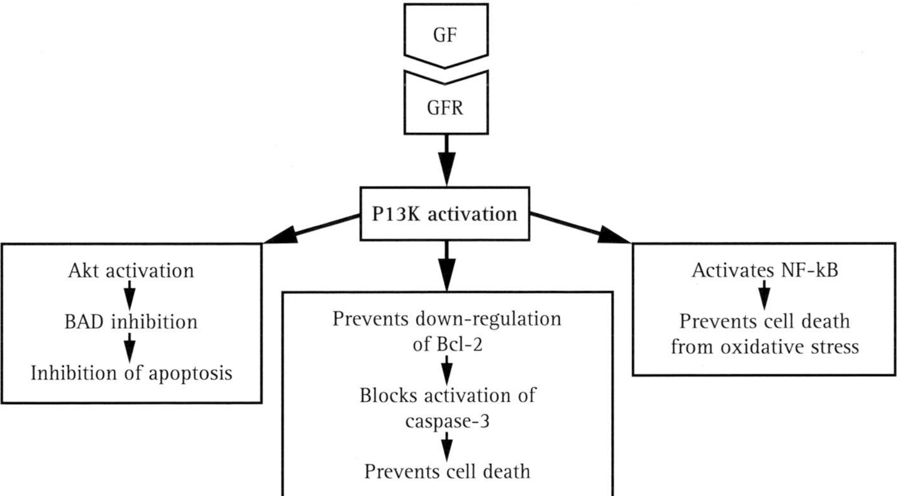


**Figure 28.5** Possible mechanisms by which growth factors may inhibit cell death. Binding of the ligand to the receptor tyrosine kinase results in phosphorylation of tyrosine residues, which leads to activation of phosphoinositide 3-kinase (PI3K). This can then result in the activation of several intracellular signaling pathways that may block apoptosis. Polyphosphoinositide products of the PI3K activity can bind to the PH domain of Akt (a protein kinase) with subsequent translocation to the membrane. Inhibition of PI3K by wortmannin also blocks the growth-factor-related activation of Akt. Cell survival and suppression of apoptotic signals are mediated via Akt-regulated phosphorylation of the pro-apoptotic protein BAD, which sequesters BAD in the cytoplasm and thereby blocks the apoptotic activity of this protein. Alternatively, growth factors may prevent neuronal death by preventing the down-regulation of the anti-apoptotic protein Bcl-2 and thereby blockage of caspase-3 activity. Caspase-3 protease inhibitors do not inhibit the down-regulation of Bcl-2 protein, suggesting that the caspase-3 activation is downstream of the Bcl-2 step. Thirdly, growth factors protect rat primary cerebellar neurons from oxidative stress ($H_2O_2$) by the induction of the transcriptional activity and the DNA-binding activity of NF-kB. The pathway leading to NF-kB activation also involves PI3K since wortmannin can block this effect as well.

toxicity, endotoxin and pro-inflammatory cytokines is characterized by a paucity of recruitment of polymorphonuclear leukocytes (PMN) and a delay before monocytes/microglia are activated (Anderson *et al.* 1991), and major insults with vast destruction of tissue components are needed to elicit an acute inflammatory reaction as it occurs in non-CNS tissues. Such a resistance to inflammation is, however, a property limited to the adult CNS as injection of endotoxin into the immature (7-day-old mice) brain induces a considerable recruitment of PMN and a rapid mononuclear response (Lawson & Perry 1995) suggesting a time-window during development when the immature brain is highly susceptible to the damaging consequences of inflammation. Microglial cell activation occurs early also following hypoxia–ischemia in the immature rat CNS, being more rapid in white matter than in gray matter (McRae *et al.* 1995), whereas the PMN accumulation is restricted to capillaries and post-capillary venules (Hudome *et al.* 1997; Bona *et al.* 1999). A limited accumulation of lymphocytes (CD4+ and CD8+) was detected during the late phase after hypoxia–ischemia (Bona *et al.* 1999). The mechanisms by which these cells are activated in response to different insults are not known, but cytokines/chemokines are believed to be involved.

### Cytokines

Cytokines constitute a heterogenous group of proteins (polypeptides or glycoproteins; 5000–30 000 Da) with various functions including trophic influences on hematopoiesis and acting as transmitters within the immune system and between the nervous and the immune system (Thomson 1998). IL-1β and TNF-α exert pro-inflammatory action as they activate microglia/macrophages and stimulate production of adhesion molecules on the endothelial surface (P-selectins; intercellular adhesion molecule-1, ICAM-1) and neutrophil surface [L-selectin; β2-integrins (CD11/CD18)] and thereby promote the PMN–endothelial interaction (Akopov *et al.* 1996). The sensitivity to IL-1β is highly age-related as 500× higher dose (intracerebrally administered) was required to elicit an inflammatory response in adult rats as compared to juvenile or neonatal rats whereas the response to TNF-α was not as dependent on stage of postnatal development (Anthony *et al.* 1997).

Chemokines represent a subgroup of cytokines being produced by a variety of immune and non-immune cells showing chemotactic activity for specific types of leukocytes. The α-chemokines (CXC) mainly attract PMN, whereas β-chemokines attract and activate macrophages/microglia and other immune cells besides PMNs. Interleukin (IL)-8, MIP-2 and GRO (α,β,γ) are examples of α-chemokines, and MCP-1, RANTES, and MIP-1α/β are β-chemokines. MIP-1α may be responsible for the entry of mononuclear cells during CNS maturation.

Cytokines/chemokines are expressed in the immature brain in response to a variety of insults. IL-1β and MCP-1 are expressed after intracerebral injection of NMDA (Hagan *et al.* 1996; Szaflarski *et al.* 1998), and IL-1α, IL-1β, TNF-α, IL-6, MIP-1α, MIP-1β, MIP-2, RANTES, GRO, and MCP-1 are all induced after hypoxia–ischemia in 7-day-old rats (Szaflarski *et al.* 1995; Hagberg *et al.* 1996; Ivacko *et al.* 1997; Bona *et al.* 1999). IL-6, IL-8, and, in some infants, IL-1β, immunoreactive proteins were increased in the CSF after asphyxia and the levels correlated to the degree of newborn encephalopathy (Sävman *et al.* 1998), whereas TNF-α, IL-10, and GM-CSF were unaffected.

### Cytokines – brain injury (see also p. 376)

The contribution of microglia in the process leading to brain injury has not been evaluated in immature animals, but anti-proliferative treatment (chlorochine + cholchicine) in adult rabbits reduced microgliosis after spinal cord ischemia, which was associated with a reduction of delayed injury (Giulian & Vaca 1993). Anti-neutrophil serum administered to 7-day-old rats reduced edema and brain injury after hypoxia–ischemia provided that treatment was started before the insult (Hudome *et al.* 1997).

It has been demonstrated that TNF-α induces apoptosis in oligodendroglia (Leist & Nicotera 1998) which may be mediated by activation of the TNF receptor 1 (p55) leading to activation of the caspase cascade directly via caspase-8 (Cohen 1997). Repeated injections of endotoxin, which releases TNF-α, cause white-matter injury in kittens (Gilles & Kerr 1997). In the adult brain, TNF-binding protein reduced ischemic (Nawashiro *et al.* 1997) brain injury, and TNF-α antibodies attenuated ischemic damage (Lavine *et al.* 1998), offering further support for the assumption that TNF-α exerts injurious effects. Contrary to these findings, TNF-α protects cultured neurons from the toxicity of β-amyloid, and TNF-knock out mice are more prone to extensive inflammation and demyelination (Liu *et al.* 1998). Furthermore, genetic deletion of both TNF receptors (p55 and p75) increased the extent of ischemic and excitotoxic injury (Bruce *et al.* 1996), suggesting that TNF-α is cytoprotective. There are no simple explanations for these paradoxical findings, but TNF may have different effects on the two TNF receptors. TNF or TNF receptor knock-out mice may also compensate for their molecular deficits during development by mechanisms such as increased IL-1β production (Rothwell & Luheshi 1996).

Administration of the endogenous IL-1 receptor antagonist (IL-1 ra) systemically (Martin *et al.* 1994) or intracerebrally (Hagberg *et al.* 1996) reduced brain injury in immature rats subjected to hypoxia–ischemia. Adenovirus-mediated overexpression of IL-1 ra effectively reduced injury induced by injection of NMDA (Hagan *et al.* 1996), suggesting that IL-1 has toxic properties. Platelet activating factor (PAF) is a proinflammatory mediator that promotes interactions between endothelial and immune cells and stimulates production of pro-inflammatory cytokines and OFR. The PAF-antagonist, BN52021, reduces brain injury in neonatal rats after hypoxia–ischemia (Liu *et al.* 1996), which offers further support to the idea that inflammation contributes to the pathogenesis of immature brain injury.

Chemokines induce a number of important changes in leukocytes such as the production of oxygen radicals and bioactive lipids, and the release of cytotoxic proteases (Baggiolini 1998). Injection of MIP-2 has been shown to overide the CNS resistance to PMN infiltration induced by endotoxin with concurrent rupture of the blood–brain barrier (Bell *et al.* 1996). Transgenic mice for the α-chemokine KC under the control of myelin basic protein promoter in oligodendroglia resulted in recruitment of PMNs, activation of microglia, disruption of the blood–brain barrier, and severe neurological symptoms (Tani *et al.* 1996).

## POSSIBILITIES OF CEREBROPROTECTION

Immature brain lesions in both preterm and term infants often involve both gray and white matter (see Chapters 20–22). Therefore, it is important to recognize that most types of interventions have been evaluated with regard to selective neuronal necrosis or infarction in the gray matter, and the effect on white matter is usually unknown. Drugs like NMDA receptor antagonists would not be expected to prevent lesions in white matter, whereas sodium channel blockers may exert axonoprotective effects as well. Trophic factors, anti-inflammatory agents, or hypothermia may be anticipated to exert beneficial effects on both gray and white matter.

### EXCITATORY AMINO ACIDS: RECEPTOR ANTAGONISTS AND SODIUM CHANNEL/EAA RELEASE INHIBITORS

Because of the critical role of NMDA receptors in the cascade leading to injury, receptor antagonists have been suggested for use as neuroprotective treatment in humans (Lees 1997). However, non-competitive and competitive NMDA receptor antagonists have been shown to have psychomimetic actions and to cause vacuolar/degenerative changes in the retrosplenial and cingulate cortex in adult animals (Olney 1994). These side-effects do not appear in immature animals (Gilland *et al.* 1997), but the NMDA receptor is crucial for CNS development, and NMDA-receptor antagonists induce CNS malformations during early gestation (Andaloro *et al.* 1998). Furthermore, it has recently been discovered that moderate doses of NMDA receptor antagonists induce widespread apoptotic cell death in the brain of 7-day-old rats, i.e. at a developmental age corresponding to the near-term infant (Ikonomidou *et al.* 1999).

There are data suggesting that some of the adverse effects seen with EAA agonist-site or channel-site antagonists can be avoided by modulation of other sites of the NMDA receptor complex. Glycine antagonists do not cause vacuolar cell changes in the retrosplenial cortex and exert fewer cardiovascular and behavioral disturbances (Dannhardt & Kohl 1998). There is also an ongoing development of NR2B subunit type specific antagonists that are preferentially active only in situations of pathological NMDA receptor stimulation with much less interference with physiological NMDA-mediated functions (Chenard & Menniti 1999). However, there is no evidence at present to suggest that the proapoptotic effects in immature animals can be avoided by these alternative pharmacological strategies.

The neuroprotective effect of voltage-dependent sodium channel blockers (e.g. phenytoin, lidocaine, tetrodotoxin, and lamotrignine-like substances) has been evaluated in a number of adult and immature animal models [see Hagberg (1997) for a review]. Generally, these drugs are neuroprotective, provided that they are administered before hypoxia–ischemia in the immature animal (Hagberg *et al.* 1985), whereas the efficacy is considerably reduced if administered after the insult. Voltage-dependent sodium channel blockers delay anoxic depolarization, attenuate extracellular accumulation of glutamate, and reduce ATP depletion during ischemia, which may explain their cerebroprotective potency.

### HYPOTHERMIA

For many centuries, hypothermia has been used to treat various diseases and, more recently, has also been considered as a therapeutic agent for brain injury. Numerous studies in animal models of both global and focal cerebral ischemia have examined the neuroprotective effects of hypothermia, with the hypothermia induced either during or after the ischemic episode. Further variables include the depth and duration of the temperature reduction and whether systemic or selective head cooling is induced. Some of the recent studies performed in immature animals are shown in Table 28.1. In summary, these experiments have shown that cooling during hypoxia–ischemia, even when relatively mild hypothermia is induced, results in long-term neuroprotection in immature rats (Yager *et al.* 1993). In contrast, brief periods of cooling started immediately after reperfusion show variable results (Thoresen & Wyatt 1997). In some cases, protection of hypothermia (for 3 h) was seen in the short-term but not in the long-term (Trescher *et al.* 1997). However, hypothermia administered directly after hypoxia–ischemia sustained for 6 h reduced injury (but not functional outcome) up to 6 weeks after the insult. Recent studies in fetal sheep suggest that the therapeutic window after the insult can be extended to 6 h, provided that the cooling period was extended to 72 h (Table 28.1).

Several of the factors and mechanisms that are presumed to contribute to brain injury are altered by hypothermia, at least if it is induced during the ischemic period (Wagner *et al.* 1999). Neurotransmitter release, including glutamate, is temperature-dependent and is reduced at lower temperatures. Hypothermia also reduces metabolic rate, resulting in a slower depletion of energy stores and reduced cerebral oxygen consumption, preserves tissue pH during impaired cerebral blood flow, and attenuates changes in some of the protein kinases that have been implicated in cerebral ischemia. Several studies have demonstrated that oxygen free-radical production may be inhibited by a reduction in temperature. In particular, there appear to be a reduction in the release of hydroxyl radicals, which may be partly through

**Table 28.1** Treatment effects of hypothermia after hypoxic–ischemic injury in immature animals

| Model | Hypothermic treatment | Outcome after hypothermia | References |
|---|---|---|---|
| 7-day-old rats, unilateral carotid artery ligation + 8% $O_2$ for 3 h | Environmental temperature was reduced from 37 to 34 or 31°C for 3 h; hypothermia induced either during the hypoxia or immediately after hypoxia | Brief reductions in temperature of 3–6°C had neuroprotective effects if initiated during, but not after, the insult | Yager *et al.* (1993) |
| 7-day-old rats, unilateral carotid artery ligation + 8% $O_2$ for 3 h | 30°C vs. 37°C started immediately after insult | Percentage damage in the ipsilateral hemisphere was reduced from 45.5 to 0% in hypothermic animals | Saeed *et al.* (1993) |
| 9-day-old piglets, neck compression + hemorrhagic hypotension (15 min) | Intraischemic temperature reduced from 38 to 35°C (rectal temperature) | Partial neuroprotection with reduced damage in areas of cerebral cortex and caudate nucleus | Laptook *et al.* (1994) |
| 7-day-old rats, unilateral carotid artery ligation + 8% $O_2$ for 60 min | Focal cooling with ipsilateral scalp temp of 22–35°C vs. 37°C for 2 h during the hypoxia | Cooling of less then 28°C completely protected the brain from damage, neuropathology 3–4 days after insult | Towfighi *et al.* (1994) |
| 1-day-old piglet, bilateral carotid artery occlusion + hypoxia | 34.9°C vs. 38.5°C (tympanic membrane temperature) for 12 h, initiated immediately after resuscitation | No difference in necrotic cell numbers, but the number of apoptotic cells was reduced | Edwards *et al.* (1995) |
| Newborn piglet, transient bilateral carotid artery occlusion + hypoxia (45–98 min) | Hypothermia (35°C, tympanic) initiated at the time of resuscitation and maintained for 12 h | Energy ratios 24–48 h after insult were maintained at a similar level to sham control animals, no pathology | Thoresen *et al.* (1995) |
| 21-day-old rats, unilateral carotid artery ligation + 8% $O_2$ for 15 min | Animals were treated with post-ischemic environmental hypothermia (22°C) for either 0–6 h, 6–72 h or 0–72 h. This resulted in a 2°C reduction in brain temperature (38–36°C). | Neuroprotection was only seen after prolonged (0–72 h) post-ischemic hypothermia. Protection was still evident after 3 weeks | Sirimanne *et al.* (1996) |
| 7-day-old rat, bilateral carotid artery ligation + 8% $O_2$ for 2 h | Hypothermia (from 38°C to 32°C, rectal temperature) for 3 h, started immediately, after hypoxia–ischemia | Hypothermic animals had a 65% reduction in histological brain damage | Thoresen *et al.* (1996) |
| Piglets (< 2 week old), 15 min hemorrhage and four-vessel occlusion | Hypothermia: 36°C vs. 38°C (rectal) for 1 h, started immediately after the insult | Reduced neuronal damage at 72 h in temporal and occipital cortex and caudate nucleus | Laptook *et al.* (1997) |
| Newborn piglets | Hypothermia: 35°C vs. 39°C, initiated on resuscitation | Reduced release of excitatory amino acids and NO in the cortex after hypothermia | Thoresen *et al.* (1997) |
| Newborn piglets, $Fi_{O_2}$ 6% or higher, depending on arterial pressure and pulse rate aiming at low-voltage EEG. Total hypoxic duration approximately 45 min | Cooling for 3 h (35°C vs. 39°C), started immediately after the insult | After 3 days, there was no overall improvement in histological outcome. Hypothermia was, however, protective after adjustments for differences in severity of insult and posthypoxic seizures. Hypothermia improved neurologic score and recovery of EEG at some time-points | Haaland *et al.* (1997) |
| 7-day-old rats, unilateral carotid artery ligation + 8% $O_2$ for 75 min | 32°C vs. 35°C vs. 38°C for 3 h started immediately after HI | The brain damage was delayed but was similar to normothermic animals after > 1 week recovery | Trescher *et al.* (1997) |
| Newborn piglets, bilateral carotid artery ligation + hypoxia (31–98 min) | Cooling (rectal temperature 35°C) began at the time of resuscitation and was maintained for 12 h | Reduced rise of lactate during secondary phase as measured by MRS | Amess *et al.* (1997) |
| 7-day-old rats, bilateral carotid artery oclusion + 7.7% $O_2$ for 70 min | Hypothermia (rectal temperature 32°C) was induced for 6 h immediately after hypoxia–ischemia | Long-term (6-week) 30% reduction of injury was observed in cerebral cortex, hippocampus, basal ganglia and thalamus. No effect on sensory–motor function. | Bona *et al.* (1998) |
| Fetal sheep, 30 min bilateral carotid artery occlusion | Delayed cooling from either 1.5–72 h or from 5–72 h after ischemia, i.e. hypothermia started before postischemic seizures. Extradural temperature reduced from 39 to 30–33°C. | Reduction in neuronal loss in cerebral cortex from 40 to 99% | Gunn *et al.* (1997), Gunn *et al.* (1998) |
| Fetal sheep, 30 min bilateral carotid artery occlusion | Delayed cooling from 8 to 72 h after ischemia, i.e. hypothermia started after postischemic seizures. Selective head cooling 39°C vs. 30–33°C (extradural temperature) | No neuroprotective effects were observed | Gunn *et al.* (1999) |

a reduction in NO production. There is also evidence to suggest that the inflammatory system is affected by hypothermia, so that the expression of the pro-inflammatory cytokine IL-1β, for example, is reduced. Furthermore, hypothermia has been suggested to inhibit events leading to apoptosis after hypoxia–ischemia. Clinical data from adult patients suggest that hypothermia started soon after traumatic brain injury or in comatose patients may improve neurological outcome. Few studies have examined the effects of hypothermia in neonates. Studies some years ago showed that preterm babies born with a low Apgar score had an increased mortality after systemic hypothermic treatment. However, more recent studies in newborns with signs of HIE indicate that carefully managed mild systemic hypothermia in combination with selective head-cooling appears safe, at least in the term baby (Gunn *et al.* 1998). Further clinical trials are needed to evaluate the efficacy of this treatment.

## ALLOPURINOL

Post-treatment with allopurinol, a xanthine oxidase inhibitor and OFR scavenger, has been shown to reduce hypoxic-ischemic brain injury in immature rats (Palmer *et al.* 1993) and improve electrocortical activity in newborn sheep (Shadid *et al.* 1998). There are also some data in post-asphyxiated infants suggesting a beneficial effect on free-radical formation and electrical brain activity, without any toxic side-effects (Van Bel *et al.* 1998), and a randomized controlled trial is on-going (F. van Bel personal communication).

The presumed mechanism of allopurinol would be to inhibit xanthine oxidase (XO) and thereby reduce the production of OFR during reperfusion after hypoxia–ischemia (see Fig. 28.3). However, XO is not likely to be the major generator of OFR after ischemia, and much higher doses of allopurinol are needed to attain protection than to inhibit XO. Therefore, it is believed that allopurinol may act as a scavenger of OFR, chelator of transition metals, and inhibitor of neutrophil release of lysosomal enzymes (Palmer *et al.* 1993).

## GLUCOCORTICOSTEROIDS

It is now well established that antenatal treatment with corticosteroids (e.g. 12 mg + 12 mg betamethasone) in cases with threatening preterm birth (<32 gestational weeks) reduces respiratory distress syndrome and perinatal mortality (Perlman 1998). Furthermore, antenatal corticosteroids have been shown to reduce intraventricular/periventricular hemorrhage and periventricular leukomalacia and thereby exhibit cerebroprotective actions (Baud *et al.* 1999). See also Chapters 21 and 22.

In experimental studies, glucocorticoids administered acutely before or after hypoxia–ischemia worsen, or do not affect, brain injury. By contrast, even low doses of dexamathasone (0.01–0.5 mg/kg) administered 4 h to 3 days prior to hypoxia–ischemia *prevent* the development of brain injury in 7–14-day-old rats (Barks *et al.* 1991), i.e. corticosteroids induce tolerance to hypoxia–ischemia, which is often referred to as preconditioning. The mechanism for this dramatic preconditioning effect of glucocorticoids is not known, but a decrease of basal metabolic energy requirements and/or increase of the availability of energy substrates seems to be important, whereas hypothermia, increased cerebral blood flow, fasting, antioxidants or improved cardiorespiratory functions do not appear to contribute (Tuor 1997).

Even though a single course of corticosteroids exerts cerebroprotection, there is no evidence to support multiple courses of corticosteroids, and there are even some data implicating adverse effects. Repeated doses of corticosteroids have been shown to reduce growth (including head circumference) and to be associated with an increased risk of neurobehavioral abnormalities (French *et al.* 1999; Lampe *et al.* 1999) See p. 381 for a discussion of the potential adverse effects of early postnatal dexamethasone on brain development in preterm infants.

### Key Points

- Brain injury after hypoxia–ischemia typically develops with a delayed pattern ('secondary brain injury'), which may open a therapeutic window after the insult.
- Activation of excitatory amino acid receptors during and after hypoxia–ischemia leads to an increased intracellular $Ca^{2+}$ concentration, which triggers the production of oxygen free radicals/nitric oxide and activation of proteases and lipases.
- All cells have the biochemical machinery required to commit suicide (apoptosis). Even though the morphology of hypoxic–ischemic cell death often is different from that of apoptosis, hypoxic–ischemic and apoptotic cell death seem to share critical mechanisms, e.g. activation of a family of cysteine proteases called caspases. Inhibitors of caspases may constitute a future means of therapeutic intervention.
- Trophic factors inhibit apoptosis, promote cell survival and support reparative processes in the brain. A multitude of trophic proteins are expressed in response to hypoxia–ischemia, probably as part of a protective response. Pharmacological or genetic enhancement of the growth factor response has been shown to improve outcome after experimental hypoxia–ischemia, and is currently being explored as a target for cerebroprotective treatment in humans.
- Mitochondria appear to play a key role in brain injury. Impairment of mitochondrial function during the recovery phase may lead to cell death either secondary to energy failure or as a result of the release of pro-apoptotic proteins from the mitochondrial intermembrane space.
- Immuno-inflammatory cells and cytokines are activated after hypoxia–ischemia and contribute to the development of brain injury.
- Other than glucocorticoids, there are no cerebroprotective agents presently approved for clinical use in perinatal medicine. Regimens that have been attempted or that are being currently investigated include hypothermia, excitatory amino acid antagonists/sodium channel inhibitors and allopurinol.

## REFERENCES


✪ Akopov S, Sercombe R & Seylaz J (1996). Cerebrovascular reactivity: role of endothelium/platelet/leucocyte interactions. *Cerebrovasc Brain Metab Rev* 8:11–94.

Andaloro V J, Monaghan D T & Rosenquist T H (1998). Dextromethorphan and other N-methyl-D-aspartate receptor antagonists are teratogenic in the avian embryo model. *Pediatr Res* 43(1):1–7.

Andersson P B, Perry V H & Gordon S (1991). The kinetics and morphological characteristics of the macrophage-microglial response to kainic acid-induced neuronal degeneration. *Neuroscience* 42:201–214.

Andiné P, Sandberg M, Bågenholm R, Lehmann A & Hagberg H (1991). Intra- and extracellular changes of amino acids in the cerebral cortex of the neonatal rat during hypoxia-ischemia. *Dev Brain Res* 64:115–120.

Anthony D C, Bolton S J, Fearn S & Perry V H (1997). Age-related effects of interleukin-1 beta on polymorphonuclear neutrophil-dependent increases in blood-brain barrier permeability in rats. *Brain* 120:435–444.

Armstead W M, Mirro R, Thelin O P *et al.* (1992). Polyethylene glycol superoxide dismutase and catalase attenuate increased blood-brain barrier permeability after ischemia in piglets. *Stroke* 23(5):755–62.

Azzopardi D, Wyatt J S, Cady E B *et al.* (1989). Prognosis of newborn infants with hypoxic-ischemic brain injury assessed by phosphorus magnetic resonance spectroscopy. *Pediatr Res* 25(5):445–51.

Bågenholm R, Andine P & Hagberg H (1996). Effects of the 21-amino steroid tirilazad mesylate (U-74006F) on brain damage and edema after perinatal hypoxia-ischemia in the rat. *Pediatr Res* 40(3):399–403.

✪ Bågenholm R, Nilsson U A, Götberg C W & Kjellmer I (1998). Free radicals are formed in the brain of fetal sheep during reperfusion after cerebral ischemia. *Pediatr Res* 43:271–275.

Bågenholm R, Nilsson U A & Kjellmer I (1997). Formation of free radicals in hypoxic ischemic brain damage in the neonatal rat, assessed by an endogenous spin trap and lipid peroxidation. *Brain Res* 773:132–138.

Baggiolini M (1998). Chemokines and leukocyte traffic. *Nature* 392:565–568.

Barbacid M (1995). Neurotrophic factors and their receptors. *Curr Opin Cell Biol* 7(2):148–55.

✪ Barks J D & Silverstein F S (1992). Excitatory amino acids contribute to the pathogenesis of perinatal hypoxic-ischemic brain injury. *Brain Pathol* 2(3):235–43.

✪ Barks J D E, Post M & Tuor U I (1991). Dexamethasone prevents hypoxic-ischemic brain damage in the neonatal rat. *Pediatr Res* 29(6):558–563.

Bartus R, Baker K, Heiser A *et al.* (1994). Postischemic administration of AK275, a calpain inhibitor, provides substantial protection against focal ischemic brain damage. *J Cereb Blood Flow Metab* 14(4):537–44.

Baud O, Foix-L'Helias L, Kaminski M *et al.* (1999). Antenatal glucocorticoid treatment and cystic periventricular leukomalacia in very premature infants *N Engl J Med* 341(16):1190–6.

Beal M F, Hyman B T & Koroshetz W (1993). Do defects in mitochondrial energy metabolism underlie the pathology of neurodegenerative diseases? *TINS* 16(4):125–131.

Bell M D, Taub D D & Perry V H (1996). Overriding the brain's intrinsic resistance to leukocyte recruitment with intraparenchymal injections of recombinant chemokines. *Neuroscience* 74(1):283–292.

Bickler P, Gallego S & Hansen B (1993). Developmental changes in intracellular calcium regulation in rat cerebral cortex during hypoxia. *J Cereb Blood Flow Metab* 13:811–819.

Black S M, Bedolli M A, Martinez S, Bristow J D, Ferriero D M & Soifer S J (1995). Expression of neuronal nitric oxide synthase corresponds to regions of selective vulnerability to hypoxia-ischaemia in the developing rat brain. *Neurobiol Dis* 2:145–155.

Blennow M, Ingvar M, Lagercrantz H *et al.* (1995). Early [18F]FDG positron emission tomography in infants with hypoxic-ischaemic encephalopathy shows hypermetabolism during the postasphyctic period. *Acta Paediatr* 84:1289–1295.

Blomgren K, Hallin U, Andersson A L *et al.* (1999). Calpastatin is up-regulated in response to hypoxia and is a suicide substrate to calpain after neonatal cerebral hypoxia-ischemia. *J Biol Chem* 274(20):14046–52.

Blomgren K & Karlsson J-O (1989). Developmental changes of calpain and calpastatin in rabbit brain. *Neurochemical Research* 14(1):1149–1152.

Blomgren K, McRae A, Bona E, Saido T, Karlsson J & Hagberg H (1995). Degradation of fodrin and MAP 2 after neonatal cerebral hypoxic-ischemia. *Brain Res* 684(2):136–42.

Blumberg R M, Cady E B, Wigglesworth J S, McKenzie J E & Edwards A D (1997). Relation between delayed impairment of cerebral energy metabolism and infarction following transient focal hypoxia-ischaemia in the developing rat brain. *Exp Brain Res* 113:130–137.

Bona E, Andersson A L, Blomgren K *et al.* (1999). Chemokine and inflammatory cell response to hypoxia-ischemia in immature rats. *Pediatr Res* 45(4 Pt 1):500–9.

Brock M V, Blue M E, Lowenstein C J *et al.*. Induction of neuronal nitric oxide after hypothermic circulatory arrest. *Ann Thorac Surg* 1996; 62:1313–1320.

Bruce A J, Boling W, Kindy M S *et al.* (1996). Altered neuronal and microglial responses to excitotoxic and ischemic brain injury in mice lacking TNF receptors. *Nat Med* 2(7):788–94.

Chen C-K, Silverstein F S, S.K. F, Statman D & Johnston M V (1988). Perinatal hypoxic-ischemic brain injury enhances quisqualic acid-stimulated phosphoinositide turnover. *J Neurochem* 51:353–359.

Chenard B L & Menniti F S (1999). Antagonists selective for NMDA receptors containing the NR2B subunit. *Curr Pharm Des* 5(5):381–404.

✪ Cheng Y, Deshmukh M, DaCosta A *et al.* (1998). Caspase inhibitor affords neuroprotection with delayed administration in a rat model of neonatal hypoxic-ischemic brain injury. *J Clin Invest* 101(9):1992–9.

✪ Cheng Y, Gidday J M, Yan Q, Shah A R & Holtzman D M (1997). Marked age-dependent neuroprotection by brain-derived neurotrophic factor against neonatal hypoxic-ischemic brain injury. *Ann Neurol* 41:521–529.

Choi D W (1995). Calcium: still center-stage in hypoxic-ischemic neuronal death. *Trends Neurosci* 18:58–60.

Chumas P D, DelBigio M R, Drake J M & Tuor UI (1993). A comparison of the protective effect of dexamethasone to other potential prophylactic agents in a neonatal rat model of hypoxia/ischemia. *J Neurosurg* 80:414–420.

✪ Cohen G M (1997). Caspases: the executioners of apoptosis. Biochem J 326(Pt 1):1–16.

Croall D & DeMartino G (1984). Comparison of two calcium-dependent proteinases from bovine heart. *Biochim Biophys Acta* 788(3):348–55.

Croall D E & DeMartino G N (1991). Calcium-activated neutral protease (calpain) system: structure, function, and regulation. *Physiol Rev* 71(3):813–47.

Crow J P & Beckman J S (1995). The role of peroxynitrite in nitric oxide-mediated toxicity. *Curr Top Microbiol Immunol* 196(57):57–73.

Dannhardt G & Kohl B K (1998). The glycine site on the NMDA receptor: structure-activity relationships and possible therapeutic applications. *Curr Med Chem* 5(4):253–63.

Dawson V L, Dawson T M, Bartley D A, Uhl G R & Snyder S H (1993). Mechanisms of nitric oxide-mediated neurotoxocity in primary brain cultures. *J Neurosci* 13(6):2651–2661.

D'Ercole A J, Ye P, Calikoglu A S & Gutierrez-Ospina G (1996). The role of the insulin-like growth factors in the central nervous system. *Mol Neurobiol* 13(3):227–55.

✪ Duffy T E, Kohle S J & Vannucci R C (1975). Carbohydrate and energy metabolism in perinatal rat brain: relation to survival in anoxia. *J Neurochem* 24(2):271–6.

Eliasson M J, Sampei K, Mandir A S *et al.* (1997). Poly(ADP-ribose) polymerase gene disruption renders mice resistant to cerebral ischemia. *Nat Med* 3:1089–1095.

Enari M, Sakahira H, Yokoyama H, Okawa K, Iwamatsu A & Nagata S (1998). A caspase-activated DNAse that degrades DNA during apoptosis, and its inhibitor ICAD. *Nature* 391(6662):43–50.

Ferrer I, Tortosa A, Macaya A *et al.* (1994). Evidence of nuclear DNA fragmentation following hypoxia-ischemia in the infant rat brain, and transient forebrain ischemia in the adult gerbil. *Brain Pathol* 4:115–122.

Ferriero D M, Holtzman D M, Black S M & Sheldon R A (1996). Neonatal mice lacking neuronal nitric oxide synthase are less vulnerable to hypoxic-ischemic injury. *Neurobiol Dis* 3:64–71.

Ferriero D M, Sheldon R A, Black S M & Chuai J (1995). Selective destruction of nitric oxide synthase neurons with quisqualate reduces damage after hypoxia-ischemia in the neonatal rat. *Pediatr Res* 38:912–918.

Foster A C, Gill R, Iversen L L, Kemp J A, Wong E H & Woodruff G N (1990). Therapeutic potential of NMDA receptor antagonists as neuroprotective agents. *Prog Clin Biol Res* 361:301–29.

French N P, Hagan R, Evans S F, Godfrey M & Newnham J P (1999). Repeated antenatal corticosteroids: size at birth and subsequent development. *Am J Obstet Gynecol* 180(1 Pt 1):114–21.

Friberg H, Ferrand-Drake M, Bengtsson F, Halestrap A P & Wieloch T (1998). Cyclosporin A, but not FK 506, protects mitochondria and neurons against hypoglycemic damage and implicates the mitochondrial permeability transition in cell death. *J Neurosci* 18:5151–5159.

Gilland E, Bona E, Levene M & Hagberg H (1997). Magnesium and the N-methyl-D-aspartate receptor antagonist dizocilpine maleate neither increase glucose use nor induce a 72-kilodalton heat shock protein expression in the immature rat brain. *Pediatr Res* 42(4):472–7.

Gilland E & Hagberg H (1996). NMDA Receptor-dependent increase of cerebral glucose utilization after hypoxia-ischemia in the immature rat. *J Cereb Blood Flow Metab* 16(5):1005–13.

Gilland E, Puka-Sundvall M, Andine P, Bona E & Hagberg H (1994). Hypoxic-ischemic injury in the neonatal rat brain: effects of pre- and post-treatment with the glutamate release inhibitor BW1003C87. *Dev Brain Res* 83(1):79–84.

Gilland E, Puka-Sundvall M, Hillered L & Hagberg H (1998). Mitochondrial function and energy metabolism after hypoxia-ischemia in the immature rat brain: involvement of NMDA-receptors. *J Cereb Blood Flow Metab* 18(3):297–304.

✪ Gilles F H, DR. A & Kerr C S (1977). Neonatal endotoxin encephalopathy. *Ann Neurol* 2(1):49–56.

Giulian D, Corpuz M, Chapman S, Mansouri M & Robertson C (1993). Reactive mononuclear phagocytes release neurotoxins after ischemic and traumatic injury to the central nervous system. *J Neurosci Res* 36(6):681–93.

Giulian D & Vaca K (1993). Inflammatory glia mediate delayed neuronal damage after ischemia in the central nervous system. *Stroke* 24 (suppl I):I 84–I 90.

Gluckman P, Klempt N, Guan J *et al.* (1992). A role for IGF-1 in the rescue of CNS neurons following hypoxic-ischemic injury. *Biochem Biophys Res Commun* 182(2):593–9.

✪ Gluckman P D, Guan J, Williams C *et al.* (1998). Asphyxial brain injury-the role of the IGF system. *Mol Cell Endocrinol* 140(1–2):95–9.

Golstein P (1997). Controlling cell death. *Science* 275:1081–1082.

Greenamyre T, Penney J B, Young A B, Hudson C, Silverstein F S & Johnston M V (1987). Evidence for transient perinatal glutamatergic innervation of globus pallidus. *J Neurosci* 7:1022–1030.

Groenendaal F, Veenhoven R H & Van der Grond J (1994). Cerebral lactate and N-acetyl-aspartate/choline ratios in asphyxiated full-term neonates demonstrated in vivo using proton magnetic resonance spectroscopy. *Pediatr Res* 35(2):149–151.

Guan J, Waldvogel H J, Faull R L, Gluckman P D & Williams C E (1999). The effects of the N-terminal tripeptide of insulin-like growth factor- 1, glycine-proline-glutamate in different regions following hypoxic- ischemic brain injury in adult rats. *Neuroscience* 89(3):649–59.

✪ Gunn A J, Gluckman P D & Gunn T R (1998). Selective head cooling in newborn infants after perinatal asphyxia: a safety study. *Pediatrics* 102(4 Pt 1):885–92.

Gustafson K, Hagberg H, Bengtsson B A, Brantsing C & Isgaard J (1999). Possible protective role of growth hormone in hypoxia-ischemia in neonatal rats. *Pediatr Res* 45(3):318–23.

Hagan P, Barks J D, Yabut M, Davidson B L, Roessler B & Silverstein F S (1996). Adenovirus-mediated over-expression of interleukin-1 receptor antagonist reduces susceptibility to excitotoxic brain injury in perinatal rats. *Neuroscience* 75:1033–1045.

Hagan P, Poole S, Bristow A F, Tilders F & Silverstein F S (1996). Intracerebral NMDA injection stimulates production of interleukin-1 beta in perinatal rat brain. *J Neurochem* 67(5):2215–8.

Hagberg H (1997). Cerebroprotective strategies in the neonate based on agents that are in clinical use. *Prenat Neonat Medicine* 2:3–16.

Hagberg H (1992). Hypoxic-ischemic damage in the neonatal brain: excitatory amino acids. *Dev Pharmacol Ther* 18(3–4):139–44.

Hagberg H, Andersson P, Kjellmer I, Thiringer K & Thordstein M (1987). Extracellular overflow of glutamate, aspartate, GABA and taurine in the cortex and basal ganglia of fetal lambs during hypoxia-ischemia. *Neurosci Lett* 78:311–317.

Hagberg H, Gilland E, Bona E *et al.* (1996). Enhanced expression of interleukin (IL)-1 and IL-6 messenger RNA and bioactive protein after hypoxia-ischemia in neonatal rats. *Pediatr Res* 40(4):603–9.

Hagberg H, Gilland E, Diemer N & Andine P (1994). Hypoxia-ischemia in the neonatal rat brain: histopathology after post-treatment with NMDA and non-NMDA receptor antagonists. *Biol Neonate* 66(4):205–13.

Hagberg H, Lehmann A, Sandberg M, Nyström B, Jacobson I & Hamberger A (1985). Ischemia-induced shift of inhibitory and excitatory amino acids from intra- to extracellular compartments. *J Cereb Blood Flow Metab* 5:413–419.

Halliwell B (1992). Reactive oxygen species and central nervous system. *J Neurochem* 59:1609–1623.

Hansen A J (1977). Extracellular potassium concentration in juvenile and adult rat brain cortex during anoxia. *Acta Physiol Scand* 99:412–420.

Hasegawa K, Yoshioka H, Sawada T & Nishikawa H (1993). Direct measurement of free radicals in the neonatal mouse brain subjected to hypoxia: an electron spin resonance spectroscopic study. *Brain Res* 607(1–2):161–6.

Heyes M P, Saito K, Chen C Y *et al.* (1997). Species heterogeneity between gerbils and rats: quinolinate production by microglia and astrocytes and accumulations in response to ischemic brain injury and systemic immune activation. *J Neurochem* 69:1519–1529.

Holtzman D M, Sheldon R A, Jaffe W, Cheng Y & Ferriero D M (1996). Nerve growth factor protects the neonatal brain against hypoxic-ischemic injury. *Ann Neurol* 39:114–122.

✪ Huang Z, Huang P L, Panahian N, Dalkara T, Fishman M C & Moskowitz M A (1994). Effects of cerebral ischemia in mice deficient in neuronal nitric oxide synthase. *Science* 265:1883–1885.

Hudome S, Palmer C, Roberts R L, Mauger D, Housman C & Towfighi J (1997). The role of neutrophils in the production of hypoxic-ischemic brain injury in the neonatal rat. *Pediatr Res* 41:607–616.

Iadecola C & Ross M E (1997). Molecular pathology of cerebral ischemia: delayed gene expression and strategies for neuroprotection. *Ann N Y Acad Sci* 835:203–217.

✪ Ikonomidou C, Bosch F, Miksa M *et al.* (1999). Blockade of NMDA receptors and apoptotic neurodegeneration in the developing brain. *Science* 283(5398):70–4.

Ishimaru M J, Ikonomidou C, Tenkova T I *et al.* (1999). Distinguishing excitotoxic from apoptotic neurodegeneration in the developing rat brain. *J Comp Neurol* 408(4):461–76.

Ivacko J, Szaflarski J, Malinak C, Flory C, Warren J S & Silverstein F S (1997). Hypoxic-ischemic injury induces monocyte chemoattractant protein-1 expression in neonatal rat brain. *J Cereb Blood Flow Metab* 17:759–770.

Jaffrey S R & Snyder S H (1995). Nitric oxide: A neural messenger. *Annu Rev Cell Dev Biol* 11:417–440.

Joashi U C, Greenwood K, Taylor D L *et al.* (1999). Poly(ADP ribose) polymerase cleavage precedes neuronal death in the hippocampus and cerebellum following injury to the developing rat forebrain. *Eur J Neurosci* 11(1):91–100.

Johansson B B & Grabowski M (1994). Functional recovery after brain infarction: plasticity and neuronal transplantation. *Brain Pathology* 4:85–95.

Johnson E M, Greenlund L J S, Akins P T & Hsu C Y (1995). Neuronal apoptosis: Current understanding of molecular mechanisms and potential role in ischemic brain injury. *J Neurotrauma* 12(5):843–852.

✪ Johnston M V, Trescher W H & Taylor G A (1995). Hypoxic and ischemic central nervous system disorders in infants and children. *Adv Pediatrics* 42:1–45.

Kochanek P M & Hallenbeck J M (1992). Polymorphonuclear leukocytes and monocytes/macrophages in the pathogenesis of cerebral ischemia and stroke. *Stroke* 23:1367–1379.

✪ Kroemer G, Dallaporta B & Resche-Rigon M (1998). The mitochondrial death/life regulator in apoptosis and necrosis. *Annu Rev Physiol* 60:619–642.

Lampe J B, Touch S M & Spitzer A R (1999). Repeated antenatal steroids: size at birth and subsequent development. *Clin Pediatr* 38(9):553–4.

Lavine S D, Hofman F M & Zlokovic B V (1998). Circulating antibody against tumor necrosis factor-alpha protects rat brain from reperfusion injury. *J Cereb Blood Flow Metab* 18(1):52–8.

Lawson L J & Perry V H (1995). The unique characteristics of inflammatory responses in mouse brain are acquired during postnatal development. *Eur J Neurosci* 7:1584–1595.

LeBlanc M H, Li X Q, Huang M, Patel D M & Smith E E (1995). AMPA antagonist LY293558 does not affect the severity of hypoxic-ischemic injury in newborn pigs. *Stroke* 26(10):1908–1914.

Lees K R (1997). Cerestat and other NMDA antagonists in ischemic stroke. Neurology 49(5 Suppl 4):S66–9.

Leist M & Nicotera P (1998). Apoptosis, excitotoxicity, and neuropathology. *Exp Cell Res* 239:183–201.

Lindvall O, Ernfors P, Bengzon J *et al.* (1992). Differential regulation of mRNAs for nerve growth factor, brain-derived neurotrophic factor, and neurotrophin 3 in the adult rat brain following cerebral ischemia and hypoglycemic coma. *Proc Natl Acad Sci USA* 89(2):648–52.

Liu J, Marino M W, Wong G *et al.* (1998). TNF is a potent anti-inflammatory cytokine in autoimmune-mediated demyelination. *Nat Med* 4(1):78–83.

Lorek A, Takei Y, Cady E B *et al.* (1994). Delayed ("secondary") cerebral energy failure after acute hypoxia- ischemia in the newborn piglet: continuous 48-hour studies by phosphorus magnetic resonance spectroscopy. *Pediatr Res* 36(6):699–706.

✪ MacManus J P & Linnik M D (1997). Gene expression induced by cerebral ischemia: an apoptotic perspective. *J Cereb Blood Flow Metab* 17(8):815–32.

Maisonpierre P C, Belluscio L, Friedman B *et al.* (1990). NT-3, BDNF, and NGF in the developing rat nervous system: parallel as well as reciprocal patterns of expression. *Neuron* 5(4):501–9.

Marks K A, Mallard C E, Roberts I, Williams C E, Gluckman P D & Edwards A D (1996). Nitric oxide synthase inhibition attenuates delayed vasodilation and increases injury after cerebral ischemia in fetal sheep. *Pediatr Res* 40(2):185–91.

Martin D, Chinookoswong N & Miller G (1994). The interleukin-1 receptor antagonist (rhIL-1ra) protects against cerebral infarction in a rat model of hypoxia-ischemia. *Exp Neurol* 130:362–367.

Matsumiya N, Koehler R C, Kirsch J R & Traytsman R J (1991). Conjugated superoxide dismutase reduces extent of caudate injury after transient focal ischemia in cats. *Stroke* 22:11983–12000.

Matsuo Y, Kihara T, Ikeda M, Ninomiya M, Onodera H & Kogure K (1995). Role of neutrophils in radical production during ischemia and reperfusion of the rat brain: effect of neutrophil depletion on extracellular ascorbyl radical formation. *J Cereb Blood Flow Metab* 15(6):941–7.

McDonald J W & Johnston M V (1990). Physiological and pathophysiological roles of excitatory amino acids during central nervous system development. *Brain Res Rev* 15:41–70.

✪ McRae A, Gilland E, Bona E & Hagberg H (1995). Microglia activation after neonatal hypoxic-ischemia. *Dev Brain Res* 84:245–252.

✪ Mehmet H, Yue X, Squier M V *et al.* (1994). Increased apoptosis in the cingulate sulcus of newborn piglets following transient hypoxia-ischaemia is related to the degree of high energy phosphate depletion during the insult. *Neurosci Lett* 181(1–2):121–5.

Miller R J (1987). Multiple calcium channels and neuronal function. *Science* 235(4784):46–52.

Miller R J (1991). The control of neuronal Ca2+ homeostasis. *Prog Neurobiol* 37(3):255–85.

Nath R, Raser K J, Stafford D *et al.* (1996). Non-erythroid a-spectrin breakdown by calpain and interleukin-1b-converting-enzyme.like protease(s) in apoptotic cells: contributory roles of both protease families in neuronal apoptosis. *Biochem J* 319:683–690.

Nawashiro H, Martin D & Hallenbeck J M (1997). Neuroprotective effects of TNF binding protein in focal cerebral ischemia. *Brain Res* 778(2):265–71.

Novelli A, Reilly J A, Lysko P G & Henneberry R C (1988). Glutamate becomes neurotoxic via the N-methyl-D-aspartate receptor when intracellular energy levels are reduced. *Brain Res* 451:205–212.

Olney J W (1994). Neurotoxicity of NMDA receptor antagonists: an overview. *Psychopharmacol Bull* 30(4):533–40.

Olney J W & Ho OL (1970). Brain damage in infant mice following oral intake of glutamate, aspartate and cysteine. *Nature* 227:609–611.

✪ Ostwald K, Hagberg H, Andiné P & Karlsson J-O (1993). Upregulation of calpain activity in neonatal rat brain after hypoxic-ischemia. *Brain Res* 630:289–294.

✪ Palmer C (1995). Hypoxic-ischemic encephalopathy. Therapeutic approaches against microvascular injury, and role of neutrophils, PAF, and free radicals. *Clin Perinatol* 22:481–517.

Palmer C & Roberts R L (1997). Delayed inhibition of nitric oxide production reduces post hypoxic-ischemic brain injury in neonatal rats. *Pediatr Res* 41:294A.

Palmer C, Roberts R L & Bero C (1994). Deferoxamine posttreatment reduces ischemic brain injury in neonatal rats. *Stroke* 25:1039–1045.

Palmer C, Towfighi J, Roberts R & Heitjan D F (1993). Allopurinol administered after inducing hypoxic-ischemia reduces brain injury in 7-day-old rats. *Pediatr Res* 33(4):405–411.

✪ Parsadanian A S, Cheng Y, Keller-Peck C R, Holtzman D M & Snider W D (1998). Bcl-xL is an antiapoptotic regulator for postnatal CNS neurons. *J Neurosci* 18(3):1009–19.

✪ Penrice J, Lorek A, Cady E B *et al.* (1997). Proton magnetic resonance spectroscopy of the brain during acute hypoxia-ischemia and delayed cerebral energy failure in the newborn piglet. *Pediatr Res* 41:795–802.

Perlman J M (1998). Antenatal glucocorticoid, magnesium exposure, and the prevention of brain injury of prematurity. *Semin Pediatr Neurol* 5(3):202–10.

Phillis J W (1994). A radical view of cerebral ischemic injury. *Progr Neurobiol* 42:441–448.

Portera-Cailliau C, Price D L & Martin L J (1997). Excitotoxic neuronal death in the immature brain is an apoptosis-necrosis morphological continuum. *J Comp Neurol* 378(1):70–87.

Puka-Sundvall M, Hagberg H & Andiné P (1994). Changes in extracellular calcium concentration in the immature rat cerebral cortex during anoxia are not influenced by MK-801. *Dev Brain Res* 77(1):146–50.

Puka-Sundvall M, Sandberg M & Hagberg H (1997). Brain injury after hypoxia-ischemia in newborn rats: relationship to extracellular levels of excitatory amino acids and cysteine. *Brain Res* 750(1–2):325–8.

Rosenberg A A, Murdaugh E & White C W (1989). The role of oxygen free radicals in postasphyxia cerebral hypoperfusion in newborn lambs. *Pediatr Res* 26:215–219.

Rothwell N J & Luheshi G N (1996). Brain TNF: damage limitation or damaged reputation? *Nat Med* 2(7):746–7.

Sarnat H B (1992). *Cerebral dysgenesis.* New York: Oxford University Press.

✪ Saugstad O D (1996). Mechanisms of tissue injury by oxygen radicals: implications for neonatal disease. *Acta Pediatr* 85:1–4.

Sävman K, Blennow M, Gustafson K, Tarkowski E & Hagberg H (1998). Cytokine response in cerebrospinal fluid after birth asphyxia. *Pediatr Res* 43(6):746–51.

Scheepens A, Sirimanne E, Beilharz E *et al.* (1999). Alterations in the neural growth hormone axis following hypoxic- ischemic brain injury. *Mol Brain Res* 68(1–2):88–100.

Scott R J & Hegyi L (1997). Cell death in perinatal hypoxic-ischaemic brain injury. *Neuropathol Appl Neurobiol* 23(4):307–14.

Shadid M, Moison R, Steendijk P, Hiltermann L, Berger H M & van Bel F (1998). The effect of antioxidative combination therapy on post hypoxic- ischemic perfusion, metabolism, and electrical activity of the newborn brain. *Pediatr Res* 44(1):119–24.

Sidhu R S, Tuor UI & Del Bigio M R (1997). Nuclear condensation and fragmentation following cerebral hypoxia- ischemia occurs more frequently in immature than older rats. *Neurosci Lett* 223(2):129–32.

Siesjö B K (1986). Calcium and ischemic brain damage. *Eur Neurol* 25:45–56.

Silverstein F S, Buchanan K, Hudson C & Johnston M V (1986). Flunarizine limits hypoxia-ischemia induced morphologic injury in immature rat brain. *Stroke* 17:477–482.

Silverstein F S, Torke L, Barks J & Johnston M V (1987). Hypoxia - ischemia produces focal disruption of glutamate receptors in developing brain. *Dev Brain Res* 34:33–39.

Singleton J R, Dixit V M & Feldman E L (1996). Type I insulin-like growth factor receptor activation regulates apoptotic proteins. *J Biol Chem* 271(50):31791–4.

✪ Squier M & Cohen J (1997). Calpain, an upstream regulator of thymocyte apoptosis. *J Immunol* 158(8):3690–7.

Stein D & Vannucci R (1988). Calcium accumulation during the evolution of hypoxic-ischemic brain damage in the immature rat. *J Cereb Blood Flow Metab* 8(6):834–42.

Stone R (1993). Hot field: neurotoxicology. *Science* 259:1397.

✪ Szaflarski J, Burtrum D & Silverstein F S (1995). Cerebral hypoxia-ischemia stimulates cytokine gene expression in perinatal rats. *Stroke* 26:1093–1100.

Szaflarski J, Ivacko J, Liu X H, Warren J S & Silverstein F S (1998). Excitotoxic injury induces monocyte chemoattractant protein-1 expression in neonatal rat brain. *Mol Brain Res* 55:306–314.

Tamatani M, Ogawa S & Tohyama M (1998). Roles of Bcl-2 and caspases in hypoxia-induced neuronal cell death: a possible neuroprotective mechanism of peptide growth factors. *Mol Brain Res* 58(1–2):27–39.

Tan W K M, Williams C E, During M J *et al.* (1996). Accumulation of cytotoxins during the development of seizures and edema after hypoxic-ischemic injury in late gestation fetal sheep. *Pediatr Res* 39(5):791–797.

Tandon P, Yang Y, Das K, Holmes G L & Stafstrom C E (1999). Neuroprotective effects of brain-derived neurotrophic factor in seizures during development. *Neuroscience* 91(1):293–303.

Tani M, Fuentes M E, Peterson J W *et al.* (1996). Neutrophil infiltration, glial reaction, and neurological disease in transgenic mice expressing the chemokine N51/KC in oligodendrocytes. *J Clin Invest* 98:529–539.

Thomson A W (1998). *The cytokine handbook.* (3rd ed.) San Diego: Academic Press, . .

Thoresen M, Satas S, Puka-Sundvall M *et al.* (1997). Post-hypoxic hypothermia reduces cerebrocortical release of NO and excitotoxins. *Neuroreport* 8(15):3359–62.

✪ Thoresen M & Wyatt J (1997). Keeping a cool head, post-hypoxic hypothermia – an old idea revisited. *Acta Paediatr* 86(10):1029–33.

Trescher W H, Ishiwa S & Johnston M V (1997). Brief post-hypoxic-ischemic hypothermia markedly delays neonatal brain injury. *Brain Dev* 19(5):326–38.

Trifiletti R (1992). Neuroprotective effects of NG-nitro-L-arginine in focal stroke in the 7-day old rat. *Eur J Pharmacol* 218:197–198.

Tuor U I (1997). Glucocorticoids and the prevention of hypoxic-ischemic brain damage. *Neurosci Biobehav Rev* 21(2):175–9.

✪ Tuor U I, Bigio M R D & Chumas P D (1996). Brain damage due to cerebral hypoxia/ischemia in the neonate: pathology and pharmacological modification. *Cerebrovasc Brain Metab Rev* 8:159–193.

Uchino H, Elmer E, Uchino K, Lindvall O & Siesjö B K (1995). Cyclosporin A dramatically ameliorates CA1 hippocampal damage following transient forebrain ischaemia in the rat. *Acta Physiol Scand* 155:469–471.

Van Bel F, Shadid M, Moison R M *et al.* (1998). Effect of allopurinol on postasphyxial free radical formation, cerebral hemodynamics, and electrical brain activity. *Pediatrics* 101(2):185–93.

Wagner C L, Eicher D J, Katikaneni L D, Barbosa E & Holden K R (1999). The use of hypothermia: a role in the treatment of neonatal asphyxia? *Pediatr Neurol* 21(1):429–43.

Wang K & Yuen P (1997). Development and therapeutic potential of calpain inhibitors. *Adv Pharmacol* 37:117–52.

Wang X, Zhu C, Blomgren K & Hagberg H (1999) Caspase Activation after Hypoxia-ischemia in Neonatal Rat Brain. (Submitted) .

Wasterlain C G, Adams L M, Schwartz P H, Hattori H, Sofia R D & Wichmann J K (1993). Posthypoxic treatment with felbamate is neuroprotective in a rat model of hypoxia/ischemia. *Neurology* 43:2303–2310.

Yager J, Towfighi J & Vannucci R C (1993). Influence of mild hypothermia on hypoxic-ischemic brain damage in the immature rat. *Pediatr Res* 34(4):525–9.

Yan Q, Rosenfeld R D, Matheson C R *et al.* (1997). Expression of brain-derived neurotrophic factor protein in the adult rat central nervous system. *Neuroscience* 78(2):431–48.

Zhu C, Wang X, Hagberg H & Blomgren K (1999). Markers of apoptosis and neuronal damage in neonatal cerebral hypoxia-ischemia. Submitted .

Zoratti M & Szabo I (1995). The mitochondrial permeability transition. *Biochim Biophys Acta* 1241:139–176.

# Chapter 29 Medico-legal issues – the United Kingdom perspective

R. V. Clements

## THE LEGAL CLIMATE

Since December 1997, three major events have altered significantly the climate of clinical negligence litigation in the United Kingdom. The common law in this area has been advanced by two landmark cases in the House of Lords (Bolitho v. City and Hackney Health Authority, 1998; Wells v. Wells 1999), and procedure in the Civil Courts in England and Wales (but not in Scotland) has been radically altered by the introduction of the Civil Procedure Rules 1998 which, notwithstanding their title, came in to force in April 1999. During the same period, there have been landmark decisions in the Court of Appeal concerning consent for Cesarean section (Re MB 1997; St. George's Healthcare NHS Trust v. S 1999).

## PROCEDURE

In his report on the Civil Justice System in England and Wales 'Access to Justice' Lord Woolf (1996) suggested a wide ranging reform of the system and proposed a new set of rules to bring those reforms into force. On 26 April 1999, the Civil Procedure Rules 1998 (CPR) came into effect in England and Wales. The purpose of the rules (Gumbel 1999a) was not only to effect the substantive reforms proposed but to simplify and reduce the size of the rules, simplifying the language and eliminating Latin. Part 1 of the New Rules states the overriding objective 'of enabling the courts to deal with cases justly', ensuring that the parties are on an equal footing, saving expense and dealing with cases in ways that are proportionate to the amount of money involved, the importance of the case, the complexity of the issues and the financial position of each party. The Rules impose upon the courts the duty to manage cases, a radical reform, taking the pace and control of litigation out of the hands of the parties.

The language of the Rules is simplified; amongst the changes, the instigator of a civil action is no longer called a plaintiff – but a claimant.

## THE COMMON LAW

The House of Lords' judgment in Wells v. Wells (1999) has had a significant influence on the quantum of damage recovered by successful litigants. The judgment has had its more dramatic effects upon the damages awarded to cerebral palsy victims. The result of this judgment (Gumbel 1999b) was to reduce the discount rate (the rate at which the successful litigant could be expected to receive interest on his lump sum award) from 4.5 to 3% (Gumbel 1999b). This had the affect of increasing the damages in one (Young 1999) cerebral palsy claim from £1.85 million to £2.57 million.

In professional negligence cases, the way in which the courts in the United Kingdom assess expert evidence has for 45 years been based on the landmark cases of Hunter (Hunter v. Hanley 1954) in Scotland and Bolam (Bolam v. Friern Hospital Management Committee 1957) in England and Wales. In December 1997 (Bolitho v. City and Hackney Health Authority 1998), the House of Lords considered the Bolam test for the first time in 9 years (Watt 1999). Whilst sustaining the principle upon which expert evidence is assessed by the courts, the House of Lords added an important reservation, Lord Browne-Wilkinson expressing the view that a court is not bound to hold that a defendant doctor escapes liability for negligent treatment and diagnosis just because he leads evidence from a number of medical experts genuinely of the opinion that the defendant's treatment or diagnosis accords with sound medical practice. The court must be satisfied that the exponents of the body of opinion relied upon can demonstrate that such opinion had a logical basis and that by informing those views, the experts had directed their minds to the questions of comparative risk and benefits and reached a defensible conclusion. A judge might be entitled to the view that professional opinion was not capable of withstanding logical analysis and that the body of opinion relied upon was not reasonable or responsible.

In dealing with matters of consent, courts in the British Isles, almost alone in the developed world, apply the responsible doctor test rather than the test applied throughout North America and Europe, the test of the prudent patient. That principle has not been eroded in recent judgments (save only indirectly in Bolitho (Bolitho v. City and Hackney Health Authority 1998; Watt 1999), but the courts have on several occasions been asked to intervene in circumstances involving the refusal of treatment by a pregnant woman, refusal that might have threatened the life and well-being of her fetus and herself. In every case at the first instance, and in the only case to come before the Court of Appeal in advance of the event, the courts have ruled in favor of intervention and have declared lawful Cesarean section notwithstanding the refusal of the mother. In Re MB (1997), Lady Justice Butler-Sloss, giving the leading judgement

> rejected the submission that the rights of the unborn child should be weighed in the balance and upheld the principle that

> the competent mother has the unqualified right to decide whether or not to accept surgical intervention in childbirth. However on the facts the court upheld the decision of the first instance judge who had held that the mother's phobia of the injection needle rendered her incompetent (Lord Justice Thorpe 1999a).

The only occasion on which the courts took a different view was in the case of St. George's Heathcare NHS Trust ex. Parte S (1999) in which, long after the event, the Court of Appeal was able to say that the autonomy of the woman is sacrosanct and must be preserved in future cases. In that case, the Court of Appeal laid down guidelines for the future conduct for cases, both by doctors and by lawyers, where maternal consent to intervention in pregnancy is refused. These matters, the absolute right of any adult to choose, to accept or refuse treatment and the rights of the fetus in law are discussed in detail elsewhere (Grace 1999; Lord Justice Thorpe 1999a).

## LITIGATION AND RISK MANAGEMENT

There is no doubting that the impetus for clinical risk management was provided by the increasing costs of malpractice litigation. The sums of money involved are significant. The Auditor General (1999) estimates that in total, potential liabilities within the National Health Service in England are £1.8 billion (£394 million of provisions and £1.4 billion assistance from departmental schemes), but this excludes the additional liabilities relating to incidents incurred but not yet reported and the cases where the NHS considers that there is less than 50% likelihood of a successful claim. However, these figures relate of course only to damages and legal costs. The true cost to the community is incalculable. Clinical risk management (Vincent & Clements 1995) is not primarily about the avoidance of litigation: it is about the avoidance of harm to patients. The Harvard Medical Practice Study (Brennan *et al.* 1991) and the subsequent Australian Studies (Wilson *et al.* 1995) have demonstrated that only a small proportion of negligent events result in litigation; if the focus remains with litigation, the majority of occasions on which patients are harmed will go unobserved and uncorrected.

A similar study is planned for the United Kingdom, but the results are not expected to be significantly different. The focus of clinical risk management therefore must be on the analysis of adverse events with the aim of reducing and, as far as possible, eliminating harm to the patient and dealing with the injured patient by continuity of care and swift compensation for the justified claimant. Clinical risk management is about the avoidance of harm to patients: it is not about the evasion of responsibility for that harm.

In an attempt to improve standards and reduce harm, there has been a flood of advice, in the form of guidelines, from two principal sources. The Royal College of Obstetricians and Gynaecologists (RCOG) has published 20 such guidelines, the last of which in July 1999 dealt with the management of breech presentation (RCOG 1999a). The Royal College has also recently begun a series of reports on evidence-based practice. The other source of guidelines is the clinical negligence scheme for Trusts (CNST). With very few exceptions, secondary healthcare providers have joined this scheme, introduced in 1995 by the National Health Service Litigation Authority (NHSLA) (Sanderson 1998) as a mutual 'pay as you go system' for the pooling of litigation risk. To encourage good risk-management practice, the NHSLA introduced standards, compliance with which attracted a discount for the Trust from the scheme. Of the first 11 standards issued in August 1997, only one was clinical, on maternity care. Additional standards were published in July 1999, which take effect from 1 October 1999 (NHS Litigation Authority 1999). The clinical maternity care standard (now standard 12) is extensively based upon the RCOG's own publications (RCOG 1999b) 'Maintaining Good Practice in Obstetrics and Gynaecology' and 'Towards Safer Childbirth' (RCOG 1999c) as well as on the Confidential Enquiry into Stillbirths and Deaths in Infancy and on the Confidential Enquiry into Maternal Death. It is at present unclear how the courts will view these guidelines, but one view is that

> 'With the law as it now stands, it is open to a judge to make finding of negligence even if the practitioner has carefully and conscientiously followed published guidelines – if subsequent research were, for example, to provide evidence that an accepted practice of the time was unsound, illogical, and based merely on convention and consensus' (Leigh & James 1998).

## EXPERT EVIDENCE

Part 35 of the CPR (White Book 1999), dealing with experts and assessors has two principal themes:

- the overriding duty of the expert to the court
- the proportionality of cost to the value of the claim (Clements 1999).

Following the implementation of the New Rules, it may be expected that there will be less experts, less money available for experts, less time for experts to respond and less oral evidence. The Rules favor single experts, require a standard format for expert reports, provide for written questions to experts, encourage expert discussions, and give the expert the right to ask the court for directions. Much of this is new. The practice direction to Part 35 (White Book 1999) sets out in detail the form and content of experts' reports. Perhaps the most important change for the medical expert is the requirement that '*where there is a range of opinion on the matters dealt with in the report*', the expert must summarize the range of that opinion and give reasons for his own opinion.

The practice Direction associated with Part 35 of the CPR requires that within the report, the expert must give 'details of any literature or other material which the expert has relied on in making the report'. In some jurisdictions, textbook authorities are not much favored, but in the United Kingdom courts, the expert for the claimant will be expected to support his view of the standard of care required to be supported by standard textbooks current at the time.

The report must also include a summary of the conclusions reached and a statement that the expert understands his duty to the court and has complied with that duty. The report must contain a statement of truth, the precise wording of which is set out in the practice direction. The expert must also 'state the substance of all material instructions, whether written or oral, on the basis of which the report was written'. Thus, privilege previously afforded to the exchange between solicitor and expert is explicitly ended. Once the report has been disclosed, questions may be put to the expert in writing within 28 days but '*must be for the purpose only of clarification of the report*'. Part 35 provides the court with the power to direct that evidence on a particular issue shall be given by one expert only. The 'single joint expert' may be appointed by agreement between the parties, but if the parties cannot agree, the Rules provide for the court to '*direct that the expert be selected in such a ... manner as the court may direct*'. The reality is that the courts will not, at least for the foreseeable future, impose single experts on main issues of liability in medical negligence cases. They will, however, expect the parties to agree on single joint experts in many peripheral issues, and the practice is already developing. It is not unusual now in a cerebral palsy case for a single jointly instructed expert in neuroradiology to be appointed by mutual consent. Many issues concerning quantum will be increasingly delegated to a single expert.

The practice direction refers to 'an expert's protocol' with which the expert's report should also comply. Since the rules were published, the terminology has changed, and the protocol has become a 'Code of Guidance for Experts' (Draft Code 1999). The Code of Guidance is, at the time of writing, published for consultation, but it is confidently expected that by the end of 2001, it will be published in definitive form and become a practice direction.

Part 35 encourages discussion between experts of opposing parties, to identify the issues in the proceedings and, where possible, to reach an agreement on an issue. The principle is not new, and there is a wide variation in current practice. The Clinical Disputes Forum (Burn & Scotland 1998), a body set up in the wake of the Woolf Inquiry, has recently issued guidelines on experts' discussions in the context of clinical disputes. That document, too, has been published for consultation (Guidelines 2000).

## ESTABLISHING LIABILITY

A disproportionately large percentage of the NHS liability for malpractice claims results from birth injury. When, at the beginning of the decade, the Legal Aid regulations changed so that the infant plaintiff was assessed on his/her own financial position, there was a flood of old cerebral palsy claims released into the system. Old claims continue to surface, for there is effectively no time limit. Parents are increasingly inclined, in the present climate, to seek financial remedy for an imperfect child. There is an overall increase in cerebral palsy because of the increased survival of low-birthweight infants. All of these facts make it likely that cerebral palsy claims will continue to grow and since the judgement in Wells v. Wells will be increasingly expensive for defendants.

## CEREBRAL PALSY – THE INTERNATIONAL CONSENSUS STATEMENT

In October 1999 the British Medical Journal (McLelland, 1999) published '*A template for defining a causal relationship between acute intrapartum events and cerebral palsy: International Consensus Statement*'. There were 49 authors from seven countries; similar articles had previously appeared elsewhere. Only 6 representatives from the British Isles took part and only one UK organization is listed amongst the supporters of the Consensus Statement, The Royal College of Obstetricians and Gynaecologists (RCOG). Involvement of the Royal College was somewhat informal: the document was shown to a few senior members of the College with an interest in feto-maternal medicine (but none with any great medico-legal experience), but did not pass through council or through the joint standing committee of the RCOG and the Royal College of Paediatrics and Child Health (RCPCH). Of the four obstetricians from the British Isles, three are past or present members of council of one of the medical defence organizations. No UK pediatric neurologist took part, although several were invited and declined. The RCPCH is not on the list of supporting bodies. So much for consensus! The article set out to review the literature on the link between cerebral palsy and birth events but contained no new research. Its shortcomings, both in terms of science (Dear *et al.* 2000) and law (Pickering 2000) were subsequently demonstrated elsewhere. The statement attempts to set standards for expert evidence but appears to have a poor understanding of the law, the standard of proof required by the courts or the proper conduct of expert witnesses.

## ASPHYXIAL DAMAGE BEFORE LABOR

Whilst the cause of the majority of cerebral palsy remains unknown, the commonest allegations in malpractice litigation surround hypoxia. Whilst a pre-natal origin for neurological fetal injury is thought to be common, litigation is relatively infrequent. It is difficult for the claimant to establish a causative breach of duty because the markers for this condition are somewhat imprecise.

## PRETERM LABOR

One special circumstance deserves mention. Preterm delivery and low birthweight are major risk factors for cerebral palsy

(Dite *et al.* 1998). Preterm babies who develop respiratory distress syndrome (RDS) are at particular risk because of the combination of hypoxemia and mixed acidosis that results from this condition (Dear 1999). There is little convincing evidence that labor can be delayed significantly by the use of tocolytic drugs (Thornton 1999). However, for some time, there has been some convincing evidence that the administration of glucocorticoids to the mother in preterm labor before 34 weeks has a beneficial effect in reducing the incidence and severity of respiratory distress syndrome. The initial work by Liggins and Howie (1972) was published in the early 1970s, but it was not until 1989 (Crowley 1989) that a meta-analysis, bringing together a number of large studies, provided convincing statistical evidence of the effectiveness of this treatment.

From the publication of that review, it could be supposed that it would be easy for a claimant to demonstrate breach of duty if glucocorticoids were not administered in appropriate circumstances after that date. Even after 1989, there were those who feared maternal complications, particularly in the presence of hypertension or when tocolytic drugs were being employed. There is ample evidence of the reluctance of the clinicians to use steroids in preterm labor in the published results of the open study of infants at high risk of, or with, respiratory insufficiency – the role of the surfactant (OSIRIS Collaborative Group 1992). Of the premature infants entered into the trial (all of them by definition at high risk of RDS), 15.5–23.3% had had ante-natal steroids. In some cases, there may have been anecdotal reasons for the withholding of steroids but even allowing for that, it is difficult to show that even the majority of hospitals in the United Kingdom were employing ante-natal corticosteroids in the pre-delivery management of babies at high risk of RDS.

## CHRONIC PARTIAL HYPOXIA–ISCHAEMIA

Most actions coming before the courts alleging hypoxic cause for cerebral palsy relate to intra-partum events. Spastic tetraplegia and dyskinetic cerebral palsy are the conditions most commonly associated with an asphyxial cause (Rosenbloom 1996) (see Chapter 27). Tetraplegic cerebral palsy, the consequence of prolonged partial intermittent hypoxic ischemia is the condition most likely to lead to a successful action by an infant plaintiff with cerebral palsy. Several hours of abnormal cardiotocograph trace (CTG) with no intervention by medical staff provide sufficient ammunition to establish both breach of duty and causation. But what if there is no CTG? Save only in 'high risk' labor there is at present no consensus amongst experts that CTG monitoring is mandatory. The notion persists, supported by the Dublin Study (McDonald *et al.* 1985), that listening to the baby some of the time is as effective as listening all of the time! In the absence of a CTG, the claimant has not only the difficulty of establishing that the trace would have demonstrated abnormality had it been in place but also that the defendant had a duty of care to monitor electronically. The argument cannot of course be maintained when uterotropic drugs, whether prostaglandin or oxytocin, are part of management. The abuse of Syntocinon causing excessive uterine activity and intermittent chronic hypoxia is one of the most disturbing and frequent causes of successful litigation in this field.

Failure on the part of midwives and junior doctors to recognize clear CTG abnormalities is another cause for concern. With the drastic reduction in junior doctors' working hours, resident staff are exposed to much less clinical experience than in previous years. If levels of competence are to be maintained, formal teaching programmes have to be introduced, to compensate for this lack of experience. The CNST standard 12.1.7 (NHS Litigation Authority 1999) requires all clinicians to attend six-monthly multidisciplinary in-service education and training sessions for the management of high-risk labors and CTG interpretations. This might seem a somewhat modest ambition. The involvement of consultants in the labor ward is widely acknowledged as the most effective solution to this difficulty, but at present, only lip service is paid to the notion. It is now the requirement of most consultant contracts that one or two sessions per week are dedicated to labor ward duties. Unfortunately, as might be expected, the use made of these sessions varies widely. CNST standard 12.2.3 (level 2) (NHS Litigation Authority 1999) requires that the labor ward has sufficient medical leadership and experience to provide a reasonable standard of care at all times. The guidance goes on '*It is the view of the CNST that over time there will be a greater involvement of consultants throughout the 24 hour period as this will result in better organization and clinical decision-making.*' That, too, seems to be the view of the RCOG, but its achievement is a long way off. For the moment, the guidance specifies only that '*Consultant supervision should be available for the labour ward for a minimum of 50 hours per week of scheduled sessions.*' All are somewhat modest aims; any real change is unlikely until the nettle is grasped and consultant presence guaranteed on site throughout the 24 h in all major obstetric departments.

Another area of concern is the relationship between the junior doctor and the midwife. Where senior house officers are training as general practitioners, they seldom achieve levels of competence and experience that exceed those of an experienced midwife. Yet, in many labor wards, the midwife is required to call the senior house officer, no matter how junior, if she is concerned about a CTG or any other aspect of the management of her patient. This is a recipe for delay and indecision. The senior house officer on the labor ward should be regarded as supernumerary until he/she has demonstrated a level of competence and experience appropriate for decision making.

## ACUTE NEAR-TOTAL HYPOXIA–ISCHEMIA

Dyskinetic cerebral palsy is associated with brief periods of acute near-total hypoxia–ischemia (p. 493). It may occur as the end result of a chronic asphyxial process but is more commonly seen as a result of one of the disasters of labor such as cord compromise, placental abruption, rupture of the uterus, maternal hypotension or shoulder dystocia. The claimant is more likely to succeed if it can be argued on his/her behalf that the disaster should never have been allowed to occur. In placental abruption, the claimant seeking to bring an action on the grounds of lack of expedition is usually in great difficulty, for the defendants will argue cogently that the damage was achieved within minutes of the major abruption occurring. Any subsequent culpable delay was irrelevant to causation. Famously, one plaintiff (Murphy v. Wirral Health Authority 1996) was able to persuade the judge that the mother should not have been in labor at the time the abruption occurred, and, given the competent management of desultory labor requiring augmentation, should have delivered much earlier.

When the cord prolapses without prior warning soon after admission to the delivery suite, successful litigation is unlikely, but on many occasions, the accident is not unforeseeable. The presence of variable decelerations on the CTG often provides warning of an impending cord disaster, whilst the footling breech allowed to labor is, the claimant will argue, to invite a cord accident. Acute asphyxial injury in the vaginal delivery of a second twin frequently gives rise to complaints. For many years, the courts have taken the view that both an experienced obstetrician (Bull and Another v. Devon Area Health Authority 1993) and a competent anesthetist (Kralj v. McGrath 1986) should be present for twin delivery.

Rupture of the uterus in the context of vaginal birth after Cesarean section (VBAC) is a common cause for litigation, but few cases get as far as the courts. The majority are settled at an early stage, for, in truth, the accident can seldom be defensible. The textbooks (Dickinson 1999) would suggest that any woman with one previous Cesarean section and no other adverse features is eligible for VBAC. In this regard, neither twins nor breech nor non-diabetic macrosomia count as adverse features. More than one previous Cesarean section remains controversial, and the author concedes that patient preference may influence his choice. Generally accepted contraindications include previous classical Cesarean section and the diabetic macrosomic fetus.

The textbooks do not, in my opinion, give adequate prominence to the question of consent. Since all series of VBAC report an incidence of scar rupture, it is not, in my view, acceptable to recommend this form of management to a woman without explanation of the risk of rupture and its possible consequences. Most textbooks accept that oxytocin can be used in the conduct of VBAC, but Dickinson warns that caution should be exercised. In my experience, it is the abuse of Syntocinon in such circumstances that leads to disaster. I have collected a personal series of 18 uterine ruptures, of which 17 followed Cesarean section (the other followed myomectomy). Five of the mothers were injured (above and beyond the rupture of their uterus), and 14 babies were either injured or died. In two cases, both mother and baby were injured. Of the fetal injuries, four were stillbirths, four neonatal deaths, and six survivors with athetoid cerebral palsy.

Amniotic fluid embolism (AFE) as a cause of cerebral palsy is rare. In recent years, the definition has become somewhat fudged with the introduction of the concept of an 'anaphylactoid syndrome' rather than true embolus. AFE figures too frequently in the defense of cases of unanticipated maternal collapse, probably because of its acknowledged appalling prognosis, and seems to have become again the refuge of the diagnostically destitute.

## INTRACRANIAL HEMORRHAGE (see Chapter 21)

Intracranial hemorrhage, causing neurologic injury may be the result of operative vaginal delivery. The potential for injury occurs with all manipulation of the fetal head whether by the obstetric forceps and ventouse or during delivery of the aftercoming head of the breech, by whatever means (Drife 1998). In these days of diminishing skills amongst junior doctors, the ventouse has gained in popularity because it is perceived to require less operative dexterity and to be capable of causing less harm to the fetus. Nevertheless, the instrument is capable of producing sub-galeal bleeding, cephalhematoma and primary sub-arachnoid hemorrhage (Govaert 1993).

Rotational operative vaginal delivery, particularly in inexpert hands, has the potential for inflicting severe cerebral damage. Head level is critical in such deliveries and often poorly documented. Since 1983 (Cardozo *et al.* 1983), the advice has been quite clear that Kjelland's forceps should not be applied to any head that is more than one-fifth palpable by abdominal palpation.

## SHOULDER DYSTOCIA (see Chapter 40)

Shoulder dystocia with resulting anoxic injury or peripheral nerve injury has increasingly become a subject of litigation. Only one case has to my knowledge been decided in favor of the plaintiff in the high court (Gaughan v. Bedfordshire Health Authority 1997), but many others have settled. The textbooks in the United Kingdom were not all clear on the optimum management before about 1994, and for babies delivered before that date, successful cases are difficult to bring.

## RECURRING THEMES

Throughout obstetric malpractice litigation, certain themes recur:

- communication
- delay
- cascade of events.

The junior doctor makes an error in the context of a busy labor ward, often in the middle of the night, but the fault lies only partly with that individual; to a greater extent, the fault lies with his senior colleagues who made poor decisions (or often, no decisions at all) in the antenatal clinic, the antenatal ward, or earlier in the labor. It often lies in the delay of the midwives or SHO in failing to seek help earlier. The proximal cause of the accident is easy to identify and to blame; the remote cause – the system failure which set it up – is the real target of risk management.

### Key Points

- Civil Procedure Rules, introduced following the Woolf reforms now exercise strict control over the conduct of experts.
- The House of Lords has qualified to some extent the Bolam principle in the case of Bolitho v. City and Hackney Health Authority.
- Damages continue to increase, not only because of inflation but also because of changes in the law.
- Errors leading to malpractice litigation in obstetrics are almost always the result of system failures and a cascade of error.

## REFERENCES


*Access to Justice: Final Report to the Lord Chancellor on the Civil Justice System of England and Wales* (1996) London: HMSO.

Auditor General (1999) *NHS summarized accounts (England) 1997/1998 report of the comptroller and auditor general.* London: HMSO.

Bolam v. Friern Hospital Management Committee (1995) (1957) 1WLR 582; (1957) 2All ER 118. *Clin Risk* 1:84.

Bolitho v. City and Hackney Health Authority (1998) AC 232 HL (1997) 4 All ER 771 (1997) 3WLR 1151.

Brennan T A, Leape L L, Laird N *et al.* (1991) Incidence of adverse events and negligence in hospitalised patients: results of the Harvard Medical Practice Study 1. *N Engl J Med* 324:370–386.

Bull and Another v. Devon Area Health Authority (1993) 4 Med LR.

Burn S & Scotland A D (1998) The Clinical Disputes Forum and its pre-action protocol. *Clin Risk* 4:137–138.

Cardozo L D, Gibb D M F, Studd J W W *et al.* (1983) Should we abandon Kjelland's forceps? *BMJ* 287:315–319.

Clements R V (1999) The Civil Procedure Rules: Part 35. *Clin Risk* 5:90–92.

Crowley P (1989) Promoting pulmonary maturity. In: Chalmers I, Enkin M & Mark JNC (eds) *Effective care in pregnancy and childbirth.* Oxford: Oxford University Press; Chapter 45.

Dear P R F (1999) The preterm infant. *Clin Risk* 5:7–13.

Dear P, Rennie J, Newell S & Rosenbloom L (2000) Response to proposal of a template for defining a causal relation between acute intrapartum events and cerebral palsy. *Clin Risk* 6:137–142.

Dickinson J E (1999) Previous caesarean section. In: James D K, Steer P J, Weiner C P *et al.* (eds) *High risk pregnancy management options.* Philadelphia, PA: W B Saunders; Chapter 67, 2nd edn.

Dite G S, Bell R, Reddihough D S *et al.* (1998) Ante-natal and peri-natal antecedents of moderate and severe spastic cerebral palsy. *Austral N Z J Obstet Gynaecol* 38:377–383.

Draft Code (1999) Draft Code of Guidance for Experts: for consultation. *Clin Risk* 5:168–172.

Drife J (1998) Intracranial haemorrhage in the newborn: obstetric aspects. *Clin Risk* 4:71–74.

Gaughan v Bedfordshire Health Authority (1997) 8 Med LR 182–195.

Govaert P (1993) Conclusions In: *Cranial haemorrhage in the term newborn infant.* Mac Keith Press; Chapter 12.

Grace J (1999) Should the foetus have rights in law? *Medico-Legal J* 67:57–67.

Guidelines (2000) Guidelines on experts' discussions in the context of clinical disputes: for consultation. *Clin Risk* 6:149–152.

Gumbel E A (1999a) The New Civil Procedure Rules: A First Impression. *Clin Risk* 5:86–89.

Gumbel E A (1999b) Damages in Obstetric Negligence Cases: Part IV – Calculation of Damages Following the House of Lords' Decision in Wells v. Wells. *Clin Risk* 5:14–16.

Hunter v. Hanley (1954) SC200. *Clin Risk* 5:59, 60.

Kralj v. McGrath (1986) 1 All ER 54.

Leigh T H & James C E (1998) Medico-legal commentary: shoulder dystocia. *Br J Obstet Gynaecol* 105:815–817.

Liggins G C & Howie R N (1972) A controlled trial of antepartum glucocorticoid treatment for prevention of the respiratory distress syndrome in premature infants. *Paediatrics* 50:515–525.

Lord Justice Thorpe (1999a) Consent for Caesarean section: Part 1 – development of the Law. *Clin Risk* 5:173–176.

Lord Justice Thorpe (1999b) Consent for Caesarean section: Part 2 – autonomy, capacity, best interest, reasonable force and procedural guidelines. *Clin Risk* 5:209–212.

McDonald D, Grant A, Sheridan-Pereira M *et al.* (1985) The Dublin randomized controlled trial of intrapartum fetal heart rate monitoring. *Am J Obstet Gynaecol* 152:524–539.

McLelland A (1999) A template for defining a causal relation between acute intrapartum events and cerebral palsy: international consensus statement. *BMJ* 319:1054–1059.

Murphy v. Wirral Health Authority (1996) 7 Med LR 99–107.

NHS Litigation Authority (1999) *Clinical risk management standards: additional standards effective from 1.10.99.* The NHS Litigation Authority.

OSIRIS Collaborative Group (1992) Early versus delayed neonatal administration of synthetic surfactant – the judgement of OSIRIS: the OSIRIS Collaborative Group (Open study of infants at High Risk or with Respiratory Insufficiency – the role of surfactant). *Lancet* 340:1363–1369.

Pickering J (2000) Legal comment on the internal consensus statement on causation of cerebral palsy. *Clin Risk* 6:143–144.

RCOG (1999a) Guideline No. 20. July 1999: The Management of Breech Presentation. *Obstet Gynaecol* 1:1.

RCOG (1999b) *Maintaining good practice in obstetrics and gynaecology*, April.

RCOG (1999c) *Towards Safer Childbirth.* RCOG Press, February.

Re M B (1997) 2FCR 541 AC. 38 BMLR 175–194.

Rosenbloom L (1996) Perinatal asphyxial injury: clinical sequelae. *Clin Risk* 2:43–46.

Sanderson I M (1998) The CNST: a review of its present function. *Clin Risk* 4:35–39.

St. George's Healthcare NHS Trust v. S, R v. Collins, ex pS (1999) Fam 26 CA (1998) 3WLR 936. 44 BMLR 160–196.

Thornton J M (1999) Preterm labour: obstetric aspects. *Clin Risk* 5:1–6.

Vincent C & Clements R V (1995) Clinical risk management – why do we need it? *Clin Risk* 1:1–4.

Watt J (1999) Bolitho v. City and Hackney Health Authority. *Clin Risk* 5:17–20.

Wells v. Wells, Thomas v. Brighton Health Authority & Page v. Sheerness Steel plc (1999) 1AC 345 HL (1998) 3 WLR 329. 43 BMLR 99–142.

White Book (1999) *Civil Procedure: The Civil Procedure Rules. A White Book Service.* London: Sweet & Maxwell.

Wilson R M, Runciman W B, Gibberd R W *et al.* (1995) The Quality in Australian Healthcare Study. *Med J Austral* 163:458–471.

Young M (1999) Practical Implications of the House of Lords' Decision in Wells v. Wells, Thomas v. Brighton Health Authority and Page v. Sheerness Steel plc. *Clin Risk* 5:23–24.

# Chapter 30 Medico-legal issues – the United States perspective

B. S. Schifrin and K. A. Schifrin

## INTRODUCTION

The dynamic clash between law and medicine plays out most clearly in obstetrical malpractice litigation. Exploring the facts, questions and problems found in obstetrical malpractice casts much light on the larger fields of law and medicine generally. In this review we step into two worlds of thought as the law tries to reconcile a body of science with the art of clinical practice while medicine tries to reconcile a body of laws with notions of fault and accountability.

## THE LEGAL CLIMATE

Most changes in the medical and legal professions are evolutionary, and it is often difficult to define any sea change. The last two decades, however, have witnessed several remarkable and probably enduring changes in the medico-legal climate in the United States. Many of the changes derive from an obstetric access crisis triggered in the mid-1980s when the malpractice insurance premiums charged by major insurers increased precipitously (Rosenblatt *et al.* 1990). In Washington state between 1984 and 1986, for example, malpractice premiums for obstetrics jumped approximately 100%. As a consequence, physicians marched on legislatures or joined many family physicians, obstetricians, and midwives in an exodus from obstetric practice. Those remaining in practice became more reluctant to care for high-risk obstetric patients and less willing to accept indigent patients and reduced fees. In many rural locales across the US, obstetric care became virtually unobtainable. These circumstances galvanized legislative activity in virtually every state and led to far-reaching modifications of existing tort and insurance law (Institute of Medicine 1989; Sloan & Bovbjerg 1989).

Most Liability Reform Acts had four major components: (1) a cap on non-economic damages; (2) the elimination of joint and several liability for cases in which a plaintiff found to be partially at fault becomes responsible for a disproportionate share of the damages; (3) a reduction in the length of the statute of limitations – the time during which a lawsuit can be brought; and (4) periodic payments – the latitude to pay future economic damages over time. Other initiatives legislated review panels to pass on the merit of a case prior to the institution of suit, while others attempted to remove the infant who is brain damaged during birth from the medico-legal arena by the institution of no-fault insurance. In a related move in 1988, the US Congress established a National Practitioner Data Bank authorizing the collection of data about physicians and dentists from malpractice settlements, awards and disciplinary actions, these data to be supplied by insurers, hospitals and HMOs (Cohn 1990). Queries of the Data Bank may be made by hospitals and physicians, but there is nominally no access by the public or actual or prospective litigants including patients and attorneys. This tracking has probably decreased the willingness of physicians to settle cases, but has probably not decreased the frequency of malpractice.

While premiums stabilized almost immediately, it is far from clear, however, that this was indeed the result of the tort reform legislation. Normally, it takes years before legislative tort reform has a direct impact on malpractice premiums, and several, but not all, state courts have invalidated the cap on damages, the component of the law with the greatest potential to reduce premiums (Zuckerman *et al.* 1989). Malpractice premiums are affected by a constellation of additional factors, including the general investment climate, interest rate cycles, and insurance regulations (Department of Health and Human Services 1989). Whether driven by legislation or not, it seems reasonable that stable malpractice insurance premiums offered by experienced, reputable companies are important reasons for maintaining physician availability and equilibrium.

There is no evidence that tort reform has resulted in better care or a more realistic confrontation of error. Tort reform simply 'tinkers with certain aspects of the system in a piecemeal fashion without having to grapple with fundamental reform of either the health care delivery system, the reimbursement system or physician behavior'. Despite the relative leveling off of premiums, the frequency of malpractice suits has shown no real signs of abating. Indeed, there is a seeming growth in the frequency of lawsuits for the 'bad baby', in part because of the large verdicts sometimes realized but also because of the increasing incidence of cerebral palsy (CP) related to increasing survival of low-birthweight infants (Visser & Narayan 1996). In addition, several clinical practices and media attention would seem also to be impacting on the frequency and type of lawsuit. As an example, the United States Food and Drug Administration (FDA) issued a national advisory on the risks of vacuum extractors (FDA, 1999). This was rapidly followed by a nation-wide television program emphasizing some of the disastrous results with vacuums. In turn, there has been a dramatic increase both in the reporting of adverse events associated with vacuum deliveries to the FDA and lawsuits alleging negligent care in the use of vacuums. Similarly, the methods undertaken to lower the Cesarean section rate in the US have perhaps been achieved at the expense of an increased risk of ruptured uterus, shoulder dystocia and lawsuit (Stainaker *et al.* 1997; Sachs *et al.* 1999). While all authorities would agree that any woman with one previous Caesarean section and no other adverse features may be eligible for attempted vaginal birth after Cesarean section (VBAC), some health-maintenance organizations (HMO) have required that every patient with a previous Cesarean be given a trial of labor. One institution in California was assessed almost $25 million as a result of 48 women who suffered adverse outcome as a result of this policy.

## LEGAL VULNERABILITY

The last several decades have also witnessed the development of new bases for lawsuit in reproductive matters including wrongful birth and wrongful life. In the former, the parents with an injured child may bring suit alleging that negligent treatment or advice deprived them of the opportunity to avoid conception or terminate a pregnancy. The latter, brought on behalf of the child born with birth defects, alleges that the child would not have been born but for negligent advice to, or negligent treatment of, the parents. It should be emphasized that such allegations are actionable in some states but not in others. While not strictly related to malpractice, a mother who pleaded with her hopelessly premature infant's caretakers to discontinue resuscitation was not heeded, resulting in the survival of a severely handicapped child and a provisional $42 million verdict for the plaintiff.

Perhaps the most far reaching impact on litigation will be the legislation permitting suing not the direct provider of health care, i.e. the physician, nurse or hospital, but the Health Maintenance Organization (HMO) responsible for authorizing what care is and is not available to the patient. In many instances, the HMOs have created a conflict of interest between the physician and the patient by offering incentives to physicians who limit the use of care and specialists, etc. In 1999, a nation-wide survey of 1053 primary care and specialist physicians (87%) reported that their patients had been denied coverage by their HMO and that in a number of such cases, patients' health had suffered thereby (Kaiser Family Foundation 1999). Such data combined with the litany of anecdotal complaints by individual patients has brought nation-wide attention and legislative action.

The US House of Representatives and several state legislatures have approved legislation that will allow a patient to sue their health maintenance organization (HMO). In California, a patient is able to sue their managed care organization when '[t]he failure to exercise ordinary care resulted in the denial, delay, or modification of the health care service recommended for, or furnished to, a' subscriber or enrolee causes the patient 'substantial harm' (California Civil Code Section 3428). In Shea v. Esensten, the Eighth Circuit Court of Appeals held that '[w]hen an HMO's financial incentives discourage a treating doctor from providing essential health care referrals for conditions covered under the plan benefit structure, the incentives must be disclosed' (Shea v. Esensten 1997). While certain HMOs are doubtless modifying their stances to give more free reign to the physician in the name of patient desire, there seems little doubt that such a strategy is in part designed to forestall law suits.

Even more recently has come the increasing attention of the amount of medical error that has heretofore gone unnoticed and undocumented. The AMA has created a Patient Safety Initiative, and the Federal Government is considering legislation that will likely reorient the approach to error.

## EXPERT TESTIMONY

Until 1993, federal courts had used the 'general acceptance' test, set forth in Frye v. United States, to assess the admissibility of expert scientific testimony (Frye v. United States 1923). In 1993, the United States Supreme Court modified the standard for determining the admissibility of expert scientific testimony in federal trials. In Daubert, the court stated that the Frye test did not comport with the Federal Rules of Evidence and that 'a rigid "general acceptance" requirement would be at odds with the "liberal thrust" of the Federal Rules and their "general approach to relaxing the traditional barriers to opinion testimony"' Accordingly, the court emphasized that a trial judge must screen the proposed scientific testimony to ensure that the testimony is relevant and reliable before allowing the testimony to be presented at trial. Rule 702 reflects the need for screening and provides:

> If scientific, technical, or other specialized knowledge will assist the trier of fact to understand the evidence or to determine a fact in issue, a witness qualified as an expert by knowledge, skill, experience, training, or education, may testify thereto in the form of an opinion or otherwise (Daubert v. Merrell Dow Pharmaceuticals, Inc. 1993).

The court set forth four factors that may be used to assist the trial judge in determining 'whether the expert is proposing to testify to scientific knowledge that will assist the trier of fact to understand or determine a fact in issue'. The factors that may be considered when determining the validity of a scientific theory or technique are: (1) whether the theory or technique can be tested; (2) whether the theory has been subject to peer review and publication; (3) the rate of error; and (4) the acceptance of the theory of technique within the community. The court cautioned that '[t]he focus ... must be solely on principles and methodology, not on the conclusions that they generate'. The court emphasized that these factors are not exclusive.

Thus, under Daubert, a defendant doctor may be considered negligent for treatment and diagnosis, even though he presents evidence from a number of medical experts genuinely of the opinion that the defendant's care followed customary medical practice. The court must determine for itself the appropriateness and the logic of the professional opinion and find reassurance that the body of opinion relied upon was not created for defensive purposes (see below).

While, in theory, any physician may act as an expert in court, increasingly in obstetrical cases, the role of expert is most often played by practitioners currently active in the field. Academics are less active as experts. Some universities impose restrictions on testifying within the state or for the plaintiff. In some states, experts can only be derived from immediately adjacent states. Other states require that the expert reside in any state but must obtain consultation from a physician within the state. In addition, federal rules give a judge the authority to (1) limit cumulative evidence, i.e. more than one expert testifying to the same issues unrelated to qualifications, or (2) retain experts to assist the court, or (3) with mutual consent appoint a single expert witness. Despite these available options, especially in 'bad baby cases', there is an increasing tendency to line up a broad array of qualified experts on both sides including an obstetrician, perinatologist, placental pathologist, neonatologist, neurologist, nurse, economist, neuroradiologist, etc. There is at least some evidence that this proliferation of experts (and costs), more likely driven by the defense, is counterproductive. Bors-Koffelt *et al.* (1998) found that the use of multiple defense expert witnesses decreased the chances of a successful defense.

Many jurisdictions have attempted to insinuate the expert witness into the proceedings prior to the case being filed. In several states, a report or affidavit of merit from the expert is required to launch the suit, in others only the testimony by the lawyer that he has contacted an expert is required. By and large, there is no standard format for expert reports, and they are normally quite minimal and non-specific. There is also no requirement that the 'expert' who signed the letter of merit will subsequently be involved in the case, a circumstance that we deplore. Even if he/she were later involved, there would be no mechanisms short of deposition or interrogatory to amplify on the experts' allegations. In some states, the expert cannot be deposed before trial, and indeed, his identity is unknown to the opposing side until he is called to the stand – widely referred to as 'trial by ambush'.

While the expert's opinion is normally protected by the doctrine of witness immunity, this does not protect the witness from fraud or professional malpractice liability (LLMD of Michigan, Inc. v. Jackson-Cross, Co. 1999) or from other forms of harassment. 'The goal to insuring that the path to truth is unobstructed and the judicial process is protected, by fostering an atmosphere where the expert witness will be forthright and candid in stating his or her opinion, is not advanced by immunizing the expert witness from . . . negligence in forming the opinion.' (idem.) In one instance an expert was sued for failing to testify on behalf of the plaintiff when he believed that causation could not be proven satisfactorily. In an effort to increase the accountability of the expert, numerous initiatives to make expert testimony accountable in a medical forum have been floated – none have taken hold. At least in Federal Court, the expert's legal activities over the last 5 years must be listed with the court prior to his appearance. The process of accountability sometimes gets out of hand when pre-trial challenges to the expert witness (that he or she is a purveyor of 'junk science') creates the spector of a trial within a trial and adds greatly to the expense of litigation.

## MEDICAL RECORDS

Unfortunately, the expert's early opinions that serve to launch malpractice proceedings are most often based on medical records that are frequently silent on the intentions of the provider or their exercise of 'medical judgement'. As a result, medical records, which represent both a medical document and a legal document, often promote and perpetuate cases and confound their defense. A cost analysis of 3205 multi-specialty claims showed an average cost per claim of $22 584 (Richards & Thomasson 1992). Deficits in the medical record, e.g. inadequate instructions, delayed entries, inadequate notes, and consent-form issues, more than double the average cost. System failures nearly tripled the average cost. Thus, while an erroneous decision may be defensible if the reasons leading to it are recorded in the chart (Richards), the changed record and the contradictory record are almost impossible to defend.

COMMENT: Until medical records objectively communicate the findings, the attention paid, the comprehension that was achieved, and offer a reasonable plan followed by appropriate and consistent action, their appearance in court will continue to be an uphill battle for the physician and he/she will get little credit for the thought process or use to his/her advantage the testimony of 'a witness whose memory never dies'. As an aside, the reader is invited to compare the two enclosed notes regarding a midforceps procedure (Tables 30.1a,b). In the first example, the note invites lawsuit if there is an adverse outcome. The note provides no indication for, or detail about, the procedure. It is more a personal memorandum than a responsible medical description relevant for decisions about care in future pregnancies, for example. The second note, however, would seem to protect against lawsuit in several ways. The note (1) clearly bespeaks thoughtfulness, (2) bespeaks understanding of the medical issues and alternatives, and (3) underscores the physician's efforts to provide a forthright explanation to the patient and her husband – all powerful disincentives to lawsuit.

## MEDICAL CLIMATE

Today in medicine there is considerable enthusiasm for 'evidence-based medicine;' epidemiologically-driven decisions; and structured reimbursement. These initiatives to narrow the variation in medical care seem driven as much by motives of cost control as by the hope for better health

**Table 30.1a Operative delivery note**

| Operative delivery note | Translation |
|---|---|
| MF, OP >> OA, Mid epis, no lac | Midforceps, Occiput anterior to Occiput anterior |
| Apgar 8,9 P and M intact | Midline episiotomy, no lacerations |
| EBL 400, M and B left DR in good cond. | Apgar scores 8, 9 at 1, 5 min |
| | Placenta and membranes expressed intact |
| | Estimated blood loss 400 ml |
| | Mother and infant left the delivery room in good condition |

**Table 30.1b Operative delivery note**

| | Operative delivery note: |
|---|---|
| Procedures | Trial of forceps, midforceps rotation, episiotomy repaired |
| Findings | Gyneocoid pelvis, normal active phase, +3 station, minimal molding, direct OP, epidural anesthesia, second stage = 2.5 h, pushing inadequate, patient tired. EFW = 3000; Prev. baby = 2800 |
| Indications | Persistent occiput posterior, prolonged second stage, secondary arrest of descent, tired patient. Discussed options with patient and husband who agree and understand that if any difficulty is encountered, the forceps will be abandoned and Cesarean section undertaken. Operating room alerted |
| Methods | Kielland forceps – direct application to OP without difficulty. Gentle rotation ROT >> OA. Kiellands removed, Simpson forceps applied. Gentle traction = Delivered over midline episiotomy |
| Fetal outcome | 3200-g male infant APGAR 8; infant examined by pediatrician, sent to regular nursery |
| Resuscitation | Oxygen only, no evidence of trauma to infant |
| Mother outcome | Perineum intact, episiotomy repaired, no lacerations. Placenta and membranes intact. Estimated blood loss: 300 ml. Mother left delivery room in good condition |

care services. It seems important to emphasize that the true objective of medical care is to raise the mean (improve outcome); the impact on the variance is secondary.

## CLINICAL PRACTICE GUIDELINES

A clinical practice guideline is any guide to the clinical management of a patient. The specificity of these will vary, as will the purpose for which they are written and who has been selected to write them. They may be driven by medico-legal issues, by the cost of care, or by the quality of care. While great emphasis has now been placed on the process of writing guidelines, may providers have become concerned with the basic precepts of guidelines, including the possible emergence of 'cookbook' medicine, the effect of patient variability, and the need to keep guidelines flexible, current, and credible (Meeter 1992). The notion that compliance with guidelines renders the clinician immune from lawsuit has not been upheld. Consensus, after all, is not necessarily wisdom.

One of the most widely quoted and misunderstood guidelines requires that institutions be capable of instituting an emergency Cesarean section within 30 min of decision (American College of Obstetricians and Gynecologists 1990). Some institutions cannot meet these guidelines reliably, while others maintain a standard that can result in an emergency Cesarean section in 10 min or less. While there have been several studies of the reasonableness of 'the 30 minute rule', neither the studies nor the 'guidelines' take into account certain realities or certain remedies.

COMMENT: The '30 minute rule' is shorthand designation for a more encompassing principle that under certain conditions, performance of a Cesarean section shall be carried out as quickly as possible consistent with concern for the health and well-being of the mother and fetus, preferably within 30 min. What is the standard if there is already one Cesarean section in progress, or two? If a physician is late in realizing the need for Cesarean section or is ready to operate within 20 min but fritters away 10 min beforehand, his conduct cannot possibly comport with a reasonable standard of care, even if the patient is delivered within 30 min. Further, it stands to reason that institutions normally unable to consistently meet the 30-min rule must modify their practices and exhibit a willingness to prepare for Cesarean sections early (even if it proves unnecessary) in anticipation of problems and make special arrangements for unique situations such as VBAC.

There is frequent debate over whether 'official' pronouncements such as the '30-minute rule' are to be construed as 'standards of care'. It seems to us that irrespective of whether these writings are entitled practice parameters, guidelines, standards, apocrypha, hints, clues, etc., the imprimatur of an official body, gives any statement about care the force of a standard. Guidelines, whatever their provenance, become 'medico-legally binding' *only* in the instance when there is no thoughtful (and annotated) alternative.

## MALPRACTICE MYTHOLOGY – THE FAILURE OF MEDICO-LEGAL EDUCATION

An enduring feature of malpractice is the mythological proportions to the ignorance of malpractice doctrine in the medical community, especially in obstetrics. Not only is there widespread fear of being sued, there is a great misperception of the requirements for proof of malpractice, the outcomes of lawsuits, the reasons patients sue, and little appetite to deal with the real litogen (a factor promoting lawsuit) – physician behavior.

Some current mythology: 'Malpractice relates to the incompetence of a few bad physicians'. 'Anyone can sue, everyone wins'. 'The system is unfair and favors the plaintiff'. 'Patients who sue are greedy ingrates'. 'Judges and juries cannot understand medicine'. 'Losing a lawsuit raises premiums and besmirches my name in the community'. 'The plaintiff's attorney and expert are the enemy, along with the judge, jury, insurance company, etc'. 'Malpractice doesn't make care better'. There is abundant refutation of these myths.

A poll of ACOG members showed that about 66% of the fellows had been sued once. This can hardly be related to 'a few bad physicians'. With the allegation of medical negligence, the law gives health-care providers considerable advantage. They are advantaged by the presumption of non-negligence. They do not have to be right in their care, just reasonable. The law denies the jury the right to decide medical issues and even requires 'expert witnesses' from the profession itself. There is almost universal belief that the injured child's appearance in the courtroom elicits the greatest sympathy from the jury. Physicians win ~80% of lawsuits that go to court. It is naïve to believe that these were the cases in which the plaintiff attorney forgot to bring the affected child into the courtroom. More reasonably, it is the thoughtful, compassionate physician who maintains his sympathy and compassion that most easily obtains the jury's favor and a favorable verdict.

The defendant is often unaware of the statistics that about 40% of cases are dropped, about 50% settle, sometimes as befitting the merits of the case and sometimes as a calculated strategy that limits exposure of assets. The physician who is terrified by an *ad-damnum* clause (demand for damages) that greatly exceeds his reasonable policy is rarely in our experience reassured by his own attorney that the risk of such an eventuality is essentially nil. Despite counseling, the frightened obstetrician does 'not want to be the first one'. To some extent, the defense attorney may be excused for failing to understand how impoverished is the medico-legal education of the physician. Medical and legal organizations have long recognized the importance of legal medicine and have repeatedly recommended its study by physicians in training – with minimal success. In 1952, the AMA advised that 'No medical student should be permitted to receive his medical degree without instruction in legal duties'. Four decades later, less than 50% of medical schools had medico-legal courses, considering the subject too unimportant to teach. Kollas (1997) studied the medico-legal knowledge base of senior residents in internal medicine. Only 28% felt they had been adequately trained in the subject. Only 26% could list the requirement for people of (1) duty, (2) deviation from the standard of care, (3) damages, and (4) direct causation.

It is our belief that the most devastating myth or fiction is that allegation of malpractice represents the allegation of incompetence, or misanthropy, or malice when it really represents the allegation of fallibility. Imagine the response of the physician who believes that he or she is being accused of malice – the intention to do harm. This allegation of malice is precluded by the precepts of tort law. Nevertheless, it is this fiction that fuels the lawsuits, the media scandal, the demonization of error, of lawyers and experts and infects our educational system and our care of patients.

## WHY DO PATIENTS SUE?

Many physicians find it easier to believe that patients who sue are greedy and ungrateful. In reality, patients want a forthright explanation of what happened and want to understand if they played a role in it. They are real people, and whether the injury was the result of negligence or not, they, and not the physicians burdened with a lawsuit, are the real victims. When asked, 'What was wrong with the care you or your child received?' or 'What complaints do you have about physicians?', patients respond rather specifically (Table 30.5) (JAMA 1992). As underscored by these data, the attorney is often the last person who is contacted, not the first. Most often, patients are directed to an attorney by a member of the medical community.

## PATIENT CONSENT

In dealing with matters of informed consent, courts in the United States use the test of the prudent patient. The courts have on several occasions been asked to intervene in circumstances involving the refusal of treatment by a pregnant woman, a refusal that nominally threatens the life and well-being of her fetus and herself. While the courts' responses have been varied, there is general consensus amongst the specialities that these ethical (not legal) issues should *not* be resolved in court and that considerable ethical weight be given to the mother's decision as long as the consent has been proper and there has been no coercion. Lawsuits based entirely on informed consent are quite uncommon, but most seem to involve vaginal birth after cesarian (VBAC).

**Table 30.2 Why patients sue**

| | |
|---|---|
| Cited deficiencies of care | |
| Recognizing fetal distress | 53% |
| Managing fetal distress | 57% |
| Timely Cesarean section | 35% |
| Physician unavailable | 29% |
| Birth injury (forceps) | 28% |
| Consultation or transfer | 10% |
| What prompted lawsuit? | |
| Person outside family | 33% |
| Medical personnel | 23/41 (56%) |
| Lawyer | 8/41 (20%) |
| Money for long-term care | 24% |
| Physician deception | 24% |
| Child would have no future | 20% |
| Find out what happened | 20% |
| Deter malpractice/revenge | 19% |
| Complaints about physicians | |
| Not informed about injury potential | 70% |
| Misled patient | 48% |
| Would not talk or answer questions | 32% |
| Would not listen | 13% |

*Source*: *JAMA* (1992).

In one VBAC case (Schreiber), a patient with a history of two previous Cesarean sections, the first undertaken for arrest of labor after 17 h (the second was elective), had agreed prior to labor to attempt VBAC (Schreiber v. Physicians Insurance Company of Wisconsin 1996). During labor, in the face of slow progress and severe abdominal pain, she changed her mind and repeatedly requested a Cesarean section. Just as often, the obstetrician maintained that it was unnecessary. The obstetrician commented that if he performed Cesarean section on every woman who wanted one, all deliveries would be by Cesarean section. Intimidated, the patient no longer requested Cesarean section. Ultimately, the uterus ruptured, and the child was hopelessly injured despite delivery within 30 min. The physician defended his conduct on the ground that the original informed consent should prevail throughout the labor and that the standard of care had been met by the 'timely' delivery. He noted that the patient had reaffirmed upon admission her earlier willingness to undergo a trial of labor and the fact that they continued to manage labor 'without objection'. The court rejected the defense position that the patient's resignation implied acceptance of a continued trial of labor. The court did not comment on the change in the medical situation (dysfunctional labor, unexplained abdominal pain) that required medical reconsideration of the case and updating of the informed consent. The court did maintain that the legal situation had changed. Where two or more medically acceptable options for treatment are present, the 'competent patient has the absolute right to select from among those treatment options after being informed of the relative risks and benefits of each approach'. But consent, once given, is not categorically immutable, and the patient was entitled to withdraw her consent to VBAC. That indisputable withdrawal placed the patient and her physician in their original position – a blank slate on which the parties must again diagram their plan, which, in this case, would have resulted in Cesarean section.

COMMENT: If the 'informed consent' document in such cases is to truly represent 'informed consent,' it must reveal the patient's understanding that she may either undergo an elective repeat Cesarean section or, if she is a suitable candidate, attempt a VBAC. She must understand that not all patients are candidates for VBAC and that not all VBAC attempts will result in successful vaginal delivery. She must be aware that some of the determinable clinical factors that affect the success of VBAC become apparent only in labor. The patient must also understand that all pregnancies carry a small risk to both mother and fetus, whether or not the

**Table 30.3 Experience with 169 closed obstetrical cases**

| | Number | Percentage of total |
|---|---|---|
| Total cases | 5,197 | 100% |
| Obstetrical cases | 169 | 3% |
| Obstetrical expenses | $10,506,768 | 10% |
| Obstetrical indemnity | $60,082,728 | 18% |

| Disposition | Number | Average indemnity | Average costs | Average totals | Total indemnity | Total charges | Total dollars |
|---|---|---|---|---|---|---|---|
| Indemnity – settled | 124 | $484,272 | $53,343 | $537,615 | $60,049,728 | $ 6,614,532 | $66,664,260 |
| Indemnity – lost in court | 1 | $ 33,000 | $20,000 | $ 53,000 | $ 33,000 | $ 20,000 | $ 53,000 |
| Won in court | 43 | $ | $90,052 | $ 90,052 | $ – | $ 3,872,236 | $ 3,872,236 |
| | 169 | $517,272 | $62,170 | $680,667 | $60,082,728 | $10,506,768 | $70,589,496 |

From Bors-Koefoed

mother has had a previous Cesarean section. In patients with a previous Cesarean section, the risk of uterine rupture during a VBAC is approximately 1%, and this occasionally may result in serious, potentially life-threatening complications for the mother or the baby. If the patient initially agrees to attempt VBAC, she needs to understand that she is entitled to an updating of the likelihood of success and to change her mind at any reasonable time and to obtain a Cesarean section, even during labor. Finally, the patient should understand that no decision, however thoughtfully made or reasonably pursued, guarantees a normal outcome for the mother or the infant.

## COMPLICATION OR ERROR?

The 'recognized risk defense', asserts that the undesirable outcome or injury in question is nothing more than an unavoidable complication – an understandable and acceptable risk of a properly considered and provided treatment. Accordingly, so long as the patient is reasonably apprised of the more serious and commonplace risks and participates in the decision, then in theory, there can be no issue of negligence. A typical example is subgaleal or intracranial hemorrhage in the newborn following vacuum extraction assisted delivery. Indeed, every obstetrical text devotes significant space to such complications but only rarely do they include a full discussion about preventability or even the distinction between complication and negligence. Is intracranial/subgaleal hemorrhage following vacuum extraction an unavoidable risk or simply the result of negligence, and how would that be determined? (see below)

## TORT REFORM AND FINANCES – LITIGATION AND RISK MANAGEMENT

There is universal agreement that the medical needs of those with adverse outcome need more attention, whether it is related to negligence or not. There is also universal agreement that the present medico-legal system is neither efficient nor error-free in reaching settlement or that the distribution is equitable. In the United States, only about 28 cents of every premium dollar goes to injured patients after an average delay of 4.9 years to dispose of a case.

The surviving, handicapped infant continues to represent the highest payout/case. There are numerous representative reviews of closed cases. An analysis of 353 closed claims involving obstetrician–gynecologists revealed that the 40 highest-paid claims (11.3%) accounted for 88.7% of the total dollars spent. The majority of these, 23 (57.5%), were obstetrical, including the five highest claims and 17 of the first 20 highest-paid awards. Obstetrical negligence represented over $5 million (76.5%) of the total expense. Of the 40 cases, 23 (60%) were resolved with a compromise settlement, nine claims (22.5%) resolved with indemnity payment on the basis of verdict or pre-trial compromise; seven (17.5%) had no indemnity payment because of a jury verdict or voluntary dismissal. These seven were in the highest-paid claims group only because of expenses (Rosenblatt 1989).

Of the 40, 28 (70%) were judged to be meritorious, and 12 (30%) were judged to be non-meritorious. Seven of the latter 12 settled without indemnity costs, including four that went to trial with a defense verdict and three that were dismissed, leaving five others in this group with proper treatment and indemnity costs. Expenses to defend all 12 cases of proper treatment totaled over $500 000. Irrespective of the absence of strict negligence, each of these 'non-meritorious claims' illustrated substantial deficits with the medical record or system failures – inviting the allegation of negligence and lawsuit. These analyses clearly reveal that bad outcomes may not be the fault of the physician, but that physician behaviour in the conduct of the case and the conduct of the record contribute heavily to successful allegations of malpractice.

Is no fault insurance better? To determine whether Florida's implementation of a no-fault system for birth-related neurological injuries reduced lawsuits and total spending associated with such injuries, and whether no fault was more efficient than customary tort procedures in distributing compensation, Sloan *et al.* (1998) compared claims and payments before and after implementation of a no-fault system in 1989. They found that the number of tort claims for permanent labor-delivery injury and death indeed fell by about 16–32%. However, when no-fault claims were added to tort claims, the total claims frequency rose by 11–38%. Further, of the estimated 479 children who suffered birth-related injuries annually, only 13 were compensated under no fault. Total combined payments to patients and all lawyers did not decrease, but under no fault, a much larger portion of the total went to patients. Thus, less than 3% of total payments went to lawyers under no fault versus 39% under tort – a new equilibrium. Some claimants with birth-related injuries were winners, taking home a larger percentage of their awards than their tort counterparts. Lawyers clearly lost under no fault, but so did many children with birth-related neurologic injuries who did not qualify for coverage because of the narrow statutory definition.

In a survey reported by the ACOG, physicians reported wholesale changes in their practices (Table 30.4) and their

**Table 30.4 Malpractice-induced activities**

| Modality | Percentage |
|---|---|
| Testing | 76.2 |
| Monitoring | 73.3 |
| Documenting | 72.2 |
| Informed consent | 61.6 |
| Consulting MDs | 58.0 |
| Patient information | 51.2 |
| Referrals | 47.2 |
| Staff presence | 21.8 |

*Source*: ACOG (1990).

fees as a result of malpractice. The specter of malpractice has galvanized the medical profession in this area to also modify its vocabulary and its accountability. A series of 'scientific initiatives' have appeared, not for the purpose of answering clinical questions or directing therapy, but for the purpose of counteracting plaintiff testimony in court. The ACOG has recommended the elimination of such universally applied terms of art as 'fetal distress', 'perinatal asphyxia', 'stat Cesarean section' and have modified the definitions of 'low forceps' and 'mid forceps' (ACOG 1994, 1998). Various articles have created definitive, unyielding requirements for the diagnosis of birth related injury and suggest that labor-related injury is rare and perhaps irreducible (ACOG 1992; MacLennan 1999; Towner 1999). Irrespective of motivation, these publications have not been accompanied by any decrease in lawsuits, any improvement in outcome, or any less defensive posture on the part of the obstetrical community. These efforts to make our specialty 'fair of speech' and litigation-proof, discount important mechanisms of injury, diminish notions of medical judgement, inhibit scientific inquiry into the timing and mechanism of fetal injury, and delay the testing of new paradigms for dealing with adverse outcome.

A number of factors increase the risk of birth injury (Table 30.5). From a California database of 583 340 live-born singleton infants born to nulliparous women between 1992 and 1994 and weighing between 2500 and 4000 g, Towner *et al.* evaluated the relation between the mode of delivery and various measures of immediate morbidity including intracranial hemorrhage (Towner 1999). In general, the highest rate of complications was found after a failed attempt at operative vaginal delivery (whether ultimately delivered vaginally or by Cesarean section), an intermediate risk was found after uncomplicated operative vaginal delivery after onset of labor (vacuum, forceps or Cesarean section), and the lowest risk in non-operative vaginal delivery or Cesarean section prior to labor. Reasonably, the authors concluded that a substantial portion of the morbidity previously thought to be a function of operative vaginal delivery may actually represent an effect of labor itself. They offer, further, that the injuries associated with vacuum and forceps represent the 'irreducible component of morbidity among infants of normal birth weight because the rate of intracranial injuries was not significantly lower in infants born by Cesarean section during labor than in those delivered by vacuum extraction or with the use of forceps'. This unfortunate conclusion is useful legally by defense attorneys who will surely underscore the word 'irreducible'.

The analysis suffers from both a lack of understanding of fetal risks and obstetrical decisions. It is well known that the risk of adverse outcome with vaginal delivery increases as a function of fetal weight above 4000 g. Neonatal weight cannot be determined reasonably before delivery. There are clearly infants within this range, for example, whose estimated weights were deemed to be higher who received elective Cesarean section. The data also fail to provide information on the indications and the techniques used for attempted operative vaginal delivery, or indeed whether the patients ever reached full dilatation or not. With regard to the second stage, we have no data on the duration, the amount of contractions, the amount of pushing, the position and station of the fetal head, the use of fundal pressure, the use of oxytocin, or epidural and the course of labor up to complete dilatation. It is well known that the risk of injury increases with a higher station of the fetal head and that vacuum more commonly fails in the OP position than with other positions. The data offer no long-term consequences of the obvious injuries.

Underreporting is likely, especially in the number of failed vacuums/forceps as well as the number of infants with intracranial hemorrhage as only those with immediate symptoms are included. Subgaleal hemorrhage (p. 364) – one of the major concerns of the FDA advisory is not included as a measure of outcome. The most serious deficiency of the study, however, is the lack of data on the mechanism and timing of fetal neurological injury other than the fact that some injury precedes delivery.

Several widely distributed 'Guidelines' require certain clinical findings in order to begin to propose any relationship between intrapartum events and subsequent neurological handicap (ACOG 1992; MacLennan 1999) and have doubtless had an impact on the frequency and defense of malpractice cases.

Both manifestos require a unique definition of 'asphyxia' – it must be progressive and be operational at the moment of delivery, a 'terminal asphyxial model' of injury. They permit no event (not even a sentinal one) to occur early in labor that injures the fetus but from which the fetus recovers metabolically prior to delivery. In addition, in this model, the fetus diverts blood flow away from less vital organs (skin, skeleton, lungs, kidneys and viscera) in an effort to protect the placenta, brain, heart, and adrenals. As a result, if the brain is injured, the other organs must be severely compromised first. In this model, injury from cerebral ischemia represents the final, failing output of the compromised fetal heart.

For this model to be operative, however, blood flow to the brain and the placenta must be maintained without interfer-

**Table 30.5 Factors predisposing to birth injury**

| | |
|---|---|
| Dystocia | Precipitate or prolonged labor, macrosomia/CPD |
| Fetal distress | Hypoxia, trauma |
| Infection/hemorrhage | Amnionitis, placenta previa/abruptio |
| Preterm labor/delivery | Infection/trauma/hypoxia |
| Obstetric procedures | Version/extraction, forceps, vacuum, amniocentesis/PUBS/CVS |
| Malpresentation | Face/brow/breech/OP |
| Fetal anomalies | Hydrops/hydrocephalus *et al.* |
| Multiple gestation | Esp monozygous twins |

ence. However, head and umbilical cord compression, with their frequent restriction of regional blood flow during labor, diminish the relevance of this model. In addition, severe metabolic acidosis has no specificity for brain injury; indeed, most severely asphyxiated infants are not injured. The requirement that numerous systems be involved including the brain seems to relate better to systemic hypoxia than to injury. Finally, the Template requires profound depression of the Apgar score and neonatal behavior, irrespective of whether the area of the injured brain is involved with respiration or behavior.

Furthermore, if this model were correct, (1) there would be a strong correlation between low pH (acidosis) and outcome, (2) EFM, and pH would predict all injured fetuses, (3) preventing acidosis would prevent injury, and (4) most injury would be preventable. Clinical and experimental data fail to support these notions (Shields & Schifrin 1988; Vannucci 1993; Phelan & Ahn 1994; Ikeda *et al.* 1998).

There can be little doubt that the prime motivation of these articles is an attempt to influence the undertaking and outcome of litigation. There is no consideration given to brain injuries seen in infants born prior to 34–36 weeks of gestation. The template contains no analysis of legal cases of their own or meta-analysis of those published by others. They attempt to influence the defense in these cases in two ways: They declare that 'it is not possible to ascertain retrospectively whether earlier obstetric intervention could have prevented cerebral damage in any individual case where no detectable sentinel hypoxic event occurred'. However, the more practical inference for the defense is simply: DO NOT OBTAIN A BLOOD GAS IN THE IMMEDIATE NEONATAL PERIOD. Because of the importance of timely blood gases to the diagnosis of intrapartum injury, failing to obtain early blood gases in a severely compromised newborn (apparent negligence) would eliminate possible litigation. Finally, the authors of the Template spend some time defining the qualifications of the expert witness suitable to testify about these matters. We believe that it is for the court, not the medical establishment, to decide the suitability of any witness.

It is well to compare these pronouncements with a widely respected authority of neonatal brain injury.

> Brain injury in the intrapartum [period] does occur, [it] effects a large absolute number of infants worldwide ... and represents a large source of potentially preventable neurological morbidity. Among the many adverse consequences of the explosion in obstetrical litigation has been a tendency in the medical profession to deny the importance or even existence of intrapartum brain injury (Volpe 1995).

Although the Template and TB#163 discount the value of both electronic fetal monitoring (by inference) and neuroimaging (specifically) in defining the timing of injury, most 'bad baby' litigation alleging an intrapartum injury revolves around the interpretation of the fetal monitoring tracing and neuroimaging. In part because of the pivotal role they play in malpractice cases, there have been attacks on fetal monitoring that have come both from within the profession and from without. In an article in the Stanford University Law Review, Margaret Lent (1999), a young defense lawyer, argues that the widespread use of EFM is both medically and legally unsound. Ms Lent points to selected clinical trials to demonstrate that EFM does not reduce fetal mortality, morbidity, or cerebral palsy rates (see Chapter 25). She argues that because EFM has a very high false positive rate and its usage correlates strongly with a rise in Cesarean section rates, it offers no medical advantage over auscultation. Similarly, she argues, EFM provides no protection in the courtroom. Though obstetricians believe that they should use EFM because its status as the standard of care will protect them from liability, Ms Lent argues that given its failings, it may in fact expose them to liability. She further argues that auscultation, at least as safe and effective as EFM, is also more likely to protect physicians from liability. Ms Lent concludes that obstetricians have an obligation to their patients and to themselves to adopt auscultation as the new standard of care. She finds 'no excuses left to defend the continued use of EFM'.

An obvious problem with electronic fetal heart rate monitoring, of course, is the lack of a consistent nomenclature. Numerous articles attest to the wide range of inter- and intra-observer variation in the interpretation of fetal heart rate patterns, even among experts. Even the so-called randomized controlled trials failed to provide any consistent, unambiguous definitions of the FHR patterns upon which the evaluations and management were based. To correct this problem of nomenclature, the NIH Research Planning Workshop proposed a 'standardized and rigorously unambiguously described set of definitions which can be quantified, etc'. (JOGNN 1997). In actuality, the Committee simply defined a series of isolated cardiotachometric phenomena without any effort to provide a physiologic or circumstantial context for the evaluation of heart rate patterns. It offers little benefit to the clinician or the lawyer who reasonably might argue that after 25 years of use, tens of millions of tracings, tens of thousands of articles and experiments, it is too late to make 'no assumptions [about] patterns or their relationship to hypoxemia or metabolic acidemia'.

Both Ms Lent and the NIH select panel fail to deal with certain fundamental pitfalls of fetal monitoring beyond the nomenclature. Both accept that the original rationale for the introduction of fetal heart rate monitoring was that it could 'serve as a screening test for asphyxia which is severe enough to cause neurological damage'. By this notion, fetal heart rate patterns would alert clinicians to potential problems, enabling them to intervene more quickly ('rescue') and to prevent more fetal deaths and irreversible brain injuries than could be prevented with auscultation (American College of Obstetricians and Gynecologists). This notion has failed because of a failure to understand the mechanism and rapidity with which injury may occur and the appropriate role of fetal monitoring.

Fetal monitoring works in great measure by limiting potentially harmful techniques to the demonstrably normal fetus. As widely acknowledged, monitoring is unerring in defining the normally responsive fetus. Monitoring surely deserves credit for reducing intrapartum death, one of the original rationales for its development. However, by contributing to a lowered death rate, especially in the premature, it may, in fact, be contributing to the increasing severity and incidence of cerebral palsy (Visser & Narayan 1996). Fetal monitoring, however, may also be increasing the risk of adverse outcome in another way when the normal tracing is allowed to override normal obstetrical judgment. For example, may the second stage of labor be extended indefinitely with relentless expulsive efforts from the mother, but without progress, as long as the tracing is normal? It is our belief that the role of the tracing is to keep the fetus out of harm's way, not, as the original precept dictated, to effect rescue.

Nevertheless, FHR patterns afford significant insight into the timing of fetal injury. The association of abnormal patterns and CP has been repeatedly demonstrated (Vannucci 1993; Pheran & Ahn 1994; Schifrin *et al.* 1994; Nelson *et al.* 1996; Ikeda *et al.* 1998; Spencer 1997). As shown by Ikeda, the prediction of neurological injury following an ischemic event is related, not to the lowest pH, but to the duration of the hypoxia and the fetal heart-rate pattern after recovery from the ischemic event (Ikeda *et al.* 1998). Schifrin *et al.* have defined rigorous criteria for the purpose of identifying the ischemic/asphyxial event, and in certain circumstances, fetal neurological injury (Table 30.6). Others have reported rather specific CTG patterns associated with fetal seizures (Westgate 1999). These data support the notions that a fetus may be injured during labor without being globally asphyxiated, that a fetus may be globally asphyxiated during labor without suffering injury, and that injury may develop so rapidly that it may be impossible to prevent, irrespective of the speed of intervention. These studies also support the notion that injury that does occur during labor often develops without the 'required' constellation of signs and symptoms of total systemic collapse required by ACOG TB#163 or the Template.

When applied to a large series of malpractice cases near term, the analysis indeed confirms that the majority of CP cases coming to suit suffer injury before labor (Shields *et al.*) The majority of those injured prior to labor were often injured in the week preceding entrance into labor, frequently in association with oligohydramnios, postdate pregnancy and the mother's complaint of decreased fetal movement. They do not profit from Cesarean section. Most fetal injury during the 1st stage of labor results from catastrophic events, uterine rupture, abruptio, ruptured vasa previa, etc. (the sentinel events of the Template) and is often not preventable. Most 2nd-stage injury is probably preventable. It most often results from exuberant pushing especially in the OP position but sometimes in relationship to extraordinary efforts at operative delivery (Ennis 1990; Towner 1999).

These newer studies further suggest no compelling association between acidosis and injury or necessary multi-system organ failure. Indeed, most acidotic and injury fetuses were injured antepartum. Regional ischemia, as might develop from cord compression or head compression (in the second stage), not systemic asphyxia, is the most common mechanism of fetal injury. The timing of injury cannot be deduced from the duration or the severity of the IUGR (Schifrin *et al.*), nor can the severity of the injury cannot be deduced from the severity of the FHR pattern. The absence of the CTG makes the problem of the timing and mechanism of injury quite difficult and entirely dependent upon 'clinical circumstances' without a reliable definition of the condition of the individual fetus at the time in question. This is illustrated in the Registry data from Australia by Blair & Stanley (1988) not necessarily related to malpractice (Table 30.7). In this widely quoted study the majority of injury cannot be timed. The definition of intrapartum hypoxia rested with the determination of low Apgar scores, time to sustained respiration and the presence of neonatal encephalopathy in the neonate. CTG tracings were not used.

**Table 30.6 Electronic fetal monitoring and the timing of injury (all must apply)**

A. Demonstrably normal fetus
   - Reactive NST
   - Normal tracing intrapartum

B. Identifiable event or episode
   - Deceleration(s) (occasionally absent)
   - Sudden change in baseline, variability
   - Loss of fetal movement (antepartum)

C. Recovery to persistently
   - Higher baseline (usually)
   - Absent variability (occasionally bizarre pattern)
   - Variable decelerations with overshoot

## THE VACUUM EXTRACTOR (VX) STUDY

In a retrospective review, we compared over 200 adverse fetal/neonatal outcomes (neurological injury or death) associated with vacuum extractions (VX) derived from malpractice cases to a random group of 50 VX with normal outcomes. The use of oxytocin and epidural were common in both, as were the indications for intervention (fetal distress, maternal exhaustion). Study-group patients had larger fetuses, longer labors including 2nd stage, and a higher incidence of occiput posterior position (OP) than control patients. In 60% of the study group, forceps or Cesarean section was required to effect delivery compared to less than 5% of the control group. Shoulder dystocia occurred in about 15% of the study group and 5% of the control group. The risk of low Apgar scores, neonatal trauma, fetal acidosis,

**Table 30.7 Relationship of birth asphyxia/trauma to CP**

| Status at birth | Not possible | Possible | Probable | Definite | Number |
|---|---|---|---|---|---|
| FD–, Neuro– | 124 | 0 | 0 | 0 | 124 |
| FD–, Neuro+ | 22 | 3 | 5 | 0 | 30 |
| FD+, Neuro+ | 10 | 3 | 7 | 9 | 29 |
| Total | 156 | 6 | 12 | 9 | 183 |
| Percentage | 85.2 | 6.6 | 3.3 | 4.9 | 100 |
| Definition of 'asphyxia' | | | | | |
| Group | Apgar 1 <7 or TSR >2 | | | | |
| Infants with CP (%) | 33.5 | | | | |
| Controls (%) | 18.0 | | | | |

*Key*: FD– = absent 'fetal distress'; FD+ = 'Fetal distress' present; Neuro– = absent neonatal encephalopathy; Neuro+ = neonatal encephalopathy. NB – Fetal distress as determined by auscultation/EFM. (From Blair & Stanley, 1988).

cephalhematoma, subgaleal hemorrhage, and admission to the NICU were all markedly increased in the study group.

Analysis of the FHR patterns according to the above algorithms revealed that about 6% were injured prior to the onset of labor, and about 60% of the study group were injured in labor *prior to* the application of the vacuum. About 25% were injured during delivery (vacuum or forceps), usually in association with prolonged attempts or misapplication of the device. About 10% of the cases of subgaleal hemorrhage (all from the study group). Most appeared to have at least some neurological damage at the time the vacuum was applied. In about 40% of the study group, including three with uterine rupture, 'terminal bradycardia' prompted vacuum extraction. This indication was present in 10% of the control group. In the majority of these patients in both groups, the FHR changes were deemed inappropriate indicators of distress and likely recoverable with conservative measures.

These data suggest that injury (and lawsuit) associated with vacuum extraction often developed in association with a constellation of obstetrical abnormalities (OP, high station, etc.) that often contraindicated VX or strongly suggested that it would be unsuccessful (Bofill *et al.* 1997). When the study and control groups were analyzed for these features, the most pertinent difference between the two groups was the obstetrician's availability and the unwillingness to abandon the procedure in a timely fashion. Several vacuum applications in this study lasted over an hour; the largest number of discreet applications was 16. There are few data in this study to suggest an inherent defect in the VX itself.

These findings are somewhat similar to those reported by Ennis and their colleagues in the UK (Ennis *et al.* 1990). Of the 64 litigations reviewed by senior clinicians involving perinatal death, CNS damage, or maternal death, they found examples of inadequate fetal heart monitoring, mismanagement of forceps, and inadequate supervision by senior staff. They found multiple attempts at forceps in one-quarter of the cases, and abandonment of forceps in favor of Cesarean section in almost half.

## THE CTG IN COURT

While failure on the part of the health-care provider to recognize clear FHR abnormalities is frequently alleged in malpractice cases, to isolate the CTG tracing under these circumstances frequently oversteps its permissive role in obstetrical care. A normal CTG pattern permits ongoing labor only as long as the safe vaginal delivery is a reasonable option. If the pattern turns abnormal (rising baseline, decreasing variability along with variable/late decelerations), especially in the second stage, then the questions are several. Can the pattern be ameliorated (by reducing the oxytocin, moderating the pushing efforts)? If the pattern cannot be ameliorated, what is the feasibility of safe vaginal delivery, given the estimated fetal weight, previous obstetrical history, position, presentation of the fetal head, and progress in labor to this point? In our experience, the vast majority of cases hinge far more on the reasonableness of the obstetrical care than on the interpretation of the fetal monitor.

The presence of experienced readers throughout the day in all major obstetric departments seems quite unachievable. Here, however, advances in technology might provide a solution. CTG can now be read directly via modem or transmitted rapidly by means of FAX to an awaiting consultant who might serve many hospitals. It should be emphasized that not all the problems are solved in this way. There are also problems in interpretation that are revealed only in retrospect when correlation with ultimate outcome becomes possible. Most hospitals have neither automatic mechanism for review nor the ready access of authoritative interpretation.

## SOLVING THE MALPRACTICE PROBLEM

The Harvard Medical Practice Study (Brennan *et al.* 1991) and subsequent ones have demonstrated that only a small proportion of negligent events result in litigation. If anything, they concluded there are too few lawsuits. Further, they wrote that 'Physicians tended to equate a finding of negligence with a judgment of incompetence. Thus, although willing to admit that "all doctors make mistakes" physicians were often unwilling to label substandard care as negligent and were opposed to compensation for iatrogenic injury'.

While the focus of clinical risk management intuitively rests on the analysis of adverse events, it seems clear that this is a most inefficient way of reducing or eliminating harm to the patient. In the current climate, risk management tends to deal more with avoidance of blame and litigation than in the avoidance of harm to patients. In 1997, a highly publicized article recommended that when doctors make a mistake that harms a patient, they should tell the patient what happened, apologize, and do whatever it takes to repair the damage (Finkelstein *et al.* 1997). Basic professional ethics aver that patients have a right to know what happened to them. It should seem like the right thing to do as part of the physician's responsibility to his patient. It may be therapeutic for the physician who may feel guilt and distress. Telling the truth may also strengthen the patient's faith in the doctor, while cover-up that fails, as many do, may anger the patient and make them more inclined to sue. Cover-ups also antagonize juries. Medicine is a human enterprise, and error (i.e. fallibility) is part of being human. 'We are programmed for error'.

Understandably, the notion of admitting error has drawn skeptical reviews from the medical community, the insurance companies and the defense bar (Grody 1997). They fear that admitting mistakes will leave them open to lawsuits and hurt their reputations and careers. Indeed, the communications director for the PIAA (Jack Pope) said that urging doctors to confess their mistakes was 'asking them to commit professional suicide'. 'Without tort reform to decrease the number of malpractice suits and large settlements', he continued, 'few doctors could risk owning up to errors. If you tell the truth, apologize and reach out to a family in grief, you can defuse some of the anger and polarization that characterize a typical lawsuit. But every word you utter is an admission that can be used against you in a court of law'. Lawyers then order doctors to say nothing until all the facts have been in, and then to say nothing.

Medicine is different from industry in that the medical system has not adjusted to the realities of human fallibility. Often, the ultimate failure is not the individual provider but the systemic error in failing to understand that most error is systemic. This state of affairs benefits neither the patient nor, in the long run, the physician. While, in some instances, the fear of lawsuit has increased the amount of surveillance and may have even had a salutary effect on outcome, there is little argument that the present format for dealing with allegations of negligence provides any incentive to the profession to practice better medicine, to provide a better peer review, or, in the occasional instance, restrict the future practice of the physician, whatever his conduct. True reform will require a systemic approach to error in medicine, as elsewhere, and some refinement of our ethics and an appreciation of the paradoxes of contemporary malpractice. To lower the risk of malpractice, we must continue to attempt to raise the standard of care. We must increase communication with the patient and remain their advocate. We must not squander our greatest asset – the medical record – and stop acting the role of victim. Finally, we must be willing to participate in the process of uncovering error.

As Goethe wrote:

> The most fruitful lesson is the conquest of one's own error. Whoever refuses to admit error may be a great scholar but he is not a great learner. Whoever is ashamed of error will struggle against recognizing and admitting it, which means that he struggles against his greatest inward gain. Goethe, Maxims and Reflections

## REFERENCES


ACOG (1990) *Professional liability and its effect: Report of 1990 survey of ACOG membership.* Washington, DC: American College of Obstetricians and Gynecologists.

ACOG (1992) *ACOG Technical Bulletin, No. 163, January 1992 – Fetal and neonatal neurologic injury.*

ACOG (1994) *ACOG Technical Bulletin, No. 196, August 1994 – Operative vaginal delivery*

ACOG (1998) *ACOG Committee Opinion No. 197, February 1998 – Inappropriate use of the terms fetal distress and birth asphyxia.*

ACOG, *Technical Bulletin No. 207, fetal heart rate patterns: monitoring, interpretation, and management.*

Alastair Maclennan for the International Cerebral Palsy Task Force (1999) A template for defining a causal relation between acute intrapartum events and cerebral palsy: international consensus statement. *BMJ* 319:1054–1059.

Blair E & Stanley F J (1988) Intrapartum asphyxia: a rare cause of cerebral palsy. *J Pediatr* 112:515–519.

Bofill J A, Rust O A, Devidas M *et al.* (1997) Neonatal cephalohematoma from vacuum extraction. *J Matern Fetal Med* 6:220–224.

Bors-Koefoed R, Zylstra S & Resseguie L J *et al.* (1998) Statistical models of outcome in malpractice lawsuits involving death or neurologically impaired infants. *J Matern – Fetal Med* 7:124–131.

Brennan T A, Leape L L, Laird N *et al.* (1991) Incidence of adverse events and negligence in hospitalised patients: results of the Harvard Medical Practice Study 1. *N Engl J Med* 324:370–386.

Bush M & Schifrin B S (in press) Fetal injury associated with vacuum extractors cause or coincidence.

California – see text.

Cohn S D (1990) National Practitioner Data Bank. *J Nurse – Midwifery.* 35:385–390.

Daubert v. Merrell Dow Pharmaceuticals, Inc. (1993) 509 U.S. 579 [see Kumbo Tire Co., Ltd. V. Carmichael, 119 S. Ct. 1167 (1999).

Department of Health and Human Services (1988) *Report of the Task Force on Medical Liability and Malpractice, August 1987.* Washington, DC: United States Government Printing Office, 519-216/63040.

Ennis M *et al.* (1990) Obstetric accidents: a review of 64 cases *BMJ* 300:1365–1367.

FDA (1999) *Advisory on vacuum extractor devices.* Food and Drug Administration.

Finkelstein D *et al.* (1997) When a physician harms a patient by a medical error: ethical, legal, and risk-management considerations. *J Clin Ethics* 8:330–335.

Fry v. United States (1923) 293 F. 1013.

Grady D (1997) Doctors urged to Admit Mistakes' *NY Times* 12/9/97.

Institute of Medicine (1989) *The effects of medical professional liability on the delivery of obstetrical care.* Washington, DC: Institute of Medicine, National Academy Press.

Ikeda T, Murata Y, Quilligan E J *et al.* (1998) Fetal heart rate patterns in postasphyxiated fetal lambs with brain damage. *Am J Obstet Gynecol* 179:1329–1337.

JOGNN (1997) Electronic fetal heart rate monitoring: research guidelines for interpretation. *JOGNN* 26: 635–640.

Kaiser Family Foundation/Harvard School of Public Health Study (1989) July.

Kollas C D (1999) What the book says. *Ann Int Med* 127:238–239.

Lent M (1999) The medical and legal risks of the electronic fetal monitor *Stanford Law Rev* 51.

Meeker C I (1992) A consensus-based approach to practice parameters. *Obstet Gynecol* 79(Pt 1): 790–793.

Nelson K B, Dambrosia J M, Ting T Y *et al.* (1996) Uncertain value of electronic fetal monitoring in predicting cerebral palsy. *N Engl J Med* 334:613–618.

Phelan J P & Ahn M O (1994) Perinatal observations in forty-eight neurologically impaired term infants. *Am J Obstet Gynecol* 171:424–431.

Richards B C & Thomasson G (1992) Closed liability claims analysis and the medical record. *Obstet Gynecol* 80:313–316.

Rosenblatt R A (1989) An analysis of closed obstetric malpractice claims. *Obstet Gynecol* 74: 710–713.

Rosenblatt R A, Whelan A & Hart L G (1990) Obstetric practice patterns in Washington State after tort reform: has the access problem been solved? *Obstet Gynecol* 76:1105.

Sachs B P, Kobelin C & Castro M A *et al.* (1999) The risks of lowering the cesarean-delivery rate. *N Engl J Med* 340:54–57.

Schifrin *et al.* Outcome data.

Schifrin B S, Hamilton-Rubinstein T & Shields J R (1994) Fetal heart rate patterns and the timing of fetal injury. *J Perinatol* 14:174–181.

Schreiber v. Physicians Insurance Company of Wisconsin (1996) 223 Wis. 2d 417.

Shea v. Esensten (1997) 107 F, 3d 625 m 629 (8th Cir.)

Shields J R & Schifrin B S (1988) Perinatal antecedents of cerebral palsy. *Obstet Gynecol* 71:899–905.

Sloan F A & Bovbjerg R R (1989) *Medical malpractice: Crises, response and effects.* Washington, DC: Research Bulletin, Health Insurance Association of America.

Sloan F A, Whetten Goldstein K, & Stout E M *et al.* (1998) No-fault system of compensation for obstetric injury: winners and losers. *Obstet Gynecol* 91:437–443.

Spencer J A, Badawi N, Burton P, Keogh J, Pemberton P & Stanley F (1997) The intrapartum CTG prior to neonatal encephalopathy at term: a case-control study. *Br J Obstet Gynaecol* 104:25–28.

Stalnaker B L, Maher J E & Kleinman G E *et al.* (1997) Characteristics of successful claims for payment by the Florida Neurologic Injury Compensation Association Fund. *Am J Obstet Gynecol* 177:268–271.

Towner D, Castro M A, Eby-Wilkens E & Gilbert W M (1999) Effect of mode of delivery in nulliparous women on neonatal intracranial injury. *N Engl J Med* 341:1709–1714.

Vannucci R C (1993) Mechanisms of perinatal hypoxic-ischemic brain damage. *Semin Perinatol* 17:330–337.

Visser G H A & Narayan H (1996) The problem of increasing severe neurological morbidity in newborn infants: Where should the focus be? *Prenat Neonat Med* 1:2–15.

Volpe (1995) Neurology of the newborn, 3rd edn.

Westgate J A, Bennet L & Gunn A J (1999) Fetal seizures causing increased heart rate variability during terminal fetal hypoxia. *Am J Obstet Gynecol* 181:765–766.

Why patients sue (1992) *JAMA* 267:1359–1363.

Zuckerman S, Bovbjerg R R & Sloan F (1989) *Effects of tort reform and other factors on medical malpractice insurance premiums. Working paper 3677–11.* Washington, DC: The Urban Institute.

- Pyrimethamine is a folic acid antagonist. It can therefore depress the bone marrow and cause a macrocytic anemia, neutropenia, or thrombopenia. It should therefore be associated with folinic acid that only the human cells can use. Folinic acid does not reduce the efficacy of pyrimethamine against toxoplasma.
- Sulfadiazine, associated with pyrimethamine and folinic acid, is the treatment of choice in active infection.
- Corticosteroids are used in chorioretinitis to limit the inflammatory process.
- Clindamycine (Lakhanpal *et al.* 1983).
- Trimethoprim associated with sulfamethoxazole (cotrimoxazole).
- Spiramycin is the classical macrolide used to prevent the placenta passage of toxoplasma in mothers who seroconverted. It is not effective in fetuses already infected and does not prevent, for example, neurotoxoplasmosis in immunosuppressed patients (Leport *et al.* 1986).
- Azithromycin and clarithromycin, recent macrolides, are effective on toxoplasma gondii and increase the effectiveness of associations like pyrimethamine–sulfadiazine, at least *in vitro* (Araujo *et al.* 1988; Derouin *et al.* 1992; Cantin & Chamberland 1993; Alder *et al.* 1994; Derouin 1995). Moreover, azithromycin was found to be effective on the cyst form *in vitro* (Huskinson-Mark *et al.* 1991).

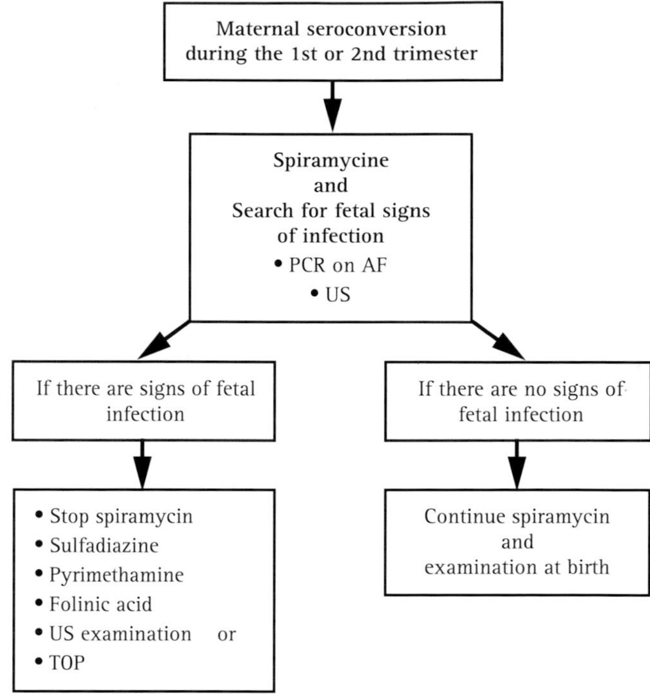


Figure 31.3 During the pregnancy if the maternal seroconversion occurred during the 1st or 2nd trimesters. US = ultrasound; PCR = polymerase chain reaction; AF = amniotic fluid; TOP = termination of pregnancy.

## MATERNAL INFECTION IN THE 1ST AND 2ND TRIMESTERS (Fig. 31.3)

If the vertical transmission occurs during the 1st or 2nd trimester, the risk of severe fetal infection is important. Nevertheless, this transmission is rare. It is therefore important to make the diagnosis of fetal infection. This is done by PCR on amniotic fluid after amniocentesis and ultrasound examination.

If the fetus is infected, there are two possibilities:

- Termination of pregnancy, but there is a probability of terminating a fetus who would have had no clinical symptom, only subclinical anomalies.
- Fetal intrauterine therapy given to the mother could reduce the severity of the fetal disease and is targeted at the fetus itself as well as to the mother. This treatment is by pyrimethamine and sulfadiazine in association with folinic acid. These drugs can cross the placenta and can be found at high concentrations in the blood of the neonate of a treated mother (Dorangeon *et al.* 1990). This treatment reduces the concentration of the parasite in the placenta, as well as that of the specific fetal IgM and IgG, and it probably reduces the number of severe infections (Couvreur *et al.* 1993). More recent data show that the administration of antibiotics to the mother of an infected child reduces the appearance of severe sequelae in the neonates (Foulon *et al.* 1999). In the study of Hohlfeld *et al.* (1989) the only child with severe congenital toxoplasmosis, out of 52 cases, did not receive 'therapeutic' drugs during the pregnancy. For example, in a follow-up of 12 cases of treatment of the mother by sulfadoxine or sulfadiazine in combination with pyrimethamine, no hematological abnormality was found in the neonates (Daffos *et al.* 1988).

If the fetus is not infected:

- Spiramycin is the drug most widely used in this situation. It seems to reduce the frequency of placentitis, thus reducing the number of infected fetuses. Studies support that the frequency of infected fetuses was lower in each trimester of the pregnancy among treated mothers than among non-treated mothers (Desmonts & Couvreur 1974). In this study, using prevention by spiramycin, only 24% of the fetuses from infected mothers where infected, and a total of 11% of fetuses had a clinical disease. Spiramycin is said not to be curative for the fetus. The prevention of fetal toxoplasmosis by spiramycin, or other drugs, is not well established for all. By reviewing several studies, Wallon *et al.* (1999) conclude that there are 'no good comparative data measuring the potential harms and benefits of antiparasitic drugs used for presumed antenatal toxoplasma infection'. This statement was confirmed by Foulon *et al.* (1999) in a large multicentric study who found that the materno-fetal transmission of the infection depended more upon the gestational age at which the infection occurred than upon the treatment given to the mother. This is probably because the placentitis occurs very early after the maternal infection before any treatment is given.

## MATERNAL INFECTION IN THE THIRD TRIMESTER (Fig. 31.4)

The frequency of vertical transmission is important here. The probability of severe neurological involvement is rare, but the risk of chorioretinitis is important *in utero* and after birth. The diagnosis of fetal infection is also made by combining PCR on amniotic fluid and ultrasound findings, but there is a risk of false negative. We can either treat these fetuses as if they were infected or perform amniocentesis and serial ultrasound examinations after starting spiramycin treatment. This will be continued up to delivery, and placenta and cord blood will be examined for infection.

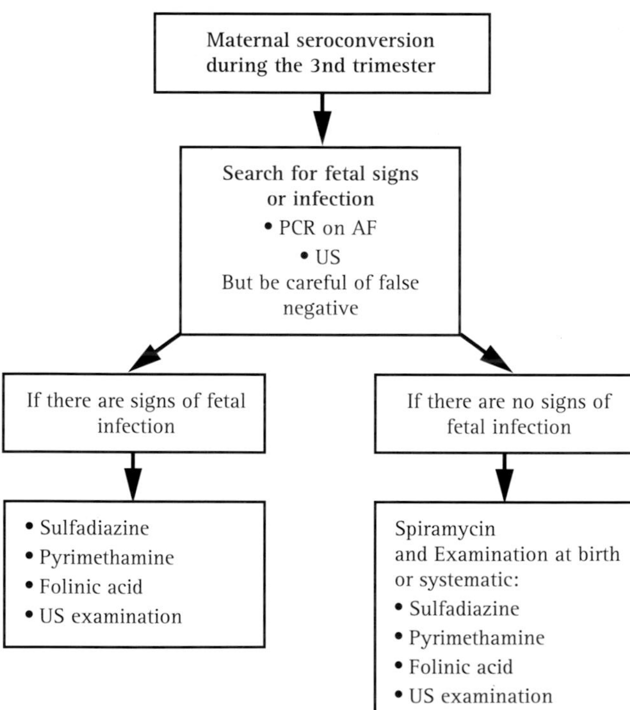


**Figure 31.4** During the pregnancy if the maternal seroconversion occurred during the 3rd trimester. US = ultrasound; PCR = polymerase chain reaction; AF = amniotic fluid; TOP = termination of pregnancy.

## TERMINATION OF PREGNANCY

This is a possibility in severely affected cases, when legally and ethically possible. It is mainly done when fetal infection occurs during the 1st or 2nd trimester of pregnancy, in 30–50% of the cases of infected fetuses (Daffos *et al.* 1988; Hohlfeld *et al.* 1989). Looking at recent and well-documented studies, 60% of children born with congenital toxoplasmosis had no clinical or laboratory abnormality, and of the 40% left, only 4% have symptoms at follow-up (Berrebi *et al.* 1994). It is therefore very difficult to assess the potential of handicap of an infected fetus to justify a termination of pregnancy.

## AT BIRTH

The attitude depends on the infectious status of the fetus and the results of the neonatal examination.

If the diagnosis of fetal infection is negative:

- parasitology of the placenta and the fetal blood
- neurologic and ophthalmologic examination
- ultrasound examination of the central nervous system
- neonatal immunologic status.

False negative results on amniotic fluid may occur when sampled in the third trimester of pregnancy. An infected neonate, whether symptomatic or asymptomatic, will be treated by alternate treatment of pyrimethamine–sulfadiazine–folinic acid for 3–4 weeks, followed by 4–6 weeks of spiramycin, and so on, for at least a year. Pyrimethamine–sulfadiazine–folinic acid can also be used alone for a year. Fewer new observed lesions of chorioretinitis seem to develop during the first year of life in children receiving several courses of treatment (Couvreur *et al.* 1984). The long-term follow-up study to 10 years of the Chicago Collaborative Treatment Trial (McAuley *et al.* 1994) suggested that after 1 year of treatment, up to 70% of the infants with severe central nervous system and ophthalmologic involvement at birth developed normally. Delay in diagnosis and therapy is indicative of a poor prognosis. It is noteworthy that only one infant was diagnosed with congenital toxoplasmosis *in utero* and all others after birth. Treatment is also known to diminish the occurrence and development of intracranial calcifications.

The pyrimethamine–sulfadiazine association during pregnancy when the fetus is infected decreases immunologic reaction to infection in the first year of life more than spiramycin alone (Fortier *et al.* 1997). The pyrimethamine, sulfadiazine and corticosteroids association seems to be more efficient than the association of clindamycine-corticosteroids, cotrimoxazole-corticosteroids or no treatment in chorioretinits (Rothova *et al.* 1993). The treatment should be followed for at least 1 year and the follow-up continued until adolescence.

## IF THE DIAGNOSIS OF FETAL INFECTION IS POSITIVE

The most important point here is not the diagnosis but the prognosis. Neonatal examination is usually easy:

- neurologic and ophthalmologic examination
- ultrasound examination of the central nervous system.

The treatment started *in utero* will be continued, and there will be a long-term follow-up.

**Key Points**

- There is a large variation in seroprevalence for toxoplasmosis amongst pregnant women from country to country and the value of screening is dependent on local factors
- Primary prevention in susceptible women may be possible by advice about not eating poorly cooked meat, avoidance of cats and their litter and not gardening whilst pregnant
- The rate of vertical transmission from mother to fetus is 40% overall and increases with gestation
- Fetal diagnosis is made by PCR on amniotic fluid and intra-uterine treatment with pyrimethamine and sulfadiazine in association with folinic acid may be effective in curing the infection
- Treatment of the infected infant comprises cycles of alternating pyrimethamine–sulfadiazine–folinic acid for 3–4 weeks followed by 4—6 weeks of spiramycin for at least a year

## REFERENCES


Ades A E & Nokes D J (1993) Modeling age- and time-specific incidence from seroprevalence: toxoplasmosis. *Am J Epidemiol* 137:1022–1034.

Alder J, Hutch T, Meulbroek J A *et al.* (1994) Treatment of experimental *Toxoplasma gondii* infection by clarithromycin-based combination therapy with minocycline or pyrimethamine. *J Acquired Immune Deficit Syndrome* 7:1141–1148.

Allain J P, Palmer C R & Pearson G (1998) Epidemiological study of latent and recent infection by *Toxoplasma gondii* in pregnant women from a regional population in the U.K. *J Infect* 36:189–196.

Araujo F G, Guptill D R & Remington J S (1988) Azithromycin, a macrolide antibiotic with potent activity against *Toxoplasma gondii. Antimicrobial Agents Chemother* 32:755–757.

Ashrafunnessa, Khatun S, Islam *et al.* (1998) Seroprevalence of toxoplasma antibodies among the antenatal population in Bangladesh. *J Obstet Gynaecol Res* 24:115–119.

Bader T J, Macones G A & Asch D A (1997) Prenatal screening for toxoplasmosis. *Obstet Gynecol* 90:457–464.

Berrebi A, Kobuch W E, Bessieres M H *et al.* (1994) Termination of pregnancy for maternal toxoplasmosis. *Lancet* 344:36–39.

Buffolano W, Gilbert R E, Holland F J *et al.* (1996) Risk factors for recent toxoplasma infection in pregnant women in Naples. *Epidemiol Infect* 116:347–351.

Buxton D (1998) Protozoan infection (*Toxoplasma gondii, neospora caninum* and *sarcocystis* spp) in sheep and goats: recent advances. *Vet Res* 29:289–310.

Buxton D, Thompson K M, Maley S *et al.* (1993) Experimental challenge of sheep 18 months after vaccination with a live (S48) *Toxoplasma gondii* vaccine. *Vet Rec* 33:310–312.

Cantin L & Chamberland S (1993) *In vitro* evaluation of the activities of azithromycin alone and combined with pyrimethamine against *Toxoplasma gondii. Antimicrobial Agents Chemother* 37:1993–1996.

Couvreur J (1999) Le problème de la toxoplasmose congénitale. *La Presse médicale* 28:753–757.

Couvreur J, Desmonts G, Aron-Rosa D (1984) Le pronostic oculaire de la toxoplasmose congénitale: rôle du traitement. *Annales de Pédiatrie* 31:855–858.

Couvreur J, Thulliez P, Daffos F *et al.* (1993) *In utero* treatment of toxoplasmic fetopathy with the combination pyrimethamine–sulfadiazine. *Fetal Diag Ther* 8:45–50.

Daffos F, Forestier F, Capella-Pavlovsky M *et al.* (1988) Prenatal management of 746 pregnancies at risk for congenital toxoplasmosis. *N Engl J Med* 318:271–275.

Dannemann B R, Vaughan W C, Thulliez P *et al.* (1990) Differential agglutination test for diagnosis of recently acquired infection with *Toxoplasma gondii. J Clin Microbiol* 28:1928–1933.

Decalvas G, Papapetropoulou M, Giannoulaki E *et al.* (1990) Prevalence of *Toxoplasma gondii* antibodies in gravidas and recently aborted women and study of risk factors. *Eur J Epidemiol* 6:223–226.

Derouin F (1995) Les nouveaus pathogènes et le mode d'action de l'azithromycine: *Toxoplasma gondii. Pathologie Biologie* 43:561–564.

Derouin F, Almadany R, Chau F *et al.* (1992) Synergistic activity of azithromycin and pyrimethamine or sulfadiazine in acute experimental toxoplasmosis. *Antimicrobial Agents Chemother* 36:997–1001.

Desmonts G & Couvreur J (1974) Congenital toxoplasmosis: a prospective study of 378 pregnancies. *N Engl J Med* 290:1110–1116.

Desmonts G & Couvreur J (1984) Histoire naturelle de la toxoplasmose congénitale. *Annales de Pediatrie* 31:799–802.

Desmonts G & Couvreur J (1984) Toxoplasmose congénitale. Etude prospective de l'issue de la grossesse chez 542 femmes atteintes de toxoplasmose acquise en cours de gestation. *Annales de Pédiatrie* 31:805–809.

Desmonts G, Forestier F, Thulliez P *et al.* (1985) Prenatal diagnosis of congenital toxoplasmosis. *Lancet* 1:500–504.

Desmonts G, Couvreur J & Thulliez Ph (1990) Toxoplasmose congénitale: cinq cas de transmission à l'enfant d'une infection maternelle antérieure à la grossess. *La Presse médicale* 19:1445–1449.

Dorangeon P H, Fay R, Marx-Chemla C *et al.* (1990) Passage transplacentaire de l'association pyrimethamine–sulfadoxine lors du traitement anténatal de la toxoplasmose congénitale. *Presse Médicale* 19:22–29.

Editorial (1990) Antenatal screening for toxoplasmosis in the UK. *Lancet* 336:346–348.

Eskild A, Oxman A, Magnus P *et al.* (1996) Screening for toxoplasmosis in pregnancy: what is the evidence of reducing a health problem? *J Med Screen* 3:1888–1894.

Fortier B, Coignard-Chatain C, Dao A *et al.* (1997) Etude des poussées cliniques évolutives et des rebonds sérologiques d'enfants atteints de toxoplasmose congénitale et suivis durant les 2 premières années de vie. *Archives de Pédiatrie* 4:940–946.

Foulon W, Naessens A, Vilckaert M *et al.* (1984) Congenital toxoplasmosis: a prospective survey in Brussels. *Br J Obstet Gynaecol* 91:419–423.

Foulon W, Naessens A, Lauwers S *et al.* (1988) Impact of primary prevention on the incidence of toxoplasmosis during pregnancy. *Obstet Gynecol* 72:363–366.

Foulon W, Villena I, Stray-Petersen B *et al.* (1999) Treatment of toxoplasmosis during pregnancy: a multicenter study of impact on fetal transmission and children's sequelae at 1 year. *Am J Obstet Gynecol* 180:410–415.

Gilbert R E, Tookey P A, Cubitt W D *et al.* (1993) Prevalence of toxoplasma IgG among pregnant women in west London according to country of birth and ethnic group. *Br Med J* 306:185.

Guerina N G, Hsu H W, Meissner H C *et al.* (1994) Neonatal screening and early treatment for congenital *Toxoplasma gondii* infection. *N Engl J Med* 330:1858–1863.

Hohlfeld P, Daffos F, Costa J M *et al.* (1994) Prenatal diagnosis of congenital toxoplasmosis with a polymerase-chain-reaction test on amniotic fluid. *N Engl J Med* 331:695–699.

Hohlfeld P, Daffos F, Thulliez P *et al.* (1989) Fetal toxoplasmosis: outcome of pregnancy and infant follow-up after *in utero* treatment. *J Pediatr* 115:765–769.

Huskinson-Mark J, Araujo G & Remington J S (1991) Evaluation of the effects of drugs on the cyst form of *Toxoplasma gondii. J Infect Dis* 164:170–177.

Jeannel D, Niel G, Costagliola D *et al.* (1988) Epidemiology of toxoplasmosis among pregnant women in the Paris area. *Int J Epidemiol* 17:595–602.

Jenum P A, Stray-Pedersen B & Gundersen A G (1997) Improved diagnosis of primary *Toxoplasma gondii* infection in early pregnancy by determination of antitoxoplasma immunoglobulin G avidity. *J Clin Microbiol* 35:1972–1977.

Jenum P A, Kapperud G, Stray-Pedersen B *et al.* (1998) Prevalence of *Toxoplasma gondii* specific immunoglobulin G antibodies among pregnant women in Norway. *Epidemiol Infect* 120:87–92.

Koppe J G, Loewer-Sieger D H, de Roever-Bonnet H (1986) Results of 20-year follow-up of congenital toxoplasmosis. *Lancet* 1:254–255.

Lakhanpal V, Schocket S S & Nirankari V S (1983) Clindamycin in the treatment of toxoplasmic retinochoroidis. *Am J Ophthalmol* 95:605.

Lappalainen M, Koskela P, Koskiniemi M *et al.* (1993) Toxoplasmosis acquired during pregnancy: improved serodiagnosis based on avidity of IgG. *J Infect Dis* 167:691–697.

Lebech M, Andersen O, Christensen N C *et al.* (1999) Feasibility of neonatal screening for toxoplasma infection in the absence of prenatal treatment. *Lancet* 353:1834–1837.

Leport C, Vilde J L, Katlama C *et al.* (1986) Failure of spiramycine to prevent neurotoxoplasmosis in immunosuppressed patients. *JAMA* 17:2290.

Ljungström I, Gille E, Nokes J *et al.* (1995) Seroepidemiology of *Toxoplasma gondii* among pregnant women in different parts of Sweden. *Eur J Epidemiol* 11:149–156.

Lynfield R, Hsu H W & Guerina N G (1999) Screening methods for congenital toxoplasma and risk of disease. *Lancet* 353:1899–1900.

Marty P, Le-Fichoux Y, Deville A *et al.* (1991) Toxoplasmose congéniale et toxoplasmose ganglionnaire maternelle préconceptionnelle. *La Presse médicale* 20:387.

McAuley J, Boyer K M, Patel D *et al.* (1994) Early and longitudinal evaluations of treated infants and children and untreated historical patients with congenital toxoplasmosis: the Chicago Collaborative Treatment trial. *Clin Infect Dis* 18:38–72.

McCabe R, Remington J S (1988) Toxoplasmosis: the time has come. *N Engl J Med* 318:313–315.

Miller M J, Aronson W J & Remington J S (1969) Late parasitemia in asymptomatic acquired toxoplasmosis. *Ann Intern Med* 71:139–145.

Mombro M, Perathoner C, Leone A *et al.* (1995) Congenital tosoplasmosis: 10-year follow up. *Eur J Pediatr* 154:635–639.

Naot Y, Desmonts G & Remington J S (1981) IgM enzyme-linked immunosorbent assay test for the diagnosis of congenital toxoplasma infection. *J Pediatr* 98:32–36.

Patel V D, Holfels E M, Vogel N P *et al.* (1996) Resolution of intracranial calcifications in infants with treated congenital toxoplasmosis. *Radiology* 199:433–440.

Peyron F, Wallon M, Bernardoux C (1996) Long-term follow-up of patients with congenital ocular toxoplasmosis. *N Engl J Med* 334:993–994.

Pinon J M, Chemla C, Villena I *et al.* (1996) Early neonatal diagnosis of congenital toxoplasmosis: value of comparative enzyme-linked immunofiltration assay immunological profiles and anti-*Toxoplasma gondii* immunoglobulin M (IgM) or IgA immunocapture and implications for postnatal therapeutic strategies. *J Clin Microbiol* 34:579–583.

Pons J C, Sigrand C, Grangeot-Keros L *et al.* (1995) Toxoplasmose congénitale: transmission au fœtus d'une infection maternelle antéconceptionnelle. *La Presse médicale* 24:179–182.

Pratlong F, Boulot P, Issert E *et al.* (1994) Fetal diagnosis of toxoplasmosis in 190 women infected during pregnancy. *Prenatal Diag* 14:191–198.

Pratlong F, Boulot P, Villena I *et al.* (1996) Antenatal diagnosis of congenital toxoplasmosis: evaluation of the biological parameters in a cohort of 286 patients. *Br J Obstet Gynaecology* 103:552–557.

Remington J S, McLeod R & Desmonts G (1995) Toxoplasmosis. In: Remington J S & Klein J O (eds) *Infectious disease in the fetus and newborn infant.* Philadelphia, PA: WB Saunders, 4th edn; pp. 140–267.

Roizen N, Swisher C N, Stein M A *et al.* (1995) Neurologic and developmental outcome in treated congenital toxoplasmosis. *Pediatrics* 95:11–20.

Roos T, Martius J, Gross U *et al.* (1993) Systematic serologic screening for toxoplasmosis in pregnancy. *Obstet Gynecol* 81:243–250.

Rothova A, Meenken C, Buitenhuis H J *et al.* (1993) Therapy for ocular toxoplasmosis. *Am J Ophtalmol* 115:517–523.

Stepick-Biek P, Thulliez P, Araujo F G *et al.* (1990) IgA antibodies for diagnosis of acute congenital and acquired toxoplasmosis. *J Infect Dis* 162:270–273.

Thulliez P, Remington J S, Santoro F *et al.* (1986) Une nouvelle réaction d'agglutination pour le diagnostic du stade évoluif de la toxoplasmose acquise. *Pathologie Biologie* 34:173–177.

Valcavi P P, Natali A, Soliani L *et al.* (1995) Prevalence of anti-*Toxoplasma gondii* antibodies in the population of the area of Parma (Italy). *Eur J Epidemiol* 11:333–337.

Velin P, Dupont D, Barbot D *et al.* (1991) Double contamination materno-fœtale par le VIH et le toxoplasme. *La Presse médicale* 20:960.

Wallon M, Liou G, Garner P *et al.* (1999) Congenital toxoplasmosis: systematic review of evidence of efficacy in pregnancy. *Br Med J* 318:1511–1514.

Wastling J M, Harkins D & Buxton D (1994) Western blot analysis of the IgG response of sheep vaccinated with S48 *Toxoplasma gondii* (Toxovax). *Res Vet Sci* 57:384–386.

Wilson C B, Remington J S, Stagno S *et al.* (1980) Development of adverse sequelae in children born with subclinical congenital toxoplasma infection. *Pediatrics* 66:767–674.

Zuber P L F, Jacquier P, Hohlfeld P *et al.* (1995) Toxoplasma infection among pregnant women in Switzerland: a cross-sectional evaluation of regional and age-specific lifetime average annual incidence. *Am J Epidemiol* 141:659–666.

Chapter 32

# Viral infections

C. S. Peckham and M.-L. Newell

## INTRODUCTION

Viral infections of the fetus or neonate may result in sustained or progressive neurologic damage (Table 32.1). Infection may be acquired before birth, during the process of delivery or in the postnatal period. Intrauterine infection follows invasion of the maternal bloodstream by microorganisms with resultant placental infection and/or transplacental transmission to the fetus. Sometimes, the placenta may be infected without fetal spread. Infections may also reach the fetus from the genital tract by the cervical amniotic route, or they may be acquired following exposure to infected cervical secretions or to maternal blood or feces during delivery. Infection acquired in the neonatal period may have been transmitted via breast milk, transfused blood, by hands or instruments, or via the respiratory route from infected contacts such as the mother, other babies, medical attendants, or other family members.

Some viruses and protozoa that cross the placenta may cause fetal damage in the form of congenital abnormalities and/or tissue invasion and destruction, both of which may involve the central nervous system (CNS). Tissue destruction may also continue after birth because of the persistence of viable organisms. Such chronic infection occurs with rubella, cytomegalovirus (CMV), herpes simplex virus (HSV), varicella-zoster (V-Z) virus, and human immunodeficiency virus (HIV).

Most infants congenitally infected by these agents have no clinical illness at birth but later may develop neurological signs and symptoms in infancy, childhood, or adult life because of the persistence and activity of the microorganism (Peckham 1972). It is usually not possible to identify the cause of these late manifestations, because microbiologic investigations at this stage alone cannot distinguish congenital from postnatally acquired infection. The difficulty is compounded by the non-specific nature of the symptoms. For example, it is not possible to diagnose a congenital infection in a 3-year-old child presenting with global retardation who is excreting CMV in the urine, if no information is available on tests carried out in the neonatal period.

**Table 32.1 Viruses known to infect the human fetus or newborn and cause damage to the nervous system**

| |
|---|
| Rubella |
| Cytomegalovirus |
| Varicella-zoster |
| Herpes virus hominis |
| Human immunodeficiency virus |
| Lymphocytic choriomeningitis virus |
| Non-polio enteroviruses |
| Polio virus |

*Source*: From Miller *et al.* (1991) © Cambridge University Press.

Some viruses, such as measles, mumps, and enteroviruses, may cause intrauterine infection but do not persist. Transplacental transmission of human serum parvovirus (B19) is also well documented [Knott & Welply 1984, PHLS (Public Health Laboratory Service) Working Party on Fifth Disease 1990], but it is not known whether infection persists postnatally as it does with animal parvoviruses. B19 is, however, known to persist in immunocompromised humans who acquire the infection postnatally (Kurtzman *et al.* 1988), and there is some evidence of limited prenatal persistence in the fetus and/or placenta in gestational infection (PHLS Working Party on Fifth Disease 1990). It is clear that the effects of this virus on the fetus are still only partially known.

Apart from congenital poliomyelitis, any neurological damage associated with prenatal infection with the non-persisting viruses appears to be non-specifically due to prematurity (Young & Gershon 1983; Cherry 1990). Demonstrating the possible role of viruses as a cause of fetal damage and/or neurological sequelae can be difficult and is open to misinterpretation. Maternal infection may be missed, because it is subclinical or non-specific and mild (CMV and HIV infection are examples). There is little precise information available on the overall frequency of infection in pregnancy, but in a prospective study of 30 000 pregnancies, carried out in the USA, about 5% were complicated by at least one clinically recognizable illness, the majority of which were non-specific and 'viral' (Sever & White 1968). In such cases, it is unlikely, if the infant is normal at birth or has non-specific symptoms, that investigations for evidence of infection will be carried out. If symptoms suggestive of congenital infection later present in the older infant or child, it may no longer be possible to reach a conclusive diagnosis. However, it has recently become possible to use the filter-paper samples, collected routinely in the neonatal period for the diagnosis of inborn errors of metabolism, for the retrospective diagnosis of specific congenital infections (Fischler *et al.* 1999). In the future, these stored samples could be used to test for the presence of congenital infection in a child presenting with problems such as cerebral palsy later in life.

Any study of the gestational effects of a microorganism known to cause mild or subclinical maternal infection must be prospective. This necessitates the serological follow-up of women through pregnancy to identify those who become infected and to investigate appropriate fetal or neonatal samples for evidence of congenital infection. Where the sensitivity of the laboratory investigation of the neonate is in doubt or unknown, infants must be followed clinically and serologically for at least the first year, until passively acquired maternal antibodies will no longer be present. The significance of non-specific outcomes such as abortion, prematurity, neurologic, or sense organ sequelae can only be interpreted by comparison with a control group of pregnancies matched for confounding variables such as age, parity, social class, and ethnic background. Large numbers of women have to be studied because even the most common congenital infection, CMV, occurs in only 1% of susceptible pregnant women, and in only a proportion of these pregnancies will transplacental infection take place.

Associating a particular infection with fetal damage may be difficult if the infection is uncommon in pregnancy, even if the maternal infection is symptomatic. Examples include mumps, chicken-pox, and measles. The likelihood of an association is increased if the organism can be recovered from the fetus or infant, or if there is serological evidence of infection in the neonate. However, unless a series of cases with similar defects or with a characteristic syndrome is reported, as with congenital varicella, evidence of transplacental transmission does not necessarily confirm that the agent was responsible for the defects.

Mumps is an example of an infection whose gestational effects are still a matter of debate. A study of placental infection following mumps vaccine in pregnancy demonstrated that fetal infection could occur (Yamauchi *et al.* 1974). Experimentally acquired hydrocephalus due to aqueduct stenosis may also develop in suckling hamsters infected with mumps virus at birth; similar defects have been reported in infants following early childhood mumps (Johnson 1968). The virus readily invades the meninges and brain, and insufficient attention has been given to the possibility of fetal mumps infection damaging the CNS. This concern may become academic in countries with an effective childhood vaccination program including measles, mumps, and rubella vaccine. However, such programs, if uptake is poor or not maintained, may lead to a change in age distribution with more cases occurring in adults.

Another example of a virus that may be embryopathic with CNS involvement is human herpesvirus type 6 (HHV-6), an agent first described in 1986. It is the cause of exanthem subitum, and seroprevalence is about 80% among children and adults. Although there are differences, it shares some biologic and morphologic characteristics with other herpes viruses, including the capacity for latency and reactivation. It is mainly trophic for T lymphocytes, but *in vitro*, it also infects other cell types, including glial cells. Its role as a cause of congenital infection is still to be elucidated, but there are at least three reports of intrauterine transmission. In one 26-week fetus (obtained through induced abortion from an HIV-1 seropositive woman), HHV-6-specific DNA sequences were detected in brain and cerebrospinal fluid, although there was no apparent clinical abnormality (Ando *et al.* 1992; Aubin *et al.* 1992; Dunne & Demmler 1992).

This chapter reviews viral infections, which, if acquired during pregnancy or the neonatal period, are known to infect the CNS and to result in neurologic sequelae. Organisms whose neuropathic effect is speculative or non-specific will not be considered.

## RUBELLA

When rubella infection is acquired in early pregnancy, the risk of fetal infection with damage is high, and a substantial number of infants are severely affected with multiple defects and neurological abnormalities. Most congenitally infected infants are damaged as a result of primary maternal infection, although damage resulting from maternal reinfection in women with previous infection or successful rubella immunization has also been described (Miller 1990). Following exposure to rubella, laboratory evidence of reinfection occurs in about 5% of individuals with natural rubella immunity (Horstmann *et al.* 1970), but clinically apparent maternal reinfection is rare, and the risk to the fetus of subclinical reinfection and damage is likely to be very small. There is no evidence that rubella immunization in pregnancy poses a risk to the fetus.

Fetal infection or damage does not inevitably follow maternal infection in pregnancy. Prospective studies carried out in the 1960s, to estimate the risk of damage and to characterize the abnormalities associated with maternal rubella, were based on clinical recognition of maternal rubella and long-term follow-up of infants born to those mothers. Taken together, these studies suggested that the risk of damage following maternal infection was about 21% following exposure to infection in the first 8 weeks of pregnancy, declining to about 6% at 12–16 weeks of gestation (Dudgeon 1976). As these early studies relied on a clinical diagnosis of maternal rubella, they are likely to have underestimated the true risk of damage because women presenting with rashes not due to rubella, but due to infections such as parvovirus, would have been included. Indeed, in a more recent study based on laboratory reports of confirmed infection in pregnancy, substantially higher estimates of fetal damage were reported (Miller 1991). Over 1000 women for whom the dates of the last menstrual period and rash were known were followed up. Over 90% of women infected in the first trimester of pregnancy and half of those infected between 13 and 16 weeks of gestation chose to have a therapeutic abortion. Table 32.2 shows the risk of defects in children with proven infection and the overall risk of damage in a pregnancy complicated by rubella. Infections after 16 weeks of gestation are only occasionally associated with defects,

**Table 32.2 Risk of congenital rubella defects following confirmed maternal infection at successive stages of pregnancy**

| Infected infants | | Overall risk of defect[a] | |
|---|---|---|---|
| Stage of pregnancy (weeks) | Number examined | Number with rubella defect[b] (%) | Following maternal rubella (%) |
| 2–10 | 20 | 18 (90) | 90 |
| 11–12 | 12 | 6 (50) | 34 |
| 13–16 | 36 | 12 (33) | 17 |
| 17–18 | 15 | 1 (7) | 3 |
| >19 | 58 | 0 | – |

*Source*: From Miller *et al.* (1991) © Cambridge University Press.

[a] Overall risk of defect = fetal infection rate (from table) × risk of defect if infected.

[b] All infants had sensorineural deafness; eight infants infected earlier than 8 weeks also had congenital heart disease.

although cases of deafness have been reported up to 22 weeks of gestation. Well-designed prospective studies of children born after later infection have shown that although rubella infection after this period can result in fetal infection, there is no increased risk of defects (Miller *et al.* 1982; Grilner *et al.* 1983). Exposure to infection early in pregnancy is likely to result in fetal infection with multiple defects, whereas damage following fetal infection in the third and fourth month usually results in a single defect, sensorineural deafness.

Although there have been isolated reports of possible congenital defects following maternal rubella before conception, in none of these cases was the maternal or fetal infection confirmed by adequate laboratory tests. In a prospective study, Enders *et al.* (1988) found no risk associated with exposure to rubella before conception.

In addition to cataracts, congenital heart disease, deafness and non-specific manifestations presenting in the newborn such as failure to thrive, hepatomegaly, splenomegaly, jaundice, and thrombocytopenic purpura, the CNS is a common site for the infection, and neurologic defects may be present. These include microcephaly, mental retardation, cerebral palsy, defects of hearing and speech, features of autism, retinal changes, and visual disturbances due to cataract and microphthalmos. Seizures and hydrocephalus are rare. With the exception of deafness, CNS involvement rarely occurs in the absence of manifestations involving other systems. Chess (1971) has drawn attention to the high incidence of autistic features in children with congenital rubella deafness, and a small number with normal hearing have also been observed with classic autism.

Sensorineural hearing loss is the most frequent rubella defect. It may be moderate or severe, bilateral, or unilateral and is often associated with pigmentary retinopathy. Epidemiological studies carried out in the UK before the introduction of rubella vaccination suggested that rubella accounted for at least 16% of cases of moderate to severe sensorineural deafness (Martin & Moore 1979; Peckham *et al.* 1979) and 2% of cases of congenital heart disease among British children (Peckham 1985). However, it is difficult to establish the full impact of congenital rubella on a population, as there is not always a history of maternal infection, and defects may not manifest or even develop until weeks, months, or years after birth when a retrospective diagnosis of congenital infection is usually no longer possible. The most important example of late-onset disease is sensorineural deafness (Peckham 1972), but other more unusual forms of late-onset disease include pneumonitis, diabetes mellitus, hypothyroidism, growth hormone deficiency, and encephalitis (Marshall 1973).

Meningoencephalitis may present occasionally in infancy or early childhood, and rubella virus has been isolated from the cerebrospinal fluid (CSF), which may contain raised protein levels and show pleocytosis (Desmond *et al.* 1967). Infection at this site may be a factor causing further damage to the nervous system. The chronic nature of congenital rubella is demonstrated by the small number of individuals with congenital rubella in whom severe progressive neurologic disease resembling subacute sclerosing panencephalitis (SSPE) of measles has been reported in the second decade of life (Johnson 1975; Townsend *et al.* 1975). The clinical features of this disorder are characterized by progressive cerebellar ataxia, spasticity, mental retardation, and seizures. In one case, rubella virus was isolated from the brain, and high levels of antibody were present in the CSF (Weil *et al.* 1975). The panencephalitis and severe degeneration of the white matter are similar to the lesions seen in SSPE, but in rubella encephalitis, vascular deposits are also observed (Singer *et al.* 1967).

## DIAGNOSIS

In the newborn period, a diagnosis of congenital rubella depends on isolation of the virus from urine or nasopharynx or by the demonstration of IgM-specific antibodies. Serological tests for rubella-specific IgG are of little value at this age because no distinction can be made between maternal and fetal antibody. The test should therefore be repeated at 6–8 months, when maternal antibody will have declined. Prenatal diagnosis has been attempted by direct puncture of the umbilical cord with determination of rubella-specific IgM on fetal blood prior to 18 weeks of gestation (Daffos *et al.* 1984), with the recommendation for termination of pregnancy in some cases based on these results.

## PREVENTION

With the development of live attenuated rubella vaccines, rubella in pregnancy has become a preventable condition. There are two possible strategies for vaccination. The first involves the immunization of all infants of both sexes to eliminate the risk of exposure of pregnant women to rubella by interrupting the transmission of infection among children. The second involves selective immunization of adolescent girls to eliminate the risk of rubella occurring in pregnancy. This strategy does not aim to interrupt the transmission of infection within the population, but to 'mop up' those who have escaped childhood infection. This approach allows for the boosting of vaccine-induced antibody by circulating virus. Universal immunization, the policy adopted in the USA in 1969, has a more immediate effect on the prevention of congenital rubella, but there is a potential danger. If high rates of vaccine coverage are not achieved and maintained, the program may slow the rate of viral transmission, thereby increasing the peak age of infection with an increase in the proportion of susceptible women of child-bearing age (Panagiotopoulos *et al.* 1999).

The success of current policies in countries using the rubella vaccine has been considerable. In the UK, rubella vaccine was introduced in 1970 for schoolgirls between 11 and 14 years of age. This was soon extended to include susceptible women of childbearing age, particularly those working with children. Pregnant women found to be susceptible to rubella were offered vaccine postpartum. In 1988, the program was extended to include measles, mumps, and rubella (MMR) vaccine for both boys and girls in their second year of life. Since the introduction of rubella vaccine, there has been a marked decline in notifications of congenital rubella and terminations of pregnancy for maternal rubella (Miller *et al.* 1997). However, the need for continued surveillance is essential, as demonstrated by the small increase in cases of congenital rubella reported in 1997 to the UK surveillance scheme following a rise in cases among young adults (Tookey & Peckham 1999).

## PARVOVIRUS INFECTION

Maternal B19 infection may present with a generalized maternal rash clinically identical to that of rubella. Fetal exposure to maternal parvovirus infection in the first 20 weeks of pregnancy can lead to intrauterine death with an excess risk of about 9%, and if infection occurs between 9 and 20 weeks' gestation, there is a 3% risk of hydrops fetalis (Miller *et al.* 1998). Although fetal infection occurs in 20–50% of exposed infants (Koch *et al.* 1994; Miller *et al.* 1998), the proportion increasing with increasing gestational age, there is no evidence of B19-associated congenital abnormality in the newborn or developmental abnormalities appearing later in childhood.

## CYTOMEGALOVIRUS INFECTION

CMV is one of the herpes group of viruses, which includes HSV, V–Z virus and the Epstein–Barr virus. A characteristic of the herpes virus group is the ability to establish latent infection after a primary infection. Periodic episodes of reactivation can occur throughout life. CMV is the most common cause of congenital viral infection. The incidence of congenital CMV infection varies in different parts of the world from 0.2 to 2.2% of live births with no evidence for a seasonal variation (Stagno *et al.* 1983). As maternal infections are nearly always asymptomatic, and over 90% of congenitally infected infants have no clinically recognizable signs of infection at birth, the vast majority of congenital infections pass unrecognized. Initial studies, largely based on children admitted to hospital, suggested that the prevalence of defects associated with congenital infection was high (Weller & Hanshaw 1964; McCracken *et al.* 1969). However, in subsequent large prospective studies, where children were systematically screened for congenital CMV, the incidence of adverse sequelae at follow-up was not as high as originally estimated (Ahlfors *et al.* 1979; Saigal *et al.* 1982; Peckham *et al.* 1983). Congenital CMV disease can occur following fetal exposure throughout pregnancy, although it appears that severe adverse neurologic outcome may be greater when a primary maternal infection occurs before 27 weeks' gestation.

It has been estimated that 33 000 infants are born with congenital CMV in the USA each year (Stagno & Whitley 1985) and 1800 in England and Wales (Preece *et al.* 1984). Fewer than 10% of congenitally infected infants are symptomatic at birth (Hanshaw & Dudgeon 1978), but the risk of CNS damage in this group is high. The majority will present with visual, cognitive, or auditory sequelae. Of the remaining 90% of children with no apparent symptoms or signs of CMV at birth, the prognosis is much better, and only 10–15% will develop long-term neurological sequelae.

### SYMPTOMATIC CONGENITAL INFECTION

The clinical manifestations of congenital infection at birth include pneumonitis, prolonged neonatal jaundice, hepatomegaly, splenomegaly, petechiae, low birthweight, microcephaly, and thrombocytopenia, and periventricular intracranial calcifications may be present also. On follow-up, symptomatic neonates are almost invariably found to have permanent brain damage, which may include signs of cerebral palsy, epilepsy, mental retardation, chorio-retinitis, optic atrophy, delayed psychomotor development, expressive language delay, and learning disability. Sensorineural deafness is the most frequent defect.

likely to be due to direct damage by HIV, rather than secondary to reactivated opportunistic infections such as toxoplasma, which are more common in HIV-infected adults (Epstein *et al.* 1987). However, the incidence of neurologic disease in vertically infected children is not known with precision, and heterogeneity in findings from different studies is common.

HIV encephalopathy is an AIDS indicator disease. It may present with developmental delay or loss of milestones in young children, cognitive impairment, axial hypotonia, and abnormal reflexes in infants, impairment of expressive language over receptive language in 2–4-year-old children, and behavioral abnormalities with loss of concentration and memory in the older child (Brouwers *et al.* 1991). A characteristic facial appearance has been described as an alert, wide-eyed expression with a paucity of spontaneous facial movements (Belman 1990). Progressive motor signs, particularly spastic diplegia and oral motor dysfunction, are a marked feature, particularly in early-onset encephalopathy (Epstein *et al.* 1986). Ataxia, mononeuropathies, and convulsions also may occur but are less common.

Non-progressive encephalopathy has been reported in approximately 25% of HIV-infected children, although some of these children later develop progressive neurologic deterioration. Many children with progressive encephalopathy have an episodic course, with periods of deterioration interrupted by periods of relative neurological stability. In others, neurologic deterioration occurs more rapidly (over a period of a few months), resulting in mental impairment and quadriparesis (Belman *et al.* 1988).

The exact timing and mechanism of HIV invasion into the CNS in infants and children are not known. In the early form of HIV encephalopathy, invasion of the CNS has probably occurred early in the infection, possibly *in utero*. At the onset of encephalopathy, affected infants usually already have other severe clinical manifestations of HIV infection and profound immunodeficiency (European Collaborative Study 1991). Basal ganglia calcification seen on computerized axial tomography or magnetic resonance scanning may be present as early as 2–3 months of age. Cerebral atrophy and ventricular dilatation are other features of the scan that usually develop later. In most patients, motor impairment remains more severe than intellectual impairment (Belman *et al.* 1988).

CNS manifestations also can be due to infections by other pathogens, cerebral abscess, or lymphoma. Primary CNS B-cell lymphoma have been reported in HIV-infected children, but is rare. Systemic lymphoma with brain metastases, and leukaemia with epidural infiltration, are other possible causes of malignant CNS complications and can be excluded by radiology. Analysis of the CSF is rarely helpful in the diagnosis of encephalopathy but may be useful in excluding other conditions.

It may be difficult to differentiate signs of early encephalopathy from poor functioning due to chronic illness and poor social and emotional circumstances, particularly in the older child where memory loss, poor concentration and behavioral changes may predominate. Confounding gestational and postnatal factors include *in utero* exposure to drugs, maternal illness during pregnancy, the child's nutritional status, chronic infections, and frequent or prolonged hospitalization. Regular monitoring of the child's neurodevelopment is an important part of management for children with HIV infection.

Based on 392 infected children enrolled in two European prospective studies of infants born to HIV-infected women, HIV disease progression in the first 6 years of life was documented, using the 1994 CDC paediatric HIV classification. Most children had developed minor or moderately severe illness in the first 4 years of life, although usually, it was transient in nature. Progression to AIDS or death was estimated to be between 16 and 24% in the first year of life, and between 3.5 and 6.5% annually thereafter, reaching a cumulative incidence of 36% by 6 years (Fig. 32.1). A quarter of infected children had died before the age of 6. Rapid progression to serious disease was associated with encephalopathy. The proportion of children who developed encephalopathy was similar in the two studies, although the diagnosis tended to be made earlier in the French cohort than in the European Collaborative Study (French Paediatric HIV Infection Study Group and European Collaborative Study 1997). None of the children were treated at an early stage.

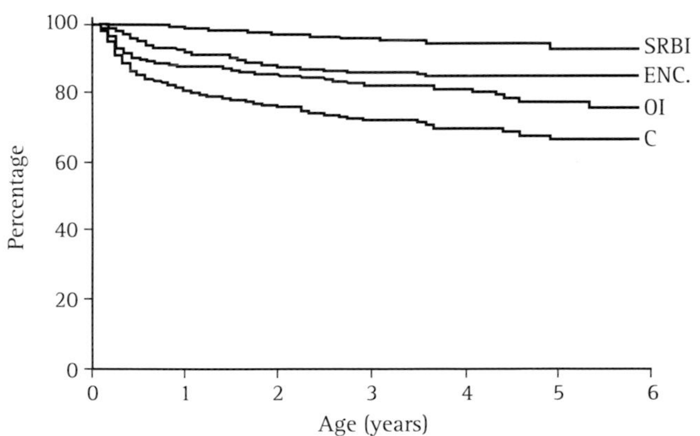


**Figure 32.1** Progression to serious disease in vertically HIV-infected children. SRBI = serious recurrent bacterial infections, ENC = encephalopathy, OI = opportunistic infections, C = all C-defining illness (French Pediatric HIV infection group and European Collaborative Study, 1997).

## DIAGNOSIS

The serological diagnosis of HIV infection in an infant born to an HIV-infected mother is problematic due to the passive transfer of maternal HIV antibodies. These antibodies may persist until well into the second year of life, although infection can be excluded in about half of the uninfected children by 10 months of life (European Collaborative Study 1991).

However, an earlier diagnosis of HIV infection can now be made using methods such as virus isolation, or the polymerase chain reaction (PCR) (Consensus Workshop on Early Diagnosis of HIV Infection 1992). It has been shown that nearly all vertically infected children, in non-breast-feeding populations, will have a positive DNA PCR test by 2 weeks of age (Dunn *et al.* 1995). RNA PCR, which measures quantitatively replicating virus, is also a sensitive diagnostic tool in infants suspected of being HIV-infected. In experienced hands, and using a multiplicity of tests, a diagnosis can usually be reached by 2 months. However, for most children, even in developed countries, diagnosis is still usually confirmed by the persistence or disappearance of antibodies beyond 15 or 18 months of age.

### THERAPY

With increased knowledge about the dynamics of HIV infection, antiretroviral therapy to delay progression of disease is now commonly initiated at an earlier stage in the infection (Centers for Disease Control and Prevention 1998). Antiretroviral therapy is complemented by supportive care and the prevention, and treatment, of opportunistic infections.

A range of drugs are currently available for use in children including the nucleoside reverse transcriptase inhibitors (NRTI) AZT (zidovudine), ddl, 3TC (lamivudine) and d4T (stavudine), the protease inhibitors (PI) saquinavir, nelfinavir, and retonavir, and the non-nucleoside reverse transcriptase inhibitors (NNRTI) such as nevirapine. It is recognized that monotherapy with any one of these drugs is no longer the recommended approach, and usually, two or three drugs are given in combination (two NRTIs with one PI or one NNRTI). The optimal therapeutic combination and timing of initiation are not clearly determined, and experience with the Pls and NNRTIs in children is limited (Bernardi *et al.* 2000). Strict adherence to complex triple therapy regimens is needed to avoid the development of viral resistance.

## LYMPHOCYTIC CHORIOMENINGITIS VIRUS

Lymphocytic choriomeningitis virus (LCMV) is acquired principally from rodents and has been described as a 'neglected pathogen of man' (Jahrling & Peters 1992). Mice and hamsters have been the most frequently implicated sources of infection, and apparently healthy animals may shed the virus in feces and urine for months (Smadel & Wall 1942). A survey conducted in an urban area in the USA between 1984 and 1989 discovered a seroprevalence of about 13% of LCMV antibody among house mice trapped from one inner-city residential site (Childs *et al.* 1992). Serosurveys on healthy humans have demonstrated rates of between 2 and 5% – the variation being ascribed to geographic differences in exposure to infected mice (Stephenson *et al.* 1992).

It is not widely appreciated that, like other arenaviruses, LCMV is a significant and undiagnosed fetal pathogen: there have been reports of LCMV infection in pregnancy associated either with abortion or hydrocephalus, and with chorioretinitis in surviving infants (Sheinbergas 1976; Sheinbergas *et al.* 1984). Perinatal acquisition from a mother infected at full term associated with neonatal meningitis has also been described (Komrower *et al.* 1955).

In recent years, a number of proven cases of congenital infection have been reported (Wright *et al.* 1997; Barton *et al.* 1999; Enders *et al.* 1999). In a series of 33 infected infants described in the US by Barton & Mets (1999), symptomatic maternal illness was documented in half, and there was known rodent exposure in one-third. Chorioretinitis, microcephaly or macrocephaly, and hydrocephalus were seen in the vast majority of infected infants, and 75% of the children had neurologic sequelae. LCM virus infection is an unrecognized cause of congenital disease that mimics congenital toxoplasmosis and congenital CMV infection. A diagnosis of congenital infection should be considered in infants with hydrocephalus and/or chorioretinitis, especially if there is a history of a severe influenza-like illness in pregnancy and/or of rodent contact. Although no specific drug treatment is available, a diagnosis is helpful in the further management of the child.

The diagnosis of infection is made by isolation of the virus, by the detection of the nucleic acid using PCR, or by serological tests. Both enzyme-linked immunosorbent assay (ELISA) and immunofluorescent antibody tests have been developed to detect LCMV-specific IgG and IgM (Stephenson *et al.* 1992; Larsen *et al.* 1993) and may be positive as early as the first day of symptoms.

## ENTEROVIRUSES

The enteroviruses include polioviruses 1–3, echoviruses 1–34, coxsackieviruses A1–24, coxsackieviruses B1–6, and the recently identified enteroviruses 68–71. The most recently classified enterovirus, type 72, is hepatitis A virus. Following infection, enteroviruses are excreted in feces and are present in the pharynx – often for several weeks. Spread, therefore, is principally via the fecal–oral route and also, to a lesser extent, by droplets or aerosols from coughing or sneezing.

Although hepatitis A has rarely been implicated in congenital infections (Leikin *et al.* 1996), isolated cases have been reported.

Hepatitis E (HEV) is a small RNA virus. Like hepatitis A, it is transmitted oro-fecally, is endemic in parts of all developing countries, and causes acute viral hepatitis. The course of the disease is usually benign with production of protective antibodies, and little risk of chronic infection and cirrhosis. However, in pregnant women, HEV is associated with a high rate of fulminant hepatitis (Hamid *et al.* 1996; Hussaini *et al.* 1997), which is often fatal in developing countries. Immune serum globulins have not been found to be effective for prevention (Arankalle *et al.* 1998), and transmission of HEV has been observed but is thought to be unusual. In a study from India (Khuroo *et al.* 1995), six of eight babies born to mothers infected with hepatitis E during the third trimester had evidence of hepatitis E infection, and two of them died within 24 h. However, the incidence of vertical transmission and the clinical course of congenital HEV infection remain to be determined.

## NON-POLIO ENTEROVIRUSES

Although transplacental transmission of echoviruses and coxsackieviruses occurs (because of the viremia that can accompany these infections), there is no published evidence of an association with CNS malformations. One survey demonstrated three cases of intrauterine echoviral disease in which all three fetuses died (Garcia *et al.* 1990). The virus was isolated from multiple fetal organs, including brain, in two of these cases. There were no macroscopic abnormalities; however, the histologic appearance was not described. All of the mothers had been asymptomatic, and it is likely that congenital infection with these viruses is under-recognized, although transplacental passage is thought not to occur readily (Amstey *et al.* 1988).

The importance of enteroviral infections lies in their effects on the neonate, which include meningitis and encephalitis. Enteroviral illness presenting in the first 5 days of life will almost certainly have been acquired from the mother, transplacentally or intranatally. The risk of an infected mother transmitting to her infant is probably high (29–56%) (Modlin & Kinney 1987). Infections occurring later are likely to have been nosocomially acquired, and outbreaks in hospital nurseries have been well documented (Nagington *et al.* 1983). Transmission is thought to be via virus on the hands of health-care personnel, the source being themselves or another infected infant (Sutherland 1992).

### EPIDEMIOLOGY

Enteroviruses accounted for 94% of cases of neonatal viral meningitis in England and Wales reported between 1975 and 1992 (Public Health Laboratory Service 1993, unpublished data). The mean annual total number of cases in England and Wales reported by laboratories between 1975 and 1992 was 14 (range 3–31), and between 1990 and 1999, 40 cases were reported.

In a 2-year prospective survey of infantile meningitis in England and Wales between 1985 and 1987, viruses accounted for 16 cases (4%) of neonatal meningitis (de Louvois *et al.* 1991).

In a review of 177 cases of neonatal meningitis treated at a center in Texas over a 15-year period (1974–1988), Shattuck & Chonmaitree (1992) reported that while the incidence of bacterial meningitis had decreased, that of aseptic meningitis had remained stable; the diagnosis of enteroviral meningitis increased in frequency. Between 1984 and 1988, these organisms were the commonest causes of meningitis in neonates older than 7 days and accounted for one-third of all cases of neonatal meningitis.

### CLINICAL FEATURES AND DIAGNOSIS

Enterovirus infections may be subclinical, mild, and non-specific, or may present with fever, rashes, generalized hemorrhagic features, respiratory illness, gastroenteritis, myocarditis, hepatitis, and pancreatitis. In addition, all enterovirus types can invade the meninges and CNS, although coxsackievirus B types are more likely to be the cause of encephalitis.

The clinical diagnosis of neonatal viral meningitis is difficult because the symptoms are non-specific and may resemble those of bacterial sepsis (Wilfert *et al.* 1983). Fever, anorexia, lethargy, jaundice, vomiting and, occasionally, apnea, tremors, increased tone, and seizures may occur. CSF examination is not always helpful because the changes can overlap those of bacterial meningitis; for example, polymorphonuclear leukocytosis and hypoglycorrhachia may be present. Diagnostic suspicion would be heightened if: (1) there was a recent pre- or postpartum maternal history of a non-specific febrile illness often accompanied by upper respiratory symptoms or abdominal pain; or one of the more characteristic enteroviral syndromes such as aseptic meningitis or hand, foot and mouth disease; (2) there was a history of such an illness in neonatal nursery staff, or family members; (3) there was a concurrent enteroviral epidemic in the nursery or community; (4) the season of onset in a temperate climate was in late summer or autumn (although these infections can occur all year round).

### LABORATORY DIAGNOSIS

Laboratory diagnosis depends principally on virus isolation and can be undertaken only in laboratories with tissue-culture facilities. Isolation from CSF provides conclusive diagnostic evidence of enteroviral NNVM, but the organism may be present for only a short time (Spector & Straube 1983). It is important, therefore, to take specimens from multiple sites. Virus can be isolated from nose, throat, urine, and buffy coat, but excretion persists for the longest time in stools. One practical difficulty with virus isolation is that it may be a week or more before a definitive result can be given.

The large number of possible serotypes and the need to examine acute and convalescent sera contemporaneously mean that serologic antibody studies to identify specific enteroviral infections are impractical. However, examination of paired sera may be useful in an outbreak where one particular prevalent enterovirus is suspected. Assays to measure enterovirus-specific IgM have been developed (Day *et al.* 1989; Glimaker *et al.* 1992) to provide a rapid, non-specific diagnosis of acute enteroviral infection. As an adjunct to virologic investigation, one survey found the complete blood count differential profile a useful means of distinguishing bacterial from viral meningitis in neonates (Bonadio & Smith 1989).

## MANAGEMENT AND PREVENTION

Management of neonatal meningitis and encephalitis is mainly non-specific and directed towards correction of fever, fluid and electrolyte balance, convulsions, and cerebral edema. Steroids are not advised (Cherry 1990). Human normal immunoglobulin (HNIG) has been used for both therapy and prevention in outbreaks of enterovirus infection in neonatal nurseries (Nagington *et al.* 1983). However, its effectiveness has has been debated, and it has not been formally evaluated. Its efficacy may depend on the titer of the appropriate neutralizing antibody in the HNIG and on its early administration (Kinney *et al.* 1986). In severe cases, a high-dose preparation should be given intravenously (Cherry 1990). A single dosage of 750 mg/kg has been recommended for neonates in whom any type of overwhelming infection is suspected (Hill 1993). It can be repeated in 5–7 days if an adequate response is not observed. For prophylaxis, intramuscular HNIG at standard dosages should be used; it would be indicated for sudden and virulent nursery outbreaks of enteroviral infection.

As non-polio enteroviral vaccines are not available, prevention is principally directed towards control of spread of infection (Kinney *et al.* 1986; Cherry 1990; Sutherland 1992). Any hospitalized infant with a known or suspected enterovirus infection should be isolated and strict enteric precautions taken. Staff and parents should not enter the nursery if they develop a feverish illness. In nosocomial outbreaks, cohorting of infants and personnel should be undertaken.

## NEUROLOGIC SEQUELAE

Enteroviral meningitis acquired early in infancy may result in long-term neurodevelopmental sequelae. It is difficult to compare results of different follow-up studies because of the different methods used. Some studies do not use appropriate controls, some are restricted to infection acquired in the neonatal period (Farmer *et al.* 1975), while others include infection acquired at any time during the first year of life (Sells *et al.* 1975; Wilfert *et al.* 1981; Chamberlain *et al.* 1983). Different viral types, degrees of severity of the initial illnesses, lengths of follow-up, and methods of assessment of neurologic and developmental outcome also make comparisons difficult. There is little information from well-conducted large studies on the long-term outcome because the condition is rare.

However, in a 6-year follow-up study of neonatally acquired coxsackievirus B meningoencephalitis, two of three infants with neurologic symptoms during their acute illness had severe neurodevelopmental sequelae, whereas the physical development, intelligence, and visual perception of the 12 without such symptoms was similar to controls (Farmer *et al.* 1975). In another study, 45 of 48 survivors of infant viral meningitis (40 enteroviral) followed for more than 5 years were in normal schools, but their mean performance IQ was 6 points lower than that of the matched controls (Chamberlain *et al.* 1983). Although this difference was statistically significant, its practical significance is questionable. The other three survivors had severe sequelae, but only one had had an enteroviral infection. In a third, controlled study of infants infected in the first 3 months of life and followed for 4 years, there were no differences in the IQ, but their receptive language functioning was significantly lower than the controls (Wilfert *et al.* 1981). This substantiated an earlier study in which delayed language and speech development was the only consistent problem observed (Sells *et al.* 1975).

Bergman *et al.* (1987) compared 33 survivors of enteroviral NNVM in infancy with their siblings. None had any major neurological sequelae, and there was no evidence of any more subtle psychomotor defects. The six cases identified in the Oxford regional survey (Hristeva *et al.* 1993) were followed for between 3 months and 3 years and had no discernible sequelae.

Although the evidence for long-term sequelae is conflicting, it seems reasonable to conclude that children with a history of enteroviral neonatal meningitis/encephalitis need careful surveillance in their preschool years.

# POLIOVIRUS INFECTION

The World Health Organization's goal for the global eradication of poliomyelitis by the end of 2000 is rapidly becoming a reality. A strategy of national immunization days has been successful in reducing the incidence of poliomyelitis to very low levels with few cases of polio now being reported, even in low-income countries.

The incidence of neonatal poliomyelitis in the pre-vaccine era is not known but is thought to be uncommon because of protection provided by maternal polioviral antibodies. Of 182 cases of paralytic disease admitted to hospital during an epidemic in Delhi in 1971, the youngest was 2 months but the 7–12-month group accounted for one-third of all the cases (Sehgal & Oberoi 1977). Nevertheless, paralytic poliomyelitis presenting in the first month of life and acquired perinatally is well documented (Bates 1955; Sathy *et al.* 1984).

## CLINICAL FEATURES AND DIAGNOSIS

There is no evidence to suggest that transplacentally transmitted poliovirus causes malformations (Cherry 1990). Furthermore, while live virus vaccine is contraindicated in pregnancy, there is no evidence to suggest that polio vaccine causes fetal malformations or neonatal disease (Harjulehto *et al.* 1989; Cherry 1990), although one report described irreparable damage to the anterior horn cells of a 20-week-old fetus whose mother was immune to poliomyelitis before conceiving, but who was inadvertently given an oral polio vaccine (OPV) at 18 weeks of gestation (Burton *et al.* 1984).

Poliomyelitis presenting in the first 5 days of life is likely to have been acquired transplacentally or intranatally. It has been estimated that the risk of an infant developing the infection when born to a woman with clinical disease at delivery is 40% (Wyatt 1979). Although asymptomatic neonatal infection probably occurs, most case reports describe severe disease resulting in death (about 50% of cases) or residual paralysis (about 50% of survivors). Fever, listlessness, dysphagia, and flaccid paralysis should suggest the diagnosis, which can be confirmed by viral isolation. Suitable specimens would be nose and throat swabs, stool, blood, and CSF; antibody tests can be undertaken on paired sera. Non-polio enteroviruses should be excluded as coxsackieviruses B and enterovirus 71 can also cause paralytic disease (Chonmaitree *et al.* 1981; Cherry 1990).

## MANAGEMENT AND PREVENTION

Management and prevention are as described for the non-polio enteroviruses with the addition of positive-pressure ventilation if respiratory paralysis occurs. Survivors will require a full course of immunization against poliomyelitis because the serotype with which they have been infected does not prevent subsequent infection with the other two. The principal thrust towards prevention of neonatal poliomyelitis is, of course, the World Health Organization's target of global eradication of this infection by the year 2000.

### Key Points

- Viruses remain important pathogens for neonatal CNS disease.
- The frequent lack of maternal history and the non-specific presentations make the differential diagnosis difficult.
- Improved laboratory tests are becoming available that make a rapid diagnosis more feasible, and with the development of antiviral drugs, it will become increasingly important to initiate therapy as early as possible in the course of the infection to reduce the incidence of serious neurologic sequelae.
- Vaccines for some of these virus infections are under development and offer scope for prevention, and the success of the polio eradication program is encouraging.

## REFERENCES


Adler S P, Chandrika T, Lawrence L *et al.* (1983) Cytomegalovirus infections in neonates acquired by blood transfusions. *Pediatr Infect Dis* 2:114–118.

Ahlfors K, Ivarsson S, Johnsson T *et al.* (1979) A prospective study on congenital and acquired cytomegalovirus infections in infants. *Scand J Infect Dis* 11:177–178.

Ahlfors K, Ivarsson S-A, Harris S (1999) Report on a long-term study of maternal and congenital cytomegalovirus infection in Sweden. Review of prospective studies available in the literature. *Scand J Infect Dis* 31:443–457.

Amstey M S, Miller R K, Menegus M A *et al.* (1988) Enterovirus in pregnant women and the perfused placenta. *Am J Obstet Gynecol* 158:775–782.

Ando Y, Kakimoto K, Ekuni Y *et al.* (1992) HHV-6 infection during pregnancy and spontaneous abortion. *Lancet* 340:1289.

Arankalle V A, Chadha M S, Dama B M *et al.* (1998) Role of immune serum globulins in pregnant women during an epidemic of hepatitis E. *J Viral Hepat* 5:199–204.

Arvin A M, Yeager A S, Bruhn F W *et al.* (1982) Neonatal herpes simplex infection in the absence of mucocutaneous lesions. *J Pediatr* 100:715–721.

Aubin J-T, Poirel L, Agut Henri *et al.* (1992) Intrauterine transmission of human herpesvirus 6. *BMJ* 340:482–483.

Ballard R A, Drew W L & Hutnagle K (1979) Cytomegalovirus infection in preterm infants. *Am J Dis Children* 133:482–485.

Barton L L & Mets (1999) Lymphocytic choriomeningitis virus: pediatric pathogen and fetal teratogen. *Pediatr Infect Dis J* 18:540–541.

Bates T (1955) Polio in pregnancy, the fetus and the newborn. *Am J Dis Children* 90:189–195.

Belman A L (1990) AIDS and pediatric neurology. *Neurol Clin* 8:571–603.

Belman A L, Diamond G, Dickson D *et al.* (1988) Paediatric acquired immunodeficiency syndrome. *Am J Dis Children* 142:29–35.

Bergman I, Painter M J, Wald E R *et al.* (1987) Outcome in children with enteroviral meningitis during the first year of life. *J Pediatr* 110:705.

Bernardi S, Thorne C, Newell M L *et al.* (2000) The use of therapeutic interventions for children with HIV-1 infection in Europe. *Eur J Padediatr* 159:170–175.

Bonadio W A & Smith D S (1989) CBC differential profile in distinguishing etiology of neonatal meningitis. *Pediatr Emerg Care* 5:94–96.

Boppana S B, Fowler K B, Britt W J *et al.* (1999a) Symptomatic congenital cytomegalovirus infection in infants born to mothers with preexisting immunity to cytomegalovirus. *Pediatrics* 104:55–60.

Boppana S, Pass R F, Jeffries D J *et al.* (eds) (1999b) Cytomegalovirus. In: *Viral infections in obstetrics and gynaecology.* London: Arnold; pp. 35–56.

Boucher F D, Yasukawa L L, Bronzan R N *et al.* (1990) A prospective evaluation of primary genital herpes simplex virus type 2 infections acquired during pregnancy. *Pediatric Infectious Disease Journal* 9:499–504.

Bradford Hill A, Doll R, Galloway T M *et al.* (1958) Virus diseases in pregnancy and congenital defects. *Br J Prevent Social Med* 12:1–7.

Bray P F, Bale J F & Anderson R E (1981) Progressive neurological disease with cytomegalovirus infection. *Ann Neurol* 9:449–502.

Brazin S A, Simkowich J W & Johnson T (1979) Herpes zoster during pregnancy. *Obstet Gynecol* 513:175–181.

Brouwers P, Belman A L & Epstein L G (1991) Central nervous system involvement: manifestations and evaluation. In: Pizzo P A & Wilfert C M (eds) *Pediatric AIDS.* Baltimore, MD: Williams and Wilkins, Chapter 22. pp. 318–335.

Brown Z A, Vontver L A, Benedetti J *et al.* (1987) Effects on infants of a first episode of genital herpes during pregnancy. *N Engl J Med* 317:1246–1250.

Brown Z A, Selke S, Zeh J *et al.* (1997) The acquisition of herpes simplex virus during pregnancy. *N Engl J Med* 337:509–515.

Brunell P A (1967) Varicella zoster infections in pregnancy. *JAMA* 199:315–317.

Burton A E, Robinson E T & Harper W F (1984) Fetal damage after accidental polio vaccination of an immune mother. *J Roy College Gen Prac* 34:390–393.

Centers for Disease Control and Prevention (1998) Guidelines for the use of anti-retroviral agents in pediatric HIV infection. *Morbid Mortal Weekly Rec* 47:1–43.

Chamberlain R N, Christie P N & Holt K S (1983) A study of school children who had identified virus infections of the central nervous system during infancy. *Child Care Health Dev* 9:29–47.

Cherry J D (1990) Enteroviruses. In: Remington J S & Klein J (eds) *Infectious diseases of the fetus and newborn infant.* Philadelphia, PA: W B Saunders, 3rd edn; pp. 326–366.

Chess S (1971) Autism in children with congenital rubella. *J Autism Childhood Schizophr* 1:33–47.

Childs J E, Glass G E, George W *et al.* (1992) Lymphocytic choriomeningitis virus infection and house mouse (*Mus musculus*) distribution in urban Baltimore. *Am J Trop Med Hyg* 47:27–34.

Chonmaitree T, Menegus M A, Schervish-Swierkosz E M *et al.* (1981) Enterovirus 71 infection: report of an outbreak with two cases of paralysis and a review of the literature. *Pediatrics* 67:489–492.

Committee on Fetus and Newborn (1980) Perinatal herpes simplex virus infection. *Pediatrics* 66:147–148.

Conboy T, Pass R, Stagno S *et al.* (1986) Intellectual development in school-aged children with asymptomatic congenital cytomegalovirus infection. *Pediatrics* 77:801–806.

Consensus Workshop for Early Diagnosis of HIV Infection (1992) *J Aquired Immune Defic Syndr* 5:1169–1178.

Corey L & Spear P G (1986) Infections with herpes simplex viruses. *N Engl J Med* 314:749–757.

Daffos F, Forestier F, Grangeot-Keros L *et al.* (1984) Prenatal diagnosis of congenital rubella. *Lancet* ii:1–3.

Dahle A J, McCoflister F P, Stagno S *et al.* (1979) Progressive hearing impairment in children with congenital cytomegalovirus infection. *J Speech Hearing Disord* 44:220–229.

Davis G L (1981) *In vitro* models of viral-induced congenital deafness. *Am J Otolaryngol* 3:156–160.

Day C, Cumming H & Walker J (1989) Enterovirus-specific IgM in the diagnosis of meningitis. *J Infect* 19:219–228.

de Louvois J, Blackbourne J, Hurley R, Harvey D (1991) Infantile meningitis in England and Wales: a two year study. *Arch Dis Child* 66:603–607.

Desmond M M, Wilson G S, Melrick J J *et al.* (1967) Congenital rubella encephalitis. *J Pediatr* 71:311–331.

Dudgeon J A (1976) Congenital rubella. *Br Med Bull* 32:77–83.

Dunn D T, Brandt C D, Krivine A *et al.* (1995) The sensitivity of HIV-1 DNA polymerase chain reaction in the neonatal period and the relative contributions of intra-uterine and intra-partum transmission. *AIDS* 9:F7–F11.

Dunne W M & Demmler G J (1992) Serological evidence for congenital transmission of human herpesvirus 6. *Lancet* 340:121–122.

Dworsky M, Whitley R & Alford C (1980) Herpes zoster in early infancy. *Am J Dis Children* 134:619.

Enders G (1984) Varicella-zoster virus infection in pregnancy. *Prog Med Virol* 29:166–196.

Enders G (1985) Varicella zoster virus infection in pregnancy. *Prog Med Virol* 29:166–196.

Enders G, Nickerl-Pacher U, Miller E *et al.* (1988) Outcome of confirmed periconceptional maternal rubella. *Lancet* i:1445–1447.

Enders G, Miller E, Cradock-Watson J *et al.* (1994) Consequences of varicella and herpes zoster in pregnancy: prospective study of 1739 cases. *Lancet* 343:1548–1551.

Enders G, Varho-Gobel M, Lohler J *et al.* (1999) Congenital lymphocytic choriomeningitis virus infection: an underdiagnosed disease. *Pediatr Infect Dis J* 18:652–655.

Epstein L G, Leroy R, Sharer L R *et al.* (1986) Neurological manifestations of human immunodeficiency virus infection. *Pediatrics* 78:678–687.

Epstein L G, Goudsmit J, Paul D A *et al.* (1987) Expression of human immunodeficiency virus in cerebrospinal fluid of children with progressive encephalopathy. *Ann Neurol* 21:397–401.

European Collaborative Study (1991) Children born to women with HIV-1 infection: natural history and risk of transmission. *Lancet* 337:253–260.

European Collaborative Study (1999) Maternal viral load and vertical transmission of HIV-1: an important factor but not the only one. *Aids* 13:1377–1385.

European Mode of Delivery Collaboration (1999) Elective caesarean-section versus vaginal delivery in prevention of vertical HIV-1 transmission: a randomised clinical study. *Lancet* 353:1714.

Farmer K, MacArthur B A, Clay M M (1975) A follow-up study of 15 cases of neonatal meningoencephalitis due to Coxsackie virus B5. *J Pediatr* 87:568–571.

Fischler B, Rodensjö, Nemeth A *et al.* (1999) Cytomegalovirus DNA detection on Guthrie cards in patients with neonatal cholestasis. *Arch Dis Children Fetal Neonatal Edition* 80:F130–F134.

Forsgren M (1990) Genital herpes simple virus infection and incidence of neonatal disease in Sweden. *Scand J Infect Dis Suppl* 69:37–41.

Fowler K B, Stagno P H S, Pass R F *et al.* (1992) The outcome of congenital cytomegalovirus infection in relation to maternal antibody status. *N Engl J Med* 326:663–667.

Fowler K B, Dable A J, Boppana S B *et al.* (1999) Newborn hearing screening: Will children with hearing loss caused by congenital cytomegalovirus infection be missed. *J Pediatr* 135:60–64.

French Pediatric HIV Infection Study Group and European Collaborative Study (1997) Morbidity and Mortality in European Children vertically infected by HIV-1. *J AIDS Hum Retrovirol* 14:442–450.

Garcia A G P (1963) Fetal infection in chickenpox and alastrim, with histopathologic study of the placenta. *Pediatrics* 32:895–901.

Garcia A G P, Basso N G D S, Fonseca M E F *et al.* (1990) Congenital Echo virus infection morphological and virological study of fetal and placental tissue. *J Pathol* 160:123–127.

Garnet G P, Cox M J, Bundy D A *et al.* (1993) The age of infection with varicella-zoster virus in St Lucia, West Indies. *Epidemiol Infect* 110:361–372.

Gershon A A (1990) Chickenpox, measles and mumps. In: Remington J S & Klein J O (eds) *Infectious diseases of the fetus and newborn infant.* Philadelphia, PA: W B Saunders; pp. 395–445.

Glimaker M, Samuelson A, Magnius L *et al.* (1992) Early diagnosis of enteroviral meningitis by detection of specific IgM antibodies with a solid-phase reverse immunosorbent test (SPRIST) and mu-capture EIA. *J Med Virol* 36:193–201.

Gray G C, Palinkas L A & Kelley P W (1990) Increasing incidence of varicella hospitalisations in the United States Army and Navy personnel: are today's teenagers becoming more susceptible? Should recruits be vaccinated? *Pediatrics* 86:867–873.

Grilner L, Forsgren M, Barr B *et al.* (1983) Outcome of rubella during pregnancy with special reference to the 17th–24th weeks of gestation. *Scand J Infect Dis* 15:321–325.

Hamid S S, Jafri S M, Khan H *et al.* (1996) Fulminant hepatic failure in pregnant women: acute fatty liver or acute viral hepatitis? *J Hepatol* 25:20–27.

Hammerberg O, Watts J, Chernesky M *et al.* (1983) An outbreak of herpes simplex virus type 1 in an intensive care nursery. *Pediatr Infect Dis* 2:290–294.

Hanshaw J B & Dudgeon J A (1978) Congenital cytomegalovirus. *Major Prob Clin Paediatr* 17:97–152.

Hanshaw J, Scheiner A, Moxley A *et al.* (1976) School failure and deafness after 'silent' congenital cytomegalovirus infection. *N Engl J Med* 295:468–470.

Hanshaw J B, Dudgeon J A & Marshall W C (1985) Congenital cytomegalovirus. In: *Viral diseases of the fetus and newborn.* Philadelphia, PA: W B Saunders; pp. 92–131.

Harjulehto T, Aro T, Hovi T *et al.* (1989) Congenital malformations and oral poliovirus vaccination during pregnancy. *Lancet* i:771–772.

Hayes K, Danks D M, Gila S H *et al.* (1972) Cytomegalovirus in human milk. *N Engl J Med* 287:177–178.

Hill H R (1993) Intravenous immunoglobulin use in the neonate: role in prophylaxis and therapy of infection. *Pediatr Infect Dis J* 12:549–595.

Horstmann D M, Liebhaber H, Le Bouvier G L *et al.* (1970) Rubella: reinfection of vaccinated and naturally immune persons exposed in an epidemic. *N Engl J Med* 283:771–778.

Hristeva L, Booy R, Bowler I *et al.* (1993) Prospective surveillance of neonatal meningitis. *Arch Dis Childhood* 69:14–18.

Hussaini S H, Skidmore S J, Richardson P *et al.* (1997) Severe hepatitis E infection during pregnancy. *J Viral Hepat* 4:51–54.

Hutto C, Arvin A, Jacobs R *et al.* (1987) Intrauterine herpes simplex virus infections. *J Pediatr* 110:97–101.

International Perinatal HIV Group (1999) The mode of delivery and the risk of vertical transmission of HIV-1 – a meta analysis of 15 cohort studies. *N Engl J Med* 340:997–987.

Jahrling P B & Peters C J (1992) Lymphocytic choriomeningitis virus. *Arch Pathol Lab Med* 116:486–489.

Johnson R T (1968) Hydrocephalus following viral infection: the pathology of aqueductal stenosis developing after experimental mumps virus infection. *J Neuropathol Exp Neurol* 27:591–606.

Johnson R T (1975) Progressive rubella encephalitis. *N Engl J Med* 292:1023–1024.

Jones C A, Issacs D, McIntyre P *et al.* (1999) In: *Australian Pediatric Surveillance Unit Sixth Annual Report 1998.* Royal Australian College of Physicians.

Khuroo M S, Kamili S & Jameel S (1995) Vertical transmission of hepatitis E virus. *Lancet* 345:1025–1026.

Kinney J S, McCray E & Kaplan J E (1986) Risk factors associated with echovirus 11 infection in a hospital nursery. *Paediatr Infect Dis* 5:192–197.

Knott P D & Welply G A C (1984) Serologically proved intrauterine infection with parvovirus. *BMJ* 289:1660.

Koch W C, Harger J H, Barnstein B *et al.* (1994) Serologic and virologic evidence for frequent intrauterine transmission of human parvovirus B19 with a primary maternal infection during pregnancy. *Pediatr Infect Dis J* 17:489–494.

Komrower G M, Williams B L & Stones P B (1955) Lymphocytic choriomeningitis in the newborn. *Lancet* i:697–698.

Kumar M L, Nankervis G A, Jacobs I B *et al.* (1984) Congenital and postnatally acquired cytomegalovirus infection: long-term follow up. *J Pediatr* 104:674–679.

Laforet E G & Lynch C L (1947) Multiple congenital defects following maternal varicella: report of a case. *N Engl J Med* 236:534–537.

Larsen P D, Chartrand S A, Tomashek K M *et al.* (1993) Hydrocephalus complicating lymphocytic choriomeningitis virus infection. *Pediatr Infect Dis J* 12:528–531.

Leikin E, Lysikiewicz A, Garry D *et al.* (1996) Intrauterine transmission of hepatitis A virus. *Obstet Gynecol* 88:690–691.

Leroy V, Newell M L, Dabis F *et al.* (1998) International multicentre pooled analysis of late postnatal mother-to-child transmission of HIV-1 infection. *Lancet* 352:597–600.

Linneman C C, Buchman T C, Light I J *et al.* (1978) Transmission of herpes simplex virus type I in a nursery for the newborn: identification of viral isolates by DNA 'fingerprinting'. *Lancet* i:964–966.

Logan G S (1993) Personal communication.

McCracken G H, Shinefield M R, Cobb K *et al.* (1969) Congenital cytomegalic inclusion disease: a longitudinal study of 20 patients. *Am J Dis Children* 117:522–539.

Manson M M, Logan W P O & Loy R M (1960) *Rubella and other virus infections in pregnancy. Reports on public health and medical subjects, No. 101.* London: HMSO.

Marshall W C (1973) The clinical impact of intrauterine rubella. In: *Intrauterine infections. Ciba Foundation, 10 (new series).* Amsterdam: Associated Scientific Publishers (Elsevier Excerpta Medica, North Holland); pp. 3–22.

Martin J A M & Moore W J (1979) *Childhood deafness in the European Community. Medicine EUR 6413.* Luxemburg: Commission of the European Communities.

Meyers J D (1974) Congenital varicella in term infants: risk reconsidered. *J Infect Dis* 129:215–217.

Miller E (1990) Rubella reinfection. *Arch Dis Childhood* 65:820–821.

Miller E (1991) Rubella in the United Kingdom. *Epidemiol Infect* 107:31–42.

Miller E, Craddock-Watson J E & Pollock T M (1982) Consequences of confirmed maternal rubella at successive stages of pregnancy. *Lancet* ii:781–784.

Miller E, Cradock-Watson J E & Ridehalgh K S (1989) Outcome in newborn babies given anti-varicella-zoster immunoglobulin after perinatal maternal infection with varicella-zoster virus. *Lancet* ii:371–373.

Miller E, Marshall R & Vurdien J (1993) Epidemiology, outcome and control of varicella-zoster infection. *Rev Med Microbiol* 4:222–230.

Miller E, Vurdien J & Farrington P (1993) Shift in age in chickenpox. *Lancet* 341:308–309.

Miller E, Waight P, Gay N *et al.* (1997) The epidemiology of rubella in England and Wales before and after the 1994 measles and rubella vaccination campaign: fourth joint report from the PHLS and the National Congenital Rubella Surveillance Programme. *Communicable Disease Report 7 review 2,* R26–R32.

Miller E, Fairley C K, Cohen B J *et al.* (1998) Immediate and long term outcome of human parvovirus B19 infection in pregnancy. *BMJ* 105:174–178.

Modlin J F & Kinney J S (1987) Perinatal entrovirus infections. *Adv Paediatr Infect Dis* 2:57–78.

Mouly F, Mirlesse V, Meritet J F *et al.* (1997) Prenatal diagnosis of fetal varicella-zoster virus infection with polymerase chain reaction of amniotic fluid in 107 cases. *Am J Obstet Gynecol* 177:894–898.

Myers E N & Stool S (1968) Cytomegalic inclusion disease of the inner ear. *Laryngoscope* 78:1904–1915.

Nagington J, Walker J, Candy G *et al.* (1983) Use of normal immunoglobulin in an Ecovirus II outbreak in a special care baby unit. *Lancet* ii:443–446.

Nahmias A J, Josey W E, Naib Z M *et al.* (1971) Perinatal risk associated with maternal genital herpes simplex virus infection. *Am J Obstet Gynecol* 110:825–828.

Nahmias A J, Keyserling H H & Kerick G (1983) Herpes simplex. In: Remington J S & Klein J O (eds) *Infectious diseases of the fetus and newborn infant.* Philadelphia, PA: W B Saunders; pp. 156–190.

Ndumbe P M, Macqueen S, Holzel H *et al.* (1985) Immunity to varicella-zoster virus in a normal adult population. *J Med Microbiol* 20:105–111.

Nelson C T, Istas A S, Wilkerson M K *et al.* (1995) PCR detection of cytomegalovirus DNA in serum as a diagnostic test for congenital cytomegalovirus infection. *J Clin Microbiol Dec* 33:3317–3318.

Newell M L (1998) Mechanims and timing of mother-to-child transmission of HIV-1. *AIDS* 12:831–837.

Nigro G, Scholz H & Bartmann U (1994) Ganciclovir therapy for symptomatic congenital cytomegalovirus infection in infants: a two regime experience. *J Pediatr* 124:318–322.

Panagiotopoulos T, Antoniadou I & Adam E V (1999) Increase in congenital rubella occurrence after immunisation in Greece: retrospective survey and systematic review. *BMJ* 319:1462–1466.

Parvey L S & Ch'ien L (1980) Neonatal herpes simplex virus infection introduced by fetal monitor scalp electrodes. *Pediatrics* 65:1150–1153.

Pass R F, Stagno S, Myers G J *et al.* (1980) Outcome of symptomatic congenital cytomegalovirus infection: results of long-term longitudinal follow-up. *Pediatrics* 66:758–762.

Pastuszak A L, Levy M, Schick B *et al.* (1994) Outcome after maternal varicella infection in the first 20 weeks of pregnancy. *N Engl J Med* 13:901–905.

Pearl K, Preece P, Ades A *et al.* (1986) Neurodevelopmental assessment after congenital cytomegalovirus infection. *Arch Dis Childhood* 61:323–326.

Peckham C S (1972) A clinical and laboratory study of children exposed *in utero* to maternal rubella. *Arch Dis Childhood* 47:571–577.

Peckham C S, Martin J A M, Marshall W C *et al.* (1979) Congenital rubella deafness: a preventable disease. *Lancet* i:258–261.

Peckham C S (1985) Congenital rubella in the United Kingdom before 1970: the prevaccine era. *Rev Infect Dis* 7:S11–S16.

Peckham C S (1986) Hearing impairment in childhood. *Br Med Bull* 42:145–149.

Peckham C, Coleman J C, Hurley R, Chin K S, Henderson K (1983) Cytomegalovirus infection in pregnancy: preliminary finding from a prospective study. *Lancet* i:1352–1356.

Peckham C S, Johnson C, Ades A *et al.* (1987) The early acquisition of cytomegalovirus infection. *Arch Dis Childhood* 62:780–785.

PHLS Working Party on Fifth Disease (1990) Propective study of human parvovirus (B19) infection in pregnancy 1990. *Br Med J* 300:1166–1170.

Plotkin S A (1999) Vaccination against cytomegalovirus, the changeling demon. *Pediatr Infect Dis J* 18:313–326.

Preece P, Pearl K & Peckham C (1984) Congenital cytomegalovirus. *Arch Dis Childhood* 59:1120–1126.

Prober C G, Sullender W M, Yasukawa L L *et al.* (1987) Low risk of herpes simplex virus infections in neonates exposed to the virus at the time of vaginal delivery to mothers with recurrent genital herpes simplex virus infections. *N Engl J Med* 316:240–244.

Ramsay M E B, Miller E & Peckham C S (1991) Outcome of confirmed symptomatic congenital cytomegalovirus infection. *Arch Dis Childhood* 66:1068–1069.

Reynolds D W, Stagno S & Stubbs K G (1974) Inapparent congenital cytomegalovirus infection with elevated cord IgM levels. *N Engl J Med* 290:291–296.

Reynolds D W, Stagno S & Mosty T S (1980) Maternal cytomegalovirus excretion and perinatal infection. *N Engl J Med* 302:1073–1076.

Saigal S, Lunyk O, Larke R P B *et al.* (1982) The outcome in children with congenital cytomegalovirus infection. *Am J Dis Children* 136:896–905.

Sathy N, Nair P M, Phillip E *et al.* (1984) Neonatal poliomyelitis. *Indian J Pediatr* 51:413–414.

Sehgal H & Oberoi M (1977) A clinical study of severe form of acute poliomyelitis in children. *Indian J Pediatr* 14:47–52.

Seigel M (1973) Congenital malformations following chickenpox, measles, mumps and hepatitis. *JAMA* 226:1521–1524.

Sells C J, Carpenter R L & Ray C G (1975) Sequelae of central nervous system enterovirus infection. *N Engl J Med* 293:1–4.

Sever J & White L R (1968) Intrauterine viral infections. *Annu Rev Med* 19:471–486.

Shattuck R E & Chonmaitree T (1992) The changing spectrum of neonatal meningitis over a fifteen-year period. *Clin Pediatr* 31:130–136.

Sheinbergas M M (1976) Hydrocephalus due to prenatal infection with lymphocytic choriomeningitis virus. *Infection* 4:185–191.

Sheinbergas M M, Kilchauskiene V V & Tulevichiene J P (1984) Prenatal lymphocytic choriomeningitis (LCM): three new cases. *Infection* 12:65–66.

Singer D B, Rudolph A J, Rosenberg H S *et al.* (1967) Pathology of the congenital rubella syndrome. *J Pediatr* 71:665–675.

Smadel J E & Wall M J (1942) Lymphocytic choriomeningitis in the Syrian hamster. *J Exp Med* 75:581–591.

Spector S A & Straube R C (1983) Protean manifestations of perinatal enterovirus infections. *Western J Med* 138:847–851.

Stagno S & Whitley R J (1985) Herpes virus infections in pregnancy. 1. Cytomegalovirus and Epstein-Barr virus infections. *N Engl J Med* 313:1270–1274.

Stagno S, Reynolds D W & Amos C S (1977) Auditory and visual defects resulting from symptomatic and subclinical cytomegalovirus and toxoplasma infection. *Pediatr* 59:669–678.

Stagno S, Reynolds D W, Pass R F *et al.* (1980) Breast milk and the risk of cytomegalovirus infection. *N Engl J Med* 302:1073–1076.

Stagno S, Brasfield D M & Brown M B (1981) Infant pneumonitis associated with cytomegalovirus, chlamydia, pneumocystis and ureaplasma – a prospective study. *Pediatrics* 68:322–329.

Stagno S, Pass R & Dworsky M (1982) Congenital cytomegalovirus infection: the relative importance of primary and recurrent maternal infection. *N Engl J Med* 306:945–949.

Stagno S, Pass R F, Dworsky M E *et al.* (1983) Congenital and perinatal cytomegalovirus infections. *Semin Perinatol* 7:31–42.

Stephenson C B, Blount S R, Lanford R E *et al.* (1992) Prevalence of serum antibodies against lymphocytic choriomeningitis virus in selected populations from two US cities. *J Med Virol* 38:27–31.

Sutherland S (1992) Enteroviruses. In: Greenough A, Osborne J & Sutherland S (eds) *Congenital, perinatal and neonatal infections.* London: Churchill Livingstone; pp. 63–70.

Tookey P & Peckham C S (1996) Neonatal herpes simplex virus infection in the British Isles. *Paediatr Perinat Epidemiol* 10:432–442.

Tookey P & Peckham C S (1999) Surveillance of congenital rubella in Great Britain, 1971–96. *BMJ* 318:769–770.

Townsend J J, Baringer J R & Wolinsky J S (1975) Progressive rubella parencephalitis: late onset after congenital rubella. *N Engl J Med* 292:990–993.

Weil M L, Habashi H H, Cromer N E *et al.* (1975) Chronic progressive parencephalitis due to rubella virus simulating sclerosing panencephalitis. *N Engl J Med* 292:994–998.

Weller T H & Hanshaw J B (1964) Virologic and clinical observations on cytomegalic inclusion disease. *N Engl J Med* 266:1233–1244.

Whitley R J, Nahmias A J, Soong S J *et al.* (1980a) Vidarabin therapy of neonatal herpes simplex virus infection. *Pediatrics* 66:495–501.

Whitley R J, Nahmias A J, Visintine A M *et al.* (1980b) The natural history of herpes simplex virus infection of mother and newborn. *Pediatrics* 66:489–494.

Whitley R J, Corey L, Arvin A M *et al.* (1988) Changing presentation of herpes simplex virus infection in neonates. *J Infect Dis* 158:109–116.

Whitley R J, Arvin A, Prober C *et al.* (1991) Predictors of morbidity and mortality in neonates with herpes simplex virus infections. *N Engl J Med* 324:450–454.

Whitley R J & Arvin A M (1995) Herpes simplex virus infections. In: Remington J S & Klein J O (eds) *Infectious diseases of the fetus and newborn infant.* Philadelphia, PA. W.B. Saunders; 2nd edn, pp. 354–374.

Whitley R J, Cloud G, Gruber W *et al.* (1997) Ganciclovir Treatment of Symptomatic Congenital Cytomegalovirus Infection: Results of Phase II Study. *J Infect Dis* 175:1080–1086.

Wilfert C M, Thompson R J J, Sunder T R *et al.* (1981) Longitudinal assessment of children with enteroviral meningitis during the first three months of life. *Pediatrics* 67:811–815.

Wilfert C M, Lehrman S N & Katz S L (1983) Enteroviruses and meningitis. *Pediatric Infect Dis* 2:333–341.

Wilkins A, Ricard D, Todd J *et al.* (1993) The epidemiology of HIV infection in a rural area of Guinea-Bissau. *AIDS* 7:1119–1122.

Williams K A B, Scott J M, MacFarlane D E *et al.* (1981) Congenital toxoplasmosis: a prospective survey in the west of Scotland. *J Infect* 3:219–229.

Williamson W D, Desmond M M, LaFevers N *et al.* (1982) Symptomatic congenital cytomegalovirus: disorders of language learning and hearing. *Am J Dis Children* 136:902–905.

Wilson C B, Remington J S, Stagno S *et al.* (1980) Development of adverse sequelae in children born with subclinical congenital toxoplasma infection. *Pediatrics* 66:767–776.

World Health Organization (1993) Reported polio – 1992. *Epidemiol Alert* 7:1–5.

Wright R, Johnson D, Neumann M *et al.* (1997) Congenital lymphocytic choriomeningitis virus in twins. *Pediatrics* 100:1–6.

Wyatt H V (1979) Poliomyelitis in the fetus and the newborn. *Clin Pediatr* 18:33–38.

Xu W *et al.* (1993) Diagnosis of cytomegalovirus infections using polymerase chain reaction, virus isolation and serology. *Scand J Infect Dis* 25:311–316.

Yamauchi T, Wilson C & St Geme J W (1974) Transmission of live attenuated mumps virus to human placenta. *N Engl J Med* 290:710–712.

Yeager A S (1983) Viruses uncommonly associated with infection of the fetus and newborn infant. In: Remington J S & Klein J (eds) *Infectious diseases of the fetus and newborn infant.* Philadelphia, PA: W B Saunders; pp. 544–554.

Yeager A S, Arvin A M, Urbani L J *et al.* (1980) Relationship of antibody to outcome in neonatal herpes simplex virus infections. *J Infect Immun* 29:532–538.

Yeager A S, Grumet F C, Hafleigh E B *et al.* (1981) Prevention of transfusion-acquired cytomegalovirus infection in newborn infants. *J Pediatr* 98:281–287.

Young N N, Gershon A A (1983) Chickenpox, measles and mumps. In: Remington J S, Klein J O (eds) *Infectious diseases of the fetus and newborn infant.* W B Saunders, Philadelphia, p 375–427.

# Chapter 33 Bacterial and fungal infections

P. McMaster and D. Isaacs

## INTRODUCTION

Neonatal central nervous system (CNS) infections due to bacteria, viruses or fungi should be considered in the differential diagnosis whenever a clinician is confronted with a sick neonate, even one without neurologic signs or symptoms. Unfortunately, there seems to be little sign of CNS infections becoming less common, particularly in non-industrialized countries. One exception is the decrease in the incidence of group B streptococcal infection described due to the use of intrapartum antibiotics. There is ever more being learnt about the pathogenesis and pathologic mechanisms of CNS infections. New diagnostic tests are being assessed to circumvent the lack of reliability of clinical signs and our difficulty with interpreting the wide range of 'normal' CSF findings. Indications for lumbar puncture are being refined, as ventricular tapping becomes less common. Improvements in neonatal intensive care push the boundaries of supportive care, whilst new antibiotics struggle to keep pace with rapidly developing resistance of organisms infecting the CNS. The role of new imaging modalities is being assessed. Despite these advances, CNS infections still have a high mortality.

## EPIDEMIOLOGY

### INCIDENCE

Meningitis is more common in the first month after birth than at any other age and more common in the first week than later. Population-based studies in the United States have consistently shown 0.2–0.5 cases of bacterial meningitis per 1000 live births (Klein *et al.* 1995) (see Table 33.1). The incidence of neonatal bacterial meningitis has remained

**Table 33.1 Incidence (per 1000 live births) and number of cases of bacterial meningitis in neonates**

| Country | Incidence | *n* | GBS | GNR | Predominant organisms | Reference |
|---|---|---|---|---|---|---|
| USA | 0.27 | 257 | 53% (136) | 31% (80) | *E. coli* 16% (42)<br>*L. monocytogenes* 7% (18) | Yatsyk (1998) |
| England | 0.25 | 23 | 47% (7) | 40% (6) | *K. oxytoca* 13% (2) | Hristeva *et al.* (1993) |
| England & Wales | 0.32 | 423 | 38% (118) | 34% (106) | *E. coli* 25% (78)<br>*L. monocytogenes* 7% (23) | de Louvois *et al.* (1991) |
| Northern Ireland | 0.54 | 41 | 7% (2) | 62% (18) | *E. coli* 56% (15)<br>*S. aureus* 22% (6) | Bell *et al.* (1989) |
| UK | | 1846 | 34% (633) | 42% (775) | *E. coli* 29% (526)<br>*L. monocytogenes* 7% (125) | Synnott *et al.* (1994) |
| Australia | 0.17 | 116 | 35% (41) | 36% (42) | *E. coli* 22% (22)<br>*L. monocytogenes* 3% (3) | Francis & Gilbert (1992) |
| Israel | 0.5 | 32 | 19% (6) | 53% (17) | *Klebsiella* + *E. coli* 13% (4)<br>*Proteus* 6% (2) | Greenberg *et al.* (1997) |
| S. Africa | – | 60 | 35% (21) | – | *K. pneumoniae* 28% (17)<br>*E. coli* 17% (10) | Adhikari *et al.* (1995) |
| Nigeria | 1.9 | 36 | 0 | 35% (9) | *S. aureus* 42% (11)<br>*Klebsiella* spp. 15% (4) | Airede (1993) |
| Jordan | 1.1 | 53 | 4% (2) | 81% (43) | *K. pneumoniae* 36% (19)<br>*Enterobacter* spp. 19% (10) | Daoud *et al.* (1996) |
| Trinidad | 2.9 | 54 | 56% (5) | 33% (3) | *Enterobacter* 11% (1)<br>*E. coli* 11% (1) | Ali (1995) |
| Thailand | | 77 | 12% (9) | 51% (39) | *Ps. aeruginosa* 17% (13)<br>*E. coli* 10% (8) | Chotpitayasunondh (1994) |

*Key*: GBS = group B streptococcus; GNR = Gram-negative rods. Of the positive bacterial isolates, the frequency of GBS, GNR and predominant organisms are given as a percentage and number of positive isolates.

constant in England and Wales at 0.25–0.32 cases per 1000 live births, from 1969 until the early 1990s (de Louvois *et al.* 1991; Hristeva *et al.* 1993). In Germany, the incidence has also remained unchanged in a group born between 1962 and 1974 compared with those born from 1975 to 1982, at 0.5 per 1000 live births. The incidence of verified bacterial meningitis decreased from 0.36 to 0.19 per 1000 livebirths in Sweden. The minimum incidence in Australia was reported as 0.17 per 1000 (Francis & Gillbert 1992). In Oxford, the incidence of neonatal bacterial meningitis was 0.25 per 1000; viral meningitis was 0.11 per 1000, and fungal meningitis 0.02 per 1000 live births (Hristeva *et al.* 1993). About 10–30% of cases of early-onset neonatal septicemia and about 10% of late-onset cases are complicated by bacterial meningitis (Klein *et al.* 1993).

### Developing countries

In non-industrialized countries, the incidence of neonatal bacterial meningitis is usually higher than that in industrialized countries. In Nigeria, the incidence was 1.9 per 1000 (Airede 1993); it was 2.9 per 1000 in Trinidad, West Indies (Ali 1995), while in Ethiopia, the incidence in preterm neonates over a 10-year period in the capital Addis Ababa was 3.66 and in term newborns was 0.97 per 1000 live births.

### High-risk groups

The incidence of neonatal bacterial meningitis is higher in infants of low birthweight; the reported incidence will, therefore, vary according to the population being studied. Certain groups of babies are at greatly increased risk of meningitis, irrespective of birthweight. Babies with open myelomeningoceles are particularly likely to develop bacterial meningitis, especially caused by Gram-negative enteric bacilli. CSF shunts are highly likely to become infected with skin organisms, such as coagulase negative staphylococci. Dermal sinuses overlying the CSF anywhere from the bridge of the nose, over the skull, and down the back to the sacrum may penetrate through to the dura and give rise to meningitis. If a dermal sinus is missed (and they can be very small and hidden under the hair), then recurrent meningitis can occur.

## ORGANISMS

### Group B streptococcus

In most industrialized countries, group B streptococcus (GBS) is the commonest cause of neonatal bacterial meningitis (see Table 33.1). The incidence of early-onset GBS sepsis increased in the UK after the 1970s, but was found in Oxford, UK to have remained steady from 1985 to 1996, with an annual incidence of 0.5 per 1000 live births, of whom 15% had meningitis (Moses *et al.* 1998). In contrast, the incidence was higher in the USA (Platt *et al.* 1999) and Australia, where the peak incidence of early-onset GBS sepsis reached 2.0 per 1000 live births or even greater, of whom 7–10% had meningitis (Isaacs & Royle 1999). However the incidence has fallen substantially to 0.5 cases per 1000 in Australia (Isaacs & Royle 1999) and even lower in Boston (Platt *et al.* 1999), almost certainly due to the widespread use of intrapartum antibiotics.

### Gram-negatives

After group B streptococcus, Gram-negative rods (GNR) are the next most common group of organisms causing neonatal meningitis in industrialized countries (see Table 33.1). Of the GNRs, *Escherichia coli* is the most frequently isolated. However, several other enteric GNRs can cause meningitis, including *Pseudomonas, Proteus, Klebsiella* and *Enterobacter. Neisseria meningitidis* and *Haemophilus influenzae* also cause neonatal meningitis occasionally.

### Other organisms

*Listeria monocytogenes* is the third most prevalent organism in most industrialized countries, causing <10% of cases of meningitis (see Table 33.1). These are followed by various Gram-negative and Gram-positive cocci (*Streptococcus pneumoniae* and other streptococci). Anaerobic meningitis is rare. A list of organisms causing bacterial meningitis is given in Table 33.2, based on the studies of de Louvois *et al.* (1991) and Synnott *et al.* (1994), in the approximate order of frequency for the United Kingdom (approximate because bacterial meningitis is under-reported).

**Table 33.2 Organisms causing neonatal bacterial meningitis in approximate order of frequency for United Kingdom**

| |
|---|
| Group B streptococcus |
| *Escherichia coli* |
| *Listeria monocytogenes* |
| *Streptococcus pneumoniae* |
| *Enterococci* |
| Other streptococci |
| *Proteus* species |
| *Neisseria meningitidis* |
| *Staphylococcus aureus* |
| *Klebsiella* species |
| *Haemophilus influenzae* |
| *Pseudomonas* species |
| *Enterobacter* species |
| *Citrobacter* species |
| *Serratia* species |
| *Salmonella* species |
| Other Gram-negative bacilli |
| Anaerobes |
| *Mycobacterium tuberculosis* |
| *Campylobacter* species |
| Coagulase-negative staphylococci (shunt infections) |

*Source*: From de Louvois & Lambert (1991), Hristeva *et al.* (1993), and Synnott *et al.* (1994).

### Non-industrialized countries

Typically, the pattern of organisms causing bacterial meningitis in non-industrialized countries is very different from those in industrialized countries. For example, group B streptococcal infection is generally rare in non-industrialized countries. There were no cases of GBS meningitis over 3 years in Nigeria where the most common causative organisms were *S. aureus* and *Klebsiella* (Airede 1993). GBS caused 11.7% of cases in Thailand (Chotpitayasunondh 1994), the other main organisms being *Pseudomonas aeruginosa* (16.9%), *Klebsiella pneumoniae* (13.0%), *E. coli* (10.4%) and *Enterobacter* species (10.4%). In Mexico, 61% of CSF isolates were GNR, and in Ethiopia, 67% of isolates were *Klebsiella pneumoniae, E. coli,* or *Enterobacter* species (Rios-Reategui *et al.* 1998). In the 1980s, *Klebsiella* was the commonest cause in Durban, South Africa, followed by *E. coli* and GBS. More recently, in South Africa, GBS has caused more cases (35%) than *Klebsiella* (28%) and *E. coli* (17%). GBS is now the predominant organism in Trinidad, West Indies, with a mean age at presentation of 4 days (Ali 1995), and in Zimbabwe, GBS was the predominant organism (61%).

### High-risk groups

Shunt infections are most commonly due to coagulase-negative staphylococci. A specimen of CSF should always be obtained in suspected shunt infections because *Staphylococcus aureus*, Gram-negative bacilli or fungi may also cause these. Meningitis complicating myelomeningocele is usually caused by Gram-negative enteric bacilli.

The isolation of certain organisms should alert the physician to special problems. For example, *Citrobacter* meningitis is frequently associated with brain abscess, although abscess may occur with other organisms such as *Proteus*. Other important pathogens are *Salmonella* species and rare, but important, *Mycobacterium tuberculosis*.

Fungal meningitis almost exclusively affects babies <1500 g birthweight, and as survival of this group increases with improved neonatal care, the incidence of fungal meningitis also increases. It is still extremely rare compared with bacterial meningitis: one-tenth as common in Oxford (Hristeva *et al.* 1993). *Candida* is the most commonly isolated yeast infection, but other fungi such as *Trichosporon beigelii* are rare CNS pathogens.

### Summary of epidemiology

- Bacterial meningitis is more common in the first month than at any other age.
- About 10–30% of babies with early-onset septicemia and 10% with late-onset septicemia have meningitis.
- Group B streptococcus is the commonest cause of early-onset meningitis in industrialized countries.
- Gram-negative enteric bacilli are the commonest cause of late-onset meningitis.

## PATHOGENESIS

Organisms reach the subarachnoid space most commonly by bacteremia seeding within the choroid plexus. The magnitude of bacteremia correlates strongly with the probability of meningitis. Less commonly, meningitis can be due to direct spread, either from an infected scalp lesion with spread through skull sutures and thrombosed veins or from otitis media. CSF environmental factors such as pH and osmolality have been shown experimentally to affect bacterial ability to invade brain microvascular endothelial cells.

Low birthweight is the most significant risk factor for meningitis: in a recent prospective study, meningitis was 10 times more common in neonates with a birthweight under 2 kg than those >2 kg (de Louvois *et al.* 1991). Other host factors include prematurity (risk ratio 17.8), ventriculo-peritoneal shunts, myelomeningocele, maternal sepsis, multiple pregnancy, prior infant sepsis, and invasive procedures on the neonate (Francis & Gilbert 1992). Other risk factors are also associated with sepsis and meningitis such as infants requiring resuscitation, intubation, male sex, and socio-economic deprivation (Klein & Marcy 1995).

The most common associated site of infection outside the CNS is the lung (pneumonia or empyema). There may also be otitis or omphalitis (which have occasionally been the original source of sepsis), peritonitis, pyelonephritis, enterocolitis, osteomyelitis, septic arthritis and abscesses in other organs (skin, liver, etc.).

## ORGANISMS

### *Escherichia coli*

Certain organisms are far more likely to cause bacterial meningitis than others, so that the virulence of the invading organism as well as host factors are important in determining whether or not meningitis occurs. The K1 capsular antigen of *Escherichia coli*, which is similar to the capsular polysaccharide of Group B *Neisseria meningitidis*, is important in facilitating bloodstream survival. More than 80% of cases of neonatal *Escherichia coli* meningitis are caused by strains carrying the K1 antigen. The relative pathogenetic importance of predisposing host factors and virulence-associated bacterial characteristics of *E. coli*, such as possession of P-fimbriae, O and K antigens and hemolysins has been studied. Bacterial factors were more important in neonatal meningitis and UTI, whereas host factors contributed to septicemia or bacteremia. Certain genetic markers have been found to be more common in *E. coli* strains from neonates with meningitis than in *E. coli* in blood or commensals. The specific outer membrane protein (OmpA), which contributes to *E. coli* K1 membrane invasion, has been experimentally shown to be inhibited by wheat-germ agglutinin. Specific gene locations have been identified in the serotype O18:K1:H7 (the most virulent *E. coli* in newborn meningitis), which are associated with its ability to penetrate the blood–brain barrier and invade the brain microvascular endothelial cells. This may give rapid-identification genotyping organisms, which can be instructive regarding epidemiology. For example, despite concurrent urine and CSF isolation of *E. coli* in one study, the two were proved to be different genotypes.

### Group B streptococcus

In a study of neonatal meningitis in Australia (Francis & Gilbert 1992), 80% of neonates with GBS infections had no risk factors for sepsis. This is because late-onset GBS meningitis predominantly affects full-term babies when they are 2–6 weeks old. Risk factors in these babies are virtually confined to having low levels of transplacental antibodies to the type III GBS capsular polysaccharide. Group III GBS strains are disproportionately likely to cause late-onset meningitis (>80% of cases), compared with early-onset sepsis when strains I, II and III are equally common. Thus, early onset GBS meningitis typically involves a high-risk baby who acquires maternal GBS at the time of delivery, develops high-level septicemia and hence meningitis. In contrast, late-onset meningitis usually occurs in an apparently healthy full-term baby whose nasopharynx is colonized (at birth or subsequently) with serotype III GBS and who lacks antibody to the capsule.

### Staphylococci

Other organisms that are common causes of neonatal septicemia virtually never cause meningitis. Coagulase-negative staphylococci are one of the commonest causes of late-onset septicemia in industrialized countries, but meningitis virtually only occurs if there is a CSF shunt. *Staphylococcus aureus* is another common cause of septicemia, but a rare cause of meningitis unless there has been surgery, a shunt, or seeding from bacterial endocarditis. A polysaccharide capsule is one characteristic of the organisms causing meningitis that is lacking in staphylococci.

### *Listeria*

*Listeria monocytogenes*, like GBS, can cause early and late-onset forms of bacterial meningitis. The early form may be acquired transplacentally (granulomatosis infantiseptica) or by inhalation of infected amniotic fluid, whereas the late-onset form follows nasopharyngeal colonization and later invasion of the blood and meninges, usually at 2–6 weeks of age.

## PATHOLOGY

Toxic products of the bacterial cell wall, peptidoglycans and teichoic acid from Gram-positive and lipopolysaccharide (endotoxin) from Gram-negative organisms, cause substantial damage to the endothelial cells of the cerebral capillaries, which form the so-called 'blood–brain barrier'. Disruption of the tight junctions between the endothelial cells increases the permeability and allows entry of bacteria and white cells, and leakage of protein (see Fig. 33.1).

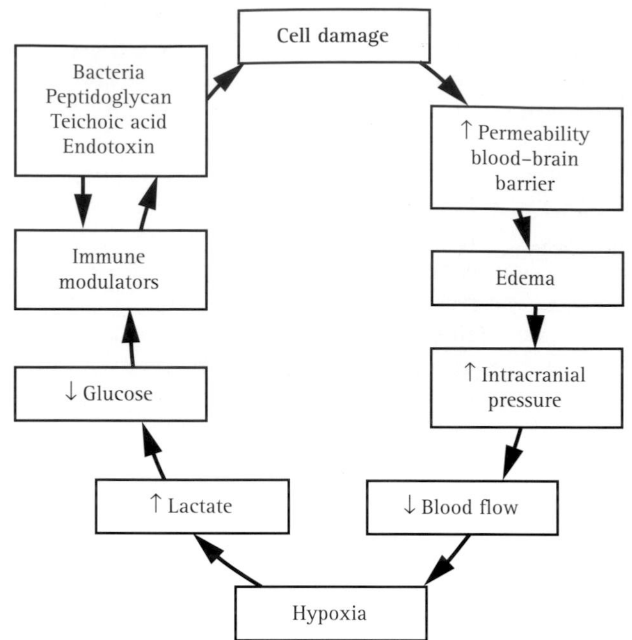


**Figure 33.1** Pathophysiology of bacterial meningitis.

The host immune response causes damage to the central nervous system. High levels of tumor necrosis factor (TNFα) and interleukin-1 and 6 (IL1β and IL6) in the CSF have been correlated with prolonged fever, fits, spasticity, and death. These cytokines from mononuclear cells may damage endothelial cells and lead to raised intracranial pressure and cerebral edema. Oxygen free radicals have also been found to be released in association with meningitis-causing strains of *E. coli* in healthy full-term neonates. These could harm surrounding tissue and potentiate the inflammatory process. Arachidonic acid metabolites from platelets are also probably important in pathogenesis. Levels of prostaglandin $E_2$, a potent vasoactive substance, rise in the CSF in experimental meningitis, and this contributes to cerebral edema; both the increased levels and cerebral edema can be blocked by indomethacin. Complement may be important in opsonizing organisms, but can also lyse host cells if bacterial cell-wall products are incorporated into them. Soluble CD14 from intrathecal leucocytes is massively released into the CSF and may play an important role in the pathogenesis of meningitis.

Intracranial pressure (ICP) is always elevated in bacterial meningitis; the possible mechanisms include cerebral edema, vasodilatation of cerebral veins and capillaries, loss of autoregulation of cerebral blood flow, and impaired circulation of CSF. Reduced cerebral blood flow produces regional hypoxemia, increased metabolism of arachidonic acid, and anaerobic glycolysis with increased production of lactate. There is also decreased carrier-mediated transport of glucose into CSF, and this is probably the main cause of the characteristic low CSF glucose (hypoglycorrhachia) seen in bacterial meningitis. Consumption of glucose by bacteria or white cells is unlikely to be a major cause of low CSF glucose, since the CSF sugar can be low, even zero, for weeks after acute bacterial meningitis, without causing any symptoms.

The outcome in neonatal meningitis is generally worse than that in older children. The relatively poor neonatal immune response, permitting rapid bacterial multiplication, is one possible reason. Severe ventriculitis, a hallmark of neonatal meningitis, is rarely seen outside the newborn period. Fever is relatively uncommon in neonatal meningitis, and this may contribute to the poor outcome, since CSF bacterial multiplication in experimental pneumococcal meningitis is far more rapid at normal body temperatures than when animals are febrile.

### SUMMARY OF PATHOLOGY

- Ventriculitis is common in neonatal bacterial meningitis, particularly Gram-negative meningitis, and there may be collections of pus in the ventricles and subarachnoid space.
- Subdural effusions are rarely of a sufficient size to cause raised intracranial pressure.
- Hydrocephalus may develop secondary to purulent exudate obstructing the arachnoid granulations over the surface of the brain, or as a result of exudate in the ventricles obstructing the foramina of Magendie and Luschka or the aqueduct.
- Intraventricular hemorrhage may occur and contribute to hydrocephalus.
- Vasculitis is common and may lead to venous thrombosis; there may be infarcts and focal necrosis.
- Neuronal damage is often widespread in severe cases and leads to necrotic liquefaction or cerebral atrophy.
- Abscesses may develop: they often lack the capsule seen in older children and are multiple.

## CLINICAL FEATURES

The classic clinical features of bacterial meningitis are frequently absent, and there may be no apparent distinction between the newborn with sepsis with or without meningitis. A body temperature greater than 38°C or less than 36.7°C is an indication for further investigation and consideration of lumbar puncture. However, in one series of 223 proven cases of neonatal bacterial meningitis, only nine cases had a temperature greater than 38.0°C (de Louvois & Lambert 1991). The neonate may even appear well yet still be found to have meningitis. A bulging fontanelle strongly suggests meningitis but may be absent with dehydration. Group B streptococcal sepsis can present with respiratory distress within a few hours of birth that may be confused with hyaline membrane disease, and will progress rapidly to meningitis if untreated. The majority of Gram-negative meningitis associated with obstetric complications occurs in the first 2 weeks. The more premature and the younger the baby, the less specific the symptoms and signs. Klein and Marcy (1995) summarized the clinical signs in 255 neonates with bacterial meningitis in six centers (see frequencies in Table 33.3).

**Table 33.3 Clinical signs of bacterial meningitis**

| Symptoms | Percentage | Signs | Percentage |
|---|---|---|---|
| Lethargy | 50 | Fever or hypothermia | 61 |
| Anorexia | | Respiratory distress | 47 |
| Vomiting | 49 | Irritability | 32 |
| Diarrhea | | Jaundice | 28 |
| Convulsions | 40 | Full/bulging fontanelle | 28 |
| Apnea | 7 | Neck stiffness | 15 |
| Altered sleep pattern | | Hypotonia | |
| High-pitched cry | | Petechiae | |
| | | Hypotension, shock | |
| | | Bradycardia | |

*Source*: Frequencies from Klein & Marcy (1995).

### LUMBAR PUNCTURE

#### Indications

Because of the difficulty in making a clinical diagnosis of meningitis, it is vital that if sepsis is suspected, either an LP is performed or, if the LP is delayed because of the baby's unstable condition, blood cultures are taken, and antibiotics started that will adequately cover the organisms likely to cause bacterial meningitis. The wide range of possible pathogens makes empirical antimicrobial therapy without a lumbar puncture far more difficult. Up to one-third of all cases of early-onset meningitis are associated with negative blood cultures (Visser & Hall 1980), so if antibiotics are started for suspected early-onset sepsis without performing a lumbar puncture, the LP should be done later, particularly if blood cultures are positive. However, occasionally meningitis may be present with normal CSF microscopy, while an intraventricular hemorrhage may complicate the later interpretation of the CSF white-cell count. However, in a study of 728 LPs performed in the first week of life on babies with early-onset respiratory distress, bacteria were isolated from the CSF of nine, but only one had a clinical course consistent with meningitis.

The indications for lumbar puncture are controversial. They range from inclusion of LP as part of a routine septic work-up in asymptomatic neonates based on maternal risk factors, to restricting LP to those who have signs and symptoms of severe sepsis. In one study, 43 cases of meningitis were reviewed retrospectively by application of selective criteria for performing LP only if CNS symptoms or signs were present, and the diagnosis of bacterial meningitis would have been delayed or missed in 37% of them. Of admission lumbar punctures for respiratory distress, only one of over 1700 infants had an organism identified in the CSF that was not isolated in the blood. A prospective study of lumbar punctures for suspected sepsis in 148 neonates found that five had CSF white-cell counts > 130 (Kumar *et al.* 1995). In Australia, a survey of neonatalogists revealed that none performed an LP routinely for a preterm neonate with respiratory distress and 83–85% if the blood culture was positive (Joshi & Barr 1998).

### Technique

Neonates can decompensate rapidly with handling during lumbar puncture, due to hypoxia, hypercapnea and hypertension. The LP should be delayed if there is respiratory distress or labile blood pressure. Preoxygenation can help prevent desaturation. Local anesthesia decreases the amount of struggling but not physiological changes. The risk of coning of the medulla oblongata into the foramen magnum is small, and papilledema is rare, even with raised intracranial pressure. Topical local anesthetic mixtures reduce pain and are safe in term neonates but cause raised methemoglobin in preterm infants, although this has not been shown to have any clinical consequences. Performing the LP with the neonate in the sitting position has been shown to reduce the degree of hypoxia. The rate of coning in neonates has been reported as 1% (four out of 423 neonates) (de Louvois *et al.* 1991).

Lumbar puncture should be performed with a needle with a stylet in preference to a hypodermic needle. This is to prevent the risk of an epidermoid tumor in the spinal canal from a fragment of skin. This may not present for many years after neonatal LP. There has been some suggestion that the stylet should be reinserted before the needle is removed to reduce CSF leak. The success rate in 181 neonates using different types of needle has been shown to be the same, and the traumatic taps did not result in pleocytosis on repeat LP. A formula for the depth of insertion of the lumbar puncture needle has been calculated in centimeters as 0.03 × height of child (cm). A sterile technique should be used to prevent introduction of infection and contamination of the specimen. Contamination is particularly important when a shunt is being tapped, as the organisms causing shunt infections are often skin flora. However, iodine containing disinfectants should not be used to prevent transient hypothyroidism. Chlorhexidine is a suitable disinfectant. The opening pressure should be measured, as this would be high in meningitis. The normal pressure in neonates is 0–5.7 mmHg (7.6 cm water) with the head deflexed, and the baby horizontal and quiet.

### Other tests

The larger the specimen of CSF, the more chance of isolation of organisms that are present in small numbers such as mycobacteria and fungi. CSF should also be sent for protein and glucose assay with simultaneous blood glucose assay. The measurement of CSF lactate is not routinely useful in meningitis, though it may be of use in the investigation of the neonate with seizures or suspected metabolic abnormality. Further tests may be of use such as latex agglutination test for group B streptococcus, which is commercially available. However, it is possible to have a false-negative result when excess antigen is present (prozone effect) and false positive with skin contamination. Urinary antigen testing is not generally useful because of high false-positive and false-negative rates. Newer methods of ultrasound-enhanced particle agglutination show improved detection rates. The sensitivity of latex agglutination for infants with group B streptococcal meningitis varies between 73 and 100% for CSF and 75 and 84% for urine.

If syphilis is suspected, a non-treponemal test such as VDRL should be performed on the CSF. The CSF should be examined by microscopy and a differential cell count. A Gram stain should be performed, even if there are no white cells as meningitis can occur in the absence of pleocytosis. The spun CSF should be cultured on blood agar and chocolate agar routinely. If there is a shunt, this should be brought to the attention of the microbiology laboratory so that the CSF can be cultured in enrichment broth. A viral culture should also be performed when indicated clinically and, if appropriate, specific viral PCR such as for HSV or enterovirus.

Inflammatory markers can also be useful in diagnosing infection. C-Reactive Protein (CRP) can be measured in the CSF and blood. The result of a meta-analysis suggests that only a negative CRP test is highly informative in the diagnosis of bacterial meningitis. Interleukin-1 receptor antagonist (IL-1ra) and interleukin-6 (IL-6) levels have been found to rise in serum 2 days before clinical manifestation of infection in neonates. However, an LP is effectively a biopsy, giving a rapid diagnosis of the condition and the likely cause, whereas no acute phase reactant will have 100% specificity, nor will it distinguish septicemia from meningitis.

## INTERPRETATION OF CSF FINDINGS

### Normal CSF white-cell count

In general, CSF white-cell count and protein levels are higher and CSF glucose levels lower in normal neonates than in older children and adults (see Table 33.4). These differences are even more marked in preterm infants. In normal preterm infants, the mean CSF white-cell count is up to 27/μl, about one-half neutrophils, with a range of 0–112. In normal-term infants, the mean white-cell count is lower (5–10/μl) in most studies, but again the range is up to 130 (Ahmed *et al.* 1996). There is no difference in CSF findings between term and preterm infants at high risk of infection but without meningitis. The mean CSF white-cell counts were 8 and 9/μl and the ranges 0–32 and 0–29 for term and preterm babies, respectively. Sixteen babies with septicemia without meningitis had a mean CSF white count of 20/μl

**Table 33.4 Normal CSF combined values from selected studies**

| | Number of infants | White cells ($\times 10^6$/l) Mean (range) | Protein (g/l) Mean (range) | Glucose (mg/l) Mean (range) |
|---|---|---|---|---|
| Preterm | 188 | 12 (0–112) | 1.09 (0.31–2.69) | 7.1 (2.4–10.6) |
| Term | 409 | 8.8 (0–130) | 0.72 (0.17–1.74) | 5.0 (2.6–24.8) |

*Source*: From Klein & Marcy (1995) and Isaacs & Moxon (1999).

(range: 0–112). Traumatic taps are common, but interpretation of the ratio of white to red cells is not reliable. A repeat lumbar puncture after a traumatic tap may also be misleading as the blood can cause an inflammatory response, or red cells can lyse giving a falsely low RBC count.

### CSF white-cell count in meningitis

Of 21 babies with proven group B streptococcal meningitis and of 98 babies with Gram-negative enteric meningitis, 29 and 4%, respectively, had CSF white counts <32 μl. This shows that there is considerable overlap between the CSF white-cell count in babies with and without meningitis. Bacteria may sometimes be cultured from the CSF of babies with normal CSF microscopy (no white cells and no organisms seen). Nine per cent of a UK series of 223 neonates with meningitis had less than 10 white cells in the CSF (de Louvois & Lambert 1991). Ahmed *et al.* (1996) closely examined a cohort of 108 full-term neonates and excluded meningitis using the most stringent criteria, including performing PCR for enteroviruses. The mean CSF white-blood-cell count was 7.3/μl (95% confidence interval 6.6–8.0). The SD was 14, so 2SD above the mean would be 35. The median was 4, and most babies had CSF white counts from 0 to 20 (90% had <11). However, there was one baby with a CSF white count of 130 and one with a count of 62. Clearly, this degree of overlap between apparently uninfected babies and babies with meningitis makes interpretation of white counts in the 20–130 range problematic. Leucocyte aggregation is a feature of bacterial meningitis, which distinguishes it from viral or aseptic meningitis.

Because of overlap, a CSF wite-cell count alone does not always distinguish the baby with meningitis from the baby without. The CSF white count should always be considered in conjunction with CSF protein and sugar, CSF red-cell count, baby's age, etc. As a useful rule, however, a CSF white-cell count over 20, in the absence of raised red cells, should be considered suggestive of meningitis.

### CSF protein

The mean CSF protein in preterm babies without meningitis is about 100 mg/dl (1.0 g/l) with the normal range approximately 50–290 mg/dl (0.5–2.9 g/l). For term babies, the mean is about 60 mg/dl (0.6 g/l) and the range 30–240 mg/dl (0.3–2.4 g/l). The CSF protein is often raised in bacterial meningitis but in one study was within the normal range of 20–170 mg/dl (0.2–1.7 g/l) in 47% of babies with group B streptococcal meningitis and 23% with Gram-negative enteric bacillary meningitis. Elevated CSF protein in the absence of pleocytosis may be seen in parameningeal infections, congenital infections and intracranial hemorrhage.

### CSF glucose

Mean absolute CSF glucose concentrations in normal babies have varied from 50 to 80 mg/dl (2.7–4.4 mmol/l) with a range of 24–100 mg/dl (1.5–5.5 mmol). The CSF glucose is generally low in bacterial meningitis and may be zero, but in some cases may be higher than the lower limit of the 'normal range'. As CSF and blood glucose concentrations are both lower in healthy newborn infants than in older children, it has been suggested that the ratio of CSF to blood glucose is a useful indicator of neonatal meningitis. In the study by Sarff *et al.* (1976), the mean CSF:blood glucose ratio was 81% (range: 44–248) in preterm infants without meningitis and 74% (range: 55–105) in term infants. However, 45% of infants with group B streptococcal meningitis and 15% with Gram-negative bacillary meningitis had CSF:blood glucose ratios >44%, showing that the CSF:blood glucose ratio is relatively poor at discriminating babies with and without meningitis.

In viral meningitis, the CSF glucose level is usually normal, although low glucose levels may occur, the protein level is often elevated, and the mean CSF white cell count is usually <1000/μl, although it may be up to 4500 with a neutrophil predominance. Thus, in the absence of organisms on Gram staining, it can be extremely difficult to distinguish viral from bacterial meningitis.

### Gram's stain

Of the 117 babies with neonatal meningitis (Sarff *et al.* 1976), only one had completely normal CSF microscopy and biochemistry. The Gram stain reveals organisms in about 80% of cases of meningitis. The CSF white-cell count is generally higher in Gram-negative enteric bacillary than in group B streptococcal meningitis [median number more than 2000/μl and less than 100/μl respectively (Klein & Marcy 1995)]. Although neutrophils usually predominate in bacterial meningitis, the same is also true in early viral meningitis.

### VENTRICULAR TAP

Ventriculitis is present in most babies with Gram-negative enteric meningitis and many with group B streptococcal meningitis. The diagnosis can be made by finding >100 white cells/μl in ventricular CSF obtained by ventricular tap. However, ventricular taps can result in intracerebral cysts, and ventriculitis is so common that it can almost be assumed to be present, particularly in Gram-negative bacillary meningitis. Ventriculitis can sometimes be diagnosed on cerebral ultrasound imaging by seeing unusual fibrin strands in the ventricles. Ventricular or cisternal taps may have a role in specific circumstances such as suspected meningitis in a child with spinal bifida or other local contraindication to lumbar puncture. However, they are not justifiable as routine following traumatic lumbar puncture, particularly as the blood from the LP can be seen in the ventricles. Intracranial hemorrhage itself can result in pleocytosis, low CSF glucose and raised CSF protein.

#### Summary of indication for LP

- Definite sepsis (positive blood culture), early or late onset.
- Suspected severe sepsis, early or late onset.
- Early-onset respiratory distress if associated with signs of sepsis.
- Suspected late-onset sepsis.

## MANAGEMENT

### CLINICAL ASSESSMENT

When meningitis is 'proven' (organisms seen on CSF Gram's stain) or probable (raised CSF white-cell count, but no organisms seen), a careful clinical assessment is the first priority. The baby should be examined for a source of infection, notably otitis, omphalitis, and osteomyelitis of the skull and also for midline CNS anomalies such as congenital dermal sinuses. These can occur anywhere in the midline from the bridge of the nose, on the scalp under the hairline and down the spine to the sacrum.

Skin rashes – erythematous, maculopapular or purpuric – may accompany bacterial meningitis, while a fine, macular rash may occur in enteroviral meningitis. The eyes should be examined for the characteristic retinal or vitreous lesions of fungal meningitis. The head circumference should be measured, both to see if there has been a marked increase from the last measurement and to act as a baseline for serial measurements during treatment.

A full clinical examination is, of course, essential, both to look for other foci of infection and to assess the overall clinical state. The blood pressure should be measured but may be artificially maintained due to raised intracranial pressure and peripheral vasoconstriction. Thus, an assessment for shock should also include an assessment of peripheral perfusion (capillary return and core-peripheral temperature difference), pulse character, heart rate, and urinary output.

### SUPPORTIVE THERAPY

The same basic principles for supportive therapy apply as for systemic sepsis. The first priority is to support the systemic circulation with fluid. The choice of fluid has been recently reviewed with concerns about human albumin, which is not now recommended as the first line in neonatal hypovolemia. Crystalloid has been shown in randomized controlled trials of hypotensive preterm infants to be as effective as colloid. Fresh frozen plasma (FFP) is not immediately available, as it needs to be matched and thawed. FFP may raise IgG levels but does not change opsonic activity in neonates with coagulase negative staphylococcal septicaemia.

Exchange transfusion with fresh whole blood improves survival in scleremic neonates with sepsis. Immunomodulating drugs may have a role in the future as pentoxifylline has been found to decrease serum levels of tumor necrosis factor and interleukin-1 and to reduce mortality in a randomized double-blind trial of sepsis in premature infants. Recombinant human granulocyte colony-stimulating factor (G-CSF) in preterm neonates with neutropenia is effective at preventing infection if given prophylactically. However, there are conflicting results regarding its effectiveness if given after the onset of suspected sepsis. A Cochrane review (Ohlsson *et al.* 1998) found that although prophylactic intravenous immunoglobulin (IVIG) has been shown to reduce sepsis in preterm neonates, it did not significantly reduce mortality or other morbidities (NEC, IVH, length of hospital stay). IVIG has been given as therapy for late-onset sepsis, but the numbers studied have been too small to show a significant reduction in mortality, although there is a strong trend to reduced mortality (a halving). IgM-enriched IVIG may be more effective, with a significant difference in mortality found in a Saudi study with 3/44 (6.8%) mortality with IgM-enriched IVIG and 11/43 (25.5%) in a control group.

The hypotension associated with sepsis unresponsive to fluids and inotropes has also been improved with the use of methylene blue as an inhibitor of guanylate cyclase, which causes vascular smooth muscle dilation in the presence of excess nitric oxide in septic shock. Although inappropriate secretion of antidiuretic hormone (ADH) and cerebral edema are common in bacterial meningitis, the only prospective randomized trial of fluid restriction versus maintenance fluids with a clinical end point in acute meningitis showed a trend towards lower mortality in the group receiving full maintenance fluids. There is also experimental data from *E. coli* meningitis in rabbits that found that fluid restriction causes higher levels of CSF lactate and lower levels of CSF glucose but has no effect on cerebral edema.

Phenobarbitone is the anticonvulsant of choice for convulsions associated with meningitis in neonates. A loading dose of 15–20 mg/kg followed by a maintenance dose of 5 mg/kg once daily is appropriate. The levels of chloramphenicol may be reduced if this antibiotic is being used (as in developing countries), in which case, ampicillin and gentamicin may be a better empiric combination. Diazepam can cause hypotension but is an appropriate first-line anticonvulsant for ongoing seizure activity at a dose of 0.1 mg/kg, repeated if necessary. Steroids have not been shown to be of benefit in neonatal meningitis.

## ANTIBIOTIC THERAPY

The choice of antibiotic therapy will depend on which organisms are prevalent in the community, and which are seen on a Gram stain and culture. There may be an initial suggestion from the Gram staining: Gram-positive cocci (most probably group B streptococcus, enterococcus or pneumococcus), Gram-positive bacilli (*Listeria*) or Gram-negative bacilli (most likely *E. coli, Pseudomonas*, coliforms or *Haemophilus influenzae*), or no bacteria at all. The situation is completely different for infected ventricular shunts and is considered later in this chapter. However, empiric antibiotic treatment should be continued until the organism is positively identified by culture and sensitivity rather than on Gram's stain, which is sometimes misleading.

It is generally acknowledged that all antibiotics should be given parenterally for the entire duration of therapy of neonatal meningitis. Oral absorption of antibiotics is extremely erratic in the neonatal period. Aminoglycosides are sometimes given intramuscularly because intravenous boluses can give rise to high serum peak levels, but recent evidence suggests that high peak levels do not cause toxicity, and IV therapy is safe and kinder. All antibiotics used for treating bacterial meningitis should be given intravenously because muscle perfusion may be poor.

For rapid sterilization of the CSF, drug concentrations of at least ten times MIC are required. The entry of hydrophilic antibacterials such as beta-lactams (penicillins and cephalosporins) and glycopeptides (e.g. vancomycin) into the CSF is poor with an intact blood–brain barrier (BBB) but increases with meningeal inflammation. Lipophilic antibacterials such as chloramphenicol or rifampicin penetrate well across the BBB and are not inflammation-dependent.

### Developing countries

Third-generation cephalosporins are very expensive in terms of the poorest countries' health budgets. Historically, chloramphenicol was widely used in the United Kingdom. There has been a high rate of side-effects attributed to its use in neonates. In a study of 64 neonates treated with chloramphenicol in ten UK hospitals, five developed 'gray baby syndrome', four of whom had cardiovascular collapse, one baby became 'very gray', and four more had reversible hematological abnormalities. However, in the treatment of neonates with meningitis, serious toxicity has been associated only with dosages higher than recommended and none if serum levels are kept between 15 and 25 mg/l. Chloramphenicol is bacteriostatic for most Gram-negative enteric bacilli. Although glucuronide conjugation is depressed by immaturity, chloramphenicol is metabolized by other pathways.

### Streptococci

For Group B streptococcal meningitis, penicillin and an aminoglycoside is the treatment of choice. Even throughout the 1990s, GBS remained sensitive to penicillin G. Recommendations for the dose of penicillin G for treating GBS meningitis vary from 50 000 units/kg per dose to 240 mg/kg/day. The dose frequency varies with age (see Table 33.5). There is experimental evidence advocating synergism of an aminoglycoside with the penicillin until the CSF is sterile, although there are no clinical data to suggest that this increases survival.

Isolates of *Streptococcus pneumoniae*, particularly those causing invasive disease, are increasingly being found to be relatively resistant to penicillin and third-generation cephalosporins. In the USA between 1993 and 1996, 12.7% of pneumococci causing meningitis in children had intermediate sensitivity to penicillin, and 6.6% were completely resistant; 4.4% had intermediate resistance to ceftriaxone, and 2.8% were resistant. There have been treatment failures using third-generation cephalosporins to treat pneumococcal meningitis, which has responded to vancomycin. Hence, empiric treatment with vancomycin may be appropriate if *Streptococcus pneumoniae* is suspected from Gram's stain or culture from another site. However, vancomycin is not an appropriate first-line empiric therapy in neonates, in whom meningitis is rarely caused by pneumococci.

Group D streptococci (enterococci) can cause meningitis, sometimes in association with shunt infections. They are resistant to cephalosporins and should be treated with ampicillin, if sensitive, or vancomycin.

### Staphylococci

Staphylococcal neonatal meningitis is rare, but occasional cases do occur. Vancomycin may be necessary when there are Gram-positive cocci in bunches suggestive of staphylococci seen in the CSF. Local prevalence of methicillin-resistant *Staphylococcus aureus* (MRSA) will determine the choice of flucloxacillin or vancomycin pending sensitivity testing. The true incidence of coagulase negative staphylococcal meningitis in the absence of a foreign body is difficult to determine, as opposed to contamination of CSF culture, which is relatively common. However, if there is a ventriculo-peritoneal shunt *in situ*, then vancomycin is a reasonable first-line therapy to cover coagulase negative staphylococci.

Vancomycin penetration into the CSF of premature infants with meningitis ranges from 26 to 68% of serum levels, which is a higher proportion than for older infants and children. Serum vancomycin levels should be measured pre-dose (trough) and 30 min after a 1-h infusion (peak). Vancomycin appears safe in neonates, even with

**Table 33.5 Summary of antibiotic therapy**

| | | Dose (mg/kg/day) | Age (days) | Interval comment | |
|---|---|---|---|---|---|
| Group B Strep | Penicillin G | 240 | ≤ 7 | 12 h | |
| | | | > 7 | 6 h | |
| *S. aureus* | Flucloxacillin | 200 | ≤ 7 | 12 h | |
| | | | > 7 | 8 h | |
| Coagulase neg staph | Vancomycin | 20 | ≤ 7 | Daily | ≤ 1500 g |
| | | 30 | ≤ 7 | 12 h | > 1500 g |
| | | 30 | > 7 | 8 h | ≤ 1500 g |
| | | 45 | > 7 | 8 h | > 1500 g |
| *Listeria monocytogenes* | Ampicillin | 200 | ≤ 7 | 12 h | |
| | | 400 | > 7 | 8 h | |
| Gram-negative bacilli | Cefotaxime | 150 | ≤ 7 | 12 h | Prem |
| | | | | 8 h | Term |
| | | 200 | > 7 | 8 h | Prem |
| | | | | 8 h | Term |
| | Gentamicin | 2 | ≤ 7 | Daily | <800 g |
| | | 3 | ≤ 7 | Daily | 800–1499 g |
| | | 4 | ≤ 7 | 18 h | 1500–2000 g |
| | | 5 | ≤ 7 | 12 h | >2000 g |
| | | 3–5 | > 7 | Daily | <800 g |
| | | 3–5 | > 7 | 18 h | 800–1499 g |
| | | 3–5 | > 7 | 12 h | 1500–2000 g |
| | | 7.5 | > 7 | 8 h | >2000 g |
| *Pseudomonas* | Ceftazidime | 150 | | 8 h | |
| Anaerobes | Metronidazole | 15 | ≤ 7 | 12 h | |
| | | 30 | > 7 | 12 h | |
| *Candida, Aspergillus* | Amphotericin | 0.5 | | Daily | Day 1 |
| | | 1.0 | | Daily | Day 2+ |
| | 5-Fluorocytosine | 100 | | 6–12 h | Prem |
| | | 200 | | | Term |
| Multi-resistant | Meropenem | 45–60 | | 8 h | |

vancomycin serum concentrations >40 µg/ml, without causing nephrotoxicity.

### Listeria

For meningitis attributable to *Listeria monocytogenes*, ampicillin and an aminoglycoside is the regimen for which there are most data. *Listeria* is susceptible to ampicillin, gentamicin, cotrimoxazole, vancomycin, and meropenem *in vitro*. There is little to choose between penicillin and ampicillin. There have been a few reports of treatment failures using penicillin G and an aminoglycoside, but there are many successes, and ampicillin is not always successful either. The third-generation cephalosporins are inactive against *Listeria*.

### Gram-negative bacilli

Cefotaxime is now the preferred antibiotic therapy for Gram-negative bacillary meningitis (except *Pseudomonas*). Although this choice is that of the majority of experts polled in the USA in 1992, cefotaxime has never been compared to previous antibiotic regimens, such as ampicillin and gentamicin in controlled trials. However, cefotaxime achieves good CSF levels, whereas aminoglycosides only penetrate inflamed meninges. Cefotaxime is not effective for *Pseudomonas*: for proven or suspected *Pseudomonas meningitis*, ceftazidime should be used. The addition of an aminoglycoside to cefotaxime or ceftazidime may improve outcome.

Studies from McCracken's group showed that ampicillin and gentamicin sterilized the CSF of most cases of Gram-negative meningitis, even when due to ampicillin-resistant *E. coli* (McCracken *et al.* 1980). Clearance of septicemia plus some CSF penetration of inflamed meninges are the probable mechanisms. Cephalosporins and aminoglycosides act by different mechanisms, and synergy might be expected. As prognosis depends on the speed of sterilization of CSF, we recommend using both a third-generation cephalosporin and an aminoglycoside for Gram-negative bacillary meningitis, unless the latter is contra-indicated.

In 1971–1975, the mortality for Gram-negative enteric meningitis was 30%, and half the survivors were felt to be normal. In order to improve CSF delivery of antibiotics, McCracken studied intrathecal administration of aminoglycosides, which did not alter the outcome. He then studied intraventricular administration of aminoglycosides, which actually increased the mortality (McCracken *et al.* 1980).

The advent of the third-generation cephalosporins was heralded as solving the problem of CSF penetration of antibiotics. Ceftriaxone has been used in the USA, but caution is needed in the neonatal period because it can displace bilirubin bound to albumin and aggravate hyperbilirubinemia. Trimethroprim-sulfamethoxazole (cotrimoxazole) can be very useful against multi-resistant Gram-negative bacilli.

### Multi-resistant organisms

One exception to the above antibiotic recommendations is if the baby with meningitis is known to be infected with a cefotaxime-resistant Gram-negative bacillus or if there is widespread colonization of other babies with resistant organisms. In such a case, the baby should be treated with an antibiotic with good CSF penetration to which the organism is sensitive, e.g. meropenem. Imipenem has good CSF penetration, but causes convulsions in older children with meningitis, so meropenem should be used in preference. However, either carbapenem should only be used if there are no alternatives. Experience with meropenem is limited but when used to treat 15 neonates (8 preterm) there were no side-effects recorded (Unhanand *et al.* 1993). Although imipenem is more effective in the treatment of multi-resistant Gram positive bacteria, meropenem has good activity against cephalosporin-resistant pneumococci. Multi-resistant *Acinetobacter baumannii* presents a particular challenge in its ability to survive on fomites and develop resistance to carbapenems, but treatment with ampicillin/sulbactam has been successful. Fourth-generation cephalosporins (e.g. cefpirome) have been used in children with bacterial meningitis, and CSF penetration is good, but there are currently no data on neonates.

### Duration of therapy

The duration of therapy for neonatal meningitis has not been well studied, is ignored in some textbooks, and is largely empirical. Relapses are not uncommon from Gram-negative and, more rarely Gram-positive, meningitis; however, the histories of those babies who have more than one relapse suggest that the relapses are not due to inadequate duration of therapy, but rather to sequestration of organisms.

Ventriculitis is almost invariable in Gram-negative enteric meningitis. It may be diagnosed by showing a pleocytosis in CSF obtained by ventricular tap or, less invasively, by showing fibrin strands on a cerebral ultrasound scan. Gram-negative enteric meningitis should be treated for at least 3 weeks because of the difficulty of treating ventriculitis. It is usually stated that GBS meningitis can be treated for 2 weeks. As ventriculitis rarely complicates GBS meningitis, we prefer to obtain an ultrasound. We treat for 2 weeks if there is no evidence of ventriculitis but for at least 3 weeks if fibrin strands are seen.

### Summary of treatment

- Treatment of early-onset meningitis should be with ampicillin and an aminoglycoside (unless Gram-negative bacilli are seen on a Gram stain).
- Treatment of Gram-negative meningitis should be with cefotaxime (or ceftazidime for *Pseudomonas*) and an aminoglycoside.
- Empirical therapy for neonatal meningitis (organism unknown) should be with ampicillin and cefotaxime.
- Gram-negative meningitis should be treated for at least 3 weeks.
- Neither fluid restriction nor steroids have been shown to be of benefit in neonatal meningitis.

## COMPLICATIONS

### MONITORING

Regular neurological examination is, of course, essential. Close monitoring of vital parameters is essential in order to minimize morbidity and mortality, and newborns with bacterial meningitis should ideally be looked after in a tertiary referral centre. For shocked babies, continual monitoring of arterial and central venous pressure allows better fluid balance management. Urine output, urine and serum osmolality, and serum electrolytes should be monitored to permit anticipation of problems with inappropriate ADH secretion. Hematological parameters, including clotting, should be regularly measured. Serial serum CRP measurements can be a useful indicator of progress, low levels showing resolution, and elevated levels suggesting continuing infection. Drug levels of antibiotics and anticonvulsants may need to be measured. Head circumference should be measured at least daily, as should the baby's weight.

### REPEAT LUMBAR PUNCTURES

Some textbooks recommend daily lumbar puncture, particularly for Gram-negative infections, until it is clear that the meningitis is improving. However, others recommend only repeating the lumbar puncture if there is a failure to respond to treatment (de Louvois & Lambert 1991). CSF cultures remain positive in Gram-negative bacillary meningitis (mean: 6 days, range: 2–11 days) for longer than in GBS meningitis, in which CSF cultures are usually sterile within 2–3 days of starting treatment. It has not been shown to be useful to do a lumbar puncture just before stopping therapy.

Babies with no cells may relapse, while babies with persistent CSF pleocytosis may recover if therapy is stopped. Persisting or recurrent fever may be due to persistence of meningitis, to subdural or intracerebral abscess, to infection in other sites (pleural empyema, septic arthritis, and osteomyelitis), or to intercurrent infection.

Recurrences of both Gram-positive and Gram-negative meningitis may occur after stopping apparently successful treatment. A careful search, both clinical and radiographic, should be made for persisting foci of infection, but these are rarely found.

We have seen a baby with two recurrences of *E. coli* meningitis, despite apparently adequate and successful treatment with cefotaxime; no underlying cause was found, and the baby was finally cured using intravenous trimethoprim-sulfamethoxazole. One small study from Australia reported that five (21%) of 24 babies with Gram-negative meningitis relapsed when treatment with chloramphenicol and gentamicin (three babies) or cefotaxime (2) was stopped. However, in a national study, only two (5%) of 40 babies with Gram-negative and one of 41 with GBS meningitis relapsed (Francis & Gilbert, 1992). A relapse rate of 8% was reported in another large study of neonatal meningitis from Sweden.

## INTRACRANIAL PRESSURE (p. 482)

Intracranial pressure (ICP) is rarely monitored in the newborn period, but cerebral perfusion pressure (arterial blood pressure minus ICP) may be an important determinant of outcome. The measurement of fontanelle pressure by fontanometer, although non-invasive, is less reliable than invasive ICP monitoring. Invasive monitoring of ICP by subdural catheter or intraventricular catheter is rarely performed in newborns, but might be indicated when there is evidence (e.g. rising blood pressure, falling heart rate) of a significantly raised ICP.

## EEG (see also Chapter 11)

Continuous EEG monitoring, particularly of comatose babies and those receiving muscle relaxants, may reveal clinically unrecognized convulsions, which can impair cerebral perfusion. Where this facility is not available, serial EEGs can be helpful. Seizures may be clinically evident; they may present insidiously with apneic attacks or episodes of hypoxia, or may be subclinical and only diagnosed by EEG. In general, the presence of seizures is a poor prognostic feature, particularly if they are not controlled by anticonvulsants. If the EEG appearance is considered in conjunction with the history of seizures and level of consciousness, a reasonably accurate prediction of neurological outcome can be made.

## ULTRASOUND (see also Chapter 6)

Ultrasound detects complications requiring neurosurgical intervention such as empyema, brain abscess or hydrocephalus in infants with bacterial meningitis. Small subdural effusions may be difficult to detect by ultrasound but occur often in bacterial meningitis and very rarely need any intervention. Larger effusions may cause persistent fever and midline shift of the brain with symptoms of raised intracranial pressure. Such effusions may show up on transillumination of the skull. Hydrocephalus is more likely after neonatal meningitis than after meningitis in infancy or in childhood.

## CT AND MRI (see also Chapter 6)

The role of computed tomography (CT) in detection of the complications of neonatal meningitis is limited when ultrasound has advantages of accessibility and lack of radiation. However, contrast-enhanced CT is useful in diagnosis and follow-up of cerebral candidiasis (see Fig. 33.2). Ring enhancement seen on CT may be due to infarction as reported with *Enterobacter* mimicking abscess formation. Magnetic resonance imaging (MRI) may rarely have a role in detecting brainstem or spinal-cord complications, but it has not been shown to correlate well with prognosis for seizures. Recurrent meningitis may need investigation with scintigraphic CSF leak studies, particularly if it follows neurosurgery.

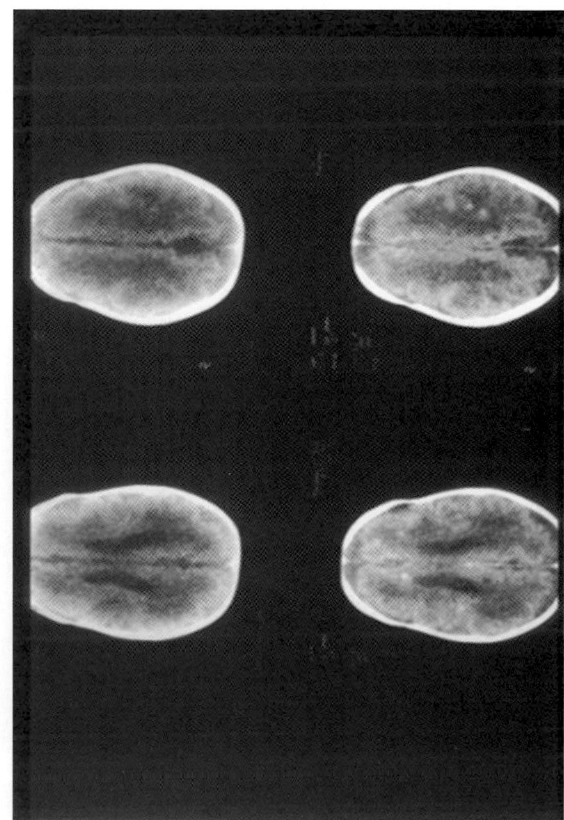

Figure 33.2 CT changes of fungal meningitis.

## BRAIN ABSCESS

Brain abscess, although still rare, is more common in the neonatal period, particularly in association with *Citrobacter* and *Proteus* meningitis (see Fig. 33.3). Other organisms associated with brain abscess include *Serratia marcescens, Salmonella enteritidis, Morganella morganii, Haemophilus influenzae* and *Escherichia coli. Citrobacter* can be rapidly fatal and has been associated with omphalitis. *Staphylococcus aureus* brain abscesses may originate from intravenous cannula sites in premature infants. In brain abscess, there may be a moderate increase in CSF white-cell count, with up to a few hundred cells, mostly mononuclear, and raised CSF protein. Organisms are not usually seen on Gram's stain nor grown from the CSF. Abscesses are often multiple, which makes surgical drainage more complicated. Ultrasound-guided needle aspiration can be used with local anesthetic to drain single abscesses. They may resolve with medical treatment alone. Brain abscess is associated with a mortality of around 50%. Neurosurgical management of brain abscess is discussed in p. 780.

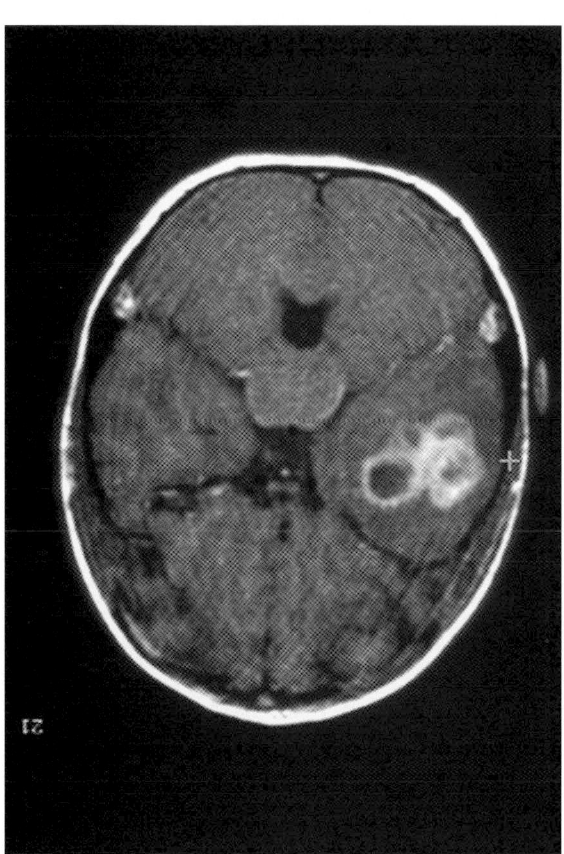

Figure 33.3 MRI showing multifocal brain abscess.

## MORTALITY

The mortality of neonatal meningitis still remains high at 20–30%, whether the meningitis is of early or late onset (see Table 33.6). The mortality increases with prematurity and low birthweight. The fatality rate for Gram-negative neonatal meningitis has been reported as 17% (of 72) over a 21-year period in the USA (Unhanand *et al.* 1993) to 31% (of 93) in the UK and 33% (of 40) in Australia. The mortality for Group B streptococcus in the same studies in the UK was 24% (of 112) and 29% (of 41) in Australia. The number of cases of *Listeria* meningitis was small, and the number of deaths was two out of 19 and one out of three, respectively.

## MORBIDITY

Neonatal meningitis results in a high rate of long-term sequelae such as hydrocephalus and neurodevelopmental problems. Although it is not always clear to what extent meningitis and other predisposing factors such as extreme prematurity have contributed to the outcome, significant neurologic sequelae develop in 20–60% of all survivors of neonatal bacterial meningitis caused by any organism (Klein & Marcy 1995). These sequelae include major neurodevelopmental handicap, hemiparesis, spastic paraparesis, cranial nerve palsies, hydrocephalus, hearing loss, visual handicap, convulsions, and speech and hearing disorders.

The rate of hydrocephalus has been reported as 41% (29/71) and gross abnormalities in the neurological examination 62% (44/71) from a study in Brazil. Another study from Brazil of term neonates with meningitis followed up for a mean of 5 years, showed neurological sequelae in 64% (35/55), cerebral palsy 58% (severe 24%), hydrocephalus 46% and convulsions 35%. From the UK, three of 11 survivors of neonatal bacterial meningitis developed hydrocephalus, and one had significant neurologic sequelae.

**Table 33.6 Mortality rates for neonatal bacterial meningitis**

| Years | Country | Cases | Deaths | Reference |
|---|---|---|---|---|
| 1970–1980 | USA | 26 | 5 (19%) | Franco *et al.* (1992) |
| 1973–1986 | N. Ireland | 41 | 20 (49%) | Bell *et al.* (1989) |
| 1977–1987 | Brazil | 109 | 38 (35%) | Feferbaum *et al.* (1993) |
| 1985–1987 | UK | 423 | 79 (20%) | de Louvois *et al.* (1991) |
| 1987–1989 | Australia | 116 | 30 (26%) | Francis & Gilbert (1992) |
| 1984–1991 | UK | 23 | 6 (26%) | Hristeva *et al.* (1993) |
| 1990–1995 | Mexico | 31 | 9 (29%) | Rios-Reategui *et al.* (1998) |

### Group B streptococcal meningitis

The risk factors associated with poor outcome in 61 neonates with group B streptococcal meningitis between 1974 and 1979 included presentation comatose or semicomatose, decreased perfusion, total peripheral white-cell count less than $5 \times 10^9$/1, absolute neutrophil count less than $1 \times 10^9$/l, and CSF protein greater than 3 mg/l. Of 38 survivors followed up for at least 3 years, 29% had severe neurologic sequelae and 21% minor deficits. From another study with follow-up at 3–18 years old, 12% (9/34) had major neurologic sequelae.

### Gram-negative meningitis

Of survivors of Gram-negative neonatal meningitis, 56% (24/43) had permanent neurologic sequelae (the same percentage in term neonates as preterm neonates): hydrocephalus (13), seizure disorder (13), cerebral palsy (11), developmental delay (14) and hearing loss (7) (Unhanand *et al.* 1993). Significant poor prognostic factors included platelets <100 (× $10^9$/l), CSF leucocytes >2000 (× $10^6$/l), CSF/blood glucose ratio <0.5, CSF protein 2 (g/l), and positive CSF culture for > 48 h after the start of treatment. The rates of sequelae may vary with the organism: the rate for *Escherichia coli* was reported as 43% (13/30) and for *Klebsiella–Enterobacter* species 67% (6/9). Complications are significantly more common in Gram-negative, than Gram-positive, meningitis (6/10 vs. 13/76; $p$=0.014; 1987–1989 in Australia) (Francis & Gilbert 1992).

### Hearing loss (see also p. 686)

Otoacoustic emissions are a useful screening test for hearing loss that can be performed in neonates before discharge from hospital. Auditory brainstem responses (ABR) may be considered the gold standard for testing hearing after meningitis in neonates. However, interpretation of ABR requires expertise, and it can be time-consuming and expensive. Furthermore, young children sometimes require sedation, or even general anesthesia, before ABR can be performed. Insertion of cochlear implants in infancy is possible for profound sensorineural deafness.

### Rare neurologic sequelae

Reported rare neurologic complications from meningitis include ischemia of the spinal cord resulting from vasculitis associated with *Escherichia coli* meningitis. A transverse myelitis with development of spinal cord cavitation and destruction of the cerebellum developing posterior cysts has been reported in a preterm neonate with *Streptococcus agalactiae* (GBS) meningitis. Sagittal sinus thrombosis has been reported with *Streptococcus pyogenes* meningitis in a neonate, which is of particular interest as the incidence of Group A streptococcal infections is increasing. Central diabetes insipidus as a complication of hypothalamic damage can occur with hemorrhage and hydrocephalus subsequent to Group B streptococcal meningitis.

### Endophthalmitis

This rare infection of the orbit of the eye has been reported, complicating meningitis in the neonate. It is usually secondary to trauma, such as with face masks or eye pads for phototherapy. However, it can also be hematogenous and may be associated with meningitis. Responsible organisms include *Serratia marcescens* and *Pseudomonas aeruginosa* associated with sepsis and *Escherichia coli* with meningitis. It has also been described congenitally and with *Candida albicans* and *Aspergillus fumigatus*. The diagnosis should be suspected when a hypopyon is seen, and confirmation can be obtained by ultrasound if an anterior uveitis obstructs vision of the retina. The treatment includes urgent intraocular antimicrobials, e.g. antibiotics such as vancomycin and intravenous antibiotics such as ceftriaxone that penetrate the globe (more so than cefotaxime). Vitrectomy may also be necessary.

### Summary of complications

- Lumbar puncture before stopping antibiotics is not necessary.
- Babies with GBS meningitis should have a cerebral ultrasound: treat with at least 2 weeks of antibiotics, but at least 3 weeks if ventriculitis is present.
- Bacterial meningitis has a mortality of 10–25%, and 20–60% of survivors have major neurodevelopmental sequelae.
- Endophthalmitis is often associated with meningitis in neonates and requires urgent intra-ocular antibiotics.

## SHUNT INFECTIONS

Infections of ventriculoperitoneal (VP) or ventriculoatrial (VA) shunts should be considered separately from bacterial meningitis. These occur in between 3 and 27% of shunts, with a mean of 11% (Anonymous 1989). Although shunt infections may present like classic bacterial meningitis, they commonly present more insidiously. VP shunt infections cause vomiting, lethargy and irritability with or without fever, whereas VA shunt infections may cause low-grade fever, progressive anemia, and hematuria and hypertension secondary to shunt nephritis. Infection of a newly placed shunt is highly likely if there is significant infection of the skin overlying the reservoir, a situation that readily occurs in small preterm neonates when the skin of the scalp is stretched over the reservoir.

Coagulase-negative staphylococci, such as *Staphylococcus epidermidis*, are the commonest cause of shunt infections, but these may also be caused by *Staphylococcus aureus* and, particularly in babies of low birthweight, by Gram-negative bacilli (e.g. *Pseudomonas*), by low-grade pathogens such as diphtheroids, and by fungi (see Table 33.7). In a study from Germany, 22 of 28 (79%) were Gram-positive cocci and two were Gram-negative bacilli. *Staphylococcus epidermidis* produces an extracellular slime

**Table 33.7 CSF shunt infection rates**

| Year | Country | Infection rate per Case | Procedure | Reference |
|---|---|---|---|---|
| 1978–1983 | UK | 19% (23/155) | 12% (46/380) | Casey *et al.* (1997) |
| 1981–1992 | Italy | 17% (14/81) | 7.8% (15/191) | Dallacasa *et al.* (1995) |
| 1985–1990 | Croatia | 18% (36/201) | 9.4% (36/382) | Rotim *et al.* (1997) |
| 1991–1995 | Croatia | 8% (6/75) | 5.3% (6/112) | Rotim *et al.* (1997) |
| 1986–1989 | Germany | (25 patients) | 8% (28/350) | Kontny *et al.* (1993) |
| 1990–1996 | USA | 13% (20/145) | 11% (29/268) | Mancao *et al.* (1998) |

that enables it to adhere to implantable devices and resist antibiotic therapy. *Bacillus cereus* has also been reported, causing shunt infections. *Propionibacterium acnes*, a low-grade pathogen, has been associated with 15% of shunt infections (distinguished from being a contaminant by presence in CSF of Gram-positive rods and white cells), presenting as gradual shunt malfunction, nausea, headache and malaise, though infrequently fever.

Of 23 cases of Gram-negative shunt infections from one center in the USA, 87% (20) occurred within 4 weeks of shunt revision (median 10 days). The most frequent symptoms were fever, lethargy, and irritability, but most patients appeared relatively well. *E. coli* was isolated from 52% (12) and *Klebsiella pneumoniae* from five. Four patients had persistence of the bacteria in the CSF despite immediate shunt removal, and all had CSF glucose <1 mmol/l and a positive CSF Gram stain on admission. All were cured with no recurrence.

The first priority in suspected shunt infection is to obtain a specimen of CSF for microscopic examination by tapping the shunt reservoir. Measurement of serum CRP has been helpful in identifying whether babies with non-specific symptoms have shunt infections.

If shunt infection is confirmed, the entire shunt usually needs to be removed. In a review of several trials (Yogev 1985), the success rate of antibiotics alone was 36% (71/195); antibiotics and immediate replacement with a new shunt had a 65% (75/116) success rate; and antibiotics, shunt removal, external ventricular drain, or repeat ventricular aspirates had a 96% (154/161) success rate. The appropriate antibiotics can be given intravenously. When the protocol was changed in Zagreb to include complete shunt revision and prophylactic antibiotics, the infection rate was reduced from 18% per case to 8%.

Because an intraventricular reservoir or external ventricular drain is usually inserted to drain CSF until the shunt infection is cleared (p. 756), antibiotics can be given directly into the ventricles (e.g. vancomycin, gentamicin) if there is a problem with severe infection or infection with a multiply resistant organism. Intraventricular antibiotics themselves can cause a chemical meningitis, so when the CSF is sterile and organisms are no longer seen, intraventricular antibiotics should not be continued merely because of a raised CSF white-cell count and protein.

Prophylactic antibiotics at the time of shunt insertion have been shown to be associated with a significant reduction in shunt infections in only one study, but when 12 studies were combined in a meta-analysis, on aggregate, the approximate risk reduction was 50%, $p = 0.0002$ (Langley *et al.* 1993). In a prospective study from Italy, a single dose of ceftriaxone was given preoperatively i.v. in 100 cases, and no shunt infections were observed over a 4-year follow up period.

Although one-half of our isolates of coagulase-negative staphylococci are cloxacillin (methicillin)-resistant, we start empiric antibiotic therapy of shunt infections in which Gram-positive cocci are seen on the Gram's stain of the CSF, using flucloxacillin and aminoglycoside, rather than vancomycin, because these infections are rarely fulminant, and symptoms often resolve simply with removal of the shunt. Teicoplanin has been used intraventricularly for *Staphylococcus aureus*, *Staphylococcus epidermidis*, and *Enterococcus faecalis* shunt infections, though it was not effective given intravenously alone as an alternative to vancomycin for organisms resistant to other penicillins.

Of children with meningomyelocele, 11.5% (20/170) in a study from Italy presented within the first year following shunting with shunt infection. Infections were associated with higher meningomyeloceles, degree of ventricular dilatation, age of meningomyelocele repair, CSF shunting before repair, and abnormal CSF values.

In Taiwan, 17% (8/48) of shunt infections were attributed to fungi isolated from the CSF and not thought to be contaminants. All were in infants who had been born prematurely. The presentation was subtle and insidious, and the CSF only showed a mild pleocytosis and raised CSF protein, but only in half was the CSF glucose low.

## SUMMARY OF SHUNT INFECTIONS

- Shunt infections should usually be managed by complete removal of the tubing, external ventricular drain and antibiotics

## FUNGAL CNS INFECTIONS

Neonatal central nervous system infection with fungi is a rare, but serious, condition (see Table 33.8). In a retrospective study from Texas, *Candida albicans* accounted for 2% of all positive CSF cultures in neonates. One-third of neonates (three out of nine) in that study and three-quarters (six out of eight) of premature neonates in a retrospective study from Canada with *Candida* meningitis had candidemia. In the Canadian study, of 23 neonates with candidemia, six (26%) had *Candida* meningitis. A similar rate was found in a prospective study from Slovakia, where, of 40 neonates with *Candida* isolated from the blood, eight (20%) had candida meningitis or meningoencephalitis.

Treatment with amphotericin alone in the Texas study resulted in recovery of five out of seven babies with *Candida* meningitis. In Canada, using amphotericin and 5-flucytosine, five out of eight recovered. In Slovakia, using fluconazole alone, four out of eight recovered, and in a study in Italy, five out of six treated with liposomal amphotericin recovered. Beyond the neonatal age group, with an intact blood–brain barrier, the penetration of amphotericin into the CSF is relatively poor, and the addition of 5-flucytosine allows the use of lower doses of amphotericin. This combination is particularly useful for species other than *Candida albicans*. In adults, the starting dose of amphotericin is 0.25 mg/kg once daily by intravenous infusion. For *Candida albicans*, the dose is increased to 1 mg/kg/day. Infants tolerate amphotericin better than adults do, and in *Candida* meningitis in neonates, it is appropriate to start at 0.5–1.0 mg/kg/day. The side-effects of renal toxicity, fever, gastrointestinal upset, bone marrow suppression, anaphylaxis and severe electrolyte disturbances including hypokalemia and hypomagnesemia have been reported in infants. Liposomal amphotericin allows higher doses to be given without increasing toxicity. Because of the ten times greater cost of the liposomal preparation, it is reasonable to reserve it for neonates with renal impairment or those developing side-effects or who are refractory to amphotericin B. Occasional babies with *Candida parapsilosis* do not respond to amphotericin but do respond to fluconazole. Fluconazole is an effective alternative to amphotericin for *Candida albicans* meningitis and has the advantage it can be used orally to complete a course of antifungal therapy if intravenous access is a problem.

The mortality rate in three recent studies (see Table 33.8) was 36% (9/25). Of the five survivors followed up in the Canadian study, three had motor scales >3SD below the mean, two had intelligence scales >3SD below the mean, two had hearing loss, and one had vision loss. The mortality rate of *Candida albicans* is higher than that of *Candida parapsilosis*.

Neonates acquire *Candida albicans* through vertical transmission most commonly, but *Candida parapsilosis* and *Candida lusitaniae* are most often nosocomially acquired infections. The incidence of *Candida parapsilosis* infection is increasing, and it has now been reported as the main cause of candidemia in a NICU in the USA. Contrast-enhanced CT scanning can be useful in the diagnosis of neonatal cerebral candidiasis (see Fig. 33.2).

Apart from *Candida* species, there are other fungal infections, including *Trichoporon beigelii*, reported as causing invasive neonatal infections and shunt infections. This organism can be successfully treated with amphotericin. Other rare case reports of neonatal CNS infections include the fungi *Cryptococcus neoformans*, *Torulopsis glabrata*, and *Aspergillus sydowi* and *A. fumigatus*.

### SUMMARY OF FUNGAL MENINGITIS

- Use amphotericin B (±5-flucytosine).
- Fluconazole is an acceptable alternative to amphotericin B.
- Fluconazole can be given orally if IV access is a problem late in course.
- Treat for at least 4 weeks.

## INFANTILE BOTULISM (see also p. 705)

Infantile botulism is caused by ingestion of spores followed by gut colonization. In a case–control study from the USA of 68 infants with laboratory-confirmed infantile botulism, the main risk factor for infants under 2 months of age was living in a rural area or on a farm. Eleven of the 68 cases had consumed honey.

*Clostridium botulinum* spores are ubiquitous in the soil.

**Table 33.8 Fungal CNS infections**

| Study group | Reference | Country | Total | M:F | Age (days) Mean (range) | CSF WCC Mean (range) | CSF +ve culture | Blood +ve culture | Died |
|---|---|---|---|---|---|---|---|---|---|
| *Candida fungaemia* | Huttova *et al.* (1998) | Slovakia | 8 | 6:2 | 27 (15–29) | – | 6 | 8 | 4 |
| Premature candiasis | Lee *et al.* (1998) | Canada | 8 | – | – | 175 (1–529) | 5 | 6 | 3 |
| CSF candida | Arisoy *et al.* (1994) | USA | 9 | 2:7 | 12 (5–26) | 184 (0–1120) | 9 | 3 | 2 |

Breast-feeding may generate the optimal conditions for germination of the spores. The organism colonizes the gut and produces a powerful exotoxin. The toxin is absorbed into the bloodstream via the gut and carried hematogenously to cholinergic nerve synapses, particularly neuromuscular junctions. Here, it binds irreversibly to receptors on the presynaptic nerve terminal, blocking acetylcholine release. This explains the atropinic manifestations of the disease such as pupillary dilatation and constipation, as well as the muscular hypotonia and cranial-nerve palsies. The disease is characterized by a descending paralysis of the cranial nerves followed by paralysis of the nerves to the axial and truncal muscles. The presentation can also be acute with a sepsis-like illness and respiratory arrest. Recovery invariably occurs after some days or weeks due to sprouting of new nerve terminals.

The diagnosis is confirmed by intra-peritoneal injection of purified stool from the patient into two mice, one of which is also given the antitoxin. Death of the mouse without the antitoxin and survival of the other confirms the diagnosis. Otherwise, there are commercial assays for type A neurotoxin. Isolation of *Clostridium botulinum* from the stool and the characteristic electromyogram (EMG) also support the clinical diagnosis.

The management of infantile botulism is to protect the airway and support respiration, if necessary, until spontaneous recovery occurs. Tracheostomy prolongs hospitalization. Nasogastric feeds are usually well tolerated and obviate the need for parenteral nutrition. There is no indication for antimicrobial therapy (except for aspiration or hypostatic pneumonia). Penicillin does not speed recovery from infantile botulism, and gentamicin may exacerbate the condition, due to its effect on neuromuscular transmission. Botulinum immune globulin is available but not in routine use. Equine botulinum immune globulin is more readily available, but again not routinely necessary. The prognosis nowadays is excellent, although relapses can occur. A proposed association between infantile botulism and sudden infant death syndrome is totally unproven. Other species of clostridium including *C. barati* have also been recognized as causing infantile botulism.

### SUMMARY OF INFANTILE BOTULISM

- Classic triad of clinical features:
  - Bulbar palsies (slow/absent pupil response)
  - Alert
  - Absent fever.
- Also commonly presents with constipation, ptosis and poor feeding.

## NEONATAL TETANUS

Neonatal tetanus still causes significant mortality in developing countries despite the World Health Organization's goal of global elimination of the disease by the year 2000. The disease is caused by the neurotoxin produced by *Clostridium tetani*, a ubiquitous spore forming bacterium found in high concentrations in soil and animal excrements. The anaerobic conditions of the necrotic cord allow the spores to germinate. The cord becomes contaminated by non-hygienic practices of cutting the cord or traditional practices. In Turkey from 1991 to 1997, 55 babies with neonatal tetanus had all been delivered by untrained birth attendants in rural areas. The cord had been cut with a razor blade (55%), scissors (27%), or knife (18%). In KwaZulu-Natal, cow dung has been used to staunch the blood flow from the severed cord, and in Pakistan, neonatal tetanus has been associated with the practice of bundling, where the infant is wrapped for prolonged periods in a sheepskin cover after dried cow dung is applied.

The incidence in developing countries may not be accurately known, for example, when the infant dies before reaching medical help, and the diagnosis has to be made from care-givers' interviews. In Bangladesh, the sensitivity and specificity of particular combinations of signs are >80% for neonatal tetanus. In 1997, there were an estimated 277 400 deaths world-wide due to neonatal tetanus, but 20 years ago, there were an estimated 800 000 deaths annually. In the USA, there has only been one case from 1989 to 1997. Several studies have shown a male predominance: 78% (161/207) and 76% (42/55).

The mean age of onset of symptoms is 5–6 days (range 1–21 days) with the fatal cases presenting significantly earlier in reviews of cases from 1976 to 1994 and 1991 to 1997. The most common symptoms are spasticity (76%), lack of sucking (71%), trismus (60%), fever (49%), omphalitis (44%), irritability (24%), risus sardonicus (22%), and opisthotonus (15%).

Treatment includes intravenous human tetanus immunoglobulin. The dose required for neonates is not well established. Four thousand international units (IU) is probably appropriate for neonates. The infusion should be started slowly and increased as tolerated (e.g. from 0.1 ml/min for 30 min increased to 0.2 ml/min). If this is not available intramuscular tetanus immune globulin (TIG) should be given. A dose of 500 IU has been effective in neonates, part of the dose traditionally being injected around the umbilicus, though this is not of proven value. If neither is available, equine tetanus antitoxin (TAT) can be given after a test dose because 10–20% develop serum sickness. Ten thousand international units has been found to be an adequate dose. Alternatively intravenous gammaglobulin can be given, though the dose has not been evaluated.

The umbilicus should be debrided if there is necrotic tissue, but wide excision of the umbilical stump is not recommended. Metronidazole (30 mg/kg/day given at six-hourly intervals) is effective at reducing the number of vegetative forms of *C. tetani* and is the antibiotic of choice. Penicillin G (100 000 U/kg/day) given at 4–6-h intervals is an alternative treatment. The antibiotics should be continued for 10–14 days. High-dose diazepam (40 mg/kg/day), phenobarbitone, and chlorpromazine have been found to lower the mortality significantly compared to less sedation.

The mortality remains high, even when intensive care is available. The mortality rate was 47% in the older study and 40% in the more recent study without any equipment for mechanical ventilation. In Nigeria, a mortality rate of 59% was reported, and in South Africa, where ventilation in a pediatric intensive care setting was available, the mortality rate was 22%. The mean age at death is 9 days and 5 days from admission. In those ventilated, the mean duration of ventilation was 23 days (range 17–60 days) and ICU stay 35 days (range 13–87 days).

The World Health Organization's major strategy for prevention of neonatal tetanus is the administration of at least two properly spaced doses of tetanus toxoid to women of child-bearing age in high-risk areas to passively protect their newborns at birth. Part of the failure to reach the goal of elimination of neonatal tetanus has been subpotent vaccine, as well as a failure to immunize. Other strategies have been the provision of 'safe-birth kits' with a sterile razor blade (or half blade so that it is not taken for use for other purposes!); teaching birth attendants hand washing (OR 0.64 $p$=0.005); and application of topical antibiotics and disinfectants to the cord.

### SUMMARY OF NEONATAL TETANUS

- WHO aims to eliminate neonatal tetanus, but cases still occur, even in industrialized countries.

## CONGENITAL NEUROSYPHILIS

A dramatic increase in syphilis, which occurred in the late 1980s and early 1990s in the USA, has subsequently declined. In the UK, there were nine presumptive cases of congenital syphilis reported between 1994 and 1997. Acute syphilitic leptomeningitis usually appears between 3 and 6 months of age. Infants present with symptoms and signs of acute bacterial meningitis, including a stiff neck, progressive vomiting, a positive Kernig's sign, bulging of the fontanelles, separation of the sutures, and hydrocephalus. The CSF shows a monocytosis, with up to 200 cells/mm$^3$, a modest increase in protein (0.5–2 g/l), and a normal glucose level. The CSF VDRL is positive. This form of CNS syphilis responds to penicillin.

Late manifestations of involvement of the central nervous system usually occur after 1–2 years of age. Chronic meningovascular syphilis may have a protracted course with progressive communicating hydrocephalus due to obstruction in the basilar cisterns. It may also cause VIIth cranial nerve palsies (occasionally III, IV or VI), optic atrophy, and gradual intellectual deterioration. Vascular lesions of the brain have been described, with endarteritis causing convulsions and an acute hemiplegia.

For the diagnosis of neurosyphilis, a raised neonatal CSF protein (>1.8 g/l) and raised CSF white-cell count (>25 × 10$^6$ WBC/l) in the presence of maternal evidence of inadequately treated syphilis is sufficient for treatment of the infant for neurosyphilis. The CSF white-cell count and protein can be normal in neurosyphilis. The only serological test that should be performed on the CSF is the non-treponemal Venereal Disease Research Laboratory (VDRL) slide test. The other non-treponemal tests such as rapid plasma reagin (RPR) or the automated reagin test (ART) should not be used on the neonatal CSF. The treponemal test such as fluorescent treponemal antibody absorption (FTA-ABS) test or the microhemagglutination test for *T. pallidum* (MHA-TP or TPHA) measure IgG and IgM. IgG can be detected coincidentally in the neonatal CSF after the mother has been successfully treated before pregnancy. IgM detection by immunoblot from CSF of neonates has been found to be positive in two out of six cases of neurosyphilis [defined by Rabbit Infectivity Testing (RIT)]. *T. pallidum* DNA PCR was positive in five out of the six cases. A negative CSF VDRL does not exclude neurosyphilis, and the CSF VDRL can be falsely positive by transplacental acquisition of antibody from a mother with high titer. Specific IgM to *T. pallidum* has been found in infants with congenital syphilis and is being evaluated as an alternative diagnostic tool. However, in developing countries where congenital syphilis is most common, the IgM is often not available.

The American Pediatric Association recommends that a lumbar puncture and CSF VDRL, cell count, and protein be performed on the infants of mothers with a positive syphilis treponemal test who have not had appropriate treatment documented or if the treated mother has not had an adequate decrease in non-treponemal antibody titer over 1 month. However, the need for lumbar puncture in asymptomatic infants is debatable, e.g. 329 infants from two Washington hospitals in 1990–1993 met the APA criteria for LP, but the CSF was normal, and CSF protein and glucose were not significantly different from normal controls.

The treatment for neurosyphilis is penicillin G 200 000 to 300 000 U/kg/day (50 000 U/kg every 4–6 h) for 10–14 days, possibly followed by benzathine penicillin, 50 000 U/kg/dose in three weekly doses. CSF concentrations of penicillin reach treponemicidal concentrations when given as aqueous penicillin G at 100 000 U/kg/day and were not significantly increased when the dose was raised to 200 000 U/kg/day. They were significantly higher than using procaine penicillin 50 000 U/kg/day, which did not reach treponemicidal levels in CSF in a third of infants.

### SUMMARY OF NEUROSYPHILIS

- Consider LP if maternal VDRL is positive and inadequate documentation of maternal treatment.
- LP mandatory if neonate has signs of syphilis.
- CSF dark ground microscopy, WCC and protein.
- CSF VRDL (± *T. pallidum* PCR, IgM if available).

## Key Points

- Bacterial meningitis is more common in the first month than at any other age.
- About 10–30% of babies with early-onset septicemia and 10% with late-onset septicemia, have meningitis.
- Group B streptococcus is the commonest cause of early-onset meningitis in industrialized countries.
- Gram-negative enteric bacilli are the most common cause of late-onset meningitis
- Ventriculitis is common in neonatal bacterial meningitis, particularly Gram-negative meningitis, and there may be collections of pus in the ventricles and subarachnoid space.
- Vasculitis is common and may lead to venous thrombosis; there may be infarcts and focal necrosis.
- Treatment of early-onset meningitis should be with ampicillin and an aminoglycoside (unless Gram-negative bacilli are seen on Gram-stain).
- Treatment of Gram-negative meningitis should be with cefotaxime (or ceftazidime for *Pseudomonas*) and an aminoglycoside.
- Empirical therapy for neonatal meningitis (organism unknown) should be with ampicillin and cefotaxime.
- Gram-negative meningitis should be treated for at least 3 weeks.
- Bacterial meningitis has a mortality of 10–25%, 20–60% of survivors have major neurodevelopmental sequelae.
- Shunt infections should usually be managed by complete removal of the tubing, external ventricular drain and antibiotics.
- In fungal meningitis, use amphotericin B (± 5-flucytosine) or fluconazole as an alternative; treat for at least 4 weeks.

## REFERENCES


Adhikari M, Coovadia Y M & Singh D (1995) A 4-year study of neonatal meningitis: clinical and microbiological findings. *J Trop Pediatr* 41:81–85.

Ahmed A, Hickey S M, Ehrett S *et al.* (1996) Cerebrospinal fluid values in the term neonate. *Pediatr Infect Dis J* 15:298–303.

Airede A I (1993) Neonatal bacterial meningitis in the middle belt of Nigeria. *Dev Med Child Neurol* 35:424–430.

Ali Z (1995) Neonatal meningitis: a 3-year retrospective study at the Mount Hope Women's Hospital, Trinidad, West Indies. *J Trop Pediatr* 41:109–111.

Anonymous (1989) Cerebrospinal fluid shunt infections. *Lancet* 1:1304–1305.

Arisoy E S, Arisoy A E & Dunne W M, Jr. (1994) Clinical significance of fungi isolated from cerebrospinal fluid in children. *Pediatr Infect Dis J* 13:128–133.

Bell A H, Brown D, Halliday H L *et al.* (1989) Meningitis in the newborn – a 14 year review. *Arch Dis Childhood* 64(6):873–874.

Casey A T, Kimmings E J, Kleinlugtebeld A D *et al.* (1997) The long-term outlook for hydrocephalus in childhood. A ten-year cohort study of 155 patients. *Pediatr Neurosurg* 27:63–70.

Chotpitayasunondh T (1994) Bacterial meningitis in children: etiology and clinical features, an 11-year review of 618 cases. *Southeast Asian J Trop Med Public Health* 25:107–115.

Dallacasa P, Dappozzo A, Galassi E *et al.* (1995) Cerebrospinal fluid shunt infections in infants. *Childs Nerv Syst* 11:643–648.

Daoud A S, al-Sheyyab M, Abu-Ekteish F, *et al.* (1996) Neonatal meningitis in northern Jordan. *J Trop Pediatr* 42:267–270.

✪ De Louvois J & Lambert H P (eds) (1991) Infections of the central nervous system. In: *Neonatal meningitis.* Philadelphia, PA: B.C. Decker, Chapter 13; pp. 161–174.

✪ De Louvois J, Blackbourn J, Hurley R *et al.* (1991) Infantile meningitis in England and Wales: a two year study. *Arch Dis Childhood* 66:603–609.

Feferbaum R, Vaz F A, Krebs V L *et al.* (1993) Bacterial meningitis in the neonatal period. Clinical evaluation and complications in 109 cases. *Arquivos de Neuro-Psiquiatria* 51:72–79.

Francis B M & Gilbert G L (1992) Survey of neonatal meningitis in Australia: 1987–1989. *Med J Aust* 156:240–243.

Franco S M, Cornelius V E & Andrews B F (1992) Long-term outcome of neonatal meningitis. *Am J Dis Children* 146:567–571.

Greenberg D, Shinwell E S, Yagupsky P *et al.* (1997) A prospective study of neonatal sepsis and meningitis in southern Israel. *Pediatr Infect Dis J* 16:768–773.

✪ Hristeva L, Booy R, Bowler I *et al.* (1993) Prospective surveillance of neonatal meningitis. *Arch Dis Childhood* 69:14–18.

Huttova M, Hartmanova I, Kralinsky K *et al.* (1998) *Candida fungemia* in neonates treated with fluconazole: report of forty cases, including eight with meningitis. *Pediatr Infect Dis J* 17:1012–1015.

Isaacs D & Moxon E R (1999) Meningitis. In: *Handbook of neonatal infection: a practical guide.* London: WB Saunders, Chapter 8; p. 134.

Isaacs D & Royle J (1999) Intrapartum antibiotics and early onset neonatal sepsis caused by group B *Streptococcus* and by other organisms in Australia. *Pediatr Infect Dis* 18:524–528.

Joshi P & Barr P (1998) The use of lumbar puncture and laboratory tests for sepsis by Australian neonatologists. *J Paediatr Child Health* 34(1):74–78.

✪ Klein J O, Marcy S M, Remington J S *et al.* (eds) (1995) Infectious diseases of the fetus and newborn infant. In: *Bacterial sepsis and meningitis.* Philadelphia, PA: W.B. Saunders, 4th edn, Chapter 21; pp. 835–890.

Kontny U, Hofling B, Gutjahr P *et al.* (1993) CSF shunt infections in children. *Infection* 21:89–92.

Kumar P, Sarkar S & Narang A (1995) Role of routine lumbar puncture in neonatal sepsis. *J Paediatr Child Health* 31:8–10.

Langley J M, LeBlanc J C, Drake J *et al.* (1993) Efficacy of antimicrobial prophylaxis in placement of cerebrospinal fluid shunts: meta-analysis. *Clin Infect Dis* 17:98–103.

Lee B E, Cheung P Y, Robinson J L *et al.* (1998) Comparative study of mortality and morbidity in premature infants (birth weight, < 1,250 g) with candidemia or candidal meningitis. *Clin Infect Dis* 27:559–565.

Mancao M, Miller C, Cochrane B *et al.* (1998) Cerebrospinal fluid shunt infections in infants and children in Mobile, Alabama. *Acta Paediatr* 87:667–670.

McCracken G H J, Mize S G & Threlkeld N (1980) Intraventricular gentamicin therapy in gram-negative bacillary meningitis of infancy. Report of the Second Neonatal Meningitis Cooperative Study Group. *Lancet* 1:787–791.

Moses L M, Heath P T, Wilkinson A R *et al.* (1998) Early onset group B streptococcal neonatal infection in Oxford 1985–96. *Arch Dis Childhood Fetal Neonatal Ed* 79:F148–F149.

Ohlsson A, Lacy J B, Sinclair J C *et al.* (eds) (1998) Neonatal module of the Cochrane Database of Systematic Reviews. In: *Intravenous immunoglobulin for suspected or subsequently proven neonatal infection.* Oxford: The Cochrane Collaboration.

Platt R, Adleson-Mitty J, Weissman L *et al.* (1999) Resource utilization associated with initial hospital stays complicated by early onset group B streptococcal disease. *Pediatr Infect Dis* 18:529–533.

Rios-Reategui E, Ruiz-Gonzalez L & Murguia-de-Sierra T (1998) Neonatal bacterial meningitis in a tertiary treatment center. *Revista de Investigacion Clinica* 50(1):31–36.

Rotim K, Miklic P, Paladino J *et al.* (1997) Reducing the incidence of infection in pediatric cerebrospinal fluid shunt operations. *Childs Nerv Syst* 13:584–587.

Sarff L D, Platt L H & McCracken G H, Jr (1976) Cerebrospinal fluid evaluation in neonates: comparison of high-risk infants with and without meningitis. *J Pediatr* 88:473–477.

✪ Synnott M B, Morse D L & Hall S M (1994) Neonatal meningitis in England and Wales: a review of routine national data. *Arch Dis Childhood* 71:F75–F80.

✪ Unhanand M, Mustafa M M, McCracken G H J *et al.* (1993) Gram-negative enteric bacillary meningitis: a twenty-one-year experience. *J Pediatr* 122:15–21.

Visser V E & Hall R T (1980) Lumbar puncture in the evaluation of suspected neonatal sepsis. *J Pediatr* 96(6):1063–1067.

Yatsyk G V (1998) Use of meropenem in the treatment of severe infections in newborns. *Antibiotiki i Khimioterapiia* 43:32–33.

Yogev R (1985) Cerebrospinal fluid shunt infections: a personal view. *Pediatr Infect Dis* 4:113–118.

# Section VII
# Metabolic disorders

Chapter 34

# Prenatal diagnosis of inborn errors of metabolism

J. E. Wraith

## INTRODUCTION

Despite the advances made in the therapy of inherited metabolic disease, for many, the prognosis remains poor, and the best that can be offered to the family is a prenatal test aimed at preventing the disorder occurring in future pregnancies. The advances in obstetric practice combined with the desire for earlier prenatal diagnosis have led to a wide range of options for parents with pregnancies at risk. It is appropriate to consider these developments in the context of human biochemical genetics, and the following is a general review of the available techniques and the disorders studied.

Before discussing individual procedures, it is important to state a few general principles that apply to prenatal diagnosis for inherited metabolic disease:

1. The majority of inborn errors result from a specific enzyme deficiency, but in some, the primary defect is in a transport protein or enzyme cofactor. In some conditions, the biochemical defect is limited to specific tissues, and this restricts the material available for prenatal diagnosis for these disorders. Fortunately, for many, the defect is generalized, and both amniotic and chorionic villus cells can be used as diagnostic tissue.
2. The reliability of the test is of paramount importance, and for biochemical defects, assays should only be performed in specialized laboratories that have extensive experience of the pre- and postnatal diagnosis of inherited metabolic disease. A firm biochemical diagnosis must be established in the index case. It is unsafe to rely on clinical or histologic diagnosis, as many of the inherited metabolic disorders share a similar phenotype. To make interpretation of the results easier, it is often helpful to know the heterozygote levels of activity in the parents; occasionally, these are remarkably low and can lead to difficulties in ascribing fetal genotype.
3. The properties of some enzymes are appreciably different when studied at different times of gestation. In addition, the activity obtained from chorion villus material may be very different from that obtained on amniotic fluid cells. It is essential that the correct tissue is collected at the appropriate time. Liaison with the laboratory staff performing the test is mandatory if mistakes are to be avoided.
4. Advances in molecular knowledge are beginning to impact in this area. For a number of conditions, prenatal diagnosis by direct DNA analysis is the method of choice and is certainly possible for a lot more in the future. This will replace invasive procedures such as fetal liver biopsy in those disorders where the enzyme deficiency is limited to liver, e.g. urea cycle defects. It is of paramount importance to collect a DNA sample from each positive metabolic patient and to make enquiries about possible mutation analysis.
5. If a pregnancy is terminated following a positive prenatal diagnosis, it is important to confirm the test result on the products of conception as a check on the efficiency of the diagnostic procedure.

## PREIMPLANTATION DIAGNOSIS

*In vitro* fertilization has introduced the opportunity for genetic diagnosis before implantation. The major advantage is obvious – parents at risk no longer have to decide to terminate abnormal offspring, as the fetus is screened prior to placement in the uterus. This technique has recently been employed successfully in a number of single gene disorders (Lissens *et al.* 1996) and in pregnancies at risk of producing chromosomal imbalance (Iwarsson *et al.* 1998), and, with our increasing knowledge of the molecular defects responsible for metabolic disorders, is likely to be requested more often in the future. There are, however, some problems associated with the technique, including technical failure, cost, risk to the embryo of biopsy and the relatively low chance of completing a pregnancy (Simpson & Carson 1992). Unquestionably, experience will remove many of these doubts about technique, but in a health-care system constrained by lack of resources, preimplantation diagnosis and its very high cost are unlikely to be high priorities for most purchasers of health care.

## PRENATAL DIAGNOSIS

### METHODS USED IN OBTAINING SAMPLES

#### Chorion villus biopsy (CVB)

In this technique, cells are removed from the developing placenta for enzyme or molecular analysis by either aspiration or biopsy using small forceps. The method has been used increasingly since 1984 and is now the most common prenatal technique employed for the diagnosis of inborn errors of metabolism. The transcervical approach at 8–10 weeks' gestation, under the assistance of ultrasound control, is favored by most centres in the UK. In 90% of cases, sampling is successful after a single passage of the instrument, and the fetal loss following the procedure is just over 2% (Jackson *et al.* 1992).

Recently, there have been concerns about the possibility of inducing fetal limb abnormalities by chorion villus biopsy (Firth *et al.* 1991; Burton *et al.* 1992). A vascular etiology has been suggested as the causative factor, and defects have been reported after both transcervical and transabdominal biopsies. This remains controversial, with other groups suggesting that the limb defects are due to a combination of inexperience and early biopsy (Simpson & Carson 1992).

Transabdominal biopsy at 10–12 weeks' gestation is an alternative to the transcervical technique. The advantages of the method are a lower risk of infection, ease of learning as it is similar to amniocentesis, and accuracy of biopsy as the needle can be 'aimed' at the tissue of interest. The technique is successful in 94% of cases with first passage of the instrument, and fetal loss after the procedure is less than after a transcervical approach (Jackson *et al.* 1992).

The amount of tissue removed after chorion villus biopsy, 15–40 mg wet weight, is sufficient for most diagnostic procedures. The material must be studied carefully under the dissecting microscope and any contaminating maternal decidua removed. A result from direct enzyme analysis can usually be available within 24–48 h. For some defects, a culture of the biopsy must be made, and the result would then be available in 2–3 weeks. In addition to direct enzyme assay, the villus material can be used as a source of DNA for molecular diagnoses.

### Amniocentesis

Amniocentesis under ultrasound control, with the removal of 15–20 ml of amniotic fluid, at 15–16 weeks' gestation is a reliable and safe procedure. Cell-free fluid can be used to study metabolite excretion in fetal urine, and a culture of the amniocytes can be used for enzyme assay. The risk of fetal loss following the procedure is less than 1%, but the major disadvantage is the time taken to culture cells for assay (3–4 weeks). The end result is a late termination of an affected pregnancy, and for this reason, chorion villus biopsy has almost completely replaced amniocentesis as the method of obtaining fetal material for prenatal testing.

Because of increased awareness of the problems associated with cytogenetic prenatal diagnoses following chorion villus biopsy, attempts have been made to perform amniocentesis earlier in pregnancy (Djalali *et al.* 1992). This has also led to attempts at metabolic diagnoses on samples removed by amniocentesis at 11–13 weeks' gestation. Successful culture can be obtained at this stage, and hence enzyme diagnosis, but there are no normal ranges for metabolite excretion at this early stage of pregnancy. In addition, there is an increase in fetal loss when compared to abdominal CVB, and for these reasons, CVB remains the method of choice if prenatal diagnosis is needed in the first trimester (Nagel *et al.* 1988). It is unlikely that this technique will make a major impact on the prenatal diagnosis of metabolic disease.

### Fetal blood sampling

Fetal blood can be obtained in the second trimester from puncture of vessels in the chorionic plate, umbilical cord, or fetal intrahepatic umbilical vein. The needle can be guided by ultrasound or fetoscope, and the technique is usually performed at 18–20 weeks' gestation, by which time, the fetal blood volume is sufficiently large to withstand the withdrawal of the 1–3 ml of blood necessary for diagnosis. Fetoscopy carries a relatively high risk of complication, including fetal loss, amniotic fluid leakage, infection, and preterm labor. Percutaneous umbilical cord sampling (cordocentesis) under ultrasound control has become the method of choice and appears to be a much safer procedure (Suzumori 1992). In cases where the placental cord insertion is difficult to sample, the intrahepatic umbilical vein is preferred (Nicolini *et al.* 1988).

Fetal blood sampling has a very small role to play in the prenatal diagnosis of inherited metabolic disease and is reserved for women at risk who present very late in pregnancy for prenatal testing.

### Fetal organ biopsy

In some metabolic disorders, the primary enzyme deficiency cannot be demonstrated in either chorion villus cells or amniocytes. In these disorders, the enzymes are usually expressed only in liver tissue. Fetal needle liver biopsy taken by aspiration via the fetoscope or under ultrasound control at 18–20 weeks' gestation has been used for the prenatal diagnosis of several liver-specific defects, including ornithine carbamoyltransferase deficiency, carbamoylphosphate synthase deficiency, glucose-6-phosphatase deficiency and alanine:glyoxylate aminotransferase deficiency. As more becomes known about the mutations responsible for these disorders, it is likely that fetal organ biopsy will be replaced by direct DNA analysis.

## METHODS USED IN OBTAINING A DIAGNOSIS

Many different laboratory techniques have been used to achieve a prenatal diagnosis; the following, however, are used frequently.

### Direct enzyme assay

By far the commonest method of prenatal testing is by direct enzyme assay, and there have been many detailed reports of individual positive cases diagnosed by this method (see Table 34.1). Direct analysis of enzyme activity on fresh, uncultured villus tissue usually allows a result to be available within 24–48 h of the procedure. In all cases, the level of enzyme activity obtained on testing is related to the protein content of the sample and/or to the activity of a comparable, unaffected enzyme with the same subcellular location.

**Table 34.1 Prenatal diagnosis of metabolic disorders**

| Condition | Enzyme deficiency | Prenatal diagnosis |
|---|---|---|
| **1. Carbohydrate metabolism** | | |
| *a. Galactose* | | |
| Galactokinase deficiency | Galactokinase | AF, CVB |
| 'Classical' galactosemia | Galactose-1-phosphateuridyltransferase | AF, CVB |
| Epimerase deficiency | UDP galactose 4-epimerase | Poss. CC |
| *b. Fructose* | | |
| Hereditary fructose intolerance | Aldolase B | Poss. DNA |
| Fructose 1,6-bisphosphatase deficiency | Fructose 1,6-bisphosphatase | Poss. DNA |
| *c. Glycogen storage disease* | | |
| Ia Von Gierke | Glucose 6-phosphatase | Poss. DNA |
| Ib Von Gierke | Glucose-6-phosphatase translocase ($T_1$) | Poss. DNA |
| Ic Von Gierke | Glucose-6-phosphatase translocase ($T_2$) | Poss. DNA |
| II Pompe | Lysosomal-acid glucosidase | AF, CVB |
| III Debrancher enzyme deficiency | Amylo-1,6-glucosidase | AF, CVB |
| IV Brancher enzyme deficiency | 1,4-Glucan 6-glycosyltransferase | AF, CVB |
| V McArdle | Muscle phosphorylase | No |
| VI Liver phosphorylase deficiency | Liver phosphorylase | Poss. FT |
| VII Phosphofructokinase deficiency | Phosphofructokinase | No |
| IXa Phosphorylase kinase (recessive) | Phosphorylase kinase | Poss. FT |
| IXb Phosphorylase kinase (X-linked) | Phosphorylase kinase | Poss. FT |
| **2. Amino acid metabolism** | | |
| *a. Phenylalanine* | | |
| 'Classical' phenylketonuria | Phenylalanine hydroxylase | DNA |
| Tetrabiopterin homeostasis | Dihydropteridine reductase | AF, CVB |
| Tetrabiopterin synthesis | Guanosine-triphosphate cyclohydrolase | Met. |
| | 6-Pyruvoyltetrahydropterin synthase | Met. |
| *b. Methionine* | | |
| Homocystinuria | Cystathionine synthase | AF, CC |
| *c. Tyrosine* | | |
| Tyrosinemia I | Fumarylacetoacetate hydrolase | AF, CVB |
| Tyrosinemia II | Tyrosine aminotransferase | No |
| *d. Valine, leucine, isoleucine* | | |
| Maple-syrup urine disease | Branched-chain keto-acid dehydrogenase | AF, CVB |
| *e. Glycine* | | |
| Non-ketotic hyperglycinemia | Gylcine cleavage system | CVB |
| *f. Lysine* | | |
| Hyperlysinemia | Aminoadipic-semialdehyde synthase | AF |
| *g. Proline* | | |
| Hyperprolinemia I | Proline oxidase | Unk. |
| Hyperprolinemia II | Pyrroline-5-carboxylate dehydrogenase | Unk. |
| Hyperimidodipeptiduria | Prolidase | Poss. CC |
| *h. Ornithine* | | |
| Gyrate atrophy of the choroid and retina | Ornithine aminotransferase | Poss. CC |
| Hyperornithinemia–hyperammonemia–homocitrullinemia (HHH syndrome) | Basic defect unknown | No |
| **3. Urea cycle disorders** | | |
| *N*-Acetylglutamate synthetase deficiency | *N*-Acetylglutamate synthetase | Unk. |
| Carbamyl-phosphate synthetase (CPS) deficiency | Carbamyl-phosphate synthetase | Poss. DNA/FT |
| Omithine carbamyltransferase (OCT) deficiency | Ornithine carbamyltransferase | Poss. DNA/FT |
| Citrullinemia | Argininosuccinic-acid synthetase | AF, CVB |
| Argininosuccinic aciduria (ASA) | Argininosuccinate lyase | AF, CVB |
| Argininemia | Arginase | Poss. DNA/FT |

| Condition | Enzyme deficiency | Prenatal diagnosis |
|---|---|---|
| **4. Organic acid disorders** | | |
| *a. Propionate and methylmalonate metabolism* | | |
| Propionic acidemia | Propionyl-CoA carboxylase | AF, CVB |
| | α-subunit | AF, CVB |
| | β-subunit | AF, CVB |
| Multiple carboxylase deficiency | Holocarboxlase synthetase | Met. |
| | Biotinidase | Met. |
| Methylmalonic acidemia | Methylmalonyl-CoA mutase | AF, CVB |
| | Adenosylcobalamin synthesis: | |
| | cblA | AF, CVB |
| | cblB | AF, CVB |
| | (see also Cobalamin metabolism) | |
| *b. Pyruvate and lactate metabolism* | | |
| Lactate dehydrogenase deficiency | Lactate dehydrogenase | Unk. |
| Pyruvate dehydrogenase deficiency | Pyruvate dehydrogenase complex | [a] |
| | $E_1$ (decarboxylase) component | Poss. DNA |
| | $E_2$ (dihydrolipoyl transacylase) component | |
| | $E_3$ (dihydrolipoyl dehydrogenase) component | |
| | Pyruvate-dehydrogenase phosphatase | |
| Pyruvate carboxylase deficiency | Pyruvate carboxylase | AF |
| Phosphoenolpyruvate carboxykinase deficiency | Phosphoenolpyruvate carboxykinase | Unk. |
| *c. Respiratory transport chain defects* | | |
| The components of the respiratory transport chain are composed of many polypeptide subunits, some of which are encoded by mitochondrial DNA | | |
| Complex I | NADH-CoQ reductase | [b] |
| Complex II | Succinate-CoA reductase | |
| Complex III | $CoQH_2$-cytochrome-c reductase | |
| Complex IV | Cytochrome oxidase | AF, CVB |
| Complex V | Oligomycin-sensitive ATPase | |
| *d. Branched-chain organic acidemias* | | |
| Isovaleric acidemia | Isovaleryl-CoA dehydrogenase | Met, AF |
| Isolated 3-methylcrotonyl-CoA carboxylase deficiency | 3-Methylcrotonyl carboxylase | Poss. CC |
| 3-Methylglutaconic aciduria | 3-Methylglutaconic hydratase | Poss. CC |
| 3-Hydroxy-3-methylglutaryl-CoA lyase deficiency | 3-Hydroxy-3-methylglutaryl-CoA lyase | AF, CVB |
| Mevalonic aciduria | Mevalonate kinase | AF, Poss. CVB |
| 2-Methylacetoacetyl-CoA thiolase deficiency | 2-Methylacetoacetyl-CoA thiolase | Poss. CC |
| *e. Disorders of the γ-glutamyl cycle* | | |
| 5-Oxoprolinuria | Glutathione synthetase | Poss. CC |
| γ-Glutamylcysteine synthetase deficiency | γ-Glutamylcysteine synthetase | Poss. CC |
| γ-Glutamyl transpeptidase deficiency | γ-Glutamyl transpeptidase | Poss. CC |
| 5-Oxoprolinase deficiency | 5-Oxoprolinase | Poss. CC |
| *f. Other organic acid disorders* | | |
| Alkaptonuria | Homogentisic-acid oxidase | Unk. |
| Glutaric aciduria type I | Glutaryl-CoA dehydrogenase | Poss. CC, CVB |
| Glutaric aciduria type II | Electron transfer flavoprotein (ETF) | |
| | ETF:ubiquinone oxidoreductase | Poss. CC, CVB |
| Glycerol kinase deficiency | Glycerol kinase | AF, CVB |
| Hyperoxaluria type I (glycolic aciduria) | Alanine: glyoxylate aminotransferase | FT |
| Hyperoxaluria type II (glyceric aciduria) | Glyceric dehydrogenase | Unk. |
| Canavan's disease | Aspartoacylase | Poss. Met.<br>Poss. CVB |
| **5. Fatty acid oxidation defects** | | |
| Carnitine palmitolytransferase deficiency | CPT I and CPT II | Poss. CC |
| Carnitine/acyl carnitine translocase | Carnitine/acyl carnitine translocase | Poss. CC |

| Condition | Enzyme deficiency | Prenatal diagnosis |
|---|---|---|
| Short-chain acyl-CoA dehydrogenase (SCAD) deficiency | Short-chain acyl-CoA dehydrogenase | Poss. CC |
| Medium-chain acyl-CoA dehydrogenase (MCAD) deficiency | Medium-chain acyl-CoA dehydrogenase | DNA/CVB |
| Long-chain acyl-CoA dehydrogenase (LCAD) deficiency | Long-chain acyl-CoA dehydrogenase | Poss. CC |
| Very-long-chain acyl-CoA dehydrogenase (VLCAD) deficiency | Very-long-chain acyl-CoA dehydrogenase | Poss. CC |
| Long-chain 3-OH-acyl-CoA dehydrogenase (LCHAD) deficiency | Long-chain 3-OH-acyl-CoA dehydrogenase | Poss. CC/DNA |
| Trifunctional protein deficiency | Long-chain 2-enoyl-CoA hydratse<br>Long-chain 3-OH-acyl-CoA dehydrogenase<br>Long-chain 3-ketoacyl-CoA thiolase | Poss. CC |
| **6. Lysosomal enzyme defects** | | |
| *a. Mucopolysaccharidoses* | | |
| Type IH (Hurler's syndrome) | Iduronidase | AF, CVB |
| Type IS (Scheie's syndrome) | Iduronidase | |
| Type II (Hunter's syndrome) | Iduronate sulphatase | AF, CVB |
| Type III (Sanfilippo's syndrome) | | |
| A | Heparan *N*-sulphatase | AF, CVB |
| B | *N*-Acetylglucosaminidase | AF, CVB |
| C | Acetyl-CoA-glucosaminide acetyltransferase | AF, CVB |
| D | *N*-Acetylglucosamine 6-sulphatase | Poss. CC |
| Type IV (Morquio's syndrome) | | |
| A | Galactosamine 6-sulphatase | AF, CVB |
| B | β-Galactosidase | Poss. CVB |
| Type VI (Maroteaux-Lamy's syndrome) | *N*-Acetylgalactosamine 4-sulphatase | AF, CVB |
| Type VII (Sly's disease) | β-Glucuronidase | Poss. CC |
| *b. Mucolipidoses* | | |
| Mucolipidosis II (I-cell disease) | UDP-*N*-acetylglucosamine:lysosomal enzyme phosphotransferase | AF, CVB |
| Mucolipidosis III (pseudo-Hurler polydystrophy) | Same as mucolipidosis II | AF, CVB |
| *c. Glycoproteinoses* (p. 631) | | |
| α-Mannosidosis | α-Mannosidase | AF, CVB |
| β-Mannosidosis | β-Mannosidase | Poss. CC |
| Fucosidosis | α-Fucosidase | AF, CVB |
| Aspartylglycosaminuria | Aspartylglycosaminidase | AF, CVB |
| Sialidosis type I (cherry-red spot–myoclonus syndrome) | Neuraminidase | AF, CVB |
| Sialidosis type II | | |
| Congenital and infantile | Neuraminidase | AF, CVB |
| Juvenile | Combined neuraminidase and β-galactosidase | AF, CVB |
| *d. $GM_2$ gangliosidoses* (p. 629) | | |
| Tay–Sachs's disease (variant B) | Hexosaminidase α-subunit | AF, CVB |
| Sandhoff's disease (variant O) | Hexosaminidase β-subunit | AF, CVB |
| $GM_2$, activator deficiency (variant AB) | $GM_2$ activator protein | Poss. CC |
| *e. Other lysosomal storage disorders (see Chapter 36)* | | |
| Metachromatic leukodystrophy | Arylsulphatase A | AF, CVB |
| Multiple sulphatase deficiency | Multiple lysosomal sulphatases | AF, CVB |
| Niemann–Pick's disease | | |
| Type A | Sphingomyelinase | AF, CVB |
| Type B | Sphingomyelinase | AF, CVB |
| Type C | Cholesterol esterification | AF, CVB |
| Farber's disease | Ceramidase | AF, CVB |
| Gaucher's disease | | |
| Type 1 (non-neuronopathic) | Glucocerebrosidase | AF, CVB |
| Type 2 (acute neuronopathic) | Glucocerebrosidase | AF, CVB |
| Type 3 (Norrbottnian) | Glucocerebrosidase | AF, CVB |
| Krabbe's disease | Galactocerebrosidase | AF, CVB |
| Fabry's disease | α-Galactosidase | AF, CVB |

| Condition | Enzyme deficiency | Prenatal diagnosis |
|---|---|---|
| Schindler's disease | α-*N*-Acetylgalactosaminidase | Poss. CC |
| $GM_1$ gangliosidosis | β-Galactosidase | AF, CVB |
| Wolman's disease | Acid lipase | AF, CVB |
| Cholesterol ester storage disease | Acid lipase | AF, CVB |
| Mucolipidosis type IV | Unk. | Hist. Poss. DNA |
| **7. Peroxisomal disorders** (p. 634) | | |
| Zellweger's syndrome | Peroxisome biogenesis | AF, CVB |
| Neonatal adrenoleukodystrophy | Peroxisome biogenesis | AF, CVB |
| Infantile Refum's syndrome | Peroxisome biogenesis | AF, CVB |
| (For disorders of peroxisome biogenesis, a peroxisomal enzyme – dihydroxyacetone phosphate acyltransferase – can be assayed) | | |
| Isolated dihydroxyacetone-phosphate acyltransferase (DHAP-AT) deficiency | DHAP-A/T | Poss. CVB |
| Rhizomelic chondrodysplasia punctata | Multiple peroxisomal enzymes | AF, CVB |
| Pseudo-Zellweger's syndrome | 3-Oxoacyl-CoA thiolase | AF, CVB |
| Pseudo-neonatal adrenoleukodystrophy | Acyl-CoA oxidase | Poss. CC |
| Bifunctional enzyme defect | Bifunctional enzyme | Poss. CVB |
| Glutaric aciduria type III | Glutaryl-CoA oxidase | Poss. CVB |
| X-linked adrenoleucodystrophy | Very-long-chain fatty-acid ligase | AF, CVB |
| Acatalasia | Catalase | Unk. |
| **8. Purine and pyrimidine metabolism** (p. 632) | | |
| Lesch–Nyhan's syndrome | Hypoxanthine phosphoribosyltransferase | AF, CVB |
| Adenine phosphoribosyltransferase deficiency | Adenine phosphoribosyltransferase | AF, CVB |
| Adenosine deaminase deficiency | Adenosine deaminase | AF, CVB |
| Purine nucleoside phosphorylase deficiency | Purine nucleoside phosphorylase | AF, CVB |
| Myoadenylate deaminase deficiency | Myoadenylate deaminase | No |
| Xanthinuria | Xanthine oxidase | Unk. |
| Orotic aciduria | Uridine-5′-monophosphate synthase | Poss. CC |
| Pyrimidine-5′-nucleotidase deficiency | Pyrimidine-5′-nucleotidase | Unk. |
| **9. Trace metal metabolism** | | |
| Wilson's disease | Copper transport ATP-ase | Poss. DNA |
| Menke's disease (p. 633) | Copper transport ATP-ase | AF, CVB |
| Hemachromatosis | Basic defect unknown | Unk. |
| Molybdenum cofactor deficiency | Molybdenum cofactor | AF, CVB |
| Isolated sulfite oxidase deficiency (p. 630) | Sulfite oxidase | Poss. CC |
| **10. Lipid metabolism** | | |
| Abetalipoproteinemia | Abnormal handling of apolipoprotein B | Unk. |
| Lipoprotein lipase deficiency | Lipoprotein lipase | Unk. |
| Lecithin:cholesterol acyltransferase (LCAT) deficiency | Lecithin:cholesterol acyltransferase | DNA |
| Familial hypercholesterolemia (hyperlipidemia type IIA) | Deficient low-density lipoprotein (LDL) receptors | AF |
| Dysbetalipoproteinaemia (hyperlipidemia type III) | Defective apolipoprotein E | Unk. |
| Tangier disease | ATP-binding cassette transporter 1 (ABC1) | Unk. |
| Cerebrotendinous xanthomatosis | Mitochondrial 26-hydroxylase | Poss. AF, CC |
| Phytosterolemia | Basic defect unknown | Unk. |
| **11. Vitamin metabolism** (p. 635) | | |
| *a. Folic acid* | | |
| Methylene tetrahydrofolate reductase deficiency | Methylene tetrahydrofolate reductase | AF, CVB |
| Glutamate formiminotransferase deficiency | Glutamate formiminotransferase | No |
| *b. Vitamin $B_{12}$* (cobalamin) | | |
| Transcobalamin II deficiency | Transcobalamin II | Poss. CC |
| Defects in adenosylcobalamin (AdoCbl) synthesis: | | |
| cbl A mutation | Basic defect unknown | AF, CVB |
| cbl B mutation | ATP:cob(I)alamin adenosyltransferase | AF, CVB |

| Condition | Enzyme deficiency | Prenatal diagnosis |
|---|---|---|
| (Both of the above defects cause methylmalonic acidemia as AdoCbl is an essential cofactor for the mutase enzyme) | | |
| Defects in methylcobalamin (MeCbl) synthesis: | | |
| cbl E mutation | Basic defect unknown | AF |
| cbl G mutation | Basic defect unknown | Poss. CC |
| (Both of the above disorders lead to a functional deficiency of $N_5$-methyltetrahydrofolate:homoxysteine methyltransferase, leading to homocystinuria, hypomethioninemia without methylmalonic acidaemia) | | |
| cbl C mutation | Basic defect unknown | Poss. CC |
| cbl D mutation | Basic defect unknown | Poss. CC |
| cbl F mutation | Cobalamin transport from lysosome | Poss. CC |
| **12. Defects in the synthesis and degradation of hemeproteins** | | |
| *a. Porphyrias* | | |
| δ-Aminolevulinic acid dehydratase deficiency | δ-Aminolevulinic acid dehydratase | Unk. |
| Acute intermittent porphyria | Porphobilinogen deaminase | AF |
| Congenital erythropoietic porphyria | Uroporphyrinogen III cosynthase | Met. |
| Porphyria cutanea tarda | Uroporphyrinogen decarboxylase | No |
| Hereditary coproporphyria | Coproporphyrinogen oxidase | Poss. CC |
| Variegate porphyria | Protoporphyrinogen oxidase | Poss. CC |
| Erythropoietic protoporphyria | Ferrochelatase | Poss. CC |
| *b. Bilirubin metabolism* | | |
| Crigler–Najjar's syndrome type I | UDP glucuronyltransferase | Poss. DNA |
| Crigler–Najjar's syndrome type II | UDP glucuronyltransferase | Poss. DNA |
| Gilbert's syndrome | UDP glucuronyltransferase | Poss. DNA |
| Dubin–Johnson's syndrome | Defect in anion transporter | Poss. DNA |
| Rotor syndrome | Basic defect unknown | No |
| **13. Disorders of membrane transport** | | |
| Cystinuria | Renal and intestinal transport defect | No |
| Lysinuric protein intolerance | Defect of cationic amino acid transport | No |
| Hartnup's disease | Defect of neutral amino acid transport | No |
| Cystinosis | Lysosomal cystine transport | AF, CVB |
| Infantile free sialic acid storage disease | Lysosomal sialic acid transport | AF, CVB |
| Salla's disease | Lysosomal sialic acid transport | AF |
| **14. Miscellaneous disorders** | | |
| Lowe's syndrome | Phosphatidyl inositol phosphatase | Poss. DNA |
| Congenital disorder of glycosylation Ia (p. 634) | Phosphomannomutase | Poss. DNA |
| Congenital disorder of glycosylation Ib | Phosphomannose isomerase | Poss. DNA |
| Carbonic anhydrase II deficiency | Carbonic anhydrase II | Poss. DNA |
| Refsum's disease | Phytanic acid hydroxylase | Poss. CC |
| Steroid sulphatase deficiency | Steroid sulphatase | AF, CVB |
| Hypophosphatasia | Alkaline phosphatase | AF |
| Fumaric aciduria | Fumarase | Poss. CC |
| Sjögren–Larsson's syndrome (p. 636) | Fatty alcohol NAD oxidoreductase | Poss. CC |

*Key*: AF = cell-free amniotic fluid or cultured amniocytes; CVB = assay performed on either uncultured or cultured villus cells; Hist. = histological changes (usually abnormal lysosomal storage) within amniocytes have been used as a diagnostic test; Met. = metabolites in fetal urine are detected in samples obtained after amniocentesis at 15–16 weeks' gestation; Poss. CC = as far as author is aware, prenatal diagnosis has not been performed for these disorders. However, as the enzyme is expressed in fibroblast cells, prenatal diagnosis should be possible; CC = cultured cells; Poss. DNA = the mutations causing these disorders have been established and may be the most appropriate approach to prenatal testing; Poss. FT = the enzyme defect can only be demonstrated in fetal tissue. This would usually require a fetal liver biopsy, but in some circumstances, direct fetal blood sampling by cordocentesis; UDP = uridine diphosphate; Unk. = as far as the author is aware, prenatal diagnosis has not been attempted. In a number of cases, the exact biochemical defect is yet to be established. [a] Assay of the total activity of the pyruvate dehydrogenase complex is possible, but partial deficiencies are common leading to difficulty in interpreting results. [b] Only one component of the respiratory transport chain (complex IV, cytochrome oxidase) has been studied prenatally. In families with a deletion of mitochondrial DNA, a molecular approach may be more appropriate.

The potential problems associated with enzyme diagnosis utilizing chorion villus samples have been the subject of review (Fowler *et al.* 1989).

### Metabolite accumulation

Stable isotope dilution gas chromatography – mass spectrometry with selected ion monitoring can be used for the direct analysis of metabolites excreted by the fetus into the amniotic fluid at 12–18 weeks' gestation. The technique offers the advantage of a rapid and reliable prenatal diagnosis in the second trimester of pregnancy, and a number of disorders have been studied in this way, especially organic acid defects and aminoacidopathies (Jakobs *et al.* 1990).

In a similar way, two-dimensional electrophoresis of extracted glycosaminoglycans from cell-free amniotic fluid can be used to rapidly diagnose mucopolysaccharidoses (Mossman & Patrick 1982).

For most of these disorders, however, enzyme diagnosis is available, and the technique will be reserved for the few conditions where the primary enzyme defect is not expressed in chorion villus material or the enzyme assay is fraught with technical difficulty, as in Canavan's disease, for example.

### Gene tracking

For many inherited disorders, the exact genetic defect within a family remains unknown. In these circumstances, it is still possible to detect the mutant gene by linkage analysis based on DNA polymorphisms. As normal variation occurs frequently in the human genome, polymorphisms are common, producing alleles that give rise to different lengths of DNA when digested by restriction enzymes. The restriction-fragment-length polymorphisms (RFLPs) can be used to track the mutant gene if a polymorphism is present in the chromosome containing the abnormal gene, but not in the normal chromosome or vice versa. As polymorphisms are common, there are usually several tightly linked to, or within, the gene of interest itself.

This technique has been used for the prenatal diagnosis of a number of inborn errors of metabolism, including phenylketonuria (Woo 1984) and ornithine carbamoyltransferase deficiency (Pembrey *et al.* 1985).

### Direct mutation analysis

For those disorders, where the genetic defect has been characterized, an attempt at prenatal diagnosis can be made by looking for the specific mutation in fetal DNA. In this way, both gross alterations of a gene (e.g. deletions, rearrangements and insertions) and point mutations can be detected using gene-specific probes. Amplification of DNA by the polymerase chain reaction, coupled with the use of allele-specific oligonucleotides, is a very rapid method for detecting point mutations within a family where the genetic defect is known precisely. This technique is being increasingly used as a means of prenatal diagnosis for metabolic disorders.

## SPECIFIC METABOLIC DISORDERS

Table 34.1 lists a number of inborn errors, the associated biochemical defect, and the test used for prenatal diagnosis. Where prenatal diagnosis has been successfully achieved, the method used is clearly shown. For some conditions, prenatal diagnosis is theoretically possible although, to the author's knowledge, not as yet successfully performed. In this case, the most likely tissue and method are indicated with the rider 'possible'. The abbreviations used are defined in a footnote to the table.

**Key Points**

- An exact biochemical diagnosis must be established in the index case.
- Direct enzyme assay on material obtained by chorion villus biopsy is the commonest method used in establishing a prenatal diagnosis. For some disorders cultured cells are necessary and this takes longer. It is important to check with the laboratory the exact time it takes to obtain a result before discussing with parents.
- An increasing number of disorders are being characterized at a molecular level. Check with the metabolic laboratory for the up to date position of the disorder you are interested in excluding.

## REFERENCES


Burton B K, Schulz C J & Burd L I (1992) Limb anomalies associated with chorionic villus sampling. *Obstet Gynecol* 79:726–730.

Djalali M, Barbi G, Kennerknecht *et al.* (1992) Introduction of early amniocentesis to routine prenatal diagnosis. *Prenatal Diag* 12:661–669.

Firth H V, Boyd P A, Chamberlain P *et al.* (1991) Severe limb abnormalities after chorion villus sampling at 56–66 days' gestation. *Lancet* 337:762–763.

Fowler B, Giles L, Cooper A *et al.* (1989) Chorionic villus sampling: diagnostic uses and limitations of enzyme assays. *J Inherit Metab Dis* 12(suppl 1):105–117.

Harper J C, Pergament E & Delhanty D A (2000) Preimplantation genetics and diagnosis. *Prenatal Diag* 2.

Iwarsson E, Ahrlund-Richter L, Inzunza J *et al.* (1998) Preimplantation genetic diagnosis of DiGeorge syndrome. *Mol Hum Reprod* 4:871–875.

Jackson L G, Zachary J M, Fowler S E *et al.* (1992) A randomized comparison of transcervical and transabdominal chorionic-villus sampling. *N Engl J Med* 327:594–598.

Jakobs C, Ten Brink H J & Stellaard F (1990) Prenatal diagnosis of inherited metabolic disorders by quantitation of characteristic metabolites in amniotic fluid: facts and future. *Prenatal Diag* 10:265–271.

Lissens W, Sermon K, Staessen C *et al.* (1996) Review: preimplantation diagnosis of inherited disease. *J Inherit Metab Dis* 19:709–723.

Mossman J & Patrick A D (1982) Prenatal diagnosis of mucopolysaccharidosis by two-dimensional electrophoresis of amniotic fluid glycosaminoglycans. *Prenatal Diag* 2:169–176.

Nagel H T, Vandenbussche F P, Keirse M J *et al.* (1998) Amniocentesis before 14 completed weeks as an alternative to transabdominal chorionic villus sampling: a controlled trial with infant follow-up. *Prenatal Diag* 18:465–475.

Nicolini U, Santolaya J, Ojo O E *et al.* (1988) The fetal intrahepatic umbilical vein as an alternative to cord needling for prenatal diagnosis and therapy. *Prenatal Diag* 8:665–671.

Pembrey M E, Old J M, Leonard J V *et al.* (1985) Prenatal diagnosis of ornithine carbamoyl transferase deficiency using a gene specific probe. *J Med Gene* 22:462–465.

Simpson J L & Carson S A (1992) Preimplantation genetic diagnosis. *N Engl J Med* 327:951–953.

Suzumori K (1992) The role of fetal blood sampling in prenatal diagnosis. *Early Hum Dev* 29:155–159.

Woo S L C (1984) Prenatal diagnosis and carrier detection of classic phenylketonuria by gene analysis. *Pediatrics* 74:412–423.

Chapter 35

# Inborn errors of metabolism – postnatal diagnosis and management

J. E. Wraith

## INTRODUCTION

Although individually rare, as a group, inborn errors of metabolism constitute a significant problem in neonatal practice, and few pediatricians will have avoided the predicament of being faced with a desperately ill neonate for whom a diagnosis is not immediately obvious. The majority of such infants will have comparatively common neonatal problems such as systemic infection or congenital heart disease. An appreciable minority, however, will have a potentially treatable inborn error of metabolism, and in these patients, rapid diagnosis and institution of appropriate treatment are essential if a good outcome is to be achieved. Important practice points related to the investigation and management of these conditions are summarized in Table 35.1.

**Table 35.1 Practice points in the investigation and management of suspected metabolic disease**

- The outcome for an individual child is directly related to the speed at which diagnosis is established and effective treatment started.
- Investigate and treat aggressively in the initial stages of presentation – decisions with regard to treatment can always be reassessed later.
- Whilst consulting the dysmorphology databases, always think of the possibility of an underlying metabolic defect in any dysmorphic neonate.
- The key to early diagnosis is to maintain a high index of suspicion about the possibility of metabolic disease being the cause of the infant's condition. Be prepared to investigate many to unmask the few affected.
- A basic metabolic screen should include a sample of blood for DNA analysis as well as blood spots for acyl-carnitine profile. Discuss the patient with your regional metabolic service to ensure that the correct samples are collected.
- The key to treatment is to make the infant anabolic as quickly as possible; toxin removal and other measures are secondary to this important goal.
- Biopsies are of limited value. If a diagnosis is not established on samples taken during life, diagnosis after death is possible in only very few cases. Never forget the pathologist – do not snap freeze all biopsy material, but ensure some is kept for histology.

Before considering individual disorders, a few general points about diagnosis and management need to be made. Individual conditions are rare, and experience is important if diagnosis and treatment are to proceed smoothly. Expert laboratory services are essential, but results require interpretation by clinicians specializing in inherited metabolic disease. As a result, prompt clinical consultation is important and will generally lead to transfer of the infant to a specialized hospital unit. Initial screening tests must be readily available in each region, and clinicians should be encouraged to use such tests freely. More specialized tests are needed in only a small number of supraregional or national reference laboratories.

Throughout this chapter, a policy of very aggressive investigation and management will be supported. Some clinicians feel concerned about this approach, and occasionally, we are accused of taking the risk of keeping alive a grossly handicapped infant. In our experience, this is very rarely a problem. After a short period of very energetic treatment, one can generally judge the prognosis accurately. If the prospect of return to normal cerebral function is poor, one can refrain from employing 'heroic' measures in the next acute episode of deterioration. The episodic nature of most inborn errors ensures that treatment can be reassessed at frequent intervals. There is the risk of producing survivors with minor degrees of brain damage, but this is true in all acute neonatal illnesses and in all inborn errors that can affect the brain.

## PRESENTATION OF INBORN ERRORS OF METABOLISM

Infants affected by inborn errors may come to notice in several ways.

### ACUTE, SEVERE ILLNESS IN THE NEWBORN PERIOD

The greater part of this chapter will concentrate on those inborn errors that present with life-threatening illness in the early neonatal period. A number of clues can be obtained from a careful history, examination and simple bedside tests.

### SUBACUTE PRESENTATION

A number of infants, especially those with lysosomal storage disease, present outside the newborn period. In these infants, visceromegaly and skeletal dysplasia are often associated features. Whilst a life-threatening presentation is rare, there is considerable overlap between the two groups, and a number of conditions placed in the subacute group can have dramatic neonatal presentation, e.g. hydrops fetalis in the lysosomal storage disorders and profound hypotonia in Zellweger's syndrome (Burton 1987).

The disorders that tend to present in a subacute manner are indicated in Table 35.2, and most of the disorders are discussed elsewhere (see Chapter 36). Intrauterine protection is not a feature of most of these conditions, and in the storage disorders, the storage product accumulates throughout gestation. The time of onset of clinical features and their rate of progression vary between and within the conditions.

## DYSMORPHIC FEATURES OR MULTIPLE CONGENITAL ABNORMALITIES

Many inborn errors of metabolism are associated with dysmorphic manifestations, and a metabolic work-up should be considered in any undiagnosed infant with multiple congenital anomalies or dysmorphic appearance.

In one variant of glutaric aciduria type II (multiple acyl-CoA dehydrogenase deficiency), congenital anomalies include a 'Potter-like' facial appearance, abnormal kidneys, genitalia and anterior abdominal wall (Colevas *et al.* 1988). In addition, severe hypoglycemia and acidosis lead to death in the first week of life in most affected infants.

In Smith–Lemli–Opitz syndrome, a clear defect in the biosynthesis of cholesterol has been identified, and this has led to the discovery of other malformation syndromes associated with aberrant sterol metabolism (Clayton 1998).

Inherited disorders of peroxisomal biogenesis such as Zellweger's syndrome or rhizomelic chondrodysplasia punctata have a characteristic dysmorphic presentation, allowing an easy neonatal 'syndromic' diagnosis (Theil *et al.* 1992). It is important to establish the biochemical defect in such patients as prenatal diagnosis becomes an option in future pregnancies.

3-Hydroxyisobutyryl-CoA deacylase deficiency (Brown *et al.* 1982) and 3-hydoxyisobutyric aciduria (Chitayat *et al.* 1992) are associated with brain dysgenesis due to migrational defects as well as other congenital anomalies. In both of these disorders of valine metabolism, a build-up of a teratogenic intermediary compound may be responsible for the defects.

Finally, a relatively newly described group of disorders resulting from abnormal protein glycosylation, the congenital disorders of glycosylation, can produce dysmorphism as well as dramatic clinical disease in the newborn period (Krasnewich & Gahl 1997).

## MASS SCREENING OF THE NEWBORN POPULATION

In addition to the more dramatic presentations noted above, a large number of infants with inborn errors will be detected in newborn screening programmes. The only inborn error of metabolism that has achieved universal acceptance for mass screening is phenylketonuria. The characteristics of phenylketonuria make it ideal for screening. Treatment is relatively easy and inexpensive. It is relatively frequent (1 in 10 000), and there are a number of simple laboratory methods using microsamples of blood developed for the detection of raised phenylalanine. Detection and treatment within the first 3 weeks of life give a very good outcome when compared to symptomatic diagnosis. Similar arguments justify screening for hypothyroidism, but it is not an inborn error of metabolism.

Mass screening has been suggested for a number of other inborn errors, but none of these has achieved universal acceptance (Sardharwalla & Wraith 1989). This advice, however, may change with the development of new technology (Bartlett *et al.* 1997). Tandem mass spectrometry is a powerful diagnostic tool that allows for a metabolic profiling of amino acids and acylcarnitines from neonatal blood spots. The method can be automated to produce a high-throughput suitable for a newborn screening method (Rashed *et al.* 1997). In addition to amino acid disorders such as phenylketonuria and tyrosinemia, fat oxidation defects, some organic acid disorders and urea cycle defects could also be identified from the screening blood spot. The implementation of this technology is currently subject to intense debate in a number of different countries.

Screening for galactosemia is carried out by a number of communities. It is much less common (1 in 60 000) than phenylketonuria, and a number of babies will have developed acute neonatal disease before the screening test result is back from the laboratory. In addition, the intellectual outcome of presymptomatic babies appears to be no better than that of babies diagnosed quickly after the onset of symptoms. The same criticisms apply to maple syrup urine disease but are increased by the even lower frequency (1 in 250 000) and the outcome, which is often poor even with optimal treatment.

## METABOLIC DISEASE CAN BE ANTICIPATED BECAUSE OF PREVIOUS HISTORY

Some parents who have had previously affected infants find prenatal diagnosis and termination of pregnancy unacceptable. In this situation, it is important to plan treatment before birth. In some vitamin-responsive disorders, it is possible to treat the fetus before birth by giving large doses of the relevant vitamin to the mother (e.g. in vitamin $B_{12}$-responsive methylmalonic acidemia).

In other situations, a couple may have lost a previous baby in circumstances suggestive of an inborn error, but with no firm diagnosis established. Then, we would arrange transfer of the newborn to the metabolic unit 6–12 h after delivery. This period allows for some bonding to occur between mother and baby, knowing that most inborn errors do not produce symptoms for 24–48 h. On arrival, the infant is investigated and maintained on a low-protein intake until the results are known. If investigations are negative, a normal diet is started, and the tests are repeated 48 h later.

**Table 35.2 Clinical features and biochemical findings in metabolic disease**

| | Clinical features | | Biochemical findings |
|---|---|---|---|
| **1. Carbohydrate metabolism** | | | |
| *a. Galactose* | | | |
| Galactokinase deficiency | (Sa.) | Cataracts | Galactosuria (U) (1) |
| 'Classical' galactosemia | (A) | See text | $\uparrow$ Galactose 1-phosphate (B) (1) |
| Epimerase deficiency | (A) | Identical to classical galactosemia | (1) |
| *b. Fructose* | | | |
| Hereditary fructose intolerance | (A) | Lethargy, sweating, seizures, liver failure | After exposure to fructose – abnormal |
| | | LFTs (B) (1) | |
| Fructose 1,6-bisphosphatase deficiency | (A) | Acidosis, hypoglycemia | $\uparrow$ Lactate, $\downarrow$ Glucose (B) (1) |
| *c. Glycogen storage disease* | | | |
| Ia Von Gierke | (A) | Seizures, short stature, massive hepatomegaly | $\downarrow$ Glucose, $\uparrow$ urate (2) |
| Ib Von Gierke | | Ib = neutropenia | $\uparrow$ Lactate, $\uparrow$ lipids (B) |
| Ic Von Gierke | | | |
| II Pompe | (Sa.) | Hypotonia, cardiac failure | $\downarrow$ $\alpha$-Glucosidase (B) (2) |
| III Debrancher enzyme deficiency | (Sa.) | As type I but milder | Fasting: $\downarrow$ glucose, $\downarrow$ lipids (B) |
| IV Brancher enzyme deficiency | (Sa.) | Liver failure | Abnormal LFTs (B) (2) |
| V McArdle | (Sa.) | Muscle cramps | No rise in lactate after exercise (B) (2) |
| VI Liver phosphorylase deficiency | (Sa.) | As type I but milder | (1) |
| VII Phosphofructokinase deficiency | (Sa.) | As type V | (2) |
| IXa Phosphorylase kinase (recessive) | (Sa.) | Asymptomatic hepatomegaly | Usually no $\downarrow$ glucose (1) |
| IXb Phosphorylase kinase (X-linked) | | | |
| **2. Amino acid metabolism** | | | |
| *a. Phenylalanine* | | | |
| 'Classical' phenylketonuria | See text | | (1) |
| Tetrabiopterin homeostasis | (A) | Hypotonia, feeding difficulties, seizures, spasticity | $\downarrow$ Phenylalanine (B) (2) |
| Tetrabiopterin synthesis | | | Abnormal pterins (U) |
| *b. Methionine* | | | |
| Homocystinuria | (Sa.) | Mental retardation, dislocated eye lenses, osteoporosis, premature arteriovenous thrombosis | $\uparrow$ Methionine (B) Homocystinuria (U) (1) |
| *c. Tyrosine* | | | |
| Tyrosinemia I | (A) | Liver necrosis | Abnormal LFTs (B), $\uparrow$ succinyl acetone (U) (1) |
| Tyrosinemia II | (Sa.) | Corneal erosions, hyperkeratosis | $\uparrow$ Tyrosine (B) (1) |
| *d. Valine, leucine, isoleucine* | | | |
| Maple syrup urine disease | (A) | See text | $\uparrow$ Branched chain amino acids (B, U), $\uparrow$ $\alpha$-keto acids (U) |
| *e. Glycine* | | | |
| Non-ketotic hyperglycinemia | (A) | See text | $\uparrow$ glycine (B, CSF) |
| *f. Lysine* | | | |
| Hyperlysinemia | | None | $\uparrow$ Lysine (B) (U) |
| *g. Proline* | | | |
| Hyperprolinemia I | | None | $\uparrow$ Proline (B) (U) |

**Table 35.2 (continued)**

| | Clinical features | | Biochemical findings |
|---|---|---|---|
| Hyperprolinemia II | | None | ↑ Proline (B) (U) |
| Hyperimidodipeptiduria | (Sa.) | Skin lesions, mental retardation, frequent infections | ↑ Prolidase (B)<br>Immune defects (2) |
| *n. Ornithine* | | | |
| Gyrate atrophy of the choroid and retina | (Sa.) | Progressive visual loss | ↑ Ornithine (B) (2) |
| Hyperornithinemia–hyperammonaemia–homocitrullinemia (HHH syndrome) | (A) | Lethargy, vomiting, coma | ↑ Ammonia, ↑ ornithine (1) (B) |
| **3. Urea cycle disorders** | | | |
| N-Acetylglutamate synthetase deficiency | (A) | Lethargy, vomiting, coma | ↑ Ammonia (B) (2) |
| Carbamyl-phosphate synthetase (CPS) deficiency | (A) | Lethargy, vomiting, coma | ↑ Ammonia, ↓ citrulline (B) (2) |
| Ornithine carbamyltransferase (OCT) deficiency | (A) | As CPS deficiency, X-linked | ↑ Ammonia, ↑ orotic acid (2)<br>(B) (U) |
| Citrullinemia | (A) | As CPS deficiency | ↑ Ammonia ↑ citrulline (B) (1) |
| Argininosuccinic aciduria (ASA)<br>*Trichorrhexis nodosa* | (A) | As CPS deficiency but milder | ↑ Ammonia, ↑ argininosuccinic acid (B) (1) |
| Argininemia | (A) | As CPS deficiency but milder | ↑ Ammonia, ↑ arginine (1) (B) |
| **4. Organic acid disorders** | | | |
| *a. Propionate and methylmalonate metabolism* | | | |
| Propionic acidemia | See text | | |
| Multiple carboxylase deficiency | (A) | Acidosis, alopecia, skin rash | ↑ Lactate, ↓ biotinidase (1) (B) |
| Methylmalonic acidemia | See text | | |
| *b. Pyruvate and lactate metabolism* | | | |
| Lactate dehydrogenase deficiency | (Sa.) | Muscle fatigue | ↑ Pyruvate after exercise (B) (2) |
| Pyruvate dehydrogenase deficiency | (A) (Dys.) | Hypotonia, seizures, cerebral malformations | ↑ Lactate (B) (2) |
| Pyruvate carboxylase deficiency | (A) | Acidosis, mental retardation, 'Leigh's syndrome' | ↑ Lactate (B) (2) |
| Phosphoenolpyruvate carboxykinase deficiency | (A) | Vomiting, drowsiness, hepatomegaly | ↑ Lactate, ↓ sugar (B) (2) |
| *c. Branched-chain organic acidemias* | | | |
| Isovaleric acidemia | (A) | Acidosis, lethargy, coma, 'sweaty feet' smell | ↑ Isovaleric acid and glycine conjugates (U) (1) |
| Isolated 3-methylcrotonyl-CoA carboxylase deficiency | (A) | Acidosis, lethargy, apnea | ↑ 3-Hydroxyisovaleric acid<br>↑ 3-methylcrotonyl glycine (U) (1) |
| 3-Methylglutaconic aciduria | (A) or (Sa.) | Variable – many phenotypes | ↑ 3-Methylglutaconic acid (2) (U) |
| 3-Hydroxy-3-methylglutaryl-CoA lyase deficiency | (A) | Vomiting, hypotonia, coma | ↑ Ammonia, abnormal LFTs, ↓ ketones<br>↓ Glucose, ↑ 3-hydroxy-3-methylglutarate (U) |
| Mevalonic aciduria | (A) (V) | Acidosis, diarrhea, fever | ↑ Mevalonic acid (U) (2) |
| 2-Methylacetoacetyl-CoA thiolase deficiency | (Sa.) | Vomiting, ketoacidosis | ↑ 2-Methyl-3-hydroxybutyric acid (1) (U) |
| *d. Disorders of the γ-glutamyl cycle* | | | |
| 5-Oxoprolinuria | (A) | Acidosis, hemolytic anemia, developmental delay | ↓ Glutathione synthetase (B) (2) |

| | | | |
|---|---|---|---|
| γ-Glutamylcysteine synthetase deficiency | (Sa.) | Hemolytic anemia, spinocerebellar degeneration | Generalized aminoaciduria (U) (2) |
| γ-Glutamyl transpeptidase deficiency | (Sa.) | Mental retardation | ↑ γ-Glutamyl cystine (U) (2) |
| 5-Oxoprolinase deficiency | (Sa.) | Renal stones (?) | ↑ 5-Oxoproline (U) |
| *e. Other organic acid disorders* | | | |
| Alkaptonuria | (Sa.) | Dark urine, ochronosis, arthritis | ↑ Homogentisic acid (U) (2) |
| Glutaric aciduria type I | (Sa.) | Dystonia, dyskinesia | ↑ Glutaric acid (not all) (U) (2) |
| Glutaric aciduria type II | (A) (Dys.) | See text | ↓ Glucose, ↓ pH, ↑ ammonia (B)<br>↑ Dicarboxylic acids, ↑ 2-hydroxyglutaric acid (U) (2)<br>↓ 3-Hydroxybutyric acid |
| Glycerol kinase deficiency | | | |
| Glycerol kinase deficiency is X-linked. Can occur as a microdeletion syndrome associated with congenital adrenal hypoplasia and/or Duchenne muscular dystrophy. Isolated deficiency may present in childhood or adult life with vomiting, lethargy and acidosis. Hypoglycemia and seizures are common. | | | |
| Hyperoxaluria type II (glyceric aciduria) | (Sa.) | Renal stones | ↑ Oxalic acid, ↑ glyceric acid (U) (1) |
| Canavan's disease | (Sa.) | Large head, neurodegeneration | ↑ *N*-Acetylaspartic acid (U) (2) |
| **5. Fatty acid oxidation defects** | | | |
| Defects in mitochondrial β-oxidation of fatty acids leading to hypoglycemia and fatty liver. Cardiomyopathy is a feature of some (e.g. LCHAD and carnitine transporter defect). A clinical picture similar to Reye's syndrome can occur in older children. All are diagnosed by a combination of urine organic acids, plasma acyl-carnitine profile and DNA analysis. | | | |
| Carnitine transporter defect | | Hypoglycemia, cardiomyopathy | ↓ carnitine (B) |
| Carnitine/acyl carnitine translocase | | As above | As above |
| Hepatic carnitine palmitoyl transferase (CPTI) | | Hypoglycemia, liver disease | Abn. acyl-carn. (B) |
| Long-chain acyl CoA dehydrogenase (LCAD) | | Hypoglycemia, cardiomyopathy | As CPT I |
| Medium-chain acyl CoA dehydrog. (MCAD) | | Hypoglycemia | As CPT I, DNA |
| Short-chain acyl CoA dehydrog. (SCAD) | | As CPT I | As CPT I |
| Long-chain OH-acyl CoA dehydrog. (LCHAD) | | As carnitine transporter | As CPT I |
| Trifunctional protein deficiency | | As LCHAD | As LCHAD |
| **6. Mitochondrial disorders (see text)** | | | |
| Mitochondrial disorders include defects in the components of the respiratory transport chain. These are composed of many polypeptide subunits, some of which are encoded by mitochondrial DNA. Diagnosis usually relies upon recognizing a suggestive clinical presentation plus abnormal CNS imaging and muscle histology. The biochemical marker for this group of disorders is a persistent lactic acidosis. DNA analysis of mitochondrial DNA can reveal characteristic point mutations, deletions, depletions and rearrangements in certain mitochondrial symptoms. For a review of mitochondrial disease, including presentation and diagnosis, see Chinnery & Turnbull (1997). | | | |
| **7. Lysosomal enzyme defects** | | | |
| *a. Mucopolysaccharidoses* | | | |
| Type IH (Hurler's syndrome) | (Sa.) (Dys.) (V) | Corneal clouding, mental retardation | ↑ Heparan and dermatan sulfate (U) (2) |
| Type IS (Scheie's syndrome) | (Sa.) mild (Dys.) (V) | No mental retardation | As type IH (2) |
| Type II (Hunter's syndrome) | (Sa.) (Dys.) (V) | No corneal clouding, X-linked | As type IH (2) |
| Type III (Sanfilippo's syndrome | (Sa.) | Identical clinical phenotype | ↑ Heparan sulfate (U) (2) |
| A | | Mild somatic features but very severe | |
| B | | neurodegenerative disease | |
| C | | | |
| Type IV (Morquio's syndrome) | (Sa.) (Dys.) | Severe skeletal dysplasia, risk of | ↑ Keratan sulfate (U) (2) |
| A | | cervical myelopathy, normal intelligence | |
| B | | | |

**Table 35.2 (continued)**

| | Clinical features | | Biochemical findings |
|---|---|---|---|
| Type VI (Maroteaux–Lamy's syndrome) | (Sa.) | As mucopolysaccharidosis type IH but milder and normal intelligence quotient | ↑ Dermatan sulfate (U) (2) |
| Type VII (Sly's disease) | (Sa.) | As mucopolysaccharidosis type IH | ↑ Dermatan and heparan sulfate (U) (2) |
| *b. Mucolipidoses* | | | |
| Mucolipidosis II (I-cell disease) | (A) or (Sa.) | As mucopolysaccharidosis type IH but symptoms from birth, gingival hyperplasia | Multiple lysosomal enzyme deficiencies (SF) (2) |
| Mucolipidosis III (pseudo-Hurler's polydystrophy) | (Sa.) | Joint stiffness, short stature | As mucolipidosis II (2) |
| *c. Glycoproteinoses* | | | |
| α-Mannosidosis | (Sa.) (V) (Dsy.) | As mucopolysaccharidosis type IH but milder | Abnormal mannose-rich urinary oligosaccharides (U) (2) |
| β-Mannosidosis | (Sa.) (V) (Dys.) | As mucopolysaccharidosis type IH but much milder, epileptic encephalopathy | As above (2) |
| Fucosidosis | (Sa.) (V) (Dys.) | As mucopolysaccharidosis type IH but milder | Abnormal fucose-rich urinary oligosaccharides (U) (2) |
| Aspartylglycosaminuria | (Sa.) (V) | Mental retardation | ↑ Aspartylglucosamine (U) (2) |
| Sialidosis type I (cherry-red spot–myoclonus syndrome) | (Sa.) (V) (CRS) | Mental retardation | ↓ Neuraminidase (SF) (2) |
| Sialidosis type II | | | |
| Congenital and infantile | (A) (Dys.) (V) | Mental retardation | ↓ Neuraminidase (SF) (2) |
| Juvenile | (Sa.) | | |
| *d. $GM_2$ gangliosidoses* | | | |
| Tay–Sachs's disease (variant B) | (Sa.) (CRS) | Large head, seizures, hyperacusis, spasticity | ↓ Hexosaminidase A (WBC) (2) |
| Sandhoff's disease (variant O) | (Sa.) (CRS) | As Tay-Sach's disease | ↓ Hexosaminidase A and B (WBC) (2) |
| GM, activator deficiency (variant AB) | (Sa.) (CRS) | As Tay-Sach's disease | ↓ $GM_2$ activator (SF) (2) |
| *e. Otner lysosomal storage disorders* | | | |
| Metachromatic leukodystrophy | (Sa.) | Blindness, loss of speech, gait disturbance, spasticity, seizures | ↓ Arylsulfatase A (WBC) (2) |
| Multiple sulfatase deficiency | (Sa.) (Dys.) (V) | As above plus ichthyosis, coarse facial features | ↓ Multiple sulphatase enzymes (WBC) (2) |
| Niemann–Pick's disease | | | |
| Type A | (Sa.) (V) (CRS) | Hepatosplenomegaly, neurodegeneration | ↓ Sphingomyelinase (WBC) (2) |
| Type B | (Sa.) (V) | Hepatosplenomegaly alone | ↓ Sphingomyelinase (WBC) |
| Type C | (A) or (Sa.) | Neonatal hepatitis plus neurodegenerative disease | Abnormal cholesterol esterification (SF 2) |
| Farber's disease | (Sa.) | Swollen joints, hoarseness, developmental delay, nodules | ↓ Acid ceramidase (SF) (2) |

| | | | |
|---|---|---|---|
| Gaucher's disease | | | |
| Type 1 (non-neuronopathic) | (Sa.) (V) | Hepatosplenomegaly, bone marrow infiltration, fractures | ↓ Glucocerebrosidase (WBC) (1) |
| Type 2 (acute neuronopathic) | (Sa.) (V) | Head retraction, strabismus, trismus, neurodegeneration | ↓ Glucocerebrosidase (WBC) (2) |
| Type 3 (Norrbottnian) | (Sa.) (V) | Ataxia, myoclonus, seizures, dementia | ↓ Glucocerebrosidase (WBC) (2) |
| Krabbe's disease | (Sa.) | Irritability, spasticity, seizures, neurodegeneration | ↓ Galactocerebrosidase (WBC) (2) |
| Fabry's disease | (Sa.) | Angiokeratoma, nerve pain, corneal opacity, renal failure | Proteinuria, ↓ α-galactosidase (WBC) (2) |
| Schindler's disease | (Sa.) | Myoclonic seizures, neurodegeneration | ↓ *N*-Acetylgalactosaminidase (WBC, SF) (2) |
| $GM_1$ gangliosidosis | (Sa.) (Dys.) (CRS) (V) | Neurodegeneration, macroglossia, seizures | ↓ β-Galactosidase (WBC) (2) |
| Wolman's disease | (Sa.) (V) | Malabsorption, failure to thrive, adrenal calcification | ↓ Acid esterase (WBC) (1) |
| Cholesterol ester storage disease | (Sa.) (V) | Premature atherosclerosis | ↓ Acid esterase (WBC) (1) |
| Mucolipidosis type IV | (Sa.) | Corneal clouding, mental retardation | Primary defect unknown (2) |
| **8. Peroxisomal disorders** | | | |
| Zellweger's syndrome | (A) (Dys.) | Hypotonia, seizures, mental retardation, epiphyseal dysplasia | ↑ VLCFA (P), ↓ DHAP-AT (T) (2) |
| Neonatal adrenoleukodystrophy | (A) | Hypotonia, seizures | ↑ VLCFA (P), ↓ DHAP-AT (T) (2) |
| Infantile Refsum's syndrome retinopathy, deafness | (Sa.) (V) (Dys.) | Hepatomegaly, mental retardation, | ↑ VLCFA (P), ↓ phytanic acid (P) (2) |
| Isolated DHAP-AT deficiency | (A) (Dys.) | As rhizomelic chondrodysplasia punctata | ↓ DHAP-AT (T) (2) |
| Rhizomelic chondrodysplasia punctata | (A) (Dys.) | Epiphyseal stippling, short limbs, cataracts | ↓ DHAP-AT (T), ↑ phytanic acid (P) (2) |
| Pseudo-Zellweger's syndrome | (A) (Dys.) | As Zellweger's syndrome | ↓ VLCFA (P), ↓ 3-oxoacyl-CoA thiolase (SF) (2) |
| Pseudo-neonatal adrenoleukodystrophy | (A) | As neonatal adrenoleukodystrophy | ↑ VLCFA (P), ↓ acyl-CoA oxidase (SF) (2) |
| Bifunctional enzyme defect | (A) | As neonatal adrenoleukodystrophy | ↑ VLCFA (P), ↓ bifunctional enzyme (SF) (2) |
| X-linked adrenoleukodystrophy | (Sa.) | Dementia, adrenomyeloneuropathy | ↑ VLCFA (P), ↓ VLCFA ligase (SF) (1) |
| Acatalasia | (Sa.) | Ulcerating oral lesions (Japan) | ↓ Catalase (RBC) (2) |
| Hyperoxaluria type I (glycolic aciduria) | (Sa.) | Renal stones, arthritis | ↑ Oxalic acid (U) (1) |
| **9. Purine and pyrimidine metabolism** | | | |
| Lesch–Nyhan's syndrome | (Sa.) | Self-mutilation, gouty tophi, renal stones, mental retardation | ↑ Uric acid (B) (2) |
| Adenine phosphoribosyltransferase deficiency | (Sa.) | Renal stones | ↑ 2,8-Dihydroxyadenine (U) (1) |
| Adenosine deaminase deficiency | (Sa.) | Subacute combined immune deficiency, lymphopenia | ↓ Adenosine deaminase (RBC) (1) |
| Purine-nucleoside phosphorylase deficiency | (Sa.) | Cellular immune defect | ↓ Purine-nucleoside phosphorylase (RBC) (2) |
| Myoadenytate deaminase deficiency | (Sa.) | Muscle fatigue, myalgia, myoglobinuria | ↑ Creatine phosphokinase (B) (2) |
| Xanthinuria | (Sa.) | Renal stones (1/3) | ↑ Xanthine (U) (1) |
| Orotic aciduria | (Sa.) | Megaloblastic anemia, crystalluria | ↑ Orotic acid (U) (1) |
| Pyrimidine-5′-nucleotidase deficiency | (Sa.) | Hemolytic anemic | ↑ Uracil and thymidine (U) (2) |

**Table 35.2 (continued)**

| | Clinical features | | Biochemical findings |
|---|---|---|---|
| **10. Trace metal metabolism** | | | |
| Wilson's disease | (Sa.) | Recurrent hepatitis, dystonia, Kayser–Fleischer rings, hemolysis | ↑ Copper (U), ↑ copper (liver) (1) |
| Menke's disease vascular rupture | (Sa.) (Dys.) (P) (2) | Kinky hair, neurodegeneration, | ↓ Copper (B), ↓ ceruloplasmin |
| Hemachromatosis | (Sa.) (V) | Lethargy, diabetes mellitus, arthralgia, pigmentation, cirrhosis | ↑ Ferritin (P) (1) |
| Molybdenum cofactor deficiency | (Sa.) | Mental retardation, seizures, lens dislocation | ↑ Xanthine, ↑ sulfocysteine (U) |
| Isolated sulfite oxidase deficiency | (Sa.) | As molybdenum cofactor deficiency | ↑ sulfocysteine (U) |
| **11. Lipid metabolism** | | | |
| Abetalipoproteinemia | (Sa.) | Fat malabsorption, acanthocytes, spinocerebellar ataxia, peripheral neuropathy | ↓ Cholesterol (B) (1)<br>↓ β-Lipoproteins (B) |
| Lipoprotein lipase deficiency | (Sa.) (V) | Recurrent pancreatitis, xanthomata | ↑ Chylomicrons (B) (1) |
| Lecithin:cholesterol acyltransferase (LCAT) deficiency | (Sa.) | Corneal opacities, anemia, atherosclerosis, renal failure | Proteinuria, abnormal lipoproteins (B) (2) |
| Familial hypercholesterolemia (hyperlipidemia type II) | (Sa.) | Xanthomata, premature atherosclerosis, arcus cornea | ↑ Low-density lipoproteins (B) (1) |
| Dysbetalipoproteinemia (hyperlipidemia type III) | | Xanthomata, premature atherosclerosis | ↑ Cholesterol, ↑ triglycerides (B) (1) |
| Cerebrotendinous xanthomatosis | (Sa.) | Dementia, ataxia, paresis, xanthomata, atherosclerosis | Abnormal bile acids (B) (U) (2) |
| Tangier disease | (Sa.) (V) | Orange tonsils, splenomegaly, neuropathy | ↓ High-density lipoproteins (B) (2) |
| Phytosterolemia | (Sa.) | Xanthomata, arcus cornea, premature atherosclerosis, hemolysis | ↑ Phytosterols (B) (1) |
| **12. Vitamin metabolism** | | | |
| *a. Folic acid* | | | |
| Methylene-tetrahydrofolate reductase deficiency | (Sa.) | Developmental delay, seizures, ataxia | ↑ Homocystinuria (2) |
| Glutamate formiminotransferase deficiency | (Sa.) | Unclear | ↑ Formiminoglutamic acid (U) (2) |
| *b. Vitamin $B_{12}$* (cobalamin) | | | |
| Transcobalamin II deficiency | (A) | Failure to thrive, glossitis, megaloblastic anemia | ↓ Transcobalamin II (B) (2) |
| Defects in adenosylcobalamin (AdoCbl) synthesis:<br>cbl A mutation<br>cbl B mutation | See text: methylmalonic acidemia | | |
| Both of the above defects cause methylmalonic acidemia as AdoCbl is an essential cofactor for the mutase enzyme. | | | |
| Defects in methylcobalamin (MeCbl) synthesis:<br>cbl E mutation<br>cbl G mutation | | | |

| | | | |
|---|---|---|---|
| Both of the above disorders lead to a functional deficiency of *N*-methyltetrahydrofolate: homocysteine methyltransferase leading to homocystinuria, hypomethioninemia without methylmalonic acidemia. | | | |
| cbl C mutation<br>cbl D mutation<br>cbl F mutation | Lead to impaired synthesis of both AdoCbl and MeCbl. Therefore, deficient activity of both methylmalonyl mutase and *N*-methyltetrahydrofolate:homocysteine methyltransferase | | |
| **13. Defects in the synthesis and degradation of haem proteins** | | | |
| *a. Porphyrias* | | | |
| δ-Aminolevulinic acid dehydratase deficiency | (Sa.) | Vomiting, limb pains, abdominal pain, neuropathy | ↑ Aminolevulinic acid (U) (2) |
| Acute intermittent porphyria | (Sa.) | Vomiting, abdominal pain, neuropathy affecting peripheral autonomic or central nervous system | ↑ Aminolevulinic acid (1)<br>↑ Porphobilinogen (U) |
| Congenital erythropoietic porphyria | (Sa.) | Cutaneous hypersensitivity, hemolysis | ↑ Urinary porphyrins (2) |
| Porphyria cutanea tarda | (Sa.) | Cutaneous hypersensitivity, hemolysis | ↑ Uroporphyrin I (U) (1) |
| Hereditary coproporphyria | (Sa.) | Abdominal pain, neuropathy, photosensitivity | ↑ Fecal coproporphyrin (1) |
| Variegate porphyria | (Sa.) | As acute intermittent porphyria plus photosensitivity | ↑ Fecal protoporphyrin (1) |
| Erythropoietic protoporphyria | (Sa.) | Cutaneous hypersensitivity | ↑ Protophophyrin (B) (P) (1) |
| *b. Bilirubin metabolism* | | | |
| Crigler–Najjar's syndrome type I | (A) | Severe non-hemolytic jaundice kernicterus | ↑ Unconjugated bilirubin (B) |
| Crigler–Najjar's syndrome type II | (A) | As type I but mild | ↑ Unconjugated bilirubin (B) |
| Gilbert's syndrome | (Sa.) | Mild, chronic non-hemolytic jaundice | ↑ Unconjugated bilirubin (B) (2) |
| Dubin–Johnson's syndrome | (Sa.) | Mild conjugated hyperbilirubinemia | ↑ Conjugated bilirubin (B) (U) (2) |
| Rotor syndrome | (Sa.) | As Dubin–Johnson's syndrome | |
| **14. Disorders of membrane transport** | | | |
| Cystinuria | (Sa.) | Renal stones | ↑ Cystine basic amino acids (U) (1) |
| Lysinuric protein intolerance | (Sa.) (V) | Failure to thrive, hypotonia, sparse hair, osteoporosis | ↑ Ammonia (B), ↑ orotic acid (U)<br>↑ Glutamine (B), ↑ lysine (U) |
| Hartnup's disease | (Sa.) | Photosensitivity, ataxia, psychosis | ↑ Urine excretion of neutral amino acids, e.g. alanine, serine, threonine, etc. |
| Cystinosis | (Sa.) | Corneal crystals, Fanconi's syndrome, renal failure, hypothyroidism | ↑ Cystine (WBC) (2) |
| Infantile free sialic acid storage disease | (A) or (Sa.) (V) (Dys.) | Severe mental retardation, ascites, fair skin, pale hair | ↑ Sialic acid (U) (2) |
| Salla's disease | (Sa.) (V) (Dys.) | Developmental delay, ataxia | ↑ Sialic acid (U) (2) |
| **15. Miscellaneous disorders** | | | |
| Lowe's syndrome | (Sa.) | Cataracts, mental retardation, Fanconi's syndrome | ↑ Aminoaciduria, proteinuria (2)<br>Phosphaturia and acidosis |
| Carbonic anhydrase II deficiency | (Sa.) | Osteoporosis, cerebral calcification, renal tubular acidosis, mental retardation | As Lowe's syndrome (2) |
| Refsum's disease | (Sa.) | Retinitis pigmentosa, neuropathy, cerebella ataxia | ↑ Phytanic acid (B) (1) |

**Table 35.2 (continued)**

| | Clinical features | | Biochemical findings |
|---|---|---|---|
| Congenital disorders of glycosylation (CDG syn) | (A) or (Sa.) (Dys) | Fat pads, inverted nipples, pericardial effusion, liver disease (see text) | Abnormal transferrin electrophoresis (B) |
| Steroid sulfatase deficiency | (Sa.) | Ichthyosis, corneal opacity | $\downarrow$ Steroid sulphatase (WBC) (1) |
| Hypophosphatasia | (A) or (Sa.) | Nephrocalcinosis, premature loss of teeth, fractures | $\uparrow$ Calcium (B), $\uparrow$ phosphoethanolamine (U) $\downarrow$ Alkaline phosphatase (P) (2) |
| Fumaric aciduria | (A) or (Sa.) | Lethargy, failure to thrive, mental retardation | Acidosis, $\uparrow$ fumaric acid (U) |
| Sjögren–Larsson's syndrome | (Sa.) | Ichthyosis, spasticity, hypoplastic teeth, mental retardation | $\downarrow$ Fatty-alcohol oxidoreductase (SF) (2) |

*Key*: A = acute; B = blood; CRS = cherry red spot; DHAP-AT = dihydroxyacetone-phosphate acyltransferase; Dys. = dysmorphic; LFT = liver function test; P = plasma; RBC = red blood cells; SA = subacute; SF = s<in fibroblasts; T = thrombocytes; U = urine; V = visceromegaly; VLCA = very-long-chain fatty acids; WBC = white blood cells 1 = outcome good after early treatment; 2 = outcome variable or uncertain.

This approach allows biochemical diagnosis before symptoms are apparent (Danks 1974).

## CLUES TO THE DIAGNOSIS OF AN INBORN ERROR OF METABOLISM PRESENTING AS A SEVERE NEONATAL ILLNESS

The diagnosis of a metabolic disorder in a seriously ill neonate depends largely on the awareness of the clinicians, but a number of clues can be obtained from the history, clinical examination, and simple bedside tests.

Table 35.3 outlines the essential points to be noted in the history of any child presenting with an unusual illness in the newborn period. With one or two important exceptions [e.g. ornithine carbamyltransferase (OCT) deficiency], inheritance is autosomal recessive. A family history of neonatal death or of parental consanguinity is an important clue. In OCT deficiency, there may be a history of male deaths on the maternal side of the family.

Most affected infants are delivered at, or near, term in good condition with a normal birth weight and remain well in the early days of life. Intrauterine protection from the effects of inherited metabolic disease is due to a number of factors. The fetus is in an anabolic state, and this minimizes flux through amino-acid degradative pathways and the urea cycle. The placenta effectively hemodialyses the fetus, removing toxic metabolites, and the fetus is not yet in contact with substances in the diet toxic to infants with a mutant genotype. There are some important exceptions to the general rule of intrauterine protection. In non-ketotic hyperglycinemia, features appear before, at, or soon after birth. The neurotransmitter disturbance in this disorder is not greatly influenced by placental function. In a similar way, disorders that interfere with fetal energy metabolism, e.g. primary disorders of pyruvate metabolism, can produce symptoms either *in utero* or at birth. The prognosis in such conditions is very poor as most of the damage is irreversible by the time the child is born.

Intense catabolism during the first few days of life, together with the initiation of protein-containing feeds, unmasks the metabolic lesion. A change in feeding may be an important precipitating event, e.g. a change from breast-feeding to a higher protein-containing formula. In those infants who escape severe disease in the newborn period, catabolic stress such as infection, surgery or prolonged fasting can precipitate symptoms at some later time. If the infant improves when protein is removed from the diet, only to relapse when milk feeds are recommenced, a metabolic disorder should be suspected.

**Table 35.3 Questions to ask when metabolic disease is suspected**

1. Is there a history of previous stillbirths or neonatal deaths?
2. Is there a history of parental consanguinity?
3. Was there a period of normality after birth?
4. Has there been a change of feed since birth?
5. Is there any evidence of infection?
6. Has the baby been subjected to a fast or surgical procedure?
7. Did the baby improve when feeds were discontinued?
8. Was there a relapse on restarting milk feeds?

## CLINICAL FEATURES OF INBORN ERRORS OF METABOLISM PRESENTING AS SEVERE NEONATAL ILLNESS

The clinical features and main biochemical findings of those disorders presenting acutely in the neonatal period are shown in Table 35.2.

In general, the neonate with a metabolic disorder presents with very non-specific features mimicking a host of more common neonatal problems such as sepsis, necrotizing enterocolitis and intracerebral hemorrhage. The correct interpretation of the clinical signs depends upon a high index of suspicion of a metabolic disease in the mind of the clinician managing the patient. Rarely, the typical odor of isovaleric acidemia, glutaric aciduria type II, or maple syrup urine disease will be noted. Infants with galactosemia may develop cataracts in the first week of life, but with other disorders, signs and symptoms are non-specific, and usually one is faced with a neurologically abnormal, convulsing infant who rapidly proceeds to a comatose state.

## INVESTIGATION OF THE SEVERELY ILL NEONATE FOR METABOLIC DISEASE

Metabolic investigations should proceed urgently, in parallel with other tests for infections and other common neonatal illnesses in sick infants.

Some clues can be obtained from 'bedside' tests. All severely ill neonates will have routine biochemical and hematological tests carried out. These generally include a full blood count and film, estimations of bilirubin, electrolyte and blood glucose concentrations as well as acid–base studies. A true metabolic acidosis can easily be missed unless acid–base testing is carried out promptly. A mixed metabolic and respiratory acidosis is common in a severely ill neonate, and the metabolic component may be further masked by mechanical ventilation.

In suspected metabolic disease, emphasis has been placed on urine 'spot' testing for various compounds. These tests have many shortcomings and should not be relied upon to make or refute a diagnosis. Urine testing for reducing substances is still considered important by many referring clinicians for the diagnosis of galactosemia. We have seen a number of neonates with galactosemia whose urine did not show any reducing substances despite severe illness. In others, severe renal tubular disease limits the value of urine testing. A specific screening test for classical galactosemia must be carried out as a matter of urgency on all infants suspected of having the disease, and this test must be readily available in all regions.

A urine test for ketones can be useful. Heavy ketonuria is unusual in the neonatal period, and its detection should be immediately followed by organic acid analysis.

In patients with acidosis, calculation of the anion gap – the sum of the serum concentrations of sodium and potassium minus the sum of the serum concentrations of chloride and bicarbonate – can be helpful. Patients with an increased anion gap, and especially those with a value greater than 25 mmol/l (normal range 12–16 mmol/l), are likely to have a specific organic acidemia. Patients with a normal anion gap and acidosis are most likely to have renal tubular acidosis or intestinal bicarbonate loss (Gabow *et al.* 1980).

## THE METABOLIC SCREEN

Occasionally, we are asked to give advice after an infant's death, and although we are able to perform some metabolic investigations (see below), early suspicion and collection of the appropriate tissues and fluids from a living child permit a more comprehensive screen for metabolic disease.

Although techniques vary, most laboratories will require a sample of blood (1–2 ml in a heparinized tube) and urine (5–10 ml in a sterile container with no preservatives) for a metabolic screen. In addition, one should ask for a number of blood spots to be collected onto a newborn screening filter paper.

It is essential that these basic samples be supplemented by a sample of blood (5 ml in an EDTA tube) for subsequent DNA analysis. This is particularly important for infants suspected of having MCAD deficiency where analysis for the common mutation is often the quickest way of establishing the diagnosis and will detect 90% of mutant alleles within the white population (Matsubara *et al.* 1992). It is a good principle to save and freeze all urine passed by the infant for future analysis. If an urgent result is required, it is essential that the referring clinician contact the laboratory in advance to indicate the urgency. Full details of drugs and diet must be included, and the samples should be transported rapidly to the laboratory. Where possible, blood must be taken before any blood transfusions, as this will interfere with the screening test most laboratories use to exclude galactosemia. If this is not possible, the laboratory personnel must be told about the transfusion so that an alternative test can be used. It is good clinical practice to save a sample of blood from all infants who require exchange transfusion in case screening for galactosemia is later thought to be necessary.

In our laboratory, amino acid concentrations are estimated in blood and urine by one-dimensional paper chromatography. Abnormal results are then characterized quantitatively. Gas–liquid chromatography with mass spectrometry is used for urinary organic acid analyses, and in most centers, this would be supplemented by an acylcarnitine profile performed on one of the blood spots. Blood ammonia should be measured and a portion of urine kept for orotic acid estimation if the ammonia concentration is high. Occasionally, more specialized investigations will be required, e.g. amino acid analysis on cerebrospinal fluid, and if this is the case, it is best to discuss the clinical problem with the laboratory to ensure that the appropriate samples are collected.

Infants with lactic acidosis present a difficult problem, which is also discussed on p. 637. It is difficult to distinguish primary lactic acidosis caused by a defect in pyruvate metabolism from secondary lactic acidosis caused by hypoxia, cardiac disease, infection or convulsions. It is necessary to treat possible underlying causes aggressively, while trying to separate the two groups. Plasma lactate and pyruvate are extremely sensitive to the method of collection, and venous obstruction by crying, tourniquet or restraint can cause a two- to fivefold increase in concentrations. The urinary lactate concentration is useful in monitoring if blood lactate is greater than 6 mmol/l. In those patients with secondary lactic acidosis, the urinary lactate falls as the underlying disorder improves, while infants with a primary defect are unresponsive to most treatments. Often the child dies before a clear distinction is made, and one has to rely on a formal assay of the enzymes known to cause lactic acidoses. This is an unsatisfactory approach as many patients with strong evidence of a primary defect have no biochemical abnormality on testing. Lactic acidosis is a heterogeneous group of disorders, and it is possible that many defects have not been fully defined or are tissue-specific, e.g. limited to muscle or the central nervous system (Robinson 1989).

With other disorders, we would expect to confirm the diagnosis of a urea cycle defect, amino acid disorder, fat oxidation defect or organic acidaemia within 6 h of receiving the appropriate samples (and often sooner).

## MANAGEMENT WHILST AWAITING RESULTS

The severity of symptoms dictates the aggressiveness of management. In infants who have mild symptoms, it is appropriate to discontinue milk feeds once the specimens necessary for the screen have been collected. For infants with more severe symptoms, active treatment is required, and the infant should be transferred to a specialized unit. General measures will include correcting electrolyte imbalance and treating acidosis with sodium bicarbonate. Often, large doses of the latter will be necessary, and we prefer to give it in a steady intravenous infusion over 24 h rather than as individual bolus dosages. There is always a risk of inducing hypernatremia, but with acidosis so resistant to treatment, dialysis should be considered early. Mechanical ventilation is usually required for severely affected infants.

The key to treatment is to induce an anabolic state as quickly as possible. A high energy intake, using 15–20% dextrose together with insulin (1 unit/3 g glucose or approximately 0.05 unit/kg/h), and lipid solutions may help to initiate anabolism. It is prudent to insert a central venous line, as this regimen quickly damages peripheral veins and adequate venous access is of vital importance. Although this regimen is suitable for most disorders, patients with a primary lactic acidosis may be made worse by a carbohydrate load, and for these infants, the next phase of treatment (removal of toxic metabolites) becomes of paramount importance.

A number of studies have compared the efficacy of exchange transfusion, hemodialysis, and peritoneal dialysis in the acute management of inborn errors. A positive move has now been made towards using continuous arteriovenous hemofiltration (CAVH) with peritoneal dialysis being used in those infants in whom vascular access proves impossible. The beneficial effects of exchange transfusion are at best transient, and its use cannot be recommended for the management of acute disease.

In most infants with hyperammonemia or an organic acidemia, CAVH will be needed for at least 72 h and, once established, protein should be introduced cautiously to the diet, starting at 0.5 g/kg/day and increased as tolerated to 1.2–1.5 g/kg/day. In addition, at least 120 kcal/kg/day are supplied, and this combination is usually sufficient to achieve anabolism and promote growth.

Infants with hyperammonemia respond rapidly to treatment with sodium benzoate, ammonia nitrogen being diverted away from the defective urea cycle by being conjugated with glycine to form hippurate, which is excreted in the urine. Sodium phenylbutyrate can also be utilized in a similar way to conjugate with glutamine to form phenylacetyl glutamine, and together, a rapid reduction in blood ammonia can be achieved. Sodium benzoate and butyrate should be used together with CAVH in infants with hyperammonemia greater than 600 μmol/l or alone in infants with a more moderate increase. The effects are transient, and bolus dosages of 0.25–0.5 g/kg/day should be followed by a steady infusion of 0.25 g/kg/day (Brusilow & Horwich 1989).

A number of metabolic disorders are known to have vitamin-responsive forms, and it has become traditional to administer a combination of vitamins in pharmacological dosages to sick infants whilst awaiting results. This 'blunderbuss' approach to therapy can no longer be justified. The ready availability of metabolic investigations in most regions allows for diagnosis to proceed rapidly with the use of the appropriate vitamin (in a dose approximately 100 times the daily requirement) once diagnosis has been confirmed.

## SPECIFIC MANAGEMENT AFTER DIAGNOSIS

For the majority of disorders, treatment is non-specific and relies upon protein restriction. In some, more specific regimes are available.

### UREA CYCLE DISORDERS

After CAVH or dialysis has been used to reduce plasma ammonia concentrations rapidly, protein restriction with supplementary essential amino acids forms the basis of treatment. Long-term oral sodium benzoate is often necessary, and in all the disorders except arginase deficiency, arginine supplementation becomes essential if chronic hyperammonemia is to be avoided (Brusilow 1984).

### ORGANIC ACID DISORDERS

Acute management includes correction of acidosis, toxin removal and protein restriction. In addition, the build-up of acyl coenzyme esters within the cells further compromises their normal metabolic pathways. Carnitine plays an important role by conjugating these compounds to form acylcarnitine esters, which are excreted through the kidney. This leads to secondary carnitine deficiency and has led to the use of carnitine supplementation in both the acute and chronic management of organic acidemias (Stanley 1987).

In isovaleric acidemia, isovaleryl-CoA accumulates, and the isovaleryl groups can be conjugated effectively to glycine. Glycine supplementation can therefore increase the excretion of isovaleryl glycine, leading to metabolic correction (Naglak *et al.* 1988).

Antimicrobials (e.g. metronidazole) have been used to sterilize the gut in an attempt to reduce substrate production from gut organisms in some organic acid defects (Bain *et al.* 1985).

## MANAGEMENT WHEN DEATH SEEMS INEVITABLE OR THE CHILD DIES DESPITE TREATMENT

Aggressive treatment is justified even if no diagnosis is established as some defects will be transient, e.g. transient hyperammonemia of prematurity. If death seems inevitable, it is important to gain as much information as possible about the child. Autopsy is essential, and careful thought is needed to ensure that the correct samples are collected. A post-mortem must be carried out as soon after death as possible so that biochemical studies can be made on tissues that have not yet undergone autolysis. The need for autopsy should be discussed with the parents before death and permission obtained at that time. Many couples find it easier to discuss this matter before rather than after death. If possible, 1 ml of plasma should be collected before death and frozen together with as much urine as possible (even a few drops can be useful). As our knowledge of the molecular pathology of disease has increased, it has become vital to collect a sample of blood in an EDTA tube for subsequent DNA analysis. If metabolic investigations are considered for the first time after death, one can try and retrieve samples from routine pathology laboratories. Blood from cardiac puncture can be collected, separated, and stored. Cerebrospinal fluid can be obtained after death by cisternal puncture and used for amino acid and organic acid analyses. Skin fibroblast cultures should be established for subsequent enzyme assays if metabolic disease is suggested by autopsy findings.

If permission to perform a full autopsy is not given (perhaps for religious reasons), it is important to ask the parents to agree to a limited biopsy study, e.g. liver and muscle. Many (but not all) enzymes can be accurately assayed many hours after death, and even if more than 12 h have elapsed, it is still worth collecting samples for measurement of metabolites resistant to autolysis, e.g. for diagnosis of fatty acid oxidation defects. Biopsies should be shared with the pathologist, who will require material for essential histology, histochemistry and electron microscopy. Samples for biochemical studies should be snap-frozen in dried ice or liquid nitrogen and stored frozen until assayed.

## LONG-TERM MANAGEMENT

This can involve a specific therapy such as a diet low in branched-chain amino acids in maple syrup urine disease or a non-specific low-protein diet in infants with vitamin-unresponsive forms of the organic acid defects. In the latter situation, the crucial factor is whether or not the child is able to grow within the confines of protein tolerance. A number of infants are in precarious balance, tolerating just enough protein to allow growth, but the latitude is so slight that any trivial intercurrent infection can produce acute metabolic imbalance. Good judgement is critical in treating these babies. A slightly excessive protein intake may cause a metabolic imbalance, which arrests growth. Then, a reduction in protein intake may restore growth. At other times, excessive protein restriction may stop growth, with consequent metabolic instability.

To test tolerance, it is important to increase protein intake slowly as an in-patient under close biochemical control. After discharge, the child should be admitted during the first two or three episodes of intercurrent illness. This allows one to assess the usefulness of simple therapies such as diluting feeds and supplementing with oral carbohydrates during mild exacerbations. Severe decompensation needs to be treated as aggressively as the presenting episode. Both parents and doctors gain experience of the individual child's response to catabolism and are thus able to judge when hospitalization is necessary in future episodes. The parents are finally given an 'emergency regimen' for their child to be followed during episodes of intercurrent infection. Access to the metabolic unit must be available at all times.

## SPECIFIC CONDITIONS

### PHENYLKETONURIA (see also p. 809)

There are a number of conditions associated with an elevation of plasma phenylalanine levels, and almost all are detected by the newborn screening program. Of practical importance are 'classical' phenylketonuria due to phenylalanine hydroxylase deficiency and those cases caused by a deficiency of the tetrabiopterin cofactor due to defects in synthesis or recycling. One can no longer assume that a positive result on screening indicates phenylalanine hydroxylase deficiency and that one need only decide whether the deficiency is sufficiently severe to require dietary treatment (classical phenylketonuria), or not (hyperphenylalaninemia, HPA). This is further complicated by the fact that infants with cofactor defects may have only marginally elevated phenylalanine levels, which would not warrant dietary treatment in phenylalanine hydroxylase deficiency. In cofactor-deficient cases, dietary treatment has to be supplemented with neurotransmitter precursors if neurological damage is to be avoided. Specific enzyme assay for cofactor defects combined with tetrabiopterin loading and urine pterin analysis are needed to characterize these disorders.

The long-term prognosis of 'classical' phenylketonuria is currently contentious. Whilst a detailed discussion of intellectual and neurological outcome of early diagnosed 'classical' phenylketonuria patients is beyond the scope of this chapter, a few points can be made. Late-onset neurological disease associated with white-matter changes on magnetic resonance imaging has led to a change in policy with regard to dietary therapy. Most units are persisting with tighter biochemical control into adult life, and many operate a 'diet for life' policy. There has been a reawakening of interest in adult phenylketonuria (Thompson *et al.* 1990) concentrating on the imaging abnormalities that are almost universal in adult patients (Cleary *et al.* 1994). These changes, which are reversible (Walter *et al.* 1997), possibly represent local increased water content of the brain secondary to the amino acid imbalance that occurs in phenylketonuria.

Also of relevance to this chapter is the syndrome of mental retardation, microcephaly, cardiac defects, and poor growth observed in infants born to phenylketonuria mothers (Lenke & Levy 1980). In families with a number of abnormal children, it is essential to check the mother for metabolic disease as part of the investigations.

### UREA CYCLE DEFECTS

The urea cycle defects illustrate one or two points that require expansion. OCT deficiency is one of the few conditions presenting as an acute illness in the newborn period that is inherited in an X-linked manner. In affected families, there is often a history of early male deaths on the maternal side. Female heterozygotes have a variable degree of illness. Many develop an aversion to protein-rich foods, and some develop serious episodes of hyperammonemia that cause brain damage or even death. Pregnancy seems a particularly vulnerable time.

The remainder of the urea cycle defects show autosomal recessive inheritance and occur as severe forms, lethal in the newborn period, or as less severe forms presenting later.

Long-term management is an extension of the measures used during the acute phase (see earlier) combined with a low-protein diet. Prognosis for mental development in severe cases remains poor.

Transient hyperammonemia in the newborn period is

worthy of mention. The biochemical basis of the disorder is unknown. It is more common in premature infants and important to recognize because aggressive treatment has led to normal recovery in infants whose presenting blood ammonia levels have been greater than 1000 μmol/l. Subsequently, affected infants tolerate a normal diet, illustrating the transient nature of some metabolic disorders (Giacoia & Padilla-Lugo 1986).

## MAPLE SYRUP URINE DISEASE

A defect in the mitochondrial multienzyme complex branched-chain keto-acid dehydrogenase results in an increased concentration of the branched-chain amino acids (leucine, isoleucine and valine) and keto-acids in blood and body fluids. The urine has the characteristic smell of maple syrup, and in the affected infant, signs and symptoms of an encephalopathic illness are present by the end of the first week of life. Untreated, progressive stupor and, ultimately, coma and death are the usual outcome. Survivors exhibit a severe brain dysfunction with dystonic posturing and profound mental retardation. A number of variants occur, including transient and thiamine-responsive defects.

Dietary treatment is difficult as one has to adjust the level of three amino acids in a coordinated manner. Overtreatment leads to catabolism and further metabolic instability.

The prognosis in maple syrup urine disease diagnosed after the first week of life is disappointing. Even with early diagnosis and treatment, the clinical course is one of frequent readmission to hospital over the early years of life for restabilization, but very good results have been achieved in some patients (Kaplan *et al.* 1991).

## NON-KETOTIC HYPERGLYCINEMIA (see also p. 638)

Glycine encephalopathy, or non-ketotic hyperglycinemia, is one of the few disorders in which intrauterine protection does not occur. Large amounts of glycine accumulate in body fluids due to a defect in the glycine cleavage system, a multienzyme complex responsible for the breakdown of glycine to ammonia, carbon dioxide, and formyltetrahydrofolate.

The metabolic defect produces a clinical picture dominated by severe neurological dysfunction with hypotonia, myoclonic seizures, and opisthotonic posturing. Some mothers have reported decreased fetal movements, suggesting a prenatal onset of symptoms in some patients. The EEG shows a characteristic 'burst-suppression' pattern.

The elevation of glycine is most marked in cerebro-spinal fluid, reflecting a primary disturbance of neuronal glycine metabolism. There is no associated increase in urinary organic acids, distinguishing the condition from the various ketotic hyperglycinemias.

Symptoms appear to be due to overstimulation of the excitatory *N*-methyl-D-aspartate receptor by allosteric glycine activation; treatments that modify plasma glycine have little effect on the disease. A number of different treatments have been suggested, including blocking the appropriate receptors with dextromethorphan (Hamosh *et al.* 1992). The prognosis remains very gloomy, and in the severe neonatal form of the disease, it is debatable whether treatment has any effect on outcome, and death usually results in the early months of life.

## ORGANIC ACIDEMIAS (see also p. 639)

A number of disorders are characterized by impaired catabolism of low-molecular-weight organic acids (see Table 35.2). These conditions present with a pattern of biochemical abnormality that includes severe metabolic acidosis, hyperglycinemia, hyperammonemia and hypoglycemia. Clinical features include vomiting, lethargy and convulsions leading to apnea and coma. The early management of these disorders has been outlined earlier, and a brief summary of two of the more frequent conditions is presented below.

### Methylmalonic acidemia

Methylmalonic acidemia can be subdivided into a number of different categories, depending on whether the primary defect is in the methylmalonyl-CoA mutase enzyme or in one of the steps in the formation of its cofactor, adenosylcobalamin. If the defect is in the early steps of cobalamin synthesis, there is associated homocystinuria and megaloblastic anemia. Responsiveness of the defect to vitamin $B_{12}$ needs to be assessed as treatment is very effective in those with vitamin-responsive forms of the disease, and prognosis is excellent, providing large oral (10 mg/day) or intramuscular (1000 μg three times a week) dosages of $B_{12}$ are maintained. In unresponsive forms, treatment relies on protein restriction. Frequent exacerbations are common during the early years of life, and necrosis of the basal ganglia is recognized as a complication of such episodes (Heidenreich *et al.* 1988).

Prognosis in non-$B_{12}$-responsive methylmalonic acidemia is further compromised by the development of renal tubulo-interstitial nephritis in most affected patients (D'Angio *et al.* 1991). Successful combined liver and kidney transplantation has been performed for this disorder (Van't Hoff *et al.* 1998). As with all organic acid disorders, mild variants occur, and presentation can be at any age.

### Propionic acidemia

Propionic acidemia shares many features in common with methylmalonic acidemia but has a much worse prognosis. Hyperammonemia can be a persistent problem, and the majority of affected children are anorexic and require gavage feeding. During the acute presentation and subsequent exacerbations, the affected infant is usually neutropenic and thrombocytopenic due to toxic bone marrow suppression. Treatment with a low-protein diet is only moderately successful, and almost all infants are significantly handicapped (Surtees *et al.* 1992).

## FAT OXIDATION DEFECTS

The fat oxidation defects are probably the most rapidly expanding group of metabolic disorders (Eaton *et al.* 1996). Although presentation in infancy is usual in the most common fat oxidation defect – medium chain fatty acyl-CoA dehydrogenase deficiency (MCAD) – some disorders, e.g. carnitine transporter deficiency (Rinaldo *et al.* 1997), can present with dramatic neonatal illness and sudden death. The introduction of acyl-carnitine profiling in dried blood spots has made diagnosis of this group of disorders easier, and already, much is known about the genetic mutations associated with the various disorders. Treatment relies on the avoidance of fasting and the provision of a very carefully produced emergency regimen for the parents. The latter includes instructions of how the parents should respond to intercurrent infections and how and when to contact the metabolic team for help and advice.

### GALACTOSEMIA

The clinical features of 'classical' galactosemia are due to a deficiency of the enzyme galactose-1-phosphate uridyltransferase. An identical clinical picture can be produced by a generalized deficiency of uridine-diphosphate-galactose 4-epimerase (deficiency of this enzyme in red cells alone is harmless). Affected infants fail to thrive, vomit, and develop progressive liver disease during the first weeks of life. Neurological symptoms are common, and a significant number develop *Escherichia coli* sepsis. Cataracts often appear during the first week of life, hepatomegaly is usual, and renal tubular damage leads to a gross generalized aminoaciduria.

Long-term treatment with a galactose-free diet quickly leads to a reversal of all the clinical signs. Intellectual outcome is usually in the borderline to mildly retarded range (intelligence quotient 60–80), even in those diagnosed and treated early. Speech delay is particularly common. Ovarian failure is frequent in female patients (80%) and is thought to be due to a toxic intrauterine effect of galactose or one of its metabolites. Large surveys of long-term outcome have recently been reported (Waggoner *et al.* 1990; Schweitzer *et al.* 1993).

### PYRIDOXINE-DEPENDENT SEIZURES (see also p. 651)

Pyridoxine-dependent seizures usually present in the first 24 h of life. Typically, they are generalized and intractable to normal anticonvulsants. Onset *in utero* has been reported. However, pyridoxine-dependent seizures may start some days after birth and may fluctuate in severity and/or respond temporarily to standard anticonvulsants (Bankier *et al.* 1983). Exclusion of this diagnosis is necessary in all infants with seizures. This requires administration of 100 mg of pyridoxine by intravenous injection with careful observation or EEG control. Severe drowsiness and depression may follow cessation of the convulsions in patients who truly have the condition.

### MITOCHONDRIAL DISORDERS (see also p. 637)

In recent years, an increasing number of disorders have been described where the primary genetic defect is not in the nuclear genome, but in the genetic material present within the mitochondrion – mitochondrial DNA (mtDNA) (Clarke 1992). The mtDNA differs in many aspects from nuclear DNA, e.g. it is much smaller and contains only a few genes arranged as a circular 'chromosome', which contains no introns. The genetic code of mtDNA is different from the universal code, making the nuclear and mtDNA reciprocally untranslatable. As a result, expression of mitochondrial genes relies upon mitochondrial-specific protein synthesis within the mitochondrial inner compartment.

The most important feature of mtDNA genetics is the non-Mendelian transmission of the mitochondrial genotype – mitochondrial inheritance proceeds entirely from the mother (as only the head of the sperm penetrates the egg at fertilization), leading to problems in the genetic counseling of couples with affected children.

Deletions, point mutations, duplications, rearrangements, and mtDNA depletion can all be associated with a variety of clinical disorders, some of which can present in the newborn period. Almost any organ of the body can be affected, although muscle and brain seem to be particularly vulnerable (mitochondrial encephalomyopathies) (see p. 637). Cardiomyopathy and liver failure starting in the early neonatal period have also been reported (Tulinius *et al.* 1991a, b).

Lactic acidosis is the biochemical clue to diagnosis, indicating impairment of the respiratory transport chain. The diagnosis can be supported by detecting mitochondrial structural abnormalities on electron microscopy of skeletal muscle. Specific assay of the components of the respiratory transport chain will lead to an enzyme diagnosis in a number of patients, and in others, analysis of the mtDNA will reveal the genetic abnormality.

#### Key Points

- Think metabolic – individual disorders may be rare but as a whole they are an important cause of morbidity and mortality.
- Investigate quickly and aggressively – outcome is often related to speed of diagnosis.
- All metabolic disorders are genetic – diagnosis has important future implications for the family.
- Investigation begins with a careful study of the obstetric case notes.
- Involve the metabolic consultant early in the illness and always discuss with the laboratory the urgency of the problem.
- It is possible in some cases to make a diagnosis after death as long as appropriate samples are collected.
- Long term management is specialized and patients should be refered to the nearest metabolic unit for care.

## REFERENCES


Bain M, Borriello S P, Reed P J *et al.* (1985) Therapeutic potential of antibiotics in methylmalonic acidaemia. *Pediatr Res* 19:1083.

Bankier A, Turner M & Hopkins I J (1983) Pyridoxine dependent seizures – a wider clinical spectrum. *Arch Dis Childhood* 58:415–418.

Bartlett K, Eaton S J & Pourfarzam M (1997) New developments in neonatal screening. *Arch Dis Childhood* 77:F151–F154.

Brown G K, Hunt S M, Scholem R *et al.* (1982) β-Hydroxy isobutyryl coenzyme A deacylase deficiency. A defect in valine metabolism associated with physical malformations. *Pediatrics* 70:532–538.

Brusilow S (1984) Arginine, an indispensible amino acid for patients with inborn errors of urea synthesis. *J Clin Invest* 74:2144–2148.

Brusilow S & Horwich A L (1989) Urea cycle enzymes. In: Scriver C R, Beaudet A L, Sly W S *et al.* (eds) *The metabolic basis of inherited disease.* New York, NY: McGraw-Hill; pp. 629–624.

Burton B K (1987) Inborn errors of metabolism: the clinical diagnosis in early infancy. *Pediatrics* 79:359–369.

Chinnery P F & Turnbull D M (1997) Clinical features, investigation, and management of patients with defects of mitochondrial DNA. *J Neurol Neurosurg Psychiatry* 63:559–563.

Chitayat D, Meagher-Villemure K, Mamer O A *et al.* (1992) Brain dysgenesis and congenital intracerebral calcification associated with 3-hydroxyisobutyric aciduria. *J Pediatr* 121:86–89.

Clarke L A (1992) Mitochondrial disorders in pediatrics. *Pediatr Clin N Am* 39:319–334.

Clayton P T (1998) Disorders of cholesterol biosynthesis. *Arch Dis Childhood* 78:185–189.

Cleary M A, Walter J H, Wraith J E *et al.* (1994) Magnetic resonance imaging of the brain in phenylketonuria. *Lancet* 344:87–90.

Colevas A D, Edwards J L, Hruban R H *et al.* (1988) Glutaric acidemia type II. *Arch Pathol Lab Med* 112:1133–1139.

D'Angio C T, Dillon M J & Leonard J V (1991) Renal tubular dysfunction in methylmalonic acidaemia. *Eur J Pediatr* 150:259–263.

Danks D M (1974) Management of newborn babies in whom serious metabolic illness is anticipated. *Arch Dis Childhood* 49:576–578.

Eaton S, Bartlett K & Pourfarzam M (1996) Mammalian mitochondrial β-oxidation. *Biochem J* 320:345–357.

Fernandes J, Sandubray J-M, van den Berghe G (eds) (2000) *Inborn metabolic diseases*, 3rd edition. Springer: Berlin.

Gabow P A, Kaeburg W D, Fennessey P V *et al.* (1980) Diagnostic importance of an increased anion gap. *N Engl J Med* 303: 854–858.

Giacoia G P & Padilla-Lugo A (1986) Severe transient neonatal hyperammonaemia. *Am J Perinatol* 3:249–254.

Hamosh A, McDonald J W, Valle D *et al.* (1992) Dextromethorphan and high dose benzoate therapy for nonketotic hyperglycinemia in an infant. *J Pediatr* 121:131–135.

Heidenreich R, Natowicz M, Hainline B E *et al.* (1988) Acute extrapyramidal syndrome in methylmalonic acidemia: 'metabolic stroke' involving the globus pallidus. *J Pediat* 113:1022–1027.

Kaplan P, Mazur A, Field M *et al.* (1991) Intellectual outcome in children with maple syrup urine disease. *J Pediatr* 119:46–50.

Krasenewich D & Gahl W A (1997) Carbohydrate-deficient glycoprotein syndrome. *Adv Pediatr* 44:109–140.

Lenke R R & Levy H L (1980) Maternal phenylketonuria and hyperphenylalaninemia. An international survey of the outcome of untreated and treated pregnancies. *N Engl J Med* 303:1202–1208.

Matsubara Y, Narisawa K, Tada K *et al.* (1992) Prevalence of K329E mutation in medium-chain acyl-CoA dehydrogenase gene determined from Gutherie cards. *Lancet* 338:552–553.

Naglak M, Salvo R, Madsen K *et al.* (1988) Treatment of isovaleric acidemia with glycine supplement. *Pediatr Res* 24:9–13.

Rashed M S, Bucknall M P, Awad A *et al.* (1997) Screening blood spots for inborn errors of metabolism by electrospray tandem mass spectrometry with a microplate batch process and a computer algorithm for automated flagging of abnormal profiles. *Clin Chem* 43:1129–1124.

Rinaldo P, Stanley C A, Hsu B Y L *et al.* (1997) Sudden neonatal death in carnitine transporter deficiency. *J Pediat* 131:304–305.

Robinson B H (1989) Lactic acidemia. In: Scriver C R, Beaudet A L, Sly W S *et al.* (eds) *The metabolic basis of inherited disease.* New York, NY: McGraw-Hill; pp. 869–888.

Sardharwalla I B & Wraith J E (1989) A clinician's view of the mass screening of the newborn for inherited diseases: current practice and future considerations. *J Inher Metab Dis* 12(suppl 1):55–63.

Schweitzer S, Shin Y, Jakobs C *et al.* (1993) Long-term outcome in 134 patients with galactosaemia. *Eur J Pediatr* 152:36–43.

Stanley C A (1987) New genetic defects in mitochondrial fatty acid oxidation and carnitine deficiency. *Adv Pediatr* 34:59–88.

Surtees R A H, Matthews E E & Leonard J V (1992) Neurologic outcome of propionic acidemia. *Pediat Neurol* 8:333–337.

Theil A C, Schutgens R B H, Wanders R J A *et al.* (1992) Clinical recognition of patients affected by a peroxisomal disorder: a retrospective study in 40 patients. *Eur J Pediat* 151:117–120.

Thompson A J, Smith I & Brenton D (1990) Neurological deterioration in young adults with phenylketonuria. *Lancet* 336:602–605.

Tulinius M H, Holme M, Kristiansson B *et al.* (1991a) Mitochondrial encephalomyopathies in childhood. I. Biochemical and morphological investigations. *J Pediatr* 119:242–250.

Tulinius M H, Holme M, Kristiansson N *et al.* (1991b) Mitochondrial encephalomyopathies in childhood. II. Clinical manifestations and syndromes. *J Pediatr* 119:251–259.

Van't Hoff W G, Dixon M, Taylor J *et al.* (1998) Combined liver-kidney transplantation in methylmalonic acidemia. *J Pediatr* 132:1043–1044.

Waggoner D D, Buist N R M & Donnell G N (1990) Long-term prognosis in galactosaemia: results of a survey of 350 cases. *J Inher Metab Dis* 13:812–818.

Walter J H, White F, Wraith J E *et al.* (1997) Complete reversal of moderate/severe brain MRI abnormalities in a patient with classical phenylketonuria. *J Inher Metab Dis* 20:367–369.

Chapter 36

# Degenerative disorders of the infant central nervous system

S. H. Green and R. G. F. Gray

## INTRODUCTION

There are thousands of different degenerative diseases affecting the central nervous system (CNS) (McKusick 1998), but only a limited number of these are likely to present in early infancy. The diseases described in this chapter are those where the main presenting features are likely to appear well within the first year of life (Brett 1997). These conditions are listed in Table 36.1. The aminoacidurias and organic acidurias have already been discussed in Chapter 35.

It is always difficult to date the onset of degenerative disease, but those diseases where the presentation is essentially in the second or third year of life or where there may have been some early symptoms towards the end of the first year are excluded.

The problem confronting the pediatrician when faced with an infant with an acute or sub-acute neurological presentation is to 'think' that it might be a neurometabolic disease. The acute presentation, possibly triggered by an infection, may be mistaken for a viral or toxic encephalopathy, especially if partial or temporary recovery takes place, e.g. Leigh's encephalopathy. A history of intermittent episodes of coma, ataxia, or seizures may be a clue to this condition or an organic acidemia. Even within a single disease entity, its age of onset may vary substantially. Dysmorphism present at birth can be a manifestation of some inborn errors of metabolism, e.g. Zellweger's syndrome. The MRI may be abnormal with cysts in the cortex in non-ketotic hyperglycinemia and glutathione synthetase deficiency.

## SYMPTOMS

The normal clues to the history of degenerative disease include a period of normality followed by slowing down of progress, plateauing, and the regression of skills, and these may be very difficult to detect in early life. Firstly, the degeneration may start before there is any certainty about a period of normality; secondly, there may be confusion about the early history, especially if this is compounded by perinatal problems (and neonatal encephalopathy might occasionally be metabolic in origin); and, thirdly, mental degeneration, a feature of some of the gray-matter degenerations, may not be so obvious in the first year of life, except to an astute observer. Occasionally, degeneration may be noted after immunization and wrongly attributed to it.

Visual deficit may not be obvious for quite a few months in the absence of abnormal eye movements. Deafness likewise may not be diagnosed until later in the first year. The pace of forward development is such that it may mask the degenerative process for a while.

Sometimes, a particular pattern of signs gives a clue, e.g. the presence of squint, head retraction and swallowing problems in Gaucher's disease. In other cases, a known associated finding, e.g. herniae in the mucopolysaccharidoses, may suggest the diagnosis presymptomatically.

Broadly speaking, the amino acid disorders and organic acid disorders present acutely, often in the newborn period (Chapter 35). The lysosomal storage diseases tend to manifest themselves a little later with sub-acute or chronic symptoms, but there is substantial overlap. Peroxisomal disorders may present in the newborn period with symptoms, e.g. hypotonia, which are not obviously progressive and previously might have been misdiagnosed as non-neurometabolic stationary encephalopathies. Diseases associated with respiratory chain defects (nuclear or mitochondrial DNA encoded) may present in the first year of life (and almost at any age), and the signs may be only slowly progressive. There are a wide range of described symptoms, including hypotonia, ophthalmoplegia, ptosis, other brainstem signs, and seizures. Cardiomyopathy, renal tubular disorders, endocrine disorders, liver disease, and failure to thrive may also be features. These conditions may present both acutely and sub-acutely as well as having a chronic course. The range of these diseases and the various subtypes is gradually being defined (Powers & Moser 1998).

In general, however, a history of slow development without specific signs, intermittent episodes of hypotonia, coma and ataxia, failure to achieve expected milestones, unexplained visual problems, coordination difficulties, and seizures should alert one to the possibility of a neurometabolic disease in infancy.

There are some major clinical features, which, by themselves, should alert one to the possibility of specific degenerative CNS diseases in the absence of any other obvious cause. These include:

- acousticomotor response (Tay–Sachs' disease)
- swallowing difficulties (Gaucher's disease)
- respiratory irregularities (Leigh's disease)
- gaze palsies (Niemann–Pick C disease)
- cherry-red spot (Tay–Sachs' disease)
- ophthalmoplegia (mitochondrial DNA abnormalities)
- buttock wasting, poor social development and microcephaly (carbohydrate deficient glycoprotein syndrome).

**Table 36.1 Degenerative disorders of the CNS with onset in infancy**

| Disorder | Symptoms | Primary biochemical defect | Cells, tissue or fluid for definitive diagnosis |
|---|---|---|---|
| *Lipidoses* | | | |
| GMI generalized gangliosidosis (pseudo-Hurler's syndrome) | Hypotonia, poor sucking, developmental delay, hepatosplenomegaly, coarse features, CRS | β-Galactosidase | Leukocytes<br>Fibroblasts |
| GM2 gangliosidosis 'Tay–Sachs' disease | Irritability, hypotonia, hyperacusis, regression, CRS, seizures, blindness, spasticity | Hexosaminidase A | Leukocytes<br>Plasma<br>Fibroblasts |
| Sandhoff's disease | As Tay–Sachs' disease | Hexosaminidase A and B | Leukocytes<br>Plasma<br>Fibroblasts |
| Niemann-Pick disease Type A | Hepatosplenomegaly, FTT, developmental delay, later neurological signs, CRS, neonatal hydrops | Sphingomyelinase | Leukocytes |
| Niemann-Pick disease Type C | Transient neonatal hepatitis, hypotonia, developmental delay, lateral gaze defects | Cholesterol esterification | Fibroblasts |
| Gaucher's disease Type II | Developmental delay and regression, squint, neck retraction, swallowing difficulties, splenomegaly, CRS | β-Glucocerebrosidase | Leukocytes<br>Fibroblasts |
| Farber's disease | Developmental regression, puffy hands and feet, generalized arthropathy, subcutaneous nodules | Acid ceramidase | Leukocytes<br>Fibroblasts |
| Metachromatic leukodystrophy | Progressive retardation, spasticity or hypotonia | Arylsulfatase A | Leukocytes<br>Fibroblasts |
| Krabbe's leukodystrophy | Irritability, stiffness, opisthotonus, regression, seizures, later hypotonia | β-Galactocerebrosidase | Leukocytes<br>Fibroblasts |
| Multiple sulfatase deficiency (mucosulfatidosis) | Developmental delay, spasticity with depressed reflexes, seizures, coarse features, hepatomegaly | Arylsulfatase A, B, C | Leukocytes<br>Fibroblasts |
| *Mucopolysaccharidoses* | | | |
| Mucopolysaccharidosis I (Hurler's syndrome) | Developmental delay, hernia, corneal clouding | α-Iduronidase | Fibroblasts<br>Leukocytes |
| Mucopolysaccharidosis VII (Sly's syndrome) | Coarse features, dwarfism, developmental delay, hepatosplenomegaly, hydrops fetalis | β-glucuronidase | Leukocytes<br>Fibroblasts |
| *Glycoproteinosis* | | | |
| Mucolipidosis II (I-cell disease) | Coarse features, cloudy cornea, gingival hyperplasia, restricted joint movements. | Gross elevation of many plasma lysosomal enzymes | Plasma |
| α-Mannosidosis | Developmental delay, sensorineural hearing loss, frequent infections | α-Mannosidase | Leukocytes<br>Fibroblasts |
| α-Fucosidosis | Coarse features, developmental delay, spasticity | α-Fucosidase | Leukocytes<br>Fibroblasts |
| Mucolipidosis I | Visceromegaly, coarse features, myoclonus, CRS, mental retardation | α-Neuraminidase | Fibroblasts |
| Schindler's disease | Developmental delay, seizures, strabismus, regression | α-*N*-Acetylgalactosaminidase | Leukocytes<br>Fibroblasts |
| Sialic acid storage diseases | FTT, hypotonia, dysmorphic features, hydrops fetalis | Impaired sialic acid transport | Urine<br>Fibroblasts (sialic acid quantitation) |

| Disorder | Symptoms | Primary biochemical defect | Cells, tissue or fluid for definitive diagnosis |
|---|---|---|---|
| Mucolipidosis IV | Psychomotor retardation, strabismus | Unknown | Histological analysis of conjunctival biopsy |
| *Amino acid disorders* | | | |
| Serine biosynthesis defects | Growth and psychomotor retardation, bilateral cataracts, seizures, hyperexcitability | 3-phosphoglycerate dehydrogenase | CSF (amino acids) |
| *Purine and pyrimidine disorders* | | | |
| Lesch–Nyhan syndrome | X-linked developmental delay, hypotonia, athetosis | Hypoxanthine-guanine phosphoribosyltransferase<br>Uric acid in blood | Fibroblasts<br>Erythrocytes |
| Purine nucleoside phosphorylase deficiency | Headlag, irritability, susceptibility to infection | Purine-nucleoside phosphorylase | Urine (purines)<br>Erythrocytes |
| Dihydropyrimidine dehydrogenase deficiency | Psychomotor retardation, seizures, hypertonia | Dihydropyrimidine dehydrogenase | Urine (pyrimidines)<br>Leukocytes<br>Liver<br>Fibroblasts |
| Dihydropyrimidinase deficiency | Seizures, developmental delay, microcephaly | Dihdropyrimidinase | Urine (pyrimidines) |
| Adenylosuccinase deficiency | Psychomotor retardation, seizures, autistic features | Adenylosuccinase | Urine (succinyladenosine)<br>Fibroblasts |
| Hereditary orotic aciduria | Developmental delay, strabismus, megaloblastic anemia | Uridine↔monophosphate synthetase | Erythrocytes |
| Phosphoribosyl-pyrophosphate synthetase superactivity | Sensorineural deafness, mental and motor retardation, early gout | Phosphoribosylpyrophosphate synthetase (in some cases, this may be a secondary abnormality) | Erythrocytes |
| *Peroxisomal disorders* | | | |
| Zellweger's syndrome | Dysmorphic features, hypotonia, seizures, deafness, FTT, liver disease, retinal dysfunction, patella calcification | Deficiency of multiple peroxisomal functions | Plasma or serum (very-long-chain fatty acids and bile acids)<br>Erythrocytes<br>Platelets |
| Pseudo-Zellweger's syndrome and related disorders | As above | Deficiency in a single enzyme of peroxisomal fatty and oxidation and/or bile acid biosynthesis | Plasma or serum (very-long-chain fatty acids and bile acids)<br>Fibroblasts |
| Rhizomelic chondroplasia punctata | Growth retardation, FTT, dysmorphic features, psychomotor retardation, hypotonia, limb shortening, patella calcification | Deficiency of peroxisomal plasmalogens biosynthesis and phytanic acid metabolism | Erythrocytes<br>Platelets<br>Fibroblasts |
| Pelizaeus–Merzbacher disease | X-linked, nystagmus, hypotonia, titubation, ataxia of upper limbs, Developmental delay | Myelin proteolipid protein | DNA analysis (blood) |
| Sjögren–Larssen syndrome | Developmental retardation, ichthyosis, spasticity | Fatty aldehyde oxidase | Fibroblasts (enzyme assay) or histochemically on a skin biopsy |
| Pyruvate dehydrogenase deficiency | Males generally have a more severe form of the disease with acidosis<br>Females: hypotonia, feeding difficulties, psychomotor delay, microcephaly, slight dysmorphic features | Pyruvate dehydrogenase (complex of several different subunits) | Muscle<br>Fibroblasts |
| Electron transport chain | As above but with no sex limitation | Electron transport chain functions (many different subunits) | Muscle<br>Liver |

| Disorder | Symptoms | Primary biochemical defect | Cells, tissue or fluid for definitive diagnosis |
|---|---|---|---|
| Mitochondrial DNA disorders | Multiple symptoms affecting CNS, heart, kidney, gastro-intestational system, liver, blood-forming cells | Mutations, deletions, insertions and depletions of mitochondrial DNA | Any affected tissue cell type |
| Krebs-cycle defects | As for electron transport chain disorders | Specific Krebs cycle enzyme | Muscle<br>Liver |
| *Battens disease* | | | |
| Early infantile Battens (Hagberg–Santavouri) | Developmental regression, blindness, seizures | Palmitoyl protein thioesterase | Leucocytes<br>Fibroblasts |
| *Neurotransmitter disorders* | | | |
| GABA transaminase deficiency | Psychomotor retardation, hypotonia, hyperreflexia, growth acceleration | γ-Aminobutyrate transaminase deficiency | CSF (GABA and β-alanine)<br>Liver<br>Lymphocytes |
| Succinate semi-adehyde dehydrogenase deficiency | Hypotonia, ataxia, psychomotor retardation | Succinate semi-aldehyde dehydrogenase | Urine (4-hydroxy-butyrate) |
| Tyrosine hydroxylase deficiency | Progressive motor retardation, truncal hypotonia, extrapyramidal symptoms | Tyrosine hydroxylase | CSF (neurotramsmitters)<br>Leukoyctes |
| Aromatic amino acid decarboxylase deficiency | Hypotonia, developmental delay, oculogyric crises, choreoathetosis | Aromatic amino acid decarboyxlase | CSF (neurotransmitters)<br>Plasma (L-DOPA decarboyxlase) |
| Non-ketotic hyperglycinaemia | Intractable seizures, psychomotor delay, hypotonia | Glycine cleavage enzyme (complex of different subunits) | Liver |
| Canavan's disease | Developmental delay, hypotonia, optic atrophy, seizures, macrocephaly, excessive crying | *N*-Acetylaspartoacylase | Urine (*N*-acetyl aspartate)<br>Fibroblasts |
| Biopterin defects | Developmental delay, hypotonia | Defects of biopterin biosynthesis and reduction | Plasma (phenylalanine)<br>Urine (biopterins) |
| *Organic acid disorders* | | | |
| 3-Methylglutaconic aciduria | Developmental delay, movement disorders, retinitis pigmentosa, cataracts | 3-Methylglutaconyl-CoA hydratase (some forms only) | Urine (3-methylglutaconic acid)<br>Fibroblasts (some forms only) |
| L-2-hydroxyglutaric aciduria | Developmental delay | Unknown | Urine (L-2-hydroxy-glutaric acid) |
| D-2-hydroxyglutaric aciduria | Epilepsy, hypotonia, visual failure, developmental delay, seizures, leukodystrophy | Unknown | Urine (organic acids) |
| Mevalonic aciduria | Hepatosplenoemgaly, cataracts, dysmorphic features | Mevalonate kinase | Urine (mevalonic acid)<br>Fibroblasts |
| *Carbohydrate metabolism disorders* | | | |
| Triose phosphate isomerase | Diffuse weakness, hypotonia, areflexia, limb flexion, deformities, hemolytic anemia | Triose phosphate isomerase | Erythrocytes |
| *Vitamin metabolism disorders* | | | |
| Methylene tetra-hydrofolate reductase deficiency | Psychomotor retardation | Methylene tetra-hydrofolate reductase | Liver<br>Lymphocytes<br>Fibroblasts |
| Biotinidase deficiency | Seizures and skin rashes, alopecia | Biotinidase | Plasma<br>Fibroblasts |
| Transcobalamin II deficiency | Developmental delay, peripheral neuropathy, myelopathy, megaloblastic anemia | Plasma transcobalamin II | Plasma |

| Disorder | Symptoms | Primary biochemical defect | Cells, tissue or fluid for definitive diagnosis |
|---|---|---|---|
| *Other disorders* | | | |
| Menkes disease | X-linked, hypotonia, myoclonic, seizures, kinky hair | Serum copper and ceruloplasmin | Fibroblasts (copper uptake studies) |
| Sulfite oxidase deficiency | FTT, hypothermia, seizures, muscular spasms, opisthotonos | Sulfite oxidase | Fibroblasts<br>Liver<br>Urine (sulfite and thiosulfate) |
| Molybdenum cofactor deficiency | As above | Sulfite oxidase<br>Xanthine oxidase | As above |
| Carbohydrate-deficient glycoprotein syndrome (CDGS) | Hypotonia, reduction in spontaneous movements, abnormal eye/head movements, reduction in muscle mass, dysmorphic features | Absence of terminal carbohydrate unit on glycoproteins | Plasma or serum (transferrin isoelectric focusing) |
| Smith–Lemli–Opitz syndrome | Dysmorphic features, genital disorders, micrognathia, endocrine abnormalities | 7-Dehydrocholesterol reductase | Plasma-7-dehydrocholesterol |
| *Disorders of uncertain origin* | | | |
| Leigh's encephalopathy | Variable hypotonia, abnormal movements, sighing, irregular respirations, dysphagia, FTT, cranial nerve palsies, abnormal ocular movements | In some cases, defects of pyruvate metabolism and electron transport chain functions have been described | Brain MRI scan may be helpful (holes in basal ganglia) |
| Alpers disease | Seizures, developmental delay or regression, epilepsia partialias continuans, liver failure | In a few cases, defects of electron transport chain functions of fatty acid oxidation have been described | Liver and brain hisology |
| Alexander's disease | Developmental delay, macrocephaly, seizures, CRS, cherry red spot, FTT, failure to thrive. | Unknown | MRI scan<br>Brain biopsy |

Acute (intermittent) coma, collapse, hypotonia, and respiratory problems are much more likely to be due to organic acidurias, amino acidurias or urea cycle disorders than lysosomal disorders.

## EXAMINATION AND INVESTIGATION

A full general, neurological and developmental examination is necessary. Individual features do not necessarily give an answer (at an early stage, they may be non-specific, and at a later stage, they may be too diffuse), but a constellation may (*vide supra*) do so. Particular attention should be paid to the following possible clinical features:

- the acuteness of onset of the condition
- extra CNS signs, e.g. hernia, dermatological lesions
- hepatosplenomegaly
- general developmental level
- head size
- visual attention, oculomotor function, ophthalmoscopy
- hair abnormalities
- hypotonia, spasticity, dystonia
- auditory responses, especially to startle
- myoclonus
- abnormal movements, tremor, ataxia, choreoathetosis
- deep tendon reflexes
- dysmorphism
- respiratory difficulty
- failure to thrive
- cardiomyopathy.

The following range of tests may be useful and will be referred to in more detail:

- Biochemical: Acid–base, CSF and blood lactate, plasma and urine urate, urine oxalate, urine-reducing substances, blood ammonia, urine oligosaccharides and glycosaminoglycans, urine organic acids and amino acids, white-cell lysosomal enzymes, plasma very-long-chain fatty acids (VLCFAs), and plasma transferrin electrophoresis.
- Biopsies: Skin or rectal (for Batten's disease), liver or muscle for mitochondrial cytopathy, conjunctival biopsy for neuraxonal dystrophy, and blood and tissue samples for DNA and RNA analysis.

- Radiology: Skull radiography, skeletal survey, magnetic resonance imaging (MRI) may be specifically helpful for some of the mitochondrial diseases, showing, for example, abnormalities of the basal ganglia (Aicardi *et al.* 1998).
- Electrophysiological: Electroencephalogram (EEG), electromyogram (EMG), nerve conduction velocity (NCV), electroretinogram (ERG), visual evoked responses (VERs), and auditory evoked responses (AERs) (helpful in Pelizaeus Merzbacher).

There is no perfectly satisfactory classification for the neurometabolic diseases. As far as possible, it is best to classify them according to the primary biochemical abnormality, but some diseases are still poorly understood biochemically, and there is not always a one-to-one correspondence between a particular biochemical defect and a symptom complex. The situation is even more complex with respiratory chain disorders.

The classification proposed is shown in Table 36.1. A number of different genetic mutations may cause an enzyme to be defective in different ways. In some situations, this will cause variations in severity of the disease. No absolutely agreed classification is possible at this stage because the origin of a number of diseases is uncertain: some presenting similarly may have different enzyme defects, and some with apparently identical enzyme defects may have different manifestations.

There are a number of diseases that may have their onset in the later part of the first year with mild signs of development retardation but do not show any characteristic features until the second year of life or later (e.g. late infantile Batten's disease); these diseases are not discussed in any detail.

It is always possible to make a clinical diagnosis very much earlier than usual if the disease is suspected from a family history. In these diseases, it is often the mother who makes this observation.

The classical distinction clinically between gray-matter diseases presenting with mental degeneration and seizures and white-matter disease presenting with spasticity, ataxia and optic atrophy is not easily made in early infancy.

## LYSOSOMAL DISEASES

Lysosomes (Scriver *et al.* 1995) are one of a number of subcellular organelles (others are mitochondria and peroxisomes). They degrade some endogenous and exogenous products of cellular metabolism mainly by hydrolysis of certain carbohydrates, lipids, proteins, and lipoproteins. If an enzyme is defective in function, the substrate for the reaction accumulates within the cell. This accumulation damages the cell. In the group of disorders under discussion, the CNS is involved either on its own or with other organ systems, depending on the distribution in the body of the non-degradable substrate (Watts & Gibbs 1986).

## GANGLIOSIDOSES

The gangliosidoses are a group of neurodegenerative disorders of gray matter in which a group of complex lipids, called gangliosides, accumulate within the nerve cells. Gangliosides consist of a short carbohydrate chain attached to a complex alcohol (sphingosine) to which is attached a long-chain fatty acid (VLCFA). There are a number of sialic acid residues attached to the carbohydrate chain. Three major gangliosides are found in man, namely $GM_1$, $GM_2$ and $GM_3$. Disorders of this group are classified according to the type of accumulating ganglioside.

### $GM_2$ gangliosidosis, Tay–Sachs' and Sandhoff's diseases

A deficiency of hexosaminidase results in accumulation of $GM_2$ ganglioside in the CNS and other tissues. A number of diseases are described in which subunits of hexosaminidase (A or B) are deficient (Gray *et al.* 1990).

Hexosaminidase A deficiency results in classical Tay–Sachs' disease, and hexosaminidase A and B deficiency results in Sandhoff's disease; both may present early in infancy with a similar clinical picture.

Tay–Sachs' disease occurs relatively more frequently in Ashkenazi Jews, but overall in the UK, any infant with the disorder is much more likely to be non-Jewish because of the relatively small percentage (1%) of Ashkenazi Jews in the UK.

Presentation often occurs before 6 months but not in the immediate neonatal period. Irritability, hyperacusis, a slowing down of acquired skills, and hypotonia are the early signs. A cherry-red spot in the fundus is to be expected but is not pathognomonic as it occurs in other conditions. There is no visceromegaly. Further deterioration is accompanied by frequent seizures and spasticity. Blindness supervenes (the ERG is retained, and the VER becomes abnormal). The head becomes large, and death usually occurs before the age of 3 years. Confirmation of the diagnosis is by demonstrating the absence of hexosaminidase A activity in the plasma, leucocytes, or fibroblasts. There is no specific therapy.

Sandhoff's disease, which is due to a deficiency in hexosaminidase A and B activity, has a similar clinical picture but may have a slight visceromegaly. Many late-onset variants occur (Adams & Green 1986).

### Generalized gangliosidosis ($GM_1$)

This disease is due to β-galactosidase deficiency (O'Brien *et al.* 1965) and occurs in three forms, only one of which is likely to be present in the first 6 months of life. In $GM_1$ gangliosidosis type 1 (pseudo-Hurler's syndrome), there may be hypotonia and poor sucking early in infancy. Development is slow with the appearance of hepatosplenomegaly. Coarsening of facial features resembles that in Hurler's disease (hence the name). There is skeletal dysplasia and occasionally a cherry-red spot. Other variants occasionally occur, e.g. with dystonia, but these do not usually present early. Urinary oligosaccharide thin-layer chromatography is often useful in detecting this disorder. Diagnosis is confirmed by demonstrating the absence of β-galactosidase activity in leukocytes or cultured fibroblasts. As with Tay–Sachs's disease, prenatal diagnosis is possible by the analysis of uncultured chorionic villus or cultured cells from amniotic fluid.

## NIEMANN–PICK DISEASE (SUBTYPES A AND C)

### Niemann–Pick A

In this condition, there is a deficiency of sphingomyelinase with accumulation of sphingomyelin in the CNS and elsewhere. There are a number of subtypes with varying clinical pictures, some non-neurological and occurring at different ages. The infantile type is one of the most commonly encountered forms. There may be a very slow development from birth with hepatosplenomegaly and a failure to thrive. Sphingomyelinase can be assayed in leucocytes or fibroblasts.

### Niemann–Pick C

Unlike the other varieties of Niemann–Pick disease, sphingomyelinase activity is normal in most tissues. There is a defect of intracellular cholesterol metabolism leading to impaired cholesterol esterification and the accumulation in the cell of free cholesterol (Vanier *et al.* 1991). Usually, these children present with jaundice and hepatomegaly in the neonatal period, often described as neonatal hepatitis. This jaundice usually disappears within a few months of age. Although some patients may die in this period, others show developmental problems with rapid deterioration, hypotonia, delay in development and spasticity, but usually no intellectual deterioration in the first year of life. The classic vertical supranuclear ophthalmoplegia is not usually seen in the first year of life. Squints are common, and the retinae may show a cherry-red spot in 25% of cases. Corneal and lens opacities occur. Hypotonia becomes apparent, progressing to spasticity and accompanied by myoclonic seizures. Death may occur within the first year, but on average, these children survive until about 2 years of age. However, milder forms exist.

In both the above disorders, there is a generalized distribution of lipid-laden foam cells throughout the CNS and reticulo-endothelial system. A bone marrow aspirate may show such lipid-laden cells that stain specifically. Diagnosis is by measurement of the rate of cholesterol esterification in fibroblasts and by staining them *in situ* for free cholesterol.

## GAUCHER'S DISEASE

There are several forms presenting at different ages. They all have a defect in β-glucocerebrosidase. The so-called type II disease is the one that may occur in infancy (Verity & Montasir 1977). Delayed development from the start or psychomotor retardation after a few months may be apparent. The spleen is usually more enlarged (but occasionally, there may be no splenomegaly) than the liver. Squints, swallowing problems, and head retraction occur (Fig. 36.1). Fits occur but not as a major feature. Again, as with Niemann–Pick disease, a cherry-red spot may be seen. Anemia and thrombocytopenia occur. Gaucher cells may be found in the bone marrow and can be easily distinguished from Niemann–Pick cells. There is a strongly positive acid phosphatase reaction within the cells, and the acid phosphatase level is sometimes elevated in blood. A neonatal form exists presenting with fetal hydrops that has been shown to be due to null alleles on both chromosomes (Tayebi *et al.* 1997). The definitive diagnosis is made by demonstrating β-glucocerebrosidase deficiency in leukocytes or fibroblasts. Prenatal diagnosis is possible. Apart from correcting anemia and control of fits, there is no specific treatment for the neurologic form, and death occurs early. Splenectomy is not of any proven value.

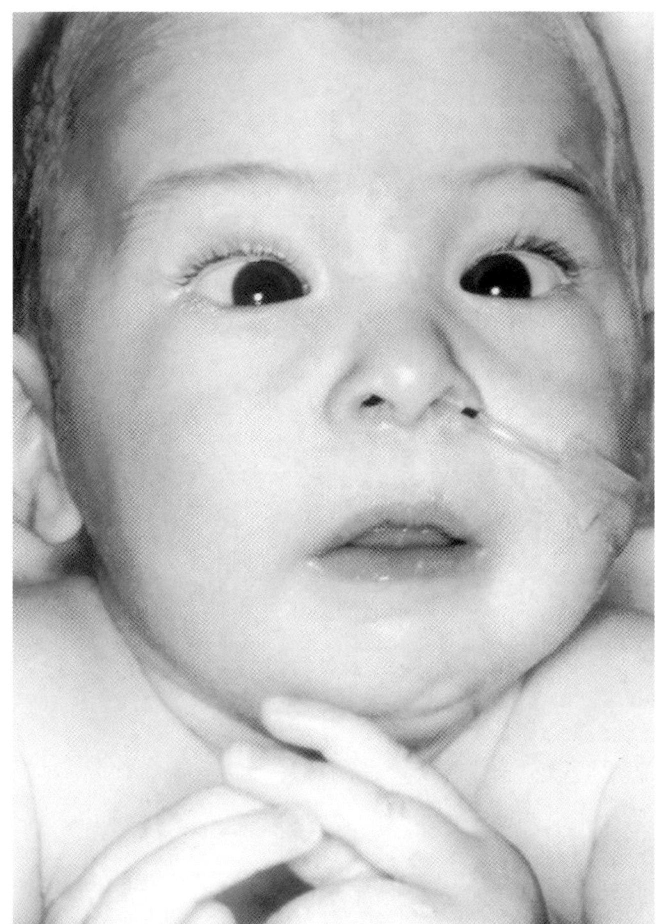

**Figure 36.1** Gaucher's disease.

## FARBER'S DISEASE

This rare metabolic disease is an inborn error of ceramide metabolism (Pavone *et al.* 1980). Onset is in the first few weeks of life. There is swelling of the hands and feet, a hoarse cry, a generalized arthropathy, and subcutaneous nodules over bony parts. Mental and motor deterioration occur. Pyramidal signs may come later. Diagnosis is suggested by the clinical picture and confirmed by biopsy of the nodules, which show granulomas with periodic acid–Schiff (PAS)-positive material. A deficiency of acid ceramidase has been found, and prenatal diagnosis is available (Scriver *et al.* 1995). Death occurs in early infancy.

## METACHROMATIC LEUKODYSTROPHY

Although, in some ways, the archetypal leukodystrophy and one of the most common of the lysosomal disorders, metachromatic leukodystrophy (MLD), presents very rarely in early infancy (McFaul *et al.* 1982), it is mentioned because it is one of the common disorders in this group. The disease is known to be due to a deficiency of arylsulfatase A (cerebroside sulfate sulfatase), which results in the accumulation of sulfatide in the CNS. The pathological picture is one of diffuse demyelination with metachromatic staining. The classical presentation with hypertonia progressing to hypotonia with depressed reflexes is not usually seen in infancy. However, it is worth considering the diagnosis in any infant with progressive retardation, and spasticity or hypotonia, without any other explanation.

Prenatal diagnosis is available for this condition. Recently, some success has been reported with marrow transplantation as a therapeutic measure, but the results are too early to assess definitely (Krivit *et al.* 1999).

All cases in which MLD is diagnosed should have another sulfatase assayed to exclude multiple sulfatase deficiency. Furthermore, since a pseudodeficiency allele exists in the general population at a high frequency, this should be excluded by DNA analysis.

## KRABBE'S DISEASE

The leukodystrophies classically present with more long tract involvement and less in the way of psychomotor retardation than does gray-matter degeneration. In the first year of life, this distinction is not so clear-cut. Nevertheless, the presentation of Krabbe's disease is different from that of the other neurovisceral storage diseases.

The most typical picture in infancy is of an irritable child who cries excessively. The child is stiff, and this progresses to episodes of opisthotonos. Regression becomes more obvious towards 6 months, with head retraction, stiffness and, occasionally, exaggerated startle to noise. Later in the first year, hypotonia with depressed reflexes may supervene and be associated with a gross demyelinating peripheral neuropathy. Seizures are not common. Pathologically, there is widespread demyelination of the CNS and peripheral nervous system with globoid cells occurring in pericapillary areas.

Diagnostic suspicion is raised in an infant with progressive CNS degeneration, depressed reflexes, slow nerve conduction, and a raised cerebrospinal fluid (CSF) protein level. The definitive test is the demonstration of deficiency of β-galactocerebrosidase in fibroblasts or leukocytes (Martin *et al.* 1981). Death occurs early in the infantile form. Prenatal diagnosis is available.

## MULTIPLE SULFATASE DEFICIENCY (MUCOSULFATIDOSIS, AUSTIN'S VARIANT)

This condition can be regarded as a variant of metachromatic leukodystrophy in which more than one specific sulfatase is deficient. This gives rise to an accumulation of sulfatide, acid mucopolysaccharides and cholesterol sulfate in the brain, liver, and kidney. The presenting features can occur much earlier than in MLD and have clinical features more akin to the mucopolysaccharidoses.

The condition is rare, and development may be normal for the first year or may be very slow from the start. A neonatal case has been described (Vamos *et al.* 1981). As in other leukodystrophies, there may be a combination of spasticity with depressed reflexes (and slowed nerve conduction). Seizures are not a particular feature. Early coarsening of the facial features may be noted, hands may be stubby with short fingers, and there is hepatomegaly. Radiography of the thoracolumbar spine shows mild changes of dysostosis. Early on, there is a fine ichthyosis due to a deficiency of the steroid sulfatase.

There is slow progression with bulbar paresis, spasticity, deafness, and optic atrophy. The patient may survive in this state for a number of years.

There are sometimes abnormalities of mucopolysaccharides in the urine and metachromatic staining in a nerve biopsy of Schwann cells. Confirmation is by demonstrating a deficiency of at least two sulfatases. Prenatal diagnosis is available in specialized centers.

## DISORDERS OF MUCOPOLYSACCHARIDE AND GLYCOPROTEIN METABOLISM

The mucopolysaccharidoses, the glycoproteinoses, and the sialic acid storage diseases show some features in common.

These are all storage diseases, mostly autosomal recessive with a relatively slow evolution of psychomotor retardation, coarsening of the features, and hepatomegaly. Seizures are not a major feature of the majority, although there are exceptions. The early signs are often more subtle than some of the diseases so far discussed, and often, the time of onset is only realized retrospectively to be relatively early in infancy.

## MUCOPOLYSACCHARIDOSES

There are seven different subtypes within this well-known clinical group according to McKusick's classification (McKusick 1998). Few of these are recognized in early infancy, but the following may present as early as 6 months.

### Hurler's disease (mucopolysaccharidosis I)

This autosomal recessive condition is due to a deficiency of α-iduronidase (Bach *et al.* 1972) and has been estimated to have an incidence of 1 in 100 000 (Lowry & Renwick 1971). Dermatan and heparan sulfate accumulate in the CNS and elsewhere. The early signs may be snorting breathing, snoring, inguinal and umbilical herniae, a barrel-shaped chest, and psychomotor slowing. The classical gargoyle-like features are not usually present before 1 year of age. Hepatomegaly may or may not be present early. Clouding of the corneas may be apparent on slit-lamp examination.

There may be early radiological changes, a J-shaped sella, rounded dorsolumbar vertebral bodies, broad ribs, and wide shafts of long bones, but these signs may be subtle in infancy.

Confirmation of the diagnosis is by determining the pattern of urinary excretion of mucopolysaccharides (dermatan and heparan sulfate in Hurler's disease) or by the demonstration of the absence of α-iduronidase in fibroblasts or leukocytes. It is in this group of diseases that enzyme replacement therapy has been tried (marrow transplant) with, it is claimed, limited success (Krivit *et al.* 1999). Prenatal diagnosis is available.

### Sly's disease (mucopolysaccharidosis VII)

This disease has a very wide clinical phenotype (Beaudet *et al.* 1975; Sheets Lee *et al.* 1985). When symptoms occur in the first year of life, they present with fetal hydrops, coarse features, dwarfism, hernias, developmental delay, and hepatosplenomegaly. Corneal clouding is a variable feature. In the most severe form, it is associated with hydrops fetalis. This disorder is due to a deficiency of β-glucuronidase, which can be measured in leukocytes or fibroblasts.

## GLYCOPROTEINOSES

These disorders combine certain features of the gangliosidoses and the mucopolysaccharidoses, and resemble the latter clinically. They are all inherited in an autosomal recessive manner (Scriver *et al.* 1995). Although abnormal mucopolysaccharides are not excreted in the urine, there is in most cases the excretion of abnormal oligosaccharides. These oligosaccharides accumulate due to defects in glycoprotein degradation. In some cases, abnormal complex lipids may also accumulate, giving some features of some of the lipidoses.

### Mucolipidosis II (I-cell disease)

This condition is clinically similar to Hurler's disease but is often apparent from birth. The coarse features are evident early in life with gingival hyperplasia, congenital dislocation of the hips, restricted joint movements, and thickened skin. Nasal discharge is common, corneas are cloudy, and kyphosis, cardiomyopathy, and hepatomegaly may appear later. Retardation is less easy to detect in the first year of life, although this becomes evident later on. There is slow progression of the disease with death in early childhood.

Whilst a number of different lysosomal hydrolases are deficient in fibroblasts, these enzymes are grossly elevated in plasma (α-iduronidase, β-glucuronidase, β-galactosidase). As with other diseases in this group, prenatal diagnosis is available. The primary defect is an enzyme, *N*-acetylglucosamine-1-phosphotransferase, which is responsible for phosphorylating mannose residues on lysosomal enzymes to allow their uptake into the lysosome. An absence of this target signal leads to a deficiency of many enzymes in the tissues and their secretion into the intercellular spaces.

### α-mannosidosis

This is a disorder of glycoprotein degradation due to the absence of α-mannosidase. The early clinical features are of developmental delay, sensorineural hearing loss, and frequent respiratory and ear infections. These sometimes occur towards the end of the first year of life. Later, coarse facial features, skeletal dysplasia, angiokeratoma, and hepatosplenomegaly develop. It is a rare condition. Vacuolated lymphocytes may be seen, and urinary oligosaccharide thin-layer chromatography is often useful in detecting this disease. The definitive diagnosis is the assay of α-mannosidase in leukocytes or fibroblasts (Taylor *et al.* 1975).

### α-fucosidosis

This disease, due to the deficiency of α-fucosidase, may present at 6–9 months of age with hypotonia, repeated respiratory infections, and feeding difficulties. This then progresses with developmental delay, progressive hypertonicity, and spasticity. There may be mild coarse facies and slight hepatosplenomegaly. As with cystic fibrosis, there is a marked increase in the chloride of the sweat, and the child may 'taste' salty. There is rapid progression to death over the next few years. Urinary oligosaccharide thin-layer chromatography may be useful in detecting this disorder, and the deficiency in α-fucosidase may be detected in cultured fibroblasts or leukocytes. Again, this is a very rare condition.

### Sialidosis (mucolipidosis I)

Another disorder of glycoprotein degradation is sialidosis. This disease (Lowden & O'Brien 1979) exists in two forms, sialidosis type II (mucolipidosis type I) being an infantile form. The basic deficiency is of the enzyme α-neuraminidase.

Clinical presentation may be at birth with hydrops, visceromegaly and coarse features, or, rarely in the first year of life, with mental retardation, myoclonus, ataxia, a cherry-red spot, and dyostosis multiplex. The features of neuraminidase deficiency are variable, and a number of different symptoms have been described. Urinary oligosaccharide thin-layer chromatography is often useful in detecting this disease. In some patients there is a coexisting deficiency of β-galactosidase.

### Schindler's disease

This is a recently discovered disorder of glycoprotein metabolism due to a defect in the enzyme α-*N*-acetylgalactosaminidase. Very few cases have been described. There are two reports to date of onset in the first year of life. One was in siblings with developmental delay, strabismus, grand mal seizures, and regression. Clinically and histologically, they resembled Seitelberger's infantile neuroaxonal dystrophy. A further case was milder with an onset of seizures at 11 months of age, with slight psychomotor retardation. The disorder cannot be consistently detected by analysis of urine oligosaccharides. However, the enzyme can be assayed in leukocytes or cultured fibroblasts (Schindler *et al.* 1989).

### Sialic acid storage diseases

There is a group of diseases in which there are increased concentrations in tissues, urine, and blood of free sialic acid (*N*-acetylneuraminic acid) (Mancini *et al.* 1991). The infantile form of this disease presents in the first 3 months of life with failure to thrive, generalized hypotonia, and coarse dysmorphic features. There is usually also hepatosplenomegaly and bony dysplasia. More severe forms can present with hydrops fetalis, ascites at birth, or a neonatal nephrotic syndrome. The disease progresses to death within 5 years of age. This form is not to be confused with another sialic acid storage disease – Salla's disease. This disorder presents at 3–6 months of age with hypotonia, ataxia, and, in some cases, ocular nystagmus. It is a slowly progressive disease with an evolving dysarthria and dyspraxia. Dysmorphic features become apparent, but there is no hepatosplenomegaly, and although the life span is usually shortened, patients may survive to adulthood. The primary cause of these disorders is unknown. They can be detected by the measurement of the free sialic acid concentration in urine or by urine oligosaccharide chromatography with resorcinol staining.

### Mucolipidosis IV

This disorder presents in the first year of life with psychomotor retardation, visual impairment (with a diminished ERG), corneal opacities, strabismus, and physical retardation (Amir *et al.* 1987). They also may develop achlorrhydria. The course of the disease is protracted, and the corneal opacity may improve with age. There is accumulation of various sialic acid-containing compounds in tissues, but no primary defect has yet been elucidated. Laboratory diagnosis is purely by histological analysis.

## AMINO ACID DISORDERS

Amino acid disorders that have an acute clinical presentation in the first months of life are dealt with in Chapters 34 and 35 or in other categories in this chapter. However, one group of disorders that has recently been identified that may show slow progressive neurological symptoms over the neonatal period are the defects of serine biosynthesis.

### SERINE BIOSYNTHESIS DEFECTS

3-Phosphoglycerate dehydrogenase is the first step in the biosynthesis of serine. Infants with a deficiency of this enzyme present with congenital microcephaly, bilateral cataracts, severe growth and psychomotor retardation, hypogonadism, epilepsy, hypertonia, and hyperexcitability. The diagnostic test for the disorder is quantitation of CSF amino acids, which reveal a markedly decreased serine (Jaeken *et al.* 1996). Oral treatment with L-serine and glycine been proved to be beneficial in controlling seizures (De Koning *et al.* 1998).

3-Phosphoserine phosphatase deficiency has been reported in a patient with Williams's syndrome. CSF serine concentrations were reduced, and there was some response to serine treatment (Jaeken *et al.* 1996).

## DISORDERS OF PURINE AND PYRIMIDINE METABOLISM (SIMMONDS 1987)

### LESCH–NYHAN SYNDROME

This well-known disorder of purine metabolism is due to deficiency of hypoxanthine–guanine phosphoribosyltransferase (HGPRT), leading to hyperuricemia (Lesch & Nyhan 1964). A number of genetic varieties are now known (Wilson *et al.* 1983). It is an X-linked recessive condition, and the classical feature in the older child is that of self-destructive biting. However, the condition may present earlier with signs that are more subtle. Motor and mental retardation, hypotonia, and athetosis may manifest as early as 6–9 months. It is the presence of early athetosis of unexplained origin that should be the clue to investigation. Orange-stained nappies due to crystals of urate should also arouse suspicion.

Uric acid concentrations in plasma and urine should be routinely measured for all males with developmental delay, especially with movement disorders. Confirmation of the diagnosis is by finding hyperuricemia and the specific deficiency HGPRT in fibroblasts or red cells. The mechanism whereby the condition causes symptoms is unknown. Allopurinol does not affect the neurological progression but may relieve the hyperuricemia. The disease slowly progresses with severe athetosis and self-destructive behavior that causes great problems in management later on. Death usually occurs towards the end of the first or the beginning of the second decade. Prenatal diagnosis is available.

### PURINE NUCLEOSIDE PHOSPHORYLASE DEFICIENCY

This disorder can present with head lag and excessive irritability at 3 months of age, but subsequently, the patient develops susceptibility to repeated infections due to a T-cell immunodeficiency. The disorder is inherited in an autosomal recessive mode. The plasma and urine uric acid concentrations are below normal limits for age, whilst the urinary total purine level is increased.

## DIHYDROPYRIMIDINE DEHYDROGENASE DEFICIENCY

The early symptoms of this disorder are of psychomotor delay followed by seizures and muscular hypertonia. MRI reveals a severe delay in myelination. Urinary concentrations of thymine and uracil are grossly elevated due to the deficiency of this pyrimidine-degradative enzyme.

## DIHYDROPYRIMIDINASE DEFICIENCY

This disorder presents with seizures in the first weeks of life and progresses to developmental delay and microcephaly. The clinical features, however, vary considerably. There are gross increases in urinary thymine, uracil, dihydrothymine, and dihydrouracil concentrations. A defect of dihydropyrimidinase, an enzyme of pyrimidine catabolism, was inferred from the nature of the accumulating metabolites.

## ADENYLOSUCCINASE DEFICIENCY

This disorder often presents in the first year of life with severe psychomotor retardation and seizures. Later, autistic features may develop. There is accumulation of succinyladenosine in the urine due to a deficiency of adenylosuccinase – one of the enzymes of the purine nucleotide cycle.

## HEREDITARY OROTIC ACIDURIA

This disorder can present in the first year of life with developmental delay and strabismus. A crucial clinical finding is a marked megaloblastic anemia with normal or raised serum vitamin $B_{12}$ and folate concentrations. Biochemically, there are grossly elevated urine concentrations of orotic acid, an intermediate in the biosynthetic pathway for pyrimidines, but normal blood ammonia concentrations. This is due to a deficiency of the bifunctional enzyme uridine-monophosphate (UMP) synthase. It is important to diagnose the disorder at an early stage as it can be successfully treated by oral doses of uridine. It is inherited in an autosomal recessive manner.

## PHOSPHORIBOSYLPYROPHOSPHATE SYNTHETASE SUPERACTIVITY

This is an X-linked disorder in which there is overactivity of the key enzyme regulating purine biosynthesis. This results in increased concentrations of uric acid and hypoxanthine in plasma and urine. Only a limited number of patients have been described, some with early symptoms of gout. Sensorineural deafness was an early feature in one case. In two siblings, there was neonatal diabetes mellitus with mental and motor retardation, absent speech development, cerebellar ataxia, polyneuropathy with areflexia, and dysmorphic features. The enzyme surfeit, in some cases, has been shown to be due to a defect in regulatory sites on the enzyme.

# MENKES' DISEASE

This is a degenerative disease of gray matter due to a defect in copper metabolism (Danks *et al.* 1972). Copper levels are low in the liver and brain but raised in other tissues. The defect is in a copper transport protein. Copper becomes unavailable for the synthesis of ceruloplasmin and the normal functioning of other enzymes. This sex-linked condition has an incidence of between one and two per 100 000 and may present very early in infancy. Hypotonia in the newborn period followed soon by refractory myoclonic-like seizures should arouse suspicion. These children feed poorly, and hypothermia may be a problem, so they fail to thrive. The typical facial appearance is not always obvious for a few months, and the steely or kinky hair is not usually noted to be abnormal for a few weeks (Fig. 36.2). It is the stubbliness and roughness of the hair that should arouse suspicion. The abnormalities monilethrix, pili torti and trichorrhexis nodosa are very characteristic although not specifically pathognomonic. They are best demonstrated by scanning electron microscopy (Taylor & Green 1981). Radiographs show metaphyseal spurring of the long bones.

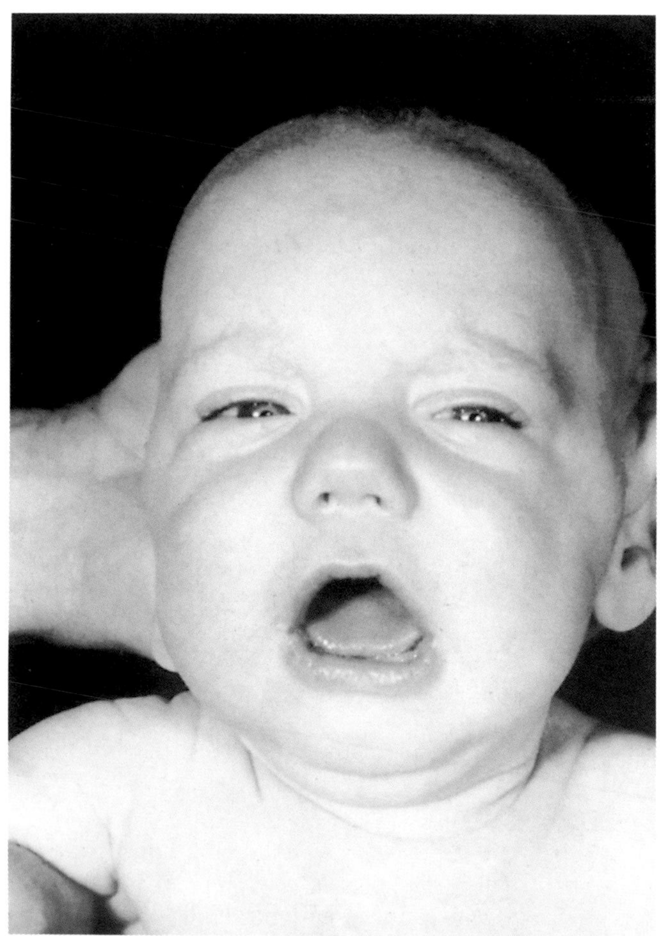

**Figure 36.2** Menkes' disease.

The evolution of the condition includes profound developmental retardation, hypotonia and further refractory seizures. These children may fail to thrive and often succumb in the first year of life, although some survive longer. Diagnosis is by the clinical history, confirmation of low serum copper and ceruloplasmin levels, and the typical scanning electron microscopic appearance of the hair.

The defect has been found to be in a cell copper transport protein (ATP7A) involved in transport of copper across the gut. The associated systemic copper deficiency leads to the clinical symptoms (Turner & Horn 1998).

Copper metabolism studies and DNA analysis have been used in prenatal diagnosis and carrier detection (Tonnesen *et al.* 1987). It may also be possible to detect carriers by examining the hair of the affected child's mother by electron microscopy (Collie *et al.* 1978; Taylor & Green 1981), but more reliable molecular biology techniques are now available.

Therapy of the condition by copper infusion has been tried with variable success (Grover & Scrutton 1975; Garnica 1984; Guitet *et al.* 1999). Death usually occurs in late infancy, but occasionally, cases have been reported with a relatively prolonged survival.

## SULFITE OXIDASE DEFICIENCY

This is a rare metabolic disease (Aukett *et al.* 1988). Only a few cases have been reported, but the condition may present in the neonatal period with seizures, muscular spasms, lens dislocation, and opisthotonos. Sulfite and thiosulfate are markedly increased in the urine. Amino acid screening shows *S*-sulphocystine in the urine, but this is not primarily an amino acid disorder. Sulfite oxidase is dependent on molybdenum as a cofactor, and there is also a disorder where there is a defect in the cofactor leading to a similar clinical and biochemical picture, but with a decreased urine and serum uric acid concentration. The latter is due to a parallel deficiency in xanthine oxidase, which also requires this cofactor. In this disorder, plasma urate levels are substantially reduced.

This disease should be considered in early onset of seizures with reduced responses where other routine screening is negative.

## SMITH–LEMLI–OPITZ SYNDROME

In the neonatal period, this disorder presents with characteristic dysmorphic facies (anteverted nares, ptosis and micrognathia), limb abnormalities, genital disorders, cataracts, endocrine abnormalities, heart and kidney malformations, and mental retardation (Ryan *et al.* 1998). The disorder is due to a defect in the 7-dehydrocholesterol reductase, which is the penultimate step of cholesterol biosynthesis. As a result, plasma cholesterol concentrations may be low. However, the diagnostic test is the quantitation of 7-dehydrocholesterol in plasma. Prenatal diagnosis is available.

## CARBOHYDRATE-DEFICIENT GLYCOPROTEIN SYNDROME (JAEKEN'S SYNDROME)

This is a newly recognized, usually generally slowly progressive, disorder, characterized by a number of clinical features (Jaeken *et al.* 1997). Hypotonia and reduction in spontaneous movements are often seen in the neonatal period. Alternating esotropia and a bilateral ocular abduction defect are early signs. There is a progressive reduction in muscle mass, particularly in the buttocks. Other features that may be present are olivopontocerebellar atrophy, retinitis pigmentosa, cardiomyopathy, stroke-like episodes, nephrotic syndrome, gastrointestinal disorders, hydrops fetalis, and liver disease. There are usually characteristic dysmorphic features. Patients can survive until adulthood, but some die at various ages from cardiomyopathy, infection, liver disease or cerebral hemorrhage. The disorder is heterogeneous, and various subtypes have been defined, based on variations in clinical and biochemical abnormalities. It can be detected by the presence of an abnormal pattern of transferrin subtypes on isoelectric focusing or gel electrophoresis of plasma or serum. This is due to abnormalities of the terminal carbohydrate chains (containing sialic acid) on the transferrin glycoprotein. This has also been found in a number of other plasma glycoproteins, including thyroxine-binding globulin. A low concentration of thyroxine-binding globulin may be indicative of this disease, and this disorder has been detected in a neonatal screening program because of a low total thyroxine concentration. The primary defect lies in the pathway for the synthesis of N-linked carbohydrate chains in glycoproteins, and a number of enzyme defects in this pathway have been defined (Young & Driscoll 1999). This newly described disorder may be relatively common and is probably easily missed.

## PEROXISOMAL DISORDERS

Although not all are truly degenerative, these disorders give rise to a group of symptoms very similar to those discussed above. They are a group of conditions that have been described by Moser & Goldfischer (1985) in which there is a defect in the functioning of a group of subcellular organelles, termed peroxisomes. These structures were first reported in 1969 (DeDuve 1969), and their relationship to a variety of human diseases is unfolding at the moment of writing. Some of these diseases give rise to progressive CNS degeneration in infancy, so it is important to recognize the symptom complexes that may lead to their diagnosis.

Although the purpose of this chapter is not basically biochemical, peroxisomal functions will be briefly listed. They include:

- breakdown of very long-chain fatty acids (VLCFAs)
- biosynthesis of ether phospholipids (plasmalogens)
- biosynthesis of bile acids
- catabolism of long- and medium-chain fatty acids

- catabolism of phytanic acid
- hydrogen peroxide degradation
- metabolism of prostaglandins
- catabolism of oxalic acid.

A number of different disorders affecting the CNS, not previously thought to be connected, have been shown to be due to peroxisomal disorders. Some of these are due to impairment of a single peroxisomal function, and others are due to multiple defects. Those due to a single or dual impairment include X-linked adrenoleukodystrophy, pseudo-Zellweger's syndrome, pseudo-neonatal adrenoleukodystrophy, bifunctional protein deficiency, acatalasemia, and rhizomelic chondrodysplasia punctata.

Those peroxisomal disorders that have multiple defects include Zellweger's syndrome, infantile Refsum's disease, and neonatal adrenoleukodystrophy and have been found to be due to defects of peroxisomal membrane assembly (Powers & Moser, 1998).

For the clinician, the main features that should draw attention to this group of conditions are:

- neonatal hypotonia
- seizures
- psychomotor retardation
- dysmorphic features
- hepatic enlargement
- failure to thrive
- retinal dysfunction – suspected because of blindness
- nystagmus.

## ZELLWEGER'S SYNDROME AND RELATED DISORDERS

Zellweger's syndrome is the archetype of this group of disorders and was known for some considerable time before it was realized that it was a peroxisomal disorder (Bowen *et al.* 1964).

The main features are hypotonia present from birth, seizures that may be early in onset and refractory, failure to thrive, and variable hepatomegaly. The dysmorphic features are subtle, but, as in many syndromes, after seeing a case, they become easier to recognize. They include a high-domed forehead, external ear abnormalities, large fontanelle, flat occiput, micrognathia, shallow supraorbital ridges, epicanthic folds, low broad nasal root, and periorbital edema with redundant neck folds (Fig. 36.3). These children usually die in early infancy. The brain at post-mortem shows an abnormal convolutional pattern with microgyria, heterotopic cortex, ectopic neurons and olivary dysplasia.

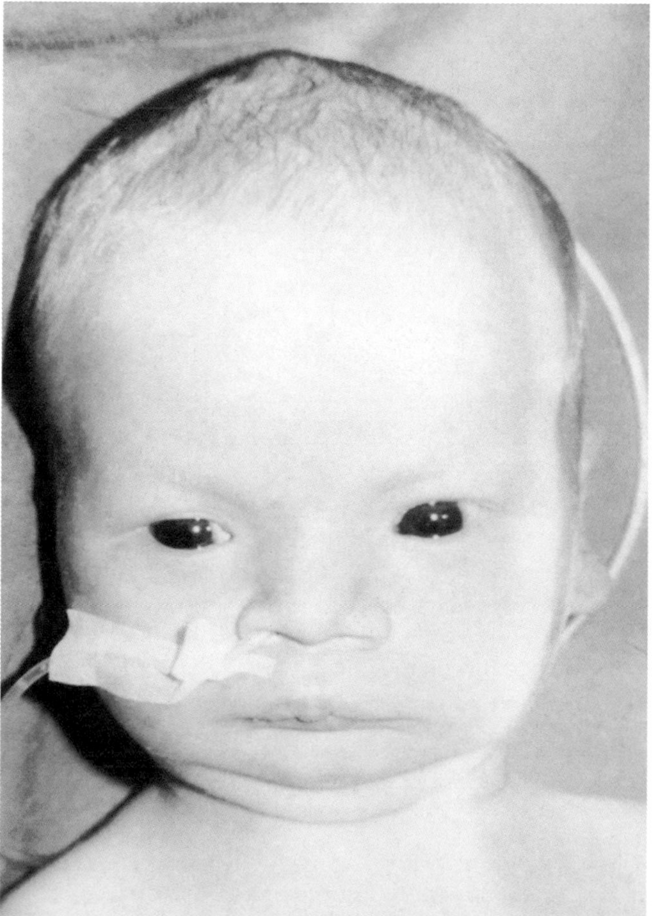

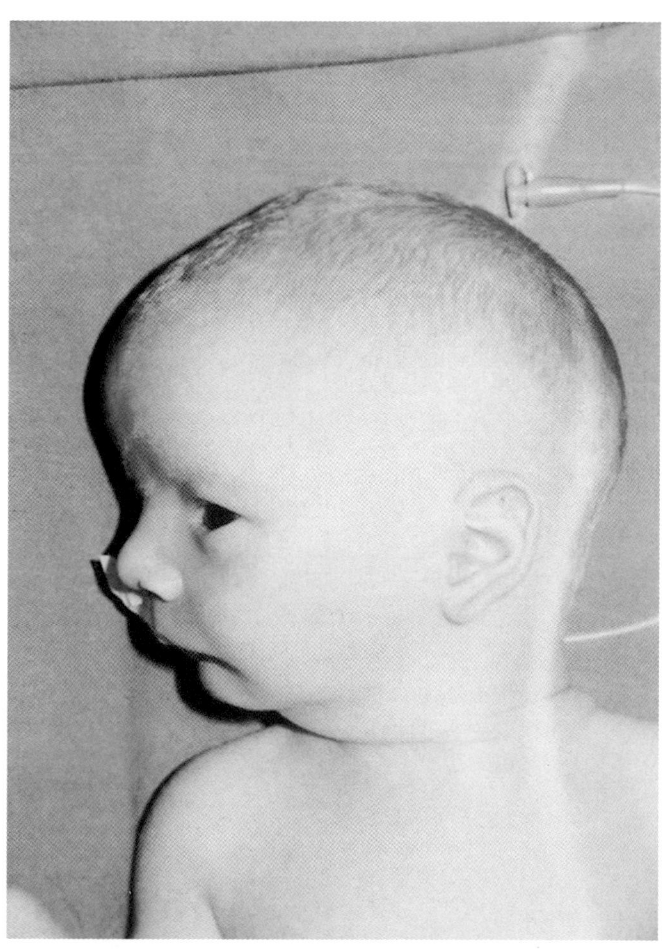

**Figure 36.3** Zellweger's syndrome.

Investigations at a first line level that are helpful include radiography of the knees, which sometimes show patella calcification, liver function tests, and electroretinography.

Biochemically, the patients show very high concentrations of plasma VLCFAs (> $C_{22}$) due to a deficiency of the enzymes of peroxisomal fatty acid β oxidation. Plasma bile acid (cholic and chenodeoxycholic acids) concentrations are often reduced, and intermediates of the bile acid biosynthetic pathway, normally not detectable, are present in greatly increased amounts. The proportion of membrane plasmalogens in erythrocytes and cultured cells is also reduced due to a deficiency of two enzymes involved in the biosynthesis of these ether lipids. In liver tissue, the peroxisomes, as visualized by catalase staining, are absent due to a selective deficiency of peroxisomal catalase.

Infantile Refsum's disease (Schutgens *et al.* 1986) exhibits the same biochemical abnormalities as Zellweger's syndrome but of a milder clinical phenotype. Retinopathy is often a major feature that may manifest itself as visual dysfunction (a depressed ERG would be a confirmatory finding). There is usually hepatic fibrosis. The plasma phytanic acid concentration is often raised in these children, but usually not until after 6 months of age. Variants of Zellweger's syndrome exist with phenotypes intermediate between the classical form and infantile Refsum's disease.

### SINGLE PEROXISOMAL OXIDATION DEFECTS

A number of disorders exist that can be clinically identical to the various forms of Zellweger's syndrome but only have abnormalities in plasma VLCFAs, and/or plasma bile acids. Pseudo-Zellweger's syndrome and pseudoneonatal adrenoleukodystrophy exhibit abnormalities in VLCFAs and bile acids. The patients with a bifunctional protein defect have shown elevated VLCFA but normal bile acid concentrations. In trihydroxycoprostanoic acidemia, only plasma bile acid concentrations are abnormal.

### RHIZOMELIC CHONDRODYSPLASIA PUNCTATA

This is a disorder that presents at birth with rhizomelic limb shortening and punctate calcification of the patella. Growth retardation, failure to thrive, dysmorphic features, and psychomotor retardation with truncal hypotonia develop within the first few months. Variants, however, have been found with no limb-shortening or without marked patella calcification. In this disorder, there is a deficiency of erythrocyte membrane plasmalogens and in the dihydroxyacetone-phosphate:acyl-CoA transferase enzyme involved in their biosynthesis. In most forms, there is also a gross elevation of the plasma phytanic acid concentration. The primary defect in this disorder is in a gene (PEX7) encoding a receptor required for the import of some peroxisomal matrix proteins. Cases of this disorder have also been found without increased phytanic acid and are due to specific defects in gene coding for enzymes of plasmalogen biosynthesis (Braverman *et al.* 1997).

### INVESTIGATION OF PEROXISOMAL DISORDERS

The most useful first-line test for the investigation of these disorders is the measurement of plasma VLCFA concentrations, although this will not detect rhizomelic chondrodysplasia punctata or trihydroxycoprostanoic acidaemia. There is no specific therapy for this group of disorders, although it has been suggested that reduction of VLCFAs by diet and Lorenzo's oil, and oral bile acid therapy to normalize the plasma bile acid concentration, may be of value. All the disorders discussed show an autosomal recessive mode of inheritance. Prenatal diagnosis is available for all the disorders mentioned.

## PELIZAEUS–MERZBACHER DISEASE

This leukodystrophy is due to a deficiency of a major lipoprotein component of the myelin sheath (proteolipid protein). The clinical picture of the classical type I form is essentially of a male infant (the disease is considered to be X-linked recessive) who presents in infancy with abnormally jerky eye movements. Horizontal nystagmus and tracking difficulties are seen (and should be distinguished from the wandering eye movements of the blind and the more bizarre movements of Leigh's encephalopathy). These are accompanied or followed by hypotonia, titubation, and ataxic movements of the arms. Sitting may be delayed or never achieved. Degeneration is slow, and although visual failure, spasticity, and mental deterioration occur, these are not usually noted in infancy. Children may survive with this condition for many years, and progressive degeneration is slow. The original observations were in fact in adults. MRI may be helpful in identifying a mother who is a carrier, but usually is not abnormal in the first year of life.

There exists a more severe variety (type II Seitelberger) (Ulrich & Herschkowitz 1977) where presentation is in the neonatal period. Nystagmus, gross involuntary movements and spasticity of the lower limbs are the main features. There is little developmental progress. This type may be X-linked recessive. Sporadic transitional types may occur.

Pathologically, there is atrophy of the cerebellum and cortex with accumulation of sudanophilic lipid. MRI scanning may help by confirming atrophy, but the diagnosis is essentially clinical after the exclusion of other known diseases. The primary defect has been shown to be due to duplications or point mutations in the proteolipid protein gene expressed in oligodendrocytes (Wang *et al.* 1997).

## SJÖGREN–LARSSON SYNDROME (RIZZO & CRAFT 1991)

Patients with this autosomal recessive disorder classically exhibit a clinical triad of congenital ichthyosis, spasticity, and mental retardation. The disorder can often present as early as the first year of life, with developmental delay particularly affecting speech or motor functions. This progresses to spastic diplegia or quadriplegia with moderate to profound mental retardation. However, unlike the lipid storage diseases, it does not show regression, and the patients can survive to adulthood. The crucial clinical finding in the early stages is icthyosis, which can occur at birth or up to 1 year of life. Clinically, it resembles lamellar ichthyosis or congenital icthyosiform erythyroderma and shows a generalized distribution. A further diagnostic finding is the presence of glistening white dots on the fundus of the retina, although their absence does not exclude the disease. This disorder has been found to be due to a defect in the oxidation of fatty alcohols. Fatty alcohols are important constituents of skin and nerve-cell membranes. The primary defect lies in fatty-aldehyde dehydrogenase, which is a component of the fatty-alcohol:NAD oxidoreductase complex. The disorder has been diagnosed biochemically by the measurement of fatty alcohol oxidation in cultured fibroblasts and histologically by staining for fatty alcohol activity in skin or jejunal biopsies.

## LACTIC ACIDEMIA

Disorders affecting the metabolism of pyruvic acid cause a lactic acidosis that generally results in an acute presentation. These have been dealt with in Chapter 35.

However, when the blood lactic acid level is only moderately elevated or when the disorder primarily resides in the brain so that only the CSF lactate concentration is significantly raised, they may present with a chronic form.

### PYRUVATE DEHYDROGENASE DEFICIENCY

The pyruvate dehydrogenase enzyme consists of three components, one of which (E1) consists of $\alpha$ and $\beta$ subunits. The $\alpha$ subunit is coded for on the X chromosome. A defect in the E1 $\alpha$ subunit will result in very low activity of the enzyme in males with the abnormal gene. However, the clinical expression of the disease in heterozygous females can vary considerably and unpredictably due to variations in X chromosome inactivation. Females have been found who present with hypotonia and feeding problems in the neonatal period, often with evidence of intrauterine growth failure (Brown *et al.* 1988). This progresses to developmental delay and microcephaly, and there may be mild dysmorphic features. Blood lactate concentrations are normal or moderately raised, whilst CSF lactate levels are usually markedly elevated. Studies on cultured fibroblasts have revealed that these patients are heterozygous for a defect in the E1 $\alpha$ subunit and have unfavorable X chromosome inactivation. As well as females, there may exist males with partial defects who may present with similar clinical features to these females.

### ELECTRON TRANSPORT CHAIN DISORDERS (see also Chapter 35)

The electron transport chain is responsible for transferring reducing equivalents generated by pyruvate dehydrogenase. Krebs-cycle enzymes, the fatty-acid oxidation system and other enzyme systems to oxygen, producing water and energy in the form of ATP. There are five complexes incorporated into the mitochondrial membrane, and each complex contains many subunits and cofactors. Defects in these subunits can lead to defective complex functions and hence defective transfer of reducing equivalents. The net effect of this is accumulation of pyruvic acid and hence lactic acid. Partial defects in biochemically less essential subunits can produce a clinical course resembling pyruvate dehydrogenase deficiency, Leigh's syndrome or even Alper's syndrome (Tulinius *et al.* 1991). As in pyruvate dehydrogenase deficiency, blood lactate concentrations may not always be markedly raised, whilst, if the brain is affected, CSF lactate concentrations are usually elevated. Diagnosis of this group of disorders is by muscle or liver biopsy with measurement of the electron transport chain complexes, preferably in fresh unfrozen tissue. However, it has to be remembered that if the brain is primarily affected, the muscle or liver may not show clear abnormalities. In fact, normal electron chain complex assay results in these tissues do not totally exclude a partial defect of this system.

#### Mitochondrial DNA disorders (see also p. 620)

The electron transport chain complex subunits can be coded either on nuclear DNA or on the mitochondrial DNA (Tulinius *et al.* 1991). Defects in the mitochondrial DNA can lead to a bewildering range of clinical symptoms varying in type and relative severity, even between affected siblings. Some, however, may present (as a slowly progressive disorder) in the first year of life with multisystem disease including hypotonia, ophthalmoplegia, seizures, developmental delay, cardiomyopathy, gastrointestinal disturbances, and failure to thrive. Blood lactate concentrations are not always elevated, nor are ragged red fibers always observed in muscle in the non-acute forms. In some cases, the mutations that cause particular clinical syndromes are known and the mitochondrial abnormalities can be detected in muscle, liver, or blood. However, in many cases, only sequencing of the entire mitochondrial DNA genome can reveal underlying abnormalities. Some patients have been reported with structurally normal mitochondrial DNA, which is present in substantially reduced quantities (mtDNA depletion disorders) (Vu *et al.* 1998). They are usually of a severe early onset and often show hepatological, as well as neurological, symptoms as well as hypoglycemia. Respiratory chain assay results may be normal or only marginally reduced. These are believed to be due to defects in as-yet untyped nuclear genes that control mitochondrial DNA replication.

Mitochondrial neurogastrointestinal encephalomyopathy (MNGIE) is a syndrome characterized by gastrointestinal dysmotility, ophthalmoparesis, peripheral neuropathy, and myopathy that results in reductions and multiple deletions in the mitochondrial DNA. It has been found to be due to mutations in the nuclear thymidine phosphorylase gene, which is believed, in some way, to be important in mitochondrial DNA replication (Nishino *et al.* 1999).

### Nuclear encoded disorders

There are many more nuclear genes encoded for in the respiratory chain than in the mitochondrial genome.

As well as genes coding for subunits, there are also many more nuclear genes responsible for the import, assembly, and regulation of the subunits and complexes. In the neonatal disorders, the nuclear encoded forms are believed to be much more frequent than the mitochondrially encoded disorders. However, to date, only a few nuclear encoded genes have been screened for mutations. Recently, defects have been found in the SURF1 gene, which is believed to be involved in the assembly of the cytochrome oxidase complex (Zhu *et al.* 1998). As a result, the defect is expressed generally, particularly in cultured fibroblasts and cultured chorionic villus cells. This latter fact is important as it is one of the few respiratory chain disorders to date where antenatal diagnosis is feasible.

### KREBS CYCLE DEFECTS

Recently, defects in some of the enzymes of the Krebs Cycle (Tricarboxylic acid cycle) have been described. Fumarase deficiency can present in the first day of life with cyanosis and hypothermia progressing to microcephaly, failure to thrive with cerebral atrophy (Remes *et al.* 1992). Blood lactate concentrations can be elevated, and the urinary concentration of fumaric acid is grossly increased.

## NEUROTRANSMITTER DISORDERS

These are a group of disorders in which the defect is in the biosynthesis or degradation of a neurotransmitter (Jaeken 1990). Not surprisingly, these can present with progressive neurological problems in infancy.

### GABA TRANSMINASE DEFICIENCY

Defects in the catabolism of γ-aminobutyric acid (GABA) can lead to psychomotor retardation. GABA transminase deficiency also results in hypotonia, hyperreflexia and growth acceleration. The disorder is confirmed by the measurement of the CSF concentration of GABA, which is grossly elevated.

### SUCCINATE SEMI-ALDEHYDE DEHYDROGENASE DEFICIENCY

Succinate semi-aldehyde dehydrogenase is the second enzyme in the pathway for GABA degradation, and a defect in this enzyme leads to hypotonia, a non-progressive ataxia, and mild to marked psychomotor retardation. Less frequently, hyperactivity, choreoathetosis, autistic features, convulsions, hyporeflexia, nystagmus, and oculomotor apraxia may occur. The disorder is diagnosed by the measurement of the accumulating urinary 4-hydroxybutyric acid. The CSF GABA level is usually also elevated.

### AROMATIC AMINO ACID DECARBOXYLASE DEFICIENCY

Aromatic amino acid decarboxylase catalyses the conversion of L-DOPA to dopamine and 5-HTP to serotonin (Hyland & Clayton 1990). The patients presented with hypotonia with developmental delay and seizures at the age of 2 months with an absence of spontaneous movements but with preserved tendon reflexes. Oculogyric crises and choreoathetoid movements have been described. Marked decreases in CSF HVA and HIAA with raised concentrations of L-DOPA were found. The patients responded favorably to treatment with a monoamine oxidase inhibitor, a dopamine agonist and pyridoxine

### TYROSINE HYDROXYLASE DEFICIENCY

Tyrosine hydroxylase is the rate-linking step in the pathway for catecholamine biosynthesis. Patients present in the first months of life with hypokinesia, progressive motor retardation, truncal hypotonia, and extrapyramidal symptoms (Wevers *et al.* 1999). Diagnosis is by measurement of CSF catecholamines, which show generalized reductions. The patients respond to treatment with L-DOPA and carbidopa.

### NON-KETOTIC HYPERGLYCINEMIA (see also p. 619)

Glycine is known to be an important neurotransmitter. Non-ketotic hyperglycinemia exists in a severe form that exhibits intractable seizures with death in the first weeks of life. However, a milder form exists that can exhibit symptoms as early as 2 months of age and presents with psychomotor delay with or without seizures, apneic attacks and muscular hypotonia. The disorder can be diagnosed by the measurement of CSF and plasma glycine concentrations. Confirmation of the diagnosis can be made by the assay of the activity of liver glycine cleavage enzyme, which is defective in this disorder.

### CANAVAN'S DISEASE

In this disorder, there is early onset of developmental delay with hypotonia, visual failure due to optic atrophy, and seizures. Symptoms may start in the first few months, and macrocephaly is a striking feature. The developmental delay, visual problems, and large head often make the clinician suspect hydrocephalus. Nystagmus may be a clue to optic atrophy. Excessive, apparently unprovoked, crying may be a striking feature. Hypotonia and listlessness give way to spasticity and relentless progress to a decorticate state. These children regress with gross deterioration, blindness, and spasticity. It is said to be most common in Ashkenazi Jews, but non-Jewish children may be affected. A characteristic finding is the MRI scan, which shows widespread attenuation of subcortical white matter, external and internal capsules and thalami. In urine, plasma, and CSF, there is the accumulation of *N*-acetylaspartate – an important neurotransmitter. This is due to a deficiency of the enzyme *N*-acetylaspartoacylase (Matalon *et al.* 1992). Prenatal diagnosis is available.

### BIOPTERIN DEFECTS

Tetrahydrobiopterin is a cofactor for the enzymes tryptophan hydroxylase and tyrosine hydroxylase, which are responsible for the biosynthesis of serotonin, adrenaline, and noradrenaline. Defects or reduction in its biosynthesis produce non-specific developmental delay, psychomotor retardation, and hypotonia in the first months of life. It is also a cofactor for phenylalanine hydroxylase, and such defects can be detected by measurement of the plasma phenylalanine concentration. However, plasma samples taken in the first weeks of life may not show a raised phenylalanine level. Confirmation and delineation of the primary defect may require the measurement of the concentration of CSF, plasma or urine biopterins and erythrocyte enzymes. It is important to diagnose this group of disorders as early as possible as some are treatable by the administration of biopterins.

## ORGANIC ACID DISORDERS (see also p. 619)

Whilst the majority of organic acid disorders show static or intermittently progressive neurological dysfunction, a few can present with slow progressive problems. Often, there is no evidence of a metabolic acidosis or of bouts of decompensation associated with other illnesses.

### 3-METHYLGLUTACONIC ACIDURIA

This disorder presents in four forms, of which only one (type I) has been to date associated with an enzyme defect (Gibson *et al.* 1991). Type IV 3-methylglutaconic aciduria presents with moderate to severe neurological problems in the first year of life. There are seizures, developmental delay, movement disorders, minor malformations, retinitis pigmentosa, optic atrophy, and cataracts. The disorder is detected by the measurement of the urinary 3-methylglutaconic acid concentration.

### L-2-HYDROXYGLUTARIC ACIDURIA

This disorder can present early in life with hypotonia, psychomotor retardation, ataxia, macrocephaly, and leukodystrophy. It is detected by the measurement of the concentration of urinary L-2-hydroxyglutaric acid, which must be distinguised from its D-isomer, the excretion of which is associated with another disorder (Divry *et al.* 1992).

### D-2-HYDROXYGLUTARIC ACIDURIA

This disorder may present in the first months of life with epilepsy, hypotonia, cerebral visual failure, and profound developmental delay. Patients often have a cardiomyopathy. Diagnosis is by urine organic acid analysis for D-2-hydroxyglutaric acid, which must be distinguished from its L-isomer (Van der Knaap *et al.* 1999).

### MEVALONIC ACIDURIA

This disorder presents in the neonatal period or later with hepatosplenomegaly, cataracts, and dysmorphic features. Severe developmental delay and hypotonia develop with repeated respiratory infection, febrile episodes, and gastrointestinal problems. The disorder is diagnosed by urine organic acid analysis to detect the accumulating mevalonic acid (Hoffman *et al.* 1986).

## CARBOHYDRATE METABOLISM DISORDERS

Most disorders of carbohydrate metabolism that affect the brain have an acute or intermittently progressive nature. However, triosephosphate isomerase deficiency presents with severe progressive neurological dysfunction as early as 6 months of age. There is diffuse weakness, hypotonia, absent limb reflexes and unintelligible speech with flexion deformities of the limbs. A key feature is a marked non-spherocytic hemolytic anemia. This disorder is diagnosed by the measurement in erythrocytes of the glycolytic enzyme triosephosphate isomerase.

## VITAMIN METABOLISM DISORDERS

There are a number of inherited disorders involving defects in the absorption transport and metabolism of vitamins. Some of these present without neurological problems, and some present with acute neurological features. However, some disorders can present with a progressive neurological picture.

### BIOTINIDASE DEFICIENCY

This disorder is due to a deficiency of an enzyme (biotinidase) that is present in body fluids and recycles biotin from biotinylated amino acids. A defect in the enzyme leads to a systemic biotin deficiency with its associated symptoms. Whilst they usually present at several months of age, they can present at 8 weeks of age with seizures and a slow progressive course reminiscent of Leigh's syndrome (q.v.) often with skin rashes and alopecia and sensorineural hearing loss (Collins *et al.* 1994). It is important to recognize this disorder early as it is effectively treated with biotin administration, and without treatment, residual damage may occur.

### METHYLENE TETRAHYDROFOLATE REDUCTASE DEFICIENCY

This disorder can present in the first year of life with psychomotor retardation, which may progress later in life to hypertonicity, seizures, and demyelination. The disorder results in increased plasma homocystine and low methionine concentrations due to a failure of methylation of homocystine to methionine. This is due to a deficiency of methylene tetrahydrofolate reductase, an enzyme responsible for producing 5-methyltetra-hydrofolate, which is an important methylating agent. Despite the fact that the defect lies in folic acid metabolism, serum folate concentrations are not significantly reduced, and anemia is not a feature of the disease.

### TRANSCOBALAMIN II DEFICIENCY

Children with this disorder can present with developmental retardation with peripheral neuropathy, myelopathy, and encephalopathy. However, this is usually preceded by a failure to thrive and a marked megaloblastic anemia. The disorder is due to a deficiency of one of the circulating vitamin $B_{12}$ transport proteins – transcobalamin II. However, plasma vitamin $B_{12}$ concentrations are not significantly reduced due to the presence of other transporter proteins. The disorder is treatable by administration of vitamin $B_{12}$, so an early diagnosis is important. This is done by the specific measurement of the concentration of transcobalamin II in plasma. The disorder is usually initially detected by the accumulation of methylmalonic acid and homocystine in the plasma and urine.

## BATTEN'S DISEASE

There is some variation in terminology in this group of CNS degenerative diseases. The term 'Batten's disease' is best used for the whole group – alternatively known as neuronal ceroid lipofuscinosis because of the storage material found in the CNS and elsewhere. The major forms are early infantile (CLN1), late infantile (CLN2), and juvenile (CLN3). The genes for these disorders have been identified, and enzyme or molecular biological tests are now routinely available for their diagnosis. The primary defects lie in protein catabolism in the lysosome. Histological analysis, however, still remains a useful test for the exclusion and typing of the disorder (Bennett & Hofmann, 1999).

### EARLY INFANTILE BATTEN'S DISEASE (HAGBERG–SANTAVUORI DISEASE)

This variety of Batten's disease (neuronal ceroid lipofuscinosis) is the rarest of the three variants in the UK, although it is relatively more common in Finland (Haltia *et al.* 1973). It may present in the second half of the first year of life with progressive psychomotor retardation without any obvious features. Blindness may slowly supervene (the ERG is extinguished and the VER diminished). The head stops growing, and myoclonic jerks appear, although sometimes, these do not present until the second year of life.

It is a relatively rare disease in the UK, and as the signs early on are not very specific, it is easily missed. The EEG is abnormal before seizures appear – it is chaotic and irregular and gradually becomes lower in amplitude as the disease progresses.

The disorder is due to a deficiency of lysosomal palmitoyl-protein thioesterase 1 (PPT1), which can be measured in leukocytes and fibroblasts, and prenatal diagnosis is now available. Histological analysis of a rectal or skin biopsy shows electron dense bodies known as 'Finnish Snowballs'.

## DISEASES OF UNCERTAIN ORIGIN

### LEIGH'S DISEASE

Although Leigh's disease represents a number of different genetic entities, including mitochondrial disorders and pyruvate dehydrogenase deficiency, at the moment, it serves the purpose of describing a clinical picture that although variable, is important to recognize, not least because of possible therapeutic intervention. The pathology of this condition is that of symmetrical vascular lesions throughout the brainstem, basal ganglia and thalamus (Dayan *et al.* 1970); the origin of this is unknown. Some infants with Leigh's disease have been found to have defects in the metabolism of pyruvate. Pyruvate carboxylase (Hommes *et al.* 1968) and pyruvate dehydrogenase (Robinson & Sherwood 1975) have been shown in individual cases to be deficient, and cases have been shown to be associated with respiratory chain dysfunction (Pfeiffer *et al.* 1988).

Of the degenerative diseases seen in the first year of life, Leigh's disease is one of the most common, although experience varies from country to country. The onset is nearly always in the first year, often by months of age, and may even present in the neonatal period. There is a wide variety of presenting symptoms, and the initial features may be acute, apparently triggered by non-specific infection. The condition may be self-limiting or may be followed by deterioration, which may be chronic or show a stepwise downhill progress with varying plateaux. This is a relatively unusual pattern and should make one suspect Leigh's disease.

The typical features include hypotonia, abnormal movements (later becoming athetoid), sighing, or irregular respirations with periods of hyperventilation and apnea, swallowing difficulties that may contribute to failure to thrive, and other cranial nerve palsies. Abnormal eye movements occur. These are not simply the wandering nystagmoid eye movements of the blind but include complex nystagmoid movements that may be horizontal, rotary or vertical, ocular flutter, gaze palsies, and oculomotor paresis. Seizures are not a common feature in infancy, optic atrophy may develop later, and there may be evidence of a peripheral neuropathy (depressed reflexes and delayed nerve conduction studies). MRI scans may show hypodense symmetrical lesions in the region of the basal ganglia.

Lactate and pyruvate concentrations are sometimes elevated in the blood and CSF. A number of specific tests have been suggested in the past, but none have proved very useful. Final confirmation is only by the typical post-mortem findings.

Most cases of the disease are likely to be autosomal recessive, and as yet, there is no prenatal test. The course of the disease may be very prolonged with periods of stabilization.

Various cofactors, lipoic acid, vitamin $B_6$, thiamine, have been tried without any proof of success. The natural history of the disease makes assessment of therapy difficult.

It is likely that this condition represents a syndrome complex with more than one cause. The literature is confused because of different definitions of the syndrome, some pathological and some clinical, and in only a few have specific enzyme defects been determined.

### ALPERS DISEASE

Like Leigh's disease (see above) Alpers disease (progressive degeneration of cerebral gray matter; Alpers 1960) probably represents more than one neurological disorder, and in a few cases, a biochemical defect in the electron transport chain or fatty acid oxidation has been found (Tulinius *et al.* 1991). The literature on Alpers disease is sometimes confusing and conflicting, but in general, the presentation is in infancy with seizures and an intermittent downhill course, and there is diffuse non-specific destruction of cortical neurons. However, a condition has been described, known as 'progressive neuronal degeneration with hepatic failure' (Harding *et al.* 1986), which seems to be a specific entity within the Alpers spectrum. This condition presents with seizures that start suddenly and may have a myoclonic or generalized pattern. These seizures progress over months and are often refractory to therapy. Epilepsia partialis continuans may appear (this sign is otherwise very unusual in neurometabolic disease), there is progressive psychomotor retardation, and in the preterminal phase, hepatic involvement becomes apparent. The liver may be noticeably enlarged, and jaundice supervenes. Liver failure may be a terminal event. Serum enzyme concentrations indicative of liver damage (alanine transaminase and aspartate transaminase) become raised.

It has been suggested that liver involvement may be the result of antiepileptic drugs (Green 1984), but there is no evidence that drugs are responsible for the whole disease. The pathology of the liver shows a microvesicular steatosis, and in the brain, there is widespread proliferation and loss of neurons particularly affecting the visual cortex.

### INFANTILE NEURAXONAL DYSTROPHY

The clinical picture is that of CNS degeneration with mental retardation and long tract signs accompanied by hypotonia and peripheral wasting. Facial nerve paresis, oculomotor paresis, and optic atrophy may occur. Deterioration with dementia follows. Nerve conduction studies and EMG show denervation but relatively normal speeds of conduction, and the CSF protein level is raised. Both the central neuraxis and the peripheral nerves are involved. The latter may be shown on biopsy to have specific swellings (spheroid bodies) along the length of the axons. Three different clinical pictures emerge, only one of which, Seitelberger's disease (Seitelberger 1971) presents in infancy. Diagnosis is usually by conjunctival biopsy, which may demonstrate the spheroid bodies in nerve endings (Arsenio-Nunes & Goutières 1978). The disease is slowly progressive with death in early childhood. There is a report of infantile neuroaxonal dystrophy in which there was a defect of the lysosomal enzyme α-*N*-acetylgalactosaminidase (Schindler's disease) (Schindler *et al.* 1989). No prenatal diagnosis is yet available, unless the above deficiency is present.

### SPONGY DEGENERATIONS

Both Canavan's disease and Alexander's disease are examples of spongiform leukodystrophies that may present early in infancy. Canavan's disease is autosomal recessive, and due to a deficiency of *N*-acetylaspartoacylase (q.v.), whilst the genetic origin of Alexander's disease is unclear.

### ALEXANDER'S DISEASE

This disease is probably rarer than Canavan's disease. There are few symptoms other than psychomotor retardation amounting to an arrest of development; seizures and spasticity may supervene. An enlarged head is a constant sign. CT shows a low attenuation of white matter, particularly in the frontal areas, and ventricular dilatation.

There is no specific marker that can be identified in life. Seizures become more prominent later on, and death occurs early in childhood. This condition is one of the few where it may be justified to do a brain biopsy. The typical findings include the so-called 'Rosenthal' fibers (Boltshauser & Wilson 1976).

## DIFFERENTIAL DIAGNOSIS

Other non-metabolic causes of CNS degeneration must be considered in the differential diagnosis of the metabolic diseases. Progressive epilepsy, particularly myoclonic, may be due to a number of different epileptic encephalopathies (Aicardi *et al.* 1998). Progressive psychomotor retardation with hypotonia or spasticity may occasionally be due to diffuse tumors of the CNS. Postinfective (viral) encephalopathies may occasionally be progressive, e.g. progressive polio encephalitis.

Rett's syndrome, probably a relatively common condition in girls, causing developmental regression, loss of communication skills, ataxia, and abnormal hand movements, may just be recognized at 6–9 months, although classically, it presents in the second year of life. The cause is probably a gene on the distal arm of Xq28 (Ellaway & Christodoulou 1999).

## SPECIFIC THERAPIES

There are very few specific therapies available for most of these metabolic disorders. Copper therapy has been tried in Menkes' disease without any clear evidence of success. (Guitet *et al.* 1999).

Marrow transplantation has been performed in a few centers in different countries (Krivit *et al.* 1999). Claims have been made for limited success with MLD. The most experience, however in the UK, is with the mucopolysaccharides. Not all the data of analysis are yet available, and the results are not yet clear. Although some success has been claimed with Hurler's disease (Vellodi *et al.* 1997), it is our impression from the literature and from colleagues that there is no hard and fast evidence that the transferred enzyme enters the CNS and persists to sufficient levels of affect neurological progression. Physical reduction of liver size and clearing of corneal clouding have been shown (Hobbs *et al.* 1981). It is much more difficult to evaluate the improvement of intellectual status over a short period. Moreover, the procedure is available in only a few specialized centers, requires a compatible donor, is expensive, and has a very high morbidity and mortality. At the moment, it must be considered an experimental therapy.

However, it must be remembered that in a few cases, e.g. the neurotransmitter disorders, biotinidase deficiency, hereditary orotic aciduria, and transcobalamin II deficiency, treatment can be very effective and needs to be started early.

## CONCLUSION

Even though there is as yet no evidence of any specific therapy in most of the CNS degenerative diseases discussed, it is very important to try and make a diagnosis and to do this accurately, efficiently, and as early as possible. Diagnosis is important for management, prognosis, and counseling and is essential for prenatal diagnosis. It may serve later on as a starting point for therapy should that become available.

The management of the progressive diseases is fraught with difficulty for the clinician. Firstly, the time from symptoms to diagnosis may be prolonged, causing anxiety in the family. This may occur because of the confusing clinical picture that presents and the rarity of individual diseases that have to be thought about before they can be diagnosed. Sometimes, the symptoms are wrongly ascribed to perinatal encephalopathies or the consequence of infantile spasms. Some diseases in this group are only slowly progressive without gross symptomatology, and development masks psychomotor retardation. An acute deterioration may be, for example in Leigh's disease, wrongly attributed to a viral encephalopathy.

The very act of diagnosis sometimes gives relief to some parents (at least to those who have been aware that there is something wrong). Supportive therapy must include management of seizures, often very difficult, reduction of spasticity, and sometimes sedation. Most important is an excellent standard of nursing care both in hospital and at home. Facilities for shared care and respite care should be provided. The management problems of the dying child with all the social, emotional, and nursing implications have been a concern of those working in the field over the last few years. This has led to a number of approaches based on support groups, specialized home nursing, and hospices for children.

The diagnosis of this group of conditions should always be confirmed pathologically or biochemically. As these tests are not available in non-specialized laboratories, the diagnosis should be confirmed by a specialist laboratory, and ideally, the same laboratory should be involved in the prenatal diagnosis of any further pregnancies. To some extent, this will avoid any difficulties caused by variations of the methodology of enzyme assays amongst laboratories.

### Key Points

- Degenerative disorders, unlike disorders of amino and organic acids, usually present after a period of normality followed by slowing down of progress and plateauing of skills before regression occurs
- Non-neurologic signs of these disorders include hernias, dermatologic disorders, hair abnormalities, dysmorphism, failure to thrive and cardiomyopathy.
- Specialized laboratory investigations are required for diagnosis in most cases and will require expert advice in their performance and interpretation
- Individual causes of degenerative disorders are rare, but diagnosis is important for management, prognosis and counseling and is essential for prenatal diagnosis

## REFERENCES


Adams C & Green S (1986) Late-onset hexosaminidase A and hexosaminidase A and B deficiency: family study and review. *Dev Med Child Neurol* 28:236–243.

Aicardi J, Gillberg C, Ogier H *et al.* (1998) *Diseases of the nervous system in childhood (clinics in developmental medicine)*. Cambridge: Cambridge University Press, 2nd edn.

Alpers B J (1960) Progressive cerebral degeneration of infancy. *J Men Nerv Dis* 130:442–448.

Amir N, Zlotogora J & Bach G (1987) Mucolipidosis type IV: clinical spectrum and natural history. *Paediatrics* 79:953–959.

Arsenio-Nunes M L & Goutières F (1978) Diagnosis of infantile neuraxonal dystrophy by conjunctival biopsy. *J Neurol Neurosurg Psychiatry* 41:511–515.

Aukett A, Bennett M J & Hosking G P (1988) Molybdenum co-factor deficiency: an easily missed inborn error of metabolism. *Dev Med Child Neurol* 30:531–535.

Bach G, Friedman R, Weissman B *et al.* (1972) The defect in the Hurler and Schele syndromes: deficiency of alpha-L-iduronidase. *Proc Natl Acad Sci USA* 69:2048–2051.

Beaudet A L, DiFerrante N M, Ferry G D *et al.* (1975) Variation in the phenotype expression of beta-glucuronidase deficiency. *J Pediatr* 86:338–394.

Bennett M J & Hoffmann S L (1999) The neuronal ceroid-lipofuscinosis (Battens disease): A new class of lysosomal storage diseases. *J Inher Metab Dis* 22:535–544.

Boltshauser E & Wilson J (1976) Value of brain biopsy in neurodegenerative disease in childhood. *Arch Dis Childhood* 51:260–268.

Bowen P, Lee C S N, Zellweger H *et al.* (1964) A familial syndrome of multiple congenital defects. *Bull Johns Hopkins Hosp* 114:402–414.

Braverman N, Steel G, Obje C *et al.* (1997) Human PEX7 encodes the peroxisomal PTS2 receptor and is responsible for rhizomelic chondrodysplasia punctata. *Nat Genet* 15:369–370.

Brett E M (ed) (1997) *Paediatric neurology*. Edinburgh: Churchill Livingstone. 3rd edn.

Brown G K, Haan E A, Kirkby D M *et al.* (1988) Cerebral lactic acidosis: defects in pyruvate metabolism with profound brain damage and minimal systemic acidosis. *Eur J Paediatr* 147:10–14.

Collie W R, Moore C M, Goka T J *et al.* (1978) Pill torti as marker for carriers of Menkes' disease. *Lancet* i:607–608.

Collins J E, Nicholson N S & Dalta Bm Leonard J V (1994) Biotinidase deficiency: early neurological presentation. *J Dev Med Child Neurol* 36:263–270.

Danks D M, Campbell P E, Stevens B J *et al.* (1972) Menkes' kinky hair syndrome: an inherited defect in copper absorption with widespread effects. *Pediatrics* 50:188–201.

Dayan A D, Ockenden B G & Crome L (1970) Necrotising encephalomyelopathy of Leigh: neuropathological findings in 8 cases. *Arch Dis Childhood* 45:39–48.

DeDuve C (1969) The peroxisome: a new cytoplasmic organelle. *Proc Roy Soc Lond* (B) 173:71–83.

De Koning T J, Duran M, Dorland L *et al.* (1998) Beneficial effects of L-serine and glycine in the management of seizures in 3-phosphoglycerate dehydrogenase deficiency. *Ann Neurol* 44:261–265.

Divry P, Vianey-Saban C, Jakobs C *et al.* (1992) L-2-Hydroxyglutaric aciduria: a further case. In: *Abstracts of Free Communications of the 30th Annual Symposium of the Society for the Study of Inborn Errors of Metabolism* 72.

Ellaway C & Christodoulou J (1999) Review article: Rett syndrome: Clinical update and review of recent genetic advances. *J Paediatr Child Health* 35:419–426.

Garnica A D (1984) The failure of parenteral copper therapy in Menkes' kinky hair syndrome. *Eur J Pediatr* 142:98–102.

Gibson K M, Sherwood W G, Hoffman G F *et al.* (1991) Phenotypic heterogeneity in syndromes of 3-methylglutaconic aciduria. *J Paediatr* 118:885–890.

Gray R G F, Green A, Rabb L *et al.* (1990) A case of the B1 variant of GM2-gangliosidosis. *J Inher Metab Dis* 13:280–282.

Green S H (1984) Sodium valproate and routine liver function tests. *Arch Dis Childhood* 59:813–814.

Grover W D & Scrutton M C (1975) Copper infusion therapy in trichopoliostrophy. *J Pediatr* 86:216–220.

Guitet M, Campistol J & Medina M (1999) Menkes disease: experience in copper salts therapy. *Rev Neurol* 29: 127–130.

Haltia M, Rapola J & Sabtavouri P (1973) Infantile type of so called neuronal ceroid lipofuscinosis. *Acta Neuropathol* 26: 157–170.

Harding B N, Egger J, Portman B *et al.* (1986) Progressive neuronal degeneration of childhood with liver disease. *Brain* 109: 181–206.

Hobbs J R, Hugh-Jones K, Barrett A J *et al.* (1981) Reversal of clinical features of Hurler's disease and biochemical improvement after treatment by bone-marrow transplantation. *Lancet* ii:709–712.

Hoffman G, Gibson K, Brandt I K *et al.* (1986) Mevalonic aciduria – an inborn error of cholesterol and nonsterol isoprene biosynthesis. *N Engl J Med* 314:1610–1614.

Hommes F A, Polman H A & Reerink J D (1968) Leigh's encephalo-myelopathy: an inborn error of gluconeogenesis. *Arch Dis Childhood* 43:423–426.

Hyland K, Clayton P (1990) Aromatic amino acid decarboxylase deficiency in twins. *J Inher Metab Dis* 13: 301–304.

Jaeken J (1990) Disorders of neurotransmitters. In: Fermandez J, Saudubray J M & Tada K (eds) *Inborn metabolic diseases*. Berlin: Springer; pp. 637–648.

Jaeken J, Detheux M, van Maldergen L *et al.* (1996) 3-phosphoglycerate dehydrogenase deficiency and 3-phosphoserine phosphatase deficiency; inborn errors of serine biosynthesis. *J Inher Metab Dis* 19:223–226.

Jaeken J, Matthijs G, Barone R *et al.* (1997) Carbohydrate deficient glycoprotein (CDG) syndrome type 1. *J Med Genet* 34:73–76.

Krivit W, Auborg P, Shapiro E *et al.* (1999) Bone marrow transplantation globoid cell leukodystrophy, adrenoleukodystrophy, metachromatic leukodystrophy and Hurler syndrome. *Curr Opin Haematol* 6:377–382.

Lesch M & Nyhan W L (1964) A familial disorder of uric acid metabolism and central nervous system function. *Am J Med* 36:561–570.

Lowden J A & O'Brien J S (1979) Sialidosis: a review of human neuraminidase deficiency. *Am J Hum Genet* 31: 1–18.

Lowry R B & Renwick H G (1971) Relative frequency of the Hurler and Hunter syndromes. *N Engl J Med* 28: 221–222.

McFaul R, Cavanagh N, Lake B D *et al.* (1982) Metachromatic leucodystrophy: review of 38 cases. *Arch Dis Childhood* 57:168–175.

McKusick V A (1998) *Mendelian inheritance in man: a catalog of human genes and genetic disorders.* Baltimore, MD: Johns Hopkins University Press, 12th edn.

Mancini G M S, Verheijen F W, Beerens C E M T *et al.* (1991) Sialic acid storage disorders: observations on clinical and biochemical variation. *Dev Neurosci* 13:327–330.

Martin J J, Leroy J G, Centerick C *et al.* (1981) Fetal Krabbe's leukodystrophy: a morphological study of two cases. *Acta Neuropathol* 53:87–91.

Matalon R, Michals K, Gashkoff P *et al.* (1992) Prenatal diagnosis of Canavan's disease. *J Inher Metab Dis* 15: 392–394.

Moser H W & Goldfischer S L (1985) The peroxisomal disorders. *Hosp Prac (office edn)* 20:61–70.

Nishino I, Spinazzola A & Hirano M (1999) Thyrimidine phosphorylase gene mutations in MNGIE, a human mitochondrial disorder. *Science* 283:689–692.

O'Brien J S, Stern M B, Landing B H *et al.* (1965) Generalised gangliosidosis: another inborn error of ganglioside metabolism? *Am J Dis Children* 109:338–346.

Pavone L, Moser H W, Mollica F *et al.* 1980 Farber's lipogranulomatosis: ceramide deficiency and prolonged survival in three relatives. *Johns Hopkins Med J* 147:193–196.

Pfeiffer J, Kustermann-Kuhn B, Mortier W *et al.* (1988) Mitochondrial myopathies with necrotizing encephalopathy of the Leigh type. *Pathol Res Prac* 183:706–716.

Powers J M & Moser H W (1998) Peroxisomal disorders: genotype, phenotype, major neuropathological lesions and pathogenesis. *Brain Pathol* 18:101–120.

Remes A M, Rantala H, Hiltunen *et al.* (1992) Fumarase deficiency: two siblings with enlarged cerebral ventricles and polyhydramniosis *in utero*. *Paediatrics* 89:730–734.

Rizzo W B & Craft D A (1991) Sjogren-Larsson syndrome-deficient activity of fatty alcohol: NAD oxidoreductase in cultured fibroblasts *J Clin Invest* 88:1643–1648.

Robinson B H & Sherwood W G (1975) Pyruvate dehydrogenase phosphatase deficiency: a cause of congenital chronic lactic acidosis in infancy. *Pediatr Res* 9:935–939.

Ryan A K, Bartlett K, Clayton P *et al.* (1998) Smith-Lemli-Opitz syndrome: a variable clinical and biochemical phenotype. *J Med Gene* 35:558–565.

Schindler D, Bishop D F, Wolfe D E *et al.* (1989) A neuroaxonal dystrophy due to lysosomal alpha-*N*-acetylgalactosaminidase deficiency. *N Engl J Med* 320:173–174.

Schutgens R B H, Heymans H S A, Wanders R J A *et al.* (1986) Peroxisomal disorders: a newly recognised group of genetic diseases. *Eur J Pediatr* 1:430–440.

Scriver C R, Beaudet A L & Sly W S (eds) (1995) *The metabolic and molecular bases of inherited disease*. New York, NY: McGraw Hill, 7th edn.

Seitelberger F (1971) Neuropathological conditions related to neuraxonal dystrophy. *Acta Neuropathol* (suppl) 5:17–19.

Sheets Lee J E, Falk R E, Ng W G *et al.* (1985) Beta-glucuronidase deficiency: a heterogeneous mucopolysaccharidosis. *Am J Dis Childhood* 139:57–59.

Simmonds A (1987) Purine and pyrimidine disorders. In: Holton J (ed.) *The inherited metabolic diseases.* Edinburgh: Churchill Livingstone.

Tayebi N, Cushner S R, Kleijer E K *et al.* (1997) Prenatal lethality of a homozygous null mutation in the human glucocerebrosidase gene. *Prenatal Diag* 73:41–47.

Taylor C J & Green S H (1981) Menkes' syndrome (trichopoliodystrophy): use of scanning electron-microscope in diagnosis and carrier identification. *J Dev Med Child Neurol* 23:361–368.

Taylor H A, Thomas G H, Aylsworth A *et al.* (1975) Mannosidosis: deficiency of a specific alpha-mannosidase component in cultured fibroblasts. *Clin Chim Acta* 59:93–99.

Tonnesen T, Horn N, Sondergaard F *et al.* (1987) Experience with first trimester prenatal diagnosis of Menkes disease. *Prenatal Diag* 7:497–509.

Tulinius M H, Holme E, Kristiansson B *et al.* (1991) Mitochondrial encephalomyopathies in childhood 11 – clinical manifestations and syndromes. *J Paediatr* 119:251–258.

Turner Z & Horn N (1998) Menkes disease: underlying genetic defect and new diagnostic possibilities. *J Inherit Metab Dis* 21:604–612.

Ulrich J & Herschkowitz N (1977) Seitelberger's connatal form of Pelizaeus–Merzbacher disease: case report; clinical, pathological and biochemical findings. *Acta Neuropathol* 40:129–136.

Vamos E, Liebaers I, Bousard N *et al.* (1981) Multiple sulphatase deficiency with early onset. *J Inherit Metab Dis* 4:103–104.

Van der Knaap M S, Jakobs C, Hoffman G F *et al.* (1999) D-2-Hydroxyglutaric aciduria; Biochemical marker or clinical disease entity? *Ann Neurol* 45:111–119.

Vanier M-T, Pentchev P, Rodriguez-Lufrasse C *et al.* (1991) Niemann-Pick C disease type C: an update. *J Inher Metab Dis* 14:580–595.

Vellodi A, Young E P, Cooper A *et al.* (1997) Bone marrow transplantation for mucopolysaccharidosis type I: experience of two British centres. *Arch Dis Childhood* 76:92–99.

Verity M A & Montasir M (1977) Infantile Gaucher's disease: neuropathology, acid hydrolase activities and negative staining observations. *Neuropaediatrie* 8:89–100.

Vu T H, Sciacco M, Tanji K *et al.* (1998) Clinical manifestations of mitochondrial DNA depletion. *Neurology* 50:1783–1790.

Wang P J, Hwu W L, Lee W T *et al.* (1997) Duplication of proteolipid protein gene, a possible major cause of Pelizaeus–Merzbacher disease. *Pediatr Neurol* 17:125–128.

Watts R W E & Gibbs D A (1986) *Lysosomal storage diseases: biochemical and clinical aspects.* London: Taylor and Francis.

Wevers R A, de Rijk van Adel J F, Bräutigam C *et al.* (1999) A review of biochemical and molecular genetic aspects of tyrosine hydroxylase deficiency including a novel mutation (291delC). *J Inher Metab Dis* 22:364–373.

Wilson J M, Young A B & Kelley W N (1983) Hypoxanthine-guanine phosphoribosyltransferase deficiency: the molecular basis of the clinical syndromes. *N Eng J Med* 309:900–910.

Young G & Driscoll M C (1999) Coagulation abnormalities in the carbohydrate-deficient glycoprotein syndrome: case report and review of the literature. *Am J Haematol* 166:66–69.

Zhu Z, Yao J, Johns T *et al.* (1998) SURF1 encoding a factor involved in the biogenesis of cytochrome C oxidase, is mutated in Leigh syndrome. *Nat Genet* 20:337–343.

# Section VIII
# Seizure disorders

# Chapter 37 Seizure disorders of the neonate and infant

A. Arzimanoglou and J. Aicardi

## INTRODUCTION

Epileptic phenomena are the most frequent of the overt manifestations of neonatal neurologic disorders (Fenichel 1985; Aicardi 1994; Volpe 1995; Mizrahi & Kellaway 1998). Early diagnosis of neonatal epileptic seizures is a crucial and clinically significant issue, since it often reveals the presence of serious neurologic abnormalities, including structural or acquired brain lesions. Furthermore, particularly in neonates, seizures may interfere with important supportive measures such as feeding and may in themselves be dangerous by interfering with vital functions or being directly or indirectly a cause of brain injury.

Yet, paroxysmal phenomena in neonates may be difficult to recognize. Spectacular features, similar to those observed in older patients, are usually absent, and atypical manifestations are frequent. In fact, any type of bizarre or unusual transient event in the neonatal period may be a seizure, especially if stereotyped and periodically recurring. However, some of these phenomena may prove to be non-epileptic in nature and may represent 'release' phenomena of subcortical origin. The differential diagnosis may be very difficult or even impossible, although separation of epileptic and nonepileptic events is important to define a therapeutic strategy. The presence or absence of ictal EEG activity is of great help although not always sufficient. The response of the infant to stimulation and restraint is of importance, but more importantly, the clinician must consider the neurological context within which the paroxysmal phenomena are observed.

This chapter mainly deals with seizures of epileptic mechanism but will include the discussion of other more dubious phenomena, the knowledge of which may be of value to the physician for bedside differentiation of paroxysmal attacks. The relationship of the various clinical phenomena with EEG events will then be considered, and a syndromic approach to the diagnosis will be attempted. Etiology, prognosis, and therapeutic strategies will be discussed.

## EPIDEMIOLOGY

The precise frequency of neonatal seizures is difficult to determine from available information. The difficulty of identifying the various mechanisms of paroxysmal events as epileptic or non-epileptic and the frequent occurrence of electrical discharges without clinical manifestations in neonates are in part responsible for the discrepant figures given for incidence of neonatal seizures. Different referral patterns and/or factors inherent in the populations studied have to be considered. Incidence figures vary between 0.15 and 1.4% (Bergman *et al.* 1983; Goldberg 1983; Legido 1988; Aicardi 1992). The reported incidence in the general population of neonates was 3.5/1000 live births in Lanska's retrospective cohort study (Lanska *et al.* 1995), and 2.5/1000 live births in the prospective study reported by Ronen & Penney (1995). The very high incidence figure (up to 22.7%) reported in premature infants by Bergman *et al.* is probably due in part to a high frequency of non-epileptic events in this group. Stratification of data according to birthweight (Lanska *et al.* 1995) shows a much higher incidence in very-low-birthweight (<1500 g) infants, estimated at 57.5 cases for 1000 live births. Scher *et al.* (1993) estimated that 2.3% of all infants cared for in an intensive care unit experienced seizures.

The problem of seizure incidence in the neonatal period is further compounded by the frequent occurrence of electrical discharges without clinical manifestations (Hellstrom-Westas *et al.* 1985; Clancy *et al.* 1988). Although they may precede, follow, or alternate with electroclinical attacks, they may also occur in isolation and may sometimes be more common than electroclinical seizures. The converse phenomenon of typical clinical seizures without electrical concomitants has also been reported.

## PATHOPHYSIOLOGY

Neonatal paroxysmal events may be of an epileptic or non-epileptic nature. For those events that suggest involvement of an epileptic mechanism, the differences between epileptic attacks in newborn babies and those in older children probably reflect the incomplete neuroanatomic and neurophysiologic development of the neonatal brain (Aicardi 1994). Changes in the receptors of both excitatory (glutamate and aspartate) and inhibitory (GABA) circuits play a major role in the modulation of cortical excitability, and their differential rate of maturation with age may explain the changing susceptibility to epilepsy at various ages (Moshé 1987; Johnston 1996; Holmes 1997) and the variability in clinical expression of seizures.

A detailed study of the mechanisms supposed to be responsible for the generation and propagation of epileptic discharges in neonates is beyond the scope of this chapter (for a review, see Volpe (1995); Schwartzkoin (1994)). Experimental data suggest that early in development, excitatory activity, mediated primarily by glutamate receptors, especially in the hippocampus, predominates. In the immature brain, there is an increased density of NMDA-gated channels, and they are less voltage-dependent (Hablitz 1987; Ben-Ari *et al.* 1988). Inhibitory systems are relatively underdeveloped. In particular, GABA A receptors seem to play an excitatory role as a result of the differences in concentration of intracellular chloride in the immature brain (Ben-Ari *et al.* 1989; Cherubini *et al.* 1991).

However, a number of clinical observations (better prognosis after status epilepticus as compared to adults) and laboratory findings (less histological damage and fewer behavioural deficits after prolonged seizures induced by several convulsants) suggest that the immature brain is less vulnerable than the mature brain to seizure-related brain damage. This may be the result of some physiologic features of the immature brain (Holmes 1997) suggesting decreased excitability and the development of inhibition at a faster pace than excitation. A definitive answer to the question of seizure susceptibility and to seizure-induced damage has yet to be given. As stressed by Holmes, 'it is important to recognize the limitations of some of the techniques used in experimental studies' and to remember that 'the degree of seizure-related damage may be related to the species of the animal model studied'.

Clinical and laboratory evidence proves that prolonged and recurrent seizures can be harmful to the immature brain. Subtle deficits may be difficult to detect at this age but may be manifested only later in life. The impact of those subtle changes on natural evolution needs to be studied further. For some of the clinical phenomena observed in neonates (mainly tonic and subtle seizures), the mechanisms involved are uncertain. Although it cannot be excluded that some may be associated with cortical epileptic discharges that are not picked up on the scalp, such an explanation is unlikely to apply to a majority of cases (Aicardi 1990). Such events may be of subcortical origin and may be related to liberation of tonic influences from brainstem origin as a result of the loss of cortical inhibition due to diffuse cortical damage or dysfunction (Kellaway & Hrachovy 1983; Camfield & Camfield 1987). Such a mechanism is in agreement with the fact that 'release phenomena' are frequently graded rather than all-or-none phenomena, can be elicited by stimulation, inhibited by restraint, and may demonstrate spatial and temporal summation. Similar features have been demonstrated in animal models of reflex physiology, supporting the suggestion that these clinical phenomena are non-epileptic in origin and are exaggerated reflex behaviors in affected neonates (Mizrahi & Kellaway 1998).

## CLINICAL AND EEG FEATURES

The variable terminology used in the literature when referring to neonatal paroxysmal events (convulsions, seizures, epileptic seizures, non-epileptic seizures, muscular twitching, and motor automatisms) reflects the difficulty in recognizing and interpreting motor phenomena and autonomic signs in the newborn. Such difficulties may result either in overdiagnosis of epileptic seizures or in delay in the diagnosis of true 'epileptic' attacks, as not all paroxysmal neonatal events are epileptic seizures. The variable clinical manifestations and EEG features of seizures result from the incomplete synaptic organization, the different balance between excitation and inhibition related to different development of receptors, age-related differences in response to pharmacologic agents, and developmental regional variability (see also Chapter 11).

Early diagnosis of neonatal seizures and their differentiation from similar non-epileptic phenomena, essential for current management, can be suspected on the clinical features but, in the majority of cases, requires neurophysiologic confirmation. The etiologic context and the results of neurological evaluation are of crucial importance in determining diagnosis and management.

However, the absence of typical EEG paroxysms does not preclude an epileptic mechanism since even typical clonic seizures may not be accompanied by typical EEG discharges. As noted by Volpe (1995), 'the electrical discharges that are so readily generated in neonatal brain, particularly in hippocampus, may not propagate sufficiently to be observed by surface EEG, and even when synchronous discharges do appear at the surface near the end of the seizure, behavioural phenomena may not correlate well because of deficient myelination of cerebral efferent systems'. EEG monitoring, and even better video-EEG, is desirable even if it does not answer all the questions. Therefore, interictal EEG is useful in assessing brain maturation and prognosis, but its value for the diagnosis of neonatal seizures is limited (Volpe 1995; Mizrahi & Kellaway 1998).

The stereotyped nature of the events, the absence of sensitivity to stimuli and to restraint (Aicardi 1992; Mizrahi & Kellaway 1998), the etiologic context, and global neurologic evaluation favor the diagnosis of epileptic seizures. Video-EEG documents might be used to seek advice from an experienced examiner.

Seizures in the neonatal period are only rarely an isolated event. In most cases, they tend to recur for periods of variable duration, from a few minutes to several hours or even days. Individual seizures are almost always brief events lasting seconds to minutes (Clancy *et al.* 1988). The term 'serial seizures' is probably more precise than that of status epilepticus because long continuous seizures are rare, and assessment of the level of awareness and responsiveness is often impossible at this age, due to the underlying condition and the depressive effects of drug therapy. Whatever the repetition rate and duration of the seizure period, the occurrence of several seizure patterns in the same patient, including subtle seizures or other paroxysmal events of uncertain pathophysiology, is frequent.

## TYPES OF SEIZURES

Four main types of seizures are usually described: clonic, tonic, myoclonic, and subtle seizures. Increasing use of EEG-polygraphic-video monitoring techniques during the last decade allowed for a more precise description and classification of neonatal seizures and for a better understanding of their pathophysiology. However, it should be emphasized that many infants will experience several seizure types, rendering classification difficult. In one study, 22% of neonates with seizures experienced more than one type of seizure (Mizrahi & Kellaway 1987; Aicardi 1994)

- Clonic seizures. These may be focal or multifocal. They are described as repetitive, rhythmic contractions of muscle groups of the limbs, face, or trunk; they may occur simultaneously but asynchronously and involve any part of the body or both sides but rarely a whole side. Localized clonic movements may also shift quite rapidly to another body part or to the opposite side, in a disordered fashion. Several segments can be simultaneously involved, simulating a generalized seizure (multifocal seizures). When seizures shift rapidly from one region to another, they are termed 'migratory' or 'erratic'. They usually do not indicate the presence of a fixed focal lesion, as this may be the case with unifocal seizures, but may be related to metabolic disorders.
- Tonic seizures. These may be focal or generalized. When generalized, they consist of a tonic symmetric extension of all limbs, trunk and neck. This type of tonic stiffening, particularly when isolated, is more commonly unassociated with EEG ictal discharges and is often considered as a 'release' non-epileptic phenomenon, mimicking 'decorticate' posturing. Associated, stereotyped, partial manifestations such as sustained eye deviation or sustained posturing of one limb and opening or closing movements of the eyelids may be clues in favor of an epileptic mechanism.
- Myoclonic seizures. These are random, single, rapid contractions of muscle groups of the limbs, face, or trunk. They can be erratic or fragmentary, typically not repetitive. They are usually generalized and may be associated with tonic contractions. They may be provoked by stimulation and, from a pathophysiologic point of view, they may or may not be epileptic in origin.
- Subtle or minimal seizures. These comprise various behavioral phenomena, especially oral–buccal–lingual movements (chewing, swallowing, sucking, lip-smacking, and grimacing), ocular and periocular movements (eye-opening, staring, and repetitive blinking), movements of progression (stepping, pedalling, swimming-like movements, or combinations of these), and complex purposeless movements. Mizrahi & Kellaway (1998) prefer the term 'motor automatisms' to describe these phenomena that they consider as non-epileptic in nature. Although this may be true for a number of cases, the use of video-EEG suggests caution when interpreting such phenomena. In fact, these manifestations may also be partial epileptic seizures, due to a focal lesion (ex. dysplasia). When the clinical manifestations persist, are stereotyped in clinical expression, and are insensitive to stimuli, it is reasonable to recommend a video-EEG/polygraphy recording and neuroimaging.

Autonomic phenomena such as vasomotor changes, salivation, or modification of heart rate can also be observed as isolated phenomena but are more often associated with motor automatisms.

Apneic seizures may be isolated or associated with other autonomic manifestations. They are often associated with subtle seizures, especially abnormal ocular movements (Willis & Gould 1980; Watanabe *et al.* 1982). Although isolated apnea has been documented with electrical seizure activity, especially in the full-term newborn (Fenichel *et al.* 1980; Watanabe *et al.* 1982), the vast majority of apneic episodes in the premature infant are not epileptic in nature (Radvanyi-Bouvet *et al.* 1985). Fenichel *et al.* (1980) found that epileptic apneas are not associated with bradycardia, showing the interest in always recording the ECG simultaneously.

Epileptic spasms (Dulac *et al.* 1994) are sudden, usually bilateral tonic contractions of the muscles of the neck, trunk, and extremities, which may be flexor, extensor, or mixed. Each spasm usually lasts less than 2 s, may be followed by a less intense contraction and/or behavioral arrest lasting about 10 s, and recurs in series. Although they can occur in the neonatal period, they are most often observed in the first year of life as the main seizure manifestation of West syndrome. The repetitive character of the spasms is an important diagnostic clue, especially as the individual spasms may have a very limited expression (slight head-nodding, elevation of the eyeballs, and shrugging of the shoulders).

## EEG FEATURES (see also Chapter 11)

The combination of both EEG and clinical criteria more accurately diagnoses and classifies seizures in neonates. As pointed out by Mizrahi & Kellaway (1998), 'the best application of EEG is to help answer specific clinical questions'. Interpretation must take into account gestational age, consideration of developmental milestones, analysis of wake/sleep cycles, the presence of lateralizing features, and/or focal abnormalities. EEG findings must be correlated with medical history, state of alertness, and relevant laboratory data. The maturational aspects, the normal and abnormal features of neonatal EEG, and the features that may be of uncertain significance are beyond the scope of this chapter (Dreyfus-Brisac & Curzi-Dascalova 1979; Hrachovy *et al.* 1990). Almost all electrical activity in the neonate begins focally, except for the more generalized activity associated with myoclonic jerks or infantile spasms.

Interpretation of interictal sharp-wave transients may be difficult. Isolated sharp waves do occur in normal neonates, but they are not usually sufficient evidence for a focal epileptogenic brain abnormality. Ictal discharges in the newborn are exceedingly variable in appearance, voltage, frequency, and polarity. Changes may occur between different discharges in the same infant and even within the same discharge. The modification in rhythm and polarity may be progressive, usually with slowing of the rhythm toward the end of a discharge, or quite sudden, with abrupt changes in the frequency, morphology, and amplitude of the paroxysmal complexes. Generalized symmetrical discharges are very rare. Two main elements, commonly associated, constitute the EEG discharges in newborns: abnormal paroxysmal rhythms and repetitive spikes or sharp waves.

Abnormal paroxysmal rhythms consist of rhythmic wave forms resembling alpha, theta, beta or delta activity or a mixture of these. They usually remain focal, but hemispheric extension or even diffusion to the contralateral side is possible. More commonly, unrelated discharges, at different rhythms, may occur in different locations. The frequency and morphology of a given discharge usually remain constant throughout the seizure, but a change in appearance may be recorded. Duration is quite variable. Most authors require that a discharge last at least 10 s to be considered ictal (Radvanyi-Bouvet *et al.* 1985; Clancy & Legido 1988). Focal discharges of sharp waves may be relatively fast (2–4 Hz) or occur at a slow rate (~1 Hz), a pattern that resembles the periodic lateralized discharges (PLEDs) of older patients (Lombroso 1982; Holmes 1985).

Some ictal patterns occur especially in neonates with severe encephalopathies:

- Electrical seizures in the depressed brain are typically low in voltage, long in duration, and narrowly localized, usually seen in EEGs whose background activity is low in amplitude and undifferentiated (Mizrahi & Kellaway 1998);
- 'alpha seizure activity' or 'paroxysmal alpha pattern' (Knauss *et al.* 1978; Watanabe 1982) is characterized by the sudden appearance of rhythmic 8- to 12-Hz, 20- to 70-μV activity in one temporal or central region and is usually indicative of a severe encephalopathy, suggesting a poor prognosis.

In premature infants, the EEG findings tend to be more stereotyped, and purely EEG discharges are especially common. Sharp waves are uncommon. They were observed in only five of 12 prematures by Radvanyi-Bouvet *et al.* (1985), whereas they were present in 13 of their 15 full-term babies. The most typical discharge in preterm infants is a rhythmic delta activity with a steeply ascending initial deflection. Focal low-frequency discharges and multifocal spikes or sharp-wave rhythmic discharges are also observed. The ictal discharges tend to be more synchronous over one hemisphere in premature infants than in term neonates. The duration of ictal discharges is quite variable, from a few seconds to several minutes. Their diffusion remains, in most cases, fairly restricted.

### THE PROBLEM OF PURE EEG DISCHARGES

The practice of long-duration EEG monitoring in newborns has shown that many EEG seizure discharges, even long-lasting discharges remain without detectable clinical manifestations. This is especially frequent in small, ill babies and may be particularly common after repetition of prolonged seizures. This dissociation may be in part the result of drug administration ('decoupling' of the clinical from the electrical seizure), particularly phenobarbital. The clinical seizures may then be controlled while the electrical seizure persists. The role of long EEG records is therefore difficult to assess as the significance of isolated discharges is unclear, and their potential to produce brain damage is unknown. In a recent study (McBride *et al.* 2000), the outcome of neonates with electrographic seizures were compared to those that were at risk but did not have electrographic seizures recorded. The authors' data indicated an association between the amount of electrographic seizure activity and subsequent mortality and morbidity in at risk infants in general and in infants with perinatal asphyxia.

## ETIOLOGY

There is a wide range of causes for neonatal convulsions. In addition, apparently idiopathic seizures are found in up to one-third of all cases (Levene 1985). The major known causes include diffuse hypoxic–ischemic encephalopathy (HIE), intracranial infections, and localized ischemic or hemorrhagic events, metabolic disorders, and developmental brain abnormalities (Table 37.1). Prenatal factors play an even more important role than perinatal injury. In recent years, the role of HIE has been discussed, and the importance of prenatal events has been emphasized. Some investigators have proposed to abandon the term HIE and to replace it by the non-committal term of neonatal encephalopathy. Clearly, prenatal factors are important, and acute birth hypoxia may be more damaging when chronic prenatal unfavorable conditions were present. It seems, indeed, likely that many infants with HIE have already suffered harm *in utero*, as shown by the frequency of prenatal placental damage (Gaffney *et al.* 1994; Burke & Tannenberg 1995).

Changes in the incidence of specific etiologies (especially HIE) in recent years are mainly due to increasing sophistication of neonatal care, new developments in diagnostic or preventative techniques, and increased recognition of different etiological agents and disorders. Mizrahi & Kellaway (1998) discussed the changes in etiological factors, as reported in four studies conducted at the Texas Children's Hospital between 1962 and 1995. For example, hypocalcemia was reported in 31% of cases in 1971 and only in 4% in 1995, while the percentage of 23% with unknown etiology in 1971 was reduced to 9%. The percentage of diagnosed infectious disease increased from 4 to 14%.

Seizures related to hypoxic–ischemic encephalopathy (see Chapter 27) are regularly associated with other neurological signs and occur within the first 24–48 h of life. Infections may be frequently due to prenatal viral disease (see Chapter 32), but, in the absence of an obvious cause, bacterial infections remain an important cause, and lumbar puncture is justified, given the relatively high frequency of meningitis (see

**Table 37.1 Main causes of neonatal seizures**

| |
|---|
| Hypoxic–ischemic encephalopathy (may produce both clearly epileptic attacks and seizures probably non-epileptic in nature) |
| Intracranial hemorrhage |
| Subarachnoid hemorrhage (clonic seizures in term infants 1–5 days of age) |
| Intraventricular hemorrhage (mainly tonic seizures and episodes of apnea without EEG correlates, occasionally typical EEG discharges) |
| Intracerebral hematoma (fixed localized clonic seizures) |
| Intracranial infections |
| Bacterial meningitis and/or abscess |
| Viral meningoencephalitis |
| Cerebral malformations |
| Metabolic causes |
| Hypocalcemia (clonic, multifocal seizures) |
| Hypoglycemia |
| Hyponatremia |
| Inborn errors of amino acids or organic acids and $NH_3$ metabolism (often atypical, mostly unassociated with EEG discharges) |
| Molybdenum cofactor deficiency |
| Bilirubin encephalopathy (atypical, no EEG discharges) |
| Pyridoxine dependency |
| Biotinidase deficiency |
| Carbohydrate-deficient glycoprotein syndrome |
| Toxic or withdrawal seizures (probably non-epileptic phenomena in most cases) |
| Familial neonatal convulsions |
| 'Benign' neonatal seizures of unknown origin ('fifth-day fits') |

Source: From Aicardi (1998).

Chapter 33). Hypocalcemia and hypoglycemia are much less common, but treatable, conditions. Early hypocalcemia is usually associated with other problems (e.g. diabetes, intrauterine growth restriction, toxemia, etc.), so another cause for the seizures should be sought in such patients. Rare metabolic causes include pyridoxine dependency (see p. 620), biotine deficiency and familial folinic-acid responsive seizures. In the absence of an obvious cause, systematic administration of vitamin $B_6$, biotin, and perhaps folinic acid is advised, as this may be the simplest and sometimes the only way of making the diagnosis. Localized ischemic events resulting from obstruction of major arterial branches are increasingly being recognized as a cause (see Chapter 22). In such patients, the seizures appear between a few hours and 4–5 days after birth. They are mostly focal clonic in type, and usually remain localized to the same territory, even when they persist for hours. The neurologic status is fairly well preserved, and some babies recover without sequelae, even when residual cavitation is evident on later neuroimaging. In other cases, hemiplegia or other localized deficits eventually appear.

Although the diversity of mechanisms responsible for neonatal paroxysmal behavioral events makes it difficult to determine whether some types of seizures are more or less specifically related to certain etiologic factors (Aicardi 1994), some rough correspondence may exist. Subtle seizures (motor automatisms) are often associated with a picture of neonatal encephalopathy and with depressed awareness, hypotonia, and autonomic symptoms. It seems likely that most such seizures in this context are 'release' phenomena, but some are associated with epileptic discharges. Seizures associated with metabolic disorders are often also subtle, and features like 'pedalling' or 'boxing' have been frequently described in maple syrup urine disease or organic acidemias. However, erratic myoclonus is particularly suggestive of non-ketotic hyperglycinemia, although it may be observed with other, including metabolic, disorders. Clonic partial seizures repeated in a fixed location are suggestive of focal ischemic lesions. Late hypocalcemic seizures are usually multifocal and occur in a newborn in good general condition and with a ravenous appetite.

## NEONATAL SEIZURES IN THEIR OVERALL CONTEXT (SYNDROMES)

The ILAE classification recognizes four syndromes, two of them classified within the group of idiopathic epilepsies (Benign idiopathic familial and non-familial neonatal convulsions) and the remaining two within the group of symptomatic epilepsies (Early Myoclonic Epileptic Encephalopathy and Early Epileptic Encephalopathy with suppression bursts). Some other epilepsy syndromes such as West syndrome, Benign Myoclonic Epilepsy of Infancy, Severe Myoclonic Epilepsy of infancy (Dravet syndrome) and Migrating Partial Seizures of Infancy, do not really belong to the neonatal period and as such will not be described here, even though their onset may be as early as the end of the first month of life.

The different sets of circumstances and associated clinical pictures depend at least in part on cause. Therefore, ILAE criteria for definition of syndromes, i.e. seizure type and EEG features, are not easily applicable. In all cases, it may be more in conformity to clinical practice to consider the circumstances of presentation and major clinical features, particularly the neurological context. Two groups can be schematically distinguished: early-onset seizures in severely affected neonates and seizures in relatively well babies.

### SUBGROUP OF NEUROLOGICALLY IMPAIRED NEONATES WITH EARLY-ONSET SEIZURES

In this group, neonates present with signs of severe neurologic impairment and altered vigilance. Hypotonia, sucking difficulties, lack of reactivity, and absent primary reflexes are almost regularly associated. Seizures that occur during the first 3 days of life, frequently the result of HIE or inborn errors of metabolism, are often fragmentary or subtle in type and tend to occur in long series. Subtle seizures, myoclonic jerks, or tonic spasms are frequent. Very abnormal interictal

EEG patterns are usually recorded. The electrolytic disturbances (hypoglycemia, hypocalcemia or hypomagnesemia) that may be observed usually are not the primary cause. Such an electroclinical picture may also be the result of an intraventricular hemorrhage. Interestingly, local-anesthetic intoxication from inadvertent injection into the infants' scalp at the time of placement of a paracervical, pudendal, or epidural block produces a similar picture of hypotonia, bradycardia and hypoventilation. The pupils are fixed to light, and the vestibular reflex (doll's head) is abolished. Seizures occur within 6 h of birth. Despite the apparent severity, the prognosis is excellent when the diagnosis is made, and early vigorous supportive treatment is given resulting in complete recovery.

Within this general category, two syndromes have been more clearly described and included in the ILAE classification: Early Myoclonic Encephalopathy or Neonatal Myoclonic Encephalopathy (NNME), first described by Aircardi & Goutières in 1978 and Early-infantile epileptic encephalopathy (EIEE) with suppression burst described by Ohtahara. The neurological status of infants with NNME is always very poor, even at birth, or as soon as the onset of the seizures occurs, with marked hypotonia of truncal muscles and progressive deterioration. More than half of these babies die before one year of age. The main ictal manifestations include partial or fragmentary erratic myoclonus, massive myoclonias, partial motor seizures, and tonic infantile spasms. The EEG features associated with NNME are very distinctive (suppression–burst pattern). The normal background activity is absent. Complex bursts of spikes and irregular, arrhythmic sharp waves lasting for 1–5 s and alternating with flat periods of 3–1 s, during which there is practically no activity, are recorded. Familial cases are frequent. Several associated causes have been reported, including non-ketotic hyperglycinemia. Similar findings have been reported in infants with D-glyceric acidemia (Brandt *et al.* 1974) and in a case with propionic acidemia (Vigevano *et al.* 1981). The relationship between NNME and EIEE described by Ohtahara has given rise to some nosological controversy. EIEE consistently includes tonic spasms and does not feature erratic myoclonus. The condition seems to remain static over time. The main causes are thought to be malformative or clastic brain lesions, but metabolic causes have been recently reported. The paroxysmal bursts seem to be longer in EIEE than in NNME, and the periods of suppression shorter. There is a tendency in the course of EIEE to evolve into West syndrome, which may be regarded as an early form. NNME, however, is characterized by erratic myoclonus and partial seizures and may also evolve to infantile spasms. It may thus be difficult to make a clear-cut distinction between the two conditions.

## SUBGROUP OF NEUROLOGICALLY WELL NEONATES

This is a relatively infrequent pattern. The seizures can be either symptomatic or idiopathic. In the symptomatic group, seizures are often the result of an infarct or of primary subarachnoid hemorrhage or of localized intracerebral bleeding. They are commonly observed on the second day of life, may be focalized to the same site, particularly when due to an infarct, or shift from one area to another. Interictally, neurologic examination is normal. The EEG may also be practically normal. As discussed above, although localized deficits may follow intra-parenchymal hemorrhage, the prognosis for this group is rather favorable.

Two syndromes were identified in the ILAE classification within the idiopathic group (Familial and Non-familial Benign Idiopathic Neonatal Convulsions). The main difference between these two syndromes is the presence or absence of a family history of neonatal convulsions of unknown etiology and both have a favorable outcome. In individual patients, the initial diagnosis may be difficult, since the 'benign evolution', which is often wrongly thought to be part of the definition of the syndrome, can only be suspected but not confirmed until after an undetermined lapse of time.

### Benign familial neonatal convulsions (BFNC)

The prevalence of the syndrome is unknown. Plouin (1994) reviewed the data from 334 cases of BFNC belonging to 38 families published since the initial description by Rett & Teubel (1964). Seizures, usually clonic, have their onset within 2–15 days of life, are frequently recurrent, but stop spontaneously within a few days or weeks. The neonates are neurologically normal. Interictal EEG is either normal or shows minimal focal or multifocal abnormalities or a pattern of 'theta pointu alternant'. Patterns suggestive of a poor prognosis, such as paroxysmal or inactive EEG, have never been reported. Further psychomotor development is favorable. The overall rates of secondary epilepsy and febrile convulsions were 11 and 5%, respectively. The rate of febrile convulsions is comparable to that of the general population. The syndrome is classified among idiopathic generalized epilepsies, but some authors (Mizrahi & Kellaway 1998) consider that the electroclinical presentation suggests an age-dependent partial idiopathic epilepsy. Diagnosis from BINC rests entirely on the occurrence of similar events in relatives, consistent with an autosomal dominant transmission. The first gene related to BFNC was identified on chromosome 20 (20q13.2) in 1989, and a second locus was found on chromosome 8q. In some families, no linkage was found either with chromosome 20 or with chromosome 8, confirming genetic heterogeneity. Mutations in two potassium channels have been defined (see also Bates & Gardiner 1999).

### Benign idiopathic neonatal convulsions (BINC)

Since the first report by Dehan *et al.* (1977), several authors have reported on BINC (Plouin 1994; Hirsch *et al.* 1993). Because of their usually late occurrence, these seizures were also referred to as 'fifth day fits'. Plouin (1994) reviewed the literature on 299 cases. Clinical seizures consist of repeated seizures, mostly clonic and/or apneic, with onset between 3 and 7 days of age. The EEG discharges of sharp waves or spikes occur on a relatively normal background tracing. The pattern described as 'theta pointu alternant' is present in almost 60% of the cases but is not specific for the syndrome. It is characterized by a dominant theta activity, alternating or discontinuous, unreactive, with sharp waves. The natural course of the seizures is self-limited, and there is no identifiable etiology. However, clinicians must be aware of the fact that the definition of the syndrome is rather loose and that BINC remains a diagnosis of exclusion, and all possible causes should have been ruled out. It is important to keep in mind that late in such cases, even long-repeated seizures without severe interictal EEG abnormality are usually of a favorable prognosis. Similar seizures may take place later in life and are difficult to separate clearly from the partial infantile seizure syndrome described by Vigevano *et al.* (1981).

## COURSE AND PROGNOSIS

The uncertainties, mentioned many times above, regarding the true nature of neonatal epileptic seizures and related paroxysmal events as well as the various etiologies, explain why it is impossible to assign an overall prognosis to neonatal seizures. In addition, there is still no consensus as to whether epileptic seizures *per se* are responsible for a compromised long-term outcome. As a result, the significance of reported neurologic outcomes is rather difficult to assess because of the considerable variations, in different studies reported, in the timing and description of neurologic evaluation, categorization of the results, and etiologies considered. Both acute and chronic sequelae must be considered.

With the evolution of obstetric management and neonatal intensive care facilities, a decrease in mortality rates from 40 to 15–20% has been reported. However, the incidence of neurologic sequelae in survivors remained approximately the same, usually quoted as 30–35% (for discussion, see Aicardi 1994; Volpe 1995; Mizrahi & Kellaway 1998). Such stability may simply express the fact that, in recent years, more sophisticated and detailed criteria are used to evaluate these babies. The possibility of late perceptual or specific learning difficulties in children with neonatal seizures remains to be explored.

All authors agree that the cause of the seizures is the most important determinant of prognosis. In fact, it is the degree of brain injury and nature of brain damage responsible for the seizures that influences outcome. Other prognostic factors such as age at onset of seizures or type, repetition, and duration of seizures are largely consequent upon the nature and extent of damage. The recognized prognostic value of the interictal EEG also reflects the depth and extent of cerebral insult. A normal background EEG pattern with well-organized sleep stages is associated with a 75% or greater chance of the infant being normal by 5 years (Lombroso 1983). Legido *et al.* (1991) reported that infants with electrographic seizures frequent enough to be detected on 'randomly timed EEG examinations' had an unfavorable prognosis.

Whether the occurrence of the seizures themselves can produce or augment the brain damage that is originally responsible for the seizures remains a controversial point. It is well known that even prolonged and/or repeated seizures occurring with hypocalcemia or even because of an unknown cause have a favorable outcome. Recent data suggest that hippocampal injury following prolonged seizures may be observed in mature brains, but whether such phenomena occur in the immature brain continues to be debated (Holmes *et al.* 1999). Similar controversies concern seizure-induced excessive release of excitatory amino acids and their resulting effects. If it were confirmed that neonatal seizures are harmful above and beyond their cause, then the need for anticonvulsant treatment would be more rationally founded.

Few studies have specifically studied the relationship between neonatal seizures and the eventual development of epilepsy later in life. Late epilepsy occurs in 10–26% of patients but may be as high as 81% when brain malformation is the cause. Following EEG-confirmed seizures, Legido *et al.* (1991) found that epilepsy developed in 15 of 27 survivors of a group of 40 patients, most of whom had hypoxic–ischemic encephalopathy. The first postnatal seizure occurred at an average corrected age of 12.7 months, despite ongoing anticonvulsant treatment in nine of the 15. Predictors of recurrent seizures included the presence of coma at the time of neonatal events, a duration of neonatal seizures of more than 10 h, and an abnormal background EEG in 68% of cases. The age of onset of the neonatal seizures, Apgar score at birth, and gestational age were not indicative of the risk of later epilepsy. Late seizures were infantile spasms in seven of 15 (47%), complex partial seizures in four, and generalized tonic–clonic seizures in four. Recurrent seizures are only uncommonly isolated sequelae. In most cases, later seizures are associated with cerebral palsy and mental retardation. Infantile spasms associated with tetraplegia and microcephaly are observed in a small proportion of infants with repeated neonatal convulsions of anoxic origin.

When a precise diagnosis of a syndrome is possible, a more accurate prognosis can be proposed. Otherwise, particularly during the acute period, predicting outcome can be rather challenging. Prognosis should be determined not only on the basis of presence or absence of seizures but also on the basis of global neurologic evaluation, consideration of etiologic factors, neuroimaging study results, and EEG data. All authors agree that the essential predictor of prognosis for infants with neonatal seizures is the cause of the convulsions.

## TREATMENT

Management of paroxysmal events should depend, at least theoretically, on the mechanism of the attacks. Accurate diagnosis, characterization of the nature of the paroxysmal phenomena, and correlation with the EEG data are of importance. It has been argued that, when dealing with non-epileptic attacks such as release brainstem phenomena, administration of anti-epileptic drugs might be potentially dangerous by increasing cortical depression, thus facilitating brainstem tonic discharges (Camfield & Camfield, 1987).

Therapy of neonatal seizures has a triple objective: support of vital functions, treatment of the cause(s) of the attacks and control of the seizures by antiepileptic drugs, when epileptic in origin. Initial general management measures are the first indispensable step, independently of the nature and etiology of the paroxysmal events. Monitoring of vital constants, such as respiration and heart rate, body temperature, or blood pressure, is essential. Continuous EEG recording is desirable and extremely useful, but when dealing with recurring seizures, obtaining an EEG should not delay initiation of treatment. An intravenous line should be established for rapid correction of any metabolic derangement. Administration of dexamethasone or the use of osmotic agents is indicated for the treatment of established cerebral edema remains controversial (see p. 491), while the necessity of prophylactic treatment remains in dispute. Severely disturbed infants may require therapeutic respiratory muscle paralysis to facilitate assisted ventilation. This will prevent clinical manifestations of seizures, thus necessitating EEG monitoring. Levels of electrolytes, pH, calcium, and magnesium should be obtained and fluid administration restricted to 75% of that normally required amount to avoid dilutional hyponatremia.

Specific treatment is immediately indicated whenever a treatable cause for the seizures is found. If hypoglycemia is present, 2–4 ml/kg of a 20–30% solution of glucose is given intravenously. A slow intravenous injection of 2.5–5% calcium gluconate is administered with electrocardiographic monitoring to neonates with hypocalcemia. Magnesium sulfate, 2–8 ml of a 2–3% solution, intravenously, or 0.2 ml/kg of a 50% solution, intramuscularly, is added when there is associated hypomagnesemia. Serum levels of magnesium should be monitored to avoid its potential curare-like effect. A trial of pyridoxine (a slow injection of a single dose of 100 mg for all neonates) should be administered, but excessively high doses should be avoided as hypotonia and apnea can result. Other metabolic derangements are uncommon and are more often responsible for non-epileptic movements than for true seizures.

There is no agreement as to which seizures require antiepileptic drug treatment, what are the drugs to be used first, the timing for starting them, or the duration. Whether electrical discharges without clinical manifestations justify antiepileptic treatment has not been established. Although it is not possible to be dogmatic, it seems that only moderate efforts at suppressing purely electrographic seizures are justified. However, further controlled studies are needed to better determine the indication of treating electrographic seizures (McBride *et al.* 2000).

Phenobarbitone or phenytoin are commonly used, particularly by those who recommend immediate therapy with large doses of long-acting anticonvulsants. Large loading doses are usually prescribed (phenytoin, a single i.v. dose of 20 mg/kg, not to be repeated – further doses can be administered under the control of blood level to reach a level of 15–20 μg/ml; phenobarbitone, 20–25 mg/kg/day intravenously to reach a blood level of at least 20 μg/ml). For both drugs, the maintenance dose used of the order of 3–5 mg/kg/day. For phenytoin, the loading dose should be administered slowly at a rate not exceeding 50 mg/min to avoid disturbances of cardiac rhythm. Fosphenytoin, a new phenytoin pro-drug, offers advantages over phenytoin for IV administration. Clinical studies with IV and IM fosphenytoin demonstrate that the efficacy, safety and pharmacokinetics of this drug are similar in 5- and 18-year-old children and young adults. The safety and pharmacokinetic profiles of IV and IM fosphenytoin in neonates and infants is currently being investigated (Pellock 1996). For phenobarbitone, pharmacokinetics at this age demand close monitoring of blood levels to permit rapid dosage adjustment. Data concerning the use of other drugs such as valproate, primidone or carbamazepine are limited.

Anticonvulsant agents may have deleterious effects on the neonatal brain (Mikati *et al.* 1994), and their efficacy has not been established. In one study, the apparent effectiveness of phenobarbitone and phenytoin was the same and did not exceed 38% (Painter *et al.* 1994). More importantly, they found that the seizure decreased on treatment, mainly when a decreasing trend had been observed previously, and that the drugs failed to prevent the onset of subsequent seizures, to delay the time of onset of recurrent seizures, or to attenuate the severity of recurrence.

Those investigators who believe that only repeated seizures are harmful tend to postpone initiation of long-acting antiepileptic agents until diagnosis is clarified, unless there is evidence of systemic effects. Lombroso (1983) favors the initial use of short-acting drugs, especially in cases in which seizures seem likely to be transient, such as mild hypoxic–ischemic encephalopathy, sepsis, or cryptogenic seizures. Our own practice is to use benzodiazepines as first drugs, which often avoids the use of other drugs. The benzodiazepines, especially lorazepam, may be satisfactory as a first line or even as the only treatment (Deshmukh *et al.* 1986; Hakeem & Wallace 1990). Lorazepam is rapidly effective and has the advantage of a longer action and absence of secondary release from brain and fat tissue. The usual dose of 0.05 mg/kg can be repeated at 6-h intervals. Diazepam can be used intravenously or rectally at doses of 0.5–1 mg/kg, repeatable at 4- to 6-h intervals, for 24–48 h. Alternatively, continuous infusion at a rate of 0.7–2.7 mg/h for up to 24 h followed by slow tapering has yielded good results. Clonazepam has also been used successfully in neonates.

The optimal duration of therapy for neonatal seizures has not been determined. Some investigators advise discontinuation of drug treatment as soon as the seizures have stopped, while others advocate continuation of therapy until all neurologic abnormalities have disappeared. Intermediate approaches take into account the likelihood of recurring seizures after discontinuation of treatment, but this is difficult to predict. Moreover, continuation of treatment does not regularly prevent later epilepsy, even though few data are available in this regard. Our opinion is that continuation of antiepileptic treatment for more than a few weeks is justified when there is a high likelihood of recurrent seizures, specifically in cases of a dysgenetic brain defect. For acute conditions such as hemorrhages, mild or moderate hypoxic-ischemic encephalopathy, and cryptogenic neonatal seizures, there is no need to continue therapy. Waiting for epilepsy to appear, thus avoiding the potential risks of chronic antiepileptic drug administration to developing infants, is perhaps a safer alternative.

Although it is hoped that successful antiepileptic drug treatment of neonatal seizures will either prevent adverse sequelae or improve the long-term outcome, specific criteria for selection of individuals to be treated and even more to be kept under long-term treatment remain controversial. Most clinicians use personal judgement and experience in management of neonatal seizures (Mizrahi & Kellaway 1998). Much remains to be done to evaluate therapy – taking into account the nature of the seizures observed, the epilepsy syndromes, and the most frequent etiological factors – and to establish objective protocols of drug administration and assessment of results.

### Key Points

- Early diagnosis of neonatal seizures and their differentiation from similar nonepileptic phenomena, essential for current management, can be suspected from the clinical features. Neurophysiological confirmation is usually required.
- The etiological context and the results of neurological evaluation are of crucial importance in determining diagnosis and management.
- The recognized prognostic value of the interictal EEG also reflects the depth and extent of cerebral insult.
- The stereotyped nature of the events, the absence of sensitivity to stimuli and to restraint, favor the diagnosis of epileptic seizures. Video-EEG documents might be used to seek advice from an experienced examiner.
- Clonic seizures may be focal or multifocal. Tonic seizures may be focal or generalized.
- Myoclonic jerks may be provoked by stimulation and, from a pathophysiological point of view, they may or may not be epileptic.
- Subtle or minimal seizures comprise various behavioral phenomena that may or may not be epileptic.
- Two main elements, commonly associated, constitute the EEG discharges in newborns: *abnormal paroxysmal rhythms* and *repetitive spikes or sharp waves*. Abnormal paroxysmal rhythms consist of rhythmic wave forms resembling alpha, theta, beta or delta activity, or a mixture of these. Focal discharges of sharp waves may be relatively fast (2–4 Hz) or occur at a slower rate (~1 Hz), a pattern that resembles the periodic lateralized discharges (PLEDs) of older patients.
- In premature infants, the EEG findings tend to be more stereotyped and purely EEG discharges are especially common. Sharp waves are uncommon.
- The practice of long-duration EEG monitoring in newborns has shown that many EEG seizure discharges, even long-lasting ones, remain without detectable clinical manifestations.
- ILAE criteria for definition of syndromes, i.e. seizure type and EEG features, are not easily applicable. In all cases, it may be more in conformity to clinical practice to consider the circumstances of presentation and major clinical features, particularly the neurological context. Two groups can be schematically distinguished: early-onset seizures in severely affected neonates and seizures in relatively well babies.
- Whether the occurrence of the seizures themselves can produce or augment the brain damage that is originally responsible for the seizures remains a controversial point.
- Therapy of neonatal seizures has a triple objective: support of vital functions; treatment of the cause(s) of the attacks; and control of the seizures by AEDs, when epileptic in origin.

## REFERENCES


Aicardi J (1990) Neonatal seizures. In Dan M & Gram L (eds) *Comprehensive Epileptology*. New York, Raven Press, pp. 99–112.

Aicardi J (1994) *Epilepsy in Children*, 2nd edition, New York: Raven Press.

Aicardi J (1998) Epilepsy and other seizure disorders. In: *Aicardi's Diseases of the Nervous System in Childhood*. London: MacKeith Press, 2nd edn; pp. 575–637.

Bates L & Gardiner M (1999) Genetics of inherited epilepsies. *Epileptic Disord* 1:7–20.

Ben-Ari Y, Cherubini E, Corradetti R & Gaiarsa J L (1989) Giant synaptic potentials in immature rat CA3 hippocampal neurons. *J Physiol* 416:303–325.

Ben-Ari Y, Cherubini E & Krnjevic K (1998) Changes in voltage dependence of NMDA currents during development. *Neurosci Lett* 94:88–92.

Bergman I, Painter M J, Hirsch R P *et al.* (1983) Outcome of neonates with convulsions treated in an intensive care unit. *Ann Neurol* 14:642–647.

Brandt N J, Rasmussen K, Brandt S & Schonheyder F (1974) D-glyceric acidemia with hyperglycinemia: A new inborn error of metabolism. *BMJ* 4:334–336.

Burke C J & Tannenberg A E (1995) Prenatal brain damage and placental infarction – an autopsy study. *Dev Med Child Neurol* 37:555–562.

Camfield P R & Camfield C S (1987) Neonatal seizures: A commentary on selected aspects. *J Child Neurol* 2:244–251.

Cherubini E, Galarsa J L & Ben-Ari Y (1991) GABA: an excitatory transmitter in early postnatal life. *Trends Neurosci* 14:515–519.

Clancy R R, Legido A & Lewis D (1988) Occult neonatal seizures. *Epilepsia* 29:256–261.

Dehan M, Quilleron D, Navelet Y *et al.* (1977) Les convulsions du cinquième jour de vie: un nouveau syndrome? *Arch Franç Pédiatr* 34:730–742.

Deshmukh A, Wittert W, Schnitzler E & Mangurten H H (1986) Lorazepam in the treatment of refractory neonatal seizures: a pilot study. *Am J Dis Child* 140:1042–1044.

Dreyfus-Brisac C & Curzi-Dascalova L (1979) The EEG during the first year of life. In: Remond A. (ed.) *Handbook of Electroencephalography and Clinical Neurophysiology*. Amsterdam: Elsevier; Vol. 6, Part B, pp. 24–30.

Dulac O, Chugani H & Dalla Beranrdina B (eds) (1994) *Infantile Spasms and West Syndrome*. London: W B Saunders.

Fenichel G M (1985) Seizure in newborns. In: *Neonatal Neurology*, edited by G M Fenichel, pp. 25–52. Churchill Livingstone, Edinburgh.

Fenichel G M, Olson B J & Fitzpatrick J E (1980) Heart rate changes in convulsive and nonconvulsive neonatal apnea. *Ann Neurol* 7:577–582.

Gaffney G, Sellers S, Flavell V *et al.* (1994) Case control study of intra-partum care, cerebral palsy, and perinatal death. *BMJ* 308:743–750.

Goldberg H J (1983) Neonatal convulsions – a 10 year review. *Arch Dis Childh* 58:976–978.

Hablitz J J (1987) Spontaneous ictal-like discharges and sustained potential shifts in the developing rat neocortex. *J Neurophysiol* 58:1052–1065.

Hakeem V F & Wallace S J (1990) EEG monitoring of therapy for neonatal seizures. *Dev Med Child Neurol* 32:858–864.

Hellstrom-Westas L, Rosen I & Svenningsen S W (1985) Silent seizures in sick children in early life. *Acta Paediatr Scand* 74:741–748.

Hirsch E, Velez A, Sellal F *et al.* (1993) Electroclinical signs of benign neonatal familial convulsions. *Ann Neurology* 34:835–841.

Holmes G L (1985) Neonatal seizures. In: Pedley T A & Meldrum B S (eds) *Recent Advances in Epilepsy*. Edinburgh: Churchill Livingstone; pp. 207–237.

Holmes G L (1997) Epilepsy in the developing brain: lessons from the laboratory and clinic. *Epilepsia* 38:12–30.

Holmes G L, Sarkisian M, Ben-Ari Y, Chevassus-Au-Louis N (1999) Effects of recurrent seizures in the developing brain. In: Nehlig A, Motte J, Moshé S L, Plouin P, (eds) *Childhood Epilepsies and Brain Development*. John Libbey; pp. 263–276.

Hrachovy R A, Mizrahi E M & Kellaway P (1990) Electroencephalography of the newborn. In: Daly D & Pedley T A (eds) *Current practice of clinical electroencephalography*. New York, NY: Raven, 2nd edn; pp. 210–242.

Johnston M V (1996) Developmental aspects of epileptogenesis. *Epilepsia* 37, Suppl. 1:S2–S9.

Kellaway P & Hrachovy R A (1983) Status epilepticus in newborns: A perspective on neonatal seizures. In: *Advances in Neurology, Vol. 34: Status Epilepticus*, edited by A V Delgado-Escueta, C G Wasterlain, D M Treiman and R J Porter, pp. 93–99. Raven Press, New York.

Knauss T A, Thomas A, Coldevin B *et al.* (1978) Neonatal paroxysmal monorrhythmic alpha activity. *Arch Neurol* 35:104–107.

Kroll J S (1985) Pyridoxine for neonatal seizures: an unexpected danger. *Dev Med Child Neurol* 27:377–379.

Lanska M J, Lanska D J & Baumann R J *et al.* (1995) A population-based study of neonatal seizures in Fayette County, Kentucky. *Neurology* 45:724–732.

Legido A, Clancy R R & Berman P H (1988) Recent advances in the diagnosis, treatment and prognosis of neonatal seizures. *Pediatr Neurol* 4:79–86.

Legido A, Clancy R R & Berman P H (1991) Neurologic outcome after electroencephalographically proven neonatal seizures. *Pediatrics* 88:583–596.

Levene M (1985) Aetiology of neonatal seizures. In: Ross E & Reynolds E (eds) *Paediatric perspectives on epilepsy*. Chichester, UK: Wiley; pp. 11–22.

Lombroso C T (1982) Neonatal electroencephalography. In: Niedermeyer E & Lopes de Silva F (eds) *Electroencephalography*. Baltimore, MD: Urban & Schwarzenberg; pp. 599–637.

Lombroso C T (1983) Prognosis in neonatal seizures. In: Delgado-Escueta A V, Wasterlain C G, Treiman D M *et al.* (eds) *Advances in neurology, Vol. 34, status epilepticus*. New York, NY: Raven Press.

McBride M C, Laroia N, Guillet R (2000) Electrographic seizures in neonates correlate with poor neurodevelopmental outcome. *Neurology* 55:506–513.

Mikati M A, Holmes G L & Chronopoulos A *et al.* (1994) Phenobarbital modifies seizure-related brain injury in the developing brain. *Ann Neurology* 36:425–433.

Mizrahi E M & Kellaway P (1987) Characterization and classification of neonatal seizures. *Neurology* 37:1837–1844.

Mizrahi E M & Kellaway P (1998) *Diagnosis and Management of Neonatal Seizures*. New York: Lippincott-Raven.

Moshé S L (1987) Epileptogenesis and the immature brain. *Epilepsia*, 28:S3–S15.

Ogier H & Aicardi J (1998) Metabolic diseases. In: *Aicardi's diseases of the nervous system in childhood*. London: MacKeith Press, 2nd edn; pp. 245–323.

Painter M J, Scher M S, Paneth N S *et al.* (1994) Randomized trial of phenobarbital vs phenytoin treatment of neonatal seizures. *Pediatric Research* 35, 384A.

Pellock J M (1996) Fosphenytoin use in children. *Neurology* 46 (suppl 1): S14–S16.

Plouin P (1994) Benign idiopathic neonatal convulsions (familial and non-familial). Open questions about these syndromes. In: Wolf P (Ed.) *Epileptic Seizures and Syndromes*. London: John Libbey, pp 193–202.

Radvanyi-Bouvet M F, Vallecalle M H, Morel-Kahn F *et al.* (1985) Seizures and electrical discharges in premature infants. *Neuropediatrics* 16:143–148.

Rett A & Teubel R (1964) Neugeborenen Krampfe im Rahmen einer epileptisch belasten Familie. *Wien Klin Wschr* 76:609–613.

Ronen G M & Penney S (1995) The epidemiology of clinical neonatal seizures in Newfoundland, Canada: a five year cohort. *Ann Neurol* 38:518–519.

Scher M S, Aso K, Beggarly M, Hamid M Y, Steppe D A & Painter M J (1993) Electrographic seizures in pre-term and full-term neonates: clinical correlates, assoicated brain lesions, and risk for neurologic sequelae. *Pediatrics* 91:128–134.

Schwartzkoin P A (1994) Cellular electrophysiology of human epilepsy. *Epilepsy Res* 17:185–192.

Vigevano F, Bosman C, Giscondi A, Maccagnami F, Sevanti G & Sergo M (1981) Neonatal myoclonic epileptic encephalopathy without hyperglycinemia. *Electroencephalogr Clin Neurophysiol* 52:52–53.

Volpe J J (1995) Neonatal seizures. In: Volpe J J (ed.) *Neurology of the newborn*. Philadelphia, PA: WB. Saunders, 3rd edn; pp. 172–207.

Watanabe K, Hara K, Miyazaki S *et al.* (1982) Apneic seizures in the newborn. *Am J Dis Child* 15:584–596.

Willis J & Gould J B (1980) Periodic alpha seizures with apnea in the newborn. *Dev Med Child Neurol* 22:214–222.

# Section IX
# The special senses

# Chapter 38

# Disorders of vision

A. R. Fielder

## INTRODUCTION

This chapter is primarily concerned with the neuro-ophthalmology of the first 6 months of life. Thus, ocular disorders such as infantile cataract, glaucoma, or retinopathy of prematurity are not considered here. In view of the rapid maturation occurring during infancy, various aspects of normal development are reviewed before considering the abnormal. Individual conditions are covered only briefly, and referencing commences with a bibliography of major texts, followed by a list of the cited articles.

## EYE MOVEMENTS

### NORMAL EYE MOVEMENTS

In this section, a brief description of the various types of eye movements is given. For more detailed accounts, there are several reviews (Hoyt *et al.* 1982; Boothe *et al.* 1985; Fielder 1985; Harris 1997a, b).

#### Embryology of the extraocular muscles

The extraocular muscles are formed as condensations of mesoderm that commence differentiation at 6 weeks of gestation and are fully formed by 12 weeks. By this time, the ocular motor nerves have reached their destination. The supranuclear eye movement system, which is responsible for feeding information to the brainstem ocular motor nuclei, is not fully developed until after full term.

#### Fetal eye movements

Eye movements can be detected, using ultrasonography, from 16 weeks of gestation (Birnholz 1981; Prechtl & Nijhuis 1983; Inoue *et al.* 1986). These are discussed in detail in Chapter 4. Eye movements commence as slow changes in eye position, but these later become faster. Rapid eye movements are seen between 30 and 33 weeks of gestational age (GA[1]) and are organized into periods of activity, which after 36 weeks GA are related to fetal behavioural state.

[1] Gestational age (GA) is the period *in utero* and is calculated from the first day of the last menstrual period. Once birth has occurred, the term 'gestational age' is inappropriate, and postnatal age (PNA), postmenstrual age (PMA), and postconceptual age (PCA) are used. PMA is preferred to denote GA plus postnatal age, in weeks. PCA is also used inaccurately and synonymously to PMA.

### TYPES OF EYE MOVEMENT

Conjugate eye movements are movements of both eyes in the same direction and are also called versions. In dysjugate movements, the two eyes move in opposite directions, and these are called vergence movements. Conjugate movements include pursuit, saccadic, optokinetic, and vestibulo-ocular eye movements. Pursuit movements enable the eyes to follow a relatively slow-moving target and hold the image on the fovea of the retina so that the target is seen clearly. If the object moves too fast for the pursuit system, a catch-up saccade is required to refixate the image back on to the fovea. Saccades are fast movements that allow us to change our direction of visual interest and direct the object of interest on to the fovea. Both optokinetic and vestibulo-ocular movements coordinate head and eye movements during body movements. Each type of eye movement is subserved by a separate supranuclear system, but all share a final common infranuclear pathway from the ocular motor nuclei to the eye muscles.

Finally, eye movement control requires a neural integrator that enables a chosen and eccentric eye position (gaze) to be maintained, even in the dark (absence of vision). The neural substrates include brain stem and cerebellar components (Harris 1997b).

#### Eye movements in infancy

The distinction between normal and abnormal eye movements in the neonatal period is not always easy to determine.

##### Ocular alignment and excursion

The eyes of neonates commonly appear divergent (Fig. 38.1), particularly if they are born prematurely (Rethy 1969). This has been studied by Nixon *et al.* (1985) and Archer *et al.* (1989), and while most neonates appear to be divergent, by 3 and 6 months of age, 75 and 97%, respectively, had no deviation. These authors suggested that in the normal course of development, the eyes are initially divergent, but this diminishes over the ensuing few weeks. This view has been challenged by Thorn *et al.* (1994) and Horwood (1993), who say that in many instances, the divergent appearance is due, in part, to the shape of the neonatal eye (large angle κ) and absence of convergence until around 3 months of age.

Horizontal gaze probably develops before vertical (Jones, quoted by McGinnis 1930).

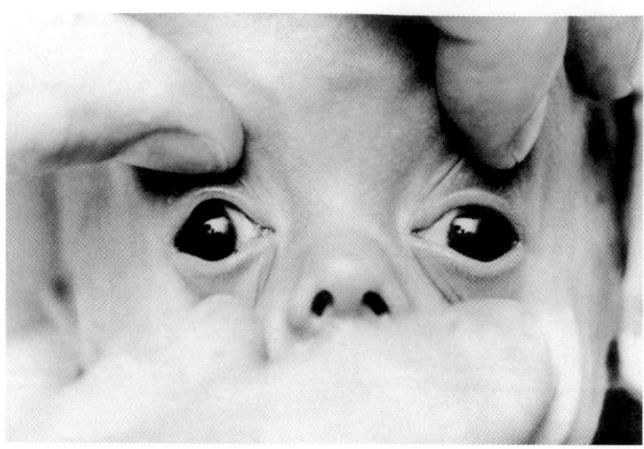

Figure 38.1 The divergent appearance of the eyes of a preterm neonate.

### Pursuit movements

The pursuit system enables the eyes to follow a moving target accurately and smoothly while maintaining foveal fixation, so that during a pursuit movement, clear vision is maintained. The neonate can only make slow smooth eye and head movements (Kremenitzer *et al.* 1979; Roucoux *et al.* 1983; Harris 1997b).

Tests of pursuit involve following a slow-moving target, or the slow phase of optokinetic nystagmus (see below).

### Saccadic movements

The saccadic system allows us to change our direction of visual interest and place the new object of regard on to the fovea. An everyday example is the shifting of gaze from the end of one line to the beginning of the next whilst reading. Saccades are rapid movements, and the example given is a voluntary movement, but saccades also include reflex changes of fixation and the fast phases of all forms of nystagmus (vestibular and optokinetic nystagmus). In contrast to pursuit, vision is partially suppressed during a saccade. For instance, the reader is not aware of the fixational shift when gaze switches from the end of one line to the beginning of the next line of text.

The infant achieves refixation by means of multiple hypometric saccades (Aslin & Salapatek 1975; Regal *et al.* 1983; Roucoux *et al.* 1983; Harris *et al* 1993). Infants rely more on coordinated head and eye movements than do adults when shifting gaze. By the age of 1 year, the saccadic system has developed, enabling a change of fixation on to an eccentric target to be achieved by using a single saccade. Clinically, these changes are easily observed: for example, it takes much longer to attract the visual interest of a neonate to a novel stimulus in the periphery of the visual field compared with a 9-month-old infant.

Tests of saccadic function involve inducing refixation eye movements, and voluntary and command movements.

### Optokinetic nystagmus

This response is elicited by moving a striped tape or drum across the field of vision. It is characterized by a slow (following) phase in the direction of the moving stripe followed by a fast corrective phase, which returns the eye to its original position. The amplitude of the optokinetic nystagmus (OKN) response is about 15°. Functionally, OKN is part of the vestibulo-ocular reflex (VOR) and coordinates head and eye movements, ensuring clear vision during body movements. OKN can be elicited from the first day of life in the full-term infant (McGinnis 1930; Gorman *et al.* 1957).

Before the age of 3 months, an OKN response can be obtained when the tape is moved in a temporal-to-nasal direction but not in a nasal-to-temporal direction when each eye is tested separately. In early infancy, vision may be subserved largely at a subcortical level (Atkinson 1992), and after 3 months, this OKN asymmetry disappears due to the establishment of cortical vision (Braddick & Atkinson 1983). For the preterm infant, the transition from asymmetrical to symmetrical OKN occurs later postnatally, corresponding to about 3 months of corrected age (van Hof-van Duin & Mohn 1984a). Persistence of monocular OKN asymmetry beyond this age may be associated with strabismus and an absence of binocular function.

The pathways involved in the OKN response are poorly understood (Braddick & Atkinson 1983; van Hof-van Duin & Mohn 1983). The temporal-to-nasal response is probably mediated to a large extent subcortically, whereas the nasal-to-temporal response requires a functioning cortex. Responses have been obtained in cortical blindness (van Hof-van Duin & Mohn 1983), while more recently, OKN could not be elicited in the absence of a cortex (Braddick *et al.* 1992).

#### *Tests of OKN*

The OKN tape or drum should be moved slowly in both horizontal and vertical directions, the responses being recorded separately in each direction, graded 0 to ++++. Its clinical uses include:

1. Vision assessment. A valuable but crude indication that vision is present. However, this is a test of visibility, not resolution (see later). Be aware of the extremely rare possibility of a positive response in severe visual cortical damage (van Hof-van Duin & Mohn 1983).
2. Eye movements. OKN is a test of both pursuit (slow phase) and saccadic (fast phase) systems, and binocular eye movements. This is also a simple means of detecting subtle slowness of the adducting eye in internuclear ophthalmoplegia.
3. Nystagmus. In infantile (congenital) nystagmus, the OKN responses along the horizontal meridian are characteristically inverted (see later) but normal when the stripes are presented vertically. This is a useful diagnostic aid and helps to differentiate infantile

nystagmus from the variable nystagmus associated with reduced vision. In the latter, OKN response cannot be elicited in any direction.

4. The OKN test procedure may permit the best close-up, hands-off view of the infant's eye and its movements.

### Vestibulo-ocular reflexes

The VOR ensures that the image remains stationary on the retina during head and body movements. Acceleration induces a movement of endolymph in the semicircular canals from which impulses are conveyed by the vestibular nerve to the brainstem and via the medial longitudinal fasciculus to the ocular motor nuclei. The VOR is vital for everyday activities, so that eye movements adapt to, and vision is not disrupted by, body movements.

#### *Tests of the VOR*

There are three clinical tests: the doll's head maneuver, rotation of the infant, and caloric testing.

1. Doll's head maneuver. In the unconscious adult and conscious infant, head rotation induces a conjugate ocular deviation towards the opposite side; head to the left, eyes to the right (Fig. 38.2) – the Doll's head movement. This is only observed in infancy before vision has developed sufficiently to suppress this response, or in the comatose adult patient. A normal response indicates an intact vestibular apparatus and ocular motor system – including the nuclei and peripheral nerves. The doll's head maneuver can therefore be used to detect limitation of ocular movements due to a gaze or cranial nerve palsy. This test is not informative about the pursuit or saccadic systems.
2. Rotational tests. These fall into two groups which induce different responses:

   a. Barany chair rotation. In this laboratory technique, the infant is held upright and is rotated about his or her own vertical axis. This induces an ocular deviation in the direction opposite to the direction of rotation, as in the doll's head maneuver (Eviatar *et al.* 1974). In the premature infant, only a slow tonic deviation is induced, but with increasing gestational age, a recovery fast phase develops, thereby inducing nystagmus.
   b. Rotation at arm's length. For this method, the infant is held upright at arm's length with the head inclined slightly forward and then rotated. This procedure, commonly used in clinical practice, induces a tonic ocular deviation in the direction of the movement (as if the infant is looking ahead of the movement), i.e. rotation to the right, eyes deviate to the right (Fig. 38.3); in the older infant, nystagmus also occurs. This response using a different axis of rotation induces a movement in the opposite direction to that seen using the Barany method.

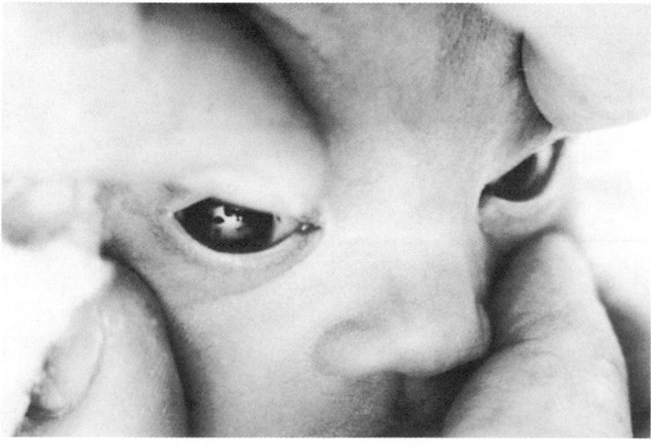

Figure 38.2 Doll's head maneuver: head turn to the left induces a deviation of the eyes to the right.

Whichever method is used, rotation of the premature infant induces a tonic deviation alone, and the fast

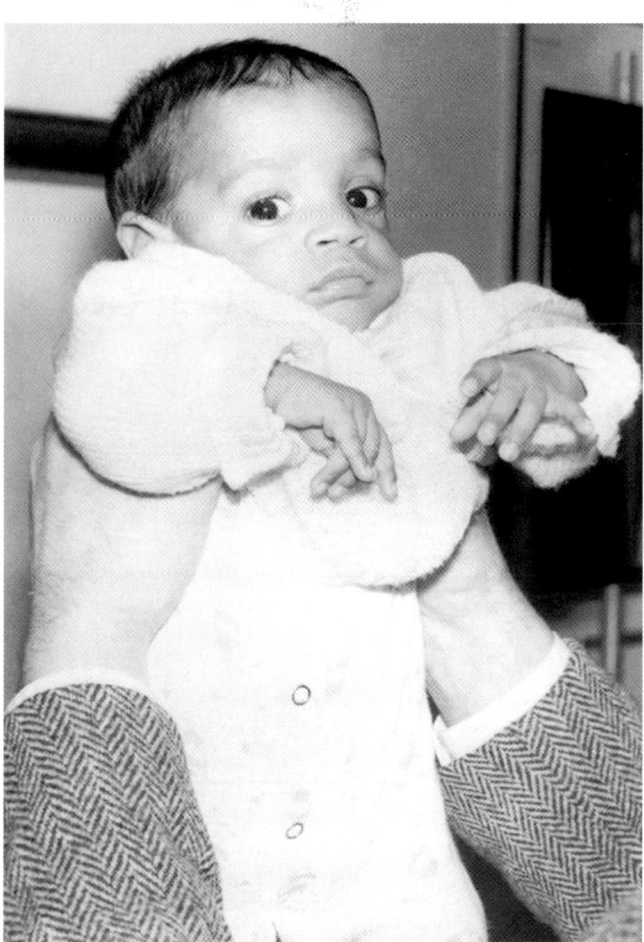

Figure 38.3 Rotation at arm's length. This baby is being rotated to his right, and his eyes deviate to the right – the opposite direction to that seen in the doll's head maneuver.

phase (nystagmus) does not develop until about 45 weeks postmenstrual age (PMA) (Mitchell & Cambon 1969; Eviatar *et al.* 1979; Ornitz *et al.* 1979; Rossi *et al.* 1979; Donat *et al.* 1980; Cordero *et al.* 1983). The behavioral state can influence this test: a fast phase elicited when the infant is awake may not be present when drowsy.

Once the age at which nystagmus occurs has been reached, post-rotatory nystagmus, in the opposite direction to that occurring during rotation, is seen. Its duration depends upon PMA, behavioral state, whether the test is performed in the dark, and the stage of visual development (Mitchell & Cambon 1969; Ornitz *et al.* 1979; Cordero *et al.* 1983), but in the alert sighted infant, post-rotational nystagmus should cease within 5 s.

Rotation at arm's length is simple to perform and provides a great deal of clinically useful information on vision, the saccadic system, the vestibular system, ocular motor nuclei, and infranuclear pathways.

Thus, rotation of the premature infant induces a full ocular deviation, because at this age, vision is not sufficiently developed to modify the VOR. Later, vision dampens the VOR, and hence the per-rotational excursion decreases – these maturational changes are very simple to demonstrate. In clinical terms, severely reduced vision can be suspected if rotation after 3 months of age induces an inordinately large rotational excursion and post-rotatory nystagmus persists for more than 5 s. This test is also a simple method of evaluating the range of eye movements in infancy and enables a sixth nerve palsy to be differentiated from a concomitant convergent squint.

3. Caloric tests. Donat *et al.* (1980) confirmed the observation that the preterm infant cannot generate the fast phase of nystagmus. They observed, on caloric testing, an internuclear ophthalmoplegia in some normal premature infants, indicating immaturity of the medial longitudinal fasciculus, i.e. the brainstem communication between the vestibular apparatus and the ocular motor nuclei. As the doll's head maneuver always induced complete excursion, they considered caloric testing to be a sensitive test of brainstem interconnections.

### Vergence movements

The eye movements considered so far have all been conjugate. Convergence to near targets is clearly dysjugate and cannot be consistently demonstrated until between 2 and 4 months of age (Ling 1942; Aslin 1977, 1993; Thorn *et al.* 1994; Hainline 1998), and accommodation and convergence are both inaccurate before about 4 months of age (Aslin 1993). Fusion, the response to a base-out prism, is not established until 6 months (Aslin 1977). Preterm infants probably show a delay in the development of fusion commensurate with GA (Coakes *et al.* 1979). The onset of sensory (fusion and stereopsis) and motor binocularity (convergence) at the same time indicate the development of cortical function (Thorn *et al.* 1994).

#### *Tests of vergence*

Observe convergence and divergence when an object is brought nearer or taken further away.

## ABNORMAL EYE MOVEMENTS

Many of these conditions have important neurologic or ophthalmologic associations. Some of these disorders persist throughout life, but the emphasis will be directed towards those aspects relating particularly to the neonatal period and early infancy. Details of examination are adequately covered in other texts. Eye movement disorders can be divided into three groups: nuclear and infranuclear disorders, supranuclear disorders, nystagmus, and related oscillations.

### Nuclear and infranuclear disorders

These disorders limit the movement of one eye, whereas supranuclear abnormalities affect the movement of both eyes. Conditions involving the peripheral nerves, in the cavernous sinus, orbit, and the extraocular muscles, as in myasthenia, are all included in this category. This section concentrates on strabismus.

#### Strabismus

Strabismus (squint) may be the first sign of a serious ocular or systemic disorder, and this possibility must always be borne in mind.

It has already been noted that neonates are, or appear to be divergent (see Fig. 38.1) (Rethy 1969; Nixon *et al.* 1985; Archer *et al.* 1989; Thorn *et al.* 1994). With time, this appearance resolves over the ensuing few weeks.

So-called congenital esotropia (concomitant convergent strabismus) is rarely, if ever, present at birth (Nixon *et al.* 1985) but develops within the first 6 months of life and is therefore more appropriately called infantile esotropia. Abduction is often initially considered to be limited, but by rotation, full excursions are generated, so differentiating infantile esotropia from a sixth nerve palsy.

Paralytic squints, either congenital or acquired, are not frequent in early infancy. Congenital palsies may be due to maldevelopment of the cranial nerve nuclei or nerves, or prenatal infection, although in most, the etiology is unknown. The role of birth trauma as a cause of nerve palsy has been greatly overemphasized. A sixth nerve palsy can rarely present at birth as a very large-angle esotropia. If an isolated anomaly, as it usually is, it characteristically resolves spontaneously over a few weeks. While third or sixth nerve palsies are relatively obvious, a congenital fourth nerve palsy, which may have no systemic connotations, can easily be missed for some years until a compensatory head tilt is noted.

In contrast, an acquired cranial nerve palsy frequently denotes a significant neurological disorder such as hydrocephalus, intracranial inflammation, tumor, neurodegenerative disorder and trauma and as such may develop at any age (Fielder 1989).

- Squint may be the presenting feature of an infant with severe neurologic or ophthalmic pathology. A blind eye may diverge or, less commonly, converge (Fig. 38.4), although this usually becomes apparent later in childhood.

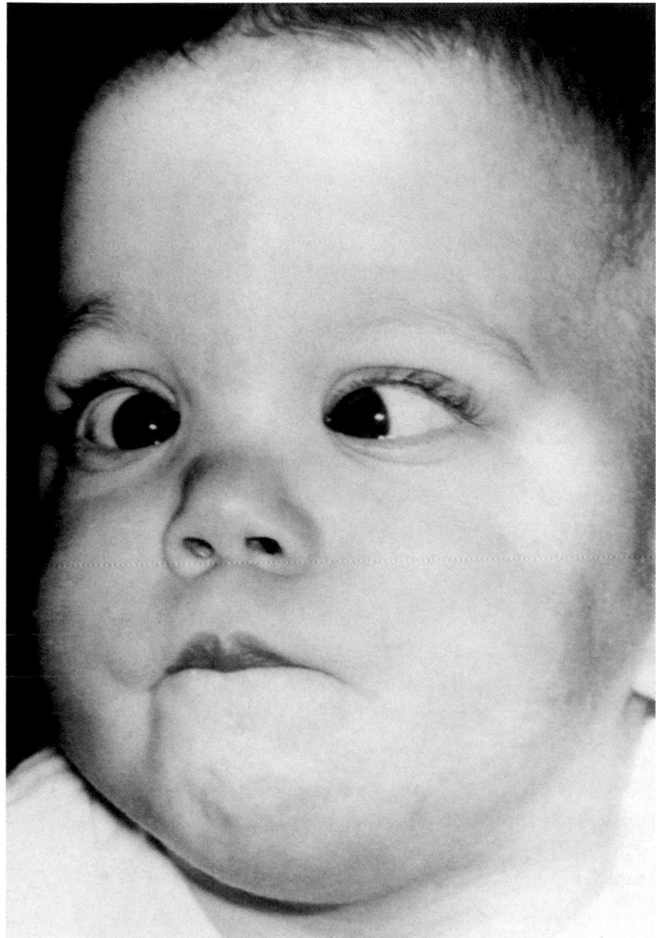

Figure 38.4 Left convergent squint due to ocular pathology. Cicatricial retinopathy of prematurity has severely affected the vision of the left eye.

The prevalence of concomitant squint in the general population is about 2–3% but occurs more commonly in children who have suffered brain damage (von Noorden 1990), or are experiencing neurodevelopmental problems (Bankes 1974). Preterm birth is also associated with an increased incidence of squint from 11 to >30% (Burgess & Johnson 1991; McGinnity & Bryars 1992; Laws *et al.* 1992; Page *et al.* 1993; Bremer *et al.* 1998; Holmstrom *et al.* 1999). Gibson *et al.* (1990) in a follow-up of infants of 1500-g birthweight and below reported strabismus in 50% of those with cystic periventricular leukomalacia and 70% of those with posterior cysts, while Pike *et al.* (1994) reported an incidence of 49%.

- Because of the possibility of coexistent or causative neurologic or ophthalmic pathology, every infant should have a detailed ophthalmic assessment and neurologic work-up, as indicated (Fielder 1989).

## Supranuclear disorders

The supranuclear eye movement system governs the movements of both eyes in unison: pursuit, saccadic, vestibulo-ocular, OKN, and vergence movements. According to the site of the lesion, the various types of movement are affected differentially, but retention of some infranuclear movement and bilaterality, which characterize the supranuclear disorder, differentiates it from a lesion of the infranuclear pathways. Currently, it is impossible to fully differentiate the possible influences on the development of strabismus of: prematurity *per se*, ROP, or neurological insults. Indeed, in many infants, more than one of these COH exist.

### Saccadic palsy

This is not uncommon in infancy and is usually the result of an intracranial hemorrhage in the neonatal period affecting either the frontal cortex or the frontomesencephalic pathway as this descends to the brainstem (Trounce *et al.* 1985). In saccadic palsy, the eyes deviate to the side of the lesion (Fig. 38.5); thus ipsilateral, but not contralateral, saccades can be elicited. Pursuit and the slow phase of the VOR are both unaffected if the lesion is above the brainstem.

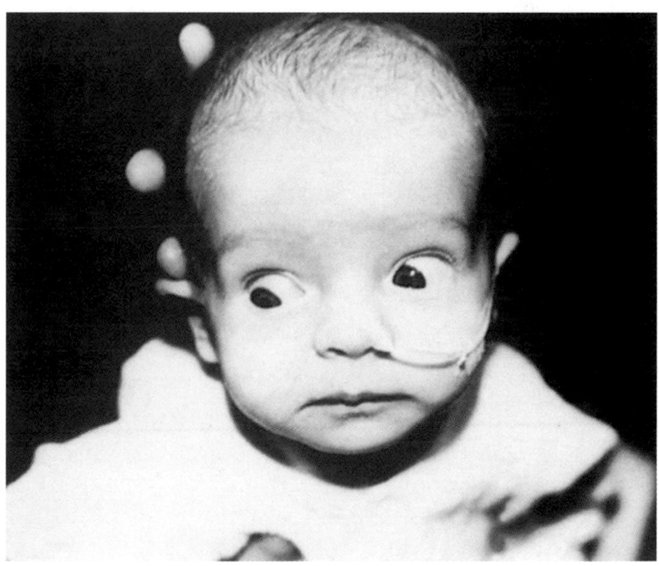

Figure 38.5 Neonatal thalamic hemorrhage (see p. 361). Ocular signs include 'sunsetting', skew deviation (left eye is higher than the right), and a tonic deviation of the eyes to the right (saccadic paresis).

### Pursuit disorders

Isolated abnormalities of pursuit that do not also involve saccades are exceptionally rare.

### Disorders of OKN

OKN can be affected by disorders of pursuit, saccades, brainstem connections (internuclear ophthalmoplegia) or a muscle paresis. OKN is often abnormal in parietal lobe lesions with a hemianopia. OKN is often abnormal in infantile nystagmus and neurological lesions affecting the brain stem, cerebellum, or cortex.

### Gaze palsy

In gaze paresis, both saccadic and pursuit functions are affected and, depending on the site of the lesion, also the VOR. Most gaze palsies are caused by brainstem pathology where the various supranuclear eye movement pathways are close together. Horizontal gaze palsy may be congenital, as an isolated anomaly (Hoyt *et al.* 1977), or in association with other abnormalities, e.g. in the Klippel–Feil or Möbius syndromes. Brainstem glioma may produce an acquired palsy. In neonates, vertical gaze palsies are more common than horizontal. Up-gaze is usually affected more than down-gaze, and the eyes may deviate down – a 'sunsetting' sign (Fig. 38.5). Eyelid retraction is common, although occasionally, ptosis is present. Transient downward deviation of the eyes can occur in healthy neonates (Hoyt *et al.* 1980), but an up-gaze abnormality is usually indicative of a midbrain lesion, e.g. tumor, neurodegenerative disorder, encephalitis, or hydrocephalus. This last is the most common cause of an up-gaze paresis in early infancy, and the signs, according to Swash (1976), are due to hydrocephalic distortion of the posterior commissure. Paroxysmal tonic upgaze, which lasts a few months, has also been described (Campistol *et al.* 1993). Up-gaze palsy has been reported in preterm infants who sustained intraventricular haemorrhages (Tamura & Hoyt 1987). These infants showed tonic downward ocular deviations and convergent squints due to hemorrhage in thalamic and mesencephalic structures. Unilateral congenital vertical gaze palsy (double-elevator palsy) was observed affecting the left eye of identical prematurely born twins (Bell *et al.* 1990). Rarely, a periodic alternating gaze deviation has been reported in infants in association with hindbrain anomalies (Legge *et al.* 1992).

### Congenital ocular motor apraxia

In congenital ocular motor apraxia (COMA), horizontal saccades to command are defective, hence the alternative term saccadic initiation failure. The affected child cannot shift gaze to either side voluntarily and, in order to look from one object to another, has to insert a jerky head thrust characteristic of COMA (Cogan 1952, 1966). The head thrust, which is in the direction of the target, uses the VOR to drive the eyes to the opposite side of the orbit. This head movement carries on past the target, dragging the eyes with it until they are aligned on the target; the head then moves slowly back as the eyes remain fixed on the object of interest. While COMA is a defect of saccades, slow pursuit and the VOR are also affected, especially in early infancy, as at this age, no eye movements at all can be elicited along the horizontal meridian. In COMA, vertical movement are unaffected.

Before the head thrust develops around 5 months of age, the infant may be suspected to be blind as he or she will not show any visual interest in objects placed to one side, and no horizontal following movements can be demonstrated. At this early age, the diagnosis can be suspected if the OKN response is absent horizontally but normal vertically. Also, rotation induces nystagmus if performed in the vertical, but not the horizontal, meridian. After the head thrust has developed, the diagnosis is obvious, although over the years signs subside considerably. A degree of asymmetry is common.

In COMA, motor delay is probably universal in infancy and lessens, but does not necessarily completely resolve, with time. Delay in other spheres, particularly with speech, is common (Fielder *et al.* 1986a; Rappaport *et al.* 1987; Harris 1997b).

Structural CNS abnormalities are common, particularly agenesis of the corpus callosum and cerebellum. However, in view of the occurrence of these anomalies without COMA, it is possible that COMA forms part of a spectrum of neurologic malformation, which may at times involve the corpus callosum and/or the cerebellum. However, these may simply be markers indicative of early CNS maldevelopment and not an integral part of the mechanism of COMA.

The range of neurologic associations with COMA is now extensive, including the aforementioned developmental abnormalities, neurodegenerative disorders (e.g. infantile Gaucher's disease), acquired disease such as posterior fossa tumors, and herpetic encephalitis (Harris 1997b).

### Neonatal eye movements

As already mentioned, eye movements, which would be considered abnormal and even warrant urgent neuro-ophthalmic investigation in the older child, are quite common in the neonate, particularly if preterm. Bursts of eye movements may be seen through closed eyelids but are most commonly seen when the infant is turned or disturbed. Tonic downward deviation, up- or down-beat nystagmus and nystagmus in other directions are commonly observed. Ocular flutter, opsoclonus (bursts of saccades) and skew deviations are less commonly seen. There is essentially no information on the prevalence and possible significance of these neonatal eye movements, or indeed whether they should even be considered abnormal. Dubowitz *et al.* (1981) reported a strong correlation between intraventricular hemorrhage and roving eye movements. Hoyt *et al.* (1980) examined 242 full-term neonates, without any neurologic abnormalities, and observed downward deviations (five infants), opsoclonus (nine), and skew deviation (22). Five of those with a skew deviation later developed a squint. Archer

& Helveston (1994) commented on the rarity of skew deviation as they had not observed it once in 2271 examinations.

Clinicians should have a low threshold for investigating an abnormal eye movement if it persists more than a 'few weeks', especially if associated with other signs.

## Nystagmus

The reader is referred to the reviews of nystagmus by Archer & Helveston (1994) and Harris (1997a).

### Physiologic nystagmus

The various types of physiologic nystagmus, including rotational, caloric, and optokinetic nystagmus, have already been discussed.

### CNS conditions – neurologic nystagmus

Nystagmus can occur in many CNS conditions such as cerebellar, brainstem, and vestibular lesions. In the adult, these often produce predictable specific types of nystagmus, which point to a particular anatomical location, whereas in the infant, features tend to be more variable and have less diagnostic value (Dell'Osso *et al.* 1990). Clearly, nystagmus due to a CNS cause may be apparent at any age, in contrast to the so-called congenital nystagmus (see later). Thus, nystagmus observed within the first week or so of life is more likely to have a CNS basis. Dubowitz *et al.* (1981) observed roving eye movements some time after the development of germinal matrix hemorrhage–intraventricular hemorrhage in preterm infants.

### Sensory deprivation nystagmus

Bilaterally reduced vision in infancy and early childhood leads to nystagmus, but only if the lesion involves the anterior visual pathway. Consequently, nystagmus is not a feature of cortical blindness (Whiting *et al.* 1985; Fielder & Evans 1988). Any condition of the anterior visual pathway sufficient to preclude normal visual development will cause sensory deprivation nystagmus. These conditions include: corneal scarring, albinism, achromatopsia, aniridia, congenital cataracts, and optic nerve pathology, including atrophy and hypoplasia. Occasionally bilateral nystagmus may result from a uniocular condition (Good *et al.* 1997).

Nystagmus due to a visual deficit does not develop until about 3 months of age, and presents clinically in two forms:

1. wandering eye movements associated with blindness
2. nystagmus, which is clinically indistinguishable from or very similar to congenital nystagmus.

It should be recognized that these may simply represent different ends of a single spectrum and not two distinct entities (Fielder & Evans 1988).

- *Blindness.* As mentioned above, severe visual deprivation before the age of 2 years, and sometimes later, results in nystagmus. As a very crude guide, the better the vision, the faster the oscillation. In complete blindness, the eye movements are slow, large in amplitude, and variable in direction – nystagmoid movements of the blind.
- *Nystagmus indistinguishable from congenital nystagmus.* Conditions such as albinism, achromatopsia, and aniridia cause a visual defect, but not blindness, and result in nystagmus, which is either similar or identical to that seen in congenital nystagmus. As mentioned above, the oscillation usually starts at about 3 months. Occasionally, the movement may be vertical on presentation (Hoyt & Gelbart 1984; Fielder & Evans 1988), but this subsequently becomes horizontally directed, as is the rule in congenital nystagmus. The ocular findings in many of these conditions are subtle and easily missed, so it is essential that congenital nystagmus is a diagnosis of exclusion, made only after all other possibilities have been excluded (see later). The clinical severity of certain conditions may vary between patients: thus, Leber's congenital amaurosis or optic nerve hypoplasia may both cause either blindness and nystagmus of the blind or, if less severe, reduced vision and a congenital nystagmus picture. Two conditions deserve special mention: albinism and achromatopsia.
- *Albinism.* This is straightforward to diagnose in most instances but can be difficult, especially in the infant from a blond family or the X-linked ocular form. Albinos may present in early infancy with reduced vision, which subsequently improves (delayed visual maturation) around the time that the nystagmus commences. Slit-lamp examination reveals iris transillumination, and the foveal reflex is absent. The finding of the typical carrier retinal picture in the mother or sister of a suspected ocular albino is diagnostic. The definitive test for albinism is the visually evoked potential (VEP) by which visual pathway misrouting at the optic chiasm, characteristic of this condition, is identified (Apkarian & Tijssen 1992).
- *Achromatopsia.* This is a congenital absence of retinal cones and is inherited as an autosomal recessive trait. Retinal cones function optimally in bright light and subserve fine discrimination (acuity) and color vision, so the infant with achromatopsia (complete color blindness) presents with photosensitivity and poor vision, particularly under conditions of bright illumination. Visual function is reduced especially in sunlight, and color vision is absent. Nystagmus in achromatopsia closely resembles congenital nystagmus, but its amplitude is less (Yee *et al.* 1981). Ocular examination is essentially negative in infancy except for two subtle clues: paradoxical pupil response and a significant refractive error (Evans *et al.* 1989). Neither of these is diagnostic, as both signs are also seen in Leber's congenital amaurosis Color vision testing is impossible at this age, and the diagnosis can only be established definitively be electroretinography at 30 Hz (Figs 38.6 and 38.7). Unsurprisingly, achromatopsia is rarely diagnosed correctly in the first year of life.

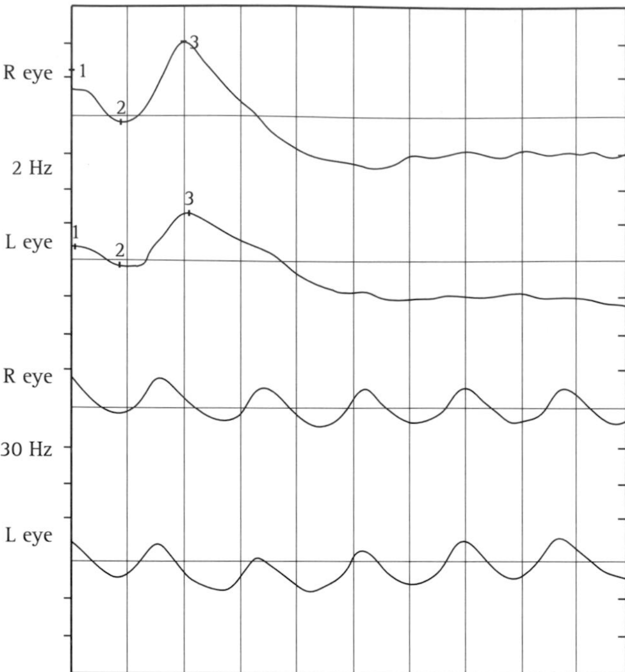


Figure 38.6 Electroretinogram (ERG) traces at 2 Hz (rod and cone response) and 30 Hz (cone response alone). These are normal responses obtained from a 2-year-old child without sedation using skin electrodes.

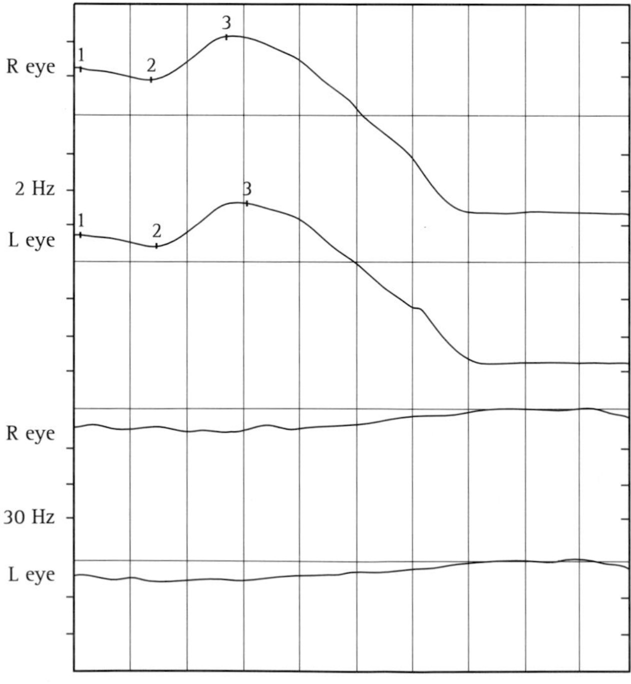


Figure 38.7 ERG traces from a child with achromatopsia. A response is obtained at 2 Hz, indicating the presence of rod photoreceptors, but not at 30 Hz, due to an absence of retinal cones.

## Infantile (congenital) nystagmus

The term 'infantile' nystagmus should be reserved for nystagmus presenting in infancy that is not associated with any other ocular abnormality (Dell'Osso *et al.* 1990). The words 'congenital' and 'infantile' are used interchangeably with reference to nystagmus. The term 'motor nystagmus' is sometimes used to avoid confusion with nystagmus due to a sensory defect. The condition may be inherited as a dominant, recessive, or X-linked disorder. While familial congenital nystagmus is free of neurodevelopmental problems, this is often not so for non-familial types (Jan *et al.* 1992). Infantile is preferred to congenital as the onset is usually at about 6 weeks of age, although very occasionally, it is observed immediately after birth. Sometimes, if associated with delayed visual maturation (see later), it does not develop for a few months, until around the time when vision develops.

In infantile nystagmus, the oscillation is binocular, symmetrical, and horizontally directed in all positions of gaze, except for the rare vertical variant. In early infancy, the oscillation is slow and of large amplitude, and may be horizontal, vertical, or rotatory, but with increasing age, the movement becomes more rapid, fine, and horizontal (Reinecke *et al.* 1988). The movement is dampened by convergence and often increases on lateral gaze. Vertical OKN is normal, but horizontal OKN is commonly absent. Compensatory head-nodding, the null position, and the compensatory head posture will not be covered here as they develop after infancy. Making a diagnosis of infantile nystagmus can be difficult, particularly as during early infancy, it may be variable, and the aforementioned characteristics may not be apparent. Furthermore, as many other forms of nystagmus with ocular or neurologic associations mimic this condition to the extent that they are clinically indistinguishable, the diagnosis of infantile nystagmus must be one of exclusion (Weiss & Biersdorf 1989).

## Spasmus nutans

This syndrome consists of the triad nystagmus, head-nodding, and torticollis, and commences between 4 and 18 months of age. Not all features are present at one time; thus, the head nod may be present before the nystagmus and vice versa. Although the nystagmus is usually bilateral, it can be grossly asymmetrical and may be either horizontal or vertical. Like congenital nystagmus, spasmus nutans is a diagnosis of exclusion. Infants with these signs can harbor intracranial tumors (Antony *et al.* 1980; Arnoldi & Tycheson 1995), full neurologic assessment is mandatory, all the more important because there are no clinical features that distinguish those infants with and without CNS lesions (Gottlob *et al.* 1990, 1992). Spasmus nutans resolves spontaneously usually within 1–2 years.

## Asymmetric nystagmus

Nystagmus, which is either totally monocular or significantly asymmetric between the two eyes, may be seen in infancy, as in spasmus nutans. Farmer & Hoyt (1984) emphasized the frequency of monocular nystagmus in infants with chiasmal tumors. Monocular blindness can cause monocular nystagmus, but the latter usually develops after infancy. Unfortunately, as there are no clinical features that distinguish infants with spasmus nutans absolutely from those with chiasmal tumors, full neurologic and neuroradiologic investigations are necessary (Gottlob *et al.* 1990).

Conversely, occasionally monocular visual defects are associated with binocular nystagmus (Good *et al.* 1997).

#### Special nystagmus types

Many other types of nystagmus not considered here may have important neurologic implications – such as downbeat, upbeat, see-saw, dissociated (e.g. in internuclear ophthalmoplegia), ocular bobbing, and retraction nystagmus (Dell'Osso *et al.* 1990; Harris 1997a).

#### The investigation of nystagmus

Nystagmus must always be taken seriously as it may signify a serious neurologic or ocular disorder. The pattern of eye movement must be carefully evaluated, in each eye individually, by recording the direction (convention dictates this to be in the direction of the fast phase), amplitude, and frequency of the nystagmus in the nine positions of gaze. The distinction between pendular and jerk nystagmus is not diagnostically helpful as both may exist in the same patient in different positions of gaze. Accurate diagnosis is rarely possible from the observation of the pattern of nystagmus alone. Because the incidence of neurologic and visual pathway disorders is high and these cannot always be differentiated on a clinical basis (Weiss & Biersdorf 1989; Jan *et al.* 1992), all infants with nystagmus should have a full ophthalmic and pediatric-neurologic assessment that includes electrophysiologic investigations. The latter may be performed simply without sedation in most infants, and the stimulus frequencies should be 2 Hz (which elicits a combined rod and cone response) and 30 Hz (cone response alone) (Figs 38.6 and 38.7).

## VISION

### NORMAL DEVELOPMENT

The rapid development of vision in the first few months of life is one of the most rewarding features of infancy, although its quantitative assessment remains a major clinical challenge. In this section, only brief mention is made of the qualitative assessment of visual function, emphasis being on the quantitative measurement of visual acuity, particularly the adaptation of the preferential looking technique – the acuity card procedure.

As described by Slater (1998), infants exhibit 'natural' preferences for:

- patterned, rather than unpatterned, visual stimuli
- horizontal, rather than vertical, stripes
- moving, compared to stationary, targets
- three-dimensional, rather than two-dimenstional, stimuli
- curvilinear, rather than rectilinear, patterns
- objects in the fronto-parallel plane rather than at an angle
- high-contrast, rather than low-contrast, stimuli
- optimally sized objects
- face-like stimuli

#### Qualitative aspects of visual development

Many infants' responses have a visual basis and consequently provide a useful, qualitative indication of visual development (van Hof-van Duin & Mohn, 1984a; Isenberg 1994; Vital-Durand *et al.* 1996; Taylor 1997; Slater 1998).

#### Blink reflex

The blink reflex to a bright light is said to be present from 28 weeks PMA (Robinson 1966) and in almost all full-term and preterm babies at 40 weeks PMA (Kurtzberg *et al.* 1979). A response does not invariably indicate the presence of vision, as a blink reflex has been observed in hydranencephaly with absence of the visual cortex (Aylward *et al.* 1978).

#### Eyelid opening

Eyelid opening is a function of PMA. Thus, babies have their eyes shut for over 90% of the time at 28 weeks PMA, but by 34 weeks, they are open for 40% (Robinson *et al.* 1989)

#### Awareness and fixation

From 30 weeks PMA, there are periods of awareness during which visual fixation occurs, and these periods naturally increase with increasing age (Hack *et al.* 1981).

Visual attention is not considered here, but it is pertinent to many of the behavioral tests currently used to measure a range of visual functions. Before about 54 weeks PMA, the latency of phasic orientation (attention getting) is stable but decreases thereafter. Similarly, the duration of tonic orientation (attention holding) exhibits a plateau until around 54 weeks PMA and then decreases (Foreman *et al.* 1991). These alterations of attention getting and holding with age are obvious during all tests of preferential looking (see later), both as the speed of response by the neonate compared to the older infant to a peripherally located stimulus and the duration of looking at the stimulus, respectively. Indeed, understanding of these changes is required to avoid misinterpretation. Infants at 1 month, compared to those of 3 months of age, are more disrupted by, and respond slower to, a competitive stimulus consisting of two stimuli (Atkinson *et al.* 1992). It has also been suggested that in certain neurologic impairments, attention may be selectively affected compared to VEP measures (Hood & Atkinson 1990).

#### Orientation

Head-turning to a diffuse light can be demonstrated from about 32 weeks PMA (Robinson 1966) and is elicited in most by full term (Goldie & Hopkins 1964). After 36 weeks PMA, there is no significant difference between preterm and full-term infants (Robinson 1966), although Ferrari *et al.* (1983) have reported that preterm infants examined around 40 weeks PMA are significantly poorer in orientation. Anderson *et al.* (1989) noted that infants with intraventricular hemorrhage may have a poor orientation.

### Following

Using a red ball, Brazelton *et al.* (1966) detected following in 57% of normal infants at full term. Dubowitz *et al.* (1980) found a red woollen ball to be a better stimulus and were able to elicit following from 31 weeks PMA. Vehrs & Baum (1970), in testing preterm and full-term neonates around full term, considered a flashing light to be a more effective stimulus than either a red ball or diffuse light.

### Optokinetic nystagmus

Responsiveness to an OKN stimulus can be elicited at full term (Kremenitzer *et al.* 1979).

### Visual threat response

Eyelid closure to an approaching threatening object does not develop until about 16 weeks of corrected age for full-term and preterm infants and is thought to be a cortical response. When performing this test, it is important to avoid tactile stimulation, e.g. a rush of air (van Hof-van Duin & Mohn 1984a).

### Reaching

Visually directed reaching with one hand is first seen from about 2 months (White *et al.* 1964; Cavanagh 1997).

### Smiling

Vision can be an important component of this response, so failure to smile by 6 weeks of age may signify a serious visual defect.

## Other visual functions

### Pupil reactions

The onset of the pupillary response to light is between 30 and 34 weeks GA (Robinson & Fielder 1990). These reactions are clinically difficult to assess in infants, and care must be taken to ensure that light and near reactions are not also active.

The pupillary response to light is one of the best known reflexes, but whether the pupil reacts to other visual stimuli such as its spatial structure, color and movement, is less well known. Thus, the subtle pupillary constriction to a grating stimulus, the pupil grating response (PGR) and measured by infrared pupillometry, can be used to quantify visual acuity (Cocker *et al.* 1994). The PGR in contrast to the pupil light response (PLR) is cortically mediated and is not present until 1 month of age, by which age, behavioral responses have been obtainable for several weeks (Fig 38.8).

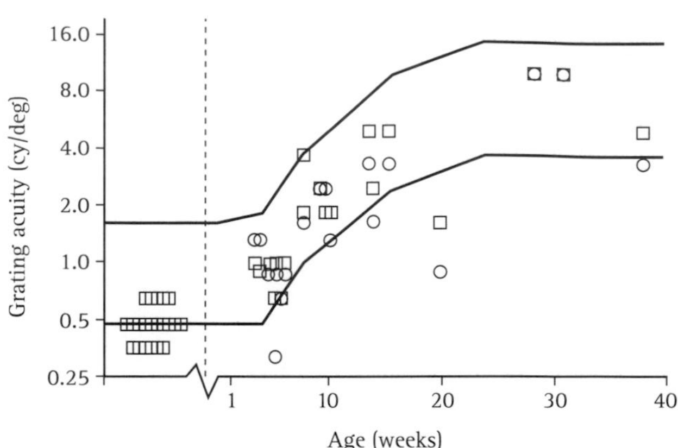


**Figure 38.8** Visual acuities obtained by pupillometry and behavioral (ACP) methods. Binocular age norms are indicated by the solid lines. Open squares: behavioral acuities. Open circles: pupil acuities. No pupil acuites were measurable during the neonatal period, following which, they correlated well with ACP values.

### Color vision

At 1 month of age, infants do not discriminate between colors (Hainline 1998), but this has developed by 2 months, and by 3 months, color vision is similar to that in adults (Boothe *et al.* 1985; Mercer *et al.* 1991, Teller 1998). Infants are probably more sensitive to brightness than color cues (Hainline 1998)

### Visual field

At birth, the visual field is approximately 30° on either side of the horizontal, and this reaches adult proportions after 3 years of age (Mohn *et al.* 1986; Dobson *et al.* 1998) and is not greatly influenced by preterm birth (van Hof-van Duin *et al.* 1992). Lewis & Maurer (1992) have also studied the development of the visual field and discuss the relative merits of kinetic (stimulus location moves, intensity constant) and static (stimulus stationary, its intensity increases) perimetry. The application of perimetry to the infants and children is reviewed by Mayer & Fulton (1993).

# DEVELOPMENT OF VISUAL ACUITY – METHODS OF MEASUREMENT

## Resolution, recognition, and visibility – types of visual acuity

A prerequisite to evaluating a patient's history or tests of visual function is an understanding of the parameter being measured. This topic bewilders clinicians of all disciplines, particularly those who attempt to correlate measurements obtained by different methods. No clinician would dream of equating X-ray, CT, and MRI scans, as they measure different parameters. Thus, the various stimuli are used to assess vision. There are three stimulus types in common usage:

- *Visibility:* the assessment of vision using a single object containing no detail, such as a sweet or white ball. Tests include the Catford drum, Stycar balls, or sweets.
- *Resolution acuity:* the ability to distinguish two separate points such as stripes in a grating or the squares of a checker board. Tests include preferential-based tests and the visually evoked potential.
- *Recognition acuity:* the ability to distinguish the detail of letters or pictures. For the older child and adult, these are the tests used in everyday clinical practice. Tests include the Snellen, Sheridan, and Gardiner letter tests, Cardiff cards, and today's gold standard – the logMAR chart.

In infancy, resolution and visibility tests are used, but as the figure shows (Fig 38.9), the correlation between the two is poor (Atkinson *et al.* 1981; van Hof-van Duin 1989). Tests of visibility seriously overestimate vision when compared with resolution acuities (Atkinson *et al.* 1981; van Hof-van Duin 1989). Thus, a parent's observation that a child can see a very small sweet is merely a comment on visibility and does not preclude a serious resolution defect, to the extent that in this writer's opinion, visibility tests are so misleading that they should not be used.

## BEHAVIORAL METHODS – PREFERENTIAL LOOKING

Parents are rewarded by their infant's visually directed look or smile; and in the absence of accurate methods of measuring visual acuity, this has been the mainstay of clinical assessment of visual performance. Fantz in the 1950s transferred this subjective response to a test of visual acuity based on the infant's preference to look at a patterned rather than a non-patterned stimulus. In the 1970s, this was taken further, and forced-choice preferential looking was developed, mainly by Teller and associates. Techniques based on the preferential looking (PL*) (Pearson *et al.* 1989; Dobson 1994) are tedious and time-consuming and have not been incorporated into routine clinical use. Nevertheless, these laboratory studies have added greatly to our knowledge of normal and abnormal visual development (Teller 1997).

The situation changed completely with the latest PL modification – the acuity card procedure (ACP) (McDonald *et al.* 1985) (and a similar test employed by Dubowitz *et al.* 1980; Morante *et al.* 1982). This is a portable apparatus, it is relatively simple and quick to perform and suitable for use in everyday practice, and it permits the evaluation of a population who could not be studied by traditional means (e.g. Fielder *et al.* 1992) (Figs 38.10 and 38.11).

Although ACP is more adaptable than formal PL, it is potentially more subjective, as the tester may know the location of the grating. For all PL tests, the following issues can be problematic: judging looking patterns in the presence of nystagmus, congenital ocular motor apraxia, a field defect, or strabismus. In these situations, holding the cards vertically rather than horizontally is helpful.

PL-based studies indicate that vision develops at a rate of one cycle per degree per month and does not reach adult levels of 30 cycles until 3–5 years of age (Atkinson & Braddick 1983; Boothe *et al.* 1985; Teller *et al.* 1986). Grating acuities are measured in cycles per degree, i.e. the number of pairs of black and white stripes per degree of visual angle. Thus, the infant whose vision is developing normally sees 3 cycles/degree (6/60) at 3 months, 6 cycles/degree (6/30) at 6 months and 12 cycles/degree (6/18) at 1 year of age. It is interesting to note that PL-based tests enable the effect of dietary intake on visual development to be quantified. Birch *et al.* (1993) observed significantly better acuities in infants fed ω-3 fatty acids (human milk) compared to those fed a corn-oil-based formula low in these substances.

The success rate for binocular testing by ACP is around 95% in the first 2 years of life (Teller *et al.* 1986; Sebris *et al.* 1987; Chandna *et al.* 1988; Fielder & Moseley 1988; Courage & Adams 1990; Salomao and Ventura 1995). This level is obtained throughout childhood by experts, although lower success rates, around 80% between 2 and 3 years of age, have been reported in less rigorous clinical settings (Fielder & Moseley 1988). Monocular testing is more difficult, but even so, success rates range from 66 to 96% under 3 years (Chandna *et al.* 1988; Mayer *et al.* 1995) and 5 years (Sebris *et al.* 1987) of age. The maximum acuity difference between the two eyes in the normal infant is about 0.5 octaves (Chandna 1991; Raye *et al.* 1992).

### Optokinetic nystagmus

This response has been used to measure visual acuity (Gorman *et al.* 1957), although recently, this technique has attracted relatively little interest.

### Visual evoked potentials

Having already been dealt with in Chapter 12, only a few aspects need to be mentioned here. Both the flash (Fielder *et al.* 1983) and pattern VEP (Moskowitz & Sokol 1983) reflect visual pathway maturation (Birch & Petrig 1996; Crognale *et al.* 1997). However, only the latter, as it contains an edge, can be used to measure acuity. Pattern reversal VEP estimates of infant visual acuity indicate that adult levels are reached by about 6–12 months (Marg *et al.* 1976; Sokol 1978). However, in a study by de Vreis-Khoe & Spekreijse (1982), using a pattern onset stimulus, this level was not achieved until about 4 years of age. Apkarian *et al.* (1991) have shown that the behavioral state dramatically affects all VEP components, resulting in considerable intra- and intersubject variability. Recently, the sweep visually evoked potential has been introduced to measure resolution acuity in infants. This technique employs a rapidly reversing sinusoidal grating (steady-state VEP) that changes its spatial frequency every 5–10 s. This enables a range of spatial frequencies to be 'swept' in a short time and an acuity estimate derived (Norcia *et al.* 1987; Kriss & Thompson 1997).

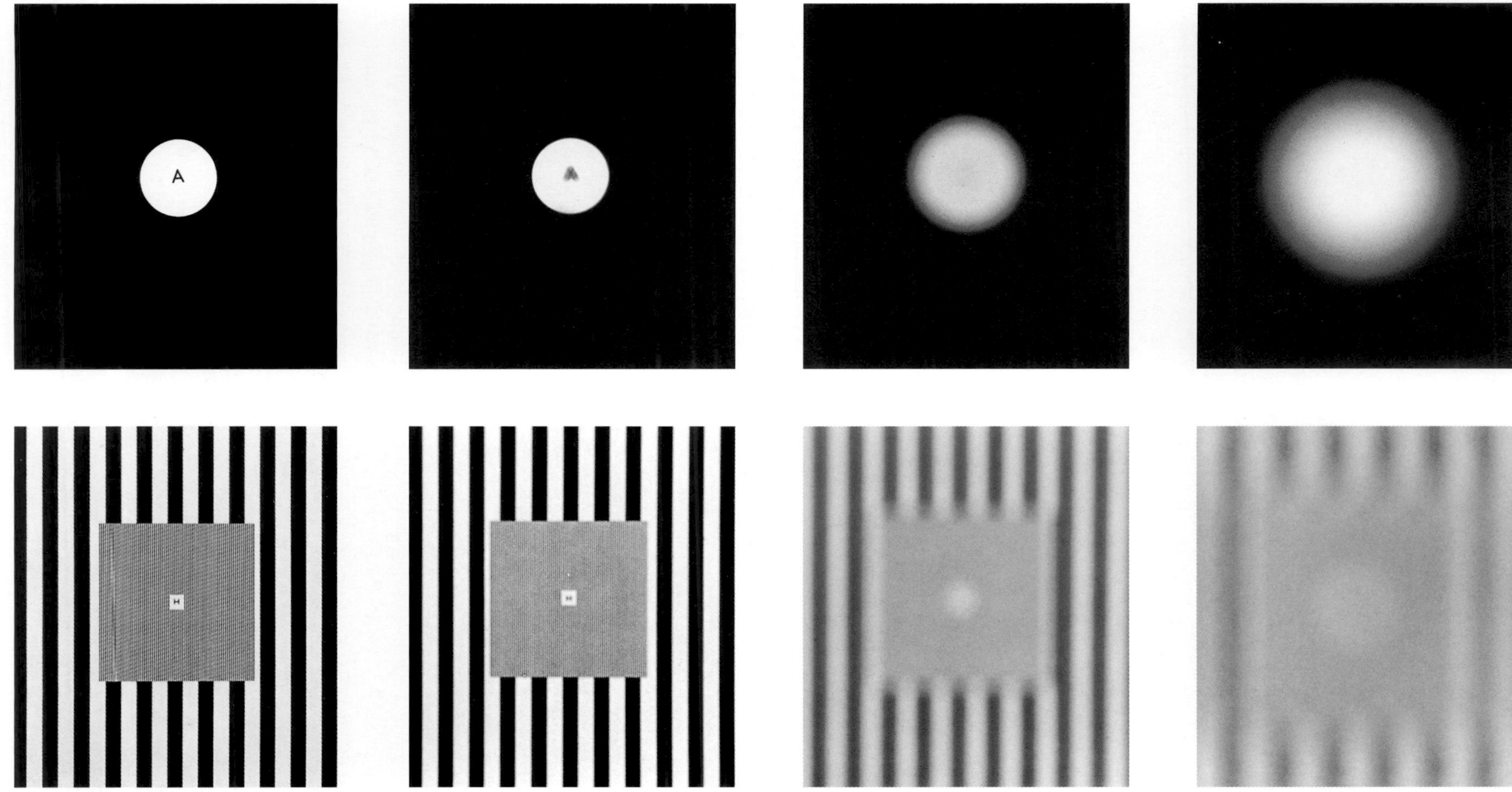

**Figure 38.9** Visibility (white ball) and recognition (letter A) (top line) and resolution (grating) (bottom line) stimuli. All three elements are blurred by the same amount: defocus affects in order of sensitivity – fine gratings, the letter A, coarse gratings, while the white ball remains visible and indeed enlarges with increasing blurr. At an early stage of blur, the fine gratings are invisible as such, while the letter A, although indistinct, remains recognizable as either an A or an upside down V. This figure provides the explanation for how a severely visually impaired child can still see a sweet! PL* will be used here to cover all tests based on the preferential looking principle, although ACP will be used specifically for the acuity card procedure.

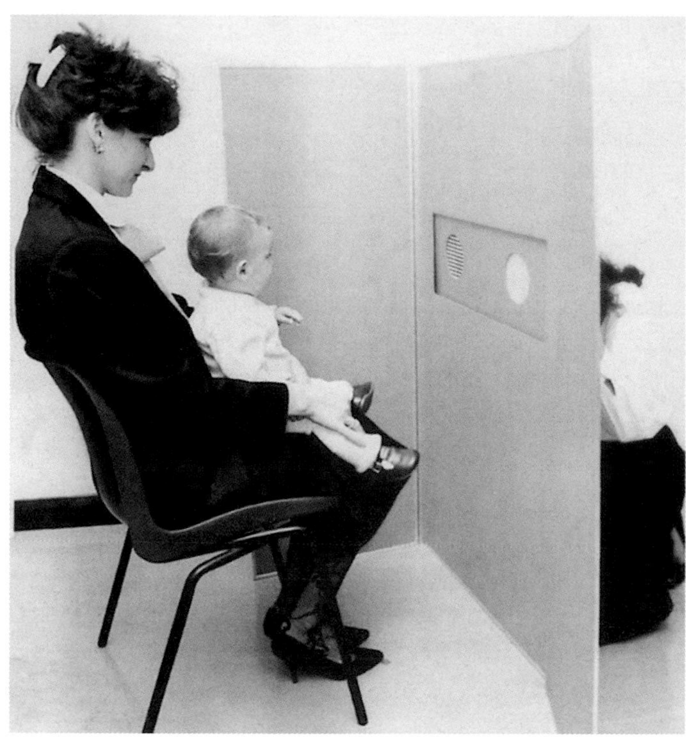

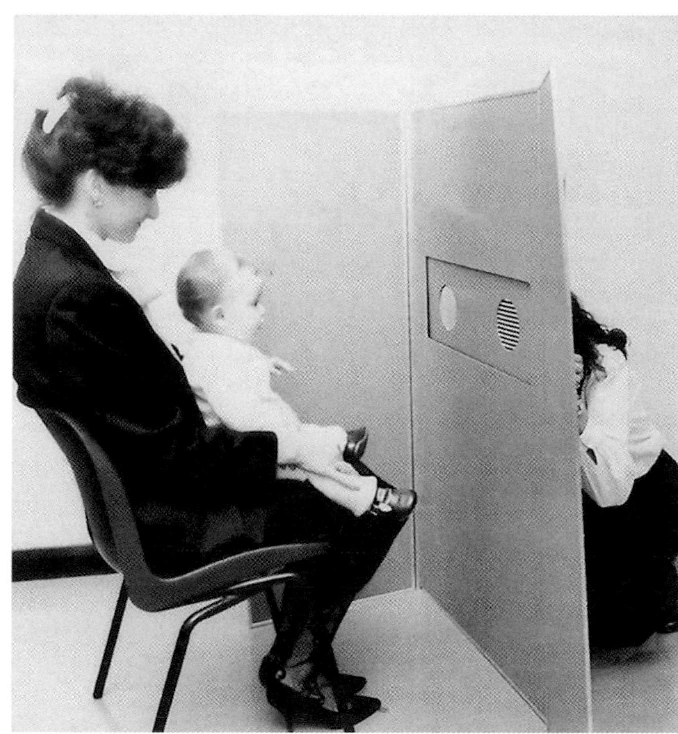

**Figure 38.10** Acuity card procedure. The infant is clearly looking towards the grating (the near-side panel has been turned sideways for the photograph).

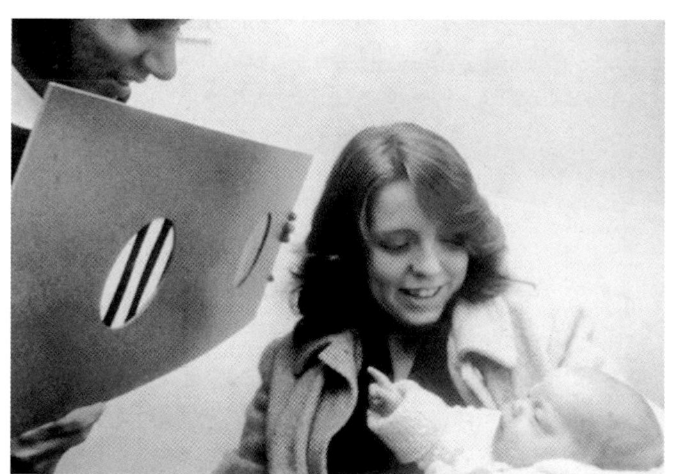

**Figure 38.11** Acuity card procedure. In certain circumstances, the stimulus cards may be used without the surrounding apparatus.

### The VEP:PL discrepancy

For each age VEP acuity estimates are higher than those obtained by PL. The basis of this discrepancy has not been fully resolved, but it is interesting to note that foveal development takes much longer than originally thought, maturity not being reached until between 15 and 45 months after birth (Hendrickson & Youdelis 1984), corresponding closer to PL than VEP results. One exception is the VEP study of de Vreis-Khoe & Spekreijse (1982), which correlates with both anatomic and PL data. Sokol *et al.* (1992) reported a smaller discrepancy if phase-alternating gratings were used to estimate both VEP and PL, compared to the usual method, which employs phase-alternating gratings to estimate the VEP and stationary gratings to estimate PL.

### The PL:Snellen acuity discrepancy

The clinician, already confused by the discrepancy between behavioral (ACP) and evoked potential acuity estimates, is now confronted with another discrepancy: that between PL and Snellen estimates. Acuities obtained by PL are not always directly comparable to those obtained by Snellen or other recognition targets. Thus, PL grating acuities may be significantly better than Snellen acuities in certain clinical conditions, particularly amblyopia (Mayer *et al.* 1984). This difference is not fully understood (Fielder *et al.* 1992) but may be due partly to methodologic differences in measuring PL and Snellen acuities (Moseley *et al.* 1988). While it does not negate the value of PL, it does reduce its value as a method of determining the precise magnitude of amblyopia and also its sensitivity as a screening tool (Fielder *et al.* 1992). However, PL tests are of value in amblyopia as the interocular acuity difference can be used both to identify this defect and to monitor the effect of treatment (Catalano *et al.* 1987; Birch & Stager 1988; Mayer *et al.* 1989).

Despite these problems it should not be forgotten that the ACP is the only quantitative test of vision that can be used simply and rapidly in the clinical situation and provides far more information than existing qualitative tests. Its value in recording visual development and assessing the infant who appears not to see well is not in question (Fielder *et al.* 1992).

### Pupil grating response

The subtle pupillary constriction to sinusoidal gratings of varying frequency can be used to measure visual acuity and correlates well with levels obtained by behavioral methods by 4–6 weeks after birth (Cocker *et al.* 1994). The use of pupillometry is currently confined to clinical research.

### Visual development of preterm infants

It is now pertinent to consider the effect of preterm birth on the visual system (Fielder *et al.* 1988). What is the effect of removal from the protective milieu of the uterus and early exposure to the harsh neonatal environment? Is visual development hastened, retarded or unaffected (Fielder & Moseley 2000)?

This is not the place to consider retinopathy of prematurity, but it should be borne in mind that most neonates with a birthweight below 1000 g will have developed at least minor stages of this condition.

The ERG can be recorded from around 32 weeks PMA (Mactier *et al.* 2000), and Kennedy *et al.* (1997) did not detect any effect with light reduction by goggling.

At full term, the vision of the preterm infant is lower than that of his or her full-term counterpart (Morante *et al.* 1982) and remains so until about 30 weeks, if postnatal age is used as the parameter (van Hof-van Duin *et al.* 1983; van Hof-van Duin & Mohn 1984a). However, when corrected for the degree of prematurity, preterm and full-term infants develop similarly as assessed by behavioral techniques (Dobson *et al.* 1980; Morante *et al.* 1982; van Hof-van Duin *et al.* 1983; van Hof-van Duin & Mohn 1984a; Brown & Yamamoto 1986; Roy *et al.* 1995; Weinacht *et al.* 1999). In contrast to the above, some VEP studies show mild hastening of acuity development in preterm infants (Sokol & Jones 1978; Norcia *et al.* 1987). All these results show that, very broadly speaking, premature birth neither hastens nor retards visual development in infancy, i.e. the visual acuity maturation is controlled predominantly by innate, rather than environmental, processes.

Neurologically abnormal preterm infants may show a delay in visual acuity maturation (Dubowitz *et al.* 1983; Placzek *et al.* 1985; Norcia *et al.* 1987; Groenendaal *et al.* 1989). Shepherd *et al.* (1999) showed that the flash VEP in preterm neonates has some predictive value for both survival and cerebral palsy. Harvey *et al.* (1997a) reported that grating acuity is affected by IVH, but this is not related to its grade or presence of PVL, and visual field development is reduced only before 17 months. For children with bronchopulmonary dysplasia, uncomplicated by neurologic problems, their grating and field development is normal, but recognition acuity may be affected (Harvey 1997b).

## ABNORMALITIES OF VISION

One of the most difficult clinical problems is the assessment of the infant or child who might be harboring a visual deficit. A carefully taken history can be more informative than the subsequent clinical examination. Concern voluntarily expressed by a parent must always be taken seriously as this is rarely unfounded and usually more reliable than most qualitative tests of vision. A seeming lack of concern must, however, be treated with caution as it does not necessarily indicate that all is well. This attitude can be adopted for a number of reasons. First, a low expectancy is generally held for vision in very early infancy. Second, anxiety may be hidden until the parent's fear that their baby has defective vision is either allayed or confirmed by medical staff, following which they may pour out a detailed account accurately describing reduced vision dating back to very early infancy. Third, information may be withheld for fear of biasing the professional towards an unfavorable verdict.

The visual pathway abnormalities to be considered in this section are divided into those affecting the anterior (eye to optic chiasm) and posterior (optic tracts to visual cortex) portions. Only neuro-ophthalmic conditions are considered, and problems such as cataract and retinopathy of prematurity are omitted.

While the above two paragraphs represent the current situation, the situation is changing rapidly. Thus, we are now aware of certain patterns of acuity development (Fielder *et al.* 1992), which are shown in a stylized form in Figs 38.12–38.14. This information has introduced a degree of complexity hitherto unsuspected, but it does offer the clinician insight into fundamental mechanisms and provides valuable information for patient care and for counseling.

### Disorders of the anterior visual pathway

Lesions of the anterior visual pathway (i.e. eye to the lateral geniculate nucleus) sufficient to reduce vision bilaterally in early life lead to nystagmus and afferent pupillary defects. The latter can be difficult to test clinically in infants and children.

#### Electroretinography in infancy

For several conditions, ophthalmoscopic signs are either minimal or absent. In this situation, an ERG is essential to distinguish retinal pathology from that elsewhere in the visual pathway (Weleber & Palmer 1991). Clinicians must have a low threshold for arranging this test. As a general rule, it should be performed on all infants and children with unexplained low vision, nystagmus, myopia, or optic atrophy, i.e. where there is a possibility of retinal disease.

As mentioned, an ERG can be obtained without sedation, using lid, fiber, gold foil or, even, contact lens electrodes.

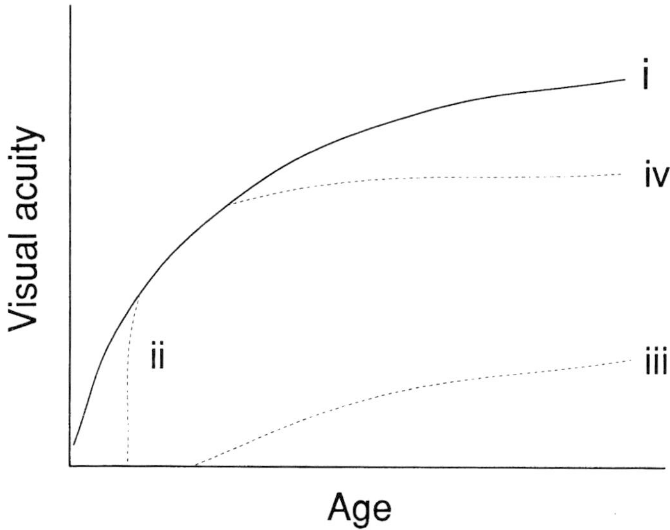


Figure 38.12 Normal visual development is shown by line i. Early delayed visual development may be followed by rapid (ii) or slow (iii) improvement. These patterns are seen in delayed visual maturation types 1 and 4 (see later). Following normal or delayed development, acuity may plateau or become asymptotic (iv). The level at which this occurs depends on the severity of the visual pathway abnormality, but is seen in infantile nystagmus.

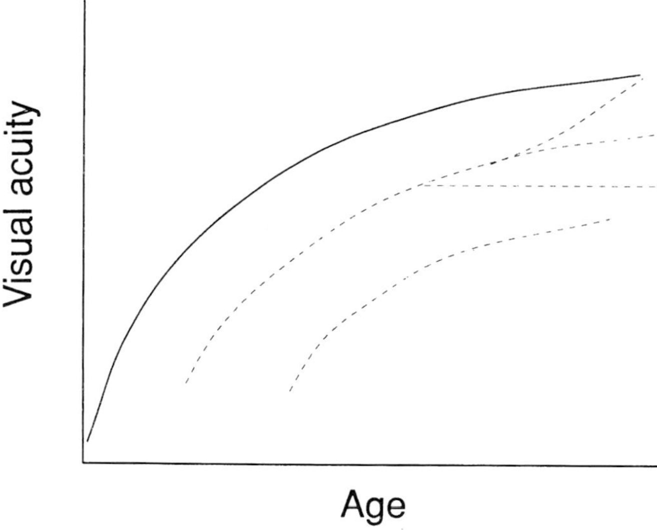


Figure 38.13 Parallel visual development. This is seen after surgery for congenital cataract surgery or severe retinopathy of prematurity. Late catch-up does not always occur.

Stimulus rates of 2 Hz (generating both rod and cone responses) and 30 Hz [generating only a cone response (see Fig. 38.6)]. Performed this way, it is probably advisable to consider the ERG obtained as qualitative rather than quantitative, but in most clinical instances, this is adequate.

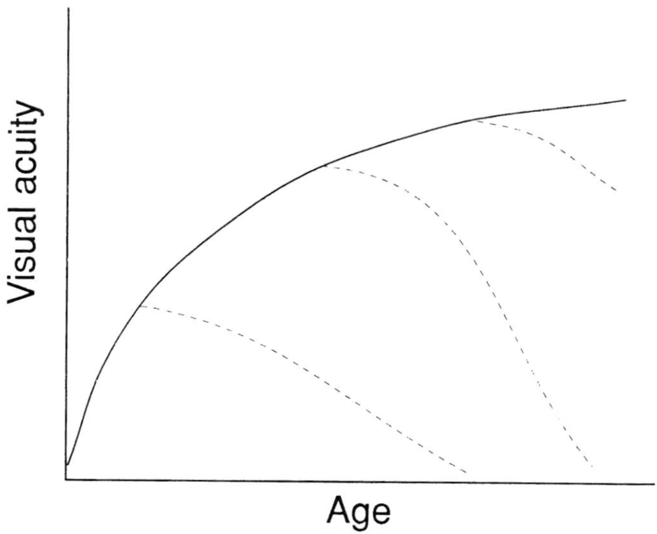


Figure 38.14 Regression. This may occur in a large range of progressive ophthalmic or neuro-ophthalmic disorders.

## Retinal disorders

Many retinal disorders produce a severe visual defect. Some of these are ophthalmoscopically obvious such as retinopathy of prematurity or chorioretinal scarring. Other conditions such as achromatopsia (see p. 665) and the tapetoretinal degenerations (including Leber's congenital amaurosis) are frequently not associated with ophthalmoscopically visible signs, at least in early infancy. In these conditions, a precise diagnosis can only be established by an ERG.

### The cherry-red spot

This classic, but rarely seen sign, results from storage of abnormal substances in the retinal ganglion cells. As these cells are abundant around the macula but are absent from the very center, the fovea is red and its surround white. This subtle sign, which fades with time, is seen in a number of conditions, including Tay–Sach's, Sandhoff's, Niemann–Pick and Farber's diseases, metachromatic leukodystrophy, and the mucolipidoses. These are discussed in detail in Chapter 36.

## Optic nerve disorders

### Optic atrophy

Optic atrophy is a sign and not a diagnosis, which can be difficult to identify if mild. The appearance of the optic disc alone does not indicate the amount of visual function. Optic atrophy (particularly if associated with retinal arteriolar attenuation) may be the only visible sign of serious retinal disease, for instance in Leber's congenital amaurosis or the Laurence–Moon–Biedl (Biedl–Bardet) syndrome. Only by an ERG can retinal involvement be confirmed or eliminated.

Optic nerve damage secondary to retinal disease is termed consecutive or ascending atrophy. Damage to the optic radiation and visual cortex can cause trans-synaptic degeneration and a descending type of optic atrophy, but this response is confined to visual-pathway insults before and during early infancy.

- *Hereditary optic atrophy.* Behr's optic atrophy is an autosomal recessive condition in which optic atrophy is associated with mild mental retardation, hypertonia, and ataxia. Onset may be within the first year of life. Whether isolated recessive optic atrophy is a true entity is uncertain. Other hereditary optic atrophies such as Leber's optic neuropathy, dominant optic atrophy, and the DIDMOAD syndrome all present after the first year of life and are not considered here.
- *Retinal disease.* Tapetoretinal degenerations such as Leber's congenital amaurosis, and Laurence–Moon–Biedl (Biedl–Bardet) and Zellweger's syndromes, may all cause optic atrophy.
- *Intrauterine disease.* Optic atrophy may occur following intrauterine infections, asphyxia, and cerebral malformations (described elsewhere).
- *Perinatal damage.* It is well established that optic atrophy can result from neonatal events but, even following very premature birth, is infrequent. The mechanism(s) by which this occurs is poorly understood. Birth trauma very rarely leads to unilateral nerve damage. Birth asphyxia is sometimes associated with optic atrophy, which may be trans-synaptic, resulting from damage to the postgeniculate pathway (Hellström *et al.* 1997). This is a feature of the immature visual system alone and may result from perinatal brain asphyxia or malformation, e.g. holoprosencephaly, porencephaly, and hydranencephaly.
- *Inflammatory.* Severe meningoencephalitis in infancy may cause optic atrophy.
- *Compression.* Hydrocephalus, by stretching or compression, can lead to optic atrophy. Tumors may compress the chiasm or nerve (e.g. craniopharyngioma) or involve the anterior visual pathway (glioma).
- *Metabolic.* This includes the lipid storage diseases (e.g. Tay–Sachs's disease), Leigh's subacute necrotizing encephalopathy, and osteopetrosis.

## Optic nerve hypoplasia

This is a congenital anomaly of the optic nerve (Brodsky 1991; Taylor & Scott 1997), whose incidence may be increasing (Robinson & Jan 1987). Typically, the optic disc is small, surrounded by a peripapillary pigmented ring (Fig. 38.15), the retinal vessels are slightly tortuous, and the nerve fiber layer is thinned (Frisen & Holmegaard 1978; Skarf & Hoyt 1984). As none of these signs are pathognomonic, mild optic-nerve hypoplasia (ONH) may be difficult to diagnose – the disc may be of normal size, and examination of the nerve fiber layer is not feasible in infancy. To add to this difficulty, the double-ring sign is quite common in the 'normal' premature infant.

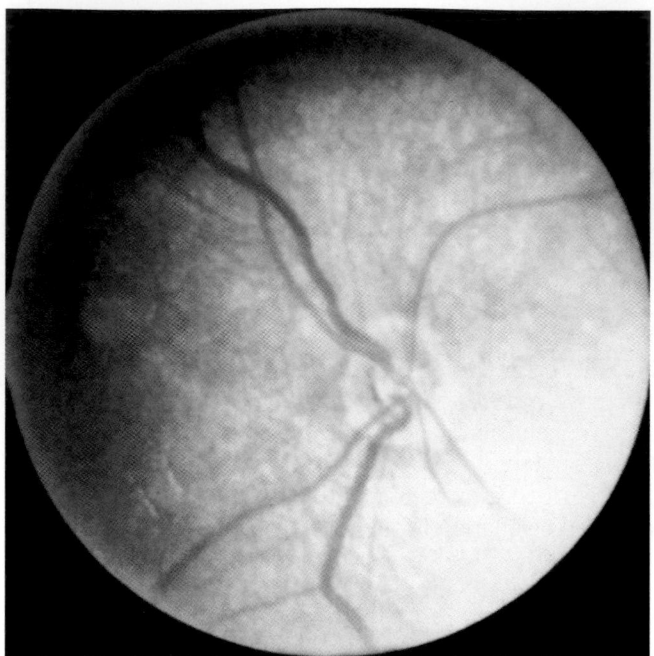

**Figure 38.15** Optic-nerve hypoplasia.

The pathogenesis of optic-nerve hypoplasia is not known but it may represent a non-specific manifestation of damage to the developing visual system (Frisen & Holmegaard 1978). Not surprisingly, therefore, a degree of optic atrophy often coexists. Thus, optic-nerve hypoplasia may be associated, particularly if bilateral, with a large variety of ocular or systemic abnormalities (Margalith *et al.* 1984; Skarf & Hoyt 1984). Structural CNS abnormalities associated with optic-nerve hypoplasia include absence of the septum pellucidum, hydranencephaly, porencephaly, holoprosencephaly, cerebral atrophy, and cystic subcortical leukomalacia, and may therefore be occasionally detected on routine examination of neurologically abnormal neonates (Fielder *et al.* 1986b). Optic-nerve hypoplasia has recently been described in infants exposed to cocaine *in utero* (Good *et al.* 1992).

Neuroendocrine dysfunction occurs in 20–30% of cases of optic-nerve hypoplasia, with or without a structural neurologic anomaly. As this often does not become apparent until about 2–5 years of age, continued surveillance is necessary. Growth, thyroid, and gonadotrophin hormones may all be affected, and diabetes insipidus has been reported (Margalith *et al.* 1984, 1985; Skarf & Hoyt 1984; Costin & Murphree 1985). Transient neonatal cholestatic jaundice and hypoglycemia are reported associations (Stanhope *et al.* 1984), but it is not known whether these are the patients liable to develop other neuroendocrine problems later. Absence of a septum pellucidum is not in itself associated with intellectual, behavioral, or neurologic deficits (Williams *et al.* 1993).

CT or ultrasound scanning may determine the extent of, and anticipate, possible future neurodevelopmental problems. Also, MRI spectroscopy may predict neuroendocrine problems (Brodsky & Glasier 1993).

### Other congenital abnormalities of the optic disc

Abnormalities such as coloboma, the morning glory syndrome, and pits are not considered here.

## Posterior visual pathway disorders

Disorders of the posterior visual pathway, in contrast to those of the anterior visual pathway, do not affect the pupil responses, and nystagmus is not a feature. As a caveat to the last comment, many posterior visual pathway disorders are the consequence of widespread neurological damage. Thus, a few jerks of nystagmus may be present, but this is not the sustained oscillation in the straight ahead position, which is due to the visual deficit *per se*.

### Delayed visual maturation

Parents and clinicians have known for years that the sight of a blind infant may later improve. First described by Beauvieux (1926), the term 'delayed visual maturation' (DVM) was introduced by Illingworth (1961). This is probably the most common cause of a severe bilateral visual defect in early infancy, and, at its simplest, DVM is an isolated defect with subsequent complete and permanent visual improvement. Unfortunately, as Beauvieux (1947) recognized, not all infants with DVM do so well. Although a degree of visual improvement by definition occurs in all, some with associated ocular and/or neurologic problems behave differently clinically and suffer a permanent visual defect dependent upon the underlying pathology.

Expanding upon Beauvieux's observations, DVM has been classified by Uemera *et al.* (1981), Fielder *et al.* (1985), and, most recently, Fielder & Mayer (1991):

- Type 1. DVM as an isolated anomaly:
  A. Normal perinatal period
  B. With perinatal problems
- Type 2. DVM associated with obvious and persistent neurodevelopmental problems
- Type 3. DVM associated with nystagmus and albinism
- Type 4. DVM with severe congenital, bilateral structural ocular abnormalities.

The spectrum is becoming increasingly broad, as Russell-Eggitt *et al.* (1998) stated DVM is not a single condition but a feature common to neurologic abnormalities affecting several areas of the brain.

*DVM as an isolated anomaly – types 1A and 1B* In this type of DVM, the infant presents with severely reduced or absent vision. There are no abnormal signs on examination, other than those attributable to the visual defect (e.g. ocular divergence). Nystagmus is never present. The ERG is always normal, and the flash VEP may range from absent to normal. The time of visual improvement ranges from about 10 to 18 weeks for type 1A, although for type 1B, this may not occur for up to 24 weeks. Characteristically, this change is rapid, often occurring over only a few days or a week or so, and the subsequent visual acuity development is normal (Fig. 38.16). Although DVM is considered the sole abnormality in this group, a significant number are either born prematurely or suffer perinatal problems (type 1B), on occasion resulting in permanent, usually mild, neurologic sequelae, including squint (Tresidder *et al.* 1990).

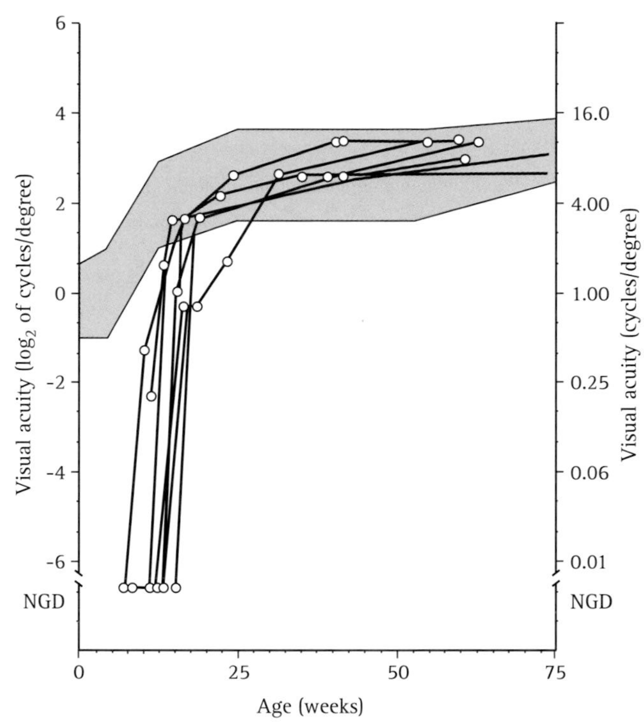


**Figure 38.16** Delayed visual maturation type 1A. Visual acuities recorded by the ACP. [Reprinted, with permission, from Tresidder *et al.* (1990)]

*DVM associated with obvious and persistent neurodevelopmental problems – type 2* That blind infants with severe neurodevelopmental problems may later improve visually is well known. However, in contrast to the first type of DVM, the improvement is often slow, occurring over weeks and months rather than days (Fig. 38.17). The eventual level of vision achieved is obviously governed by the amount of visual pathway damage but does not reach normal levels. Nystagmus, consequent upon associated neurologic damage, may be present in this group, but this is rarely sustained. Again, the ERG is always normal and the VEP variably affected, and may be normal during the period of amaurosis (Lambert *et al.* 1989).

*DVM associated with infantile nystagmus and albinism – type 3* For over a century, it has been known that infants with

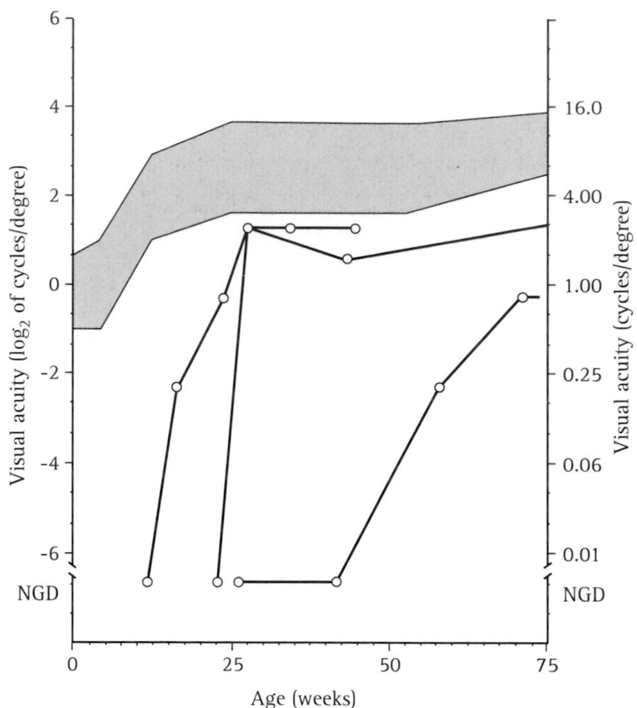


Figure 38.17 Delayed visual maturation type 2. No infant achieved normal acuity. [Reprinted, with permission, from Tresidder *et al.* (1990).]

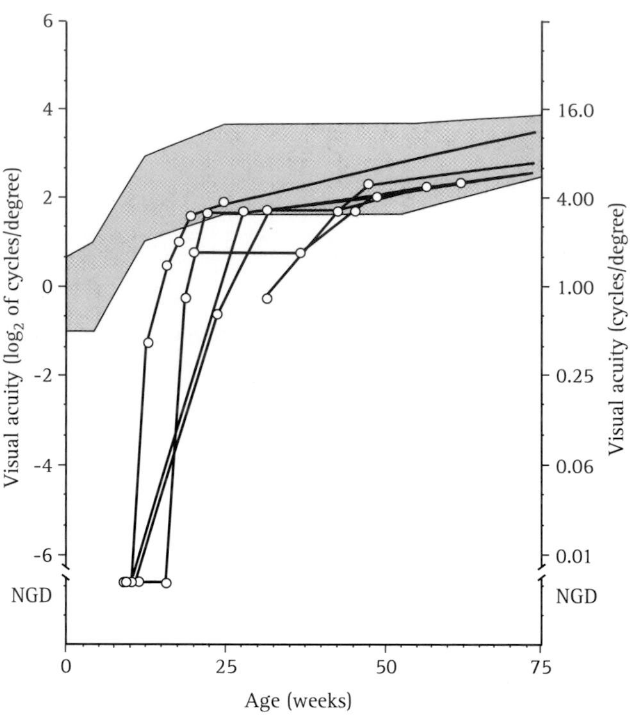


Figure 38.18 Delayed visual maturation type 3. Although normal acuity (ACP data) was achieved during infancy, if the measurements had continued, plateauing would have become apparent in early childhood as children with nystagmus have subnormal acuity (see Fig. 33.10). [Reprinted, with permission, from Tresidder *et al.* (1990).]

albinism may be blind in early infancy and then subsequently improve. This also occurs in congenital/infantile nystagmus. It is interesting to note that during the period of blindness, nystagmus is not a feature, and this oscillation commences around the time of (or slightly before) the development of vision (it was stated earlier that nystagmus rarely commences at birth). Vision improves in this group between 13 and 21 weeks (Tresidder *et al.* 1990) (Fig. 38.18), and the pattern of change is quite different from that seen in type 4 DVM, which is slow and extremely limited.

*Delayed visual maturation with severe congenital, bilateral structural ocular abnormalities (excluding albinism) – type 4* Clinicians have known for years that some infants who are blind due to severe ocular abnormalities may exhibit a degree of improvement (Fielder & Mayer 1991) (Fig. 38.19). Type 4 DVM is seen in optic nerve hypoplasia, Leber's congenital amaurosis, and coloboma (Fielder *et al.* 1991; Good *et al.* 1992). While the functional importance of this improvement must not be underestimated, it is nevertheless limited, and all children remain visually impaired and probably legally blind. Initially confusing, in clinical practice, differentiating between types 3 and 4 is not a problem. In type 3, DVM dominates the clinical picture, whereas in type 4, the ocular abnormality is the major feature and the improvement relatively modest.

*Summary of the clinical features of DVM* All infants show a reduced or absent visual responsiveness from birth that subsequently improves. The degree of improvement is governed by any coexisting visual pathway or CNS pathology but in the absence of these is complete. Nystagmus is not a feature during the period of blindness but becomes apparent in type 3 around the time of visual improvement. The possible exception to the last comments is type 4, in which the early natural history is unknown.

*Pathogenesis of DVM* This cannot be discussed in detail here (Tresidder *et al.* 1990; Fielder & Mayer 1991; Hoyt & Good 1993; Russell-Eggitt *et al.* 1998). With a normal ERG, a retinal origin is improbable, and a defect in myelination is unlikely to be the whole story. The evidence at present points either to a cortical and/or subcortical defect, the latter is currently favored as vision in early infancy may be subserved on a subcortical basis (Atkinson 1992), and the onset of vision coincides with the emergence of cortical vision (Cocker *et al.* 1998). In connection with the latter, it is interesting to note the suggestion that the VEP in early infancy may have a subcortical origin (Dubowitz *et al.* 1986). As a number of these infants have experienced problems in the neonatal period, there is a possibility that a

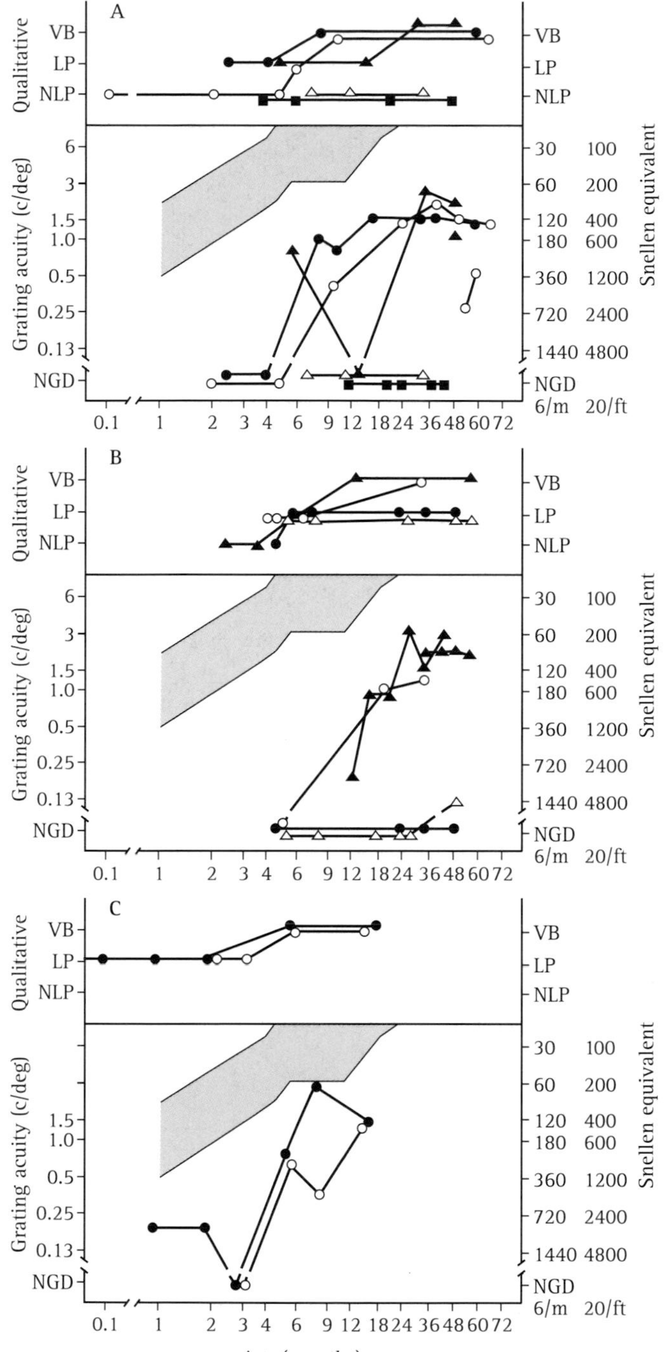


**Figure 38.19** Delayed visual maturation type 4. Qualitative visual responses (upper) and ACP acuities (lower). **(A)** Five patients with Leber's congenital amaurosis. **(B)** Four with optic nerve hypoplasia and **(C)** two infants with bilateral colobomata. NLP = no light perception; VB = visually guided behavior; NGD = no grating detection. [Redrawn, from Fielder *et al.* (1991) Copyright 1991, with permission from Elsevier Science].

subtle neurologic insult may be a factor in some cases of DVM, and it is pertinent to recall the observation that neurologically abnormal preterm infants may show delayed acuity maturation (Placzek *et al.* 1985). It is unlikely that the full spectrum of DVM, ranging from DVM as an isolated anomaly to associated involvement with other ocular and neurologic conditions, has the same basis. For DVM type 1 with its tight clinical course, we have postulated a discrete rather than a widespread structural abnormality (Cocker *et al.* 1998), which may impinge on parietal cortex function (Russell-Eggitt *et al.* 1998).

## Periventricular leukomalacia (see Chapter 22)

This ischemic neurologic lesion, which may complicate birth at term or before, is dealt with in detail elsewhere in this book. A cause of cortical blindness, it is considered separately first to cover aspects other than the visual acuity deficit, which will be dealt with below. Visual pathway involvement is probably frequent in periventricular leukomalacia (PVL), particularly if the lesion is located posteriorly (Gibson *et al.* 1990). These include low acuity, delayed visual field and acuity development, strabismus, and supranuclear disorders of eye movement (Weindling *et al.* 1985; Calvert *et al.* 1986; de Vries *et al.* 1987; Lambert *et al.* 1987; Scher *et al.* 1989; Gibson *et al.* 1990; Cioni *et al.* 1992; Pike *et al.* 1994). The mechanism of visual pathway involvement is not known, but it is interesting to note that infants who experience recurrent hypoxia (bronchopulmonary dysplasia) but who do not have PVL show normal development of both grating acuity and visual field (Luna *et al.* 1992). As mentioned previously, subtle optic nerve abnormalities that may represent trans synaptic degeneration have been reported (Hellström *et al.* 1997)

## Cortical visual impairment

The term 'cortical blindness' describes a patient totally and permanently blind but with a normal ocular examination including preservation of the pupillary responses. Fortunately for the infant and child, these comments are incorrect, as a degree of visual recovery is the rule, so the term 'cortical visual impairment' (CVI) is preferred (in future editions of this book, this may be further modified to cerebral vision impairment as objective signs of visual cortex damage are not always present).

The child with CVI has often suffered widespread brain damage and may exhibit many diverse CNS and ocular signs (Whiting *et al.* 1985; Jan & Wong 1991; Good *et al.* 1994; Cioni *et al.* 1996; Lambert 1997; Dutton *et al.* 1999).

The causes of CVI include:

- *Prenatal*: malformations, intrauterine infection, and toxemia
- *Perinatal*: hypoxic–ischemic episodes as in neonatal asphyxia and intracerebral hemorrhage, hypoglycemia, meningitis, and encephalitis
- *Acquired*: meningitis, encephalitis, cardiac arrest, neurodegenerative disorders, trauma, cortical vein thrombosis, and shunt failure.

Clinical assessment of these patients is often difficult, and as many have suffered diffuse brain damage, coexistent ophthalmic and neurologic signs are common (van Hof-van Duin & Mohn 1984b; Whiting *et al.* 1985; Huo *et al.* 1999). The absence of nystagmus is an important clue to cortical involvement, with the qualification already made that there may be multiple pathology and that poorly sustained CNS nystagmus may be present.

The VEP to a flash stimulus is not always abnormal in CVI and was so in less than half of the patients reported by Whiting *et al.* (1985). Frank & Torres (1979) were unable to detect any significant difference between the VEPs of normal and cortically blind children. These findings have reduced the value of this test as a means of investigation in cortical visual problems; however, the presence of a normal VEP is helpful in predicting those infants and children who may subsequently improve.

The clinical course of cortical blindness is extremely variable and is determined to a certain extent by its etiology. Hoyt (1986b) was unable to establish any correlation between the duration of the blindness and the extent of the visual recovery. However, total recovery within a few hours has been observed in children who suffered 'trivial' head trauma (Griffith & Dodge 1968). Visual improvement is obviously not anticipated in patients with neurodegenerative disorders, and the prognosis following bacterial meningitis is worse than for other causes (Ackroyd 1984). Thus, complete recovery has been reported following head injury (Griffith & Dodge 1968) and cardiac arrest (Weinberger *et al.* 1962) but in only 50% of patients with bacterial meningitis (Ackroyd 1984). Chen *et al.* (1992) reported a lack of improvement only with hypoxia. Martin & Barkovich (1995) reported a good correlation between MRI taken before 3 days and outcome.

Complete blindness is rarely permanent in CVI (Lambert *et al.* 1987; Jan & Wong 1991; Good *et al.* 1994), although it should be emphasized that the degree of improvement is often incomplete (Hoyt 1986b); for this reason, the designation cortical visual impairment (CVI) is more appropriate (Whiting *et al.* 1985). The relationship between CVI and DVM needs to be clarified, as almost by definition, DVM type 2 falls into the CVI complex. It is possible that in many instances, the distinction is one of timing and degree rather than the site of the lesion. According to Schenk-Rootlieb *et al.* (1992), a degree of CVI is frequent, albeit often 'mild' in children with cerebral palsy and may remain so, unless vision is quantified by tests such as the ACP. Visual improvement may take from a few hours to more than 2 years, and begins first with light perception and then the ability to follow objects. Eye-to-eye contact is often lacking, and visual function may vary from hour to hour. Most children achieve at least navigational vision, although severe visual-perceptual difficulties sometimes persist (Dutton *et al.* 1999).

### Investigation and management of the visually inattentive infant

Each infant should have a detailed ophthalmic and pediatric assessment, the extent of which is governed by clinical findings. Nowadays, this should include both qualitative and quantitative assessment of visual functions. In view of the varied natural history of many of these disorders and the absence in many conditions of ophthalmoscopically visible signs, the clinician should have a very low threshold to undertake electrophysiologic investigations, particularly the ERG. Excepting the vision deficit, should the infant be normal in all respects, the likelihood of some improvement of vision occurring is very high and should be conveyed to parents. In general, however, caution is recommended in counseling, for misplaced optimism results in considerable and unnecessary parental anxiety and turmoil.

## Conclusion

The past couple of decades have been some of the most exciting with respect to the basic and clinical research on the developing visual system. Our understanding of the ophthalmic associations with neurologic disorders has also greatly increased, and hopefully, these will pave the way to tease out mechanisms.

**Key Points**

- Distinction between normal and abnormal eye movements in the neonatal period may be very difficult
- Eye movement disorders are divided into either nuclear/infranuclear, supranuclear or nystagmus/related oscillations
- The neurologic site of severe visual impairment must be investigated. This includes disorders of the anterior visual pathway, retinal disorders, optic nerve disorders and posterior visual pathway disorders
- Delayed visual maturation is probably the most common cause of severe bilateral visual defect in early infancy. If isolated, subsequent complete and permanent visual improvement is expected

## REFERENCES


Ackroyd R S (1984) Cortical blindness following bacterial meningitis: a case report with reassessment of prognosis and aetiology. *Dev Med Child Neurol* 26:227–230.

Anderson L T, Coll C G, Vohr B R *et al.* (1989) Behavioural characteristics and early temperature of premature infants with intracranial haemorrhage. *Early Hum Dev* 18:273–283.

Antony J H, Ouvrier R A & Wise G (1980) Spasmus nutans: a mistaken identity. *Arch Neurol* 37:373–375.

Apkarian P, Mirmian M & Tijssen R (1991) Effects of behavioural state on visual processing in neonates. *Neuropediatrics* 22:85–91.

Apkarian P & Tijssen R (1992) Detection and maturation of VEP albino asymmetry: an overview and a longitudinal study from birth to 54 weeks. *Behav Brain Res* 49:57–67.

Archer S M & Helveston E M (1994) Strabismus and eye movement disorders. In: Isenberg I (ed.) *The eye in infancy*. St. Louis, MO: Mosby; 2nd edn, pp. 254–274.

Archer S M, Sondhi N & Helveston E M (1989) Strabismus in infancy. *Ophthalmology* 96:133–137.

Arnoldi K A & Tycheson L (1995) Prevalence of intracranial lesions in children initially diagnosed awith disconjugate nystagmus (Spasmus nutans). *J Pediatr Ophthalmol Strabismus* 32:296–301.

Aslin R & Salapatek P (1975) Saccadic localization of visual targets by the very young human infant. *Percept Psychophys* 17:293–302.

Aslin R N (1977) Development of binocular fixation in human infants. *J Exp Psychol* 23:133–150.

Aslin R (1993) Infant accommodation and convergence. In: Simons K (ed.) *Early visual development: normal and abnormal*. Oxford: Oxford University Press; pp. 30–38.

Atkinson J (1992) Early visual development: differential functioning of parvocellular and magnocellular pathways. *Eye* 6:129–135.

Atkinson J & Braddick O (1983) Assessment of visual acuity in infancy and early childhood. *Acta Ophthalmol (Copenhagen)* 157 (suppl):18–26.

Atkinson J, Braddick O J, Pimm-Smith E *et al.* (1981) Does the Catford drum give an accurate assessment of acuity? *Br J Ophthalmol* 66:652–656.

Atkinson J, Hood B, Wattam-Bell J *et al.* (1992) Changes in infants' ability to switch visual attention in the first three months of life. *Perception* 21:643–653.

Aylward G P, Lazzara A & Meyer J (1978) Behavioural characteristics of a hydranencephalic infant. *Dev Med Child Neurol* 20:211–217.

Bankes J L K (1974) Eye defects of mentally handicapped children. *BMJ* ii:533–535.

Beauvieux J (1926) La pseudo-atrophie optique des nouveaux-nes (dysgenesie myelinique des voies optiques). *Annales d'Oculistique* 163:881–921.

Beauvieux M (1947) La cecite apparente chez le nouveau-ne la pseudoatrophie grise du nerf optique. *Archives Ophthalmologie (Paris)* 7:241–249.

Bell J A, Fielder A R & Viney S A (1990) Congenital double elevator palsy in identical twins. *J Clin Neuro-ophthalmol* 10:32–34.

Birch E E, Birch D, Hoffman D *et al.* (1993) Breast-feeding and optimal visual development. *J Pediatr Ophthalmol Strabismus* 30:33–38.

Birch E E & Stager D R (1988) Prevalence of good visual acuity following surgery for congenital unilateral cataract. *Arch Ophthalmol* 106:40–43.

Birch E & Petrig B (1996) FPL and VEP measures of fusion, stereopsis and stereoacuity in normal infants. *Vis Res* 36:1321–1327.

Birnholz J C (1981) The development of human fetal eye movement patterns. *Science* 213:679–681.

Boothe R G, Dobson V & Teller D Y (1985) Postnatal development of vision in human and nonhuman primates. *Ann Rev Neurosci* 8:495–545.

Braddick O & Atkinson J (1983) Some recent findings on the development of human binocularity: a review. *Behav Brain Res* 10:141–150.

Braddick O, Atkinson J, Hood B *et al.* (1992) Possible blindsight in infants lacking one cerebral hemisphere. *Nature* 360:461–463.

Brazelton T B, Scholl M L & Robey J S (1966) Visual responses in the newborn. *Pediatrics* 37:284–290.

Bremer D L, Palmer E A, Fellows R R *et al.* (1998) *Arch Ophthalmol* 116:329–333.

Brodsky M C (1991) Septo-optic dysplasia: a reappraisal. *Semin Ophthalmol* 6:227–232.

Brodsky M & Glasier C (1993) Optic nerve hypoplasia: clinical significance of associated central nervous system abnormalities in magnetic resonance imaging. *Arch Ophthalmol* 111:66–74.

Brown A M & Yamamoto M (1986) Visual acuity in newborn and preterm infants measured with grating acuity cards. *Am J Ophthalmol* 102:245–253.

Burgess P & Johnson A (1991) Ocular defects in infants of extremely low birthweight and low gestational age. *Br J Ophthalmol* 75:84–87.

Calvert S A, Hoskins E M, Fong K W *et al.* (1986) Periventricular leukomalacia: ultrasound diagnosis and neurological outcome. *Acta Paediatr Scand* 75:489–496.

Campistol J, Prats J M & Garaizar C (1993) Benign paroxysmal tonic upgaze of childhood with ataxia. A neuro-ophthalmological syndrome of familial origin. *Dev Med Child Neurol* 35:436–438.

Catalano R A, Simon J W, Jenkins P L *et al.* (1987) Preferential looking as a guide for amblyopia therapy in monocular cataracts. *J Pediatr Ophthalmol Strabismus* 24:56–63.

Chandna A (1991) Natural history of the development of visual acuity in infants. *Eye* 5:20–26.

Chandna A, Pearson C M & Doran R M L (1988) Preferential looking in clinical practice: a year's experience. *Eye* 2:488–495.

Chen T C, Weinberg M H, Catalano R A *et al.* (1992) Development of object vision in infants with permanent cortical visual impairment. *Am J Ophthalmol* 114:575–578.

Cioni G, Bartalena L, Biagioni E *et al.* (1992) Neuroimaging and functional outcome of neonatal leukomalacia. *Behav Brain Res* 49:7–19.

Cioni G, Ipata A E, Canapicchi R *et al.* (1996) MRI findings in children with cerebral visual impairment. In: Vital-Durand F, Atkinson J & Braddick O J (eds) *Infant vision*. Oxford: Oxford University Press; pp. 373–382.

Coakes R L, Clothier C & Wilson A (1979) Binocular reflexes in the first 6 months of life: preliminary results of a study of normal infants. *Child Care, Health Dev* 5:405–408.

Cocker K D, Moseley M J, Bissenden J G *et al.* (1994) Visual acuity and pupillary responses to spatial structue in infants. *Invest Ophthalmol Vis Sci* 35:2620–2625.

Cocker K D, Moseley M J, Stirling H F *et al.* (1998) Delayed visual maturation: pupillary responses implicate subcortical and cortical visual systems. *Dev Med Child Neurol* 40:160–162.

Cogan D G (1952) A type of congenital ocular motor apraxia presenting jerky head movements. *Trans Am Acad Ophthalmol Otolaryngol* 56:853–862.

Cogan D G (1966) Congenital ocular motor apraxia. *Can J Ophthalmol* 1:253–260.

Cordero L, Clark D L & Urrutia J G (1983) Postrotatory nystagmus in the full-term and premature infant. *Int J Pediat Otorhinolaryngol* 5:47–57.

Costin G & Murphree A L (1985) Hypothalamic-pituitary function in children with optic nerve hypoplasia. *Am J Dis Children* 139:249–254.

Courage M L & Adams R J (1990) Visual acuity assessment from birth to three years using the acuity card procedure: cross-sectional and longitudinal samples. *Optometry and Vis Sci* 67:713–718.

Crognale M A, Kelly J P, Chang S *et al.* (1997) Development of pattern visual evoked potentials: longitudinal measurements in human infants. *Optometry Vis Sci* 74:808–815.

Dell'Osso L F, Daroff R B & Todd Troost B (1990) Nystagmus and saccadic intrusions and oscillations. In: Glaser J S (ed.) *Neuro-ophthalmology*. Hagerstown: Harper and Row; pp. 325–356.

De Vries-Khoe L H & Spekreijse H (1982) Maturation of luminance and pattern EPs in man. In: Niemayer G (ed.) *Documenta Opthalmologica Proceedings Series* 31:461–475.

De Vries L S, Connell J A, Dubowitz L M S *et al.* (1987) Neurological electrophysiological and MRI abnormalities in infants with extensive cystic leukomalacia. *Neuropediatrics* 18:61–66.

Dobson V (1994) Visual acuity testing by preferential looking techniques. In: Isenberg I (ed.) *The eye in infancy*. St. Louis, MO: Mosby; 2nd edn, pp. 131–156.

Dobson V, Brown A M, Harvey E M *et al.* (1998) Visual field extent in children 3.5–30 months of life tested with a double-arc LED perimeter. *Vis Res* 38:2743–2760.

Dobson V, Mayer D L & Lee C P (1980) Visual acuity screening of preterm infants. *Invest Ophthalmol Vis Sci* 19:1498–1504.

Dobson V, Schwartz T L, Sandstrom D J *et al.* (1987) Binocular visual acuity of neonates: the acuity card procedure. *Dev Med Child Neurol* 29:199–206.

Donat J F G, Donat J R & Lay K S (1980) Changing response to caloric stimulation with gestational age in infants. *Neurology* 30:776–778.

Dubowitz L M S, Dubowitz V, Morante A *et al.* (1980) Visual function in the preterm and fullterm newborn infant. *Dev Med Child Neurol* 22:465–475.

Dubowitz L M S, Levene M I, Morante A *et al.* (1981) Neurologic signs in neonatal intraventricular hemorrhage: a correlation with real-time ultrasound. *J Pediatr* 99:127–133.

Dubowitz L M S, Mushin J, de Vries L *et al.* (1986) Visual function in the newborn infant: is it cortically mediated? *Lancet* i:1139–1141.

Dubowitz L M S, Mushin J, Morante A *et al.* (1983) The maturation of visual acuity in neurologically normal and abnormal newborn infants. *Behav Brain Res* 10:39–45.

Dutton D N, Day R E & McCulloch D M (1999) Who is a visually impaired child? A model is needed to address this question for children with cerebral visual impairment. *Dev Med Child Neurol* 41:211–213.

Evans N M, Fielder A R & Mayer D L (1989) Ametropia in congenital cone deficiency – achromatopsia: a defect of emmetropisation? *Clin Vis Sci* 4:129–136.

Eviatar L, Eviatar A & Naray (1974) Maturation of neurovestibular responses in infants. *Dev Med Child Neurol* 16:435–446.

Eviatar L, Miranda S, Eviatar A *et al.* (1979) Development of nystagmus in response to vestibular stimulation in infants. *Ann Neurol* 5:508–514.

Farmer J & Hoyt C S (1984) Monocular nystagmus in infancy and early childhood. *Am J Ophthalmol* 98:504–509.

Ferrari F, Grosoli M V, Fontana G *et al.* (1983) Neurobehavioural comparison of low-risk preterm and fullterm infants at term conceptual age. *Dev Med Child Neurol* 25:450–458.

Fielder A R (1985) Neonatal eye movements: normal and abnormal. *B Orthop J* 42:10–15.

Fielder A R (1989) The management of squint. *Arch Dis Childhood* 64:413–418.

Fielder A R, Dobson V, Moseley M J *et al.* (1992) Preferential looking – clinical lessons. *Ophthal Paediatr Genet* 13:101–110.

Fielder A R & Evans N M (1988) Is the geniculostriate system a prerequisite for nystagmus? *Eye* 2:628–635.

Fielder A R, Foreman N, Moseley M J *et al.* (1993) Prematurity and visual development. In: Simons K (ed.) *Early visual development: normal and abnormal.* New York: Oxford University Press; pp. 485–504.

Fielder A R, Fulton A B & Mayer D L (1991) Visual development of infants with severe ocular disorders. *Opthalmology* 98:1306–1309.

Fielder A R, Gresty M A, Dodd K L *et al.* (1986a) Congenital ocular motor apraxia. *Trans Ophthalmol Soc UK* 105:589–598.

Fielder A R, Harper M W, Higgins J E *et al.* (1983) The reliability of the VEP in infancy. *Ophth Paediatr Genet* 3:73–82.

Fielder A R, Levene M I, Trounce J Q *et al.* (1986b) Optic nerve hypoplasia in infancy. *J Roy Soc Med* 79:25–29.

Fielder A R & Mayer D L (1991) Delayed visual maturation. *Semin Ophthalmol* 6:182–193.

Fielder A R & Moseley M J (1988) Do we need to measure the vision of children? *J Roy Soc Med* 81:380–383.

Fielder A R & Moseley M J (2000) Environmental light and the preterm infant. *Semin Perinatol* 24:291–298.

Fielder A R, Moseley M J & Ng Y K (1988) The immature visual system and premature birth. *Br Med Bull* 44:1093–1118.

Fielder A R, Russell-Eggitt I R, Dodd K L *et al.* (1985) Delayed visual maturation. *Trans Ophthalmol Soc UK* 104:653–661.

Foreman N, Fielder A, Price *et al.* (1991) Tonic and phasic orientation in full-term and preterm infants. *J Exp Child Psychol* 51:407–422.

Frank Y & Torres F (1979) Visual evoked potentials in the evaluation of 'cortical blindness' in children. *Ann Neurol* 6:126–129.

Frisen L & Holmegaard L (1978) Spectrum of optic nerve hypoplasia. *Br J Ophthalmol* 62:7–15.

Gibson N A, Fielder A R, Trounce J Q *et al.* (1990) Ophthalmic findings in infants of very low birthweight. *Dev Med Child Neurol* 32:7–13.

Goldie L & Hopkins I J (1964) Head turning towards diffuse light in the neurological examination of newborn infants. *Brain* 87:665–672.

Good W V, Ferriero D M, Golabi M *et al.* (1992) Abnormalities of the visual system in infants exposed to cocaine. *Ophthalmology* 99:341–346.

Good W V, Jan J E, Desa L *et al.* (1994) Cortical visual impairment in children. *Surv Ophthalmol* 38:351–364.

Good W V, Jan J E, Hoyt C S *et al.* (1997) Monocular vision loss can cause bilateral nystagmus in young children. *Dev Med Child Neurol* 39:421–424.

Gorman J J, Cogan D G & Gellis S S (1957) An apparatus for grading the visual acuity of infants on the basis of opticokinetic nystagmus. *Pediatrics* 19:1088–1092.

Gottlob I, Zubcov A, Catalano R A *et al.* (1990) Signs distinguishing spasmus nutans (with and without central nervous system lesions) from infantile nystagmus. *Ophthalmology* 97:1166–1175.

Gottlob I, Zubcov A A, Wizow S S *et al.* (1992) Head nodding is compensatory in spasmus nutans. *Ophthalmology* 99:1024–1031.

Griffith J G & Dodge P R (1968) Transient blindness following head injury in children. *N Engl J Med* 278:648–651.

Groenendaal F, van Hof-van Duin J, Baerts W *et al.* (1989) Effects of perinatal hypoxia on visual development during the first year of (corrected) age. *Early Hum Dev* 20:267–279.

Hack M, Muszynski S Y & Miranda S B (1981) State of awakeness during visual fixation in preterm infants. *Pediatrics* 68:87–92.

Hainline L (1998) The development of basic visual abilities. In: Slater A (ed.) *Perceptual development: visual, auditory and speech perception in infancy.* Hove: Psychology Press; pp. 5–50.

Harris C M (1997a) Nystagmus and eye movement disorders. In: Taylor D (ed.) *Paediatric ophthalmology.* Oxford: Blackwell Science; 2nd edn, pp. 869–896.

Harris C M (1997b) Other eye movement disorders. In: Taylor D (ed.) *Paediatric ophthalmology.* Oxford: Blackwell Science; 2nd edn, pp. 897–924.

Harris C M, Jacobs M, Shawkat F *et al.* (1993) The development of saccadic accuracy in the first 7 months. *Clin Vis Sci* 8:85–96.

Harvey E M, Dobson V, Luna B *et al.* (1997a) Grating acuity and visual-field development in children with intraventricular hemorrhage. *Dev Med Child Neurol* 39:305–312.

Harvey E M, Dobson V & Luna B (1997b) Long-term grating acuity and visual-field development in preterm children who experienced bronchopulmonary dysplasia. *Dev Med Child Neurol* 39:167–173.

Hellström A, Chen Y H & Svenson E (1997) Optic disc size and retinal vessel characteristics in healthy children. *Arch Ophthalmol* 115:1263–1269.

Hendrickson A E & Youdelis C (1984) The morphological development of the human fovea. *Ophthalmology* 91:603–612.

Holmstrom G, el-Azazi M & Kugelberg U (1999) Ophthalmological follow up of preterm infants: a population based, prospective study of visual acuity and strabismus. *Br J Ophthalmol* 83:143–150.

Hood B & Atkinson J (1990) Sensory visual loss and cognitive deficits in the selective attentional system of normal infants and neurologically impaired children. *Dev Med Child Neurol* 32:1067–1077.

Horwood A M (1993) Maternal observations of ocular alignment in infants. *J Paediatr Ophthalmol Strabismus* 30:100–105.

Hoyt C S (1986a) Objective techniques of visual acuity assessment in infancy. In: *Pediatric ophthalmology and strabismus: Transactions of the New Orleans Academy of Ophthalmology.* Raven Press: New York, NY: pp. 7–13.

Hoyt C S (1986b) Cortical blindness in infancy. In: *Pediatric ophthalmology and strabismus: Transactions of the New Orleans Academy of Ophthalmology.* New York, NY: Raven Press, pp.235–243.

Hoyt C S, Billson F A & Taylor H (1977) Isolated unilateral gaze palsy. *J Pediat Ophthalmol* 14:343–345.

Hoyt C S & Gelbart S S (1984) Vertical nystagmus in infants with congenital ocular abnormalities. *Ophthal Paediatr Genet* 4:155–162.

Hoyt C S & Good W V (1993) Visual factors in developmental delay and neurological disorders in infants. In: Simons K (ed.) *Early visual development: normal and abnormal.* New York: Oxford University Press; pp. 505–512.

Hoyt C S, Mousel D K & Weber A A (1980) Transient supranuclear disturbances of gaze in healthy neonates. *Am J Ophthalmol* 89:708–713.

Hoyt C S, Nickel B L & Billson F A (1982) Ophthalmological examination of the infant: developmental aspects. *Surv Ophthalmol* 26:177–189.

Huo R, Burden S K, Hoyt C S *et al.* (1999) Chronic cortical visual impairment in children: aetiology, prognosis, and associated neurological deficits. *Br J Ophthalmol* 83:670–675.

Illingworth R S (1961) Delayed visual maturation. *Arch Dis Childhood* 36:407–409.

Inoue M, Koyanagi T, Nakahara H *et al.* (1986) Functional development of human eye movement *in utero* assessed quantitatively with real-time ultrasound. *Am J Obstet Gynecol* 155:170–174.

Isenberg I (ed.) (1994) *The eye in infancy.* St. Louis, MO: Mosby; 2nd edn.

Jan J E, Carruthers J D & Tillson G (1992) Neurodevelopmental criteria in the classification of congenital nystagmus. *Can J Neurosci* 19:76–79.

Jan J E & Wong P K H (1991) The child with cortical visual impairment. *Semin Ophthalmol* 6:194–200.

Kennedy K A, Ipson M A, Birch D G *et al.* (1997) Light reduction and the electroretinogram of preterm infants. *Arch Dis Childhood* 76:F168–F173.

Kremenitzer J P, Vaughan H G, Kurtzberg D *et al.* (1979) Smooth-pursuit eye movements in the newborn infant. *Child Dev* 50:442–448.

Kriss A & Thompson D (1997) Visual electrophysiology. In: Taylor D (ed) *Paediatric ophthalmology.* Oxford: Blackwell Science; pp. 93–121.

Kurtzberg D, Vaughan H G Jr, Daum C, Grellong B A, Albin S, Rotkin L (1979) Neurobehavioral performance of low-birthweight infants at 40 weeks conceptional age: comparison with normal fullterm infants. *Dev Med Child Neurol* 5: 590–607.

Lambert S (1997) Brain problems. In: Taylor D (ed.) *Paediatric ophthalmology.* Oxford: Blackwell Science; pp. 740–750.

Lambert S R, Hoyt C S, Jan J E *et al.* (1987) Visual recovery from hypoxic cortical blindness during childhood: computed tomographic and magnetic resonance imaging predictors. *Arch Ophthalmol* 105:1371–1377.

Lambert S R, Kriss A & Taylor D (1989) Delayed visual maturation in infancy: a longitudinal study – clinical and electrophysiological assessment. *Ophthalmology* 96:524–528.

Laws D, Shaw D E, Robinson J *et al.* (1992) Retinopathy of prematurity: a prospective study. Review at six months. *Eye* 6:477–483.

Legge R H, Weiss H S, Hedges T R *et al.* (1992) Periodic alternating gaze deviation in infancy. *Neurology* 42:1740–1743.

Lewis T L & Maurer D (1992) The development of the temporal and nasal visual fields during infancy. *Vis Res* 32:903–911.

Ling B-C (1942) A genetic study of sustained visual fixation and associated behaviour in the human infant from birth to six months. *J Genet Psychol* 61:227–277.

Luna B, Dobson V & Guthrie R D (1992) Grating acuity and visual field development of infants with bronchopulmonary dysplasia. *Dev Med Child Neurol* 34:813–821.

McDonald M A, Dobson V, Sebris S L *et al.* (1985) The acuity card procedure: a rapid test of infant acuity. *Invest Ophthalmol Vis Sci* 26:1158–1162.

McGinnis J M (1930) Eye-movements and optic nystagmus in early infancy. *Genet Psychol Monogr* 8:321–427.

McGinnity F G & Bryars J H (1992) Controlled study of ocular morbidity in school children born preterm. *Br J Ophthalmol* 76:520–524.

Mactier H, Hamilton R, Bradnam M S *et al.* (2000) Contact lens electroretinography in preterm infants from 32 weeks after conception: a development in current technology. *Arch Dis Childhood* 82:F233–F236.

Marg E, Freeman D N, Peltzman P *et al.* (1976) Visual acuity development in human infants: evoked potential measurements. *Invest Ophthalmol* 15:150–153.

Margalith D, Jan J E, McCormick A Q *et al.* (1984) Clinical spectrum of congenital optic nerve hypoplasia: a review of 51 patients. *Dev Med Child Neurol* 26:311–322.

Margalith D, Tze W J & Jan J E (1985) Congenital optic nerve hypoplasia with hypothalamic-pituitary dysplasia. *Am J Dis Children* 139:361–366.

Martin E & Barkovich A J (1995) Magnetic resonance imaging in perinatal asphyxia. *Arch Dis Childhood* 72:62–70.

Mayer D L, Beiser A S, Warner A F *et al.* (1995) Monocular acuity norms for the Teller Acuity Cards between ages one month and four years. *Invest Ophthalmol Vis Sci* 36:671–685.

Mayer D L & Fulton A B (1993) Development of the visual field. In: Simons K (ed.) *Early visual development: normal and abnormal.* New York: Oxford University Press; pp. 117–129.

Mayer D L, Fulton A B & Rodier D (1984) Grating and recognition acuities of pediatric patients. *Ophthalmology* 91:947–953.

Mayer D L, Moore B & Robb R M (1989) Assessment of vision and amblyopia by preferential looking tests after early surgery for unilateral cataracts. *J Pediatr Ophthalmol Strabismus* 26:61–67.

Mercer M E, Courage M L & Adams R J (1991) Contrast/color card procedure: a new test of young infants' color vision. *Optometry Vis Sci* 68:522–532.

Mitchell T & Cambon K (1969) Vestibular response in the neonate and infant. *Arch Otolaryngol* 90:40–41.

Mohn G, Dobson V, Schwartz T *et al.* (1986) The visual field of human infants: kinetic perimetry. *Behav Brain Res* 20:122.

Morante A, Dubowitz L M S, Levene M I *et al.* (1982) The development of visual function in normal and neurologically abnormal preterm and fullterm infants. *Dev Med Child Neurol* 24:771–784.

Moseley M J, Fielder A R, Thompson J R *et al.* (1988) Grating and recognition acuities of young amblyopes. *Br J Ophthalmol* 72:50–54.

Moskowitz A & Sokol S (1983) Developmental changes in the human visual system as reflected by the latency of the pattern reversal VEP. *Electroencephalogr Clin Neurophysiol* 56:1–15.

Nixon R B, Helveston E M, Miller K *et al.* (1985) Incidence of strabismus in neonates. *Am J Ophthalmol* 100:798–801.

Norcia A M (1994) Vision testing by visual evoked potential techniques. In: Isenberg I (ed.) *The eye in infancy.* 2nd edition; Chicago: Mosby; pp. 157–173.

Norcia A M, Tyler C W, Piecuch R *et al.* (1987) Visual acuity development in normal and abnormal preterm human infants. *J Pediatr Ophthalmol* Strabismus 24:70–74.

Ornitz E M, Atwell C W, Walter D O *et al.* (1979) The maturation of vestibular nystagmus in infancy and childhood. *Acta Otolaryngol* 88:244–256.

Page J M, Schneeweiss S, Whyte H E A *et al.* (1993) Ocular sequelae in premature infants. *Pediatrics* 92:787–790.

Pearson C M, Chandna A & Doran R M L (1989) Preferential looking: the state of the art. *Br Orthop J* 46:66–72.

Pike M G, Holmstrom G, de-Vries L S *et al.* (1994) Patterns of visual impairment associated with lesions of the preterm infant brain. *Dev Med Child Neurol* 36:849–862.

Placzek M, Mushin J & Dubowitz L M S (1985) Maturation of the visual evoked response and its correlation with visual acuity in preterm infants. *Dev Med Child Neurol* 27:448–454.

Prechtl H F R & Nijhuis J G (1983) Eye movements in the human fetus and newborn. *Behav Brain Res* 10:119–124.

Rappaport L, Urion D, Strand K *et al.* (1987) Concurrence of congenital ocular motor apraxia and other motor problems: an expanded syndrome. *Dev Med Child Neurol* 29:85–90.

Raye K, Pratt E, Beiser A *et al.* (1992) Normative Teller acuity card study: II. Test-retest reliability. *Invest Ophthalmol Vis Sci* 33(suppl):717.

Regal D M, Ashmead D H & Salapatek P (1983) The coordination of eye and head movements during early infancy: a selective review. *Behav Brain Res* 10:125–132.

Reinecke R D, Guo S & Goldstein H P (1988) Waveform evolution in infantile nystagmus: an electro-oculo-graphic study of 35 cases. *Binoc Vis* 3:191–202.

Rethy I (1969) Development of the simultaneous fixation from the divergent anatomic eye-position of the neonate. *J Pediatr Ophthalmol* 6:92–96.

Robinson R J (1966) Assessment of gestational age by neurological examination. *Arch Dis Childhood* 41:437–447.

Robinson J & Fielder A R (1990) Pupillary diameter and reaction to light in preterm neonates. *Arch Dis Childhood* 65:35–38.

Robinson G C & Jan J E (1987) Congenital ocular blindness in children, 1945 to 1984. *Am J Dis Children* 141:1321–1324.

Robinson J, Moseley M J, Thompson J R *et al.* (1989) Eyelid opening in preterm neonates. *Arch Dis Childhood* 64:943–948.

Rossi L N, Pignataro O, Nino L M *et al.* (1979) Maturation of vestibular responses: preliminary report. *Dev Med Child Neurol* 21:217–224.

Roucoux A, Culee C & Roucoux M (1983) Development of fixation and pursuit eye movements in human infants. *Behav Brain Res* 10:133–140.

Roy M S, Barsoum-Homsy M, Orquin J *et al.* (1995) Maturation of binocular pattern visual evoked potentials in normal full-term and preterm infants from 1 to 6 months of age. *Pediatr Res* 37:140–144.

Russell-Eggitt J, Harris C M & Kriss A (1998) Delayed visual maturation: an update. *Dev Med Child Neurol* 40:130–136.

Salomao S R & Ventura D F (1995) Large sample population age norms for visual acuities obtained with Vistech-Teller Acuity Cards. *Invest Ophthalmol Vis Sci* 36:657–670.

Schenk-Rootlieb A J F, van Nieuwenhuizen O, van der Graff Y *et al.* (1992) The prevalence of cerebral visual disturbance in children with cerebral palsy. *Dev Med Child Neurol* 34:473–480.

Scher M S, Dobson V, Carpenter N A *et al.* (1989) Visual and neurological outcome of infants with periventricular leukomalacia. *Dev Med Child Neurol* 31:353–365.

Sebris S L, Dobson V, McDonald M A *et al.* (1987) Acuity cards for visual acuity assessments of infants and children in clinical settings. *Clin Vis Sci* 2:45–58.

Shepherd A J, Saunders K J, McCulloch D L *et al.* (1999) Prognostic value of flash visual evoked potentials in preterm infants. *Dev Med Child Neurol* 41:9–15.

Simons K (ed.) (1993) *Early visual development: normal and abnormal.* Oxford: Oxford University Press.

Skarf B & Hoyt C S (1984) Optic nerve hypoplasia in children. *Arch Ophthalmol* 102:62–67.

Slater A (1998) The competent infant: innate organisation and early learning in infant visual perception. In: Slater A (ed.) *Perceptual development: visual, auditory and speech perception in infancy.* Hove: Psychology Press; pp. 105–130.

Sokol S (1978) Measurement of infant visual acuity from pattern reversal evoked potentials. *Vis Res* 18:33–39.

Sokol S & Jones K (1978) Implicit time of pattern evoked potentials in infants: an index of maturation of spatial vision. *Vis Res* 19:747–755.

Sokol S, Moskowitz A & McCormack G (1992) Infant VEP and preferential looking acuity measured with phase alternating gratings. *Invest Ophthalmol Vis Sci* 33:3156–3161.

Stanhope R, Preece M A & Brooke C G D (1984) Hypoplastic optic nerves and pituitary dysfunction. *Arch Dis Childhood* 59:111–114.

Swash M (1976) Disorders of ocular movement in hydrocephalus. *Proc Roy Soc Med* 69:480–483.

Tamura E E & Hoyt C S (1987) Oculomotor consequences of intraventricular hemorrhages in premature infants. *Arch Ophthalmol* 105:533–535.

Taylor D (ed.) (1997) *Paediatric Ophthalmology.* Oxford: Blackwell Science; 2nd edn.

Taylor D & Scott A (1997) Optic nerve: congenital abnormalities. In: Taylor D (ed.) *Paediatric ophthalmology.* Oxford Blackwell Science; 2nd edn, pp. 660–700.

Teller D Y (1997) First glances: the vision of infants: the Friedenwald lecture. *Invest Ophthalmol Vis Sci* 38:2183–2203.

Teller D Y (1998) Spatial and temporal aspects of infant color vision. *Vis Res* 38:3275–3282.

Teller D Y, McDonald M A, Preston K *et al.* (1986) Assessment of visual acuity in infants and children: the acuity card procedure. *Dev Med Child Neurol* 28:779–789.

Thorn F, Gwiazda J, Cruz A A V *et al.* (1994) The development of eye alignment, convergence, and sensory binocularity in young infants. *Invest Ophthalmol Vis Sci* 35:544–553.

Tresidder J, Fielder A R & Nicholson J (1990) Delayed visual maturation: ophthalmic and neurodevelopmental aspects. *Dev Med Child Neurol* 32:872–881.

Trounce J Q, Dodd K L, Fawer C-L *et al.* (1985) Primary thalamic haemorrhage in the newborn: a new clinical entity. *Lancet i*:190–192.

Uemera Y, Oguchi Y & Katsumi O (1981) Visual developmental delay. *Ophthal Paediatr Genet* 1:49–58.

Van Hof-van Duin J (1989) The development and study of visual acuity. *Dev Med Child Neurol* 31:543–552.

Van Hof-van Duin J, Heersema D J, Groenendaal F *et al.* (1992) Visual field and grating acuity development in low-risk preterm infants during the first 2½ years after term. *Behav Brain Res* 49:115–122.

Van Hof-van Duin J & Mohn G (1983) Optokinetic and spontaneous nystagmus in children with neurological disorders. *Behav Brain Res* 10:163–176.

Van Hof-van Duin J & Mohn G (1984a) Vision in the preterm infant. *Clin Dev Med* 94:93–114.

Van Hof-van Duin J & Mohn G (1984b) Visual defects in children after cerebral hypoxia. *Behav Brain Res* 14:147–155.

Van Hof-van Duin J & Mohn G (1986) The development of visual acuity in normal fullterm and preterm infants. *Vis Res* 26:909–916.

Van Hof-van Duin J, Mohn G, Petter W P F *et al.* (1983) Preferential looking in preterm infants. *Behav Brain Res* 10:47–50.

Vehrs S & Baum D (1970) A test of visual responses in the newborn. *Dev Med Child Neurol* 12:772–774.

Vital-Durand F, Atkinson J & Braddick OJ (eds) (1996) *Infant vision.* Oxford: Oxford University Press.

Von Noorden G K (1990) In: *Burian von Noorden's binocular vision and ocular motility: theory and management of strabismus.* St. Louis, MO: C V Mosby.

Weinacht S, Kind C, Monting J S *et al.* (1999) Visual development in preterm and full-term infants: a prospective masked study. *Invest Ophthalmol Vis Sci* 40:346–353.

Weinberger H A, Van der Woude R & Maier H C (1962) Prognosis of cortical blindness following cardiac arrest in children. *JAMA* 179:126–129.

Weindling A M, Rochefort M J, Calvert S A *et al.* (1985) Development of cerebral palsy after ultrasonographic detection of periventricular cysts in the newborn. *Dev Med Child Neurol* 27:800–806.

Weiss A H & Biersdorf W R (1989) Visual sensory disorders in congenital nystagmus. *Ophthalmology* 96:517–523.

Weleber R G & Palmer E A (1991) Electrophysiological evaluation of children with visual impairment. *Semin Ophthalmol* 6:161–168.

White B L, Castle P & Held R (1964) Observations on the development of visually-directed reaching. *Child Dev* 35:349–364.

Whiting S, Jan J E, Wong F K H *et al.* (1985) Permanent cortical visual impairment in children. *Dev Med Child Neurol* 27:730–739.

Williams J, Brodsky M C, Griebel C M *et al.* (1993) Septo-optic dysplasia: the clinical significance of an absent septum pellucidum. *Dev Med Child Neurol* 35:490–501.

Yee R D, Baloh R W & Honrubia V (1981) Eye movement abnormalities in rod monochromacy. *Ophthalmology* 88:1010–1018.

# Chapter 39

# Disorders of hearing

V. E. Newton

## DEVELOPMENT OF THE EAR AND RESPONSES TO SOUND

The ear is formed from three germ layers and consists of the external ear, middle ear, and inner ear. The external auditory meatus develops around the fourth to fifth week from the first pharyngeal groove, which deepens and then opens up to form the external auditory canal. The tympanic membrane forms at the point where this meets the middle ear cleft. Several small hillocks arise around the first pharyngeal groove about the sixth week, and these coalesce to form the pinnae. The external ear is initially low set upon the developing embryo but becomes less so as the fetus develops.

The development of the middle ear starts during the third week. It is formed from the first pharyngeal pouch, which also gives rise to part of the Eustachian tube. The ossicles develop from the first and second bronchial arches from the fourth week and are ossified by the 30th week.

The neural crest, an early and transitory developmental structure, gives rise to the auditory and vestibular ganglia and to cells that are the precursors of the melanocytes found in the inner ear. The otic placode, which becomes the inner ear, starts as a thickening in the surface ectoderm at about the third week of embryonic life. The placode invaginates into the ectoderm and then becomes separate to form an otocyst, which is closely linked with cells of the neural crest. The otocyst differentiates to form the membranous labyrinth, and this process is complete by the tenth week of gestation. The inner ear is adult-sized by the end of the 20th week.

Further development takes place after birth with growth of the temporal bone. The direction of the external auditory canal changes, and the tympanic membrane, which is horizontal in the neonate, develops at an angle to the horizontal plane. The Eustachian tube also starts more horizontally in the neonate compared to its adult direction.

An agent that causes damage to the ear at an early stage of development may result in structural abnormalities that are demonstrable radiologically. More frequently, however, the damage affects the membranous, rather than the bony, labyrinth. An absent or vestigial vestibulocochlear nerve is rare.

### DEVELOPMENT OF HEARING

Development of hearing begins in intrauterine life with low- to middle-frequency discrimination (Lippe & Rubbel 1983). Evidence from animal experiments indicates that the basal end of the cochlea matures first and that, initially, this region responds to low-frequency sounds. With increasing maturity, there is a shift in frequency coding along the basilar membrane so that in the mature animal, low-frequency sounds are coded at the apex (Hyson & Rudy 1987).

The neonate responds to loud sound with a startle reaction but does not respond to quiet sounds. As the infant matures, there develops the ability to respond to quieter sound intensities. By 4 months, an infant would be expected to turn when his/her name is called, but a sound that is above the physiologic threshold is required to elicit this response. By the time the infant is 6–7 months old, he/she can respond to very quiet sounds and can locate the direction from which the sounds have come in the horizontal plane.

## CAUSES OF PERMANENT HEARING IMPAIRMENT

Normal hearing is defined as having pure tone audiometric thresholds better than, or equal to, 15 dB HL across the main speech frequency range of 250–4 kHz, though many would accept 20 db HL as being within the normal range at the lower frequency of 250 Hz. In distraction testing, responses of 30/35 dBA are usually accepted as indicative of normal hearing. The 'A' weighting on a sound level meter used to measure the intensity of the sounds indicates that the response of the instrument resembles the response of the human ear in being less sensitive in the low frequencies.

Hearing impairment in babies and very young children may be the result of congenital or acquired disorders. The site of origin of the hearing impairment determines whether or not the hearing impairment is described as conductive, sensorineural, or mixed. In a conductive hearing impairment, the defect is in the external or middle ear or both. Sensorineural hearing loss results from defects affecting the cochlea, vestibulocochlear nerve or the auditory pathways, i.e. it may be cochlear or retrocochlear, but a cochlear site is the more common. A mixed hearing loss indicates that both conductive and sensorineural components are present.

Most conductive hearing impairment is acquired, whereas sensorineural hearing loss in this young age group is mainly the result of prenatal factors. Genetic causes account for at least 50–60% of congenital hearing impairment and are believed to be the cause of most isolated hearing losses. Congenital uterine infections, chromosomal abnormalities, and ototoxic drugs account for most of the remainder. A very small group of children are born with congenital defects of unknown origin but which may be due to a combination of genetic and environmental factors. Adverse perinatal events may lead to a sensorineural hearing loss, particularly in babies of low gestation, whereas postnatally, infections are important causes of hearing impairment in young children (Table 39.1)

**Table 39.1 Causes of permanent hearing impairment**

| |
|---|
| Genetic |
| Autosomal dominant |
| Autosomal recessive |
| X-linked |
| Mitochondrial |
| Chromosomal abnormalities |
| Infections |
| Congenital abnormalities |
| Perinatal factors |
| Ototoxic medication |
| Unknown causation |

## GENETIC CAUSES

Genetic hearing impairment is 70% autosomal recessive, 25% autosomal dominant, and 5% X-linked or due to mitochondrial inheritance. Most are non-syndromal. Around 60 loci have been discovered for non-syndromal genes, and around 15 genes have been identified. Connexin 26 mutations have been found in DNA samples from a proportion of sib pairs with non-syndromal hearing impairment (Lench *et al.* 1999). Two genes that cause non-syndromal hearing impairment have been found also to underlie syndromic conditions.

Some of the syndromal conditions are described according to their mode of inheritance.

### Autosomal dominant syndromes

The prevalence of Waardenburg syndrome is believed to be around one in 10–20 000 of the population. Various pigmentary defects are found, including white forelock, iris heterochromia, and skin hypo/hyper-chromia associated with congenital sensorineural hearing loss or normal hearing (Read & Newton 1997). Four types have been described. Types 1 and 2 are most often encountered and are distinguished by Type 1 having an eyelid defect and lateral displacement of the inner canthi. Type 1 is a neural crest defect and has been shown to be due to loss-of-function mutations in the PAX3 gene on chromosome 2. This gene encodes a DNA-binding transcription factor. No relationship has been found between genotype and phenotype, and the expression of the gene is highly variable, even within families.

Type 2 is a heterogeneous group, and in about 15% of families, it is caused by mutations in MITF on chromosome 3. Hearing loss is more prevalent in Type 2 than Type 1 (Newton 1990).

Type 3, in which upper-limb abnormalities are associated with the eyelid defect and lateral displacement of the inner canthi found in Type 1, has been shown to be due to a mutation in Pax3. Type 4 has the clinical features of Type 2 and is associated with Hirschsprung's disease. Mutations in EDN3 and SOX 10 genes give rise to this phenotype.

#### Branchio-oto-renal syndrome

Prevalence of this syndrome is estimated as one in 40 000, and hearing impairment is the most common feature. Hearing loss is usually mixed but may be sensorineural or conductive (Chen *et al.* 1995). Preauricular pits are the most common external feature. Other features include branchial fistulae and a cup-shaped pinna and renal dysplasia, which varies in degree of severity. Cochlear hypoplasia and a dilated vestibular aqueduct may be demonstrated radiologically. Branchio-otic syndrome is similar phenotypically but differs in the absence of renal abnormalities. A gene causative of branchio-oto-renal syndrome has been identified on chromosome 8.

#### Stickler or Marshall–Stickler syndrome

This is a connective tissue disorder in which eye conditions, particularly myopia, are associated with congenital sensorineural or mixed hearing impairment and cleft palate. The mid-face may be underdeveloped and the nose short and saddle-shaped. When a hearing loss is present, the high frequencies are usually affected most, and the hearing loss can be progressive (Lucarini *et al.* 1987). Collagen genes have been identified as causative of this condition.

#### Treacher Collins syndrome (mandibular dysostosis)

This disorder arises from a defect of the first arch, and it is sometimes called the first arch syndrome. It gives rise to a conductive hearing impairment. The clinical features are symmetric and include anti-mongoloid slant to the eyes, coloboma, low set ears, external and middle ear abnormalities, hypoplasia of mid-facial structures, micrognathia, and cleft palate. Gene expression is very variable, and not all of those affected have a hearing impairment. A causative gene, TREACLE, has been found on chromosome 5.

### Autosomal recessive syndromes

#### Usher syndromes

In these syndromes, retinitis pigmentosa (RP) is associated with congenital bilateral sensorineural hearing loss. In type 1, the hearing impairment is profound, RP appears in the first decade, and vestibular function is absent (Smith *et al.* 1994). Children usually have a history of delayed motor milestones. Six gene locations have been found, and one gene for Usher syndrome type 11 (USH2B) has been identified. This is the myosin VIIA gene, which is expressed in both the retina and the cochlea. In type 2, there is a moderately severe to severe hearing impairment worse in the higher frequencies than in the lower-frequency range, vestibular function is normal, and RP appears in the second decade. A causative gene has been identified on chromosome 1. In type 3, the hearing loss is progressive, and the time of onset of RP and the pattern of vestibular function are variable.

#### Pendred syndrome

Congenital sensorineural hearing impairment is associated with an organification defect of the thyroid gland. A goiter usually appears after the age of 8 years but occasionally may be present in infancy. Those affected are usually euthyroid but may become hypothyroid. They may have a Mondini defect on radiologic examination or dilated vestibular aqueducts (Phelps *et al.* 1998). A positive perchlorate test supports the diagnosis but is not specific to this condition. A causative gene has been identified on chromosome 7, and the protein encoded is believed to be involved in ion transportation.

#### Jervell and Lange-Neilsen syndrome

A congenital sensorineural hearing impairment is found in association with a cardiac conduction defect. This is a rare, but important, cause of sensorineural hearing impairment as the cardiac defect, untreated, can lead to ventricular fibrillation and death. There may be brief episodes of altered consciousness or syncopal attacks lasting a few minutes as a result of arrhythmias. These may be precipitated by exercise or stress. Bradycardia is found and may be detected in the fetus *in utero* (Splawsky *et al.* 1997). The ECG in this syndrome typically shows a prolonged QT interval and T-wave inversion. ECG abnormalities may also be identified in the heterozygote. Homozygous KVLQTI mutations have been found in affected persons.

#### Mucopolysaccharidoses

Most of the mucopolysaccharidoses are inherited as a result of autosomal recessive inheritance. The most common of this group of lysosomal storage diseases is Hurler's disease (MPS1), which is due to an alpha-L-iduronidase deficiency. Glycosamines accumulate in the tissues and are excreted in the urine. Hearing loss, when present, is usually mixed (Briedencamp *et al.* 1992) Bone-marrow transplantation can result in stabilization of hearing, or, in some instances, there may be an improvement in auditory thresholds (Griffon *et al.* 1998; Papsin *et al.* 1998).

## X-LINKED SYNDROME

#### Alports syndrome

A glomerular nephritis precedes the appearance of a sensorineural hearing loss, which affects the high frequencies initially and is progressive. Eighty-five per cent of Alport's syndrome is X-linked and the remainder either autosomal recessive (10%) or dominant. The syndrome is caused by mutations in COL4A3, COL4A4, and COL4A5 genes. These are found in the basilar membrane, parts of the spiral ligament, and the stria vascularis, but the mechanism by which they cause a hearing impairment is not known.

## MITOCHONDRIAL INHERITANCE

A mutation in the 12S rRNA gene has been found in families with maternally inherited non-syndromic hearing loss and in individuals and families with a non-syndromal hearing loss, which develops after treatment with aminoglycoside antibiotics (Prezant *et al.* 1993). The level of aminoglycoside, which is ototoxic in these individuals, is below that which usually is required to cause a hearing impairment. A second mitochondrial mutation was found subsequently in a family where a progressive sensorineural hearing loss was associated with palmoplantar keratoderma.

## CHROMOSOMAL ABNORMALITIES

Various chromosomal defects are associated with sensorineural, conductive, or mixed hearing loss. The commonest are Down syndrome and Turner syndrome.

### Down syndrome

Most hearing loss found in association with Down syndrome is conductive, mainly as a result of otitis media with effusion. The conductive element is contributed to by the fact that the external ear is frequently narrow, and, in a small proportion, there may be ossicular abnormalities usually affecting the stapes. Affected individuals may have pinna abnormalities.

Congenital sensorineural hearing loss is found in about 5% of children born with Down's syndrome. A shorter cochlea than normal has been described, and there may be a Mondini defect on radiologic examination (Bilgin *et al.* 1996).

### Turner syndrome

The XO genotype has clinical features, which include short stature, a webbed neck, nuchal lymphedema, shield-shaped chest, cubitus valgus, ovarian dysgenesis, and congenital heart disease. Renal abnormalities are found, including horseshoe kidney. The ears are low set with rotation, and the external auditory canals may have an abnormal downward slope.

Progressive sensorineural hearing loss has been described, which is usually in the high frequencies but may be mid-frequency. In the early years, there is frequently a history of otitis media, which may disguise the development of a sensorineural hearing loss.

Benazzo *et al.* (1997) examined 62 patients with Turner syndrome aged between 5 and 32 years. Thirteen of these were found to have a bilateral symmetric sensorineural hearing loss. Nine had a progressive high-frequency impairment and the remaining four a dip in the mid-frequency range.

## INFECTIONS

### Intrauterine infections (see Chapters 31 and 32)

Sensorineural hearing impairment may result from congenital infections with rubella, cytomegalovirus, toxoplasmosis, and syphilis – the TORCH conditions. The two former infections are the commonest, although hearing impairment resulting from rubella has almost been eliminated in some countries as a result of MMR immunization.

Rubella virus crosses the placental barrier and, if it affects the fetus early in the first trimester, usually results in defects of the heart and eye as well as the ear, and may give rise to microcephaly. Infections later in the first trimester or in the second trimester may cause hearing impairment as a single defect. The hearing defect may be bilateral or unilateral and can be progressive. A small proportion of babies develop language disorders unrelated to a hearing impairment. The typical rubella retinopathy or 'salt and pepper' appearance may be present.

Cytomegalovirus is believed to have its major effects in the first trimester. Hearing loss is more prevalent after a symptomatic, rather than an asymptomatic, infection. Hearing loss is usually bilateral but may be unilateral and is frequently progressive. Periventricular radiolucencies or calcifications seen on a CT scan indicate an increased risk for hearing loss (Williamson *et al.* 1992).

### Postnatal infections (Chapter 33)

Infants suffering from meningitis in the neonatal period and subsequently are at risk for hearing impairment. About 10% of children acquire a hearing loss after meningitis (Fortnum 1992). Hearing loss occurs after both bacterial and viral meningitis, but particularly the former. Causative organisms include *Streptococcus pneumoniae, Streptococcus type B, Haemophilus influenzae* and *Neisseria meningitidis.*

Hearing loss and balance disturbance occur early in the illness (Vienny *et al.* 1984) Hearing loss is three times more common in children treated >24 h after the onset of the illness (Richardson *et al.* 1997). In this prospective multicenter study, 10.5% had a reversible hearing loss, and the majority had reversed within 2 days. It was suggested that there may be a critical period around the second day of the illness in which treatment may result in reversal. Guiscafre *et al.* (1984) noted that severe initial hearing losses tended to be permanent, whereas mild and moderate hearing losses were likely to be reversible.

Studies have come to differing conclusions regarding the role of early treatment of meningitis upon the incidence of hearing loss (Fortnum 1992). There is evidence that dexamethasone results in a lower prevalence of hearing loss or hearing loss of milder degree (Kuhlahli *et al.* 1997).

## CONGENITAL ABNORMALITIES

### CHARGE association

CHARGE is an acronym for Coloboma, Heart, Atretic choanae, Retarded growth, Genital hypoplasia and Ear abnormalities. Additional abnormalities that may be found include orofacial cleating and facial weakness. The condition is usually sporadic, but familial cases have been reported (Metlay *et al.* 1987). The ears are typically low-set and cup-shaped. Hearing impairment is frequently present and is usually severe. On the whole, a mixed hearing loss is the most common type of hearing impairment, but sensorineural and conductive hearing impairment have been described. A characteristic feature radiologically is an absence of the semicircular canals (Morgan *et al.* 1993).

### The Klippel–Feil anomalad

Congenital hearing loss is associated with variable degrees of fusion of the spine in the cervical, thoracic, and sometimes lumbar regions. When severe, the neck is short, and there is a low posterior hairline. Hearing loss may be sensorineural, conductive, or mixed, and unilateral, as well as bilateral, hearing loss has been described. Ossicular abnormalities are the cause of the conductive hearing impairment. In Wildervanck syndrome, the Klippel Feil anomalad is associated with Duane's syndrome.

## PERINATAL FACTORS

Babies of a low gestation and birthweight are more prone to develop a hearing impairment than full term babies. Veen *et al.* (1993) investigated hearing in a geographically defined population of preterm and very-low-birthweight babies when they reached the age of 5 years and could cooperate in pure tone audiometry. Eight-hundred and ninety children were assessed, and 15.3% had a unilateral or bilateral hearing impairment. Thirteen children had a sensorineural hearing impairment, the majority bilateral and ranging from moderately severe to profound. A significant relationship was found between intermittent positive pressure ventilation (IPPV) and SNHL and/or continuous positive airway pressure (CPAP), intracranial hemorrhage, and sepsis. The prevalence of hearing impairment >50 dB in the infants was ten times higher than that of 8 year olds in the population.

SNHL has been attributed to hypoxia in several investigations. Das (1991) described 17 preterm and five term infants with a SNHL of which 14 in the preterm group had respiratory distress syndrome, and eight had a history of apneic episodes. Eleven had required assisted ventilation. Fifteen of this group of infants had a hearing loss averaging more than 80 dB. The five term/post term infants all had severe birth asphyxia, and all five had a hearing loss in this severe category.

Jiang (1995) investigated hearing levels in children exposed to perinatal and postnatal asphyxia, and hearing loss was found more frequently in those who suffered neurodevelopmental deficits (17.1%) than those without (6.3%), although the difference was not statistically significant. None of those with postnatal asphyxia had a permanent hearing loss. It was suggested that there was a critical period for the effects of hypoxia on the auditory system, which ranged from some time prenatally to a short time after birth, possibly the third postnatal month.

In a prospective study by Graziani *et al.* (1997) of 223 infants treated with neonatal extracorporeal membrane oxygenation (ECMO), it was noted that profound hypocarbia before ECMO and delayed ECMO treatment were associated with a significant increased risk for hearing loss. Borg (1997) reviewed the literature with respect to birth asphyxia, ischemia and hearing loss and noted that hypoxia was less likely to cause a hearing impairment than hypoxic ischemia.

Hyperbilirubinemia is associated with hearing loss with and without the presence of kernicterus. In de Vries *et al.*'s (1987) study of the relationship between serum bilirubin levels and hearing impairment in newborns weighing less than 1500 g, sensorineural hearing loss was strongly associated with hyperbilirubinemia greater than 240 μmol/l. Low-gestation babies are more prone to develop hyperbilirubinemia and more prone to its effects. However, hyperbilirubinemia >200 μmol/l was not significantly related to SNHL in Veen *et al.*'s (1993) cohort of preterm and very-low-birthweight infants.

In an animal study, Silver *et al.* (1995) found that neither asphyxia nor elevated bilirubin levels, when occurring alone, were associated with hearing impairment. Only when these were in combination in 10-day-old rats was there any evidence of hearing loss. It was suggested that this could have some significance for neonates with jaundice and hypoxia perhaps as a result of respiratory distress syndrome.

### Ototoxic medication

Infants may be exposed to ototoxic drugs through medication given to the mother during pregnancy or as a result of treatment they themselves require after birth. Aminoglycosides, used to treat Gram-negative infections, are both ototoxic and nephrotoxic but differ with regard to the degree to which they affect the cochlea and the vestibular system. In the cochlea, the outer hair cells of the basal turn are destroyed initially, but later, the damage extends to the apex of the cochlea, and the inner hair cells become affected. As these drugs are excreted through the kidney, infants with renal damage are particularly at risk for ototoxic damage. Monitoring peak and trough levels is necessary to prevent potentially harmful serum levels. Frusemide is ototoxic, and, when given together with an aminoglycoside, the ototoxic effects are potentiated.

### Unknown causation

In spite of investigations, the cause of a hearing loss is not always identified. Recently, in some of this group of children, it has been possible to identify mutations in the Connexin 26 gene on chromosome 13, indicating that the cause of the hearing loss is autosomal recessive inheritance (Lench *et al.*, 1999).

## DETECTION OF HEARING IMPAIRMENT

The prevalence of permanent hearing impairment in a population study in the UK was found to be 1.33/1000 live babies, and 1.12/1000 were congenital (Fortnum & Davies 1997). Hearing impairment should be detected as soon as possible after the defect has occurred to facilitate early habilitation and avoid the problems experienced by the child and their families as a result of a late diagnosis. Concern has been expressed that detection too early could adversely affect maternal–child bonding. Mothers asked for their views indicated that they were generally in favor of early tests (Watkins *et al.* 1997).

In the first few months of life, normal-hearing babies already learn to distinguish the sounds of their own language from that of another language. This was demonstrated by Kuhl *et al.* (1992) in 6-month-old babies from the United States and Sweden using computer-synthesized phonemes in speech.

That the exposure to sound in these early months is important for speech and language development is also being shown by studies of hearing impaired children. Downs (1995) found that infants habilitated before the age of 3 months scored higher on the expressive language component of the Minnesota Child Development Inventory test than children habilitated between the ages of 6 and 12 months when each was compared to normal. Those with a severe hearing impairment particularly benefited from early habitation.

Yoshinaga *et al.* (1998) examined the language abilities of 72 children whose hearing impairment was diagnosed before the age of 6 months and 78 children whose hearing impairment was diagnosed after this time. The children had mild to profound hearing impairments affecting both ears and had received early intervention services within an average of 2 months after diagnosis. They were compared in relation to the size of their receptive and expressive language scores on the Minnesota Child Development Inventory. Children with normal cognitive function who had been habilitated before the age of 6 months had significantly better receptive and expressive language scores than those whose hearing impairment was detected and habilitated at a later age.

## NEONATAL SCREENING TESTING METHODS

Methods are available to examine a baby's hearing in the neonatal period. These include an auditory response cradle, an auditory brainstem response test, and otoacoustic emissions. The tests provide information about different parts of the auditory system.

### The auditory response cradle

The cradle examines behavioral responses to sound and, therefore, tests the auditory system from the periphery to the auditory cortex. It requires a loud stimulus to elicit a response from a neonate, and the cradle, in using a loud stimulus, could miss detecting a moderate hearing impairment. This method of screening hearing in neonates was one of the earliest methods introduced but is now little used.

### Auditory Brainstem Response Test

The Auditory Brainstem Response Test (ABR) examines the auditory system to brainstem level and can be carried out manually; an automated test is also available (Mason *et al.* 1998). The test investigates the presence or absence of a pattern of waveforms in response to a stimulus (Fig. 39.1). The infant needs to be still in order to obtain accurate readings, and testing is performed with the infant asleep. The test can also be performed using sedation or general anesthesia.

The stimulus that is usually used to elicit a response is a click sound. This includes a wide range of frequencies, but as high-frequency neurons fire more synchronously than those of a lower frequency, the response is only informative about hearing in the high frequencies around 3 kHz. Tone pips have been used to elicit responses in the mid-frequencies but are thought to be less useful in providing specific information about low frequencies, and the test is time-consuming. More recently, the use of steady-state potentials has been shown to be useful in providing information about a wider range of frequencies (Lins *et al.* 1995; Rance *et al.* 1998).

### Otoacoustic emissions

Otoacoustic emissions (OAEs) are responses of outer hair cells in the organ of Corti in the cochlea to a stimulus. They are absent in ears with a hearing loss of 30 dB or more and in ears with fluid in the middle ear. Most screening programs use transient evoked emissions (TEOAEs), which are elicited with a click stimulus. The test involves the placement of a small soft probe at the opening of the ear canal. The tests can then be performed manually; automated test devices are also available. Distortion product otoacoustic emissions (DPOAEs), which are elicited by pure tones that vary only very slightly in frequency, can also be used for screening (Ochi *et al.* 1998).

Otoacoustic emissions develop during the first few days of life, and some babies if tested on the first day after birth may have absent emissions. In a small proportion of children, otoacoustic emissions may be present in the absence of an ABR or an abnormal ABR. This has been labelled 'auditory neuropathy'. Hyperbilirubinemia is one of the causes and indicates the need for caution in the management of babies with this history who are found to have a hearing impairment on auditory brainstem testing. All should be additionally tested with otoacoustic emissions.

Screening programs have used OAEs for initial screening and ABR testing for those babies with unsatisfactory results on screening (Watkins & Baldwin 1999). Babies are usually screened at term before leaving hospital, with low-gestation babies tested prior to leaving hospital or brought back when their adjusted age is term-equivalent.

### Targeted versus universal screening

Initial screening programs were based upon targeted screening. This involved identification of at-risk factors (Table 39.2). The groups initially tested were the SCBU population. Later, this group was increased by the addition of those with a relevant family history and babies with craniofacial abnormalities. At-risk factors succeed in detecting only about 50% of those with a significant hearing impairment. Those missed by selective screening are those with an autosomal recessive hearing loss but where the babe is the first affected child born in the family. Missed from the 'at risk' group would be those in which a new dominant mutation had occurred leading to non-syndromic hearing impairment or those infants infected *in utero* after a maternal sub-clinical infection.

**Table 39.2 At-risk factors for hearing impairment**

- Family history of hereditary hearing loss of childhood onset
- Intrauterine infections
- Craniofacial abnormalities
- Birthweight <1500 g
- Hyperbilirubinemia sufficient to require exchange transfusion
- Ototoxic medication
- Apgar 0–4 at 1 min or 0–6 at 5 min
- Bacterial meningitis
- Mechanical ventilation lasting 5 days or longer
- Features of a syndrome involving hearing loss

*Source*: Adapted with permission from Joint Committee on Infant Hearing 1994 Position Statement, American Speech and Hearing Association.

To avoid missing the children not identified as being at risk for hearing impairment, universal screening has been advocated. The Position Statement put out by the Joint Committee on Infant Hearing, USA was that the goal was for all infants with hearing loss to be identified before the age of 3 months and that they should receive intervention by the age of 6 months (JCIH 1994). Mehl & Thomson (1998) screened 41 796 neonates 1992–1996 and concluded that universal newborn hearing screening was feasible, beneficial, and justified.

## SCREENING AT A LATER AGE

### Questionnaires

Some babies will miss having their hearing screened as neonates or will develop a hearing loss subsequently. Some genetic hearing loss is not manifest until after the neonatal period, and babies who have had an intrauterine infection could suffer a progression of their hearing loss. A method for detecting hearing impairment after the neonatal period is needed, and questionnaires have been used. These depend upon the observations of parents or carers, and it is likely that a mild hearing impairment and a unilateral hearing loss would be missed. Some Health Districts use distraction testing by Health Visitors as a second screen to detect children with a previously unsuspected hearing impairment.

Children who develop conditions such as meningitis, where there is a known risk for hearing impairment, need to be referred for testing at an audiology clinic whilst still in hospital.

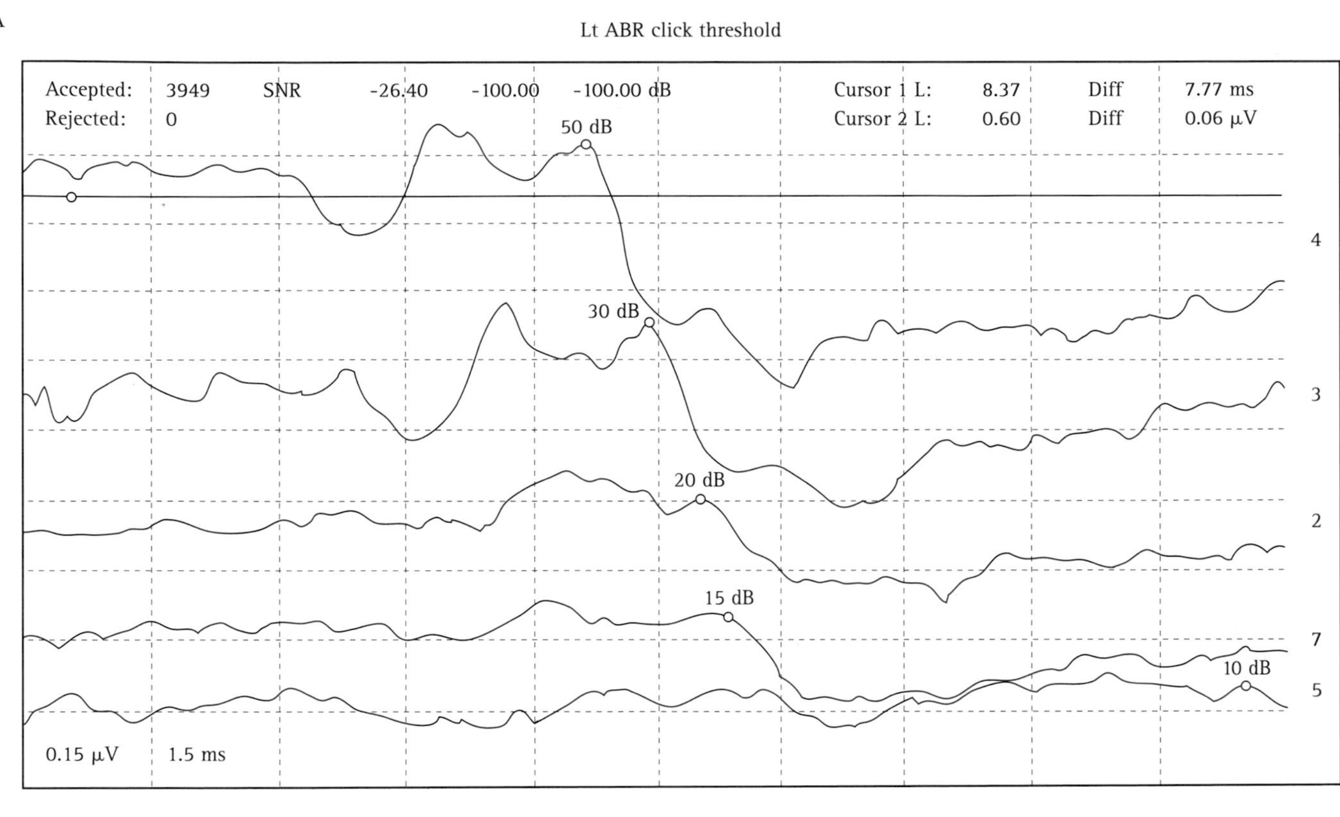


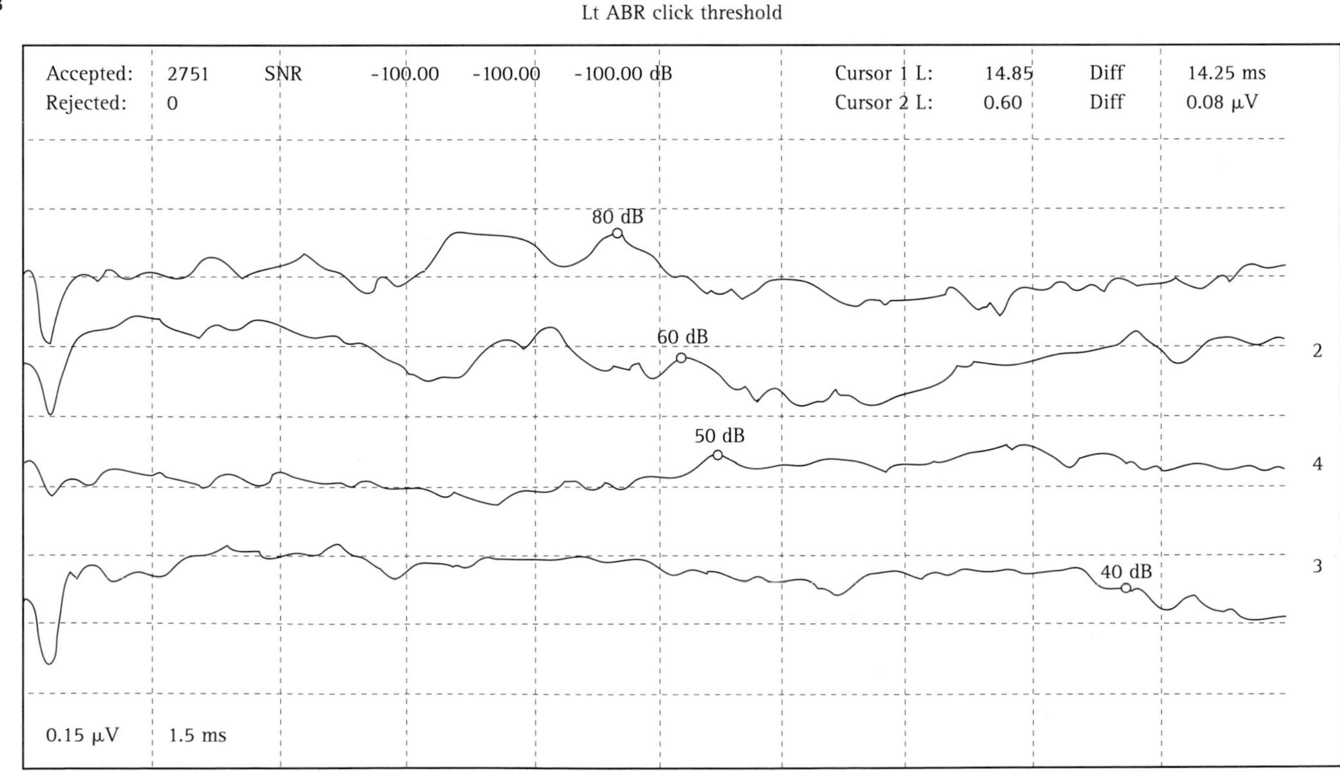


**Figure 39.1** An auditory brainstem response test showing (a) a normal threshold of 15 dBnHL and (b) a threshold of 50 dBHL indicating a moderate hearing loss.

### Behavioral tests of hearing

After screening, babies found to be hearing-impaired need to have the degree of hearing loss measured. A diagnostic ABR test can be performed, and both air and bone conduction thresholds can be measured as necessary. The information obtained should be supplemented as soon as possible using insert earphones and visual reinforcement audiometry (VRA). This is possible when babies are developmentally able to turn towards a stimulus, and it enables information to be obtained at low, middle, and high frequencies.

VRA involves conditioning an infant to turn to a sound by showing a lit-up toy or revolving light as a reinforcer at the same time as the sound is introduced. When the infant has been conditioned, the sound is introduced alone and the reinforcer switched on subsequently as a reward. The use of insert earphones enables hearing levels to be measured in each ear separately (Fig 39.2). The results of VRA testing correlated well with pure tone audiometry in a longitudinal study carried out by Talbott (1987).

Where VRA is not available, the infant can be tested using distraction methods, but this test is less frequency-specific and does not give ear-specific information. Full information about the threshold of hearing in each ear will not be available until masking procedures can be performed.

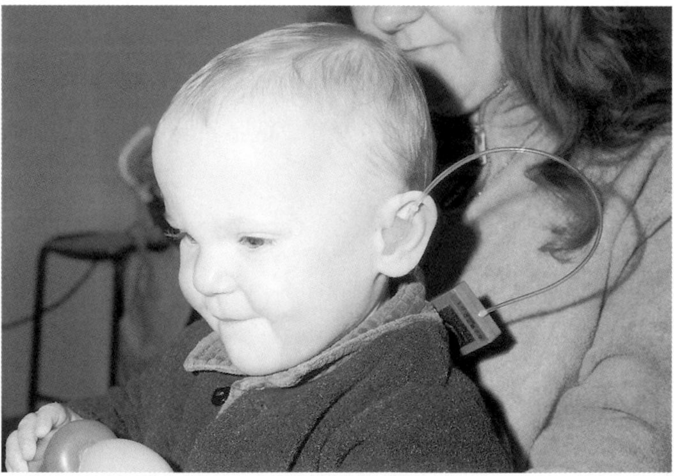

**Figure 39.2** Child with insert earphones ready for Visual Reinforcement Audiometry.

## MANAGEMENT OF HEARING IMPAIRMENT

This will depend upon the type of hearing loss and whether or not it is permanent. Otitis media with effusion in a young baby will usually resolve spontaneously. In the small proportion in which the effusion persists for at least 6 months, there may eventually be a need for myringotomies and grommet insertion. Children with Down's syndrome and those with a cleft palate have a tendency to have persistent 'glue ear', and management with hearing aids may be the preferred option.

For the child with a significant (>30dB) sensorineural or permanent conductive or mixed hearing loss, management will involve a series of steps. Investigations into the cause of the hearing loss, identification of any additional problems, and genetic counseling for the parents need to be carried out as soon as possible. As well as a general pediatric examination, etiological investigations need to be undertaken. These will include tests to detect any evidence of an intrauterine infection having taken place and tests to detect signs indicative of a genetic syndrome. Hearing aids need to be provided for the baby as soon as possible after diagnosis of the hearing loss. The National Deaf Children's Society have set a standard for hearing aids to be provided within 1 month of detection of the hearing loss (NDCS 1996).

Management of the child is a partnership between parents and professionals. Parents provide the habilitative support needed by the baby, and in order for them to do this effectively, their own needs as parents have to be provided for. They may experience feelings akin to those experienced in bereavement and need to be able to express these to an empathetic listener. The local Hearing Impaired services should be involved with the family as soon as possible after diagnosis so that a teacher visits to give support to the parents and to the child.

## HEARING-AID SERVICES

Hearing aids are an important provision for the hearing-impaired baby, but the extent to which they can alleviate the effects of a hearing impairment depends upon the type of hearing loss. A conductive hearing impairment results in loss of sensitivity to sound, and this can be overcome by the use of amplification with the result that the child can hear satisfactorily. A sensorineural hearing loss results in more than a loss of sensation. The ability to differentiate between sounds of different frequency arriving at the same time and consecutively and to resolve time of arrival differences are important additional cochlear functions that affect reception of speech. Amplification in a sensorineural hearing loss helps to lessen the effects of reduced sensitivity but not the additional functional deficits, with the result that normal hearing is not restored.

Hearing aids may be body-worn, worn behind the ear (BTE), or worn in the ear (ITE). For the majority of babies, BTEs are provided, but if some babies are too small and do not have a pinna that is able to support these initially, a body-worn hearing aid may be supplied. Special features provide for safety and for ensuring that the hearing-aid fittings are not inadvertently altered from those intended. These include locks on the battery chamber and covers on the gain control of the hearing aid.

Good hearing aids are available for all degrees of hearing loss and the technology for making well-fitting earmoulds. Unless earmoulds fit well, children will be unable to maximize the benefits of the output of the hearing aid as the sound leaks out and, when fed back through the microphone of the hearing aid, gives rise to a screeching noise. This may necessitate the gain of the hearing aid being reduced for it to stop. Small babies growing rapidly need to have new earmoulds made every few weeks to ensure that a good fit is constantly achieved.

Fitting of hearing aids in babies is different from fitting adults. The degree to which information is available about a baby's hearing is less precise. The acoustic properties of children's ears are different. Not only is the external auditory canal much smaller, but the peak resonances in the canal are different. Babies are unable to provide feedback as to the quality of the sound input and indicate whether or not they are experiencing loudness discomfort. Information about the performance of hearing aids is based upon adult ears, and measurements need to be made upon individual baby ears to ensure an optimal fit. Evaluation of amplification provision subsequently is a continual process as the child grows and as acquired conditions such as otitis media with effusion affect the hearing thresholds.

Infants with bilateral external ear abnormalities will need to be fitted with bone conduction hearing aids and, at an older age, may be candidates for bone-anchored implants.

### COCHLEAR IMPLANTS

Hearing aids are provided initially for most children with a profound sensorineural hearing impairment, but some children with this degree of hearing loss do not benefit at all from hearing aids, or the amplification achieved is not adequate to enable them to hear speech at conversational levels. The children may benefit from a cochlear implant. This is an implanted device with electrodes that are inserted into the cochlea and stimulate nerve endings directly. The device is attached to a speech processor worn outside the body. Implantation is followed by a habilitative program, which is essential for the infant or child to derive benefit from the implant.

Babies who have had meningitis and have developed a profound sensorineural hearing loss are implanted as soon as possible afterwards. This is because of the ossification process that may take place within the cochleae and is variable as to time of onset. MRI is useful in indicating whether or not this process is underway. A young age does not preclude implantation, as the bony cochleae are an adequate size at the time of birth.

In the case of a congenital hearing impairment, investigations include imaging of the cochleae with MRI, and occasionally, MRI has revealed a congenital absence of the vestibulocochlear nerve or its cochlear branch. Not all degrees of cochlear dysplasia prevent the use of an implant, and children with a Mondini defect have been implanted.

### UNILATERAL HEARING IMPAIRMENT

The term unilateral hearing loss (UHL) is used when one ear is hearing-impaired, and the other is normal hearing. A permanent UHL is usually acquired but can be caused as a result of an intrauterine infection or genetic conditions, as indicated earlier in the chapter. A permanent UHL can be identified at birth, but the degree of difference between the two ears may not be identifiable at this early age.

There is mounting evidence that children with UHL experience difficulties in school. This is because they lack the acoustic information available to the binaural listener, and this places them at a disadvantage against a noisy background and in reverberant surroundings. Problems are greater for those with a right-ear impairment than an impairment affecting the left ear. Children with UHL need to have a favorable class position in which they sit in front of the teacher or with their better ear towards the teacher. Classroom amplification can be of benefit to these children.

## CONCLUSION

A severe hearing impairment is a major childhood disability, and measures to prevent its occurrence should be carried out wherever possible. Most significant hearing loss in infancy is present in the neonatal period and is not always indicated by 'at-risk' factors. For this reason, universal neonatal hearing screening should be performed wherever practical, as this enables the habilitation of the infant to commence as early as possible. Congenital hearing impairment should be both detected and habilitated within the first 6 months of life to optimize the opportunity for infants to develop speech and language. Hearing-service provision should take into account the need for early detection of any hearing loss that develops at a later age.

### Key Points

- Hearing impairment is a significant cause of childhood disability
- Most congenital hearing impairment is sensorineural in origin
- Genetic factors account for at least half of congenital hearing impairment
- At risk factors detect only about half of those with a hearing loss
- Universal neonatal hearing screening is both feasible and desirable
- There is a need to provide services to detect hearing loss developed subsequently
- Habilitation in the first six months of life significantly improves speech and language development
- Hearing aids alleviate a hearing impairment but do not restore hearing to normal
- Children with a hearing loss have a higher risk than normal of having additional abnormalities
- Unilateral hearing loss can be a disabling condition especially in a noisy environment

## REFERENCES


Benazzo M, Lanza L, Cerniglia M *et al.* (1997) Otological and audiological aspects in Turner syndrome. *J Audiol Med* 6:147–159.

Bilgin H, Kasemsuwan L, Schachern P A *et al.* (1996) Temporal bone study of Down's syndrome. *Arch Laryngol Head Neck Surg* 122:271–275.

Borg E (1997) Perinatal asphyxia, hypoxia, ischaemia and hearing loss. An overview. *Scand Audiol* 19:77–91.

Briedenkamp J K, Smith M E, Dudley J P *et al.* (1992) Otolaryngologic manifestations of the mucopolysaccharidoses. *Ann Otol Rhinol Laryngol* 101:472–478.

Chen A, Francis M, Ni L *et al.* (1995) Phenotypic manifestations of branchio-oto-renal syndrome. *Am J Med Genet* 58:365–370.

Das V K (1991) Adverse perinatal factors in the causation of sensorineural hearing impairment in young children. *Int J Pediatr Otorhinolaryngol* 21:121–125.

✪ Davis A, Bamford J, Wilson I *et al.* (1997) A critical review of the role of neonatal screening in the detection of congenital hearing impairment. *Health Technol Assess* 1:1–196.

De Vries L S, Lary S & Whitelaw A G (1987) Relationship of serum bilirubin levels and hearing impairment in newborn infants. *Early Hum Dev* 15:269–277.

Downs M P (1995) Universal newborn hearing screening – the Colorado story. *Int J Pediatr Otorhinolaryngol* 32:257–259.

Fortnum H (1992) Hearing impairment after bacterial meningitis: a review. *Arch Dis Childhood* 67:1128–1133.

Fortnum H & Davis A (1997) Epidemiology of permanent hearing impairment in Trent Region, 1985–93. *Br J Audiol* 31:409–446.

Graziani L J, Ringlas M & Baumgart S (1997) Cerebrovascular complications and neurodevelopmental sequelae of neonatal ECMO. *Clin Perinatol* 24:655–675.

Griffon N, Souillet G, Maire I *et al.* (1998) Follow up of nine patients with Hurler syndrome after bone marrow transplantation. *J Pediatr* 133:119–125.

Guiscafre H, Martinez M C, Benitez-Diaz L *et al.* (1984) Reversible hearing loss after meningitis. Prospective assessment using auditory evoked responses. *Ann Otol Rhinol Laryngol* 93:229–232.

Hyson R I & Rudy J W (1987) Ontogenic change in the analysis of sound frequency in the infant rat. *Dev Psychobiol* 20:187–207.

JCIH (1994) Joint Committee on Infant Hearing position statement. *ASHA* 36:38–41.

✪ Jiang Z D (1995) Long term effect of perinatal and postnatal asphyxia on developing human auditory brainstem responses: peripheral hearing loss. *Int J Pediatr Otorhinolaryngol* 33:225–238.

Kuhl P K, Williams K A, Lacerda F *et al.* (1992) Linguistic experience alters phonetic perception in infants by six months of age. *Science* 255:606–608.

Kuhlali I, Ozturk M, Bilen C *et al.* (1997) Evaluation of hearing loss with auditory brainstem responses in the early and late period of bacterial meningitis in children. *J Laryngol Otol* 111:223–227.

Lench L, Houseman M, Newton V *et al.* (1999) Connexin-26 mutations in sporadic non-syndromal deafness, *Lancet* 351:415.

Lins O G, Picton P E & Picton T W (1995) Auditory steady-state responses to tones amplitude-modulated at 80–110 Hz. *J Acoust Soc Am* 97:3051–3063.

Lippe W R & Rubbel E W (1983) Development of the place principle: tonotopic organisation. *Science* 219:514–516.

Lucarini J W, Liberfarb R M, Eavey R D (1987) Otological manifestations of the Stickler syndrome. *Int J Pediatr Otorhinolaryngol* 14:215–222.

Mason S, Davis A, Wood S *et al.* (1998) Field sensitivity of targetted neonatal hearing screening using the Nottingham ABR screener. *Ear Hear* 19:91–102.

Mehl A L & Thomson V (1998) Newborn hearing screening: the great omission. *Pediatrics* 101: E4.

Metlay L A, Smythe P S & Miller M E (1987) Familial CHARGE syndrome: Clinical report with autopsy findings. *Am J Med Genet* 26:577–581.

Morgan D, Bailey M, Phelps P *et al.* (1993) Ear-nose-throat abnormalities in the CHARGE Association. *Arch Otolaryngol Head Neck Surg* 119:49–54.

NDCS (1996) *Quality standards in paediatric audiology. Vol. 11: the audiological management of the child with permanent hearing loss.* London: National Deaf Children's Society.

Newton V E (1990) Hearing loss and Waardenburg syndrome: Implications for genetic counselling. *J Laryngol Otol* 104:97–103.

Newton V E, Liu X Z & Read A P (1994) The association of sensorineural hearing loss and pigmentation abnormalities in Waardenburg syndrome. *J Audiol Med* 3:69–77.

Ochi A, Yasuhara A & Kobayashi (1998) Comparison of distortion product otoacoustic emissions with auditory brain-stem response for clinical use in neonatal intensive care unit. *Electroencephalogr Clin Neurophysiol* 108:577–583.

Papsin B C, Vellodi A, Bailey C M *et al.* (1998) Otologic and laryngologic manifestations of mucopolysaccharidoses after bone marrow transplantation. *Otolaryngol Head Neck Surg* 118:30–36.

Phelps P D, Coffey R A & Trembath R C *et al.* (1998) Radiological manifestations of the ear in Pendred's syndrome. *Clin Radiol* 53:268–273.

Prezant T R *et al.* (1993) Mitochondrial ribosomal RNA mutation associated with both antibiotic-induced and non-syndromic deafness. *Nat Genet* 4:289–294.

Rance G, Dowell R C & Rickards F W (1998) Steady-state evoked potential and behavioural hearing thresholds in a group of children with absent click-evoked auditory brain stem response. *Ear Hear* 19:48–61.

Read A P & Newton V E (1997) Waardenburg Syndrome. *J Med Genet* 34:656–665.

Richardson M P, Reid A & Tarlow M J *et al.* (1997) Hearing loss during bacterial meningitis. *Arch Dis Childhood* 76:134–138.

Silver S, Kapitulnik J & Sohmer H (1995) Contribution of asphyxia to the induction of hearing impairment in jaundiced Gunn rats. *Pediatrics* 95:579–583.

Smith R J H, Berlin C I, Hejtmancik J F *et al.* (1994) Clinical diagnosis of the Usher syndromes, Usher Syndrome Consortium. *Am J Med Genet* 50:32–38.

Splawsky I, Timothy K W, Vincent G M *et al.* (1997) Molecular basis of the Long-QT syndrome associated with deafness. *N Engl J Med* 336:1562–1567.

Talbott C B (1987) A longitudinal study comparing responses of hearing impaired infants to pure tones using visual reinforcement and play audiometry. *Ear Hear* 8:175–179.

✪ Veen S, Sassen M L, Schreuder A M *et al.* (1993) Hearing loss in very preterm and low birthweight infants at the age of 5 years in a nationwide cohort. *Int J Pediatr Otorhinolarynogol* 26:11–28.

Vienny H, Despland P A, Lutchg J *et al.* (1984) Early diagnosis and evolution of deafness in childhood bacterial meningitis: a study using brainstem auditory evoked potentials. *Pediatrics* 73:579–586.

✪ Watkins P M & Baldwin M (1999) Confirmation of deafness in infancy. *Arch Dis Childhood* 81:380–389.

Watkins P M, Baldwin M, Dixon R *et al.* (1997) Maternal anxiety and attitudes to universal neonatal screening. *Br J Audiol* 32:27–37.

Williamson W D, Demmler G J, Percy A K *et al.* (1992) Progressive hearing loss in infants with asymptomatic congenital cytomegalovirus infection. *Pediatrics* 90:862–866.

✪ Yoshinaga-Itano C, Sedey A L, Coulter D K *et al.* (1998) Language of early and later identified children with hearing loss. *Pediatrics* 102:1161–1171.

# Section X
# Disorders of the nerve and muscle

# Chapter 40

# Disorders of the spinal cord, cranial, and peripheral nerves

M. I. Levene

## INTRODUCTION

As a group of disorders, those affecting the spine, cranial, and peripheral nerves are not common but are important because of the risk of severe sequelae in terms of permanent neurologic disability. Although trauma is the commonest underlying pathology, it is clear that, in a minority, other poorly understood mechanisms are important in their etiology.

## CRANIAL NERVES

The seventh cranial nerve is most commonly recognized to be abnormal in the newborn period because its dysfunction is most obvious in its effect on facial symmetry. Although congenital or acquired abnormalities of other cranial nerves occur, they may not be recognized as such in the neonatal period because loss of function is less obvious or, if present, may be part of a much more severe neurologic disturbance as the result of massive injury such as birth asphyxia. An example of this is bulbar palsy in the presence of a grossly neurologically abnormal infant. Involvement of cranial nerves, other than VII, is rarely described in the literature as a pure entity. Multiple cranial nerve involvement is generally considered in the diagnostic category of the Möbius sequence (see below).

### FACIAL PALSY

Facial palsy has been reported to occur with an incidence of 0.23% (McHugh *et al.* 1969), but more recent figures are not available.

#### Etiology

The etiology of facial palsy can be considered as either developmental or traumatic (Table 40.1). It may be difficult to distinguish between these two major categories in the neonatal period, but the developmental problems tend not to improve, unlike traumatic facial palsy. Congenital facial nerve palsy due to a developmental disorder is often associated with other features, including the Möbius sequence (see below) and may be due to dysplasia of central nuclei. Rarely has bilateral facial palsy together with other developmental problems been related to abnormalities occurring very early in pregnancy such as bilateral infarction of the anterior operculum (Gropman *et al.* 1997).

Trauma accounts for the majority of cases of neonatal facial palsy; Smith *et al.* (1981) reported trauma to account for 78% of all cases. The extracranial course of the facial nerve is very superficial as it leaves the stylomastoid foramen and is particularly liable to neuropraxia as a result of pressure either from impaction of the head against the pelvic outlet or as the result of forceps application. Forceps delivery was reported to be associated with facial palsy in 75% of cases (Smith *et al.* 1981). In a large study of 53 children with permanent facial palsy, there was no statistically increased risk of this condition if the baby was delivered with the aid of forceps (Laing *et al.* 1996). They suggest that cases of long-standing facial palsy are due to prenatal factors. An alternative cause of acquired 'traumatic' injury is as the result of pressure from the maternal sacrum on the facial nerve. To support this, Hepner (1951) showed that

**Table 40.1 Classification of causes of facial nerve palsy**

| |
|---|
| Developmental |
| Agenesis/dysplasia of the facial nerve nuclei |
| Primary |
| Associated with other defects |
| Möbius sequence |
| Hemifacial microsomia |
| Oculoauriculovertebral dysplasia |
| Cardiofacial syndrome |
| Poland's syndrome |
| Degeneration of the facial nerve nuclei |
| Ischemia and infarction |
| Brainstem hemorrhage |
| Teratogenesis |
| Thalidomide embryopathy |
| Viruses (rubella) |
| Dystrophia myotonica |
| Acquired |
| Birth trauma |
| Forceps injury |
| Maternal sacral compression |
| Intracranial hemorrhage |
| Otitis media |
| Meningitis |
| Viral infections |
| Congenital varicella |
| Infectious mononucleosis |
| Poliomyelitis |

*Source*: Adapted from Harris *et al.* (1983) © American Medical Society.

those babies with transient facial palsy who were born without forceps had a left-sided palsy if they were delivered from a left occipitoanterior position and vice versa for those presenting right occipitoanteriorly. Supranuclear facial palsy is also rarely associated with intracranial hemorrhage (Paine 1957).

### Clinical features

The lesion is most obvious when the baby cries. The baby's lower lip fails to move downward and outward on the affected side, and there may be an inability to close the eye on the ipsilateral side (Fig. 40.1). This condition must be distinguished from asymmetric crying facies (see below). The child should be carefully examined for evidence of abnormalities in other cranial nerves or other congenital malformations/deformations. Examination of the ear may reveal a hematotympanum that supports a traumatic origin (Harris *et al.* 1983).

### Investigations

Neurophysiologic assessment may help in determining whether the lesion is congenital or acquired. Investigations include a maximal stimulation test as well as evoked and standard electromyograms (EMGs). If the nerve is non-stimulatable on maximum impulse and has a silent EMG, then it is very likely that there is a developmental cause (Harris *et al.* 1983). Auditory brainstem responses (see Chapter 12) may be useful as the auditory pathways lie close to the facial nerve nuclei in the brainstem, and abnormalities may indicate a more widespread dysplastic process involving these structures.

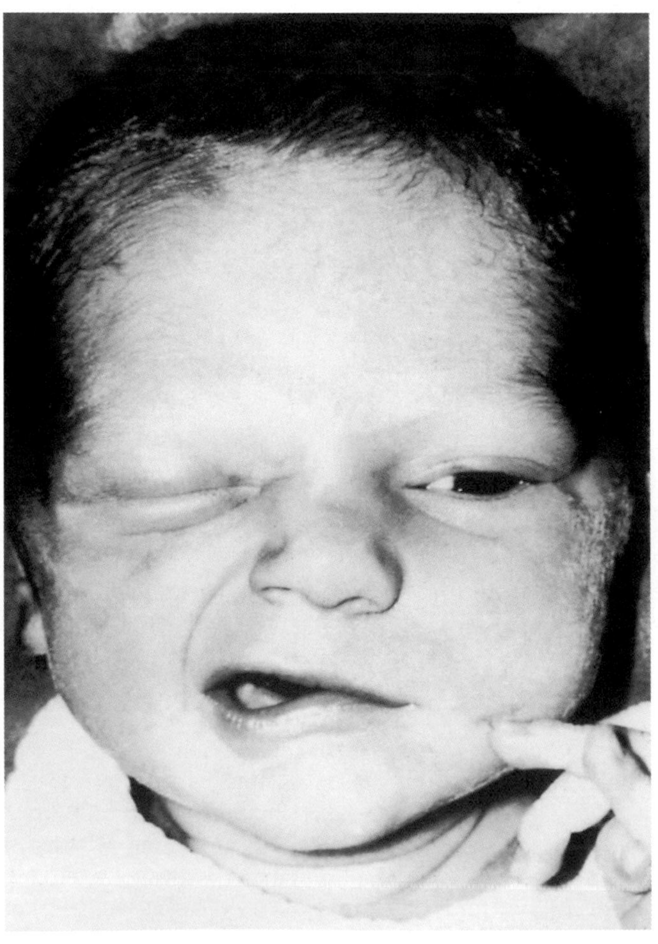

**Figure 40.1** Left-sided facial nerve palsy. On crying, the baby is unable to close the left eye or open the mouth normally on the left side.

### Management

Ninety per cent of facial nerve palsies show signs of spontaneous recovery within 4 weeks of birth (Smith *et al.* 1981). Surgical exploration is therefore unwarranted in the majority of cases. Indications for surgical decompression of the nerve (Bergman *et al.* 1986) include:

1. hematotympanum with a displaced fracture of the petrous bone
2. no recovery of function either clinically or electrophysiologically at 5 weeks of age.

It is suggested that the initial surgical approach should be directed towards the intraparotid portion of the nerve in the stylomastoid region. Inability to locate the nerve suggests agenesis, and further surgery is unwarranted (Narcy *et al.* 1982).

## Möbius sequence

The first report of an abnormality of multiple cranial nerves was by Graefe in 1880, and further cases were reported by Möbius in 1888 and 1892 (for a review, see Pitner *et al.* 1965). The sequence is best described by the minimum combination of facial palsy (usually bilateral) together with involvement of at least one cranial nerve controlling eye movement. The abducent nerve (VI) is reported to be affected in 68–85% of cases (Carr *et al.* 1997; Abramson *et al.* 1998), and involvement of other cranial motor nerves (including III, IV, V, IX, X and XII) is more variable. Other associated malformations are seen in about one-third of cases (Smith 1982). These involve the lower limb (talipes equinovarus), upper limbs, facial structures (microtia, micrognathia, and microphthalmia), and chest-wall anomalies, as seen in Poland's anomaly (Sugarman & Stark 1973). Familial cases have been reported, and a variety of gene loci have been identified on chromosome 3 and 10 (Verzijl *et al.* 1999), as well as a 1;2 reciprocal translocation (Nishikawa *et al.* 1997). It has also been reported to occur as the result of an autosomal dominant gene (Baraitser 1977).

The underlying pathologic abnormality has been much debated and still remains unclear. In the majority of cases, the Möbius sequence is not due to any one pathologic insult, and it is to be expected that multiple etiologies exist for this sequence of abnormalities. Degenerative and dysplastic causes have both been described. Calcification of the brainstem, pons, and medulla has been reported at autopsy (Thakkar *et al.* 1977) and on computerized tomography (CT)

(Govaert *et al.* 1989), supporting a prenatal ischemic brainstem insult hypothesis. The associated non-cranial abnormalities seen in this condition also support a more systemic circulatory insult. Other studies where there has been careful inspection of the brain, facial nerves, and involved muscles have not revealed any evidence of acquired disorders. A peripheral muscular dysplastic disorder with secondary atrophy of brainstem nuclei has been suggested to be one cause (Pitner *et al.* 1965).

Recently, it has been shown that in Brazil, the use of misoprostol as an attempted abortifacient in early pregnancy increased the risk of the baby being born with the Möbius sequence by almost 30-fold (Pastuszak *et al.* 1998). Others have suggested that induction of uterine contractions with drugs such as misoprostol or ergotamine at 6–7 weeks of pregnancy induces this abnormality as the result of vasocontriction (Graf & Shepard 1997).

### Asymmetric crying facies

This condition may be easily confused with facial nerve palsy. The term 'asymmetric crying facies', which describes the condition well, was coined by Pape & Pickering (1972), but is also known by the term 'congenital unilateral lower lip palsy' (CULLP) (Kobayashi 1979). This is a relatively common minor cosmetic disorder with a unilateral abnormality of the muscle, which draws down the lower lip. It affects the left side more commonly than the right (Pape & Pickering 1972; Kobayashi 1979). When the child cries, the normal side of the mouth is pulled down, and the abnormal side remains horizontal. This is the opposite of facial nerve palsy.

Approximately 40% have other abnormalities, of which minor ear anomalies were the most common; 7% had associated cardiac defects (Kobayashi 1979). The cause is unknown, but there are reported cases of familial grouping (Perlman & Reisner 1973). The disorder causes no disability, and no treatment is necessary. The asymmetry appears to improve with age.

## RECURRENT LARYNGEAL NERVE INJURY

The recurrent laryngeal nerve is a branch of the vagus and, on the left side, loops under the aortic arch and behind the ductus arteriosus at its junction with the aorta. It innervates the larynx. Its anatomic proximity to the ductus arteriosus renders it very vulnerable to accidental transection during ductal ligation or coarctation repair. Left laryngeal palsy has been reported to occur in 4% of cases following this operation in children and 8% in infants with a birthweight below 1500 g (Fan *et al.* 1989). A large ductus arteriosus aneurysm has been reported to cause recurrent laryngeal nerve and phrenic nerve palsy, which was reversible after resolution of the aneurysm following surgery (Hornung *et al.* 1999). Persisting symptoms include stridor and hoarseness, and spontaneous recovery of laryngeal nerve paresis is rare.

## HYPOGLOSSAL NERVE INJURY

This may be associated with the Möbius sequence (see above). Damage to the hypoglossal nerve has rarely been reported as the result of birth injury (Greenberg *et al.* 1987; Haenggeli & Lacourt 1989). It results from excessive lateral flexion of the neck with torsion affecting the brainstem. Brachial plexus is usually the major clinical feature. Hypoglossal nerve injury causes ipsilateral paralysis of the tongue with immobility and bulging on the affected side. When the tongue is extended, it curves towards the affected side, and this is associated with difficulties in sucking. Swallowing remains normal. Spontaneous recovery is reported in affected cases.

# THE SPINAL CORD

The embryologic development of the spinal cord is discussed in detail in Chapter 3, and some inherited disorders of the spinal cord such as spinal muscular atrophy, which may cause confusion with other neuromuscular problems, are discussed in Chapter 41. Abnormalities of the spinal cord may be classified as either malformations or deformations, acquired as the result of an insult occurring after a stage of normal development. Pathology affecting the spinal cord can be classified, as is shown in Table 40.2. By far the most common abnormalities involving the spinal cord involve disorders of the neural tube, and many of these are discussed in detail in Chapter 45. Spinal-cord pathology in the neonatal period is usually overt and presents with either major clinical neurologic signs such as paresis, or associated with obvious anatomic maldevelopment. Less obvious neural tube disorders may have a cutaneous marker of spinal abnormality such as spina bifida occulta (p. 199). Other congenital anomalies of the spine or spinal cord rarely present in the neonatal period, and diagnosis may be delayed until growth and neurologic development unmask the functional effects of the abnormality (see below). The most important in this respect are lipomatous infiltration of the cord, tethered cord, diastematomyelia, hemangiolipomata, dermoid cysts, and enterogenous cysts. Very rarely, tumors of the cord may cause neurologic problems in the neonate.

## DEVELOPMENTAL DISORDERS

### Caudal regression syndrome (CRS)

This acquired anomaly is due to an insult occurring very early in intrauterine life and usually involves the lower spinal cord. Its incidence is 0.01–0.05 per 1000 births, and 16% of cases are seen in association with maternal diabetes (Egelhoff 1999). An inherited form of partial sacral agenesis has been described (Say & Coldwell 1975). CRS may be ischemic in nature, and the timing and nature of the insult may cause associated abnormalities in other organs that develop rapidly at that time. The baby presents with a neurogenic bladder and anal flaccidity, possibly paraplegia depending on the level of cord involvement with arthrogryposis. The lumbar spine is abnormal in about 25% of cases and can be best evaluated by MR imaging.

### Segmental spinal dysgenesis

Segmental spinal dysgenesis (SSD) is a very rare disorder with localized agenesis or dysgenesis of the lumbar or thoracolumbar cord and associated spinal column disruption. This usually includes severe congenital kyphosis or kyphoscoliosis of the thoracolumbar, lumbar, or lumbosacral spine present at birth. Rarely, complete aplasia of the cord below the affected level may be seen. It has been suggested that the caudal regression syndrome is a variant of SSD affecting the lower caudal segments (Tortori-Donati *et al.* 1999).

MR imaging shows a normal upper cord, a markedly abnormal section (thinned or apparently absent) with a bulky, thickened and low-lying lower cord (Tortori-Donati *et al.* 1999). Clinically, the infant shows severe flaccid paralysis below the level of the affected spinal cord with orthopedic abnormalities of the lower limbs.

Surgery is indicated if there is compression of the remaining cord from the abnormally formed bony elements of the spine.

### Split notocord syndrome

This rare condition may present either with spina bifida in its posterior–anterior form or with intact skin and underlying posterior structures, but visceral malformations (neurenteric cyst). In this latter case, there is a posterior cyst that can be either mediastinal or abdominal and extends into the spinal canal causing anterior cord compression. It may be associated with diastematomeyelia (partial or complete clefting of the spinal cord). Cord compression requires neurosurgical treatment.

### Anterior sacral meningocele

In this condition, there is anterior herniation of a dural sac through a bony sacral or coccygeal defect. Presentation may be with neurologic disruption of bladder and/or bowel function or a pelvic mass. The diagnosis is confirmed on MR scanning, which shows a CSF filled pelvic mass in continuity with the distal thecal sac through a narrow neck (Egelhoff 1999). Neurosurgical excision is required.

## INTRASPINAL TUMORS (see also p. 783)

These are very rare in the neonate, and those reported to occur in infancy are listed in Table 40.2. The baby may present with swelling over the spine or with more insidious progression of neurologic signs with bladder distension or reduced movement of the lower limbs. Tumors arising from non-spinal origins such as teratoma, neuroblastoma, and hamartoma are rarely associated with neurologic complications, and this will only occur if there is infiltration into the spinal canal with cord compression.

**Table 40.2 Classification of abnormalities of the spinal cord presenting within the neonatal period**

| |
|---|
| **Malformations** |
| Neural tube defects |
| Meningocele |
| Myelomeningocele |
| Spina bifida occulta |
| Diastematomyelia |
| Segmental spinal dysgenesis |
| Caudal regression syndrome |
| Split notocord syndrome |
| Anterior sacral meningocele |
| **Intraspinal tumor** |
| Ependymoma |
| Teratoma |
| Histiocytosis - X |
| Neuroblastoma |
| Ganglioneuroma |
| Harmartoma |
| Neurenteric cyst |
| **Trauma** |
| Cord transection |
| Extradural hemorrhage and compression |
| **Vascular injury** |
| Watershed insult |
| Focal ischemic damage secondary to trauma |
| Emboli |

## TRAUMATIC CORD LESIONS

The incidence of trauma to the cord is unknown, particularly when it is not severe enough to cause persisting neurologic abnormalities. It is certainly less common now that it was before modern intrapartum care became of a consistently high standard in developed countries. Trauma to the spinal cord resulting in permanent disability is now a rare, but devastating, condition.

### Etiology

The neonatal spine is particularly vulnerable to stretching, and Towbin (1969) has reported that autopsy studies have found that the spinal cord can only be stretched by 6 mm before tearing occurs, whereas the vertebral column can be stretched to 5 cm without disruption. This explains why major cord disruption may occur in the absence of bony damage or dislocation. Traction due to excessive neck rotation damages higher cervical structures and breech delivery with excessive rotation, flexion, or hyperextension of the spine may cause cervico-thoracic or thoracolumbar damage.

Bony damage has also been reported in cases of cord trauma, with fractures of the odontoid peg and dislocation of the atlas vertebra (Schulman *et al.* 1971). Severe over-extension of the neck may also cause occipito-osteodiastasis (see p. 355), which has been reported to cause medullary transection and tearing of the tentorium (Pape & Wigglesworth 1979). The asphyxiated infant appears to be particularly prone to cord injury. It is suggested that asphyxia-induced hypotonia predisposes the baby to greater tractional and rotational forces to the unprotected neck (Clancy *et al.* 1989).

Case reports of infants with major cord trauma describe functional damage either in the upper cervical cord (above C4) or lower in the region of the cervico-thoracic or thoraco-lumbar spine. MacKinnon *et al.* (1993) describe 22 babies who had sustained spinal cord injury at birth from five Canadian centers. Fourteen had upper cervical lesions, and all were delivered cephalically after attempted forceps rotation of the head. All the babies with lesions below C4 were born by the breech.

The fetus presenting by the breech with hyperextension of the head (the 'stargazing' or 'flying' fetus) is at particular risk of cord damage after vaginal delivery (Abroms *et al.* 1973; Bhagwanani *et al.* 1973; Maekawa *et al.* 1976). Abroms *et al.* (1973) estimate that 25% of fetuses delivered vaginally in this position will have permanent neurologic deficit, and Cesarean section may not protect the fetus fully from permanent spinal cord injury (Maekawa *et al.* 1976). In these cases, the cord lesion is probably of prenatal onset due to vascular compromise (Maekawa *et al.* 1976).

### Pathology

Towbin (1969) examined the spinal cord in a large number of neonatal deaths and found that 10% had evidence of trauma to the cord or adjacent structures. Pathology included:

1. meningeal damage, the commonest form of injury, with bleeding into the subarachnoid and epidural spaces
2. nerve root laceration or avulsion (see brachial plexus injury)
3. cord injury ranging from relatively minor lacerations to complete transection
4. dislocation or fracture of vertebral bodies.

The pattern of pathologic findings relate to the duration of time from injury to pathologic examinations. Early changes include hemorrhage, which may lead to severe hematomyelia with blood filling the dura at the site of laceration, cord edema, and acute neuronal damage. Bleeding and edema may lead to progressive neuronal necrosis due to compression. If death does not occur in the first few days following the injury, then severe cord atrophy develops at the level of the injury, with cystic degeneration, loss of axons, myelin, and gliosis. Proliferation of Schwann cells in the remaining cord tissue has been described (Babyn *et al.* 1988). The 'dying back' phenomenon is associated with degeneration of descending corticospinal tracts and ascending spinothalamic tracts above the level of cord transection, which extends up into the pons.

### Clinical features

Loss of spontaneous movement of the upper and/or lower limbs may take some days to be clinically apparent, particularly when the infant is ill, and consequently, the diagnosis of spinal cord injury is often delayed. Bladder distension is usually present and should alert the clinician to the need for a more careful neurologic inspection. Concurrent asphyxia with severe hypoxic–ischemic encephalopathy is reported in 64% of babies with high cervical lesions (MacKinnon *et al.* 1993), and this may obscure the neurologic signs of associated cord damage.

The infant with an acute cord injury will initially show 'spinal shock' with hypotonia and reduced or absent tendon reflexes. The baby will often not breathe spontaneously for several days, even in the absence of a high cervical cord lesion (MacKinnon *et al.* 1993). Signs of recovery within the first few days of life indicate less severe neurologic damage. Regular reassessment is necessary in the first week of life. Neurologic evaluation of a motor and sensory level should be documented, although this may initially be patchy and asymmetric. Flexion withdrawal of the lower limbs to painful stimuli may represent a spinal reflex and should not be confused with spontaneous recovery. In one study, five of six babies with lower cord lesions breathed spontaneously by 20 days of age (MacKinnon *et al.* 1993), but babies with high cervical lesions will remain dependent on mechanical ventilation indefinitely.

Some infants with early features of lower limb paralysis may show progressive signs of ascending involvement, with paresis of the upper limbs within 24 h due to hemorrhage or edema of the cord. Similarly, babies who initially breathe spontaneously may show ascending involvement of respiratory muscles with progressive hypoventilation and respiratory arrest. A markedly asymmetric motor level may be seen, which is most likely to be due to a relatively low spinal lesion with unilateral brachial plexus injury.

A sensory level is usually detected on careful clinical examination, but this may not necessarily correlate with the level of motor involvement. An asymmetric sensory level is not uncommon. A neurogenic bladder with distension and urine dribbling from the urethra is usually seen in severe cord trauma together with paralysis of the anal sphincter. Tendon and grasp reflexes are lost, but touch or painful stimuli to the limbs or body may elicit vigorous withdrawal reflexes, which may be confused with spontaneous movement. Horner's syndrome may be present (see p. 701).

Differential diagnosis includes spinal muscular atrophy (see p. 717), HIE (see p. 476), bilateral brachial plexus injury (see p. 699) and respiratory disease.

### Investigations

Plain X-ray of the spine should be performed in all suspected cases to assess evidence of bony damage or vertebral instability. Imaging the cord in the acute phase is important to establish the level of injury and the extent of associated hemorrhage and edema. Ultrasound examination of the spinal canal and cord is possible up to the age of 6 months due to poor ossification of the vertebral spines and serial real-time scanning at the cotside appears to be the most sensitive modality in the acute phase of cord injury. Demonstration of acute cord injury, hematomyelia, and hemorrhage around the cord has been reported (Jequier *et al.* 1984; Babyn 1988, MacKinnon *et al.* 1993; de Vries *et al.* 1995; Simon *et al.* 1999). It has been suggested that serial ultrasound scanning is the most accurate imaging technique for diagnostic purposes (MacKinnon *et al.* 1993). In the later stages of recovery when atrophy has developed, ultrasound examination may demonstrate myelomalacia and a decrease in cord diameter.

Magnetic resonance is becoming widely used to image the spine but appears to be more sensitive after the acute phase of spinal cord injury for localizing the site and type of damage (Lanska *et al.* 1990). False-negative findings with MR have been reported in the acute stages of cord injury (MacKinnon *et al.* 1993; Simon *et al.* 1999). There is no place for myelography, and CT scanning is the least useful of the imaging techniques.

Electrophysiologic assessment may also help confirm the diagnosis and determine the level of cord trauma. Motor and sensory nerve conduction times will be normal for peripheral nerves. Electromyography may reveal changes of acute denervation, which include no spontaneous electrical activity, polyphasic motor unit potentials of small amplitude and short duration, and spontaneously occurring fibrillation potentials. These may be intermixed with larger-amplitude, longer-duration motor unit potentials (Clancy *et al.* 1989). Somatosensory evoked potentials have also been used to confirm the level of the cord injury (Bell & Dykstra 1985).

### Prognosis

In general, the prognosis both for survival and functional outcome is very poor (MacKinnon *et al.* 1993; Simon *et al.* 1999) but is dependent on the level of the cord lesion and the rate of clinical recovery over the first few weeks of life. MacKinnon *et al.* (1993) have reported that all infants with an upper cervical lesion had a very poor prognosis. Fifty per cent died early, and all but one of the survivors remained partially or wholly dependent on mechanical ventilation. The child who came off the ventilator showed rapid signs of neurologic recovery and was weaned from the ventilator at 19 days. In patients with lesions lower than C4 (MacKinnon *et al.* 1993), all but one showed some spontaneous breathing activity on day 1 (the other commenced breathing on day 8). In fact, only two children in this group survived, both of whom were described as having paraplegia on follow-up, and one required mechanical ventilation at night. MacKinnon *et al.* (1993) recommend withdrawal of mechanical ventilation if there has been no spontaneous respiratory activity by 3 weeks after birth. Koch & Eng (1979) reported that in surviving infants, flaccidity in the neonatal period led to spastic paraplegia in the majority of cases. In contrast to this, others have found that neonatal flaccidity and areflexia persisted into infancy and childhood in one-half of survivors (Burcher *et al.* 1979).

### Management

Damage to the bony vertebral structures rarely requires surgical stabilization. If a fracture occurs, it is usually through the epiphyseal plate of the vertebral body, and management by positioning in extension is all that is required. Extradural hemorrhage may cause compression or spinal block, but there is little evidence that neurosurgical drainage improves outcome. Management of the nerve injury of the spine is expectant.

## VASCULAR ACCIDENTS OF THE CORD

### Aetiology

It is proposed that some neonates with paraplegia without an obvious traumatic etiology have sustained hypoxic–ischemic injury to the spinal cord (Clancy *et al.* 1989; Singer *et al.* 1991). The anterior horn cells of the spinal cord may be particularly susceptible to hypoxic–ischemic insult, which causes marked transient weakness, flaccidity and areflexia in affected babies. This may be confused with, or be a major part of, signs of severe hypoxic–ischemic encephalopathy (Clancy *et al.* 1989).

The spinal cord has a rich anastomotic blood supply from both extraspinal and intraspinal sources. The extraspinal vessels arise from the aorta or vertebral arteries via the anterior spinal artery (Fig. 40.2) supplying segments C1–T3, the dorsal radicular artery supplying segments T4–T8, and the artery of Adamkiewcz, which is the main branch of the lower anterior spinal artery supplying T9–L1. There is some inconstancy as to the precise levels of origin of these three arteries. There is therefore a potentially vulnerable watershed area between these vascular territories, which may predispose to focal spinal cord infarction.

Sladky & Rorke (1986) have described two distinct sites for cord damage as the result of vascular injury. The commonest type involved injury to the lumbosacral region. In these cases, there was more severe damage to central, rather than peripheral, regions, suggesting a radial artery watershed distribution. Another study has shown a selective vulnerability of some cellular elements in the lumbar cord but not suggestive of a vascular distribution (DeGirolami & Zivin 1982). Less commonly, Sladky & Rorke (1986) found infarction to be limited to dorsal gray matter in the mid- and upper-thoracic regions, and this may correspond to the thoracic watershed territory.

Jacobs *et al.* (1987) have shown that ligation of the abdominal aorta in an animal model caused complete hind limb paralysis with functional recovery 4 h after release of the ligature. From 12 to 18 h following the ischemic insult, a secondary and permanent loss of hind-limb function occurred, and it has been suggested that this is due to a secondary impairment of blood flow to the spinal cord. Infarction of the cord may occur as a result of obstruction to

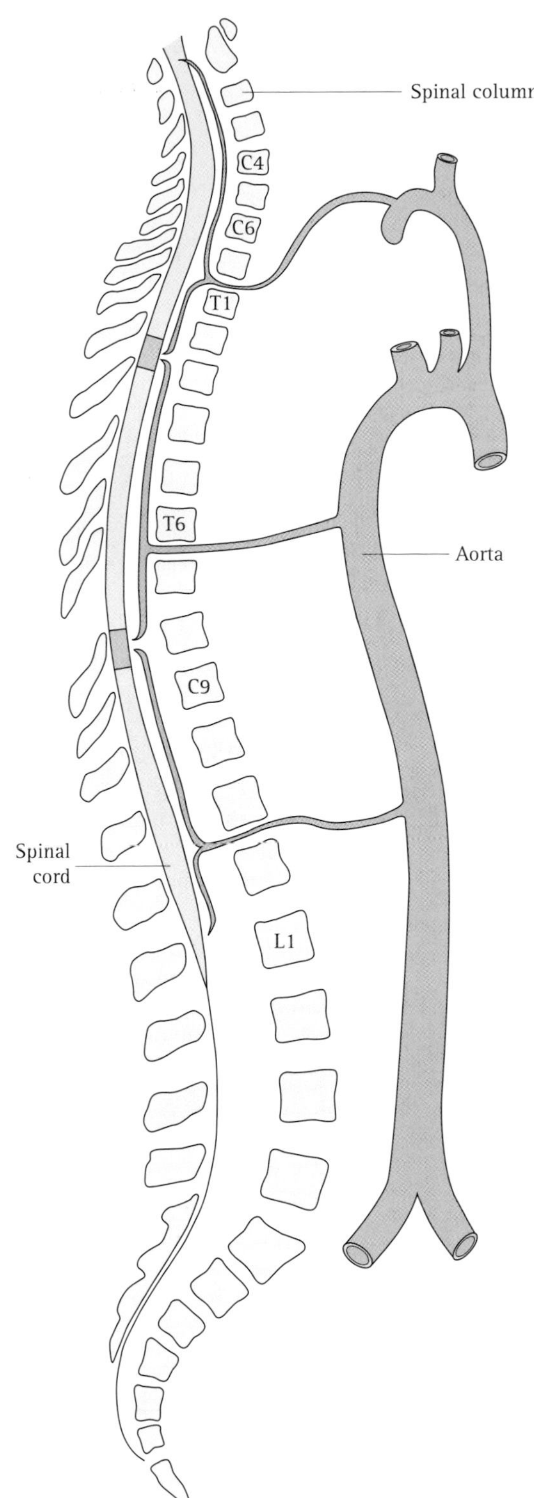


Figure 40.2 Arterial supply of the spinal cord. The shaded areas within the spinal cord represent watershed regions susceptible to potential underperfusion.

flow through the feeding vessels arising from the aorta by a umbilical artery catheter placed in the aorta.

The spinal cord appears to be a more resistant structure to ischemic insults than the brain, and consequently, global ischemia or asphyxia is more likely to damage the brain than the spinal cord alone. Ischemic lesions of the spinal cord alone therefore are most likely to have a more focal etiology such as local impairment of blood flow in the aorta or emboli from an arterial catheter placed in the lower aorta.

Three major etiological factors for ischemic cord lesions have been reported.

1. Acute spinal cord infarction as a complication of generalized hypoxic/ischemic lesions. This has been described as occurring after cardiac arrest or severe asphyxial insults (Schneider *et al.* 1975; Sladky & Rorke 1986). Basal ganglia and brainstem abnormalities occur commonly in association with spinal cord damage (Schneider *et al.* 1975) similar to that which has been described after acute total asphyxial insult (p. 474). This was the most commonly described form of spinal infarction in a group of neonates who came to autopsy examination (Sladky & Rorke 1986).
2. Localized infarction of the spinal cord secondary to a traumatic lesion such as transection or extradural spinal hemorrhage in which regional blood supply is compromised (Sladky & Rorke 1986). Focal infarction has also been reported to occur prenatally (Darwish *et al.* 1981; Farrell & McGillivray 1983; Young *et al.* 1983).
3. Embolic infarction associated with the placement of an umbilical artery catheter in the descending aorta (Aziz & Robertson 1973; Dulac & Aicardi 1975; Krishnamoorthy *et al.* 1976). A catheter tip position between T10 and L2 may predispose to embolic damage to the lower cord through the artery of Adamkiewcz. An alternative mechanism for irreversible spinal injury is catheter-induced, prolonged spinal-artery spasm. Cardiac surgery requiring prolonged clamping of the descending aorta has been reported to cause spinal cord injury in infants but rarely in the neonate.

## BRACHIAL PLEXUS PALSY

The brachial plexus is a web of nerves emerging from the lower cervical and upper thoracic roots. These may be damaged by stretching during delivery, but there is increasing evidence that in some, the injury to the brachial plexus may predate the birth process. Although the majority of babies with brachial plexus injury recover spontaneously, surgical intervention may improve the functional outcome of some of the more severe cases.

### CLASSIFICATION

The brachial plexus comprises the conjunction and subsequent disjunction of spinal nerves from C4–C8 and T1.

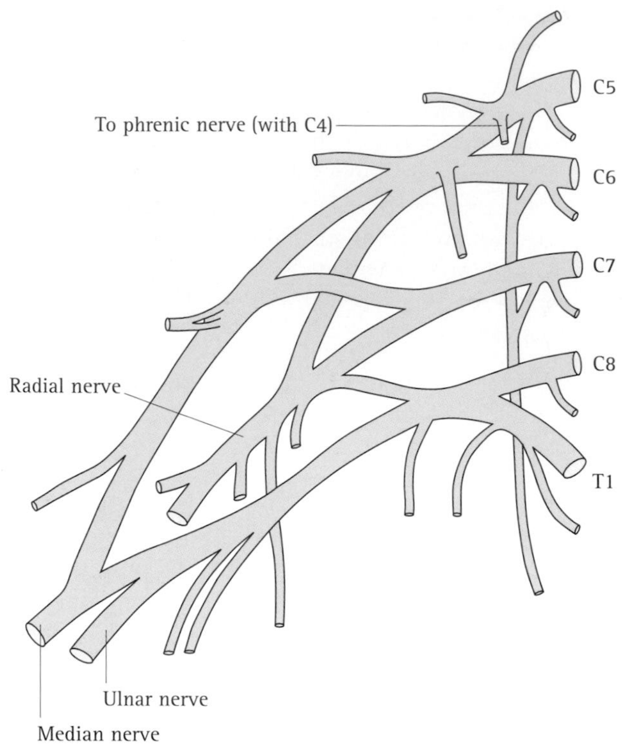


**Figure 40.3** The components of the brachial plexus showing the formation of the major nerves of the arm.

Combinations of these spinal nerves unite to form the major nerves of the upper limb (Fig. 40.3). Tearing or damage to these spinal nerves will cause functional disability to the arm depending on the level at which the damage has occurred. Clinically, two main types of brachial plexus lesions are recognized:

1. upper (C5–7) and described as Erb's palsy
2. upper and lower (C5–T1) and described as Klumpke's palsy.

## Incidence

The incidence of brachial plexus injury in 11 centers was reviewed by Gherman *et al.* (1998). He describes an overall incidence from these studies of 1.8 per 1000 live-born births. There have been two large geographically based cohorts from the state of California (1994–1995) and the whole of Sweden (1980–1989) (Bager 1997). The reported incidence from these studies were 1.5 and 1.6 per 1000, respectively.

Prospectively collected Swedish data show that there has been a statistically significant increase in the incidence of this condition in a 10-year period from 1980 (1.3/1000) to 1994 (2.2/1000) (Bager 1997). Data from the US (Graham *et al.* 1997) show no significant increase over a 30-year period in one institution when the period 1954–1959 (1.2/1000) was compared with 1987–1991 (1.0/1000), although there had been a fourfold increase in Cesarean section rates over this same period of time.

## Etiology

Shoulder dystocia and macrosomia are the two most commonly recognized risk factors for this condition, but there are increasing numbers of reports of cases due to factors other than severe neck traction at delivery. The classic insult reported to cause brachial plexus palsy is excessive downward traction on the neck during attempted delivery of the anterior shoulder during vaginal delivery. Fetal macrosomia is an important risk factor for shoulder dystocia, which is the underlying cause for excessive neck traction resulting in damage to the anterior plexus. Gherman *et al.* (1998) have estimated from their data that 18% of patients with shoulder dystocia requiring the McRobert's maneuver to facilitate delivery resulted in brachial plexus injury. In Sweden, half the infants with brachial plexus lesions were large for gestational age, and for those of birthweight >4500 g, the incidence was 45 times higher than for those with birthweight <3500 g (Bager 1997).

A second group at risk of obstetric trauma at delivery are those born by the breech where the posterior arm is used to rotate the baby. Geutjens *et al.* (1996) reviewed 36 babies with brachial plexus injury who had been born by the breech. They had a different pattern of injury, with 81% having avulsion of the upper cervical roots with poor prognosis for complete recovery.

It is now well recognized that brachial plexus injury occurs in the absence of shoulder dystocia. In some studies, almost 50% of cases occur without a history of difficult delivery (Koenigsberger 1980; Dunn & Engle 1985; Jennett *et al.* 1992; Graham *et al.* 1997; Ouzounian *et al.* 1997; Gherman *et al.* 1998 for a review), and these babies have a significantly lower birthweight than the dystocic group and a worse prognosis for full recovery. In one report, fracture of the clavicle was only seen with Erb's palsy occurring in the absence of shoulder dystocia (Gherman *et al.* 1998). Interestingly, the posterior shoulder was more likely to be affected when the baby was born without shoulder dystocia compared with the anterior shoulder in dystocic deliveries (Gherman *et al.* 1998). It is suggested that in these cases of brachial plexus injury without shoulder dystocia, there is an intrapartum etiology, possibly pressure of the shoulder against the sacral promontory, or symphasis pubis. Cases of Erb's palsy with transient facial palsy have been cited to add weight to this hypothesis (Gherman *et al.* 1998). A case has been reported of proven prenatal onset of brachial plexus injury associated with a bicornuate uterus (Dunn & Engle 1985).

Right-sided palsy occurs more commonly than lesions on the left (Gilbert *et al.* 1991), and this appears to be due to the more common cephalic left occipital anterior presentation, which predisposes the right shoulder to a higher risk of impaction. Bilateral brachial plexus palsy is more commonly seen following difficult breech extraction.

Rarely families have been reported with brachial plexus palsy in multiply affected children (Gordon *et al.* 1973; al-Qattan & al-Kharfy 1996; Brett 1991). Other reported causes include neonatal hemangiomatosis (Lucas *et al.* 1995), and late-onset group-B streptococcal osteomyelitis (Sadleir & Connolly 1998).

### Pathology

The injury involves a number of the brachial plexus roots comprising $C_5$–$T_1$. The roots may be stretched, totally ruptured, or avulsed from the spinal cord. Avulsion rarely occurs in the region of $C_5$ and $C_6$ and is much more common at the level of $C_8$ and $T_1$. Lesions confined to the lower roots are rare. Traumatic meningoceles may develop at the site of root avulsion.

### Clinical assessment

The clinical diagnosis of brachial plexus injury is made by observing loss of active movement of the upper limb together with a full range of passive movements. Attention must be given to the diagnosis of Horner's syndrome (see below), phrenic nerve involvement (chest X-ray may show an elevated diaphragm), and associated fracture of the ipsilateral humerus or clavicle. A full neurologic examination should evaluate spontaneous movement of all limbs to exclude a cerebral (hemiplegia) or spinal (tetraplegia) cause for loss of spontaneous movement.

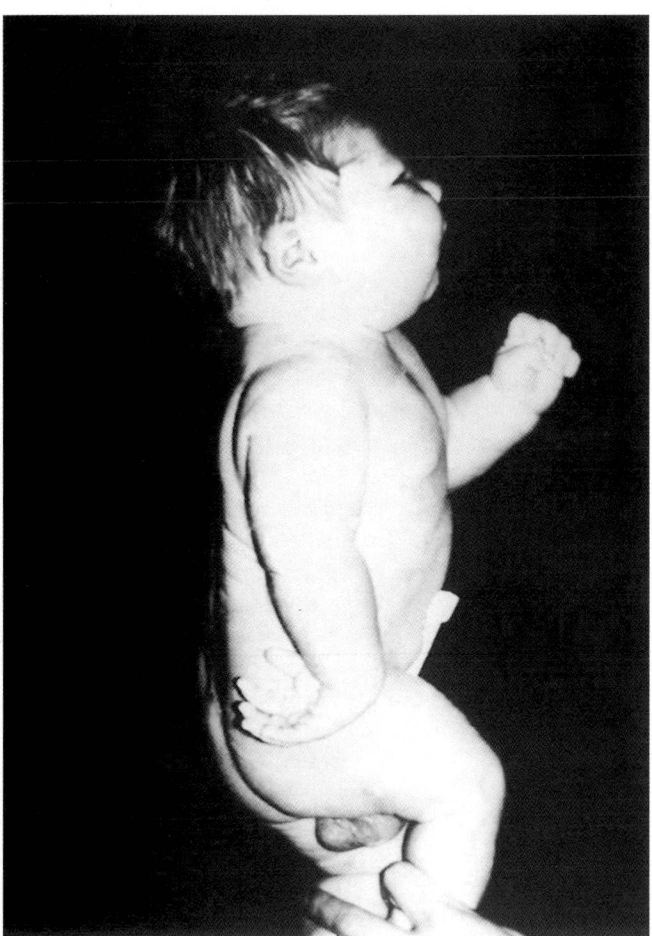

**Figure 40.4** Erb's palsy. The infant's right arm is adducted and internally rotated with the elbow extended and pronated. The wrist and fingers are flexed.

#### Erb's palsy

The arm is adducted and internally rotated at the shoulder, and the elbow is extended with pronation of the forearm. The wrist and fingers are flexed. This produces the classic 'waiter's tip' position (Fig. 40.4). Involvement of $C_7$ causes the elbow to be slightly flexed. Tendon reflexes (biceps, triceps, brachioradialis) are usually absent or markedly reduced in the affected limbs.

#### Klumpke's palsy

There is damage to all nerve roots, and the arm is flail with a claw hand. There is often vasomotor disturbance with mottling of the arm. Diaphragmatic palsy may occur, and a Horner syndrome (see below) may be a variable finding. Although the majority of cases of Klumpke's palsy are apparent immediately after birth, Rossi *et al.* (1982) reported that five of 36 cases were not diagnosed until some weeks after birth. It is not clear whether these children were entirely asymptomatic prior to diagnosis.

If improvement occurs, it starts distally, and a total paralysis may regress to involve only the upper roots over a number of weeks. In patients who improve to a complete recovery, the biceps and deltoid muscle are the first to show contraction, and this has been found to occur by 1 month with normal contractions by 2 months (Gilbert *et al.* 1991). Incomplete, but adequate, recovery of the shoulder musculature was seen if the biceps and deltoid muscles started to show spontaneous contractions by 3 months. If there was no recovery in biceps or triceps by 3 months, then the prognosis for adequate recovery was poor.

#### Horner's syndrome

This is due to a lesion of the cervical sympathetic nerve fibers. Preganglionic fibers emerge from the spinal cord in the upper thoracic roots and travel superiorly in the paravertebral sympathetic chain to the superior cervical ganglion. This long course makes them particularly vulnerable to traumatic forces similar to those that produce brachial plexus injury. Rarely, congenital neuroblastoma of the neck can cause Horner's syndrome.

Horner's syndrome involves abnormalities in motor and sweating function over the face. The most obvious features are ptosis due to weakness of the levator palpebrae muscles of the eye, pupillary constriction, and absence of sweating over the affected side of the face (Fig. 40.5). If the lesion occurs as the result of a prenatal lesion or birth insult, then enophthalmos and heterochromia may result due to lack of sympathetic innervation of the pupil, which affects pigmentation.

### Investigations

EMG and nerve-conduction studies may be useful in determining the timing of the brachial plexus injury (see below)

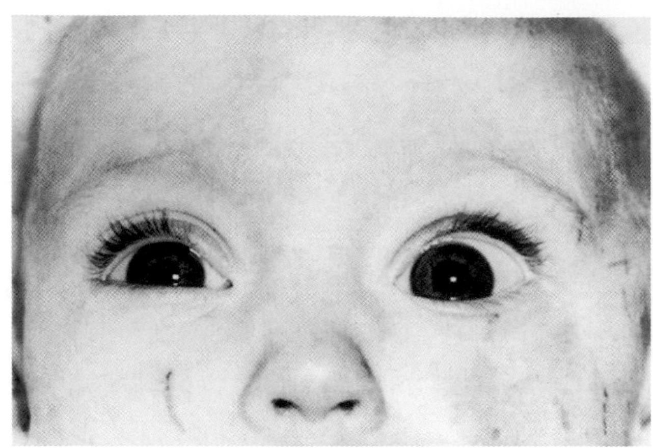

**Figure 40.5** Horner's syndrome. Note the ptosis and pupillary constriction on the affected right side.

and for determining the need for and timing of surgery but are unlikely to be of clinical value in the first few weeks of the injury.

Imaging with MR or intrathecally enhanced CT myelography has been described (Medlock & Hanigan 1997), but there are very few indications for this in the majority of cases. MRI has been shown to be useful in delineation of nerve-root avulsion with development of pseudomeningocele (Popovich *et al.* 1989).

### Prognosis

The prognosis of brachial plexus injury is generally good, and the following general points can be made with regard to the eventual outcome of brachial plexus lesion:

1. If complete recovery has not occurred by 3–4 months, eventual full recovery is very unlikely.
2. Complete recovery is much more likely in lesions involving $C_5$ and $C_6$.
3. Full recovery in lesions involving the lower roots is unlikely.

Two recent studies from Sweden have carefully evaluated the neurologic and functional outcome in groups of children with perinatal brachial plexus injury. Bager (1997) reported 41 children born in 1980–1989. Forty-nine per cent had no long-term impairment, and 22% were judged to have severe impairment. Sundholm *et al.* (1998) reviewed the progress of 105 children examined at 5 years of age. In this study, 34% were considered to show no residual symptoms, and 23% had severe impairment involving both arm and hand function.

Sundholm *et al.* (1998) describe the extensive variation in disability despite apparently similar neuroanatomic lesions. Hand function was remarkably good, even in children with residual weakness around the shoulder, although approximately half of these children were shown to have some reduction in hand-grip strength on formal testing with a Vigorimeter (Bager 1997; Sundholm *et al.* 1998). Sensation was preserved in almost all the children. In one study of overall functional ability, children were generally not seriously limited in their day-to-day activities (Sundholm *et al.* 1998), but in another study, Bager (1997) reported that 22% had a severe functional impairment. Shoulder weakness was associated with difficulties in inserting the arm into a sleeve and reaching the handlebars of a bike. Reduced grip strength made activities requiring both hands such as doing up buttons, zips, and putting on gloves difficult.

Surprisingly, almost all reports on children with less than optimal recovery from perinatal brachial plexus injury suggest that additional disability due to cerebral palsy or mental retardation is very uncommon (Gordon *et al.* 1973; Sjoberg *et al.* 1988; Bager 1997).

It has been suggested that phrenic nerve palsy in association with Erb's palsy is a marker of adverse outcome, but a recent report (al-Qattan *et al.* 1998) has shown that diaphragmatic palsy poorly predicts adverse outcome in motor power of the affected limb with a sensitivity of only 2% and a positive predictive value of 13%.

### Management

The initial management is expectant as spontaneous recovery almost always occurs to some extent. Physiotherapy is important to prevent contractures, particularly of the shoulder. Splinting of the affected arm is not recommended.

Recently, the role of microsurgical reconstruction of the brachial plexus has been reassessed. The role of surgery has been well reviewed by Kay (1998) and remains controversial. To date, no randomized controlled trials have been undertaken. In general, there is reasonable consensus that surgery for the majority of lesions should not be undertaken prior to 3–4 months from birth as significant spontaneous recovery is likely to occur during this time. Those infants with signs of a lower root injury (C5–T1 with Horner's syndrome) may benefit from surgery at about 2 months of age. Kay (1998) concludes that 'the present justification for surgery is based on the comparison of surgical outcomes with studies of the natural history and at present there are no incontrovertible indicators for surgery in the absence of direct or indirect evidence of root avulsion'.

## PERIPHERAL NERVE PALSIES

Sporadic injuries to peripheral nerves usually arise as the result of trauma, which is often avoidable. Peripheral nerve injury may occur as the result of prenatal compression of which amniotic bands are most commonly reported. Rarely, fetal embolic phenomenon may cause extensive tissue necrosis (aplasia cutis congenita) with the involvement of peripheral nerves. In general, the earlier in pregnancy the insult occurred, the poorer the prognosis.

## INFANT BOTULISM (see also p. 588)

This condition is due to the toxin produced by the spores of *Clostridium botulinum*. The organism is ingested orally and colonizes the bowel. The toxin is absorbed through the gut mucosa and binds irreversibly with cholinergic synapses, causing peripheral neuromuscular paralysis. Recovery requires regeneration of new motor end plates in the nerve endings.

Infant botulism was first reported in 1976, and since then, over 900 cases have been described in the literature (see Cochrane & Appleton 1995 for a review). The vast majority of these are from the USA, where the spores may be more endemic in the soil. The major etiological factors are breast-feeding (almost universal), and consumption of honey and corn syrup contaminated with botulinum spores. The observation that breast feeding is highly associated with the condition is interesting. This may be because breast milk actually confers some protection on the baby, thereby delaying the speed of onset and progression of the disease so that the child is recognized to be unwell and admitted to hospital. Sudden infant death syndrome due to infant botulinum toxin is well described in non-breast-fed infants.

### Clinical features

The presenting features are usually insidious and remarkably constant (Cochrane & Appleton 1995). These include weakness (90%), poor feeding (88%), and constipation (75%). On physical examination, the baby is found to be hypotonic, often with a bulbar palsy, decreased gag reflex, and dilated, poorly constricting, pupils. The condition may progress to respiratory failure requiring mechanical ventilation. Autonomic dysfunction may be present with urinary retention, labile blood pressure, and flushing.

The diagnosis depends on demonstrating *C. botulinum* in the stool and abnormal electrodiagnostic tests. Many of the children are severely constipated due to a loss of bowel motility, and rectal washout may be required to obtain a stool specimen for bacteriology. A mouse neutralization test confirms the presence of toxin and its type, most commonly B or A. Electrodiagnostic tests include repetitive nerve stimulation and electromyography and may show presynaptic dysfunction. Graf *et al.* (1992) suggest that these tests may remain negative in affected children, but this is not the experience of others in a review of 57 cases from the Children's Hospital of Philadelphia (Schreiner *et al.* 1991).

The differential diagnosis is wide, and the condition is commonly confused in its early stages with sepsis, meningoencephalitis, and dehydration. The two neurologic conditions commonly confused with infant botulism are myasthenia gravis and poliomyelitis.

### Management

The management is entirely supportive. Severe cases will require mechanical ventilation, and this may need to be prolonged. Oral feeding may not be possible for many weeks. Antibiotics do not hasten the resolution of the condition, and there is a theoretical concern that it may increase toxin release. With careful supportive management, the prognosis is excellent.

## RADIAL NERVE PALSY

Radial nerve palsy is rare and is usually associated with prolonged labor or complicated delivery (for a review, see Ross *et al.* 1983). The infants present with isolated flaccid paralysis of wrist and finger extensor muscles, and this may be easily confused with brachial plexus injury. It is often not present in the first few days of life and develops following local trauma. It is associated with localized subcutaneous fat necrosis overlying the course of the radial nerve proximal to the radial epicondyle. Radial nerve palsy has also been caused by constriction of the upper arm with damage to the nerve as it winds around the humerus. This has been reported to be due to intermittent blood pressure monitoring by a tight cuff (Tollner *et al.* 1980) and tight splinting of the arm to maintain an intravenous cannula *in situ* (Goel *et al.* 1989). Swelling of the shoulder due to bacterial sepsis may cause radial nerve palsy with recovery after aspiration of pus (Lejman *et al.* 1995). The prognosis for most causes is good, and spontaneous recovery occurs in the majority of cases.

## MEDIAN NERVE PALSY

Damage to the median nerve has been described as the result of repeated needle sampling of the brachial artery in the antecubital fossa (Pape *et al.* 1978). They reviewed 139 infants with a birth weight of 1500 g and below, and found that 13% showed persistent median nerve damage. Anatomic dissection of the antecubital fossa showed varying degrees of perineural sheath hemorrhage and Wallerian degeneration of the median nerve. The affected infants were found to have mild to moderate impairment of pincer grasp at 18 months. There was also a reduction in flexion of the lateral two or three fingers when the hand was held in the 'position of rest'. Spontaneous recovery occurs in some cases, although a persisting disability at 3 years has been reported (Pape *et al.* 1978).

## SCIATIC NERVE PALSY

The sciatic nerve is most commonly damaged either by intragluteal injection or as a result of an errantly placed umbilical artery catheter. The common peroneal division of the sciatic nerve is most frequently involved. Palsy rarely arises as a result of direct trauma from the needle to the nerve but more commonly as the result of inflammation associated with the injected substance (Gilles & Matson 1970). Others have suggested that sciatic nerve damage occurs through thrombosis of the inferior gluteal artery, which supplies the nerve following injection of a hypertonic solution into the buttock. These lesions are entirely avoidable by giving intramuscular injections into the anterior thigh. Ramos-Fernandez *et al.* (1998) reviewed 21 cases of neonatal sciatic nerve palsy, and in all cases, there was spontaneous recovery with independent ambulation by 14 months of age. They suggest that the outcome is better after umbilical artery cannulation than for drug-injection-induced inflammation.

Misplacement of an aortic catheter into the internal iliac artery may cause ischemic infarction of the structures supplied by this artery, including the sciatic nerve (Cumming & Burchfield 1994). The inferior gluteal artery has also been reported to have been thrombosed following injection of a hypertonic solution (50% glucose) into the umbilical artery. This caused extensive deep and superficial damage to the buttock as well as severe sciatic nerve involvement secondary to the thrombosis (San Agustin *et al.* 1962). Full recovery was not reported in any of the 13 patients with peroneal nerve (a branch of the sciatic nerve) palsy as a result of drug injection into the umbilical vessel (de Sanctis *et al.* 1995).

### Key Points

- Facial palsy recovers spontaneously in 90% of cases and surgical exploration is usually unnecessary.
- Spinal cord injury is rare but must always be considered as a cause of impoverished spontaneous limb movement.
- Trauma to the cervical cord and focal vascular insults are the commonest cause of acute cord lesions.
- Prognosis after brachial plexus injury is generally good. If complete recovery has not occurred by 3–4 months, eventual recovery is very unlikely.
- At present, there are no incontrovertible indications for surgery in the absence of evidence for direct or indirect route avulsion.

## REFERENCES


Abramson D L, Cohen M M & Mulliken J B (1998) Mobius syndrome: classification and grading system. *Plastic Reconstruct Surg* 102:961–967.

Abroms I F, Bresnan M J, Zuckerman J E *et al.* (1973) Cervical cord injuries secondary to hyperextension of the head in breech presentations. *Obstet Gynecol* 41:369–378.

Al-Qattan M M & al-Kharfy T M (1996) Obstetric brachial plexus injury in subsequent deliveries. *Ann Plastic Surg* 1996; 37:545–548.

Al-Qattan M M, Clarke H M & Curtis C G (1998) The prognostic value of concurrent phrenic nerve palsy in newborn children with Erb's palsy. *J Hand Surg (Br Eur Vol)* 23B:225.

Aziz E M & Robertson A F (1973) Paraplegia: A complication of umbilical artery catheterization. *J Pediatr* 82:1051–1052.

Babyn P S, Chuang S H, Daneman A *et al.* (1988) Sonographic evaluation of spinal cord birth trauma with pathologic correlation. *Am J Roentgenol* 151:763–766.

✪ Bager B (1997) Perinatally acquired brachial plexus palsy – a persisting challenge. *Acta Paediatr* 86:1214–1219.

Baraitser M, Stewart F, Winter R M, *et al.* (1997) A syndrome of brachyphalangy, polydactyly and absent tibiae. *Clin Dysmorphol* 6:111–21.

Bell H J & Dykstra D D (1985) Somatosensory evoked potentials as an adjunct to diagnosis of neonatal spinal cord injury. *J Pediatr* 106:298–301.

✪ Bergman I, May M, Wessel H B *et al.* (1986) Management of facial palsy caused by birth trauma. *Laryngoscope* 96:381–384.

Bhagwanani S G, Price H V, Laurence K M *et al.* (1973) Risks and prevention of cervical cord injury in the management of breech presentation with hyperextension of the fetal head. *Am J Obstet Gynecol* 115:1159–1162.

Brett E M (ed.) (1991) *Paediatric neurology.* Edinburgh: Churchill Livingston; 2nd edn.

Burcher H U, Bolthauser E, Friderich J *et al.* (1979) Birth injury to the spinal cord. *Helv Paediatr Acta* 34:517–527.

Carr M M, Ross D A & Zuker R M (1997) Cranial nerve defects in congenital facial palsy. *J Otolaryngol* 26:80–87.

✪ Clancy R R, Sladky J T & Rorke L B (1989) Hypoxic-ischemic spinal cord injury following perinatal asphyxia. *Ann Neurol* 25:185–189.

Cochrane D P & Appleton R E (1995) Infant botulism – is it that rare? *Dev Med Child Neurol* 37:274–278.

Cumming W A & Burchfield D J (1994) Accidental catheterization of internal iliac artery branches: a serious complication of umbilical artery catheterization. *J Perinatol* 14:304–9.

Darwish H, Sarnat H, Archer C *et al.* (1981) Congenital cervical spinal atrophy. *Muscle and Nerve* 4:106–110.

DeGirolami U & Zivin J A (1982) Neuropathology of experimental spinal cord ischemia in the rabbit. *J Neuropathol Exp Neurol* 41:129–149.

De Sanctis N, Cardillo G & Nunziata Rega A (1995) Gluteoperineal gangrene and sciatic nerve palsy after umbilical vessel injection. *Clin Orthopaed Relat Res* 316:180–184.

De Vries E, Robben S G & van den Anker J N (1995) Radiologic imaging of severe cervical spinal cord birth trauma. *Eur J Pediatr* 154:230–232.

Dulac O & Aicardi J (1975) Paraplegia complicating umbilical artery catheterization. *Archives Francaises de Pediatrie* 32:659–64.

Dunn D W & Engle W A (1985) Brachial plexus palsy: intrauterine onset. *Pediatr Neurol* 1:367–369.

Egelhoff J C (1999) MR imaging of congenital anomalies of the pediatric spine. *MRI Clin N Am* 7:459–479.

Fan L L, Campbell D N, Clarke D R *et al.* (1989) Paralyzed left vocal cord associated with ligation of patent ductus arteriosus. *J Thorac Cardiovasc Surg* 98:611–613.

Farrell K & McGillivray B C (1983) Arthrogryposis following maternal hypotension. *Dev Med Child Neurol* 25:648–650.

✪ Geutjens G, Gilbert A & Helsen K (1996) Obstetric brachial plexus palsy associated with breech delivery. A different pattern of injury. *J Bone Joint Surg (Br Vol)* 78:303–306.

Gherman R B, Ouzounian J G, Miller D A *et al.* (1998) Spontaneous vaginal delivery: a risk factor for Erb's palsy? *Am J Obstet Gynaecol* 178:423–427.

Gilbert A, Brockman R & Carlioz H (1991) Surgical treatment of brachial plexus birth palsy. *Clin Orthopaed Relat Res* 264:39–47.

Gilles F H & Matson D D (1970) Sciatic nerve injury following misplaced gluteal injection. *J Pediatr* 76:247–254.

Goel S P, Agarwal R P, Garg B K *et al.* (1989) Nerve injuries in neonates. *J Ind Med Assoc* 87:132–134.

Gordon M, Rich H, Deutschberger J *et al.* (1973) The immediate and long-term outcome of obstetric birth trauma. I. Brachial plexus paralysis. *Am J Obstet Gynecol* 117:51–56.

Govaert P, Vanhaesebrouck P, De Praeter C *et al.* (1989) Moebius sequence and prenatal brainstem ischemia. *Pediatrics* 84:570–573.

Graf W D, Hays R M, Astley S J *et al.* (1992) Electrodiagnosis reliability in the diagnosis of infant botulism. *J Pediatr* 120:747–749.

Graf W D & Shepard T H (1997) Uterine contraction in the development of Mobius syndrome. *J Child Neurol* 12:225–227.

Graham E M, Forouzan I & Morgan M A (1997) A retrospective analysis of Erb's palsy cases and their relation to birth. *J Maternal–Fetal Med* 6:1–5.

Greenberg S J, Kandt R S & D'Souza B J (1987) Birth injury-induced glossolaryngeal paresis. *Neurology* 37:533–535.

Gropman A L, Barkovich A J, Vezina L G *et al.* (1997) Pediatric congenital bilateral perisylvian syndrome: clinical and MRI features in 12 patients. *Neuropediatrics* 28:198–203.

Haenggeli C A & Lacourt G (1989) Brachial plexus injury and hypoglossal paralysis. *Pediatr Neurol* 5:197–198.

Harris J P, Davidson T M, May M *et al.* (1983) Evaluation and treatment of congenital facial paralysis. *Arch Otolaryngol* 109:145–151.

Hepner W R (1951) Some observations on facial paresis in the newborn infant. Etiology and incidence. *Pediatrics* 8:494–497.

Hornung T S, Nicholson I A, Nunn G A *et al.* (1999) Neonatal ductus arteriosus aneurysm causing nerve palsies and airway compression: surgical treatment by decompression without excision. *Pediatr Cardiol* 20:158–160.

Jacobs T P, Shohami E & Baze W (1987) Deteriorating stroke model: histopathology, edema, and eicosanoid changes following spinal cord ischemia in rabbits. *Stroke* 18:741–750.

Jennett R J, Tarby T J & Kreinick C J (1992) Brachial plexus palsy: an old problem revisited. *Am J Obstet Gynecol* 166:1673–1677.

Jequier S, Cramer B & O'Gorman A M (1984) Ultrasound of the spinal cord in neonates and infants. *Annales de Radiologie* 28:225–231.

✪ Kay S P J (1998) Obstetrical brachial palsy. *Br J Plastic Surg* 51:43–50.

Kobayashi T (1979) Congenital unilateral lower lip palsy. *Acta Otolaryngol* 88:303–309.

Koch B M & Eng G M (1979) Neonatal spinal cord injury. *Arch Phys Med Rehab* 60:378–381.

✪ Koenigsberger M R (1980) Brachial plexus palsy at birth: intrauterine or due to delivery trauma? *Ann Neurol* 8:228.

Krishnamoorthy K S, Fernandez R J, Todres I D *et al.* (1976) Paraplegia associated with umbilical artery catheterization in the newborn. *Pediatrics* 58:443–445.

Laing J H E, Harrison D H, Jones B M *et al.* (1996) Is permanent congenital facial palsy caused by birth trauma? *Arch Dis Childhood* 74:56–58.

Lanska M J, Roessmann U & Wiznitzer M (1990) Magnetic resonance imaging in cervical cord birth injury. *Pediatrics* 85:760–764.

Lejman T, Strong M & Michno P (1995) Radial-nerve palsy associated with septic shoulder in neonates. *J Pediatr Orthop* 15:169–171.

Lucas J W, Holden K R, Purohit D M *et al.* (1995) Neonatal hemangiomatosis associated with brachial polexus palsy. *J Child Neurol* 10:411–413.

✪ MacKinnon J A, Perlman M, Kirpalani H *et al.* (1993) Spinal cord injury at birth: Diagnostic and prognostic data in twenty-two patients. *J Pediatr* 122:431–437.

McHugh H, Sowaen K A & Levitt M N (1969) Facial paralysis and muscle agenesis in the newborn. *Arch Otolaryngol* 89:157–168.

Maekawa K, Masaki T & Kokubun Y (1976) Fetal spinal cord injury secondary to hyperextension of the neck: no effect of caesarean section. *Dev Med Child Neurol* 18:229–238.

Medlock M D & Hanigan W C (1997) Neurologic birth trauma. *Clin Perinatol* 24:845–857.

Narcy P, Tran-Ba-Huy E, Margoloff B *et al.* (1982) Indications therapeutiques dans les paralysies faciales du nouveau-ne. A propos de 9 observations. *Annales d'Otolaryngologie* 99:377–382.

Nishikawa M, Ichiyama T, Hayashi T, Furukawa S (1997) Mobius-like syndrome associated with a 1;2 chromosome translocation. *Clin Genet* 51:122–3.

Ouzounian J G, Korst L M & Phelan J P (1997) Permanet Erb palsy: A traction-related injury? *Obstet Gynaecol* 89:139–141.

Paine R S (1997) Facial paralysis in children. *J Pediatr* 19:303–315.

Pape K E, Armstrong D L & Fitzhardinge P M (1978) Peripheral median nerve damage secondary to brachial arterial blood gas sampling. *J Pediatr* 93:852–856.

Pape K E & Pickering D (1972) Asymmetric crying facies: an index of other congenital anomalies. *J Pediatr* 81:21–24.

Pape K E & Wigglesworth J S (1979) Haemorrhage, ischaemia and the neonatal brain. *Clin Dev Med* 69/70:85–99.

Pastuszak A L, Schuler L, Speck-Martins C E *et al.* (1998) Use of misoprostol during pregnancy and Mobius' syndrome in infants. *N Engl J Med* 338:1881–1885.

Perlman M & Reisner S H (1973) Asymmetric crying facies and congenital anomalies. *Arch Dis Childhood* 48:627–630.

Pitner S E, Edwards J E & McCormick W F (1965) Observations on the pathology of the Mobius syndrome. *J Neurol Neurosurg Psychiatry* 28:362–374.

Popovich M J, Taylor F C & Helmer E (1989) MR imaging of birth-related brachial plexus avulsion. *Am J Neurol Res* 10:S98.

Ramos-Fernandez J M, Oliete-Garcia F M, Roldan-Aparicio S *et al.* (1998) Neonatal sciatic palsy: etiology and outcome of 21 cases. *Revista de Neurologia* 26:752–755.

Ross D, Royden Jones H, Fisher J *et al.* (1983) Isolated radial nerve lesion in the newborn. *Neurology* 33:1354–1356.

Rossi L N, Vassella F & Mumenthaler M (1982) Obstetrical lesions of the brachial plexus. Natural history in 34 cases. *Eur Neurol* 21:1–7.

Sadleir L G & Connolly M B (1998) Acquired brachial-plexus neuropathy in the neonate: a rare presentation of late onset group-B streptococcal osteomyelitis. *Dev Med Child Neurol* 40:496–499.

San Agustin M, Nitowsky H M & Borden J N (1962) Neonatal sciatic palsy after umbilical vessel injection. *J Pediatr* 60:408–413.

Say B & Coldwell J G (1975) Heriditary defect of the sacrum. *Humangenetik* 27:231–234.

Schneider H, Ballowitz L & Schachinger H (1975) Anoxic encephalopathy with predominant involvement of basal ganglia, brainstem and spinal cord in the perinatal period. *Acta Neuropathol* 32:287–238.

Schreiner M S, Field F & Ruddy R (1991) Infant botulism: A review of 12 years experience at the Children's Hospital of Philadelphia. *Pediatrics* 87:159–165.

Schulman S T, Madden J D, Esterly J R *et al.* (1971) Transection of spinal cord. A rare obstetrical complication of cephalic delivery. *Arch Dis Childhood* 46:291–294.

Simon L, Perreaux F, Devictor D *et al.* (1999) Clinical and radiological diagnosis of spinal cord birth injury. *Arch Dis Childhood Neonatal Ed* 81: F235–F236.

Singer R, Joseph K, Gilai A N *et al.* (1991) Nontraumatic, acute neonatal paraplegia. *J Pediatr Orthoped* 11:588–593.

✪ Sjoberg I, Erichs K & Bjerre I (1988) Cause and effect of obstetric (neonatal) brachial plexus palsy. *Acta Paediatr Scand* 77:357–364.

✪ Sladky J T & Rorke L B (1986) Perinatal hypoxic/ischemic spinal cord injury. *Pediatr Pathol* 6:87–101.

Smith D W (1982) *Recognizable patterns of human malformation.* Philadelphia, PA: W B Saunders; 3rd edn, 168–169.

Smith J D, Crumley R C & Harker L A (1981) Facial paralysis in the newborn. *Otolaryngol Head Neck Surg* 89:1021–1024.

Sugarman G I & Stark H H (1973) Mobius syndrome with Poland's anomaly. *J Med Genet* 10:192–196.

✪ Sundholm L K, Eliasson A C & Forssberg H (1998) Obstetric brachial plexus injuries: assessment protocol and functional outcome at age 5 years. *Dev Med Child Neurol* 40:4–11.

Thakkar N, O'Neil W & Duvally J (1977) Moebius syndrome due to brainstem tegmental necrosis. *Arch Neurol* 34:124–126.

Tollner U, Bechinger D & Pohlandt F (1980) Radial nerve palsy in a premature infant following long-term measurement of blood pressure. *J Pediatr* 96:921–922.

Tortori-Donati P, Fondelli M P, Rossi A *et al.* (1999) Segmental spinal dysgenesis: neuroradiologic findings with clinical and embryologic correlation. *Am J Neuroradiol* 20:445–456.

Towbin A (1969) Latent spinal cord and brain stem injury in newborn infants. *Dev Med Child Neurol* 11:54–60.

Verzijl H T, van den Helm B, Veldman B *et al.* (1999) A second gene for autosomal dominant Mobius syndrome is localized to chromosome 10q, in a Dutch family. *Am J Hum Genet* 65:752–756.

Young R K, Towgighi J & Marks K H (1983) Focal necrosis of the spinal cord *in utero. Arch Neurol* 40:654–655.

# Chapter 41 Neuromuscular disorders

E. Mercuri, J. Heckmatt and V. Dubowitz

## INTRODUCTION

Although the neuromuscular disorders in infancy and childhood have had extensive coverage (Dubowitz 1980, 1985, 1995), this chapter concentrates on those specific to the neonatal period, and provides a problem-oriented approach as well as dealing with each disorder individually.

## CLINICAL PROBLEMS

### CLINICAL PRESENTATION

Table 41.1 details the main features of the various neuromuscular disorders that present in infancy with hypotonia plus other problems and contrasts them with the non-neuromuscular disorders that might present in a similar fashion. In the table, an attempt has been made to indicate the relative importance of various signs and laboratory abnormalities. A neuromuscular disorder should be suspected when the infant has a problem, such as hypotonia, feeding difficulty or persistent ventilatory failure but an insufficient central nervous system (CNS) or lung involvement to apparently account for it. Important clues are: (1) delayed quickening and poor fetal movements throughout the pregnancy or normal movements initially but reduction later; (2) polyhydramnios suggesting involvement of the muscles of swallowing; (3) a family history of neonatal death and stillbirth; (4) a history of possible or definite neuromuscular disease in the mother and other members of the family; and (5) thin ribs on the chest radiograph, suggesting poor respiratory muscle movement *in utero*.

On examination of the baby, there may be important associated abnormalities, such as overt facial weakness, ophthalmoplegia, limited limb movement, and lack of antigravity power on stimulation of the limbs. These physical signs may be difficult to assess on one single occasion if the baby is severely ill (e.g. on a ventilator), and repeated examination is often useful. It is not always easy to differentiate a CNS from a neuromuscular disorder, especially as the baby may have overt CNS involvement (e.g. seizures, hydrocephalus, intraventricular hemorrhage/periventricular leukomalacia) in association with a neuromuscular disorder, and this may not always relate to severe birth asphyxia. Furthermore, a baby with neuromuscular disease may have reasonable power in the limbs and still have severe respiratory muscle weakness.

#### The timing of the clinical onset

Some disorders may already have an antenatal onset, others present in the immediate newborn period, and others are delayed for hours or days after birth. For example, myotonic dystrophy is associated with an antenatal onset (Table 41.1), while neonatal myasthenia usually presents a few hours after birth, and the mitochondrial myopathies present a few days or weeks after birth. Spinal muscular atrophy (Werdnig–Hoffman disease) may be present at birth or present after a period of normality before the onset of weakness.

#### The family

Most neuromuscular disorders are genetic, and establishing a pattern of inheritance is important in the differential diagnosis. There may be subclinical manifestations in dominant and X-linked disorders. For example, myotonic dystrophy is inherited as an autosomal dominant trait. In many cases, the mother, who is always affected, and other affected family members may be mildly affected and unaware that they have the disease. It is therefore important to inquire about any family history that would indicate myotonic dystrophy, in particular presenile cataract, muscle stiffness, progressive weakness, frontal baldness, and early death from cardiorespiratory disease. In addition, family members should be examined personally for abnormal physical signs, such as facial weakness (which may consist only of an inability to bury the eyelashes), wasting of the facial muscles (especially the temporalis and the sternomastoids), percussion myotonia of the tongue and hands, and relaxation myotonia of the hands. It is important to alert all affected persons to the risk of anesthesia.

The other neuromuscular disorder that should be excluded in the mother is myasthenia gravis, which may lead to transient neonatal myasthenia due to passive transfer of antibody across the placenta. Severe centronuclear myopathy, which is characterized by a similar clinical presentation to myotonic dystrophy in the newborn, is X-linked recessive, and there may be a family history of stillbirth and neonatal death stretching back several generations.

### CLINICAL EXAMINATION

Overt facial weakness is characteristic of myotonic dystrophy and centronuclear myopathy, but also often occurs in other congenital myopathies such as nemaline myopathy and congenital muscular dystrophy. External ophthalmoplegia is a feature of centronuclear myopathy.

**Table 41.1 Differential diagnosis of neuromuscular disease in the neonatal period presenting as hypotonia and other problems**

| | Diminished fetal movements | Polyhydramnios | Birth asphyxia | Persistent ventilatory failure | Distribution of respiratory muscle weakness | Facial weakness | Ptosis | Ophthalmoplegia | Proximal muscle paralysis | Fixed bilateral talipes | Arthrogryposis | Feeding difficulties | Tendon jerks | Distended bladder | Seizures | Hepatomegaly | Persistent metabolic acidosis | Hyperammonemia | Abnormal smell | Genetics |
|---|---|---|---|---|---|---|---|---|---|---|---|---|---|---|---|---|---|---|---|---|
| Muscular dystrophy | | | | | | | | | | | | | | | | | | | | |
| Myotonic | ++ | ++ | ++ | + | G/D | ++ | ++ | (+) | + | + | (–) | ++ | (–) | – | (–) | – | – | – | – | AD(m) |
| Congenital | + | (+) | (+) | (+) | G/D | + | (+) | – | + | ++ | ++ | + | (–) | – | (+) | – | – | – | – | (AR) |
| Myasthenia gravis | | | | | | | | | | | | | | | | | | | | |
| Neonatal | – | – | (+) | * | G/D | + | (+) | (+) | + | – | – | + | (–) | – | – | – | – | – | – | –(m) |
| Congenital | (+) | (–) | – | (*) | (–) | + | + | + | (+) | – | – | (+) | (–) | – | – | – | – | – | – | (AR) |
| Familial | (+) | (+) | (+) | * | G/D | (+) | (+) | – | + | – | – | + | (–) | – | – | – | – | – | – | (AR) |
| Congenital myopathy | | | | | | | | | | | | | | | | | | | | |
| Nemaline | + | + | + | (+) | G/D | + | (+) | (–) | + | (+) | (–) | + | (–) | – | – | – | – | – | – | (AR) |
| Centronuclear | ++ | ++ | ++ | ++ | G/D | ++ | ++ | + | ++ | + | (–) | ++ | (–) | – | (–) | – | – | – | – | (XLR) |
| Mitochondrial | (–) | – | – | * | G | + | + | (+) | + | – | (+) | + | (+) | – | (+) | + | ++ | – | – | AR/XLR |
| Neurogenic weakness | | | | | | | | | | | | | | | | | | | | |
| Spinal muscular atrophy | + | (–) | (–) | (–) | I/G | (–) | – | – | ++ | (–) | – | (+) | – | – | – | – | – | – | – | AR |
| Spinal cord transection | – | – | ++ | (+1) | I/G(1) | – | – | – | +(1) | – | – | + | – | ++ | (–) | – | – | – | – | – |
| Non-neuromuscular | | | | | | | | | | | | | | | | | | | | |
| Prader–Willi syndrome | (+) | (+) | – | – | – | (+) | – | – | – | – | – | ++ | + | – | – | – | – | – | – | –(15) |
| Organic acidurias | – | – | – | * | (G) | (+) | (+) | – | (+) | – | – | ++ | (–) | – | + | + | ++ | + | + | AR |
| Urea cycle defects | – | – | – | * | (G) | – | – | – | (+) | – | – | + | (–) | – | + | – | (–) | ++ | – | AR |
| Peroxisomal disorders | – | – | (–) | (–) | – | – | – | – | (+) | – | – | + | (–) | – | ++ | (+) | – | – | – | AR |
| Neonatal sepsis | – | – | (+) | * | – | – | – | – | – | – | – | + | + | – | (+) | (–) | (+) | (+) | – | – |
| IVH/PVH/PVL | – | – | (+) | * | – | – | – | – | – | – | – | + | + | – | (+) | – | – | – | – | – |

*Key*: Ventilatory failure: * = may present with sudden collapse.
Distribution of respiratory muscle weakness: G = global; D = diaphragmatic; I = intercostal.
Genetics: AR = autosomal recessive; XLR = X-linked recessive; AD = autosomal dominant; (15) = deletion or translocat chromosome 15; (m) = mother affected.
Clinical and laboratory features: ++ = frequently present and striking; + = often present; (+) = sometimes pr (–) = usually absent; – = always absent.
IVH = intraventricular hemorrhage; PVH = periventricular hemorrhage; PVL = periventricular leukomalacia; (1) = depend on the level of the spinal cord lesion.

In the severe type of spinal muscular atrophy, the facies are usually normal, and the infant is likely to be quite bright and able to follow with the eyes, despite being very weak generally. Tongue fasciculation at rest is a characteristic feature of spinal muscular atrophy. While spinal muscular atrophy is highly likely to be associated with severe paralysis, other neuromuscular disorders such as myotonic dystrophy and congenital muscular dystrophy are more variable.

The distribution of the respiratory muscle weakness is important. The weakness may be diaphragmatic, with abdominal paradox, in congenital muscular dystrophy or in some of the congenital myopathies such as myotubular, nemaline, and minicore, and in congenital myasthenia. In contrast, in spinal muscular atrophy, the weakness is mainly intercostal, the breathing pattern is abdominal, and the rib cage moves paradoxically with the abdomen.

Fixed bilateral talipes is associated with congenital myotonic dystrophy and myotubular myopathy. Arthrogryposis (i.e. contractures of several joints) is associated with congenital dystrophy and certain neurogenic disorders. Fixed-joint contractures are not usually a feature of severe spinal muscular atrophy, but may occur in a recently recognised more severe form with prenatal onset.

## INVESTIGATIONS

The serum creatine kinase (CK) activity is normally increased in cord blood up to 1000 units (normal levels for adults <200 IU/l). This increased activity reflects muscle damage during labor and usually comes down in the first 10 days of life. Measurement of serum CK activity is likely to be of most value in preclinical Duchenne's muscular dystrophy, where it will be markedly elevated (several thousand units); in congenital muscular dystrophy, the elevation is moderate and variable and only occurs in about half the patients. A motor nerve conduction study will reveal an absent motor action potential in spinal muscular atrophy due to the extensive denervation. If myasthenia gravis is suspected, then repetitive stimulation of the peripheral nerve may show a decrement in the motor action potential. A slow nerve conduction velocity may point to a hereditary motor neuropathy, which may present rarely in early infancy.

An electromyogram (EMG) can be useful in diagnosis and differential diagnosis of neuromuscular disorders in infancy. However, in the neonatal period, interpretation can be difficult as the severely weak baby often makes little spontaneous movement. If there is any suggestion that the infant may have myotonic dystrophy, then one should obtain EMGs from both parents (and particularly the mother), looking for myotonic discharges. The favored site for this is the first dorsal interosseus muscle of the hand.

Ultrasound imaging of muscle can help to demonstrate striking selective involvement, such as sparing of the rectus femoris and marked involvement of the vasti within the quadriceps muscle. This is of considerable practical importance when taking a biopsy. Muscle biopsy is done using a 4-mm Bergstrom needle. The success rate is as high as in older children, despite the small size of the patient. This is because there has been no time for muscle atrophy, nor extensive replacement of muscle by fat and connective tissue to occur, and also because the size of the individual muscle fibers is small, and only a relatively small sample is needed. Needle muscle biopsy is carried out under a local anesthetic in the cot or incubator, and the critically sick newborn can readily be examined with minimal disturbance. A detailed description of the technique is given in Heckmatt *et al.* (1984).

It is important to be aware of the value and limitations of muscle biopsy in the newborn period. Muscle biopsy will show an unequivocal abnormality in the congenital myopathies, which have specific structural changes, but may appear normal in spinal muscular atrophy (prepathologic stage) or show a universal atrophy (i.e. very small fibers at about 10 μm) without the characteristic large fibers. Muscle biopsy is usually normal in infants with myotonic dystrophy but may show identical appearances to centronuclear myopathy (Dubowitz 1995).

Brain imaging (cranial ultrasound and/or brain magnetic resonance imaging) can help to identify intracranial abnormalities, such as structural brain lesions, hemorrhage, and/or ischemic lesions or ventricular dilatation, which is a common associated feature in myotonic dystrophy and centronuclear myopathy.

## MANAGEMENT

The major problem of management presented by these disorders is that of ventilatory failure and deciding a prognosis and how long to continue giving ventilatory support. It will be necessary to take into account any CNS complication, such as progressive ventricular dilatation. In myotonic dystrophy, there is a trend for improvement in muscle power and a reasonable chance of the infant becoming independent of the ventilator (see later). The respiratory failure may be compounded by premature delivery, which is more common in these cases. If an infant with spinal muscular atrophy is put on a ventilator, it may be extremely difficult to wean him or her off, but most infants with this disorder have sufficient diaphragm function to cope without ventilatory support. The other disorders are more variable, but in myotubular myopathy and congenital muscular dystrophy, there is a trend for improvement, although it is slow, and a tracheostomy may be necessary for long-term respiratory management.

## THE MUSCULAR DYSTROPHIES

### CONGENITAL MYOTONIC DYSTROPHY

The first description of congenital myotonic dystrophy was by Vanier (1960) of six children between the ages of 9 months and 13 years, all of whom had presented as floppy infants; four had feeding difficulty, and three had bilateral talipes. Vanier pointed out the severe facial muscle weakness and wasting (particularly of the sternomastoids leading to a long 'swan-like' neck), nasal speech and mental retardation. The mothers in all the cases were affected but only had minimal signs of the disease. In two families, the maternal uncles were severely affected, and in one family, both the mother and maternal grandmother had presenile cataracts.

Another important early report was that by Dodge *et al.* (1965) of five definite cases. The bilateral facial weakness had led to severe feeding difficulties in infancy, and this was accompanied by marked generalized weakness and hypotonia. One girl had an affected 4-year-old brother, who had been admitted at the age of 2 months for eventration of the diaphragm associated with partial collapse of the right lung; he had been cyanosed as an infant but had sucked better than his sister and had good limb strength and reflex activity.

Harper (1975a,b) reported an extensive survey of all available cases in Britain. He emphasized the polyhydramnios and reduced fetal movements and suggested a high incidence of missed cases as there was an elevated neonatal mortality (16%) in liveborn siblings. Of the 70 cases in his study, the mean intelligence quotient was only 66. However, there was no correlation with respiratory problems, suggesting a prenatal cause for the mental deficiency. In all cases, the mother was affected, and Harper postulated that an intrauterine factor must be operating, in addition to the gene that has to be present to have the disease.

Outside the neonatal period, most cases with the congenital type survive but few become independent. Of 46 congenital cases followed up retrospectively, only four had died, but of the 42 survivors, only two were in normal education, and only one was gainfully employed. Testicular atrophy was evident in all affected males at puberty (O'Brien & Harper 1984).

Table 41.2 summarizes our experience of ten patients who presented in the neonatal period. In general, these were more severely affected than previously reported cases, which perhaps reflects selective referral to our neonatal intensive care unit. The extent of the weakness was variable, but most had some antigravity power in the limbs. There was no direct relationship between limb power and degree of respiratory muscle involvement, and the baby with the best limb power was the longest on the ventilator (112 days) because of elevation of the diaphragm, which required plication. The eight infants who had cranial ultrasound showed ventricular dilatation. In three of these, this was present on the first day of life, without any evidence for intraventricular hemorrhage, suggesting an antenatal cause (Regev *et al.* 1987). Three of the infants had gastrointestinal stasis, with bile-stained aspirate, requiring a period of intravenous feeding (duration 2–7 weeks). A typical case is illustrated in Fig. 41.1.

Percussion myotonia of the tongue, facial weakness, and myotonic discharge on the EMG were demonstrated in all ten mothers. Clinical myotonia of the hands was more variable. Three mothers had been previously diagnosed, two on the basis of an affected baby, one born to the same mother and one to an aunt. In only one case had the mother previously presented with symptoms of myotonia, and this had led to the diagnosis in other members of her family. In all cases, there was a strongly suggestive family history, apart from evidence of disease in the mother. In these ten families, we were personally able to confirm the diagnosis beyond doubt in seven previously undiagnosed adults, apart from the mothers, and were suspicious about a further five, either on the basis of presenile cataract (three cases), or frontal baldness with probable facial muscle wasting (two cases) but without any other physical signs or abnormalities on the EMG.

### Molecular genetics

The abnormality of the gene in myotonic dystrophy on chromosome 19 has been shown to be an expansion of the DNA with an increase in the number of CTG trinucleotide repeats. In normal people, there may be up to 30 or so of these

**Table 41.2 Congenital myotonic dystrophy: presenting features**

| Patient | Gestation (weeks) | Birth weight (kg) | Fetal movements | Hydramnios | Apgar score (1/5/10 min) | IPPV[a] (days) | Talipes |
|---|---|---|---|---|---|---|---|
| 1 | 32 | 1.8 | ? | – | | – | – |
| 2 | 34 | 1.7 | Reduced | + | 4/5 | 31 | + |
| 3 | 34 | 1.8 | ? | + | | 16 | + |
| 4 | 34 | 2.2 | ? | + | 1/5/10 | 1 | + |
| 5 | 35 | 1.3 | Reduced | – | 2/4 | 112 | – |
| 6 | 35 | 2.3 | Reduced | + | 4/5/5 | 12 | – |
| 7 | 36 | 1.9 | Reduced | + | 6/7/8 | >49 | + |
| 8 | 38 | 2.7 | Reduced | – | 0/3/4 | 1 | – |
| 9 | 40 | 2.7 | ? | – | 1/7/5 | – | – |
| 10 | 40 | 4.0 | Reduced | + | 1/7/4 | – | + |

[a]IPPV = intermittent positive-pressure ventilation.

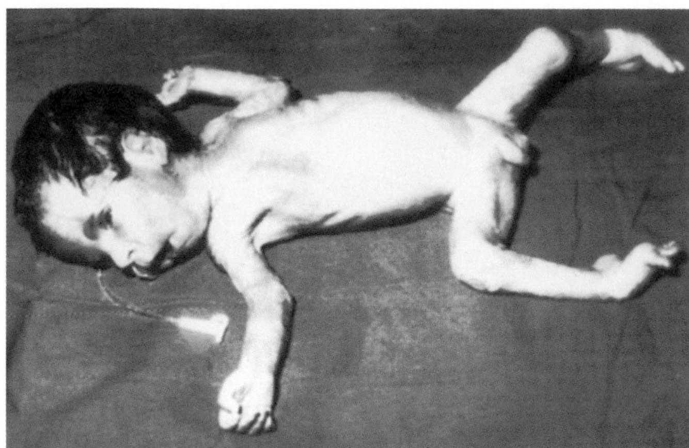

A

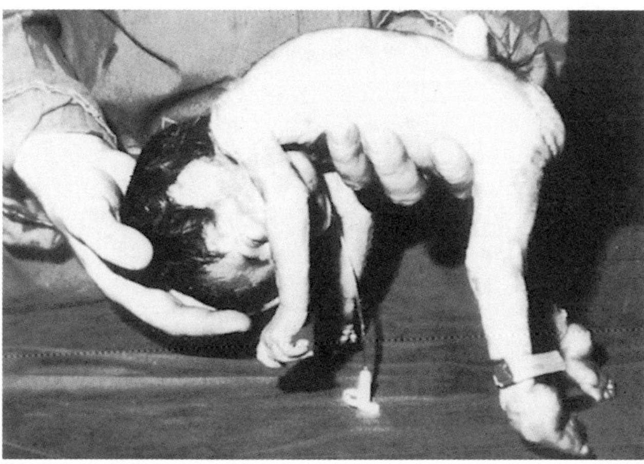

B

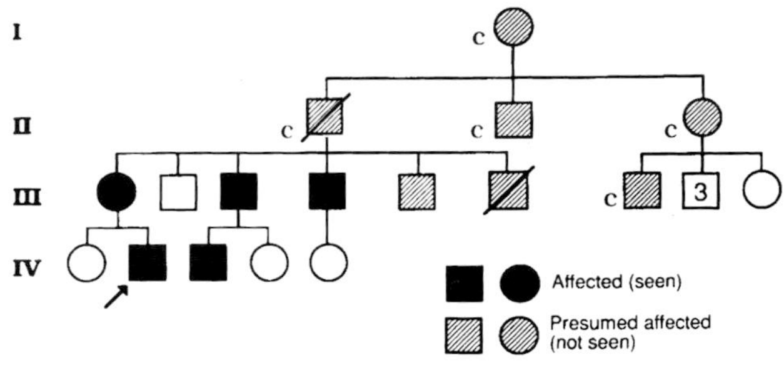


C

**Figure 41.1 (A,B)** Infant with congenital myotonic dystrophy admitted at the age of 20 days, having been ventilator-dependent from birth till 15 days without overt lung problem. He was born at 34 weeks of gestation (birth weight 1.8 kg), by elective Cesarian section for breech presentation. On examination, he was generally hypotonic with fixed bilateral talipes equinovarus. He had a large head with wide open fontanelles and parted sutures, and ultrasound scan showed bilateral ventricular dilatation. The mother had definite signs of the disease although she had not been previously diagnosed. **(C)** On investigation of the family, two maternal uncles (III 3 and 4) and one cousin (IV 3) were affected with facial weakness, myotonia and a positive EMG. Two uncles (III 5 and 6) were not available, but one was said to have frontal baldness and the other to have some stiffness of the hands. One of these uncles subsequently died following dental anesthesia, possibly due to undue sensitivity to muscle relaxants and an unsuspecting anesthetist. There was a history of presenile cataract in several relatives on the maternal grandfather's side of the family.

repeats, but in affected patients, it usually seems to be beyond about 50, and some may have several thousand repeats. The cases of congenital myotonic dystrophy have in general had a much greater expansion of the gene than other members of the family with later onset (Buxton *et al.* 1992). This new advance provides an additional method for confirming the diagnosis in an individual case and in identifying subclinical cases within a family. It also provides the opportunity for prenatal diagnosis on chorionic villus biopsy early in pregnancy (Aslanidis *et al.* 1992).

## CONGENITAL MUSCULAR DYSTROPHY

This is an important group of neuromuscular disorders characterized by weakness, usually from birth, and a muscle biopsy showing striking pathologic changes similar to muscular dystrophy (Dubowitz 1995). An International Consortium in 1993 separated three well-defined syndromes (Fukuyama congenital muscular dystrophy, Walker–Warburg syndrome, muscle–eye brain disease), all associated with structural brain changes, from a 'pure' or classical form of congenital muscular dystrophy, not associated with structural brain changes (Dubowitz 1994; Dubowitz & Fardeau 1995). Since then, numerous other phenotypes have been identified. Tome *et al.* (1994) reported that a proportion of children with pure congenital muscular dystrophy showed a deficiency of the laminin α2 chain (merosin), an extracellular membrane protein normally present in skeletal muscle.

### Clinical presentation

Generalized weakness and hypotonia are usually present at birth. Facial weakness is frequently present but not as severe or striking as that in congenital myotonic dystrophy (Fig. 41.2). Many affected infants will have contractures at birth, sometimes extensive arthrogryposis (see later), and will show a tendency to develop contractures during infancy. It is particularly important to recognize these patients and start a program of active treatment of the contractures in infancy to try and improve the range of joint mobility. A few patients have respiratory involvement at birth. A feature of this condition is that the disease process may pick out certain muscles, including those of respiration, leaving others relatively spared (Fig. 41.3). A further group presents later in the first or second years of life with motor delay, having not apparently had any recognized problem in infancy.

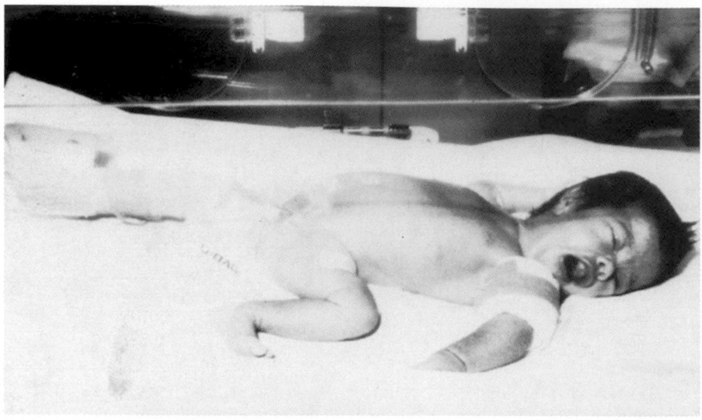

A

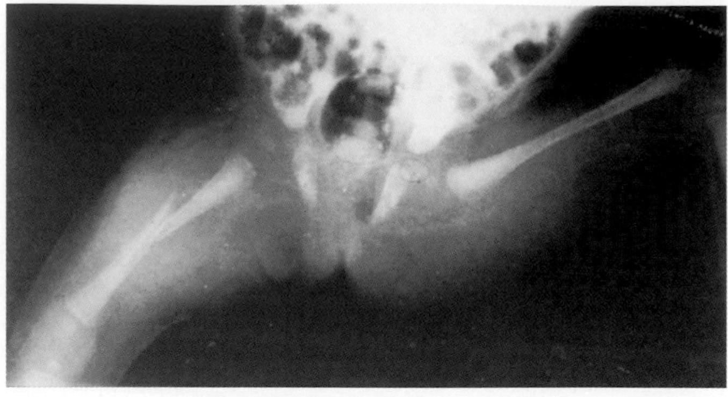

B

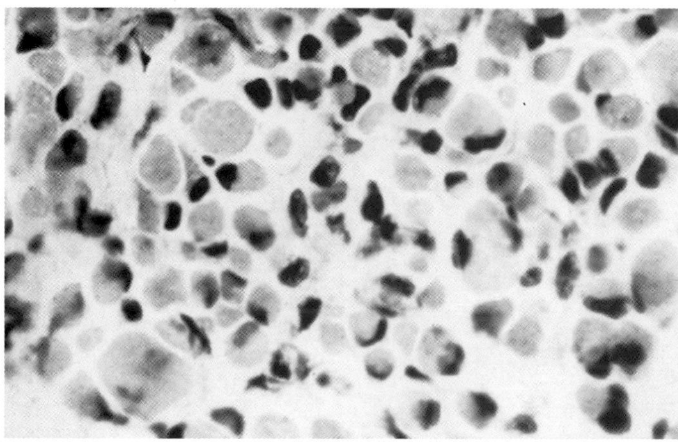

C

**Figure 41.2** **(A)** A 5-day-old girl with congenital muscular dystrophy. She was born by elective Cesarean section at 39 weeks of gestation and sustained a fracture of the femur during delivery (birth weight 2.3 kg), and subsequently a fracture of the left humerus during normal nursing care. On examination she had mild facial weakness and no antigravity power in the limbs. A brother had also been affected, had been born with fractures of all four limbs and had died on the first day of life of intracranial hemorrhage. He had been suspected of having osteogenesis imperfecta. **(B)** The girl's radiograph shows slender bones but only minimal osteoporosis. Her serum CK level was normal (28 IU/l). **(C)** Needle muscle biopsy at 5 days of age showed unequivocal pathological change with variability in fiber size, proliferation of endomyseum and some cellular infiltration. The poor bone development was presumably secondary to the weak muscles. Following an intensive program of regular passive stretching of all joints and early mobilization in a standing frame, she was walking independently by the age of 4 years in light-weight knee-ankle-foot orthoses, and subsequently unaided, and there were no further fractures.

The spectrum of clinical signs in the neonatal period, however, can be quite variable, and in some of the congenital muscular dystrophy syndromes, the involvement of the CNS can dominate the clinical picture. Table 41.3 illustrates the classification of congenital muscular dystrophy based on clinical and MRI findings, and, when known, on protein and molecular data.

## MEROSIN-NEGATIVE CONGENITAL MUSCULAR DYSTROPHY

Children with merosin deficiency generally have a more severe clinical course than the children with merosin positive congenital muscular dystrophy. They are usually symptomatic at birth or in the first few weeks of life with hypotonia, muscle weakness, and weak cry, and, in 10–30% of cases, present with contractures.

Diffuse white-matter changes on MRI are a constant feature in these children. These changes, however, are not obvious on the scans performed in the first months of life and become more evident around 6 months (Mercuri *et al.* 1996). Despite their dramatic appearance on imaging, these changes are not usually associated with clinical signs of CNS involvement. The only sign of the involvement of the central nervous system is epilepsy, which has been observed in 10–30% of children (Voit 1998). Recent studies have demonstrated that other patterns of brain lesions, such as cerebellar hypoplasia and/or cortical dysplasia, can be observed in some of these patients with merosin-deficient congenital muscular dystrophy.

## MEROSIN POSITIVE CONGENITAL MUSCULAR DYSTROPHY

The clinical picture of children with merosin positive congenital muscular dystrophy is very heterogeneous. Children affected by merosin positive CMD show a milder phenotype compared to those with merosin deficiency (Philpot *et al.* 1995). The infantile hypotonia can be variable, as opposed to that observed in merosin-deficient CMD,

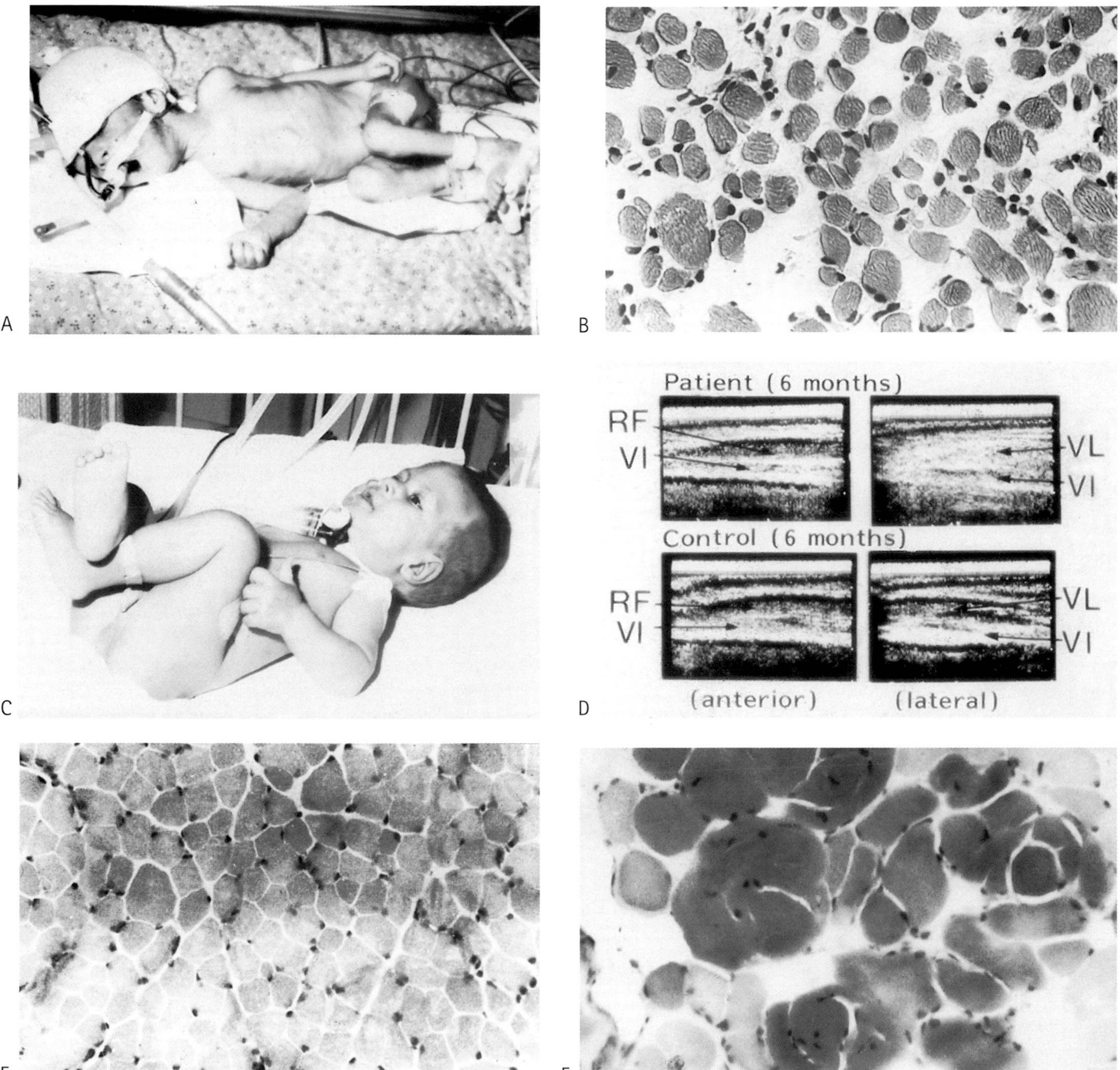


**Figure 41.3** **(A)** An 8-day-old boy with congenital muscular dystrophy presenting with persistent ventilatory failure. Pregnancy was complicated by polyhydramnios and reduced fetal movements. He was born at 34 weeks of gestation (birth weight 1.6 kg). He was severely asphyxiated and needed immediate intubation and intermittent positive-pressure ventilation. His serum CK level was normal (66 IU/l). **(B)** Needle muscle biopsy (vastus lateralis) at 8 days of age showed variability in fiber size and proliferation of connective tissue. **(C)** There was a marked improvement in limb power by 6 months of age but he still needed ventilation and had had a tracheostomy. **(D)** Real-time ultrasound scans of the thigh (longitudinal views) at that time showed a normal appearance of the rectus femoris (RF) and marked echogenicity of the vastus lateralis (VL) and of the vastus intermedius (VI). A second needle muscle biopsy was performed, taking a piece concurrently from the rectus femoris and the vastus lateralis. This showed that **(E)** the rectus was normal while **(F)** the vastus was abnormal, with adipose and connective tissue proliferation and variability in fiber size, including some large whorled fibers with multiple internal nuclei (hematoxylin and eosin staining, H and E). This suggested that the respiratory muscles were selectively affected in the same way as the vastus lateralis. By 13 months he only needed ventilatory support at night, could sit unsupported and stand with support, and vocalize with a speaking tube *in situ*. At 15 months of age he had a sudden respiratory and cardiac arrest while having tracheostomy care, suffering irreversible brain damage, and died the following day.

**Table 41.3 Classification of the congenital muscular dystrophies (CMD)**

| Form | Clinical features | MRI findings | Protein and molecular data |
|---|---|---|---|
| Fukuyama CMD | Severe mental retardation, epilepsy, eye involvement | Micropolygyria, pachygyria, cerebellar involvement, abnormal signal in white matter | Fukutin 9q31 |
| Walker–Warburg syndrome | Severe mental retardation, epilepsy, eye involvement | Type II lissencephaly, hydrocephalus, brainstem and cerebellar hypoplasia | |
| Muscle–eye–brain disease | Severe mental retardation, epilepsy, eye involvement | Pachygyria and polymicrogyria. Brainstem and cerebellar hypoplasia, periventricular white matter frequent but not constantly observed. | Chromosome 1p |
| Merosin negative CMD: | No severe mental retardation, | | 6q2 |
| • typical form | epilepsy 20% | Diffuse white matter changes. | Laminin a2 (merosin) |
| • with cortical dysplasia | Severe mental retardation, | WM changes and cortical dysplasia | |
| • with cerebellar hypoplasia | epilepsy (frequent) | WM changes and cerebellar hypoplasia | |
| Merosin positive CMD: | | | |
| • typical form | | Normal or non-specific changes | |
| • + mental retardation | | Normal or non-specific changes | |
| • + cerebellar hypoplasia | | Cerebellar hypoplasia | |
| Ulrich syndrome | | Normal | |

WM = white matter

which is often severe. Both respiratory problems and developmental delay can also be variable. Serum CK is generally mildly elevated. Classically, normal merosin has been associated with normal MRI, but recent studies have shown that a proportion of these children can show brain changes, ranging from non-specific localized white-matter changes, probably due to antenatal or perinatal distress, to the presence of structural abnormalities, such as cerebellar hypoplasia (Echenne *et al.* 1997; Trevisan *et al.* 1997).

## THE CONGENITAL MYOPATHIES

These disorders are associated with a structural abnormality within the muscle fiber. They can all present in the neonatal period as a floppy infant. Only centronuclear and nemaline myopathy are described here, however, because of their propensity to severe respiratory problems.

### MYOTUBULAR (CENTRONUCLEAR) MYOPATHY

There are three clinical and genetic subtypes: (1) a severe X-linked type, presenting in the neonatal period, (2) a less severe infantile type, which is probably autosomal recessive, and (3) a mild juvenile or adult type, which is autosomal dominant in some cases. The X-linked type is the most severe and has the earliest onset with severe hypotonia and weakness at birth, associated with persistent ventilatory failure and often with feeding difficulties. These infants usually have an antenatal history of polyhydramnios (Heckmatt *et al.* 1985; Wallgreen-Petterson and Thomas 1994; Dubowitz 1995). The majority of these infants die within the first days or weeks of life, and few survive into adulthood (Dubowitz 1995; Wallgreen Petterson *et al.* 1995). Intracranial ventricular dilatation was a feature in these infants, as it is in congenital myotonic dystrophy. The autosomal dominant and recessive types of myotubular myopathy show a milder course, and their onset is generally after the neonatal period.

The principal pathologic feature (irrespective of the genetics) is the presence of large central nuclei in fibers of both types. Only a proportion of the fibers show the central nuclei in transverse section because they are spaced out along the fibers with gaps in between them. The central area of the fibers is devoid of myofibrils but occupied by mitochondria and glycogen. Histochemical stains show a large proportion of fibers with central aggregation of stain with the NADH-TR and periodic acid–Schiff (PAS) reactions and 'holes' in the center of the fibers on the ATPase reaction due to the absence of myofibers.

#### Molecular genetics

The gene for the severe X-linked form of congenital myotubular myopathy has been localized on Xq28 (Thomas *et al.* 1990) and numerous mutations have been identified. The gene has been called MTM1 and encodes the tyrosine phosphatase myotubularin. This has allowed not only to confirm the diagnosis but also to perform prenatal diagnosis (Tanner *et al.* 1999).

### NEMALINE MYOPATHY

This congenital myopathy is of variable severity and inheritance and may present in the neonatal period. The ENMC international consortium on nemaline myopathy, formed in 1996, has agreed on the following, broad definition: 'nemaline myopathy is a neuromuscular disorder characterized by muscle weakness and the presence in the muscle fibres of nemaline (rod) bodies', in the absence of other known conditions sometimes associated with nemaline bodies (Wallgren-Petterson & Laing, 1996). The rods are easily overlooked on the hematoxylin and eosin section and readily demonstrated with the Gomori trichrome stain, being a striking red color in contrast to the blue-green of the muscle fibers. There may be two populations of fibers, one hypertrophic and the other atrophic, and the rods are mainly in the atrophic fibers.

The most common mode of inheritance is autosomal recessive, and the spectrum of clinical phenotypes within the autosomal recessive nemaline myopathy is quite heterogeneous (Wallgren-Patterson & Laing 1996; Wallgren-Petterson 1998). The most common form is the 'typical' or mainstrea form. In this form, the onset is generally in infancy with pronounced facial and proximal weakness.

A severe perinatal form has also been described and is often fatal. The first severe infantile case was reported by Shafiq *et al.* (1967) in a 15-week-old male infant, who presented with generalized hypotonia and difficulty in feeding. The infant's main problem was the accumulation of secretions, which tended to obstruct and compromise his airway. His face was expressionless but moved symmetrically on crying. He had had multiple episodes of pneumonitis and atelectasias, and at 4 months, a feeding gastrostomy was performed. Subsequently, his muscle power improved, but he died at the age of 10 months from a fulminating pneumonia. Post-mortem examination showed involvement of the tongue, diaphragm, and pharynx, in addition to variable involvement of the skeletal muscles.

Kuitunen *et al.* (1972) described two unrelated children who had been weak from birth with sucking difficulty – both improved and had eventually became ambulant. Neustein (1973) reported three affected siblings who had been floppy from birth. The first had died at 3 months of age, the second at 2 days, and the third at 11 months, probably from respiratory causes in each case. All had reduced fetal movements *in utero*. The third sibling had a detailed autopsy, and involvement of skeletal muscle was widespread.

There have also been reports of nemaline myopathy presenting as ventilatory failure in the newborn. Norton *et al.* (1983) reported two infants: one of which was a girl born at 35 weeks of gestation who had persistent ventilatory failure with no improvement, and ventilatory support was discontinued after 3 months. Tsujihata *et al.* (1983) reported a female infant, born at 37 weeks of gestation, who was hypotonic from birth, failed to establish effective respiration, required ventilatory support, and subsequently died at the age of 3 months. Autopsy again revealed widespread involvement of skeletal muscles, particularly the diaphragm.

#### Molecular genetics

Our understanding of the genetic aspects of nemaline myopathy has dramatically improved over the last few years. It has been demonstrated that there are at least three genes mutated in several types of nemaline myopathy: mutations in the gene for tropomyosin, TPM3, on chromosome 1q21 have been found in both dominant and recessive nemaline myopathies (Tan *et al.* 1998; Wallgren-Petterson 1998); mutations localized on chromosome 2q22, in a region harboring the gene for the muscle protein nebulin, have been found in typical non- or slowly progressive forms (Wallgren-Petterson 1995). More recently, mutations in the a-actin gene have also been demonstrated in patients with a variable severity of phenotype (Nowak *et al.* 1999)

## MYASTHENIA GRAVIS

### AUTOIMMUNE

Neonatal myasthenia gravis is a transient disorder occurring in about 12% of the offspring of myasthenic mothers. Namba *et al.* (1970) gave a detailed review of 82 cases from the literature and included two of their own. The infants presented usually within a few hours of birth or, at the very latest, the first 72 h, with feeding difficulty, generalized weakness, poor respiratory effort, and inability to handle pharyngeal secretions (Figs 41.4 and 41.5). At least half had facial weakness characterized by 'mask-like' faces and infrequent blinking and staring; 15% had ptosis, and 8% had decreased ocular movements. Virtually all cases reviewed responded to anticholinesterases. Some of the patients had repetitive stimulation, at 5–20 Hz, which showed a decrement in the amplitude of the motor action potential. Nine died, and in six who came to autopsy, the cause was respiratory failure, with atelectasis and pneumonia. The mean duration of illness was 18 days, with a maximum of 7 weeks.

Neonatal myasthenia cannot be related to duration or severity of maternal disease, to any alteration in the maternal symptoms during pregnancy, or to thymectomy. It is associated with acetylcholine receptor (ACHR) antibody, which is passively transferred across the placenta in both affected and unaffected babies but is more persistent in the serum of affected babies. Exchange transfusion is said to be of no value in the management of the baby (Lefvert & Osterman 1983), which is contrary to what might be expected, considering the undoubted response to plasma exchange in most adults.

### NON-AUTOIMMUNE

The term 'congenital myasthenic syndromes' includes a heterogeneous group of hereditary disorders affecting the neuromuscular junction. Conomy *et al.* (1975) reported an 18-month-old boy with familial infantile myasthenia who had recurrent episodes of choking from the age of 2 weeks, who responded dramatically to edrophonium, and whose sister had had delayed motor milestones and 'bedroom eyes' and had died suddenly during a respiratory infection at the age of 15 months. Robertson *et al.* (1980) reported a 14-year-old boy who had had repeated episodes of severe apnea

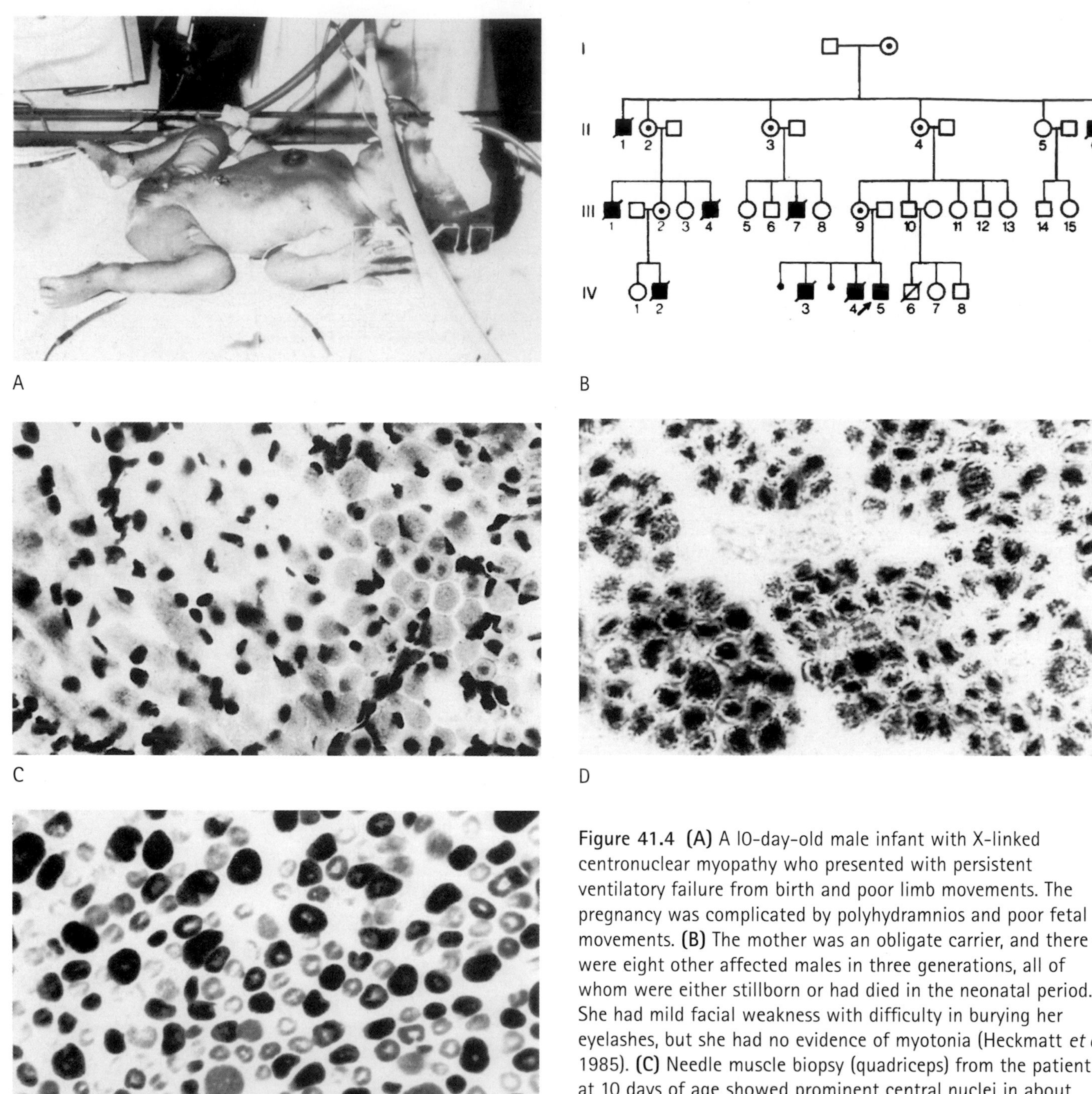


Figure 41.4 **(A)** A 10-day-old male infant with X-linked centronuclear myopathy who presented with persistent ventilatory failure from birth and poor limb movements. The pregnancy was complicated by polyhydramnios and poor fetal movements. **(B)** The mother was an obligate carrier, and there were eight other affected males in three generations, all of whom were either stillborn or had died in the neonatal period. She had mild facial weakness with difficulty in burying her eyelashes, but she had no evidence of myotonia (Heckmatt *et al* 1985). **(C)** Needle muscle biopsy (quadriceps) from the patient at 10 days of age showed prominent central nuclei in about 40% of fibers (H and E). **(D)** The NADH-TR reaction showed central aggregation of stain in virtually all fibers. **(E)** The ATPase 9.5 showed a clear zone in the center of many fibers.

from the neonatal period, which resolved at around the age of 2 years. Marked fatiguability had persisted, and there was mild proximal weakness. He had responded to prostigmine, which was first tried at the age of 4 years. An older brother had had similar episodes of apnea, which also ceased at the age of 2 years. On repetitive stimulation, there was a marked decrement in the size of the motor action potential in the biceps. Albers *et al.* (1984) reported a clinically atypical infant who had to be ventilated from 1 week of age and who failed to respond to anticholinesterase but showed a striking decrement in the motor action potential on repetitive stimulation at 2 Hz. The baby died at the age of 8 months of pneumonia. The authors suggested a failure of resynthesis, mobilization, or storage of acetylcholine.

Vincent *et al.* (1981) reported five male patients, including two brothers, aged 13–25 years with congenital myasthenia

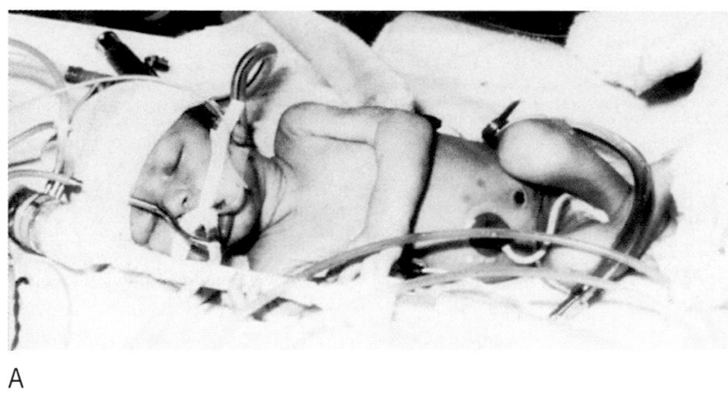

A

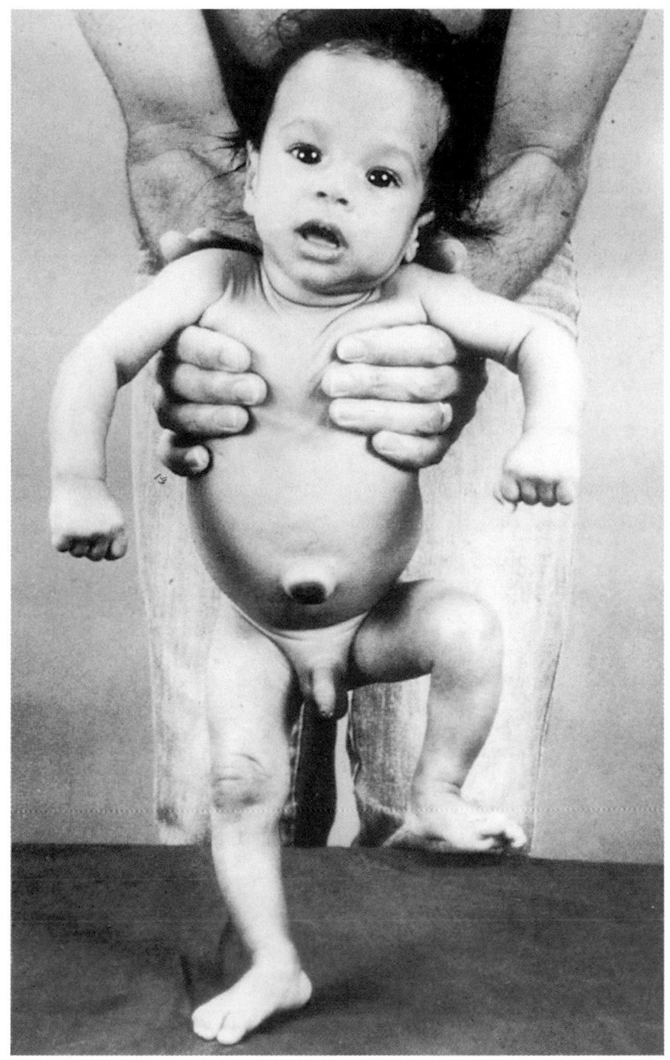

B

Figure 41.5 (A) A 10-day-old boy with transient neonatal myasthenia. Atypical presentation at birth with diaphragmatic and pharyngeal paralysis in the presence of normal limb and facial movements. The mother had a similar pattern of muscle involvement and developed ventilatory failure postpartum, due to severe diaphragm weakness, responding eventually to plasma exchange and immunosuppressive medication. The baby presented at birth because the mother was not on anticholinesterase medication; this is transferred passively across the placenta and has some transient protective effect. Magnetometry of the rib cage and abdomen, and repetitive stimulation of the peripheral nerve, were both suggestive of muscle fatigue (Heckmatt *et al* 1987). By 6 weeks of age the baby had made a complete recovery. (B) The infant attempting to stand at the age of 6 months.

gravis. Three had an onset at birth with feeding difficulty, ptosis, and facial involvement and two had an onset before 2 years. Four had oculomotor paralysis, but none had major respiratory involvement. The response to anticholinesterases was variable, but three showed a definite improvement. The authors performed end-plate electrophysiology on intercostal muscle biopsies and found a variety of pre- and post-synaptic defects, suggesting that congenital myasthenia is a heterogeneous condition.

Historically, two clinical types of non-autoimmune myasthenia, so-called 'familial' and 'congenital', have been described (Vincent *et al.* 1981). The familial infantile type is characterized by episodes of severe respiratory and feeding difficulties at birth or during infancy and normal extraocular movements. Patients show a good response to anticholinesterase treatment and a high remission rate. The disease occurs frequently in siblings, and inheritance is probably autosomal recessive. Congenital myasthenia usually develops before the age of 2 years, and in many cases, symptoms have been present at birth or *in utero*. Males tend to be affected more than females, and affected siblings are frequently encountered, which also suggests autosomal recessive inheritance. Ocular muscles are the most commonly affected, but severe weakness of bulbar, trunk, and limb muscles can occur. The symptoms tend to be non-progressive, and, in contrast to the familial type, anticholinesterase is not always beneficial, and remission is unusual. It is occasionally associated with congenital arthrogryposis (Smit & Barth 1980; Teyssier *et al.* 1982).

This distinction, however, was somehow confusing as congenital myasthenia is also familial. An ENMC international workshop on congenital myasthenic syndromes in 1995 suggested a new classification based on the modality of inheritance, with type i including the autosomal recessive forms, type ii the autosomal dominant and type iii the sporadic cases. Each type was further subdivided in further subtypes (Middleton 1996). According to this classification, the form classically called familial is a subtype of the type I congenital myasthenic syndromes (Ia), and this has created some confusion between the old and new terminology

(Deymeer *et al.* 1999). In recent years, the forms have been reclassified according to whether the defect is present at a presynaptic, synaptic, or postsynaptic level. Recent studies have been able to demonstrate the defect at the molecular level, identifying several mutations in the gene encoding the collagenic tail subunit of the endplate species of acetylcholinesterase (Donger *et al.* 1998; Ohno *et al.* 1999) and from mutations in acetylcholine receptor (AChR) subunit genes (Ohno *et al.* 1999).

## OTHER NEUROMUSCULAR DISORDERS

### ARTHROGRYPOSIS

This disorder is defined as congenital non-progressive limitation of movement in two or more joints in different body areas (Hageman & Willemse 1983). It is not a diagnosis as such but a symptom complex, and the potential end result of several different types of pathologic process. There is general agreement that the final mechanism is immobility *in utero*. This might be produced by restriction of the fetus or inability of the fetus to move due to some failure of the motor system (Fig. 41.6).

Hall (1985) stated that affected limbs are, on average, 20% shorter than expected for gestational age, while the trunk and head are of normal size, which suggests that part of normal limb growth relates to forces engendered by use. Catch-up may occur during vigorous use of limbs and also a return to normal size of lungs, and cranial–facial structures. Hall (1985) states that return of range of motion could occur up to 1 year (in our experience, this is a conservative estimate) and relative increases in strength of the muscle for many years.

Prolonged oligohydramnios or a bicornuate uterus might be a cause in some cases (Fig. 41.6). It has been generally assumed that very few are due to primary muscle disease. After an extensive review of the literature, Swinyard (1982) estimated that the proportion was only 10–15%. In a study of the spinal cord of 11 infants with arthrogryposis, Clauren & Hall (1983) found a reduction in the number of a motor neurons, an increase in the numbers of small neurons in all but one, and CNS involvement in three. These results cannot be applied to all arthrogryposis patients, as those who die may be a selected population. The Pena–Shokeir syndrome of multiple ankyloses, facial abnormalities, pulmonary hypoplasia, and cryptorchidism has been associated with problems in brain formation and loss of anterior horn cells in the spinal cord, but a primary muscle disorder could also have the same clinical end-result (Moerman *et al.* 1983).

There have been relatively few reports of EMG and muscle studies done systematically in arthrogryposis, particularly with modern histochemical techniques. One such study was by Strehl & Vanasse (1985) in 22 patients, and they found ten with a neurogenic cause (five with a spinal origin, two of cerebral origin and three mixed), and nine myopathic (three congenital muscular dystrophy, three congenital myotonic dystrophy, one fibre-type disproportion, and two non-specific myopathy). One had an inherited malformation syndrome, and in two, the cause was unknown. They stated that precise diagnosis would have been impossible without needle muscle biopsy. This is more in accord with our own experience, where the most common associated neuromuscular disorder is congenital muscular dystrophy (Fig. 41.7).

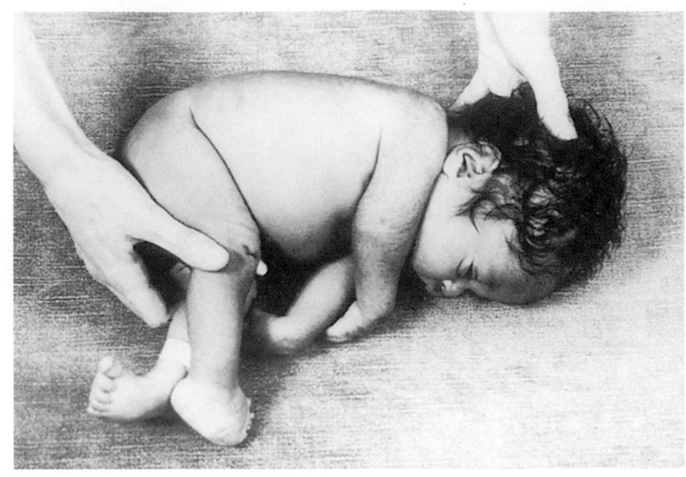

A

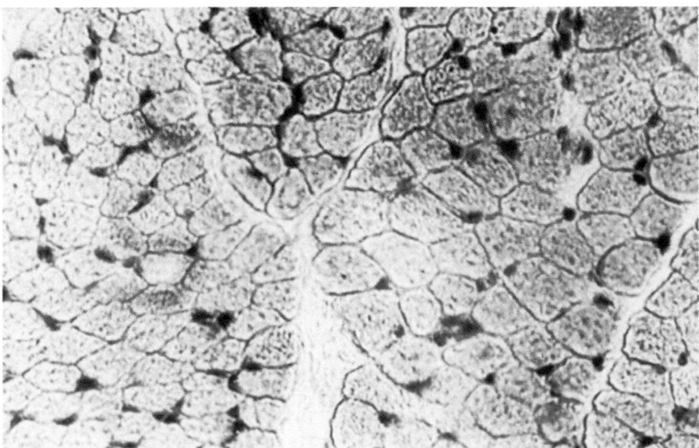

B

**Figure 41.6** **(A)** A 2-day-old boy, born at full term with arthrogryposis. Continuous drainage of liquor occurred from the sixth month of pregnancy and fetal movements diminished from that time. He was delivered at full term. Note the flexion deformities of the fingers and wrists and equinus deformities of the feet but no hip and knee contractures. Shoulder abduction was limited and elbows were held in extension. The muscles of the shoulders were atrophic but there seemed to be reasonable power of the hip and thigh muscles. The trunk seemed normal but there was excessive head lag. The facies was normal. **(B)** Needle muscle biopsy at 2 days of age (quadriceps) was normal. The arthrogryposis was thought to be due to intrauterine restriction secondary to the oligohydramnios.

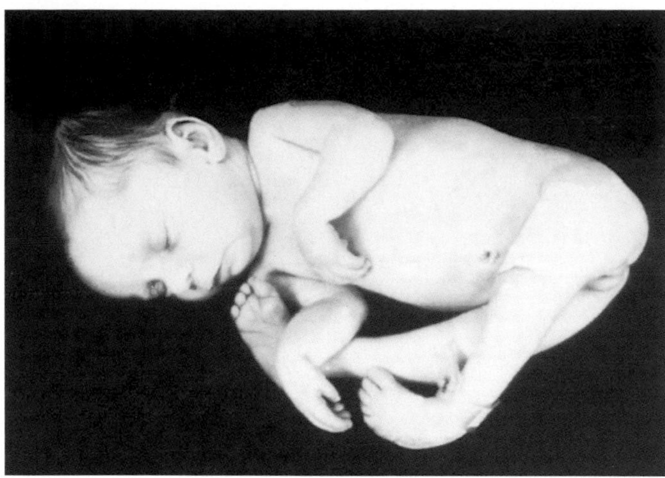

A

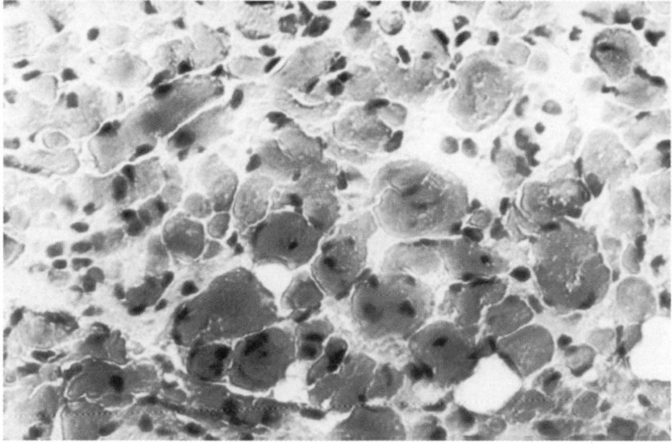

B

**Figure 41.7** **(A)** A 2-week-old girl with arthrogryposis and generalized hypotonia. Fetal movements were reduced throughout pregnancy; there was oligohydramnios and poor fetal growth. The baby was delivered at full term (birth weight 2 kg) and adopted a 'fetal' position with the arms tucked under the chin and the legs flexed at the hips, the left against the chest and the right along the trunk behind the arm. There were no spontaneous movements of the limbs. She sucked well, however, and there were no breathing difficulties. She had fixed flexion contractures of both elbows, 30° flexion contractures of both wrists, dislocated right hip, right genu recurvatum and severe bilateral talipes. Her serum CK was normal (107 IU/l). **(B)** Needle muscle biopsy at 2 weeks of age (quadriceps) showed dystrophic change. She had bilateral talectomy to correct the talipes at the age of 19 months and is now standing regularly in a frame.

## SPINAL MUSCULAR ATROPHY

This important group of disorders can be divided into three clinical subtypes: (1) severe, in which the infant is very weak, never acquires the ability to sit, has severe respiratory muscle weakness, and dies usually before the age of 1 year of an intercurrent respiratory infection; (2) intermediate, in which the infant acquires the ability to sit and usually survives but with complications such as scoliosis; and (3) mild, in which the child is able to walk (for a detailed discussion of the clinical classification, see Dubowitz 1995, 1999). In general, those presenting in the neonatal period will have the severe type, but the age of onset of symptoms is not an absolute guide to disease severity. Classically, infants with type 1 show a very consistent phenotype characterized by general hypotonia, with axial and limb weakness. The legs are more affected than the arms, and proximal muscles more than distal. There is little spontaneous activity, mainly limited to the feet and hands. Facial muscles are spared, and the infants show a normal bright expression (Fig. 41.8). The intercostal muscles are always affected, but the diaphragm is spared. In addition to the extensive paralysis of the limbs and distinctive breathing pattern, other useful pointers to the diagnosis are the characteristic 'jug-handle' posturing of the upper limbs with internal rotation of the shoulders and pronation of the forearms, tongue fasciculation, and the bright alert facies (Fig. 41.8). MacLeod *et al.* (1999) have recently documented some cases of prenatal onset spinal muscular atrophy with reduced fetal movements, severe weakness and asphyxia at birth, and short survival time (MacLeod *et al.* 1999). This form, confirmed by gene deletion studies, suggests that the phenotype of SMA is still expanding (Dubowitz 1999).

When there is a short history of weakness and the muscle biopsy is normal or shows only universal atrophy, the nerve conduction study is useful because it will show an absent or greatly diminished amplitude of the motor action potential, whereas in the myopathies, the motor action potential is usually of a reasonable size (> 0.5 mV). The EMG may show some fibrillation potentials at rest and isolated motor units of normal size and configuration on volition, but will not show the classical changes of reinnervation (i.e. large isolated motor units).

Spinal muscular atrophy is autosomal recessive, and the severity in affected siblings is usually similar, but occasionally, there may be marked discordance in severity. Infants with Werdning–Hoffman disease generally do not show central nervous system involvement, but non-specific changes such as cerebral atrophy or other ischemic changes have been observed in some of these children, mainly associated with prematurity or birth asphyxia (Rudnick-Schoneborn *et al.* 1996).

### Molecular genetics

The gene for the autosomal recessive, proximal symmetric spinal muscular atrophies has been localized to chromosome 5q11–q13. In 1995, the gene defect for SMA (deletion of the telomeric copy of the SMN gene) was identified and homozygous deletion of SMN exon 7 has been found in more than 98% of SMA patients. This has provided a very useful and rapid diagnostic tool.

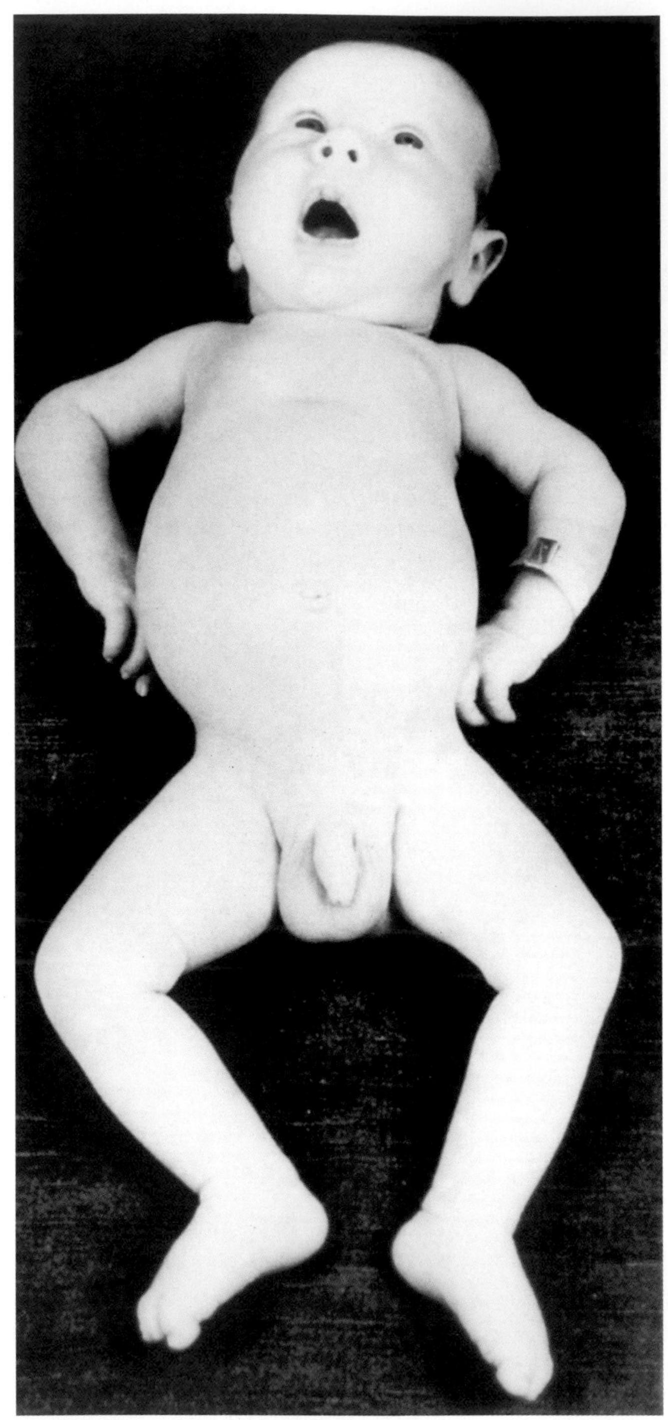

A

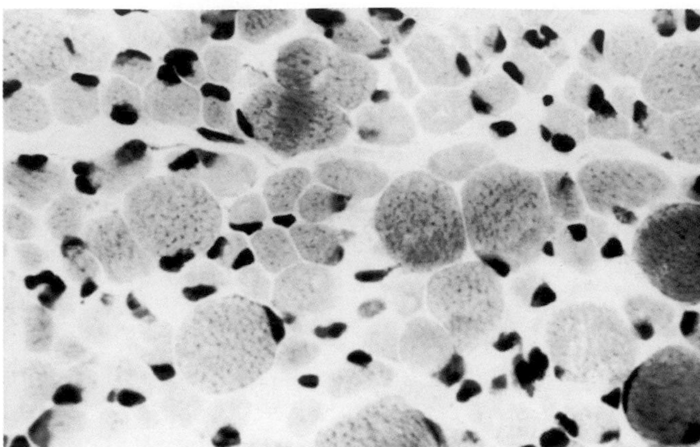

B

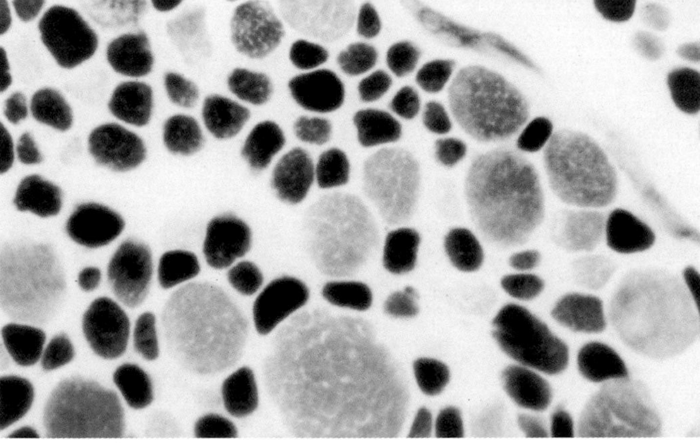

C

**Figure 41.8** **(A)** A 4-week-old boy with severe spinal muscular atrophy. There was insidious onset of weakness with poor limb movement and internal rotation of the arms. Fetal movements were normal, and movements seemed normal at birth. Note the typical frog posture, together with the jug-handle posture of the arms and internal rotation at the shoulders, and the alert facies. There is also a narrow chest with poor intercostal movement and a distended abdomen, reflecting the well-preserved diaphragmatic function. With inspiration there is further expansion of the abdomen and costal retraction. Tongue fasciculation was present. Motor nerve conduction (peroneal nerve) showed a markedly reduced motor action potential at 0.05 mV (normal >0.5 mV). Electromyography of the quadriceps showed fasciculation potentials at rest but no activity on volition. **(B)** Needle muscle biopsy (quadriceps) at 4 weeks of age showed variability in fiber size (H and E) **(C)** The larger fibers were all type 1, suggestive of some reinnervation (ATPase 9.5).

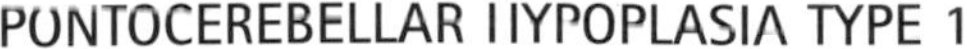

## PONTOCEREBELLAR HYPOPLASIA TYPE 1

Motor neuron involvement is also found in another condition, called pontocerebellar hypoplasia type 1, in which spinal muscular atrophy is associated with hypoplasia of the cerebellar vermis, and often also of the cerebellar hemispheres, associated with a thin brainstem and pons (Barth 1993). Infants affected by this form show a combination of clinical signs related to both motoneuron disorder and central nervous system involvement. The clinical course is progressive, and respiratory and feeding difficulties, already present at birth or in early infancy, become more severe.

### Molecular genetics

This form is not allelic to SMA (Dubowitz *et al.* 1995), and the gene responsible for this form has not yet been identified. The differential diagnosis is with other forms, such as the carbohydrate-deficient glycoconjugate syndromes, which show cerebellar and brainstem hypoplasia and peripheral nerve involvement. The carbohydrate-deficient glycoconjugate syndromes include a group of genetic disorders characterized by a deficiency of the carbohydrate moiety of glycoconjugates (Jaeken *et al.* 1991; Jaeken & Casaer 1997). Type 1 is the most common and has been related to a deficit in phosphomannomutase. Infants present with dysmorphic features, hypotonia and hyporeflexia, abnormal eye movements, and poor feeding. Other signs, such as skeletal abnormalities, hepatomegaly, proteinuria, and cardiomyopathy are also frequent. The involvement of the peripheral nerves is shown by abnormal motor and sensory nerve conduction velocity. Brain MRI shows brainstem and cerebellar hypoplasia (Jaeken 1991; Akaboshi *et al.* 1995; Jaeken & Casaer 1997).

## NON-NEUROMUSCULAR DISORDERS

### PRADER–WILLI SYNDROME

This is a relatively common disorder with an estimated incidence of one in 10 000, and it occurs in all races. It was originally described by Prader *et al.* (1956), who reported five patients with adiposity, short stature, mental subnormality, and undescended testes in the males. The presentation is frequently in the neonatal period with extreme hypotonia and lethargy. There is also a marked swallowing defect in the absence of any associated respiratory problems, in contrast to conditions such as myotonic dystrophy or myotubular myopathy, which have both. With time, the hypotonia resolves, and all these children become ambulant. The problems with hyperphagia and obesity usually start after that. There is a characteristic facies, with a high forehead, narrow bifrontal diameter, up-slanting almond-shaped palpebral fissures, and a triangular mouth with a thin upper lip. Squint is present in approximately two-thirds, and there are small hands and feet, which may be more apparent in later childhood. The facies may be more distinctively abnormal when the infant is crying, as these infants tend to screw up the face in a particular way (Fig. 41.9) The striking feature about these infants, in comparison with those with neuromuscular disorders, is that the severity of the hypotonia is disproportionate to the intermittently good antigravity movements that may be observed.

There is no neuromuscular involvement, the EMG, nerve conduction velocity, and muscle biopsy are normal, and diagnosis is primarily clinical. Routine chromosome analysis is usually normal in these patients, but with high-resolution techniques, a deletion has been demonstrated on the long arm of chromosome 15 (15q12) in about 50% of cases (Ledbetter *et al.* 1982; Fear *et al.* 1985). A further important observation was that the deletion appears to be of paternal origin (Butler & Palmer 1983). Recent advances with molecular genetic techniques have shown that those cases without an overt deletion usually have maternal disomy, with two copies of the maternal chromosome and a corresponding absence of the paternal contribution. This is thus equivalent to a deletion of the paternal contribution for that part of the chromosome. A number of laboratories are currently searching for a candidate gene. Initially, it was thought that possibly a $\gamma$-aminobutyric acid receptor, which is located in that region, might be the likely candidate, but this has now been shown to be some way from the Prader–Willi locus.

## METABOLIC DISORDERS

### MITOCHONDRIAL DISORDERS (see also Section 7)

Only a few of the mitochondrial disorders affecting children and adults have neonatal onset, and these are mainly related to deficiency of complex I and III and, more commonly of complex IV of the respiratory chain. Lactic acidosis is the landmark of most of these forms. Other myopathies that present in the first few weeks of life and can be divided into three clinical and genetic subtypes are: a 'benign' type, of unknown genetic etiology, and two progressive, fatal or 'severe' types, one autosomal recessive and one X-linked recessive. In general, presentation is with progressive muscle weakness after a period of apparent normality, and these infants may be mistakenly diagnosed as spinal muscular atrophy. There have been descriptions of a fatal infantile form with cardiac and renal involvement, seizures, hypotonia and respiratory distress with cortical and subcortical atrophy and dysmyelination on brain imaging (Aicardi 1998). The muscle can be normal or reveal lipid–glycogen storage.

### POMPE'S DISEASE (GLYCOGENOSIS TYPE 2)

This is a fatal autosomal recessive disorder characterized by a deficiency of acid $\alpha$-glucosidase and lysosomal accumulation of glycogen. Presentation is usually between the ages of 3 and 6 months with either cardiorespiratory failure or severe progressive hypotonia, but abnormality may extend back to the neonatal period, in particular the cardiomegaly (Burton 1987). There is likely to be skin pallor, hepatomegaly, macroglossia, and possibly some skeletal muscle hypertrophy. Electromyography is a useful screening investigation showing pseudomyotonic discharges; peripheral blood leukocytes should show the presence of glycogen granules.

Muscle biopsy shows marked vacuolation of the muscle fibers and increased glycogen but no lipid accumulation. The enzyme can be assayed in skin fibroblasts, amniotic fluid cells, and trophoblasts (Besancon *et al.* 1985). Rapid prenatal diagnosis can also be made by electron microscopy of uncultured amniotic fluid cells (Hug *et al.* 1984).

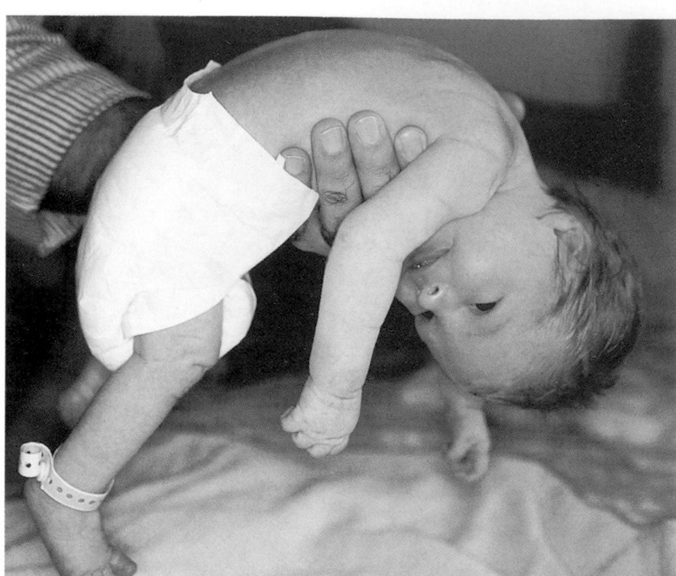

A

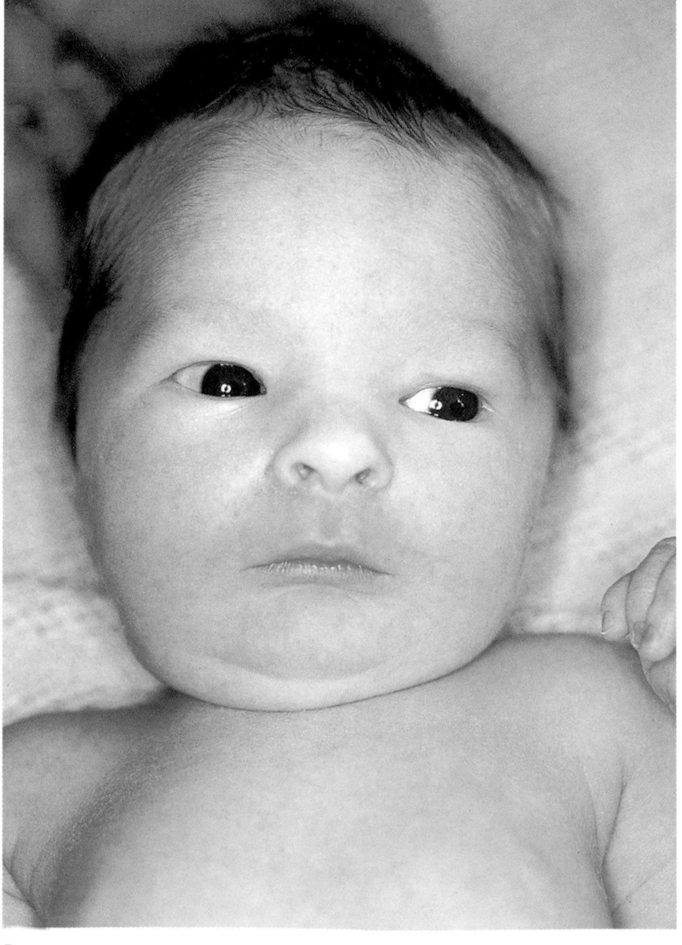

B

C

**Figure 41.9** Male infant with Prader–Willi syndrome (A) The baby was clearly hypotonic on day 4. (B) The facies show dysmorphic features at rest. (C) There is excessive wrinkling of the forehead when crying.

## GLYCOGENOSIS TYPE 3

This disorder presents with hepatomegaly, hypoglycemia, and ketosis. The time of presentation is variable but may be at birth. The defective enzyme is the glycogen debrancher amylo-1,6-glucosidase. There is usually mild hypotonia, and muscle biopsy is likely to show some glycogen accumulation. It seems to be unusual for muscle manifestations to be detected before the patient is ambulant (Slonim *et al.* 1984).

Metabolic disorders not primarily involving muscle are the other large group of conditions that present as the floppy infant. It is not possible to give more than a brief outline here, and they are also listed in Table 41.1 (see also Section 7).

## ORGANIC ACIDURIAS AND UREA-CYCLE DEFECTS (see also Chapter 35)

In the neonatal period, these disorders may present acutely with a weak cry and suck, seizures and diminishing level of consciousness, and rapid progression with shallow respirations, cyanosis and hypotonia, sometimes alternating with decerebrate posturing and opisthotonus. There is a symptom-free interval varying from one to several days before presentation, and the signs are often precipitated by the onset of protein intake or any condition associated with catabolism such as infection. There will be a metabolic acidosis, usually a ketoacidosis, hypoglycemia and hyperammonemia (found particularly in disorders of the urea cycle). The odor of the urine can be diagnostic, e.g. in maple syrup urine disease or isovalericacidemia.

## PEROXISOMOPATHIES (see also p. 634)

This is a group of genetic disorders, associated with cranial-facial dysmorphism (often present at birth in Zellweger's syndrome), severe hypotonia, a poor suck, epileptic seizures, and hepatomegaly. There is progressive deterioration, and if presentation is in early infancy, survival beyond a year is unusual. Diagnosis may require detailed examination of serum bile acids, but it is worth estimating white-cell dihydroacetonephosphate acetyltransferase activity and performing a radiograph of the knee for calcification as a diagnostic screen (Schutgens *et al.* 1986).

### Key Points

1. A neuromuscular disorder should be suspected if infants show hypotonia, feeding difficulty or persistent ventilatory failure, with or without evidence of central nervous system involvement.
2. Other important signs suggesting a possible neuromuscular involvement can be obtained from a detailed clinical history. Important clues are:
   - poor fetal movements throughout the pregnancy or in the last few months,
   - polyhydramnios
   - a family history of possible or definite neuromuscular disease, or of neonatal death and stillbirth.
3. The clinical examination can provide other important clues:
   - limited limb movement and lack of antigravity power on stimulation of the limbs
   - facial weakness and/or ophthalmoplegia
   - contractures
   - distribution of the respiratory muscle weakness
   - thin ribs on the chest radiograph
4. It is not always easy to differentiate a neuromuscular from a CNS disorder, especially as CNS involvement (e.g. hydrocephalus, hemorrhages and periventricular or diffuse white matter changes) can be present in infants with a neuromuscular disorder.
5. Serum creatine kinase levels, muscle ultrasound and EMG can help to identify possible muscle involvement. When indicated, in most cases muscle biopsy will provide more specific information on the type of muscle disorder.

## REFERENCES


Aicardi J (1998) *Diseases of the nervous system in childhood.* Mac Keith Press; London.

Akaboshi S, Ohno K, Takeshita K (1995) Neuroradiological findings in the carbohydrate-deficient glycoprotein syndrome. *Neuroradiology* 37:491–495.

Albers J W, Faulkner J A, Dorovini-Zis K *et al.* (1984) Abnormal neuromuscular transmission in an infantile myasthenic syndrome. *Ann Neuro* 16:28–34.

Aslanidis C, Jansen G, Amemiya C *et al.* (1992) Cloning of the essential myotonic dystrophy region and mapping the putative defect. *Nature* 355:1253–1255.

Barth P G (1993) Pontocerebellar hypoplasia. An overview of a group of inherited neurodegenerative disorders with fetal onset. *Brain Dev* 15:411–422.

✪ Barth P G, Scholte H R, Berden J A *et al.* (1983) X-linked mitochondrial disease affecting cardiac muscle, skeletal muscle and neutrophil leukocytoses. *J Neurol Sci* 62:327–355.

Besancon A-M, Castelnau L, Nicolesco H *et al.* (1985) Prenatal diagnosis of glycogenosis type 11 (Pompe's disease) using chorionic villi biopsy. *Clin Genet* 27:479–482.

✪ Boustany R N, Aprille J R, Halperin J *et al.* (1983) Mitochondrial cytochrome deficiency presenting as a myopathy with hypotonia, external ophthalmoplegia, and lactic acidosis in an infant and as fatal hepatopathy in a second cousin. *Ann Neurol* 14:462–470.

Burton B K (1987) Inborn errors of metabolism: the clinical diagnosis in early infancy. *Pediatrics* 79:359–369.

Butler M G & Palmer C G (1983) Parental origin of chromosome 15 deletion in Prader–Willi syndrome. *Lancet* i:1285–1286.

Buxton J, Shelbourne P, Davies J *et al.* (1992) Detection of an unstable DNA specific to individuals with myotonic dystrophy. *Nature* 355:547–548.

Clauren S K & Hall J G (1983) Neuropathological findings in the spinal cords of 10 infants with arthrogryposis. *J Neurol Sci* 58:89–102.

Conomy J P, Levinsohn M & Fanaroff A (1975) Familial infantile myasthenia gravis: a cause of sudden death in young children. *J Pediatr* 87:428–430.

Deymeer F, Serdaroglu P & Ozdemir C (1999) Familial infantile myasthenia: confusion in terminology. *Neuromusc Disord* 9:129–130.

Dodge P R, Gamstorp I, Byers R K *et al.* (1965) Myotonic dystrophy in infancy and childhood. *Pediatrics* 35:3–19.

Donger C, Krejci E, Pou Serradell A *et al.* (1998) Mutation in the human acetylcholinesterase-associated collagen gene, COLQ, is responsible for congenital myasthenic syndrome with end-plate acetylcholinesterase deficiency (Type Ic) *Am J Hum Genet* 63:967–975.

✪ Donner M, Rapola J & Somer H (1975) Congenital muscular dystrophy: a clinicopathological and follow-up study of 15 patients. *Neuropediatrie* 6:239–258.

Dubowitz V (1980) *The floppy infant.* London: Heinemann; 2nd edn.

Dubowitz V (1985) *Muscle biopsy, a practical approach.* London: Baillière Tindall.

Dubowitz V (1994) Workshop report on 22nd ENMC-sponsored meeting on congenital muscular dystrophy held in Baarn, The Netherlands, May 14–16 1993. *Neuromusc Disord* 4:75–81.

Dubowitz V (1995) *Muscle disorders in childhood.* London: Saunders; 2nd edn.

Dubowitz V (1999) Very severe spinal muscular atrophy (SMA type 0): an expanding clinical phenotype. *Eur J Paediatr Neurol* 3:49–52.

Dubowitz V, Daniels R J & Davies K E (1995) Olivopontocerebellar hypoplasia with anterior horn cell involvement (SMA) does not localize to chromosome 5q. *Neuromusc Disord* 5:25–29.

Dubowitz V & Fardeau M (1995) Workshop report on 27th ENMC-sponsored meeting on congenital muscular dystrophy held in Baarn, The Netherlands, April 22–24 1994. *Neuromusc Disord* 4:253–258.

Echenne B, Rivier F, Jellali A J *et al.* (1997) Merosin positive congenital muscular dystrophy with mental deficiency, epilepsy and MRI changes in the cerebral white matter. *Neuromusc Disord* 7:187–190.

Fear C N, Mutton D E, Berry A C *et al.* (1985) Chromosome 15 in Prader-Willi syndrome. *Dev Med Child Neurol* 27:305–311.

Hageman G & Willemse J (1983) Arthrogryposis multiplex congenita. *Neuropediatrics* 14:6–11.

Hall J G (1985) *In utero* movement and use of limbs are necessary for normal growth: a study of individuals with arthrogryposis. *Prog Clin Biol Res* 200:155–162.

Harper P S (1975a) Congenital myotonic dystrophy in Britain. 11. Genetic basis. *Arch Dis Childhood* 50:514–521.

Harper P S (1975b) Congenital myotonic dystrophy in Britain. 1. Clinical aspects. *Arch Dis Childhood* 50:505–513.

✪ Heckmatt J Z & Dubowitz V (1987) Ultrasound imaging and directed needle biopsy in the diagnosis of selective involvement in neuromuscular disease. *J Child Neurol* 2:205–213.

Heckmatt J Z, Moosa A, Hutson C *et al.* (1984) Diagnostic needle muscle biopsy, a practical and reliable alternative to open biopsy. *Arch Dis Childhood* 59:528–532.

Heckmatt J Z, Sewry C A, Hodes D *et al.* (1985) Congenital centronuclear (myotubular) myopathy: a clinical and genetic study in eight children. *Brain* 108:941–964.

Hug G, Soukup S, Ryan M *et al.* (1984) Rapid prenatal diagnosis of glycogen-storage disease type 11 by electron microscopy of uncultured amniotic-fluid cells. *N Engl J Med* 310:1018–1022.

Jaeken J & Casaer P (1997) Carbohydrate-deficient glyconjugate (CDG) syndromes: a new chapter of neuropaediatrics. *Eur J Paediatr Neurol* 2/3:61–66.

Jaeken J, Stibler H & Hagberg B (1991) The carbohydrate-deficient glycoprotein syndrome: a new inherited multisystemic disease with severe nervous system involvement. *Acta Paediatr Scand Suppl* 375: monograph.

Kuitunen P, Rapola J, Noponen A L *et al.* (1972) Nemaline myopathy. *Acta Paediatr Scand* 61:353–361.

Ledbetter D H, Mascarello J T, Riccardi V M *et al.* (1982) Chromosome 15 abnormalities and the Prader-Willi syndrome: follow-up report of 40 cases. *Am J Hum Genet* 34:278–285.

Lefvert A K & Osterman P O (1983) Newborn infants to myasthenic mothers: a clinical study and an investigation of acetylcholine receptor antibodies in 17 children. *Neurology* 33:133–138.

MacLeod M J, Taylor J E, Lunt P W *et al.* (1999) Prenatal onset spinal muscular atrophy. *Eur J Paediatr Neurol* 3:65–72.

✪ Melki J, Abdelhak S, Sheth P *et al.* (1990b) Gene for chronic proximal spinal muscular atrophies maps to chromosome 5q. *Nature* 344:767–768.

✪ Melki J, Sheth P, Abdelhak S *et al.* (1990a) Mapping of acute (type 1) spinal muscular atrophy to chromosome 5q12–q14. *Lancet* 336:271–273.

Mercuri E, Pennock J, Goodwin F *et al.* (1996) Sequential study of central and peripheral nervous system involvement in an infant with merosin-deficient CMD. *Neuromusc Disord* 6:425–429.

✪ Meyers K R, Golomb H M, Hansen J L *et al.* (1974) Familial neuromuscular disease with 'myotubes'. *Clin Genet* 5:327–337.

Middleton L T (1996) Report on the 34th ENMC International workshop – congenital myasthenia syndromes. *Neuromusc Disord* 6:133–136.

Moerman P H, Fryns J P, Goddeeris P *et al.* (1983) Multiple ankyloses, facial anomalies, and pulmonary hypoplasia associated with severe antenatal spinal muscular atrophy. *J Pediatr* 103:238–241.

Namba T, Brown S B & Grob D (1970) Neonatal myasthenia gravis: report of two cases and review of the literature. *Pediatrics* 45:488–504.

Neustein H B (1973) Nemaline myopathy, a family study with three autopsied cases. *Arch Pathol* 96:192–195.

Norton P, Ellison P, Sulaiman A R *et al.* (1983) Nemaline myopathy in the neonate. *Neurology* 33:351–356.

Nowak K J, Wattanasirichaigoon D & Goebel H H *et al.* (1999) Mutations in the skeletal muscle alpha-actin gene in patients with actin myopathy and nemaline myopathy. *Nat Genet* 23:208–212.

O'Brien J A & Harper P S (1984) Course prognosis and complications of childhood onset myotonic dystrophy. *Dev Med Child Neurol* 26:62–67.

Ohno K, Anlar B & Engel A G (1999) Congenital myasthenic syndrome caused by a mutation in the Ets binding site of the promoter region of the acetylcoline receptor ε subunit gene. *Neuromusc Disord* 9:131–135.

Philpot J, Sewry C, Pennock J *et al.* (1995) Clinical phenotype in congenital muscular dystrophy: correlation with expression of merosin in skeletal muscle. *Neuromusc Disord* 5:301–305.

Prader A, Labhart A & Willi H (1956) Ein Syndrom von Adipositas, Kleinwuchs, Kryptorchismus und Oligophrenie nach Myatonieartigm zustand im Neugeborenenatter. *Schweizerische Medizinische Wochenschrift* 86:1260–1261.

Regev R, de Vries L S, Heckmatt J Z *et al.* (1987) Cerebral ventricular dilation in congenital myotonic dystrophy. *J Pediatr* 111:372–376.

Robertson W C, Chun R W M & Kornguth S E (1980) Familial infantile myasthenia. *Arch Neurol* 37:117–119.

✪ Rowland I P (1955) Prostigmine responsiveness and the diagnosis of myasthenia gravis. *Neurology* 5:612–624.

Rudnick-Schoneborn, Forkert R, Hahnen E *et al.* (1996) Clinical spectrum and diagnostic criteria of infantile spinal muscular atrophy: further delineation on the basis of SMN deletion findings. *Neuropediatrics* 27:8–15.

Schutgens R H B, Heymans H S A, Wanders R J A *et al.* (1986) Peroxisomal disorders: a newly recognised group of genetic diseases. *Eur J Pediatr* 144:430–440.

Shafiq S A, Dubowitz V, Hart de C Peterson *et al.* (1967) Nematine myopathy: report of a fatal case, with histochemical and electron microscopic studies. *Brain* 90:817–828.

Slonim A E, Coleman R A & Moses W S (1984) Myopathy and growth failure in debrancher enzyme deficiency: improvement with high-protein nocturnal enteral therapy. *J Pediatr* 105:906–911.

Smit L M E & Barth P G (1980) Arthrogryposis multiplex congenita due to congenital myasthenia. *Dev Med Child Neurol* 22:371–373.

Strehl E & Vanasse M (1985) EMG and needle muscle biopsy studies in arthrogryposis multiplex congenita. *Neuropediatrics* 16:225–227.

Swinyard C A (1982) Concepts of multiple congenital contractures in man and animals. *Teratology* 25:247–258.

Tan P, Briner J, Bolthauser E *et al.* (1998) Homozygosity for a nonsense mutation in the alpha-tropomyosin gene TPM3 in a patient with severe congenital nemaline myopathy. *Neuromuscular Disord.* 9:573–579.

Tanner S M, Laporte J, Guiraurd-Chaumeil C *et al.* (1998) Confirmation of prenatal diagnosis results of X linked recessive myotubular myopathy by mutational screening and description of three new mutations in the MTM1 gene. *Hum Mutat* 11:62–68.

Teyssier G, Damon G, Bertheas M F *et al.* (1982) Congenital myasthenia and arthrogryposis: apropos of 2 cases manifesting at birth. *Pediatrie* 37:295–298.

Thomas N S T, Williams H, Cole G *et al.* (1990) X-linked neonatal centronuclear/myotubular myopathy: evidence for linkage to Xq28 DNA marker loci. *J Med Genet* 27:284–287.

Tome F M, Evangelista T, Leclerc A *et al.* (1994) Congenital muscular dystrophy with merosin deficiency. *C R Acad Sci Paris Science de la vie/Life Sciences* 317–351.

Trevisan C P, Martinello F & Armani M *et al.* (1997) Brain involvement in a series of cases with merosin-positive congenital muscular dystrophy. *Neuromusc Disord* 7:433.

Tsujihata M, Shimomura C, Yoshimura T *et al.* (1983) Fatal neonatal myopathy; a case report. *J Neurosurg Psychiatry* 46:856–859.

Vanier T M (1960) Dystrophia myotonica in childhood. *Br Med J* ii:1284–1288.

Vincent A, Cull-Candy S Q, Newsom-Davis J *et al.* (1981) Congenital myasthenia: end plate acetylcholine receptors and electrophysiology in five cases. *Muscle and Nerve* 4:306–318.

Voit T (1998) Congenital muscular dystrophies: 1997 update. *Brain Dev* 20:65–74.

Wallgren-Petterson C (1998) Genetics of the nemaline myopathies and the myotubular myopathies. *Neuromusc Disord* 8:401–404.

Wallgreen-Petterson C, Avela K, Marchmand S *et al.* (1995) A gene for autosomal recessive nemaline myopathy assigned to chromosome 2q by linkage analysis. *Neuromusc Disord* 5:441–443.

Wallgreen-Petterson C & Laing N G (1996) Nemaline myopathy. *Neuromusc Disord* 6:389–391.

Wallgreen-Pettersson C & Thomas N S T (1994) A report on the 20th ENMC sponsored workshop: myotubular/centronuclear myopathy. *Neuromusc Disord.* 4:71–74.

# Section XI
# Hydrocephalus and neurosurgery

# Chapter 42 Fetal neurosurgical interventions

M. Y. Chan, R. W. Jennings and B. Westerburg

## INTRODUCTION

Fetal neurosurgical intervention is the natural sequelae of advances in sonography and invasive diagnostic procedures that have dramatically changed the understanding and management of many congenital neurological anomalies. Prenatal sonographic detection and serial examinations have made it possible not only to define their natural history, but also to determine the features that most affect clinical outcome. Sonography can now identify a growing number of disorders at a stage of development early enough to plan management strategies to improve prognosis. Fetal surgery can now be considered if: (1) prenatal diagnostic methods can accurately identify fetuses that would most benefit; (2) the pathophysiology and natural history of the disease are well understood; (3) the natural history can be altered by intervention; and (4) the risk to thc mother is small (Harrison 1993). From the fetus' perspective, the risk of the procedure is weighed against the benefit of correcting a fatal or debilitating defect. The risks and benefits for a mother are more difficult to assess. She must incur the risk of surgery and preterm labor while not deriving any direct health benefits. If the uterus is opened, the mother may require a Cesarean section for all subsequent births to prevent the possibility of uterine rupture. While most prenatally diagnosed neurological malformations are best managed by medical and surgical therapy after term delivery, *in utero* intervention for hydrocephalus and myelomeningocele, although currently experimental, may potentially offer superior outcomes.

## TREATMENT OF FETAL HYDROCEPHALUS

### ANIMAL STUDIES

The successful treatment of neonatal hydrocephalus with postnatal CSF shunting generated considerable enthusiasm in attempting prenatal treatment of fetal hydrocephalus. Experimentally, Michejda & Hodgen (1981) created a fetal rhesus monkey model of fetal hydrocephalus by administering the teratogen triamcinolone acetonide to pregnant females during the first several weeks of gestation resulting in hydrocephalus and neural tube defects in 90% of fetuses. They followed the neural tube defects and development of hydrocephalus using ultrasonography, α-fetoprotein levels, and fetoscopy. Untreated hydrocephalic monkeys developed severe, progressive ventricular enlargement, marked growth retardation, poor coordination, and frequent seizures; most died within 2 weeks of delivery. The monkeys that received antenatal CSF shunts at the beginning of the 3rd trimester not only survived, but also demonstrated markedly superior postnatal development of motor skills and grew at near-normal rates (Michejda & Hodgen 1981). Glick and Harrison, working with fetal lambs and monkeys, created animal models of hydrocephalus uncomplicated by concomitant neurological abnormalities by injecting kaolin into the cisterna magna during the third trimester (Glick *et al.* 1984). They reported that shunting, 21–25 days later, improved gross ventriculomegaly and overall survival.

### HUMAN STUDIES

The first human trial of *in utero* treatment of hydrocephalus was described by Birnholz & Frigoletto (1981) in a fetus with progressive hydrocephalus diagnosed at 24 weeks. Six serial, atraumatic, cephalocenteses were performed between weeks 25 and 32 under ultrasound guidance (Fig. 42.1 A–D). After the 28th week, cranial puncture became increasingly difficult because of advanced ossification. Delivered at 35 weeks of gestation, the infant received a postnatal ventricular-peritoneal shunt; however, at 16 months of age, it remained severely developmentally retarded. It was later discovered that the infant had Becker's muscular dystrophy and unrecognized intracranial abnormalities (Cromblehome 1994). Nevertheless, it was felt that intermittent serial cephalocentesis would not be able to deliver consistent ventricular decompression (Milhorat 1978; Lorber & Grainger 1983).

This led to the development of experimental ventriculo-amniotic shunt systems. Clewell *et al.* (1982) described the first ventriculo-amniotic shunt placement for hydrocephalus in a human fetus in 1982 (Fig. 42.2A–C).

The fetus carried a diagnosis of X-linked aqueductal stenosis, and the treatment plan was conceived and performed by a multispecialty team of perinatologists, radiologists, a neurosurgeon, a bioengineer, and a geneticist. After the procedure, there was a decrease in the ventricular size, LVH/HW, and biparietal diameter, with a concomitant increase in cortical mantle thickness. The infant was delivered at 32 weeks of gestation, and a standard ventriculo-peritoneal shunt was placed postnatally. Several other groups reported similar decreases in ventricular size after shunt placement (Duncan *et al.* 1982; Frigoletto *et al.* 1982; Depp *et al.* 1983).

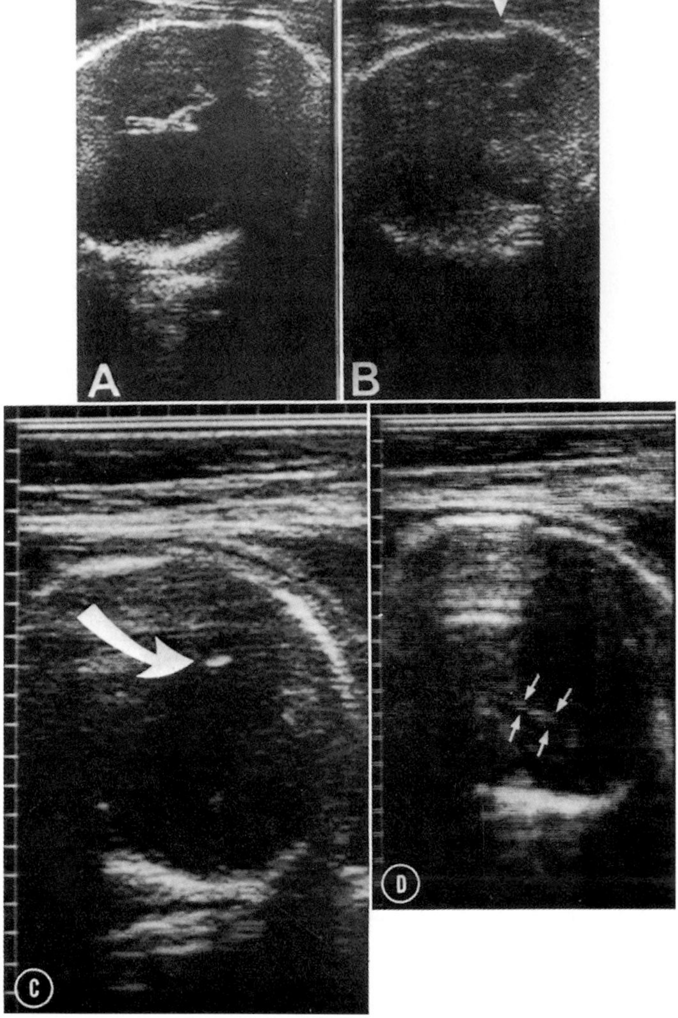


Figure 42.1 (A) Sonogram of fetal head prior to cephalocentesis. (B) Sonogram of fetal head after cephalocentesis with arrow pointing to overlapping cranial sutures. (C) Sonogram of fetal head with arrow pointing to tip of 18-gauge needle in dilated ventricle. (D) Sonogram of fetal head after cephalocentesis, with arrows outlining stream of blood.

The following guidelines for fetal hydrocephalus patient selection were recommended by Frigoletto *et al.* 1981 (Birnholz & Frigoletto 1981).

1. The hydrocephalus should be detected sufficiently early that delivery and postnatal shunting are not realistic options.
2. The hydrocephalus should appear as a simple obstructive variety without associated major dysmorphic brain development.
3. The hydrocephalus should not be associated with other major malformations that are themselves incompatible with survival or that indicate an irremediable malformation syndrome.
4. Each pregnancy should be evaluated for chromosomal abnormalities and associated neural tube defects during initial work-up.
5. The ventricular dilatation should be progressive.
6. Pretreatment evaluation should include a multidisciplinary team's consultation with physicians in perinatology, neonatology, ultrasonography, neurosurgery, and genetics.

The consensus in the early 1980s was that the ideal patient for intervention was one with progressive ventriculomegaly that was isolated from any concomitant congenital anomalies.

Subsequently, the international Fetal Surgery Registry was established in 1982 with the dual goal of (1) providing updated information on cumulative results to all inquiring institutions and (2) accumulating data to assess treatment efficacy and safety (Clewell *et al.* 1982; Manning *et al.* 1986). In 1986, the results of 44 procedures for obstructive hydrocephalus reported to the registry over the preceding 3 years were published (Table 42.1) (Manning *et al.* 1986).

These cases were drawn from a large number of centers but had no consistent selection criteria for intervention. In this series of patients, the survival after *in utero* shunt placement was 83%. However, the overall mortality was 19%, over half of which were procedure-related (10.25%) (Fig. 42.3A–C). Even more troubling was that 53% of survivors were left with

**Table 42.1 Fetal obstructive hydrocephalus: distribution by primary diagnosis and survival in 41 treated cases**

| Primary diagnosis (postnatal) | No of cases | Percentage of total cases | No of deaths | Percentage mortality by diagnosis | No of survivors | Percentage survival by diagnosis |
|---|---|---|---|---|---|---|
| Aqueductal stenosis | 32 | 76.9 | 4 | 13.3 | 28 | 87.5 |
| Associated anomalies | 5 | 12.7 | 2 | 40 | 3 | 60 |
| Holoprosencephaly | 1 | 2.6 | 0 | 0 | 1 | 100 |
| Dandy-Walker syndrome | 1 | 2.6 | 0 | 0 | 1 | 100 |
| Parencephalic cyst | 1 | 2.6 | 0 | 0 | 1 | 100 |
| Arnold-Chiari syndrome | 1 | 2.6 | 0 | 0 | 1 | 100 |
| Total | 41 | 100 | 7 | 17 | 34 | 83 |

*Source*: Adapted from Harrison *et al.* (1990).

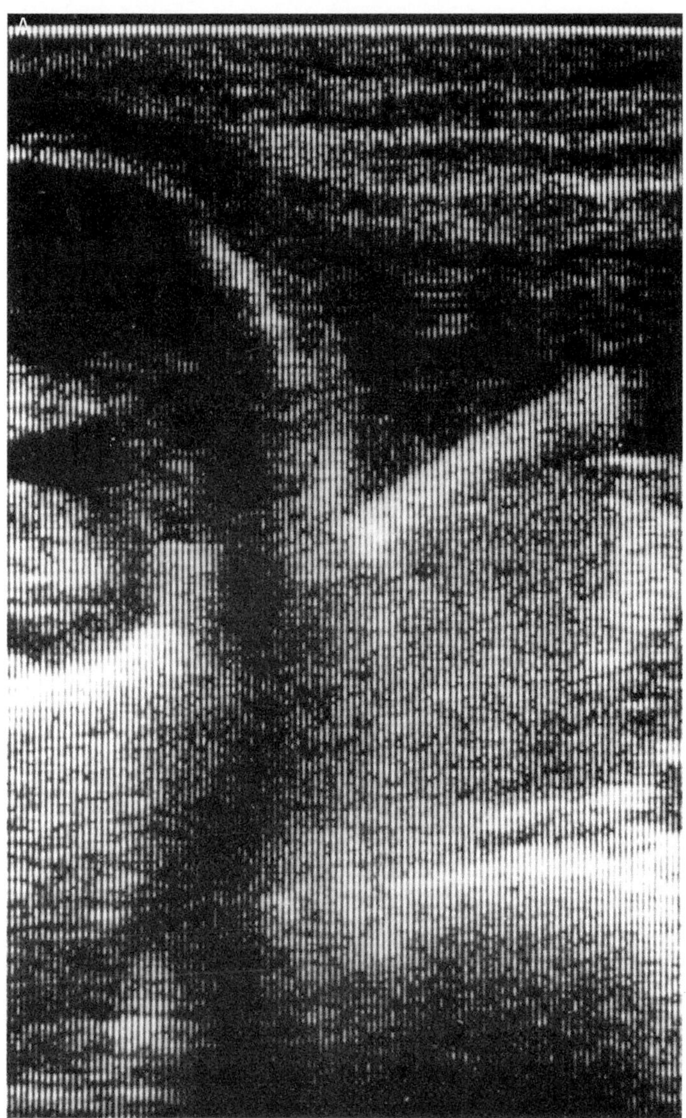

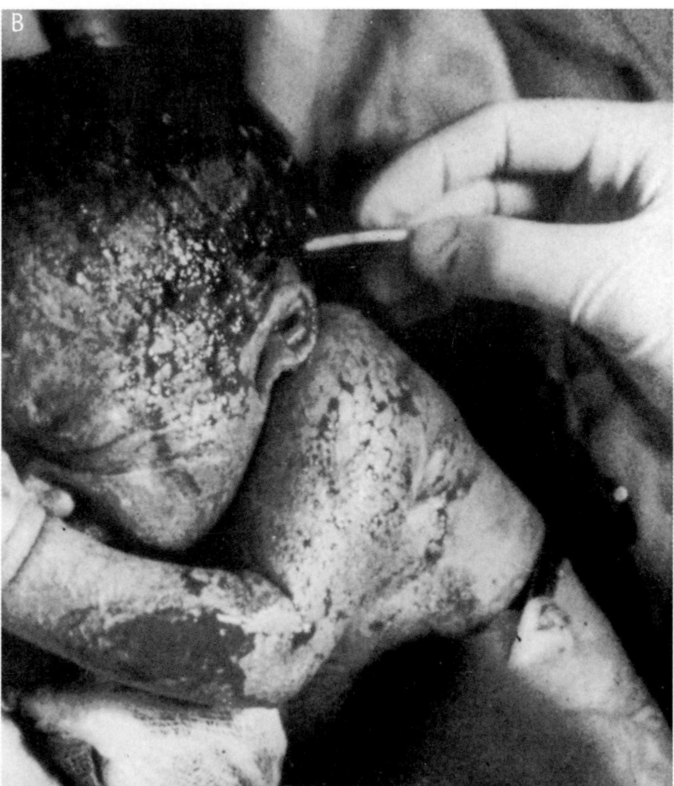

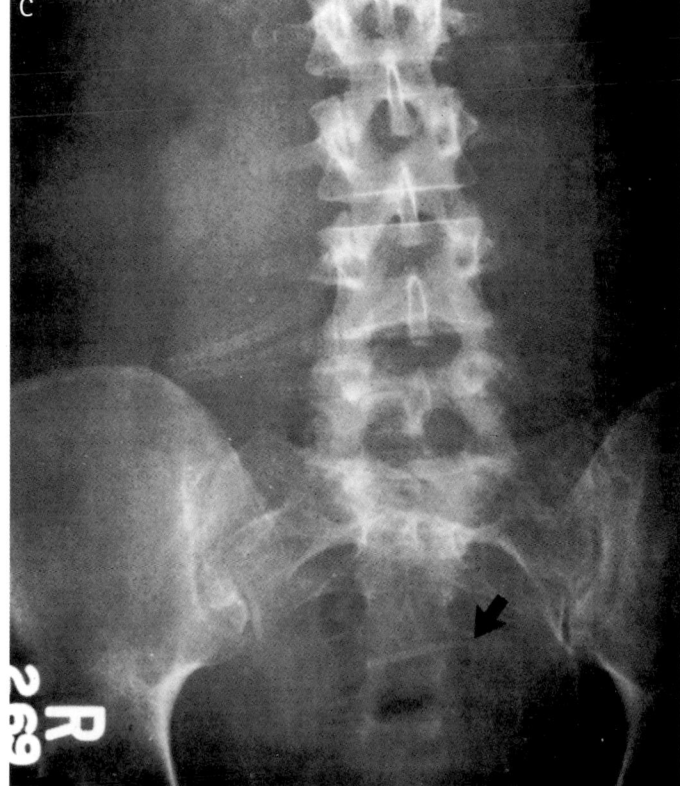


Figure 42.2 (A) Cranial sonogram demonstrating ventriculoamniotic shunt protruding from fetal skull. (B) Ventriculoamniotic shunt protruding from skull of newborn infant. (C) Radiograph demonstrating ventriculoamniotic shunt entering fetal skull (arrow).

moderate to serious neurological handicaps, and only 12% developed normally (Manning *et al.* 1986).

Although these shunt systems had sparked considerable enthusiasm, it became clear that the results were poor (Cromblehome 1994). This was primarily because many of these patients had CNS and non-CNS anomalies that went undetected. In fact, the associated comorbidities, rather than the degree of ventriculomegaly, overwhelmingly determined

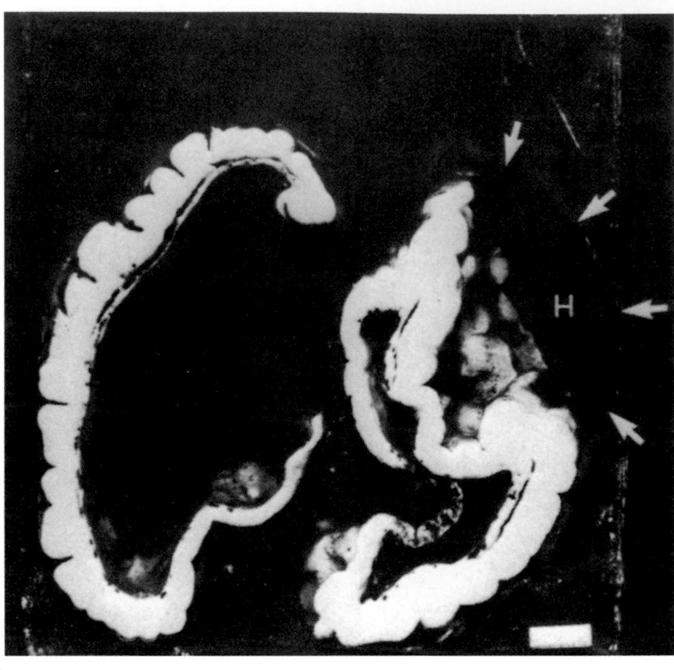


A

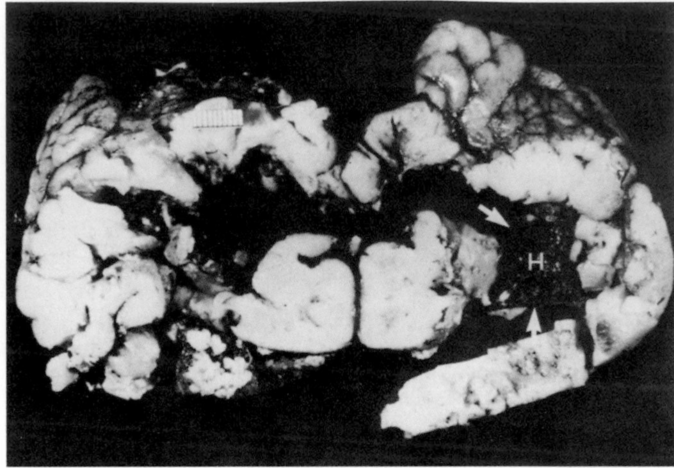


B

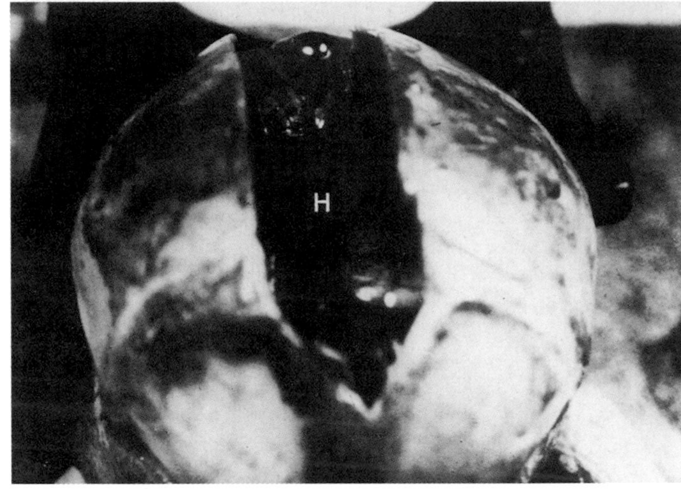


C

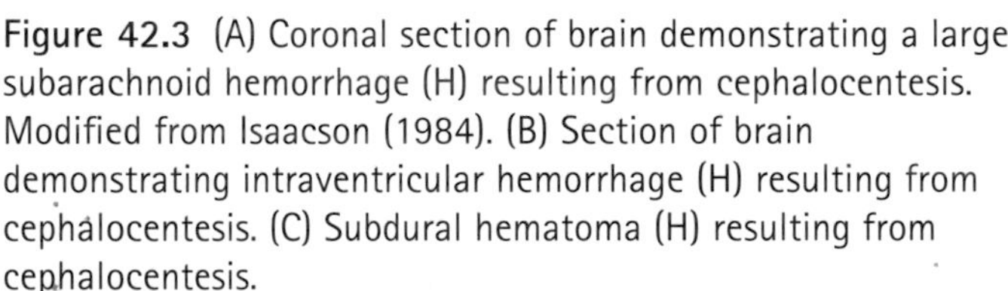

**Figure 42.3** (A) Coronal section of brain demonstrating a large subarachnoid hemorrhage (H) resulting from cephalocentesis. Modified from Isaacson (1984). (B) Section of brain demonstrating intraventricular hemorrhage (H) resulting from cephalocentesis. (C) Subdural hematoma (H) resulting from cephalocentesis.

prognosis. Furthermore, the shunts failed to deliver consistent ventricular decompression due to clogging and migration (Manning *et al.* 1986). As a result of this 1986 report and the inadequacies in diagnosis and shunting technique, the Fetal Medicine and Surgery Society recommended that intrauterine treatment of obstructive hydrocephalus be considered of unproven efficacy and an experimental procedure to be attempted only at highly specialized centers (Manning 1986; Adzick & Harrison 1994).

In June 1999, Bruner and Tulipan in Vanderbilt performed an open fetal surgical placement of ventricular shunt for fetal X-linked hydrocephalus. It remains to be seen how the infant will develop neurologically; however, the case has spurred renewed public interest in the possibility of fetal treatment for hydrocephalus.

## TREATMENT OF MYELOMENINGOCELE AND THE CHIARI II MALFORMATION (see also p. 205)

Myelomeningocele (MMC), the most severe form of spina bifida, is defined as a herniation of the meninges, spinal cord, and nerve roots through a cleft in the spinal column (Harrison *et al.* 1980; Reigel 1982; Longaker *et al.* 1991). All children born with MMC develop an associated Chiari II malformation that is characterized by a low-lying tentorium, small posterior fossa, and abnormal cerebellum with downward displacement of the vermis through the foramen magnum (Cottron *et al.* 1999; Guin 1999) (see Table 42.2).

## ANIMAL STUDIES

Although it is accepted that the congenital defect of MMC contributes significantly to neurological dysfunction, growing experimental evidence suggests major damage to the exposed spinal cord as a result of environmental factors occurring during gestation. Drewek *et al.* (1997) showed that after 34 weeks of gestation, the amniotic fluid became toxic to cultured rat spinal cord tissue. Studies of surgically induced neural tube defects in fetal animals have demonstrated that prenatal repair of the lesion may preserve neurological function (Heffez *et al.* 1990). Mueli *et al.* (1995a,b) created a spina bifida-type defect at 75 days of gestation in

**Table 42.2 Chiari classification of hindbrain hernias**

| Chiari class | Pathologic changes |
|---|---|
| Chiari I | Caudal movement of the cerebellar tonsils<br>Impaction of the tonsils through the foramen magnum (usually >3 mm)<br>Tip of the tonsils is rarely below C-2<br>Commonly associated with syringohydromyelia |
| Chiari II | Caudal movement of the cerebellar vermis through the foramen magnum<br>Commonly, the lower brainstem and 4th ventricle migrate caudally as well<br>Seen almost exclusively in association with MMC |
| Chiari III | Displacement of the cerebellum and brainstem into a high cervical pouch<br>Patients generally have a guarded prognosis with regard to eventual level of function |

*Source*: Adapted from Ranzzino *et al.*

fetal lambs. Four weeks later, the developing MMC lesions were repaired *in utero*. Unrepaired lambs were characterized by complete sensorimotor paraplegia and urinary and stool incontinence. Evaluation of the sagittal brain sections revealed that lambs undergoing the creation of a myelomeningocele-type lesion developed distinct signs of the Chiari II malformation (Fig. 42.4). Repaired lambs, however, demonstrated near-normal neurological function with only mild paraparesis and no signs of incontinence.

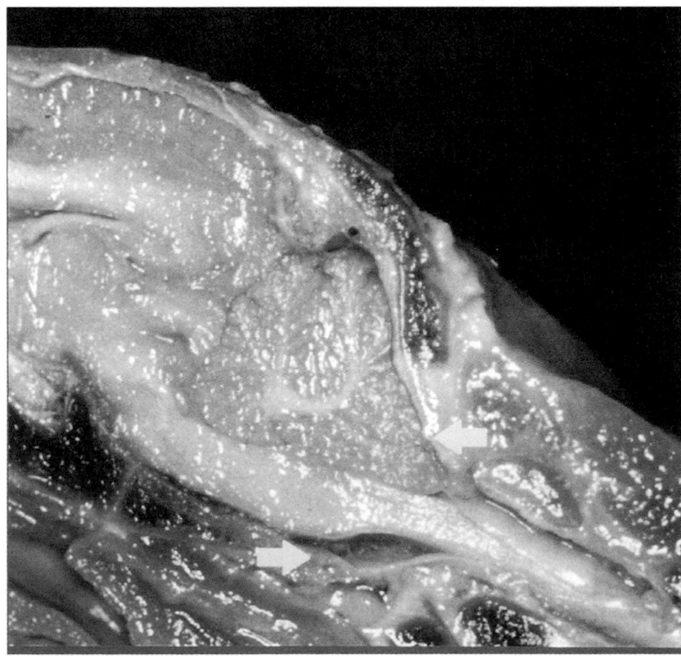

**Figure 42.4** Development of the Chiari II malformation in the unrepaired myelomeningocele-type lesion.

Additionally, all animals that had undergone repair of the lesion either by coverage with Alloderm or by primary neurosurgical repair did not show any signs of a Chiari II malformation (Fig. 42.5A–C). The posterior fossa was of normal size, and the medulla and vermis of the cerebellum were located well above the foramen magnum.

Similarly, Michejda (1984) created a spina bifida-like lesion in eight Macaca mulatta fetuses by performing intrauterine lumbar laminectomies and displacing the spinal cords from the central canals. In five monkeys, this condition was repaired *in utero*. At delivery, the five repaired animals developed normally, while those with open lesions were paraplegic with lower extremity somatosensory loss and incontinence. Heffez *et al.* (1990) reproduced similar results in a rat model. It is now hypothesized that the neurological defects seen in children with MMC result from both congenital myelodysplasia and progressive intrauterine spinal cord injury (Hoffman *et al.* 1987).

## PATHOGENESIS

The development of the fetal brain and calvaria are interlinked and exquisitely dependent on fluid pressures. In the normally developing fetal CNS, the CSF develops in the lateral and 3rd ventricles and passes through the aqueduct into the 4th ventricle. From here, the fluid flows through the lateral recesses into the posterior fossa to bathe the developing fetal cerebellum. This gentle fluid distention enlarges the size of the fetal posterior fossa as the fluid works its way around the tentorium, separating the cerebellum from the cranial fossa. Upon reaching the vein of Galen, the fluid is reabsorbed. Of note, the CSF also flows around the developing spinal cord. However, within the central spinal canal, the CSF is essentially stagnant. The fluid access to the spinal canal is via the obex located on the anterior surface of the 4th ventricle.

Early views suggested that the Chiari II malformation was a result of a tethered spinal cord pulling the posterior fossa structures downward (Fig. 42.6). In the 1960s, Gardner proposed the hydrodynamic hypothesis in which alteration in CSF dynamics at the craniospinal junction arises from a failure of the primitive rhombic roof to be permeable during fetal development (Caban & Bentson 1982). Accordingly, obstruction of the foramen of Magendie results in hydrocephalus and caudal displacement of the tentorium and hindbrain (Carmer 1982).

An alternative hypothesis is that fluid drainage from the posterior fossa creates a low-pressure situation so that the posterior cranial fossa is not induced to increase its capacity (Fig. 42.7). This leakage of low-pressure fluid can occur through an open MMC. In such a case, CSF in the 4th ventricle flows into the obex, down the central canal, and out into the amniotic fluid. This creates a low-pressure circuit with concomitant lower posterior fossa distention pressures. Because of this low-resistance circuit, there is little fluid accumulation in the posterior fossa. As the fetal

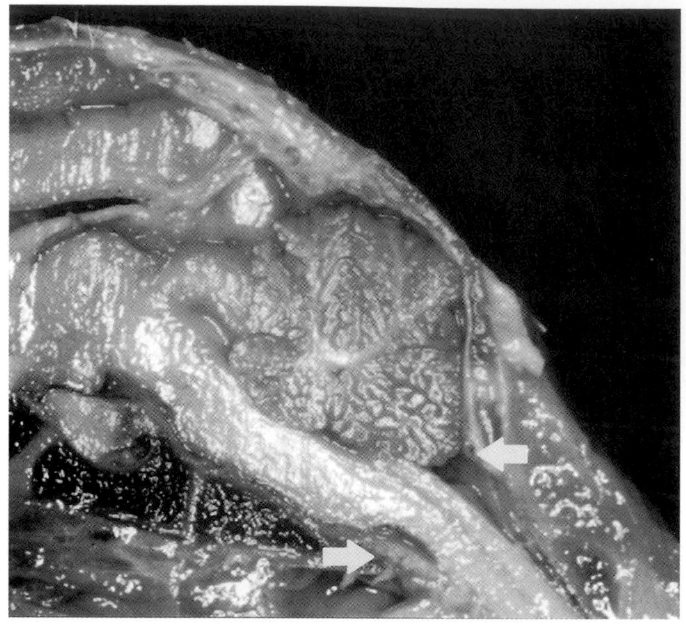
A

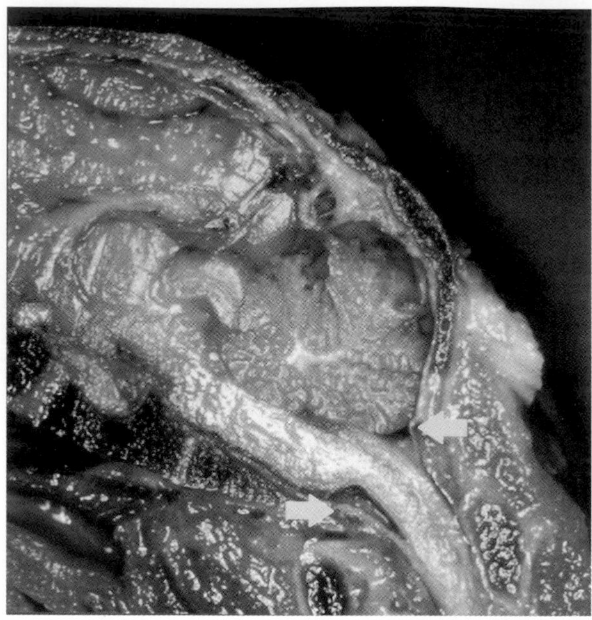
C

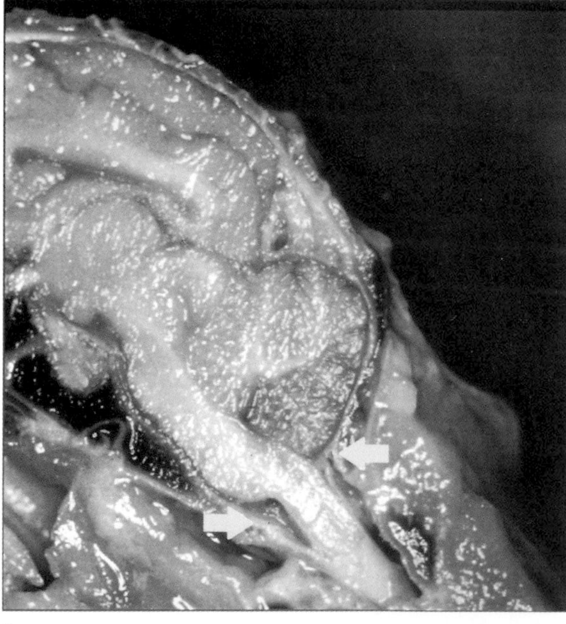
B

Figure 42.5 Absence of Chiari II malformation. Arrows indicate level of foramen magnum. (A) Control lamb without creation of a surgical myelomeningocele-type lesion. (B) Lamb with standard neurosurgical repair. (C) Lamb with synthetic Alloderm used as coverage.

cerebellum develops, it is forced to fill a smaller volume, resulting in a higher resistance to flow around the cerebellum in order to get the outside of the cerebellum into the posterior fossa.

Due to the unique anatomy of the fetal brain, even when the cerebellum essentially obstructs fluid flow around and into the posterior fossa, the fluid still flows out through the obex and down the central canal into the amniotic fluid. It is only later in the development of the brain that fluid egress is inhibited to create the hydrocephalus that results from increased fluid build-up within the ventricles. In this theory, hydrocephalus is a consequence of hindbrain herniation, rather than the cause. Based on this relatively simple hydrodynamic theory of fetal brain development, correction of the MMC lesion may prevent some or all elements of impending Chiari II malformation.

## CURRENT PREVENTION AND TREATMENT

Although approximately 25% of MMCs can be prevented by adequate dietary folic acid intake during pregnancy (see Chapter 19), a significant number will still develop despite adequate replacement. With widespread maternal serum α-fetoprotein screening and the use of high-resolution ultra-

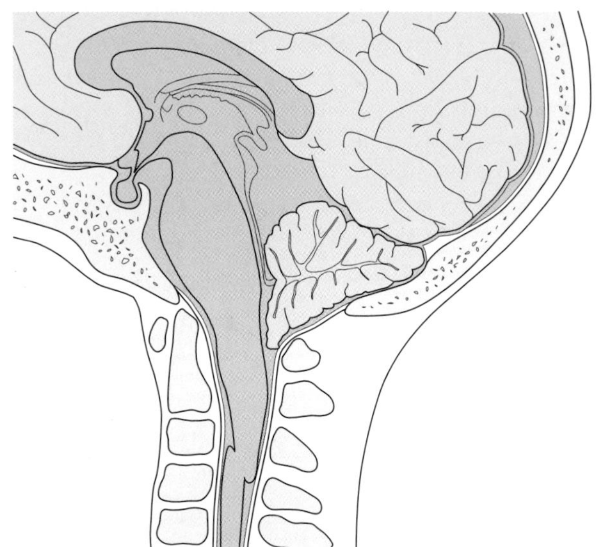

**Figure 42.6** Chiari II malformation.

sonography, over 80% of the cases of fetal MMC are now detectable in the mid-2nd trimester of pregnancy. Nevertheless, despite early detection, management options have been limited to either termination or continuation of the pregnancy with neonatal therapy. In light of this, the concept of *in utero* surgery to correct the defect of MMC before the open spinal cord can be damaged remains extremely attractive.

## PROSPECTS FOR FETAL SURGERY

Recently, open fetal surgery for myelomeningocele has emerged as a viable solution to prevent neurological dysfunction in the newborn. Adzick *et al.* (1998) reported the first clinical case of fetal surgery for MMC in a 23-week infant who later demonstrated improved distal neurological function. Subsequently, Tulipan and Brunner have shown that, despite a significant risk of preterm labor and preterm delivery, patients treated with *in utero* repair had a significantly decreased need for ventriculo-peritoneal shunting and hindbrain herniation compared to cohort controls (Tulipan & Bruner 1998; Tulipan *et al.* 1998). Recently, they have published a single-institution, non-randomized observation study comparing 29 patients with isolated fetal MMC repaired between 24 and 30 weeks to 23 historical controls (Bruner *et al.* 1999). Cases were matched for diagnosis, level of lesion, practice parameters, and calendar time, and all infants were followed up for a minimum of 6 months after delivery. Not only did they find an older median age at shunt placement (50 vs. 5 days), but they reported a 35% reduction in the need for VP shunting after *in utero* repair. They suggested that this may be explained by a 60% reduction in the incidence of hindbrain herniation among study infants. It should be noted, however, that patients were at a significantly higher risk of oligohydramnios and preterm labor compared to controls. Concurrently, Adzick *et al.* reported on a series of ten patients undergoing MMC closure between 22 and 25 weeks (Sutton *et al.* 1999). No controls were utilized. Using serial MRI scans at 19–24 weeks (prior to fetal

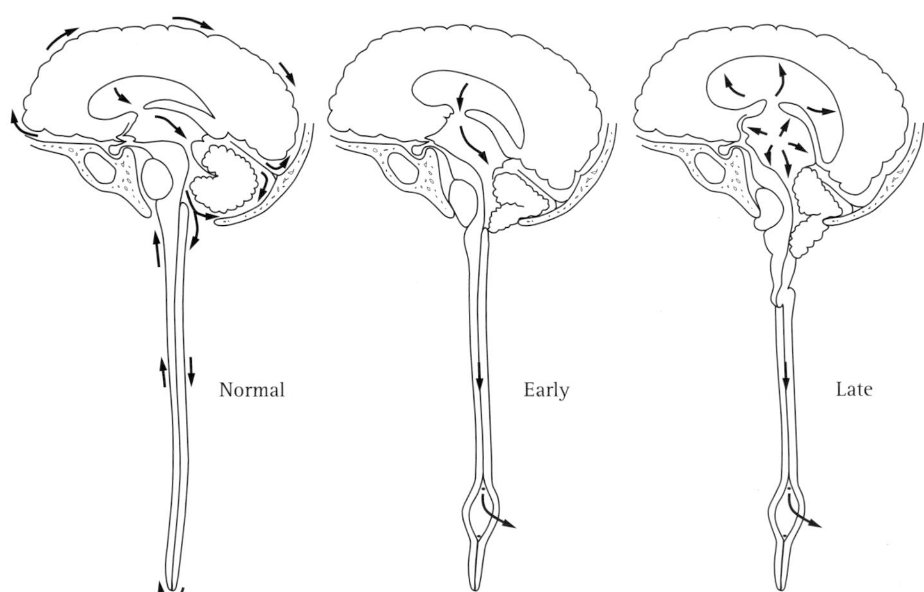


**Figure 42.7** Development of the Chiari II malformation. Normal development of the brain and the skull, in particular the posterior fossa, is thought to be dependent upon gentle distention of the embryonic ventricles. Decrease of pressure due to loss of spinal fluid through a myelomeningocele lesion induces the development of an abnormally small posterior fossa. This malformation causes the herniation of brainstem and cerebellum through the foramen magnum and tentorium. As the cerebellum herniates through the foramen magnum, the normal circulation of CSF is obstructed. Hydrocephalus subsequently develops.

surgery) and 3 and 6 weeks after fetal surgery, they demonstrated serial improvement in hindbrain hernation.

## HORIZONS IN FETAL NEUROSURGERY

Although these early reports are encouraging, fetal surgery remains an innovative treatment strategy and is not currently the standard of care for any neurological anomalies. The principal obstacle still encountered in fetal surgery is maternal morbidity and fetal morbidity and mortality from pre-term labor. To minimize the risks of inducing pre-term labor, fetal endoscopic techniques, also known as FETENDO, are being increasingly utilized at several fetal treatment centers for a variety of cases. Ultimately, however, the decision to apply *in utero* surgical techniques widely for neurological anomalies as well as for other organ system anomalies will depend on the long-term effectiveness of the treatment protocols and their ethical acceptability in terms of safety for the mother and quality of life for the affected infant (Wilberg & Baghai 1983).

### Key Points

- Fetal surgery can now be considered if: prenatal diagnostic methods can accurately identify fetuses that would most benefit, the pathophysiology and natural history of the disease are well understood, the natural history can be altered by intervention, and the risk to the mother is small.
- The successful treatment of *neonatal* hydrocephalus with postnatal CSF shunting generated considerable enthusiasm to attempt *prenatal* treatment of fetal hydrocephalus, but results to date have not been encouraging.
- Approximately 25% of MMCs can be prevented by adequate dietary folic acid intake during pregnancy; a significant number will still develop despite adequate replacement.
- With widespread maternal serum alpha-fetoprotein screening and the use of high-resolution ultrasonography, over 80% of the cases of fetal MMC are now detectable in the mid-second trimester of pregnancy.
- Despite early detection, management options have been limited to either termination or continuation of the pregnancy with neonatal therapy.
- Open fetal surgery for myelomeningocele has emerged as a viable solution to prevent neurological dysfunction in the newborn.
- Fetal surgery remains an innovative treatment strategy and is not currently the standard of care for any neurological anomalies.
- The principal obstacle still encountered in fetal surgery is maternal morbidity and fetal morbidity and mortality from pre-term labor.
- To minimize the risks of inducing pre-term labor, fetal endoscopic techniques, also known as FETENDO, are being increasingly utilized at several fetal treatment centers for a variety of cases.
- Ultimately, the decision to widely apply *in utero* surgical techniques for neurological anomalies as well as for other organ system anomalies will depend on the long term effectiveness of the treatment protocols and their ethical acceptability in terms of safety for the mother and quality of life for the affected infant.

## REFERENCES


Adzick N S, Harrison M R (1994) Fetal surgical therapy. *Lancet* 343:897–902.

Adzick N S, Sutton L N, Crombleholme T M *et al.* (1998) Successful fetal surgery for spina bifida [letter]. *Lancet* 352[9141]:1675–1676.

Birnholz J C, Frigoletto F D (1981) Antenatal treatment of hydrocephalus. *N Engl J Med* 303:1021–1023.

Birnholz J C, Frigoletto F D (1981) Antenatal treatment of hydrocephalus. *N Engl J Med* 303:1021–1023.

Bruner J P, Tulipan N, Pachal R L *et al.* (1999) Fetal surgery for myelomeningocele and the incidence of shunt-dependent hydrocephalus. *JAMA* 282:1819–1825.

Caban L, Bentson J (1982) Considerations in the diagnosis and treatment of syringomyelia and the Chiari malformation. *J Neurosurg* 57:24–31.

Carmel P (1982) *The Arnold-Chiari malformation. Pediatric neurosurgery of the developing nervous system.* New York, NY: Grune & Stratton pp. 61–77.

Clewell W H, Johnson M L, Meier P R *et al.* (1982) A surgical approach to the treatment of hydrocephalus. *N Engl J Med* 306:1320–1325.

Clewell W H, Johnson M L, Meier P R *et al.* (1982) A surgical approach to the treatment of hydrocephalus. *N Engl J Med* 306:1320–1325.

Coltran R S, Kumars V & Collins T (1999) *Robbins pathologic basis of disease.* Philadelphia, PA: WB Saunders, 6th edn; pp 1301–1302.

Cromblehome T M (1994) Invasive fetal therapy: Current status and future directions. *Semin Perinatol* 18:385–397.

Depp R, Sabbagha R E, Brown J T *et al.* (1983) Fetal surgery for hydrocephalus: successful *in utero* ventriculoamniotic shunt for Dandy-Walker syndrome. *Obstet Gynecol* 61:710–714.

Drewek M J, Bruner J P, Whetfell W O *et al.* (1997) *Pediatr Neuro Surg* 27:190–193.

Duncan C C, Berkowitz R L, Hobbins J C (1982) Fetal hydrocephalus: An approach to management. Presented at the 32nd Annual Meeting of the Congress of Neurological Surgeons. Toronto, Canada, October 3–8.

Frigoletto F D, Birnholz J C, Greene M F (1982) Antenatal treatment of hydrocephalus by ventriculoamniotic shunting. *N Engl J Med* 248:2496–2497.

Glick P L, Harrison M R, Halks-Miller M *et al.* (1984) Correction of congenital hydrocephalus *in utero.* II. Efficacy of *in utero* shunting. *J Pediatr Surg* 19:870–881.

Guin P R (1999) *Arnold-Chiari malformation. A closer look.* World Arnold-Chiari Association.

Harrison M R, Jester J A, Ross N A (1980) Correction of congenital diaphragmatic hernia *in utero*. The model: intrathoracic balloon produces fetal pulmonary hypoplasia. *Surgery* 88:174–182.

Harrison M (1993) Fetal surgery. *West J Med* 159:341–349.

Heffez D S, Aryanpur J, Hutchins G M *et al.* (1990) The paralysis associated with myelomeningocele: clinical and experimental data implicating a preventable spinal cord injury. *Neurosurgery* 26:987–992.

Heffez D S, Aryanpur J, Hutchins G M *et al.* (1990) The paralysis associated with myelomeningocele: clinical and experimental data implicating a preventable spinal cord injury. *Neurosurgery* 26:987–992.

Hoffman H J, Neill J, Crone K R *et al.* (1987) Hydrosyringomyelia and its management in childhood. *Neurosurgery* 21:347–351.

Longaker M T, Golbus M S, Filly R A *et al.* (1991) Maternal outcome after open fetal surgery. A review of the first 17 human cases. *JAMA* 265:737–741.

Lorber J, Grainger R G (1983) Cerebral cavities following ventricular puncture in infants. *Clin Radiol* 14:98–109.

Manning F A (1986) International fetal surgery registry: 1985 update. *Clin Obstet Gynecol* 29:551–557.

Manning F A, Harrison M R, Rodeck C *et al.* (1986) Catheter shunts for fetal hydronephrosis and hydrocephalus. Report of the International Fetal Surgery Registry. *N Engl J Med* 315:336–340.

Michejda M (1984) Intrauterine treatment of spina bifida: primate model. *Z Kinderchir* 39:259–261.

Michejda M, Hodgen G D (1981) *In utero* diagnosis and treatment of non-human primate fetal skeletal anomalies. I. Hydrocephalus. *JAMA* 246:1093–1097.

Milhorat T H. *Pediatric neurosurgery.* Philadelphia, PA: FA Davis; pp. 112–121.

Mueli M, Mueli-Simmen C, Yingling C D *et al.* (1995a) Creation of myelomeningocele *in utero*: A model of functional damage from spinal cord exposure in fetal sheep. *J Pediatr Surg* 30:1028–1032.

Mueli M, Meuli-Simmen C, Hutchins G M *et al.* (1995b) In utero surgery rescues neurological function at birth in sheep with spina bifida. *Nat Med* 1:342–347.

Reigel D H (1982) *Spina bifida in pediatric neurosurgery, surgery of the developing nervous system.* Section of Pediatric Neurosurgery of the American Association of Neurological Surgeons. New York, NY: Grune & Stratton; Chapter 2, pp. 23–47.

Sutton L N, Adzick N S, Bilaniuk L T *et al.* (1999) Improvement in hindbrain herniation demonstrated by serial fetal magnetic resonance imaging following fetal surgery for myelomeningocele. *JAMA* 282:1826–1831.

Tulipan N & Bruner J P (1998) Myelomeningocele repair *in utero*: a report of three cases. *Pediatr Neurosurg* 28:177–180.

Tulipan N, Hernanz-Shulman M, Bruner J P (1998) Reduced hindbrain hernation after intrauterine myelomeningocele repair: a report of 4 cases. *Pediatr Neurosurg* 29:274–278.

Wilberg J E & Baghai P (1983) *Neurosurgery* 13:596–600.

# Chapter 43

# Neonatal hydrocephalus – clinical assessment and non-surgical treatment

A. Whitelaw

## DEFINITION

Hydrocephalus is defined as excessive accumulation of cerebrospinal fluid (CSF) accompanied by excessive growth of the head. Ventricular dilatation occurs before head enlargement, as the first stage of hydrocephalus, but not all ventricular dilatation progresses to hydrocephalus. Ventricular dilatation can be reversible, may become static without accelerated enlargement, and may be due to cerebral atrophy and not to CSF accumulation.

## CSF CIRCULATION AND ABSORPTION

The mechanism of hydrocephalus is nearly always obstruction somewhere along the pathways to CSF absorption. The choroid plexus in the lateral and third ventricles is the major site of CSF production. The fluid then has to flow through the aqueduct of Sylvius to the fourth ventricles. From here, the fluid leaves through the foramina of Luschka and Magendie into the cisterna magna, from whence it flows through the subarachnoid space around the cerebral hemispheres to be reabsorbed into the blood via the cranial venous sinuses (Fig. 43.1).

In adults and in children, there is good evidence that reabsorption occurs through the arachnoid granulations with their microscopic villi projecting into the venous sinus (Davson *et al.* 1987). Two mechanisms for CSF reabsorption have been proposed: (1) passage through pores on the arachnoid villi; and (2) an energy-consuming pinocytotic process by which intracytoplasmic vacuoles are transported from one side of the arachnoid membrane to the other. The principal advantage of the growth of arachnoid granulations and villi is thought to be the greatly increased surface area available for reabsorption. However, newborn infants do not have visible arachnoid granulations, and microscopic examination has not yet demonstrated any structure corresponding to arachnoid villi in the neonate. The absence of such structures may mean that CSF is absorbed by different mechanisms in the neonate or that the maximum capacity for reabsorption is less than in the adult.

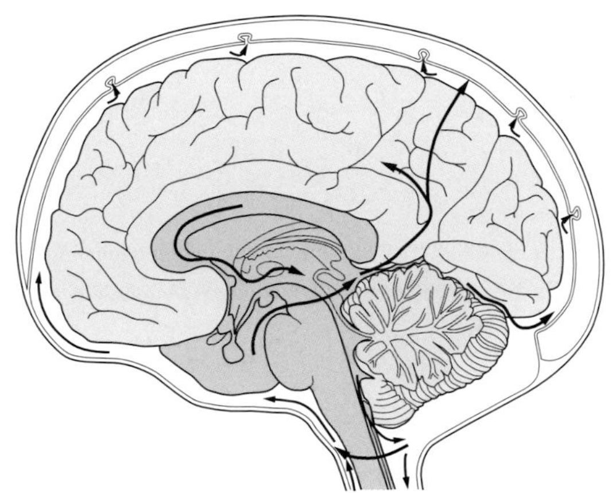

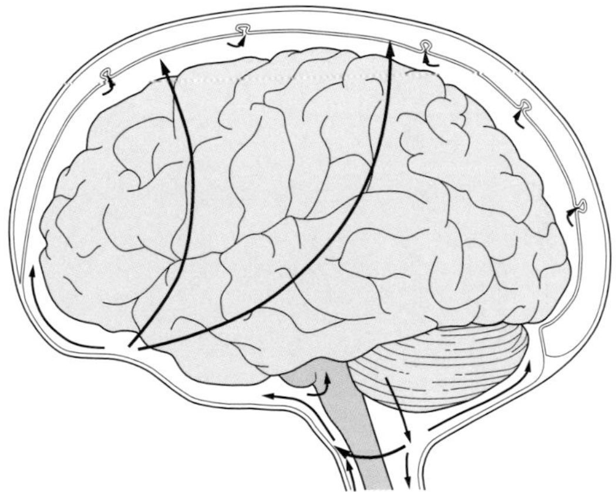

**Figure 43.1** Pathways of CSF flow. (Reproduced, with permission, from Milhorat 1972).

## ETIOLOGY

The overall incidence of infantile hydrocephalus is given as three to four per 1000 live births, but this is almost certainly an underestimate. As an isolated congenital disorder, the incidence is 0.9–1.5 per 1000 births, and when associated with myelomeningocele, it is 1.3–2.9 per 1000 births (Myrianthopoulos & Kurland 1961).

A classification into those cases due to, or associated with, a cerebral malformation, as opposed to those cases due to an acquired lesion, is given in Table 43.1. Hydrocephalus has been noted in a larger number of syndromes (see p. 238), but a genetic etiology for this condition is uncommon. The etiology of the acquired lesions is usually self-evident.

## CONGENITAL OBSTRUCTION OF THE VENTRICULAR SYSTEM

The majority of cases of congenital hydrocephalus are due to narrowing of the aqueduct of Sylvius. Aqueductal

**Table 43.1 Causes of neonatal hydrocephalus**

1. Congenital malformation
   - Aqueduct stenosis:
     - Gliosis
     - Forking of the aqueduct
     - Aqueductal septum
     - 'True' narrowing of the aqueduct
     - X-linked aqueductal stenosis
   - Arnold–Chiari malformation type 2 (hydrocephalus and meningomyelocele)
   - Atresia of the foramina of Luschka and Magendie (Dandy–Walker malformation)
   - As part of a major cerebral malformation, e.g. encephalocele and holoprosencephaly
   - As part of an inherited metabolic disease, e.g. achondroplasia or Hurler's disease
2. Posthemorrhagic
   - Intraventricular hemorrhage:
     - Intrauterine bleeding because of thrombocytopenia or coagulation factor deficiency
     - Respiratory distress syndrome after preterm birth
   - Birth trauma:
     - Subdural hemorrhage
     - Subarachnoid hemorrhage
3. Postinfection
   - Neonatal ventriculitis/meningitis, especially when due to Gram-negative bacilli
   - Intrauterine virus infection, e.g. cytomegalovirus
   - Intrauterine *Toxoplasma gondii*
4. Neoplastic and vascular malformations
5. Benign external hydrocephalus
6. Overproduction of CSF
   - Choroid plexus papilloma
7. Others
   - Craniofacial dysmorphisms
   - Platybasia
   - Osteogenesis imperfecta

stenosis may be due to gliosis, forking of the aqueduct, a septum across the aqueduct, or true narrowing. A small minority of cases of aqueduct stenosis have an X-linked inheritance and this has been associated with mutations in the gene encoding the neural cell-adhesion molecule L1 (Jouet *et al.* 1995). Congenital obstruction of the foramina of Luschka and Magendie leads to gross enlargement of the fourth ventricles into the cisterna magna. The Dandy–Walker malformation is described on p. 240.

The majority of cases of meningomyelocele have hydrocephalus with an associated malformation of the brain. This is referred to as the type 2 Arnold–Chiari malformation (Carmel 1982). The features are caudal dislocation of the medulla oblongata and cerebellar vermis, and the majority have a kink in the medulla. The disturbed anatomy of the fourth ventricle and cisterna magna is thought to be the main reason for hydrocephalus. Arachnoid cysts, congenital tumors, and vascular malformations may produce hydrocephalus by expanding to the extent that they distort and obstruct the aqueduct or fourth ventricle.

## ACQUIRED HYDROCEPHALUS AFTER HEMORRHAGE OR INFECTION

Hydrocephalus may follow either intraventricular or subarachnoid hemorrhage into the CSF (Fig. 43.2). Multiple small clots may obstruct the ventricular system or the channels of reabsorption initially but lead to a chronic arachnoiditis of the basal cisterns involving the deposition of extracellular matrix proteins and obstruction of the foramina of the fourth ventricles or the subarachnoid space over the cerebral hemispheres (Larroche 1972).

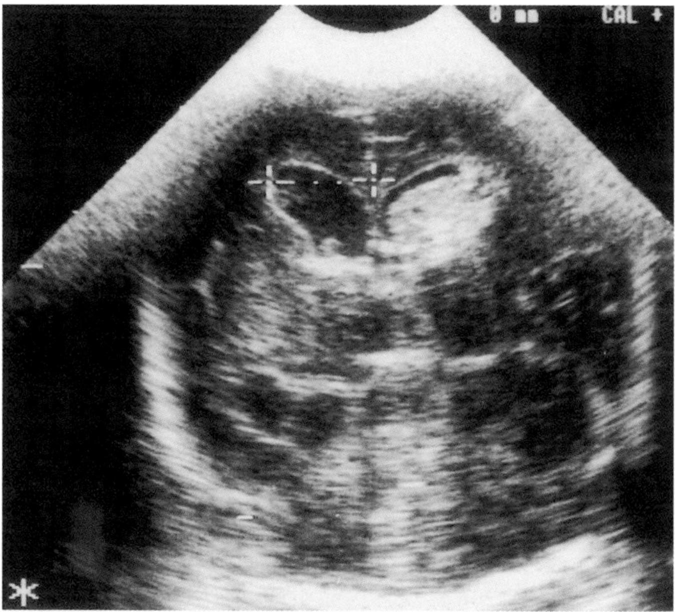


**Figure 43.2** Cerebral ultrasound (coronal view) showing a large intraventricular hemorrhage in the right ventricle. The contralateral ventricle has begun to dilate, and there is CSF visible above the clot. The two caliper marks indicate where the ventricle width was from the midline to the lateral border of the ventricle.

Traumatic hemorrhage into the tentorium or falx may also lead to hydrocephalus by displacement of the aqueduct (Fig. 43.3).

Ventriculitis can give rise to hydrocephalus by inflammatory obstruction of the aqueduct or foramina, and meningitis can produce chronic thickening of the leptomeninges with fibrin deposition (Stewart 1964).

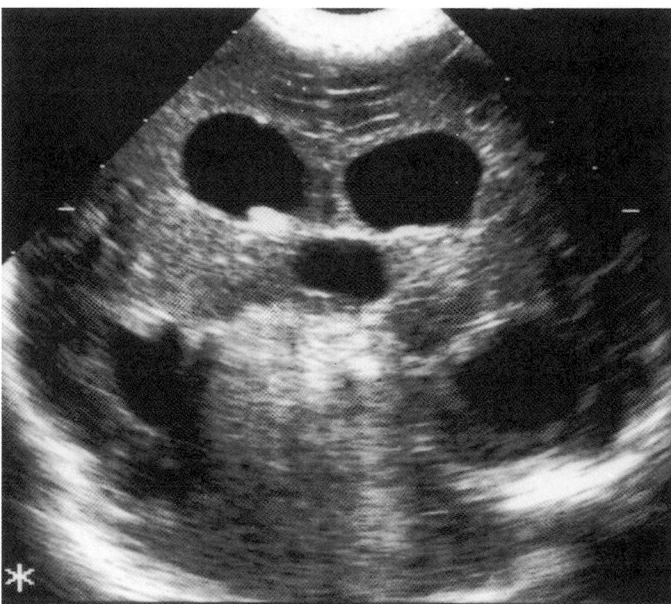

A

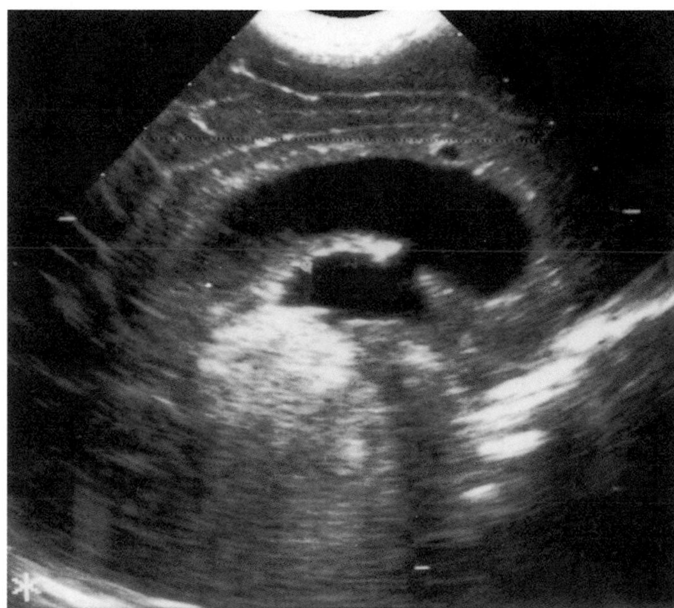

B

Figure 43.3 (A) Cerebral ultrasound (coronal view) showing marked dilatation of both lateral ventricles and the third ventricle with a hemorrhage just below the third ventricle obstructing the aqueduct. (B) Cerebral ultrasound scan (sagittal view) of the same infant as in (A) showing the dilated third ventricle with a hemorrhage below it. The hemorrhage was due to birth trauma.

## TRANSFORMING GROWTH FACTOR-β1 AND POST-HEMORRHAGIC HYDROCEPHALUS

There is mounting evidence that transforming growth factor-β1 (TGF-β1) is involved in the pathogenesis of posthemorrhagic hydrocephalus. TGF-β1 is a cytokine that is chemotactic for fibroblasts and upregulates the expression of genes encoding fibronectin, collagen, and other extracellular matrix proteins. TGF-β1 is involved in wound healing, scar formation, and a variety of pathologic processes including fibrosis in the lung, liver cirrhosis, and glomerulonephritis. TGF-β1 can be synthesized by virtually all cells, and nearly all cells have been shown to have receptors for TGF-β1. It is a 25-kDa disulfide-linked peptide that is secreted bound to a latency associated peptide and requires activation by separation from the latency-associated peptide before it is biologically active. TGF-β1 is synthesized by leptomeningeal cells and is stored in granules of platelets, and these mechanisms may explain how the cytokine could have gained access to the cerebrospinal fluid following IVH. It has been shown that lysis of blood clot *in vitro* releases TGF-β1. TGF-β1 has been demonstrated in the CSF of adults with subarachnoid hemorrhage, and those with elevated levels went on to hydrocephalus (Kitisawa & Tada 1994). Intrathecal administration of TGF-β in mice has produced ventricular dilatation and reduced the number of cilia on the ependyma (Tada *et al.* 1994). Whitelaw *et al.* (1999) showed that TGF-β1 is detectable at very low concentrations in neonatal CSF, infants with transient PHVD have increased CSF concentrations of TGF-β1, and infants who later develop permanent hydrocephalus have even higher CSF concentrations of TGF-β1.

## BENIGN EXTERNAL HYDROCEPHALUS

Ment *et al.* (1981) described 18 infants with transient enlargement of the subarachnoid space without any evidence of subarachnoid hemorrhage. The prognosis is good, but the cause is not understood. A transient disturbance in CSF reabsorption has been postulated. It is important to distinguish the condition from subdural effusion and posthemorrhagic hydrocephalus. There is initially excessive head growth, and CSF pressure may be moderately raised. These two features distinguish it from cerebral atrophy. We have seen seven infants with this condition, and all had a good outcome without surgery (Fig. 43.4).

## OVERPRODUCTION OF CSF

Since the choroid plexus is the main site of CSF production, it is not surprising that enlargement of the plexus (choroid plexus papilloma) can overproduce CSF to a greater extent than it can be absorbed (Milhorat 1982).

## COMMUNICATING AND NON-COMMUNICATING HYDROCEPHALUS

It is conventional to classify hydrocephalus according to whether there is normal communication between the ventricular system and the subarachnoid space. In non-communicating hydrocephalus, a lumbar puncture yields only a few drops of CSF, usually less than 2 ml. In communicating hydrocephalus, a lumbar puncture usually produces

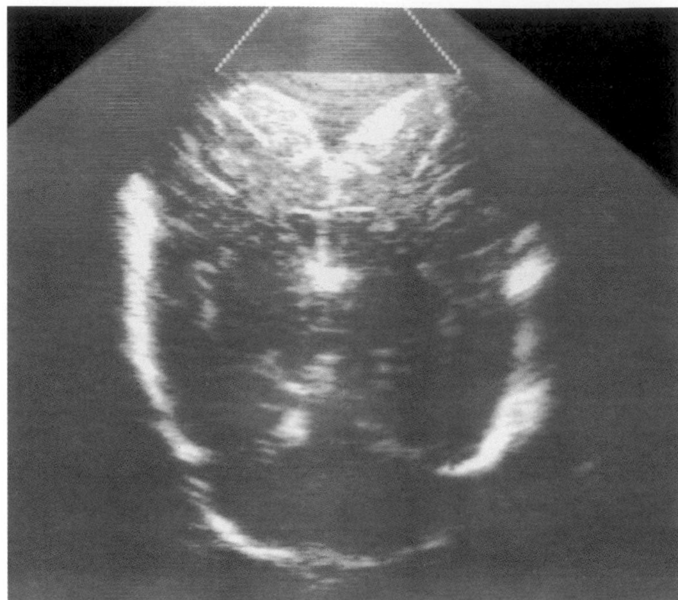

A

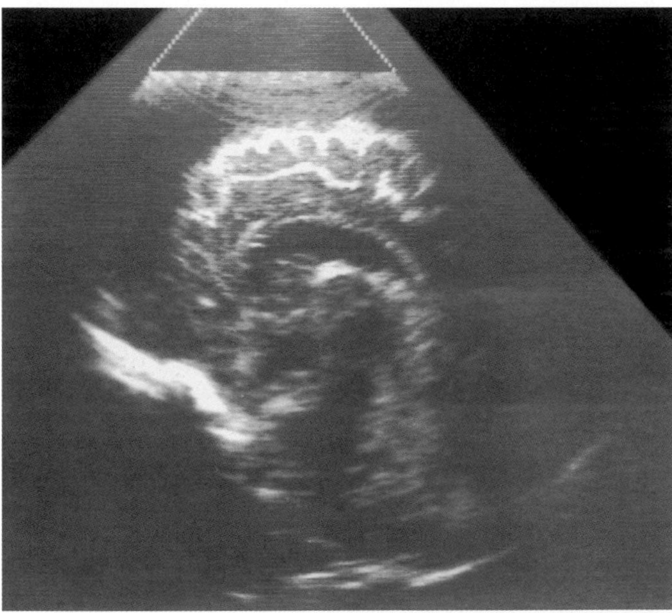

B

Figure 43.4 (A) Cerebral ultrasound scan (coronal view) showing external hydrocephalus. The subarchnoid space is enlarged over the cerebral hemispheres. (B) Cerebral ultrasound scan (parasagittal view) of the same infant as in (A). The subarachnoid space over the cerebral hemisphere is enlarged.

at least 5 ml of CSF and can produce much more. Non-communicating hydrocephalus tends to give a higher CSF pressure and a more rapid rate of ventricular enlargement and therefore requires more urgent investigation and treatment. Communicating hydrocephalus tends to be less rapid in its course, and some cases may be appropriately managed by non-surgical treatment. Isotope cisternography, by which an isotope is injected into the lumbar CSF and its spread to the ventricular or cisternal spaces is followed by gamma camera imaging, is rarely used in infants to determine management. Post-hemorrhagic and postinfectious hydrocephalus may begin as communicating and then become non-communicating after several months.

## HYDROCEPHALUS AND NEUROPATHOLOGIC CHANGES

Animal models of hydrocephalus have demonstrated that progressive ventricular dilatation driven by raised CSF pressure produces flattening and destruction of the ependymal lining, as well as edema and necrosis of the periventricular white matter (Weller *et al.* 1971). There is evidence from neuropathologic studies that a similar process occurs in the developing brain of the human infant (Weller & Shulman 1972). Such periventricular damage would be likely to lead to motor deficits, but mental and sensory functions of the brain might also be damaged and epileptic foci initiated if the effects of edema and pressure were more widespread in the small immature brain.

## DIAGNOSIS

Hydrocephalus may be considered at birth on the basis of a disproportionately large head with bulging fontanelles, wide sutures, and congested scalp veins. In many other cases, hydrocephalus becomes gradually apparent weeks or months after birth. The presence of spina bifida or evidence of previous intracranial hemorrhage or infection further increases the index of suspicion. The confirmation of hydrocephalus requires (1) the demonstration of enlargement of the ventricular system and (2) the demonstration that excessive head enlargement has occurred (head circumference over the 97th centile) or that the rate of head growth is excessive.

### HEAD CIRCUMFERENCE

Head circumference should be measured with a paper tape measure around the largest part of the occiput and the mid-frontal area of the brow without exerting enough pressure to actually compress the head. The head circumference must be plotted on a centile chart that is appropriate for the gestational and postnatal age, sex, and ethnic group of the infant. Most countries have compiled their own centiles for full-term infants. A useful centile chart for preterm infants was compiled by Gairdner & Pearson (1971).

### CRANIAL ULTRASOUND

Cranial ultrasound is by far the quickest, cheapest, and most convenient method of demonstrating ventricular enlargement. Ventricular width measured from the midline to the lateral border of the lateral ventricle in the mid-coronal view is the measurement with the least interobserver variability,

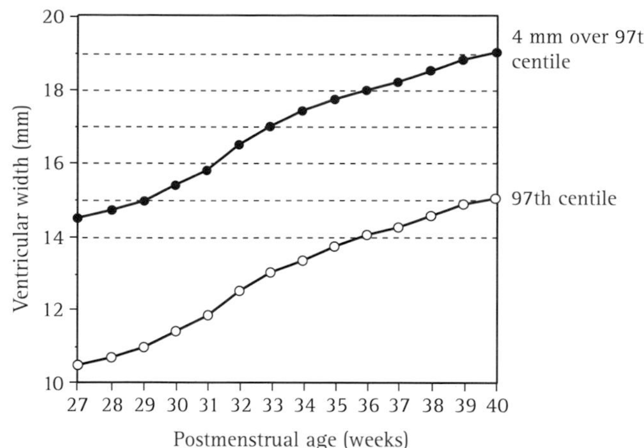


**Figure 43.5** The lower line is the 97th centile for ventricular width of Levene (1981). The upper line defines ventricular dilatation severe enough to be treated (Kaiser & Whitelaw 1985).

and centiles for postmenstrual (gestational) age have been compiled (Levene 1981). We have found 4 mm over the 97th centile (Fig. 43.5) to be a useful criterion for defining genuinely pathologic ventricular enlargement.

Ultrasound has the enormous advantages of portable equipment, brief examination time without sedation, and no irradiation, and remains the first choice for imaging in preference to computerized tomography (CT) or magnetic resonance imaging (MRI).

Ultrasound can demonstrate abnormalities such as a Dandy–Walker cyst (Fig. 43.6), third ventricle clot (Fig. 43.7), and intracerebral calcification or intraventricular fibrin strands after ventriculitis (Fig. 43.8).

CT or MR may be needed to better define atypical cases or to show a tumor or subdural hematoma. The role of different imaging techniques is discussed in Chapter 6.

## WHEN IS VENTRICULAR DILATATION DUE TO ATROPHY OR MALFORMATION?

It is important to distinguish ventricular dilatation due to atrophy from hydrocephalus due to excessive CSF under pressure. Cerebral atrophy can result in enlargement of the ventricles, but the ventricular outline is usually irregular, and there may be other features of cerebral atrophy such as widening of the interhemispheric fissure. Observation over time will show whether the head is growing excessively or not. In pure cerebral atrophy, the head growth is usually slower than normal and certainly does not grow excessively. Loss of cerebral substance following hemorrhagic infarction or periventricular leukomalacia may coexist with progressive hydrocephalus. Some infants with midline cerebral defects such as agenesis of the corpus callosum or holoprosencephaly have dilated cerebral ventricles without raised CSF pressure or excessive head growth.

## NEUROLOGIC EXAMINATION

As well as establishing the diagnosis, it is important to document the infant's necrologic state (Chapter 8). Raised intracranial pressure may be associated with irritability,

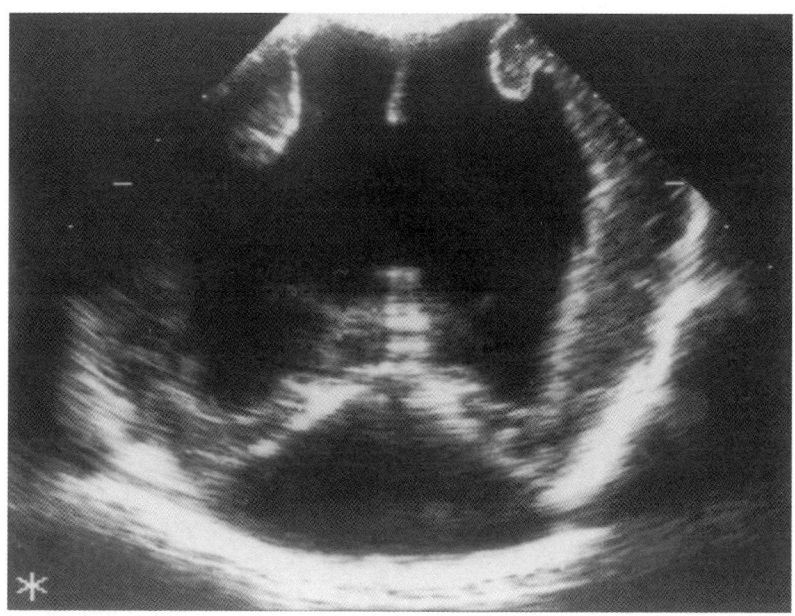

**Figure 43.6** Cerebral ultrasound scan (coronal view). There is hydrocephalus associated with a midline defect (holoprosencephaly) and a large fluid space posterior to the cerebellum due to obstruction of the foramina (Dandy–Walker cyst).

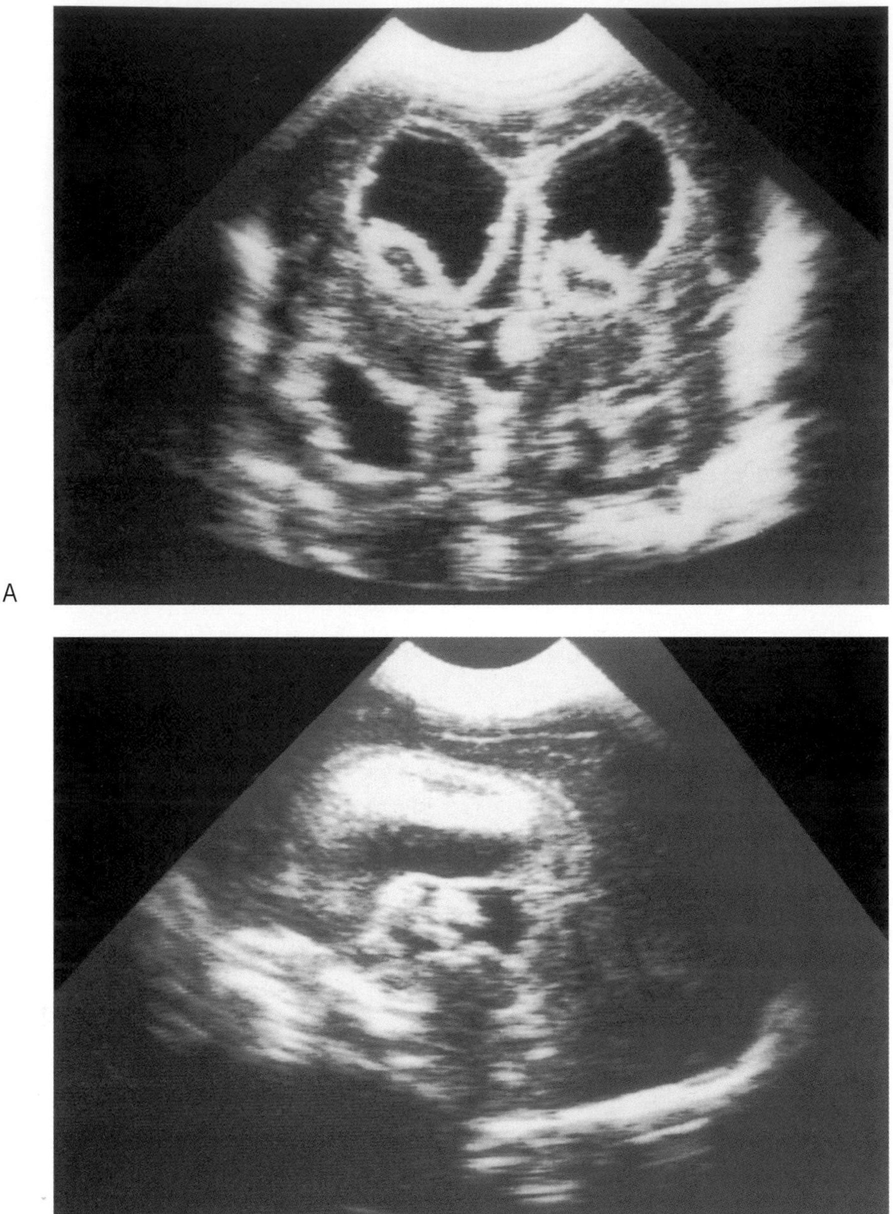


Figure 43.7 (A) Cerebral ultrasound scan (coronal view) showing large clots in both lateral ventricles. In addition, the third ventricle is dilated and contains several clots. (B) Cerebral ultrasound scan (sagittal view) showing the dilated third ventricle containing several clots in addition to the normal massa intermedia.

vomiting, and increased extensor tone in the limbs with increased tendon reflexes. However, some infants with definite hydrocephalus exhibit no such signs. The hydrocephalus may have developed slowly, and the splaying of the sutures may have prevented the intracranial pressure from rising considerably. Some infants with hydrocephalus after intraventricular hemorrhage may show hypotonia with a disproportionately tight popliteal angle. Asymmetry is unusual. In neonates, visual fixation to a target may be impaired, but the hearing response is usually normal. Eye movements may be abnormal, but sunsetting, so often quoted as a sign of hydrocephalus, is relatively non-specific in our experience. An objective means of recording the neurologic examination is helpful in comparing examinations (Dubowitz & Dubowitz 1981).

After a full review of the pregnancy, delivery, and immediate neonatal period, together with a clinical examination and a careful ultrasound examination, it is usually possible to classify the baby into one of the etiological groups above. If no obvious explanation for the hydrocephalus can be given, intrauterine infection should be investigated, and a careful family history should be taken. Coagulation factor

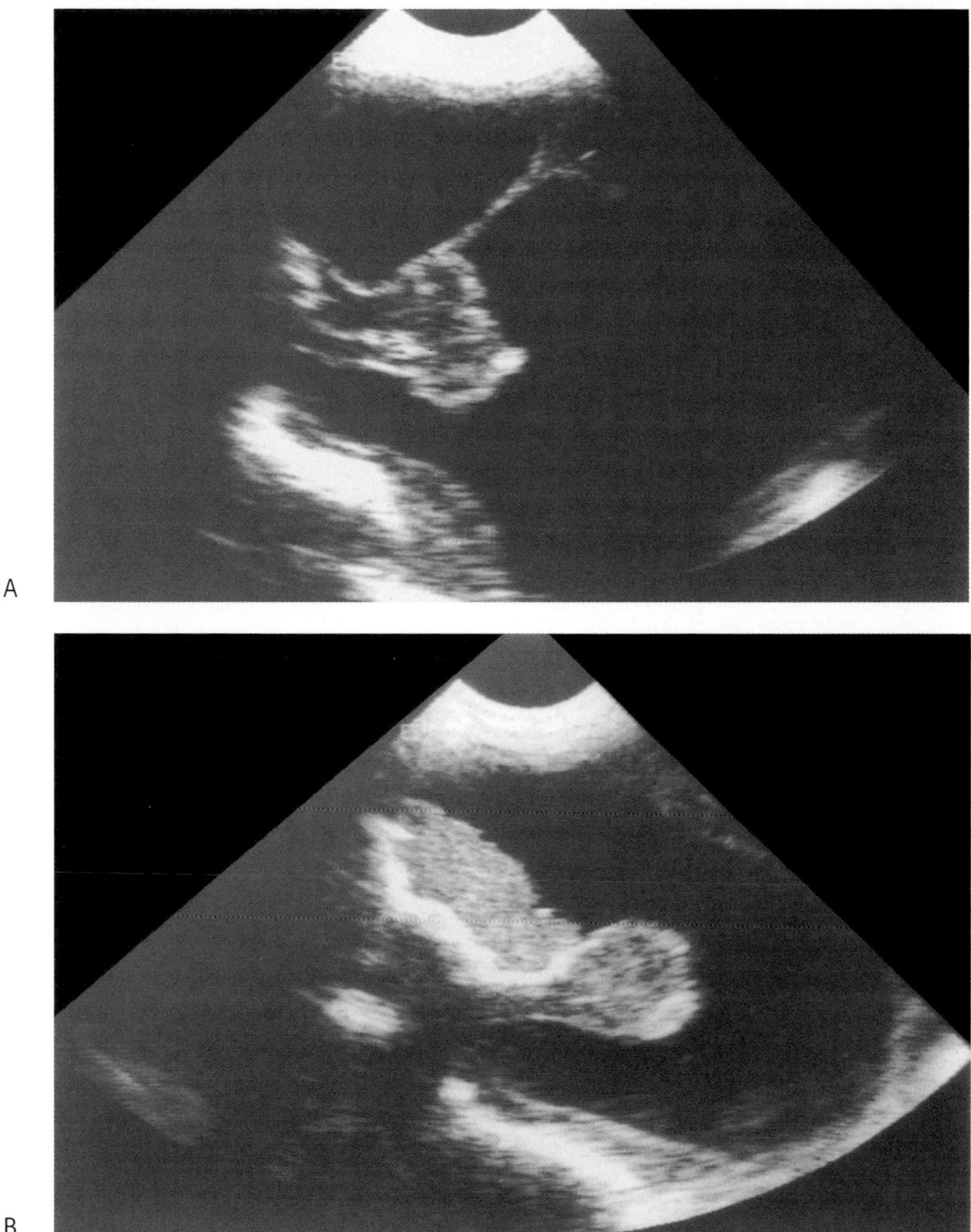


Figure 43.8 (A) Cerebral ultrasound scan (sagittal view) showing marked ventricular dilatation with a fibrinous septum across the ventricle. The infant had chronic bacterial ventriculitis. (B) The same infant as in (A) with chronic ventriculitis. Parasagittal view of one dilated ventricle showing necrotic material on a layer of calcification.

deficiency as well as thrombocytopenia should be excluded before any surgery is undertaken. Isoimmune thromocytopenia and coagulation factor V deficiency can present as congenital hydrocephalus resulting from antenatal intraventricular hemorrhage (see Chapters 20 and 21).

## CSF PRESSURE MEASUREMENT

### Technique of CSF pressure measurement

CSF pressure measurement can be helpful in distinguishing hydrocephalus from other causes of ventricular dilatation, in assessing the acuteness of the process and in deciding treatment. We have not found non-invasive invasive measurement of intracranial pressure by a fontanometer to correlate well with directly measured ventricular pressure (Kaiser & Whitelaw 1987). Changes in intracranial pressure appeared to be well represented, but the absolute values in millimeters of mercury (mmHg) were disappointingly inaccurate. CSF pressure can be measured with a conventional fluid-filled manometer, but an electronic pressure transducer gives a trace on the monitor screen that is useful for demonstrating that the measurement is stable and can also demonstrate the

CSF pulse pressure (Kaiser & Whitelaw 1986). The transducer must be carefully zeroed before the measurement, and the position of the transducer during the measurement should be level with the middle of the head. The infant should be horizontal and not forcefully restrained during the measurement. A wide pulse pressure is a sign that the limits of cranial compliance have been reached and the inflow of blood with each contraction of the heart is enough to increase intracranial pressure.

### CSF pressure in normal neonates and infants with posthemorrhagic ventricular dilatation

Kaiser & Whitelaw (1986) have studied CSF in neonates undergoing lumbar puncture to exclude sepsis and who were retrospectively classified as neurologically normal. When the infant was horizontal, at rest, and had no pressure on the abdomen, neck, or head, the lumbar CSF pressure had a mean of 2.8 mmHg, and the upper limit was 6 mmHg. Kaiser & Whitelaw (1985) studied CSF pressure in a group of infants with progressive posthemorrhagic ventricular dilatation. Many of the infants had communicating ventricular dilatation and could be studied with lumbar puncture. In cases of non-communicating ventricular dilatation, the CSF pressure was measured at the time of ventricular puncture. Infants who were actively expanding their ventricles after intraventricular hemorrhage had a mean CSF pressure of 8.8 mmHg (three times the normal) but with a wide scatter. Some preterm infants could dilate their lateral ventricles and expand their heads at pressures that were still within the normal range, whereas few generated pressures over 15 mmHg. Probably because infants with communicating hydrocephalus rarely generate dangerously high pressures, we have never encountered acute herniation of the brainstem (coning), despite having lumbar punctured many infants with CSF pressures considerably above the normal range. It has not been easy to define the level of CSF pressure at which action should be taken to lower pressure, but 12 mmHg has been used as the trigger pressure (Ventriculomegaly Trial Group 1990).

### NEUROPHYSIOLOGIC ASSESSMENT IN HYDROCEPHALUS

De Vries *et al.* (1990) have shown that the latency of somatosensory evoked potentials (SEPs) in infants with hydrocephalus correlates well with CSF pressure and improved when treatment lowered pressure. As clinical neurologic examination correlates poorly with CSF pressure measurement, SEPs (see Chapter 12) may prove to be a valuable way of demonstrating the effect of pressure on cerebral function and thus help in prognosis and treatment decisions.

### CEREBRAL BLOOD FLOW VELOCITY WAVEFORMS IN HYDROCEPHALUS

Serial measurements of pulsatility index and resistance index by Doppler on the middle cerebral artery or anterior cerebral artery tend to increase as ICP increases. In other words, the diastolic part of the pulse becomes reduced in relative terms. However, Hanlo *et al.* (1995) have made simultaneous long-term transcranial Doppler and invasive ICP recordings. Although pulsatility and resistance indices tended to go down after successful shunt surgery, there was much variability between the Doppler and ICP measurements, and they concluded that Doppler indices are inadequate for monitoring dynamic changes in patients with raised ICP. Taylor & Madsen (1996) confirmed the poor correlation between baseline resistive index and ICP but found that fontanelle compression (which increased ICP) changed the Doppler measurement in an informative way. A large change in Doppler resistive index had a 0.8 correlation with elevated intracranial pressure.

## PROGNOSIS

### PROGNOSIS OF UNCOMPLICATED HYDROCEPHALUS

Eighty survivors of 'pure' hydrocephalus operated on between 1956 and 1976 in Cleveland were reviewed by Nulson & Rekate (1982). These were infants with hydrocephalus not complicated by primary brain disease or spina bifida. Of these, 43 had aqueduct stenosis, 13 had blockage at the fourth ventricle outlets and 24 had communicating hydrocephalus. There was a good correlation between intelligence quotient (IQ) and the thickness of the frontal cerebral mantle (determined at follow-up). Normally, the cerebral mantle is 5.0–5.5 cm. The children with a cerebral mantle of 3.0 cm or more had an IQ distribution approaching normal. All eight patients failing to achieve a cerebral mantle of 2.0 cm were not adequately shunted until after 6 months of age. Six cases with a final mantle of 2.0–3.0 cm (IQ 63–95) were all first adequately shunted after 5 months of age. All cases adequately shunted before 5 months had a mantle measurement over 3.0 cm, including nine cases with initial mantles of less than 1.0 cm. No increase in mantle size occurred in any of the five children first operated after age 18 months. The authors concluded that if infantile hydrocephalus is severe with a frontal mantle of less than 2.0 cm, the opportunity for a good developmental result diminishes with time. The outcome for fetal ventriculomegaly is discussed in Chapter 42.

### PROGNOSIS OF HYDROCEPHALUS WITH MYELOMENINGOCELE

The relationship between frontal cerebral mantle thickness and IQ is much less predictable than in 'pure' hydrocephalus. These children are identified at birth because of the myelomeningocele, and hydrocephalus is to be expected. Very few are operated on late because of a delay in diagnosis. Thus, it is relatively unusual to fail to develop at least a 3-cm-thick frontal mantle. The IQ distribution in the Cleveland series was much lower than for the corresponding group of children with pure hydrocephalus and a 3-cm-thick mantle (Nulsen & Rekate 1982). Over 50% had an IQ below 80 (versus 15%), and only 15% were above 100 (versus 51%). Clearly, some children in this group have a considerable degree of paraplegia that affects many of their activities, and this, plus the frequency of CSF infection, may have an adverse effect on development and thus IQ.

### PROGNOSIS OF POSTHEMORRHAGIC VENTRICULAR DILATATION

Preterm infants who develop a large intraventricular hemorrhage are at risk of developing progressive ventricular dilatation leading to hydrocephalus. This condition has a worse prognosis than congenital hydrocephalus.

Epidemiologic surveillance of neurologic disabilities in south-west Sweden has shown a disturbing increase in the numbers of preterm infants surviving with posthemorrhagic hydrocephalus and multiple severe disabilities. Of these infants requiring shunt surgery, 78% subsequently developed cerebral palsy, 72% had a developmental quotient or IQ below 70, and 56% had epilepsy (Fernell *et al.* 1990). In a group of 33 infants with posthemorrhagic ventricular dilatation (PHVD) followed to a mean age of 50 months, 58% had delayed motor development, and 52% had delayed mental development (Shankaran *et al.* 1989).

The Ventriculomegaly Trial Group (1990, 1994) studied 157 infants with PHVD: 32 infants died after entry to the study using the entry criterion of ventricular width 4 mm over the 97th centile, 13 were lost to follow-up, and 112 survivors were examined by one neurodevelopmental pediatrician at 30 months postterm. Overall, 54% scored below 70 on the Griffith's developmental scales, 90% had neuromotor impairment, and 76% had marked disability. Fifty-six per cent had multiple impairments. Vision was severely affected in 9%, and 27% had a field defect. Six per cent had a sensorineural hearing loss, and 14% were taking regular anticonvulsants. An important factor affecting prognosis in PHVD was the presence or absence of parenchymal cerebral lesions in the neonatal period. Parenchymal hemorrhagic infarction with subsequent formation of a porencephalic cyst or periventricular leukomalacia substantially worsened the prognosis.

An important study by Fletcher *et al.* (1997) compared the outcome at an average age of 8.5 years of a group of prematurely born children with and without hydrocephalus. Four groups were studied: preterm no hydrocephalus, preterm arrested hydrocephalus, preterm shunted hydrocephalus, and term children. Those born preterm who developed hydrocephalus had an equal severity of underlying parenchymal involvement. The only significant difference in these groups on later performance was that the shunted preterm group were significantly poorer in motor performance and visual-spatial tests, but not language tests. This study adds further weight to the independent adverse effect of hydrocephalus on non-verbal cognitive skills

## NON-SURGICAL TREATMENT OF HYDROCEPHALUS

### REPEATED TAPPING OF CSF

The experimental hydrocephalus findings and the moderately elevated CSF pressure suggested that early CSF tapping by lumbar puncture or ventricular puncture might benefit babies with PHVD by (1) reducing pressure, thus reducing periventricular tissue damage and (2) removing excess protein and blood in the CSF, thus preventing permanent blockage of the CSF pathways. Mantovani *et al.* (1980) and Anwar *et al.* (1985) carried out randomized trials of serial lumbar punctures in babies with a large intraventricular hemorrhage. Both studies concluded that these measures did not reduce the progression to hydrocephalus and eventual surgical shunting. Dykes *et al.* (1989) carried out a randomized trial of repeated lumbar puncture in infants with asymptomatic large IVH and found that there was no significant reduction in either the numbers of infants shunted, the mortality, or single or multiple disabilities.

The hypothesis that early tapping of infants with PHVD by either the lumbar or ventricular route might reduce neurodevelopmental impairment and disability was tested in the Ventriculomegaly Trial Group's (1990) multicenter trial, which recruited 157 infants in England, Ireland, and Switzerland from 1984 to 1987. Infants fulfilling the diagnostic criteria described above were randomized to either early CSF tapping to prevent further ventricular enlargement or conservative management. The survivors were examined at 12 and 30 months post-term by one developmental pediatrician. The mean CSF pressure was 9 mmHg in both treatment groups, and early tapping did succeed in reducing the rate of ventricular and head expansion. The mean gestational age in the infants randomized was 28 weeks, and the mean birth weight was just over 1200 g. Of the survivors, 62% received ventriculoperitoneal shunts, the same percentage in each treatment group.

At 12 months past term, 85% of survivors had abnormal neuromotor signs and 77% had disability, with no difference between the treatment groups (Ventriculomegaly Trial Group 1990). The proportion of children with neuromotor impairment plus other types of disability, such as mental retardation and visual or hearing loss, was not significantly different between the two treatment groups. There was a suggestion that infants who had already had a parenchymal cerebral lesion at the time of entry to the trial had a lower proportion of multisystem impairments at the 12-month follow-up examination, but the level of significance was only 5% (39), and this finding was not confirmed at the 30-month examination (Ventriculomegaly Trial Group 1994). The high frequencies of single and multiple impairments were the same for both treatment groups. Repeated CSF tapping was followed by CSF infection (ventriculitis) in 11 infants (7%). An additional complication of repeated ventricular tapping is the production of needle track lesions through the cerebral hemisphere (Fig. 43.9).

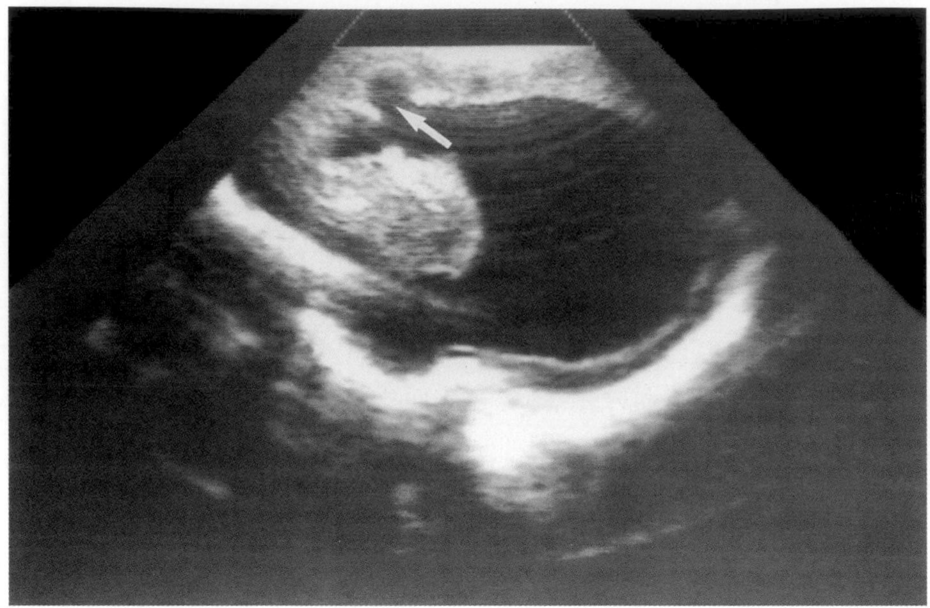

**Figure 43.9** Cerebral ultrasound (parasagittal view) showing a needle track lesion (arrow) in the roof of the lateral ventricle after repeated ventricle taps.

The Cochrane Collaboration have published a systematic review of repeated lumbar or ventricular puncture after IVH, and the meta-analysis (in Table 43.2) shows that there is no significant effect on shunt surgery, disability, or multiple disability (Whitelaw 1998).

Because of the lack of any consistent neurodevelopmental benefit, the absence of any reduction in surgical shunt dependence, and the significant risk of serious infection, early treatment by CSF tapping cannot be recommended for PHVD.

We reserve CSF tapping for relief of symptoms associated with excessive pressure or excessive head expansion. We consider 12 mmHg to be an excessive CSF pressure. This is four times the normal mean and 100% over the upper limit

**Table 43.2 Comparison: repeated lumbar or ventricular punctures (Expt) vs. conservative management (Cont) for PHVD**

| Outcome | Expt | Cont | RR (95% CI) |
|---|---|---|---|
| Ventriculoperitoneal shunt | | | |
| Anwar *et al.* (1985) | 10/24 | 9/23 | 0.57 (0.41, 0.78) |
| Dykes *et al.* (1989) | 9/22 | 8/16 | 0.65 (0.39, 1.08) |
| Mantovani *et al.* (1980) | 4/19 | 3/19 | 1.33 (0.34, 5.17) |
| Ventriculomegaly Trial Group (1990) | 41/79 | 42/78 | 0.96 (0.72, 1.30) |
| Total | 64/144 | 62/136 | 0.97 (0.76, 1.25) |
| Major disability in survivors | | | |
| Dykes *et al.* (1989) | 8/15 | 10/14 | 0.75 (0.42, 1.33) |
| Ventriculomegaly Trial Group (1990) | 47/59 | 41/53 | 1.03 (0.85, 1.25) |
| Total | 55/74 | 51/67 | 0.98 (0.81, 1.18) |
| Multiple disability in survivors | | | |
| Dykes *et al.* (1989) | 4/15 | 5/14 | 0.75 (0.25, 2.23) |
| Ventriculomegaly Trial Group (1990) | 32/59 | 31/53 | 0.93 (0.67, 1.28) |
| Total | 36/74 | 36/67 | 0.90 (0.66, 1.24) |

0.1 1 10

Relative risk (95% CI fixed effects model)

*Source*: Adapted from a systematic review (Whitelaw 1998).

of normal. This pressure is not necessarily associated with specific signs, but we have often noted irritability and a tense fontanelle at this level. If tapping is carried out, then CSF should be allowed to drip out without suction as rapid suction with a syringe usually causes discomfort in the baby and may precipitate fresh intraventricular bleeding. Fluid can be removed until the normal mean of 3 mmHg is reached. The volume we have found to be effective is 10–20 ml CSF/kg.

## DRUGS TO REDUCE CSF PRODUCTION

Because of the risks and lack of benefit from repeated tapping, non-invasive treatment to reduce the production of CSF was an attractive alternative.

### Acetazolamide

Acetazolamide (Diamox) reduces CSF production by inhibiting the enzyme carbonic anhydrase and has been used in many centers for treatment of PHVD. Frusemide has an inhibitory effect on CSF production in experimental animals. Shinnar *et al.* (1985) described a selected uncontrolled group of infants with hydrocephalus, some of whom were below 1500 g, in whom 100 mg/kg/day of acetazolamide was combined with 1 mg/kg/day of frusemide. The authors concluded that they avoided shunt insertion in 50% of the babies who would otherwise have been candidates for surgery.

The International PHVD Drug Trial Group (1998) reported the results of a randomized controlled trial of acetazolamide 100 mg/kg/day and frusemide 1 mg/kg/day in infants with posthemorrhagic ventricular dilatation using identical eligibility criteria to the Ventriculomegaly Trial. Forty-nine out of 75 (65%) infants receiving drug treatment died or required shunt insertion, and 35 out of 76 (46%) infants in the control group died or required shunt insertion (relative risk 1.42, confidence interval 1.06–1.9) Twenty-one out of 151 (14%) infants developed CNS infections with no difference between the two treatment groups. Thirty-eight out of 48 (79%) infants in the drug treatment group were impaired or disabled at 1 year, whereas 30 out of 57 (53%) in the control group were impaired or disabled at 1 year. The trial was stopped by the data-monitoring committee before the planned completion, as the results clearly showed a worse outcome in the drug-treated infants. These findings could not be explained by differences between the groups of infants at trial entry, delays in shunt surgery, or an increase in infections in the drug-treated group.

Acetazolamide has a number of effects on important physiologic systems that may be relevant to the findings of this trial. Cerebral blood flow is increased substantially for several hours following 50 mg/kg of acetazolamide. Blood pressure does not change, but the cerebral vasodilatation can give a transient rise in intracranial pressure before the reduced production of CSF has time to reduce the intracranial pressure (Cowan & Whitelaw 1991). These effects on the cerebral circulation are not thought to increase the risk of intraventricular hemorrhage in stable infants who are several weeks or months old.

The effects on $PCO_2$ can be clinically significant. Carbonic anhydrase is necessary for the rapid conversion of circulating bicarbonate to carbon dioxide, which is exhaled as blood flows through the alveolar capillaries of the lungs. Acetazolamide inhibits pulmonary carbon dioxide elimination. In newborn piglets which had been tracheostomized, ventilated and paralysed to hold the $PCO_2$ constant, intravenous acetazolamide produced an immediate reduction in end-tidal $PCO_2$ measured by tracheal catheter and a rise in arterial $PCO_2$ of 1.5 kPa within 10 min (Fig. 43.10) (Thoresen & Whitelaw 1990).

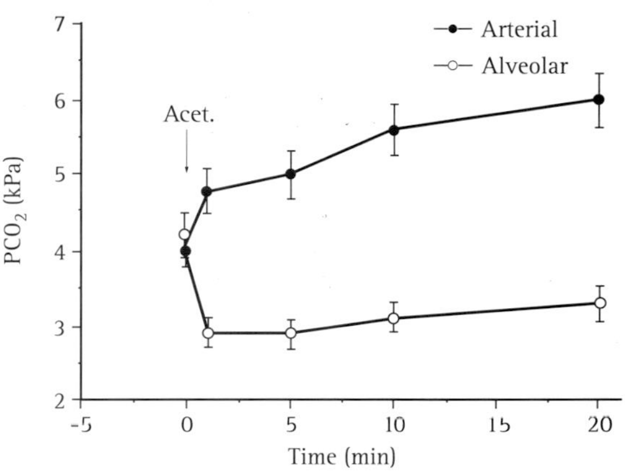


Figure 43.10 Changes in arterial and end-tidal $PCO_2$ (mean + SEM) after administration of acetazolamide 50 mg/kg to tracheostomized and ventilated newborn pigs. (Reproduced, with permission from S. Kerger AG, Basel, from Thoresen 1990).

This inhibition of $CO_2$ elimination is not a clinical problem in infants with normal lungs as they can compensate by breathing faster, thus holding $PCO_2$ constant. However, infants who are ventilator-dependent or who have significant bronchopulmonary dysplasia cannot compensate (Cowan & Whitelaw 1991). In four such infants, acetazolamide produced a median increase of 2.0 kPa (range 0.6–3.4 kPa) with a corresponding reduction in pH such that acetazolamide had to be discontinued and mechanical ventilation increased (Fig. 43.11).

Many preterm infants with PHVD are also likely to have chronic lung disease. Acetazolamide also has a mild diuretic effect and increases urinary excretion of bicarbonate. Thus, it is normally necessary to give 4 mmol/kg/day of sodium bicarbonate and, if frusemide is used as well, 1 mmol/kg/day of potassium chloride, as replacement for urinary losses. A considerable proportion of infants under 1500 g with PHVD are also likely to have chronic lung disease and immature renal function and may therefore be at risk of acid–base, blood-gas and electrolyte disturbances. Aplastic anemia has

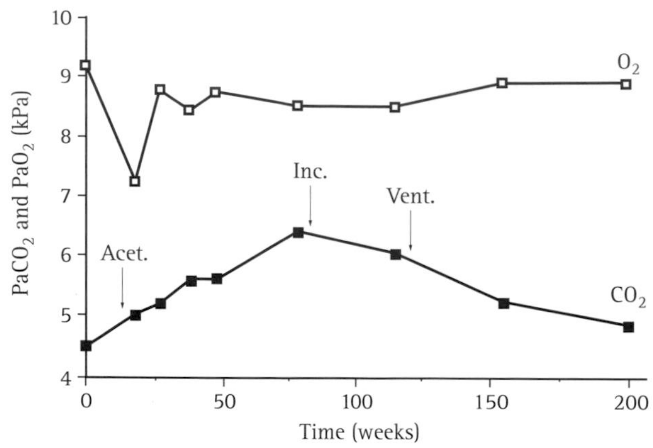


Figure 43.11 Changes in arterial $PCO_1$ and $PO_2$ after the intravenous administration of 50 mg/kg of acetazolamide to an infant with posthemorrhagic hydrocephalus and bronchopulmonary dysplasia. 'Inc vent' = the times when the respirator rate was increased; Acet = acetazolamide. (Reproduced, with permission, from Cowan & Whitelaw 1991.)

been associated with acetazolamide therapy (Keisu *et al.* 1990).

### Isosorbide

Isosorbide reduces CSF production by an osmotic effect, but a high incidence of side-effects such as vomiting has been reported (Liptak *et al.* 1992).

### Glycerol

Glycerol is another osmotic agent that has been used for control of hydrocephalus. There is no published experience with small preterm infants.

For all of the above reasons, drug therapy to reduce CSF production cannot be recommended.

## VENTRICULAR RESERVOIR

If there is persistent intracranial hypertension and excessive head growth, despite attempts at medical management, surgical treatment becomes the only option. Excessive head growth is arbitrarily defined as an increase of 15 mm per week or crossing from below the 50th centile to 2 cm over the 90th centile on the Gairdner growth chart (Gairdner & Pearson 1971). A ventricular catheter can be inserted through a burr hole and connected to a subcutaneous reservoir. Such a reservoir can be used to measure CSF pressure and remove CSF as often as is necessary to control pressure and head growth. This can be done even in the presence of blood-stained, protein-rich or infected CSF. Such CSF tapping does require sterile technique, and there is a small risk of introducing infection, but it is considerably easier than ventricular or lumbar puncture. Another possible advantage is that fresh needle tracks are not made through the brain every time CSF is removed. Thus, a ventricular reservoir is an alternative to repeated ventricular punctures. The surgical procedure is shorter and simpler than a full shunt, and many infants below 1000 g have been treated in this way (Anwar *et al.* 1986). A ventricular reservoir provides temporary control in hospital while waiting for (1) the PHVD to resolve spontaneously, (2) protein and blood to clear from the CSF, and (3) growth and recovery of the infant from lung disease before insertion of a permanent shunt. The details of shunt surgery and its complications are discussed in Chapter 44.

## INTRAVENTRICULAR FIBRINOLYTIC THERAPY

### Urokinase and streptokinase in hydrocephalus after ventriculitis

Fibrin deposition can also lead to hydrocephalus after ventriculitis and streptokinase and urokinase have been given intraventricularly to infants with ventriculitis to prevent hydrocephalus (Stewart 1964). The effectiveness of this approach cannot be judged as no controlled trials have been carried out.

### Streptokinase and urokinase in posthaemorrhagic hydrocephalus

Obstruction of the ventricular foramina by multiple small blood clots is part of the mechanism of PHVD, and the presence of X oligomer (a fibrin degradation product) in the CSF of infants with PHVD is evidence of endogenous fibrinolysis in the CSF (Whitelaw *et al.* 1991). We have also been able to demonstrate fibrinolytic activity in the CSF of infants with PHVD by a fibrin plate assay. Because none of the existing treatment methods are free of serious complications and because of the unsatisfactory outcome of PHVD, it seems logical to try to augment the natural fibrinolysis with a plasminogen activator in the CSF. A controlled trial in dogs showed that intraventricular urokinase given after intraventricular injection of blood significantly reduced the risk of hydrocephalus (Pang *et al.* 1986). An open study of six adult patients with intraventricular hemorrhage showed that repeated intraventricular injections of urokinase gave a lower incidence of hydrocephalus than a group of historical control patients (Todo *et al.* 1991). In a pilot, non-randomized study, nine infants with PHVD (with the same diagnostic criteria as described above (ventricular width 4 mm over the 97th centile) received intraventricular infusions of streptokinase at 1000 units/h for about 48 h via a ventricular catheter inserted percutaneously through the lambdoid suture. They were nearly all very-low-birthweight preterm infants and were treated between 7 and 28 days of age. Secondary bleeding occurred in only one infant, and the proportion of infants subsequently requiring shunt surgery was much lower than expected (Whitelaw *et al.* 1992). Intraventricular streptokinase increases fibrin degradation products in the CSF. Luciano *et al.* (1997) carried out a randomized trial of intraventricular streptokinase in 12 infants developing posthemorrhagic ventricular dilatation.

Twenty thousand units of streptokinase/day were given for 4 days via a ventricular reservoir. Three out of six infants in each group had to be shunted, and one died in each group. One of the infants in the streptokinase group developed secondary intraventricular hemorrhage and meningitis.

### Recombinant human tissue plasminogen activator

Recombinant human tissue plasminogen activator (rtPA) activates all the available plasminogen to plasmin and has the additional advantage of not being antigenic. Many adult patients with subarachnoid or intraventricular hemorrhage have been treated with intrathecal or intraventricular rtPA. The overall conclusion of these uncontrolled observations was that intrathecal fibrinolytic therapy had helped to reduce vasospasm and clear blood from the CSF. We have carried out a phase 1 open trial of intraventricular tPA (0.5 mg for infants below 1000 g and 1.0 mg for infants 1000 g or more) in 22 infants with PHVD using the same inclusion criteria as the Ventriculomegaly and PHVD Drug trials. The tPA was given by bolus injection, and the median number of doses was two. Twelve of the 22 infants survived without shunt surgery, nine infants required shunts, and one infant died with hydrocephalus. One definite case of secondary intraventricular hemorrhage was observed. There was no secondary infection (Whitelaw 1996). These results were only marginally better than historical controls, and this method of treatment cannot be recommended.

We are currently evaluating a procedure that involves insertion of two intraventricular catheters, one frontal on the right, and one occipital on the left. tPA (0.5 mg) is given intraventricularly, and after 2 h, the ventricular system is irrigated with isotonic artificial CSF (without protein) at 20 ml/h for 72 h. The second catheter is attached to a drainage system that can be positioned to increase or decrease the rate of drainage (usually at least 20 ml/h), and a pressure transducer on the infusion line provides continuous intracranial pressure. This procedure is called DRIFT (DRainage, Irrigation and Fibrinolytic Therapy). The objectives are to remove old blood and cytokines, particularly TGF-$\beta$1. Of nineteen infants with PHVD treated with this protocol, fourteen have survived without a shunt. This highly invasive and experimental intervention cannot be recommended until a more objective evaluation provides positive evidence.

## SUMMARY OF MANAGEMENT OF PHVD

There are few randomized controlled trials to guide the best management of PHVD, but the current advice on the principles of management is summarized in below.

### Key Points

- Use recognized diagnostic criteria, e.g. 4 mm over 97th centile for ventricular width
- Differentiate cerebral atrophy or leukomalacia from CSF-driven ventricular enlargement
- Note the presence, location, and extent of any parenchymal cerebral lesions
- Do a neurologic examination and assess the rate of head enlargement and intracranial pressure effects
- If there is symptomatic raised pressure or rapid enlargement at 15 mm or more/week, the pressure should be normalized (to $< 7$ mmHg) and the effects on neurologic signs and physiologic parameters documented. This may be achieved by lumbar puncture/ventricular puncture/ventricular reservoir or external ventricular drain depending on local expertise and availability of a neurosurgeon.
- If there is no evidence of signs or symptoms from raised intracranial pressure, observe without intervention
- Progressive and persistent enlargement of the ventricles together with accelerated head enlargement (8–14 mm/week) without obvious symptoms over 4 weeks should prompt careful assessment for neurologic and physiologic deterioration, and this may shift the baby into the symptomatic group
- Progressive and persistent enlargement of ventricles and accelerated head growth over 6 weeks, even without symptoms, should prompt evaluation for shunt surgery. The surgeon may wish to defer if the CSF is still blood-stained or has a protein content over 2 g/l, if there is infection, or if the baby's cardiorespiratory condition is poor
- Elective use of early repeated lumbar punctures is not recommended
- Acetazolamide and furosemide are not recommended.

## REFERENCES


Anwar M, Dolye A J, Kadam S *et al.* (1986) Management of post-haemorrhagic hydrocephalus in the preterm infant. *J Pediatr Surg* 21:334–337.

✪ Anwar M, Kadam S, Hiatt I M *et al.* (1985) Serial lumbar punctures in prevention of posthaemorrhagic hydrocephalus in preterm infants. *J Pediatr* 107:446–449.

Carmel P W (1982) The Arnold-Chiari malformation. In: *Pediatric neurosurgery. Section of Pediatric Neurosurgery of the American Association of Neurological Surgeons.* New York, NY: Grune and Stratton.

Cowan F & Whitelaw A (1991) Acute effects of acetazolamide on cerebral blood flow velocity and $PCO_2$, in the newborn infant. *Acta Paediatr Scand* 80:22–27.

Davson H, Welch K & Segal M B (1987) The physiology and pathophysiology of the cerebrospinal fluid. Edinburgh: Churchill Livingstone.

De Vries L S, Pierrat V, Minami T *et al.* (1990) The role of short latency somatosensory evoked responses in infants with rapidly progressive ventricular dilatation. *Neuropediatrics* 21:136–139.

Dubowitz L M S, Dubowitz V & Mercuri E (1999) The neurological assessment of the preterm and full-term newborn infant. *Clin Dev Med*: No. 148.

✪ Dykes F D, Dunbar B, Lazarra A *et al.* (1989) Posthemorrhagic hydrocephalus in high risk infants: Natural history, management and long term outcome. *J Pediatr* 114:611–618.

Fernell E, Hagberg G & Hagberg B (1990) Infantile hydrocephalus – the impact of enhanced preterm survival. *Acta Paediatr Scand* 79:1080–1086.

Fletcher J M, Landry S H, Bohan T P *et al.* (1997) Effects of intraventricular hemorrhage and hydrocephalus on the long-term neurobehavioural development of preterm very-low-birthweight infants. *Dev Med Child Neurol* 39:596–606.

Gairdner D & Pearson J (1971) A growth chart for premature and other infants. *Arch Dis Childhood* 46:783–787.

Hanlo P W, Gooskens R H, Nijhuis I J *et al.* (1995) Value of transcranial Doppler indices in predicting raised ICP in infantile hydrocephalus. *Childs Nerv Syst* 11:595–603.

Hansen A R, Volpe J J, Goumnerova L C *et al.* (1997) Intraventricular urokinase for the treatment of posthaemorrhagic hydrocephalus. *Pediatr Neurol* 17:213–217.

International PHVD Drug Trial Group (1998) International randomised controlled trial of acetazolamide and furosemide in posthaemorrhagic ventricular dilatation in infancy. *Lancet* 352:433–440.

Jouet M, Moncia A, Paterson J *et al.* (1995) New domains of neural cell-adhesion molecule L1 implicated in X -linked hydrocephalus and MASA syndrome. *Am J Hum Genet* 56:1304–1314

Kaiser A & Whitelaw A (1985) Cerebrospinal fluid pressure in infants with post-haemorrhagic ventricular dilatation. *Arch Dis Childhood* 60:920–924.

Kaiser A & Whitelaw A (1986) Normal cerebrospinal fluid pressure in the newborn. *Neuropediatrics* 17:100–102.

Kaiser A & Whitelaw A (1987) Non-invasive measurement of intracranial pressure. Fact of fancy. *Dev Med Child Neurol* 29:320–326.

Keisu M, Wiholm B E, Öst A *et al.* (1990) Acetazolamide-associated aplastic anaemia. *J Intern Med* 228:627–632.

Kitisawa K & Tada T (1994) Elevation of transforming growth factor-β-1 level in cerebrospinal fluid of patients with communicating hydrocephalus after subarachnoid hemorrhage. *Stroke* 25:1400–1404.

Larroche J C (1972) Posthaemorrhagic hydrocephalus in infancy. *Biologia Neonatorum* 20:287–299.

✪ Levene M I (1981) Measurement of the growth of the lateral ventricles in pretem infants with real time ultrasound. *Arch Dis Childhood* 56:900–940.

Liptak G S, Gellerstedt M E & Klionsky N (1992) Isosorbide in the medical management of hydrocephalus in children with myeodysplasia. *Dev Med Child Neurol* 34:150–154.

✪ Luciano R, Velardi F, Romagnoli C *et al.* (1997) Failure of fibrinolytic endoventricular treatment to prevent neonatal post-haemorrhagic hydrocephalus. *Childs Nerv System* 13:73–76.

✪ Mantovani J F, Pasternak J F, Mathew O P *et al.* (1980) Failure of daily lumbar punctures to prevent the development of hydrocephalus following intraventricular haemorrhage. *J Pediatr* 97:278–281.

Ment L R, Duncan C C & Geehr R (1981) Benign enlargement of the subarachnoid spaces in the infant. *J Neurosurg* 54:504–508.

Milhorat T H (1972) *Hydrocephalus and the cerebrospinal fluid.* Baltimore, MD: Williams & Wilkins.

Milhorat T H (1982) Hydrocephalus: historical notes, etiology and clinical diagnosis. In: *Pediatric neurosurgery. Section of Pediatric Neurosurgery of the American Association of Neurological Surgeons.* New York, NY: Grune and Stratton.

Myrianthopoulos N C & Kurland L T (1961) Present concepts of the epidemiology and genetics of hydrocephalus. In: Fields W J, Demond M M (eds) *Disorders of the developing nervous system.* Springfield, IL: Charles C Thomas; pp. 187–702.

Nulsen F E & Rekate H L (1982) Results of treatment for hydrocephalus as a guide to future management. In: *Pediatric neurosurgery. Section of Pediatric Neurosurgery of the American Association of Neurological Surgeons.* New York, NY: Grune and Stratton.

Pang D, Sclabassi R J & Horton J A (1986) Lysis of intraventricular blood clot with urokinase in a canine model: part 3. *Neurosurgery* 19:553–572.

Shankaran S, Koepke T, Woldte E *et al.* (1989) Outcome after posthaemorrhagic ventriculomegaly in comparison with mild haemorrhage without ventriculomegaly. *J Pediatr* 114:109–114.

Shinnar S, Gammon K, Bergman E W *et al.* (1985) Management of hydrocephalus in infancy: use of acetazolamide and furosemide to avoid cerebrospinal fluid shunts. *J Pediatr* 107:31–63.

Stewart G T (1964) Fibrinolytic therapy in meningitis and ventriculitis. *J Clin Pathol* 17:355–359.

Tada T, Kanaji M & Kobayashi S (1994) Induction of communicating hydrocephalus in mice by intrathecal injection of human recombinant transforming growth factor-β-1. *J Neuroimmunol* 50:153–158.

Taylor G A & Madsen J R (1996) Neonatal hydrocephalus: hemodynamic response to fontanelle compression – correlation with intracranial pressure and need for shunt placement. *Radiology* 201:685–689.

Thoresen M & Whitelaw A (1990) Effect of acetazolamide on cerebral blood flow velocity and $CO_2$ elimination in normotensive and hypotensive newborn piglets. *Biol Neonate* 58:200–207.

Todo T, Usui M & Takakura K (1991) Treatment of severe intraventricular hemorrhage by intraventricular infusion of urokinase. *J Neurosurg* 74:81–86.

✪ Ventriculomegaly Trial Group (1990) Randomised trial of early tapping in neonatal posthaemorrhagic ventricular dilatation. *Arch Dis Childhood* 65:3–10.

✪ Ventriculomegaly Trial Group (1994) Randomised trial of early tapping in neonatal posthaemorrhagic ventricular dilatation: results at 30 months. *Arch Dis Childhood* 70:F129–F136.

Weller R & Shulman K (1972) Infantile hydrocephalus: clinical, histological, and ultrastructural study of brain damage. *J Neurosurg* 36:255–265.

Weller R, Wisnieski H, Shulman K *et al.* (1971) Experimental hydrocephalus in young dogs: histological and ultrastructural study of the brain tissue damage. *Neuropathol Exp Neurol* 30:613–627.

Whitelaw A (1998) *Repeated lumbar or ventricular punctures in newborns with intraventricular haemorrhage.* Oxford: The Cochrane Library, Update Software. Disk Issue 4.

✪ Whitelaw A, Christie S & Pople I (1999) Transforming Growth Factor Beta: a possible signal molecule for post-hemorrhagic hydrocephalus. *Pediatr Res* 46:576–580.

Whitelaw A, Creighton L & Gaffney P (1991) Fibrinolytic activity in cerebrospinal fluid after intraventricular haemorrhage. *Arch Dis Childhood* 66:808–809.

Whitelaw A, Rivers R, Creighton L *et al.* (1992) Low dose intraventricular fibrinolytic therapy to prevent posthaemorrhagic hydrocephalus. *Arch Dis Childhood* 67:12–14.

Whitelaw A, Suliba E, Fellman V, Mowinckel M C, Acolet D, Marlow N (1996) Phase 1 study of intraventricular recombinant tissue plasminogen activator for treatment of post haemorrhagic hydrocephalus. *Arch Dis Child* 75: F20–26.

# Chapter 44 Neurosurgical management of hydrocephalus

J. Punt

## INTRODUCTION

Hydrocephalus is an abnormal accumulation of cerebrospinal fluid (CSF) within the cerebral ventricles and cranial subarachnoid space due to an imbalance between production and absorption of CSF, or to an obstruction to the flow of CSF. In practice, virtually all cases of hydrocephalus seen in humans are due to an obstructive lesion (Russell 1949). The term 'non-communicating' hydrocephalus describes those conditions in which the obstructive lesion is so placed that there is no free communication between the ventricular system and the subarachnoid space. The term 'communicating' hydrocephalus describes those conditions in which the obstructive lesion is outside the brain, thus allowing communication between the cerebral ventricles and at least part of the subarachnoid space. These distinctions are of importance with regard to the different etiologies, the radiologic appearances, and the therapeutic possibilities. Posthemorrhagic ventricular dilatation, which, in some cases, progresses to hydrocephalus, is discussed separately in Chapter 43.

## CLINICAL FEATURES

The first clinical indication is usually discovery of an abnormally large head circumference at or shortly after birth; or abnormally rapid increase in head growth during the neonatal period, either in an otherwise normal baby, or one that is known to be at risk of developing hydrocephalus. It is important to realize that such a finding merely indicates the possibility of raised intracranial pressure; it does not allow any assumptions to be made about the cause of the raised intracranial pressure, whatever the clinical background. Furthermore, both constitutional macrocephaly and the acceleration in head growth seen in previously undernourished babies who are 'catching up' may be clinically indistinguishable from the macrocephaly of raised intracranial pressure. The absence of any apparent clinical disturbance, neurologic deficit, or developmental delay does not exclude the possibility of hydrocephalus (Kirkpatrick *et al.* 1989). Megalencephaly, hydranencephaly, and certain degenerative disorders, notably Alexander's disease, all display macrocephaly.

Later symptoms include bulging of the anterior fontanelle, sutural diastasis, dilatation of scalp veins, irritability, vomiting, sixth nerve palsies, downward deviation of the eyes, and, in advanced cases, bradycardias and bradypneas. Premature babies, especially those who have suffered early respiratory difficulties, frequently appear to display cardiorespiratory changes that seem to be disproportionate to the degree of intracranial hypertension. It must be repeated that these symptoms merely indicate a state of raised intracranial pressure, and not the underlying cause.

If the diagnosis is not made in the neonatal period, then relative spasticity of the lower limbs or an ataxia of the trunk with poor sitting balance and, later unsteady gait, may be seen in infancy and childhood. Papilledema, with or without consecutive optic atrophy, is not usually a major feature in the neonatal period.

Hydrocephalus in the neonate rarely causes rapidly progressive raised intracranial pressure; indeed, the baby who displays severe, or rapidly advancing, features or who appears disproportionately sick should be regarded as having a more sinister condition such as partially treated meningitis, brain abscess, brain tumor or subdural effusion. Epileptic seizures are only very rarely a feature of hydrocephalus *per se*.

Increasingly, hydrocephalus is discovered by cranial ultrasound scanning in asymptomatic babies in the pre- and post-natal period. Furthermore, ultrasound is used to follow those children that are at risk of developing progressive ventriculomegaly following germinal matrix or other intracranial hemorrhage, meningitis, or closure of myelomeningocele or encephalocele.

## DIAGNOSIS

The great majority of cases can be diagnosed immediately and simply by ultrasound scanning (US) through the anterior fontanelle. The ease and safety with which this investigation can be performed make it mandatory in all cases of macrocephaly and in those babies with failure to thrive associated with vomiting for which there is no immediately obvious cause such as gastro-esophageal reflux (Neville 1993). Rarely, computerized tomographic (CT) scanning or magnetic resonance (MR) imaging will be required to resolve specific anatomic or diagnostic difficulties. In such cases, MR is the preferred modality as it provides more detail of the brain parenchyma coupled with multi-planar imaging, which is useful in planning surgical approaches. Occasional cases of hydranencephaly may require MR angiography to distinguish them from severe hydrocephalus. CT ventriculography, previously used to investigate certain intracranial congenital cysts, has been superseded by MR.

## MANAGEMENT

The management of hydrocephalus in the special circumstances of the child who is still *in utero*, following germinal matrix hemorrhage, and in association with meningitis and ventriculitis has been discussed in detail in Chapter 42 and will not be reiterated; neither will the non-surgical management, which is reviewed in Chapter 43. This chapter is concerned purely with the surgical management. The history of surgical endeavors in this challenging and frustrating area have recently been reviewed, and it is clear to all concerned that efforts should continue to devise better methods in terms of both efficacy and reduction of complications (Rachel 1999).

The objective of the surgical management of neonatal and infantile hydrocephalus is the symptomatic relief of raised intracranial pressure so as to minimize the risks of neurologic handicap, developmental delay, and unsightly macrocephaly. Experiments on laboratory animals showing ultrastructural changes in the periventricular tissues notwithstanding (Weller & Wisniewski 1969; Weller *et al.* 1971; Wozniak *et al.* 1975), neuronal destruction is a late consequence of hydrocephalus. The finding of ventriculomegaly on imaging is not in itself an indication for surgical intervention; there needs to be either radiologic evidence of progression or clinical evidence of adverse effects attributable to the hydrocephalus. In particular, in the case of premature babies with posthemorrhagic ventriculomegaly, it is unproven whether early surgical intervention, based purely on ultrasound appearances, influences the neurodevelopmental outcome favorably.

As essentially all human hydrocephalus is obstructive in nature, the ideal remedy would be removal of the obstruction; however, with the exception of the very occasional cerebral tumor, this is rarely appropriate in neonatal practice. A full account of all of the options for treatment is given elsewhere (Punt 1993, 1996).

### CHOROID PLEXECTOMY

This was first described in 1918 by Dandy as an open procedure but proved dangerous and unsuccessful. Endoscopic coagulation was pursued in the pre-shunt era (Putnam 1934; Scarff 1970). The advent of modern neuroendoscopy led to a revival of interest in this approach. In an analysis of results of 71 patients treated by endoscopic choroid plexectomy between 1972 and 1983, the overall success rate was 49%, and there was only one operative mortality. Success related to etiology: 18 out of 35 patients with communicating hydrocephalus, 12 out of 26 with myelomeningocele, and five out of nine with obstructive hydrocephalus were deemed successful (Griffiths & Symon 1986). A later report described a high rate of infection probably attributable to a regime of post-operative ventricular irrigation (Griffith & Jamjoom 1990). Recent technical developments notwithstanding, endoscopic choroid plexectomy will probably remain confined to that very small number of patients with genuinely hypersecreting choroid plexi (Pittman & Bucholz 1992) and the very occasional neonate in whom there are desperate reasons, such as intra-abdominal sepsis, for postponing insertion of a ventricular shunt (Bucholz & Pittman 1991).

### EXTERNAL VENTRICULAR DRAINAGE

Occasionally, intracranial pressure due to ventriculomegaly needs to be controlled on a temporary basis by external ventricular drainage. This most frequently arises as a result of intraventricular hemorrhage, ventriculitis, or an infected ventricular shunt. It is important to tunnel the drain as far as possible to an exit point at a distance from the incision used to insert the device so as to reduce the risk of infection. All incisions should be made with careful consideration so as to avoid any potential future shunt sites. CSF lost externally should be replaced by oral or intravenous routes as normal saline. With care, tunneled shunts can be maintained in neonates for a few weeks with low rates of secondary infection (Berger *et al.* 2000) or, in some hands, no complications at all (Cornips *et al.* 1997).

### NEUROENDOSCOPIC THIRD VENTRICULOSTOMY (NTV)

Although the first endoscopic third ventriculostomy was performed by Mixter in 1920 (Mixter 1923) and was actively pursued by a few neurosurgeons, notably Scarff (Scarff 1936), the technique was generally abandoned when ventricular shunts were introduced. However, stimulated by a revival of interest (Vries 1978), NTV was reintroduced. Stimulated by the long and broadly favorable experience in Sydney, Australia, and aided by advances in endoscope design, the technique has undergone a renaissance. The largest series with long follow-up is that accumulated in Sydney and extends back to 1978 with an overall success rate of 61% in a mixed series of 103 children and adults (Jones *et al.* 1994). Much smaller series have reported much higher success rates but in highly selected cases: for example, an American center recorded eight successes in 10 patients followed for up to 3 years (Cohen 1994) and a French center reported 33 successes in 35 previously untreated cases of aqueduct stenosis or posterior third ventricle tumor (Decq *et al.* 1994). Another group reported that 42 of 69 patients, of median age 16 months, were asymptomatic and shunt-free at a median interval of 20 months' follow-up (Punt & Vloeberghs 1998). It is generally stated that NTV is less successful in the very young. In one series specifically examining the very young, only six out of 27 children of median age 3.7 months had a successful outcome (Buxton & Punt 1998). In a further group of 19 babies born at a mean of 32 weeks' gestational age and all operated upon in the first year of life (mean 9 weeks), NTV was successful in six (Buxton & Punt 1998). Although this was a low overall rate of success, the benefit of a shunt-free existence in the successful cases is not to be underrated. NTV is therefore a reasonable approach in the first year of life, especially in patients with obstructive hydrocephalus, providing that morbidity is low. NTV has been employed in the *in utero* treatment of hydrocephalus but with a fatal outcome for the baby due to intracranial hemorrhage (Vloeberghs personal communication).

## VENTRICULAR SHUNTING

The mainstay of modern management of infantile hydrocephalus remains the ventricular shunt, introduced in 1951 (Nulsen & Spitz 1951; Pudenz 1980). The decision to insert a shunt should result from a close collaboration between the physician and the surgeon, who should agree that the benefit that may accrue outweighs the risk of complications for any particular child. Similarly, the timing of operation is a point of good clinical judgment, especially in the premature baby with posthemorrhagic ventriculomegaly or the child with neonatal meningitis.

In the period immediately before shunt insertion, it is crucial that the condition of the child's skin is carefully considered. Scalp vein needles must be avoided, especially in the region of the proposed operative site. Napkin rashes and, in particular, any oral or cutaneous candidal infections must be eradicated. The skin along the proposed path of the shunt, usually the anterior chest and abdominal wall, must be left entirely free of monitoring electrodes, as these damage the epidermis and increase bacterial contamination. Any other focus of infection must be controlled, as all of these factors greatly increase the risk of shunt infection (Renier *et al.* 1984).

The physician, and indeed the inexperienced surgeon, may be justifiably bewildered by the wide variety of shunt devices now available and by lengthy debates on the physical characteristics of their performance (Portnoy 1982). These deliberations, although intellectually stimulating to some, have generally failed to lead to the production or selection of any device that is free of the common complications of blockage and infection. Manufacturers' claims of novel properties are essentially marketing devices. Shunts are big business estimated at US$100 million of the United States' national health-care expenditure per annum, nearly half of which is on revisional procedures (Bondurant & Jimenez 1995). The surgeon should gain familiarity with one, preferably simple, shunt and stick with it. Of much greater importance is the choice of the route of shunting. Although ventriculoatrial shunting was the first to be regularly successful, the need for revision due to growth of the child and the serious nature of the complications experienced with the intravascular end, especially nephritis, systemic sepsis, venous thrombosis, and fatal pulmonary hypertension (Strenger 1963; Nugent *et al.* 1966; Forrest & Cooper 1968), render this route highly undesirable unless exceptional circumstances exist, rendering the peritoneum inaccessible. Ventriculoperitoneal shunts require fewer revisions, and the late complications are much less serious. This is the only route that should be employed in babies and infants (Keucher & Mealey 1979). In children aged over about 5 years, a ventriculopleural shunt can be inserted if the peritoneum is not available.

The operative surgery of shunt insertion will not be considered, as it is described in detail elsewhere (Marlin 1996; Punt 1996), except to state a personal opinion that shunt surgery should be carried out by interested and experienced neurosurgeons, preferably those with a special commitment to pediatric practice. The potential for serious complications, many of which can be avoided by attention to detail, makes shunt insertion a procedure that is poorly suited to delegation to unsupervised trainees. In well-developed health-care systems, it is no longer appropriate for shunt surgery to be performed by general pediatric surgeons. Operations should be conducted swiftly so as to minimize the risk of bacterial colonization of the shunt and to reduce heat loss from the baby. Operations should be performed in an appropriately equipped operating room with facilities for continuing neonatal intensive care, including respiratory support. As with all neonatal surgery, the highest anesthetic skills are mandatory, and anesthesia should only be provided by those with specific pediatric expertise in the context of 'children only' operating sessions. A surgical isolator has been employed by some surgeons, but there are no data to confirm that infection rates are reduced, although it does maintain the baby's temperature (James & Murphy 1998).

Lumboperitoneal shunting has been advocated by some for the treatment of children with communicating hydrocephalus (Hoffman *et al.* 1976). Early complications are relatively few, but late complications can be tiresome, including spinal deformity, arachnoiditis, slit ventricles, and hindbrain herniation (Chumas *et al.* 1993). Although some of these complications may have related to the use of early polythene shunts, as opposed to more modern silastic devices, it is a route that is best avoided in childhood.

Postoperatively, the child is handled and fed normally. Some premature babies who have only recently become independent of ventilatory support may require a period of assisted ventilation. Indeed, it is a sound practice to plan to ventilate these babies electively, if only for a few hours. This also makes transport between the operating room and the neonatal unit safer. Routine follow-up imaging is not required if the child remains well and without signs of recurrent intracranial hypertension. The shunt track is examined daily for the first week; some bruising is permissible, but any inflammation indicates an acute infection, and only immediate removal will prevent ascending infection and damaging ventriculitis. Malnourished premature babies should be provided with protection for several weeks when lying on the side of the shunt, and prolonged pressure on the cranial end should be avoided, otherwise decubitus ulceration may result with inevitable shunt infection.

Follow-up should occur jointly with the neurosurgeon and physician. Specific serial neurodevelopmental evaluation is likely to be required and the need for special educational provision considered. In cases where multiple handicaps are envisaged, enrolment in a child development clinic is advisable. The family should be instructed throughout on the probable symptoms of shunt malfunction that might be expected as the child develops and matures. In the first 2 years of life, symptoms may be non-specific, but a combination of irritability, vomiting, and reduced responsiveness is very suggestive. Head circumference should be monitored and, charted as chronic shunt failure in the first 5 years of life, may well manifest itself simply as progressive disproportionate head growth. There is of course nothing about a shunt that protects a child from the usual childhood upper respiratory tract and gastro-intestinal illnesses, or the acute specific fevers. There is a natural tendency to attribute all symptoms to the shunt, however improbable. A useful guideline is that illnesses that are predominantly febrile, or in which repeated vomiting is the principle feature, are unlikely to be shunt-related. For every new 'shunt family', there is always an element of learning what is, and what is unlikely, to be a symptom of shunt malfunction. It is mutually advantageous for all involved in the child's care to learn together. Particular problems may arise with those children who have severe neurodevelopmental handicaps, and of these children especially, it is sensible to be guided by the family and other carers as to what represents unusual patterns of behavior. Certain children with a regular shunt malfunction develop stereotyped patterns of presentation, and it is a foolish doctor who ignores the family's observations. Shunt revision is only undertaken for symptomatic malfunction. Routine digital pumping by carers and attendants is unnecessary and undesirable as it provides no reliable information and is potentially hazardous in terms of promoting overdrainage and aspirating brain of choroid plexus into the ventricular catheter.

Follow-up should be for life so that guidance can be given to the child, the family, and relevant parties as to the effects of hydrocephalus on everyday activities and social aspects. Families should be offered contact with a support group such as the UK Association of Spina Bifida and Hydrocephalus (ASBAH). Some families find written information of value. Although some surgeons have questioned the need for regular neurosurgical review at intervals of less than 2 years (Colak *et al.* 1997) and others have suggested that it may not be needed at all for non-tumoral cases (Kimmings *et al.* 1996), it is more generally accepted that there is a responsibility incumbent upon the neurosurgeon to continue follow-up (Hayden *et al.* 1983; Rekate 1991). This is important if the risks of additional disabilities, especially visual loss, are to be avoided. Failure of follow-up may have expensive medico-legal consequences (Hockley 1999) and may cause otherwise avoidable deaths (Buxton & Punt 1998). In one study of 28 children with shunts who died of shunt-related causes, at least ten had experienced typical symptoms of shunt malfunction for days or weeks prior to presentation; five of these ten had not had adequate follow-up (Iskandar *et al.* 1998a). Furthermore, complications continue into adult life, with 16% of revisions occurring after the age of 16 years in one institutional series (Sgouros *et al.* 1995). The purpose of follow-up is, however, not just concerned with chance detection of shunt malfunction; the likelihood of detecting this at a routine annual appointment is improbable. It relates as much to the requirements of continuing education of the parents, or other carer, and later, the patient into those features of shunt malfunction that should trigger medical attention. Of equal importance is the provision of the advice and support needed to enable maximum fulfillment of potential, including neuropsychologic evaluations and interaction with other agencies, in particular education authorities and employers. It is the need to care for the child rather than just the condition that is one of the hallmarks and ambitions of pediatric neurosurgery (James 1998). Whatever arrangements are made for follow-up, it is crucial that the carers, and later the child, are afforded a rapid and effective route of return to specialist care, and this author advocates an 'open door' policy of return direct to the neurosurgical unit: in this respect, the invention that is likely to save most time, distress, unnecessary hazard, and indeed lives is not the CT but that devised by Alexander Graham Bell a century before – the telephone!

Pediatricians and adult physicians seeing patients with shunts should appreciate that the diagnosis of shunt malfunction relies heavily on careful attention to the clinical features as neither CT nor MR can reliably confirm or negate a diagnosis of shunt malfunction (Iskandar *et al.* 1998b). There can be normal shunt malfunction with dilated ventricles and dangerously raised intracranial pressure with small ventricles. Helpful clues include poor position of the ventricular catheter, obliterated basal cisterns and cortical sulci, and extravasation of CSF along the track of the ventricular catheter. If the shunt is functioning, the ventricle containing the catheter is typically smaller than the contralateral ventricle. Despite a variety of tests proposed from time to time (Howman-Giles *et al.* 1984), shunt independence can be a dangerous and, on occasion, life-threatening false assumption (Hemmer & Boehm 1976; Vaishnav & Mackinnon 1986; Punt 1993).

## COMPLICATIONS

The failure of ventricular shunts to be the answer to the maiden's prayer is expressed by the universal experience that 25–40% fail by 1 year after insertion (Drake & Sainte-Rose 1995). The probability of later failure accrues to 81% by 12 years (Sainte-Rose *et al.* 1991) and 83% by 20 years (Sgouros *et al.* 1995). The catalog of shunt complications is extensive and well documented elsewhere (Keucher & Mealey 1979; Punt 1993). It includes: obstruction; infection; fracture, disconnection, and distraction of shunt components; overdrainage leading to subdural effusions, slit ventricle syndrome or secondary synostosis with craniocerebral disproportion; ulceration; CSF ascites; perforation of viscera; and many others. Only the most frequently encountered and the most significant will be considered here. A prospective 10-year single-institution observational study, in which there were 1183 shunt failures in 839 patients, demonstrated that age under 40 weeks' gestation and age between 40 weeks and 1 year were both risk factors for failure. A most interesting finding from the same study was that the time interval since previous shunt surgery was also an important independent predictor, an interval of less than 6 months correlating with an increased risk of failure (Tull *et al.* 2000).

## OBSTRUCTION

In one series, 30% of shunt malfunctions occurred within 1 year of insertion, and thereafter, the rate of failure was 2–5% per annum (Sainte-Rose *et al.* 1991). Another major review reported the prevalence of failure to be 39% at 1 year and 53% at 2 years from initial insertion (Drake *et al.* 1998). Most early shunt obstructions relate to the ventricular catheter (Kast *et al.* 1994). Obstruction of the shunt occurring soon after insertion most frequently results from poor positioning of the ventricular catheter. Early reopening of the wound, within 10 days of surgery, is to be deprecated, as infection of the shunt is the almost inevitable result: it is preferable to insert a second shunt through fresh incisions. Early obstruction of the peritoneal end may result from inadvertent extraperitoneal placement of the tubing. Late obstruction of the peritoneal end will occur with growth if only short lengths of peritoneal catheter are inserted: the author employs the same total length of peritoneal catheter into all children, regardless of size or age, as into older patients, and has not encountered any disadvantages from this practice. It has been suggested that multiple shunt failures may result from unidentified biologic factors (Lazareff *et al.* 1998).

Whereas the symptoms are most usually those of raised intracranial pressure, less frequent features include neck pain, spinal cord dysfunction in association with hydromyelia, lower cranial nerve palsies in patients with myelomeningocele, and loss of upgaze with paralysis of convergence (Lee *et al.* 1999). As noted above, some patients can have symptoms that are very particular to them. In general, epileptic seizures are not due to blocked shunts and are more likely to relate to the underlying cerebral pathology (Johnson *et al.* 1996; Keene & Ventureyra 1999). Indeed, in every case, it is important to go through the exercise of considering whether the presenting symptoms are consistent with shunt malfunction or are more likely to arise from a background condition. Investigations should include plain radiographs of the head, trunk, and abdomen to check the position of the shunt and to confirm its continuity; specific imaging can be by US if the anterior fontanelle is still open, or by CT or MR. The purpose of the imaging is to demonstrate ventricular size and the position of the ventricular catheter, and to exclude any recurrence of underlying pathology, such as brain tumor, or any intercurrent condition, such as subdural effusion. Ventricular size alone does not indicate whether the shunt is, or is not, functioning (Iskandar *et al.* 1998b).

More recently, it has been demonstrated that shunt obstruction can be treated satisfactorily by NTV in up to 71% of cases (Mallucci *et al.* 1997), and this should be considered the treatment of choice whenever possible (Cinalli *et al.* 1998). Thirty-seven of 47 patients with childhood hydrocephalus, whose median age at the time of initial shunt insertion was 3 months, and who underwent NTV at the time of symptomatic shunt malfunction at a median age of 118 months, were relieved of their symptoms. There were only three significant adverse events. It is noteworthy that the median number of previous shunt procedures was two, but with a range of one to 18 (Mallucci *et al.* 1997).

## INFECTION (see also p. 586, Chapter 33)

This is the most serious complication encountered in infancy as, even in the absence of frank ventriculitis, it relates strongly to poor ultimate intellect (McLone *et al.* 1982). Overall infection rates of up to 20% (Renier *et al.* 1984) are reported, and for premature babies, the author has encountered those who privately acknowledge rates of up to 50%. In the most fortunate hands, the incidence has, however, declined, and rates of less than 3% are now achieved by some specialist pediatric neurosurgeons (O'Brien *et al.* 1979). Few can emulate the remarkable feat of reducing the infection rate from 7.75% per procedure to 0.17% per procedure attained by one major pediatric neurosurgery service, but it is noteworthy that this was achieved through attention to peri-operative care as well as to surgical technique (Choux *et al.* 1992). Prophylactic antibiotics were employed, but their role remains uncertain (Haines & Walters 1994). Identifiable etiological factors include very young age (Dallasca *et al.* 1995), poor skin condition, sites of intercurrent sepsis, and technical inexperience on behalf of the surgeon (Renier *et al.* 1984; Lund-Johansen *et al.* 1994; Borgbjerg *et al.* 1995). Some have not found any correlation with age: Davis *et al.* (1999) analyzed 2325 ventriculoperitoneal shunt procedures in 1193 patients and found an infection rate of 4% in those aged under 1 month compared to an overall rate of 3.2%. The same authors also found no correlation with prematurity.

Acute postoperative infection is heralded by malaise, fever, and, occasionally, seizures. It is confirmed by examination of CSF aspirated from the shunt reservoir. Chronic colonization most frequently presents masquerading as intermittent shunt malfunction, perhaps accompanied by mild fever. CSF taken from the shunt may be sterile in up to 50% of cases, and the causative microorganism may only be obtained by culture of the shunt components themselves. The finding of CSF ascites or a localized peritoneal cyst around the tip of the peritoneal catheter is highly suggestive of shunt colonization. It is again important to appreciate that culture of CSF may be sterile and that it is culture of the shunt components that is required. Of 18 children with abdominal CSF pseudocysts, culture of CSF was positive in only eight cases out of 11 from whom culture of the abdominal catheter tip was positive (Salomao & Leibinger 1999). Frequent unexplained episodes of apparent shunt malfunction are also suggestive of colonization. Except in the very young, blood tests such as the full peripheral blood picture, erythrocyte sedimentation rate, C-reactive protein, and blood cultures are generally unhelpful in the diagnosis of colonized ventriculoperitoneal shunts. They may be of value in infected ventriculoatrial shunts. The finding of a pleural effusion is indicative of ventriculopleural shunt malfunction, which may, or may not, be colonized.

Although treatment of shunt infection by intensive intravenous and intra-shunt antibiotics without shunt removal has been successful for some surgeons (Ward & McLaurin 1980), most practitioners have found the technique to be associated with an unacceptably high failure rate (Forward *et al.* 1983). The most successful approach is shunt removal with interval external ventricular drainage; systemic antibiotics supplemented by intraventricular antibiotics if necessary; and then shunt reinsertion through fresh incisions when the cerebrospinal is sterile. It is important to obtain an accurate microbiologic diagnosis and to employ high doses of antibiotics likely to penetrate the blood–CSF barrier (Frane & McLaurin 1982). For the occasional child in whom further surgery would be particularly undesirable, medical treatment may be attempted. The essential prerequisites are that the shunt is functioning; that there are no loose or free-floating, or non-functioning items of shunt hardware in place; and that accurate microbiologic diagnosis and antibiotic sensitivities are available. Antibiotics in high doses are given intravenously and into the shunt until the CSF becomes bactericidal to the infecting organism at a titer of 1:8 when tested *in vitro*. At least two antibiotics should be used and treatment continued for 3 weeks from the time of achieving bactericidal levels in the CSF. Traditional therapy by removal, interval drainage, antibiotics, and reinsertion is frequently simpler, quicker, and cheaper. It has been suggested that infection with Propionibacterium acnes can be treated more simply by antibiotics and shunt replacement without interval external drainage in view of the broad sensitivity to antibiotics, the relatively benign nature of the micro-organism, and the rapidity of achieving a sterile CSF (Thompson & Albright 1998). The infecting organism is usually *Staphylococcus epidermidis*; occasionally *Staphylococcus aureus*; and, less frequently, coliforms, *Pseudomonas*, *Klebsiella*, or *Candida*. Premature babies on neonatal intensive care units may well harbor multiply resistant organisms. It is self evident from the complexity and seriousness of the condition that a close collaboration between neurosurgeon and microbiologist is central to success.

## SLIT VENTRICLE SYNDROME

There are many debates as to the precise incidence and significance of so-called overdrainage, usually attributed to insertion of a system working at a pressure deemed to be too low (Folz & Blanks 1997). True slit ventricle syndrome, in which the ventricles appear to lose the capacity to expand, even in the face of shunt blockage, is probably quite a rare and relatively late complication of ventricular shunting occurring in no more than about 5% of children. Those shunted in very early life and who have sustained parenchymal brain injury seem to be at particular risk. Whether it is actually chronic overdrainage or the periventricular white-matter damage that leads to the stiffening of the ventricular wall is debatable; as it is improbable that most shunts do not overdrain under the effects of gravity, the fault may lie in the brain, rather than in the shunt hardware. The effect is that ventricular enlargement does not occur, or occurs minimally, even when the shunt blocks. These children present with recurrent episodes of transient intracranial hypertension that may be of such a frequency that they erode the quality of life and interfere with education. They may deteriorate very rapidly, losing consciousness. Vision may be lost. One approach is to change the shunt for one working at a different pressure or for a variable type that can be adjusted after insertion. An alternative is to introduce an anti-siphon device into the shunt. It is a manifestation of the relative lack of success of these tactics that shunt manufacturers have produced a plethora of technical solutions. A more useful strategy is subtemporal decompression (Epstein *et al.* 1974, 1978). A portion of the squamous temporal bone is removed beneath the temporalis muscle. The operation is performed ipsilateral to the ventricle that contains the tip of the shunt catheter. The frequency of episodes of symptomatic intracranial hypertension is reduced, as is the need for shunt revision. The insertion of future ventricular catheters is facilitated (Buxton & Punt 1995, 1999). An alternative approach is to replace the shunt with an external ventricular drain and then promote expansion of the ventricles by progressively raising the level of the drain until they are of a size that will accommodate a neuroendoscope such that a third ventriculostomy can be made. Particular care has to be taken not to irrigate too fiercely during the endoscopy lest cardiac dysrhythmias are precipitated (Handler *et al.* 1994).

## MULTICOMPARTMENTAL HYDROCEPHALUS

Multicompartmental, or multiloculated hydrocephalus, arises when one ventricle, or part of a ventricle, becomes isolated from the rest of the ventricular system, is no longer effectively drained, and consequently becomes dilated or 'trapped'. It occurs under a number of circumstances that are particularly common in neonates: namely, posthemorrhagic hydrocephalus (Eller & Paternak 1985); neonatal meningitis (Kalsbeck *et al.* 1980); in association with myelomeningocele (Scotti *et al.* 1980); neonatal brain abscess with intraventricular rupture; ventriculitis in association with ventricular shunt infection; and after intraventricular surgery. Multicompartmental hydrocephalus is a singularly unpleasant state. The symptoms may be those of intracranial hypertension but may also include accentuation of pre-existing focal neurologic signs. Patients with a trapped fourth ventricle may present with vomiting, eye movement disorder, and lower cranial nerve signs amounting to bulbar palsy and ataxia. The management is difficult and the outcome frequently poor in terms of multiple shunt revisions, neurologic disability, and mortality (McLone *et al.* 1987; Bindal *et al.* 1990). These patients can often end up with multiple shunts. Neuroendoscopy can be usefully employed to marsupialize the loculated compartments into the main ventricular system and thereby simplify the shunt required. Imaging may make such procedures look deceptively attractive, but they are actually very difficult in execution as there is a paucity of normal anatomic features to aid navigation, and the walls between the chambers may be thick and surprisingly vascular. The trapped fourth ventricle is especially dangerous because of its tendency to adversely affect brainstem function, sometimes irreversibly or even fatally. The very nature of the condition is such that many of the sufferers already have major neurodevelopmental handicaps and compromised brain function, making them especially vulnerable to additional insults. Fourth-ventricle shunts are notoriously difficult to maintain. It is best to avoid conjoined shunts. The anatomic complexity of the condition emphasizes the importance of full evaluation by MR. Endoscope-assisted shunt placement may be helpful in achieving optimal positioning of the fourth-ventricle catheter (Sandberg & Souweidane 1999). The alternative strategy of suboccipital craniectomy and open fenestration has some advocates (Villavicencio *et al.* 1998) but the circumstances that predispose to a trapped fourth ventricle might be thought to mitigate success, and that has certainly been the present author's observed experience. Overdrainage of the fourth ventricle may precipitate cranial nerve palsies by irritation of the floor of the ventricle by the shunt catheter. Shortening of the catheter, endoscope-assisted placement and a flow-regulated or high-pressure valve may prevent or relieve the complication (Eder *et al.* 1997).

## ABDOMINAL SURGERY

Intuitively, it seems probable that abdominal or pelvic surgery in shunted patients must carry a risk to the shunt, yet no standard or commonly accepted protocol exists to deal with this eventuality. In one report of six children with ventriculoperitoneal shunts in place, who developed acute appendicitis, the shunts were left in place. There were no cases of ascending shunt infection, but one child did develop an intra-abdominal CSF collection, necessitating removal of the older shunt. The authors therefore suggested that when there is frank abdominal or pelvic disease that requires surgery, the peritoneal catheter should be left in place (Pumberger *et al.* 1998). Alternatively, the opportunity might be taken to perform a NTV and to remove the shunt completely. For cold, clean abdominal or pelvic surgery, this would seem a little extreme, although there is some evidence for gastrostomy being associated with a risk of shunt infection. Laparoscopy can cause a rise in intracranial pressure in shunted patients (Uzzo *et al.* 1997), and it has been suggested that these patients should have the peritoneal catheter exposed through a separate incision over the chest wall, occluded, and that every 30 min during the laparoscopy the abdomen should be desufflated and the valve pumped 25–50 times to allow drainage (Gaskill *et al.* 1998). For children with peritoneal shunts who require gastrostomy, it may be a sensible precaution to consider diversion of the shunt elsewhere, such as the pleura, or NTV and shunt removal prior to the gastrostomy to avoid the risk of the shunt becoming infected.

## OUTCOME

Natural-history studies demonstrate that, untreated, 46% of children with hydrocephalus survive infancy, only 38% of these have normal intelligence, and the actuarial survival to adult life is 20–23% (Laurence & Coates 1962). With the introduction of modern shunting devices, and with a greater understanding of shunt complications and management, one early series found that 95% of shunted children survived for 10 years and 70% of them had normal intelligence, if significant numbers of infants shunted for posthemorrhagic hydrocephalus were excluded (Milhorat 1972). Of those who have impaired intellect, neurodevelopmental delay, or frank neurologic handicap, the deficits relate either to shunt complications, especially infection (McLone *et al.* 1987), or to the process that has produced the hydrocephalus. In this regard, neonates who have suffered grade III or grade IV intraventricular hemorrhage, or pyogenic meningitis, fare relatively badly. Children with aqueductal stenosis have an excellent prognosis, while those with the Dandy–Walker syndrome do badly; 70% have learning difficulties, with an intelligence quotient (IQ) of less than 83 (Sawaya & McLaurin 1981). Although the thickness of the cerebral mantle correlates variably with ultimate intellectual function, it appears that for most children with hydrocephalus uncomplicated by other factors, the IQ will be normal if a cerebral mantle of 3 cm or more is achieved by the age of 4 or 5 months (Nulsen & Rekate 1982).

Although intelligence quotient (IQ) is an index of outcome, 53% of children achieving an IQ greater than 80 (Dennis *et al.* 1981), it may disguise the cognitive difficulties associated with discrepancies between verbal and non-verbal performance, the former typically exceeding the latter. It may also hide problems relating to failure to make age-appropriate progress in the more challenging arena of secondary education. The ability to attend normal school is a better measure (Hirsch 1994) and is of greater practical relevance to families. This was recognized in one 10-year cohort study of 155 children initially shunted between 1978 and 1983 that reported that 59% of those surviving to school age attended mainstream school. The outlook was better for those with congenital hydrocephalus, of whom 29% required special education, than for those with post-meningitic or post-hemorrhagic hydrocephalus of whom 52% and 60%, respectively, required special education. Forty-four per cent did not require revisional surgery. The first year was the most frequent time to require shunt revision that was most commonly needed because of blockage (49%), infection (19%), and disconnection (13%). Mortality was 11% for those with non-tumoral hydrocephalus (Casey *et al.* 1997). Others (Hoppe-Hirsch *et al.* 1998), reporting on 129 consecutive children with non-tumoral hydrocephalus initially shunted between 1979 and 1982, found a 10-year mortality of less than 5%; although 60% attended mainstream school, half of these were experiencing difficulties. Thirty per cent had epilepsy, and this was associated with a particularly poor neuropsychologic outcome. Initial major ventriculomegaly was an adverse factor. The etiology of the hydrocephalus was also relevant, children with myelomeningocele having the best neuropsychologic outcomes and those with post-meningitic hydrocephalus the worst.

It should be fully appreciated that although many of the processes that produce hydrocephalus in the neonatal period carry a significant risk of disability, the option of not treating the hydrocephalus in the face of progressive and symptomatic ventriculomegaly is usually not realistic. The neonatal neurosurgeon must accept that relief of hydrocephalus in such children can be an important palliative measure and should not reject them out of hand because of the perceived likelihood of a less-than-perfect developmental outcome.

## REFERENCES


Berger A, Weninger M, Reinprecht A *et al.* (2000) Long-term experience with subcutaneously tunneled external ventricular drainage in preterm infants. *Child's Nerv Syst* 16:103–110.

Bindal A K, Storrs B B & McLone D G (1990) Management of the Dandy-Walker malformation. *Pediatr Neurosurg* 16:163–169.

Bondurant C P & Jimenez D F (1995) Epidemiology of cerebrospinal fluid shunting. *Pediatr Neurosurg* 23:254–259.

Borgbjerg B M, Gjerris F, Albeck M J *et al.* (1995) Risk of infection after cerebrospinal shunt: An analysis of 884 first-time shunts. *Acta Neurochirurg (Wien)* 136:1–7.

Bucholz R D & Pittman T (1991) Endoscopic coagulation of the choroid plexus using the Nd:YAG laser: Initial experience and proposal for management. *Neurosurgery* 28:421–427.

Buxton N & Punt J (1995) The value of sub-temporal decompression in the treatment of shunt complications. *Eur J Pediatr Surg* 5(suppl 1):18.

Buxton N & Punt J (1998) Failure to follow patients with hydrocephalus shunts causes deaths. *Br J Neurosurg* 12:399–401.

Buxton N & Punt J (1999) Subtemporal decompression in hydrocephalus related raised intracranial pressure. *Neurosurgery* 44:513–519.

Caldarelli M, Di Rocco C & La-Marca F (1996) Shunt complications in the first post-operative year in children with myelomeningocele. *Child's Nerv Syst* 12:748–754.

Casey A T H, Kimmings E J, Kleinlugtebeld A D *et al.* (1997) The long-term outlook for hydrocephalus in childhood. *Pediatr Neurosurg* 27:63–70.

Choux M, Genitori L, Lang D *et al.* (1992) Shunt implantation: reducing the incidence of shunt infection. *J Neurosurg* 77:875–880.

Chumas P D, Kulkarni A V, Drake J M, Hoffman H J, Humphreys R P, Rutka J T (1993) Lumboperitoneal shunting: a retrospective study in the pediatric population. *Neurosurgery* 32:376–83.

Cinalli G, Salazar C, Mallucci C *et al.* (1998) The role of endoscopic third ventriculostomy in the management of shunt malfunction. *Neurosurgery* 43:1323–1329.

Cohen A R (1994) Ventriculoscopic surgery. *Clin Neurosurg* 41:546–562.

Colak A, Albright A L & Pollack I F (1997) Follow-up of children with shunted hydrocephalus. *Pediatr Neurosurg* 27:208–210.

Cornips E, Van Calenbergh F, Plets C *et al.* (1997) Use of external drainage for posthemorrhagic hydrocephalus in very low birth weight premature infants. *Child's Nerv Sys* 13:369–374.

Dallasca P, Dappozzo A, Galassi E *et al.* (1995) Cerebrospinal fluid shunt infections in infants. *Child's Nerv Syst* 11:643–648.

Dandy W E (1918) Extirpation of the choroid plexus of the lateral ventricles in communicating hydrocephalus. *Ann Surg* 68:569–579.

Dandy W E (1922) An operative procedure for hydrocephalus. *Johns Hopkins Hosp Bull* 33:189.

Davis L (1939) *Neurological surgery*. Philadelphia, PA: Lea and Febiger p. 405.

Davis S E, Levy M L, McComb J G *et al.* (1999) Does age or other factors influence the incidence of ventriculoperitoneal infections? *Pediatr Neurosurg* 30:253–257.

Decq P, Yepes C, Anno Y *et al.* (1994) L'endoscopie neurochirurgicale. Indications diagnostiques et therapeutiques. *Neurochirurgie* 40:313–321.

Dennis M, Fitz C R & Netley C T (1981) The intelligence of hydrocephalic children. *Arch Neurol* 38:607–615.

Drake J M, Kestle J R W, Milner R *et al.* (1998) Randomised trial of cerebrospinal fluid shunt valve design in pediatric hydrocephalus. *Neurosurgery* 43:294–305.

Drake J M & Sainte-Rose C (1995) *The shunt book*. Cambridge, MA: Blackwell Science; pp. 123–192.

Eder H G, Leber K A & Gruber W (1997) Complications after shunting isolated IV ventricles. *Child's Nerv Syst* 13:13–16.

Eller T W & Paternak J F (1985) Isolated ventricles following intraventricular haemorrhage. *J Neurosurg* 62:357–362.

Epstein F, Marlin A E & Wald A (1978) Chronic headache in the shunt-dependent adolescent with nearly normal ventricular volume: diagnosis and treatment. *Neurosurgery* 3:351–335.

Epstein F J, Fleischer A J, Hochwald G M *et al.* (1974) Subtemporal craniectomy for recurrent shunt obstruction secondary to small ventricles. *J Neurosurg* 41:29–31.

Folz E L & Blanks J P (1997) Symptomatic low intracranial pressure in shunted hydrocephalus. *J Neurosurg* 86:401–408.

Forrest D M & Cooper D G N (1968) Complications of ventriculo-atrial shunts: a review of 455 cases. *J Neurosurg* 29:506–512.

Forward K R, Fewer D & Stiver H G (1983) Cerebrospinal fluid shunt infections: a review of 35 infections in 32 patients. *J Neurosurg* 59:389–394.

Frane P T & McLaurin R L (1982) Antibiotic therapy in central nervous system infections. In: *Paediatric neurosurgery: surgery of the developing nervous system.* New York, NY: Grune and Stratton; pp. 591–599.

Gamache F W J (1995) Treatment of hydrocephalus in patients with myelomeningocele or encephalocele: A recent series. *Child's Nerv Syst* 11:487–488.

Gaskill S J, Cossman R M, Hickman M S *et al.* (1998) Laparoscopic surgery in a patient with a ventriculoperitoneal shunt: a new technique. *Pediatr Neurosurg* 28:106–107.

Griffith H B (1986) Endoneurosurgery: endoscopic intracranial surgery. In: Griffith H B & Symon L (eds) *Advances and technical standards in neurosurgery*. New York, NY: Springer; pp. 2–24.

Griffith H B & Jamjoom A B (1990) The treatment of childhood hydrocephalus by choroid plexus coagulation and artificial cerebrospinal fluid perfusion. *Br J Neurosurg* 4:95–100.

Haines S J & Walters B C (1994) Antibiotic prophylaxis for cerebrospinal fluid shunts: a metanalysis. *Neurosurgery* 34:87–93.

Handler M H, Abbott R & Lee M (1994) A near-fatal complication of endoscopic third ventriculostomy: case report. *Neurosurgery* 35:525–528.

Hayden P W, Shurtleff D B & Stuntz T J (1983) A longitudinal study of shunt function in 360 patients with hydrocephalus. *Dev Med Child Neurol* 25:334–337.

Hemmer R & Boehm B (1976) Once a shunt, always a shunt? *Dev Med Child Neurol* 18 (suppl 37):69–73.

Hirsch J F (1994) Consensus statement. Long-term outcome in hydrocephalus. *Child's Nerv Syst* 10:64–69.

Hockley A D (1999) Congenital anomalies of the central nervous system. In: Garfield J & Earl C (eds) *Medical negligence. The cranium, spine and nervous system.* Oxford: Blackwell Science, pp. 237–252.

Hoffman H J, Harwood-Nash D & Gilday D L (1980)

Percutaneous third ventriculoscopy in the management of non-communicating hydrocephalus. *Neurosurgery* 7:313–321.

Hoffman H J, Harwood-Nash D, Gilday D L *et al.* (1981) Percutaneous third ventriculostomy in the management of non-communicating hydrocephalus. In: *Concepts in paediatric neurosurgery.* Basel: Karger, vol. I; pp. 87–106.

Hoffman H J, Hendrick E B & Humphreys R P (1976) New lumboperitoneal shunt for communicating hydrocephalus (technical note). *J Neurosurg* 44:258–261.

Hoppe-Hirsch E, Laroussinie F, Brunet L *et al.* (1998) Late outcome of the surgical treatment of hydrocephalus. *Child's Nerv Syst* 14:97–99.

Howman-Giles R, McLaughlin A, Johnston I *et al.* (1984) A radionuclide method of evaluating shunt function and CSF circulation in hydrocephalus. Technical note. *J Neurosurg* 61:604–605.

Iskandar B J, Tubbs S, Mapstone T B *et al.* (1998a) Death in shunted hydrocephalic children in the 1990s. *Pediatr Neurosurg* 28:173–176.

Iskandar B J, McLaughlin C, Mapstone T B *et al.* (1998b) Pitfalls in the diagnosis of ventricular shunt dysfunction: Radiology reports and ventricular size. *Pediatrics* 101:1031–1036.

James H (1998) Follow-up of children with shunted hydrocephalus. *Pediatr Neurosurg* 28:327.

James H E & Murphy K G (1998) The Surgical Isolation Bubble System and patient temperature during ventriculoperitoneal shunt insertion in preterm and term newborn infants. *Child's Nerv Syst* 14:26–29.

Johnson D, Conry J & O'Donnell R (1996) Epileptic seizures as a sign of cerebrospinal fluid shunt malfunction. *Pediatr Neurosurg* 24:223–228.

Jones R F C, Kwok B C T, Stening W A *et al.* (1994) Neuroendoscopic third ventriculostomy. A practical alternative to extracranial shunts in non-communicating hydrocephalus. *Acta Neurochirurg* (suppl 61):79–83.

Jones R F C, Stening W A S & Bryden M (1990) Endoscopic third ventriculostomy. *Neurosurgery* 26:86–92.

Jones R F C, Teo C, Stening W A *et al.* (1992) Neuroendoscopic third ventriculostomy. In: Mainwaring K H & Crone K R (eds) *Neuroendoscopy.* Liebert, New York, NY: Liebert vol. 1; pp. 63–77.

Kalsbeck J E, De Souza A L, Kleiman M B *et al.* (1980) Compartmentalization of the cerebral ventricles as a sequel of neonatal meningitis. *J Neurosurg* 52:547–552.

Kast J, Duong D, Norwazi F *et al.* (1994) Time-related patterns of ventricular shunt failure. *Child's Nerv Syst* 10:524–528.

Keene D L & Ventureyra E C G (1999) Hydrocephalus and epileptic seizures. *Child's Nerv Syst* 15:158–162.

Keucher T R & Mealey J Jr (1979) Longterm results after ventriculoatrial and ventriculoperitoneal shunting for infantile hydrocephalus. *J Neurosurg* 50:179–186.

Kimmings E, Kleinlugtebeld A, Casey A T H *et al.* (1996) Does the child with shunted hydrocephalus require long-term neurosurgical follow-up? *Br J Neurosurg* 10:77–81.

Kirkpatrick M, Engelman H & Minns R A (1989) Symptoms and signs of progressive hydrocephalus. *Arch Dis Childhood* 64:124–128.

Laurence K M & Coates S (1962) The natural history of hydrocephalus. *Arch Dis Childhood* 37:345–362.

Lazareff J A, Peacock W, Holly L *et al.* (1998) Multiple shunt failures: an analysis of relevant factors. *Child's Nerv Syst* 14:271–275.

Lee T T, Uribe J, Ragheb J *et al.* (1999) Unique clinical presentation of pediatric shunt malfunction. *Pediatr Neurosurg* 30:122–126.

Lund-Johansen M, Svendsen F & Wester K (1994) Shunt failures and complications in adults as related to shunt type, diagnosis, and the experience of the surgeon. *Neurosurgery* 35:839–844.

McLone D, Czyzewski D & Raimondi A J (1982) The effects of complications on intellectual function in 173 children with myelomeningocele. Cited by: Reigel D J 1982 Spina bifida. In: *Paediatric neurosurgery: surgery of the developing nervous system.* New York, NY: Grune and Stratton; pp. 23–47.

McLone D G, Naidich T P & Cunningham T (1987) Posterior fossa cysts: Management and outcome. *Concepts Pediatr Neurosurg* 7:134–141.

Mallucci C L, Vloeberghs M & Punt J A (1997) Neuroendoscopic III ventriculostomy: the first-line treatment for blocked ventriculo-peritoneal shunts? *Child's Nerv Syst* 13:498.

Marlin A E (1996) Shunting In: Cheek W R (ed.) *Atlas of pediatric neurosurgery.* Philadelphia, PA: WB Saunders; pp. 65–71.

Milhorat T H (1972) In: *Hydrocephalus and the cerebrospinal fluid.* Baltimore, MD: Williams and Wilkins.

Mixter W J (1923) Ventriculoscopy and puncture of the floor of the third ventricle. *Boston Med Surg J* 188:277–278.

Neville B G R (1993) Clinical features of hydrocephalus in childhood and infancy. In: Schurr P H & Polkey C E (eds) *Hydrocephalus.* Oxford: Oxford Medical Publications; pp. 100–118.

Nugent G R, Lucas R, Judy M *et al.* (1966) Thromboembolic complications of ventriculoatrial shunts: angiographic and pathologic correlation. *J Neurosurg* 24:34–42.

Nulsen F E & Rekate H L (1982) Results of treatment for hydrocephalus as a guide to future management. In: *Paediatric neurosurgery: surgery of the developing nervous system.* New York, NY: Grune and Stratton; pp. 229–241.

Nulsen F E & Spitz E B (1951) Treatment of hydrocephalus by direct shunt from ventricle to jugular vein. *Surg Forums* 2:399–403.

O'Brien M, Parent A & Davis B (1979) Management of ventricular shunt infections. *Child's Brain* 5:304–309.

Pittman T & Bucholz R D (1992) Endoscopic choroid plexectomy. In: Mainwaring K H & Crone K R (eds) *Neuroendoscopy.* New York, NY: Liebert, vol. 1; pp. 97–102.

Portnoy H D (1982) Hydrodynamics of shunts. *Monogr Neural Sci* 8:173–183.

Pudenz R H (1980) The surgical treatment of hydrocephalus: an historical view. *Surg Neurol* 15:15–26.

Pumberger W, Lobl M & Geissler W (1998) Appendicitis in children with a ventriculoperitoneal shunt. *Pediatr Neurosurg* 28:21–26.

Punt J (1993) Principles of CSF diversion and alternative treatments. In: Schurr P H & Polkey C E (eds) *Hydrocephalus.* Oxford: Oxford Medical Publications; pp. 139–160.

Punt J (1996) Management of hydrocephalus in new-born infants. *Semin Neonatol* 1:203–210.

Punt J & Vloeberghs M (1998) Endoscopy in neurosurgery. *Min Invas Ther Allied Technol* 7:159–170.

Putnam T J (1934) Treatment of hydrocephalus by endoscopic coagulation of the choroid plexus. *N Engl J Med* 210:1373–1376.

Rachel R A (1999) Surgical treatment of hydrocephalus: a historical perspective. *Pediatr Neurosurg* 30:296–304.

Rekate H L (1991) Shunt revision: Complications and their prevention. *Pediatr Neurosurg* 17:155–162.

Renier D, Lacombe J, Pierre-Kahn A *et al.* (1984) Factors causing shunt infection: computer analysis of 1174 operations. *J Neurosurg* 61:1072–1078.

Russell D S (1949) *Observations on the pathology of hydrocephalus. Special reports and services of the Medical Research Council, No. 265.* London: HMSO.

Sainte-Rose C (1992) Third ventriculostomy. In: Mainwaring K H & Crone K R (eds) *Neuroendoscopy.* New York, NY: Liebert vol. 1, pp. 47–62.

Sainte-Rose C, Piatt J H, Renier D *et al.* (1991) Mechanical complications in shunts. *Pediatr Neurosurg* 17:2–9.

Salomao J F & Leibinger R D (1999) Abdominal pseudocysts complicating CSF shunting in children. *Pediatr Neurosurg* 31:274–278.

Sandberg D I & Souweidane M M (1999) Endoscopic-guided proximal catheter placement in treatment of posterior fossa cysts. *Pediatr Neurosurg* 30:180–5.

Sawaya R & McLaurin R L (1981) Dandy–Walker syndrome: clinical analysis of 23 cases. *J Neurosurg* 55:89–98.

Scarff J E (1936) Endoscopic treatment of hydrocephalus. Description of a ventriculoscope and preliminary report of cases. *Arch Neurol Psychiatry* 35:853–861.

Scarff J E (1970) The treatment of non-obstructive (communicating) hydrocephalus by endoscopic cauterization of the choroid plexuses. *J Neurosurg* 33:1–18.

Scotti G, Musgrave M A, Fitz C R *et al.* (1980) The isolated fourth ventricle in children: CT and clinical review of 16 cases. *Am J Radiol* 135:1233–1238.

Sgouros S, Mallucci C, Walsh R *et al.* (1995) Long-term complications of hydrocephalus. *Pediatr Neurosurg* 23:127–132.

Strenger L (1963) Complications of ventriculovenous shunts. *J Neurosurg* 20:219–224.

Thompson T P & Albright A L (1998) Propionibacterium acnes infections of cerebrospinal fluid shunts. *Child's Nerv Syst* 14:378–380.

Tull S T, Drake J, Lawless J *et al.* (2000) Risk factors for repeated cerebrospinal shunt failures in pediatric patients with hydrocephalus. *J Neurosurg* 92:31–38.

Uzzo R G, Bilsky M, Mininberg D T *et al.* (1997) Laparoscopic surgery in children with ventriculoperitoneal shunts: Effect of pneumoperitoneum on intracranial pressure – Preliminary experience. *Urology* 49:753–757.

Vaishnav A & MacKinnon A E (1986) Progressive hydrocephalus in teenage spina bifida patients. *Zeitschrift für Kinderchirurgie* 41 (suppl 1):36–37.

Villavicencio A T, Wellons J C III & George T (1998) Avoiding complicated shunt systems by open fenestration of symptomatic fourth ventricular cysts associated with hydrocephalus. *Pediatr Neurosurg* 29:314–319.

Vries J K (1978) An endoscopic technique for third ventriculostomy. *Surg Neurol* 9:165–168.

Ward S L & McLaurin R L (1980) Cerebrospinal fluid antibiotic levels during treatment of shunt infections. *J Neurosurg* 52:41–46.

Weller R O, Kida S & Harding B N (1993) Aetiology and pathology of hydrocephalus. In: Schurr P H & Polkey C E (eds) *Hydrocephalus.* Oxford: Oxford Medical Publications; pp. 48–99.

Weller R O & Wisniewski H (1969) Histological and ultrastructural changes with experimental hydrocephalus in adult rabbits. *Brain* 92:819–828.

Weller R O, Wisniewski H, Shulman K *et al.* (1971) Experimental hydrocephalus in young dogs: histological and ultrastructural study of the brain tissue damage. *J Neuropathol Exp Neurol* 30:613–627.

Wozniak M, McLone D G & Raimondi A J (1975) Micro- and macrovascular changes as the direct cause of parenchymal destruction in congenital murine hydrocephalus. *J Neurosurg* 43:535–545.

# Chapter 45 Surgical management of neural-tube defects

J. Punt

## INTRODUCTION

The spectrum of neural tube defects spans some of the most minor to the most devastating congenital malformations encountered. An understanding of the possible implications, the probable outcome, and the range of appropriate neurosurgical management is essential knowledge for all of those who may be in a position to identify these lesions, whether they be obstetrician, radiologist, neonatologist, general pediatrician, neonatal nurse specialist, or health visitor. This chapter reviews current management and prognosis of open and closed neural tube defects.

## ENCEPHALOCELE

Encephaloceles are congenital hernias that may contain meninges, cerebrospinal fluid (CSF), and, on occasion, varying amounts of cerebral parenchyma. They are classified according to site (Suwanwela & Chaturaporn 1966; see Table 45.1): 70% are occipital, and 15% are frontoethmoidal. In certain Far Eastern countries, notably Thailand, Burma, and Malaysia, this ratio is reversed, and frontoethmoidal lesions predominate (Rapport *et al.* 1981). In Thailand, the incidence reaches one per 6000 live births (Rahman 1979), and the ratio of frontal to occipital sites is 9.5:1 (Charoonsmith & Suwanwela 1974).

**Table 45.1 Classification of encephalocele according to Suwanwela & Chaturaporn (1966)**

| |
|---|
| Cranial vault |
| Occipital |
| Interfrontal |
| Parietal |
| Anterior or posterior |
| Temporal |
| Frontoethmoidal (sincipital) |
| Nasofrontal |
| Nasoethmoidal |
| Naso-orbital |
| Basal |
| Transethmoidal |
| Sphenoethmoidal |
| Transsphenoidal |
| Spheno-orbital |

The diagnosis usually declares itself at birth, though larger lesions may be recognized prenatally by ultrasound from around 16 weeks of gestational age. Management commences with a general examination to exclude other congenital anomalies, especially cardiac (dextrocardia), respiratory (pulmonary hypoplasia and laryngomalacia), genito-urinary (renal agenesis), and the occasional concomitant myelomeningocele (Reigel 1982a–c). Anterior lesions may be associated with complex bone defects in the skull base and also with arhinencephaly and anophthalmia (Rapport *et al.* 1981). The site and size of the mass and the condition of the overlying skin are noted, and the occipito-frontal circumference is charted. For occipital encephaloceles, the only special investigation required is ultrasound scanning (US) of the lesion, the cranium, and the craniocervical junction. This will define the contents of the sac, the ventricular size and configuration, and the presence of any major concomitant cerebral malformation such as holoprosencephaly, Dandy–Walker malformation, and Chiari malformation. If readily available, magnetic resonance imaging (MRI) is also performed, as it provides more information. Brain tissue is present within the sac in 25–80% of cases (Mealey *et al.* 1970); the viability and functional capacity of such brain tissue are questionable, but on occasion, cerebral angiography may be justified to establish whether there is a useful blood supply. Anterior lesions demand more exacting imaging with computerized tomography (CT) and MRI to define the extent of abnormality of the skull base and of the brain. Particular attention should be paid to the position of the pituitary gland and optic chiasm. Except in cases of severe underdevelopment of the brain itself, neurologic examination is usually normal at birth. Particular attention should be paid to visual function in cases of large occipital encephaloceles, although it is recognized that assessment is difficult in the neonatal period and relies very much on the baby's behavior and degree of co-ordination of eye movements. Unlike myelomeningocele, the risk of infection in the neonatal period is low. That notwithstanding, large occipital encephaloceles are repaired shortly after birth, the general condition of the baby permitting, as they are distressing to behold and make handling, feeding, and the positioning of the baby for sleep difficult. Small occipital lesions may be left for a few weeks to enable the child to weather any other perinatal crises and to allow bonding with the parents. Frontal and basal encephaloceles are repaired after the first few weeks of life when the child has regained birthweight and is thriving, or may even be delayed until such time as definitive craniofacial corrective procedures are contemplated. The objectives of surgery are removal or replacement of the herniated cranial contents; watertight dural closure; repair of major bone defects; and adequate, cosmetically acceptable skin cover and craniofacial contours. With occipital lesions, these aims can usually be achieved with a single definitive procedure, although large skull defects may have to await further growth of the skull and secondary repair by bone grafting taken from elsewhere on the cranial vault. It is best to wait until the child's skull has grown sufficiently for the skull vault to be thick enough to permit split calvarial grafts to be harvested, usually from the parietal regions. An intact cranium can therefore be achieved within the primary school years. Frontal and basal lesions have often been dealt with as staged procedures, but the development of modern craniofacial surgery has brought the possibility of one-stage repair with later cosmetic adjustments as required (Sargent *et al.* 1988). The surgical techniques involved have been well described (Reigel 1982a–c; Hendrick 1985; Goodrich *et al.* 1991). All of these procedures should be performed by surgical, anesthetic, and nursing teams accustomed to the requirements of neonatal operations and post-operative care. Closure of an occipital encephalocele is performed with the child in the prone position, and both the surgeon and the anesthetist should be prepared to deal with blood loss from major venous sinuses around the torcula, as well as venous air embolism and cardiovascular irregularities if the brainstem is disturbed. Although attempts should be made to preserve the contents of an occipital encephalocele (Guthkelch 1970), this is often impractical, and the contents are frequently not functional (Ulrich 1976). Some surgeons have devised elaborate procedures to retain the contents of even the largest occipital encephaloceles in the fear of losing functioning tissue, but those children have a poor prognosis anyway. The herniated tissue in frontal encephaloceles and most basal encephaloceles can be sacrificed. Care is, needed, however, to identify and preserve hypothalamic and pituitary tissue and the anterior visual pathways. Postoperatively, the child is held and fed normally. A careful watch is kept for the development of hydrocephalus both by clinical monitoring with regular measurements of occipitofrontal circumference and by serial cranial US scans. Sixty to 70% of babies with occipital encephaloceles will require placement of a hydrocephalus shunt device, but this is rare with frontal and basal lesions. No information is yet available on the feasibility of neuroendoscopic third ventriculostomy (NTV) in the neonatal period for this population.

There is no realistic option, but to repair these lesions as, except for the occasional baby with a lethal extracranial anomaly, the condition untreated is rarely fatal. The family is afforded appropriate counseling and genetic advice. Follow-up entails monitoring of head growth and serial multi-disciplinary developmental assessments to identify any potential handicaps. This is best provided through a team approach at a child development center. Evaluation of visual function is important in both occipital and anterior basal lesions. Endocrine assessments are important with frontobasal anomalies.

### OUTCOME

In frontal and basal encephaloceles, the prognosis for neurodevelopmental progress is usually excellent (Nakamura *et al.* 1974); for occipital lesions, it is much more guarded (Matson 1969). For the latter, outcome relates to four factors: the presence or absence of brain tissue in the sac; the development of hydrocephalus; the state of development of the brain, often well indicated by coexistent microcephaly, which is an unfavorable feature; and the presence of concomitant cerebral malformations such as microgyria, holoprosencephaly, heterotopias, agenesis of the corpus callosum, and optic pathway dysgenesis. Of children with no brain tissue in the sac, 60–80% develop normally (Lorber 1967; Guthkelch 1970), as opposed to only 10–25% when brain tissue is present in the sac. Only 30% of those with hydrocephalus, but no herniated neural tissue, have normal intellect (Mealey *et al.* 1970). The 20% of children with microcephaly nearly all show developmental delay if the occipitofrontal circumference remains below the tenth centile (Lorber 1967; Guthkelch 1970).

## MYELOMENINGOCELE (see also Chapters 16 and 19)

Myelomeningocele, 'the most complex, treatable, congenital anomaly consistent with life' (Bunch *et al.* 1972), may first become apparent at birth but is more frequently recognized from elevated levels of α-1-fetoprotein in maternal serum and by prenatal US scanning. The real incidence is steadily falling in most parts of the world; for example, in the UK, there has been a reduction by one-third over a 20-year period (Cuckle *et al.* 1985). The true incidence of myelomeningocele in England and Wales, including cases diagnosed prenatally and aborted, fell from 215/100 000 in 1972 to 38/100 000 in 1991. Since 1992, this decline has stabilized (Kadir *et al.* 1999).

### PRENATAL MANAGEMENT

The diagnosis is usually made *in utero* at around 16–18 weeks' gestational age. Careful US examination is essential to detect any concomitant lesions and to assess ventricular size (see Chapters 17 and 18). It is preferable for the parents to be given the opportunity of consultation with a pediatric neurosurgeon rather than for the responsibility for providing accurate advice to be left purely with the obstetrician or pediatric physician. Indeed, it is frankly unwise for obstetricians or non-specialist pediatricians to be the sole doctors to advise the parents, even when the parents are already decided as to whether they wish the pregnancy to continue. Based upon the level of the lesion, the pediatric neurosurgeon can give a rough estimate of the minimum likely disability in terms of motor and sphincter function, explain the complex and multi-faceted nature of the condition, and describe the 'second lesions' that may develop and the treatments that may be available. It is important for the parents to understand that the condition is for life and that as complications can arise throughout childhood and adult life, there will be a permanent need for, and commitment to, ongoing health care. Such consultations must occur in an appropriate environment, such as a pregnancy assessment center, and must be unhurried and structured so that the parents feel enabled to make decisions with which they can be comfortable. It is crucial to record very clearly the information given together with a statement regarding the limitations of pre-natal prognosis in order to protect against any future claim for 'wrongful birth' based upon allegations of inadequate consultation. For those pregnancies that proceed, there are obvious advantages to all involved if the various issues have been discussed pre-natally at a time when emotions are more collected and when there are no great pressures of time. Ventricular size should be monitored by US from around 32 weeks' gestational age, but there is no indication for early delivery unless hydrocephalus advances very rapidly from 34 weeks. Vaginal delivery is perfectly acceptable. Ideally, the baby should be born in a maternity unit with, or closely adjacent to, a neonatal neurosurgery facility so that transfer, or separation of mother from baby, in the immediate post-natal period is avoided.

The possibility of prenatal surgery has been recently proposed, and successful closure of a thoraco-lumbar myelomeningocele has been reported at 23 weeks' gestational age (see Chapter 42). Of particular interest was that at birth, the baby had good motor function, and that hydrocephalus and a hindbrain hernia seen *in utero* had resolved (Adzick *et al.* 1998). The theoretical basis for such surgery is that there is evidence from some rodent models and from human fetal material that the neural placode is initially still capable of neuronal differentiation but is subsequently damaged by amniotic fluid (Copp *et al.* 1990; Keller-Pack & Mullen 1993). However, not all animal models have demonstrated deterioration of the exposed neural tube (McLone *et al.* 1997). In an artificial ovine model, neuronal degeneration and neurologic dysfunction were prevented by *in utero* closure (Meuli *et al.* 1995). The hypothesis is therefore that the neurologic deficits seen in human myelomeningocele are not due to the primary lesion but are secondary to the adverse physical and chemical effects of the amniotic fluid (Tulipan & Bruner 1998). The major benefit of *in utero* closure may be in avoidance of hydrocephalus rather than in preservation of spinal cord function. In one series, only 21 out of 42 children required a shunt. Interestingly intrauterine repair appeared to reverse an established hindbrain hernia in nine children who were studied with serial imaging (Tulipan *et al.* 1999a). Closure may have this effect by stopping CSF flow through the placode. Whereas this may cast light on the pathogenesis, it remains uncertain whether the reversal of the hernia prevents symptoms developing. In the series cited, only two out of 42 became symptomatic early on in life. In a further case-control study, the effect on incidence of shunt-dependent hydrocephalus was less impressive at 58% versus 92% in the historic controls (Tulipan *et al.* 1999b). Such surgery, if widely followed, may bring hazards to both mother and baby (Harrison *et al.* 1993; Adzick & Harrison 1994; Harrison *et al.* 1997). Before accepting the alleged benefits and adopting this approach, it would be appropriate to restrict this surgery to a small number of centers and to analyze the results by further careful case–control studies using contemporary, rather than historic, controls. It is essential to be clear that there are definite benefits to the baby that exceed the risks to both patients (Dias 1999).

## POST-NATAL MANAGEMENT

The first step in management is careful clinical assessment, ensuring that the baby is warm and not influenced by any sedative medications that may have been given to the mother. General examination will reveal any associated anomalies of the cardiovascular, pulmonary, or gastrointestinal systems, but these would be exceptional as myelomeningocele is unusual in being one of the few major congenital malformations that is not often coupled with anomalies in other systems.

The baby is first placed prone, and the level of the lesion and the configuration of the sac and exposed neural tissue are observed. Lesions that are very flat with little sac are more difficult to close, even if they are not particularly large. Those lesions in which a considerable craniocaudal extent of the neuraxis is exposed, with an open 'filleted' appearance of the spinal cord and visibly open central canal, are more correctly described as myeloschisis; they are associated with more severe neurologic abnormalities. The thoracolumbar junction is the most frequent level (45%), followed by lumbar (20%), lumbosacral (20%) and sacral (10%), more rostral lesions are unusual (5%). Multiple lesions do occur, as does the occasional associated encephalocele. A concomitant spinal deformity, either scoliosis, kyphosis, or 'telescoping' may be noted. Next, with the baby supine, a careful examination of motor function is made; note is taken of any spontaneous movements occurring with crying. All stimulation should be confined to the shoulders or head as purely reflex movement may result from stimulation of paralysed lower limbs and trunk and give a false impression. Muscle bulk, general development of the lower limbs and trunk, and any deformities of the lower limbs are noted. A sensory level is determined using an open nappy pin (never a hypodermic needle) moving from caudal to rostral dermatomes. Asymmetry of sensorimotor level and a sensory level more rostral than the motor level is the rule rather than the exception. Each lesion is individual and has its own peculiarities. Sphincter function is assessed by observing anal tone and noting whether urine dribbles continuously from the urethra. Anal and urethral mucosae may prolapse in severely paralyzed cases. Any orthopedic deformities of hips, knees, ankles, and feet are noted and give further clues of the functional neurologic level. Finally, the head is examined, the occipitofrontal circumference is measured and charted, and any additional features of intracranial hypertension, such as sutural diastasis or sunsetting eye posture, are sought.

Clinical examination is complimented by US scanning of the brain to determine ventricular size and of the craniocervical junction to assess the extent of the hindbrain hernia that is almost invariably present. If the neurologic level is higher or the deficit much more severe than suggested by the level of the placode, or if there is any other major discrepancy, MRI of the spine should be performed lest there be some concomitant intraspinal lesion such as a hydromyelia or more rostral tethering lesion. US examination of the kidneys, ureters, and bladder is performed but is usually normal in the neonatal period.

Clinical evaluation permits prediction of minimum disability, and unless there is gross hydrocephalus or a very dysmorphic baby, potentially normal intellect should be assumed. Parents who have not been seen in the antenatal period are then counseled as to the basic nature of the condition and its likely implications for their child in terms of the estimated minimum disability, the need for, and hazards of, treatment for hydrocephalus; the potential for deterioration in later life, the need for multidisciplinary follow-up for life, and the role of active intervention versus conservative management. Clearly, this is a vast amount of information for the new parents to absorb, and appropriate time must be allowed for the counseling to be of any value to them. It emphasizes the value of prenatal contact whenever possible. The presence of an experienced neonatal nurse to provide support and reinforcement of the information given is generally advisable. The decision to treat the child actively or otherwise involves a veritable cosmos of medical, ethical, philosophical, religious, cultural, and social variables that are well-covered elsewhere (Black 1979).

Active treatment consists of closure of the lesion within the first 24 h of birth to reduce the risk of serious infection of the central nervous system, to obtain watertight closure of the dura, and to provide good skin cover. The surgical techniques required are fully described elsewhere (Humphreys 1985; Goodrich *et al.* 1991; Reigel 1996). Before operating, the child is nursed prone with a moist saline dressing on the sac to prevent desiccation. If transfer from a distant neonatal unit to the pediatric neurosurgery unit is necessary, or if the child is to have to wait any length of time for operation, then the usual neonatal precautions against dehydration, hypoglycemia, and hypothermia are put in hand. Under general anesthesia, in the prone position, the sac is opened directly into the subarachnoid space through an incision placed at the junction between the epithelialized part of the sac and the arachnoid. The neural placode is mobilized. Dural flaps are raised and closed over the placode in a watertight fashion to create as capacious a sac as possible so as to reduce the risk of retethering. The fascial, subcutaneous layers, and skin are then closed without drainage, and a light dressing is applied. Using this technique, as opposed to the older general surgical approach of a circumferential incision around the base of the sac, elaborate skin flaps are rarely needed. Occasionally, usually for the flatter lesions, the involvement of a plastic or reconstructive surgeon will be required. This should be anticipated from the post-natal examination. Post-operatively, admission to a neonatal intensive care unit is not usually required. Feeding and handling by parents can be normal, but the baby is nursed prone in a way that minimizes soiling of the wound until it is well-healed in 7–10 days. Prophylactic antibiotics are not indicated. The occurrence of ventriculitis may relate more to wound breakdown and CSF fistulation at the site of closure than to actual delay in closure (Brau *et al.* 1990).

In the neonatal period, two further associated anomalies may manifest themselves: hydrocephalus and hindbrain herniation. Although virtually all children with myelomeningocele have ventriculomegaly, only a variable proportion develop progressive hydrocephalus requiring surgical treatment. The more rostral the lesion, the more likely and the more prominent is the hydrocephalus: overall, 80% require treatment, but only 50% of those with purely sacral lesions are affected. Hydrocephalus usually becomes clinically apparent within the first 2 weeks of life and can be monitored clinically by weekly measurement and recording of the occipitofrontal circumference and by cranial US. Treatment is usually by insertion of a ventriculoperitoneal shunt, but neuroendoscopic third ventriculostomy should be considered, especially in those aged over 6 months in whom the overall success rate is 77% (Teo & Jones 1996) (see Chapter 44). Children with pronounced hydrocephalus at birth should undergo simultaneous shunt placement and myelomeningocele closure; there is some evidence that this is less hazardous, in terms of shunt complications, than sequential procedures (Epstein *et al.* 1985). The risk of malfunction or infection is certainly not increased (Parent & McMillan 1995). Dysraphic children suffer a disproportionately high incidence of shunt infections overall (Hoffman *et al.* 1982), but first-time shunts in patients with neural tube defects are not at greater risk of becoming infected if the open spinal defect is closed early. Some studies suggest within 36 h of birth (Gamache 1995); others within 2–3 days of birth (Davis *et al.* 1999) or within the first week of life (Caldarelli *et al.* 1996).

The hindbrain hernia, or Chiari II malformation, is present in at least 95% of patients with myelomeningocele (El Gamma *et al.* 1988; Wolpert *et al.* 1988; Curnes *et al.* 1989). It may produce bulbar paresis in the neonatal period, even in the presence of a functioning shunt. The first symptoms are progressive slowing down of the child's feeding with nasal regurgitation and a change in the pitch of the cry. It is therefore the mother or the nurse who detects these symptoms, which, if not promptly recognized and acted upon, progress to stridor, quadriparesis, and respiratory arrest, following which, useful recovery is unusual (Hoffman *et al.* 1975; Park *et al.* 1983; Bell *et al.* 1987). Overall, 50% of those who become symptomatic soon after birth die (Rauzzino & Oakes 1995). Neuroradiologic investigation by US or MR confirms the presence and extent of the hindbrain hernia. Urgent neurosurgical intervention with decompressive cervical laminectomy and wide opening of the dura to a point caudal to the displaced cerebellar tonsils is required. This may entail removal of all of the cervical laminae. The dura is either left open or repaired with a graft of a dural substitute. The bone of the posterior cranial fossa should not be removed, as this is not only unnecessary but also rewards the unwary with horrendous bleeding from caudally displaced and abnormal dural venous sinuses.

Following surgical closure of the myelomeningocele and shunt placement, if required, full orthopedic and urologic evaluations are made in conjunction with pediatric orthopedic and urologic surgeons. The parents are given further instructions on the various aspects of the condition and offered the opportunity of early contact with a patients' association. Genetic counseling is suggested in view of the 2–4% recurrence risk of neural-tube defect in subsequent siblings. Thereafter, the child should be managed in a combined neurosurgery/orthopedic/urology clinic.

If conservative management is elected upon, then those surviving children will often return with progressive hydrocephalus and will then require shunt insertion and the same full neurosurgical, orthopedic, and urologic support. Secondary delayed closure of the myelomeningocele will frequently be needed and is often a complex and unpleasant procedure. Plastic surgery involvement is frequently required with implantation of tissue-expanding silicon balloons progressively inflated over several weeks in order to gain adequate skin cover.

## FURTHER FOLLOW-UP

As mentioned above, ongoing supervision in the setting of a combined clinic with full support services such as a community urology nurse specialist, a dedicated social worker, and participation from a field worker from a patients' association is essential. It is best for these children to be followed in conjunction with a child development center so that developmental assessments, physiotherapy, and occupational therapy can be coordinated with the specialist surgical aspects of follow-up. As a proportion of the children will have learning difficulties, the prompt identification of all of their special needs is important before they enter primary school so that the necessary additional support can be provided in conjunction with the local education authority. This is now generally appreciated, although services do remain patchy in extent and quality. What is still less well realized is that supervision in childhood must extend throughout adult life so that new symptoms due to other aspects of the condition (the so-called 'second lesion') can be recognized promptly and dealt with appropriately. Continuing urologic care is also required if renal complications are to be avoided.

The commonest need for further neurosurgical intervention relates to hydrocephalus and the complications of ventricular shunts. Although it is usually apparent within the first few weeks of life whether there is progressive hydrocephalus necessitating surgical intervention, there remains a lifelong risk of untreated but apparently 'arrested' hydrocephalus becoming symptomatic. This may occur spontaneously or may be precipitated by other surgical interventions, most especially spinal surgery. Indeed, the possibility of new neurologic features being due to hydrocephalus must always be considered. For this reason, a 'top down' approach to new problems is advisable. This applies not just to frank neurologic symptoms but also to spinal vertebral and even urologic problems (Jeelani *et al.* 1999). If significant ventriculomegaly is found, then consideration should be given to establishing effective ventricular drainage by shunt insertion or revision, or by neuroendoscopic third ventriculostomy, as the initial procedure. The possibility of apparently 'arrested' hydrocephalus becoming active must always be remembered when spinal surgery is performed and the patient forewarned of this risk. It is also important that non-neurosurgical medical and nursing staff are aware so that post-operative observations are appropriate.

The complications of ventricular shunts in general are dealt with elsewhere (see Chapter 44). However, those features that relate specifically to patients with myelomeningocele will be considered here. Although the symptoms and signs of shunt malfunction will most usually be those of raised intracranial pressure, patients with myelomeningocele may also present with symptoms referable to the hindbrain hernia, namely neck pain and sensorimotor dysfunction in the upper limbs (see below). Papilledema is only of value if it is present, and its absence can never be taken as evidence that there is no raised intracranial pressure. The ocular feature that is of most value in detecting shunt malfunction is the absence of upgaze, especially if the patient is known to have full upward eye movement in health. Many patients with myelomeningocele have very abnormal eye movements. These are usually abnormalities of horizontal conjugate gaze, most frequently an asymmetric, often oblique, nystagmus. It is therefore sensible to make a written record in a prominent place in the contemporary clinical notes of the character of each patient's eye movements at times of routine follow-up. Clearly, loss of previously full upward eye movement is a highly significant sign.

Traditionally, shunt malfunction has been treated by revisional surgery, but more recently, the possibility of neuroendoscopic third ventriculostomy (NTV) has been introduced. This is addressed in greater detail elsewhere (see Chapter 44). With regard to patients with shunted hydrocephalus in association with myelomeningocele, success rates for NTV of up to 80% have been achieved in those who have been previously shunted (Teo & Jones 1996; Punt & Vloeberghs 1998), and this should now be considered the treatment of choice if the anatomy is suitable. The anatomic anomalies frequently seen in the anterior part of the third ventricle have to be considered when undertaking NTV in these patients. They are well shown on MR, especially if sequences employing constructive interference in the steady state (CISS) are used. The abnormalities include unusual appearances at the floor of the anterior third ventricle that, if not recognized, could make NTV more difficult or even more dangerous (Jaspan *et al.* in press). In many cases, the anatomic peculiarities, in particular at the level of the interventricular foramen, make use of a flexible neuroendoscope preferable to a rigid instrument.

The hindbrain hernia has been mentioned as a cause of cervicomedullary compression in the neonatal period, but it can also become symptomatic at any time in life in up to 20% of patients with myelomeningocele (Rauzzino & Oakes 1995). Symptoms include progressive sensorimotor disturbance in the upper and lower limbs (Bell *et al.* 1987), increasing spasticity and scoliosis (Park *et al.* 1985). Any patient with disproportionate, progressive or severe spinal deformity, or with increasing neurologic deficits should be investigated for the possibility of hindbrain hernia. MR is the appropriate tool and will identify any hindbrain hernia, its extent, and any associated hydromyelia. If there is spinal deformity considerable expertise will be required from both neuroradiologist and radiographer in order to acquire useful images. Surgical procedures include ventricular shunt insertion or revision if there is persistent ventriculomegaly, decompression of the brainstem and upper cervical spinal cord, and exploration of the hydromyelic cavity with plugging of the obex (Hoffman *et al.* 1975; Park *et al.* 1985). The results of treatment of the hindbrain hernia are variable but are often good (Bell *et al.* 1987).

Progressive spinal deformity, usually scoliosis, eventually afflicts up to 90% of long-term survivors (Piggott 1980) and may require specialist orthopedic instrumentation; it is crucial that any coexisting neural lesion is identified and dealt with first or concomitantly. Such orthopedic surgery is best performed by spinal specialists in close conjunction with a neurosurgeon.

Other lesions include secondary tethering of the placode at the site of closure, or just rostral to the repair (Tamaki *et al.* 1988); this can produce symptoms even into the eighth decade (Wilden & Hadley 1989). Intraspinal dermoid cysts may arise at or near the original placode (Scott *et al.* 1986). Fortunately, MR can now identify most of these lesions (Fitz 1992). The general principle to follow in investigating these problems is to adopt the 'top down' approach and image the entire neuraxis, never forgetting that hydrocephalus can persist or return even after many years of apparent quiescence. There remains an unfortunate tendency for general practitioners, non-specialist physicians, and even adult neurologists to fail to appreciate the significance of new symptoms in these already disadvantaged patients. Only fastidious long-term follow-up by interested teams will provide adequate protection against needless additional disability and suffering from late neurologic, urologic or orthopedic consequences (McCarthy 1991; Jeelani *et al.* 1999).

There is an increased incidence of latex allergy in patients with myelomeningocele and the risk of developing latex IgE antibodies rises with multiple operations (Cremer *et al.* 1998). Thirty-nine of 83 children with myelomeningocele had latex-specific IgE antibodies, compared to six of 40 chronically ill controls with similar surgical histories, four of 105 medical patients and two of 75 well individuals (Pittman *et al.* 1995). In 646 operations over 18 years, there was one episode of intraoperative anaphylaxis attributable to latex allergy. Some feel that the risk justifies special measures to reduce exposure of patients with myelomeningocele and introduction of screening for latex sensitivity in view of the potentially serious sequelae (Mazagri & Ventureyra 1999).

## OUTCOME

Since the report of the London Committee in 1885 (Marsh *et al.* 1885), prolonged survival without any special active treatment has been well described. From detailed surveys in South Wales, Laurence (1966) has established the most complete natural survival history of untreated cases: namely, 30% at 1 year, 20% at 2 years, and somewhat fewer thereafter. Deaths in the first few months are mainly from meningitis and ventriculitis: subsequent mortality is due to untreated hydrocephalus and, in older children, renal failure (Laurence 1964). Only 3.5% survive without any physical handicap and with intelligence quotients (IQ) above 85 (Lawrence 1966). Personal experience over the last 16 years indicates that in developed Western communities, the survival rate of untreated cases is currently higher than that observed in the past and probably relates to changing views and practices regarding terminal care for neonates with congenital malformations. Delayed repair may be associated with 1-year survival rates of 94% (Sutton *et al.* 1986).

For reasons that are not totally clear, the prognosis for those children treated actively appears to be more favorable in North America than in Britain. The 5-year survival rates of around 50% quoted from the earlier English studies (Sharrard *et al.* 1967; Lorber 1971) have been superceded by figures of over 80% and rising in more recent North American series (Leonard & Freeman 1981; McLone *et al.* 1981), and even 100% at one year (Gross *et al.* 1983). With regard to quality of survival, the older English experience was grim: in the large unselected Sheffield series (Lorber 1971), only 1% of the total and 4% of the survivors were without handicap; 15% had a moderate handicap and 49% were severely disabled. Only 40% of the handicapped survivors could attend ordinary schools, and barely 7% were expected to become independent.

By contrast, many North American authors have found grounds for optimism (O'Brien & McLanahan 1981; Reigel

1982a–c), with most children becoming ambulatory with appropriate orthopedic and orthotic assistance (Kupka *et al.* 1978).

The prognosis for mobility relates not surprisingly to the segmental level of the lesion, especially the sensory level (Hunt *et al.* 1973). The prognosis for intellect appears to relate to the presence of hydrocephalus: 87% of those without hydrocephalus having IQs greater than 80 compared with 63% when hydrocephalus is present (Soare & Raimondi 1977). It is more likely that final intellect relates more to shunt complications, especially infections, rather than to hydrocephalus *per se* (McLone *et al.* 1982). Optimum hydrocephalus management is therefore essential.

Although the majority have a neuropathic bladder, the management has been revolutionized by the advent of intermittent catheterization by parent or patient (Lapides *et al.* 1972). Of one group aged 16–24 years, 18% were sexually active (Shurtleff & Sousa 1977). Psychosexual counseling is another area where there are almost certainly unmet needs in the adolescent and adult population with myelomeningocele.

What is absolutely clear is that there is no single approach that will be acceptable to all physicians dealing with all children of every family in a wide range of societies and cultures; there are clearly fundamentally different philosophical standpoints between those who select children to die and those who select them to live (Black 1979). It is no longer appropriate to rely upon the studies of a quarter of a century ago. Allowing for scope within individual management (McCarthy 1991), the only way forward for those health-care systems that are adequately financed, staffed, and equipped is in the direction of active intervention by dedicated and coordinated teams of specialists with the necessary knowledge, skills, support, and enthusiasm to tackle the problem in its totality for the lifetime of the patient. The problems facing 'Third World' nations are immense when faced with such potential commitments, and children borne into such societies and economies will remain disenfranchised and disadvantaged for the foreseeable future (McLone 1998).

## OCCULT SPINAL DYSRAPHISM

This term embraces all those conditions in which there has been disordered closure of the neural tube or its coverings but in which the resultant lesion is still skin covered. The older term 'spina bifida occulta' is inappropriate as 10–20% of the population have a single deficient lamina in the lumbosacral spine, and the very mention of 'a type of spina bifida' is terrifying to parents, who not unnaturally make associations with the open lesions and their more severe connotations.

The importance of this group of lesions lies in their propensity to produce neurologic, urologic and orthopedic sequelae later in childhood, adolescence, or even adult life (Till 1969; James & Lassman 1972; Park 1992). Most affected children are neurologically normal at birth, and it is the finding of a cutaneous blemish that alerts the pediatrician, nurse, or parent to their presence. All newborn children must have the midline of the neuraxis positively examined for the presence of such stigmata, which include skin-covered meningoceles, subcutaneous fatty pads, angiomatous telangiectatic patches, hairy tufts, congenital 'scars', dermoid and dermal sinuses, and skin-covered fibro-fatty tail-like appendages. Many babies have a postanal pit over the sacrococcygeal region that is of no serious import: a pathologic sinus is one that is relatively rostral in the natal cleft, or even higher, eccentrically placed, or associated with another of the aforementioned stigmata. Postanal pits are to be distinguished from the dermoid sinus, which is clearly a punctate orifice, variably tethered to the underlying tissues from which clear fluid, hairs, and dermoid matter may emerge. The majority of lesions are sited in the lumbosacral region. The finding of any of these stigmata, or suspicion of them, calls for specialist neurosurgical referral. Clinical examination usually confirms the absence of neurologic signs; concomitant orthopedic deformities of the lower limbs, especially the feet, and evidence of sphincter disturbance should be positively sought but are usually absent at birth. Such apparent normality should not deter formal neuroradiologic evaluation.

Plain spine radiographs are of very limited value in the neonatal period as the neural arches are cartilaginous and thus relatively radiolucent, so defective laminae and spinous processes will not be revealed. The aim of the investigation is to define the intraspinal anatomy and in particular to seek evidence of any lesion that might tether the spinal cord. Modern real-time US is useful in the first few weeks of life only and to be of any value must be performed conscientiously by an experienced radiographer using high-quality equipment. It is unreliable as a screening test performed by the occasional, inexpert practitioner. MR will provide the ultimate answer (Brophy *et al.* 1989; Fitz 1992). The simplest and invariably the most appropriate initial investigation is referral to a pediatric neurosurgeon. An investigation towards a definitive opinion and management strategy can then proceed within the first few months of life. The most frequently encountered intraspinal abnormalities are the thickened filum terminale in association with a conus medullaris, which is regarded as low if it is at or caudal to the body of the second lumbar vertebra; the lipomyelomeningocele, the diastematomyelia, and the dermoid cyst. Less common are fibrous bands and adhesions, hydromyelia, neurenteric cysts, hamartomatous masses, and isolated intradural lipomata and myelomeningocystoceles. The entire length of the spine should be examined, as multiple lesions are occasionally discovered. In general, however, hindbrain hernia and hydrocephalus are not concomitants of closed dysraphic states, in marked contrast to myelomeningocele in which they are almost universally present.

Any orthopedic deformities of the lower limbs or spine are formally sought and assessed. Occasionally, it is these that bring the condition to light as may features associated with multiple vertebral segmentation anomalies such as Klippel–Feil deformity and Sprengel's malformation. The urinary tracts are evaluated by US of the kidneys, ureters, and bladder and by urine microscopy and culture.

Following accurate radiologic definition of the lesion, a decision is made regarding the need for operative intervention. The generally accepted hypothesis is that the intraspinal lesion tethers the neural tissue that may then be damaged, probably more by repeated traction injury rather than by passive stretching. Prophylactic untethering in infancy may reduce or eliminate this risk. Surgery designed to untether the spinal cord is therefore indicated to prevent serious neurologic, urologic and orthopedic disabilities from developing (Till 1969; Hoffman *et al.* 1976; Yamada 1992). Whereas, previously, an expectant policy might have been adopted, there now seems little advantage to the child in allowing preventable abnormalities to develop before operating, especially as they may arise acutely and quite unpredictably and may not be correctable. Slowly evolving, subtle abnormalities, especially of sphincter control, may be difficult to detect. Although the perfect longitudinal study is yet to be achieved, it is now generally accepted that prophylactic surgery in infancy is correct for thickened filum terminale and diastematomyelia (Ander *et al.* 1997), the aim being to untether the spinal cord. Dermoid sinuses are a special case as the communication between the subarachnoid space and the exterior presents a very real risk of intercurrent infection with the development of an intraspinal dermoid abscess or meningitis. Such a complication can prove damaging or even fatal. Dermoid sinuses should therefore be referred and dealt with as a matter of urgency.

The lipomyelomeningocele remains a difficult and contentious lesion. It represents one of the more common lesions and is seen more frequently than the other closed lesions; girls outnumber boys (Bruce & Schut 1979). The role of prophylactic surgery for lipomyelomeningocele remains keenly debated in pediatric neurosurgical circles. Previously, in the distant past, the subcutaneous fatty mass has been variously regarded as of mainly cosmetic significance, or alternatively as simply not amenable to surgical intervention. More recently, it appeared that the majority of children harboring this lesion, and who are apparently normal at birth, will acquire serious disabilities by adolescence (Anderson 1975; McLone *et al.* 1983). Thus, of 56 children aged under 6 months at presentation to the Toronto Hospital for Sick Children, 35 were normal compared with 41 aged over 6 months, only 12 of whom were normal (Hoffman *et al.* 1985). As with many institutional series, it may, however, be inherent to the catchment process that the older patients are more likely to have abnormalities to justify the referral. Furthermore, whereas there are medium-term follow-up series that appear to show that children undergoing prophylactic repair in infancy fare better than those having delayed repair or conservative management (McLone *et al.* 1983; Schut *et al.* 1983; Hoffman *et al.* 1985; Kanev *et al.* 1990), there is also a large study that casts considerable doubt on the value of prophylactic surgery in the asymptomatic patient (Pierre-Kahn *et al.* 1995a–c, 1997). This is especially true for bladder function (Pierre-Kahn *et al.* 1997). Alternatively, the experience of a large North American institution taking a special interest in the field of neural tube defects has been very different (La Marca *et al.* 1997). Out of 71 asymptomatic patients undergoing operation, 66 remained normal, if nine children who required re-operation for subsequent deterioration are included. By contrast, of 87 symptomatic patients undergoing operation, 36 required second procedures for further deterioration, 20 were worse than at initial presentation, 44 were stable, and only 23 improved. The authors concluded that prophylactic surgery was required 'as soon as possible'. Comparing the American and French experiences with patients operated upon and followed for longer than 5 years, there was also a difference; five out of 30 in the American study had deteriorated, compared with 15 out of 32 in the French study. The position therefore remains unclear. What is required is a population-based natural-history study and a therapeutic trial with either a randomized or strategy-based design, or a case–control study. Unfortunately, the current somewhat entrenched opposing views mitigate against realizing such ideals. A practical and pragmatic approach for those who, like the present writer, feel that they can no longer recommend prophylactic surgery to asymptomatic patients with lipomyelomeningocele that has much to recommend it is the following strategy devised by the Paris group: MR, repeated at the age of 6 months, to define the lesion and to confirm that it is not growing; urodynamic studies and neurophysiologic examination of the lower limbs and perineum; and twice-yearly clinical review until the age of 2 years. Surgery is only advised if there are neurologic, orthopedic, or sphincter abnormalities, if the urodynamics become abnormal, if the lipoma enlarges, or if the family is opposed to expectant management (Pierre-Kahn *et al.* 1997). Whichever approach is adopted, continued follow-up into adult life is required and is ideally conducted by a multidisciplinary team as for myelomeningocele.

When surgery is undertaken, a better understanding of the surgical anatomy (Chapman 1982; Chapman & Davis 1983) has led to a rational technique, consisting of thorough untethering of the lesion, reduction of the intraspinal fatty mass, and generous duraplasty. It is firmly held by some that the fatty mass should be completely excised. Advances such as the operating microscope, the surgical laser, and reliable dural substitutes have all contributed to improved technical results, although intraoperative monitoring of somatosensory evoked potentials has not been generally helpful (Byrne *et al.* 1995).

A clinical genetic opinion should be offered to all parents of children with closed dysraphic lesions as there is a significantly enhanced risk of open neural-tube defects in subsequent siblings (Carter *et al.* 1976), which can be reduced by use of periconceptual folic acid (Wald 1994).

## SACRAL AGENESIS

This rare spinal anomaly consists of varying degrees of absence of the sacrum associated with neurologic abnormalities ranging in severity from total flaccid paraplegia with sphincter paralysis to mild foot deformities (Reigel 1982a–c; Pang 1985). It is now regarded as part of the spectrum of a caudal regression syndrome possibly due to an ischemic insult to the developing spine (Barkovich *et al.* 1989). The severely affected neonate has characteristically flattened buttocks, a short natal cleft, a narrow pelvis and prominent iliac crests with an absent sacrum on rectal examination. Motor abnormalities frequently exceed sensory features. In severe cases, there are associated anomalies in the neuraxis, axial skeleton and cardiorespiratory, gastrointestinal and genitourinary systems (Sarnat *et al.* 1976; White & Klauber 1976; Andrish *et al.* 1979; Mariani *et al.* 1979). Of affected infants, 16% are born to mothers with diabetes mellitus (Passage & Lenz 1966).

Full general, orthopedic, neurologic and urologic assessments are required, and the child is best managed in a combined clinic as for myelomeningocele. The occasional case is associated with myelomeningocele (Renshaw 1978). The condition should not be dismissed as a static one as it is now recognized that progressive neurologic deterioration can take place and that this can be arrested, reversed, or even prevented by surgery. Because there may be an associated tethered spinal cord, diastematomyelia, dural stenosis, syringomyelia, lipomyelomeningocele, or myelomeningocystocele (Williams & Nixon 1957; Pang & Hoffman 1980; Hafeez & Tihansky 1984,), all children should be investigated by MR as plain skeletal radiographs do not accurately predict the presence or absence of potentially unstable neurological lesions (O'Neill *et al.* 1995). Of 27 patients with sacral agenesis (15) or dysgenesis (12), seven had a low conus, six had intraspinal lipomas, and four had syringomyelia. The only case in which there was neurologic deterioration was amongst those with intraspinal lipomas (O'Neill *et al.* 1995). Untethering is justified in the light of several reports of improved motor and bladder function (Pang 1993; O'Neill *et al.* 1995); certainly, any child showing deteriorating neurologic or urologic function should be referred for neurosurgical and neuroradiologic evaluation. For many, the major thrust will be directed towards appropriate compensatory procedures to cope with the established orthopedic, urologic and neurologic disabilities. Children with anorectal anomalies should also be examined neurologically and investigated by MR as, although only 21% will have anomalies of the bony sacrum, 15% will have neurologic deficits, and 10% will have operable intraspinal anomalies, principally a tethered spinal cord for which surgery would be appropriate (Muthukumar *et al.* 2000).

## REFERENCES


Adzick N S & Harrison M R (1994) Fetal surgical therapy. *Lancet* 343:897–902.

Adzick N S, Sutton L N, Crombleholme T M *et al.* (1998) Successful fetal surgery for spina bifida. *Lancet* 352:1675–1676.

Andar U B, Harkness W F J & Hayward R D (1997) Split cord malformations of the lumbar region. *Pediatr Neurosurg* 26:17–24.

Anderson F M (1975) Occult spinal dysraphism: a series of 73 cases. *Pediatrics* 55: 826–835.

Andrish J, Kalanchi A & MacEwan G D (1979) Sacral agenesis: a clinical evaluation of its management, heredity and associated anomalies. *Clin Orthopaed Relat Res* 139:52–57.

Barkovich A J, Raghavan N, Chuang S H *et al.* (1989) The wedge-shaped cord terminus: a radiographic sign of caudal regression. *Am J Neuroradiol* 10:1223–1231.

Bell W O, Charney E B, Bruce D A *et al.* (1987) Symptomatic Arnold-Chiari malformation: review of experience with 22 cases. *J Neurosurg* 66:812–816.

Black P (1979) Selective treatment of infants with myelomeningocele. *Neurosurgery* 5:334–338.

Brau R H, Rodriquez R & Ramirez M V (1990) Experience of the management of myelomeningocele in Puerto Rico. *J Neurosurg* 72:726–731.

Brophy J D, Sutton L N & Zimmerman R A (1989) Magnetic resonance imaging of lipomyelomeningocele and tethered cord. *Neurosurgery* 25:336–340.

Bruce D A & Schut L (1979) Spinal lipomas in infancy and childhood. *Child's Brain* 5:192–203.

Bunch W H, Cass A S, Benson A S *et al.* (1972) *Modern management of myelomeningocele.* St. Louis, MO: Warren H Green.

Byrne R W, Hayes E A, George T M *et al.* (1995) Operative resection of 100 spinal lipomas in infants less than 1 year of age. *Pediatr Neurosurg* 23:182–187.

Caldarelli M, Di Rocco C & La Marca F (1996) Shunt complications in the first postoperative year in children with meningomyelocele. *Childs Nerv Syst* 12:748–54.

Carter C O, Evans K A & Till K (1976) Spinal dysraphism: genetic relations to neural tube malformations. *J Med Genet* 13:343–360.

Chapman P H (1982) Congenital intraspinal lipomas: anatomic considerations and surgical treatment. *Child's Brain* 9:37–47.

Chapman P H & Davis K R (1983) Surgical treatment of spinal lipomas in childhood. In: Raimondi A J (ed.) *Concepts in pediatric neurosurgery.* Basel: Karger, No. 3; pp.178–190.

Charoonsmith T & Suwanwela C (1974) Fronto ethmoidal encephalo meningocele with special reference to plastic reconstruction. *Clin Plastic Surg* 1:27–47.

Copp A J, Brooh F A, Estibeiro J P *et al.* (1990) The embryonic development of mammalian neural tube defects. *Prog Neurobiol* 35:363–403.

Cremer R, Hoppe E, Kleine-Diepenbruck U *et al.* (1998) Natural rubber latex allergy: prevalence and risk factors in patients with spina bifida compared with atopic children and controls. *Eur J Pediatr* 157:13–16.

Cuckle H S, Wald N J & Cuckle P M (1985) Prenatal screening and diagnosis of neural tube defects in England and Wales in 1985. *Prenatal Diag* 9:393–400.

Curnes J T, Oakes W J & Boyko O B (1989) MR imaging of hindbrain deformity in Chiari II patients with and without symptoms of brainstem compression. *Am J Neuroradiol* 10:293–302.

Dias M S (1999) Myelomeningocele repair *in utero. Pediatr Neurosurg* 30:108.

El Gamma T, Mark E K & Brooks B S (1988) MR imaging of the Chiari II malformation. *Am J Roentgenol* 150:163–170.

Epstein N E, Rosenthal A D & Zito J (1985) Shunt placement and myelomeningocele repair: simultaneous VS sequential shunting. Review of 12 cases. *Child's Nerv Syst* 1:145–147.

Fitz C (1992) Neuroradiology of spinal dysraphism. In: Park T S (ed.) *Contemporary issues in neurological surgery. Spinal dysraphism.* Boston, MA: Blackwell; pp. 161–182.

Gamache F W Jr (1995) Treatment of hydrocephalus in patients with meningomyelocele or encephalocele: a recent series. *Childs Nerv Syst* 11:487–8.

Goodrich J T, Post K D & Argamaso R V (1991) Plastic techniques in neurosurgery. New York, NY: Georg Thieme.

Gross R H, Cox A & Tatyrek R (1983) Early management and decision making for the treatment of myelomeningocele. *Pediatrics* 72:450–458.

Guthkelch A N (1970) Occipital cranium bifidum. *Arch Dis Childhood* 45:104–109.

Hafeez M & Tihansky D P (1984) Intraspinal tumor with lumbosacral agenesis. *Am J Neuroradiol* 5:481–482.

Harrison M R, Adzick N S, Flake A W *et al.* (1993) Correction of diaphragmatic hernia *in utero*. VI. Hard-earned lessons. *J Pediatr Surg* 28:1411–1418.

Harrison M R, Adzik N S, Bullard K M *et al.* (1997) Correction of diaphragmatic hernia *in utero.* IV. A prospective trial. *J Pediatr Surg* 32:1637–1642.

Hendrick E B (1985) Encephaloceles. In: Wilkins R H & Rengachary S S (eds) *Neurosurgery.* New York, NY: McGraw-Hill; pp. 2087–2091.

Hoffman H J, Hendrick E B & Humphreys R P (1975) Manifestations and management of Arnold–Chiari malformations in patients with myelomeningocele. *Child's Brain* 1:255–259.

Hoffman H J, Hendrick E B & Humphreys R P (1976) The tethered spinal cord: its protean manifestations, diagnosis and surgical correction. *Child's Brain* 2:145–155.

Hoffman H J, Hendrick E B & Humphreys R P (1982) Management of hydrocephalus. *Monogr Neural Sci* 8:21–25.

Hoffman H J, Taecholarn C, Hendrick E B *et al.* (1985) Management of lipomyelomeningoceles. Experience at the Hospital for Sick Children, Toronto. *J Neurosurg* 62:1–8.

Humphreys R P (1985) Spinal dysraphism. In: Wilkins R H & Rengachary S S (eds) *Neurosurgery.* New York: McGraw-Hill; pp. 2041–2052.

Hunt G, Lewin W, Gleave J *et al.* (1973) Predictive factors in open myelomeningocele with special reference to sensory level. *BMJ* iv: 197–201.

James C C M & Lassman L P (1972) *Spinal dysraphism: spina bifida occulta.* London: Butterworth.

Jaspan T, Costigan C, McConachie N *et al.* New features of the Chiari II malformation demonstrated by ultra-high resolution CISS imaging. *Am J Neuroradiol. in press.*

Jeelani N O U, Jaspan T & Punt J (1999) Tethered cord syndrome in post-myelomeningocoele repair patients. *BMJ* 318:516–517.

Kadir R A, Sabin C, Whitlow B *et al.* (1999) Neural tube defects and periconceptual folic acid in England and Wales: retrospective study. *BMJ* 319:92–93.

Kanev P M, Lemire R J, Loeser J D *et al.* (1990) Management and long-term follow-up reviews of children with lipomyelomeningocele 1952–1987. *J Neurosurg* 73:48–52.

Keller-Pack C & Mullen R J (1993) Evidence for late neuronal degeneration in the open neural tube of curly tail mutant mice. *Soc Neurosci Abstracts* 19:181.

Kupka J, Geddes N & Carroll N C (1978) Comprehensive management in the child with spina bifida. *Orthopaed Clin N Am* 9:97–113.

La Marca F, Grant J A, Tomita T & McLone D G (1997) Spinal lipomas in children: outcome of 270 procedures. *Pediatr Neurosurg* 26:8–16.

Lapides J, Diokno A C, Silber S J *et al.* (1972) Clean, intermittent self-catheterisation in the treatment of urinary tract disease. *J Urol* 107:458–461.

Laurence K M (1964) The natural history of spina bifida cystica; detailed analysis of 407 cases. *Arch Dis Childhood* 39:41–57.

Laurence K M (1966) The survival of untreated spina bifida cystica. *Dev Med Child Neurol* 11(suppl):10–19.

Laurence K M & Tew B J (1966) Follow-up of 63 survivors from the 425 cases of spina bifida cystica born in South Wales between 1956 and 1962. *Dev Med Child Neurol* 13(suppl):1–3.

Leonard C O & Freeman K M (1981) Spina bifida: a new disease. *Pediatrics* 68:136–137.

Lorber J (1967) The prognosis of occipital encephalocele. *Dev Med Child Neurol* 13(suppl):75–86.

Lorber J (1971) Results of treatment of myelomeningocele: an analysis of 524 unselected cases with special reference to possible selection for treatment. *Dev Med Child Neurol* 13:279–303.

McCarthy G (1991) Treating children with spina bifida. An individual programme for each child. *BMJ* 302:65–66.

McLone D G (1998) A boutique practice or specialist to the world. *Child's Nerv Syst* 14:630–635.

McLone D, Czyzeqski D & Raimondi A J (1982) The effects of complications on intellectual function in 173 children with myelomeningocele. In: *Surgery of the developing nervous system.* New York, NY: Grune & Stratton; pp. 49–60.

McLone D, Raimondi A J & Sommers R (1981) The results of early treatment of 100 consecutive newborns with myelomeningocele. *Kinder Chirugie* 34:115–117.

McLone D G, Dias M S, Goossens W K *et al.* (1997) Pathological changes in exposed neural tissue of fetal delayed splotch (Spd) mice. *Child's Nerv Syst* 13:1–7.

McLone D G, Mutluer S & Naidich T P (1983) Lipomyelomeningoceles of the conus medullaris. In: Raimondi A J (ed.) *Concepts in pediatric neurosurgery.* Basel: Karger, No. 3; pp. 170–177.

Mariani A J, Stern J, Khan A U *et al.* (1979) Sacral agenesis: an analysis of 11 cases and review of the literature. *J Urol* 122:684–686.

Marsh H, Gould A P, Clutton H H *et al.* (1885) Report of a committee of the society nominated Nov. 10 1882 to investigate spinal bifida and its treatment by the injection of Dr. Morton's iodo-glycerine solution. *Trans Clin Soc Lond* 18:339.

Matson D D (1969) *Neurosurgery of infancy and childhood.* Springfield, IL: Charles C Thomas; 2nd edn, pp. 61–75.

Mazagri R & Ventureyra E C G (1999) Latex allergy in neurosurgical practice. *Child's Nervous System* 15:404–407.

Mealey J Jr, Dzenitis A J & Hackey A A (1970) The prognosis of encephaloceles. *J Neurosurg* 22:209–218.

Meuli M, Meuli-Simmen C, Hutchins G M *et al.* (1995) *In utero* surgery rescues neurological function at birth in sheep with spina bifida. *Nat Med* 1:342–347.

Muthukumar N, Subramaniam B, Gnanaseelan T *et al.* (2000) A tethered cord syndrome in children with anorectal malformations. *J Neurosurg* 92:626–630.

Nakamuma T, Grant J A & Hubbard R F (1974) Nasoethmoidal meningoencephalocele. *Arch Otolaryngol* 100:62–64.

O'Brien M S & McLanahan C S (1981) Review of the neurosurgical management of myelomeningocele at a Regional Pediatric Medical Center. In: *Concepts in pediatric neurosurgery.* Basel: Karger, No. 1; pp. 202–215.

O'Neill O R, Piatt J H Jr, Mitchell P *et al.* (1995) Agenesis and dysgenesis of the sacrum: neurosurgical implications. *Pediatr Neurosurg* 22:20–28.

Pang D (1985) Sacral agenesis. In: Wilkins R H & Rengachary S S (eds) *Neurosurgery.* New York, NY: McGraw-Hill; pp. 2075–2077.

Pang D (1993) Sacral agenesis and caudal spinal cord malformations. *Neurosurgery* 32:755–779.

Pang D & Hoffman H J (1980) Sacral agenesis with progressive neurological deficit. *Neurosurgery* 7:118–126.

Parent A D & McMillan T (1995) Contemporaneous shunting with repair of myelomeningocele. *Pediatr Neurosurg* 22:132–135.

Park T S (ed.) (1992) Contemporary issues in neurological surgery. Spinal dysraphism. Boston, MA: Blackwell.

Park T S, Hoffman H S, Hendrick E B *et al.* (1983) Experience with surgical decompression of the Arnold–Chiari malformation in young infants with myelomeningocele. *Neurosurgery* 13:147–152.

Park T S, Wayne S C, Maggio W M *et al.* (1985) Progressive spasticity and scoliosis in children with myelomeningocele. Radiological investigations and surgical treatment. *J Neurosurg* 62:367–375.

Passage E & Lenz H (1966) Syndrome of caudal regression in infants of diabetic mothers: observations of further cases. *Pediatrics* 37:672–675.

Pierre-Kahn A, Zerah M & Renier D (1995a) Lipomes malformatifs intra-rachidiens. Les troubles neurologiques evolutifs. *Neurochirurgie* 41(suppl 1):63–67.

Pierre-Kahn A, Zerah M & Renier D (1995b) Lipomes malformatifs intra-rachidiens. Resultats de la chirurgie. *Neurochirurgie* 41(suppl 1):103–110.

Pierre-Kahn A, Zerah M & Renier D (1995c) Lipomes malformatifs intra-rachidiens. Attitude therapeutique. *Neurochirurgie* 41(suppl 1):114–118.

Pierre-Kahn A, Zerah M, Renier D *et al.* (1997) Congenital lumbosacral lipomas. *Child's Nerv Syst* 13:298–334.

Piggott H (1980) The natural history of scoliosis in myelodysplasia. *J Bone Joint Surg (Br)* 62:54–58.

Pittman T, Kiburz J, Gabriel K *et al.* (1995) Latex allergy in children with spina bifida. *Pediatr Neurosurg* 22:96–100.

Punt J & Vloeberghs M (1998) Endoscopy in neurosurgery. *Min Invas Ther Allied Treat* 7:159–170.

Rahman N V (1979) Nasal encephalocele. Treatment by transcranial operation. *J Neurol Sci* 42:73–85.

Rapport R L, Dunn R C & Alhady F (1981) Anterior encephalocele. *J Neurosurg* 54:213–219.

Rauzzino M & Oakes W J (1995) Chiari II malformation and syringomyelia. *Neurosurg Clin N Am* 6:293–308.

Reigel D H (1982a) Spina bifida. In: *Pediatric neurosurgery: surgery of the developing nervous system.* New York, NY: Grune and Stratton; pp. 23–47.

Reigel D H (1982b) Encephalocele. In: *Paediatric neurosurgery: surgery of the developing nervous system.* New York, NY: Grune and Stratton; pp. 49–60.

Reigel D H (1982c) Sacral agenesis and diastematomyelia. In: *Pediatric neurosurgery: surgery of the developing nervous system.* New York, NY: Grune and Stratton, pp. 79–89.

Reigel D H (1996) Myelomeningocele. In: Cheek W R (ed.) *Atlas of pediatric neurosurgery.* Philadelphia, PA: WB Saunders; pp. 1–5.

Renshaw T S (1978) Sacral agenesis: a classification and review of twenty-three cases. *J Bone Joint Surg (Am)* 60:373–383.

Sargent L A, Seyfer A E & Gunby E N (1988) Nasal encephaloceles: definitive one-stage reconstruction. *J Neurosurg* 68:571–575.

Sarnat H B, Case M E & Graviss R (1976) Sacral agenesis: neurologic and neuropathologic features. *Neurology* 26:1124–1129.

Schut L, Bruce D A & Sutton L N (1983) The management of the child with a lipomyelomeningocele. *Clin Neurosurg* 30:446–476.

Scott R M, Wolpert S M, Bartoshesky L E *et al.* (1986) Dermoid tumours occurring at the site of previous myelomeningocele repair. *J Neurosurg* 65:779–783.

Sharrard W J W, Zachary R B & Lorber J (1967) Survival and paralysis in open myelomeningocele with special reference to the time of repair of the spinal lesion. *Dev Med Child Neurol* 13(suppl):35–50.

Shurtleff D B & Sousa J C (1977) The adolescent with myelodysplasia: development, achievement, sex and deterioration. In: McLaurin R L (ed.) *Myelomeningocele.* New York, NY: Grune and Stratton; pp. 809–835.

Soare P & Raimondi A J (1977) Intellectual and perceptual motor characteristics of treated myelomeningocele children. *Am J Dis Children* 131: 199–204.

Sutton N L, Charney E B & Bruce D A (1986) Myelomeningocele – the question of selection. *Clin Neurosurg* 33:371–381.

Sutton L N, Duhaime A-C & Schut L (1992) Lipomyelomeningocele. In: Park T S (ed.) *Contemporary issues in neurological surgery. Spinal dysraphism.* Boston, MA: Blackwell; pp. 59–73.

Suwanwela C & Chaturaporn H (1966) Fronto-ethmoidal encephalocele. *J Neurosurg* 25:172–182.

Tamaki N, Shirataki K, Kojima N *et al.* (1988) Tethered cord syndrome of delayed onset following repair of myelomeningocele. *J Neurosurg* 69:393–398.

Teo C & Jones R (1996) Management of hydrocephalus by endoscopic third ventriculostomy in patients with myelomeningocele. *Pediatr Neurosurg* 25:57–63.

Till K (1969) Spinal dysraphism in a study of congenital malformations of the lower back. *J Bone Joint Surg (Br)* 51:415–422.

Tulipan N & Bruner J P (1998) Myelomeningocele repair *in utero*: a report of three cases. *Pediatr Neurosurg* 28:177–180.

Tulipan N, Hernanz-Schulman M, Lowe L H *et al.* (1999a) Intrauterine myelomeningocele repair reverses preexisting hindbrain hernia. *Pediatr Neurosurg* 31:137–142.

Tulipan N, Bruner J P, Hernanz-Schulman M *et al.* (1999b) Effect of intrauterine myelomeningocele repair on central nervous system structure and function. *Pediatr Neurosurg* 31:183–188.

Ulrich H (1976) Malformations of the nervous system, perinatal damage and related conditions in early life. In: Blackwood W & Corsellis J A W (eds) *Greenfield's neuropathology.* London: Edward Arnold, London, 2nd edn; pp. 361–469.

Wald N J (1994) Folic acid and neural tube defects: the current evidence and implications for prevention. In: Bock G & Marsh J (eds) *Neural tube defects. CIBA Foundation Symposium No. 181* Chichester, UK: Chichester; pp.191–211.

Weaver D W (1985) Genetics of developmental defects. In: Wilkins R H & Rengachary S S (eds) *Neurosurgery.* New York, NY: McGraw-Hill; pp. 2025–2040.

White R I & Klauber G T (1976) Sacral agenesis: analysis of 22 cases. *Urology* 8:521–525.

Wilden J N & Hadley D (1989) Delayed tethered cord syndrome after myelomeningocele repair. *J Neurosurg* 70:815.

Williams D I & Nixon H H (1957) Agenesis of the sacrum. *Surg Gynaecol Obstet* 105:84–88.

Wolpert S M, Scott R M, Platenberg C *et al.* (1988) The clinical significance of hindbrain herniation and deformity as shown on MR images of patients with Chiari II malformation. *Am J Neuroradiol* 9:1075–1078.

Yamada S (1992) Tethered spinal cord: patho-physiology and management. In: Park T S (ed.) *Contemporary issues in neurological surgery. Spinal dysraphism.* Boston, MA: Blackwell, pp.74–90.

# Chapter 46 Congenital defects, vascular malformations, and other lesions

J. Punt

## SCALP AND SKULL ABNORMALITIES

### APLASIA CUTIS CONGENITA

This is an unusual condition, first described in 1826. A variably sized scalp defect is associated with an underlying skull defect in 20% of cases and with skin defects on the trunk and limbs in 25% of cases (Vinocur *et al.* 1976). The etiology is unknown. The condition is usually sporadic, although familial cases, usually autosomal dominant and, more rarely, recessive, are recorded (McMurray *et al.* 1977). In those with multiple congenital anomalies, chromosomal abnormalities may be found, as in trisomy D, in which 35% have aplasia cutis. There is a known association with monozygotic fetus papyraceous (Mannino *et al.* 1977). The scalp lesions are usually 1–2 cm in size and are situated over the parietal vertex (Fig. 46.1); they may, however, be multiple and very extensive. If the skull is absent, the dura is also frequently missing, with arachnoid forming the base of the lesion. Associated anomalies may affect many systems, including the brain (holoprosencephaly, hydrocephalus), spinal cord (myelomeningocele), skull base (aplastic sphenoid wing), genitourinary system (absent or polycystic kidneys, ambiguous genitalia, double uterus), and limb bones (Cutlip *et al.* 1967).

The principal concerns are the dangers of infection and hemorrhage; the latter may prove fatal if the superior sagittal sinus is involved. Excision and primary repair, using complex full-thickness skin grafts where necessary, have been advised in the past, followed by cranioplasty at a later age to repair the skull defect. These procedures, hampered in the neonate by the limited availability of donor sites, have not infrequently been complicated by meningitis, hemorrhage, occlusion of the superior sagittal sinus, cortical damage, and a surgical mortality of up to 30%. Conservative management with dressings kept moist with sterile saline had proved successful, even for huge, full-thickness lesions, spontaneous healing of skin, and skull defects being observed (Muakkassa *et al.* 1982). This conservative approach, fastidiously avoiding desiccation, is therefore preferred. Any remaining bone defect can be repaired at the age of 5 years or beyond when the child's skull is thick enough to provide split calvarial grafts.

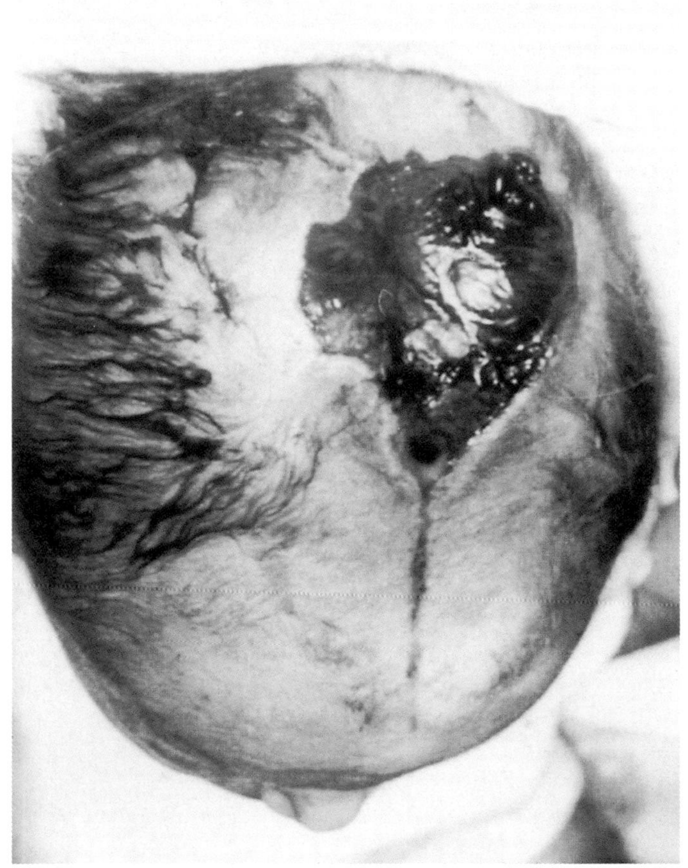

**Figure 46.1** Large scalp defect. There was also an underlying defect of the skull and agenesis of the corpus callosum.

### CONGENITAL SKULL DEFECTS

The most frequently encountered congenital skull defects are persistent parietal foramina, which occur less than once in 25 000 live births (Robinson 1962). The cause is unknown. The anomaly consists of symmetrically placed, paired defects 1–2 cm in diameter, at the site of emissary veins on either side of the midline, in the mid- to posterior parietal region. Over the first 5 years of life, the defects become relatively smaller as the res of the calvarium grows. They have no serious significance, but reassurance is required, especially if pulsatile venous channels are prominent. If parental anxiety persists, especially regarding the risk of injury, the defects can be closed at the age of 3–5 years using calvarial grafts.

Agenesis of the sphenoid wing is a rare abnormality producing painless, pulsatile, and usually mild, nonprogressive unilateral proptosis (Le Wald 1933). It occurs as a mesodermal manifestation of neurofibromatosis in 20% of cases (Matson 1969). The lesion is usually of cosmetic significance only and, if desired, can be repaired at craniotomy at, or after, the age of 5 years. Cranioplasty using autogenous ribs or, preferably split calvarium, is performed: it is crucial to plicate the underlying middle cranial fossa dura to avoid erosion of the bone graft.

## DERMOID CYSTS AND SINUSES

Incomplete separation of the epithelial ectoderm in the fourth week of gestation results in a lesion lined with stratified squamous epithelium and containing hair follicles, sebaceous and sweat glands (Lekias & Stokes 1970). Continuous production of sebaceous matter and epithelial desquamation produces a slowly expanding lesion with or without an associated discharging skin sinus. When a skin sinus is present, superadded infection produces inflammatory changes that significantly reduce the possibilities for total excision and eradication. In those with an intradural component, recurrent episodes of pyogenic or chemical meningitis may occur. Dermoids may occupy all or any of the layers of the neuraxis from the skin to the brain, and it is this possibility of intracranial extension that occasions concern and demands proper neurosurgical attention. The risk of intracranial extension relates to the site of the lesion, principally those lesions occurring over the occipital bone, at the nasion and along the midline of the nose. For lesions in these sites, nothing less than full neuroradiologic evaluation with magnetic resonance (MR) imaging of the brain and soft tissues, and occasionally complimented by computerized tomography (CT) of the skull base, is adequate. Under no circumstances should partial excision of the cutaneous element alone by a general, plastic, or nose surgeon be permitted as this regularly precipitates serious intracranial infection if an unrecognized intracranial portion is left behind. In occipital dermoid sinuses, the track always takes a caudal direction and even may traverse the brainstem. The transverse sinus at the level of the torcula is often involved as the track pierces the dura, adding another potential hazard to the exploration. Excision therefore should be performed by a neurosurgeon prepared to pursue the lesion intracranially to its full anatomic conclusion.

The most common location is over the anterior fontanelle, especially in children of Afro-Caribbean origin (Wong *et al.* 1986). Happily, dermoids at this site never extend intracranially and can be safely excised without any prior special investigation (Pannell *et al.* 1982). Care should be taken, however, to avoid damaging the superior sagittal sinus which lies in the underlying skull defect. Although typically midline, dermoids are also seen over the parietal eminence, at the lateral canthus of the orbit, and over the root of the mastoid process, usually at the site of cranial sutures (Pannell *et al.* 1982). Investigations, where indicated, and elective excision are recommended in the first few months of life. Clinically indistinguishable lesions also encountered at the anterior fontanelle include Langerhans cell histiocytosis and angiofibroma.

## CRANIOSYNOSTOSIS

Craniosynostosis describes a very wide range of conditions in which one or more of the cranial sutures becomes functionally obliterated or ossified at a premature stage in the growth of the skull with the result that, during the most rapid period of brain growth in the first 6 months of extrauterine life, the skull vault expands asymmetrically (Virchow 1851). The resultant deformity is characteristic of the pattern of suture fusion involved. In the most complex forms, the facial skeleton is also implicated, and the more correct term craniofacial dysmorphism applies. A primary abnormality of the skull base commencing *in utero* and producing abnormal tensile forces in the convexity dura was, for many years, considered responsible (Moss 1959). The role of the dura in determining fusion of the sutures is now known to be critical (Opperman *et al.* 1993) and is under genetic control, principally through fibroblast growth factors (FGF) (Alden *et al.* 1999). Mutations in the FGF receptor gene FGFR2 are found in Crouzon's disease (Bresnick & Schendel 1995) and in Apert's syndrome (Bresnick & Schendel 1998). Interaction with other genes such as those coding for MSX-2 and TWIST determine the phenotype produced (Lajeune *et al.* 1999). When the first edition of this book was published in 1988, there were 17 identified syndromes of craniofacial dysmorphism with differing genetic characteristics and a wide range of associated somatic anomalies (Hoffman & Hendrick 1979). There are currently around 140 syndromes involving craniosynostosis. Furthermore, 14% of cases of non-syndromic coronal synostosis are familial. A recurrent point mutation in FGFR3 is found in 73% of familial and 12% of sporadic cases, especially the more severe cases. The mutation, which converts proline 250 into arginine, is associated with lower IQ and less satisfactory results following surgical correction (Renier *et al.* 2000).

The overall incidence of all forms of craniosynostosis is one in 2000 of the population (Anderson 1977). Sagittal synostosis occurs four times as frequently in males as in females; coronal synostosis affects females slightly more often than males. Caucasians considerably outnumber black- and yellow-skinned children. Isolated sagittal synostosis comprises 60% of all cases, unilateral coronal synostosis 18%, bilateral coronal synostosis 12%, and metopic synostosis 4%; involvement of three or more sutures occurs in 18% of cases (Matson 1969). Genuine lambdoid synostosis is extraordinarily rare.

Management commences with recognition of the condition shortly after birth. This depends essentially upon the clinical acumen of the pediatrician, who must not succumb to the temptation to attribute the deformity to molding, forceps delivery, cephalhematoma, or prematurity through a misguided desire to reassure the parents that their newborn is normal. Plain skull radiographs will demonstrate that the affected sutures are absent or abnormal, if interpreted correctly. However, it is unreasonable to expect the non-specialist radiologist to be reliable in this respect, and the most profitable investigation is an informed pediatric neurosurgery opinion. This should be obtained in the first few weeks of life so that an accurate diagnosis is reached, the parents advised appropriately, and an optimal management plan devised.

The deformities are characteristic: sagittal synostosis produces a long scaphocephalic head, often narrow posteriorly, with bulging of the frontal bones and a palpable, often visible, midline sagittal ridge (Fig 46.2a). The anterior fontanelle is usually very small and frequently absent. Unilateral coronal synostosis leads to a variable degree of asymmetric flattening of the forehead (anterior plagiocephaly), supraorbital recession, and deviation of the nasion. The ipsilateral palpebral fissure is wide. Bilateral coronal synostosis results in symmetric foreshortening of the head (brachycephaly) with bilateral recession of the supraorbital margins (Fig 46.2b). In the craniofacial dysmorphisms, this brachycephaly is associated with variable ocular hypertelorism, proptosis, midfacial recession due to maxillary hypoplasia, and a range of concomitant peripheral anomalies such as syndactyly of hands and feet in Apert's syndrome and characteristic broad thumbs and large great toes in Pfeiffer syndrome. Metopic synostosis produces a keel-shaped forehead deformity (trigonocephaly), which may be associated with ocular hypotelorism and an extremely narrow, pinched forehead. Multiple suture closure produces complex variants of the aforementioned. In the very rare total synostosis, or craniostenosis, the head circumference is very small, and there may be severe proptosis. An equally rare variant of this condition in which the coronal, metopic, and lambdoid sutures are closed produces a bizarre cloverleaf skull deformity with a high vertex and bulging of the temporal bones (kleeblattschadel). It is usually associated with one of the named craniofacial syndromes, most frequently Pfeiffer syndrome, or with skeletal dysplasias such as thanatropic dwarfism (Yujinovsky & Nyhan 1978). It is rarely sporadic (Esmer *et al.* 2000).

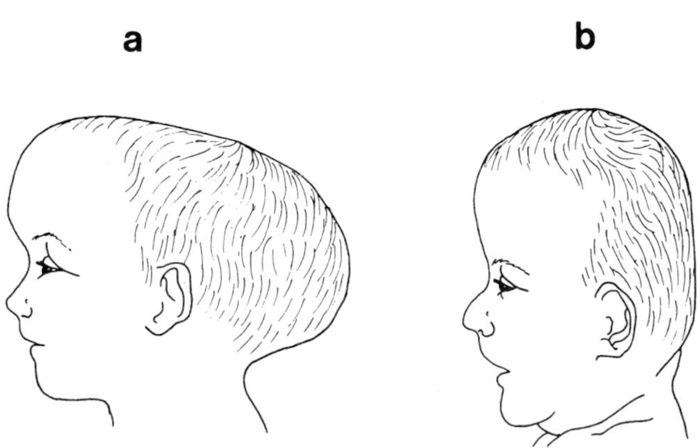


**Figure 46.2** Typical head configuration in craniosynostosis. **(a)** Sagittal craniosynostosis with scaphocephaly. **(b)** Bilateral coronal synostosis showing the characteristic brachycephalic head shape.

The term posterior plagiocephaly describes flattening of the back of the head. It is only very rarely due to genuine lambdoid synostosis. The commonest cause is probably due to lambdoid positional molding, and this may explain why it appears to have become much more frequent since the introduction of the 'back to sleep' campaign intended to reduce the risk of sudden infant death syndrome. Although the lambdoid suture is present, there may be perisutural hyperostosis on the inner table of the skull and even some frank bony bridging across the suture (Hinton *et al.* 1984; Muakkassa *et al.* 1984), lending some justification to the terms 'locked lambdoid syndrome' or functional lambdoid synostosis. There is often some anterior displacement of the ipsilateral pinna, which may also be angulated outward and even displaced downward. There may be some mild prominence of the ipsilateral forehead. The child is usually normal at birth, and the flattening appears in the first few weeks of life, increases in the first 6–10 months of life, and then regresses. There are associations with sternomastoid tumor. In one series of 121 cases seen at a single North American institution, there were only three cases of genuine synostosis, there was a highly significant male preponderance of 74%, and 72% of cases were on the right side. The authors noted torticollis in 41% of cases (Chadduck *et al.* 1997). An apparent increase in incidence has been noted in most craniofacial services since the introduction of the supine sleeping position to reduce the risk of sudden infant death syndrome. A superficially similar condition is cranioscoliosis, in which there is posterior flattening, which is more on the side of the head than at the back; the ipsilateral pinna, the forehead and the maxilla are advanced as if the head and face have been divided in the mid-sagittal plane and one half advanced upon the other.

The goal of treatment in the simple synostoses is to achieve a cosmetically acceptable head shape. In general terms, they have not been thought to be associated with any inherent risk of neurodevelopmental delay, raised intracranial pressure having been found very occasionally (Hirsch *et al.* 1981). More recently, overnight subdural pressure monitoring with single suture synostosis has demonstrated unequivocal intracranial hypertension in 13 of 74 children, most commonly with sagittal or metopic synostosis. Invasive intracranial pressure monitoring should therefore be considered in children with isolated midline synostosis aged under 1 year if the parents would not want surgery for purely cosmetic reasons, and in scaphocephalic and trigonocephalic children aged over 1 year as any surgical procedure would need to expand intracranial volume as well as produce a cosmetic result (Thompson *et al.* 1995). The principle of surgery is to release the fused suture so as to allow normal brain growth to encourage the development of a normal craniofacial contour. Surgery should therefore be carried out early and in the first year of life. This presupposes early referral. The extent of pre-operative work-up actually required is unclear. Clinical photographs to document the appearances and the opinion of a clinical geneticist are probably about the minimum. In cases of non-syndromic coronal unilateral or bilateral synostosis, it is probably advisable to check for mutations in the FGFR2 and FGFR3 genes. It is reasonable to obtain CT of the brain to exclude any major intracranial anomaly and to obtain simultaneous bone window views to confirm the extent of sutural closure; computer software packages enable the production of three-dimensional reconstructions, which some surgeons find helpful in operative planning (Marsh & Vannier 1983). Intracranial pressure monitoring is rarely indicated in the simple synostoses. The actual surgical procedures employed have become more sophisticated; sagittal synostosis is now generally no longer treated by craniectomy and insertion of silastic interposition substance (Shillito 1973) but more often by a more extensive skull vault remodeling. Coronal and metopic synostosis are treated by forehead remodeling and supraorbital advancement (Marchac 1978). Posterior plagiocephaly rarely requires active treatment, and indeed, there is no evidence to recommend any particular therapy in the absence of any Class I or II studies (Rekate 1998). Most parents simply want reassurance that the condition does not have any adverse neurodevelopmental connotations. The finding of significant intracranial pathology in up to 20% of cases of lambdoid positional molding justifies specialist consultation and careful examination (Chadduck *et al.* 1997). In very severe cases, if there is no great improvement by the age of 12 months, then intervention is justified if the parents are disturbed by the appearance to the point that it is affecting their relationship with the child. Simple procedures such as wide linear craniectomy with insertion of silastic interposition substance (Muakkassa *et al.* 1984) have been replaced with more extensive posterior vault remodeling techniques (Goodrich 1991). An alternative approach that has been advocated but never tested in a randomized trial is that of cranial remodeling by application of an external helmet.

The craniofacial syndromes require full evaluation by a specialist craniofacial team. MR is of value to give better brain detail and to look for hindbrain herniation (Hayward *et al.* 1992). This was noted in ten out of 27 cases specifically investigated at one institution (Thompson *et al.* 1997). The finding of a strong correlation with raised intracranial pressure and small posterior cranial fossa size suggested to the authors that hindbrain herniation in such cases is a consequence of brain deformation rather than a primary malformation. Anomalies in the major venous sinuses are sought by MR venography. Careful ophthalmologic examination and neurodevelopmental assessment are required. Treatment involves complex combined techniques, as introduced by Tessier (1967), in which multiple osteotomies to correct hypertelorism and the maxillary deformities are combined with forehead and supraorbital advancement The timing of operation is a subject of judgement and debate (Marchac & Arnaud 1999). Whereas forehead and supraorbital remodeling and advancement performed in the first year of life may be successful and even promote a degree of mid-face improvement (Persing *et al.* 1981), it is now understood that very early intervention may eventually fail presumably because of the fundamental genetic abnormalities. It is therefore now felt that operation is generally best postponed until later in infancy or childhood. In cases of severe exorbitism or critical intracranial hypertension, early intervention is indicated in order to protect vision and development. Holding procedures such as posterior skull vault release may be useful to relieve intracranial hypertension. Extensive, multiple sutural closure demands urgent early intervention by morcellation craniectomy often combined with forehead advancement. Tracheostomy may be required if the upper airway is critical. The value of external or implanted devices in achieving advancement of the mid-face is the subject of controversy and on-going evaluation. Serial staged procedures over many years are often required.

These interventions are all major procedures and carry the risks of dural laceration with subsequent fistulation of cerebrospinal fluid (CSF), damage to the dural venous sinuses, infection, especially if internal fixation is employed, and even death from intraoperative blood loss, post-operative intracranial hematoma, or brain swelling. The prerequisites for safe surgery are skilled pediatric neuroanesthesia, good surgical technique to minimize operating times and blood loss, and diligent postoperative nursing and medical care.

The cosmetic and functional results of appropriate management are generally good, although as is usual with corrective surgery of this nature, there is a paucity of objective outcome measures and audit of the complications of treatment is an easier, albeit lowlier, yardstick.

It is clear that the full requirements of these cases, in terms of both efficacy and safety, will only be met by early recognition by the pediatrician and referral to a specialist pediatric craniofacial team.

## INTRACRANIAL INFECTION (see also Chapter 33)

### CONSEQUENCES OF MENINGITIS

The major impacts of neonatal meningitis have been covered in Chapters 31–33, and here, only those aspects in which neurosurgical involvement is required will be considered. Such consequences are particularly frequent when pyogenic meningitis occurs in the first 2 months of life (Overall 1970), and sequelae are especially severe in the preterm and low-birthweight baby (Karan 1986).

#### Hydrocephalus

This is observed at some stage in 30% of cases of neonatal meningitis (Karan 1986). It may occur as an early phenomenon, when it is usually indicative of either a partially treated infection or infection with an unusual organism such as listeria, salmonella, active toxoplasmosis, or fungus.

Clinical recognition of an unusual degree of tenseness in the anterior fontanelle, abnormally large or accelerating head circumference, or particularly poor neurologic state indicate the need for imaging by US, CT, or MR. US will reveal ventriculomegaly but will not necessarily demonstrate alternative conditions such as subdural effusion. The management consists of establishment of an accurate microbiologic diagnosis by examination of lumbar and ventricular CSF and exhibition of intravenous antibiotics in high dosage for a prolonged course. Unless there is frank purulent ventriculitis, there is no advantage in giving intraventricular antibiotics routinely (McCracken & Mize 1976; McCracken 1977). Ventricular shunting is often not required and, in any event, should be delayed until the child is less acutely ill and preferably until the infection is controlled. If intracranial hypertension from progressive ventriculomegaly becomes a clinical problem in the acute stage, control by anterior fontanelle punctures can often be achieved. If this fails, an implanted ventriculostomy reservoir can be inserted, or an external ventricular drain can be established. When hydrocephalus is recognized early in the illness, the child should be carefully monitored by weekly measurements of head circumference and US imaging during the acute stage. If surgical intervention is not required in the acute stage, follow-up should include secure arrangements for checking head circumference in the convalescent stage and for several months thereafter.

Hydrocephalus may also develop after 1–2 weeks of intravenous chemotherapy, when it is usually associated with persistent or intermittent fever and malaise; at this stage, it is almost invariably a manifestation of ventriculitis, which, if not promptly recognized and treated appropriately, is a common cause of therapeutic failure (Salmon 1972). Assessment of the ventricular CSF in terms of cell count, glucose level, Gram stain and culture is vital, together with a review of the chemotherapy with an interested and involved microbiologist. Microorganisms may continue to multiply in, and be cultured from, the ventricular CSF, even when the lumbar CSF is sterile (Salmon 1972; McCracken 1977). Intraventricular antibiotics are given by daily instillation by anterior fontanelle puncture, via a ventriculostomy reservoir, or via an external ventricular drain. The dose and type of antibiotic are determined in consultation with the microbiologist. The ventricular CSF is examined regularly to establish that bactericidal levels of antibiotics are being achieved, that the white cell count is falling, and that bacteria are being eradicated. Treatment is usually required for about 2 weeks. The daily removal of 10–20 ml of ventricular CSF usually controls the intracranial pressure. If anterior fontanelle punctures are employed, they should generally be performed on alternate sides on alternate days; it is important to secure the cutaneous puncture sites with a suture to prevent leakage of CSF and secondary infection. It is important to avoid the use of scalp veins for administration of antibiotics, especially over the posterior part of the cranium, as this will render the scalp in a poor condition for shunt placement should this become necessary. When the clinical and laboratory features confirm that the infection has been eradicated, antibiotics are stopped. It is sensible to check the ventricular CSF 48 h later. If ventricular shunting is required to control hydrocephalus, it can now safely proceed. There may, however, be advantages to postponing shunting for a short while if there are no pressing symptoms of intracranial hypertension.

Even if there is no immediate progressive hydrocephalus, there is a significant risk for many months following successful antimicrobial chemotherapy of bacterial meningitis on account of leptomeningeal fibrosis consequent upon purulent exudate in the basal CSF cisterns in the acute phase (Volpe 1981a). The risk is particularly high with atypical forms of meningitis such as listeria and tuberculosis. Advancing hydrocephalus will usually be heralded by an abnormally rapid rate of head growth, although this is not invariable if there has been major parenchymal brain tissue loss due to the meningitis. The diagnosis can be confirmed by US, but there are advantages to obtaining MR as this will show the extent of parenchymal damage. Neuroendoscopic third ventriculostomy has been uniformly unsuccessful, and so treatment is by ventricular shunting (Buxton *et al.* 1998a,b).

The prognosis in terms of neurodevelopmental sequelae relates to the extent of cerebral infarction rather than to the occurrence of hydrocephalus (Albanese *et al.* 1981), but overall, 65% make a good recovery (McCracken & Mize 1976; McCracken 1977). The management of the hydrocephalus may be complicated by the development of compartmentalization of the ventricular system secondary to ependymitis (Berman & Banker 1966; Kalsbeck *et al.* 1980). This possibility should be considered when a child who has been shunted for post-meningitic hydrocephalus develops symptoms of recurrent intracranial hypertension. Careful attention to the clinical features, together with MR, is indicated.

### Subdural effusions

These are seen on cranial US in the convalescent phase of neonatal pyogenic meningitis in up to 50% of cases. Clinically significant effusions are, however, relatively infrequent and complicate only about 5% of cases (Milhorat 1978). They present with persistent fever, irritability, and seizures, or with signs of intracranial hypertension, or a combination of these features. Diagnosis by US may be difficult with machines, or techniques, of less than optimum caliber; near-field imaging is required. As always, it is important that the clinician gives the radiologist a clear indication of what is being sought. Gadolinium-enhanced MR is most useful in confirming the extent of the effusion and is preferable to CT.

In the first instance, the effusions are explored and drained by subdural tap through the anterior fontanelle or through a diastased coronal suture. An 18-gauge subdural needle, or, if such is unavailable, an 18-gauge adult lumbar puncture needle, is employed. The baby is wrapped in a sheet and held supine by an assistant so as to secure the head, arms, and trunk. The entry point is either at a point in line with the pupil or at the most lateral extremity of the anterior fontanelle, whichever is further from the midline. The needle is passed at a shallow angle, in an anterior direction, through the skin and then through the relatively resistant dura. The obturator is removed from the needle and any subdural fluid allowed to drain spontaneously. Aspiration is unwise as veins or even the cortex may be damaged. Drainage of up to about 80 ml of fluid may be tolerated. If too much is removed, the baby may become very pale and subdued, and although this is a transient state, it does cause alarm. If there are bilateral effusions, the procedure is performed on both sides. The needle is then withdrawn and the puncture hole in the skin closed with a suture. Subdural taps are repeated on alternate sides on alternate days until the volumes obtained are consistently 10 ml or less.

If microorganisms are seen on Gram stain or cultured, appropriate intravenous antibiotics are continued for at least a further 3 weeks. The majority of post-meningitic subdural effusions will resolve eventually with rigorously executed subdural taps. However, if they are very large and the cranium has become very expanded, it may take some considerable time, especially if brain growth is poor. If there is still a substantial effusion after 2 weeks of taps, it is usually advisable to insert a subdural shunt. A simple non-valved tube without a reservoir inserted into the peritoneal cavity is employed (Till 1968). Although the pleural cavity has also proved very effective, it is best avoided in very small babies and in those who have suffered pulmonary complications, especially pneumothorax. A unilateral shunt usually suffices. It is placed away from any site that might be needed later for placement of a ventricular shunt should hydrocephalus occur.

Outcome again relates to the extent of cerebral parenchymal damage sustained from the acute meningitis.

### Subdural empyema

This is a much less frequent consequence of neonatal meningitis than is subdural effusion. This chapter restricts the use of the term empyema to those cases in which there is frank pus in the subdural space. The condition presents during the course of antibacterial chemotherapy for pyogenic meningitis, or within 2–3 weeks of stopping treatment. The clinical features include those of raised intracranial pressure, persistent fever, seizures, hemiparesis, and poor feeding. The diagnosis can usually be made by CT, which shows a low-attenuation extracerebral collection with a characteristic enhancing rim over the surface of the brain. However, CT frequently underestimates the true extent of the collection, and MR is the preferred investigation. Subdural taps through the anterior fontanelle may produce turbid fluid containing a predominance of polymorphonuclear leukocytes on microscopy, but is often surprisingly unproductive. Gram stain and culture are usually negative. In most cases, the fluid is thin enough to be removed by subdural taps with an 18-gauge needle, and repeated taps coupled with prolonged intravenous antibiotics suffice. Occasionally, the pus is too thick to be drained in this way and can only be evacuated adequately at craniotomy. This is a major undertaking in a sick, frail neonate and demands a combination of swift surgery and skillful pediatric anesthesia. Following evacuation, antibiotics in maximum intravenous dosage are continued for 3 weeks, together with anti-epileptic drugs, if indicated on account of continuing seizures.

Often, seizures show a transient increase in the immediate post-operative period and then regress. MR is used to monitor progress but continued abnormal appearances can be expected for many weeks and even months after resolution of the clinical problem. CT can also show alarming appearances with cortical enhancement, suggesting extensive subcortical infarction, but these changes are often transient and are not necessarily indicators of severe irretrievable neurologic damage. A mortality of 50% has been recorded (Farmer & Wise 1973), but more recently, this has fallen considerably. Serious neurologic sequelae occur in about 25% of cases and include microcephaly, cerebral diplegia, and developmental delay (Jacobson & Farmer 1981), but for the majority, a good recovery is possible. Aggressive intervention is justified.

A related condition, which does not appear to feature in other texts, is one in which babies being treated for pyogenic meningitis, usually pneumococcal, develop the principal features of a subdural empyema, namely recurrence of fever and seizures, and are found to have an extracerebral collection on imaging that appears to be in the subdural space. It is often in isolated pockets. Subdural aspiration is negative, and at craniotomy, one finds a slough of amorphous yellow matter of a consistency not unlike that of institutional scrambled egg. On close inspection, the material is seen to lie in the subarachnoid space and may co-exist with clear, colorless CSF. There is only a limited amount that can be done to evacuate the material for fear of damaging the cortex. On histologic examination, the material is featureless and acellular and contains no microorganisms on Gram stain or on culture. Whereas craniotomy and maximal safe evacuation may bring resolution of the fever, this is not guaranteed, and it may persist or relapse after a short remission. Repeat imaging, especially with MR, often shows persistence of the extracerebral matter that may draw the neurosurgeon into operating again. The origin of the material is unclear. The most profitable line of management would appear to be prolonged treatment with antibiotics, possibly changing to an alternative agent that gains maximum penetration of the CSF even in the absence of inflammatory disruption of the blood–CSF barrier.

### Intracerebral abscess

Brain abscesses in neonates are the result of bacteremia occurring during, or shortly after, birth. In many cases, the source of the infecting organism is never identified. The predominance of Gram-negative organisms tends to implicate the mother's genital tract, and in one-third of cases, the same organism can be cultured both from the abscess and from the mother's urine (Renier *et al.* 1988). The occasional case can be traced to peripheral sepsis in soft tissues or the umbilicus. Spread to the brain is hematogenous. Typically, brain abscesses in neonates are large with thin walls and particularly extensive cerebral white-matter edema (Arseni *et al.* 1966). Rupture into the subarachnoid space with resultant meningitis or into the cerebral ventricles with pyocephalus may occur (Izquierdo *et al.* 1978). Although infantile brain abscess has been known for a long time (Holt 1898; Farley 1949), the condition was difficult to recognize until the advent of US and CT; previously, the diagnosis was usually made by chance in the course of performing a ventricular puncture looking for ventriculitis. The more widespread application of US in the neonatal period will undoubtedly favor earlier discovery.

The clinical features are usually a combination of seizures associated with raised intracranial pressure, with or without fever. The presentation therefore mimics meningitis, which is the most frequent initial diagnosis. Lumbar puncture is undesirable because of the considerable risk of precipitating brain shifts and deterioration (Garfield 1969), but in reality, it is almost inevitable that it will often be performed in response to an initial diagnosis of meningitis. Any neonate, who displays features that are atypical for meningitis, should undergo cranial imaging. US will exclude any large parenchymal abscess, but as the differential diagnosis will include subdural effusion or subdural empyema, it is preferable to use MR as that will give more extensive information. Any child with CSF that is not typical of pyogenic meningitis should undergo MR. The identification of *Proteus* species or *Citrobacter* species in the CSF should always raise the possibility of a brain abscess (Graham & Band 1981; Dulac *et al.* 1984,) and should be pursued by MR. *Proteus mirabilis* is the offending organism in the vast majority of cases. Most are frontal in location, and multiplicity is not unusual (Renier *et al.* 1988).

The mainstays of treatment are:

- the establishment of an accurate microbiologic diagnosis from pus obtained from the abscess or, failing that, from cultures of the baby's blood and the mother's genitourinary tract;
- control of raised intracranial pressure by aspiration of pus from the abscess, by needle aspiration either through the anterior fontanelle, through a diastased suture, or through a burr hole;
- control of sepsis by appropriate antibiotics in high intravenous dosage;
- suppression of seizures with antiepileptic drugs.

If there is a well-formed abscess cavity, repeated aspirations should continue daily until the cavity has collapsed. US guidance may be helpful in achieving optimal drainage. This can be monitored by US, CT, or MR. Both radiologic results, as judged by serial CT and functional outcome, are better following fastidious repeated tapping (Renier *et al.* 1988). Intracavitary antibiotics are not needed unless there has been rupture of the abscess into the ventricular system. Intravenous antibiotics are continued under the guidance of a microbiologist until there is satisfactory reduction in the size of the lesion and, in any event, for never less than 3 weeks. Because cerebral abscesses enlarge towards the ventricular system, intraventricular rupture is quite common; if this occurs spontaneously before antibiotics have been exhibited, the consequences can be disastrous with abrupt deterioration mimicking fulminating meningitis or spontaneous intracranial hemorrhage. If there is frank pyocephalus, there is a place for neuroendoscopic ventricular lavage and external ventricular drainage with intraventricular antibiotics. The repeated aspirations can occasionally precipitate intraventricular rupture, but if the baby is already on antibiotics, the consequences may be less severe. Hydrocephalus is, however, a frequent sequel (Hoffman *et al.* 1970), and ventriculoperitoneal shunt placement may be required once the ventricular CSF is clear and sterile. Multicompartmental hydrocephalus requiring multiple shunts or neuroendoscopic marsupialization is a distinct possibility (Renier *et al.* 1988). Early tapping of the abscess may reduce the risk of hydrocephalus. The occasional baby with septic cerebritis (Enzman *et al.* 1979, 1982) rather than a well-formed cavity, is best treated with antibiotics alone on a 'best guess' basis without surgical intervention (Daniels *et al.* 1985); repeat imaging will still be required to ensure that an abscess cavity has not developed. Multiple small abscesses and lesions in inaccessible sites such as the brainstem may be treated similarly (Rosenblum *et al.* 1980), although every effort should be made to obtain at least one sample of pus to facilitate accurate microbiologic diagnosis. Surgical excision is rarely needed in neonatal brain abscess.

Formerly, outcomes have been poor (Munslow *et al.* 1957; Hoffman *et al.* 1970; Renier *et al.* 1988) but hopefully will gradually improve with more prompt recognition through heightened clinical awareness lowering the threshold for diagnostic imaging (Rosenblum *et al.* 1978). There is some morbidity that is inherent to the condition relating to the degree of cerebral infarction (Foreman *et al.* 1984). Late epilepsy and neurodevelopmental delay are very common. Additional morbidity from shunt-related complications, especially with complex, multi-compartmental hydrocephalus, may arise at a distance from the original illness. Neonatal brain abscess remains a formidable condition in which good team work between the neonatologist, neurosurgeon, microbiologist, and neuroradiologist is central to successful management.

## VASCULAR MALFORMATIONS

The principal structural causes of spontaneous intracranial hemorrhage in the first year of life are aneurysm, arteriovenous malformation, cavernous vascular malformations, and tumors (Tekkok & Ventureyra 1997). Imaging by transfontanelle US will indicate that a structural abnormality is likely and can guide further investigation by CT, MR, and cerebral angiography.

## INTRACRANIAL ANEURYSMS

Although often presumed to be congenital in origin, presentation in childhood and especially in the neonatal period is exceptional. Interestingly, no incidental aneurysm or arteriovenous malformation was discovered in 10 000 cerebral angiograms performed at the Hospital for Sick Children, Toronto (Harwood-Nash & Fitz 1976), and none was found in an autopsy study that included 3000 children (Housepian & Pool 1958). Only a handful of cases are reported from the neonatal period (Newcomb & Munns 1949), Jones & Shearburn 1961; Pickering *et al.* 1970; Grode *et al.* 1978; McLellan *et al.* 1986) at ages ranging from a few hours (Newcomb & Munns 1949) to 6 weeks (McLellan *et al.* 1986).

Presentation is usually with spontaneous intracranial hemorrhage precipitating irritability and seizures; other features are a bulging fontanelle, retinal hemorrhages, low hemoglobin level, and bloodstained CSF obtained at lumbar puncture that has been performed to exclude meningitis. These features may misleadingly suggest non-accidental injury, but the pattern of intracranial hemorrhage on CT scan characterizes the source as spontaneous rather than traumatic (McLellan *et al.* 1986). Cerebral angiography should be performed urgently lest a further hemorrhage leads to neurologic deterioration or death (Storrs *et al.* 1982).

When the child is in a stable state, with any fits controlled, craniotomy is performed, and the aneurysm is excluded from the circulation by clipping to forestall any further hemorrhage. The advent of more technically sophisticated interventional angiography offers the prospects of transarterial obliteration of the sac by introduction of detachable metal coils (Malisch *et al.* 1997). Whereas this is being increasingly employed in adults, the extreme rarity of aneurysms in children and neonates in particular makes comparative evaluation of open and closed approaches difficult. Both involve risk, and the long-term outcome is uncertain with coils. However, the endovascular approach is intuitively appealing. The results of continuing international randomized controlled clinical trials in adults should inform the individual clinical decisions in children. The greater proportion of giant aneurysms and of posterior circulation lesions may also favor endovascular therapy (Nicholls *et al.* 1997).

The results of aggressive surgical management, including developmental follow-up, have been generally good in the few cases that have been operated upon (Grode *et al.* 1978; McLellan *et al.* 1986), although there have been some fatalities (Tan *et al.* 1998). Aneurysms have been encountered on the middle cerebral artery (Jones & Shearburn 1961; Grode *et al.* 1978; McLellan *et al.* 1986), posterior cerebral artery (Newcomb & Munns 1949) and posterior inferior cerebellar artery (Pickering *et al.* 1970). Aneurysms of the middle cerebral artery are the most frequent, comprising 45.5%, followed by the posterior cerebral artery at 13%. Approximately 70% are on the anterior circulation and 30% on the posterior circulation (Tekkok & Ventureyra 1997)

More frequent use of cranial US and CT will inevitably reveal similar cases in the future, and in this regard, the characteristics of intracranial aneurysms discovered later in childhood are noteworthy. They frequently present with seizures and are often located peripherally on the cerebral circulation rather than on the circle of Willis, and giant aneurysms, in other words a size greater than 10 mm or even 25 mm, are not unusual (Nishio *et al.* 1991).

## INTRACRANIAL ARTERIOVENOUS MALFORMATIONS

Although arteriovenous malformation is twice as common as aneurysm as a cause of spontaneous intracranial hemorrhage in childhood (Humphreys 1982), only 4% of childhood arteriovenous malformations occur in infancy (Shapiro 1985), and virtually none of these occur in the neonatal period. Intracranial arteriovenous malformations may present with congestive cardiac failure in the neonatal period if they effectively behave as arteriovenous fistulae (Silverman *et al.* 1959; Stern *et al.* 1968; Holden *et al.* 1972). Presentation may also be with spontaneous intracranial hemorrhage that may be intraventricular, intracerebral, or subdural; there are eight such cases in the literature (Wakai *et al.* 1990). Raised intracranial pressure may also lead to recognition of giant arteriovenous fistulae (Hanigan *et al.* 1990), producing hydrocephalus either by obstruction of the Sylvian aqueduct by secondary dilatation of the vein of Galen or by virtue of being intraventricular as in the case of cavernous hemangiomata of the choroid plexus (McGuire *et al.* 1954) or ventricular wall (Iwasa *et al.* 1983). Spontaneous intracranial hemorrhage in term neonates is unusual without an apparent predisposing cause such as bleeding diatheses or hypoxic–ischemic insults (Volpe 1981b), and when it does occur, further investigation is indicated (Heafner *et al.* 1985). Definitive investigation must await resolution of any hematoma as followed by US. High-definition CT or MR angiography is usually sufficient, and cerebral angiography is reserved for those cases in which suspicious abnormalities remain on CT or MR. Primary thalamic hemorrhage in full-term babies is not associated with underlying vascular malformations (Trounce *et al.* 1985). Any vascular malformation that is disclosed is treated along conventional lines by open surgery or by interventional radiology according to its own merits. Spontaneous regression has been observed (Hanigan *et al.* 1990). A cerebral tumor is a more likely structural cause of spontaneous intracranial hemorrhage in a neonate than is an arteriovenous malformation (Palma *et al.* 1979; Lacey & Terplan 1982).

## VEIN OF GALEN MALFORMATIONS

These rare congenital vascular anomalies (Johnston *et al.* 1987) result from fistulous connections that develop near the embryonic choroidal plexuses of the 20–40-mm embryo (Padget 1956). The ectatic vein is actually the median vein of the prosencephalon (Raybaud *et al.* 1989). The consequent high-flow arteriovenous shunt between branches of the anterior, middle, posterior cerebral, and superior cerebellar arteries and the vein of Galen, leads to progressive aneurysmal dilatation of the vein, whose wall becomes thick and tough. Two distinct types of malformation are recognized: a primary vein of Galen malformation, in which large arteries feed directly into the aneurysmal sac; and a secondary vein of Galen aneurysmal dilatation, in which an arteriovenous malformation in the adjacent cerebral or cerebellar hemispheres, brainstem, or tentorium drains via the Galenic vein, which becomes dilated.

The clinical features differ quite characteristically with the age at presentation (Gold *et al.* 1964). Neonates present in the first few hours after birth with severe and progressive high-output congestive cardiac failure (Silverman *et al.* 1959) soon complicated by pulmonary hypertension and myocardial ischemia. Infants present either with abnormal head size, due to hydrocephalus, and are found to have cardiomegaly, or with mild neonatal cardiac failure resolving spontaneously or with treatment, and within the first few months of life, progressive macrocephaly and a cranial bruit are observed. Children aged over 2 years with this condition may be discovered in the course of investigation of macrocephaly. In adolescence or adult life, headaches, subarachnoid hemorrhage, or the incidental finding of ring-shaped, pineal region calcification leads to the diagnosis. Cranial US, CT, or MR will confirm the diagnosis.

Until the last decade, the prognosis for neonates was abysmal, with a mortality of 96% in those managed conservatively and 77% in those undergoing surgery; half of those surviving intervention had neurodevelopmental deficits that were often severe (Johnston *et al.* 1987). The majority died of congestive cardiac failure without surgical intervention. Of those reported in the literature as having undergone surgical treatment, most died, and the survivors usually had major deficits attributed to gross ischemic damage in the surrounding brain (Norman & Becker 1974). This position has now changed with the advent of a better understanding of the pathophysiology and improved methods of endovascular therapy. The decision to intervene, and the timing of intervention, can only be reached on the basis of an objective scoring system encompassing cardiac, cerebral, hepatic, respiratory, and renal function. Transfer to a department having all the requisite skills in neonatal intensive care, pediatric interventional radiology, and neonatal anesthesia is required. Involvement of a skilled neonatal intensive care team is essential in order to optimize the disordered physiology and to participate in the evaluations. Low-scoring children, including those with severe cerebral damage, are managed conservatively; high-scoring children are operated upon at an interval of about 5 months; those in an intermediate category undergo emergency intervention. Cerebral angiography is only undertaken as a prelude to therapeutic intervention and is not required purely for diagnosis as the nature of the condition can be confirmed by MR. Obliteration of the lesion by transarterial embolization via the femoral artery is the preferred technique, employing *N*-butyl cyanoacrylate (Berenstein & Lasjaunias 1992). The transvenous route is no longer appropriate. It is important to appreciate that in those children that can be stabilized and who do not have severe cerebral damage, there is a therapeutic window of opportunity that, if missed, will lead to progressive loss of brain tissue with inevitably disastrous neurodevelopmental sequelae. It is now realized that ventricular shunting is to be avoided as it is associated with complications and poor neurologic outcome but does not provide a good solution to the very complex hydrodynamic problems that exist in these babies (Zerah *et al.* 1992).

As a result of careful analysis of the anatomic and physiologic problems and advances in endovascular surgery the results in specialist centers are now very much better (Lasjaunias 1997). In one very large series of 120 children in which logical selection criteria were applied and great attention was paid to medical care, timing of intervention and operative technique 17% were managed conservatively, and 9% of those undergoing embolization died, giving an overall case mortality of 26%. Of the 65% who underwent complete obliteration of the lesion by embolization, 66% were neurologically normal, 11.5% had mild symptoms, and 8.5% had severe permanent sequelae (Lasjaunias *et al.* 1996).

Of those diagnosed antenatally, 22% have fatal irreversible brain damage at birth and do not survive long. The outcome of those diagnosed antenatally and actively treated is better than those diagnosed postnatally, 88% having no neurologic deficits compared to 78% overall in one series. This is attributed to the better opportunity to choose the ideal moment for intervention. Cardiomegaly *in utero* is an indicator of poor prognosis, but antenatal macrocephaly has no adverse significance.

It is clear from this brief summary that this most complex lesion can now be managed with good prospects of acceptable outcome, but it is implicit that such good results will only be achieved by highly specialized teams to whom patients should be referred as early as possible so as to optimize management.

## TUMORS OF THE CENTRAL NERVOUS SYSTEM

Neoplasms of any type are very rare in the neonatal period, accounting for 6.24 deaths per million live births (Fraumeni & Miller 1969), but central-nervous-system tumors must still be remembered in the differential diagnosis of raised intracranial pressure and of paraplegia. A team approach with early involvement of a pediatric oncologist, preferably prior to any surgical intervention, is essential.

## INTRACRANIAL TUMORS

Intracranial tumors present at birth, or producing symptoms in the first few months of life, are correctly regarded as true congenital tumors (Arnstein *et al.* 1951; Solitaire & Krigman 1964), and they account for 0.5–1.9% of all childhood brain tumors (Sato *et al.* 1964; Jooma & Kendall 1982; McWhirter *et al.* 1996). This rarity notwithstanding, 200 cases have been systematically reviewed (Wakai *et al.* 1984). An incidence of 0.34 per million live births has been estimated (Fraumeni & Miller 1969).

Unlike in older children, 70% of neonatal brain tumors are supratentorial and only 30% infratentorial. The supratentorial tumors are as often hemispheric in location as midline, and the infratentorial lesions are uniformly related to the fourth ventricle. Furthermore, the cell types differ from older children in that in one series, 36.5% were teratomas, and of the rest, 50% were of neuroepithelial origin (Fig 46.3), of which the most frequent are medulloblastomas/cerebellar primitive neuroectodermal tumors (12%), astrocytomas (10%), choroid plexus tumors (8%), and ependymomas (7%) (Jooma & Kendall 1982). In a more recent series, 24 out of 45 tumors were poorly differentiated, including 12 immature teratomas, eight primitive neuroectodermal tumors and four medulloblastomas (Buetow *et al.* 1990). By contrast, only 2–9% are glioblastomas (Lee *et al.* 1999).

There is no overall sex predilection (Buetow *et al.* 1990), but females predominate with medulloblastomas and males with ependymomas (Wakai *et al.* 1984). Of affected babies, 12% have associated congenital anomalies, although there is no particular pattern except for epignathus in about 15% of those with teratomas. Neonatal medulloblastomas have been recorded in siblings of different pregnancies (Belarmaric & Chan 1969) and also in identical twins (Grienpentrog & Pauly 1957).

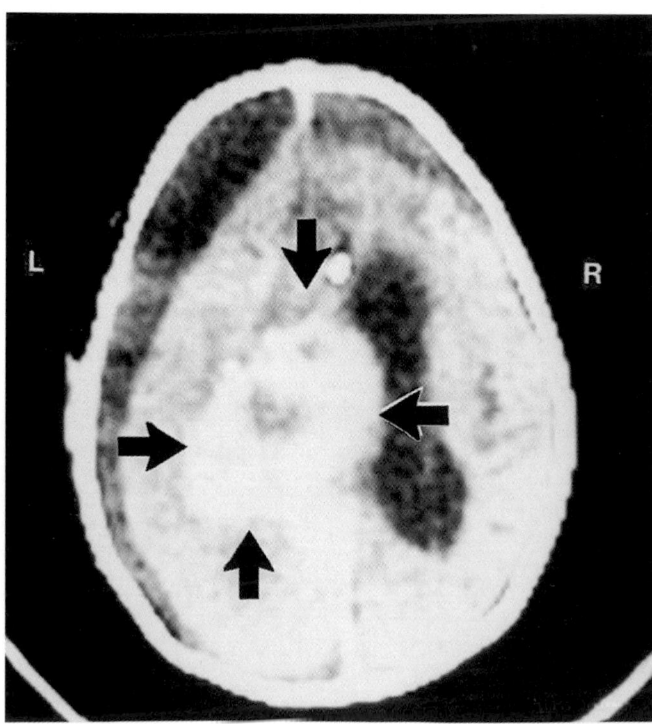


**Figure 46.3** Primitive neuroepithelial tumor (arrowed) in a young infant. There is subdural effusion on the left side. (Reproduced by courtesy of Dr Rosemary Shannon.)

Presentation is with symptoms of raised intracranial pressure that is characteristically more severe and more rapidly progressive than that encountered in non-tumoral hydrocephalus or subdural effusion. Macrocephaly may be of such a degree as to cause dystocia in 18% of cases. Fifteen to 18% present with spontaneous intracranial hemorrhage, 18% are stillborn, and 14% are premature (Wakai *et al.* 1984; Buetow *et al.* 1990).

The diagnosis of brain tumor is suggested by the appearance on US and is confirmed by CT, or preferably MR. Examination of the entire neuraxis by MR is essential to look for metastatic disease. The occasional non-tumoral congenital malformation may create diagnostic difficulty, especially if associated with hydrocephalus. Typically, these neonatal tumors are very large, heterogeneous, and variably enhancing on CT or MR. Prenatal diagnosis is occasionally suggested by fetal US when the differential diagnosis is usually of intracerebral hemorrhage; this can be resolved by MR.

Teratoma can often be diagnosed by raised germ-cell tumor markers, α-fetoprotein and human chorionic gonadotrophin, in the blood, and these should be performed in all cases. In cases that are negative for germ-cell tumor markers, the diagnosis should be established by biopsy. In those children with severely raised intracranial pressure from hydrocephalus, a ventriculoperitoneal shunt will provide a few days' respite in which to improve the child's nutritional state and thereby minimize one source of complications. In cases of midline tumors with dilatation of the lateral and third ventricles, consideration should be given to neuroendoscopic third ventriculostomy, which, in suitable cases, can be combined with tumor biopsy and sampling of CSF for germ-cell tumor markers and tumor cytology. Even if a shunt is eventually required, tumors abutting on the lateral and third ventricles can be biopsied endoscopically. In many cases, craniotomy will be required. Both the surgeon and the anesthetist must be prepared for major hemorrhage perhaps amounting to one or two whole blood volumes. Whether an attempt is made at radical resection will depend upon the site, intraoperative histology, and condition of the baby to withstand major surgery. When the diagnosis is made *in utero*, delivery by elective Cesarian section is probably the safest policy, especially if there is considerable macrocephaly, if only to minimize the risk of hemorrhage into the tumor.

In common with many infant brain tumors, neonatal brain tumors are frequently very large and vascular, and surgical excision is challenging to neurosurgeon and neuroanesthetist and hazardous. The use of chemotherapy to enable safer and more complete excision has been successful in malignant choroid plexus tumors (Greenberg 1999), and this strategy could usefully be projected to other tumor types.

The dire neurodevelopmental consequences of irradiation of the immature brain preclude the administration of radiotherapy (Jooma *et al.* 1984; Walter *et al.* 1998). The mainstay of adjuvant therapy is therefore chemotherapy in the context of an infant brain protocol, of which, many have proliferated amongst national and international children's cancer study groups since 1990 (Kellie 1999).

With the exception of benign astrocytomas of the cerebral hemispheres and choroid plexus tumors, which, in skilled hands, are amenable to curative excision, the outcome is generally poor, most babies being dead within a year: the teratomas are almost uniformly highly malignant (Jooma *et al.* 1984; Sato *et al.* 1984; Wakai *et al.* 1984). The median time to disease progression is 6–9 months (Kellie 1999). There are risks of second cancers in relation to both radiation therapy and chemotherapy as well as to genetic factors (Propp *et al.* 1998). The dual challenges of increasing efficacy of disease control while minimizing toxicity and consequent neurodevelopmental disability remain a focus of increasing interest to pediatric neuro-oncologists.

## SPINAL TUMORS (see also p. 698)

Spinal tumors are exceptionally rare in the neonatal period but should still be suspected in any child without features of spinal dysraphism who has congenital paraplegia, or who develops progressive paraparesis or sphincter disturbance. The majority are dumb-bell, or hour-glass, neuroblastomas (Punt *et al.* 1980), but occasional gliomas (Parkinson *et al.* 1954), schwannomas (Elliott 1984), and leukemic deposits (Mosberg 1951) are encountered. The occasional child with an intramedullary astrocytoma has symptoms originating in infancy, but recognition in the neonatal period is exceptional. That notwithstanding, the commonest intramedullary tumor at this age is a low-grade astrocytoma (Constantini *et al.* 1996).

Plain spine radiographs may show expansion of the spinal canal and, in the case of neuroblastomas, a paraspinal soft tissue mass that may display dystrophic tumor calcification. Definitive diagnosis of spinal tumor is made by MR and, as with intracranial tumors in this age group, all children with intradural tumors should undergo MR of the entire neuraxis in order to define accurately the extent of the disease. Urinary catecholamines should be estimated, as elevated levels will confirm a diagnosis of neuroblastoma.

Surgical decompression is indicated to forestall neurologic deterioration and to obtain tissue for histologic diagnosis. Laminotomy, in which the neural arches are replaced at the end of the spinal exploration, is preferred by many neurosurgeons to laminectomy, in the hope of reducing the risk of late spinal deformity. In the case of neuroblastoma, without rapidly progressive neurologic deterioration, treatment is initially with chemotherapy, surgical excision being reserved for any residuum.

The outcome is dependent upon the nature of the tumor and the neurologic state at presentation, those with congenital paraplegia being left with severe sensorimotor and sphincter deficits that require the same combined services of orthopedic and urologic surgeons as those with spinal dysraphism. For those with neuroblastoma, the prospects for survival are excellent, as with most children with that disease presenting in the first year of life (Punt *et al.* 1980). Late spinal deformity may require corrective surgery.

## REFERENCES


Albanese V, Tomasello F & Sampaulo S (1981) Multiloculated hydrocephalus in infants. *Neurosurgery* 8:641–646.

Alden T D, Lin K Y & Jane J A (1999) Mechanisms of premature closure of cranial sutures. *Child's Nerv Syst* 15:670–675.

Anderson H (1977) Craniosynostosis. In: Vinken P J & Bruyn G W (eds) *Handbook of clinical neurology. Congenital malformations of the brain and skull.* Amsterdam: Elsevier vol. 30, part 1; p. 219–233.

Arnstein L H, Boldrey E & Naffzigger H C (1951) A case report and survey of brain tumours during the neonatal period. *J Neurosurg* 8:315–319.

Arseni C, Horvath L & Dumitrescu L (1966) Cerebral abscesses in children. *Acta Neurochirurgica (Wien)* 14:197–224.

Belarmaric J & Chan S (1969) Medulloblastoma in newborn sisters. *J Neurosurg* 30:76–79.

Berenstein A & Lasjaunias P (1992) *Surgical neuroangioangiography volume 4: Endovascular treatment of cerebral intracranial lesions.* Berlin: Springer.

Berman P H & Banker B Q (1966) Neonatal meningitis: a clinical and pathological study of 39 cases. *Pediatrics* 38:6–24.

Bresnick S & Schendel S (1995) Crouzon's disease correlates with low fibroblastic growth factor receptor activity in stenosed cranial sutures. *J Craniofacial Surg* 6:245–248.

Bresnick S & Schendel S (1998) Apert's syndrome correlates with low fibroblastic growth factor receptor activity in stenosed cranial sutures. *J Craniofacial Surg* 9:92–95.

Buetow P C, Smirniotopoulos J G & Done S (1990) Congenital brain tumours: a review of 45 cases. *Am J Roentgenol* 155:587–593.

Buxton N, Macarthur D, Mallucci C *et al.* (1998a) Neuroendoscopy in the premature population. *Child's Nerv Syst* 14:649–652.

Buxton N, Macarthur D, Mallucci C *et al.* (1998b) Neuroendoscopic third ventriculostomy in patients less than one year old. *Pediatr Neurosurg* 29:73–76.

Chadduck W M, Kast J & Donahue D J (1997) The engima of lambdoid positional moulding. *Pediatr Neurosurg* 26:304–311.

Chumas P D, Armstrong D C, Drake J M *et al.* (1993) Tonsillar herniation: The rule rather than the exception after lumboperitoneal shunting in the pediatric population. *J Neurosurg* 78:568–573.

Constantini S, Houten J, Miller D C *et al.* (1996) Intramedullary spinal cord tumors in children under the age of 3 years. *J Neurosurg* 85:1036–1043.

Cutlip B D Jr, Cryan D M & Vineyard W R (1967) Congenital scalp defects in mother and child. *Am J Dis Child* 113:597–9.

Daniels S R, Price J K, Towbin R B & McLaurin R (1985) Nonsurgical cure of brain abscess in a neonate. *Childs Nerv Syst* 1:346–8.

Dulac O, Diebler C & Figueroa D (1984) La scanographie dans les meningites purulentes du nouveau-ne. *Presse Medicale* 13:201–204.

Elliott G R (1984) Neurofibroma complicating spina bifida. *Med Rec New York* 25:194–195.

Enzman D R, Britt R H, Lyons B *et al.* (1982) High resolution ultrasound evaluation of experimental brain abscess evolution: comparison with computed tomography and neuropathology. *Radiology* 142:95–102.

Enzman D R, Britt R H & Yeager A S (1979) Experimental brain abscess evolution: computerised tomographic and neuropathologic correlation. *Radiology* 133:113–122.

Esmer M C, Rodriguez-Soto G, Carrasco-Daza D *et al.* (2000) Cloverleaf skull and multiple congenital anomalies in a girl exposed to cocaine *in utero*: case report and review of the literature. *Child's Nerv Syst* 16:176–180.

Farley D L B (1949) Cerebral abscess in an infant followed by recovery. *Lancet* i:264–266.

Farmer T W & Wise G R (1973) Subdural empyema in infants, children and adults. *Neurology (Minneapolis)* 23:254–261.

Foreman S D, Smith E E & Ryan N J (1984) Neonatal *Citrobacter* meningitis: pathogenesis of cerebral abscess formation. *Ann Neurol* 16:655–659.

Fraumeni J F & Miller R W (1969) Cancer deaths in the newborn. *Am J Dis Children* 117:186–189.

Garfield J S (1969) Management of supratentorial abscess: a review of 200 cases. *BMJ* ii:7–11.

Gold A P, Ransohoff J & Carter S (1964) Vein of Galen malformation. *Acta Neurol Scand* 11(suppl):5–31.

Goodrich J T (1991) Craniofacial reconstruction for craniosynostosis. In: Goodrich J T, Post K D & Argamaso R V (eds) *Plastic techniques in neurosurgery*. New York, NY: Georg Thieme; pp. 75–108.

Graham D R & Band J D (1981) *Citrobacter diversus* brain abscess and meningitis in neonates. *J Am Med Assoc* 245:1923–1925.

Greenberg M L (1999) Chemotherapy of choroid plexus carcinoma. *Child's Nerv Syst* 15:571–577.

Grienpentrog F & Pauly H (1957) Intra- und extrakranielle, fruhmanifeste Medulloblastome bei erbgleichen Zwillingen. *Zentralblatt für Neurochirurgie* 17:129–139.

Grode M L, Saunders M & Carton C A (1978) Subarachnoid haemorrhage secondary to ruptured aneurysms in infants. Report of two cases. *J Neurosurg* 49:898–902.

Hanigan W C, Brady T, Medlock M *et al.* (1990) Spontaneous regression of giant arteriovenous fistulae during the perinatal period. Case report. *J Neurosurg* 73:954–957.

Harwood-Nash D C & Fitz C R (1976) In: *Neuroradiology in infants and children.* St. Louis, MO: C V Mosby, vol. 3; pp. 906–913.

Hayward R D, Harkness W, Kendall B *et al.* (1992) Magnetic resonance imaging in the assessment of craniosynostosis. *Scand Plastic Reconstruct Hand Surg* 26:292–299.

Heafner M D, Duncan C C, Kier E L *et al.* (1985) Intraventricular haemorrhage in a term neonate secondary to a third ventricular arteriovenous malformation. *J Neurosurg* 63:640–643.

Hinton D R, Becker L E, Muakkassa K F *et al.* (1984) Lambdoid suture: normal development and pathology of 'synostosis'. *J Neurosurg* 61:333–339.

Hirsch J, Renier D & Saint-Rose C (1981) *Intracranial pressure in craniostenosis. Ninth meeting of the International Society for Pediatric Neurosurgery, Budapest, Hungary, 20–22 July 1981.*

Hoffman H J, Chuang S & Hendrick E B (1983) Aneurysms of the vein of Galen. In: Raimondi A J (ed.) *Concepts in pediatric neurosurgery.* Basel: Karger, No. 3; pp. 52–74.

Hoffman H J, Hendrick E B & Hiscox J L (1970) Cerebral abscesses in early infancy. *J Neurosurg* 33:172–177.

Hoffman H J & Hendrick E B (1979) Early neurosurgical repair in craniofacial dysmorphism. *J Neurosurg* 51:796–803.

Hoffman H J & Mohr G (1976) Lateral canthal advancement of the supraorbital margin: a new corrective technique in the treatment of coronal synostosis. *J Neurosurg* 45:376–381.

Holden A M, Fyler D C, Shillito J Jr *et al.* (1972) Congestive heart failure from intracranial arteriovenous fistula in infancy. Clinical and physiologic considerations in eight patients. *Pediatrics* 49:30–39.

Holt L E (1898) A report of 5 cases of abscesses of the brain in infants, together with a summary of 27 collected cases in infants and very young children. *Arch Pediatr* 15:81.

Horowitz M E, Mulhern R K, Kun L E *et al.* (1988) Brain tumours in the very young child. Postoperative chemotherapy in combined modality treatment. *Cancer* 61:428–434.

Housepian E M & Pool J L (1958) A systematic analysis of intracranial aneurysms from the autopsy file of the Presbyterian Hospital 1914–1956. *J Neuropathol Exp Neurol* 17:409–423.

Humphreys R P (1982) Arteriovenous malformations of the brain and spinal cord. In: *Pediatric neurosurgery: surgery of the developing nervous system.* New York, NY: Grune and Stratton; pp. 625–635.

Iwasa H, Indel I & Sato F (1983) Intraventricular cavernous hemangioma. Case report. *J Neurosurg* 59:153–157.

Izquierdo J M, Sanz F & Coca J M (1978) Pyocephalus of the new-born child. *Child's Brain* 4:129–136.

Jacobson P L & Farmer T W (1981) Subdural empyema complicating meningitis in infants. *Neurology (New York)* 31:190–193.

Johnston I H, Whittle I R, Besser M *et al.* (1987) Vein of Galen malformation: diagnosis and management. *Neurosurgery* 20:747–758.

Jones R K & Shearburn E W (1961) Intracranial aneurysms in a four week old infant: diagnosis by angiography and successful operation. *J Neurosurg* 18:122–124.

Jooma R & Kendall B E (1982) Intracranial tumours in the first year of life. *Neuroradiology* 23:267–274.

Jooma R, Kendall B E & Hayward R D (1984) Intracranial tumours in neonates: a report of seventeen cases. *Surg Neurol* 21:165–170.

Kalsbeck J E, De Sousa A L, Kleiman M B *et al.* (1980) Compartmentalization of the cerebral ventricles as a sequel of neonatal meningitis. *J Neurosurg* 52:547–552.

Karan S (1986) Purulent meningitis in the newborn. *Child's Nerv Syst* 2:26–31.

Kellie S J (1999) Chemotherapy of central nervous system tumours in infants. *Child's Nerv Syst* 15:592–612.

Lacey D J & Terplan K (1982) Intraventricular hemorrhage in full-term neonates. *Dev Med Child Neurol* 24:332–337.

Lajeune E, Catala M & Renier (1999) Craniosynostosis: from a clinical description to an understanding of bone formation of the skull. *Child's Nerv Syst* 15:676–680.

Lasjaunias P (1997) *Vascular diseases in neonates, infants and children.* Berlin: Springer; 67–202.

Lasjaunias P, Alvarez H, Rodesch G *et al.* (1996) Aneurysmal malformation of the vein of Galen, follow up of 120 children treated between 1984 and 1994. *Interven Neuroradiol* 2:15–26.

Lee D-Y, Kim Y-M, Yoo S-J *et al.* (1999) Congenital glioblastoma diagnosed by fetal sonography. *Child's Nerv Syst* 15:197–201.

Lekias J & Stokes B (1970) Dermoid lesions of the central nervous system in childhood. *Austral N Z J Surg* 39:335–340.

Le Wald L T (1933) Congenital absence of the superior orbital wall associated with pulsatile exophthalmos: report of four cases. *Am J Roentgenol* 30:756–764.

McCracken G H Jr (1977) Intraventricular treatment of neonatal meningitis due to Gram-negative bacilli. *J Pediatr* 91:1037–1038.

McCracken G H Jr & Mize S G (1976) A controlled study of intrathecal antibiotic therapy in Gram-negative enteric meningitis of infancy. *J Pediatr* 89:66–72.

McGuire T H, Greenwood J & Newton B L (1954) Bilateral angioma of choroid plexus. Case report. *J Neurosurg* 11:428–430.

McLellan N H, Prasad R & Punt J (1986) Spontaneous subhyaloid and retinal haemorrhages in an infant. *Arch Dis Childhood* 61:1130–1132.

McMurray B R, Martin L W, Dignan P S *et al.* (1977) Hereditary aplasia cutis congenita and associated defects: three instances in one family and a survey of reported cases. *Clin Pediatr* 16:610–614.

McWhirter W R, Dobson C & Ring I (1996) Childhood cancer incidence in Australia, 1982–1991. *Int J Cancer* 65:34–38.

Malisch T W, Guglielmi G, Vinuela F *et al.* (1997) Intracranial aneurysms treated with Guglielmi detachable coil: midterm clinical results in a consecutive series of 100 patients. *J Neurosurg* 87:176–183.

Mannino F L, Jones K L & Benirschke K (1977) Congenital skin defects and fetal papyraceous. *J Pediatr* 91:559–564.

Marchac D (1978) Radical forehead remodelling for craniostenosis. *Plastic Reconstruct Surg* 61:823–835.

Marchac D & Arnaud E (1999) Midface surgery from Tessier to distraction. *Child's Nerv Syst* 15:681–694.

Marsh J L & Vannier M W (1983) The 'third' dimension in craniofacial surgery. *Plastic Reconst Surg* 71:759–767.

Matson D D (1969) Congenital defects of the scalp and skull. In: *Neurosurgery of infancy and childhood.* Springfield, IL: Charles C Thomas; 2nd edn, pp. 168–178.

Milhorat T H (1978) In: *Pediatric neurosurgery.* Philadelphia, PA: Davis; pp. 352–356.

Mosberg W H (1951) Spinal tumours diagnosed during the first year of life: with report of a case. *J Neurosurg* 8:220–224.

Moss M L (1959) The pathogenesis of premature cranial synostosis in man. *Acta Anatomica (Basel)* 37:351.

Muakkassa K F, Hoffman H J, Hinton D R *et al.* (1984) Lambdoid synostosis. 2. Review of cases managed at the Hospital for Sick Children 1972–1982. *J Neurosurg* 61:340–347.

Muakkassa K F, Kling R B & Stark D B (1982) Nonsurgical approach to congenital scalp and skull defects. *J Neurosurg* 56:711–715.

Munslow R A, Stovall V S, Price R D *et al.* (1957) Brain abscess in infants. *J Pediatr* 51:74–79.

Newcomb A L & Munns G F (1949) Rupture of aneurysm of the circle of Willis in the newborn. *Pediatrics* 3:769–772.

Nicholls D A, Brown R D Jr, Thielen K R *et al.* (1997) Endovascular treatment of ruptured posterior circulation aneurysms using electrolytically detachable coils. *J Neurosurg* 87:374–380.

Nishio A, Sakaguchi M, Murata K *et al.* (1991) Anterior communicating artery aneurysm in early childhood. Report of a case. *Surg Neurol* 35:224–229.

Norman M G & Becker L E (1974) Cerebral damage in neonates resulting from arteriovenous malformation of vein of Galen. *J Neurol Neurosurg Psychiatry* 37:252–258.

Opperman L A, Sweeney T M, Redmon J *et al.* (1993) Tissue interactions with underlying dura mater inhibit osseous obliteration of developing cranial sutures. *Dev Dynam* 198:312–322.

Overall J C Jr (1970) Neonatal bacterial meningitis: analysis of predisposing factors and outcome compared with matched control subjects. *J Pediatr* 76:499–511.

Padget D H (1956) The cranial venous system in man with references to development, adult configuration, and relation to arteries. *Am J Anatomy* 98:307–355.

Palma P A, Miner M E & Morriss F H Jr (1979) Intraventricular hemorrhage in the neonate born at term. *Am J Dis Children* 133:941–944.

Pannell B W, Hendrick E B, Hoffman H J *et al.* (1982) Dermoid cysts of the anterior fontanelle. *Neurosurgery* 10:317–323.

Parkinson D, Medovy H & Mitchell J R (1954) Spinal cord tumour in a newborn. *J Neurosurg* 11:629–632.

Persing J, Babler W, Winn R *et al.* (1981) Age as a critical factor in the success of surgical correction of craniosynostosis. *J Neurosurg* 54:601–606.

Pickering K, Hogan G R & Gilbert E F (1970) Aneurysm of the posterior inferior cerebellar artery: rupture in a newborn. *Am J Dis Children* 119:155–158.

Punt J, Pritchard J, Pincott J *et al.* (1980) Neuroblastoma: a review of 21 cases presenting with spinal cord compression. *Cancer* 45:3095–3102.

Raybaud C A, Strother C M & Hald J K (1989) Aneurysms of the vein of Galen: embryonic considerations and anatomical features relating to the pathogenesis of the malformation. *Neuroradiology* 31:109–128.

Rekate H L (1985) Lambdoid suture synostosis. *J Neurosurg* 62:185.

Rekate H L (1998) Occipital plagiocephaly: a critical review of the literature. *J Neurosurg* 24–30.

Renier D, E l Ghouzzi V, Bonaventure J *et al.* (2000) Fibroblast growth factor receptor 3 mutation in nonsyndromic coronal synostosis: clinical spectrum, prevalence, and surgical outcome. *J Neurosurg* 92:631–636.

Renier D, Flandin C, Hirsch E *et al.* (1988) Brain abscesses in neonates. A study of 30 cases. *J Neurosurg* 69:877–882.

Robinson R G (1962) Congenital perforations of the skull in relation to the parietal bone. *J Neurosurg* 19:153–158.

Rosenblum M L, Hoff J T, Norman D *et al.* (1980) Nonoperative treatment of brain abscesses in selected high risk patients. *J Neurosurg* 52:217–225.

Rosenblum M L, Hoff J T, Norman D *et al.* (1978) Decreased mortality from brain abscesses since advent of computerised tomography. *J Neurosurg* 49:658–668.

Salmon J H (1972) Ventriculitis complicating meningitis. *Am J Dis Children* 124:35–38.

Sato T, Shimoda A, Takahashi T *et al.* (1984) Congenital anaplastic ependymoma: a case report of familial glioma. *Child's Brain* 11:342–348.

Sato O, Tumura A & Sano K (1964) Brain tumours of early infants. *Child's Brain*:121–125.

Shapiro K (1985) Subarachnoid haemorrhages in children. In: Fein J M & Flamm E S (eds) *Cerebrovascular surgery.* New York, NY: Springer, vol. 3; pp. 941–965.

Shillito J (1973) A new cranial suture appearing in the site of craniectomy for synostosis. *Radiology* 107:83–88.

Silverman B K, Brekzt T, Craig J *et al.* (1959) Congestive failure in the newborn caused by cerebral arteriovenous fistula. *Am J Dis Children* 89:539–543.

Solitaire G B & Krigman M R (1964) Congenital intracranial neoplasm. *J Neuropathol Exp Neurol* 2:280–292.

Stern L, Ramos A D & Wigglesworth F W (1968) Congestive heart failure secondary to cerebral arteriovenous aneurysm in the newborn infant. *Am J Dis Children* 115:581–587.

Storrs B B, Humphreys R P, Hendrick E B *et al.* (1982) Intracranial aneurysms in the pediatric age group. *Child's Brain* 9:358–361.

Strauss L C & Killmond T M (1991) Efficacy of postoperative chemotherapy using cisplatin plus etoposide in young children with brain tumours. *Med Pediatr Oncol* 11:16–21.

Tan M P, McConachie N S & Vloeberghs M (1998) Ruptured fusiform cerebral aneurysm in a neonate. *Child's Nerv Syst* 14:467–469.

Tekkok I H & Ventureyra E C G (1997) Spontaneous intracranial hemorrhage of structural origin during the first year of life. *Child's Nerv Syst* 13:154–165.

Tessier P (1967) Osteotomies totales de la face, syndrome de Crouzon, syndrome d'Apert, oxycephalies, scaphocephalies, turricephalies. *Annales de Chirurgie Plastique* 12:273–286.

Thompson D N P, Harkness W, Jones B M *et al.* (1997) Aetiology of herniation of the hindbrain in craniosynostosis. *Pediatr Neurosurg* 26:288–295.

Thompson D N P, Malcolm G, Jones B M *et al.* (1995) Intracranial pressure in single-suture craniosynostosis. *Pediatr Neurosurg* 22:235–240.

Till K (1968) Subdural haematoma and effusion in infancy. *BMJ* ii:400–402.

Trounce J Q, Fawer C-L, Punt J *et al.* (1985) Primary thalamic haemorrhage in the newborn: a new clinical entity. *Lancet* i:190–192.

Van Eys J, Cangir A & Coody D (1985) Mopp regimen as primary chemotherapy for brain tumours in children. *J Neuro-Oncol* 3:237–243.

Vinocur C D, Weintraub W H, Wilensky R T *et al.* (1976) Surgical management of aplasia cutis congenita. *Arch Surg* 111:1160–1164.

Virchow R (1851) Uber den Cretisimus, Namentlich in Franken und uber pathologische Schadel formen. *Verhandlungen der Deutschen Gesellschaft fur physische Medizin (Wurzburg)* 2:230.

Volpe J J (1981a) Neurology of the newborn. Philadelphia, PA: Saunders; pp. 747–802.

Volpe J J (1981b) *Neurology of the newborn. Major problems in clinical pediatrics.* Philadelphia, PA: W B Saunders; vol. 22; pp. 239–261.

Wakai S, Andon Y, Nagai M *et al.* (1990) Choroid plexus arteriovenous malformation in a full-term neonate. Case report. *J Neurosurg* 72:127–129.

Wakai S, Arai T & Nagai M (1984) Congenital brain tumours. *Surg Neurol* 21:597–609.

Walter A, Mulhern R, Heideman R *et al.* (1998) The treatment of infants and young children with brain tumours at St Jude Children's Research Hospital: survival and neuropsychological outcome. *Child's Nerv Syst* 14:504.

Wong T, Wann S & Lee L (1986) Congenital dermoid cysts of the anterior fontanelle in Chinese children. *Child's Nerv Syst* 2:175–178.

Yujinovsky O & Nyhan W L (1978) The cloverleaf skull. *Clin Genet* 14:178–180.

Zerah M, Garcia-Monaco R, Rodesch G *et al.* (1992) Hydrodynamics in vein of Galen malformation in 43 cases. *Child's Nerv Syst* 8:111–117.

# Section XII

# Epidemiology of neurologic disability

# Chapter 47 The epidemiology of the cerebral palsies

E. Blair and F. Stanley

## DEFINITION

Cerebral palsy is an umbrella term covering a group of non-progressive, but often changing, motor impairment syndromes secondary to lesions or anomalies of the brain arising in the early stages of its development (Mutch *et al.* 1992). This latest consensus definition was written in 1990, but it has not changed substantially for decades (MacKeith & Polani 1958; Bax 1964).

It is an unusual medical definition. There is no diagnostic test for cerebral palsy, and its development cannot be reliably inferred from pathologic findings. It is defined by clinical description over time. Thus, if the clinical symptoms disappear or the lesion turns out to be progressive, it is the description of cerebral palsy that changes, not the natural history of cerebral palsy. Therefore, it is not possible to be certain that the term is correctly applied without following the patient over time. In the definition, the phrases 'non-progressive but not unchanging' and 'early stages of development' are imprecise. There is no agreement on an allowed limit for the rate of progression, nor whether the therapeutic halting of a normally progressive condition constitutes a non-progressive condition, nor the age before which an insult is considered early. In practice, the limits are determined arbitrarily, depending on the given purpose and local conditions. This is discussed below.

The label of cerebral palsy is not a diagnosis in the sense that it does not exclude another diagnosis. In the past, the term tended to be reserved for motor impairments of unknown etiology. A motor impairment with a specific diagnosis, such as a chromosomal anomaly, tended to be excluded from the cerebral palsy group. Therefore, some easily recognized diseases that fit the clinical definition of cerebral palsy have traditionally been excluded (Badawi *et al.* 1998). Conditions only recently diagnosable are less likely to be excluded.

It is clear that the cerebral palsies are heterogeneous with respect to cause and to clinical description, so a label of cerebral palsy is not useful for communicating the cause, severity, or prognosis of a child's condition. It is therefore reasonable to ask whether 'cerebral palsy' is a term worth retaining.

The usefulness of a classification depends on the aim of making the classification. The term 'cerebral palsy' groups cases of a similar clinical nature and this may be useful for health service planners. With decreasing perinatal mortality, the prevalence of cerebral palsy has been used as a measure of pregnancy outcome with a view to evaluating obstetric and neonatal care. This is of dubious validity for term infants for whom the quality of medical care is currently either not (Niswander 1985) or only weakly (Blair 1994; Gaffney *et al.* 1994; Richmond *et al.* 1994) associated with the likelihood of cerebral palsy. It may be a more reasonable measure of the care of infants born extremely preterm, though the evidence for separating motor from other central nervous system impairments is weak (Stanley *et al.* 2000). There are better grounds for using it together with other adverse pregnancy outcomes as a measure of the general health of a population.

The best reasons for retaining the term are not medical. It identifies a group at risk of severe disability and handicap in a non-pejorative manner, which is now familiar to policy-makers and to the public. Additionally, in this era of information technology it is short and unique. A keyword of cerebral palsy or even of palsy will give references almost exclusively related to non-progressive motor impairments of central origin recognized in childhood or infancy. It conveys considerable information and yet it is flexible: it can be most useful if it conveys the same information to everyone.

## DIFFERENTIAL DESCRIPTIONS

The heterogeneous clinical descriptions included under cerebral palsy necessitate standardized subclassifications, although intercenter reproducibility of description is somewhat elusive (Stanley *et al.* 2000). Traditionally, cases are differentiated by descriptions of type, topography, and severity of the motor impairment. Increasingly, descriptions of additional impairments and, more recently, details of cerebral imaging are being added.

### TYPE OF IMPAIRMENT

Spasticity is the predominant feature for approximately 80% of cases of cerebral palsy. It is characterized by abnormal muscular control, the clasp-knife effect (sudden disappearance of abnormal resistance to passive stretch), exaggerated reflexes and/or clonus and sometimes with reduced truncal tone. The enduring Babinski reflex indicates a lesion of the pyramidal tract.

Dyskinesia is more often found with spasticity than alone. It is characterized by involuntary movements that may be athetoid (writhing), dystonic (rigid posturing), or, now rarely, choreic (rapid and jerky).

Ataxia and hypotonia are seen so frequently that they are seldom explicitly described, except in the rare cases where they constitute the predominant motor impairment. Isolated hypotonia frequently accompanies intellectual impairment, and this is not traditionally classified as cerebral palsy (Badawi *et al.* 1998).

These different types of movement disorders may co-exist, and the predominant form may vary over time within an individual.

### TOPOGRAPHY

There are four commonly occurring bodily distributions of spasticity. Quadriplegia (also termed tetraplegia or double hemiplegia, though the latter implies lateral asymmetry) denotes involvement of all four limbs with the arms being equally or more affected than the legs. Diplegia denotes that the legs are more severely affected than the arms. The inter-center agreement on differentiating between quadriplegia and diplegia is poor, but together, they account for about 50% of cerebral palsy. Left and right hemiplegia denote that one side of the body is considerably more affected than the other, with the arm usually being more affected than the leg. The hemiplegias account for about one-third of cerebral palsy. Less symmetric distributions give rise to terms such as monoplegia and triplegia.

### SEVERITY

It is difficult to measure severity of motor impairment objectively because the resulting disability is so dependent on other factors, particularly cognitive ability (Jarvis & Hey 1984). It is therefore usual to report functional ability, which may now be assessed using the Gross Motor Function Measure (GMFM) (Russell *et al.* 1989) or classified using the five category Gross Motor Function Classification System (GMFCS) (Palisano *et al.* 1997). While there is debate as to whether the severity of motor impairment may be estimated by adjusting the results of the GMFCS for treatments or associated impairments, in practice, most treatments have little effect on the GMFCS. The GMFM was devised to evaluate the effects of physical therapy but tends to be rather insensitive to small changes in functional ability, particularly the unusual functional skills that may be associated with significant gains in quality of life for the severely motor impaired.

In the past, functional impairment has been somewhat subjectively assessed as: minimal (with no perceptible effect on function), mild (perceptible dysfunction, but not requiring aids other than ankle foot orthoses), moderate (requiring aids other than a wheel chair), and severe. This last category is very broad, including the relatively independent wheelchair user to the totally dependent. The minimal category is likely to be underascertained and is sometimes omitted from cerebral palsy statistics. On the Western Australian Cerebral Palsy Register, about half the cases are classified as mild, 30% as moderate and 20% as severely motor impaired. It is concerning that the proportion classified as severely impaired has increased steadily in Western Australia from 12% in the period 1973–1976 to 29% in 1989–1992.

### ADDITIONAL IMPAIRMENTS

Cerebral palsy is associated with cognitive and learning disabilities, seizure and behavioural disorders and sensory defects which can very significantly affect functional prognosis. The likelihood and severity of associated impairments increases with increasing severity of motor impairment. For cases born in Western Australia 1975–1990, severe cognitive impairment (IQ<35) was found in 4.4% of those with mild but 52% of those with severe cerebral palsy: similarly ongoing seizures were a problem in 20 and 60%, blindness was found in 3 and 24% and deafness in 0.3 and 3.7% of mild and severely motor impaired cases, respectively (Stanley *et al.* 2000).

## HETEROGENEITY AND MULTIFACTORIALITY OF CAUSE

Consideration of the definition makes it clear that any circumstances that can affect the integrity of motor areas of the brain at any time between conception and early childhood are possible causes of cerebral palsy. While there are many conceivable causes, no cause is readily apparent for many cases, while others have many risk factors that could contribute to the cause (Blair & Stanley 1993b). This confirms heterogeneity of cause and suggests the possibility of multifactorial causes (Blair & Stanley 1993a). There are a few confirmed causes of cerebral palsy, now largely confined to developing countries, such as maternal methyl mercury exposure (Takeuchi & Matsumoto 1969; Amin-Zaki *et al.* 1979), maternal rubella (Stanley *et al.* 1986), or cytomegalovirus infection (Hagberg *et al.* 1996), neonatal kernicterus secondary to maternal Rhesus iso-immunization and genetically acquired defects (Hughes & Newton 1992) responsible for an association between cerebral palsy and consanguinous marriage (Gustavson *et al.* 1969; Al-Rajeh *et al.* 1991). There are a far greater number of risk factors: these factors are associated with the occurrence of cerebral palsy, but their role in its causation is not well understood.

## RISK FACTORS FOR CEREBRAL PALSY

### GESTATIONAL AGE

Preterm (<37 completed weeks gestation) and particularly very preterm (<33 weeks) birth is very strongly associated with cerebral palsy. The risk of cerebral palsy increases dramatically with decreasing gestational age at delivery, being 30 times higher in children born before 30 weeks of gestation than among those born at term (Stanley *et al.* 2000) (Fig. 47.1). The rate is also slightly increased among post-term births. For the 1986–1992 birth cohort in Western Australia, preterm births accounted for 34.7% of cases of

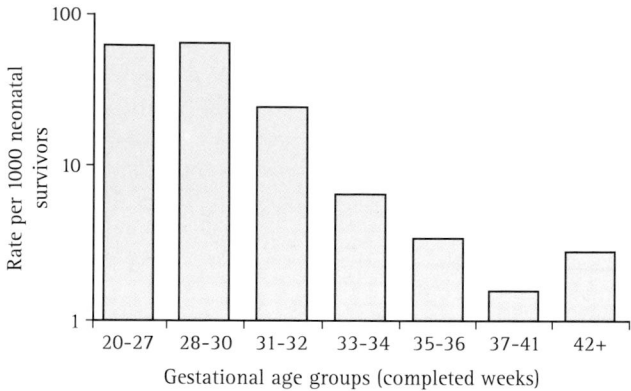


**Figure 47.1** Gestational-age-specific cerebral palsy rates (log scale) in Western Australia, 1980–1992 combined (excludes cases due to postneonatal causes).

cerebral palsy and very preterm births for 24.8%, while they only accounted for 7.5 and 1.3% of neonatal survivors. Very preterm survival is a relatively new phenomenon. It largely results from the availability of neonatal intensive care, so very preterm cerebral palsy is primarily a problem of developed countries. However, even the slightly preterm infant born at 35–36 weeks has more than double the risk of cerebral palsy than a child born at term.

Among very preterm infants, cerebral palsy is very closely associated with intraparenchymal leukomalacia (p. 386). When present, this cerebral pathology can be considered the organic basis for the movement disorder and cannot therefore be considered a cause of the cerebral palsy; it *is* the cerebral palsy. The cause of the cerebral palsy is therefore the cause of the cerebral lesions, and it is these precursors of the cerebral pathology that must be understood in order to prevent the cerebral palsy. However, not all very preterm children with cerebral palsy have parenchymal involvement, and not all very preterm born children with parenchymal involvement have cerebral palsy (Stanley *et al.* 2000). It is dangerous to use parenchymal lesions as a surrogate outcome for cerebral palsy, though it is likely to select a more etiologically homogeneous group of cases. While all very preterm born children with cerebral palsy without obvious postneonatal causes (see below) are grouped with cases likely to be of antepartum or intrapartum origin, it is quite likely that at least a proportion acquire the brain lesions responsible postnatally due to complications occurring after birth.

## APPROPRIATENESS OF INTRAUTERINE GROWTH

Appropriateness of growth is usually inferred from birthweight for gestational age, though the increasing use of serial ultrasound and Doppler flow studies provide more direct means of assessment for those fetuses considered at risk for growth restriction (Kingdom *et al.* 2000). For infants born after 33 weeks of gestation, there is a strong and consistent association between measures of growth restriction and cerebral palsy (Kyllerman *et al.* 1982; Blair & Stanley 1990; Uvebrant & Hagberg 1992; Palmer *et al.* 1994), with the risk increasing with decreasing proportion of expected birthweight and with evidence of long-standing restriction (Blair & Stanley 1990, 1992).

Since very preterm birth is always associated with pathology, it is not possible to measure a similar association in infants born before 33 weeks of gestation because there is no satisfactory (normal) control group with which to compare very preterm infants who are also growth-restricted. The associations with cerebral palsy measured by comparing very preterm infants considered small for gestational age (SGA) with equally preterm infants who are not SGA are not consistent (Blair & Stanley 1990; Uvebrant & Hagberg 1992; Murphy *et al.* 1995; Topp *et al.* 1996). This may be because the distribution of pathologies associated with very preterm birth in the comparison groups varies between studies.

There are many causes of intrauterine growth restriction. It is not clear whether associated pathologic outcomes are associated more closely with the cause of the restriction or with characteristics of the restriction. These characteristics, such as the gestational age at onset, duration and severity of restriction, are themselves associated with the cause (Blair 2000).

## MULTIPLE BIRTH

Multiple birth is a cause of both intrauterine growth restriction and preterm birth, but these are not the sole or even the primary factors increasing the risk of cerebral palsy in children resulting from multiple pregnancies. Combining the relevant studies published by 1998, the relative risk (and 95% confidence interval) of cerebral palsy is 4.5 (3.9–5.2) for each twin and 18.2 (10.4–31.9) for each triplet (Stanley *et al.* 2000). The relative risk of cerebral palsy is therefore of the order of 9 for a twin and 50 for a triplet pregnancy. Comparing twin pregnancies with singletons born at the same gestational ages, the relative risk of cerebral palsy in a twin pregnancy is most elevated for term infants 3.0 (1.9–4.9), followed by twins of 33–36 weeks' gestation, 2.3 (1.3–3.7), extremely preterm twins (<29 weeks), 1.9 (1.2–3.2) and very preterm twins (29–32 weeks) 1.0 (0.7–1.6) (Stanley *et al.* 2000), demonstrating that while the prematurity associated with twinning contributes to the risk of cerebral palsy, it is not entirely responsible for it, particularly in term and moderately preterm infants. The risk of cerebral palsy in twins is not associated with zygosity, or, in the absence of information on zygosity, with like-sex, rather than unlike-sex, twins or, in recent studies, with birth order (Grether *et al.* 1993; Petterson *et al.* 1993). Among multiple births, antenatal fetal death of one of them is a strong risk factor for cerebral palsy, with the survivor of a twin pregnancy in whom one fetus died being at 11 times the risk of cerebral palsy as twins with co-twins who survive the neonatal period. Fetal death of a co-twin is biologically a very plausible cause in monochorionic twins with placental anastomoses. It is less likely to account for the increased risk in dizygotic twins. As antenatal death of one and only one twin after 20 weeks' gestation is reasonably uncommon, fetal death of a co-twin is responsible for only a small proportion of cerebral palsy risk attributed to multiple pregnancy. Intrapartum factors were previously thought to put the second-born twin at greater risk. The lack of association with birth order throws doubt on this hypothesis. However, of a twin pair with one live and one stillbirth, it is usually the liveborn twin that is born first (Grether *et al.* 1993; Petterson *et al.* 1993). Thus, birth order is sometimes determined by factors that are themselves determinants of death or cerebral palsy and should not be considered simply as a marker for intrapartum difficulties. The role of intrapartum difficulties in twin deliveries may need re-assessment.

## GENDER

There is a tendency for males to be at somewhat greater risk of cerebral palsy in all populations studied. For example, the ratio of males to females on the Western Australian Cerebral Palsy Register born in 1956–1994 was 1.34. This ratio varies over time more than might be expected to result from random variation but has almost always been greater than the male proportion of all births. There are a few exceptions to this general rule. In the SW Swedish 1983–1986 birth cohort, the ratio of males to females was 0.9, whereas in 1987–1990, it was 1.1. The origin of the male excess is not understood: the few identified X-linked causes of cerebral palsy are not sufficiently numerous to be responsible.

## ANTEPARTUM FACTORS

Several maternal factors such as menstrual abnormalities (Nelson & Ellenberg 1986), seizure disorders (Nelson & Ellenberg 1982), advanced maternal age (Blair & Stanley 1993a,b), parity (first births and births after the third) (Blair 1996), and low social class (Dowding & Barry 1990; Dolk *et al.* 1996) have been associated with cerebral palsy.

The most consistent evidence of a strong association with suboptimal antepartum events comes from the association with fetal malformation syndromes, since the events themselves are frequently unrecorded and perhaps even unobserved. While the observed association with central nervous system anomalies might be anticipated, associations with malformations outside the central nervous system are also consistently reported (Coorssen *et al.* 1991; Miller 1991; Fletcher & Foley 1993; Palmer *et al.* 1995). The antenatal insults may consist of congenital infections, particularly those of the TORCH group (Gilbert 1996), infections of the fetal membranes (Murphy *et al.* 1995; Grether & Nelson 1997), maternal thyroid abnormalities (Blair & Stanley 1993a, Badawi 2000), iodine deficiency, which, if sufficiently severe, results in cretinism (spastic diplegia and deaf mutism) (Hetzel 1994), toxic exposures, which may include alcohol (Olegård *et al.* 1979), and even mechanical trauma (Gilles *et al.* 1996). The role of the inflammatory effects of infection, that is of infection *per se* rather than any specific infection, is coming under increasing scrutiny and suspicion as a causal factor for cerebral palsy in births of all gestational ages (Leviton 1993; Dammann & Leviton 1997; Grether *et al.* 1999).

## INTRAPARTUM FACTORS

In the middle of the 19th century, Little described 'the forms of abnormal parturition that he had observed to precede certain mental and physical derangements' (Little 1958). From that time to the beginning of the 1990s, intrapartum factors were believed to be the primary initiators of the pathway to cerebral palsy. This occurred despite both Little's paper suggesting that intrapartum factors were only one of several possible causes and could represent the final step in a multicausal pathway and Freud's suggestions in 1897 (Freud 1968) that antepartum factors may play an important role. In developed countries, during the intervening 140 years, obstetricians or public-health measures have abolished the intrapartum factors that Little mentioned as antecedents of cerebral palsy, yet the association between cerebral palsy and intrapartum and neonatal observations from which damaging asphyxia is inferred persists. The question is whether these signs *do* represent de-novo damaging asphyxia or whether they are the final straw in a multicausal pathway or the first readily observable clinical signs of cerebral malformation or damage occurring earlier in pregnancy (Blair 1993; Stanley *et al.* 2000, chapter 9). While it is plausible that obstetric malpractice could be responsible for impaired survival, available evidence suggests that it contributes very little (Niswander 1985; Blair 1994; Gaffney *et al.* 1994; Richmond *et al.* 1994), yet the concept is responsible for a crippling volume of medical litigation. In response, relevant medical fraternities have created guidelines for determining conditions under which intrapartum factors are likely to be causal (Society of Obstetricians and Gynaecologists of Canada 1996; PSANZ 1999).

## POSTNEONATAL FACTORS

A proportion of all cerebral palsy is acquired in infancy or childhood as the result of a variety of brain damaging events such as meningitis or head injury. These cases, termed 'postneonatally acquired', are often considered separately to those acquired earlier, because the immediate causes are well understood, they are considered to be independent of obstetric and neonatal care, and they may have systematic differences in their response to cerebral pathology (Carr 1996). However, their disabilities are just as severe, and in Western Australia, the rate of postneonatally acquired cerebral palsy is increasing, as is the proportion classified as severely impaired (Stanley *et al.* 2000). The decreasing trends of postneonatally acquired cerebral palsy reported from Sweden (Hagberg *et al.* 1989, 1993, 1996) suggest that this increase is not inevitable and that the precursors of the immediate causes must be investigated in order to devise rational preventive strategies.

Whichever uppermost age limit is chosen, most postneonatally acquired cerebral palsy is acquired before 1 year of age. Males are at greater risk, though there is little evidence that any other medical or biological factors predispose to cerebral injury, apart from congenital vascular or metabolic abnormalities (Morton *et al.* 1991; Badawi *et al.* 1998). Apart from cases resulting from congenital abnormalities, which may include those requiring early surgical repairs with the risk of peri-operative cerebro-vascular accident, there is a strong association with social disadvantage. It is primarily a disease of poverty and ignorance combining to create barriers to effective parenting. With increasing economic development, the profile of immediate causes changes with cerebral infection and febrile convulsions becoming less prominent and head injury, which would previously have been more likely to be fatal, becoming more prominent (Stanley *et al.* 2000).

The challenge to clinicians and epidemiologists is to understand the mechanisms by which these risk factors are related to cerebral palsy, under what circumstances they constitute causal factors, and the most effective and acceptable means of interrupting the causal pathways on which they lie (Stanley *et al.* 2000).

## FACTORS AFFECTING ESTIMATES OF PREVALENCE

Estimates of prevalence, whether over time or between populations, are the mainstay of cerebral palsy epidemiology, so it is unfortunate that there are so many barriers to obtaining estimates of rates of cerebral palsy that are directly comparable.

### DEFINITION

As is readily apparent from earlier in this Chapter, the definition of cerebral palsy does not define the severity of disability; it does not exclude any types of movement disabilities, nor does it exclude any causes. The rational approach to definition is determined by the reasons for making the definition. Thus, it is reasonable to exclude those causes that are well understood if one plans to investigate causes that are not well understood, or to exclude those with minimal disability if one is interested in providing disability services. As an aside, it is also traditional to exclude children with isolated hypotonia, particularly where this is accompanied by intellectual disability. However, if the reason for defining cerebral palsy is to compare trends over time or between populations, then the overriding requirement of the definition is that it remain stable over time or between populations (Badawi *et al.* 1998).

Mild and particularly minimal cerebral palsy is likely to be underascertained, the degree of underascertainment being very dependent on the means by which ascertainment is effected. More valid comparisons of rates are therefore likely to be achieved by confining comparisons to moderate and severe cerebral palsy, since these cases are immediately apparent and almost certain to be receiving services for their disability, at least in developed countries.

### AGE OF ACQUISITION OF THE LABEL OF CEREBRAL PALSY

There is no general agreement on either the minimum or maximum age at which the label of cerebral palsy may be applied. The minimum age is the age at which one can be confident that motor impairment exists and is not progressive. This age varies both between individual cases (earlier confidence is possible with more severely affected cases) and between individual clinicians. However, the choice of minimum age can greatly affect the estimated rate of severe cerebral palsy since death before that age removes the possibility of acquiring the label, and more severely affected children are at greatest risk of early mortality (Evans *et al.* 1990; Hutton *et al.* 1994; Crichton *et al.* 1995). The maximum age is the age at which the brain is no longer considered to be at an early stage of development. Since brain development continues at a diminishing rate throughout childhood, there is no biological rationale for the choice of any particular age. The choice has varied between 2 and 13 years of age, though the age of school entry (around 5 years) is a popular one. Since the rate of postneonatal acquisition drops rapidly with age, the differences in rate attributable to choice of maximum age are not usually very great.

### AGE AND COMPLETENESS OF ASCERTAINMENT

The age at which ascertainment is considered complete must of course be at or above the set maximum age of acquisition. Its choice is dictated by pragmatic concerns, usually centered on maximizing the completeness of ascertainment. This is responsible for the popularity of an age at which there is a routine check on each child's performance, such as the age of school entry. Completeness of ascertainment can markedly affect estimates of prevalence, which is of course the reason that the most comparable estimates are those limited to moderate and severely affected cases.

### SURVIVAL

Only children who survive to the minimum age of acquisition are at risk of being described as having cerebral palsy. Ideally, the denominator should be the total population of children surviving to that minimum age. In practice, routine statistics of all births and of live births are usually available, but routine statistics of neonatal survivors are

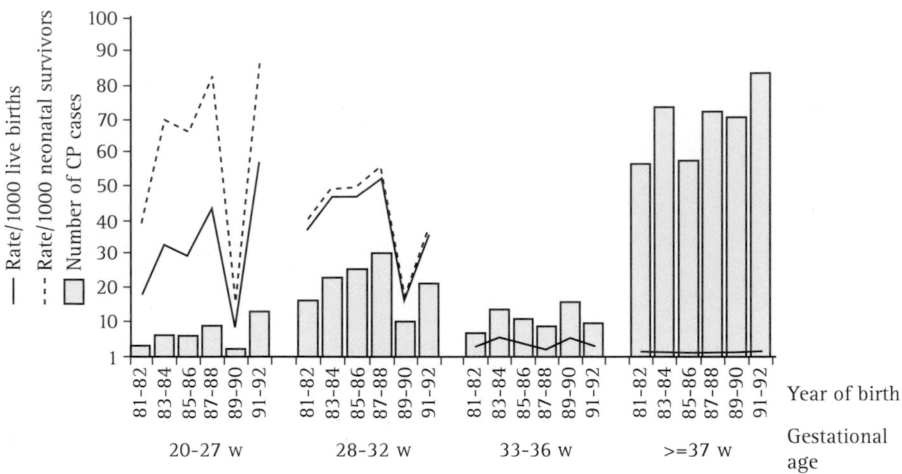


Figure 47.2 Cerebral palsy numbers and rates (excluding cases due to postneonatal causes) by gestational age in Western Australia, 1981–1992.

less likely, and routine statistics of survivors of infancy are much less likely to be available. Since neonatal and postneonatal deaths are rare in term births, the use of live births rather than infant survivors as the denominator makes little difference to estimates of rates but can markedly affect the estimates in preterm births, particularly very, and extremely, preterm births (Stanley *et al.* 2000) (Fig. 47.2).

To enable valid comparisons, it is important to report any exclusions based on cause, severity, type of disability, or age of acquisition and to define the minimum and maximum ages of acquisition and the age of complete ascertainment.

## CHANGES IN PREVALENCE OVER TIME

In view of the considerations in the section on prevalence, it is frequently invalid to make direct comparisons between different studies. The most reliable trends will be obtained from longitudinal studies that have maintained consistent methods over time in populations with sufficient numbers of births to minimize random variation. There are now registers of cerebral palsy in at least 22 geographically defined populations, all in the developed world (Stanley *et al.* 2000). However, only two (Western Sweden and Western Australia) commenced before 1960, both with annual birth cohorts of the order of 20 000. Two further registers commenced in the decade of the 1960s, one (Mersey) with an annual birth cohort in excess of 20 000. These three registers have all observed little change in overall birth prevalence over their timespans but a marked change in the birthweight and gestational age profiles with registrants tending to be born at earlier gestations and lower birthweights. These changes are concurrent with the increasing survival of very premature infants and, more recently, with the advent of neonatal intensive care.

## CONCLUSION

Decreasing rates of perinatal mortality initiated by changes in public health status have been maintained in recent decades by changes in obstetric and neonatal service provision, most recently by the availability of neonatal intensive care. While these changes may have resulted in a net gain in unimpaired survival, the high rate of cerebral palsy among surviving very premature infants is of considerable concern, particularly since the severity of impairment in these affected children is increasing, as is the occurrence of associated impairments. These observations should temper our enthusiasm for pushing the new perinatal technologies to their limits without equal enthusiasm for investigating causal pathways leading to preterm births.

### ACKNOWLEDGEMENTS

We are grateful for the support of the NH&MRC who fund cerebral palsy studies in Western Australia, also to Linda Watson, who maintains the WA Cerebral Palsy Register and the many health professionals who provide information to the Register.

### Key Points

- Cerebral palsy implies motor impairment resulting from a non-progressive brain lesion or anomaly acquired early in life.
- It is a clinical description, not a diagnosis.
- Since it cannot be applied until the motor impairment becomes apparent only neonatal survivors are at risk.
- The motor impairments are heterogeneous but 80% exhibit spasticity.
- Despite considerable efforts, inter-center agreement of description remains elusive.
- The effect on function ranges from imperceptible to total incapacitation.
- Motor impairment may be accompanied by other impairments, which may additionally limit functional attainment.
- Its causes are heterogeneous and may be multifactorial.
- Risk factors include preterm birth, restricted intra-uterine growth, multiple gestation, male gender, several antenatal factors, sentinel intrapartum events, poor condition at birth or neonatally and post neonatal cerebral infection or trauma.
- With the exception of post neonatal events, the relationships between risk factors and causes are poorly understood and no risk factor is an accurate predictor.
- Birth prevalence has changed little in the latter half of the twentieth century, but an increasing proportion are born very prematurely, concurrent with the increasing survival of premature infants particularly since the advent of neonatal intensive care.

## REFERENCES


Al-Rajeh S, Bademosi O, Awada A *et al.* (1991) Cerebral palsy in Saudi Arabia: A case-control study of risk factors. *Dev Med Child Neurol* 33: 1048–1052.

Amin-Zaki L, Majeed M A, Elhassani S B *et al.* (1979) Prenatal methylmercury poisoning. Clinical observations over five years. *Am J of Dis Childr* 133: 172–177.

Badawi N, Korinczuk J J, MacKenzie C L *et al.* (2000) Newborn encephalopathy: an association with maternal thyroid disease. *BMJ* 107: 798–801.

✪ Badawi N, Watson L, Petterson B *et al.* (1998) What constitutes cerebral palsy? *Dev Med Child Neurol* 40: 520–527.

Bax M C O (1964) Terminology and classification of cerebral palsy. *Dev Med Child Neurol* 6: 295–297.

Blair E (1993) A research definition for 'birth asphyxia'? *Dev Med Child Neurol* 35: 449–555.

Blair E (1994) Cerebral palsy and intrapartum care: Wrong denominator used (letter). *BMJ* 309: 1229.

✪ Blair E (1996) Obstetric antecedents of cerebral palsy. *Fetal Matern Med Rev* 8: 199–215.

Blair E (2000) Paediatric implications of intrauterine growth restriction with special reference to cerebral palsy. In: Kingdom J & Baker P (eds) *Intrauterine growth restriction.* London: Springer-Verlag pp. 351–366.

Blair E & Stanley F J (1990) Intrauterine growth and spastic cerebral palsy I. Association with birth weight for gestational age. *Am J Obstet Gynecol* 162: 229–237.

Blair E & Stanley F J (1992) Intrauterine growth and spastic cerebral palsy II. The association with morphology at birth. *Early Hum Dev* 28: 91–103.

✪ Blair E & Stanley F J (1993a) When can cerebral palsy be prevented? The generation of causal hypotheses by multivariate analysis of a case-control study. *Paediatr Perinatal Epidemiol* 7: 272–301.

Blair E & Stanley F J (1993b) Aetiological pathways to spastic cerebral palsy. *Paediatr Perinatal Epidemiol* 7: 302–317.

Carr L J (1996) Development and reorganization of descending motor pathways in children with hemiplegic cerebral palsy. *Acta Paediatrica* 85 (suppl 416): 53–57.

Coorssen E A, Msall M E & Duffy L C (1991) Multiple minor malformations as a marker for prenatal etiology of cerebral palsy. *Dev Med Child Neurol* 33: 730–736.

Crichton J U, Mackinnon M & White C P (1995) The life-expectancy of persons with cerebral palsy. *Dev Med Child Neurol* 37: 567–576.

Dammann O & Leviton A (1997) Maternal intrauterine infection, cytokines, and brain damage in the preterm newborn. *Pediatr Res* 42: 1–8.

Dolk H, Parkes K & Hill A E (1996) Cerebral palsy prevalence in relation to socio-economic deprivation in Northern Ireland. *Paediatr Perinatal Epidemiol* 10: A4.

Dowding V M & Barry C (1990) Cerebral palsy: social class differences in prevalence in relation to birthweight and severity of disability. *J Epidemiol Community Health* 44: 191–195.

Evans P M, Evans S J W & Alberman E (1990) Cerebral palsy: why we must plan for survival. *Arch Dis Childhood* 65: 132–133.

Fletcher N A & Foley J (1993) Parental age, genetic mutation, and cerebral palsy. *J Med Genet* 30: 44–46.

Freud S (1968) *Infantile cerebral paralysis* (translation by Russin L A of: *Die Infantile cerebrallahmung.* Wein: A. Holder, 1897). Coral Gables, FL: University of Miami Press.

Gaffney G, Sellers S, Flavell V *et al.* (1994) Case-control study of intrapartum care, cerebral palsy, and perinatal death. *BMJ* 308: 743–750.

Gilbert G L (1996) Congenital fetal infections. *Sem Neonatol* 1: 91–105.

Gilles M T, Blair E, Watson L *et al.* (1996) Maternal trauma in pregnancy and cerebral palsy – Is there a link? *Med J Austral* 164: 500–501.

Grether J, Nelson K, Dambrosia J *et al.* (1999) Interferons and cerebral palsy. *J Pediatr* 134: 324–332.

Grether J K & Nelson K B (1997) Maternal infection and cerebral palsy in infants of normal birth weight. *JAMA* 278: 207–211.

Grether J K, Nelson K B & Cummins S K (1993) Twinning and cerebral palsy: Experience in four northern California counties, births 1983 through 1985. *Pediatrics* 92: 854–858.

Gustavson K-H, Hagberg B & Sanner G (1969) Identical syndromes of cerebral palsy in the same family. *Acta Pædiatrica Scand* 58: 330–340.

Hagberg B, Hagberg G & Olow I (1993) The changing panorama of cerebral palsy in Sweden VI. Prevalence and origin during the birth year period 1983–1986. *Acta Paediatr* 82: 387–393.

Hagberg B, Hagberg G, Olow I *et al.* (1989) The changing panorama of cerebral palsy in Sweden. V. The birth year period of 1979–82. *Acta Pœdiatr Scand* 78: 283–290.

Hagberg B, Hagberg G, Olow I *et al.* (1996) The changing panorama of cerebral palsy in Sweden. VII. Prevalence and origin in the birth year period 1987–90. *Acta Paediatr* 85: 954–960.

Hetzel B S (1994) Iodine deficiency and fetal brain damage. *N Engl J Med* 331: 1770–1771.

Hughes I & Newton R (1992) Genetic aspects of cerebral palsy. *Dev Med Child Neurol* 34: 80–86.

Hutton J L, Cooke T & Pharoah P O D (1994) Life expectancy in children with cerebral palsy. *BMJ* 309: 431–435.

Jarvis S & Hey E (1984) Measuring disability and handicap due to cerebral palsy. In: Stanley F & Alberman E (eds) *The epidemiology of the cerebral palsies.* Oxford: Blackwell Scientific Publications, pp. 35–45.

Kingdom J, Baker P & Blair E (in press) Definitions of intrauterine growth restriction. In: Kingdom J & Baker P (eds) *Intrauterine growth restriction.* London: Springer-Verlag.

Kyllerman M, Bager B, Bensch J *et al.* (1982) Dyskinetic cerebral palsy I. Clinical categories, associated neurological abnormalities and incidences. *Acta Pœdiatrica Scandinavica* 71: 543–550.

Leviton A (1993) Preterm birth and cerebral palsy: Is tumor necrosis factor the missing link? *Dev Med Child Neurol* 35: 553–558.

Little W J (1958) On the influence of abnormal parturition, difficult labours, premature birth, and asphyxia neonatorum, on the mental and physical condition of the child, especially in relation to deformities. *Cerebral Palsy Bull* 1: 5–36.

MacKeith R C & Polani P E (1958) Cerebral palsy (letter). *Lancet* 1: 61.

Miller G (1991) Cerebral palsy and minor congenital anomalies. *Clin Pediat* 30: 97–98.

Morton D H, Bennett M J, Seargeant L E *et al.* (1991) Glutaric aciduria type I: common cause of episodic encephalopathy and spastic paralysis in the Amish of Lancaster County, Pennsylvania. *Am J Med Genet* 41: 89–95.

Murphy D J, Sellers S, MacKenzie I Z *et al.* (1995) Case-control study of antenatal and intrapartum risk factors for cerebral palsy in very preterm singleton babies. *Lancet* 346: 1449–1454.

Mutch L W, Alberman E, Hagberg B *et al.* (1992) Cerebral palsy epidemiology: Where are we now and where are we going? *Dev Med Child Neurol* 34: 547–555.

Nelson K B & Ellenberg J H (1982) Maternal seizure disorder, outcome of pregnancy, and neurologic abnormalities in the children. *Neurology* 32: 1247–1254.

Nelson K B & Ellenberg J H (1986) Antecedents of cerebral palsy. Multivariate analysis of risk. *N Engl J Med* 315: 81–86.

Niswander K R (1985) Quality of obstetric care and occurrence of fetal asphyxia and cerebral palsy: Is there a relationship? *Postgrad Med* 78: 57–64.

Olegård R, Sabel K-G, Aronsson M *et al.* (1979) Effects on the child of alcohol abuse during pregnancy: retrospective and prospective studies. *Acta Pædiatrica Scand* (suppl 275): 112–121.

Palisano R, Rosenbaum P, Walter S *et al.* (1997) Development and reliability of a system to classify gross motor function in children with cerebral palsy. *Dev Med Child Neurol* 39: 214–223.

Palmer L, Blair E, Petterson B *et al.* (1995) Antenatal antecedents of moderate and severe cerebral palsy. *Paediatr Perinatal Epidemiol* 9: 171–184.

Palmer L, Petterson B, Blair E *et al.* (1994) Family patterns of gestational age at delivery and growth in utero in moderate and severe cerebral palsy. *Dev Med Child Neurol* 36: 1108–1119.

✪ Perinatal Society of Australia and New Zealand (PSANZ) (1999) A template for defining a causal relationship between acute intrapartum events and cerebral palsy: a consensus statement. *BMJ* 319:1054–1059.

Petterson B, Nelson K B, Watson L *et al.* (1993) Twins, triplets, and cerebral palsy at birth in Western Australia in the 1980s. *BMJ* 307: 1239–1243.

Richmond S, Niswander K, Snodgrass C A *et al.* (1994) The obstetric management of fetal distress and its association with cerebral palsy. *Obstet Gynecol* 83: 643–646.

Russell D J, Rosenbaum P L, Cadman D T *et al.* (1989) The gross motor function measure: a means to evaluate the effects of physical therapy. *Dev Med Child Neurol* 31: 341–352.

Society of Obstetricians and Gynaecologists of Canada (1996) Policy statement: Task Force on Cerebral Palsy and Neonatal Asphyxia (Part I). *J Soc Obstet Gynaecol Canada* 18: 1267–1279.

✪ Stanley F J, Alberman E & Blair E (2000) The cerebral palsies: epidemiology and causal pathways. *Clinics in Developmental Medicine* 151. Oxford: MacKeith Press.

Stanley F J, Sim M, Wilson G *et al.* (1986) The decline in congenital rubella syndrome in Western Australia: an impact of the school girl vaccination program? *Am J Pub Health* 76: 35–39.

Takeuchi T & Matsumoto H (1969) Minamata disease of human fetuses. In: Mishimura H & Miller J R (eds) *Methods for teratological studies in experimental animals and man.* Tokyo: Igatsu Shoin, pp. 280–282.

Topp M, Langhoff-Roos J, Uldall P *et al.* (1996) Intrauterine growth and gestational age in preterm infants with cerebral palsy. *Early Hum Dev* 44: 27–36.

Uvebrant P & Hagberg G (1992) Intrauterine growth in children with cerebral palsy. *Acta Pædiatrica* 81: 407–412.

# Chapter 48

# Epidemiology of mental retardation

M. S. Durkin, N. Schupf, Z. A. Stein and M. W. Susser

## INTRODUCTION

Cognitive disability arising early in life, or mental retardation, is among the most common of disabilities observed in childhood, with prevalence rates greater than 2% in most populations (Kiely 1987; Murphy *et al.* 1995). Advances in genetics and medical technology have not resulted in lower overall prevalence rates, as their effects are often offset by simultaneous gains in survival of individuals with neurodevelopmental disorders. Down's syndrome is an example of a disorder for which, in technologically advanced societies, prevalence rates at birth have declined or remained constant at the same time that survival of children with Down's syndrome has increased steadily (Fryers 1984; Dupont *et al.* 1986; Baird & Sadovnick 1987; McGrother & Marshall 1990; Staples *et al.* 1991, Krivchenia *et al.* 1993; Mutton *et al.* 1993) (Fig. 48.1). The net effect has been a rise over the past half century in the prevalence of Down's syndrome in adolescents and adults. Nicholson & Alberman (1992) predict that, even with improved screening and assuming an increased use of selective abortion to prevent Down's syndrome births, prevalence rates will be higher during the 21st century than ever before. This trend will continue to bring increased demands for medical care and support services.

Valid generalizations regarding the frequency and causes of mental retardation in populations are difficult to ascertain for several reasons. Most studies are cross-sectional and use service records or registries to ascertain prevalent (surviving) cases. The feasibility, completeness and accuracy of this approach vary greatly over time and between populations, limiting opportunities for comparison and generalization. For the purpose of investigating etiology, an epidemiologic study would ideally include all incident (newly occurring) cases in a population, allowing causes to be distinguished from factors associated with survival. Studies of the true incidence of mental retardation, however, are not achievable because only a minority of cases survive long enough to be identified and because the onset and recognition of disability are often insidious as development unfolds (Hook 1982b; Stein & Susser 1984). Additional problems of case identification arise from reliance on standardized tests of intelligence and behavior to diagnose mental retardation in people of diverse cultural and socio-economic backgrounds; the cross-cultural appropriateness of these tests and potential for over-identification of cases in the lower social classes are ongoing controversies (Mercer 1992, Suzuki & Valencia 1997).

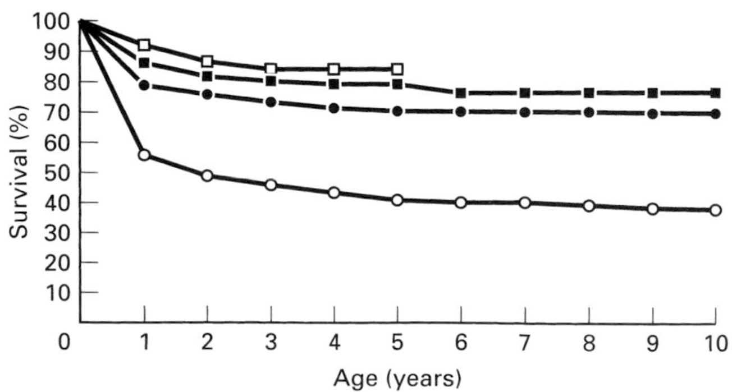


Figure 48.1 Survival rates for the first decade of life in Down's syndrome cohorts studied between 1940 and 1960 (○), and 1960 and 1980 (birth cohorts 1950–1970) (●), and in Leicestershire 1976–1985 (■) with subset 1981–1985 (□). (Redrawn, with permission from Blackwell Science Ltd, from McGrother & Marshall 1990).

Another challenge to epidemiology is the heterogeneity of specific causes and types of mental retardation. By lumping these into a single category of mental retardation, defined in terms of functional deficit, epidemiologic studies dilute the chances of finding consistent patterns and risk factors associated with a single cause. Given current knowledge, such lumping is unavoidable; in any population, most cases of mental retardation are still of unknown etiology (Yeargin-Allsopp *et al.* 1997). A related challenge to epidemiology is the rareness of each specific known cause. The most common known genetic causes of mental retardation, for example, Down's syndrome and fragile X syndrome, have crude prevalence rates at birth of about 1/800–1000 births and 1/4000 males, respectively, and account for a small proportion of all cases of mental retardation. The majority of specific causes occur much less frequently and are, consequently, difficult to study on a population basis. Table 48.1 lists the known causal categories of mental retardation along with several specific causes and estimates of their frequencies.

In spite of conceptual and methodologic difficulties, epidemiologic studies have made important contributions to our understanding of the frequency, causes, and prevention of mental retardation. This chapter summarizes selected contributions to each of these areas. We have chosen to focus on major types of mental retardation for which the etiology is fairly well understood.

**Table 48.1 Causal categories of mental retardation with examples of syndromes and estimated frequencies with each category**

| Category | Syndromes/diseases | Estimated frequency | Comments (mental retardation occurs in virtually all cases unless otherwise specified) |
|---|---|---|---|
| 1. Genetic | | | |
| *A. Chromosomal causes (autosomal) (chromosome number)* | | | |
| i. Trisomy | | | |
| (21) | Downs syndrome (common type) | 1/650–1000 live births | Risk increases with maternal age; thus, frequency depends on maternal age structure of the population |
| (18) | Edward's syndrome | 1/5000 births | Survival past infancy rare |
| (13) | Patau's syndrome | 1/10 000 births | Survival past infancy rare |
| ii. Deletion | | | |
| (5) | 'Cri du chat' syndrome | 1/20 000–50 000 births | |
| (7) | Williams syndrome | 1/10 000 births | |
| (15, paternal origin) | Prader–Willi syndrome | 1/16 000–25 000 births | Most have mild mental retardation or low normal intelligence quotient |
| (15, maternal origin) | Angelman's syndrome | | Rarer than Prader–Willi syndrome, population frequency estimate not available |
| (17) | Miller–Dieker syndrome (lissencephaly) | | Population estimates not available, very rare |
| iii. Transiocation | | | |
| (21) | Down syndrome (rare form) | 1/25 000 births | Not associated with maternal age; de-novo and inherited types occur |
| iv. Ring | | | |
| (5) | 'Cri du chat' syndrome | | Population estimates not available, extremely rare |
| *B. X-linked* | | | |
| i. Chromosomal, numeric | | | |
| Trisomy, 47XXY | Klinefelter's syndrome | 1/500 males | Mental retardation occurs in a minority of cases |
| Monosomy, 45XO | Turner's syndrome | 1/10 000 births | Mental retardation occurs in about 10% of cases |
| ii. Single gene | | | |
| | Fragile X syndrome | 1/4000–6045 males | About 80% of male and 30–50% of female carriers of the mutation have some degree of mental retardation |
| | Menkes's syndrome | 1/40 000 births (Melbourne); 1/298 000 births (several European countries) | |
| | Duchenne's muscular dystrophy | | Mental retardation occurs in approximately 30% of cases; survival into adulthood is rare |
| | Rett's syndrome | 1/10 000–15 000 girls | Phenotype occurs only in females, X-linked mutation lethal in males |

| | | | |
|---|---|---|---|
| *C. Single gene, autosomal* (*Chromosome number if mapped*) | | | |
| i. Dominant | | | |
| (9, 11, 12) | Tuberous sclerosis | 1/15 400 children <5 years (Oxford, UK), 1/12 000 children < 10 years (Scotland) | Mental retardation occurs in approximately 50% of cases |
| ii. Recessive | | | |
| (12) | Phenylketonuria (PKU) | 1/10 000–15 000 births | Mental retardation is usually prevented in populations with neonatal screening for PKU |
| (15) | Tay–Sachs disease | Ashkenazi Jews are at high risk | Fatal during childhood |
| (4) | Hurler's syndrome (mucopolysaccharidosis) | 1/144 274 births (British Columbia) | |
| II. Nutritional | | | |
| *A. Prenatal* | | | |
| Maternal iodine deficiency | Cretinism and less severe mental deficiency from iodine deficiency disorder | Estimated world-wide crude, prevalence is 20 million (1/300, all ages) | Affects up to 10% in iodine-deficient populations, may be the leading cause of preventable mental retardation world-wide |
| Maternal hyperphenylalaninemia | | | A rare and emerging cause of mental retardation; observed in offspring of women with PKU detected at birth and successfully treated, but with hyperphenylalaninemia at the time of conception and early pregnancy |
| III. Infectious | | | |
| *A. Prenatal* | | | |
| Intrauterine | Toxoplasmosis<br>Syphilis<br>Rubella<br>Cytomegalovirus<br>Herpes<br>HIV | | Frequency varies with timing and extent of infection and other factors |
| *B. Perinatal* | Syphilis<br>HIV | | |
| *C. Postnatal* | Meningitis<br>Encephalitis<br>Immunization-associated encephalopathy | | |
| IV. Environmental exposures | | | |
| *A. Prenatal* | Ionizing radiation | Sporadic occurrence | Restricted to offspring exposed between 9th and 15th weeks of pregnancy |
| Alcohol | Fetal alcohol syndrome | 1/6000 live births (US military); 1/600 live births (Gothenburg, Sweden) | |
| *B. Postnatal* | Lead poisoning | 17% of US children age 6 months to 5 years have blood levels > 15 μg/dl | Exposure varies with level of industrialization and presence of legal restrictions; negative association between blood lead levels and intellectual performance |

**Table 48.1 Continued**

| Category | Syndromes/diseases | Estimated frequency | Comments (mental retardation occurs in virtually all cases unless otherwise specified) |
|---|---|---|---|
| V. Multifactorial and other | | | |
| Interaction of genetic susceptibility and maternal folic acid intake first trimester of pregnancy | Spina bifida | 1/200 births (Dublin), 1/350 births (Sikhs in British Columbia), 1/750 (non-Sikhs, British Columbia), 1/10 000 births (Bogota) | Mental retardation occurs in about one-third of cases; large geographic/ethnic variation in frequency |
| Perinatal events | Low birthweight<br>Asphyxia | | Increased risk of mental retardation in children with cerebral palsy associated with perinatal events, underlying cause may be prenatal |
| Postnatal trauma | Closed head injury | Annual incidence 1/435 children <15 years, 1/17 adolescent boys (USA) | Neuropsychologic sequelae may occur in 10% of cases, risk of mental retardation *per se* not known |
| Neoplasm | Brain tumor | | Cognitive disability likely after radiotherapy |
| VI. Unknown cause | | | |
| | 'Cultural–familial' (mild mental retardation of unknown etiology, no coexisting neurologic or physical abnormalities) | 1/25–50 children of school age | Virtually restricted to children from economically disadvantaged households; residual category after excluding known causes |
| | Congenital hypothyroidism | 1/3500 births | Mental retardation is prevented in populations with neonatal screening for hypothyroidism |

*References*: Amir *et al.* (1999), Annegers *et al.* (1980), Burd *et al.* (1991), Bushby *et al.* (1991), Butler *et al.* (1986), Davies *et al.* (1988), Durkin *et al.* (1998c), Frankowski *et al.* (1985), Fryer *et al.* (1987), Greenberg *et al.* (1986), Hagberg (1985, 1987, 1989), Hagerman & Silverman (1991), Hetzel (1989), Hoffman *et al.* (1987), Hunt & Lindenbaum (1984), Kiely (1987), Kline *et al.* (1989), Lowry *et al.* (1990), McKusick (1998), Mattei *et al.* (1984), Miller & Ramer (1992), Pembrey *et al.* (1989), Sherman *et al.* (1991), Tangsrud & Halvorsen (1989), Tonnesen *et al.* (1991), Turner *et al.* (1986), van Essen *et al.* (1992), Waisbren *et al.* (1988), Weitzman *et al.* (1993).

## DEFINITION AND CLASSIFICATION

The distinctions between the physical dimension of impairment, the functional dimension of disability, and the social dimension of handicap (Susser & Watson 1971; World Health Organization 1980) are fundamental to defining mental retardation. Impairment is the organic abnormality of the brain or neurologic processes that is the known or presumed basis of cognitive disability. Disability, in mental retardation, refers to limitations of intellectual function and adaptive skills; these are by definition present in all cases and measurable by psychometric instruments such as intelligence quotient (IQ) tests and adaptive scales. Handicap refers to limitations of social role and opportunity imposed on people with special needs by societal and other environmental conditions.

The dominant approach to defining and classifying mental retardation is by severity of disability rather than by cause. Mental retardation is defined as a significant deficit in intelligence and adaptive skills with onset during or prior to childhood (Grossman 1983; Luckasson *et al.* 1992; American Psychiatric Association 1994). Adaptive skills include those needed for communication, self-care, home living, social interaction, academic study, leisure, work, and other domains. The tenth revision of the *International Classification of Diseases* (World Health Organization 1992) as well as the *Diagnostic and Statistical Manual* (Fourth Edition) of the American Psychiatric Association (American Psychiatric Association 1994) and former versions of the American Association on Mental Retardation (formerly the American Association on Mental Deficiency) classification (Grossman 1983) distinguish four grades of severity defined in terms of IQ (Table 48.2). The most recent version of the American Association on Mental Retardation's classification system acknowledges an IQ of 70 or 75 (approximately 2 standard deviations below the mean IQ) as an upper bound for mental retardation, but has moved away from distinguishing grades of intellectual deficit towards defining severity in terms of the level of support required for optimal functioning. Four levels of support are distinguished: (1) intermittent; (2) limited; (3) extensive; and (4) pervasive (Luckasson *et al.* 1992). These revised categories have not generally been used in epidemiologic studies. Until now, epidemiologic studies have tended to collapse moderate, severe, and profound grades of intellectual disability into a single category of severe mental retardation (IQ below 50 or 55) and distinguished this from mild mental retardation (IQ between 50 or 55 and 70).

Classification is increasingly based on etiology, as advances in cytogenetics, molecular genetics, and brain imaging improve our ability to identify specific causes of mental retardation. Etiological classifications have clear advantages for epidemiologic research and for primary prevention; they may also be useful for assessing specific needs for medical care, rehabilitation, and other services (Zigler *et al.* 1984; Durkin & Stein 1996).

**Table 48.2 Classification of mental retardation by severity based on IQ [*International Classification of Diseases, tenth revision* (ICD-10) (World Health Organization 1992)]**

| Severity | ICD-10 code | Approximate IQ range[a] |
|---|---|---|
| Mild | F70 | 50–69 |
| Moderate | F71 | 35–49 |
| Severe | F72 | 20–34 |
| Profound | F73 | <20 |

[a]Precise IQ cut-off points may vary to allow for differences between tests. Guidelines of the American Association of Mental Deficiency (Grossman 1983) and the DSM-IV of the American Psychiatric Association (1994) recommend the use of these or similar cut-off points as well as clinical judgement and assessment of adaptive skills in the diagnosis and classification of the severity of mental retardation.

## PREVALENCE

Severe and mild mental retardation are distinctive in terms of their frequency and distribution in populations. Table 48.3 contrasts the major epidemiologic characteristics of each form. In developed countries, the prevalence of severe mental retardation in childhood is consistently found to range from three to five per 1000 (see Table 48.2), and more than 50% of cases are attributed to genetic causes. Mild mental retardation in developed countries varies widely in prevalence, until recently, has been much more frequent than severe forms, and is rarely attributed to single major genes or other known causes. Prevalence estimates from Sweden are lower than in other populations, particularly for mild mental retardation, which is similar in frequency there to severe mental retardation (Hagberg *et al.* 1981).

The few estimates available from less developed countries, Bangladesh (Zaman *et al.* 1992), Jamaica (Thorburn *et al.* 1992), and Pakistan (Durkin *et al.* 1998a), point to elevated prevalence rates of severe mental retardation, possibly due to the higher frequency in those settings of nutritional, traumatic, and infectious causes of brain damage (Stein *et al.* 1986). The extent to which excess incidence in these populations is offset by increased vulnerability of disabled children to early death has not been studied. The excess of severe mental retardation observed in some south Asian populations (Table 48.4) may be related to a high prevalence of consanguineous marriage resulting in increased homozygosity for deleterious mutations. Consanguinity has been linked to elevated rates of perinatal mortality and disabling childhood conditions in a number of populations (Devi *et al.* 1987; Bittles *et al.* 1991; Bundy & Alam 1993).

In addition to prevalence rates and known etiology, severe mental retardation differs from mild in terms of average life expectancy, frequency of co-morbidity (particularly the occurrence of other neurodevelopmental disorders) and the

**Table 48.3 Epidemiologic characteristics of severe and mild mental retardation**

| | Severe mental retardation | Mild mental retardation |
|---|---|---|
| Prevalence range in childhood (per 1000) | | |
| Populations with advanced medical care | 2.5–5.0 | 2.5–40.0 |
| Less-developed countries | 5.0–25.0 | Few estimates available, 54–78 in Karachi |
| Life expectancy | Less than general population; strong negative association with presence of congenital heart disease and with severity of mental retardation and restricted mobility | Somewhat shorter than general population |
| Percentage with other neurodevelopmental, or sensory disorders | About 85% | About 30% |
| Percentage with other psychiatric disorders | Higher frequency than general population | Higher frequency than general population |
| Percentage with known genetic cause | About 50% | Small |
| Percentage with unknown cause | Minority | Majority |
| Usual age at recognition | Infancy or preschool years | School age |
| Duration | Life long | May be restricted to school age |
| Male:female ratio | Male excess (1.1–1.4:1) | Male excess (1.1–1.8:1) |
| Major demographic risk factors | Maternal age is a strong predictor of trisomies, which cause about 30% of severe mental retardation | Low socio-economic status |
| Association with social class | Prevalence is relatively even across the social classes | Occurs predominantly in children of low social class |

*References*: Alberman (1978), Durkin *et al.* (1998a,c), Eyman *et al.* (1990), Kaveggia *et al.* (1975), Kiely (1987).

**Table 48.4 Severe mental retardation in childhood: selected estimates of prevalence**

| Location | Reference | Data source | Age (years) | Prevalence/1000 |
|---|---|---|---|---|
| England | Lewis (1929) | Agency records, informants | 10–14 | 4.35 |
| Aberdeen, Scotland | Birch *et al.* (1970) | Follow-up of births | 8–10 | 3.7 |
| Isle of Wight, England | Rutter *et al.* (1970) | Population screening, evaluations | 5–14 | 3.0 |
| Quebec, Canada | McDonald (1973) | Agency records | 10 | 3.84 |
| The Netherlands | Stein *et al.* (1976b) | Birth cohort, military records | 19 | 3.73 |
| UK | Peckham & Pearson (1976) | Birth cohort, examinations, interviews | 7 | 2.4 |
| | | | 11 | 3.3 |
| | | | 16 | 3.4 |
| Uppsala County, Sweden | Gustavson *et al.* (1977a) | Registry, agency, vital, records | 11–16 | 2.88 |
| Salford, England | Fryers & Mackay (1979) | Agency records | 5–15 | 4.5 |
| Karnataka, India | Narayanan (1981) | Household survey, evaluations | 5–9 | 12.4 |
| Karachi, Pakistan | Hasan & Hasan (1981) | Household survey, evaluations | 11–15 | 24.3 |
| Kuruma City, Japan | Shiotsuki *et al.* (1984) | | 7–12 | 4.90 |
| Beijing, China | Zuo *et al.* (1986) | Household survey, evaluations | 0–14 | 2.94 |
| New Brunswick, Nova Scotia (Canada) | McQueen *et al.* (1987) | Agency records | 7–10 | 4.61 |
| | | | | 2.82 |
| North-west Spain | Diaz-Fernandez (1988) | Registry | 5–9 | 2.71 |
| | | | 10–14 | 4.08 |
| May Pen, Jamaica | Thorburn *et al.* (1992) | Household survey, evaluations | 2–9 | 17.0 |
| Bangladesh | Zaman *et al.* (1992) | Household survey, evaluations | 2–9 | 5.28 |
| Atlanta, USA | Murphy *et al.* (1995) | School and other record review | 10 | 3.60 |
| Karachi, Pakistan | Durkin *et al.* (1998a) | Household survey, evaluations | 2–9 | 19.00 |

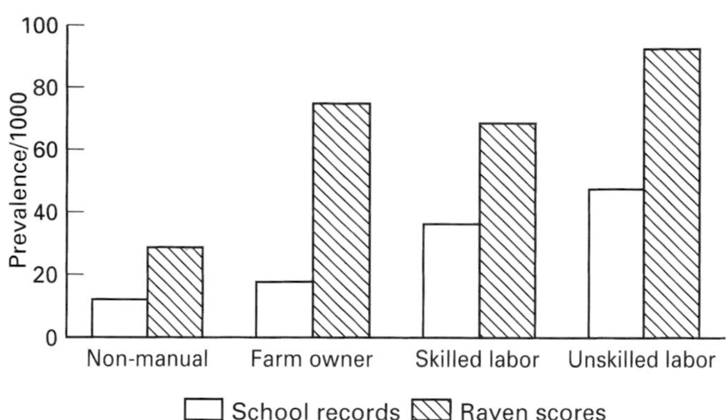


Figure 48.2 Socio-economic status and the prevalence of mild mental retardation. (From data presented in Stein *et al.* 1976a).

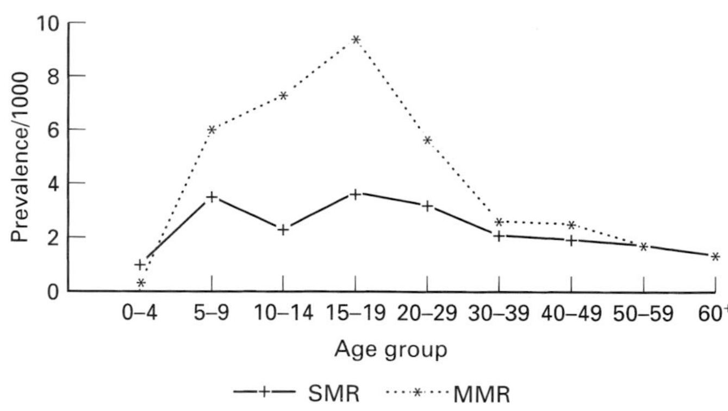


Figure 48.3 Mean age-specific prevalence of severe and mild mental retardation. (From data presented in Kiely 1987).

impact of socio-economic status (see Table 48.3). Low socio-economic status is the strongest and most consistent predictor of mild mental retardation (Fig. 48.2) but has little or no association with the prevalence of severe mental retardation (see Table 48.3) (Stein *et al.* 1976a,b). This pattern points to the role of poverty and social disadvantage in the etiology of mild mental retardation. Evidence is accumulating that preschool programs providing social and intellectual stimulation can boost IQ, improve educational outcomes, and reduce the risk of mild mental retardation in vulnerable groups (Stein & Susser 1970; McKay *et al.* 1978; Garber 1988; Ramey & Ramey 1998).

A male excess is observed in both severe and mild mental retardation, due in part to the contribution of X-linked forms of mental retardation (discussed below) and possibly to a gender bias favoring increased detection of cognitive disabilities in boys (Richardson *et al.* 1986). Several cross-sectional studies of age-specific prevalence rates conducted in different decades and populations are consistent in showing, for both severe and mild mental retardation, increasing prevalence rates with age during childhood followed by declining rates with advancing age throughout adulthood (Kiely 1987) (Fig. 48.3). The tendency for mild mental retardation to be first identified when children enter school is evident in Fig. 48.3. Severe mental retardation is much more likely than mild to be diagnosed during infancy. The increasing prevalence with age during childhood could be due to increases with age in the use of speciality services and in the probability of being included in agency records as well as the likelihood of exposure to postnatal risk factors (infections, trauma). For severe mental retardation, excess mortality is responsible for the decline in prevalence with age after childhood. For mild mental retardation, a likely explanation for the decline in prevalence during adulthood is that societies do not universally require of adults the cognitive skills that they require of schoolchildren. A degree of recovery is also probable. Thus, many persons categorized as mildly retarded in school do not carry this label into adulthood (Durkin *et al.* 1998c).

## SELECTED SPECIFIC CAUSES

### GENETIC CAUSES

Recent advances in molecular genetics have led to the identification of a number of abnormalities, of chromosomes or single genes, which are associated with mental retardation. These include trisomies resulting from non-disjunction of chromosomes during meiosis, and expanding repeat disorders involving repetitive DNA sequences, which show a length variation in normal and affected individuals. In expanding repeat disorders, the length of the repeat in genomic DNA is correlated with risk for disorder. Another class of genetic disorders has been termed segmental autosomy syndromes. Segmental autosomy syndromes result from abnormalities in gene dosage caused by structural defects (deletion, duplication) or functional imbalance (imprinting defects, uniparental disomy) of critical genes (Budarf & Emanuel 1997). Imprinting is the differential expression of genetic material, either at a chromosomal or at an alleleic level, depending on whether the genetic material was inherited from the mother or father. These differences in expression that depend on the sex of the transmitting parent are associated with differences in DNA methylation patterns that, in turn, regulate gene transcription. Imprinting defects lead to loss of expression in the normally expressed parental gene. Uniparental disomy is defined as the presence of two chromosomes of a pair, both inherited from one parent. Thus, in both imprinting and uniparental disomy, there is a functional loss of expression of genes inherited from one parent. Below, we provide examples of each of these processes.

#### Chromosomal anomalies

Chromosomal anomalies are a major cause of severe mental retardation. These anomalies may be structural or numerical. Structural changes result from the breakage and rearrangement of chromosome parts and can be induced, in animal experiments, by a variety of exposures, including ionizing

**Table 48.5 Estimates of the frequency of selected chromosomal aberrations among miscarriages, stillbirths, and live births**

| Aberration | Rates per 1000 | | | Distribution among outcomes (%) | | |
|---|---|---|---|---|---|---|
| | Miscarriage (*n*=3353) | Stillbirth (*n*=452) | Live birth (*n*=31 521) | Miscarriage | Stillbirth | Live birth |
| Autosomal trisomies | | | | | | |
| 13 | 11.0 | 2.2 | 0.1 | 93 | 2 | 5 |
| 16 | 55.8 | 0.0 | 0.0 | 100 | 0 | 0 |
| 18 | 8.4 | 13.3 | 0.2 | 78 | 12 | 0 |
| 21 | 20.0 | 8.8 | 1.1 | 71 | 3 | 26 |
| Other | 118.1 | 13.3 | 0.0 | 99 | 1 | 0 |
| Trisomies of sex chromosomes | 3.3 | 4.4 | 1.5 | 24 | 3 | 73 |
| Monosomy X | 83.5 | 0.0 | 0.1 | 99 | 0 | <1 |
| Triploidy | 57.9 | 4.4 | 0.0 | 99 | 1 | 0 |
| Tetraploidy | 23.9 | 0.0 | 0.0 | 100 | 0 | 0 |
| Total aberrant | 415.2 | 57.5 | 6.0 | 90 | 1 | 9 |

*Source*: From Kline *et al.* (1989).

radiation, certain viral infections, and toxic substances. They occur as duplications, deletions, translocations, insertions, or inversions of chromosome parts or as rings on selected chromosomes. Numerical anomalies arise through non-disjunction during meiosis or mitosis, or through lagging of chromosomes at anaphase of cell division. Among several types of abnormalities of chromosome number that occur, only trisomies play a major role in the etiology of mental retardation.

Chromosomal anomalies as a whole contribute more to fetal loss than to live births and mental retardation. Table 48.5 provides estimates of the frequency of selected chromosomal aberrations among miscarriages, stillbirths and live births. About 40% of miscarriages are chromosomally aberrant; the frequency is about 6% in stillbirths and less than 1% in live births (Kline *et al.* 1989). Kline *et al.* (1989) estimate that from 8 weeks after the last menstrual period, the proportion of chromosomal aberrations lost by miscarriage exceeds 90% for all but trisomy 21 (Downs syndrome), XXX, XXY (Klinefelter's syndrome) and XYY. In survivors after birth in developed countries, chromosomal anomalies cause more than 30% of the cases of severe mental retardation, with the majority of these having Down's syndrome (Gustavson *et al.* 1977a,b; Hagberg 1987).

## Down's syndrome

Down's syndrome is the most common genetic cause of mental retardation and the leading known cause of severe mental retardation in developed countries (Nicholson & Alberman 1992). All cases of Down's syndrome result from partial or complete duplication of chromosome 21 in the genome (Epstein 1986). The most common form (95% of cases at birth) is standard trisomy, involving duplication of chromosome 21. In over 90% of these cases, the extra chromosome is of maternal origin, due to non-disjunction during meiosis (Hassold *et al.* 1984; Stewart *et al.* 1988; Sherman *et al.* 1991). Translocation of chromosome 21 material to another chromosome (usually 13 or 18) and mosaicism (co-existence of normal and trisomic cells in variable proportions in affected persons) are rare causes of Down's syndrome (Hook 1982a; Staples *et al.* 1991).

The most striking epidemiologic characteristic of Down syndrome, and in fact all trisomic conceptions, is the marked increase in risk with increasing maternal age, from one per 1550 live births at ages 20–24 years to one per 700 live births at ages 30–34 years to one per 50 live births at ages 41–45 years (Cuckle *et al.* 1987) (Fig. 48.4). Despite this strong association with maternal age, most Down's syndrome births are to women aged under 35 years because younger women contribute the great majority of births. Thus, the crude birth rate of Down's syndrome in a population will depend on the maternal age distribution and the availability and use of prenatal diagnosis followed by selec-

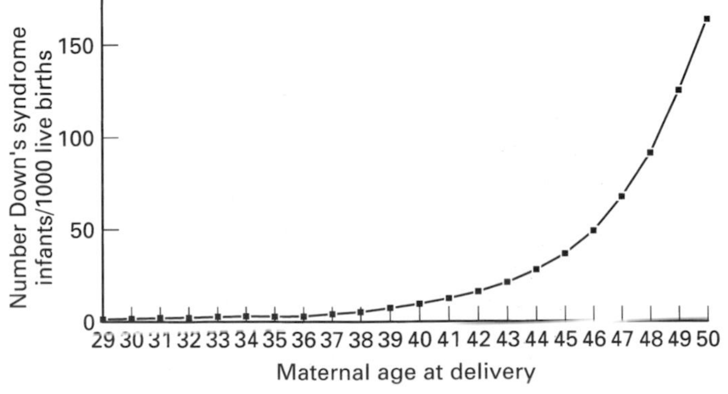


Figure 48.4 Maternal age-specific risk for Down's syndrome births. (From data presented in Cuckle *et al.* 1987).

tive abortion. In developed countries, increased availability of effective birth control in the 1960s was followed by reductions in the number and proportion of births to older women and corresponding reductions in the prevalence of Down's syndrome at birth (Staples *et al.* 1991); however, recent data suggest a rise in the numbers of pregnancies at increased maternal ages in developed countries (Alberman *et al.* 1995; O'Leary *et al.* 1996). The discovery of safe and practical methods of screening for this anomaly during the first trimester of pregnancy is, therefore, an important public-health goal.

Prenatal screening for, and diagnosis of, Down's syndrome using amniocentesis or chorionic-villus sampling alone can detect and potentially prevent no more than 20% of affected births because these procedures are currently offered only to women 35 years and over and at high risk for a Down's syndrome birth (Adams *et al.* 1991). In some developed countries, screening of all pregnant women receiving prenatal care is based on maternal serum screening during the second trimester, using α-fetoprotein, human chorionic gonadotrophin, and unconjugated estriol levels in serum in conjunction with maternal age and ultrasound estimation of gestational age. This procedure may have a sensitivity of up to 70% (Phillips *et al.* 1992; Wald & Kennard 1992). Women screening positive (serum marker levels at or above a criterion risk, e.g. at least one in 250) are then offered a diagnostic test using either amniocentesis or chorionic-villus sampling. Alternatively, screening at 10–14 weeks can be implemented using fetal nuchal translucency and studies of maternal sera (high maternal serum concentrations of the free beta subunit of human chorionic gonadotropin and low serum concentrations of pregnancy-associated plasma protein A). This first trimester screening strategy can have a sensitivity as high as 80% but is not widely used in practice (Haddow *et al.* 1998). In populations where maternal serum screening is universal, screening has resulted in an increase in the proportion of Down's syndrome pregnancies terminated (from 14% to 30–40%) and in observable declines in the birth prevalence of Down's syndrome (Lopez *et al.* 1995; O'Leary *et al.* 1996). While the sensitivity of maternal serum screening is high, specificity is moderate, and the screen is associated with a 5% false positive rate. Of additional concern, the risk of miscarriage during diagnostic testing is approximately 0.9% for amniocentesis and 1.4% for chorionic villus sampling (Wald *et al.* 1997). Wald and colleagues have proposed using an integrated test combining first- and second-trimester markers to increase the sensitivity and reduce the false positive rate of the screen (Wald *et al.* 1999). They estimate that the integrated test can yield an 85% detection rate with a false positive rate of only 0.9%, reducing the need for invasive diagnostic tests by four-fifths. To date, no single screening strategy both optimizes the detection rate of Down's syndrome and minimizes the number of procedure-related miscarriages; hence, selection of a screening policy will require consideration of social, cultural, and individual values as well as effectiveness, equity, and efficiency (Cuckle 1998; Serra-Prat *et al.* 1998).

About one-third of children with Down's syndrome have congenital heart defects, and 2–5% have duodenal obstruction. Other conditions that occur with increased frequency in Down's syndrome are childhood leukemia, recurrent infections, hypothyroidism, and seizure disorders. Virtually all persons with Down's syndrome are cognitively disabled, with the majority functioning in the moderate to profound range of intellectual disability. Observations of children living at home with their families or enrolled in infant stimulation programs suggest that the intellectual potential of children with Down's syndrome may have been underestimated (Centerwall & Centerwall 1960; Melyn & White 1973; Bennett *et al.* 1979; Sharav & Shlomo 1986; Youn & Youn 1991; Connolly *et al.* 1993; Dodd *et al.* 1994). A number of studies suggest that children with Down's syndrome who participated in early stimulation programs exhibit higher scores on tests of intellectual, motor, and adaptive functioning than controls.

Adults with Down's syndrome show a variety of age-related changes in physical and functional capacities suggestive of premature or accelerated aging (Martin 1978), including changes in skin tone, hypogonadism, increased frequency of cataracts, increased frequency of hearing loss, hypothyroidism, seizures, degenerative vascular disease, and Alzheimer's disease (Sare *et al.* 1978; Wisniewski *et al.* 1985; Oliver & Holland 1986; Zigman *et al.* 1996; Schupf *et al.* 1996). The increased life-span of individuals with Down's syndrome and accompanying age-associated morbidity impose heavy demands for medical care and community services as well as sustained support from family members, who are facing new concerns about the need for prolonged care of offspring with Down's syndrome.

### Sex-linked mental retardation

Sex-linked disorders arise from differences between males and females in the expression of genes on the sex chromosomes. Only in males are the genes located on the X chromosome fully expressed. In females, random inactivation in each cell of either the maternal or paternal X chromosome occurs early in embryonic development. Thus, if a female is heterozygous for an X-linked mutant gene, on average, approximately half her cells have the normal and half the abnormal allele as the functional member. This averaging of the effects of the two X chromosomes protects females from certain disorders transmitted on the X chromosome, such as hemophilia. Genes on the X chromosome are associated with a number of neurologic and cognitive disorders, including the Lesh–Nyan syndrome, Duchenne's muscular dystrophy, X-linked hydrocephalus, Menkes' syndrome, and fragile X syndrome. Of these, fragile X syndrome is the most common form of inherited mental retardation.

The search for X-linked genes associated with cognitive deficit began with epidemiologic studies showing a male excess in prevalence of mental retardation, especially among those with mild or moderate mental retardation (Lewis 1929;

Penrose 1938; Drillien *et al.* 1966; Turner & Turner 1974). Together with reported familial mental retardation in which males who were related only through the maternal line were retarded while females were not (Penrose 1938; Renpenning *et al.* 1962; Herbst & Miller 1980; Jacobs *et al.* 1980), these observations led Lehrke (1974) to suggest that X-linked genes were responsible for the increased prevalence of males with mental retardation. The full spectrum of X-linked mental retardation may involve many distinct pathogenic mechanisms. Current work has identified approximately 120 different X-linked learning disorders, although most are rare and have been observed only in studies of single families (Lubs *et al.* 1999). Because many X-linked learning disorders are not associated with additional phenotypic features and can only be identified by genetic mapping, the full extent and diversity of X-linked mental retardation will probably have to await genetic screening of all affected individuals.

### Fragile X syndrome

The fragile X syndrome [fra(X)], is the most common form of inherited mental retardation. In addition to cognitive disability, the phenotype includes macroorchidism, a long face, prominent jaw, large ears, thickening of the nasal bridge, and joint hypermobility. Behavioral abnormalities may include autistic-like features, repetitive speech patterns, social anxiety, perseveration, and gaze aversion (Hagerman 1991; Brown *et al.* 1982; Opitz & Sutherland, 1984; Reiss & Freund 1990). Neuroimaging has demonstrated a small posterior cerbellar vermis, and enlarged hippocampus, caudate nucleus, thalamus, and lateral ventricles, and Reiss and colleagues have shown correlations between these structural abnormalities and IQ (Reiss *et al.* 1991, 1994, 1995).

A fragile site on the X chromosome, fra(X), was first identified in males from families with X-linked mental retardation. In cytogenetic studies, Lubs (1969) described a constriction on the long arm of the X chromosome. Sutherland (1977) showed that the fragile X site could be routinely observed as a gap or break in the X chromosome when culture media deficient in folate or thymidine were used, and the site has since been localized to Xq27.3. The proportion of cells showing the fragile X site in cytogenetic studies is quite variable and may be characteristic of each individual. About 80% of male carriers of the mutation and about 30% of female carriers show some degree of mental retardation (Chudley *et al.* 1983; Sherman *et al.* 1984). An unusual pattern of inheritance emerged from segregation analysis of families affected with fra(X), which followed the intergenerational passage of the gene (Sherman *et al.* 1984, 1985). About 20% of males who carry the genotype are clinically unaffected and do not express the fra(X) site on cytogenetic testing. Mothers of these non-penetrant males are rarely affected. These non-penetrant males transmit the mutation to daughters who, although unaffected themselves, are carriers and will have affected children. Thus, grandsons of male carriers are often mentally retarded, and granddaughters may show some cognitive impairment (Sherman *et al.* 1984, 1985). That the risk of mental retardation of individuals depends upon generation position within the family is known as the Sherman paradox: mothers and daughters of non-penetrant males, both obligate carriers of the gene and phenotypically similar, have differing risks in their offspring. Brothers of non-penetrant males are at low risk (approximately 9%), while grandsons and great grandsons are at high risk (approximately 40–50%).

The molecular basis of the Sherman paradox was elucidated with the isolation of the fra(X) gene, FMR1, in 1991 (Bell *et al.*, 1991; Fu *et al.* 1991; Oberle *et al.* 1991; Kremer *et al.* 1991; Verkerk *et al.* 1991; Vincent *et al.* 1991). Understanding of the inheritance of this condition has changed accordingly and affords a unique opportunity to examine the influence of a genetic factor on development. At the molecular level, the FRAXA site contains an exon of the FMR1 gene responsible for the fragile X mental retardation, a repetitive CGG sequence, which demonstrates length variation in normal and in fra(X) individuals, and a cytidine phosphate guanosine (CpG) island that shows preferential methylation in fra(X) cases (Bell *et al.* 1991; Vincent *et al.* 1991). The length of the CGG repeat in genomic DNA is correlated with risk for the fragile X syndrome (Kremer *et al.* 1991). Normal individuals have CGG repeat lengths of six to 50 repeats, and non-penetrant males and carrier females have a permutation that is seen as a length variation of the CGG repeat in the range 50–200 repeats. Affected individuals, however, show a dramatic amplification of the CGG repeat (from 200 to 1000) and hypermethylation of the repeat and adjacent CpG region, resulting in a shut down of transcription of FMR1 and absence of the FMR1 protein (Bell *et al.* 1991; Oberle *et al.* 1991; Pieretti *et al.* 1991; Sutcliffe *et al.* 1992; Verheij *et al.* 1993). The full mutation, when fully methylated, results in cognitive disability in all males and in 50–70% of affected females (Hagerman *et al.* 1992; Rousseau *et al.* 1994; de Vries *et al.* 1996).

Expansion of the premutation to the full mutation occurs only in female meiotic transmission (Oberle *et al.* 1991; Yu *et al.* 1991; Smits *et al.* 1992): risk for expansion to the full mutation increases with the number of repeats (Fu *et al.* 1991). As amplification of the gene increases, it becomes more unstable, leading to mitotic instability as well as meiotic instability (Fu *et al.* 1991; Oberle *et al.* 1991; Pieretti *et al.* 1991). The mitotic instability of the full repeat causes longer and shorter expansions, resulting in mosaicism with respect to size (premutation together with a full mutation) or with respect to degree of methylation (from 10 to 100% of leukocytes with an unmethylated full mutation). Several cases of intellectually normal males with a high proportion of unmethylated leukocytes have been reported, suggesting that methylation is critical for a lack of transcription of the FMR1 gene and expression of the phenotype (Nolin *et al.* 1994; Hagerman *et al.* 1994a; Rousseau *et al.* 1994; de Vreis *et al.* 1998). In addition, several cases have been found with atypical mutations at the FRAXA site, two involving a deletion and one a point mutation in the FRM1 gene (Gedeon *et al.* 1992; Wohrle *et al.* 1992). Other fragile sites (FRAXE, FRAXD, FRAXF) are found close to the FRAXA site. FRAXE is associated with learning disabilities but is caused by a different expanding trinucleotide repeat (Feldman 1996).

#### Prevalence of the fragile X syndrome

Prevalence studies in defined populations have employed cytogenetic or DNA testing for fra(X) among individuals with mental retardation. Prevalence estimates from these studies have ranged from 0.5 to 4.2% of patients with mental retardation (Jacobs *et al.* 1993; Hagerman *et al.* 1994b; van den Ouweland *et al.* 1994; Meadows *et al.* 1996; Murray *et al.* 1996; Turner *et al.* 1996; de Vries *et al.* 1997). The wide range of these estimates is likely to be due to differences in the distribution of mental retardation causes in the samples studied, as well as variability in the DNA analysis. Within the general population, the prevalence of fra(X) has been estimated to range from 1/4000 to 1/6045 males (Turner *et al.* 1996; de Vries *et al.* 1997; Morton *et al.* 1997). Estimates of the prevalence of the FRAXA premutation carrier frequency among females in the general population have also ranged widely, from 1/248 women to 1/1000 women (Reiss *et al.* 1994; Holden *et al.* 1995; Rousseau *et al.* 1995; Spence *et al.* 1996; Holden *et al.* 1999).

### Autosomal genetic causes

Autosomally inherited disorders are rare, but important, causes of mental retardation (see Table 48.1). Autosomal dominant disorders causing mental retardation include tuberous sclerosis and neurofibromatosis. The more common mode of transmission is through autosomal recessives. A number of metabolic disorders transmitted in this fashion are marked by progressive mental retardation with systemic manifestations.

### Phenylketonuria (see also p. 618)

This rare defect of amino acid metabolism occurs in 1/15 000 Caucasian live births, with somewhat lower rates in other ethnic groups. Phenylketonuria (PKU) results from a mutation at the phenylalanine hydroxylase gene and is inherited in an autosomal recessive manner. Deficient metabolism of phenylalanine causes accumulation, which, untreated at birth or very soon after, leads to hyperphenylalaninemia, progressive damage to the developing brain during the neonatal and postnatal periods, and severe mental retardation in most cases. Neonatal screening permits early dietary intervention to diminish phenylalanine levels. The diet must be continued through puberty to achieve the maximum protective effect. In countries with routine neonatal screening programs and effective follow-up of affected children, the condition is rarely seen nowadays.

A problem resulting from the success of neonatal screening programs for PKU is the occurrence of maternal PKU in women successfully treated in childhood (Levy & Waisbren 1983). Themselves of normal or near-normal intelligence, at childbearing age, they still have high blood levels of phenylalanine and a raised risk of miscarriage. Their surviving offspring are at an increased risk of prenatally acquired mental retardation, microcephaly, congenital heart disease, and low birthweight (Lenke & Levy 1980; Rohr *et al.* 1987; Waisbren *et al.* 1998). Severe mental retardation and microcephaly are observed in 75–90% of children of mothers with classic PKU (defined as blood phenylalanine level > 1200 μmol/l). Less severe cognitive deficit may affect children of mothers with atypical PKU (elevations of blood phenylalanine levels to between 594 and 1194 μmol/l) (Levy & Ghavami 1996). Dietary restrictions during pregnancy to reduce maternal blood phenylalanine levels and prevent phenylalanine metabolite accumulation can improve the outcome in offspring if started prior to conception and maintained throughout pregnancy. In the United States, the Maternal Phenylketonuria Collaborative Study (MPKUCS) recommends that levels of phenylalanine be maintained below 900 μmol/l (Rouse *et al.* 1997). Routine umbilical cord blood screening, while it cannot prevent cases, can detect women with hyperphenylalaninemia and thus prevent recurrence in future pregnancies. From a public-health perspective, the problem is to identify and locate the population of women at risk prior to their first pregnancies. The experience of the New England Maternal PKU Project suggests that the majority of women with classic PKU can be found, but a much lower proportion of those with mild hyperphenylalaninemia are likely to be identified (Waisbren *et al.* 1988). Hanley and colleagues estimate the frequency of undiagnosed maternal phenylketonuria in Canada to be one per 100 000 births (Hanley *et al.* 1999).

### Segmental autosomy syndromes

Segmental autosomy syndromes result from abnormalities in gene dosage caused by structural defects (deletion, duplication) or functional imbalance (imprinting defects, uniparental disomy) of critical genes (Budarf & Emanuel 1997). Recent molecular studies have shown that a number of syndromes involving early onset cognitive disability are within this class of disorders. Three of these are Williams, Prader–Willi, and Angelman syndromes.

### Williams syndrome

Williams syndrome is a multisystem disorder characterized by developmental and language delays, pixie-like facial features, cardiovascular abnormalities, elevated calcium levels, problems in gross motor skills and a distinctive cognitive profile that includes mild mental retardation with relatively good language and face-processing skills. The frequency of Williams syndrome has been estimated to be ~ 1/10 000 live births (Williams *et al.* 1961; Beuren *et al.* 1962). Individuals with WS have an ~ 2 Mb deletion of chromosomal region 7q11.23 (Ewart *et al.* 1993; Perez-Jurado *et al.* 1996). Variability in deletion size may be related to variable phenotypic presentation. The majority of patients with Williams syndrome are hemizygous for 7q11.23, and in > 90% of cases, the deletion includes the locus for the elastin gene (*ELN*), a protein kinase LIM-kinase 1 (*LIMK1*), and a replication factor C subunit (*RFC2*) (Frangiskakis *et al.* 1996; Osborne *et al.* 1996; Peoples *et al.* 1996). Families with 'partial Williams syndrome', involving smaller deletions that include only ELN and LIMK1, show the cognitive and cardiovascular profile but lack other features of WS, suggesting that the loss of at least three genes is required for the full Williams syndrome phenotype (Frangiskakis *et al.* 1996; Budarf & Emanuel 1997). There is no evidence of imprinting in Williams syndrome, but if the gene deletion is of a maternal origin, patients have more severe growth retardation and microcephaly (Perez-Jurado *et al.* 1996).

### Prader–Willi/Angelman syndrome

Prader–Willi syndrome (PWS) and Angelman syndrome (AS) are characteristic of disorders resulting from genomic imprinting in which the phenotypic expression of the disorder depends on the parent from whom the genetic abnormality is inherited. Both syndromes involve structural or functional loss of expression of genes in the chromosome 15q11–q13 region, including deletions, uniparental disomy, and mutations in an imprinting center. Paternally inherited abnormalities result in PWS, while maternally inherited abnormalities result in AS (Ledbetter *et al.* 1981; Knoll *et al.* 1989). PWS is characterized by developmental delay, hypotonia, and feeding problems in infancy followed by excessive and rapid weight gain after 12 months and before age 6, cryptoorchidism, short stature, and mild mental retardation. The frequency of PWS is approximately 1/15 000 live births. In contrast, AS is characterized by developmental delay, severe mental retardation, microcephaly, and hypermotoric behavior with hand-flapping and jerky movements in association with outbursts of laughter, short attention span, hypopigmented skin and eyes, and seizures with onset under 3 years of age.

It appears that different genes are responsible for the two syndromes, all of them imprinted in the germ line, with preferential expression of maternal or paternal genes. The 15q11–q13 region contains four paternally expressed genes whose loss of expression causes PWS. The 15q11–q13 region also contains the gene for E6-AP ubiquitin-protein ligase 3A(UBE3A), which is biallelically expressed in somatic tissue but is imprinted with preferential maternal expression in the brain (Albrecht *et al.* 1997; Matsuura *et al.* 1997; Jiang *et al.* 1998); mutations in UBE3A are found in a small subset of patients with AS. In addition, microdeletions of the 15q11–15q13 region indicate that there is an 'imprinting center' (IC), localized to a 100-kb region close to SNRPN (Sutcliffe *et al.* 1994). Deletions centered around the IC close to SNRPN are associated with imprinting mutations causing PWS, while similar deletions that cluster slightly more centromerically are associated with imprinting mutations causing AS (Mutirangura *et al.* 1993; Saitoh *et al.* 1997). The effects of imprinting are also seen in cases of uniparental disomy (UPD) where maternal UPD represents loss of paternally expressed genes and is associated with PWS, while paternal UPD represents loss of maternally expressed genes and is associated with AS. Seventy per cent of cases in PWS are associated with a 4 Mb deletion in 15Q11–q13, an additional 27% display maternal uniparental disomy, and 1–2% of cases are associated with mutations and deletions in the imprinting center (Sutcliffe *et al.* 1994). As in PSW, 70% of AS cases have maternal deletions in the 15q11–q13 region, 3–5% have paternal uniparental disomy, 7–9% have imprinting mutations, 2–4% have mutations in UBE3A, and in 10–20% of cases, the molecular defect is still unknown (Wagstaff *et al.* 1992; Nicholls 1993).

## NUTRITIONAL CAUSES

### Iodine deficiency

For over a century, it was known in Europe that children stunted in growth, often deaf and of low intelligence were to be found where adults were seen with goiter, typically in high mountainous locations, like Switzerland. A 19th century report documented these relationships in Europe, and iodine lack in the drinking water was eventually found to be the causal factor. Later, somewhat similar associations were discovered in the Himalayas, although in some of these locations, the clinical findings in the children included motor defects, so-called pseudo-cerebral palsy. It is now known that iodine lack occurs in all continents and is associated with other adverse reproductive outcomes as well, including miscarriage, stillbirth, and perinatal mortality (Hetzel 1983). The implications of iodine deficiency are not to be measured by a count of cretins or even of goiters alone; cognitive and motor disabilities occur from prenatal exposure to maternal iodine deficiency less severe than that required to produce goiter. World-wide, iodine deficiency is estimated to affect 20 million people, making it a leading cause of mental retardation (Hetzel 1989). There are also sporadic forms of cretinism, and neonatal hypothyroidism, in which early detection (newborn screening) and thyroid hormone supplementation can prevent ensuing brain damage and mental retardation.

The correction of iodine deficiency in mothers immediately before conception is critical to prevent adverse effects on neurodevelopment and cognition in offspring. The only practical way to implement this from a public-health perspective is through universal dietary supplementation. Salt iodination, as carried out in much of the developed world, is not acceptable everywhere, partly because the salt trade in parts of the world follows a traditional market path that is not easy, or even advantageous, to modify. Iodination of drinking water has been shown to be a safe and cost-effective alternative in some settings (Elnager *et al.* 1997). Despite the availability of solutions, their implementation continues to be problematic, and iodine deficiency is still a prevalent cause of developmental disability in many settings (Bellamy 1998). Elimination of iodine deficiency has been identified as an international priority by the World Health Organization.

### Folate and neural-tube defects

This condition is discussed in detail in Chapter 19 of this book. A wide range of intellectual functions are found among survivors of infants with neural-tube defects; fewer than half have a severe intellectual disability, and many have normal levels of intelligence.

Epidemiologic studies have revealed large geographic differences in the prevalence of neural tube defects and have shown for some time that preconceptional and periconceptional vitamin, and specifically folate, consumption of the mother is associated with a reduced incidence of neural tube defects, an observation with enormous potential for prevention (Wild *et al.* 1986) (see p. 319). We now know that this association is due, at least in part, to a gene–environment interaction. Mutations of the methylenetetra hydrofolate reluctase gene in the absence of a folate-rich diet can result in elevated maternal plasma homocysteine and may contribute to the occurrence of neural tube defects in offspring (Wilcken 1997; van der Put *et al.* 1998). It appears that folate supplementation at a level of 400 µg/day is sufficient to increase the activity of the variant methylenetetra hydrofolate reluctase, correct maternal hyperhomocysteinemia, and, when initiated prior to conception or very early in pregnancy, prevent the occurrence of a substantial portion of neural tube defects (MRC Vitamin Study Group 1991; Czeizel & Dudas 1992).

Prevention currently hinges around how, and no longer about whether, to deliver the necessary supplement of folate. As with iodine supplementation, the folate should be taken at a time that the woman will not usually know she is pregnant. The strategy adopted in the United States is to supplement the whole population at a level of 100 µg/day by adding folic acid to the bread flour. Folates are present in the normal diet, in leafy vegetables, legumes, and citrus fruits, but whether dietary advice alone can result in consumption of sufficient amounts by those who need it is doubtful. Supplementation of the whole population at the level shown to prevent neural-tube defects (i.e. 400 µg folic acid/day) raises safety concerns. For example, it could mask vitamin $B_{12}$ deficiency, because folic acid supplementation protects against the pernicious anemia typical of the deficiency but may allow the characteristic neural damage to progress undetected.

It has been estimated that folate supplementation can prevent 50–70% of neural-tube defects. Thus, not all neural-tube defects will disappear given preventive policies based on current knowledge, even though we can be confident that the frequency will decrease substantially. Future research should clarify residual causes as well as the risks and benefits of various levels of folate fortification of the food supply.

### General malnutrition

The causal role of protein-calorie malnutrition in mental retardation is more contentious than that of iodine deficiency or folate supplementation. Animal studies have shown that nutritional deprivation during the phase of maximum brain growth can adversely and, under some circumstances, irreversibly affect the brain. The effects of such deprivation on behavior in animals and on mental performance in human beings, however, are still not fully understood (Susser 1989). A major difficulty in human research is that poor nutrition is typically confounded with poverty and poor education, two of the strongest predictors of poor mental performance. A careful review of the few studies (Stein *et al.* 1975; Freeman *et al.* 1980; Rush *et al.* 1980; Waber *et al.* 1981) that have been able to investigate the effects of nutrition on children's mental development independent of the effects of poverty and education led to the following conclusions (Susser 1989):

1. Nutritional changes during gestation and up to 6 months of age and between 42 and 75 months of age produced no measurable effects on mental performance later in childhood. The nutritional changes included both supplementation in chronically malnourished communities in New York City and Bogota and deprivation in previously well-nourished communities during the World War II Dutch famine.
2. Dietary supplements of undernourished children in Bogota from 6 to 36 months of age resulted in improved mental performance from 12 to 36 months (their effects after 36 months are not known). If the effect of supplementation between 6 and 36 months is shown to persist after supplementation, it might suggest a critical period of brain development when nutrition can affect mental development. Alternatively, if this effect does not persist, we might conclude that food is needed to enable a child to perform well, but that lack of food severe enough to retard physical growth does not produce long-term cognitive delay or disability. On the whole, however, these studies point to a stronger role of education than of nutrition in explaining the association between socio-economic deprivation and mental retardation.

## PERINATAL EVENTS

At a population level, perinatal events such as preterm birth, low birthweight, and birth asphyxia are associated with elevated risks of impaired mental development during infancy and childhood (Breslau *et al.* 1994). Longitudinal studies of preterm, low-birthweight infants and controls, none the less, suggest that most survivors of even very low birthweight (<1500 g) function in the normal range on later developmental and cognitive tests (Teplin *et al.* 1991; Veelken *et al.* 1991; Paneth *et al.* 1992; Stjernqvist & Svenningsen 1993; Hack & Faranoff 1999). Perinatal factors are perhaps most strongly associated with mental retardation only when accompanied by cerebral palsy (Susser 1988), though selective cognitive deficits may be present in a larger proportion of children born prematurely. The strongest predictor of which infants will develop neurocognitive impairments among those born very prematurely and/or at very low birthweight is the presence of abnormalities indicative of white-matter damage observed neonatally on cranial ultrasound or MRI (Pinto-Martin *et al.* 1995; Whitaker *et al.* 1996; see Chapter 22). The origin of neonatal white-matter damage and its relationship to perinatal infection and maternal-fetal immunology are areas of active research at the present time (Leviton & Gilles 1996; Nelson *et al.* 1998). In addition to white matter disease, transient hypothyroxinemia of prematurity, detected during newborn thyroid screening in up to one-third of very-low-birthweight survivors, is strongly predictive of cognitive and motor delay at age 2 years (Reuss *et al.* 1996).

It is important to note that in multivariate analyses, the impacts of birthweight and other perinatal factors diminish once prenatal and postnatal variables such as genetic disorders and low socio-economic status are considered (Broman *et al.* 1987). When neurodevelopmental disability of unknown etiology follows a history of perinatal complications, one cannot assume that the cause necessarily originated in the perinatal period (Nelson & Ellenberg 1986). In fact, it is not uncommon for infants with brain damage traceable to the prenatal period to manifest clinical signs indicative of birth asphyxia during the perinatal period (Paneth *et al.* 1994).

In developed countries, advances in neonatal medicine during the past three decades have led to dramatic increases in the survival of preterm infants. During the same time period, rates of preterm birth have remained constant or increased somewhat. The net effect may be an increase in the prevalence of cognitive disabilities associated with perinatal events. Prevention of cognitive disabilities originating in the perinatal period will require a better understanding of the mechanisms and prevention of premature birth and neonatal white-matter disease.

## INFECTIONS (see also Section 6)

At least 20 different infectious agents can cause brain damage and mental deficiency in children. Congenital syphilis, the first congenital disorder to be linked to an infectious cause, is now a rare and preventable cause of mental retardation. Rubella, like syphilis, is a fetal infection. It affects the fetus only if the mother contracts the disease between the eighth and 13th weeks of pregnancy. This cause of mental retardation has been virtually eliminated in successfully vaccinated populations.

Brain damage from other intrauterine infections (toxoplasmosis, cytomegalovirus, varicella) may follow either prenatal or perinatal transmission. When exposure occurs during the first or second trimester of pregnancy, several impairments are recognizable at birth and may include microcephaly, hydrocephaly, growth retardation, cataracts, seizures, rashes, jaundice, and hepatosplenomegaly (Remington *et al.* 1995; Dunn *et al.* 1999). Exposure late in pregnancy or during delivery may result in inapparent infection at birth and onset of developmental delay during infancy or childhood (Koppe *et al.* 1986). In the case of toxoplasmosis, early detection and treatment (prenatal or neonatal) with antiparasitics are believed to reduce the occurrence of hydrocephalus and cognitive sequelae, though even among treated infants, the frequency of severe mental retardation in one follow-up study of infected infants was 21% (Roizen *et al.* 1995).

Postnatally acquired meningitis and encephalitis associated with a variety of infectious agents also leave a proportion of children with permanent cognitive disability, particularly in less developed countries where access to vaccination and treatment is more limited and often delayed. Adverse reactions to the pertussis vaccine rarely lead to encephalitis and residual mental retardation in children, and the risk is likely to be lower than the risk of death from pertussis infection in unvaccinated populations (Hinman & Koplan 1984; American Academy of Pediatrics Committee on Infectious Diseases 1991).

### Human immunodeficiency virus (see also p. 564)

The human immunodeficiency virus (HIV) pandemic has emerged as an important cause of neurodevelopmental impairment, particularly in populations where it disproportionately affects childbearing women and where access to effective antiretroviral therapies and Cesarian delivery are limited or non-existent. HIV seroprevalence among unselected samples of pregnant women tested in recent years ranges from as low as 1/10 000 in Sweden to nearly 6% in Zaire. In some high-risk populations, the prevalence of infection is 20–30% in women of reproductive age (Boylan & Stein 1991; Davis *et al.* 1998; Amar *et al.* 1999).

Following the news in 1994 of the effectiveness of antiretroviral therapy (Zidovudine) in preventing perinatal transmission of HIV (Connor *et al.* 1994), the risk of vertical transmission of the virus from infected mothers to offspring has been reduced from about 25% to less than 10% in European and North American populations. When treatment is combined with delivery by Cesarian section, transmission can be reduced to as low as 2% (European Mode of Delivery Collaboration 1999; International Perinatal HIV Group, 1999). In low-income populations, which include the majority of HIV-infected women world-wide and in which prenatal screening, counseling and treatment options are limited, the probability of vertical transmission from untreated, infected mothers remains as high as 30–40%.

Once a child has been infected, the ensuring effects of pediatric acquired immunodeficiency disease (AIDS) may include central nervous system impairment, acquired microcephaly, and cognitive and movement disabilities (Belman 1992). Thus, HIV infection, has become an important, fatal cause of mental retardation in some populations. Prevention efforts must focus on cost-effective and accessible methods of preventing maternal infection as well as maternal–infant transmission. The potential for vaccine development, the role of breast-feeding, and the effectiveness of modified treatment regimens are currently areas of active research (Kuhn & Stein 1997; Wade *et al.* 1998).

## ENVIRONMENTAL TOXINS

### Lead

High concentrations of lead absorbed by children, from painted toys or paint flakes on the floor, from the fumes of burning batteries and from residential proximity to heavy lead industries, has long been known to cause the serious and often fatal condition of lead encephalopathy in children. Prior to the 1950s, survivors were regularly severely mentally retarded, and their presence could be detected in populations and institutions housing retarded persons. Neuropsychologic impairments of various kinds appeared even in children with moderately raised lead levels, well below levels that cause acute lead encephalopathy. Studies showing these impairments were typically of poor, inner-city children, often from minority groups, and the role of lead was not easy to isolate from the covariate confounders of poverty and class. The consensus of these small, often uncontrolled and cross-sectional studies was that for those with blood lead levels above 60 μg/dl, there was an association with mild mental retardation; for those with 50–60 μg/dl blood concentrations, the association was somewhat reduced. Little suspicion attached to levels lower than 40 μg/dl up to about 1980, following Needleman and colleagues' pioneering work showing an inverse association between lead levels in deciduous teeth and cognitive outcomes at age 7–8 years. Subsequent studies have demonstrated the specificity of time of exposure and of cognitive outcomes at various stages of childhood. Typical of these are the studies emanating from Port Pirie in Sydney, Australia (Baghurst *et al.* 1992) and Yugoslavia (Wasserman *et al.* 1997). Although not all studies are in agreement, evidence has strengthened that exposure prenatally as well as in toddlers reduces scores on developmental and cognitive tests. For individuals, again, deficits are small; nevertheless, the consistency in size and direction give confidence that they are real. Persistence of the effects of early lead exposure into adolescence and young adulthood has also been demonstrated (Needleman *et al.* 1990).

Today, the cumulative evidence suggests a dose–response relation of lead exposure in early childhood to mental performance and also to hyperactivity and other behavioral problems (Burns *et al.* 1999). The US government now considers levels higher than 10 μg/dl to be potentially neurotoxic. As a result of regulatory and voluntary bans enacted during the 1980s on the use of lead in gasoline, household paint, food and beverage containers, and plumbing systems, the percentage of US children with elevated blood lead levels has declined steadily, from greater than 50% in the 1970s to 4.4% according to recent survey data (Centers for Disease Control and Prevention 1997). However, the rate of decline has been uneven, and minority children in low-income households in urban areas and residents of housing built prior to the 1950s continue to be more highly exposed.

World-wide, the prevention of childhood lead poisoning should be feasible and, in the long run, is likely to be cost-effective when balanced against reduced health costs and improved school performance and quality of work (Needleman 1991). What is required is control of industrial processes, removal of lead from gasoline and paint, maintaining low lead levels in soil, and monitoring residences (many houses still have the remains of lead paint, within and without). In developing countries, especially, children continue to be exposed to lead from gasoline and industrial sources (Kumar *et al.* 1998; Khan & Khan 1999). Screening of blood lead levels in young children should be undertaken in all populations to monitor risks and identify children requiring intervention. For those with raised lead levels, removal from the source of exposure and, for those with extreme levels, possibly chelation treatment to increase the excretion level are indicated. Universal childhood screening of blood lead levels followed by intervention has been shown to be cost-effective in high-risk populations, while targeted screening based on risk factor profiles is preferable in low-risk populations (Kemper *et al.* 1998; Rolnick *et al.* 1999).

### Alcohol

Heavy alcohol abuse during pregnancy is associated with fetal alcohol syndrome in offspring (see also p. 257). This syndrome includes cognitive disability (usually mild to moderate in severity), low birthweight, microcephaly, stunting, flattened nasolabial facies, and narrow palpebral tissues. The incidence and prevalence of fetal alcohol syndrome seem to vary with the frequency of alcohol abuse in pregnancy and possibly with individual susceptibility. A frequency at birth of one per 600 was observed in Gothenburg, Sweden (Hagberg 1987), a population in which nearly 10% of the cases of mild mental retardation in schoolchildren were attributed to this cause (Hagberg *et al.* 1981). In a Canadian study, the frequency fetal alcohol syndrome was found to be as high as one per 139 live births (Williams *et al.* 1999).

Prevention is easier to prescribe than to execute. In view of evidence that alcohol consumption during pregnancy is associated with a variety of adverse fetal outcomes other than mental retardation, abstinence or restricted drinking during pregnancy has become a worthwhile public-health objective.

## TRAUMA

Within the field of mental retardation, postnatal head injury seemingly contributes a small fraction of all cognitive disability. Studies of the prevalence of mental retardation among 40 000 Swedish children, for example, found only one case due to traumatic brain injury among 171 mildly and 161 severely retarded children (Gustavson *et al.* 1977c; Blomquist *et al.* 1981). Research on incident cases of severe head injury, however, points to the importance of head injury as a preventable cause of intellectual deficiency (Chadwick *et al.* 1981; Corrigan *et al.* 1998). The annual incidence of head injury (with loss of consciousness) in childhood is estimated to be in the range of two to three per 1000 in the US (Annegers *et al.* 1980; Thurman & Guerrero 1999). The major causes are motor-vehicle collisions, falls, and assaults. Throughout childhood, boys have a twofold risk of severe head injury relative to girls. Five to 10% of all cases are fatal, and another 5–10% are estimated to result in a wide range of neuropsychologic deficits (Frankowski *et al.* 1985; Durkin *et al.* 1998b). Permanent declines in IQ and adaptive function are observed in a proportion of cases, but population-based studies of the frequency, predictors, and prevention of these outcomes have not yet been done.

### Key Points

- Epidemiologic studies have yielded a great deal of knowledge about mental retardation, including: population frequencies and the impact of improved survival; the contribution of various causes; and prospects for prevention.
- It is clear that for many of the known causes, prevention is technically and theoretically feasible, and increasingly so with each new discovery.
- Actual significant reductions in the incidence and prevalence of mental retardation will require innovative and sustained public-health efforts, particularly in low-income populations where strategies known to be effective against mental retardation are not being implemented.
- Future progress in understanding the etiology will require population studies incorporating currently valid and culturally appropriate psychometric measures and case definitions, as well as cytogenetic, molecular genetic, brain imaging, medical and family history, and environmental information.

## REFERENCES


Adams M M, Erickson J D, Layde P M *et al.* (1991) Down's syndrome: recent trends in the United States. *JAMA* 246:758–760.

Alberman E (1978) Main causes of major mental handicap: prevalence and epidemiology. *Ciba Found Symp* 59:3–16.

Alberman E, Mutton D, Ide R *et al.* (1995) Down's syndrome births and pregnancy terminations 1989 to 1993: preliminary findings. *Br J Obstet Gynaecol* 106:435–437.

Albrecht U, Sutcliffe J S, Cattanach B M *et al.* (1997) Imprinted expression of the murine Angelman syndrome gene, UBE3A, in hippocampal and Purkinje neurons. *Nat Genet* 17:75–78.

Amar H S, Ho J J & Mohan A J (1999) Human immunodeficiency virus prevalence in women at delivery using unlinked anonymous testing of newborns in the Malaysian setting. *J Paediatr Child Health* 35:63–66.

Amir R E, Van den Veyver I B, Wan M *et al.* (1999) Rett syndrome is caused by mutations in X-linked MECP2, encoding methyl-CpG-binding protein 2. *Nat Genet* 23:185–188.

American Academy of Pediatrics Committee on Infectious Diseases (1991) The relationship between pertussis vaccine and brain damage: reassessment. *Pediatrics* 88:397–400.

American Psychiatric Association (1994) Diagnostic and statistical manual of mental disorders (4th edition). American Psychiatric Association, Washington, DC.

Annegers J F, Grabow J D, Kurland L T *et al.* (1980) The incidence, causes, and secular trends of head trauma in Olmsted County, Minnesota, 1935–1974. *Neurology* 30:912–919.

Baghurst P A, McMichael A J, Wigg N R *et al.* (1992) Environmental exposure to lead and children's intelligence at the age of seven years. *N Engl J Med* 327:1279–1284.

Baird P A & Sadovnick A D (1987) Life expectancy in Down's syndrome. *J Pediatr* 110:849–854.

Bell M V, Hirst M C, Nakahori Y *et al.* (1991) Physical mapping across the fragile X: hypermethylation and clinical expression of the fragile X syndrome. *Cell* 64:861–866.

Bellamy C (1998) *The state of the world's children 1998.* Oxford: UNICEF, Oxford University Press.

Belman A L (1992) AIDS and pediatric neurology. *Neurol Clin N Am* 8:571–602.

Bennett F C, Sells C J & Brand C (1979) Influences on measured intelligence in Down's syndrome. *Am J Dis Children* 133:700–703.

Beuren A J, Apitz J & Harmajanz D (1962) Supravalvular aortic stenosis in association with mental retardation and a certain facial appearance. *Circulation* 26:1235–1240.

Birch H G, Richardson S A, Baird D *et al.* (1970) mental subnormality in the community: a clinical and epidemiologic study. Baltimore, M D: Williams and Wilkins.

Bittles A H, Mason W M, Greene J *et al.* (1991) Reproductive behavior and health in consanguineous marriages. *Science* 252:789–794.

Blomquist H K S, Gustavson K H & Holmgren G (1981) Mild mental retardation in children in a northern Swedish county. *J Men Def Res* 25:169–186.

Boylan L & Stein Z (1991) The epidemiology of HIV infection in children and their mothers – vertical transmission. *Epidemiol Rev* 13:143–177.

Breslau N, DelDotto J E & Brown G G (1994) A gradient relationship between low birth weight and IQ at age 6 years. *Arch Pediat Adoles Med* 148:377–383.

Broman S, Nichols P L, Shaughnessy P *et al.* (1987) *Retardation in young children: a developmental study of cognitive deficit.* Hillsdale, NJ: Lawrence Erlbaum Associates.

Brown W T, Jenkins E C & Friedman E (1982) Autism is associated with the fragile-X syndrome. *J Autism Dev Disord* 12:303–308.

Budarf M L & Emanuel B S (1997) Progress in the autosomal segmental aneusomy syndromes (SASs): single or multi-locus disorders? *Hum Mol Genet* 6:1657–1665.

Bundey S & Alam H (1993) A five-year prospective study of the health of children in different ethnic groups, with particular reference to the effect of inbreeding. *Eur J Hum Genet* 1:206–219.

Burd L, Vesley B, Martsolf J T *et al.* (1991) Prevalence study of Rett syndrome in North Dakota children. American Journal of Medical Genetics 38:565–568.

Burns J M, Baghurst P A, Sawyer M G *et al.* (1999) Lifetime low-level exposure to environmental lead and children's emotional and behavioral development at ages 11–13 years. The Port Pirie Cohort Study. *Am J Epidemiol* 149:740–749.

Bushby K M, Thambyayah M & Gardner-Medwin D (1991) Prevalence and incidence of Becker muscular dystrophy. *Lancet* 337:1022–1004.

Butler M G, Meaney F J & Palmer C G (1986) Clinical and cytogenetic survey of 39 individuals with Prader-Labhart-Willi syndrome. *Am J Med Genet* 23:793–809.

Centers for Disease Control and Prevention (1997) Update: blood lead levels – United States. 1991–1994. *JAMA*; 277:1031–1032.

Centerwall S A & Centerwall W R (1960) A study of children with Mongolism reared in the home compared to those reared away from the home. *Pediatrics* 678–685.

Chadwick O, Rutter M, Brown G *et al.* (1981) A prospective study of children with head injuries: II. Cognitive sequelae. *Psychol Med* 11:49–61.

Chudley A E, Knoll J, Gerrard J W *et al.* (1983) Fragile (X) X-linked mental retardation. I Retardation between age and intelligence and the frequency of expression of fragile (X) (q28). *Am J Med Genet* 14:699–712.

Connolly B H, Morgan S B, Russell F F *et al.* (1993) A longitudinal study of children with Down syndrome who experienced early intervention programming. *Phys Ther* 73:170–179: discussion 179–181.

Connor E M, Sperling R S, Gelber R *et al.* (1994) Reduction of maternal-infant transmission of human immunodeficiency virus type 1 with zidovudine treatment. *N Engl J Med* 331:1173–1180.

Corrigan J D, Smith-Knapp K & Granger C V (1998) Outcomes in the first five years after traumatic brain injury. *Arch Phys Med Rehab* 79:298–305.

Cuckle H (1998) Rational Down syndrome screening policy. *Am J Pub Health* 88:558–559.

Cuckle H S, Wald N J & Thompson S G (1987) Estimating a woman's risk of having a pregnancy associated with

Down's syndrome using her age and serum alpha-fetoprotein level. *Br J Obstet Gynaecol* 94:387–402.

Czeizel A E & Dudas I (1992) Prevention of the first occurrence of neural-tube-defects by peri-conceptional vitamin supplementation. *N Engl J Med* 327:1832–1835.

Davies K E, Smith T J, Bundy S *et al.* (1988) Mild and severe muscular dystrophy associated with deletions in Xp21 of the human X chromosome. *J Med Genet* 25:9–13.

Davis S F, Rosen D H, Steinberg S *et al.* (1998) Trends in HIV prevalence among childbearing women in the United States, 1989–1994. *JAIDS: J Acquired Immune Defic Synd* 19:158–164.

Devi A R R, Roa N A & Bittles A H (1987) Inbreeding and the incidence of childhood genetic disorders in Karnataka, south India. *J Med Genet* 24:362–365.

De Vries B B, Halley D J J, Oostra B A *et al.* (1998) The fragile X syndrome. *J Med Genet* 35:579–589.

De Vries B B, van den Ouewland A M, Mohkamsing S *et al.* (1997) Screening and diagnosis for the fragile X syndrome among the mentally retarded: an epidemiological and psychological survey. Collaborative Fragile X Study Group. *Am J Hum Genet* 61:660–667.

De Vries B B, Wiegers A M, Smits A P *et al.* (1996) Mental status of females with am FMR1 gene full mutation. *Am J Hum Genet* 58:1025–1032.

Diaz-Fernandez F (1988) Descriptive epidemiology of registered mentally retarded persons in Galicia (northwest Spain). *Am J Ment Retard* 92:385–392.

Dittrich B, Buiting K, Korn B *et al.* (1996) Imprinting switch on chromosome 15 may involve alternative transcripts of the SNRPN gene. *Nat Genet* 14:163–170.

Dodd B, McCormack P & Woodyatt G (1994) Evaluation of an intervention program: relation between children's phonology and parents' communicative behavior. *Am J Ment Retard* 98:632–645.

Drillien C M, Jameson S & Wilkinson E M (1966) Studies in mental handicaps, part I: prevalence and distribution by clinical type and severity of defect. *Arch Dis Childhood* 41:528–538.

Dunn D, Wallon M, Peyron F *et al.* (1999) Mother-to-child transmission of toxoplasmosis: risk estimates for clinical counselling. *Lancet* 353:1929–1933.

Dupont A, Vaeth M & Videbech P (1986) Mortality and life expectancy of Down's syndrome in Denmark. *J Ment Defic Res* 30:111–120.

Durkin M S, Hasan Z M & Hasan K Z (1998a) Prevalence and correlates of mental retardation among children in Karachi, Pakistan. *Am J Epidemiol* 147:281–288.

Durkin M S, Olsen S, Barlow B *et al.* (1998b) The epidemiology of urban, pediatric, neurological trauma: evaluation of, and implications for, injury prevention programs. *Neurosurgery* 42:300–310.

Durkin M S, Schupf N, Stein Z A *et al.* (1998c) Mental Retardation. In: Wallace RB (ed.) *Public health and preventive medicine.* Stamford, CT: Appleton & Lange; pp. 1049–1058.

Durkin M S & Stein Z A (1996) Classification of mental retardation. In: Jacobson J W & Mulick J A (eds) *Manual of diagnosis and professional practice in mental retardation.* Washington, DC: American Psychological Association.

Elnager B, Eltom M, Karlsson F A *et al.* (1997) Control of iodine deficiency using iodination of water in a goiter endemic area. *Int J Food Sci Nutr* 48:119–127.

Epstein C J (1986) *The consequences of chromosome imbalance.* Cambridge University Press, Cambridge

European Mode of Delivery Collaboration (1999) Elective caesarean-section versus vaginal delivery in prevention of vertical HIV-1 transmission: a randomized clinical trial. *Lancet* 353:1030–1031.

Ewart A K, Morris C A, Atkinson *et al.* (1993) Hemizygosity at the elastin locus in a developmental disorder, Williams syndrome. *Nat Genet* 5:11–16.

Eyman R K, Grossman H J, Chaney *et al.* (1990) The life expectancy of profoundly handicapped persons with mental retardation. *N Engl J Med* 323:584–589.

Feldman E J (1996) The recognition and investigation of X-linked learning disability syndromes. *J Intellect Disability Res* 40:400–411.

Frangiskakis J M, Ewart A K, Morris C A *et al.* (1996) LIM-kinase 1 hemizygosity implicated in impaired visuospatial constructive cognition. *Cell* 86:59–69.

Frankowski R F, Annegers J F & Whitman S (1985) Epidemiologic and descriptive studies part 1: the descriptive epidemiology of head trauma in the United States. In: Becker D P & Povlishock J T (eds) *Central nervous system trauma status report.* Bethesda, MD: National Institute of Neurological Diseases and Stroke; pp. 33–43.

Freeman H E, Klien R E, Townsend J W *et al.* (1980) Nutrition and cognitive development among rural Guatemalan children. *Am J Pub Health* 70:1277–1285.

Fryer A E, Conner J M, Povery S *et al.* (1987) Evidence that the gene for tuberous sclerosis is on chromosome 9. *Lancet* ii:659–661.

Fryers T (1984) *The epidemiology of severe intellectual impairment.* London: Academic Press.

Fryers T & MacKay R I (1979) The epidemiology of severe mental handicap. Early Human Development 3:277–294.

Fu Y H, Kuhl D P A, Pizzuti A *et al.* (1991) Variation of the CGG repeat at the fragile X site results in genetic stability: resolution of the Sherman paradox. *Cell* 67:1047–1058.

Garber H (1988) The Milwaukee project: preventing mental retardation in children at risk. Washington, DC: American Association on Mental Retardation.

Gedeon A K, Baker E, Robinson H *et al.* (1992) Fragile X syndrome without CGG amplification has an FMR1 deletion. *Nat Gene* 1:341–344.

Greenberg F, Stratton R F, Lockhart L H *et al.* (1986) Familial Miller–Dieker syndrome associated with percentric inversion of chromosome 17. *Am J Med Genet* 23:853–859.

Grossman H J (ed.) (1983) *Classification in mental retardation.* Washington, DC: American Association on Mental Deficiency.

Gustavson K H, Hagberg B, Hagberg G *et al.* (1977a) Severe mental retardation in a Swedish county. I. Epidemiology, gestational age, birth weight and associated CNS handicaps in children born 1959–1970. *Acta Paediatr Scand* 66:373–379.

Gustavson K H, Hagberg B, Hagberg G *et al.* (1977b) Severe mental retardation in a Swedish county: etiological and pathogenic aspects of children born 1959–1970. *Neuropadiatric* 8:293–304.

Gustavson K H, Holmgren G, Jonsell R *et al.* (1977c) Severe mental retardation in children in a northern Swedish county. *J Ment Defic Res* 21:161–177.

Hack M & Faranoff A A (1999) Outcomes of children of extremely low birth weight and gestational age in the 1990s. *Early Hum Dev* 53:193–218.

Haddow J E, Palomaki G E, Knight G J *et al.* (1998) Screening of maternal serum for fetal Down's syndrome in the first trimester. *N Engl J Med* 338:955–961.

Hagberg B (1985) Rett syndrome: Swedish approach to analysis of prevalence and cause. *Brain Dev* 7:277–280.

Hagberg B (1987) Pre- and perinatal environmental origin in mild mental retardation. *Uppsala J Med Sci* 44 (Suppl):178–182.

Hagberg B (1989) Rett syndrome: clinical peculiarities, diagnostic approach, and possible cause. *Pediatr Neurol* 5:75–83.

Hagberg B, Hagberg G, Lewerth A *et al.* (1981) Mild mental retardation is Swedish school children: prevalence. *Acta Paediatr Scand* 70:441–444.

Hagerman R J (1991) Physical and behavioral phenotype. In: Hagerman R J & Silverman A C (eds) *Fragile X syndrome: Diagnosis, treatment and research.* Baltimore, MD: Johns Hopkins University Press; pp. 3–68.

Hagerman R J, Jackson C, Amiri K *et al.* (1992) Girls with fragile X syndrome. Physical and neurocognitive status and outcome. *Pediatrics* 89:395–400.

Hagerman R J & Silverman A C (eds) (1991) *Fragile X syndrome, diagnosis, treatment and research.* Baltimore, MD: Johns Hopkins University Press.

Hagerman R J, Hull C E, Safanda J F *et al.* (1994a) High functioning fragile X males: Demonstration of an unmethylated fully expanded FMR-1 mutation associated with protein expression. *Am J Med Genet* 51:298–308.

Hagerman R J, Wilson P, Staley L W *et al.* (1994b) Evaluation of school children at high risk for fragile X syndrome utilizing bucal cell FMR-1 testing. *Am J Med Genet* 51:474–481.

Hanley W B, Platt L D, Bachman R P *et al.* (1999) Undiagnosed maternal phenylketonuria: the need for prenatal selective screening or case finding. *Am J Obstet Gynecol* 180:986–994.

Hasan Z & Hasan A (1981) Report on a population survey of mental retardation in Pakistan. *Int J Ment Health* 10:23–27.

Hassold T, Chiu D & Yamane J A (1984) Parental origin of autosomal trisomies. *Ann Hum Gene* 48:129–144.

Herbst D S & Miller J R (1980) Nonspecific X-linked mental retardation. II. The frequency in British Columbia. *Am J Med Genet* 7:461–469.

Hetzel B S (1983) Iodine deficiency disorders (IDD) and their eradication. *Lancet* ii:1126–1128.

Hetzel B S (1989) *The story of iodine deficiency: an international challenge in nutrition.* Oxford: Oxford University Press.

Hinman A R & Koplan J P (1984) Pertussis and pertussis vaccine: reanalysis of benefits, risks and costs. *JAMA* 251:3109–3113.

Hoffman E P, Brown R H & Kunkel L M (1987) The protein product of the Duchenne muscular distrophy locus. *Cell* 51:919–928.

Holden J J A, Chalifoux M, Wing M *et al.* (1995) Distribution and frequency of FMRI CGG repeat numbers in the general population. *Dev Brain Dysfun* 8:405–407.

Holden J J A, Percy M, Allingham-Hawkins *et al.* (1999) Conference Report: Eighth International Workshop on the fragile X syndrome and X-linked mental retardation, August 16–22, 1997. *Am J Med Genet* 83:221–236.

Hook E B (1982a) Epidemiology of Down syndrome. In: Pueschel S M & Rynders J E (eds) *Down syndrome: advances in biomedicine and the behavioral sciences.* Cambridge, MA: Ware Press; pp. 11–88.

Hook E B (1982b) Incidence and prevalence as measures of the frequency of birth defects. *Am J Epidemiol* 116:743–747.

Hunt A & Lindenbaum R H (1984) Tuberous sclerosis: a new estimate of prevalence within the Oxford region. *J Med Genet* 21:272–277.

International Perinatal HIV Group (1999) The mode of delivery and the risk of vertical transmission of human immunodeficiency virus type 1: a meta-analysis of 15 prospective cohort studies. *N Engl J Med* 340:977–987.

Jacobs P A, Bullman H, Macpherson J *et al.* (1993) Population studies of fragile X: a molecular approach. *J Med Genet* 30:454–459.

Jacobs P A, Glover T W, Mayer M *et al.* (1980) X-linked mental retardation: a study of 7 families. *Am J Med Genet* 7:741–489.

Jay P, Rougeulle C, Massacrier A *et al.* (1997) The human necdin gene, NDN, is maternally imprinted and located in the Prader–Willi chromosomal region. *Nat Genet* 17:357–361.

Jiang Y-H, Tsai T-F, Bressler J *et al.* (1998) Imprinting in Angelman and Prader–Willi syndromes. *Curr Opin Gene Dev* 8:334–342.

Kallen B & Knudsen L B (1989) Effect of maternal age distribution and prenatal diagnosis on the population rates of Down syndrome – a comparative study of nineteen populations. *Hereditas* 110:55–60.

Kaveggia E G, Durkin M V, Pendleton E *et al.* (1975) Genetic studies on 1,224 patients with severe mental retardation. In: *Proceedings of the Third Congress of the International Association for the Scientific Study of Mental Deficiency.* Warsaw: Polish Medical Publishers; pp. 82–93.

Kemper A R, Bordley W C & Downs S M (1998) Cost-effectiveness analysis of lead poisoning screening strategies following the 1997 guidelines of the Centers for Disease Control and Prevention. *Arch Pediatr Adoles Med* 152:1202–1208.

Khan N Z & Khan A H (1999) Lead poisoning and psychomotor delay in Bangladeshi children. *Lancet* 353:754.

Kiely M (1987) The prevalence of mental retardation. *Epidemiol Rev* 9:194–218.

Kline J, Stein Z & Susser M (1989) *Conception to birth: epidemiology of prenatal development.* New York: Oxford University Press.

Knoll J H M, Nicholls R D, Magenis R E *et al.* (1989) Angelman and Prader–Willi syndromes share a common chromosome 15 deletion but differ in parental origin of the deletion. *Am J Med Genet* 32:285–290.

Koppe J, Loewer-Sieger D & de Roever-Bonnet H (1986) Results of 20 years follow-up of congenital toxoplasmosis. *Lancet* ii:254–256.

Kremer E J, Pritchard M, Lynch M *et al.* (1991) Mapping of DNA instability at the fragile X to a trinucleotide repeat sequence p(CCG)$_n$. *Science* 252:1711–1714.

Krivchenia E, Huether C A, Edmonds L D *et al.* (1993) Comparative epidemiology of Down syndrome in two United States populations, 1970–1989. *Am J Epidemiol* 137:815–828.

Kuhn L & Stein Z (1997) Infant survival, HIV infection, and feeding alternatives in less-developed countries. *Am J Pub Health* 87:926–931.

Kumar A, Dey P K, Singla P N *et al.* (1998) Blood lead levels in children with neurological disorders. *J Trop Pediatr* 44:320–322.

Ledbetter D, Riccardi V, Airhart S *et al.* (1981) Deletions of chromosome 15 as a cause of the Prader–Willi syndrome. *N Engl J Med* 304:325–329.

Lehrke R G (1974) X-linked mental retardation and verbal disability. *Birth Defects* 10:1–100.

Lenke R R & Levy H L (1980) Maternal phenylketonuria and hyperphenylalaninemia: an international survey of the outcome of untreated and treated pregnancies. *N Enql J Med* 303:1202–1208.

Leviton A & Gilles F (1996) Ventriculomegaly, delayed myelination, white matter hypoplasia, and 'periventricular' leukomalacia: how are they related? *Pediatr Neurol* 15:127–136.

Levy H L & Ghavami M (1996) Maternal phenylketonuria: a metobolic teratogen. *Teratology* 53:176–184.

Levy H L & Waisbren S E (1983) Effects of untreated maternal phenylketonuria and hyperphenylalaninemia on the fetus. *N Engl J Med* 309:1269–1274.

Lewis E O (1929) Report on an investigation into the incidence of mental deficiency in six areas, 1925–1927. Part IV of Report of the Mental Deficiency Committee, Being a Joint Committee on the Board of Education and Board of Control. London: HMSO.

Lopez P M, Stone D & Gilmour H (1995) Epidemiology of Down's syndrome in a Scottish city. *Paediatr Perinatal Epidemiol* 9:331–340.

Lowry R B, Applegarth D A, Toone J R *et al.* (1990) An update on the frequency of mucupolysaccharide syndromes in British Columbia. *Hum Gene* 85:389–390.

Lubs H A (1969) A marker-X chromosome. *Am J Hum Genet* 21:231–244.

Lubs H, Chiurazzi P, Arena J *et al.* (1999) XLMR genes: update 1998. *Am J Med Genet* 83:237–247.

Luckasson R, Coulter D L, Polloway E A *et al.* (1992) *Mental retardation: definition, classification, and systems of supports.* Washington, DC: American Association on Mental Retardation, 9th edn.

McDonald A D (1973) Severely retarded children in Quebec: prevalence, causes and care. *Am J Ment Defic Res* 78:205–215.

McGrother C W & Marshall B (1990) Recent trends in incidence, morbidity and survival in Down syndrome. *J Ment Defic Res* 34:49–57.

McKay H, Sinisterra L, McKay A *et al.* (1978) Improving cognitive ability in chronically deprived children. *Science* 200:270–278.

McKusick V A (1998) *Mendelian inheritance in man: a catalogue of human genes and genetic disorders.* Baltimore, MD: The Johns Hopkins University Press, 12th edn.

McQueen P C, Spence M W, Garner J B *et al.* (1987) Prevalence of major mental retardation and associated disabilities in the Canadian maritime provinces. *Am J Ment Defic* 91:460–466.

Martin G M (1978) Genetic syndromes in man with potential relevance to pathobiology of aging. *Birth Defects Orig Articles Ser* 14:5–39.

Matsuura T, Sutcliffe J S, Fang P *et al.* (1997) De novo truncating mutations in E6-AP ubiquitin-protein ligase gene (UBE3A) in Angelman syndrome. *Nat Genet* 15:74–77.

Mattei M G, Soviah N & Mattei J F (1984) Chromosome 15 anomalies and the Prader–Willi syndrome: cytogenetic analysis. *Hum Genet* 66:313–334.

Meadows K L, Pettay D, Newman J *et al.* (1996) Survey of the fragile X syndrome and the fragile X E syndrome in a special education needs population. *Am J Med Genet* 64:428–433.

Melyn M A & White D T (1973) Mental and developmental milestones of noninstitutionalized Down's syndrome children. *Pediatrics* 52:542–545.

Mercer J R (1992) The impact of changing paradigms of disability on mental retardation in the year 2000. In: Rowitz L (ed.) *Mental retardation in the year 2000.* New York: Springer; pp. 15–38.

Miller G & Ramer J C (eds) (1992) *Static encephalopathies of infancy and childhood.* Raven Press, New York.

Morton J E, Bundey S, Webb T P *et al.* (1997) Fragile X syndrome is less common than previously estimated. *J Med Genet* 34:1–5.

Mowrey-Rushton P A, Driscoll D J, Nicholls R D *et al.* (1996) DNA methylation patterns in human tissues of uniparental origin using a zinc-finger gene (ZNF127) from the Angelman/Prader–Willi region. *Hum Mol Genet* 61:140–146.

MRC Vitamin Study Group (1991) Prevention of neural tube defects: results of the Medical Research Council vitamin study. *Lancet* 338:131–137.

Murphy C C, Yeargin-Allsopp M, Decoufle P *et al.* (1995) The administrative prevalence of mental retardation in 10-year-old children in metropolitan Atlanta, 1985 through 1987. *Am J Pub Health* 85:319–323.

Murray A, Youings S, Dennis N *et al.* (1996) Population screening at the FRAXA and FRAXE loci: molecular analyses of boys with learning difficulties and their mothers. *Am J Med Genet* 5:727–735.

Mutirangura A, Jayakumar A, Sutcliffe J S *et al.* (1993) A complete YAC contig of the Prader–Willi/Angelman chromosome region (15q11–q13) and refined localization of the SNRPN gene. *Genomics* 18:546–552.

Mutton D E, Ide R, Alberman E *et al.* (1993) Analysis of national register of Down's syndrome in England and Wales: trends in prenatal diagnosis, 1989–91. *BMJ* 306:431–432.

Narayanan H S (1981) A study of the prevalence of mental retardation in southern India. *Int J Men Health* 10:28–36.

Needleman H L (1991) Childhood lead poisoning: a disease for the history texts. *Am J Publ Health* 8:685–687.

Needleman H L, Gunnoe C, Leviton A *et al.* (1979) Deficits in psychologic and classroom performance of children with elevated dentine lead levels. *N Engl J Med* 300:689–695.

Needleman H L, Schell M A, Bellinger D *et al.* (1990) The long-term effects of exposure to low doses of lead in childhood: an 11-year follow-up report. *N Engl J Med* 322:83–88.

Nelson K B, Dambrosia J M, Grether J K *et al.* (1998) Neonatal cytokines and coagulation factors in children with cerebral palsy. *Ann Neurol* 44:665–675.

Nelson K B & Ellenberg J H (1986) Antecedents of cerebral palsy: multivariate analysis of risk. *N Engl J Med* 315:81–86.

Nicholls R D (1993) Genomic imprinting and candidate genes in the Prader–Willi and Angelman syndromes. *Curr Genet Dev* 3:445–456.

Nicholson A & Alberman E (1992) Prediction of the number of Down's syndrome infants to be born in England and Wales up to the year 2000 and their likely survival rates. *J Intellect Disab Res* 36:505–517.

Nolin S L, Glicksman A, Houck G *et al.* (1994) Mosaicism in fragile X affected males. *Am J Med Genet* 51:509–512.

Oberle I, Rousseau F, Heltz D *et al.* (1991) Instability of a 550-base pair DNA segment and abnormal methylation in Fragile X syndrome. *Science* 252:1097–1102.

O'Leary P, Bower C, Murch A *et al.* (1996) The impact of antenatal screening for Down syndrome in Western Australia:1980–1994. *Austral N Z J Obstet Gynaecol* 36:385–388.

Oliver C & Holland A J (1986) Down syndrome and Alzheimer's disease: A review. *Psychol Med* 16:307–322.

Opitz J M & Sutherland G R (1984) Conference Report: International Workshop on the Fragile X and X-linked mental retardation. *Am J Med Genet* 17:5–94.

Osborne L R, Martindale D, Scherer S W *et al.* (1996) Identification of genes from a 500-kb region at 7q11.23 that is commonly deleted in Williams-syndrome patients. *Genomics* 36:328–336.

Ozcelik T, Leff S, Robinsom W *et al.* (1992) Small nuclear ribonucleoprotein polypeptide N (SNRPN), an expressed gene in the Prader–Willi syndrome critical region. *Nat Genet* 9:395–400.

Paneth N, Guillemin J, Harrison H *et al.* (1992) Roundtable: survival and outcome of the extremely low-birthweight infant. *Birth* 19:154–161.

Paneth N, Rudelli R, Kazam E *et al.* (1994) *Brain damage in the preterm infant, clinics in developmental medicine No. 131.* London: Mac Keith Press.

Peckham C & Pearson R (1976) The prevalence and nature of ascertained handicap in the National Child Development Study (1958 cohort). *Publ Health* 90:111–121.

Pembrey M, Fennell S J, van den Berghe J *et al.* (1989) The association of Angelman's syndrome with deletions within 15q11–13. *J Med Genet* 26:73–77.

Penrose L S (1938) *A clinical and genetic study of 1,280 cases of mental defect. Mental Research Council Special Report Series 229,* London.

Peoples R, Perez-Jurado L, Wang Y-K *et al.* (1996) The gene for replication factor C subunit (RFC2) is within the 7q11.23 Williams syndrome deletion. *Am J Hum Genet* 58:1370–1373.

Perez-Jurado L A, Peoples R, Kaplan P *et al.* (1996) Molecular definition of the chromosome 7 deletion in Williams syndrome and parent-of-origin effects on growth. *Am J Hum Genet* 59:781–792.

Phillips O P, Elias S, Shulman L P *et al.* (1992) Maternal serum screening for fetal Down syndrome in women less than 35 years of age using alpha-fetoprotein, hCG, and unconjugated estriol: a prospective 2-year study. *Obstet Gynecol* 80:353–358.

Pieretti M, Zhang F, Fu Y H *et al.* (1991) Absence of expression of the FMR-1 gene in Fragile X syndrome. *Cell* 66:817–822.

Pinto-Martin J A, Riolo S, Cnaan A *et al.* (1995) Cranial ultrasound prediction of disabling and nondisabling cerebral palsy at age two in a low birth weight population. *Pediatrics* 95:249–254.

Power C (1992) A review of child health in the 1958 birth cohort: National Child Development Study. *Paediatr Perinatal Epidemiol* 6:81–110.

Ramey C T & Ramey S L (1998) Prevention of intellectual disabilities: early interventions to improve cognitive development. *Prevent Med* 27:224–232.

Reiss A L, Abrams M T, Greenlaw *et al.* (1995) Neurodevelopmental effects of the FMR-1 full mutation in humans. *Nat Med* 1:159–167.

Reiss A L, Aylward E, Freund L S *et al.* (1991) Neuroanatomy of fragile X syndrome: The posterior fossa. *Ann Neurol* 29:26–32.

Reiss A L & Freund L (1990) Fragile X syndrome, DSM-III-R and autism. *J Am Acad Child Adoles Psychiatry* 29:885–891.

Reiss A L, Lee J & Freund L (1994) Neuroanatomy of fragile X syndrome: The temporal lobe. *Neurology* 44:1317–1324.

Remington J S, McLeod R & Desmonts G (1995) Toxoplasmosis. In: Remington J S & Klein J O (eds) *Infectious diseases of the fetus and newborn infant.* Philadelphia, PA: W B Saunders; 4th edn, pp. 140–267.

Renpenning H, Gerrard J W, Zaleski W A *et al.* (1962) Familial sex-linked mental retardation. *Can Med Assoc J* 87:954–956.

Reuss M L, Paneth N, Pinto-Martin J A *et al.* (1996) The relation of transient hypothyroxinemia in preterm infants to neurologic development at two years of age. *N Engl J Med* 334:821–827.

Richardson S A, Katz M & Koller H (1986) Sex differences in number of children administratively classified as mildly mentally retarded: an epidemiological review. *Am J Ment Defic* 91:250–256.

Rohr F J, Doherty L B, Waisbren S E *et al.* (1987) New England Maternal PKU Project: prospective study of untreated and treated pregnancies and their outcomes. *J Pediatr* 10:391–398.

Roizen N, Swisher C N & Stein M A (1995) Neurologic and developmental outcome in treated congenital toxoplasmosis. *Pediatrics* 95:11–20.

Rolnick S J, Nordin J & Cherney L M (1999) A comparison of costs of universal versus targeted lead screening for young children. *Environ Res* 80:84–91.

Rouse B, Azen C, Koch R *et al.* (1997) Maternal Phenylketonuria Collaborative Study (MPKUCS) Offspring: Facial anomalies, malformations, and early neurological sequelae. *Am J Med Genet* 69:89–95.

Rousseau F, Heitz D, Tarleton J *et al.* (1994) A multicenter study on genotype–phenotype correlation in the fragile X syndrome, using direct diagnosis with probe StB 12.3: the first 2,253 cases. *Am J Hum Genet* 55:225–237.

Rousseau F, Rouillard P, Morel M L *et al.* (1995) Prevalence of carriers of premutation-size alleles of the FMR1 gene- and implications for the population genetics of the fragile X syndrome. *Am J Hum Genet* 57:1006–1018.

Rush D, Stein Z A & Susser M W (1980) A randomized controlled trial of prenatal nutritional supplementation. *Pediatrics* 65:683–697.

Rutter M, Tizard J & Whitmore K (eds) (1970) *Education, health and behaviour.* London: Longman.

Saitoh S, Buiting K, Cassidy S B *et al.* (1997) Clinical spectrum and molecular diagnosis of Angelman and Prader–Willi patients with an imprinting mutation. *Am J Med Genet* 68:195–206.

Sare Z, Ruvalcaba R H & Kelly V C (1978) Prevalence of thyroid disorder in Down syndrome. *Clin Genet* 14:154–158.

Schupf N, Kapell D, Zigman W B *et al.* (1996) Onset of dementia and decline in adaptive competence is associated with apolipoprotein E ε4 in Down syndrome. *Ann Neurol* 40:799–801.

Serra-Prat M, Gallo P, Jovell A J *et al.* (1998) Trade-offs in prenatal detection of Down syndrome. *Am J Publ Health* 88:551–557.

Sharav T & Shlomo L (1986) Stimulation of infants with Down syndrome: long-term effects. *Men Retard* 24:81–86.

Sherman S (1991) Epidemiology. In: Hagerman R J & Silverman A C (eds) *Fragile X syndrome diagnosis, treatment and research.* Baltimore, MD: Johns Hopkins University Press; p 69–97.

Sherman S L, Jacobs P A & Morton N E *et al.* (1985) Further segregation analysis of the fragile X syndrome with special reference to transmitting males. *Hum Genet* 69:289–299.

Sherman S L, Morton N E & Jacobs P A *et al.* (1984) The fragile X syndrome a cytogenetic and genetic analysis. *Ann Hum Genet* 48:21–37.

Sherman S L, Takaesu N & Freeman S B *et al.* (1991) Trisomy 21: association between reduced recombination and nondisjunction. *Am J Hum Genet* 49:608–620.

Shiotsuki Y, Matsuishi T & Toshimura K *et al.* (1984) The prevalence of mental retardation in Kurume City. *Brain Dev* 6:487–490.

Smits A, Smeets D, Dreesen J *et al.* (1992) Parental origin of the Fra(X) gene is a major determinant of the cytogenetic expression and the CGG repeat length in female carriers. *Am J Med Genet* 43:261–267.

Spence W C, Black S H, Fallon L *et al.* (1996) Molecular fragile X screening in normal populations. *Am J Med Genet* 64:181–183.

Staples A J, Sutherland G, Haan E A *et al.* (1991) Epidemiology of Down syndrome in South Australia, 1960–89. *Am J Hum Genet* 49:1014–1024.

Stein Z A, Durkin M S & Belmont L (1986) Serious mental retardation in developing countries: an epidemiologic approach. Mental retardation and developmental disabilities: research, education and technology transfer. *Ann NY Acad Sci* 477:8–21.

Stein Z A & Susser M W (1970) The mutability of intelligence and the epidemiology of mild mental retardation. *Rev Edu Res* 40:29–67.

Stein Z A & Susser M W (1984) The epidemiology of mental retardation. In: Butler N R & Connor B D (eds) *Stress and disability in childhood* Bristol: Wright; pp. 21–46.

Stein Z A, Susser M W, Saenger G *et al.* (1975) *Famine and human development: the Dutch hunger winter of 1944/45.* New York: Oxford University Press.

Stein Z A, Susser M W & Saenger G (1976a) Mental retardation in a national population of young men in The Netherlands: 2. Prevalence of mild mental retardation. *Am J Epidemiol* 104:159–169.

Stein Z A, Susser M W, Saenger G *et al.* (1976b) Mental retardation in a national population of young men in The Netherlands: 1. Prevalence of severe mental retardation. *Am J Epidemiol* 103:477–489.

Stewart G D, Hassold T J, Berg A *et al.* (1988) Trisomy 21 (Down syndrome): studying nondisjunction and meiotic recombination by using cytogenetic and molecular polymorphisms that span chromosome 21. *Am J Hum Genet* 42:227–236.

Stjernqvist K & Svenningsen N W (1993) Extremely low-birth weight infants less than 901 g: growth and development after one year of life. *Acta Paediatr Scand* 82:40–44.

Susser M W (1968) *Community psychiatry: epidemiologic and social themes.* Random House, New York.

Susser M W (1988) The quantification of risk factors in major neurodevelopmental disorders. In: Kubi F, Patel N, Patel N *et al.* (eds) *Perinatal events and brain damage in surviving children.* New York, NY: Springer; pp. 12–27.

Susser M W (1989) The challenge of causality: human nutrition, brain development and mental performance. *Bull NY Acad Med* 65:1032–1049.

Susser M W & Watson W (1971) *Sociology in medicine.* Oxford: Oxford University Press.

Sutcliffe J S, Jiang Y-H, Galjaard R-J *et al.* (1997) The E6-AP ubiquitin-protein ligase (UBE3A) gene is localized within a narrowed Angelman syndrome critical region. *Genome Res* 7:368–377.

Sutcliffe J S, Nakao M, Christian S L *et al.* (1994) Deletions of a differentially methylated CpG island at the SNRPN gene define a putative imprinting control region. *Nat Genet* 8:52–58.

Sutcliffe J S, Nelson D L, Zhang F *et al.* (1992) DNA methylation represses FMR-1 transcription in fragile X syndrome. *Hum Mol Genet* 1:397–400.

Sutherland G R (1977) Fragile sites on human chromosomes. Demonstration of their dependence on the type of tissue culture medium. *Science* 197:265–266.

Suzuki L A & Valencia R R (1997) Race-ethnicity and measured intelligence: educational implications. *Am Psychol* 52(10):1103–1114.

Tangsrud S E & Halvorsen S (1989) Child neuromuscular disease in southern Norway: the prevalence and incidence of Duchenne muscular dystrophy. *Acta Paediat Scand* 78:100–103.

Teplin S W, Burchinal M, Johnson-Martin N *et al.* (1991) Neurodevelopmental, health, and growth status at age 6 years of children with birth weights less than 1001 grams. *J Paediatr* 118:768–777.

Thorburn M, Desai P, Paul T J *et al.* (1992) Identification of childhood disability in Jamaica: the ten question screen. *Int J Rehab Res* 15:115–127.

Thurman D & Guerrero J (1999) Trends in hospitalization associated with traumatic brain injury. *JAMA* 282:954–957.

Tonnesen T, Kleijer W J & Horn N (1991) Incidence of Menkes disease. *Hum Genet* 86:408–410.

Turner G, Robinson H, Laing S *et al.* (1986) Preventive screening for the fragile X syndrome. *N Engl J Med* 315:607–609.

Turner G & Turner B (1974) X-linked mental retardation. *J Med Genet* 11:109–113.

Turner G, Webb T, Wake S *et al.* (1996) Prevalence of fragile X syndrome. *Am J Med Genet* 64:196–197.

Van den Ouweland A M, de Vries B B, Bakker P L *et al.* (1994) DNA diagnosis of the fragile X syndrome in a series of 236 mentally retarded subjects and evidence for a reversal of mutation in the FMR-1 gene. *Am J Med Genet* 51:482–485.

Van der Put N M J, Gabreels F, Stevens E M B *et al.* (1998) A second common mutation in the methylenetetra hydrofolate reductase gene: an additional risk factor for neural-tube-defects? *Am J Hum Genet* 62:1044–1051.

Van Essen A J, Busch H F, te Meerman G J *et al.* (1992) Birth and population prevalence of Duchenne muscular dystrophy in The Netherlands. *Hum Genet* 88:258–266.

Veelken N, Stollhoff K & Claussen M (1991) Development of very low birth weight infants: a regional study of 371 survivors. *Eur J Pediatr* 150:815–820.

Verheij C, Bakker C E, de Graff E *et al.* (1993) Characterization and localization of the FMR-1 gene product associated with fragile X syndrome. *Nature* 363:722–724.

Verkerk A J M H, Pieretti M, Sutcliffe J S *et al.* (1991) Identification of a gene (FMR-1) containing a CGG repeat coincident with a breakpoint cluster region exhibiting length variation in Fragile X syndrome. *Cell* 65:905–914.

Vincent A, Heitz D, Petit C *et al.* (1991) Abnormal pattern detected in fragile X patients by pulsed field gel electrophoreses. *Nature* 349:624–626.

Waber D P, Vuori-Christiansen L, Ortiz N *et al.* (1981) Nutritional supplementation, maternal education and cognitive development in infants at risk of malnutrition. *Am J Clin Nutr* 34:807–813.

Wade N A, Birkhead G S, Warren B L *et al.* (1998) Abbreviated regimens of zidovudine prophylaxis and perinatal transmission of the human immunodeficiency virus. *N Engl J Med* 339:1409–1414.

Waisbren S E, Chang P, Levy H L *et al.* (1998) Neonatal neurological assessment of offspring in maternal phenylketonuria. *J Inher Metab Dis* 21:39–48.

Waisbren S E, Doherty L B, Bailey I V *et al.* (1988) The New England Maternal PKU Project: identification of at-risk women. *Am J Publ Health* 78:789–771.

Wagstaff J, Knoll J H, Glatt K H *et al.* (1992) Maternal but not paternal transmission of 15q11–q13 linked nondeletion Angelman syndrome leads to phenotypic expression. *Nat Genet* 1:291–294.

Wald N J, Brock D J H & Bonnar J (1974) Prenatal diagnosis of spina bifida and anencephaly by maternal serum alpha-fetoprotein measurement. *Lancet* i:765–767.

Wald N J & Kennard A (1992) Prenatal biochemical screening for Down's syndrome and neural tube defects. *Curr Opin Obstet Gynaecol* 4:302–307.

Wald N J, Kennard A, Hackshaw A *et al.* (1997) Antenatal screening for Down syndrome. *J Med Screen* 4:181–246 [Erratum, *J Med Screen* 1998; 5:110, 166].

Wald N J, Watt H C & Hackshaw A K (1999) Integrated screening for Down's syndrome based on tests performed during the first and second trimesters. *N Engl J Med* 341:461–467.

Wasserman G A, Liu X, Lolacono N J *et al.* (1997) Lead exposure and intelligence in 7-year-old children: the Yugoslavia Prospective Study. *Environ Health Perspect* 105:956–962.

Webb T P, Bundy S, Thake A *et al.* (1986) The frequency of the fragile X chromosome among school children in Coventry. *J Med Genet* 23:396–399.

Weitzman M, Aschengrau A, Bellinger D *et al.* (1993) Lead-contaminated soil abatement and urban children's blood lead levels. *J A M A* 269:1647–1654.

Wevrick R, Kerns J A & Francke U (1994) Identification of a novel paternally expressed gene in the Prader–Willi syndrome region. *Nat Genet* 3:1877–1882.

Whitaker A H, Feldman J F, VanRossem R *et al.* (1996) Neonatal cranial ultrasound abnormalities in low birth weight infants: relation to cognitive outcomes at six years of age *Pediatrics* 98:719–729.

Wilcken D L(1997) MTHFER 677C → T mutation, folate intake, neural-tube-defects, and the risk of cardiovascular disease. *Lancet* 350:603–604.

Wild J, Read A P, Sheppard S *et al.* (1986) Recurrent neural tube defects, risk factors and vitamins. *Arch Dis Childhood* 61:440–444.

Williams J C, Barratt-Boyes B G & Lowe J B (1961) Supravalvular aortic stenosis. *Circulation* 24:1311–1318.

Williams R J, Odaibo F S, McGee J M (1999) Incidence of fetal alcohol syndrome in northeastern Manitoba. *Can J Pub Health. Revue Canadienne de Sante Publique.* 90(3):192–194.

Wisniewski K E, Wisniewski H M & Wen G Y (1985) Occurrence of Alzheimer neuropathology and dementia in Down syndrome. *Ann Neurol* 17:278–282.

Wohrle D, Kotzot D, Hirst M C *et al.* (1992) A microdeletion of less than 250 kb, including the proximal part of the FMR-1 gene and the fragile site, in a male with the clinical phenotype of fragile X sysdrome. *Am J Hum Genet* 51:299–306.

World Health Organization (1980) *International classification of impairments, disabilities and handicaps.* Geneva: World Health Organization.

World Health Organization (1992) *ICD-10 International statistical classification of diseases and related health problems, 10th revision.* Geneva: World Health Organization.

Yeargin-Allsopp M, Murphy C C, Cordero J F *et al.* (1997) Reported biomedical causes and associated medical conditions for mental retardation among 10-year-old children, metropolitan Atlanta, 1985 to 1987. *Dev Med Child Neurol* 39:142–149.

Youn G & Youn S (1991) Influence of training and performance IQ on the psychomotor skill of Down syndrome persons. *Percept Motor Skills* 73:1191–1194.

Yu S, Pritchard M, Kremer E *et al.* (1991) Fragile X genotype characterized by an unstable region of DNA. *Science* 252:1179–1181.

Zaman S S, Khan N Z, Durkin M S *et al.* (1992) *Childhood disabilities in Bangladesh.* Dhaka: Protibondhi Foundation.

Zigler E, Balla D & Hodapp R (1984) On the definition and classification of mental retardation. *Am J Ment Defici* 89:215–230.

Zigman W B, Schupf N, Sersen E *et al.* (1996) Prevalence of dementia in adults with and without Down syndrome. *Am J Ment Retard* 100:403–412.

Zuo Q H, Zhang Z X, Li Z *et al.* (1986) An epidemiological study on mental retardation among children in Chang-Qiao area of Beijing. *Chinese Med J* 99:9–14.

# Section XIII
# Ethical dilemmas

# Chapter 49 Issues for the obstetrician

F. A. Chervenak and L. B. McCullough

## INTRODUCTION

Ethics is an essential dimension of fetal neurology and neurosurgery, as it is of other specialty and subspecialty aspects of medical practice. In this chapter, we provide an account of obstetric ethics and address the important clinical concept of the fetus as a patient. With this background, we then consider the ethical and clinical dimensions of the obstetric management options for pregnancies complicated by fetal neurologic anomalies and disorders. These management options include aggressive management, abortion, termination of pregnancy during the third trimester, and non-aggressive management. We close with a consideration of cephalocentesis with its complex ethical dimensions.

## OBSTETRICS ETHICS

### ETHICS

Ethics as an intellectual discipline can be distinguished from morals or morality. Ethics is the disciplined study of morality. Morality concerns both right and wrong behaviour and good and bad character. The basic question that ethics addresses is, 'What ought morality to be?' This question entails two further questions, 'What ought our behavior to be?', and 'What virtues ought to be cultivated in our moral lives?' Ethics in obstetric practice addresses these same questions, focusing on what morality ought to be for obstetricians (McCullough & Chervenak 1994).

The bedrock for what morality ought to be in clinical practice for centuries has been the physician's obligation to protect and promote the interests of the patient (Beauchamp & Childress 1989). This is a fairly general ethical obligation. It therefore needs to be made more specific if it is to be clinically useful. This specification can be accomplished by attending to two perspectives in terms of which the patient's interests can be understood: that of the physician and that of the patient (McCullough & Chervenak 1994).

### BENEFICENCE AND RESPECT FOR AUTONOMY

In the history of Western medical ethics, the older of these two perspectives on the interests of patients is a rigorous clinical perspective. On the basis of scientific knowledge, shared clinical experience, and a careful, unbiased evaluation of the patient, the physician should identify clinical strategies that will most likely serve the health-related interests of the patient and those that should not be expected to do so. The health-related interests of the patient include preventing premature death and preventing, curing, or at least managing disease, injury, handicap, or unnecessary pain and suffering. This is because these matters are constitutive of any patient's health-related interests; they are functions of the competencies of medicine as a social institution. The identification of a patient's health-related interests should not be a function of the personal or subjective outlook of a particular physician but rather of rigorous clinical judgment about the fetal patient's condition.

The ethical principle of beneficence structures obstetric clinical judgment about the interests of the patient in that it obliges the physician to seek the greater balance of goods over harms for the health of both the pregnant woman and the fetal patient. On the basis of rigorous clinical judgment, the obstetrician should identify those clinical strategies that are reliably expected to result in the greater balance of goods, i.e. the protection and promotion of health-related interests, over harms, i.e. impairments of those interests.

The principle of beneficence in obstetrics should be clearly distinguished from the ethical principles of non-maleficence, commonly known as *Primum non nocere* or *First, do no harm* (Beauchamp & Childress 1989) Contrary to the common belief among physicians, *Primum non nocere* does not appear in the Hippocratic Oath or in the texts that accompany the Oath. The principle of beneficence was the primary consideration of the Hippocratic writers (Hippocrates 1923).

There are good reasons to be skeptical about the adequacy of *Primum non nocere* as a basic principle of obstetric ethics. If *Primum non nocere* were to become the basic principle of obstetric ethics, virtually all of obstetric practice would be unethical because virtually all medical interventions involve unavoidable risks of harm. *Primum non nocere* is therefore superseded in obstetric ethics by the principle of beneficence. The latter is sufficient to alert the physician to those circumstances in which a clinical intervention has the potential on balance to harm a patient: when a clinical intervention is on balance harmful to a patient, it should not be employed. That is, *Primum non nocere*, as a corollary of beneficence, makes it obligatory not to act in a way that is only harmful. As Strong (1987) puts it, there is a powerful beneficence-based prohibition against killing. This is obviously of direct relevance to the ethical evaluation of cephalocentesis in beneficence-based clinical judgment, as we shall see below.

The physician's perspective on the interests of the patient is only one of two legitimate perspectives on those interests. The perspective of the patient on the patient's interests is at least equally worthy of consideration by the physician (McCullough & Chervenak 1994). Each patient has developed a set of values and beliefs according to which she is to be presumed capable of making judgments about what will and will not protect and promote her interests. It is commonplace that in other aspects of her life, the patient regularly makes such judgments concerning matters of considerable complexity, e.g. choosing a professional calling, rearing and educating children, purchasing property, and writing a will of property. Despite the complexity of these and many other decisions of daily life, she is rightly assumed to be competent to make them, with the burden of proof on anyone who would challenge her competence.

The same is true about health-care decisions made by the pregnant woman. She should be assumed by her obstetrician to be competent to determine which clinical strategies serve her interests and which do not. In making such judgments, it is important to note that the pregnant woman will utilize values and beliefs that can range beyond the scope of health-related interests, e.g. religious beliefs or beliefs about how many children she wants to have. Beneficence-based clinical judgment, because it rests on the competencies of medicine, provides no authoritative basis for assessing the worth or meaning to the patient of the patient's non-health-related interests. These are matters for the patient alone to determine. Those values and beliefs help shape the patient's perspective on her interests.

The ethical significance of this perspective is expressed by the ethical principle of respect for autonomy. This ethical principle obligates the physician to respect the integrity of the patient's values and beliefs, to respect her perspective on her interests, and to implement only those clinical strategies authorized by her as the result of the informed consent process unless there is some overriding, well-established objection to doing so. Respect for autonomy is put into clinical practice by the informed consent process, which is usually understood to have three elements: (1) disclosure by the physician to the patient of adequate information about the patient's condition and its management; (2) understanding of that information by the patient; (3) a voluntary decision by the patient to authorize or refuse clinical management (Faden & Beauchamp 1986).

The physician obviously has both beneficence-based and autonomy-based obligations to the pregnant patient (McCullough & Chervenak 1994). The physician's perspective on the pregnant woman's interests provides the basis for beneficence-based obligations owed to her. Her own perspective on those interests provides the basis for autonomy-based obligations owed to her. Because of an insufficiently developed central nervous system, the fetus cannot meaningfully be said to possess values and beliefs. There is therefore no biological or conceptual basis for saying that a fetus has a perspective on its interests. There can therefore be no autonomy-based obligations to any fetus (Chervenak & McCullough 1985, 1990; McCullough & Chervenak 1994). Hence, the language of fetal rights has little or no meaning in obstetric ethics, despite its popularity in public and political discourse. This point cannot be overemphasized in obstetric ethics. This chapter, therefore, makes no further reference to fetal rights. Obviously, the physician has a perspective on the fetus's health-related interests, and the physician can have beneficence-based obligations to the fetus, but only when the fetus is a patient. Because of its importance for obstetric ethics generally and the ethics of destructive procedures in obstetrics, the concept of the fetus as a patient requires detailed consideration.

## THE CONCEPT OF THE FETUS AS A PATIENT

The concept of 'the fetus as a patient' has recently developed largely as a consequence of developments in fetal diagnosis and management strategies to optimize fetal outcome (Lorber & Zachary 1968; Rubin *et al.* 1972; Raimondi & Soare 1974; Sutton *et al.* 1980; McCullough *et al.* 1982), including those discussed elsewhere in this volume, and has become widely accepted (Fletcher 1981; Harrison *et al.* 1984; Chervenak & McCullough 1991). This obstetric-ethics concept has considerable clinical significance because, when the fetus is a patient, directive counseling, i.e. recommending a form of management, for fetal benefit would seem to be appropriate and, when the fetus is not a patient, non-directive counseling, i.e. offering, but not recommending, a form of management, would seem to be appropriate. However, these apparently straightforward roles for directive and non-directive counseling are often difficult to apply in clinical practice because of uncertainty about when the fetus is a patient. One approach to resolving this uncertainty would be to argue that the fetus is or is not a patient in virtue of personhood (Engelhardt 1986; Strong 1987), or some other form of independent moral status (Dunstan 1984; Elias & Annas 1987; Evans *et al.* 1988). We will show that this approach fails to resolve the uncertainty, and we will therefore defend an alternative approach that does resolve the uncertainty.

### THE INDEPENDENT MORAL STATUS OF THE FETUS

One fairly prominent approach for establishing whether or not the fetus is a patient has involved attempts over many centuries to show whether or not the fetus has independent moral status. The concept of the independent moral status for the fetus means that one or more characteristics that the fetus is thought to possess in and of itself and, therefore, independently of the pregnant woman or any other factor generate and therefore ground obligations to the fetus on the part of the pregnant woman and her physician.

A wide variety of characteristics have been nominated for this role in the history of the debate on the moral status of the fetus. These include the 'moment' of conception, implantation, central nervous system development, quickening, and the 'moment' of birth (Hellegers 1970; Noonan 1990; Curran 1978; Chervenak & McCullough 1987). Given the variability of proposed characteristics, there have been, and are, markedly varied views about when the fetus acquires independent moral status. Some take the view that the fetus has independent moral status from the moment of conception or implantation (Noonan 1979; Bopp 1984). Others believe that independent moral status is acquired in degrees, thus resulting in 'graded' moral status (Dunstan 1984; Evans *et al.* 1987). Still others hold, at least by implication, that the fetus never has independent moral status so long as it is *in utero* (Elias & Annas 1987).

Despite a continuing and enormous theologic and philosophical literature on this subject, stretching over more than 2000 years, there has been no closure on a single, intellectually authoritative account of the independent moral status of the fetus (Roe v. Wade 1973; Callahan & Callahan 1984). This is not a surprising outcome: given the absence of a single methodology that would be authoritative for all of the markedly diverse theologic and philosophical schools of thought involved in this endless debate, closure is impossible. For closure ever to be possible, debates about such a final intellectual authority within and between theologic and philosophical traditions would have to be resolved in a way satisfactory to all. Because this is an inconceivable event, it is best to abandon futile attempts to understand the fetus as a patient in terms of independent moral status of the fetus and turn to an alternative approach that identifies ethically distinct senses of the fetus as a patient and their clinical implications for obstetric practice.

## BENEFICENCE-BASED OBLIGATIONS TO THE FETUS

This alternative approach starts with the recognition that being a patient does not require that one possesses independent moral status. Rather, being a patient means that one can benefit from the applications of the clinical skills of the physician. Put more precisely, a human being without independent moral status is properly regarded as a patient when two conditions are met: that (a) a human being is presented to the physician, and (b) there exist clinical interventions that are reliably expected to be efficacious, in that they are reliably expected to result in a greater balance of goods over harms for the human being in question. (Of course, if the woman's body is a necessary condition, then her consent is necessary) (Chervenak & McCullough 1991; McCullough & Chervenak 1994).

The authors have argued elsewhere that beneficence-based obligations to the fetus exist when the fetus can later achieve independent moral status (McCullough & Chervenak 1994). That is, the fetus is a patient when the fetus is presented to the physician, and there exist medical interventions, whether diagnostic or therapeutic, that reasonably can be expected to result in a greater balance of goods over harms for the fetus now and/or in its future. The moral status of the fetus as a patient depends on links that can be established between the fetus *in utero* and its being reliably expected to achieve independent moral status.

One such link is viability, introducing the first application of the concept of the fetus as a patient. Viability should not be understood as an intrinsic property of the fetus because viability must be understood in terms of both biologic and technologic factors (Roe v. Wade 1973; Fost *et al.* 1980; Fletcher 1981). Both factors result in a viable fetus that can exist *ex utero* and then achieve independent moral status. It is important to note that these two factors do not exist as a function of the autonomy of the pregnant woman. When a fetus is viable, i.e. when it is of sufficient maturity so that it can survive into the neonatal period and later achieve independent moral status, given the availability of the requisite technologic support, and when it is presented to the physician, the fetus is a patient. The fetus at term is a patient when the pregnant woman presents herself to a physician or a hospital or clinic for obstetric services.

Viability exists as a function of biomedical and technologic capacities, which are different in different parts of the world. As a consequence, there is, at the present time, no world-wide, uniform gestational age to define viability. In the United States, the authors believe, viability presently occurs at approximately 24 weeks of gestational age (Chervenak & McCullough 1997). It follows directly from this sense of the fetus as a patient that destructive procedures on the at-term fetal patient, cephalocentesis in particular, must be ethically justified, a task to which we turn in the next section.

The only possible link between the previable fetus and the child it can become is the pregnant woman's autonomy, introducing the second clinical application of the concept of the fetus as a patient. This is because technologic factors cannot result in the previable fetus becoming a child. This is simply what previable means. The link, therefore, between a fetus and the child it can become, when the fetus is previable, can be established only by the pregnant woman's decision to confer the status of being a patient on her previable fetus. The previable fetus, therefore, has no claim to the status of being a patient independently of the pregnant woman's autonomy. The pregnant woman is free to withhold, confer, or, having once conferred, withdraw the status of being a patient on or from her previable fetus according to her own values and beliefs. The previable fetus is presented to the physician solely as a function of the pregnant woman's autonomy. This has important ethical implications for a range of ethical issues in obstetrics, including antenatal diagnosis and abortion (Hellegers 1970).

## MANAGEMENT OPTIONS FOR PREGNANCIES COMPLICATED BY FETAL NEUROLOGIC ANOMALIES AND DISORDERS

Before viability, the management of a pregnancy complicated by fetal neurologic anomalies and disorders is ethically straightforward. The pregnant woman is free to withhold or withdraw the moral status of being a patient from any previable fetus including that with such anomalies or disorders. When such an anomaly is detected, counseling should therefore be rigorously directive. The woman should be given the choice between abortion and continuing her pregnancy to viability and thus to term. If the woman elects an abortion, it should be performed or an appropriate referral made. If the woman elects to continue her pregnancy, she should be apprised about decisions that will need to be made later, such as Cesarean delivery for fetal indications (McCullough & Chervenak 1994).

After viability, aggressive management is the ethical standard of care. By aggressive management, we mean optimizing perinatal outcome by utilizing effective antepartum and intrapartum diagnostic and therapeutic modalities.

One important exception to aggressive management is termination of pregnancy after the usual gestational age of fetal viability. This exception applies when there is: (1) certainty of diagnosis and either (2a) certainty of death as an outcome of the anomaly diagnosed or (2b) in some cases of short-term survival, certainty of the absence of cognitive developmental capacity as an outcome of the anomaly diagnosed (McCullough & Chervenak 1994). When these criteria are satisfied, recommending a choice between non-aggressive management and termination of pregnancy is justified. Anencephaly is a classic example of a fetal neurologic anomaly that satisfies these criteria.

A second exception to aggressive management is non-aggressive management. This exception applies when there is: (1) a very high probability but sometimes less than complete certainty about the diagnosis and either (2a) a very high probability of death as an outcome of the anomaly diagnosed or (2b) survival with a very high probability of severe and irreversible deficit of cognitive developmental capacity as a result of the anomaly diagnosed (Beauchamp & Childress 1989). When these two criteria apply, both aggressive and non-aggressive management can be justified, from which it follows that a choice between aggressive or non-aggressive management, but not termination, can be recommended. Encephalocele is a classic example of a fetal neurologic anomaly that satisfies these criteria.

A third important and ethically complex exception to aggressive management is cephalocentesis.

## CEPHALOCENTESIS FOR INTRAPARTUM MANAGEMENT OF HYDROCEPHALUS

Cephalocentesis is the drainage of an enlarged fetal head, secondary to hydrocephalus (Chervenak & Romero 1984). Fetal hydrocephalus is caused by obstruction of cerebrospinal flow and is diagnosed by such sonographic signs as dilatation of the atrium or body of the lateral ventricles (Chervenak *et al.* 1993). In the third trimester, macrocephaly often accompanies the ventriculomegaly. In addition, sonography can diagnose hydrocephalus in association with gross abnormalities suggestive of poor prognosis, for example, hydranencephaly, microcephaly, encephalocele, alobar holoprosencephaly, or thanatophoric dysplasia with cloverleaf skull (Chervenak *et al.* 1993). (See chapters in Section 1 of this volume.) In the absence of defined anatomical abnormalities, however, diagnostic imaging is, at the present time, unable to predict the outcome. Although cortical mantle thickness can be measured with ultrasound, its value as a prognostic index is not established (Chervenak *et al.* 1993).

Cephalocentesis should be performed under simultaneous ultrasound guidance so that needle placement into the cerebrospinal fluid is facilitated. An 18-gauge needle is used with collapse of the cranial bones, the endpoint for this procedure. Enough fluid is drained to permit reduction of the skull diameters so that passage through the birth canal is possible (Chervenak *et al.* 1985; Clark *et al.* 1985).

Cephalocentesis is a potentially destructive procedure. Perinatal death following cephalocentesis has been reported in over 90% of cases (Chervenak & Romero 1984). The sonographic visualization of intracranial bleeding curing cephalocentesis, and the demonstration of this hemorrhage at autopsy, further emphasize the morbid nature of the procedure. However, if decompression is performed in a controlled manner, the mortality may be reduced (Birnholz & Frigoletto 1981).

Because fetal hydrocephalus is the product of varied etiologies having varied outcomes, ethical analysis must be carried out by respecting the heterogeneity of this condition (Chervenak *et al.* 1993). Therefore, we consider resolution clinical management strategies for two extremes of the continuum between isolated fetal hydrocephalus and fetal hydrocephalus with severe associated abnormalities (those incompatible with postnatal survival or those characterized by the virtual absence of cognitive function). We then consider fetal hydrocephalus with milder associated abnormalities as a middle ground on the continuum. The proposed analysis of each of these situations takes place in the following steps. First, we identify the beneficence-based and autonomy-based obligations of the physician to the pregnant woman and the fetal patient. Second, we identify the conflicts that can occur among these obligations. Third, we weigh these obligations against each other in an attempt to arrive at a balance among conflicting obligations to guide clinical judgement and intervention.

## ISOLATED FETAL HYDROCEPHALUS

We begin the clinical and ethical analysis of isolated fetal hydrocephalus by noting that there is considerable potential for normal, sometimes superior, intellectual function for fetuses with even extreme, isolated hydrocephalus (Lorber 1968; Raimondi & Soare 1974; McCullough & Balzer-Martin 1982; Sutton *et al.* 1980). However, as a group, infants with isolated hydrocephalus experience a greater incidence of mental retardation and early death than the general population. In addition, associated anomalies may go undetected, and a fetus may be incorrectly diagnosed as having isolated hydrocephalus (Chervenak *et al.* 1985; Nyberg *et al.* 1987). One thing is clear in obstetric ethics: a viable at-term fetus with isolated hydrocephalus is a fetal patient, because neither of the two exceptions described above apply, given the variable outcomes of isolated hydrocephalus.

There are compelling, beneficence-based ethical reasons for concluding that continuing existence of fetuses with isolated hydrocephalus is in their interests. Beneficence directs the physician to prevent mortality and morbidity for the fetal patient. Beneficence also directs the physician to undertake interventions that ameliorate handicapping conditions such as mental retardation. The probability of mental retardation does not diminish the interests of the fetal patient with isolated hydrocephalus in continuing existence because (1) it is impossible to predict which fetuses with isolated hydrocephalus will have mental retardation and (2) the degree of mental retardation cannot be predicted in advance.

In light of this ethical analysis of the at-term fetal patient's interests, the beneficence-based obligation of the physician caring for the fetus is to recommend strongly, and to attain, the woman's consent to perform a Cesarean delivery because this clinical intervention clearly involves the least risk of mortality, morbidity, and handicap for the fetus compared with cephalocentesis to permit subsequent vaginal delivery. Even when performed under maximal therapeutic conditions (i.e. under sonographic guidance), cephalocentesis cannot reasonably be regarded as protecting or promoting the interests of the fetal patient with isolated hydrocephalus. This procedure is followed by a high rate of perinatal mortality, fetal heart rate deceleration, and pathologic evidence of intracranial bleeding (Chervenak *et al.* 1985; Nyberg *et al.* 1987). As a consequence, cephalocentesis cannot reasonably be construed as an ethically justifiable mode of management, in so far as it is inconsistent with beneficence-based obligations to avoid increased mortality and morbidity risks for the fetal patient. Cephalocentesis, employed with a destructive intent, is altogether antithetical to these beneficence-based prohibition against killing.

It is essential in obstetric ethics that beneficence-based obligations to the fetal patient be balanced against beneficence-based and autonomy-based obligations to the pregnant woman. First, the physician has a beneficence-based obligation to avoid performing a Cesarean delivery because the possibility of morbidity and mortality for the woman is higher than that associated with vaginal delivery. Respect for autonomy obligates the physician to undertake only those interventions or forms of treatment to which the woman has given voluntary, informed consent. Informed consent is grounded in an autonomy-based right of the pregnant woman to control what happens to her body. In particular, the woman has the right to authorize or refuse operative intervention – those that are, as well as those that are not, consistent with the physician's beneficence-based obligations (McCullough & Chervenak 1994).

We are now in a position to consider the full complexity of the management of the fetal patient with isolated hydrocephalus: beneficence-based and autonomy-based obligations to the pregnant woman, as well as beneficence-based obligations to her fetus, must all be considered for clinical ethical judgment to be complete and therefore reliable. If, with informed consent, the woman authorizes Cesarean delivery, there is no conflict among these obligations. The autonomy-based obligation to act on informed consent overrides the beneficence-based obligations to the pregnant woman that were identified earlier.

By contrast, her physician faces a significant and challenging ethical conflict if the woman refuses Cesarean delivery. Two clinical interventions, each with substantial ethical justification in beneficence-based and autonomy-based clinical judgment, can be employed in intrapartum management. On the one hand, the physician has an autonomy-based obligation to the pregnant woman to perform cephalocentesis followed by vaginal delivery. On the other hand, cephalocentesis violates beneficence-based obligations to the fetal at-term patient. This conflict should be resolved in favor of the beneficence-based obligations to the fetal patient. These obligations properly override beneficence-based and autonomy-based obligations to the woman because the harm to the fetal patient is final, namely, death, and will occur with high probability. Moreover, if the fetal patient survives (death is not guaranteed by cephalocentesis), it is likely to be more damaged due to intracranial hemorrhage than if Cesarean delivery is performed. Morbidity and mortality of the pregnant woman are both minimal and therefore risks that she ought to accept to protect the fetal patient's interest (McCullough & Chervenak 1994). Such ethical conflict should be prevented by employing the preventive ethics strategies of informed consent as an ongoing dialogue, negotiation, respectful persuasion, and the proper use of ethics committees (Chervenak & McCullough 1990a; McCullough & Chervenak 1994).

If these preventive ethics strategies do not succeed and the pregnant woman continues to refuse Cesarean delivery, the physician confronts tragic circumstances. If neither Cesarean delivery nor cephalocentesis is performed, the woman is at risk for uterine rupture and death, and the fetal patient is at risk for death. This logic of beneficence-based obligations is to prevent such total and irreversible harm. Therefore, we believe that because of the grave nature of possible consequences for the woman and her fetus, because of the dangers for the woman of performing a surgical procedure on a resistant patient, and because of the pitfalls of attempted legal coercion, the physician should act on beneficence-based obligations to the woman in such an extreme circumstance. In addition, failure to respect an unwavering, voluntary, and informed refusal of a Cesarean delivery would count as a fundamental assault on the woman's autonomy. The fetal patient is at high risk for death under either alternative. The woman's death, at least, can be avoided. Serious beneficence-based obligations to the fetal patient on the part of both the physician and the pregnant woman will probably be violated, and a needless death will most probably result, however, by performing a cephalocentesis. Herein lies the tragedy of these circumstances. To avoid this tragedy, redoubled efforts of preventive ethics should be undertaken. In one author's (F.A.C.) experience, carefully explaining the fact that cephalocentesis does not guarantee death and may produce a worse outcome is very powerfully persuasive. In those rare cases in which this effort at respectful persuasion fails, cephalocentesis should be performed in the least destructive way possible or an appropriate referral made.

## HYDROCEPHALUS WITH SEVERE ASSOCIATED ABNORMALITIES

Some abnormalities that occur in association with fetal hydrocephalus are severe in nature for the child afflicted with them. We define 'severe' abnormalities as those that are either (1) incompatible with continued existence, e.g. bilateral renal agenesis or thanatophoric dysplasia with cloverleaf skull or (2) compatible with survival in some cases but result in virtual absence of cognitive function, e.g. trisomy 18 or alobar holoprosencephaly (Chervenak *et al.* 1985; Chervenak & McCullough 1990b). Because there is no available intervention to prevent postnatal death in the first group, beneficence-based obligations of the physician and the pregnant woman to attempt to prolong the life of the fetal patient are non-existent. No ethical theory and no version of obstetric ethics based on beneficence and respect for autonomy obligate the physician to attempt the impossible. For the second group, beneficence-based obligations of the physician and the pregnant woman to sustain the life of the fetal patient are minimal because the handicap imposed by the abnormality is severe. In these cases, the potential for cognitive development – and therefore the achievement of other 'good' for the child, e.g. relationships with others – are virtually absent. Such fetuses are fetal patients to which there are owed only minimal beneficence-based obligations.

In these circumstances, the woman is therefore released from her beneficence-based obligations to the at-term fetal patient to place herself at risk, because no significant good can be achieved by Cesarean delivery for the fetal patient or the child it will become. There remain only the autonomy-based and beneficence-based obligations of the physician to the pregnant woman. After the preceding analysis of these obligations, we conclude that the physician's overriding moral obligations are to the pregnant woman's voluntary and informed decision about employment of cephalocentesis.

Because there are no weighty beneficence-based obligations to the fetus in such clinical and ethical circumstances, the physician may justifiably recommend a choice between Cesarean delivery and cephalocentesis to enable vaginal delivery. Cesarean delivery permits women who wish to do so to have a live birth and satisfy religious convictions or help with the grieving process. A Cesarean delivery performed in this clinical setting is best viewed as an autonomy-based maternal indication. The strategy of offering a choice also avoids the potential negative consequences for maternal health of Cesarean delivery. Because the prognosis for infants with hydrocephalus associated with severe anomalies is poor, we believe that intrapartum fetal death resulting from cephalocentesis would not be a tragic outcome as it might be in the death of a fetal patient with isolated hydrocephalus.

## HYDROCEPHALUS WITH OTHER ASSOCIATED ANOMALIES

On the continuum between the extreme cases of isolated hydrocephalus and hydrocephalus with severe associated abnormalities, there are a variety of cases of hydrocephalus associated with other abnormalities with varying degrees of impairment of cognitive physical function. They range from hypoplastic distal phalanges to spina bifida to encephalocele (Lorber & Zachary 1968; Chervenak *et al.* 1998). Because these conditions have varying prognoses, it would be clinically inappropriate and, therefore, ethically misleading to treat this third category as homogeneous. Therefore, we propose a working distinction between different kinds of prognoses. The first we call 'probably promising', by which we mean that there is a significant possibility that the child will experience cognitive development with learning disabilities and physical handicaps that perhaps can be ameliorated to some extent. The second we call 'probably poor'. By this phrase, we mean that there is only a limited possibility for cognitive development because of learning disabilities and physical handicaps that cannot be ameliorated to a significant extent. We propose these definitions as tentative, so they are subject to revision as clinical and ethical investigations of such associated anomalies continue. As a consequence, our ethical analysis of these two categories cannot be carried out as extensively as those in the previous two sections. In essence, we propose that the clinical continuum in these cases is paralleled by an ethical continuum or progressively less weighty, beneficence-based obligations to the fetus. Such at-term fetuses are indeed fetal patients.

When the prognosis is probably promising, e.g. isolated arachnoid cyst, there are serious beneficence-based obligations to the fetal patient. However, they are not necessarily on the same order as those that occur in cases of isolated hydrocephalus. [It has been suggested that any associated anomaly may increase the possibility of a poor outcome (Chervenak *et al.* 1985)]. Therefore, in such cases with a prognosis of probably promising, we propose that the physician recommend Cesarean delivery, although perhaps not as vigorously as in cases of isolated hydrocephalus. A pregnant woman's informed refusal of Cesarean delivery should therefore be respected.

In cases when the prognosis, even though uncertain, is probably poor, e.g. encephalocele, beneficence-based obligations to the fetal patient are less weighty than those owed to the fetal patient with a promising prognosis. These cases, then, resemble ethically those of hydrocephalus with severe anomalies, with the proviso that some, albeit limited, benefits can be achieved for the fetal patient by Cesarean delivery and aggressive perinatal treatment. None the less, the physician may in these cases justifiably accept an informed voluntary decision by the woman for cephalocentesis followed by vaginal delivery. However, the physician cannot assume an advocacy role for such a decision with the same level of ethical confidence that he or she can in cases of hydrocephalus associated with severe anomalies.

## CONCLUSION

Ethics is an essential dimension of the obstetric management of pregnancies complicated by fetal neurologic anomalies and disorders. This chapter has provided an ethical framework for obstetric ethics and practical guidance, based on that framework, for the management of pregnancies complicated by such fetal anomalies and disorders. In the authors' view, managing pregnancies complicated by fetal neurologic anomalies without careful attention to their ethical dimension is clinically inappropriate.

### Key Points

- Ethics is an essential dimension of fetal neurology and neurosurgery.
- The concept of the fetus as a patient is basic to fetal medicine.
- The previable fetus is a patient solely as a function of the pregnant woman's decision to confer this status.
- The viable fetus is a patient when (a) it is presented to the physician and (b) there exist clinical interventions that are reliably expected to be effacacious.
- Before viability counseling about the management of pregnancy complicated by CNS anomalies should be non-directive.
- After viability aggressive management for fetal benefit is the ethical standard of care, with three exceptions:
  - Termination of pregnancy
  - Non-aggressive management
  - Cephalocentesis.

## REFERENCES


Beauchamp T L & Childress J F (1994) *Principles of biomedical ethics.* 4th ed. New York: Oxford University Press.

Birnholz J C & Frigoletto F D (1981) Antenatal treatment of hydrocephalus. *N Engl J Med* 104: 1021.

Bopp J (1984) *Restoring the right to life: The Human Life Amendment.* Provo: Brigham Young University.

Callahan S & Callahan D (1984) *Abortion: understanding differences.* New York: Plenum Press.

Chervenak F A & Romero R (1984) Is there a role for fetal cephalocentesis in modern obstetrics? *Am J Perinatol* 1: 170–173.

✪ Chervenak F A & McCullough L B (1985) Perinatal ethics: A practical method of analysis of obligations to mother and fetus. *Obstet Gynecol* 66: 442–446.

Chervenak F A & McCullough L B (1990) Does obstetric ethics have any role in the obstetrician's response to the abortion controversy? *Am J Obstet Gynecol* 163: 1425–1429.

Chervenak F A & McCullough L B (1990a) Clinical guides to preventing ethical conflicts between pregnant women and their physicians. *Am J Obstet Gynecol* 162: 303–307.

✪ Chervenak F A & McCullough L B (1990b) An ethically justified.clinically comprehensive management strategy for third-trimester pregnancies complicated by fetal anomalies. *Obstet Gynecol* 75: 311–316.

✪ Chervenak F A & McCullough L B (1991) The fetus as patient: implications for directive versus nondirective counseling for fetal benefit. *Fetal Diagn Ther* 6: 93–100.

Chervenak F A, Isaacson G & Campbell S (1993) *Anomalies of the cranium and its contents. Textbook of ultrasound in obstetrics and gynecology.* pp. 825–852. Boston: Little.Brown.

Chervenak F A & McCullough L B (1997) The limits of viability. *J Perinat Med* 25: 418–420.

Chervenak F A, Berkowitz R L, Tortora M *et al.* (1985) Management of fetal hydrocephalus. *Am J Obstet Gynecol* 151: 933–937.

Clark S L, DeVore G R & Platt L D (1985) The role of ultrasound in the aggressive management of obstructed labor secondary to fetal malformations. *Am J Obstet Gynecol* 152: 1042–1044.

Curran C E (1978) Abortion: Contemporary debate in philosophical and religious ethics. In Reich.WT.ed. *Encyclopedia of Bioethics.* New York: Macmillan. pp. 17–26.

Dunstan G R (1984) The moral status of the human embryo. A tradition recalled. *J Med Ethics* 10: 38–44.

Elias S & Annas G J (1987) *Reproductive genetics and the law.* Chicago: Year Book Medical Publishers.

Engelhardt H T Jr. (1986) *The foundations of bioethics.* New York: Oxford University Press.

Evans M I, Fletcher J C, Zador I E *et al.* (1988) Selective first-trimester termination in octuplet and quadruplet pregnancies: Clinical and ethical issues. *Obstet Gynecol* 71: 289–296.

Faden R R & Beauchamp T L. (1986) *A history and theory of informed consent.* New York: Oxford University Press.

Fletcher J C (1981) The fetus as patient ethical issues. *JAMA* 246: 772–773.

Fost N, Chudwin D & Wikker D (1980) The limited moral significance of fetal viability. *Hastings Cent Rep* 10: 10–13.

Harrison M R, Golbus M S & Filly R A (1984) *The unborn patient.* New York: Grune & Stratton.

Hellegers A E (1970) Fetal development. *Theological Studies* 31: 3–9.

Jones W H S (trans) (1923) *Hippocrates. Epidemics i: xi.* Loeb Classical Library.vol. 147. Cambridge: Harvard University Press.

Lorber J (1968) The results of early treatment on extreme hydrocephalus. *Med Child Neurol* (Suppl) 16: 21.

Lorber J & Zachary R B (1968) Primary congenital hydrocephalus: long-term results of controlled therapeutic trial. *Arch Dis Child* 1968 43: 516.

McCullough D C & Balzer-Martin L A (1982) Current prognosis in overt neonatal hydrocephalus. *J Neurosurg* 57: 378.

✪ McCullough L B & Chervenak F A (1994) *Obstetric ethics.* New York: Oxford University Press.

Noonan J T (1970) *The morality of abortion.* Cambridge: Harvard University Press.

Noonan J T (1979) *A Private Choice. Abortion in America in the Seventies.* New York: The Free Press.

Nyberg DA, Mack LA, Hirsch J *et al.* (1987) Fetal hydrocephalus: sonographic detection and clinical significance of associated anomalies. *Radiology* 163: 187.

Raimondi A J & Soare P (1974) Intellectual development in shunted hydrocephalic children. *Am J Dis Child* 127: 664.

Roe v. Wade, 410 US 113 (1973).

Rubin R C, Hochwald G, Liwnicz B *et al.* (1972) The effect of severe hydrocephalus on size and number of brain cells. *Dev Med Child Neurol* 14: 118.

Strong C (1987) Ethical conflicts between mother and fetus in obstetrics. *Clin in Perinatology Perinat* 14: 313–328.

Sutton L N, Bruce D A & Schut L (1980) Hydranencephaly versus maximal hydrocephalus: an important clinical distinction. *Neurosurgery* 6: 35.

Chapter 50

# Ethical dilemmas – issues for the neonatologist

T. Stephenson

## INTRODUCTION

When faced with ethical decisions in the management of newborn babies (Kennedy 1981; Stinson & Stinson 1981; Campbell 1982; Anonymous 1986; Bissenden 1986; Rhein 1992), the actions of doctors will be directed by the wishes of the parents, the doctor's conscience, the advice of the medical protection societies and the law of the country in which they practise (in this chapter, all references are to United Kingdom law). There are three important moral philosophical points (Kuhse & Singer 1985).

## THE PRINCIPLE OF THE SANCTITY OF LIFE

> Most of us think it is wrong to kill people. Some think it is wrong in all circumstances, while others think that in special circumstances (say, in a just war or in self defence) some killing may be justified. The assumption is that killing can at best only be justified to avoid a greater evil.
>
> (Glover 1977)

Doctors practising 'conviction medicine' feel that not only is it wrong to take life but it is equally wrong to withhold maximal treatment. Doctors practising 'consensus medicine' may feel that their actions are influenced by parental wishes and prognosis, and that withdrawing maximal treatment can be seen as justified in order to avoid the 'greater evil' of an unacceptable quality of life.

## QUALITY OF LIFE

> In our view the most important medical criterion is the degree of abnormality of the central nervous system. If there is little or no prospect of brain function sufficient to allow a personal life of meaning and quality or no potential for development in harmony with Fletcher's indicators of humanhood, non-treatment seems the prudent course of action.
>
> Duff & Campbell (1973)

Fletcher's 'tentative profile of man' suggests that positive criteria for humanhood would include minimal intelligence, self-awareness, self-control, a sense of time, a sense of futurity and a sense of the past, the capability to relate to others, concern for others, communication, control of existence, and curiosity (Fletcher 1972). Baby J was born very preterm and was severely brain-damaged (Re J 1990). The court held that to continue invasive treatments would not be in his best interests because he 'suffered from physical disabilities so grave that his life would from his point of view be so intolerable' that if he were able to make a sound judgement, he would not choose treatment. The Court of Appeal ruled that baby J should not be put back on a ventilator if he fell critically ill.

When faced with this kind of dilemma, some doctors take a paternalistic attitude. They would argue that the child's parents, perhaps two young lay people with no previous experience of such situations, can never be sufficiently well informed to take such a difficult decision at a time when they are deeply emotionally upset. The doctor has the experience and knowledge to take this burden (Schultz 1992). Others argue for a more democratic process.

## ACTS OF COMMISSION AND OMISSION

Switching off a ventilator when a baby has very severe brain damage may result in the death of the baby. The baby's death is hastened (i.e. the timing of death) as a result of an act of omission (Autton 1985). There is a doctrine within moral philosophy, known as the 'acts and omissions doctrine', which states that there is a moral difference between causing death to happen through an action, and allowing the same thing to happen by failing to act. Intuitively, it seems right that causing death is a greater offence than letting someone die through inaction. The strongest demand on us is that we do not harm others (the duty of non-maleficence), whereas the duty to actively help others (the duty of beneficence) is usually recognized to be weaker (Farsides 1992). Doctors may decide not to treat a child and view this as different from deciding to end the child's life actively by a lethal injection (Byrne 1990), although the intention and consequences are equivalent (Glover 1977). It has been argued that, assuming the death is morally justifiable, then this should be done in the most humane way possible, irrespective of whether this involves killing the child or letting him or her die (Rachels 1975). However, the law rarely takes such an equal view of active and passive euthanasia. The legal formalization of euthanasia is most advanced in Holland (Hellema 1992).

> Clinicians engaged in terminal care would argue that they do not withhold treatment, they change treatment. They change it from a treatment for the living, to a treatment for the dying. The

> doctor has the moral tool of the double effect. Although his primary intention is to relieve suffering, it may be that death will predictably follow from the course of treatment adopted.
>
> (Autton 1985)

The aims of treatment are changed from cure to care. Care involves controlling pain, distress, and suffering of the patient. Morphine controls pain but may also expedite death. It cannot be emphasized enough that the withdrawal of treatment does not equate with the withdrawal of care (Winter & Cohen, 1999). In a case involving an adult in a 'permanent vegetative state' (Tresch *et al.* 1991), the court took the view that nasogastric feeding constituted a medical treatment, and therefore it was lawful to withdraw this treatment. If the patient could manage to swallow food, it is likely that the legal view would be that withdrawal of food would amount to starvation (Lennard-Jones 1999). The use of enteral tube feeding for preterm infants is regarded by some as analogous to a bottle feed and thus a part of basic care (McHaffie & Fowlie 1997), but this has not been tested in a UK court. UK courts have never considered a case of withdrawing artificial nutrition or hydration from patients who are not in PVS.

Withdrawal of treatment is not an unusual situation on a neonatal intensive care unit, and the doctors involved rarely seek the advice of the courts, although the Leonard Arthur case (Anonymous 1981a) and the baby Doe case (Kopelman *et al.* 1988) drew attention to the risks of such action. Practice in the neonatal setting may be different because defining brain death criteria (Pallis 1983) and 'persistent vegetative state' (Tresch *et al.* 1991) is more difficult. For children older than 2 months, the recommendations are similar to those for adults (British Paediatric Association 1991). The guidelines apply only to children who are comatose, totally apneic and requiring ventilation, the cause of brain damage is known, and the coma cannot be explained by drugs, hypothermia, or endocrine or metabolic disturbance. For children between 37 weeks' gestation and 2 months of age, the working party concluded that it would be rarely possible to diagnose brainstem death. In infants below 37 weeks' gestation, the working party concluded that the concept of brainstem death was inappropriate, and electrophysiologic assessment had little to offer over clinical assessment.

In summary, most doctors who care for newborn babies feel that there are occasions when a baby has a right to die (Anonymous 1981b). Doctors will often claim that 'every case is different'. 'It is one thing to justify an act; it is another to justify general practice' (Beauchamp & Childress 1989). There are five situations where the withholding or withdrawal of life-prolonging treatment might be considered (Royal College of Paediatrics and Child Health 1997):

- the brain dead child
- the persistent vegetative state
- the 'no chance' situation
- the 'no purpose' situation
- the 'unbearable situation'.

## DIAGNOSIS OF NEUROLOGIC AND NEUROSURGICAL PROBLEMS IMMEDIATELY AFTER DELIVERY

Where there is reasonable uncertainty about the benefits of treatment, there should be a presumption in favor of initiating it (British Medical Association Medical Ethics Committee 1999). Clinical intervention can be discontinued later after reflection and discussion with parents, although it is often easier to withhold a treatment than to withdraw it (Winter & Cohen 1999). Misperceptions may have arisen as a result of society's acceptance of abortion for serious handicap (Leigh 1990). Some doctors and some parents believe that late termination of pregnancy because of serious handicap means that more leeway should be allowed regarding withholding or withdrawing life-prolonging treatment from handicapped newborns (British Medical Association Medical Ethics Committee,1999).

The experience of managing neural-tube defects illustrates the dilemmas for clinicians. The follow-up of a policy of operating on all children with spina bifida showed that half died (Lorber 1972). Of the 424 survivors, six had no handicap, 73 had a moderate degree of handicap, and 345 had severe physical handicaps. If selective criteria had been used for intervention (see below), not a single moderately handicapped child or one with no handicap would have been lost. One great difficulty is that some babies with the severest physical handicaps had normal intelligence. The formal criteria put forward by Lorber were: severe paraplegia, gross enlargement of the head, kyphosis, and associated gross congenital anomalies or major birth injuries. If one or more of these adverse criteria are present, the position is discussed in detail with both parents together.

Once the decision is made, whether it is to treat or to allow to die, much support will be needed in the hospital and home (Forest *et al.* 1982). It appears that withdrawal of care is perceived as easier if there is a central nervous system problem than chronic lung disease or damaged bowel (Anonymous 1981b). Distress can be caused to the family if the professional staff are unaware of their religious customs, particularly as an approach will often be made to the family for a post-mortem (Green 1989).

The question of organ donation should be handled by a professional who is outside the team caring for the infant so that it is clear to the family that there is no conflict of interests. Tests for brainstem death are not appropriate for neonates, and therefore, organs are rarely obtained from living donors. The corneas and heart valves can be obtained up to 12 h after death. A request for organ donation or post-mortem should never be made until it has been agreed with the parents that treatment has failed, and withdrawal of treatment is imminent (Working Party of the Health Department of Great Britain and Northern Ireland 1983).

## DIAGNOSIS OF NEUROLOGIC AND NEUROSURGICAL PROBLEMS AFTER PROLONGED INTENSIVE CARE

The high-technology medicine that is practised in neonatal units runs a risk of being 'disease-oriented'. Each problem as it arises is attacked with all the skill and technology that is available (Duff & Campbell 1976). There is also the danger when multiple specialists are involved. Each specialist may give the utmost attention to a particular area of expertise, but a baby is not a constellation of separate organs but is a child in his or her own right. It is important that a single senior doctor takes overall responsibility for orchestrating the actions of the several specialists involved and liaising with the family (Brahams 1988). When caring for a baby at the very limits of viability, the parents must be given realistic information about the chances of mortality and morbidity (Chiswick 1990). Of babies born at less than 26 weeks' gestation and offered intensive care, survival rates to discharge are 2, 21, 33 and 52% at 22, 23, 24 and 25 weeks, respectively (Costeloe 1998). At 2 years, half have recognized disabilities.

It has been estimated that two-thirds of all deaths in a neonatal unit result from withdrawal of therapy (Balfour Lynn & Tasker 1996). Ultrasound examination of the neonatal brain helps in making these decisions, but there remain gray areas where the long-term outcome remains unclear (Levene 1990). Moreover, doctors use words such as 'probably', 'possible', or 'likely', but the lay public's interpretation of such concepts of statistical probability is not the same as that of the physician (Shaw & Dear 1990).

If a decision is made with the parents to allow the child to die, all the equipment is disconnected at a time of the parents' choosing. The child is placed in the parents' arms in a quiet room where freedom from interruption can be guaranteed. An alternative is to elect not to resuscitate the infant when he or she next deteriorates, but this is a less satisfactory strategy for both family and staff. The ethics of making decisions not to resuscitate have been well reviewed recently (Davies & Reynolds 1992a,b; Lloyd 1993). It is very important that parents are encouraged to see and hold their child after death (Finlay & Dallimore 1991). Palliative care should be continued until the child dies.

A difficult situation arises if the parents' views are at odds with those of the doctors or nurses caring for the child. In the author's experience, this is very rare provided the parents are involved in all discussions and given time to reach a view (McCall Smith 1992). When this does happen, the doctor should ask five questions (Dunn 1990):

- Do the parents understand the prognosis?
- Should they consult with others?
- Do they require more time?
- Is their decision in the interests of the child?
- Is their decision so unreasonable in terms of benefit to the child as to request them to seek a second opinion or for the doctor to seek the advice of the courts?

Conflict may also arise within the clinical team or between the two parents (Royal College of Paediatrics and Child Health, 1997). Those with parental responsibility for a baby are, in general, legally and morally entitled to give or withhold consent to treatment. Their decision will usually be determinative unless they conflict seriously with the views of the clinical team on the child's best interests (British Medical Association Medical Ethics Committee, 1999). However, parents cannot insist on enforcing decisions based solely on their own preferences where these conflict with good medical evidence. For desperate parents to expose fatally ill children to painful, unproven, or futile treatments breaches the child's rights. The doctor's first duty is to the patient. If a conflict cannot be resolved after a reasonable time period, a court may provide guidance on whether life-prolonging treatment would benefit the child, taking into account the 1989 Children Act (Hendrick Elton *et al.* 1995; Kurtz 1995). In Re R (1993), the court invoked the Children Act to authorize blood transfusion to treat a child, against the parents' religious beliefs. However, each case is different. The High Court in the UK has both endorsed a doctor's decision to withhold ventilation and refrain from resuscitating a child against the parents wishes (Re C 1998) and also upheld the parents' refusal to consent to surgery against the advice of doctors (Re T 1997). Two babies with apparently similar medical conditions may have different decisions made about them (Sherlock 1979) because of other factors related to parental wishes and beliefs.

Finally, it is very important that a senior member of staff writes to the family after the child's death and offers to see them in privacy away from the place where the child died. By this time, the full results of the post-mortem will be available, and the intervening period also allows the parents time to decide about any issues they would like to discuss.

## CONCLUSION

In tackling the ethical dilemmas of lifesaving intervention in the newborn, the clinician must always act in the best interests of the child. Potential conflicts with this guiding principle include:

- the interests of the child versus those of the parents or the state
- ethics versus economics
- heroic management versus humanitarianism.

**Key Points**

- There are five situations where the withholding or withdrawal of life-prolonging treatment might be considered:
  - The brain dead child
  - The persistent vegetative state
  - The 'no-chance' situation
  - The 'no-purpose' situation
  - The 'unbearable' situation
- In infants below 37 weeks gestation, the concept of brain stem death is not appropriate.
- Withdrawal of treatment is a misnomer; the aims of treatment are changed from cure to care rather than total withdrawal of treatment.
- Where there is reasonable uncertainty about the benefits of treatment, there should be a presumption in favor of initiating it. Clinical intervention can be discontinued later after reflection and discussion with parents.
- It is important that a single senior doctor takes overall responsibility for orchestrating the actions of the whole team involved with the family.
- If the parents' views are at odds with those of the team caring for the child the doctor should ask the following five questions:
  - Do the parents understand the prognosis?
  - Should they consult with others?
  - Do they require more time?
  - Is their decision in the interests of the child?
  - Is their decision so unreasonable in terms of benefit to the child as to request them to seek a second opinion or for the doctor to seek the advice of the courts?
- The clinician must always act in the best interest of the child.

## REFERENCES


Anonymous (1981a) Dr. Leonard Arthur: his trial and its implications. *BMJ* 283: 1340–1341.

Anonymous (1981b) The right to live and the right to die. *BMJ* 283: 569–570.

Anonymous (1986) In the rear and limping a little: ethics and law in medicine. *BMJ* 292: 1028.

Autton N (1985) *Doctors talking.* A R Mowbray, Oxford .

Balfour-Lynn I M & Tasker R C (1996) Futility and death in paediatric medical intensive care. *J Med Ethics* 22: 279–281.

Beauchamp T L & Childress J F (1989) *Principles of Biomedical Ethics.* Oxford: Oxford University Press, pp. 120–183.

Bissenden J G (1986) Ethical aspects of neonatal care. *Arch Dis Childh* 61: 639–641.

Brahams D (1988) No obligation to resuscitate a non-viable infancy. *Lancet* i: 1176.

✪ British Medical Association Medical Ethics Committee (1999) *Witholding or Withdrawing Life-prolonging Medical Treatment – Guidance for decision making.* BMJ Books, London.

British Paediatric Association (1991) *Criteria for the diagnosis of brain death in infants and children that could be recommended for use by the medical profession as a whole.*

Byrne P (1990) The BMA on euthanasia: the philosopher versus the doctor. In: Byrne P (ed) *Medicine, medical ethics and the value of life.* Wiley, Chichester.

Campbell A G M (1982) Which infants should not receive intensive care? *Arch Dis Childh* 57: 569–571.

Chiswick M (1990) Withdrawal of life support in babies: deceptive signals. *Arch Dis Childh* 65: 1096–1097.

✪ Costeloe K (1998) EPICure: Survival and morbidity of extremely preterm infants at discharge from hospital. *Ped Res* 43: 211A.

Davies J M & Reynolds B M (1992a) The ethics of cardiopulmonary resuscitation. I. Background to decision making. *Arch Dis Childh* 67: 1498–1501.

✪ Davies J M & Reynolds B M (1992b) The ethics of cardiopulmonary resuscitation. II. Medical logistics and the potential for a good response. *Arch Dis Childh* 67: 1498–1501.

Duff R S & Campbell A G M (1973) Moral and ethical dilemmas in the special care nursery. *N Engl J Med* 289: 890–894.

Duff R S & Campbell A G M (1976) On deciding the care of severely handicapped or dying persons; with particular reference to infants. *Paediatr* 57: 487–493.

Dunn P M (1990) Life saving intervention in the neonatal period: dilemmas and decisions. *Arch Dis Childh* 65: 557–558.

Elton A, Honig P, Bentovim A *et al.* (1995) Witholding consent to lifesaving treatment: three cases. *BMJ* 310: 373–377.

Farsides C (1992) Act of impassive euthanasia – is there a distinction? *Care Crit Ill* 8(3): 126–128.

Finlay I & Dallimore D (1991) Your child is dead. *BMJ* 302: 1524–1525.

Fletcher J (1972) *Indicators of humanhood: a tentative profile of man.* Hastings Centre Report 2: 1–4.

Forest G C, Standish E & Baum J D (1982) Support after a perinatal death: a study of support and counselling after perinatal bereavement. *BMJ* 285: 1475–1479.

Glover J (1977) *Causing death and saving lives.* Penguin, London.

Green J (1989) *Death with dignity series.* Islam, 1 Feb: 56–57 Hinduism, 8 Feb: 50–51. Sikhism, 15 Feb: 56–57. Judaism, 22 Feb: 64–75. Nursing Times, London.

Hellema H (1992) Dutch issue guidelines on handicapped babies. *BMJ* 305: 1312–1313.

Hendrick J (1993) *Child Care Law for Health Professionals.* Radcliffe Medical Press, Oxford.

Kennedy I (1981) *Unmasking medicine* (Reith Lectures). Allen and Unwin, London.

Kopelman L M, Irons T G & Kopelman A E (1988) Neonatologists judge the 'baby Doe' regulations. *N Engl J Med* 318: 677–683.

Kuhse H & Singer P (1985) *Should the baby live?* Oxford University Press, Oxford.

Kurtz Z (1995) Do children's rights to health care in the UK ensure their best interests? *J Royal College Physicians London* 29: 508–516.

Leigh M A M S (1990) Capable of being born alive. *J Med Defence Union* Spring: 3.

Lennard Jones J E (1999) Giving or witholding fluid and nutrients: ethical and legal aspects. J Royal College Physicians London 33: 39–45.

Levene M I (1990) Cerebral ultrasound and neurological impairment: telling the future. *Arch Dis Childh* 65: 469–471.

Lloyd A (1993) 'Do not resuscitate' orders. *Br J Intensive Care* February: 58–62.

Lorber J (1972) Spina bifida cystica. *Arch Dis Childh* 47: 854.

McCall Smith A (1992) Consent to treatment in childhood. *Arch Dis Childh* 67(10): 1247.

McHaffie H E & Fowlie P W (1997) *Life, death and decisions: doctors and nurses reflect on neonatal practice.* Hochland and Hochland, Hale.

Pallis C (1983) *ABC of brain death.* The Devonshire Press, London.

Rachels J (1975) Active and passive euthanasia. *N Engl J Med* 292: 78–80.

Re C (Medical Treatment) [1998] 1 FLR 384.

Re J (A Minor) (Wardship: Medical Treatment) [1990] 3 All ER 930.

Re R (A Minor) (Medical Treatment) [1993] 2 FCR 544.

Re T (A Minor) (Wardship: Medical Treatment); sub nom Re C (A Minor) (Parents' Consent to surgery) [1997] 1 All ER 906.

Rhein R (1992) California says no to euthanasia. *BMJ* 305: 1175.

✪ Royal College of Paediatrics and Child Health (1997) *Witholding or Withdrawing Life Saving Treatment in Children: A Framework for Practice.* RCPCH, London.

Schultz K (1992) Treating defective neonates in Hungary. *Bull Med Ethics,* May: 20–21.

✪ Shaw N J & Dear P R F (1990) How do parents of babies interpret qualitative expressions of probability? *Arch Dis Childh* 65: 520–523.

Sherlock R (1979) Selective non-treatment of newborns. *J Med Ethics* 5: 139–142.

Stinson R & Stinson P (1981) On the death of a baby. *J Med Ethics* 7: 5–18.

Tresch D D, Sims F H, Duthie E H *et al.* (1991) Clinical characteristics of patients in the persistent vegetative state. *Arch Intern Med* 151: 930–932.

Winter B & Cohen S (1999) ABC of intensive care – withdrawal of treatment. *BMJ* 319: 306–308.

Working Party of the Health Department of Great Britain and Northern Ireland (1983) *Cadaveric organs for transplantation. A code of practice including the diagnosis of brain death.* DHSS, London.

# Index

Numbers in bold refer to tables; numbers in italics refer to illustrations


A/B (S/D) ratio, 122
Aase-Smith syndrome, **239**, **240**
Abdominal surgery, patients with shunts, 759
Abducent nerve (VI) abnormality, 696
Abetalipoproteinemia
 clinical features and biochemical findings, **612**
 prenatal diagnosis, **600**
Abscesses, 780–1
 bacterial meningitis, 577, 585
Absent fetal movements, 90
Acatalasemia, 635
Acatalasia
 clinical features and biochemical findings, **611**
 prenatal diagnosis, **600**
Acceleration of maturation, 111, 128
Accelerations, fetal heart rate, 432, 433, 452
Accidents, road-traffic, 324–5, 331
Acetazolamide, CSF reduction, 749–50
*N*-acetylaspartoacylase deficiency *see* Canavan's disease
Acetylcholine, 6
 effect on developing brain, 254
Acetylcholine receptor (ACHR) antibody, 717
α-*N*-acetylgalactosaminidase deficiency *see* Schindler's disease
*N*-acetylglucosaminidase (NAG), 486
 deficiency *see* Sanfilippo's syndrome
*N*-acetylglutamate synthetase deficiency
 clinical features and biochemical findings, **608**
 prenatal diagnosis, **597**
Achondroplasia, 283
Achromatopsia, 665, 673
 ERG traces, *666*
Acid-base status, assessment, 430
Acidemia, 460
Acidosis, 465, 472, 505
 anion gap calculation, 616
 definition, 459, 460
 effect on EEG, 161
 encephalopathy development, 407
 fetal, 421, 422, 462, 467, 472
  late decelerations on EFM, 432
 and neurological outcome, 464, 493–4
 *see also* Metabolic acidosis; Respiratory acidosis
*Acinetobacter baumannii*, multi-resistant, 583
Acoustic power, Doppler, 123
Acquired immunodeficiency syndrome (AIDS), 213, 564, 812
 HIV encephalopathy, 565
Acrania, 54, 290
Acrocallosal syndrome, 220, **241**
Actin, 510
Activated partial thromboplastin time, GMH-IVH development, 347
Active sleep, 156
 EEG recordings, *162*, *164*
 fetus, 432
Active tone, assessment, 105–6, 112
Actocardiograph, fetal, 96
Acts of commission and omission, 829–30
Acuity card procedure, 187, 667, 669, *671*
 delayed visual maturation type, 1, *675*
 delayed visual maturation type 2 and, 3, *676*
 delayed visual maturation type 4, *679*
Acute events, nursing reports, 108
Acyclovir
 herpes simplex (HSV), 564
 varicella, 562
Acyl-carnitine profiling, 620
Ad-damnum clause, 531
Adaptation of fetus, 408
ADC (apparent diffusion coefficient) maps, 63
Addictive compounds, effect on developing brain, 94, 213, 252, 255–8, **801**, 813
 *see also* Cocaine abuse; Fetal alcohol syndrome (FAS)
Adduction of thumb, non-reducible, *114*
Adenine arabinoside (Ara-A), 562
Adenine deaminase deficiency
 clinical features and biochemical findings, **611**
 prenatal diagnosis, **600**
Adenine phosphoribosyltransferase deficiency
 clinical features and biochemical findings, **611**
 prenatal diagnosis, **600**
Adenohypophysis, 27, 28
Adenosylcobalamin synthesis defects
 clinical features and biochemical findings, **612**
 prenatal diagnosis, **600–1**
Adenylosuccinase deficiency, **625**, 633
Admitting error, medical malpractice, 538
Adrenocorticotrophic responses to hypoxia, 409
Adrenoleukodystrophy, neonatal
 clinical features and biochemical findings, **611**
 prenatal diagnosis, **600**
Aerobic respiration, 327–8
Affidavit of merit, 529
Afro-Caribbean women, AFP levels, 268
Age
 fetus, postconceptual and Carnegie stage, **21**
 maternal, Down's syndrome risk, 268, 806–7
Agenesis
 cerebellar, 222, 229
 corpus callosum, 77, *78*, 219–21, 229, 743
  abdominal ultrasound, 277, *278*
  associated conditions, **219**
  genetics, 241
  transvaginal ultrasound, *309*, 311, 313
 premaxillary, 210–11
 sacral, 205, **238**, 697, 771
 sphenoid wing, 775–6
 vermis, 222–4, 277
Agglutination test, 544
Agyria-pachygyria spectrum *see* Lissencephaly
Aicardi's syndrome, 220, **240**, **241**
Alanine:glycoxylate aminotransferase deficiency *see* Hyperoxaluria
Alar plate (lamina), 23, 24, 30, 31
Albinism, 665
 delayed visual maturation, 676
Alcohol abuse, maternal, **801**, 813
 abnormal fetal behavior, 94
 effect on developing brain, 255, **256**, 257–8
  microcephaly, 213
 umbilical circulation impairment, 258
 *see also* Fetal alcohol syndrome (FAS)
Alcohol use, maternal, effect on FVEPs, 190
Alertness, states of, 100–1, 112
 deficit, 114
Alexander's disease, **627**, 641, 753
Alkaline phosphatase deficiency *see* Hypophosphatasia
Alkaptonuria
 clinical features and biochemical findings, **609**
 prenatal diagnosis, **598**
Alloimmune thrombocytopenia, 281, 363
Allopurinol
 neuroprotection in hypoxia-ischemia, 509, 517
 PVL prevention, 382
Alobar holoprosencephaly, 210, 243
 abdominal ultrasound, 275, *276*
 transvaginal ultrasound, 311
Alper's disease, **627**, 641
Alpha seizure activity, 650
Alpha-fetoprotein (AFP), 267–8, 269, 807
Alports syndrome, 685
Amacrine cells, 8
Amblyopia, 671
American Academy of Pediatrics, diagnosing brain death, **498**
American Association on Mental Retardation classification, 803
American College of Obstetricians and Gynecologists (ACOG)
 asphyxia definition, 427, 443–4
 changes in practice survey, 534
 percentage of members sued, 531
 umbilical artery pH values, 460, 464
American Medical Association (AMA)
 medico-legal education, 531, 532
 Patient Safety Initiative, 528
American Pediatric Association (APA), neurosyphilis testing, 590
Amfetamine, effect on developing brain, 254
Amino acid metabolism disorders, 623, 632, 809
 clinical features and biochemical findings, **607**, **625**
 prenatal diagnosis, **597**
Amino acids
 effect on developing brain, 254
 estimating concentrations, 616
α-amino-3-hydroxy-5-methyl-4-isoxazole-proprionic acid *see* AMPA receptors
Aminoadipic-semialdehyde synthase deficiency *see* Hyperlysinemia
Γ-aminobutyric acid (GABA), 6, 419
 A receptors, 648
 *see also* GABA transaminase deficiency
Aminoglycosides

bacterial meningitis, 581, 582, 583
ototoxicity, 685, 687
shunt infections, 587
Aminophylline, effect on CBFV, 131–2, 150
Amniocentesis, 596, 807
Amnioinfusion, intrapartum, 453, *454*
Amniotic band syndrome, 238
Amniotic fluid
cytokines in, white matter damage, 323
effect on myelomeningocele, 765
fetal swallowing, 94
infection
GMH-IVH risk, 344
PVL risk, 379
toxoplasma, 546, 550
meconium in, 429–30, 472, 493
*see also* Meconium aspiration syndrome
volume
abnormal, Doppler studies, 129
biophysical profile score, **435**
Amniotic fluid embolism (AFE), 525
AMPA receptors, 6, 505
Amphetamine *see* Amfetamine, effect on developing brain
Amphotericin, fungal meningitis, 588
Ampicillin, bacterial meningitis, 582
Amplitude-integrated EEG *see* Cerebral function monitoring (CFM)
Amygdaloid area, 26
β-amyloid precursor protein (β-APP), 375
Anaerobic glycolysis, 139, 415, 429, 505
Anaerobic metabolism, 408, 483, 484
Analgesic drugs, effect on CBFV, 131
Anaphylaxis, maternal, 331
Anatomical development of CNS, 21–36
choroid plexus, 33, 34–5
correlation with brain maturation and function, 100
cranial nerves, 32
general development, 22–4
neuroglia, 24
spinal cord, 22–4
myelination, 35–6
regional development, 24–32
association fibers, 31
commissures, 31–2
mesencephalon, 13, 14, 16, *17*, *18*, 28–9, 32, 46, 51
metenecephalon, 12, 29–31, 46
myelencephalon, 31, 46
pyramidal tract, 32
telencephalon, 24–8, 46
sulci, 27, 33, *34*, 51, 52, 53
synaptic development, 32
*see also* Ultrasound assessment, brain development
Andermann syndrome, 220, **241**
Anemia
fetal, 95, 465, 466
Doppler CBF measurments, 129
maternal, 323, 466
Anencephaly, 200, 207, 208–10, 237, 317, 319, 824
abnormal fetal movements, 90
antenatal screening, 267
abdominal ultrasound, 268, 290–1
transvaginal ultrasound, 309
clinical characteristics, 209–10
pathogenesis and pathology, 209
prevalence, 317, 318
impact, prenatal diagnosis on, 318
Anesthetics
effect on developing brain, 259, 260
effect on EEG, 161
risk, myotonic dystrophy, 709
Anesthetists, children of, 259
Aneurysms, 782
ductus arteriosus, 697
middle cerebral artery, *363*, 782
posterior cerebral artery, 782
vein of Galen, 59, 77, 79, 289, 362, 783
'Angel dust', effect on developing brain, 258
Angelman's syndrome, 213, **242**, **800**, 810
Angiography (MRA), 63, 65, 83
cerebral artery infarction, 397–8
Animal husbandry, hormonal compounds, 253
Anion gap, 616
Aniridia, 4, 665
Anlagen, eye, 3D ultrasound, 43
Anoxia, fetal, 429
Antenatal prediction of asphyxia, 427–39
fetal response to asphyxia, 429
fetal testing, 432–7
antepartum testing scheme, *436*
biophysical profile (BPP), 434–7
contraction stress test (CST), 433–4
Doppler velocimetry, 437–8
non-stress test (NST), 432–3
intrapartum fetal assessment, 438–9
key points, 439
neuroimaging, 431
pathophysiology, 427–9
perinatal mortality, 431–2
Antenatal screening, 209, 267–73
chromosomal disorders, 268–70, 807
first trimester markers, 269–70
second trimester serum markers, 268–9
genetic disorders, 270–2
Fragile X syndrome, 271–2
Tay-Sachs disease, 271
inborn errors of metabolism, 595–602
informing choice, 272–3
structural abnormalities, 267–8
impact of, 318–19
*see also* Ultrasound, antenatal assessment
Antepartum factors, cerebral palsy risk, 794
Antepartum hemorrhage, PVL risk, 379
Anterior cerebral artery
Doppler CBF measurements, 125
brain death, 499
rising ICP, 746
infarction, 393
Anterior commissure, 31–2
myelination, 36
Anterior fontanelle
as acoustic window, 57, 59, 122, 297, 298
scanning off-center, 58, 59
assessment, 102
ICP measurement, 482
punctures, 779
Anterior horn cells, spinal cord, 700
Anterior pituitary, 27, 28
Anterior spinal artery, 700
Anterior visual pathway disorders, 672–3
Anti-apoptoic genes, 419
Anti-apoptoic nuclear proteins, 418
Anti-neutrophil serum, 514
Anti-platelet antibodies, screening for, 281
Anti-varicella-zoster immunoglobuin (VZIG), 561, 562
Antibiotics
bacterial meningitis, 581–3, 779
summary, **582**
brain abscess, 781
shunt infections, 587, 757, 758
Anticholinesterases, myasthenia gravis, 719
Anticonvulsants, 175, 654
asphyxiated infants, 490–1
effect on CBFV, 131
effect on EEG, 167, 174
teratogenic effects, 251, 258
neural tube defects, 220
sexual differentiation of brain, 253
*see also* Phenobarbital; Phenytoin
Antiphospholipid antibodies, 395
α-1-antitrypsin deficiency, 362
Apert's syndrome, **239**, 776, 777
Apgar scores
asphyxia, 471, 472, 473, 492, **493**
outcome prediction, 494–5
cerebral palsy prediction, 430
GMH-IVH correlation, 344
PVL prediction, 380
Aplasia cutis congenita, 704, 775
Apnea, 395, 487, 488
Apneic seizures, 649
Apoptosis, 7, 25, 325, 327, 329, 418, 429
mechanism activation, 509–11
Aqueduct of Sylvius, 28
fetal ultrasound, 52, 53
Aqueductal stenosis, 226–7, 332, 333, 739, 740, 759
Arachidonic acid metabolites, bacterial meningitis, 576
Arachnoid cysts, 229, 740
abdominal ultrasound, 286, 288
differentiating from Dandy-Walker malformation, 225–6, 279
transvaginal ultrasound, *312*, 313
Arachnoid granulations, 739
congenital absence, 284
Arching of trunk, 103
Arginine vasopressin release, 485
Argininemia
clinical features and biochemical findings, **608**
prenatal diagnosis, **597**
Argininosuccinic aciduria
clinical features and biochemical findings, **608**
prenatal diagnosis, **597**
Arnold-Chiari malformation, 54, 202, 204, 205–7, 229, 291, 294
BAEP predictive power, 186
classification of malformations, **206**, **733**
clinical characteristics, 206–7
management, 207
pathophysiology, 206
type II deformity, 740, 778
current prevention and treatment, 734, 735
fetal neurosurgery, 735, 736
pathogenesis, 733–5, *735*
symptoms, 756–67, 768
Aromatic amino acid decarboxylase deficiency, **626**, 638
Arrhythmias, fetal, 324, 466
*see also* Bradycardia; Tachycardia
Arterial blood pressure, effect on CBFV measurements, 127
Arterial infarction, 335, 336, 358–9, 393–9, 481
diagnostic clues, **116**
Arterial spasm, blood in ventricles, 342
Arterio-venous malformations, 77, 362, 782
imaging, 79–80
abdominal ultrasound, antenatal diagnosis, 289–90
Doppler, 59
Arteriography, cerebral artery infarction, 398
Artery of Adamkiewcz, 700
Arthrogryposis, 711, 713, 720–1
Artificial ventilation *see* Mechanical ventilation
Arylsulfatase deficiency *see* Metachromatic leukodystrophy
Ashkenazi Jews, antenatal DNA screening, 271
Aspartate levels, hypoxic-ischemia, 507
Aspartoacylase deficiency *see* Canavan's disease
Aspartylglycosaminuria
clinical features and biochemical findings, **610**
prenatal diagnosis, **599**
*Aspergillus fumigatus*, 586, 588
*Aspergillus sydowi*, 588
Asphyxia
antenatal prediction, 427–39
Doppler velocimetry, 437–8
fetal gas analysis *see* Fetal gas analysis
fetal response to, 429

fetal testing, 432–7
key points, 439
markers for, 429–31
neuroimaging, 431
perinatal mortality, 431–2
at cellular level, 444
cerebral palsy risk, 794–5
classification of intrapartum, **428**
definitions, 323, 427, 443, 459–60, 471
intrapartum monitoring, 438–9, 443–55
EFM vs. traditional auscultation, 444–8
fetal pulse oximetry, 450
fetal scalp pH determination, 438, 449–50
FHR abnormalities, 444
key points, 455
management of fetal distress, 450–5
potential benefits of EFM, 448–9
potential risks of EFM, 449
medico-legal issues, 523, 535
neonatal, 471–99
'asphyxia syndrome', 471–3
brain death, 498–9
cervical cord lesions, 699
clinical features, **427**, 478–80
clinical grading system (Sarnat and Sarnat), **479**, 480
complications, 485–7
crying pattern, 101
definition, 471
hearing impairment, 686
incidence, 473–4
investigations, *142*, 187, 191, 480–5
key points, 499
neurologic assessment at birth, 113
optic atrophy, 674
outcome, 492–8, 686, **801**
pathology, 474–80
resuscitation, 487–8
spinal cord injury, 701
standard brain-orientated management, 489–92
systemic management, 488–9
neuroprotection of brain, 515–17
pathogenesis of cell death, 415–16
pathophysiology, 410–12, 427–9, 505
adaptations to fetal life, 408
brief repeated asphyxia, 413
characteristics of encephalopathy, 407–8
chronic asphyxia, 414, 415
determinants of asphyxial injury, 421–**4**
etiology of asphyxia, 408
hypoxia, 408–10
key points, 424
maturational changes in fetal response to, 413–14
phases of neuronal injury, 416–21
progessive asphyxia, 412, 413
post-asphyxiated state, 147–9
*see also* Hypoxic-ischemic brain injury
Aspiration, brain abscess, 781
Aspirin, effect on developing brain, 252, 258
Association fibers
development, 31
myelination, 36
Associative learning and synapse formation, 7, 9
Asthma, maternal, 324
Astroblasts, 24
Astrocytes, 24, 330
GFAP positive, 375
gliosis, 326
Astrocytomas, 784, 785
Asymetric tonic neck reflex (ATNR), 104, 108
Asymmetric crying facies, 697
Asymmetric nystagmus, 666–7
Asymmetric tone, 115
Ataxia, 792
Athetoid movements, 791
Atlas vertebra, dislocation, 698
ATP degradation, 484, 497
Atrophy
cerebellar, *335*
cerebral, 76, 77, 385, 386, 743
head circumference, 117
HIV infection, 565
cortical, 393
optic nerve, 673–4
pons, 397
spinal cord, 699
spinal muscular, 709, 710, 711, 721, *722*
thalamus, 395, 397
Attention deficit hyperactivity disorder, **256**, 257, 260
Attractive signals, axonal pathfinding, 5
Auditory brainstem response test (ABR), 182, 586, 688, *689*, 690
facial palsy, 696
Auditory neuropathy, 688
Auditory response cradle, 687
Auditory thresholds, 182
Auscultation, fetal heart rate, 443, 494
medico-legal issues, 535–6
versus electronic fetal monitoring (EFM), 444–8
Autism, 211
Automated auditory brainstem response (AABR), 182
*see also* Auditory brainstem respone (ABR) test
Autonomy, respect for, 821, 822, 823, 825
Autopsy
inborn errors of metabolism, 617–18
requesting, 830
Autoregulation
loss of, 346, 353
perfusion pressure-flow, 139, 144
Autosomal genetic causes, mental retardation, **801**, 809
Avidity of IgG test, 544
Awareness and fixation, 667
Axial plane, 298, 299
Axodendritic synapses, 24
Axonal guidance, neuronal migration, 5–6
Axons, formation, 23
Axosomatic synpases, 24
Azithromycin, toxoplasmosis, 549

B-cell lymphoma, 565
*Bacillus cereus*, 587
'Back-to-lying' response, 106
Background EEG abnormality, 161, 167
CFM monitoring, 178
Bacteremia, 575, 780
Bacterial meningitis, 573–86, 651, 759
clinical features, 577
complications, 583–6
brain abscess, 585
monitoring, 583
mortality and morbidity, 585–6
repeat lumbar punctures, 583–4
diagnosis, 577–80
epidemiology, 573–5
incidence, **573**
key points, 591
management, 580–3
antibiotic therapy, 581–3, 779
clinical assessment, 580
supportive therapy, 580–1
organisms, 574–5
pathogenesis, 575–6
pathology, 576–7
Bacterial shunt infections, 575, 578, 586–7, 757–8
Ballard score, 111
Banana sign, *293*, 294
Band heterotopias, 218
Barany chair rotation, 661
Barbiturates
administration, asphyxiated infants, 490
effect on developing brain, 254, 255, 256, 258
*see also* Phenobarbital
Barth microlissencephaly, **246**
Basal encephaloceles, surgery, 763, 764
Basal ganglia, 100
calcification, 81, 565
hemorrhage, 65, 477
hypoxic ischemic injury, 71, 73, 329, 330, 335, 478, 480, 481, 496
summary of MRI changes, **74**
status marmoratus, 335, 474, 476–7
Basal plate (lamina), 23, 29
motor cells arising from, 31
Basis pontis, 29
Basket cells, 31
Battens disease, **626**, 640
Bcl protein, 418
Bcl-2 gene, 419
Beat-to-beat variability
Doppler velocity signal, 126
fetal heart rate (FHR), 451
Becker muscular dystrophy, antenatal screening, 270
Beckwith-Wiedemann syndrome, 283
Behavior
fetus, 92–4
abnormal, 94
affect on Doppler CBF measurements, 126
influence on FHR, 90, **92**
twins, 95–6
neonate
anencephalic infant, 209
during feeding, 108
EEG recordings, 156–7, 171
effect of medicines on, 259
flash VEPs, 183
Behavioral tests of hearing, 690
Behr's optic atrophy, 674
Beneficence, 821, 822, 825, 829
Benign external hydrocephalus, 741
Benign extra-axial fluid collections of infancy, 77
Benign familial megalencephaly, 283
Benign Familial Neonatal Convulsions (BFNC), 652
Benign Idiopathic Neonatal Convulsions (BINC), 652–3
Benign macrocephaly of infancy, 77
Benign myoclonic jerks, 174
Benzodiazepines
effect on developing brain, 254, 257, 258
seizure disorders, 654
Benzyl alcohol in flush solutions, GMH-IVH development, 347
Betamethasone
abnormal fetal behavior, 94, 95
cerebroprotective action, 517
PVL prevention, 382
Biedl-Bardet syndrome, 673, 674
Bifunctional enzyme defect
clinical features and biochemical findings, **611**
prenatal diagnosis, **600**
Bilirubin metabolism disorders
clinical features and biochemical findings, **613**
prenatal diagnosis, **601**
Bilirubin toxicity, PVL risk, 381
Binge drinking, 257
Biochemical markers, birth asphyxia, **483**
Biochemical tests, degenerative disorders, 627
Biogenic amines, effect on developing brain, 254
Biometric parameters, fetal brain ultrasound, 51
Biophysical profile (BPP), 95, 434–7, 467
Biopsy
at autopsy, 618
degenerative disorders, 627
fetal organs, 595, 596
muscle, 711, *714*, *715*, *718*, *720*, *721*, *722*
Biopterin defects, **626**, 639
Biotinidase deficiency, **626**, 639
Biparietal diameter (BPD), 49, 50, 267, 282, 294
Bisexuality, prenatal prescribed sex hormones, 253
Bladder distension, 699
Bladder dysfunction, myelomeningocele, 203
Bladder filling, fetus, 95
Blindness
cortical, 677–8
delayed visual maturation, 675–7
nystagmus, 667

PVL infants, 391, 392
sensory deprivation nystagmus, 665
strabismus, 663
toxoplasmosis, 548
Blink reflex, 102, 667
Blood clots
intraventricular, 341, 342
lysis, TGF-β1 release, 741
Blood flow
Doppler measurements *see* Doppler ultrasound
redistribution, fetal hypoxia/asphyxia, 408, 410, 413, 414, 463
Blood pressure changes
effect on CBFV measurements, 127
fetal asphyxia, 410
fetal hypoxia, 408, 409
GMH-IVH development, 346, 347
*see also* Hypotension
Blood tests, inborn errors of metabolism, 616, 617
Blood vessel cross-sectional area, Doppler measurements, 121
Blood-brain barrier, 483, 576
Bloom syndrome, **242**
Blueberry muffin lesions, 363
BN52021, PAF-antagonist, 514
Body axis
determination of, 12
unfolding, 13
Body movements
fetus, 89–90
effect on FHR, *92*
intrafetal consistency, 90
twins, 95–6
neonate, 103
Body-worn hearing aid, 690
Bolitho v. City and Hackney Health Authority, (1998), 521
Bonding, maternal-child, hearing tests, 687
Bone conduction hearing aids, 691
Botulism, infantile, 588, 589, 705
Bovine surfactant administration, effect on CBFV, 130
Bowel, hyperechoic, toxoplasmosis, *547*
Brachial plexus palsy, 701–4, 706
classification, 701–2
etiology, 703
incidence, 702
investigations, 703–4
pathology, 703
prognosis, 704
Brachium conjunctivum, 29
Brachium pontis, 31
Brachycephaly, 777
Bradycardia
fetal, 408, 410, 429, 433, 450–1
neonatal, 488
Brain damage
clinical profile, 113–15
clues to fetal, 113, *114*
preterm infant, CBFV prediction, 132
tentative diagnosis, 115, **116**
Brain death, 498–9, 830
anencephalic infants, 209–10
intrauterine, 95
Brain development
anatomical development, 21–36, 60, 61, 63
and damage following hypoxic-ischemic injury, 328–9
early embryonic development, 11–18
epigenetic and functional organization, neuronal circuits, 3–9
ultrasound assessment of normal fetal, 45–54
Brain-derived creatinine kinase (CK-BB), 485
Brain-derived enzymes, asphyxia, 485
Brain-derived neurotrophic factor (BDNF), 5, 6, 485, 512
Brain-derived proteins, 485
'Brain-sparing' phenomenon, 111, 127, 129, 410
*see also* Blood flow: redistibution, fetal hypoxia/asphyxia
Brainstem, *18*, 32
glioma, 664
hypoxic-ischemic injury, 330, 478
necrosis, 335, *336*
Brainstem auditory evoked potentials (BAEPs), 181–2
clinical applications, 185–7, **192**
Branched-chain keto-acid dehydrogenase deficiency *see* Maple syrup urine disease
Branched-chain organic acidemias
clinical features and biochemical findings, **608**
prenatal diagnosis, **598**
Branchio-oto-renal syndrome, 684
Breast milk
cytomegalovirus transmission, 559
HIV transmission, 564
Breast and ovarian cancer susceptibility gene (BRCA1), 201, 209
Breast size, **110**
Breathing movements, fetus, 93, 94, 434
biophysical profile score, **435**
changes following asphyxia, 429
effect on Doppler CBF measurements, 125
Breech delivery
brachial plexus palsy, 702
extradural hemorrhage, 363
GMH-IVH risk, 345
occiptial osteodiastasis, 357, 360, 478
traumatic cord lesions, 698, 699
Breech presentation
cranial shape, 102
fetal eye movements, 90
ultrasound assessment, 45, 298
Bridging vein rupture, 357
Brief intermittent rhythmic discharges (BIRDS), 167
'Bright' thalamic lesions, 362, *477*
British Paediatric Association, diagnosing brain death, **498**
'Bulls' eye' method, fix and track, 101–2
Burst-suppression pattern (EEG), 155, 161, *166*, 167, 178, 497
'Bursting tendency', EEG, 160

C-Reactive Protein (CRP), 578
Cadherins, 5
Caffeine, effect on fetus and neonate, 258
Caffeine therapy, effect on CBFV, 132
Cajal-Retzius cells, 4, 15, 25, 215
Calcarine cortex, atrophy, 391
Calcarine fissure, 33, 51, 52
Calcification, intracerebral, 81, 282
capillaries, 374
cytomegalovirus infection, *327*, 557
HIV infection, 565
Möbius sequence, 696–7
toxoplasmosis, *547*, 548
Calcium antagonists, 419
Calcium gluconate, 654
Calcium, role in cell injury, 507–8
Callosal sulcus, 33, 51, 52
Caloric tests, 662
Calpains, 511
Calpastatin, 511
Canada, birth asphyxia, 474
Canavan's disease, **626**, 638, 641
prenatal diagnosis, **598**, 602
*Candida*
meningitis, 575, 586, 588
shunt infection, 758
Capillary reaction, hypoxic injury, 326
Caput succedaneum, 102
Carbamazepine
seizure management, 654
teratogenic effects, 251
Carbamoylphosphate synthetase (CPS) deficiency
clinical features and biochemical findings, **608**
prenatal diagnosis, **597**
Carbapenem, bacterial meningitis, 583
Carbohydrate metabolism disorders, 639
clinical features and biochemical findings, **607**, **626**
prenatal diagnosis, **597**
Carbohydrate-deficient glycoconjugate type I syndrome, **248**
Carbohydrate-deficient glycoprotein syndrome, 223, 606, 623, **627**, 634
prenatal diagnosis, **601**
Carbon dioxide changes, effect on CBFV measurements, 126–7, 130, 144, 145
Carbon monoxide poisoning, maternal, 213
Carbonic anhydrase II deficiency
clinical features and biochemical findings, **613**
prenatal diagnosis, **601**
'Cardiac arrest encephalopathy', 328, 335
Cardiolipin antibodies, 395
Cardiomegaly, *in utero*, 783
Cardiotocography (CTG), 464, 472
in court, 537–8
failure to recognise abnormalites, 524
and outcome, 494
*see also* Electronic fetal monitoring (EFM); Fetal heart rate (FHR)
Cardiovascular adaptation to asphyxia, 408–15, 486
summary, **420**
Carnegie staging system, **21**, 46
Carnitine palmitolytransferase deficiency
clinical features and biochemical findings, **609**
prenatal diagnosis, **598**
Carnitine supplementation, 617
Carnitine/acyl carnitine translocase deficiency
clinical features and biochemical findings, **609**
prenatal diagnosis, **598**
Carotid arteries, fetal, blood flow signals, 53
Carotid blood flow, fetal asphyxia, 410, *411*, *412*, 413, 421
Cascade testing, Fragile X syndrome, 271
Caspases, 418, 510, 514
caspase-3-mediated DNA fragmentation, 510–11
Cassette EEG, 175, 177
Catalase deficiency *see* Acatalasia
Catecholamines, 6
Caudal regression syndrome *see* Sacral agenesis
Cavitation effect, Doppler ultrasound, 123
Cavum septi pellucidi, 50, 51
persistence of, 221
ultrasound, 52, 53
transvaginal imaging, 302, *304*
Cavum vergae, 51
ultrasound, *52*
transvaginal imaging, 302
CD14, soluble, role in bacterial meningitis, 576
Cebocephaly, 210
Cefotaxime
bacterial resistance to, 582
Gram-negative meningitis, 582
Ceftriaxone
bacterial meningitis, 583
bacterial resistance to, 581
endophthalmitis, 586
prophylaxis, shunt infection, 587
Cell cycle, duration, neuronal proliferation, 4
Cell death, 325–6, 418, 428, 505
pathogenesis, 415–16
role of mitochondria, 511
*see also* Apoptosis; Necrosis
Cellular response to hypoxic ischemia, 325–7
Central fissures, 33
Central sulcus, 33, *34*, 51, 61
'Centralization' of circulation, fetal, 408
Centre for High Quality Information, NHS Executive, 273
Centronuclear myopathy, 709, 711, 716, *718*
differential diagnosis, **710**

Centrum semiovale, cysts, 384
Cephalhematoma, 102, 363, 365
Cephalic flexure, 29
Cephalocele, 207
  ultrasound detection, 291, *292*
Cephalocentesis, 729, *730*, *732*
  ethical dilemmas, 823, 824, 825, 826
Cephalosporins, bacterial meningitis, 581, 582, 583
Ceramidase deficiency *see* Farber's disease
Cerebellum, 4
  asphyxial injury, 478
  atrophy, *335*
  development, 16, *18*, 29–31, 49, 51
    genes required for, 4
  hemorrhage, 65, 68, 360–1
  malformations, 221–6, 229
    conditions associated with, **221**
    genetics, cerebellar hypoplasia, 247–8
  myelination, 36
  ultrasound, 53
    transvaginal, 303
Cerebral aqueduct, 16
Cerebral arteries
  blood flow signals
    fetal circulation, 53–*4*, 123, 124–7
    neonatal circulation, 57, 59, 126, 130–3
  infarction, 335, 336, 358–9, 393–9, 481
    diagnosis, 395–8
    etiology, 394–5
    imaging, 75–6
    incidence, 393–4
    key points, 399
    pathology, 393
    prognosis, 398–9
    timing, 394
  obstruction, 335
  *see also* Anterior cerebral artery; Middle cerebral artery; Posterior cerebral artery
Cerebral atrophy, 76, 77, 385, 386, 743
  head circumference, 117
  HIV infection, 565
Cerebral blood flow (CBF), 14, 139
  lack of regulation, ill premature infants, 346
  management, 151–2
  measurement
    in clinical practice, 150–1
    clinical research methods, 139–44
    Doppler ultrasound, 143
      *see also* Doppler ultrasound
    in hydrocephalus, 746
  outcome prediction in asphyxia, 497
  pathophysiology, 146–50
  physiological regulation, 144–5
  uncoupling from glucose metabolism in PVL, 376
Cerebral cortex
  histology, 24–6
  hypoxic-ischemic injury, 475–6
    laminar necrosis, 329, 481
    term infant, 333–4
  surface area, 33
  transvaginal ultrasound, 304, *306*
Cerebral edema, 475
  asphyxiated infants, 482, 489, 491
    imaging, 481
  bacterial meningitis, 580
  cytotoxic, 416, 428, 475
  lactic acid accumulation, 484
Cerebral energy metabolism, 139, *140*
  coupling to CBF, 144
Cerebral function monitoring (CFM), 155, 177–9, 483, 497
Cerebral hemispheres, 328
  embryonic development, 14, 15, *18*
  hemorrhage, 65, 68, *69*
  histology of cortex, 24–6
  sulci and gyri formation, 27, 33, *34*, 51, 52, 53, 61, *62*, 304, *306*
Cerebral mantle, thickness and IQ, 746, 759
Cerebral metabolic rate (CMR), 139, 144, 147
  measurement in clinical practice, 150–1
  in normal infants, 145
Cerebral optical spectroscopy, 464
Cerebral palsy, 323, 407, 422, 427, 521
  definition, 791, 795
  epidemiology, 791–7
    antepartum factors, 794
    causes other than acute intrapartum hypoxia, **530**
    changes in prevalence over time, 796
    differential descriptions, 791–2
    factors affecting estimates of prevalence, 795–6
    gender, 794
    gestational age, 792, 793, *796*
    GMH-IVH, 355
    heterogeneity and multifactorality of cause, 792
    infection, 423
    intrapartum factors, 794–5
    intrauterine growth, appropriateness of, 793
    key points, 797
    multiple birth, 793–4
    neonatal stroke, 398
    postneonatal factors, 795
    PVL, 381, 386, 387, 388, 389
  incidence, 438, 449
    in infants with biophysical profile testing, 436
  International Concensus Statement, 523
  intrapartum monitoring, 438–9, 536
  malpractice claims, 523–5
  prediction of, 188, 191, 407, 493
    Apagar scores, 430, 494
    flash VEPs, 672
  relationship with birth asphyxia, **531**
Cerebral peduncles, 16, 29
  myelination, 36
Cerebral perfusion, 139
Cerebral perfusion pressure (CPP), 482
Cerebral vein thrombosis, 76, 365–6
  imaging, 76
'Cerebro-oculo-muscular syndrome' (COMS), 216, **240**
Cerebro-oculo-skeletal syndrome (COFS), **242**
Cerebrocephaly, 275
Cerebroplacental ratio (CPR), 128
Cerebrospinal fluid (CSF)
  amino acid analysis, 616, 617
  cultures
    repeat lumbar puncture, 583–4
    in shunt infections, 757–8
  flow studies, 77, *78*, 83
  formation and circulation, 284, 302, 303, 332, 739
  glucose, 576–7, 579
  overproduction, 741
  pressure, 482, 578, 745–6
  protein, 579
  repeated tapping, 747–9
  rubella virus, 555
  ventricular, microorganisms, 779
  white cell count, 578–9
  *see also* Intracranial pressure (ICP)
Cerebrotendinous xanthomatosis
  clinical features and biochemical findings, **612**
  prenatal diagnosis, **600**
Cerebrovascular responses to asphyxia, 408–15
  in delayed phase, 419, 420
  summary, **420**
Cervical cord
  hydromyelia, 205
  myelomeningocele, 202, *203*
  syringomyelia, 205
  trauma, 699, 700
Cervical flexure, 13
Cesarean section
  '30 minute rule', 529, 530
  ethical dilemmas, 825, 826, 827
  GMH-IVH prevention, 345, 353
  informed consent, 825
  patient's refusal, 825
  poor placental function, 467
  PVL risk, 380
  rates
    amnioinfusion trials, *454*
    EFM and auscultation, trials, 445, 446, 447, 448, 449
    in US, 527
  *see also* Vaginal birth after Cesarean section (VBAC)
CHARGE association, 223, 686
Chelation, transition metals, 508
Chemical meningitis, 587
Chemokines, 514, 515
Cherry-red spot, 629, 673
Chewing movements, 103
Chiari deformity *see* Arnold-Chiari malformation
Chicken-pox *see* Varicella-zoster (V-Z) virus
Children Act 1989, 831
Chloramphenicol, bacterial meningitis, 581
Chlorimipramine, effect on developing brain, 254
Chlorisodamine, effect on developing brain, 254
Chlorophenylalanine, effect on developing brain, 254
Chlorpromazine
  effect on developing brain, 254, 258
  neonatal tetanus, 590
Cholesterol ester storage disease
  clinical features and biochemical findings, **611**
  prenatal diagnosis, **600**
Choreic movements, 791
Choreoathetosis, 493, 496
Chorioamnionitis, PVL risk, 379
Chorion villus biopsy (CVB), 595–6, 807
Chorioretinitis
  cytomegalovirus infection, 557
  lymphocytic choriomeningitis virus, 566
  toxoplasmosis, 548, 550
Choroid fissure coloboma, 210
Choroid plexectomy, 754
Choroid plexus, 48, 739
  cysts
    abdominal ultrasound, 286, *287*
    transvaginal ultrasound, 310
  development, 33, 34–5
  fourth ventricle, 16, 33, 49
  hemorrhage, 65, 343, 360
  lateral ventricles, 32, 33, 35
  papillomas, 283, 284
  telencephalic, 15, 16
  third ventricle, 32, 33
  tumors, 784, 785
  ultrasound assessment, *40*, 47, 48, 50
    transvaginal approach, 304, *305*
Chromosomal abnormalities, 200
  abnormal fetal movements, 90
  antenatal screening, 268–70
  corpus callosum agenesis, **219**, 220, 241
  Dandy-Walker syndrome, 277
  hearing loss, 685
  holoprosencephaly, 243
  lissencephaly, 216
  mental retardation, 805–9
  microcephaly, 242
  neural tube defects, 238, 319
    encephaloceles, 207
Cicatrical scars, 560
Ciclosporin-A, 511
Cingulate gyrus, 51
  ultrasound, *52*
Cingulate sulcus, 52
  transvaginal ultrasound, 304
Cingulum, myelination, 36
Circulus arteriosus of Willis, 53, *54*, 57
Cisterna magna
  macro, 224
  measuring depth, 53
  mega-cisterna, 277, 279, *280*
Cisternal tap, 580
*Citrobacter*
  brain abscess, 781
  meningitis, 575, 585
Citrulline/arginine ratio, increase after hypoxic-ischemia, 509

Citrullinemia
clinical features and biochemical findings, **608**
prenatal diagnosis, **597**
Civil Procedure Rules, 521
Part 35 (White Book 1999), 522–3
Clarithromycin, toxoplasmosis, 549
Clavicular fracture, 702
Clear cell adenocarcinoma, 252
Cleavage, disorders of, **200**, 210–11
Clindamycin, toxoplasmosis, 549
Clinical assessment, infant nervous system, 99–118
assessment of CNS function, 100–9
assessment of maturation, 109–11
brain maturation and function, physiological basis, 100
clinical clues, most common disorders, 113–15
historical background, 99
key points, 118
neurologic optimality, 40 weeks gestation, 111–13
clinical criteria defining, **112**
non-clinical investigations, integration into assessment, 115
recovery period, 115, 117
tentative diagnosis, 115, **116**
Clinical Disputes Forum, 523
Clinical maternity care standard, 522
Clinical negligence scheme for Trusts (CNST), 522, 524
Clinical practice guidelines, 529, 530
Clinical risk management, 522, 538
Clomifene citrate, teratogenic effects, 251
Clomipramine, active sleep deprivation studies, 259
Clonazepam
asphyxiated infants, 490
seizure disorders, 654
Clonic movements, 103
Clonic seizures, 648, 649
partial, 651
Clonidine
active sleep deprivation studies, 259
effect on developing brain, 254, 260
*Clostridium botulinium*, 588, 589, 705
*Clostridium tetani*, 589–90
Clots
intraventricular, 341, 342
lysis, TGF-β1 release, 741
Cloverleaf skull deformity, 777
COACH syndrome, 223, **248**
Coagulase-negative staphylococci
meningitis, 575, 576
antibiotics, 581, **582**
shunt infections, 586
Coagulation defects, 744
asphyxiated infants, 487, 489
GMH-IVH development, 347
neonatal stroke, 395
parenchymal hemorrhage, 362
Cobblestone lissencephaly, 216, **246**
genetics, 247
Cocaine abuse
effect on fetus, 252, 255, 256–7, 324
abnormal behavior, 94
microcephaly, 213
neonatal stroke, 394–5
Cochlear implants, 586, 691
'Code of Guidance for Experts' (Draft Code 1999), 523
Colliculi, 28, 29
Colloid, 580
Color flow imaging, Doppler, 59, 123, 124
Color vision, 668
Colpocephaly, 244
Combined ventricular output (CVO), fetal, 408, 409
failure of, 413
Comm gene, 5
Commission, acts of, 829, 830
Commissural plate, 31
Commissures, 27, 31–2
Common basilar artery, 53
Common Law, 521–2
Communicating hydrocephalus, 741–2, 753
CSF pressure measurement, 746
Compensatory mechanisms, fetal distress, 111
Complement, bacterial meningitis, 576
Complementary neuromotor examination, 109
Computerized tomography (CT), 57, 59–60, 83, 115
asphyxia, 75, 481
hypoxic-ischemic encephalopathy, 70, *72*
outcome prediction, 496
bright thalami, *477*
cerebral artery infarction, 395, 481
cerebral vein thrombosis, 76
focal ischemic lesions, 75
fungal meningitis, 584
hydranencephaly, *228*
intracranial hemorrhage, 65, 66, 73
GMH-IVH, 67, 348
intraparenchymal, 68
subarachnoid, 68, 69
subdural, 68, 69, 358
ulegyria, *475*
Conduct disorders, **256**, 257
Conductive hearing impairment, 683, 690
Congenital abnormalities, 59, 199–230
abnormal fetal behavior, 94, 95
antenatal screening *see* Antenatal screening
cerebellar malformations, 221–6
cerebral palsy risk, 794
cleavage and differentiation defects, 210–11
*see also* Holoprosecencephaly
diagnostic clues, **116**
EEG recordings, 167
genetics *see* Genetics
hearing impairment, 686
imaging, 77, *78*, 79
inborn errors of metabolism, 606
key points, 229
neural tube defects, 200–10
*see also* Neural tube defects
neuronal migration disorders, 211–21, 224, 283, 753
*see also* Microcephaly
optic nerve or retina, 103
pathogenesis, 199–200
postneuronal migration defects, 226–9
Congenital esotropia, 662
Congenital muscular dystrophy, 709, 711, 713–14, *715*
differential diagnosis, **710**
Congenital myopathies, 716–17
Congenital myotonic dystrophy, 709, 711–13
antenatal screening, 271
diagnostic clues, **116**
differential diagnosis, **710**
genetic inheritance, 709
molecular genetics, 712, 713
Congenital ocular motor apraxia (COMA), 664
Congenital porencephaly, 214
Congenital unilateral lower lip palsy, 697
Congential hypoplasia, 103
Congestive cardiac failure, 782, 783
Coning during lumbar puncture, 578
Conjugate eye movements, 659
Connexin 26 mutations, 684, 687
Consanguineous marriage, mental retardation, 803
Consciousness, anencephalic infants, 209
'Consensus medicine', 829
Consent *see* Informed consent
Consolability, 102
Constipation, spinal dysraphism, 204
Constructivist approach, developing brain, Purves, 9
Consultant supervision, 524
Continuous hemofiltration (CAVH), inborn errors of metabolism, 617
Continuous low voltage patterns, CFM, 178
Continuous positive airway pressure (CPAP), hearing impairment, 686
Contraction stress test (CST), 433–4
Contractions, uterine, 453, 463
Contrast agents
CT scans, 59
MRI scans, 60
Conus medullaris, 22
Convexity hemorrhages, 357, 358, 359, 364
'Conviction medicine', 829
Copper metabolism disorder *see* Menke's disease
Cord blood gases, 430, 450, 465
GMH-IVH prediction, 344
normal oxygen extraction, 461
PVL prediction, 380
Cord care, traditional practices, 589
Cord compression/occlusion, 408, 463, 472
fetal responses, 410, *411*, 412–13, 414, 421, 429, 452
maternal position, 453
Cord prolapse, 408, 453
malpractice claims, 525
Cordocentesis, 466–7, 596
determining fetal platelet count, 281
effect on CBF measurements, 129
umbilical vein lactate, 462, 463
Corneal reflex, 103
Cornelia de Lange syndrome, **242**
Corona radiata, myelination, 36, 61
Coronal plane, 298, 299
transvaginal ultrasound, subdivisons, 299, *300*, *302*
Coronal synostosis, 776, 777, 778
Corpora quadrigemina, 28, 29
Corpus callosum
agenesis, 77, *78*, 219–21, 229, 743
abdominal ultrasound, 277, *278*
associated conditions, **219**
genetics, 241
transvaginal ultrasound, *309*, 311, 313
development, 32, 33, 50, 51
myelination, 36
ultrasound, 52
transvaginal imaging, 302, *304*
Corpus striatum, 27
Cortex
histology, 24–6
hypoxic-ischemic injury, 475–6
laminar necrosis, 329, 481
term infant, 333–4
surface area, 33
susceptibility to asphyxia, 422–3
transvaginal ultrasound, 304, *306*
Cortical atrophy, 393
Cortical death, 161
Cortical dysplasia, 211, *329*
Cortical highlighting, 74, 326, 496
Cortical impedance, measuring in asphyxia, 416, *417*
Cortical plate, 15, 25, 26
Cortical visual impairment, 677–8
Corticipetal fibers, 24, 25, 26
Cortico-fugal fiber destruction, 388
Corticospinal pathways, 100, 334
Corticosteroids
asphyxiated infants, 491
effect on fetal behavior, 94, 95
GMH-IVH prevention, 344, 349
neuroprotection, hypoxic-ischemia, 517
PVL prevention, 382
respiratory distress syndrome reduction, legal considerations, 524
risks to fetal brain development, 253, 258
toxoplasmosis, 549
Corticotrophin-releasing factor (CRF), effect on developing brain, 255
Cortisol responses to hypoxia, 409–10
Cotrimoxazole, bacterial meningitis, 582
Counseling, 238, 824
antenatal screening information, 272
corpus callosum agenesis, 241
holoprosencephaly, *244*

  hydranencephaly, 240
  lissencephaly, *246*
  microcephaly, 241, 242
  multifactorial recurrence risks, NTDs, 237, **238**
  myelomeningocele, 204, 766, 767
Courtroon appearances, injured child, 531
Cover-ups, medical malpractice, 538
Coxsackieviruses, 566, 567
  meningoencephalitis, 568
Cranial nerves
  development, 32
  examination, 102–3
  myelination, 36
  nerve palsies, 662–3, 695–7
Cranial shape, 102
Craniectomy, morecellation, 778
Craniocerebello-cardiac (3C) syndrome, 223, **248**
Craniofacial dysmorphism, 776
Craniorachischisis, 209, 317
Cranioschisis, 207
Cranioscoliosis, 777
Craniostenosis, 102
Craniosynostosis, 283, 776–8
Craniotabes, 102
Craniotelencephalic dysplasia, **238**, **246**
Craniotomy
  cerebellar hemorrhage, 361
  intracranial tumors, 784
  subdural hemorrhage, 358
CRASH syndrome, 220
Creatinine kinase (CK), 485
  neuromuscular disorders, 711
Creatinine levels, asphyxiated infants, 489
Cretinism, **801**, 810
'Cri du chat' syndrome, **800**
Crigler-Najjar's syndrome
  clinical features and biochemical findings, **613**
  prenatal diagnosis, **601**
Cross-over (midline)
  axonal, 5
  callosal fibers, 32
Cross-sectional area, blood vessels, Doppler measurements, 121
Crossed extension reflex, 107, *108*
Crouzon's disease, 776
Crown-rump length (CR), **21**, **22**
Crying
  facial asymmetry, 103, 697
  pattern, 101
*Cryptococcus neoformans*, 588
Cryptophthalmos syndrome, **238**
Crystalloid, 580
Cuneate nuclei, 31
Cuneus, 51
Cup electrodes, EEG, 157
Curosurf, natural, effect on CBFV, 130–1
Cyclic AMP, 484
Cyclopia, 4, 210, 275
Cyclosporin *see* Ciclosporin-A
Cystathionine synthase deficiency *see* Homocystinuria
Cysteine levels, hypoxic-ischemia, 507
Cystinosis
  clinical features and biochemical findings, **613**
  prenatal diagnosis, **601**
Cystinuria
  clinical features and biochemical findings, **613**
  prenatal diagnosis, **601**
Cysts
  arachnoid, 225–6, 229, 279, 286, 288, *312*, 313
  centrum semiovale, 384
  choroid plexus, 286, *287*, 310
  conversion of necrotic tissue to, 326
  dermoid, 768, 776
  multicystic encephalomalacia, 74–5
  multicystic leukoencephalopathy (MCLE), 330, 331, 332, 392, 431, 478, 481
  periventricular leukomalacia (PVL), 60, 69, 70–1, 155, 330, 378, 383–4, 385, 386–9, 390, 391
  porencephalic, 214, 215, 282, 329, 393, 431
  renal, 223
  subependymal, 67, 355
Cytokine theory, PVL pathophysiology, 376–7, 382
Cytokines, 514
  levels in asphyxia, 485
  levels in bacterial meningitis, 576
  microglial expression, 419
  reducing brain injury, 514–15
  role in posthemorrhagic hydrocephalus, 741
Cytomegalovirus (CMV), 553, 554, 556–9, 812
  asymptomatic congenital infection, 557
  BAEP monitoring, 187
  diagnosis, 558–9
  hearing loss, 686
  mineral deposits, *327*
  psychomotor development, 558
  recurrent maternal infection, 558
  sensorineural hearing impairment, 556, 557–8
  symptomatic congenital infection, 556–7
  treatment and prevention, 559
Cytotoxic edema, 416, 428, 475

Dandy-Walker malformation, 54, 216, 240–1, 277, 279, *280*
Dandy-Walker syndrome, **208**, 216, 222, 224–6, 229, *280*, 759
  abdominal ultrasound, 277, 279
  clinical characteristics, 225, 226
  management, 226
  pathologic findings, 224–5
Dandy-Walker variant, 277, 279, *280*
DCX gene mutations, 244
ddI, 566
Deafness *see* Hearing impairment
Decelerations, fetal heart rate, 452–5
  early, 452
  late, 453, 454, 455
  variable, 452, 453
Decerebrate posturing, 348
Decision aids, antenatal screening, 272
Decussation, pyramidal, 32
Deep tendon reflexes, 108
  absent, 115
Deferoxamine, 509
Degenerative disorders, 623–42
  differential diagnosis, 641
  disorders
    Alexander's disease, **627**, 641, 753
    Alper's disease, **627**, 641
    amino acid disorders, **597**, **607**, 623, **625**, 632, 809
    Battens disease, **626**, 640
    carbohydrate metabolism disorders, **597**, **607**, **626**, 639
    carbohydrate-deficient glycoprotein syndrome, 223, **601**, 606, 623, **627**, 634
    infantile neuraxonal dystrophy, 641
    lactic acidemia, 637–8
    Leigh's disease, 623, **627**, 640–1
    lysosomal diseases, 605–6, 623, 628–32, 685
    Menke's disease, **600**, **612**, **627**, 634, 642, **800**
    neurotransmitter disorders, **626**, 638–9
    organic acid disorders, **598**, 606, **608**, 618, 619, 623, **626**, 639, **710**, 725
    Pelizaeus-Merzbacher disease, 636
    peroxisomal disorders, **600**, **611**, 623, **625**, 634–6
    purine and pyrimidine metabolism disorders, **600**, **611**, **625**, 632–3
    Sjögren-Larsson's syndrome, **601**, **614**, **625**, 636–7
    Smith-Lemli-Opitz syndrome, **240**, **242**, **243**, 275, 606, **627**, 634
    sulfite oxidase deficiency, **600**, **612**, **627**, 634
    vitamin metabolism disorders, **600**, **612–13**, **626**, 639–40
    Zellweger's syndrome, **241**, **600**, 606, **611**, 623, **625**, 635–6, 674, 725
  examination and investigation, 627–8
  key points, 642
  specific therapies, 642
  symptoms, 623–7
  *see also* Inborn errors of metabolism
Dekaban-Arimas syndrome, **248**
Delayed visual maturation, 675–7
  pathogenesis, 676–7
  relationship with cortical visual impairment, 678
Delivery, method of
  brachial plexus palsy, 702
  influence on GMH-IVH devlopment, 344–5
  influence on PVL development, 380
  operative vaginal delivery
    forceps, 525, 534, 535, 695
    neurologic injury, 525
    notes and translations, **532**
    vacuum extraction, 356–7, 364, 527, 534, 535
  *see also* Breech delivery; Cesarean section
'Delta brush', EEG, 160, *162*, *163*, 167
Delta-theta activity, EEG pattern, 160
Dendrites, formation, 23, 24
Dentate nucleus, 29, 31
Dentists, children of, 259
Deoxyhemoglobin, 143
Depolarization following anoxia, 507
Depressive illness, major, 11
Depressor angulae oris, 103
Dermal sinuses, meningitis, 574
Dermoid cysts, 768, 776
Dermoid sinuses, 769, 770, 776
Destructive procedures *see* Cephalocentesis
Developing countries
  bacterial meningitis, 574
    antibiotics, 581
    organisms involved, 575
  lead exposure, 813
  mental retardation prevalence, 803
  myelomeningocele, 769
  perinatal asphyxia, 474
  traditional practices, cord care, 589
Development of CNS
  anatomy, 21–36
  early embryonic brain development, 11–18
  milestones, **3**
  neuronal circuits, epigenetic and functional organization, 3–9
  ultrasound assessment, first trimester, 41–2
Dexamethasone
  asphyxiated infants, 491
    prevention of brain injury, 517
  cerebral edema, 654
  effect on CBFV, 131–2
  effect on fetal behavior, 95
  neurotoxic effect, 381–2
Dextrose administration, inborn errors of metabolism, 616
Diabetes insipidus, following GMH-IVH, 355
Diabetes mellitus, maternal
  abnormal fetal behavior, 94
  abnormal fetal body movements, 90
  AFP levels, 268
  holoprosencephaly, 275
  microcephaly, 213
Diaschisis phenomenon, 505
Diastematomyelia, 204, 698
Diazepam
  effect on CBFV, 131
  effect on developing brain, 254, 259
  effect on EEG, 167, 174
  neonatal tetanus, 590
  seizure disorders, 654
DIDMOAD syndrome, 684
Diencephalon, 26–8
  ultrasound, 41, 42, 46, 47, 49
Diet and visual development, 669

Dietary supplements, undernourished children, 811
see also Folic acid: supplementation
Diethylstilbestrol (DES), teratogenic effects, 252
Diffusion-weighted imaging, 60, 63, *64*, 65, 482
focal infarction, 75, 76, 394, 396
periventricular leukomalacia (PVL), 70, 385
Digital intravenous angiography, 398
Dihydropteridine reductase deficiency *see* Tetrabiopterin disorders
Dihydropyrimidinase deficiency, **625**, 633
Dihydropyrimidine dehydrogenase deficiency, 633
Diphenylhydantoin, effect on developing brain, 254
2,3 Diphosphoglycerate (2,3 DPG), 461
Diplegia, 792
Diplomyelia, 204–5
Direct enzyme assay, 596
Disability, definition, 803
Disconjugate gaze, 103
Discontinuous EEG, permanent or transitory, 161, 167
Disseminated intravascular coagulation (DIC), 487, 489
Distortion product otoacoustic emissions (DPOAEs), 688
Diurnal rhythm, fetal heart rate (FHR), 90
Divergent eye appearance, neonates, 659, *660*
DNA, active degradation, 418
Dobutamine administration, asphyxiated infants, 489
Dolichocephaly, 102
Doll's head maneuver, 661
Dopamine
administration, asphyxiated infants, 489
effect on CBF, 150
Dopamine neurones, 32
Doppler ultrasound, 143, 473
Doppler measurements, 121–2
equipment, 122–3
fetal cerebral circulation, 53–*4*, 123, 133
CBF in complicated pregnancies, 127–30
physiological variables affecting CBF, 125–6
technique, CBF measurement, 124–5
key points, 133
neonatal cerebral circulation, 57, 59, 133
CBFV and drugs, 130–2
CBFV and prediction, 132–3
physiological variables affecting CBFV, 126–7
technique, CBF measurement, 126
pathology
asphyxia, 467, 483, 486, 497, 498
cerebral vein thrombosis, 76
fetal arterio-venous malformations, 289
pregnancy-induced hypertension, 111
progressive hydrocephalus, 77
safety, 123
practical guidance, 123–4
umbilical vessels, 93, 437–8
Dorsal flexion in axis, 105
Dorsal radicular artery, 700
Dorsal roots, spinal nerves, 23
Dorso-ventral axis, formation, 3, 4
Doublecortin protein, 216, 244
Down-beat nystagmus, 664
Down's syndrome
antenatal screening, 273
first trimester markers, 269–70
informing choice, 272
second trimester markers, 268–9
fetal habituation, 95
hearing loss, 685, 690
mental retardation, **800**, 806–7
prevalence and survial rates, 799
DRIFT procedure, 751
Drosophila *see* Fruit fly
Drug addiction, effect on fetus, 94, 213, 252, 255–8, 260, **801**, 813
Duane's syndrome, 686
Dubin-Johnson syndrome
clinical features and biochemical findings, **613**
prenatal diagnosis, **601**
Dubowitz score, 111
Duchenne's muscular dystrophy, **800**
antenatal screening, 270–1
creatinine kinase levels, 711
Ductus arteriosus, 408
aneurysm, 697
patent (PDA)
cerebral artery infarction, 393, 394
GMH-IVH risk, 346–7
indometacin, 131
PVL risk, 381
Ductus venosus, 463
absent or reversed flow, 128–9
Duplex Doppler ultrasound, 122, 123
Dura, role in suture fusion, 776
Dural fistulae, 59
Dural sinus thrombosis, 365
Dural tears, 356–7
Dysbetalipoproteinemia
clinical features and biochemical findings, **612**
prenatal diagnosis, **600**
Dysjugate eye movements, 659
Dyskinesia, 791
Dysmature EEG, *170*, 171, *172*, 173
Dysmorphic features, inborn errors of metabolism, 606
Dystonia, late onset, 493
Dystonic movements, 791

Ear, development of, 683
Early myoclonic encephalopathy, 652
Early-infantile epileptic encephalopathy (EIEE) with suppression bursts, 652
Earmoulds, hearing aids, 690–1
Ears, form and firmness, **110**
Echoviruses, 566, 567
Edema *see* Cerebral edema
EDN3 gene mutations, 684
Edrophonium, 717
Edward's syndrome, 319, 475, **800**
maternal serum markers, 270
Electrocardiography (ECG), 157
Electrocerebral silence, 161
Electrodes
EEG, 157
needle, 177
evoked potentials, 181, 182
Electroencephalography (EEG), 115, 155–79
abnormal, 161, *166*, 167, *168–70*, 171, *172*, 173
abnormalities in organization of behavioral states and EEG indices, 171, *172*, 173
background EEG abnormality, 161, 167
classification of abnormalities, **161**
EEG transients, 167, *168–70*, 171
seizure patterns, 649–50
clinical applications, 173–5
key points, 179
maturational changes, 158–61
less than 31 weeks, 158, *159*, 160
31–32 weeks of PMA, **158**, 160
33–34 weeks of PMA, **158**, 160, *162–3*
35–37 weeks of PMA, **158**, 160
38–42 weeks of PMA, **158**, 160, *164–5*
43–44 weeks of PMA, **158**, 160–1
normal appearances, 155–*7*
behavioral states and neonatal EEG, 156–7
EEG as diagnostic tool, 156
preterm vs. full-term infants, 155–6
pathology
asphyxia, 416, *417*, 482–3, 497, 499
bacterial meningitis, 584
GMH-IVH, 348
neonatal stroke, 398
PVL, 385–6
prolonged monitoring, techniques, 175–9
recording EEG, 157
Electromyography (EMG)
neuromuscular disorders, 711
spinal cord trauma, 700
Electron transport chain disorder, **625**, 637
Electronic fetal monitoring (EFM), 432, 438, 443
guidelines for, 433
medico-legal issues, 535–6, 537
timing of injury, **536**
and outcome prediction, 494
potential benefits, 448–9
potential risks, 449
versus traditional auscultation, 444–8
randomized controlled trials, 445–8
*see also* Cardiotocography (CTG); Fetal heart rate (FHR)
Electronic pressure transducer, CSF pressure measurement, 745–6
Electrophoresis, diagnosing mucopolysaccharidoses, 602
Electroretinography (ERG), *666*, 672–3
preterm infants, 672
Embolic causes, neonatal stroke, 394
Embolic infarction, spinal cord, 701
Emboliform nuclei, 31
Embryonic development, 11–18, **21**
neural circuits, 7–8
neurons
axonal guidance, 5–6
migration, 4–5
proliferation, 4
synaptogenesis, 6–7
organogenesis, 11–17
patterning, fetal brain, 3, 4
*see also* Anatomical development of CNS; Ultrasound assessment, brain development
Emotions, maternal, effect on fetus, 94
EMX2 gene mutations, 247
EN genes, 4, 224
Encephalitis
enteroviruses, 567, 568
herpes, *82*, 83, 563
mental retardation, 812
mumps, 227
necrotizing, 81
Encephalocele, 54, 207, *208*, 237, 317, 319
associated syndromes, 207, **208**
clinical characteristics, 207
occipital, MRI imaging, 65
surgery, 763–4
ultrasound detection, 291, *292*
Encephaloclastic porencephaly, 214, 347, 356
Encephaloclastic proliferative vasculopathy, 240
Encephalomalacia, imaging, 74–5
Encephalomyelocele, 207
'*Encoches frontales*', EEG pattern, 160, 161
Endonucleases, DNA fragmentation, 418
Endophthalmitis, 586
Endoscopy
fetal, 736
neuroendoscopic third ventriculostomy (NTV), 754–5, 766, 767–8, 784
Endothelial cells, susceptibility to hypoxia, 326
Endothelial NOS (eNOS), 419, 420, 509
Endotoxin levels and PVL, 377
Engrailed (En) genes, 4, 224
Enteral tube feeding, 830
*Enterobacter* meningitis, 574, 575, 584
Enteroviruses, 553, 566–7
meningitis, 580
non-polio, 567–8

poliovirus, 568–9
Environmental influences
brain development, 4, 11
neural tube defects, 319
*see also* Teratology
Enzyme-linked immunosorbent assay (ELISA)
lymphocytic choriomeningitis virus, 566
toxoplasmosis, 544
Ependyma, 326
Ependymal cells, 23
Ependymal layer, spinal cord, 22, 23
Ependymomas, 784
Eph receptors, 5
Ephrins, 5
Epidemiology
cerebral palsies, 791–7
changes in prevalence over time, 796
differential descriptions, 791–2
factors affecting prevalence, 795–6
heterogeneity and multifactorality of cause, 792
key points, 797
risk factors, 792–5
mental retardation, 799–814
causal categories, **800–2**
definition and classification, 803
environmental toxins, 813
genetic causes, 805–10
infectious causes, 812–13
key points, 814
nutritional causes, 810–11
perinatal causes, 811–12
prevalence, 803–5
trauma, 813–14
neural tube defects, 317–18
impact of prenatal diagnosis, 318–19
Epidermoid tumor following lumbar puncture, 578
Epidural hemorrhage *see* Extradural hemorrhage
Epigenetic and functional organization, neuronal circuits, 3–9
migration of neurons, 4–5
axonal guidance, 5–6
neurotransmitters, 6
neurotrophic agents, 6
organization of brain, 8–9
patterning of fetal brain, 3–4
proliferation of neurons, 4
synaptogenesis, 6–7
wiring the brain, 7–8
Epignathus, 784
Epilepsia partialis continuans, 641
Epileptic spasms, 649
Epimerase deficiency
clinical features and biochemical findings, **607**
prenatal diagnosis, **597**
Epiphysis cerebri, 26, 27
Epithalamus, development, 26, 27
Equine botulinium globulin, 589
Equine tetanus antitoxin (TAT), 589
Erb's palsy, 702, 703, 704
Erect posture, control of, 100
Erratic seizures, 649, 651
Error, medical malpractice, admitting, 538
Erythropoietin (Epo) production, asphyxia, 485
*Escherichia coli*
meningitis, 574, 575–6, 581, 584, 585
outcome, 586
shunt infections, 587
Esotropia, 662
Estrogen, effect on developing brain, 252, 253
Etamsylate, postnatal, GMH-IVH prevention, 351–2
Ethical issues, 821–2, 829–32
acts of commission and omission, 829–30
beneficence-based obligations to fetus, 823
hydrocephalus
cephalocentesis for intrapartum management, 824
isolated fetal, 824–6
with other abnormalities, 826–7
with severe abnormalities, 826
independent moral status of fetus, 822–3
key points, 827, 832
neurologic problems
diagnosis after prolonged care, 831
diagnosis immediately after delivery, 830
management options, 823–4
quality of life, 829
sanctity of life, 829
Ethmocephaly, 210, 275
European Registration of Congenital Abnormalities and Twins (EUROCAT), 317, 318
Eustachian tube, 683
Euthanasia, 829–30
Evoked otoacoustic emissions (EOAE), 182, 688
Evoked potentials, 181–93, 497
brainstem auditory evoked potentials (BAEPs), 181–2
clinical applications, 185–7
key points, 193
somatosensory evoked potentials (SEPs), 184–5
clinical applications, 190–3, 386
visual evoked potentials (VEPs), 182–3
clinical applications, 187–90, 386
Exanthem subitum, 554
Exchange transfusion
bacterial meningitis, 580
inborn errors of metabolism, 617
Excitatory amino acids (EAAs), 32, 505–7
CSF concentration in asphyxia, 485
extracellular accumulation in ischemia, 416
receptor antagonists, 515
Excitotoxic theory, PVL pathophysiology, 376
Excitotoxicity, 505, 507
Exencephaly, 11, 207
abdominal ultrasound, 290–1
transvaginal ultrasound, 309
Exosurf, synthetic, effect on CBFV, 130, 131
Expanding repeat disorders, 805
Expert evidence
UK perspective, 522–3
US perspective, 528–9
External auditory meatus, 683
External granular layer, cerbellum, 31
External hydrocephalus, 77
External ventricular drainage, 754
External version of fetus, 298
Extracorporeal membrane oxygenation (ECMO)
abnormal BAEPs, 187
hearing impairment risk, 687
intraparenchymal hemorrhage, 362
Extradural hemorrhage, 363–4
Extraocular muscles, embryology, 659
Extravascular pressure, GMH-IVH risks, 347
Extreme low voltage EEG, 161
Eye movements
fetal, 90, 659
effect on FHR, *92*
key points, 678
neonatal, 659–67
abnormal, **662–7**
EEG measurements, 157
effect on Doppler CBF measurements, 126
normal, 659
types of, 659–62
Eye-to-eye contact, 101
Eyelids
closure, 668
opening, 667

F52 deficiency, 201
Fabry's disease
clinical features and biochemical findings, **611**
prenatal diagnosis, **599**
Facial abnormalities, holoprosencephaly, 210–11, 275, *276*
Facial bruising, GMH-IVH prediction, 344
Facial movements, assessment, 103
Facial palsy, 103, 695–6, 702, 706
Facial weakness, 709, 712
Factor V Leiden disorder, 240, 365, 395
Factor XIII concentrate, GMH-IVH prevention, 353
Falx cerebri, 48
tears, 356
Familial Dandy-Walker syndrome, 225
Familial hypercholesterolemia
clinical features and biochemical findings, **612**
prenatal diagnosis, **600**
Familial microcephaly, 212
Familial porencephaly, 240
Farber's disease, 629–30
clinical features and biochemical findings, **610, 624**
prenatal diagnosis, **599**
Fasciculation
modulation in axonal guidance, 5
of tongue, 102, 711
Fasciculus retroflexus, 29
Fastigial nuclei, 31
Fatty acid oxidation defects, 606, 618, 620
clinical features and biochemical findings, **609**
prenatal diagnosis, **598–9**
Fecal incontinence, spinal dysraphism, 204
Federal Rules of Evidence, 528
Feeding behavior, 108
Ferritin-positive cells, 376
Fetal akinesia deformation sequence, 90
Fetal alcohol syndrome (FAS), 213, **242**, 251, 257–8, **801**, 813
Fetal blood sampling, 596
cordocentesis, 281, 466–7, 596
scalp blood sampling, 438, 449–50, 452, 464, 494
herpes simplex infection, 563
toxoplasmosis, 546
Fetal distress, 90, 95, 111
controversy over term, 438
definition, 443
during labor, 472
Fetal gas analysis, 459–68
acute asphyxia
causes, 464
diagnosis with blood gases, 463–5
pathophysiology, 463
chronic asphyxia
causes, 466
diagnosis with blood gases, 466–7
pathophysiology, 465–6
impaired oxygen delivery, 462–3
key points, 468
normal oxygen delivery, 460–2
fetal respiration, 462
oxygen carriage in blood, 460–1
placental gas exchange, 461–2
Fetal heart rate (FHR), 90–2, 434, 438
asphyxia, 410, *411*, *412*, 413, 444
auscultation, 443, 494
medico-legal issues, 535–6
versus EFM, 444–8
baseline, 450
bradycardia, 408, 410, 429, 433, 450–1
computer analysis, 450
contraction stress test (CST), 433–4
effect on Doppler CBF measurements, 125
in growth-retarded fetuses, 91–2
guidelines for monitoring, 433, 450–1
hypoxia, 408, 409, 429
intrafetal consistency, 91
non-stress test (NST), 432–3
normal, 432, 450
patterns, 92
cystic PVL, 379
differential diagnosis, silent and sinusoidal FHR, **93**, 95

mouth and sucking movements, 94
periodic and episodic, 452–5
sinusoidal, **93**, 451
variability, 451–2
tachycardia, 408, 451
twins, 96
*see also* Electronic fetal monitoring (EFM)
Fetal Medicine and Surgery Society, 732
Fetal movement center, 434
Fetal movements, 89–90, *92*, 115, 432, 434
biophysical profile score, **435**
breathing movements, 93, 94, 125, 434, **435**
changes following asphyxia, 429
effect on heart rate, 452
eye movements, 90, *92*, 659
first fetal, 24
twins, 95–6
Fetal tone center, 434
FETENDO technique, 736
Fetoscopy, 596
Fetus as patient, concept of, 822–7
FG syndrome, **239**, **241**
Fibrinolytic therapy, intraventricular, 750–1
Fibroblast growth factor (FGF), suture fusion, 776
Fibroblast growth factor receptor-1 gene, 201
Filum terminale, 22
thickened, 769, 770
Fine motor skills, 100
Finger grasp reflex, 107
Finger movements, 103
Finnish muscle-eye-brain disease, **246**
'Finnish Snowballs', 640
First arch syndrome, 684
Fixation, visual, 667
fix and track, 101–2
Flash-VEPs, 183, 672
clinical applications, 187
Flavin-adenine dinucleotide (FADH) accumulation in asphyxia, 428
Flocculonodular lobes, cerebellum, 30
Floor plate, 5
Floppy infant, 95
Flucloxacillin
bacterial meningitis, 581
shunt infections, 587
Fluconazole, fungal meningitis, 588
5-flucytosine, fungal meningitis, 588
Fluid attenuated inversion recovery (FLAIR) sequences, 60
Fluids
replacement, bacterial meningitis, 580
restricting
asphyxiated infants, 489
bacterial meningitis, 580
Flunarizine, reducing hypoxic injury, 507
Fluorescent treponemal antibody absorption (FTA-ABS) test, 590
Flush solutions, benzyl alcohol in, 347
Focal ischemic lesions, 74, 75–6
seizures, 651
*see also* Infarction
Focal seizures, 649
Focal transmural dysplasia, 214
Focus settings, ultrasound imaging, 59
Fodrin, 510, 511
Folate deficiency, 251, 811
Folia, cerebellum, 30
Folic acid, 201
metabolism disorders
clinical features and biochemical findings, **612**
prenatal diagnosis, **600**
role in NTD prevention, 319–20
supplementation, 237, 251, 291, 319, 734, 810
Following, vision, 668
Fontanelles
as acoustic window, 45, 53, 57, 59, 122, 297, 298, 299
scanning off-center, 58, 59
assessment, 102
bulging, 577
pressure measurement, 584
tense, 102, 348
*see also* Anterior fontanelle
Food and Drug Administration (FDA), US, vacuum extraction risks, 527
Foot deformities, myelomeningocele, 204
Foot dorsiflexion angle, 104
Foramina of Luschka, 16, 34, 35, 58, 59
congenital obstruction, 740
Foramina of Magendie, 16, 35
congenital obstruction, 740
Foramina of Munro, 41, 47, 48
Forceps deliveries, 525, 534, 535
facial palsy, 695
Forearm recoil, 104
Forebrain *see* Prosencephalon
Forehead remodeling, 778
Fornix, 31, 32
myelination, 36
Fourth nerve palsy, 662
Fourth ventricle, 302
Dandy-Walker malformation, 277, 279
development, 16, *30*, 31
choroid plexus, 33, 34–5
trapped, 759
ultrasound, *40*, 50, 53, *304*
Fractures
clavicular, 703
congenital muscular dystrophy, *714*
odontoid peg, 698
skull, 363
Fragile X syndrome
antenatal screening, 271–2
mental retardation, 799, **800**, 808–9
prevalence, 809
France, birth asphyxia, 474
Free β-subunit of hCG, 268, 269, 270
Fresh frozen plasma (FFP)
asphyxiated infants, 489
bacterial meningitis, 580
GMH-IVH prevention, 352
'Frog facies', 290
Frontal encephaloceles, surgery, 763, 764
Frontal planes, transvaginal ultrasound, 299, *300*
'Frontal sharp transients', EEG pattern, 160
Frontofacionasal dysplasia, **238**
Fructose metabolism disorders
clinical features and biochemical findings, **607**
prenatal diagnosis, **597**
Fruit fly, 4, 5
genes, 4, 11, 16
Frusemide *see* Furosemide
Frye v. United States, 528
Fryns syndrome, 220, **240**
α-fucosidosis, 631
clinical features and biochemical findings, **610**, **624**
prenatal diagnosis, **599**
Fukuyama congenital muscular dystrophy, 216, 217, **246**, 713, **716**
Fulminant hepatitis, 566
Fumarase deficiency, 638
Fumaric aciduria
clinical features and biochemical findings, **614**
prenatal diagnosis, **601**
Fumarylacetoacetate hydrolate deficiency *see* Tyrosinemia
Functional ability, cerebral palsy assessment, 792
Functional assessment, fetal CNS, 89–96
behavioral states, 92–4
clinical implications of, 95
body movements, 89–90
breathing movements and hiccups, 94
eye movements, 90
fetal heart rate (FHR), 90–2
*see also* Fetal heart rate (FHR)
key points, 96
micturition, 94–5
mouth movements, 94
neurology, 95
sex of fetus, 95
twins, 95–6
Functional magnetic resonance imaging (MRI), 65, 143
Fundoscopy, 103
Fungal infections, meningitis, 575, 580, 586, 588
lumbar puncture, 578
Funisitis, 379
Furosemide
CSF reduction, 749
ototoxicity, 687

GABA transaminase deficiency, **626**, 638
Gadopentetate dimeglumine, 60
Gag reflex, 102
Gain settings, ultrasound imaging, 58, 59
Galactocerebrosidase deficiency *see* Krabbe's disease
Galactokinase deficiency
clinical features and biochemical findings, **607**
prenatal diagnosis, **597**
Galactosamine 6-sulfatase deficiency *see* Morquio's syndrome
Galactosemia, 606, 615, 620
blood tests, 616
clinical features and biochemical findings, **607**
prenatal diagnosis, **597**
urine testing, 615
α-galactosidase deficiency *see* Fabry's disease
Gancyclovir, cytomegalovirus, 559
Gangliosidoses, 628–9
clinical features and biochemical findings, **610**, **611**, **624**
prenatal diagnosis, **599**
Gas-liquid chromatography, 616
Gastroesophageal reflux, 103
Gastrointestinal tract
asphyxia, 444, 486
neuropeptides, 6
Gastrostomy, patients with shunts, 759
'Gastrulation' phase, 46
Gaucher's disease, 623, 629
clinical features and biochemical findings, **610–11**, 623, **624**
prenatal diagnosis, **599**
Gaughan v. Bedfordshire Health Authority (1997), 525
Gaze palsy, 664
Gender differences
BAEPs, 182
cerebral palsy risk, 794
fetal behavior, 95
mental retardation, 805
Gene tracking, 602
'General acceptance' test, federal courts, 528
Genes
anti-apoptotic, 419
in embryonic development, 8, 11, 12, 15, 16
axonal guidance, 5
fetal brain patterning, 3–4
mutations
anencephaly, 209
corpus callosum agenesis, 241
Fragile X, 808
hearing impairment, 684
holoprosencephaly, 244
hydrocephalus, 238, 239
Joubert syndrome, 224
lissencephaly, 244
neural tube defects, 237
schizencephaly, 247
sex-linked mental retardation, 807
Genetic causes
hearing impairment, 684–5
mental retardation, **800**, 805–10
Genetic determinism, 8
Genetic diseases
antenatal screening, 270–2
diagnostic clues, **116**
Genetic models, neural tube defects, 201
Genetics, 237–49
anencephaly, 209
cerebellar hypoplasia, 247–8
congenital myopathies, 716, 717
corpus callosum agenesis, 241
Dandy-Walker malformation, 240–1

fetal response to asphyxia, 429
holoprosencephaly, 242–4
hydranencephaly, 240
hydrocephalus, 238, 239
key points, 249
lissencephaly, 216, 244–7
microcephaly, 212, 241–2
myasthenia gravis, 719, 720
myotonic dystrophy, 709, 712, 713
neural tube defects, 237–8, 319
pontocerebellar hypoplasia, 723
porencephaly, 240
schizencephaly, 247
spinal muscular trophy, 721
vermian agenesis, 224
Geniculate bodies
formation, 26
layering of, 8
Genital herpes infection, 564
Genitalia, assessment, **110**
Genome, 3, 8
Gentamicin
bacterial meningitis, 582
shunt infections, 587
Germinal layer, 22, 328
hemorrhage, 150
Germinal matrix, 328, 330, 340
blood supply, 340
hemorrhages, 332, 340
EEG recordings, 174
parenchymal hemorrhagic infarction, 333
MRI appearance, *61*, *62*, 63
Germinal matrix hemorrhage-intraventricular hemorrhage (GMH-IVH), 155, 339–56
classification, grading system, **67**
diagnosis, 348
etiology, 344–7, *348*
cardiovascular factors, 346–7
coagulation defects, 347
extravascular pressure, 347
intrapartum factors, 344–5
lung disease and complications, 345–6
prenatal factors, 344
imaging, 65, 67, 68, 83
incidence, 342–3
in mature infants, 343
pathology, 339–42
prevention, 348–53
antenatal drugs, 349–50
postnatal drugs, 350–3
prognosis, 353–5
mortality, 354
neurodevelopmental outcome, 354–5
sequelae, 355–6
timing of bleed, 343–4
Gestational age, 21–2
affect on
fetal CBF, 125
neonatal CBF, 126
cerebral palsy risk factor, 792–5
choroid plexus formation, 33, 34–5
cranial nerves, 32
general development, 22–4
myelination, 35–6
PVL development, 380
regional development, 24–32
sulci and gyri formation, 33
synaptic development, 32
ultrasound assessment, 41–2
*see also* Maturation
Giant arteriovenous fistulae, 782
Giant cell tumors, 81
Gilbert's syndrome
clinical features and biochemical findings, **613**
prenatal diagnosis, **601**
Gillespie syndrome, **248**
Glia limitans, 23
Glial cells
increase in, 23
migrating, MRI appearance, *62*, 63
precursors, 330
radial, 4, 15, 23, 24, 328
reactive proliferation, 332
Glial fibrillary acidic protein (GFAP), 485
Glial neuronal heterotopias, 218–19
Glioblasts, 22, 24
Gliomas, 283, 785
brainstem, 664
nasal, 207
Gliosis, 325, 326, 330, *331*, *332*, 374, 385, 390
Globose nuclei, 31
Globus pallidus, development, 27
Glucocerebrosidase deficiency *see* Gaucher's disease
Glucose
administration, asphyxia, 489–90
CSF levels in bacterial meningitis, 577, 579
β-glucuronidase deficiency *see* Sly's disease
'Glue ear', 690
Glutamate
affect on neuronal migration, 5
excitotoxicity, 507
role in asphyxia, 419, 423, 428
Glutamate formiminotransferase deficiency
clinical features and biochemical findings, **612**
prenatal diagnosis, **600**
Γ-glutamyl cycle disorders
clinical features and biochemical findings, **608–9**
prenatal diagnosis, **598**
Glutaric aciduria
clinical features and biochemical findings, **609**
congenital anomalies, 606
prenatal diagnosis, **598**, **600**
Gluteal artery thrombosis, 706
Glycerol
asphyxiated infants, 492
hydrocephalus control, 750
Glycerol kinase deficiency
clinical features and biochemical findings, **609**
prenatal diagnosis, **598**
Glycine
increase in hypoxic-ischemia, 507
supplementation, 617
Glycine antagonists, 515
Glycine metabolism disorders
biochemical findings, **607**
prenatal diagnosis, **597**
Glycine-proline-glutamate (GPE), 512–13
Glycogen depletion, fetal asphyxia, 410, 413
Glycogen storage disease
clinical features and biochemical findings, **607**
prenatal diagnosis, **597**
Glycogenosis
type 2, 723
type 3, 725
Glycoproteinoses
clinical features and biochemical findings, **610**, **624**
prenatal diagnosis, **599**
GMU1u gangliosidoses, 628–9
clinical features and biochemical findings, **611**, **624**
prenatal diagnosis, **600**
GMU2u gangliosidoses, 628
clinical features and biochemical findings, **610**, **624**
prenatal diagnosis, **599**
Goiter, 685
Goldenhar syndrome, **208**
Gracile nuclei, 31
Gradient echo cine MRI, 77
Gram stain, bacterial meningitis, 579
Gram-negative organisms
meningitis, 574, 576, 580, 584
antibiotics, 582–3
CSF white cell counts, 579
outcome, 586
shunt infections, 586, 587
Gram-positive organisms, meningitis, 576, 581, 584
Granular layer, 16, 31
Granule cells, 31
apoptosis, 327
failure of formation, 222
'Gray baby syndrome', 581
Gray columns, spinal cord, 23
Gray matter
development, 14
spinal cord, 23
injury to, 475
Gross Motor Classification System (GMFCS), 792
Gross Motor Function Measure (GMFM), 792
Group B streptococcal meningitis, 573, 574, 575, 576, 577, 580, 581
antibiotics, 581, **582**
CSF white cell counts, 579
latex agglutination test, 578
outcome, 586
Group D streptococcal meningitis, 581
Growth charts, 102
Growth cones, axonal tips, 5
Growth factors, 419
insulin-like (IGFs), 419, 512–13
Growth hormone (GH)
asphyxiated infants, 485
IGF-I production, 513
Growth, intrauterine, cerebral palsy, 793
Growth-retarded fetuses, 111, 414–15, 423
abnormal behavior, 94
abnormal eye movements, 90
abnormal fetal body movements, 90
chronic hypoxia, 465, 467
Doppler CBF measurements, 127–9
Doppler umbilical S/D ratio elevation, 437
evoked potentials
effect on BAEPs, 186–7
effect on FVEPs, 189
effect on SEPs, 191
fetal heart rate (FHR), 91–2
metabolic disturbances, 423
white matter lesions, 328
Guanosine-triphosphate cyclohydrolase deficiency *see* Tetrabiopterin disorders
Gyrate atrophy of choroid and retina
clinical features and biochemical findings, **608**
prenatal diagnosis, **597**
Gyri, development, 14, *17*, 33, *34*, 51, 53, 61

Habenular commissure, 27, 32
Habituation, fetal, 95
*Haemophilus influenzae* meningitis, 574, 581, 585, 686
Hagberg-Santavuori disease, 640
Haloperidol, effect on developing brain, 259
Hamartomas, 81
Hand, foot and mouth disease, 567
Handicap, definition, 803
Handling of infant, blood pressure changes, 346, 353
Happy puppet syndrome *see* Angelman's syndrome
Hartnup's disease
clinical features and biochemical findings, **613**
prenatal diagnosis, **601**
Harvard Medical Practice Study, 522, 538
Havercamp *et al*, EFM vs. ausculation trials, 445, 446
Head circumference
assessment, 102
chronic shunt failure, 756
increased, 580, 753
ultrasound imaging, 77
*see also* Macrocephaly
measuring, 473, 742, 779
normal increase after birth, 117
subnormal, 113
*see also* Microcephaly
Head coils, MRI, 60
Head control, acquisition of, 117
Head growth, excessive, definition, 750
Head injury, mental retardation, **801**, 813–14
Head measurement, fetal ultrasound, 49–50
Health Maintenance Organizations (HMOs), 527
lawsuits against, 528
Health-care decisions, pregnant woman, 822
Hearing
assessment, 102, 103
BAEPs, 185–6, 187
development, 683
Hearing aids, 690–1
Hearing impairment, 623
causes of, 683–7, **688**

bacterial meningitis, 586
cytomegalovirus, 556, 557–8
rubella, 555
detection of, 687–90
key points, 691
management, 690–1
risk factors for, **185**
screening, 688, 690
Heart abnormalities, fetal, 466
Heart block, fetal, 450–1, 453
Heart rate, fetal *see* Fetal heart raate (FHR)
Heating effect, Doppler ultrasound, 123
Hedgehog genes, 4, 12, *13*, 244
Hemachromatosis
clinical features and biochemical findings, **612**
prenatal diagnosis, **600**
Hematologic manifestations of asphyxia, 444, 487
Hematomyelia, 699
Heme proteins, defects in synthesis and degradation
clinical features and biochemical findings, **613**
prenatal diagnosis, **601**
Hemiagenesis, cerebellar, 222
Hemihypertrophy of body, 283
Hemimegalencephaly, 211, 224
Hemiplegia, 792
Hemodialysis, inborn errors of metabolism, 617
Hemoglobin dissociation curve, 460, *461*
Hemoglobin, fetal, 460
Hemorrhage *see* Intracranial hemorrhage
Hemosiderin staining, 66
Heparan *N*-sulfatase deficiency *see* Sanfilippo's syndrome
Heparin
cerebral venous thrombosis thrombolysis, 366
GMH-IVH development, 347
parenchymal hemorrhage, 362
Hepatitis A virus (HAV), 566
Hepatitis E virus (HEV), 566–7
Hereditary fructose intolerance
clinical features and biochemical findings, **607**
prenatal diagnosis, **597**
Hereditary optic atrophy, 674
Hereditary orotic aciduria, 633
clinical features and biochemical findings, **611**, **625**
prenatal diagnosis, **600**
Heroin addiction, 255, **256**
Herpes encephalitis, 563
imaging, *82*, 83
Herpes simplex virus (HSV), 81, *82*, 83, 553, 562–4
clinical presentation, 563
diagnosis, 563, 564
incidence and risk, 562
intrapartum infection, 563
management, 564
transplacental infection, 562–3
Herpes zoster, 560, 561, 562
Heterotopias, 208–18, 244, 329
Hexosaminidase deficiency *see* Gangliodsidoses
β-hexosaminidase testing, 271
High frequency ventilation (HFV)
GMH-IVH risk, 346
PVL risk, 380
High-risk neonates
bacterial meningitis, 574, 575
BAEP prediction of outcome, 186
VEP prediction of outcome, 187–8
Hindbrain *see* Rhombencephalon
Hindbrain herniation *see* Arnold-Chiari malformation: type II deformity
Hippocampal commissure, 31, 32, 36
Hippocampal sulcus, 33
Hippocampus
development, 15, 16, 50, 51
hypoxia, 476
Hippocratic Oath, 821
Hirschprung's disease, 684
Histology
cerebellum, 30, 31
cerebral cortex, 24–6
spinal cord
early embryo, 22–4
late embryo and fetus, 24
Holoacrania, 290
Holocarboxylase synthetase deficiency *see* Multiple carboxylase deficiency
Holoprosencephaly, 4, 54, 77, 210–11, 229, 743
clinical characteristics, 210–11
genetics, 242–4
ultrasound
3D assessment, 42, 43
abdominal, 275–7
transvaginal, 311
Holoventricle, 243
HOM genes, 11, 12
Homeobox genes, 15, 16
EMX2 mutations, 247
Homeotic genes, 3, 4, 11, 16
Homocystinuria, 619
clinical features and biochemical findings, **607**
prenatal diagnosis, **597**
Homogentisic-acid oxidase deficiency *see* Alkaptonuria
Homonymous hemianopia, 395, 398
Homosexuality, prenatal prescribed sex hormones, 253
Horizontal gaze palsy, 664
Hormone response in asphyxia, 485
Horner's syndrome, 699, 703, *704*
HOX genes, 3, 4, 11, 12
deficiency, 209
Human albumin, 580
Human chorionic gonadotrophin (hCG), 268, 269, 807
Human herpesvirus type 6 (HHV-6), 554
Human immunodeficiency virus (HIV), 553, 564–6
diagnosis, 565–6
mental retardation, 812–13
neurologic features, 564–5
treatment, 566
Human normal immunoglobulin (HNIG), 568
Hunter's syndrome
clinical features and biochemical findings, **609**
prenatal diagnosis, **599**
Hurler's syndrome, 631, 642, 685, **801**
clinical features and biochemical findings, **609**, **624**
prenatal diagnosis, **599**
Hydranencephaly, 77, 227, *228*, 230, 336, 431, 753
abdominal ultrasound, 279, *280*, 281
genetics, 240
Hydrocephalus
antenatal assessment
abdominal ultrasound, 50, 284–6
transvaginal ultrasound, 310
clinical features, 753
complications, 756–9
abdominal surgery, 759
infection, 757–8
multicompartmental hydrocephalus, 758–9
shunt obstruction, 757
slit ventricle syndrome, 758
diagnosis, 742–6, 753
brainstem auditory evoked potentials (BAEPs), 186
CBF velocity, 132, 746
cranial ultrasound, 76, 77, 742–3
CSF flow studies, 77, *78*
CSF pressure measurement, 745–6
Doppler ultrasound, 77
flash VEPs, 189
head circumference, 742
neurologic examination, 743, 744–5
somatosensory evoked potentials (SEPs), 190, 746
ethical considerations in management, 824–6
cephalocentesis for intrapartum management, 824
hydrocephalus with abnormalities, 826–7
etiology, 226–7, 739–42
acquired after hemorrhage or infection, 740, *741*
bacterial meningitis, 577, 778–9
benign external hydrocephalus, 741
communicating and non-communicating, 226, 741–2
congenital obstruction, 739–40
cytomegalovirus infection, 557
lymphocytic choriomeningitis virus, 566
myelomeningocele, 202, 203, 205
subdural hemorrhage, 358
table of causes, **740**
TGF-β1 and post-hemorrhagic, 741
fetal eye movements, 90
fetal neurosurgery, 729–32
animal studies, 729
human studies, 729–32
genetics, 238–9
key points, 751, 760
neuropathologic changes, 742
neurosurgical management, 753–60
choroid plexectomy, 754
external ventricular drainage, 754
neuroendoscopic third ventriculostomy (NTV), 754–5
ventricular shunting, 755–6
*see also* Shunts
non-surgical treatment, 747–51
drugs, 749–50
intraventricular fibrinolytic therapy, 750–1
repeated CSF tapping, 747–9
ventricular reservoir, 750
prognosis and outcome, 759–60
hydrocephalus with myelomeningocele, 746–7
optic atrophy, 674
posthemorrhagic ventricular dilatation, 747
uncomplicated hydrocephalus, 746
Hydrocephaly/VATER association, **239**
Hydrolethalus, **239**, **240**
Hydromyelia, 205
Hydrops
fetalis, 466, 606
non-immune, 324
3-hydroxy-3-methylglutaryl-CoA lyase deficiency
clinical features and biochemical findings, **608**
prenatal diagnosis, **598**
Hydroxybutyrate dehydrogenase (HBDH), 485
L-2-hydroxyglutaric aciduria, **626**
D-2-hydroxyglutaric aciduria, **626**
L-2-hydroxyglutaric aciduria, 639
D-2-hydroxyglutaric aciduria, 639
3-hydroxyisobutyryl-CoA deacylase deficiency, 606
Hydroxyl radicals, 508, 515, 517
'Hyperalertness', 480
Hyperammonemia, 486–7, 617, 618, 619
Hyperbilirubinemia
evoked potentials
BAEPs, 187
FVEPs, 189
SEPs, 192, 193
hearing loss, 687, 688
PVL risk, 381
Hypercapnia, 462
asphyxiated infants, 488
effect on CBFV measurements, 126–7
fetal, 410
and GMH-IVH development, 345, 347, 353
PVL risk, 381
Hypercarbia, PVL risk, 381
Hyperexcitability, 101, 114
Hyperexplexia, 175
Hyperglycemia, 328, 423
Hyperglycinemia, non-ketotic, 615, 619, **626**, 638
biochemical findings, **607**
prenatal diagnosis, **597**
seizures, 651, 652
Hyperimidodipeptiduria
clinical features and biochemical findings, **608**
prenatal diagnosis, **597**

Hyperlysinemia
biochemical findings, **607**
prenatal diagnosis, **597**
Hyperornithinemia-hyperammonemia-homocitrullinemia (HHH syndrome)
clinical features and biochemical findings, **608**
prenatal diagnosis, **597**
Hyperoxaluria
clinical features and biochemical findings, **611**
prenatal diagnosis, **598**
Hyperoxia, effect on CBFV measurements, 126
Hyperperfusion following asphyxia, 147, 151, 419
Hyperphenylalaninemia, 618
Hyperplasia, cerebellar, 224
Hyperprolinemia
biochemical findings, **607**, **608**
prenatal diagnosis, **597**
Hyperpyrexia following GMH-IVH, 355
Hypertelorism, 'physiological', *40*, 42
Hypertension, maternal, 323, 324
*see also* Pregnancy-induced hypertension
Hyperthermia, role in asphyxia, 424
Hypertonia, 104
Hyperventilation, 149, 150
controlled, asphyxiated infants, 491
GMH-IVH prevention, 353
Hypocalcemia, seizures, 651
treatment, 654
Hypocapnia, 150
Hypocarbia
PVL risk, 381
reduction in CBF after, 376
Hypoglossal nerve injury, 697
Hypoglycemia, 139
asphyxiated infants, 473, 490, 651
CBF and cerebral metabolism, 149
evoked potentials, 193
hypoxic-ischemic injury, 336
optic nerve hypoplasia, 674
treatment, 654
Hypomagnesemia, 654
Hyponatremia, 486
Hypoperfusion
animal studies of PVL, 375–6
post-asphyxial, 414, 416, 421, 422
Hypophosphatasia
clinical features and biochemical findings, **614**
prenatal diagnosis, **601**
Hypophysis cerebri, 27–8
Hypoplasia
cerebellum, 222
genetics, 247–8
limb, varicella infection, 560, 561
optic nerve, 665, 674–5
pontocerebellar, 222, **248**, 722–3
Hypotension
fetal asphyxia, 410, *411*, *412*, *413*, 414, 421, 429, 463
'watershed' distribution of neuronal loss, 421, 422
GMH-IVH risk, 346, 347
maternal, 453, 463
neonatal asphyxia, 489
PVL risk, 381
Hypothalamic sulcus, 27
Hypothalamic-pituitary disturbance, 227
Hypothalamus, 26, 27, 32
Hypothermia
preventing, 488
therapeutic, 515, **516**, 517
Hypothyroidism
mental retardation, **801**, 810
SEPs
preterm infants, 190–1
term infants, 192
Hypothyroxinemia
of prematurity, 812
in PVL, 381
Hypotonia, 104, 114, 480, 496, 606
cerebral palsy, 792
severe global, 114, 115
traumatic cord lesions, 699
Hypoxanthine (Hx), 484, 485
Hypoxanthine-guanine phosphoribosyltransferase deficiency *see* Lesch-Nyhan syndrome
Hypoxemia, 459, 462
maternal, 466
Hypoxia, 471
acute intrapartum event criteria, **530**
definition, 323, 443, 459
fetal, 408–10, 429, 463
60 minutes, responses in fetal sheep, *409*
adaptation to, 408
effect on biophysical profile, *435*
maturational changes in response, 410
prolonged, 410
Hypoxic-ischemic brain injury, 395, 473, 505
cerebral blood flow (CBF), 146–7
Doppler CBFV prediction of, 132–3
definition, 427, 459
diagnostic clues, **116**
EEG recordings, 155, 161, *166*, 171, 174, *176*
evoked potentials, *191*
normal BAEPs, 186
VEPs/SEPs predicting outcome, 188, 191–2
fetal, 323–36
brain development and damage patterns, 328–9
cellular responses, 325–7, 415
damage early gestation 0–28 weeks, 329–30
damage late gestation 36 weeks to term, 333–5
damage mid-gestation 24–36 weeks, 330–3
damage occuring at any age, 335–6
pathogenesis, 323–5
pathologic outcome, factors influencing, 327–8
global hypotonia, 114
imaging, 69–75, 83, 431
preterm infant, PVL, 69–71
term infant, 71–5
incidence, 474
key points, 336
malpractice claims, 524–5
outcome, 495
pathogenesis, 323–5
pathophysiology, 146–7
seizures, 650, 651
severity of encephalopathy, grading, **479**, 480
terminology, 323
tongue fasciculation, 102

I-cell disease, 631
Iatrogenic causes, GMH-IVH, 347
Ictal EEG discharges, 649–50
Iduronate sulfatase deficiency *see* Hunter's syndrome
Iduronidase deficiency *see* Hurler's syndrome
IGF-binding proteins (IGFBPs), 512
Imaging neonatal brain
care of infant, 57
choice of technique, 83
modalities
computerized tomography (CT), 59–60
*see also* Computerized tomography (CT)
magnetic resonance imaging (MRI), 60–5
*see also* Magnetic resonance imaging (MRI)
magnetic resonance (MR) spectroscopy, 65, 77, 79, 83, 142–3, 151
near infrared spectrophotometry (NIRS), 141–2, **144**, 147, 149
positron emission tomography (PET), 65, 83, 141, **144**, 147, 148
radionuclide imaging, 65, 398
ultrasound, 57–9
*see also* Doppler ultrasound; Ultrasound imaging, neonatal
Imipenem, bacterial meningitis, 583
Imipramine, hyperactivity treatment, 260
Immune globulin, maternal administration, 281
Immuno-inflammatory cells, 513, 514
Immunofluorescent antibody tests, lymphocytic choriomeningitis virus, 566
Immunoglobulin cell adhesion molecules (Ig Cams), 5
Immunohistochemistry techniques, PVL distribution, 375
Immunosorbent agglutination assay (ISAGA), 544
Impairment, definition, 803
Imprinting, genetic, 805
*In-vitro* fertilization, 595
Inappropriate antidiuretic hormone secretion (IADHS), 355, 486, 489, 580
Inborn errors of metabolism, 553
key points, 620
management
after diagnosis, 617
long-term, 618
when death seems inevitable, 617–18
whilst awaiting results, 616–17
postnatal diagnosis, 605–20
clinical features and biochemical findings, **607–14**, 615
clues to diagnosis, 615
investigation, 615–16
practice points in investigation and management, **605**
presentation, 605–6, 615
prenatal diagnosis, 595–602
conditions, **597–601**
general principles, 595
key points, 602
methods used to obtain diagnosis, 596, 603
methods used to obtain samples, 595–6
preimplantation diagnosis, 595
specific conditions, 618–20
fat oxidation defects, 620
maple syrup urine disease, 619
non-ketotic hyperglycinemia, 619
organic acidemias, 619
phenylketonuria, 618–20
urea cycle defects, 618–19
*see also* Degenerative disorders
Incisor, single central, 210, 275, 277
Independent moral status, fetus, 822–3
India, perinatal asphyxia, 474
Indirect fluorescent antibody test (IFA), 544
Indirect hemagglutination test (IHA), 544
Indocyanine green, 141
Indometacin
cystic PVL risk, 379
effect on CBFV, 131, 150, *151*
GMH-IVH prevention, 350, 351
GMH-IVH risk, 347
Inducible NOS (iNOS), 419, 420, 509
Infantile free sialic acid storage disease
clinical features and biochemical findings, **613**
prenatal diagnosis, **601**
Infantile neuraxonal dystrophy, 641
Infantile nystagmus, 666
delayed visual maturation, 676
Infantile Refsum's syndrome, 636
clinical features and biochemical findings, **611**
prenatal diagnosis, **600**
Infarction, 428, 476, 477
cerebral arteries, 75–6, 335, 336, 358–9, 393–9, 481
diagnostic clues, **116**
following asphyxia, 431
mineral deposits, 326
spinal cord, 700–1
venous, 67, 341–2, 394
Infection
amniotic fluid
cystic PVL risks, 379
GMH-IVH risk, 344
toxoplasma, 346, 550

  - asphyxiated infants, 489
  - bacterial, 573–87
  - fetal, 323
    - cerebral palsy risk, 423, 794
    - congenital malformations, **199**, 200
    - IFN-α detection, 285
    - microcephaly, 212, 282
  - fungal, 575, 578, 580, 586, 588
  - hearing impairment, 686
  - imaging, 81–3
  - importance in PVL pathophysiology, 376–7
  - mental retardation, **801**
  - mineral deposits, 327
  - seizures, 651
  - shunt, 575, 578, 586–7, 757–8
  - toxoplasmosis, 543–51
  - viral, 553–69
- Inferior olive, 30
- Information aids, antenatal screening, 272
- Informed consent, 822
  - Cesarean delivery, 825
  - UK, 521–2, 525
  - US, 532–3
- Infranuclear eye movement disorders, 662–3
- Infundibular stem, 28
- Infundibulum, 27, 28
- Inherited disorders of oxidative phosphorylation, 79
- Inherited metabolic disease *see* Inborn errors of metabolism
- Inhibin A, 268, 270
- Iniencephaly, 210, 237
  - ultrasound detection, 291
- Injured child in courtroom, 531
- Inner ear, development, 683
- Insula, 33, *34*, 48, 53
- Insulin levels, asphyxiated infants, 485
- Insulin-like growth factors (IGFs), 419, 512–13
- Insurance
  - insurance premiums, malpractice, 527
  - no-fault insurance, 527, 533–4
- Intellectual outcome, discussing with parents, 117
- Intelligence quotient (IQ)
  - asphyxiated infants, 493
  - cerebral mantle thickness, 746, 759
  - cytomegalovirus outcome, 558
  - hydrocephalus outcome, 759–60
  - lead exposure, 813
  - mental retardation, 803
  - myelomeningocele with hydrocephalus, 746–7, 769
  - preschool programs boost in, 805
- Intercostal-to-phrenic inhibitory reflex (IPIR), fetal, 95
- Interferon-α (IFN-α), fetal serum, 285
- Interhemispheric asymmetry, EEG, 167, *168*
- Interhemispheric asynchrony, EEG, 167, *168*, *169*
- Interleukin-1 receptor antagonist (IL-1 ra)
  - bacterial meningitis, 578
  - hypoxic ischemic injury reduction, 514
- Interleukin-1β (IL-1β)
  - bacterial meningitis, 576
  - hypoxic-ischemic injury, 514
  - in PVL, 377, 382
- Interleukin-6 (IL-6)
  - bacterial meningitis, 576, 578
  - in PVL, 377, 382
- Intermittent positive pressure ventilation (IPPV), hearing impairment, 686
- Internal capsule, myelination, 36, 61, *62*
- Internal carotid arteries, fetal, 53
  - Doppler measurements, 53, 124
    - abnormal amniotic fluid volume, 129
    - IUGR fetuses, 127, 128
- International Classification of Diseases (ICD-10), mental retardation, **803**
- International Committee of Radiation Protection, 143
- International Concensus Statement, cerebral palsy, 523
- International Fetal Surgery Registry, 730
- International PHVD Drug Trial Group, 749
- Interparietal sulcus, 51
- Interventricular foramen, 46
- Intracerebral abscess, 780–1
- Intracranial hemorrhage, 114, 339–66
  - basal ganglia, 65, 477
  - cephalhematoma, 102, 363, 365
  - cerebellar, 65, 68, 360–1
  - choroid plexus, 65, 343, 360
  - effect on CBF, 150
  - extradural (epidural), 363–4
  - fetal ultrasound, 281–2
    - abdominal, 281–2
    - transvaginal, 313, *314*
  - germinal matrix, 174, 332, 333
    - *see also* Germinal matrix hemorrhage-intraventricular hemorrhage (GMH-IVH)
  - hypoxic-ischemic injury, 481
  - intraparenchymal, 68, *69*, 333, 341, 343, 362–3
  - intraventricular *see* Intraventricular hemorrhage
  - key points, 366
  - legal issues, 525, 535
  - localization, **339**
  - retinal, 103
  - spontaneous, 782
  - subaponeurotic, 364–5
  - subarachnoid, *58*, 65, 68–9, 74, 359–60, 740
  - subdural, *58*, 65, 68–9, 74, 356–9
  - thalamus, 68, 343, 361–2, 365, *663*, 782
- Intracranial pressure (ICP)
  - measuring following asphyxia, 482
  - outcome prediction, 497
  - raised
    - in bacterial meningitis, 576, 584
    - correlation with Doppler CBFV measurements, 132
    - fontanelle signs, 102
- Intracytoplasmic red cells, 326
- Intrahepatic umbilical vein, blood sampling, 596
- Intraparenchymal hemorrhage, 68, *69*, 333, 341, 343, 362–3
- Intraparenchymal leukomalacia, 793
- Intraparietal sulcus, 61
- Intrapartum factors, cerebral palsy risk, 794–5
- Intrapartum monitoring for asphyxia, 443–55
  - electronic fetal monitoring (EFM), 443
    - potential benefits, 448–9
    - potential risks, 449
    - versus traditional auscultation, 444–8
    - *see also* Electronic fetal monitoring (EFM)
  - fetal heart rate (FHR)
    - abnormalities, 444
    - auscultation, 443
    - *see also* Fetal heart rate (FHR)
  - fetal scalp pH determination, 449–50
  - key points, 455
- Intrauterine growth retardation *see* Growth-retarded fetuses
- Intravenous human tetanus immunoglobulin, 589
- Intravenous immunoglobulin (IVIG), bacterial meningitis, 580
- Intraventricular antibiotics, 779
- Intraventricular fibrinolytic therapy, 750–1
- Intraventricular hemorrhage (IVH), 65, 328, 339
  - bacterial meningitis, 577
  - BAEP latencies, 186
  - diagnostic clues, **116**
  - EEG recordings, 174
  - following asphyxia, 423
  - with hydrocephalus, 740, *741*, 744
    - intraventricular fibrinolytic therapy, 750–1
    - outcome, 759
    - prognosis, 747
    - repeated CSF tapping, 747, 748
  - imaging
    - CT scan, *66*
    - MRI scan, 66, *68*
    - ultrasound, 65, *66*
  - transient ventricular dilatation, 77
  - up-gaze palsy, 664
  - *see also* Germinal matrix hemorrhage-intraventricular hemorrhage (GMH-IVH)
- Intraventricular rupture, 781
- Iodine deficiency, **801**, 810–11
- Iodine skin disinfectants, 578
- Iranian Jews, NTDs, 237
- Ischemia, 74, 75–6, 471
  - definition, 323
  - myocardial, 486
  - spinal cord, 701
  - *see also* Infarction
- Ischemic penumbra, 416
- Isoelectric EEG, 161, 178, 497, 499
- Isoimmune thrombocytopenia, 362
- Isolated holoprosencephaly, 243, 244
- Isolated lissencephaly sequence (ILS), 244
- Isolated microcephaly, 242
- Isonation, angle of, 121, 124
- Isorbide, reduction in CSF production, 750
- Isotretinoin, 200, 225
- Isovaleric acidemia
  - clinical features and biochemical findings, **608**, 615
  - management, 617
  - prenatal diagnosis, **598**
- Isthmus prosencephali, 49
- Isthmus rhombencephali, 29
  - ultrasound, 41, 42, *46*, 49

- Jaeken's syndrome *see* Carbohydrate-deficient glycoprotein syndrome
- Jarcho-Levin syndrome, **238**
- Jaundice, transient cholestatic, 674
- Jervell syndrome, 685
- Jewish population
  - Ashkenazi, 271
  - Iranian, 237
- Joubert syndrome, **208**, 222–4, **240**, **248**
- 'Jug-handle' posturing, 721, *722*
- Jugular veins, 53
  - blood flow measurements, 143
- Junior doctors, reduction in hours, 524

- Kainate receptors, 505
- Karyohexis, 418
- Kelso *et al* EFM vs. auscultation trial, **445**, 446
- Kernicterus, 114
- Ketonuria, 616
- Kety-Schmidt method, 139, 140
- Kidneys, asphyxial injury, 444, 486
- Kjellands forceps, 525
- *Klebsiella*
  - meningitis, 574, 575
    - outcome, 586
  - shunt infections, 587, 758
- Kleeblattschädel, 777
- Klinefelter's syndrome, **800**
- Klippel-Feil anomalad, 686, 770
- Klippel-Feil syndrome, 664
- Klumpke's palsy, 702, 703
- Knobloch syndrome, 207, **208**, **238**
- Krabbe's disease, 630
  - clinical features and biochemical findings, **611**, **624**
  - prenatal diagnosis, **599**
- Krebs cycle defects, **626**, 638
- Krox-20 gene, 4, 12
- Kyphoscoliosis, 291

- Labor
  - asphyxia during contractions, 413
  - effect on Doppler CBF measurements, 129, 130
  - fetal injury during, 536, **537**
  - normal hypoxia during contractions, 450
  - trial of, 527, 533
  - *see also* Delivery, method of
- Lactate
  - CSF, bacterial meningitis, 578
  - MRI resonances, cerebral artery infarction, 397

production, 430, 483
umbilical vein, 462, 463
Lactate dehydrogenase (LDH) deficiency
clinical features and biochemical findings, **608**
prenatal diagnosis, **598**
levels in asphyxia, 485
Lactic acid accumulation in asphyxia, 428
Lactic acidemia, 637–8
Lactic acidosis, 616, 617, 620, 723
Lambdoid postional molding, 777, 778
Lambdoid synostosis, 777
Lamin, 510
Lamina dissecans, 16, 31
Lamina terminalis, 31, 32
Laminar heterotopias, 218
Laminar necrosis, 329
Laminin deficiency, 11
Laminotomy, 785
Lamivudine (3TC), 566
Lange-Neilson syndrome, 685
Language development, hearing impairment, 687
Lanugo, **110**
Laparoscopy, patients with shunts, 759
Late-onset GMH-IVH, 344
Latent phase, energy failure in hypoxic-ischemia, 415
Lateral fissures, 33
Lateral geniculate body, formation, 26
Lateral occipital sulcus, 51
Lateral striae arteries, 340
Lateral sulcus, 33, 52, 61
Lateral ventricles, 51
choroid plexus, 32, 33, 35
hemorrhage, ultrasound imaging, 67
ultrasound
developmental assessment, 41, 42, 46, 47, 48, 49, 50
fetal size assessment, 284
three-horn view (3HV), 3-D neuroscan, 307
transvaginal imaging, 302, 303–4
Latex agglutination test, 578
Latex allergy, myelomeningocele patients, 768
Laurence-Moon-Biedl syndrome, 673, 674
Lead exposure, 252, **801**, 813
Learning and synapse formation, 7, 9
Leber's congenital amaurosis, 223, 665, 673, 674
Lecithin cholesterol acyltransferase deficiency
clinical features and biochemical findings, **612**
prenatal diagnosis, **600**
Legal Aid regulations, UK, 523
Legal issues *see* Medico-legal issues
Leigh's disease, 623, **627**, 640–1
Lemon sign, 291, *293*, 294
Lennox-Gastaut syndrome, 218
Lenticulostriate branches, infarction, 398
Leptomeningeal fibrosis, 779
Leptomeningeal heterotopias, 218–19
Lesch-Nyhan's syndrome, 632
clinical features and biochemical findings, **611**, **625**
prenatal diagnosis, **600**
Lethargy, abnormal, 101, 480
Leucocyte aggregation, bacterial meningitis, 579
Leukoencephalopathy, 211, 377
Leukomalacia *see* Periventricular leukomalacia (PVL)
Lhermitte-Duclos syndrome, 224
Liability, medico-legal issues, 523–4
Liability Reform Acts (US), 527
LICAM gene mutations, 220, 238, 239
Lidocaine (lignocaine), asphyxiated infants, 490, 491
Light sensitivity, testing, 187
Light-emitting diode (LED) goggles, 183
LIM Homeobox gene Lhx5, 15, 16
Limbs
assessment
active tone, 105–6, 112
passive tone, 103–5
paralysis, spinal cord lesions, 699
Linear sebaceous nevus syndrome, **239**
Lingual gyrus, 51
Lipid metabolism disorders, 674
clinical features and biochemical findings, **612**
prenatal diagnosis, **600**
Lipid peroxidation, 508
Lipidoses, **624**
Lipomas
intracranial, 277, 283, 284
intraspinal, 201, *202*
Lipomyleomeningocele, surgery, 770
Lipoprotein lipase deficiency
clinical features and biochemical findings, **612**
prenatal diagnosis, **600**
Liposomal amphotericin, fungal meningitis, 588
LIS-1 gene, 215, 216, 244
Lissencephaly, 215–17, 229, 244
malformation syndromes with, **246**
type I, 215, 216
genetics, 244
type II, 216
genetics, 247
type III, 216
X-linked
lissencephaly/subcortical band heterotopias, 216–17, *245*
*Listeria monocytogenes* meningitis, 574, 576, 581, 779
antibiotics, 582
Litigation, 522
optimal neurologic assessment at birth, 113
Liver biopsy, fetal, 595, 596
Liver function tests, asphyxia, 486
Lobar holoprosencephaly, 211, 243
abdominal ultrasound, 275, 277
transvaginal ultrasound, *310*, 311
Local anesthetics, lumbar puncture, 578
'Locked lambdoid syndrome', 777
Locus coeruleus, 32
London Dysmorphology Database, 237, 241, 242
Long-chain polyunsaturated fatty acids (LCP), dietary and FVEPs, 189
Longitudinal fissure, 33
Lorazepam, seizure disorders, 654
Low velocity car accidents, 324–5
Low voltage irregular EEG pattern (LVI), 160
Lowe's syndrome
clinical features and biochemical findings, **613**
prenatal diagnosis, **601**
Lumbar puncture, 480–1
bacterial meningitis, 577–9
indications, 577–8
interpretation, CSF findings, 578–9
repeat, 583–4
technique, 578
repeated CSF tapping, 747–8
*see also* Cerebrospinal fluid (CSF)
Lumboperitoneal shunts, 755
Lungs, asphyxia manifestations, 444, 486
Luthy *et al* EFM vs. auscultation trial, **445**, 447–8
'Luxury perfusion', 147, 151, 419
Lymphocytes
accumulation, late phase hypoxia-ischemia, 514
lymphocyte count, asphyxia, 430
Lymphocytic choriomeningitis virus (LCMV), 566
Lymphoma, HIV infected infants, 565
Lysine metabolism disorders
biochemical findings, **607**
prenatal diagnosis, **597**
Lysinuric protein disease
clinical features and biochemical findings, **613**
prenatal diagnosis, **601**
Lysosomal diseases, 605–6, 623, 628–32, 685
Lysosomal enzyme defects
clinical features and biochemical findings, **609**
prenatal diagnosis, **599**

MacDonald *et al* EFM vs. auscultation trial, **445**, 446–7
MacMARKS gene, 209
McRobert's maneuver, 702
Macrocephaly, 77, 211, 566, 753, 783, 784, 824
antenatal diagnosis, abdominal ultrasound, 283
etiology, **213**
Macrocerebellum, 224
Macrocrania, 76, 77
Macroglia, 24
Macrophages
meconium transportation, 429–30
role in neuronal injury, 326, 419, 420
Macrosomia, 702
Magnesium sulfate, 654
GMH-IVH prevention, 349, 350
PVL prevention, 382
Magnetic resonance imaging (MRI), 57, 60–3, 83, 115
arachnoid cysts, *225*
Arnold-Chiari malformation, *206*
cerebellar vermian hypoplasia, *223*
cerebral artery infarction, 396–8
cerebral vein thrombosis, 76
congenital malformations, 77, *78*, 79
focal ischemic lesions, 75–6
herpes encephalitis, *82*, 83
hydrocephalus, 753
hypoxic ischemic encephalopathy (HIE), 73–5, 481–2, 496–7
intracranial hemorrhage, 66, **67**
germinal matrix, *340*
GMH-IVH, 68, 348
intraparenchymal, 68
intraventricular, *68*
subarachnoid, 68
subdural, 68, 358
thalamus, 361, *362*
lipoma, intraspinal, *202*
lissencephaly, *215*, *245*
meningitis, 584, *585*
meningoencephalocele, *208*
multicystic leukoencephalopathy, *479*
myelomeningocele, *203*
periventricular heterotopias, 218
periventricular leukomalacia (PVL), 70–1, 385, *390*
polymicrogyria, *228*
sacral agenesis, *205*
special techniques
angiography (MRA) and venography, (MRV), 64, 65, 83, 397–8
diffusion weighted imaging, 63, *64*, 65, 70, 75, 76, 385, 394, 396
spinal cord injury, 700
subcortical cystic leukomalacia, *392*
tethered spinal cord, *202*
third ventriculostomy, 77
tuberous sclerosis, *80*
vascular malformations, 79, 80
venous sinus thrombosis, *365*
ventricular dilation, 77
Magnetic resonance (MR) spectroscopy, 65, 77, 79, 83, 142–3, 151
asphyxiated infants, 147, *149*, 484, 497–8
cerebral artery infarction, 397
periventricular leukomalacia(PVL), 385
Maladaption at birth, 472
Male-mediated drug effects, 259
Malnutrition, mental retardation, 811
Mamillotegmental tract, 29
Mammillary bodies, 27
Mammilothalamic tract, myelination, 36
Mandibular dysostosis, 684
Mannitol, asphyxiated infants, 492
Mannosidosis, 631

  clinical features and biochemical findings, **610**, **624**
  prenatal diagnosis, **599**
Mantle layer (intermediate layer), 14, 23
Maple syrup urine disease, 606, 615, 619
  biochemical findings, **607**
  long-term management, 618
  prenatal diagnosis, **597**
  seizures, 651
Marginal layer, 15
Marginal zone, 23, 24, 25
Marijuana, effect on developing brain, 255, **256**, 257
Maroteaux-Lamy's syndrome
  clinical features and biochemical findings, **610**
  prenatal diagnosis, **599**
Marrow transplantation, degenerative disorders, 642
Marshall-Stickler syndrome, 684
MASA syndrome, 238, 239, **241**
Mass screening, inborn errors of metabolism, 606
Massa intermedia, 26, 50
Mastoid fontanelle, as acoustic window, 57, 59
Maternal causes, fetal circulatory insults, 323, 324
Mathl gene, 222
Maturation
  acceleration of, 111, 128
  assessment of fetus and embryo, 21
    change of state variables, 93
  changes in fetal response to asphyxia, 413–14, 422–3
  delayed visual, 187, 675–7
  EEG recordings, 156, 158–61, *162–5*
    dysmature EEG, *170*, 171, *172*, 173
  evoked potentials, 181–5
  influence on asphyxial lesions, 474
  in motor control, 100
  MRI assessment, 60, *61–3*
  neurologic maturation, 109–10
  physical maturation, non-CNS, 110–11
Mean arterial blood pressure (MAP), asphyxia, 421
Measles, 553, 554
  subacute sclerosing panencephalitis (SSPE), 555
Mechanical ventilation
  asphyxiated infants, 488
  effect on CBF, 150
  GMH-IVH risk, 346, 347
  hearing impairment, 686
  PVL risk, 380
Meckel's syndrome, 207, **208**, 220, **238**, **240**, **242**, **243**, 275, 291, 319
Meconium in amniotic fluid, 429–30, 472, 493
Meconium aspiration syndrome, 429, 486, 488
  prevention, 453
Media attention, medical malpractice, 527
Medial geniculate body, formation, 26
Median cleft face syndrome, **208**
Median nerve palsy, 705
Median nerve SEPs, 184–5
  clinical applications, 190, 191
Median plane, transvaginal ultrasound, 299, *301*, 302, *303*, *304*
Medical records, malpractice claims, 529
Medical Research Council trial, prevention of neural tube defects, 319
Medico-legal issues, 113
  UK perspective, 521–6
    establishing liability, 523–5
    expert evidence, 522–3
    key points, 526
    legal climate, 521–2
    litigation and risk management, 522
  US perspective, 527–38
    clinical practice guidelines, 529, 530
    complication or error, 533
    CTG in court, 537–8
    expert testimony, 528–9
    legal climate, 527–8
    medico-legal education, failure of, 530–2
    solving the malpractice problem, 538
    timing of injury in term fetus, **537**
    tort reform and finances, 533–7
    vacuum extraction study, 537
    why patients sue, **531**, 532–3
Medium chain fatty acyl-CoA dehydrogenase deficiency (MCAD), 620
Medroxyprogesterone, prenatal, 253
Medulla oblongata, 31, 32
Medulloblastoma, 31, 784
Megalencephaly, 211, 753
  antenatal diagnosis, abdominal ultrasound, 283
  hemimegalencephaly, 211, 224
Megaloblastic anemia, 619
Melanin pigment cells, pineal gland, 27
Membrane transport disorders
  clinical features and biochemical findings, **613**
  prenatal diagnosis, **601**
Meningitis, 480, 481
  bacterial *see* Bacterial meningitis
  consequences of, 778–81
  crying pattern, 101
  fungal, 575, 578, 580, 586, 588
  hearing impairment, 686, 688
    cochlear implants, 691
  mental retardation, 812
  neurosyphilis, 590
  recurrent, 201
  viral, 567–8, 580
Meningocele, 200, 201, 202, *203*, 237, 291, *293*, 317
  anterior sacral, 698
Meningoencephalitis, rubella, 555
Meningoencephalocele, *208*
Menke's disease, 633–4, 642, **800**
  clinical features and biochemical findings, **612**, **627**
  prenatal diagnosis, **600**
Mental retardation, epidemiology, 792, 799–814
  causal categories, **800–2**
  characteristics of severe and mild, **804**
  definition and classification, 803
  key points, 814
  prevalence, 803–5
  specific causes
    environmental toxins, 813
    genetic, 805–10
    infections, 548, 812–13
    nutritional, 810–11
    perinatal, 811–12
    trauma, 813–815
Mercury poisoning, teratogenic effects, 251
Meroacrania, 290
Meroanencephaly, 209, 210
Meropenem, bacterial meningitis, 582, 583
Merosin-negative congenital muscular dystrophy, 714, **716**
Merosin-positive congenital muscular dystrophy, 714, 716
Mesencephalon, 13, 14, 16, *17*, *18*, 28–9, 32, 46, 51
  ultrasound, *39*, *40*, 41, 42, 43, 47, 48, 49
Mesenteric vessels, resistance in asphyxia, 486
Mesmetencephalic sulcus, 29
Metabolic acidemia, venous flow abnormalities, 128
Metabolic acidosis
  cord blood gases, 465
  during resuscitation, 488
  fetal, 410, 415, 421, 429, 430, 459, 463
  GMH-IVH development, 345
  neonatal, 615
  neurodevelopmental outcome, 483
  placental dysfunction, 466
Metabolic disorders *see* Inborn errors of metabolism
Metabolic problems
  asphyxiated infants, 486–7
  encephalopathy, MR spectroscopy, 77, 79
  GMH-IVH, 355
Metabolite accumulation, analysis in metabolic disorders, 602
Metabotrophic receptors, 505, *506*
Metachromatic leukodystrophy, 630
  clinical features and biochemical findings, **610**, **624**
  prenatal diagnosis, **599**
Metencephalon, 12, 29–31, 46
Methadone, effect on developing brain, 255, **256**
Methicillin-resistant *Staphylococcus aureus* (MRSA), 581
Methionine metabolism disorders
  clinical features and biochemical findings, **607**
  prenatal diagnosis, **597**
Methionine synthase reductase (MTRR) polymorphism, 320
*N*-methyl-D-aspartate *see* NMDA receptors
2-methylacetoacetyl-CoA thiolase deficiency
  clinical features and biochemical findings, **608**
  prenatal diagnosis, **598**
Methylcobalamin synthesis defects, **612**
3-methylcrotonyl-CoA carboxylase deficiency
  clinical features and biochemical diagnosis, **608**
  prenatal diagnosis, **598**
α-methyldopa, 260
  effect on developing brain, 254, 258, 260
Methylenetetrahydrofolate (MTHFR) gene mutations, 237
Methylenetetrahydrofolate reductase deficiency, 639–40
  clinical features and biochemical findings, **612**, **626**
  prenatal diagnosis, **600**
3-methylglutaconic aciduria, 639
  clinical features and biochemical diagnosis, **608**, **626**
  prenatal diagnosis, **598**
Methylmalonic acidemia, 606, 619
  clinical features and biochemical findings, **608**
  prenatal diagnosis, **598**
Methylthioninium chloride (methylene blue), bacterial meningitis, 580
Methylxanthines, effect on CBFV, 131–2, 150
Metopic synostosis, 777, 778
Metronidazole
  neonatal tetanus, 589
  organic acid disorders, 617
Mevalonic aciduria, 639
  clinical features and biochemical findings, **608**, **626**
  prenatal diagnosis, **598**
Micrencephaly, 215
  vera, 212
Microangiomata, 361
Microcephaly, 4, 102, 211, 212, 217, 275
  antenatal diagnosis, abdominal ultrasound, 282–3
  cytomegalovirus infection, 557
  genetics, 241, 242, **243**
  lymphocytic choriomeningitis virus, 566
  maternal/prenatal disorders with, 212, 213
  postnatal disorders with, 213
  secondary, 473
  toxoplasmosis, 548
Microglia, 24, 326
  activation, 514
    in apoptosis, 419
  quinolinic acid production, 507
Microgyria, 229
Microhemagglutination test for *T. pallidum*, 590
Microphthalmia, 210
Microvenography, deep periventricular white matter, *341*
Micturition, fetus, 93, 94–5
Mid-coronal planes, transvaginal ultrasound, 299, *300*
Mid-sagittal plane *see* Median

Spontaneous gasping, 487
Spontaneous intracranial hemorrhage, 782
Spontaneous movement, neonate, 103, 112
  loss of, 699
Spontaneous respiration
  delay in, 492–3
  onset of, outcome prediction, 495
Sprengel's malformation, 770
Squint, 662–3
  PVL infants, 390, 391
Stable isotope dilution gas chromatography, 602
Stable xenon-enhanced computed tomography, 141
Stanford University Law Review, 535
Staphylococcal meningitis, 575, 576
  antibiotics, 581, 582
*Staphylococcus aureus*
  meningitis, 575, 585
  shunt infection, 758
*Staphylococcus epidermis*, shunt infection, 586–7, 758
Startle responses, 174, 683
Statoacoustic system, myelination, 35
Status epilepticus
  maternal, 324
  neonatal, 648
    electroclinical correlations, 175, *176*
Status of fetus, 822–3
  previable fetus, 823, 824
Status marmoratus, 335, 474, 476–7
Stavudine (d4T), 566
Sternocleidomastoid muscle, examination, 103
Sternomastoid tumor, 777
Steroid sulfatase deficiency
  clinical features and biochemical findings, **614**
  prenatal diagnosis, **601**
Stickler syndrome, 684
Stiff-baby syndrome, 175
Stimulation, importance of, 7–8
Strabismus, 662–3
  PVL infants, 391, 392
*Streptococcus agalactiae* meningitis, 586
*Streptococcus pneumoniae* meningitis, 574, 686
  antibiotics, 581
*Streptococcus pyogenes* meningitis, 586
Streptokinase, intraventricular, 750–1
Stress, maternal, effect on fetus, 253
Striatal nuclei, neuronal loss in asphyxia, 422
Stroboscopic flashlights (Flash VEPs), 183
Stroke, neonatal *see* Cerebral arteries: infarction
Sturge-Weber disease, 81
Subacute hemorrhage, imaging, 66
Subacute sclerosing panencephalitis (SSPE) of measles, 555
Subaponeurotic hemorrhage, 364–5
Subarachnoid catheter insertion, ICP measurement, 482
Subarachnoid cysts, 286
Subarachnoid hemorrhage, 359–60
  hydrocephalus, 740
  imaging, *58*, 65, 68–9, 74
Subarachnoid space, empyema, 780
Subcommissural organ, 26, 28
Subcortical band heterotopias, 216–17, 244, 329
Subcortical leukomalacia, 391–3, 481
Subcortical structures, asphyxia, 476
Subcortical white matter heterotopias, 218
Subdural effusions, bacterial meningitis, 577, 779–80
Subdural empyema, 780
Subdural hemorrhage, 356–9
  clinical findings, 357
  complications, 358–9
  diagnosis, 358
  etiology, 356–7
  imaging, *58*, 65, 68–9, 74
  treatment and prognosis, 358
Subdural tap, 358, 779–80
Subependymal cyst, 67
Subependymal heterotopias *see* Periventricular heterotopias
Subependymal pseudocyst, 355
Subgaleal hemorrhage, 535, 537
Submental muscle activity (EMG), 157
Subpial hemorrhage, 359
Subpial layer (marginal zone), 23, 24
Subplate neurones, 25
Substance P, effect on developing brain, 255
Substantia nigra, 16, 28, 29, 32
Subtemporal decompression, slit ventricle syndrome, 758
Subtle seizures, 648, 649, 651
Succinate semi-aldehyde dehydrogenase deficiency, **626**, 638
Suck-swallow reflex, 108
Sucking movements, fetus, 94
Sucking reflex, 102, 103
  weak or absent, 480
Sudden infant death syndrome, 255
  'back to sleep' campaign, 777
  infantile botulism, 705
  'near miss', 479
Sulci formation, 27, 33, *34*, 51, 52, 53
  MRI imaging, 61, *62*
  transvaginal ultrasound, 304, *306*
Sulcus limitans, 23, 29
Sulfadiazine, toxoplasmosis, 549, 550
Sulfite oxidase deficiency, 634
  clinical features and biochemical findings, **612**, **627**
  prenatal diagnosis, **600**
'Sunsetting' sign, 361, *663*, 664
Superficial cortical heterotopias, 218–19
Superior cerebellar arteries, 125
Superior frontal sulcus, 51
Superior sagittal sinus, ultrasound imaging, 58
Superior temporal sulcus, 51, 53
Superoxide dismutase (SOD), 508, 509
Superoxide radical, 508
Supine sleeping position, posterior plagiocephaly, 777
Supranuclear disorders, 663–4
Supranuclear facial palsy, 696
Supraorbital remodeling, 778
Supraventricular tachycardia, fetal, 324, 466
Surfactant administration
  effect on CBFV, 130–1
  GMH-IVH prevention, 353
Sutures
  assessment, 102
  cranial ridges on, *114*, 117
  craniosynostosis, 283, 776–8
Swallowing reflex, 103
Sweden, birth asphyxia, 473, 474
Sylvian fissure, 33, 52, 61
Synaptic development, 32
Synaptic transmission, immature brain, 6
Synaptogenesis, 6–7, 11, 24, 36, 329
Syndromal holoprosencephaly, 243
Syndromal microcephaly, 242
Syntocinon administration, abuse of, 524, 525
Syphilis
  meningitis, 578, 590
  mental retardation, 812
Syringomyelia, 205

Tachycardia, fetal, 324, 408, 451, 466
Talipes, fixed bilateral, 711
Tandem mass spectroscopy, 606
Tangier disease
  clinical features and biochemical findings, **612**
  prenatal diagnosis, **600**
Tay-Sach's disease, 628, **801**
  clinical features and biochemical findings, **610**, 623, **624**
  prenatal diagnosis, 271, **599**
Technetium scan, cerebral artery infarction, 398
Tectocerebellar dysraphia, 222
Tectum, 4, 28, 29, 51
Tegmentum, 16, 28, 29
Teicoplanin, shunt infections, 587
Tela choroidea, 32, 35
  hemorrhage, 343
  ultrasound, *52*
Telencephalic leukoencephalopathy, 330
Telencephalic vesicles, 14, 15, *16*, 24
Telencephalon, 24–8, 46
  myelination, 36
  ultrasound, 47
Telephone helpline, antenatal screening, 273
Temperature
  cerebral, role in asphyxia, 424
  effect on hemoglobin dissociation curve, 461
  therapeutic hypothermia, 515, **516**, 517
Temporal artery catheterization, 394
Teratology, **199**, 200, 237, 251–60
  chemicals affecting brain development, 252–8
    action of, 258–9
    addictive compounds, 94, 213, 255–8, **801**, 813
    corticosteroids, 253
    neurotransmitters, 254–5
    sex hormones, 252–3
    thyroid hormones, 253
  clinical awareness and future research, 259–60
  functional teratology, 251–2
  holoprosencephaly, 275
  key points, 260
  microcephaly, 212, 213, 241
  myelodysplasia, 201
Teratomas, 283, *284*, 784, 785
'Terminal asphyxial model' of injury, 535
Termination of pregnancy
  inborn errors of metabolism, 595
  neural tube defects, 318
  toxoplasmosis, 550
Testicular cancer, DES prenatal exposure, 252–3
Tetanic uterine contractions, 453
Tetanus immune globulin (TIG), 589
Tetanus, neonatal, 589–90
Tethered spinal cord, 201, *202*, 204, 768, 770
Tetrabiopterin disorders
  clinical features and biochemical findings, **607**
  prenatal diagnosis, **597**
Tetraplegia, 524, 792
Thalamus
  atrophy, 395, 397
  development, 26–7, 42
  hemorrhage, 68, 343, 361–2, 365, 782
    ocular signs, *663*
  hypoxic-ischemic injury, 481
  infarction, 477
  status marmoratus, 335, 476–7
α-thalassaemia/mental retardation (ATR-X) syndrome, **241**
Thalidomide, 251
Thanatophoric dysplasia, **239**
Thanatropic dwarfism, 777
Theory of neuronal group selection (TNGS), Edeleman, 8
Therapeutic window, asphyxia, 428, 505
'Theta pointu alternant', 652–3
Thiopentone, asphyxiated infants, 490
Third nerve palsy, 662
Third ventricle, 26, 302, 304
  choroid plexus, 32
  neuroendoscopic ventriculostomy, MRI, 77
  ultrasound, 41, 42, 48, 50, 52
    dilatation, 284
Thoraco-lumbar spine, trauma, 699
Three-dimensional ultrasound imaging, 39–44, 45, 59, 304, 305–6
  advantages and limitations, 307–8
  embryonic anomalies, 42–3
  technique, 39–40, 306–9
Three-horn view (3HV), 3-D neuroscan, 307, 310

Thrombocytopenia
fetal, 281
neonatal, 362, 363
Thrombolic causes, neonatal stroke, 394
Thrombophilia, 240
Thrombosis, cerebral vein, 76, 365–6
Thumbs, adduction, 103
Thyroid hormones
risk to psychomotor development, 253, 258
*see also* Hypothyroxinemia
Thyrotropin-releasing hormone (TRH)
effect on developing brain, 255
GMH-IVH prevention, 350
PVL risk, 381
Tirilazad mesylate, 508, 509
Tocolysis, β-sympathomimetic, GMH-IVH risk, 344
Tone, fetal, 434
biophysical profile score, **435**
*see also* Muscular tone, neonate
Tongue
examination, 102, 103
fasciculation, 102, 711
Tonic downward eye deviation, 664
Tonic orientation, 667
Tonic posturing, 174
Tonic seizures, 648, 649
TORCH conditions, 686, 794
Toriello-Carey syndrome, **241**
Tort reform, 527, 533–7
*Torulopsis glabrata*, 588
Toxoplasmosis, *81*, 543–51
congenital toxoplasmosis, 543–4, 546–8
in fetus, 546, 548
in neonate, 548
epidemiology, 544–5
seroprevalence and incidence, **545**
immunology, 544
key points, 551
maternal infection, 543
mental retardation, 812
parasitology, 543
prevention, 545, 546
treatment, 548–51
at birth, 550
if diagnosis of fetal infection is positive, 550
maternal infection, 1st and 2nd trimesters, 549–50
maternal infection, 3rd trimester, 550
termination of pregnancy, 550
*Tracé alternant* (TA), EEG pattern, 160, *165*, 167
Trace metal metabolism disorders
clinical features and biochemical findings, **612**
prenatal diagnosis, **600**
Tranexamic acid, GMH-IVH prevention, 353
Transabdominal approach
chorion villus biopsy, 596
ultrasound scan, 45, 124, 297, 298
Transarterial embolization, 783
Transarterial obliteration, 782
Transcephalic impedance, 143
Transcervical approach, chorion villus biopsy, 595–6
Transcobalamin deficiency, 640
clinical features and biochemical findings, **612**, **626**
prenatal diagnosis, **600**
Transducers
choice of, 45
frequency, 57–8
transvaginal, 39, 45, 297
Transexualism, 253
Transfontanelle approach, 30, 45, 53, 57, 59, 122, 297, 298, 299
Transforming growth factor-β1 (TGF-β1)
role in posthemorrhagic hydrocephalus, 741
studies in PVL, 375, 376
Transient evoked emissions (TEOAEs), 688
Transillumination of skull, hydranencephaly, 227
Transpontine fibers, myelination, 35
Transported infants, GMH-IVH risk, 345
Transtemporal approach, 57, 59, 122, *123*
Transvaginal fetal neuroscan, 45, 125, 297–315
aspects of, 300, 302–6
3-D ultrasound, 39–44, 304, 305–9
equipment and technique, 297–8
key points, 313
pathology, 309–15
arachnoid cysts, *312*, 313
choroid plexus cysts, 310
corpus callosum agenesis, *309*, 311, 313
holoprosencephaly, *310*, 311
intracranial hemorrhage, 313, *314*
neural tube defects, 309–10
periventricular leukomalacia, 313
ventriculomegaly and hydrocephaly, 310
scanning planes, 298–300
newly proposed planes, 299–300, *301*, *302*
Transvaginal probes/transducers, 39, 45, 297
Transverse fissure, 33
Trauma, maternal, 324
Treacher Collins syndrome, 684
TREACLE gene, 684
Tremors, 174
persistent, 103
Treponemal test, 590
'Trial by ambush', 529
Trial of labor, previous Cesarean section, 527, 533
*Trichosporon beigelii*, 575, 588
Tricuspid atresia, 486
Trigonocephaly, 211, 777
Trimethoprim, toxoplasmosis, 549
Trimethoprim-sulfamethoxazole, Gram-negative meningitis, 583
Triose phosphate isomerase disorder, **626**
Triploidy, 270
Trisomy syndromes
Dandy-Walker malformation, 240
mental retardation, 805, 806
trisomy 13: 245, 277
trisomy 18: 288, 321
trisomy 21: 808
trisomy D, 775
*see also* Down's syndrome
Trk receptors, 512
Trochlear (IV) motor nuclei, 29
Trophic factors, neuroprotection following asphyxia, 511–13
Tropomyosin kinase receptors, 6
Tuber cinereum, 27
Tuberculous meningitis, 779
Tuberous sclerosis, *80*, 81
differentiation from X-linked periventricular heterotopias, 218
mental retardation, **801**
Tumor necrosis factor-α (TNF-α)
bacterial meningitis, 576
microglia activation, 419, 514
in PVL, 375, 377
Tumors, 783–5
epidermoid, following lumbar puncture, 578
intracranial, 784–5
antenatal diagnosis, 283, *284*
brainstem glioma, 664
mental retardation, **801**
optic atrophy, 674
parenchymal hemorrhage, 362
teratomas, 283, *284*, 784, 785
neuroblastoma, 703
spinal, 698, 785
sternomastoid, 797
Turner's syndrome, 270, **800**
hearing loss, 685
TV transducer, transvaginal ultrasound, 298
Twin-twin transfusion syndrome (TTTS), 129, 281, 394
Twins
cardiac and venous Doppler studies, 129
cerebral palsy risk, 794
death of co-twin, 324, 794
fetal behavior, 95–6
fetal body movements, **89**
fetal heart rate (FHR), 96
maternal serum markers
AFP levels, 268
second trimester, 270
periventricular leukomalacia (PVL), 379
vaginal delivery of second, malpractice claims, 525
Tympanic membrane, 683
Tyrosine hydroxylase deficiency, **626**, **638**
Tyrosine kinase receptors, 512
Tyrosine kinases, 16
Tyrosinemia, 606
clinical features and biochemical findings, **607**
prenatal diagnosis, **597**

UK
medico-legal issues, 521–6
establishing liability, 523–5
expert evidence, 522–3
legal climate, 521–2
litigation and risk management, 522
prenatal asphyxia, 473, 474
Ulegyria, 334, *335*, 474, 475
Ulrich syndrome, **716**
Ultrasound, antenatal assessment, 209, 267, 268, 269
abdominal, 275–95
arachnoid cysts, 286, 287
arterio-venous malformation, 289–90
choroid plexus cysts, 286, *287*
congenital toxoplasmosis, *547*, 548
corpus callosum, agenesis, 277, *278*
Dandy-Walker syndrome, 277, 279
holoprosencephaly, 275–7
hydranencephaly, 279, *280*, 281
hydrocephalus, 284–6
intracranial hemorrhage, 281–2
intracranial tumors, 283, *284*
key points, 295
megalencephaly/macrocephaly, 283
microcephaly, 282–3
neural tube defects, 290–4
biophysical profile (BPP), 434
transvaginal, 297–315
3-D neuroscan, 304–9
arachnoid cysts, *312*, 313
aspects of, 300, 302–4
choroid plexus cysts, 310
corpus callosum agenesis, *309*, 311, 313
equipment and technique, 297–8
neural tube defects, 309–10
scanning planes, 298–300
ventriculomegaly and hydrocephaly, 310
Ultrasound assessment, brain development, 45–54
3-D assessment, 39–44, 45, 59
embryonic anomalies, 42–3
choice of transducer and approach, 45
first trimester <14 weeks, 41–2, 46–50
2 weeks 0 days, 46
7 weeks 0–6 days, 46–7
8 weeks 0–6 days, 47–8
9 weeks 0–6 days, 48–9
early postembyronic period, 10 and 11 weeks, 42, 49–50
late first trimester 12 and 13 weeks, 50
second trimester 14 to 27 weeks, 51–3
third trimester 28 weeks to term, 53
vasculature of brain, 53–*4*
*see also* Doppler ultrasound: fetal cerebral circulation
Ultrasound imaging, neonatal, 57–9, 83, 115
bacterial meningitis, 584
cerebral artery infarction, 395, *396*, *397*
cerebral infection, 81, 83
congenital malformations, 77, *78*
focal ischemic lesions, 76
hydranencephaly, *228*

hydrocephalus, *741*, 742–3, *744*
hypoxic ischemic encephalopathy (HIE), 69, 72, *73*, 75, 481
intracranial hemorrhage, 65
cerebellum, 361
choroid plexus, *361*
GMH-IVH, 67, *342*, 343, 344, 348
intraparenchymal, 68
subarachnoid, 68, 69
subdural, 68, 69, 358
myelomeningocele, *203*, 766
neuromuscular disorders, 711
periventricular leukomalacia (PVL), 69, *70*, 382–5, *390*
spinal cord trauma, 699–700
subcortical leukomalacia, *392*
subependymal pseudocysts, *355*
vascular malformations, 79
ventricular dilatation, 77
*see also* Doppler ultrasound: neonatal cerebral circulation
Ultrasound-enhanced particle agglutination, 578
Ultrasound-guided aspiration, brain abscess, 585
Umbilical artery
blood gases *see* Cord blood gases
Doppler blood flow, 437–8, 467
fetal blood sampling, 129
IUGR fetuses, 128
pH, 430, 464, **465**, 483, 493
Umbilical artery catheters
position, GMH-IVH development, 347
spinal cord infarction, 701
Umbilical vein lactate, 462, 463
Uncal herniation, 359
Unconjugated estriol (uEU3u), 268, 269
Unilateral hearing impairment, 691
Uniparental disomy, 805
Up-beat nystagmus, 664
Up-gaze palsy, 664
Urea, asphyxiated infants, 492
Urea cycle disorders, 606, 618–19, 725
clinical features and bichemical findings, **608**
differential diagnosis, **710**
management, 617
prenatal diagnosis, **597**
Uric acid, elevated, 344
Uridine-diphosphate-galactose 4-epimerase deficiency, 620
Uridine-monophosphate (UMP) synthetase deficiency *see* Hereditary orotic aciduria
Urinary β-core hCG, 268
Urinary incontinence, myelomeningocele, 203
Urinary lactate, 616
ratio to creatinine, 484
in hypoxia, 430
Urine tests
cytomegalovirus, 559
inborn errors of metabolism, 615–16, 617
Urokinase
cerebral venous thrombosis, 366
intraventricular, 750
USA
medico-legal issues, 527–38
clinical practice guidelines, 529, 530
complication of error, 533
CTG in court, 537–8
expert testimony, 528–9
legal climate, 527–8
medico-legal education, 530–2
tort reform and finances, 533–7
why patients sue, **531**, 532–3
perinatal asphyxia, 473, 474
Usher syndromes, 684–5
Uterine blood flow, 461
Uterine hypertonus, 453, 463

Vaccines
cytomegalovirus, 559
mumps, 554
mumps, measles and rubella (MMR), 556
polio, 568, 569
rubella, 556
Vacuum extraction, injuries, 534, 535
dural tears, 356–7
media interest in, 527
subaponeurotic hemorrhage, 364
vacuum extractor study, 537
Vagal tone, modulation, 452
Vaginal birth after Cesarean section (VBAC), 527, 530, 532
uterine rupture, 525
Valproate, 654
Valproic acid, teratogenic effects, 220, 251
Values and beliefs, 822
Vancomycin
bacterial meningitis, 581, 582
endophthalmitis, 586
shunt infections, 587
Varaadi-Papp syndrome, **243**, **248**
Varicella-zoster (V-Z) virus, 553, 554, 559–62, 812
congenital varicella syndrome, 560–1
management, 561, 562
perinatal infection, 561
Vascular accidents, spinal cord, 700–1
Vascular malformations, 79, 81, 781–3
imaging, 79–80
Vascular mechanisms, neuroprotection, 513, 514
Vascular theory, PVL pathophysiology, 375–6
Vasculitis, bacterial meningitis, 577
spinal cord ischemia, 586
Vasoactive intestinal peptide (VIP) administration, PVL studies, 376
Vasodilatation, nitric oxide-induced, 145
Vasogenic edema, 475
Vasopressin, effect on developing brain, 255, 260
Vasopressin levels, asphyxiated infants, 485
Vasotocin, effect on developing brain, 255
Vein of Galen aneurysm, 59, 77, 79, 289, 362, 783
Velocardiofacial syndrome, **243**
Venereal Disease Research Laboratory (VDRL) test, syphilitic meningitis, 578, 590
Venography (MRV), 63, 65
Venous infarction, 341–2, 394
ultrasound, 67
Venous occlusion plethysmography, 143, 144
Ventouse extraction, intracranial hemorrhage, 525
Ventral flexion in axis, 105
Ventral roots, spinal nerves, 23
Ventricles *see* Fourth ventricle; Lateral ventricles; Third ventricle
Ventricular dilatation, 76, 77
*see also* Hydrocephalus; Ventriculomegaly
Ventricular hemorrhage *see* Intraventricular hemorrhage (IVH)
Ventricular layer, 14
Ventricular reservoir, 750, 779
Ventricular tap, 580, 747
versus conservative management, 748
Ventricular zone, 22, 23, 24
Ventriculitis, 81
bacterial meningitis, 577, 580, 583
hydrocephalus, 740
intraventricular fibrinolytic therapy, 750
phakomatoses, 81
Ventriculoamniotic shunts, 729, *731*
Ventriculoatrial shunts, 586, 755
Ventriculocele, 207
Ventriculofugal arteries, 374, 381
Ventriculomegaly, 51
antenatal ultrasound, 284–6
3-D neuroscan, 307
dangling choroid plexus, 304, *305*
toxoplasmosis, *547*, 548
transvaginal, 310
periventricular leukomalacia, 390
*see also* Hydrocephalus
Ventriculomegaly Trial Group, 747
Ventriculoperitoneal shunts, 215, 755, 758, 766, 781, 784
imaging, 77
infections, 586–7
Vergence movements, 659, 662
Vermis, 16, 30, 49, 51, 53
agenesis, 222–4, 277
Vertebrae, growth, 22
Vertebral arteries, fetal, 53
Vertical gaze palsy, 664
Very low birthweight (VLBW) infants
BAEPs, bilateral abnormalities, 186
posture, 103
Vesicoureteral reflux, 203
Vestibulo-ocular movements, 659
Vestibulo-ocular reflexes, 661
Viability of fetus, independent moral status, 823
Vibroacoustic stimulation (VAS), 433, 436, 438, 449
Vidarabine, HSV infection, 564
Video-EEG, 155, *176*, 648, 649
Vintzileos *et al* EFM vs. auscultation trial, **445**, 448
Viral infections, 553–69
cytomegalovirus (CMV), 187, *327*, 553, 554, 556–8, 686, 812
enteroviruses, 553, 566–7, 580
non-polio, 567–8
poliovirus, 568–9
herpes simplex (HSV), 81, *82*, 83, 562–4
herpes zoster, 560, 561, 562
human immunodeficiency virus (HIV), 553, 564–6, 812–13
key points, 569
lymphocytic choriomeningitis virus (LCMV), 566
parvovirus, 556
rubella, 554–6
varicella-zoster virus (V-Z), 553, 554, 559–62, 812
Visibility, tests of, 669, *670*
Vision
abnormalities, 623, 672–8
anterior visual pathway disorders, 672–3
cortical visual impairment, 677–8
cytomegalovirus infection, 557
delayed visual maturation, 675–7
investigation, 678
neonatal stroke, 395, 398, 399
optic nerve disorders, 673–5
periventricular leukomalacia (PVL), 390–1, 677
posterior visual pathway disorders, 675
retinal disorders, 673
toxoplasmosis, 548
assessment, 101–2, 187
key points, 678
normal development, 667–8, *673*
visual acuity, measurement of, 668–9
*see also* Eye movements
Visual evoked potentials (VEPs), 182–3, 669
clinical applications, 187–90, **192**, 386
VEP: PL discrepancy, 671
VEP: Snellen acuity discrepancy, 671–2
Visual field, 668
Visual reinforcement audiometry (VRA), 690
Visual stimulation, importance of, 7–8
Visual threat response, 668
Vitamin A
postnatal, GMH-IVH prevention, 352–3
as teratogen, 200, 251
Vitamin BU6u administration, seizure disorders, 651
Vitamin BU12u deficiency and folate supplementation, 811
Vitamin E
GMH-IVH prevention, 352
inhibition of lipid peroxidation, 508
Vitamin K
administration, asphyxiated infants, 489

deficiency
parenchymal hemorrhage, 362, 363
subaponeurotic hemorrhage, 364
GMH-IVH prevention, 350
Vitamin metabolism disorders, 639–40
clinical features and biochemical findings, **612–13**, **626**
prenatal diagnosis, **600**
Vitamin supplementation, maternal, 319
Von Hippel-Landau disease, 81

Waardenburg's syndrome, 4, 684
Walker-Warburg syndrome, **208**, 216, 217, **238**, **239**, **241**, **246**, 713, **716**
Walking reflex, 106, 107
Wallerian degeneration, 397
Weight
fetus
brain, 33
and vaginal delivery, 535
maternal, serum markers, 268, 270
neonatal brain, 21
cerebellum, 30
Wells v. Wells (1999), 521
Werdnig-Hoffman's disease, 102, 115, 709
*see also* Spinal muscular atrophy
West syndrome, 652
White Book (1999) Civil Procedure Rules, Part 35, 522–3
White cell count, CSF
bacterial meningitis, 579
neuropsyphilis, 590
normal, 578–9
White matter
CT interpretation, 59
development, 14, 15, 23
lesions, 327, 330
and mental retardation, 812
pathogenesis in asphyxia, 423, 431
in preterm infants, EEG, 173
*see also* Periventricular
ultrasound imaging, 58
'Whole body dose', radiation exposure, 143
Wildervanck syndrome, 686
Williams syndrome, 632, **800**, 809–10
Wilson's disease
clinical features and biochemical findings, **612**
prenatal diagnosis, **600**
Wiring, neural circuits, 7–8
Withdrawal of care, 499, 830, 831
Withdrawal of treatment, 830
Wolman's disease
clinical features and biochemical findings, **611**
prenatal diagnosis, **600**
Wood *et al* EFM vs. auscultation trial, **445**, 446
Woolf report, 'Access to Justice', 521
World Federation of Neurology Group, asphyxia definition, 427, 459
World Health Organization (WHO)
asphyxia, developing world, 474
tetanus eradication, 589, 590
'Wrongful birth/wrongful life' lawsuits, 528, 765

X-linked conditions, 200
adrenoleucodystrophy, **600**, **611**, 635
Alports syndrome, 685
congenital myotubular myopathy, 716, *718*
hydrocephalus, 238, 239
lissencephaly/subcortical band heterotopias, 216–17, *245*, **246**
mental retardation, **800**, 805
α-thalassaemia/mental retardation (ATR-X) syndrome, **241**
periventricular heterotopias, 217, 218
Xanthine oxidase inhibition, 517
Xanthinuria
clinical features and biochemical findings, **611**
prenatal diagnosis, **600**
Xenon clearance technique, CBF measurement, 130, 140, 144, *145*
radiation dose, **144**
XLIS gene mutations, 216, 244

Yawning, repetitive, 108

Zellweger's syndrome, 5, **241**, 606, 623, 635–6, 674, 725
clinical features and biochemical findings, **611**, **625**
prenatal diagnosis, **600**
ZIC2 gene, 244
Zidovidine (AZT), 566, 812